FOR
REFERENCE ONLY

WE 830 MAC

WE 830 MAC

Hunter - Mackin - Callahan

REHABILITATION

OF THE HAND AND

UPPER EXTREMITY

Hunter - Mackin - Callahan

REHABILITATION

OF THE HAND AND

UPPER EXTREMITY

Fifth Edition

EDITORS

Evelyn J. Mackin, L.P.T.
Executive Director
Hand Rehabilitation Foundation
Philadelphia, Pennsylvania

Anne D. Callahan, M.S., O.T.R./L., C.H.T.
Hand Therapy Consultant
Lymphedema Therapy Specialist
Philadelphia, Pennsylvania

Terri M. Skirven, O.T.R./L., C.H.T.
Director of Hand Therapy
The Philadelphia Hand Center, PC;
Associate Director, Hand Rehabilitation Foundation
Philadelphia, Pennsylvania

Lawrence H. Schneider, M.D.
Clinical Professor
Department of Orthopedic Surgery
Former Chairman, Division of Hand Surgery
Jefferson Medical College of Thomas Jefferson
    University;
Former Director, The Philadelphia Hand Center, PC,
    and Fellowship Program;
President, Hand Rehabilitation Foundation
Philadelphia, Pennsylvania

A. Lee Osterman, M.D.
Professor
Department of Orthopedic Surgery
Chairman
Division of Hand Therapy
Jefferson Medical College of Thomas Jefferson
    University;
Director, The Philadelphia Hand Center, PC, and
    Fellowship Program
Philadelphia, Pennsylvania

EDITOR EMERITUS

James M. Hunter, M.D.
Distinguished Professor of Orthopaedic Surgery
Jefferson Medical College of Thomas Jefferson
    University
Philadelphia, Pennsylvania

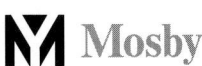

St. Louis   London   Philadelphia   Sydney   Toronto

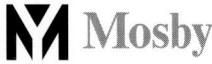

Acquiring Editor: Richard Lampert
Senior Managing Editor: Kathy Falk
Publishing Services Manager: Pat Joiner
Senior Designer: Mark A. Oberkrom

Fifth Edition

Printed in the United States of America

Mosby, Inc.
An Elsevier Science imprint
11830 Westline Industrial Drive
St. Louis, Missouri 63146

Library of Congress Cataloging in Publication Data

Rehabilitation of the hand and upper extremity / editors, Evelyn J. Mackin . . . [et al.].—5th ed.
    p. ; cm.
    Rev. ed. of: Rehabilitation of the hand. 4th ed. c1995.
    Includes bibliographical references and index.
    ISBN 0-323-01094-6
    1. Hand—Wounds and injuries. 2. Hand—Surgery. 3. Hand—Surgery—
Patients—Rehabilitation. I. Mackin, Evelyn. II. Rehabilitation of the hand.
    [DNLM: 1. Hand—surgery. 2. Arm Injuries—rehabilitation. 3. Hand
Injuries—rehabilitation. 4. Shoulder Joint—injuries. WE 830 R345 2002]
RD559 .R43 2002
617.5'7506—dc21

                                          2001055842

02 03 04 05 06 GW/MV 9 8 7 6 5 4 3 2 1

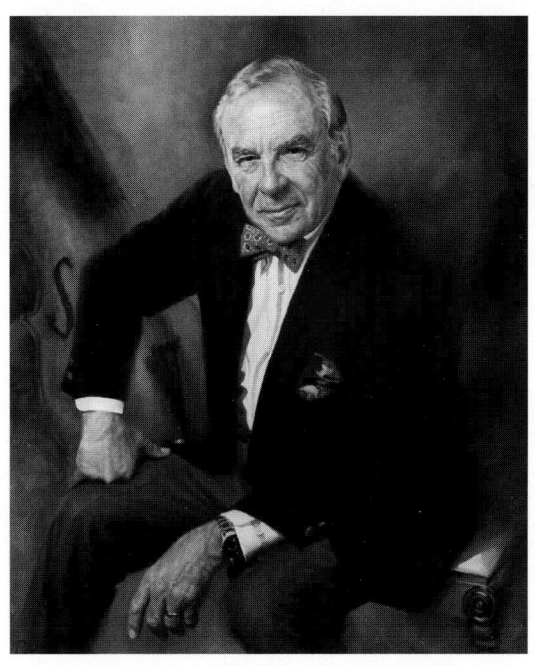

Surgeon, Mentor, Teacher, Friend

We proudly and with affection dedicate this fifth edition of *Rehabilitation of the Hand and Upper Extremity* to James M. Hunter, M.D. He served as mentor and teacher when there were few hand fellows and hand therapists in the field. His belief in the hand team—surgeon, therapist, and patient—helped shape the specialty. His philosophy led to the development of the world's first artificial tendon, the founding of the Philadelphia Hand Center, the "Philadelphia Meeting" (now in its twenty-seventh year), and the publication of four editions of *Rehabilitation of the Hand: Surgery and Therapy*. His forward vision is proof that one person can make a difference.

FIFTH EDITION EDITORS

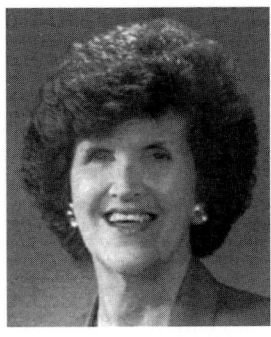

Evelyn J. Mackin, L.P.T.
Editions 1, 2, 3, 4, 5

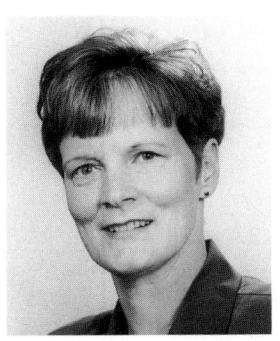

Anne D. Callahan, M.S.,
O.T.R./L, C.H.T.
Editions 2, 3, 4, 5

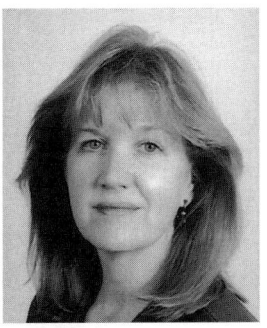

Terri M. Skirven, O.T.R./L,
C.H.T.
Edition 5

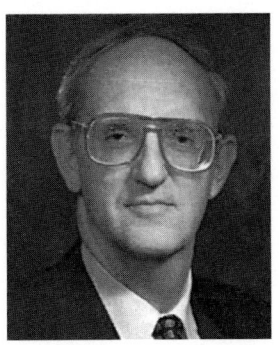

Lawrence H. Schneider,
M.D.
Editions 1, 2, 3, 5

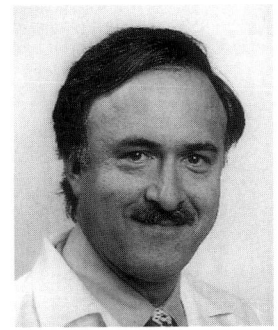

A. Lee Osterman, M.D.
Edition 5

PREVIOUS EDITORS

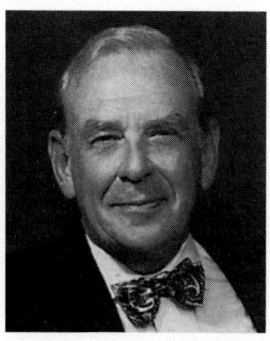

James M. Hunter, M.D.
Editions 1, 2, 3, 4

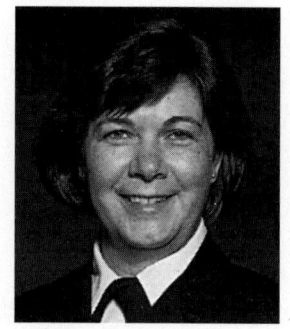

Judith A. Bell-Krotoski,
O.T.R., F.A.O.T.A., C.H.T.
Edition 1

CONTRIBUTORS

Edward Akelman, M.D.
Professor and Vice Chairman
Chief, Division of Hand
Department of Orthopedics
Rhode Island Hospital;
Brown University Medical School
Providence, Rhode Island

Christina D. Alba, M.P.T.
Department of Hand Therapy
The Philadelphia Hand Center, PC
Philadelphia, Pennsylvania

Diane M. Allen, M.D.
Hand and Microvascular Fellow
Division of Orthopedic Surgery
Duke University Medical Center
Durham, North Carolina

Steven Alter, M.D.
Hand Surgical Association
Boston, Massachusetts

Thomas J. Armstrong, Ph.D., C.I.H.
Professor
Industrial and Operations Engineering and Biomedical
    Engineering;
Director, Center for Ergonomics
University of Michigan
Ann Arbor, Michigan

Sandra M. Artzberger, M.S., O.T.R., C.H.T.
Director of Lymphedema Services
Cedar Haven Rehabilitation Agency
West Bend, Wisconsin;
Hand Therapy Consultant and Lecturer
Hartford, Wisconsin

Pat L. Aulicino, M.D.
Professor of Orthopedic Surgery
Department of Surgery
Eastern Virginia Medical School;
Adjunct Clinical Professor
Department of Community Health Professions
Old Dominion University
Norfolk, Virginia

Mark E. Baratz, M.D.
Professor
Department of Orthopedic Surgery
MCP Hahnemann University
Philadelphia, Pennsylvania;
Vice Chairman
Department of Orthopedic Surgery
Allegheny General Hospital;
Director
Division of Hand and Upper Extremity Surgery
Pittsburgh, Pennsylvania

Mary F. Barbe, Ph.D.
Associate Professor
Department of Physical Therapy
College of Allied Health Professions
Temple University;
Adjunct Associate Professor
Department of Anatomy and Cell Biology
Temple University
Philadelphia, Pennsylvania

Ann E. Barr, P.T., Ph.D.
Assistant Professor
Department of Physical Therapy
Temple University
Philadelphia, Pennsylvania

John M. Bednar, M.D.
Assistant Professor of Orthopedic Surgery
Jefferson Medical College at
    Thomas Jefferson University;
Thomas Jefferson University Hospital;
Administrative Physician
The Philadelphia Hand Center, PC
Philadelphia, Pennsylvania

Judith A. Bell-Krotoski, O.T.R., F.A.O.T.A., C.H.T.
Clinical Research Therapist and Chief
Hand and Occupational Therapy Services
Rehabilitation Research Services
National Hansen's Disease Program
Baton Rouge, Louisiana

Pedro K. Beredjiklian, M.D.
Assistant Professor of Orthopedic Surgery
Division of Hand Surgery
Department of Orthopedic Surgery
University of Pennsylvania School of Medicine
Philadelphia, Pennsylvania

Richard A. Berger, M.D., Ph.D.
Professor
Departments of Anatomy and Orthopedic Surgery
Mayo Clinic/Mayo Foundation
Rochester, Minnesota

Jeanine Biese, O.T.R., C.H.T.
Senior Therapist
Department of Hand Therapy
Rehabilitation Professionals
Grand Rapids, Michigan;
Adjunct Faculty
Grand Valley State University
Allendale, Michigan

Susan M. Blackmore, M.S., O.T.R./L., C.H.T.
Adjunct Assistant Professor
Program in Rehabilitation Sciences
MCP Hahnemann University;
The Philadelphia Hand Center, PC
Philadelphia, Pennsylvania

George P. Bogumill, M.D., Ph.D.
Distinguished Professor
Department of Orthopedic Surgery
Georgetown University School of Medicine;
Consultant, Hand Surgery
Department of Orthopedic Surgery
Walter Reed Army Medical Center;
Children's National Medical Center
Washington, DC

Paul J. Bonzani, O.T.R., C.H.T.
Coordinator of Hand Therapy Services
Division of Orthopedic Surgery
Department of Physical and Occupational Therapy
Duke University Health System
Durham, North Carolina

David J. Bozentka, M.D.
Chief, Hand Surgery
Assistant Professor of Orthopedic, Hand, & Upper
  Extremity Surgery
University of Pennsylvania
Philadelphia, Pennsylvania

Paul W. Brand, M.D.
Clinical Professor of Orthopedics, Emeritus
Department of Orthopedics
University of Washington School of Medicine
Seattle, Washington

Donna E. Breger-Stanton, M.A., O.T.R., C.H.T.
Assistant Professor
Academic Fieldworker Coordinator
Department of Occupational Therapy
Samuel Merritt College
Oakland, California

Forst E. Brown, M.D.
Professor of Surgery, Emeritus
Department of Plastic Surgery
Dartmouth Medical School
Hanover, New Hampshire;
Consultant
Department of Surgery
Veterans Administration Hospital
White River Junction, Vermont

Paul W. Brown, M.D.
Clinical Professor of Orthopedics and Rehabilitation
Clinical Professor of Plastic and Reconstructive Surgery
Yale University School of Medicine
New Haven, Connecticut

John Bucchieri, M.D.
Department of Orthopedic Surgery
Allegheny General Hospital
Pittsburgh, Pennsylvania

Sandy L. Burkart, P.T., Ph.D.
Functional Rehabilitation Associates, Inc.
Boca Raton, Florida

David C. Bush, M.D.
Director
Department of Orthopedics
Geisinger Medical Center
Danville, Pennsylvania

Nancy N. Byl, Ph.D., P.T.
Professor and Chair
Department of Physical Therapy and Rehabilitation
  Science
University of California–San Francisco
San Francisco, California

Patricia M. Byron, M.S., O.T.R./L., P.T., C.H.T.
ALTA Consultant
Student Services Division
Chester County Intermediate Unit
Exton, Pennsylvania

Anne D. Callahan, M.S., O.T.R./L., C.H.T.
Hand Therapy Consultant
Lymphedema Therapy Specialist
Philadelphia, Pennsylvania

Catherine A. Cambridge-Keeling, M.S., P.T., C.H.T.
Hand Therapy of Delaware
Wilmington, Delaware

Peter J. Campbell, M.D.
Clinical Staff, Hand Surgery
Phoenix Orthopedic Integrated Residency Program
Maricopa Medical Center;
Hand Surgery Consultants
Phoenix, Arizona

Nancy M. Cannon, O.T.R., C.H.T.
Director of Rehabilitation Services
The Hand Rehabilitation Center of Indiana
Indianapolis, Indiana

Karen Carney, O.T.R./L., C.H.T.
Co-Director
Department of Hand Therapy
University Orthopedics, Inc.
Providence, Rhode Island

Robyn Cass, P.T., C.H.T.
Certified Hand Therapist
DeRosa Physical Therapy
Flagstaff, Arizona

James Chang, M.D.
Assistant Professor and Program Director of Plastic and
    Hand Surgery
Stanford University Medical Center
Stanford, California

Jeffrey M. Chase, M.D.
Chief
Division of Orthopedic Surgery
Roy Lester Schneider Hospital;
Private Practice
Virgin Islands Orthopedics and Sports Medicine
St. Thomas, Virgin Islands

Robert A. Chase, M.D.
Emile Holman Professor of Surgery and Anatomy,
    Emeritus
Stanford University School of Medicine;
Department of Surgery
Stanford University Hospital
Stanford, California

Roberta Ciocco, O.T.R./L.
Former Director
Department of Occupational Therapy
Shriners Hospital for Children
Philadelphia, Pennsylvania;
Kinetic Rehabilitation Services, PC
New Britain, Pennsylvania

Judy C. Colditz, O.T.R./L., C.H.T., F.A.O.T.A.
Consultant in Hand Therapy
Hand Lab, A Division of Raleigh Hand
    Rehabilitation, Inc.
Raleigh, North Carolina

Ruth A. Coopee, M.O.T., O.T.R./L., C.H.T., C.K.T.I.
Per Diem Therapist and Hand Therapist
Department of Occupational Therapy
Athol Memorial Hospital;
Owner
Private Practice
Body Holistics
Athol, Massachusetts

Cynthia Cooper, M.F.A., M.A., O.T.R./L., C.H.T.
Assistant Professor of Physical Medicine and
    Rehabilitation
Mayo Medical School
Rochester, Minnesota;
Hand Therapist and Clinical Research Coordinator
Rehabilitation Services
Mayo Clinic Hospital
Phoenix, Arizona

Norman J. Cowen, M.D., P.C.
Hand and Rehabilitation Center
Washington, DC

Randall W. Culp, M.D.
Associate Professor in Orthopedic, Hand, and
    Microsurgery
Department of Orthopedic Surgery
Jefferson Medical College of Thomas Jefferson University
Philadelphia, Pennsylvania;
Owner
The Philadelphia Hand Center, PC
Philadelphia, Pennsylvania

Sylvia A. Dávila, P.T., C.H.T.
Clinical Instructor
Department of Physical Therapy
University of Texas Health Science Center;
Director
Hand Rehabilitation Associates of San Antonio, Inc.
San Antonio, Texas

Laurie Grigsby deLinde, O.T.R./L.
West Chester, Pennsylvania

Paul C. Dell, M.D.
Professor
Department of Orthopedics and Rehabilitation
University of Florida Medical Center
Gainesville, Florida

Ruth B. Dell, MHS, O.T.R., C.H.T.
Shands Rehabilitation Hand Therapy
Shands Hospital
Gainesville, Florida

Cecilia A. Devine, O.T.R., C.H.T.
Clinical Coordinator
Hand Center
Froedtert Hospital
Milwaukee, Wisconsin

James H. Dobyns, M.D.
Clinical Professor
Department of Orthopedic Surgery
University of Texas Health Sciences Center;
Consultant (Honorary)
Department of Orthopedic Surgery
Baptist Medical System Hospitals;
Consultant (Visiting)
Department of Orthopedic Surgery
University of Texas–Bexar County Hospitals
San Antonio, Texas;
Professor Emeritus
Department of Orthopedic Surgery
Mayo Medical Center
Rochester, Minnesota

Roslyn B. Evans, O.T.R./L., C.H.T.
Owner and Director
Indian River Hand and Upper Extremity Rehabilitation
Vero Beach, Florida

Jane M. Fedorczyk, M.S., P.T., C.H.T., A.T.C.
Assistant Professor
Program in Rehabilitation Sciences;
Director
Certificate Program in Hand and Upper Quarter
  Rehabilitation
MCP Hahnemann University
Philadelphia, Pennsylvania

Lynne Feehan, M.S.C., (P.T.), C.H.T.
Ph.D. Graduate Student
Interdisciplinary Studies
University of British Columbia
Vancouver, British Columbia, Canada;
Senior Hand Therapist
Hand Program
Workers Compensation Board of British Columbia
Richmond, British Columbia, Canada

Paul Feldon, M.D.
Associate Clinical Professor
Department of Orthopedic Surgery
Tufts University School of Medicine;
Hand Surgeon
Department of Orthopedic Surgery
New England Baptist Hospital
Boston, Massachusetts

Sheri B. Feldscher, O.T.R., C.H.T.
The Philadelphia Hand Center, PC
Philadelphia, Pennsylvania

John M. Fenlin, Jr., M.D.
Director, Shoulder Service
Department of Orthopedics
Rothman Institute at Jefferson Hospital
Philadelphia, Pennsylvania

Elaine Ewing Fess, M.S., O.T.R., F.A.O.T.A., C.H.T.
Hand Research
Zionsville, Indiana

Barbara G. Frieman, M.D.
Clinical Associate Professor
Department of Orthopedic Surgery
Jefferson Shoulder and Elbow Center
Thomas Jefferson University Hospital
Philadelphia, Pennsylvania

Gary K. Frykman, M.D.
Clinical Professor
Department of Orthopedic Surgery
Loma Linda University;
Chief, Hand Surgical Service
Jerry L. Pettis Veterans Hospital
Loma Linda, California

Michael C. Gartner, DO
Resident, Plastic and Reconstructive Surgery
State University of New York
Stony Brook, New York;
Nassau County Medical Center
East Meadow, New York

Eduardo Gonzalez-Hernandez, M.D.
Orthopedic Hand Surgeon
Miami Hand Center
Miami, Florida

Annabel J. Griffith, B.S., O.T.R./L.
Clinical Supervisor
Cornell Hand Rehabilitation Center
Hospital for Special Surgery
New York, New York

Brad K. Grunert, Ph.D.
Associate Professor
Department of Plastic and Reconstructive Surgery
Medical College of Wisconsin
Milwaukee, Wisconsin

Murray P. Hamlet, D.V.M.
U.S. Army Research Institute of Environmental Medicine
(Retired)
Natick, Massachusetts

Brian J. Hartigan, M.D.
Instructor of Clinical Orthopedic Surgery
Department of Orthopedic Surgery
Northwestern University Medical School
Chicago, Illinois

Edward P. Hayes, M.D.
Hand and Upper Extremity Surgery
Department of Orthopedic Surgery
Marshfield Clinic
Eau Claire, Wisconsin

Lior Heller, M.D.
Fellow in Plastic Surgery and Reconstructive Surgery
Duke University Medical Center
Durham, North Carolina

Erich E. Hornbach, M.D.
Department of Orthopedic Surgery
Edward Sparrow Hospital
Lansing, Michigan

Steven B. Huish, M.D.
Mountain Orthopedics
Bountiful, Utah

James M. Hunter, M.D.
Distinguished Professor of Orthopedic Surgery
Jefferson Medical College of Thomas Jefferson University
Philadelphia, Pennsylvania

Peter C. Innis, M.D.
Assistant Professor
Department of Orthopedic Surgery
Johns Hopkins School of Medicine;
Attending Hand Surgeon
Curtis National Hand Center
Baltimore, Maryland

Neil F. Jones, M.D.
Professor
Department of Orthopedic Surgery
Division of Plastic and Reconstructive Surgery
University of California–Los Angeles;
Chief, Hand Surgery
UCLA Medical Center
Los Angeles, California

Jesse B. Jupiter, M.D.
Professor
Department of Orthopedic Surgery
Harvard University Medical School;
Director
Orthopedic Hand Service
Massachusetts General Hospital
Boston, Massachusetts

Mary C. Kasch, O.T.R., C.H.T., F.A.O.T.A.
Executive Director
Hand and Therapy Certification Commission
Rancho Cordova, California

Parivash Kashani, O.T.R., C.H.T.
Certified Hand Therapist
Department of Rehabilitation
University of California–Los Angeles Medical Center
Los Angeles, California

Michael W. Keith, M.D.
Professor
Department of Orthopedics and Biomedical Engineering
Case Western Reserve University;
MetroHealth Medical Center;
Veterans Affairs Medical Center;
University Hospital of Cleveland
Cleveland, Ohio

Martin J. Kelley, M.S., P.T., O.C.S.
Clinical Associate Director of the Upper Extremity Center
    of Excellence
Department of Rehabilitation Medicine, Occupational and
    Physical Therapy
University of Pennsylvania Health System
Philadelphia, Pennsylvania

†**Barbara Knothe, M.O.T., O.T.R./L., C.H.T.**
Senior Occupational Therapist
Department of Physical Medicine, Rehabilitation, and
    Occupational Therapy
Temple University Hospital
Philadelphia, Pennsylvania

L. Andrew Koman, M.D.
Professor and Vice Chair
Department of Orthopedic Surgery
Wake Forest University School of Medicine
Winston-Salem, North Carolina

Scott H. Kozin, M.D.
Associate Professor
Department of Orthopedic Surgery
Temple University;
Hand Surgeon
Shriners Hospital for Children
Philadelphia, Pennsylvania

Paul N. Krop, M.D.
Virginia Beach, Virginia

Kevin A. Kucera, O.T.R./L.
Department of Physical Medicine and Rehabilitation
Cleveland MetroHealth Medical Center
Cleveland, Ohio

Georgiann F. Laseter, O.T.R., F.A.O.T.A., C.H.T.
Hand Rehabilitation Services
Dallas, Texas

†Deceased.

Paul C. LaStayo, Ph.D., M.P.T., C.H.T.
Department of Physical Therapy
Northern Arizona University
Flagstaff, Arizona

Marilyn Petersen Lee, M.S., O.T.R./L., C.H.T.
Clinical Supervisor
Hand and Upper Extremity Rehabilitation
Mercy Health System
Philadelphia and Delaware County (Havertown),
   Pennsylvania

Brian G. Leggin, P.T.
Penn Therapy and Fitness
Philadelphia, Pennsylvania

Mark S. Lemel, M.D.
Clinical Assistant Professor
Department of Orthopedics
University of Florida Health Science Center;
North Florida Hand Surgeons
Jacksonville, Florida

L. Scott Levin, M.D.
Chief
Division of Plastic, Reconstructive, Maxillofacial, and
   Oral Surgery;
Professor of Plastic and Orthopedic Surgery
Duke University Medical Center
Durham, North Carolina

John D. Lubahn, M.D., F.A.C.S.
Program Director and Chairman
Department of Orthopedics
Hamot Medical Center
Erie, Pennsylvania

Joy C. MacDermid, B.S.C.P.T., M.S.C., Ph.D.
Assistant Professor
School of Rehabilitation of Sciences
McMaster University
Hamilton, Ontario, Canada;
Co-Director, Clinical Research Lab
St. Joseph's Health Centre
Hand & Upper Limb Centre
London, Ontario, Canada

Evelyn J. Mackin, L.P.T.
Executive Director
Hand Rehabilitation Foundation
Philadelphia, Pennsylvania

Glenn A. Mackin, M.D.
Director, Neuromuscular Diseases Center
Department of Medicine (Neurology)
Lehigh Valley Hospital
Allentown, Pennsylvania;
Associate Professor of Clinical Medicine (Neurology)
Department of Medicine
Penn State and Hershey Medical Center
Hershey, Pennsylvania

Philip C. Marin, M.D.
Hand Surgery Fellow
Department of Orthopedic Surgery
Union Memorial Hospital–Curtis National Hand Center
Baltimore, Maryland

John A. McAuliffe, M.D.
Section of Hand Surgery
Department of Orthopedic Surgery
Cleveland Clinic Florida
Weston, Florida

Philip McClure, Ph.D., P.T.
Associate Professor
Department of Physical Therapy
Arcadia University
Glenside, Pennsylvania

Robert M. McFarlane, M.D., M.S.C., F.R.C.S.C.
Emeritus Professor
Department of Surgery
University of Western Ontario
London, Ontario, Canada

Kenneth D. Meadows, P.T.
Chief Therapist
Portland Hand Surgery and Rehabilitation Center
Portland, Oregon

Jeanne L. Melvin, M.S., O.T.R., F.A.O.T.A.
Program Manager
Fibromyalgia and Chronic Pain Management Programs
Rehabilitation Services
Cedars-Sinai Medical Center
Los Angeles, California

Michael M. Merzenich, Ph.D.
Professor and Vice Chair
Departments of Physiology and Otolaryngology
Keck Center for Integrative Neurosciences
University of California, San Francisco
San Francisco, California

Susan L. Michlovitz, Ph.D., P.T., C.H.T.
Associate Professor
Department of Physical Therapy
Temple University
Philadelphia, Pennsylvania

Linda T. Miller, P.T.
Clinical Director
Breast Cancer Physical Therapy Center, LTD
Philadelphia, Pennsylvania

Gregory J. Moorman, M.D.
Chief Resident
Department of Plastic and Reconstructive Surgery
Duke University Medical Center
Durham, North Carolina

Elaine Muntzer, P.T., C.H.T.
Clinical Site Coordinator
Healthsouth Hand and Rehabilitation Center
Levittown, Pennsylvania

Michael S. Murphy, M.D.
Clinical Instructor
Department of Orthopedics
Johns Hopkins School of Medicine;
Attending Hand Surgeon
Department of Orthopedics
Union Memorial Hospital
Baltimore, Maryland

Edward A. Nalebuff, M.D.
Clinical Professor
Department of Orthopedic Surgery
Tufts University School of Medicine;
Chief of Hand Surgery
New England Baptist Hospital
Boston, Massachusetts;
The Philadelphia Hand Center, PC
Thomas Jefferson University Hospital
Philadelphia, Pennsylvania

Susan Nasser-Sharif, M.D., F.R.C.S.C.
Fellow of the Philadelphia Hand Center
Thomas Jefferson University
Philadelphia, Pennsylvania

Peter A. Nathan, M.D.
Diplomate, American Board of Orthopedic Surgery
Certificate in Surgery of the Hand
Providence St. Vincent Medical Center
Portland, Oregon

Ross Nathan, M.D.
Clinical Assistant Professor
Department of Orthopedic Surgery
Harbor and UCLA Medical Center
Carson, California;
Chairman
Long Beach Memorial Medical Center
Long Beach, California

Richard N. Norris, M.D.
Director, Arts Medicine Program
Pioneer Spine and Sports Physicians, PC
Northampton, Massachusetts

James A. Nunley, M.D.
Professor and Vice Chairman of Orthopedic Surgery
Duke Medical Center
Durham, North Carolina

George E. Omer, Jr., M.D., M.S., F.A.C.S.
Professor and Chairman-Emeritus
Department of Orthopedic Surgery and Rehabilitation
University of New Mexico School of Medicine;
Professor and Chief-Emeritus
Division of Hand Surgery
Department of Orthopedic Surgery and Rehabilitation
University of New Mexico School of Medicine
Albuquerque, New Mexico

A. Lee Osterman, M.D.
Professor
Department of Orthopedic Surgery
Chairman
Division of Hand Therapy
Jefferson Medical College of Thomas Jefferson
    University;
Director, The Philadelphia Hand Center, PC, and
    Fellowship Program
Philadelphia, Pennsylvania

Nader Paksima, M.D.
Philadelphia, Pennsylvania

Stuart D. Patterson, M.D., F.R.C.S.C.
Hand and Upper Extremity Surgeon
Department of Orthopedic Surgery
Winter Haven Hospital;
Bond Clinic, P.A.
Winter Haven, Florida

Allan E. Peljovich, M.D., M.P.H.
Instructor
Department of Orthopedic Surgery
Emory University School of Medicine
Atlanta Medical Center;
The Shepherd Center
Hand Function Clinic;
The Hand Treatment Center
Atlanta, Georgia

Karen M. Stewart Pettengill, M.S., O.T.R./L., C.H.T.
Center Manager
Department of Hand Therapy
Nova Care Outpatient Rehabilitation
Springfield, Massachusetts

Cynthia A. Philips, M.A., O.T.R./L., C.H.T.
Hand Clinical Specialist
Health South Hand and Rehabilitation Center
Brookline, Massachusetts

Jean Pillet, M.D.
Pillet Hand Prostheses
New York, New York

Kevin D. Plancher, M.D., F.A.C.S., F.A.A.O.S.
Clinical Assistant Professor of Orthopedics
Albert Einstein College of Medicine
Bronx, New York;
Department of Orthopedics
Beth Israel North Hospital
New York, New York;
Stamford Hospital
Stamford, New York;
Consultant
Department of Hand Surgery
The Steadman-Hawkins Clinic
New York, New York

Bradley T. Poole, M.D.
MCP Hahnemann University
Philadelphia, Pennsylvania

William R. Post, M.D.
Clinical Associate
Department of Orthopedics
West Virginia School of Medicine
Morgantown, West Virginia

Neal E. Pratt, P.T., Ph.D.
Professor Emeritus
Department of Rehabilitation Sciences
MCP Hahnemann University
Philadelphia, Pennsylvania

James L. Price, Jr., M.D.
Hand Surgeon
Orthopedic Specialists of Charleston
Charleston, South Carolina

Beth A. Purdy, M.D.
Phoenix, Arizona

Richard L. Read, P.T., E.C.S.
Board Certified Electrophysiologic Clinical Specialist
Upper Extremity Institute
Blue Bell, Pennsylvania

Arthur C. Rettig, M.D.
Methodist Sports Medicine Center
Indianapolis, Indiana

C. Christopher Reynolds, P.T., M.H.S., C.H.T.
Owner and Director
Desert Hand Therapy
Phoenix, Arizona

Erik A. Rosenthal, M.D.
Clinical Professor of Orthopedic Surgery
Tufts University School of Medicine
Boston, Massachusetts;
Honorary Staff
Baystate Medical Center
Springfield, Massachusetts

Christopher C. Schmidt, M.D.
Director of Upper Extremity Microsurgical Reconstruction
Department of Orthopedic Surgery
Allegheny General Hospital
Pittsburgh, Pennsylvania

Lawrence H. Schneider, M.D.
Clinical Professor
Department of Orthopedic Surgery
Former Chairman, Division of Hand Surgery
Jefferson Medical College of Thomas Jefferson
    University;
Former Director, The Philadelphia Hand Center, PC,
    and Fellowship Program;
President, Hand Rehabilitation Foundation
Philadelphia, Pennsylvania

**Karen Schultz-Johnson, M.S., O.T.R.,
    F.A.O.T.A., C.H.T.**
Hand & Upper Extremity Rehabilitation
Avon, Colorado

Mark E. Schweitzer, M.D.
Thomas Jefferson University
Philadelphia, Pennsylvania

Roger L. Simpson, M.D.
Assistant Professor of Surgery (Plastic)
State University of New York
Stony Brook, New York;
Director of the Burn Center
Nassau County Medical Center
East Meadow, New York

Terri M. Skirven, O.T.R./L., C.H.T.
Director of Hand Therapy
The Philadelphia Hand Center, PC;
Associate Director
Hand Rehabilitation Foundation
Philadelphia, Pennsylvania

Beth Paterson Smith, Ph.D.
Associate Professor
Department of Orthopedic Surgery
Wake Forest University School of Medicine
Winston-Salem, North Carolina

Jennifer Smith, M.S., O.T.R., C.H.T.
Co-Director
Department of Hand Therapy
University of Orthopedics, Inc.
Providence, Rhode Island

Kevin L. Smith, M.D.
Associate Clinical Professor
Department of Plastic Surgery
University of North Carolina
Chapel Hill, North Carolina;
Charlotte Plastic Surgery Center
Charlotte, North Carolina

Thomas L. Smith, Ph.D.
Associate Professor
Department of Orthopedic Surgery
Wake Forest University School of Medicine
Winston-Salem, North Carolina

Mary K. Sorenson, P.T., C.H.T.
Director of Hand Therapy
Washington, DC

Terry Speakman, O.T.R./L
Shriners Hospital for Children
Philadelphia, Pennsylvania

Peter J. Stern, M.D.
Professor and Chairman
Department of Orthopedic Surgery
University of Cincinnati College of Medicine
Cincinnati, Ohio

Virak Tan, M.D.
Resident
Department of Orthopedic Surgery
Pavilion Presbyterian Hospital
University of Pennsylvania School of Medicine
Philadelphia, Pennsylvania

John S. Taras, M.D.
Clinical Assistant Professor
Division of Hand Surgery
Department of Orthopedic Surgery
Thomas Jefferson University
Thomas Jefferson University Hospital;
The Philadelphia Hand Center, PC
Philadelphia, Pennsylvania

Andrew L. Terrono, M.D.
Associate Clinical Professor
Department of Orthopedics
Tufts University School of Medicine;
Hand Surgeon
Department of Orthopedics
New England Baptist Hospital;
New England Bone and Joint Institute
Boston, Massachusetts

Susan M. Tribuzi, O.T.R./L., C.H.T.
Senior Therapist
Hand Rehabilitation Associates
Crystal Clinic
Akron, Ohio

Sheryl S. Ulin, Ph.D., C.P.E.
Senior Research Associate Engineer
Center for Ergonomics
University of Michigan
Ann Arbor, Michigan

Gwendolyn van Strien, P.T., M.S.C.
Course Director and Instructor
National Institute for Allied Health Post Graduate
    Education
Amersfoort, The Netherlands;
Owner and Director
Hand Rehabilitation
Den Haag, The Netherlands

June P. Villeco, M.B.A., O.T.R./L., C.H.T.
Senior Therapist
Out-Patient Occupational Therapy
Montgomery Hospital
Norristown, Pennsylvania;
Hand and UE Rehabilitation Program
Mercy Health Systems
Philadelphia, Pennsylvania

Cornelia Von Lersner-Benson, O.T., C.H.T.
Area Director of Hand Therapy
Department of Occupational Therapy
NovaCare Outpatient Rehabilitation
Cherry Hill, New Jersey

**Thomas G. Wadsworth, M.C.H., O.R.T.H., L.L. M.,
    F.R.C.S., F.A.C.S.**
Formerly Consultant Orthopedic and Hand Surgeon
St. Bartholomew's Hospital
London, England;
Associate Clinical Professor of Surgery
Michigan State University
Orthopedic Surgeon
Blodgett Memorial Hospital
Grand Rapids, Michigan

Mark T. Walsh, P.T., M.S., C.H.T.
Clinical Site Coordinator
Hand and Orthopedic Rehabilitation Center
Levittown, Pennsylvania

Jinsong Wang, M.D., Ph.D.
Clinical and Research Fellow
Division of Rheumatology
Brigham and Women's Hospital
Harvard School of Medicine;
Research Fellow
Department of Immunology and Infectious Diseases
Harvard School of Public Health
Boston, Massachusetts

Barry E. Watkins, M.D.
Instructor
Department of Orthopedic Surgery
Loma Linda University
Loma Linda, California

Stephan H. Whitenack, Ph.D., M.D.
Associate Professor
Department of Surgery
University of Philadelphia;
Chestnut Hill Hospital
Philadelphia, Pennsylvania

Diana A. Williams, M.B.A., O.T.R., C.H.T.
Georgia Hand Therapy and Upper Extremity Center
Medical Center of Central Georgia
The Macon Orthopedic and Hand Center
Macon, Georgia

Gerald R. Williams, Jr., M.D.
Associate Professor
Chief, Shoulder and Elbow Service
Department of Orthopedic Surgery
University of Pennsylvania School of Medicine;
Penn Musculoskeletal Institute
Philadelphia, Pennsylvania

Robert Lee Wilson, M.D.
Clinical Lecturer in Surgery
Department of Orthopedic Surgery
University of Arizona
Tucson, Arizona;
Consultant in Hand Surgery
Phoenix Orthopedic Residency Program
Maricopa Medical Center
Phoenix, Arizona

Jennifer Moriatis Wolf, M.D.
Clinical Instructor
Department of Orthopedics
Brown University School of Medicine;
Trauma Fellow
Rhode Island Hospital
Providence, Rhode Island

Steven L. Wolf, Ph.D., P.T.
Professor
Department of Rehabilitation Medicine;
Professor of Geriatrics
Department of Medicine;
Associate Professor
Department of Cell Biology
Emory University School of Medicine
Atlanta, Georgia

Terri L. Wolfe, O.T.R./L., C.H.T.
Director
Hand and Arthritis Rehabilitation Center
Erie, Pennsylvania

Heidi Hermann Wright, M.B.A., O.T.R., C.H.T.
President
Helping Hands Work, Wellness Spa
Indianapolis, Indiana

Thomas W. Wright, M.D.
Department of Orthopedic Surgery
University of Florida College of Medicine
Gainesville, Florida

Raymond K. Wurapa, M.D.
Department of Orthopedic Surgery
Mount Carmel Medical Center and Children's Hospital;
Greater Ohio Orthopedic Surgery, Inc.
Columbus, Ohio

David S. Zelouf, M.D.
Clinical Assistant Professor of Orthopedic Surgery
Division of Hand Surgery
Department of Orthopedic Surgery
Thomas Jefferson University
The Philadelphia Hand Center, PC
Philadelphia, Pennsylvania

FOREWORD

"Next to the Brain, the Hand is the greatest asset to man, and to it is due the development of Man's Handiwork."

(STERLING BUNNELL)

I am proud to write the foreword to the fifth edition of *Rehabilitation of the Hand and Upper Extremity*. As co-editor of four editions and editor emeritus of this edition, I would like to pay my respects to the physicians, surgeons, and therapists, here and abroad, who participated over the years in these multiple editions and in our annual "Surgery and Rehabilitation of the Hand" symposium cosponsored by the Jefferson Medical College in Philadelphia. These dedicated and giving professionals have been instrumental in integrating the philosophies of hand surgery and hand therapy and have created a roadmap to improved hand and upper extremity function.

I am privileged to pay my respects to the co-editors of previous editions: Lawrence Schneider, M.D.; Evelyn Mackin, L.P.T.; Judy Bell-Krotoski, O.T.R., F.A.O.T.A., C.H.T.; and Anne Callahan, M.S., O.T.R./L., C.H.T. They gave the time and dedication needed to see this massive project through and to build a frame for the dissemination of knowledge—a frame so strong that it authoritatively and comprehensively reflects the changes in hand surgery, hand rehabilitation, and patient care that have spanned three decades. Their vision is now shared with Terri Skirven, O.T.R./L., C.H.T., and A. Lee Osterman, M.D.

In the shadow of September 11, 2001, I see conflict in America's future. As I look into the past, almost four decades ago, I would like to give a short history lesson that occurred at the Valley Forge General Hospital during the Vietnam War, when hand rehabilitation became a partner of hand surgery.

My appointment as Hand Surgery Consultant at the Valley Forge General Hospital (VFGH) in 1964 coincided with the onset of the Vietnam conflict. This conflict grew rapidly into a major war, and casualties increased steadily. Transport systems and emergency medical treatment developed in World War II influenced how Vietnam battle casualties were handled.

Appointed by the U.S. Surgeon-General, Sterling Bunnell, M.D., was charged to establish specialized hand surgery centers in selected army hospitals in the United States and to provide expert second-phase treatment of hand injuries. One such center was established in 1941 at Valley Forge, Pennsylvania. At that time, there were no surgeons with hand surgery training in this country. Dr. Bunnell had just published the first book in hand surgery. He became the teacher of selected young surgeons at the nine army hospitals and went on to become the first president of the American Society for Surgery of the Hand (ASSH) in 1946.

Early in the Vietnam conflict, Colonel Phil Deffer was appointed Hospital Commander at VFGH. He knew Dr. Bunnell personally, had learned from Bunnell's WWII methods, and capably managed the large numbers of casualties sent by air medi-vac from the Pacific. Fortunately, by this time the specialty of hand surgery had grown. Certain medical officers who were trained in hand surgery were assigned to VFGH, which had become an orthopaedic hospital center for the eastern United States. It grew to 1100 orthopaedic beds and 150 hand and upper extremity beds, and it required more than 2000 working employees to function.

War trauma of the hand and upper extremity required comprehensive, well-planned surgery and the services of physical and occupational therapists. Physical therapists were concerned with wound care. Occupational therapists worked with open-wound amputees and early-fit plaster prostheses and provided bedside projects of leather and wood to encourage hand function. While these things were going on, the hand and upper extremity service was developing new procedures to manage the difficult high-velocity missile wounds of our casualties. Thumbs that had been lost to land mines were being rebuilt by new procedures that produced new thumb length, function, and nerve recovery with sensibility. The gliding systems of flexor and extensor tendons were often severely scarred. Passive tendon implants were used frequently with good results by the chiefs trained in hand surgery. The hand and upper extremity service became a classroom for acute surgery, reconstructive surgery, aftercare therapy, and later, rehabilitation.

About this time, 1967, Evelyn Mackin, physical therapist, joined my practice. She observed during my consulting trips to VFGH. Soon after, I was joined in my office by a second surgeon, Dr. Lawrence Schneider. This office now had two surgeons, a therapist, a whirlpool, an examining table, a splint cabinet, and a radio. We began to function as a mini-hand center, not knowing what to call our effort but enjoying our progress over the next 3 years. During this period the war casualties continued; the growth, development, and maturation of the hand surgery service continued; the orthopaedic and plastic services grew; and the rehabilitation concept continued to expand and evolve and become increasingly effective. On the civilian side, by 1971 we had grown sufficiently that we moved into a vacant bakery off campus at Thomas Jefferson University Hospital. With Evelyn Mackin overseeing therapy, we acquired an occupational therapist and an intern from the Public Health Service to do electromyographic studies, and the sign went up on the building that this was a Hand Rehabilitation Center. Shortly after this, we adopted Joe Greenberg's sculpture "Hand of Hope" as our logo.

During this same year, 1971, we held the first "Hand Symposium," entitled "Current Concepts in the Treatment of the Injured Hand," in November at Jefferson Medical College. John Madden, M.D., presented a film on a Hand Center started by Earl Peacock, M.D., in Chapel Hill, North Carolina, and he presented Irene Hollis, O.T.R., the first hand therapist at that center. Mr. George Welsh, Director of Rehabilitation of the Insurance Company of North America, spoke on programs to "minimize the disability of the working man." At the conclusion of this talk, Mr. Walsh introduced on stage the nurses and therapists who worked with him. A faculty panel entitled "Reconstruction and Rehabilitation of Peripheral Nerve Injuries" followed. The meeting was concluded for this day. Hand surgery papers and subjects had been well received, as had the presentations on rehabilitation. A pattern was developed for the future, and we realized that it was possible to bring surgery and therapy together in one forum.

The faculty and participants of this meeting were invited by Colonel Deffer to attend Grand Rounds of the hand and upper extremity service at VFGH. The guest moderators were Raoul Tubiana and J. William Littler. It was concluded by lunch at the Officers' Club and followed by a tour of the Valley Forge Battlefield.

It is time to pause and offer a "WELL DONE" tribute to Colonel Deffer and the men and women of the orthopaedic, plastic, and the hand and upper extremity services that served and aided the many casualties of the Vietnam conflict between 1964 and 1973. It was an unpopular war, and as we look back to 30 years ago, we can be proud of this medical effort. It gave hand surgery a very special opportunity to prove the importance of an organized hand and upper extremities service. The Chiefs (E. Dabezies, F. Stein, and F. Minkow) and their junior officers rose to the occasion, and they have established, forever, the importance of correlating hand surgery and hand therapy. This epic period at VFGH during the Vietnam conflict, in my opinion, heralded the beginning of hand therapy, and that is a gold nugget to be cherished from the winds of the Vietnam conflict.

Finally, the Vietnam conflict subsided with few fanfares. However, the benefits our hand center had received from an affiliation with the army hospital, and the improved results of flexor tendon surgery, gave us a boost. Our support during the Vietnam conflict assisted us in acquiring an Army Research and Development Command grant to complete our

tendon implant and prosthetic research. Even now, research continues on the development of new active tendon implants with the Wright Medical Technology, Inc.

In 1974, we held the "First Decade of Tendon Surgery" symposium, bringing together a distinguished hand surgery faculty and an audience of 400 surgeons. The meeting was reminiscent of the first tendon symposium held at Cornell Medical Center–Rockefeller Institute in 1964 and used the same dates, March 13, 14, and 15. Ever since this meeting, mid-March continues to be the time set aside for our annual symposium on "Surgery and Rehabilitation of the Hand."

With the success of the 1974 tendon meeting as a model, the first "Surgery and Rehabilitation of the Hand" symposium took place in the bicentennial year 1976 at the Benjamin Franklin Hotel in Philadelphia. Many suggested that this meeting would not be successful. However, with great efforts on the part of Dr. Schneider and Evelyn Mackin, there were 450 participants and the premiere symposium integrating hand surgery and therapy was highly successful.

This symposium became an annual affair, and the meetings of 1976 and 1977 formed the faculty that produced the first edition of *Rehabilitation of the Hand,* which was published in 1978. The editors were Hunter, Schneider, Mackin, and Bell-Krotoski. Judy Bell-Krotoski, O.T.R., had joined our group in 1976 and was already a strong force in research on sensibility evaluation in peripheral nerve neuropathies. In later years, the sensibility program at our center was further gifted by Anne Callahan. Subsequent editions of *Rehabilitation of the Hand* were edited by Hunter, Mackin, Schneider, and Callahan. Each edition presented us with an opportunity to invite recognized authorities to build on the challenging and ever-growing integration of hand surgery and therapy. The fourth edition expanded to two volumes.

This fifth edition represents a microcosm of the teaching needs learned from the Vietnam conflict, 26 "Surgery and Rehabilitation of the Hand" symposia, and the four previous editions of the text. This learned wealth of knowledge is encompassed now in two volumes and 129 chapters. This edition bonds rehabilitation of the hand to the upper extremity for now and in the future.

The fifth edition is beautifully arranged by the editors, for the reader, whoever he or she may be—something old, something new, something borrowed, and something blue.

I pay special respect to co-editor Evelyn Mackin for her contributions to hand rehabilitation for the last 35 years and to her co-editors, Anne Callahan and Terri Skirven. Special credit, too, goes to Lawrence Schneider, a review editor of great devotion, and to A. Lee Osterman, a review editor who stands in the wings and views the future.

It is now my privilege as editor emeritus, to salute this editorial team and the contributors to the first *Rehabilitation of the Hand and Upper Extremity* edition of the new millennium.

With a final drum roll, I toast our teachers and colleagues, in the words of Sir Isaac Newton:

"If I have been able to see the future, it is because I have stood on the shoulders of giants."

To the fifth edition of *Rehabilitation of the Hand and Upper Extremity,* I toast with the following thought:

This is a good ship. The human fiber in her hull and spars is tenacious and strong. The hand on the helm is thoughtful and steady. We can feel secure that this vessel is sound and will survive unknown waters and stormy seas for many years to come.

Farewell, and have a successful voyage.

JAMES M. HUNTER

PREFACE

New editions become necessary to take account of the changing concepts and advances in the treatment of hand injuries, and it is gratifying to the editors to provide the fifth edition of this book, first published in 1978 through the vision and philosophy of James M. Hunter, to whom the fifth edition is dedicated.

In his personal foreword to this fifth edition of *Rehabilitation of the Hand and Upper Extremity,* Dr. Hunter, Emeritus Editor, has well described its contents: "Something old, something new, something borrowed, and something blue."

"Something old," having kept the best and most timely topics from the previous editions; *"something new,"* recognizing that the "hand therapist" must be an "upper quarter therapist," we have added entirely new sections to the book and expanded other sections in topics covering the shoulder, elbow, and wrist; *"something borrowed,"* taking a classic chapter or two from other sources; and in the *"something blue"* category, we have added a few topics that at first glance might seem to be outside the realm of this book.

Why a fifth edition? Since the first edition appeared almost 25 years ago, the specialty of hand therapy has spread throughout the world. The International Federation of Societies for Hand Therapy now has societies in 31 countries. We are gratified that with each edition of this book, its worldwide audience has expanded accordingly, and the interest in updated editions continues. Our experience with hand surgery and hand therapy is that these specialties continue to evolve, to challenge, and to fascinate. We wanted to share these changing concepts and advances in this new edition. It was a challenge to do so and still keep the book within two volumes.

With that goal in mind, we did what we have done with each of the past four editions—we asked the best and the brightest master clinicians in hand surgery and therapy to contribute their expertise to this text. Almost without exception, these dedicated and committed professionals responded positively to our invitation. The result of their generous sharing is presented to you in this two-volume text.

Those familiar with the previous editions will recognize the "classic" topics that we have chosen to retain and will understand why—because their content is timeless. In some cases, we have retained both the chapter and author; in other cases, we have asked new authors to address an old topic with a fresh perspective.

We are excited about the 53 entirely new chapters that have been added, including Fibrocartilage Complex Injuries,

Clinical Examination of the Wrist and Elbow, Stiff Elbow, Radial Tunnel Syndrome, Nerve Injuries about the Shoulder, Focal Hand Dystonia, Electrical Injuries, Systemic Lupus Erythematosus of the Hand, Osteoarthritis, Upper Extremity Outcome Assessment, Soft Splints: Indications and Techniques, and Kinesio Taping.

Chapter topics that will serve to broaden the scope of routine practice of the hand therapist include two new chapters that address the lymphatic component in upper extremity edema: Management of Breast Cancer–Related Edemas and Manual Edema Mobilization: Treatment for Edema in the Subacute Hand. Other "out of the usual realm topics" include Focal Hand Dystonia and Rehabilitation of the Hand and Upper Extremity in Tetraplegia.

The fifth edition of *Rehabilitation of the Hand and Upper Extremity* marks a milestone for hand therapy in that the first three editors listed are hand therapists. This is a tribute to the partnership and mutual respect between hand therapy and hand surgery. Perhaps it is fitting that as James Hunter—someone who did so much to support hand therapy—retires, the editorship of this edition has passed into the hands of hand therapists.

We would like to express our appreciation first and foremost to the more than 100 surgeons and therapists who have contributed clinical expertise and academic insight to this text.

Our special thanks to James M. Hunter, who very kindly agreed to write the Foreword for this edition. It is an expression of the philosophy he established with the first edition in 1978—the surgeon and therapist together as a team.

We a owe a special debt of gratitude to Dorothy B. Kaufmann, whose loyalty and unfaltering support have resulted in much greater success for the Hand Rehabilitation Foundation than otherwise would have been achieved.

We acknowledge Thomas Jefferson University for its past and ongoing support of the educational, research, and clinical activities of the Hand Rehabilitation Foundation. This support has given us not only the credentials but also the encouragement to achieve our goals.

We continue to enjoy a close working relationship with Richard Lampert at Elsevier Science and in particular with the friendly and efficient cooperation of Kathy Falk, Senior Managing Editor, Medicine.

We especially thank Barbara G. Sielaff, Hand Rehabilitation Foundation secretary, who in addition to preparing manuscripts has also maintained lines of communication among authors, editors, and publisher contacts in the completion of this book.

Finally, we thank our spouses, Robert T. Henry, V.M.D. (EJM); Lawrence M. Matthews, Ph.D., M.D. (ADC); Charles DiGiorgio (TMS); Thelma Schneider (LHS); and Elissa Topol (ALO) for their patience, love, and encouragement always, and in particular during the 3 years it has taken to complete this book. We are pleased to present this fifth edition as a comprehensive reference for therapists and surgeons managing disorders of the hand and upper extremity caused by trauma, disease, or birth.

EVELYN J. MACKIN
ANNE D. CALLAHAN
TERRI M. SKIRVEN
LAWRENCE H. SCHNEIDER
A. LEE OSTERMAN

CONTENTS

ANATOMY OF THE UPPER EXTREMITY

Chapter 1

ATLAS ON REGIONAL ANATOMY
OF THE NECK, AXILLA,
AND UPPER EXTREMITY*

The anatomic text and illustrations in this chapter have been carefully chosen to support all of the following chapters on the hand and upper extremity.

Dr. Jack Healey's roots in the study of gross anatomy began in the Department of Anatomy at Jefferson Medical College in the 1950s. He became Professor of Anatomy at the University of Texas Graduate School of Biomedical Sciences and Chief of Experimental Surgery at the University of Texas M.D. Anderson Hospital and Tumor Institute.

*Reproduced from Healey JE Jr, Hodge J: *Surgical anatomy,* ed 2, Philadelphia, 1990, BC Decker.

Jack Healey wrote about and taught anatomy for the surgeon and graduate student all his life. In this text, we are now the beneficiaries of his gifts, in part abetted by fate, for if Jack Healey had not been stricken early with rheumatoid arthritis, he would have been a model thoracic surgeon.

The association of John Healey and Joseph Hodge, and the fine anatomic illustrations of Donald Johnson, William A. Osborn, and Jeanet Dreskin make this an excellent study for today's surgeons and hand therapists.

James M. Hunter, M.D.

THE NECK—PLATE 1
General considerations

Before examining the regional anatomy of the neck, one must know its topographic divisions and surface markings to simplify the areas of surgical importance.

Topography. (Fig. 1) The main topographic landmark in the neck is the sternocleidomastoid muscle. This muscle and the midline of the neck, along with the anterior border of the trapezius, divide the neck into an anterior and a posterior triangle.

The anterior triangle—is bounded anteriorly by the midline of the neck and posteriorly by the sternocleidomastoid muscle. Its superior boundary is formed by the lower border of the mandible and a line drawn from the angle of the mandible to the tip of the mastoid process. This triangle may be subdivided as follows:

1. Submandibular triangle
2. Submental triangle
3. Carotid triangle
4. Muscular triangle

The posterior triangle—is limited anteriorly by the sternocleidomastoid, posteriorly by the trapezius, and below by the middle third of the clavicle. This is further divided by the posterior belly of the omohyoid into the following:

5. Occipital triangle
6. Subclavian triangle

Surface markings. (see Fig. 1) In addition to the aforementioned sternocleidomastoid muscle and its bony attachments, other conspicuous and palpable structures in the neck include the following:

1. Thyroid cartilage—is especially prominent where the right and left laminae of this cartilage fuse in the upper midline of the neck, which is referred to as the *laryngeal prominence* or *Adam's apple.*

2. Hyoid bone—is located in the midline about 1 inch above the laryngeal prominence and in line with the lower border of the third cervical vertebra. If followed laterally, the greater cornu may be palpated. Its tip lies about midway between the laryngeal prominence and the mastoid process and is an important surgical landmark for the ligation of the lingual artery.

3. Cricoid cartilage—lies just below the thyroid cartilage and at the level of the sixth cervical vertebra.

Skin of the neck. The skin of the neck is of particular importance to the surgeon in regard to the cosmetic effect after incisions in this area. The fibers of the corium course predominantly in the planes of the body surface and display prevailing directions that differ strikingly in different regions of the body. These are the *Langer's lines.* In the neck, they run in a transverse direction, and incisions should be made accordingly (e.g., the collar incision for thyroidectomy).

Superficial fascia. (Fig. 2) This subcutaneous layer of the neck, like that elsewhere in the body, is made up of loose areolar connective tissue and contains superficial blood vessels and nerves. In the neck, in addition to these structures, one finds a voluntary muscle, the *platysma;* this muscle is one of facial expression, therefore innervated by the facial nerve. In incisions in the neck, the severed ends of this muscle always must be reapproximated to overcome unsightly postoperative defects. The superficial cervical veins and nerves are located deep to the platysma muscle.

1. External jugular vein—the vein descends superficial to the sternocleidomastoid muscle and pierces the deep cervical fascia in the posterior triangle to empty into the subclavian vein. The deep fascia is firmly attached to the vein wall as this vein pierces the fascia. This prevents collapse of the vein if it is accidentally cut.

2. Anterior jugular vein—begins in the suprahyoid region and descends near the midline parallel with its partner of the opposite side. Just above the clavicle, it pierces the deep fascia, passes beneath the sternocleidomastoid, and empties into the external jugular. It is often connected with the vein of the opposite side above the sternal notch, forming the *jugular venous arch.*

3. Vein of Kocher—often arises from the branches of the common facial vein, descends along the anterior border of the sternocleidomastoid, and drains into the jugular venous arch or the internal jugular. If the anterior jugular is absent, this vein usually is large.

4. Superficial cervical plexus—arises from the anterior primary divisions of cervical segments C2 to C4.

a. Lesser occipital (C2)—hooks around the spinal accessory; ascends along the posterior border of the sternocleidomastoid muscle; and terminates in auricular, mastoid, and occipital branches.

b. Great auricular (C2 to C3)—takes exit from under the middle of the posterior border of the sternocleidomastoid and extends upward posterior to and parallel with the external jugular vein.

c. Transverse cervical (C2 to C3)—exits just below the great auricular and extends across the sternocleidomastoid to the anterior triangle, where it fans out to supply the skin between mentum and sternum.

d. Supraclavicular (C3 to C4)—exits from the middle of the posterior border of the sternocleidomastoid and divides into three terminal branches:

(1) Anterior—extends downward, innervating the skin as far as the second intercostal space and the sternoclavicular joint.

(2) Middle—descends over the middle third of the clavicle, at times piercing this bone, thereby causing persistent neuralgia if involved in the callus following fractures of the clavicle.

(3) Posterior—is distributed to the skin over the upper two thirds of the deltoid and the acromioclavicular joint.

PLATE 1

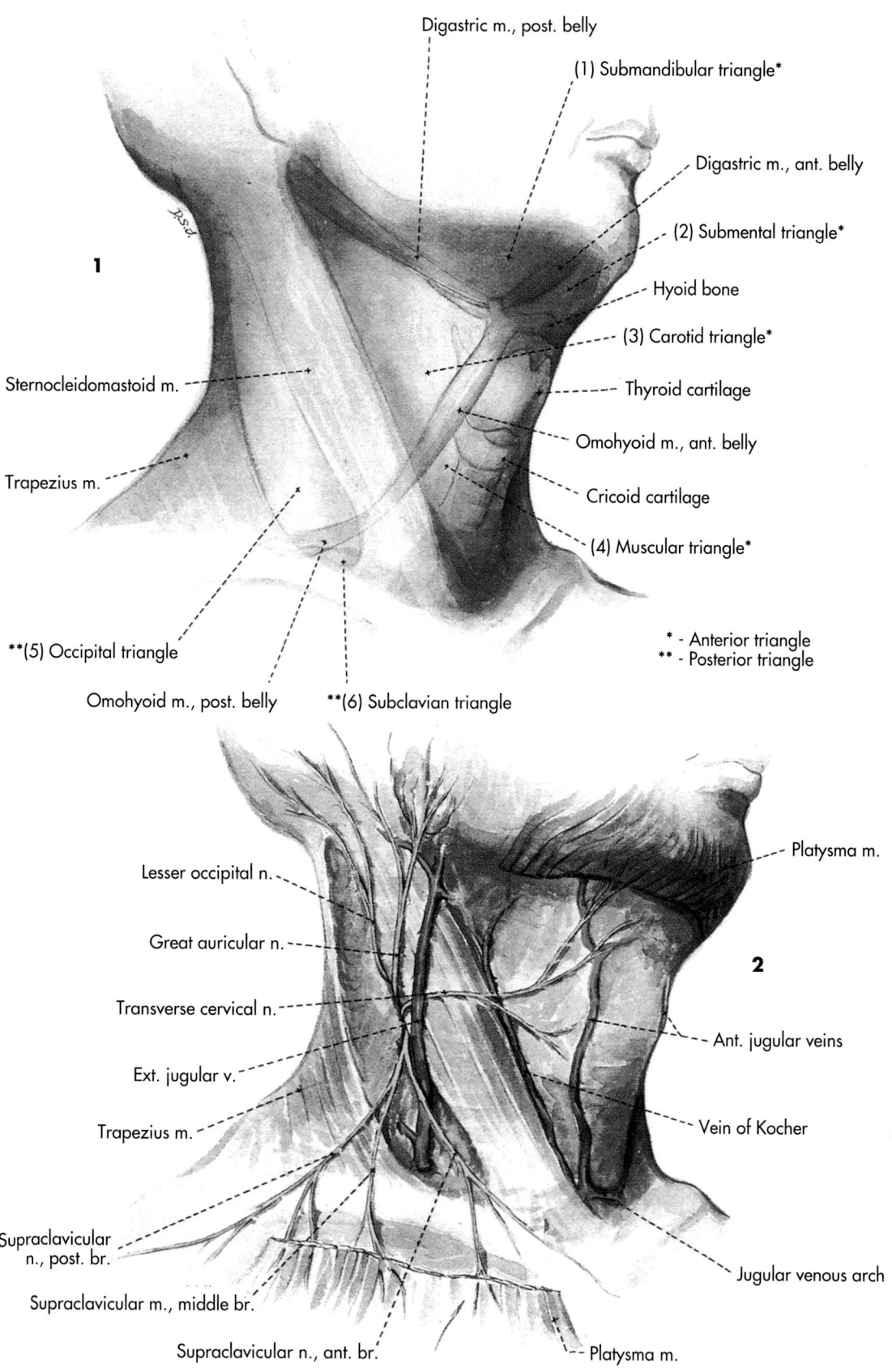

Digastric m., post. belly

(1) Submandibular triangle*

Digastric m., ant. belly

(2) Submental triangle*

Hyoid bone

(3) Carotid triangle*

Thyroid cartilage

Omohyoid m., ant. belly

Cricoid cartilage

(4) Muscular triangle*

Sternocleidomastoid m.

Trapezius m.

1

* - Anterior triangle
** - Posterior triangle

**(5) Occipital triangle

Omohyoid m., post. belly

**(6) Subclavian triangle

Lesser occipital n.

Great auricular n.

Transverse cervical n.

Ext. jugular v.

Trapezius m.

Supraclavicular n., post. br.

Supraclavicular n., middle br.

Supraclavicular n., ant. br.

Platysma m.

Ant. jugular veins

Vein of Kocher

2

Jugular venous arch

Platysma m.

THE NECK—PLATE 2
Carotid arterial system (Fig. 1)

1. Common carotid—the right common carotid arises as a terminal branch of the innominate artery, whereas the left common carotid arises directly from the arch of the aorta. In the carotid triangle, it is superficial in position and therefore readily palpable at the anterior border of the sternocleidomastoid, which partly overlaps it in the lower portion of the triangle. Only a few tributaries of the internal jugular vein, branches of the cervical plexus, and the omohyoid cross superficial to the artery. Digital compression to halt the flow of blood is placed at the anterior border of the sternocleidomastoid at the level of the cricoid, with pressure exerted posteriorly against the carotid tubercle on the transverse process of the sixth cervical vertebra *(tubercle of Chassaignac)*. The artery gives off no branches in the neck and ascends to a point ½-inch below and behind the greater cornu of the hyoid, or approximately at the upper border of the thyroid cartilage, where it terminates by dividing into the internal and external carotid arteries.

2. Internal carotid—continues upward in the carotid sheath through the submandibular and parotid spaces to enter the cranial cavity via the carotid canal. It gives off no branches in the neck.

3. External carotid—ascends through the submandibular and parotid spaces to terminate at the neck of the mandible. During its course, it gives rise to nine branches, some of which already have been described. These branches may be divided into anterior, posterior, and ascending branches:

    A. Anterior
        1. External maxillary
        2. Lingual
        3. Superior thyroid
    B. Posterior
        1. Posterior auricular
        2. Occipital
        3. Sternocleidomastoid
    C. Ascending
        1. Superficial temporal
        2. Internal maxillary
        3. Ascending pharyngeal (not illustrated)

Related structures (see Fig. 1)

1. Internal jugular vein—in the upper part of the carotid triangle, this vein receives the common facial, lingual, and superior thyroid veins. In the lower portion of the triangle, the middle thyroid vein empties into it. The venous pattern in this area is extremely variable.

2. Vagus nerve—gives off an important branch in the submandibular triangle: the *superior laryngeal,* the branches of which may be seen here. The *internal branch* may be identified piercing the thyrohyoid membrane at the lateral border of the thyrohyoid muscle. It carries sensory fibers from the larynx above the vocal cords. The *external branch* descends in association with the superior thyroid artery and innervates the cricothyroid and some fibers of the inferior constrictor.

3. Spinal accessory nerve—extends posteriorly deep to the sternocleidomastoid. Running with the nerve is the sternocleidomastoid artery, which may arise either from the external carotid or from the occipital artery.

4. Hypoglossal nerve—winds forward under the occipital artery in the upper part of the triangle and proceeds into the submandibular triangle. It appears to give off a branch to the thyrohyoid, but this is actually a branch of the deep cervical plexus, which is discussed later (Fig. 2).

5. Cervical sympathetic trunk—lies in the same position as in the submandibular triangle, posterior to the carotid sheath. This is not shown in the accompanying illustration.

Cervical plexus. (see Figs. 1 and 2) The cervical plexus arises from the anterior primary divisions of C1 to C4. The *superficial* portion of the plexus already has been described (see Fig. 2, Plate 1) and is purely sensory. The *deep cervical plexus* gives rise to some important motor nerves—mainly those to the strap muscles of the neck and the diaphragm, the latter via the phrenic nerve. Fig. 2 illustrates diagrammatically the main branches of this plexus.

1. Ansa hypoglossi—a branch from C1 joins the hypoglossal nerve and after a short course divides into a branch supplying the thyrohyoid and geniohyoid and a descending branch, the *descendens hypoglossi.* Descending branches from C2 to C3 form the *descendens cervicalis.* These two branches join to form the *ansa hypoglossi,* which usually lies anterior to the carotid sheath. It is from these cervical branches that the strap muscles receive their innervation.

2. Phrenic nerve—arises primarily from the anterior primary division of C4 but may receive slips from C3 or C5. This is discussed more fully on page 10.

PLATE 2

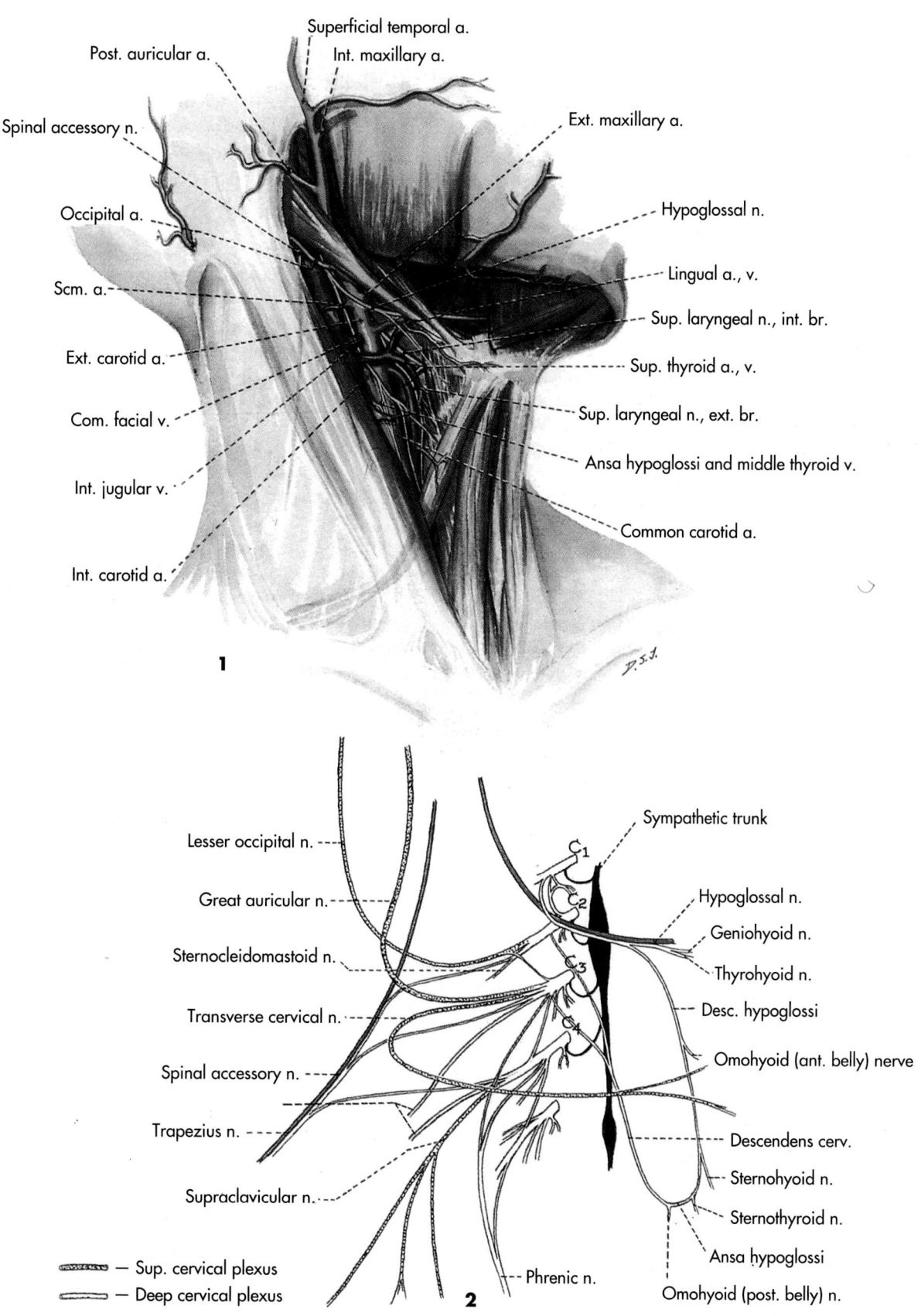

Superficial temporal a.

Int. maxillary a.

Post. auricular a.

Spinal accessory n.

Ext. maxillary a.

Occipital a.

Hypoglossal n.

Scm. a.

Lingual a., v.

Sup. laryngeal n., int. br.

Ext. carotid a.

Sup. thyroid a., v.

Com. facial v.

Sup. laryngeal n., ext. br.

Int. jugular v.

Ansa hypoglossi and middle thyroid v.

Common carotid a.

Int. carotid a.

D.S.J.

1

Lesser occipital n.

Sympathetic trunk

C_1

Great auricular n.

C_2

Hypoglossal n.

Geniohyoid n.

Sternocleidomastoid n.

C_3

Thyrohyoid n.

Transverse cervical n.

Desc. hypoglossi

C_4

Spinal accessory n.

Omohyoid (ant. belly) nerve

Trapezius n.

Descendens cerv.

Sternohyoid n.

Supraclavicular n.

Sternothyroid n.

Ansa hypoglossi

━ — Sup. cervical plexus

Phrenic n.

Omohyoid (post. belly) n.

━ — Deep cervical plexus

2

THE NECK—PLATE 3
The posterior triangle

The anterior scalene is the major landmark in this area, and the presence of the brachial plexus, phrenic nerve, and lymph nodes are of surgical importance.

Boundaries and muscular contents. (Fig. 1) The boundaries include the sternocleidomastoid, the trapezius, and the middle third of the clavicle. The posterior belly of the omohyoid divides the triangle into two smaller triangles, each of which is named according to the artery present: the *occipital* above and the *subclavian* below. Within the triangle, the following muscles may be seen, from anterior to posterior:

1. Anterior scalene—arises from the anterior tubercles of C3 to C6 and inserts on the scalene tubercle *(Lisfranc's)* on the upper surface of the first rib.

2. Middle scalene—arises by slips from the transverse processes of C1 to C6 and is the largest of the scalenes. It also inserts on the first rib on a tubercle behind the groove for the subclavian artery.

3. Posterior scalene—may be regarded as fibers of the middle scalene, which gain attachment to the lateral surface of the second rib. Like the other scalenes, these fibers are innervated by branches of the anterior rami of the cervical nerves.

4. Levator scapulae—arises from the transverse processes of the first four cervical vertebrae and inserts on the vertebral border of the scapula. It is innervated by both the deep cervical plexus and the dorsal scapular branch of the brachial plexus.

In addition to the aforementioned muscles, the *splenius capitis* and the *semispinalis capitis* are present in the apex of the occipital triangle. Both belong to the spinal group of muscles and are innervated by the posterior primary divisions of the cervical nerves.

Superficial fascia (see Fig. 2, Plate 1)

Deep fascia. (see Fig. 1) All three layers of the deep cervical fascia are present in the posterior triangle. The *superficial layer* roofs the triangle and surrounds the two bounding muscles: the trapezius and sternocleidomastoid. The *middle layer,* its anterior lamella, extends laterally to the posterior belly of the omohyoid and is therefore found only in the subclavian triangle. It is a very distinct layer, anterior to which lies a pad of brownish fat, forming an important landmark in the approach to the anterior scalene. The *deep layer* covers the muscles in the floor of the triangle and is extremely important in radical neck dissections because, as will be seen, almost all important motor nerves lie deep to this fascial plane.

Brachial plexus. (Fig. 2) The brachial plexus lies deep to the deep layer of fascia, as do all its branches. It may be divided into the following parts:

1. Anterior primary divisions—arise from C5 through T1 and are located behind the anterior scalene. Two main branches are given off from these parts: the *dorsal scapular* from C5, which innervates the rhomboids and the levator scapulae, and the *long thoracic* from C5, C6, and C7, which supplies the serratus anterior.

2. Trunks—form at the lateral border of the anterior scalene. The anterior primary divisions of C5 and C6 join to form the *upper trunk,* C7 continues as the *middle trunk,* and C8 and T1 unite to form the *lower trunk.* The upper trunk is the only one that gives rise to any branches; these are the *suprascapular,* which extends into the scapular region to supply the supraspinatus and infraspinatus, and the *subclavius,* which innervates the subclavius muscle.

3. Secondary divisions—arise just behind the clavicle, each trunk dividing into an anterior and a posterior secondary division.

4. Cords—are located in the axilla. All posterior secondary divisions join to form a posterior cord. The anterior secondary divisions of upper and middle trunks form the anterolateral cord, and the anterior secondary division of the lower trunk continues as the anteromedial cord. The cords and their terminal divisions are discussed on page 16.

PLATE 3

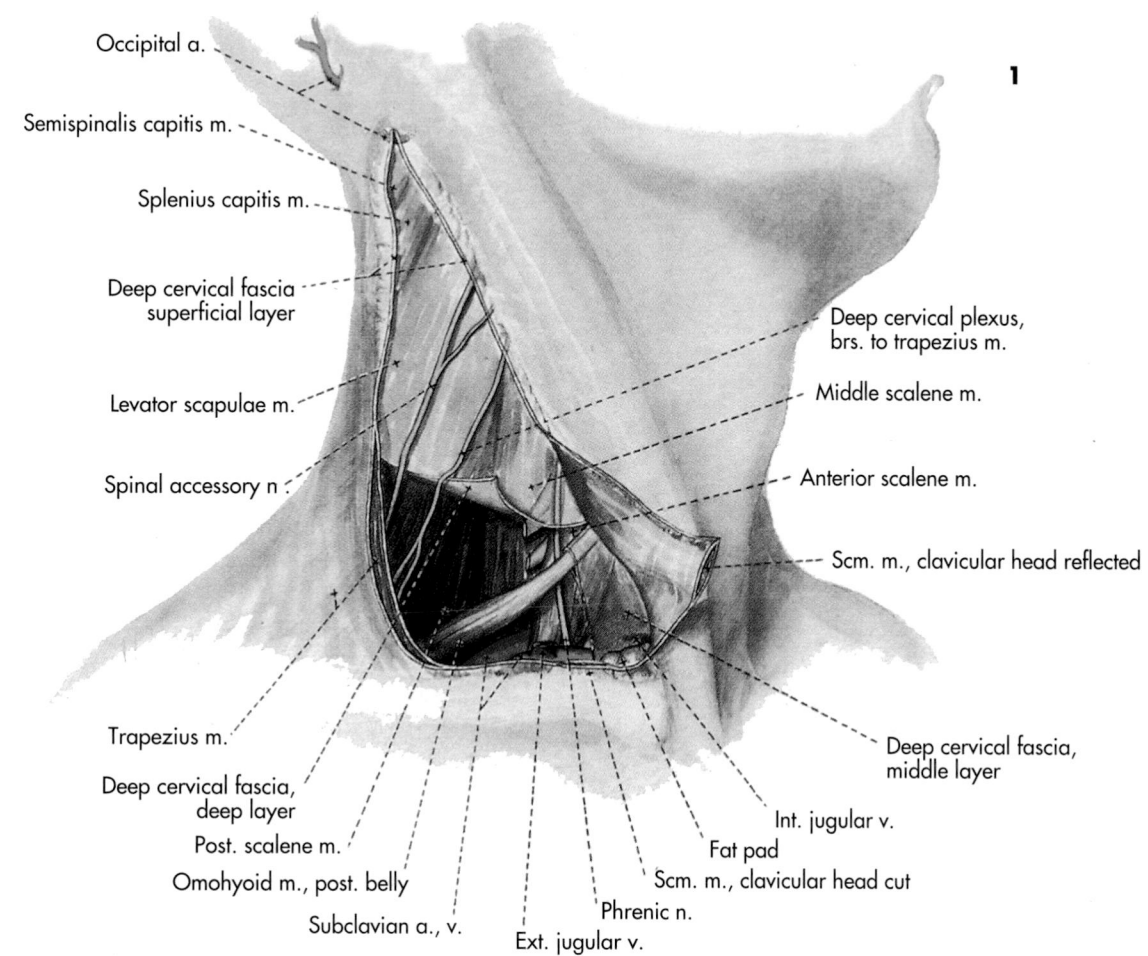

Occipital a.

Semispinalis capitis m.

Splenius capitis m.

Deep cervical fascia
superficial layer

Levator scapulae m.

Spinal accessory n

Deep cervical plexus,
brs. to trapezius m.

Middle scalene m.

Anterior scalene m.

Scm. m., clavicular head reflected

Deep cervical fascia,
middle layer

Trapezius m.

Deep cervical fascia,
deep layer

Post. scalene m.

Omohyoid m., post. belly

Subclavian a., v.

Ext. jugular v.

Phrenic n.

Scm. m., clavicular head cut

Fat pad

Int. jugular v.

1

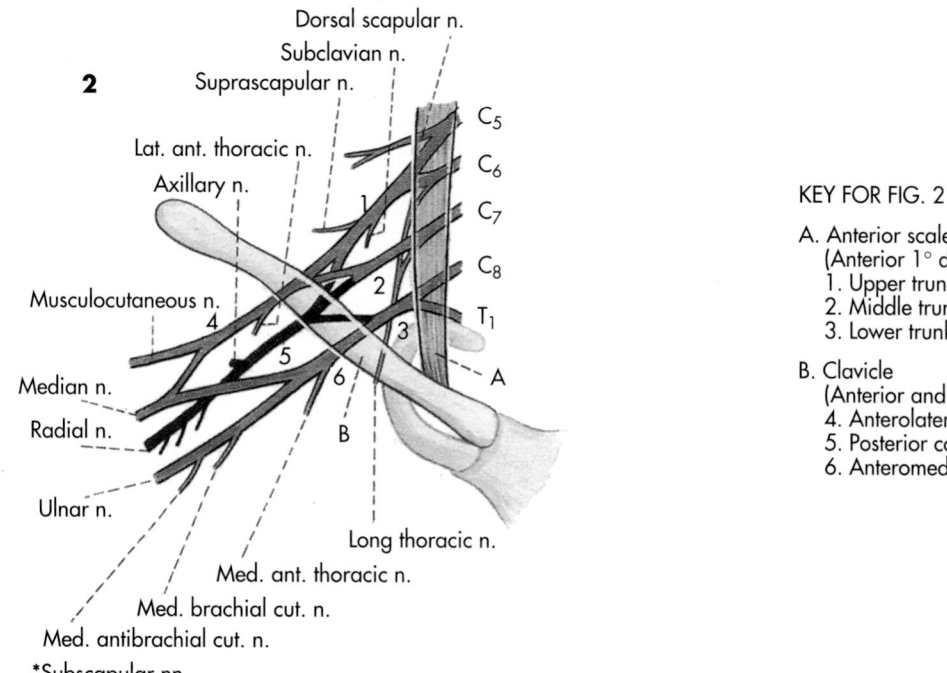

Dorsal scapular n.

Subclavian n.

Suprascapular n.

Lat. ant. thoracic n.

Axillary n.

Musculocutaneous n.

Median n.

Radial n.

Ulnar n.

Med. antibrachial cut. n.

Med. brachial cut. n.

Med. ant. thoracic n.

Long thoracic n.

*Subscapular nn.

C₅
C₆
C₇
C₈
T₁
A
B

2

KEY FOR FIG. 2

A. Anterior scalene muscle
(Anterior 1° division behind)
1. Upper trunk
2. Middle trunk
3. Lower trunk

B. Clavicle
(Anterior and posterior 2° divisions behind)
4. Anterolateral cord
5. Posterior cord
6. Anteromedial cord

THE NECK—PLATE 4

Anterior scalene muscle. (Fig. 1) This muscle has gained great clinical significance because of its relationship with such structures as the subclavian artery, brachial plexus, and phrenic nerve. Spasm or contracture of the muscle leads to circulatory and neurologic symptoms in the upper extremity that often necessitate surgical intervention. It is covered by the clavicular head of the sternocleidomastoid, and immediately in front of the muscle are the subclavian vein, the transverse cervical and transverse scapular vessels, and the phrenic nerve. Behind the muscle are the subclavian artery and the brachial plexus.

Related structures (see Fig. 1)

1. Subclavian vein—lies superficial in position in front of the anterior scalene but usually does not rise above the clavicle. It receives the external jugular in the posterior triangle, and on the left side, the thoracic duct may enter more lateral than usual, thereby passing anterior to the anterior scalene.

2. Subclavian artery—lies behind the anterior scalene, the muscle dividing the artery into three parts: the first lying medial to the muscle, the second behind, and the third lateral to the muscle.

a. First portion—gives rise to three branches: the vertebral, internal mammary, and thyrocervical trunk. The inferior thyroid branch of the thyrocervical trunk passes behind the carotid sheath to the posteromedial surface of the gland (not to the inferior pole) and sends off anastomotic branches to the superior thyroid, as well as tracheal and esophageal branches. The remaining two branches from the trunk cross in front of the anterior scalene superficial to the deep layer of cervical fascia. The transverse cervical is superior in position and extends across the posterior triangle to the anterior border of the levator scapulae muscle, where it divides into an ascending and a descending (posterior scapular) branch. The transverse scapular also passes in front of the muscle and extends laterally behind the clavicle to the supraspinatus and infraspinatus fossae.

b. Second portion—gives rise to only one branch, the costocervical trunk, which, because of its position behind the anterior scalene, is rarely of concern to the surgeon. This trunk gives rise to the deep cervical and superior intercostal arteries (not illustrated).

c. Third portion—usually has no branches. However, one may find a transverse cervical (German) arising here, which, if present along with the transverse cervical of the first portion (British), becomes the posterior scapular or descending branch.

3. Brachial plexus—anterior primary divisions of the plexus are located directly behind the anterior scalene and the trunks of the plexus at the lateral border of the muscle (page 8).

4. Phrenic nerve—is of prime importance because it supplies the muscle fibers of the diaphragm. The diaphragm develops in the cervical region and migrates downward, thus explaining its cervical innervation. The nerve arises from the anterior primary division of C4. However, it often receives fibers from C3 and C5. It takes a very characteristic course over the anterior scalene, passing downward from lateral to medial and *deep* to the deep layer of fascia. In many cases, the *accessory phrenic* is present. The three most common sites are (1) a branch from C5 passing downward lateral to the phrenic and joining it either in the root of the neck or in the subclavian triangle and thence into the thorax, (2) a branch from C5 incorporated with the nerve to the subclavius and passing into the thorax anterior to the subclavian vein (see Fig. 1), or (3) a branch from C3 incorporated in the ansa hypoglossi and joining the phrenic in the thorax.

5. Spinal accessory nerve—is not directly related to the anterior scalene but is the uppermost structure of importance in the posterior triangle. It takes exit from under the sternocleidomastoid at the junction of its upper and middle third and descends parallel with the fibers of the levator scapulae. It then disappears beneath the trapezius, which it innervates. During its course, the nerve is joined by a communicating branch from the deep cervical plexus; running below and parallel to it are muscular branches from the deep cervical plexus to the trapezius muscle (see Fig. 1, Plate 3). The latter nerves may be mistaken for the spinal accessory. The previously mentioned nerves lie in a plane between the superficial and deep layers of the cervical fascia. They are the only motor nerves that lie superficial to the deep layer of deep cervical fascia.

PLATE 4

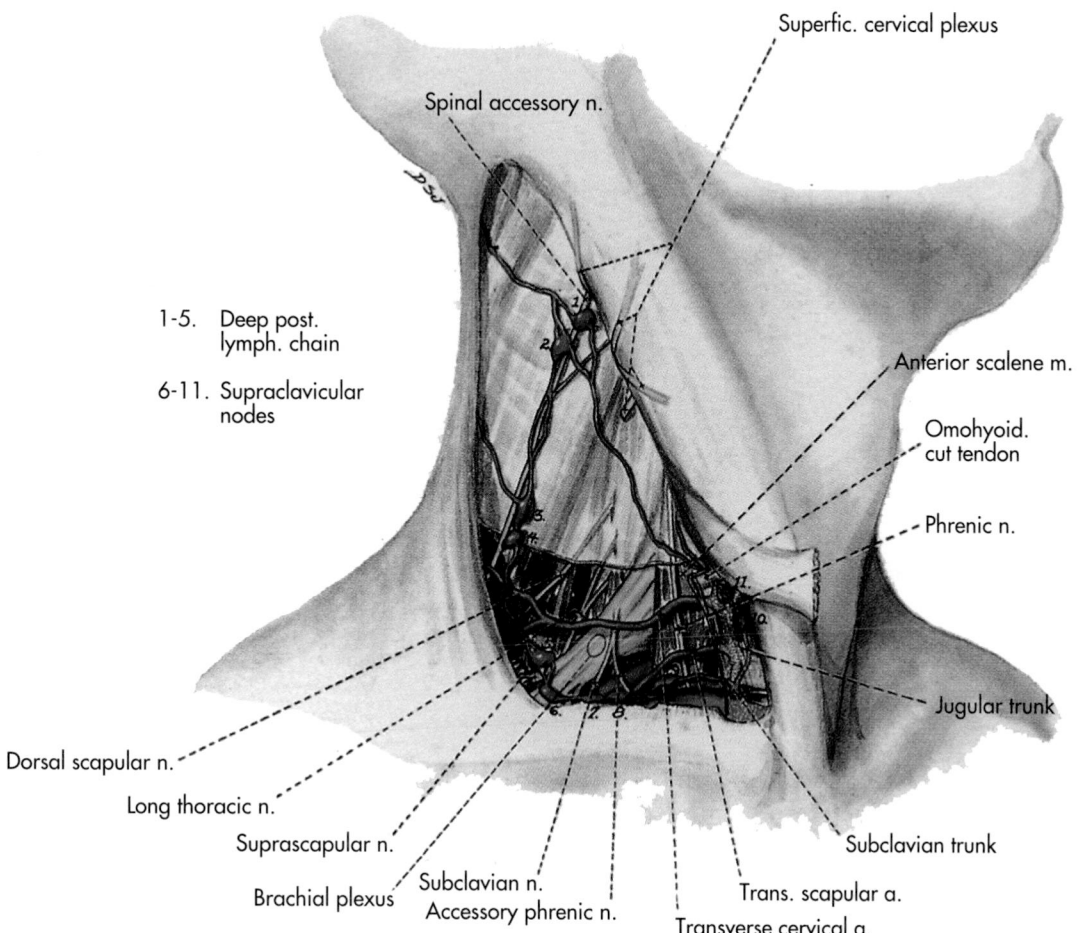

Superfic. cervical plexus

Spinal accessory n.

1-5. Deep post.
       lymph. chain

6-11. Supraclavicular
        nodes

Anterior scalene m.

Omohyoid.
cut tendon

Phrenic n.

Jugular trunk

Dorsal scapular n.

Long thoracic n.

Suprascapular n.

Subclavian trunk

Brachial plexus   Subclavian n.

Accessory phrenic n.

Trans. scapular a.

Transverse cervical a.

THE NECK—PLATE 5

Cervical rib. (Fig. 1) The incidence of cervical ribs is reported as being 1% to 2%, most of these being bilateral. The anterior extremity of a cervical rib extending from C7 may terminate in one of several ways: (1) articulate with the sternum, (2) articulate or fuse with the first rib, (3) attach to the first rib by a fibrous band, or (4) present a free end. When it is well developed, both the subclavian artery and the lower trunk of the brachial plexus groove the anterior and upper surface of the cervical rib, and symptoms of vascular or nerve compression may be produced. Poststenotic aneurysm of the third part of the subclavian artery also may result. These changes develop because of impingement of the plexus and subclavian artery between the anterior scalene muscles and the cervical rib and its fibrous band or by angulation of the plexus and vessel over the cervical rib in their exit through the superior thoracic aperture. Treatment ranges from conservative muscular reeducation to scalenotomy with or without resection of the rib.

Scalene anticus syndrome. (see Fig. 1) Although this is not a true congenital defect, it may be best mentioned here because it gives rise to symptoms identical to those of a cervical rib but results from spasm or hypertrophy of the scalene anticus muscle. Transection of the scalene at its insertion may be performed to alleviate this condition. During the procedure, one should recall the anterior relation of the subclavian vein and phrenic nerve (page 10).

Thoracic outlet syndrome. The cervical rib syndrome and the scalene anticus syndrome are two of many syndromes preferably called *thoracic outlet syndrome*. The other syndromes included are hyperabduction syndrome, first thoracic rib syndrome, pectoralis minor syndrome, and costoclavicular syndrome. The symptoms produced by all of these conditions are caused by compression of the neurovascular structures extending anywhere from the thoracic outlet to the insertion of the pectoralis minor muscle. They are characterized by neurologic deficits and/or vascular (arterial or venous) changes in the upper extremity.

Most patients are relieved by nonoperative methods, including weight reduction and muscle exercise programs. In case of vascular occlusion or aneurysmal formation in the subclavian artery, operative intervention is imperative. Operative procedures may include transaxillary resection of the first thoracic rib, division of the pectoralis minor tendon, or resection of the clavicle.

PLATE 5

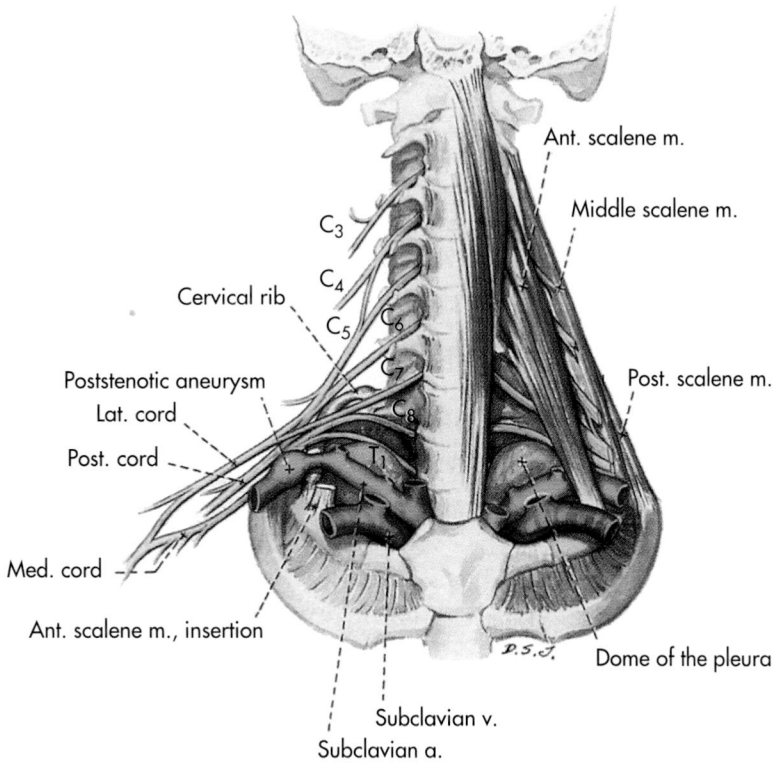

- Ant. scalene m.
- Middle scalene m.
- C₃
- C₄
- Cervical rib
- C₅
- C₆
- Poststenotic aneurysm
- Lat. cord
- C₇
- Post. scalene m.
- C₈
- Post. cord
- T₁
- Med. cord
- Ant. scalene m., insertion
- Dome of the pleura
- Subclavian v.
- Subclavian a.

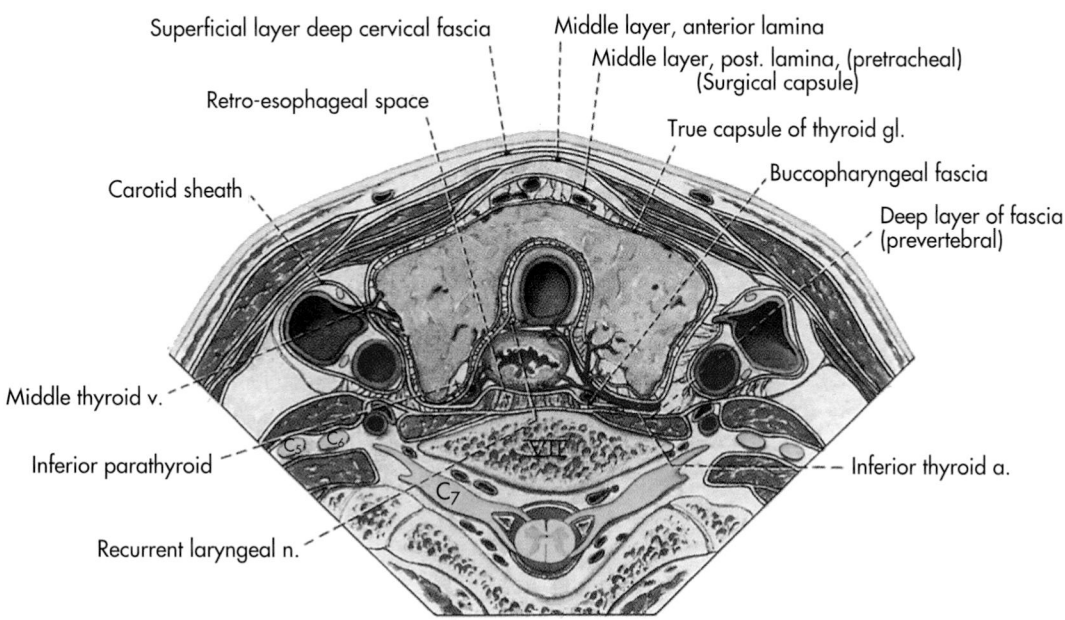

- Superficial layer deep cervical fascia
- Middle layer, anterior lamina
- Middle layer, post. lamina, (pretracheal) (Surgical capsule)
- Retro-esophageal space
- True capsule of thyroid gl.
- Carotid sheath
- Buccopharyngeal fascia
- Deep layer of fascia (prevertebral)
- Middle thyroid v.
- Inferior parathyroid
- Inferior thyroid a.
- Recurrent laryngeal n.
- C₇

THE BREAST AND AXILLA—PLATE 6
The axilla

The axilla, or armpit, is pyramidal in shape and therefore has an apex, base, and four muscular walls.

Boundaries. (Fig. 1)

1. Apex—is formed by the clavicle, the upper border of the first rib, and the superior border of the scapula.

2. Base—is made up of the skin of the axilla, the superficial fascia, and the axillary fascia, a continuation of the pectoral fascia.

3. Anterior wall—Consists of pectoralis major and minor and is innervated by the *antero*medial and *antero*lateral *cords* via medial and lateral anterior thoracic nerves.

  a. Pectoralis major—arises by a clavicular, sternal, and abdominal head and inserts into the lateral lip of the bicipital groove.

  b. Pectoralis minor—takes origin by slips from the second to fifth ribs and inserts on the coracoid process of the scapula.

4. Posterior wall—is made up of three muscles, which, from superior to inferior, are the subscapular, teres major, and latissimus dorsi, all of which are innervated by the *posterior cord* via the subscapular nerves.

  a. Subscapular—arises in the subscapular fossa and inserts into the lesser tubercle of the humerus.

  b. Teres major—takes origin from the inferior angle of the scapula and extends to the medial lip of the bicipital groove.

  c. Latissimus dorsi—has an extensive origin from the dorsum of the body and terminates in the bicipital groove.

5. Lateral wall—consists of two muscles, the coracobrachialis and the short head of the biceps, both arising from the coracoid process and innervated by the antero*lateral cord* via the musculocutaneous nerve.

  a. Coracobrachialis—extends from the coracoid process to the middle third of the shaft of the humerus.

  b. Short head of the biceps—arises in common with the coracobrachialis and inserts, after joining the long head, into the radius and the antebrachial fascia.

6. Medial wall—is formed by the upper digitations of the serratus anterius. It is innervated by the *long thoracic nerve* from anterior primary divisions of the brachial plexus.

Serratus anterius—arises from digitations from the upper nine ribs and inserts into the vertebral border of the scapula.

Deep fascia. (Fig. 2) Because the anterior wall of the axilla is made up of two muscular strata, it necessitates two distinct deep fascial layers: one covers the pectoralis major, the *pectoral fascia;* the other covers the pectoralis minor, the *clavipectoral fascia.*

1. Pectoral fascia—encloses the pectoralis major and extends from the lower border of the muscle to become *axillary* fascia extending posteriorly as the fascia of the latissimus dorsi. Laterally, it is continuous with the investing fascia of the arm.

2. Clavipectoral fascia—extends from the clavicle above to the axillary fascia below. It surrounds the subclavius and pectoralis minor muscles. Between the subclavius and pectoralis minor, this fascia is thickened to form the *costocoracoid membrane,* which is pierced by the cephalic vein, thoracoacromial vessels, and the anterior thoracic nerves. After splitting around the pectoralis minor, the fascia fuses and joins the axillary fascia to form the *suspensory ligament* of the axilla.

3. Axillary sheath—is a prolongation of the deep layer of the deep cervical fascia enclosing the axillary vessels and branches of the brachial plexus. It extends for a variable distance into the axilla.

Axillary vein (Fig. 3) With the upper extremity in the abducted position, the main structure brought into view is the axillary vein and its tributaries. More superficial, however, are the lateral cutaneous branches of the upper intercostal nerves; that from T2, passing to the medial side of the brachium, is termed the *intercostobrachial nerve.*

At the lower border of the teres major, the *basilic* vein joins the *brachial* veins to form the axillary vein, which extends upward to the lower border of the first rib. Here the vein is termed the *subclavian.* Its tributaries follow the branches of the axillary artery, except for the following:

1. Cephalic vein—arises on the dorsum of the hand, passes upward in the superficial fascia of the upper extremity, and pierces the costocoracoid membrane at the deltopectoral triangle. It empties into the axillary vein above the pectoralis minor. This vessel serves as a collateral channel for venous return from the upper extremity after occlusion of the axillary vein. It also serves as a guide to the first portion of the axillary artery.

2. Thoracoepigastric vein—connects the superficial epigastric below with the lateral thoracic branch of the axillary above, thus serving as an important collateral pathway after obliteration of the inferior vena cava.

PLATE 6

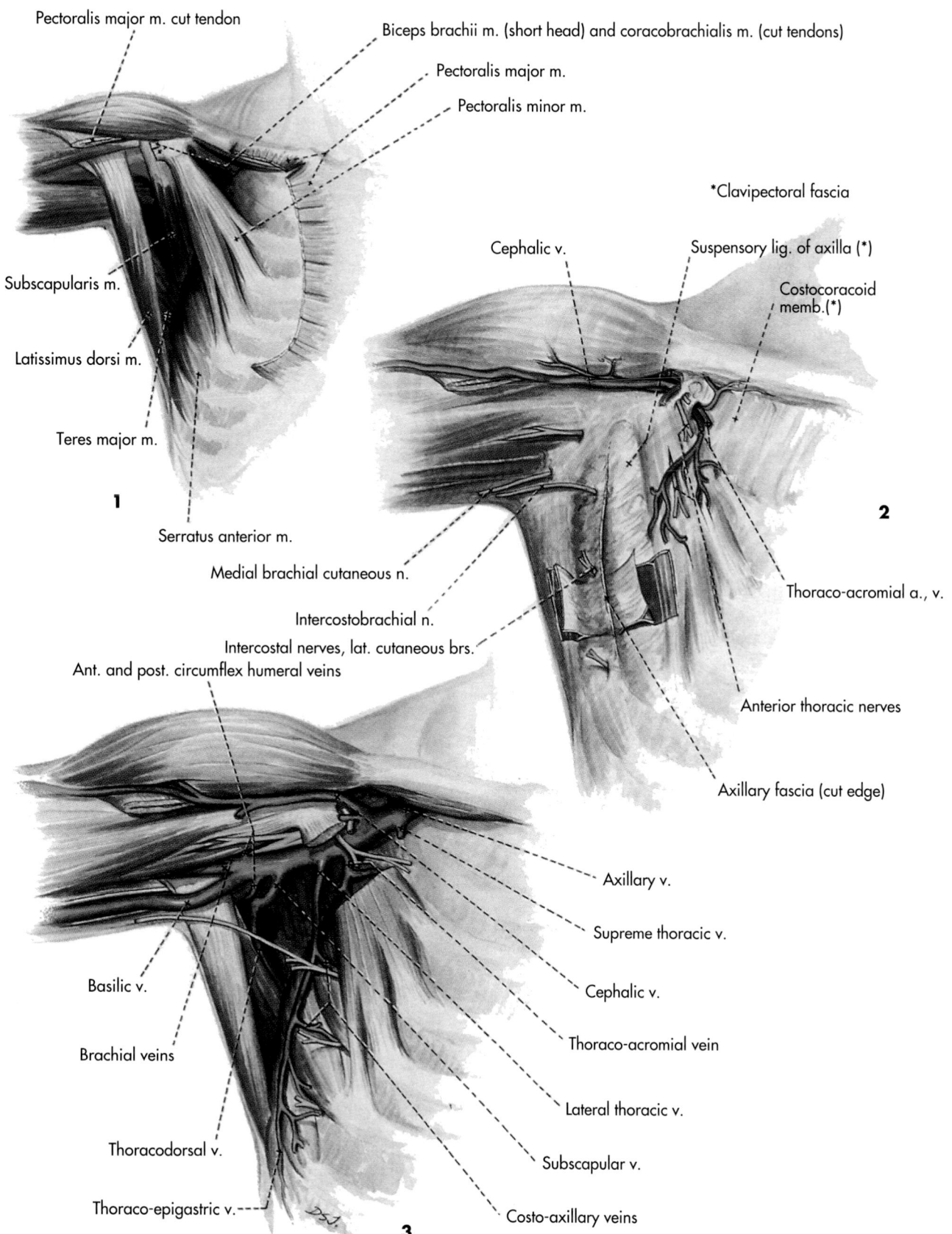

Pectoralis major m. cut tendon

Biceps brachii m. (short head) and coracobrachialis m. (cut tendons)

Pectoralis major m.

Pectoralis minor m.

*Clavipectoral fascia

Cephalic v.

Suspensory lig. of axilla (*)

Costocoracoid memb.(*)

Subscapularis m.

Latissimus dorsi m.

Teres major m.

1

Serratus anterior m.

Medial brachial cutaneous n.

Intercostobrachial n.

Intercostal nerves, lat. cutaneous brs.

Ant. and post. circumflex humeral veins

Thoraco-acromial a., v.

Anterior thoracic nerves

Axillary fascia (cut edge)

2

Axillary v.

Supreme thoracic v.

Cephalic v.

Thoraco-acromial vein

Basilic v.

Lateral thoracic v.

Brachial veins

Subscapular v.

Thoracodorsal v.

Thoraco-epigastric v.

Costo-axillary veins

3

THE BREAST AND AXILLA—PLATE 7

Axillary artery. (Figs. 1 and 2) After removal of the axillary vein, the artery is clearly visible along with the cords of the brachial plexus, which are named according to their relative position to the artery. The artery extends from the lower border of the first rib to the lower border of the teres major and is arbitrarily divided by the pectoralis minor into three parts:

1. First portion—is located between the first rib and the upper border of the pectoralis minor and gives off one branch.

SUPREME THORACIC—passes behind the axillary vein and across the apex of the axilla to supply the structures in the first intercostal space.

2. Second portion—is found behind the pectoralis minor and usually gives rise to two branches:

a. Thoracoacromial—pierces the costocoracoid membrane and divides into branches directed toward the clavicle, acromion process, and the deltoid and pectoral muscles.

b. Lateral thoracic—descends along the medial wall of the axilla to about the fifth intercostal space. It sends branches to the muscles of the anterior and medial walls of the axilla and mammary gland.

3. Third portion—extends from the lower border of the pectoralis minor to the lower border of the teres major. Three branches arise from this third portion (see Figs. 1 and 2):

a. Subscapular—extends toward the posterior wall of the axilla and terminates as the circumflex scapular and thoracodorsal. The former pierces the posterior axillary wall through a muscular interval, bounded by the subscapular, teres major, and long head of the triceps (triangular space), and reaches the infraspinatus fossa. The thoracodorsal continues through the axilla to the inferior scapular angle.

b. ANTERIOR CIRCUMFLEX HUMERAL—is a small branch that passes deep to the coracobrachial and biceps tendons and winds around the surgical neck of the humerus.

c. POSTERIOR CIRCUMFLEX HUMERAL—arises opposite the anterior circumflex branch and winds around the surgical neck of the humerus to anastomose with the anterior branch. It pierces the posterior wall of the axilla through a space bounded by the shaft of the humerus, teres minor, teres major, and long head of the triceps (*quadrilateral space*). It is accompanied in this space by the axillary nerve. The artery gives off an important anastomotic branch to the profunda brachii.

Brachial plexus. (see Figs. 1 and 2; Fig. 2, Plate 3)

1. Anterolateral cord

a. LATERAL-ANTERIOR THORACIC—pierces the costocoracoid membrane and supplies the pectoral muscles.

b. MUSCULOCUTANEOUS—is the most lateral of the terminal branches and innervates the muscles of the lateral wall of the axilla, the coracobrachialis, and the biceps. It pierces the coracobrachial as it descends to the arm.

c. LATERAL HEAD OF THE MEDIAN—forms the lateral component of the median nerve.

2. Anteromedial cord

a. MEDIAL-ANTERIOR THORACIC—joins the lateral anterior thoracic to innervate the pectoral muscles.

b. MEDIAN HEAD OF MEDIAN—passes obliquely over the third part of the axillary artery to join the lateral head from the anterolateral cord to form the median nerve. The latter lies along the lateral side of the artery.

c. ULNAR—is the largest of the medial cord branches and arises at the lower border of the pectoralis minor. It descends into the arm along the medial side of the axillary artery.

d. MEDIAL ANTEBRACHIAL CUTANEOUS—arises in close relation with the ulnar nerve.

e. MEDIAL BRACHIAL CUTANEOUS—lies medial to axillary vein in the lower axilla; pierces the deep fascia and is distributed to the skin of the medial surface of the arm.

3. Posterior cord (see Fig. 2)

a. SUBSCAPULAR NERVES—usually three in number and termed the *upper, middle,* and *lower.* They supply the muscles of the posterior wall of the axilla; the upper innervates the subscapular; the middle (thoracodorsal), the latissimus dorsi; and the lower, the teres major.

b. AXILLARY—extends dorsally and leaves the axilla via the quadrilateral space accompanied by the posterior humeral artery and innervates the deltoid and teres minor muscles.

c. RADIAL NERVE—is a direct continuation of the posterior cord lying behind the axillary artery. It is the largest terminal branch of the brachial plexus.

Long thoracic nerve. (see Fig. 1) This nerve arises from the anterior primary divisions of C5, C6, and C7. It pierces the middle scalene, then passes behind the brachial plexus into the axilla, where it runs along the medial wall, sending branches to the digitations of the serratus anterius.

Axillary lymph nodes. (Fig. 3) The axillary nodes may be arbitrarily divided into groups that are related to the four axillary walls, the apex, and the base. They are as follows:

1. Posterior (subscapular)—six or seven in number; along the subscapular vessels and thoracodorsal nerve.

2. Lateral (brachial)—four or five in number; along lower part of axillary vein.

3. Anterior (anterior pectoralis)—four or five in number; along edge of the pectoralis major.

4. Medial (posterior pectoral)—three or four; along the lateral thoracic artery and vein.

5. Central—three to five; lies at the base of the axilla in the fatty tissue.

6. Apical (infraclavicular)—four or five; at apex of triangle, closely related to axillary vein.

PLATE 7

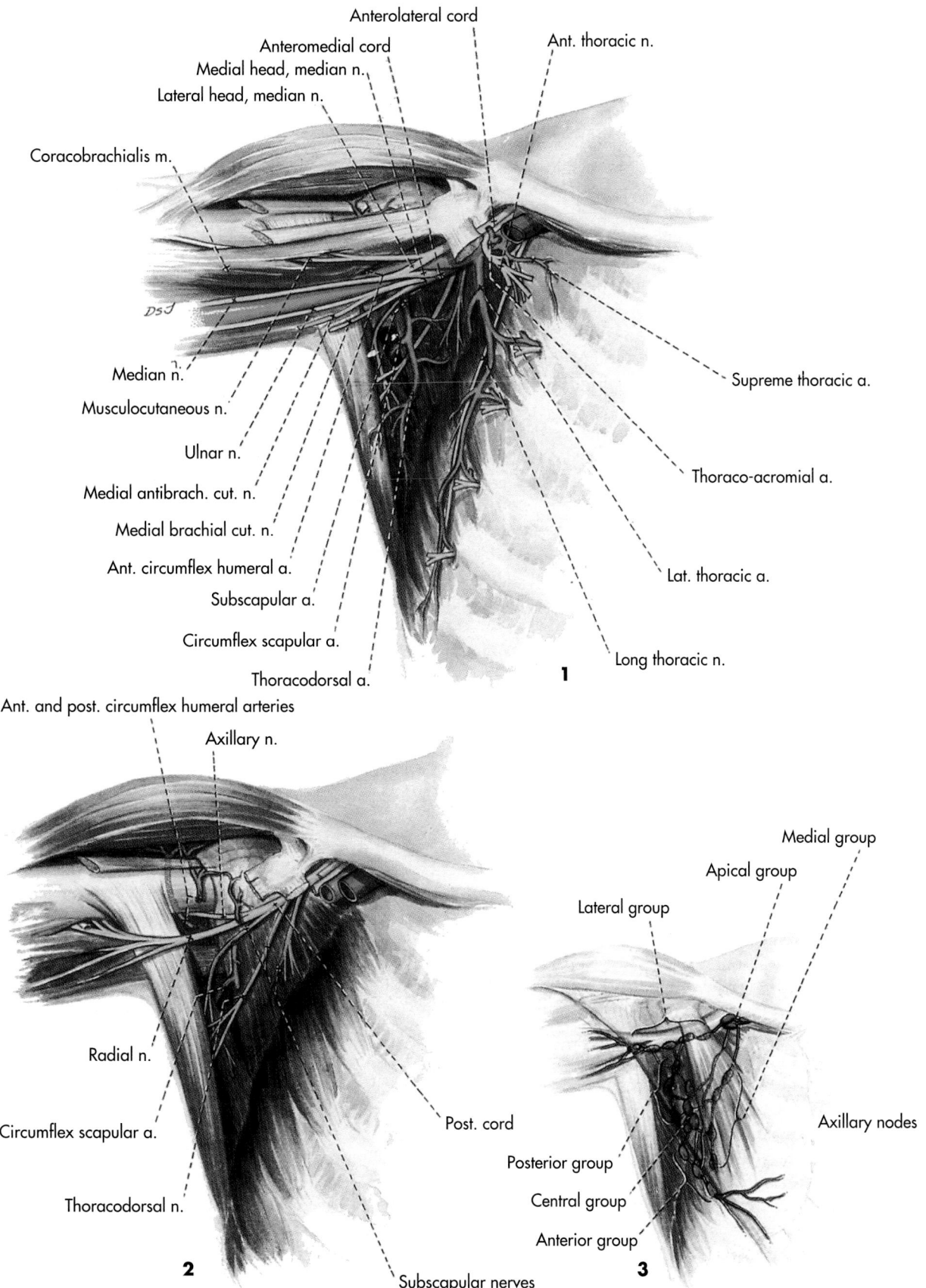

Anterolateral cord

Anteromedial cord

Ant. thoracic n.

Medial head, median n.

Lateral head, median n.

Coracobrachialis m.

Median n.

Musculocutaneous n.

Ulnar n.

Medial antibrach. cut. n.

Medial brachial cut. n.

Ant. circumflex humeral a.

Subscapular a.

Circumflex scapular a.

Thoracodorsal a.

Supreme thoracic a.

Thoraco-acromial a.

Lat. thoracic a.

Long thoracic n.

1

DsJ

Ant. and post. circumflex humeral arteries

Axillary n.

Radial n.

Circumflex scapular a.

Thoracodorsal n.

Post. cord

Subscapular nerves

2

Medial group

Apical group

Lateral group

Axillary nodes

Posterior group

Central group

Anterior group

3

THE UPPER EXTREMITY—PLATE 8
The brachium (anterior compartment)

The brachium extends from the lower border of the teres major to a line drawn through the medial and lateral epicondyles of the humerus. It contains the extensor and flexor muscles of the brachium, the terminal branches of the brachial plexus, and the brachial artery and veins.

Superficial fascia. (Fig. 1) Two main venous channels may be seen: one in the lateral bicipital groove, the *cephalic vein,* and the other in the medial bicipital groove, the *basilic.* The former already has been discussed on page 14. The basilic vein arises from the ulnar side of the dorsal venous rete of the hand and ascends through the arm in the medial bicipital groove. At the midportion of the arm, it pierces the deep brachial fascia, enters the neurovascular bundle, and joins the two brachial veins at the lower border of the teres major to form the axillary vein.

The cutaneous nerves of the arm and forearm are all direct or indirect branches of the cords of the brachial plexus. In addition to the brachial plexus, the lateral cutaneous branch of T2 *(intercostobrachial)* extends into the medial side of the arm. This explains why a brachial plexus block does not produce complete anesthesia of the arm.

Deep fascia. (Fig. 2) The brachial fascia is a tough circular encasement for the muscles of this area. It is continuous above with the axillary, pectoral, and latissimus dorsi fascial coverings; below, it is continuous with the antebrachial fascia and attaches to the epicondyles and the olecranon process. It sends septa medially and laterally to the humerus. The septa divide the brachium into two closed compartments, an anterior (flexor) and posterior (extensor), which limit effusions either hemorrhagic or inflammatory.

Muscular contents. (Figs. 3 through 5) The muscles related to the anterior compartment of the arm may be divided into two groups: an intrinsic group found within the flexor compartment and an extrinsic group that inserts into the humerus.

Extrinsic muscles

1. DELTOID—arises from the clavicle, the acromion process, and the spine of the scapula and covers the joint, producing the rounded contour of the shoulder. It inserts on a tuberosity on the lateral aspect of the middle of the humeral shaft. It is mainly an abductor of the arm and is innervated by the axillary nerve.

2. SUBSCAPULAR—arises in the subscapular fossa of the scapula, inserts into the lesser tubercle of the humerus, and forms part of the "rotator cuff" (page 40). Its chief function is medial rotation.

3. PECTORALIS MAJOR (page 14)—inserts into the lateral lip of the bicipital groove of the humerus and acts as a flexor, adductor, and medial rotator of the humerus.

4. LATISSIMUS DORSI (page 14)—inserts into the bicipital groove.

5. TERES MAJOR (page 14)—gains attachment to the medial lip of the bicipital groove and acts as a medial rotator, adductor, and extensor.

Intrinsic muscles—lie in the anterior or flexor compartment and are innervated by the musculocutaneous nerve.

1. CORACOBRACHIALIS—arises from the coracoid process of the scapula and inserts at the middle of the medial surface of the shaft of the humerus. It is pierced by the musculocutaneous nerve. This muscle acts as a flexor and adductor of the arm at the shoulder.

2. BICEPS BRACHII—the short head arises from the coracoid process; the long head takes origin from the supraglenoid tuberosity of the scapula. The biceps tendon inserts mainly into the radial tuberosity; however, some of its fibers expand medially and downward to insert in the antebrachial fascia *(lacertus fibrosus)* (see Fig. 2). Aside from its function as a flexor of the forearm, it acts as a very strong supinator.

3. BRACHIALIS—takes origin from the lower three fifths of the shaft of the humerus under cover of the biceps and inserts on the coronoid process of the ulna. In addition to its innervation by the musculocutaneous, the lower lateral fibers usually receive a twig from the radial. It serves to flex the arm at the elbow.

Neurovascular bundle. (see Fig. 5) The neurovascular bundle lies in the medial bicipital groove and contains the brachial artery and three terminal branches of the brachial plexus: the musculocutaneous, ulnar, and median nerves.

1. Musculocutaneous nerve—leaves the bundle in the upper arm, pierces the coracobrachialis, then descends between the brachialis and biceps, and continues superficially as the lateral antebrachial cutaneous. It supplies the three intrinsic muscles of the anterior compartment: the coracobrachialis, biceps, and brachialis.

2. Median nerve—is formed by the medial and lateral heads as described in the axilla (page 16). In the upper arm, the nerve lies lateral to the brachial artery, but in its descent through the arm, it crosses anterior to the artery and comes to lie on the medial side in the lower arm and cubital region. It gives off no branches in the arm.

3. Ulnar nerve—lies along the medial border of the brachial artery in the upper arm. At the insertion of the coracobrachialis, it pierces the medial intermuscular septum and enters the posterior compartment. It gives off no branches in the arm.

4. Brachial artery—supplies the entire brachium. It begins at the lower border of the teres major as a continuation of the axillary and terminates at the elbow by dividing into a radial and ulnar branch. In addition to its muscular and nutrient branches, its main trunks are as follows:

a. DEEP BRACHIAL (PROFUNDA)—is the largest branch and leaves the bundle in the upper arm to enter the posterior compartment accompanied by the radial nerve.

b. SUPERIOR ULNAR COLLATERAL—arises from the brachial about midarm, pierces the medial intermuscular septum, and accompanies the ulnar nerve into the posterior compartment.

c. INFERIOR ULNAR COLLATERAL—takes origin just above the elbow from the medial side of the brachial descending anterior to the medial epicondyle.

The brachial artery is accompanied by two brachial veins: the *venae comitantes.* At the lower margin of the teres major, these two veins join along with the basilic vein to form the axillary vein.

PLATE 8

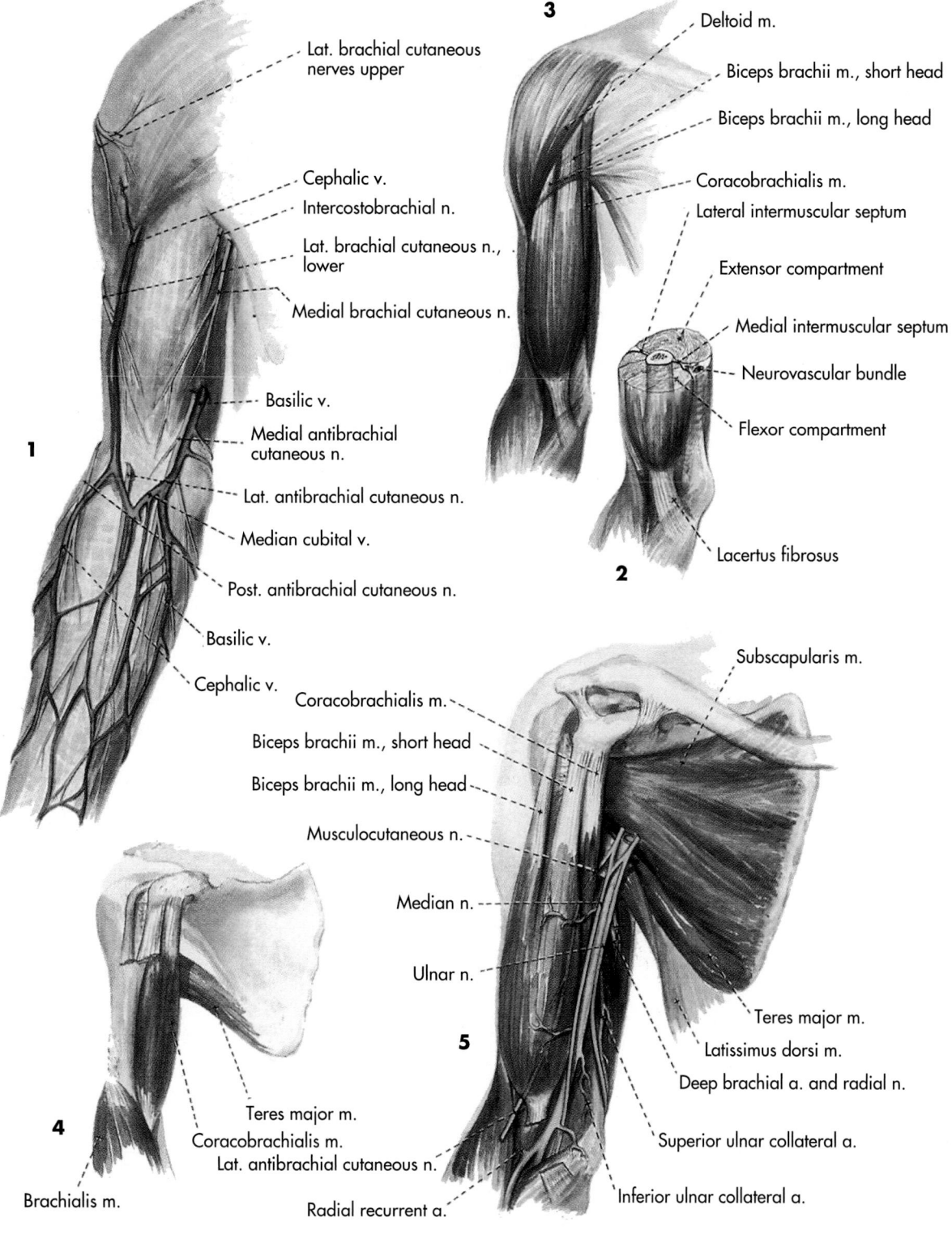

Lat. brachial cutaneous nerves upper

Cephalic v.

Intercostobrachial n.

Lat. brachial cutaneous n., lower

Medial brachial cutaneous n.

Basilic v.

Medial antibrachial cutaneous n.

Lat. antibrachial cutaneous n.

Median cubital v.

Post. antibrachial cutaneous n.

Basilic v.

Cephalic v.

1

3

Deltoid m.

Biceps brachii m., short head

Biceps brachii m., long head

Coracobrachialis m.

Lateral intermuscular septum

Extensor compartment

Medial intermuscular septum

Neurovascular bundle

Flexor compartment

Lacertus fibrosus

2

Subscapularis m.

Coracobrachialis m.

Biceps brachii m., short head

Biceps brachii m., long head

Musculocutaneous n.

Median n.

Ulnar n.

Teres major m.

Latissimus dorsi m.

Deep brachial a. and radial n.

Superior ulnar collateral a.

Inferior ulnar collateral a.

5

Teres major m.

Coracobrachialis m.

Lat. antibrachial cutaneous n.

Brachialis m.

Radial recurrent a.

4

THE UPPER EXTREMITY—PLATE 9
The brachium (posterior compartment)

The brachium contains a single muscle and is of particular importance because of the presence of the radial nerve.

Superficial fascia. (Fig. 1) The *lateral brachial cutaneous nerve,* a branch of the axillary, winds around the posterior border of the deltoid. Anesthesia in this area may be one of the early signs of injury to the axillary nerve.

Deep fascia. The brachial fascia already has been described on page 14. It is more adherent to the muscle of this compartment than in the anterior compartment.

Muscular contents. (Figs. 1 and 2) As in the anterior compartment, we may describe two groups of muscles associated with the humerus: an intrinsic (the triceps) and an extrinsic group. The latter group is made up of the deltoid and certain of the scapular muscles, the so-called SIT muscles, which insert on the greater tubercle of the humerus: the supraspinatus, infraspinatus, and teres minor. These three muscles are associated with the capsule of the shoulder joint and help form the posterior part of the "rotator cuff" (see Fig. 4, Plate 19).

Extrinsic muscles

1. DELTOID—has been described on page 18. With retraction or removal of the posterior fibers, one may see its innervation by the axillary nerve. Accompanying the nerve is the posterior humeral circumflex artery.

2. SUPRASPINATUS—arises from the supraspinatus fossa and inserts into the superior facet of the greater tubercle. It is important in initiating abduction through the first 15 degrees, the deltoid then carrying through to 90 degrees. This muscle is innervated by the suprascapular nerve from the brachial plexus.

3. INFRASPINATUS—takes origin from the infraspinatus fossa and gains attachment to the middle facet of the greater tubercle. It is the main lateral rotator of the humerus and is innervated by the suprascapular nerve. After removal of the muscle from the fossa, the circumflex scapular may be visualized with its important anastomosis with the transverse scapular forming a collateral channel between the first portion of the subclavian and the third portion of the axillary artery.

4. TERES MINOR—arises from axillary border of the scapula and inserts into the lower facet of the greater tubercle. It, too, is a lateral rotator of the numerus but is innervated by a branch from the axillary nerve.

Intrinsic muscles

TRICEPS BRACHII—is usually divided anatomically into long, lateral, and medial heads. A more practical division is into superficial and deep heads. The *superficial head* consists of the long and lateral heads. The *long head* arises from the infraglenoid tuberosity of the scapula and the lateral head of the posterior surface of the humerus above the radial groove. These two heads fuse in a V-shaped manner. The *deep head (medial head)* arises from the posterior surface of the humerus below and radial groove. The heads fuse and insert into the olecranon process of the ulna. This muscle is the extensor of the forearm and, like all extensor muscles of the upper extremity, is innervated by the radial nerve.

Neurovascular bundle. (see Fig. 2) The neurovascular bundle of the posterior compartment lies in the radial groove and consists of the deep brachial artery and the radial nerve with their main branches. It may most adequately be exposed by dividing the two portions of the superficial head (i.e., the long and lateral).

1. Deep brachial artery—the largest of the three main branches of the brachial enters the posterior compartment between the long and lateral heads of the triceps, where it gives rise to an important recurrent branch that anastomoses with the posterior humeral circumflex, forming a collateral channel between the brachial and axillary arteries. It descends laterally in the radial groove between the medial (deep) and lateral heads of the triceps accompanied by the radial nerve. In the groove, it divides into a *posterior branch (medial collateral),* which passes behind the lateral epicondyle to enter into the cubital anastomosis. The *anterior branch (radial collateral)* pierces the lateral intermuscular septum and passes in front of the lateral epicondyle and also enters into the cubital anastomosis.

2. Radial nerve—arises from the posterior cord of the brachial plexus in the axilla and enters the posterior compartment in the musculospiral (radial) groove of the humerus between the lateral and medial heads of the triceps. It may be divided into a (1) *common trunk;* (2) *superficial branch,* and (3) *deep branch.* The two latter branches are discussed on page 26.

COMMON RADIAL—innervates the three heads of the triceps and gives rise to the cutaneous branches to the posterior surface of the arm and forearm. It pierces the lateral intermuscular septum and lies between the brachioradialis and brachialis and here innervates the "lateral mobile wad" of the forearm extensors. Because of the intimate relation of the nerve to the humerus, it is commonly injured in fractures of the humeral shaft.

PLATE 9

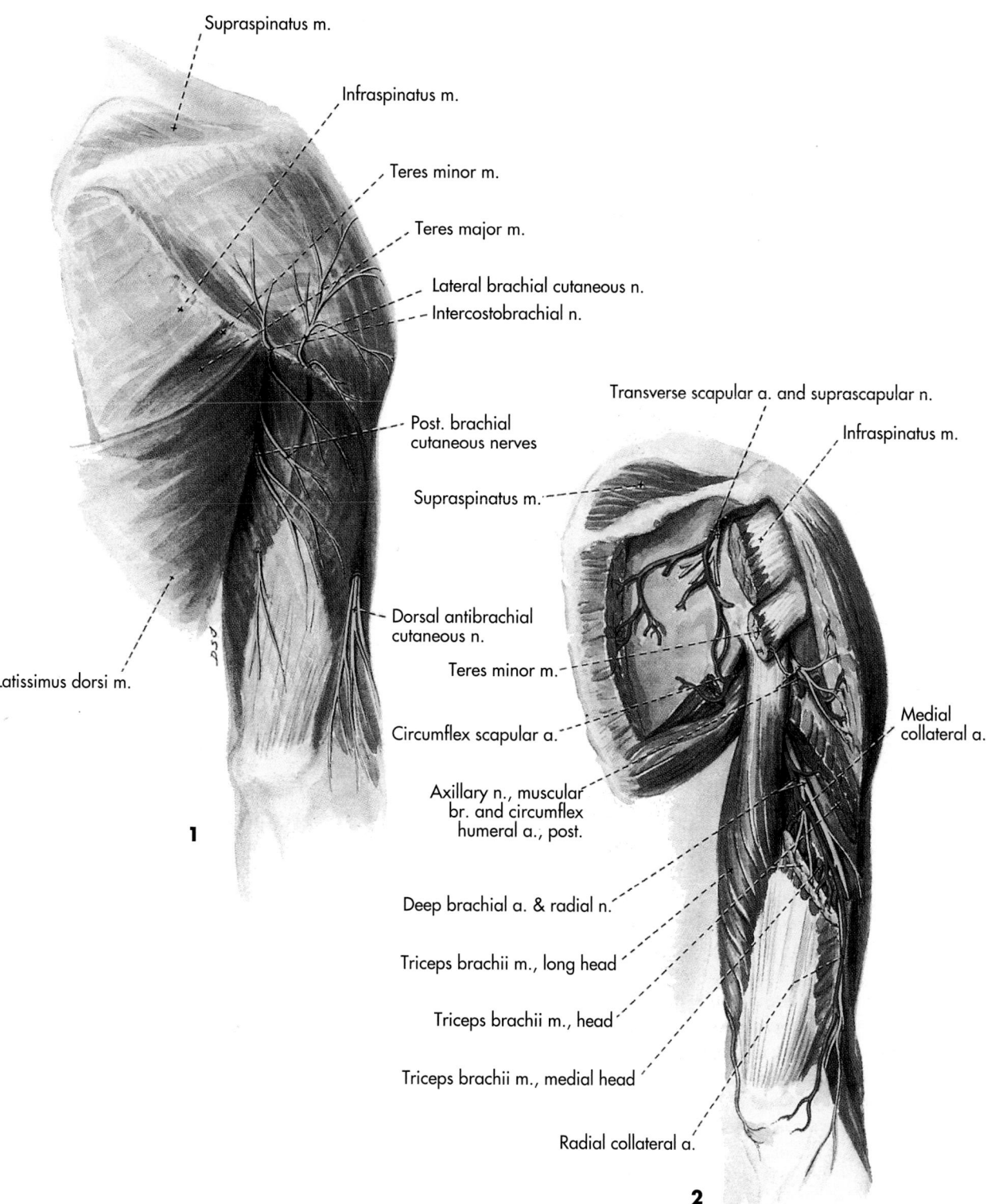

Supraspinatus m.

Infraspinatus m.

Teres minor m.

Teres major m.

Lateral brachial cutaneous n.

Intercostobrachial n.

Post. brachial
cutaneous nerves

Supraspinatus m.

Dorsal antibrachial
cutaneous n.

Latissimus dorsi m.

Circumflex scapular a.

Axillary n., muscular
br. and circumflex
humeral a., post.

Deep brachial a. & radial n.

Triceps brachii m., long head

Triceps brachii m., head

Triceps brachii m., medial head

Radial collateral a.

Transverse scapular a. and suprascapular n.

Infraspinatus m.

Teres minor m.

Medial
collateral a.

1

2

THE UPPER EXTREMITY—PLATE 10
Muscle attachments to the humerus

Because muscle pull plays such a determinant role in the displacement of fractures of the humerus and in their correct management, Fig. 1 is devoted to the important muscle attachments to this bone.

1. Supraspinatus—is inserted into the superior facet of the greater tubercle of the humerus and the capsule of the shoulder joint.

2. Subscapularis—inserts into the lesser tubercle and joint capsule as well as into the humeral shaft for about 1 inch distal to the tubercle.

3. Pectoralis major—gains attachment to the lateral lip of the bicipital groove of the humerus.

4. Latissimus dorsi—attaches to the floor of the bicipital groove.

5. Teres major—inserts into the medial lip of the bicipital groove.

6. Deltoid—inserts into the deltoid tuberosity on the middle of the lateral side of the humerus.

7. Coracobrachialis—attaches opposite the deltoid on the medial side of the shaft of the humerus.

8. Biceps brachii—although neither arising nor inserting on the humerus, influences bone displacement of fractures of that bone because of the upward pull exerted by its insertion into the tuberosity of the radius.

9. Brachialis (see Fig. 4, Plate 8)—arises from the distal three fifths of the anterior surface of the humerus and inserts on the coronoid process of the ulna.

10. Infraspinatus and teres minor (see Fig. 2, Plate 9) —insert into the middle and lower facets of the greater tubercle of the humerus, respectively.

Fractures of the upper end of the humerus

These may be grouped as follows: fractures of the anatomic neck, fracture of the tubercles, fracture of the surgical neck, and separation of the epiphysis.

1. Fractures at the anatomic neck—the anatomic neck is a narrow strip that encircles the margins of the head. The usual cause of fracture is a fall onto the shoulder, and the bony fragments are impacted rather than displaced.

2. Fractures of the tubercles—if the tubercle is separated from the humerus, the arm will be drawn in the direction of pull of the intact muscles. As an example, when the greater tubercle is detached, the supraspinatus, infraspinatus, and teres minor muscles pull the detached fragment upward and backward out of control, allowing the arm to be rotated medially by the intact subscapular muscle.

3. Fracture at the surgical neck (Fig. 2)—the surgical neck is the region immediately distal to the head and tubercles where the proximal end of the humerus and the shaft join. Fractures here usually result from falls on the elbow when the arm is abducted, but the deformity is the result of muscle pull rather than the direction of the injuring force. The fracture line occurs above the insertion of the pectoralis major, teres major, and latissimus dorsi insertions. The abducted proximal fragment is controlled mainly by the supraspinatus, which is the most powerful muscle attached to it. The distal fragment is pulled inward by the pectoralis major, teres major, and latissimus dorsi, and upward by the deltoid, biceps, and coracobrachialis muscles.

Reduction is effected by traction on the arm parallel with the body. This makes taut the tendon of the long head of the biceps, which rolls the proximal fragment of the humerus into its normal position and holds it there.

4. Separation of the upper epiphysis—normally, the epiphysis fuses by the twenty-first year; consequently, separations occur before that age. Because the epiphysis includes the tubercles, the displacement that occurs with separation is similar to that in fractures through the surgical neck.

Fractures of the shaft of the humerus

The shaft of the humerus extends from the surgical neck to the supracondylar ridges and usually is injured by a direct force resulting in a transverse fracture. Displacement of the fragments varies depending on the relation of the fracture to the insertion of the deltoid muscle. Delayed union or nonunion of fractures of the midshaft is not uncommon. This may be explained in part by the fact that the nutrient artery of the humerus enters the bone near its middle and may be ruptured in fractures in this region. Another common complication is radial nerve injury. The possibility of this complication is obvious because of the intimate relationship of the nerve to the humeral shaft (see Fig. 2, Plate 9).

1. Fracture of the shaft above the deltoid insertion (Fig. 3)—results in *adduction* of the *proximal fragment* because of the muscular pull exerted by the pectoralis major, latissimus dorsi, teres major, and subscapularis muscles. The *distal fragment* is *abducted* and pulled *upward* by the powerful deltoid.

2. Fracture of the shaft below the deltoid insertion (Fig. 4)—results in *abduction* of the *proximal fragment* by the deltoid and *elevation* of the *distal fragment* by the upward pull of the triceps, biceps, and coracobrachialis muscles.

PLATE 10

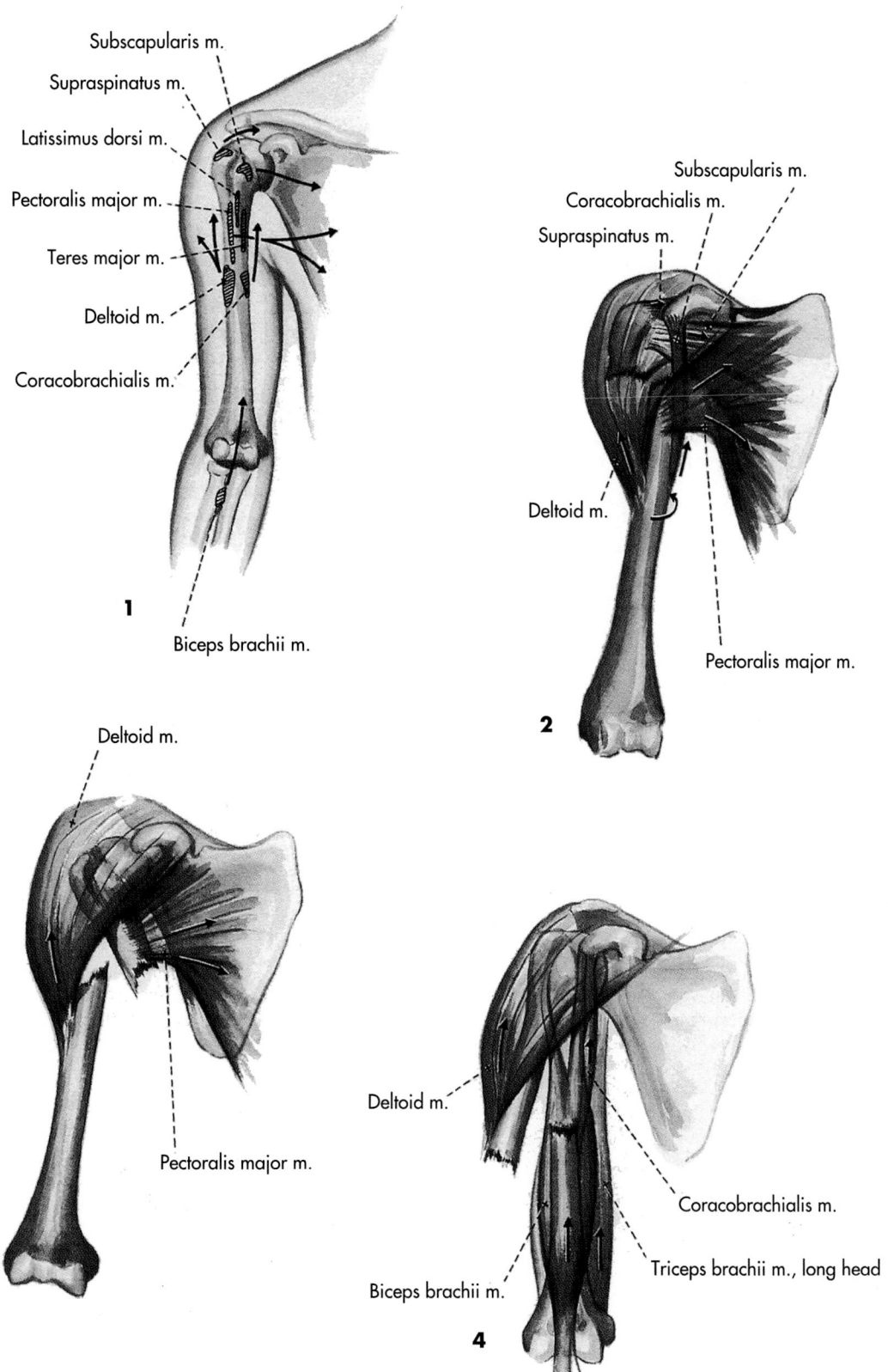

THE UPPER EXTREMITY—PLATE 11
Fractures of the lower end of the humerus

These fractures occur in great variety and in large numbers in childhood and are principally caused by falls on the outstretched hand. The force is transmitted through the bones of the forearm to the wide and flattened end of the humerus, which is weakened by the presence of the olecranon, coronoid, and radial fossae. In addition, the superficial position of the epicondyles exposes them to fracture by direct injury.

Fractures in this region include separation of the epiphyses, particularly the medial epiphysis; fracture of the epicondyles; and condylar, intercondylar, and supracondylar fractures. The mechanics of displacement and of neurovascular complications of supracondylar fractures are shown in Figs. 1, 2, and 3.

Displacement in supracondylar fractures

By far, the most common type of supracondylar fracture is the so-called extension type in which the injuring force carries the distal fragment of the humerus posteriorly, and the triceps, brachialis, and biceps muscles produce overriding of the two fragments. Not only is this more common than the so-called flexion type of supracondylar fracture, in which the distal fragment is displaced anteriorly, but it accounts for most of the neurovascular complications in association with fractures about the elbow (see Fig. 3). The fracture line often extends inferiorly through one of the fossae into the joint, resulting in T-shaped or Y-shaped fractures.

Principles of reduction in supracondylar fractures

Traction is necessary to achieve reduction, and acute flexion with the tightened triceps tendon serving as a splint is necessary to maintain it.

Because of the break in the continuity of the humerus, the strong supinating action of the biceps is lost. Consequently, the elbow joint comes under control of the pronators and is held in full pronation. Attempts to place the forearm in even slight supination result in a varus deformity because the elbow is fixed by the pronators. In the management of these fractures, the forearm is placed in full pronation during and after reduction (see Figs. 1 and 2).

Neurovascular complications in supracondylar fractures

The injuring force carries the condyles backward and strips the periosteum away from the posterior surface of the proximal fragment. The anterior edge of the proximal fragment often tears the periosteum and injures the attached soft tissues. Thus the brachial artery and the median and radial nerves may be damaged with the initial injury, or they may be compressed subsequently by fragments of bone, by blood that infiltrates the antecubital fossa, or by callus formation (Fig. 3).

Surgical exposure of the humerus

Anterior approach. Any part of the incision shown in Fig. 4 may be used to expose the underlying humerus. For example, the incision may go from the lower margin of the clavicle near the tip of the coracoid process of the scapula to the deltoid tuberosity if exposure of only the upper one third of the humerus is needed. Retraction of the deltoid laterally exposes the humerus lateral to the bicipital groove (see Fig. 3, Plate 20).

An extension of this incision distally permits exposure of the midshaft of the humerus. When carried still further, the lower one third of the shaft can be exposed in the interval between the brachioradialis laterally and the brachial and biceps muscles medially.

Posterior approach. The surgeon approaching the humerus from behind must constantly remember the relationship of the *axillary nerve* beneath the deltoid muscle to the posterior aspect of the surgical neck of the humerus, and the relation of the *radial nerve* to the posterior surface of the shaft of the humerus (see Fig. 2, Plate 9).

PLATE 11

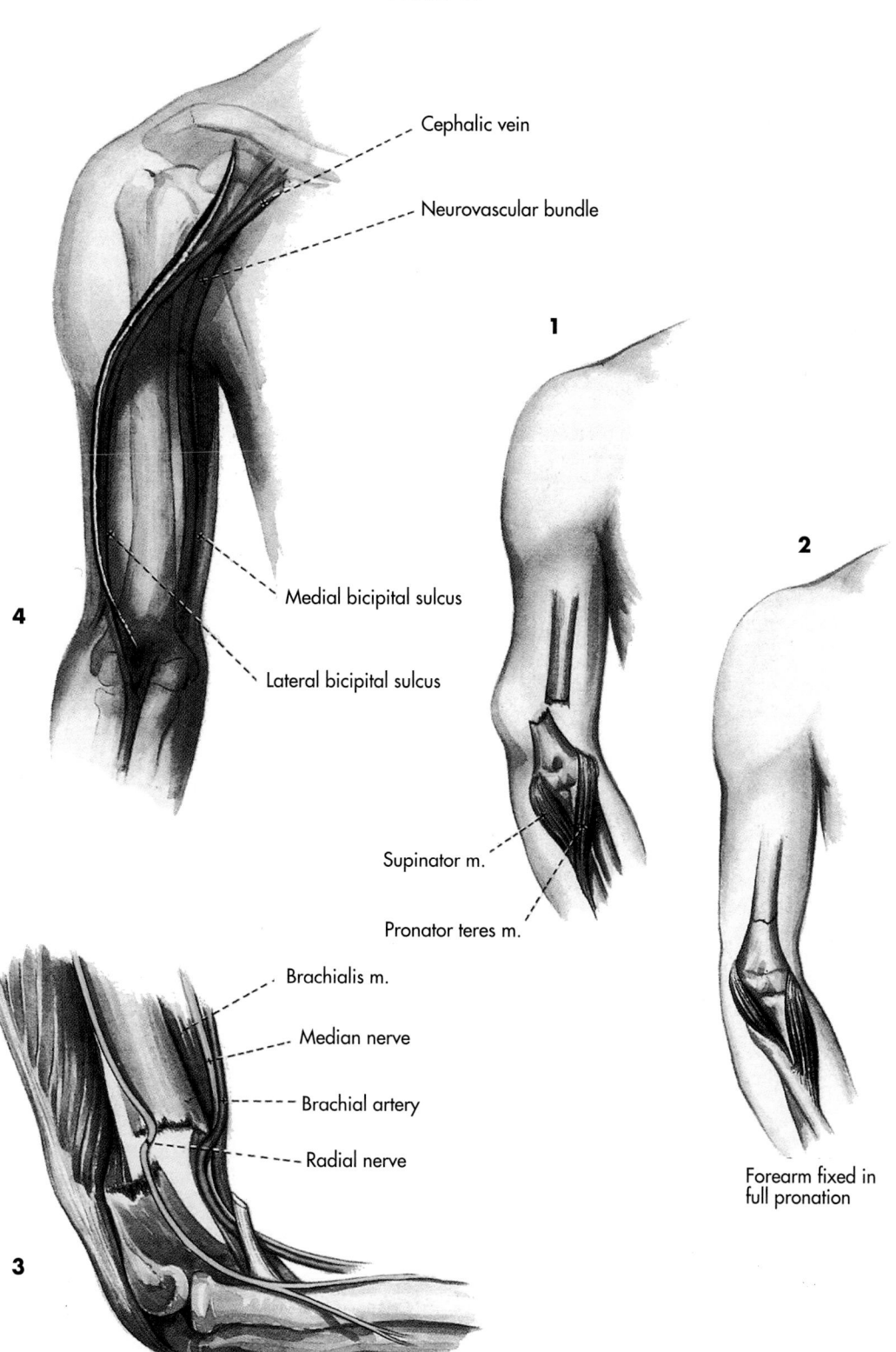

Cephalic vein

Neurovascular bundle

Medial bicipital sulcus

Lateral bicipital sulcus

Supinator m.

Pronator teres m.

Brachialis m.

Median nerve

Brachial artery

Radial nerve

Forearm fixed in
full pronation

THE UPPER EXTREMITY—PLATE 12
The antebrachium (anterior compartment)

The antebrachium extends from a line drawn between the two humeral epicondyles and terminates at the lower cutaneous fold of the wrist. Like the brachium, it may be divided into anterior (flexor) and posterior (extensor) compartments.

Deep fascia. The antebrachial fascia is thickened over the anterior surface of the wrist joint to form the *volar carpal ligament* and over its posterior surface to form the *dorsal carpal ligament* (see Fig. 1, Plate 13).

Muscular contents. The muscles of the anterior compartment may be divided into four layers. With the exception of one and a half muscles (flexor carpi ulnaris and one half of the flexor digitorum profundus), they are innervated by the median nerve.

1. First layer—all arise from the medial epicondyle and the ulna (Fig. 1).

a. PRONATOR TERES—inserts into the middle third of the lateral surface of the radius and is pierced by the median nerve.

b. FLEXOR CARPI RADIALIS—inserts into the base of the second and third metacarpals.

c. PALMARIS LONGUS—at its insertion becomes continuous with the palmar aponeurosis.

d. FLEXOR CARPI ULNARIS—gains its main attachment into the pisiform bone. It is pierced and innervated by the ulnar nerve.

2. Second layer—consists of only one muscle with an extensive origin (Fig. 2).

FLEXOR DIGITORUM SUBLIMIS—arises from the humerus, ulna, intermuscular septum, and radius. Between the humeral and septal attachments, a tendinous *sublimis tunnel* is formed, under which passes the ulnar artery and median nerve. Its four tendons insert into the shafts of the middle phalanges of the second to fifth fingers. The median nerve is adherent to its under surface.

3. Third layer—is made up of two muscles whose tendons extend into the terminal phalanx of all the fingers (Fig. 3).

a. FLEXOR DIGITORUM PROFUNDUS—takes origin from the ulna and adjacent intermuscular septum and inserts on the terminal phalanx of the second to fifth finger. The ulnar half of the muscle is innervated by the ulnar nerve; its radial half is innervated by the median nerve.

b. FLEXOR POLLICIS LONGUS—takes origin from the radius and adjacent intermuscular septum, to insert on the terminal phalanx of the thumb. It is innervated by the median nerve.

4. Fourth layer—made up of one muscle in the distal portion of the forearm (Fig. 4).

PRONATOR QUADRATUS—arises from the volar surface of the ulna and inserts into the volar surface of the radius.

Blood supply. (see Figs. 2, 3, and 4) The blood vessels of the anterior compartment are the terminal branches of the brachial artery. The latter terminates at the level of the neck of the radius by dividing into radial and ulnar branches.

1. Radial artery—is the smaller of the two terminal branches and lies superficial in position in the forearm, but it is under cover of the brachioradialis muscle in most of its course. Shortly after its origin, it gives rise to a *radial recurrent* that anastomoses with the anterior branch of the profundus. In addition to muscular branches, it gives rise to an important *superficial volar branch* and a *radial volar carpal artery* (see Fig. 2, Plate 16).

2. Ulnar artery—passes through the sublimis tunnel and immediately gives rise to two branches, the *volar* and *dorsal recurrents,* which anastomose with the inferior and superior ulnar collaterals, respectively. It then gives origin to the *common interosseous,* which in turn gives off an *interosseous recurrent,* which joins with the posterior (radial) branch of the profunda (see Fig. 1, Plate 13). In addition, the common interosseous gives rise to the *volar* and *dorsal interossei* lying on the respective surfaces of the interosseous membrane. It also supplies muscular, nutrient, and carpal branches.

Nerve supply. (see Figs. 2 and 3) The main supply to the anterior compartment is by the median nerve, innervating all but one and one half muscles.

1. Median nerve—descends into the antecubital fossa between the heads of the pronator teres and becomes adherent to the undersurface of the flexor digitorum sublimis muscle. In the lower third of the forearm, it lies superficial in position between the tendons of the palmaris longus on the ulnar side and the flexor carpi radialis on the radial side. It continues into the wrist, deep to the transverse carpal ligament. In the antecubital fossa, it sends off branches to the pronator teres, flexor carpi radialis, palmaris longus, and flexor digitorum sublimis. At the level of the radial tuberosity, it gives rise to the volar interosseous, which accompanies the artery of the same name, to innervate the muscles of the third and fourth layers.

2. Ulnar nerve—lies in a groove on the posterior aspect of the medial epicondyle at the elbow, then pierces the flexor carpi ulnaris to gain access to the flexor compartment of the forearm. It supplies the flexor carpi ulnaris and the ulnar half of the profundus. The nerve descends to the wrist, where it passes superficial to the transverse carpal ligament but deep to the volar carpal ligament.

3. Radial nerve—the *common radial* appears in the cubital region between the brachialis and brachioradialis and, after innervating the "lateral mobile wad" of muscles of the extensor group, divides into superficial and deep branches. The *deep radial* passes to the posterior compartment. The *superficial radial,* which is entirely sensory, passes through the anterior compartment under cover of the brachioradialis running parallel with the radial artery. At the lower third of the forearm, it pierces the deep fascia and appears on the dorsum of the hand.

PLATE 12

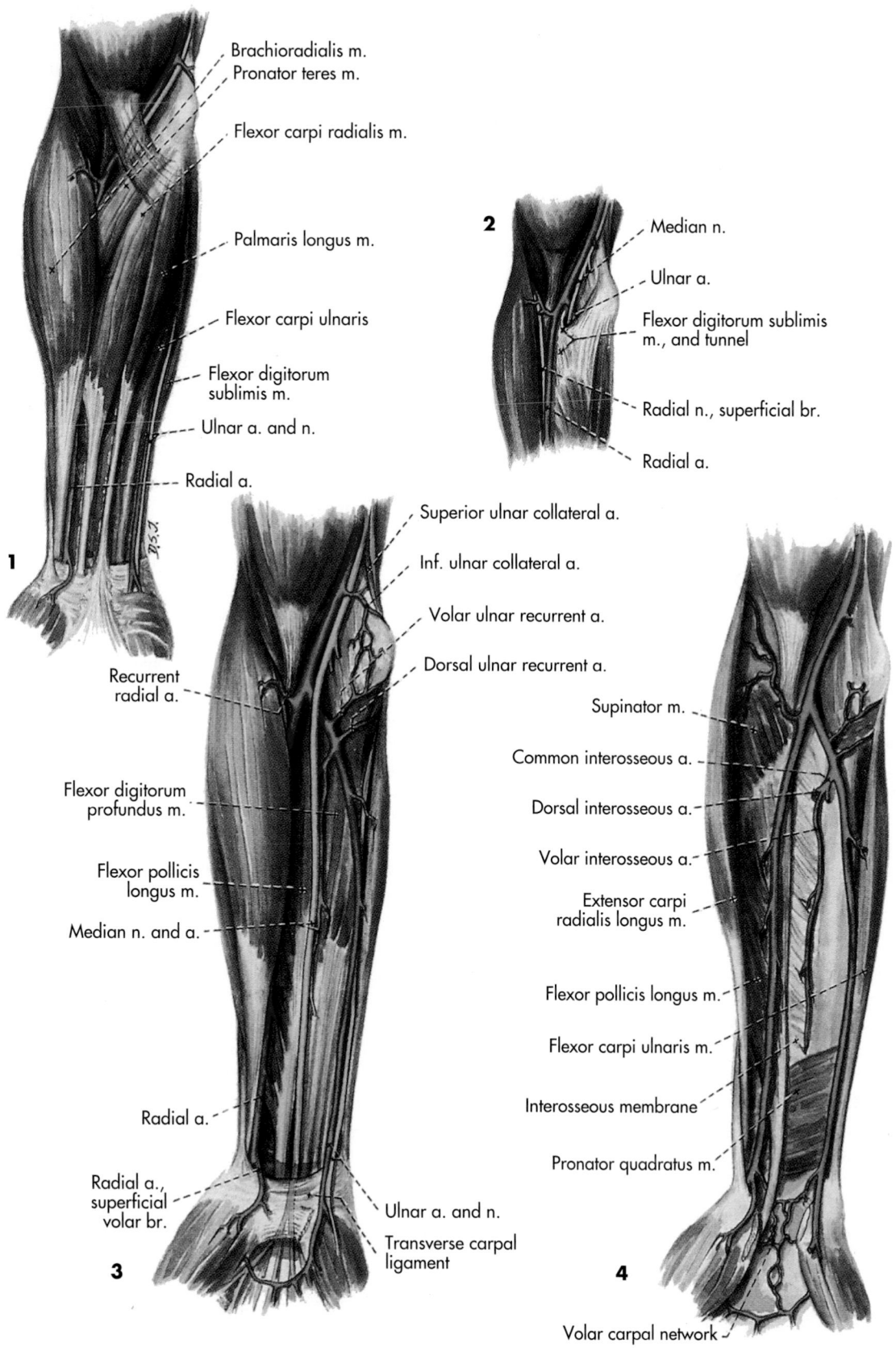

1

Brachioradialis m.
Pronator teres m.

Flexor carpi radialis m.

Palmaris longus m.

Flexor carpi ulnaris

Flexor digitorum
sublimis m.

Ulnar a. and n.

Radial a.

2

Median n.

Ulnar a.

Flexor digitorum sublimis
m., and tunnel

Radial n., superficial br.

Radial a.

3

Superior ulnar collateral a.

Inf. ulnar collateral a.

Volar ulnar recurrent a.

Dorsal ulnar recurrent a.

Recurrent
radial a.

Flexor digitorum
profundus m.

Flexor pollicis
longus m.

Median n. and a.

Radial a.

Radial a.,
superficial
volar br.

Ulnar a. and n.

Transverse carpal
ligament

4

Supinator m.

Common interosseous a.

Dorsal interosseous a.

Volar interosseous a.

Extensor carpi
radialis longus m.

Flexor pollicis longus m.

Flexor carpi ulnaris m.

Interosseous membrane

Pronator quadratus m.

Volar carpal network

THE UPPER EXTREMITY—PLATE 13
The antebrachium (posterior compartment)

The antebrachium contains the extensor muscles of the forearm, the deep (posterior interosseous) branch of the radial nerve, and the posterior interosseous branch of the ulnar artery.

Superficial fascia (see Fig. 1, Plate 9)

Deep fascia. (Fig. 1) A thickening of this layer of fascia occurs over the dorsum of the wrist and is termed the *dorsal carpal ligament.*

Muscular contents. The muscles in this compartment may be divided into two layers: superficial and deep.

1. Superficial layer (see Fig. 1)—of muscles has a closely associated origin extending from the lateral epicondylar ridge of the humerus to the lateral epicondyle. They may be subdivided into three groups: lateral (three muscles), intermediate (two muscles), and medial (one muscle).

a. LATERAL—also described as the "lateral mobile wad" because they may be grasped as a group at the lateral boundary of the cubital space. Topographically, this group may be used in the surgical approach to the radial head, the incision being placed along the posterior extension of this muscle mass. Because they are all innervated by the *common* radial nerve, their functional status is important in determining the level of injury of the radial nerve in the upper extremity.

(1) *Brachioradialis*—becomes tendinous at midforearm and inserts on the base of the styloid process of the radius. Although included with the extensor muscles and innervated by the radial nerve, it actually acts to flex the elbow (see Fig. 1, Plate 12).

(2) *Extensor carpi radialis longus*—extends to the base of the second metacarpal. It functions as an extensor and a radial abductor of the wrist.

(3) *Extensor carpi radialis brevis*—inserts into the base of the third metacarpal and acts in a fashion similar to the extensor longus.

b. INTERMEDIATE—consists of two muscles arising from the lateral epicondyle, extending to the dorsal assembly of the phalanges and innervated by the *deep* radial nerve.

(1) *Extensor digitorum communis*—divides above the wrist into four tendons that extend to the fingers as part of the dorsal assembly over the phalanges. They act mainly to extend the metacarpophalangeal joints of the fingers.

(2) *Extensor digiti quinti proprius*—supplies an additional tendon into the dorsal assembly, allowing for independent extension of the little finger.

c. MEDIAL—is made up of a single muscle that receives its nerve supply from the *deep* radial nerve.

Extensor carpi ulnaris—is inserted into the base of the fifth metacarpal and acts mainly as an ulnar deviator of the wrist and only weakly as an extensor.

2. Deep layer (Fig. 2)—these muscles arise from the radius, interosseous membrane, and ulna and insert mainly on the thumb and index finger. All are innervated by the *deep* radial nerve.

a. SUPINATOR—arises from the lateral epicondyle and upper ulna and inserts on the lateral volar surface of the upper radius. As the name suggests, it acts as a supinator of the forearm.

b. ABDUCTOR POLLICIS LONGUS—takes rise from the ulna and interosseous membrane to insert on the base of the first metacarpal and acts to abduct the thumb.

c. EXTENSOR POLLICIS BREVIS—originates from the radius and interosseous membrane and inserts on the base of the proximal phalanx of the thumb. It acts to extend the metacarpophalangeal joint.

d. EXTENSOR POLLICIS LONGUS—arises from the ulna and adjacent interosseous membrane to insert on the base of the distal phalanx of the thumb. Its main function is to extend the distal phalanx.

e. EXTENSOR INDICIS PROPRIUS—arises from the ulna and interosseous membrane and extends to the dorsal assembly of the index finger. It adds extensor power to the metacarpophalangeal joint of the index finger.

Anconeus—although located in this compartment, this muscle is morphologically and physiologically a part of the triceps. It arises from the lateral epicondyle and inserts into the olecranon process and adjacent shaft of the ulna. It receives its nerve supply from the radial trunk by a branch arising in the radial groove.

Neurovascular bundle. (see Fig. 2) The neurovascular bundle in the posterior compartment of the forearm appears between the superficial and deep layers of muscles at the lower border of the supinator muscle as it emerges under the *tendinous supinator arc.* It is made up of the dorsal interosseous artery and nerve (deep radial).

1. Dorsal interosseous artery—arises from the common interosseous branch of the ulnar artery in the anterior compartment. It emerges between the supinator and abductor pollicis longus and supplies the muscles of the compartment. It gives rise to the *interosseous recurrent artery,* which enters into the cubital anastomosis (see Fig. 1).

2. Dorsal interosseous nerve (deep radial)—takes origin from the common radial in the anterior compartment, pierces the supinator, and enters the posterior compartment. It innervates all muscles of the posterior compartment except the lateral superficial group. Injury to this nerve results in the typical "wrist drop."

PLATE 13

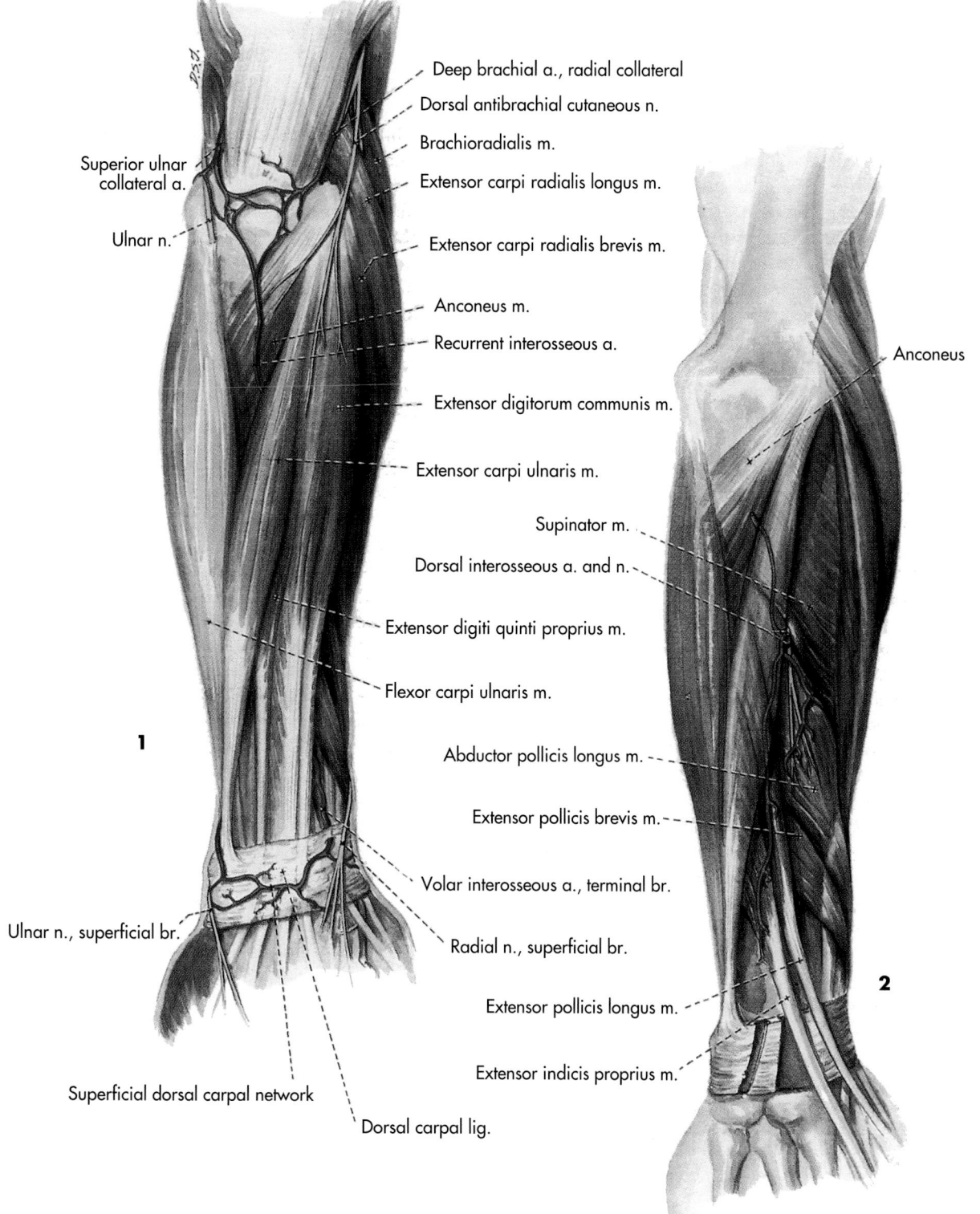

Deep brachial a., radial collateral

Dorsal antibrachial cutaneous n.

Brachioradialis m.

Extensor carpi radialis longus m.

Superior ulnar collateral a.

Extensor carpi radialis brevis m.

Ulnar n.

Anconeus m.

Recurrent interosseous a.

Extensor digitorum communis m.

Extensor carpi ulnaris m.

Supinator m.

Dorsal interosseous a. and n.

Extensor digiti quinti proprius m.

Flexor carpi ulnaris m.

Abductor pollicis longus m.

Extensor pollicis brevis m.

Volar interosseous a., terminal br.

Ulnar n., superficial br.

Radial n., superficial br.

Extensor pollicis longus m.

Extensor indicis proprius m.

Superficial dorsal carpal network

Dorsal carpal lig.

Anconeus

1

2

THE UPPER EXTREMITY—PLATE 14
Clinical considerations of the forearm (antebrachium)

The surgical anatomy of the forearm is concerned principally with fractures: the forces that account for displacement, the anatomic facts bearing on their reduction and fixation, and the surgical approach to the bones when open reduction is necessary. Occasionally, in addition, the surgeon must expose one of the bones or other structures in the forearm for the removal of a tumor or repair of an injury other than fracture.

Fractures of the bones of the forearm. From the standpoint of fractures, the shaft of the ulna may be considered a continuation of the humerus, whereas the radius is an upward continuation of the hand. With a fall on the pronated hand, the main force is communicated to the distal end of the radius and passes upward to the humerus. A fracture of the radius alone or of both the radius and ulna may result. When caused by such indirect violence, the fractures usually occur at different levels, but the fracture of the ulna is usually at the distal end.

The displacement in fractures of the bones of the forearm is usually considerable. The muscles tend to pull the distal fragments proximally. In addition, the pronator teres and pronator quadratus pull the two bones toward one another, tending to obliterate the interosseous space.

1. Isolated fractures of the ulna—are always caused by direct violence and tend to be compound because of the subcutaneous position of the posterior border of the bone. The direction of the injuring force plays a major role in displacement of the fragments of this bone.

2. Fractures of the shaft of the radius—in these, however, displacement depends largely on the pull of muscles rather than on the fracturing force. Consequently, displacement varies with the level of the fracture.

a. Fractures of the shaft of the radius above the insertion of the pronator teres (Figs. 1 and 2)—and below the insertion of the supinator result in a rotation deformity caused by the pull of the biceps and supinator on the proximal fragment (flexed and supinated) and the now-unopposed pull of the pronator teres and pronator quadratus on the distal fragment.

b. Fractures of the radial shaft below the insertion of the pronator teres (Fig. 3)—the proximal fragment is brought anteriorly (flexed) by the biceps and medially by the pronator teres, but it tends to remain in the neutral position regarding rotation because the action of the biceps and supinator opposes that of the pronator teres. The lower fragment is displaced toward the ulna by the pronator quadratus, the brachioradialis, and the extensors and abductors of the thumb. With the ulna and the inferior radioulnar joint intact, there is usually no overriding of fragments.

Surgical approach to the long bones of the forearm

1. Ulna—may be exposed along its entire length without jeopardy to any important structure by an incision along its posterior margin, which lies between the flexor carpi ulnaris and the extensor carpi ulnaris.

2. Radius—is more difficult to expose. An anterior or posterior approach may be used. The topographic landmark for either approach is the "lateral mobile wad" of muscles consisting of the brachioradialis and extensor carpi radialis longus and brevis. These three muscles can be moved as a unit across the part of the radius covered by the supinator, independent of the neighboring muscles. The anterior and posterior edges of the "wad" serve as guides for the incision.

For an anterior approach to the entire shaft of the radius, an incision is begun in the antebrachium just lateral to the biceps tendon and extended distally along the anterior border of the brachioradialis as far as the wrist. The deep fascia is divided along the length of the incision. The brachioradialis and extensor carpi radialis longus and brevis are mobilized as a unit by dividing the recurrent radical vessels (see Fig. 3, Plate 12). The supinator muscle is peeled off the radius and retracted laterally. This maneuver exposes the underlying radial shaft and protects the deep radial (dorsal interosseous) nerve, which pierces the supinator. The forearm is placed in a pronated position to expose the entire shaft of the radius.

To expose the radius via a posterior approach, one makes an incision along the posterior edge of the lateral mobile wad of muscles (Fig. 4). The antebrachial fascia is opened, and the extensor digitorum communis muscle is identified and carefully separated from the extensor carpi radialis brevis. The two muscles are then retracted to expose the deeper-lying supinator muscle (Fig. 5). Care must be taken to isolate and protect the deep radial nerve as it pierces the supinator muscle. The forearm is then supinated to locate the anterior margin of the muscle, which is cut to expose the shaft. Additional exposure of the radius is obtained by elevation and retraction of the abductor pollicis longus and the extensor pollicis brevis muscles (see Fig. 5).

PLATE 14

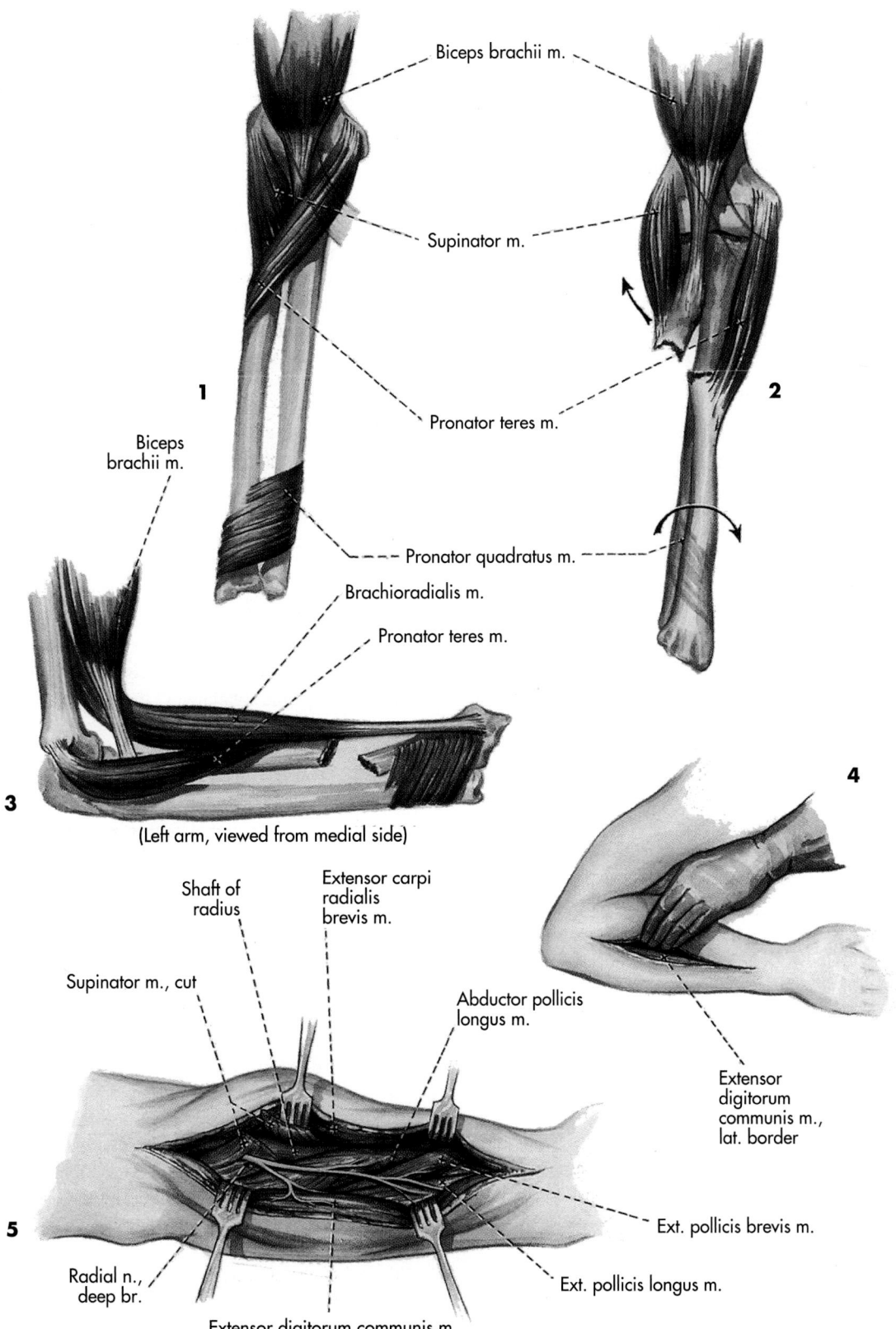

Biceps brachii m.

Biceps brachii m.

Supinator m.

Pronator teres m.

Pronator teres m.

1

Biceps brachii m.

2

Pronator quadratus m.

Brachioradialis m.

Pronator teres m.

3

(Left arm, viewed from medial side)

4

Shaft of radius

Extensor carpi radialis brevis m.

Supinator m., cut

Abductor pollicis longus m.

Extensor digitorum communis m., lat. border

Ext. pollicis brevis m.

Radial n., deep br.

Ext. pollicis longus m.

5

Extensor digitorum communis m.

THE UPPER EXTREMITY—PLATE 15
The hand (palmar or volar surface)

The two eminences are present on the palmar surface: the *thenar eminence* on the radial side and the *hypothenar eminence* on the ulnar side. These eminences correspond to the thenar and hypothenar muscular compartments. Smaller eminences are seen in the distal palm between the phalanges, the *monticuli,* beneath which the common digital arteries and nerves divide into their proper digital branches (Fig. 1).

Certain of the skin creases are of topographic importance. The proximal skin crease at the wrist marks the level of the wrist joint, and the distal crease *(rasceta),* the proximal border of the transverse carpal ligament. The creases on the phalanges overlie the interphalangeal joints. The remainder of the skin creases are of significance only in that incisions in the palm should not cross these creases.

Superficial fascia. (Fig. 2) This layer is sparse, particularly over the midpalm, where the skin is adherent to deep fascia. Three *palmar cutaneous nerves* are present in this layer in its proximal part, arising from the radial, median, and ulnar nerves. A small subcutaneous muscle also is found in this layer, the *palmaris brevis,* which is innervated by the ulnar nerve. This muscle is usually well developed when the palmaris longus is absent.

Deep (palmar) fascia. (see Fig. 2) The palmar fascia is divided into three parts: the *thenar fascia* covering the muscles of the thenar compartment; the *hypothenar fascia* covering the muscles of the hypothenar compartment; and the *palmar aponeurosis,* a thickened portion of the deep fascia over the middle compartment. The latter fibers radiate from the palmaris longus tendons to the phalanges.

Middle compartment

1. Superficial neurovascular structures (Fig. 3)—with the removal of the palmar fascia the superficial vessels and nerves of the palm are seen.

a. SUPERFICIAL VOLAR ARCH—is formed mainly by the superficial branch of the ulnar artery. This artery in turn usually joins the superficial volar branch of the radial to complete the arch. Topographically, the arch lies about three fingerbreadths distal to the rasceta. From the arch arise a number of small muscular and skin branches. One of the latter is a *proper digital* to the ulnar side of the little finger. Three *common digitals* also arise from the convexity of the arch, descend through the palm, and supply proper digital branches to all fingers except the radial side of the index finger, which is supplied by the deep arch.

b. SUPERFICIAL ULNAR NERVE—arises from the volar branch of the ulna at the wrist superficial to the transverse carpal ligament and gives off a ramus to the palmaris brevis and a communicating branch to the median nerve. It then supplies a proper digital branch to the ulnar side of the little finger and a common digital that supplies the adjacent margins of the little and ring fingers.

c. MEDIAN NERVE—passes from the forearm deep to the transverse carpal ligament, where it divides into medial and lateral divisions. The medial division receives a communicating branch from the ulnar and sends two common digital branches that supply adjacent sides of the index and middle and middle and ring fingers, respectively. The lateral division is a common digital nerve dividing into three proper digitals to supply the thumb and radial side of the index finger. An important motor nerve also arises from this lateral division, the *recurrent branch;* this nerve supplies the three thenar muscles: the abductor, flexor, and opponens pollicis. The median nerve in the palm also supplies the two radial lumbricals.

2. Superficial musculotendinous structures (Fig. 3)—in the middle compartment, deep to the superficial neurovascular structures, lie the long tendons of the phalanges, the *flexor digitorum sublimis* and *profundus.* The sublimis tendons split to attach to the middle phalanges, whereas the profundus tendons insert on the distal phalanges. The tendons enter an osseofibrous tunnel that extends from the head of the metacarpals to the distal phalanx.

The *fibrous tendon sheath* prevents the tendons from bowstringing during flexion. The sheath is thin over the joints, and the fibers are crossed *(cruciate ligament),* whereas over the phalanges the fibers are strong and transversely arranged *(annular ligament).*

The *mucous tendon sheaths* lie deep to the fibrous sheath and extend from the neck of the metacarpals to the insertion of the profundus tendon. The sheaths of the thumb and little finger extend to the carpal region as the *radial* and *ulnar bursae* (see Fig. 1, Plate 18).

The *lumbrical muscles* are four in number, arising from the tendons of the flexor digitorum profundus (see Fig. 3). These muscles pass to the radial side of the fingers and insert on the extensor assembly (see Fig. 4, Plate 17). The two lumbricals on the radial side are innervated by the median nerve; the other two are innervated by the deep ulnar nerve. These muscles along with the interossei flex the metacarpophalangeal joints and extend the interphalangeal joints.

3. Fascial spaces—between the long flexor tendons and the deep muscles of the middle compartment are located potential fascial spaces that are of surgical significance. These spaces are considered on page 38.

PLATE 15

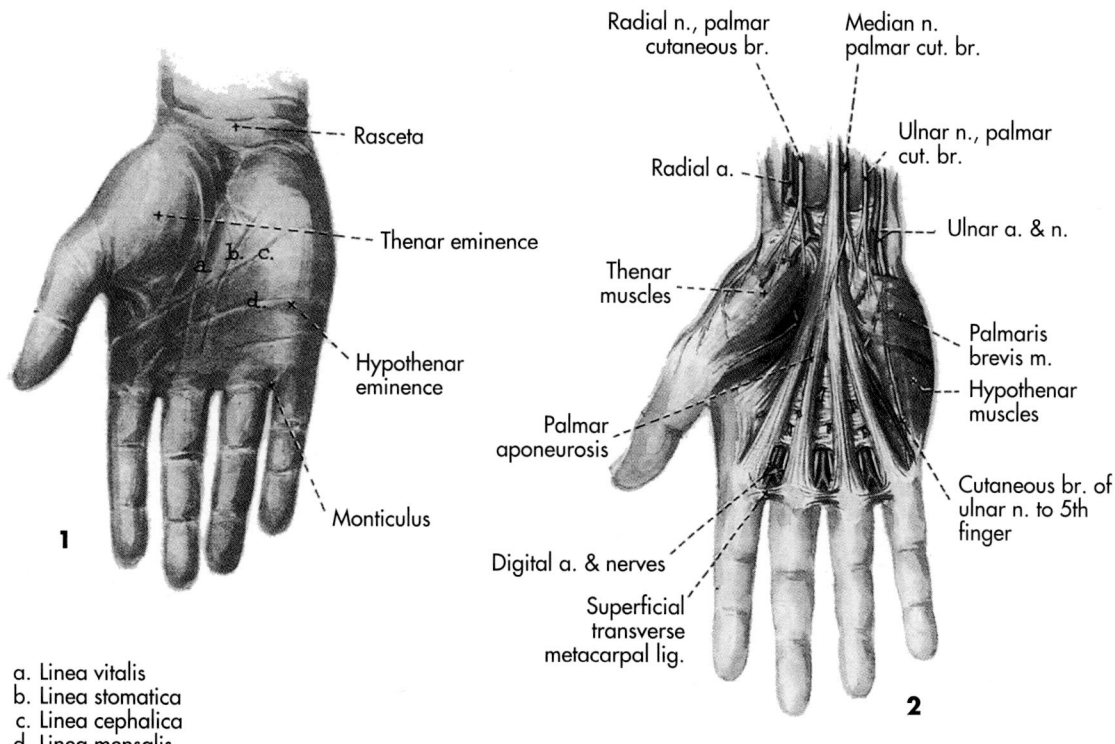

Rasceta

Thenar eminence

Hypothenar eminence

Monticulus

1

a. Linea vitalis
b. Linea stomatica
c. Linea cephalica
d. Linea mensalis

Radial n., palmar cutaneous br.

Median n. palmar cut. br.

Radial a.

Ulnar n., palmar cut. br.

Ulnar a. & n.

Thenar muscles

Palmaris brevis m.

Hypothenar muscles

Palmar aponeurosis

Cutaneous br. of ulnar n. to 5th finger

Digital a. & nerves

Superficial transverse metacarpal lig.

2

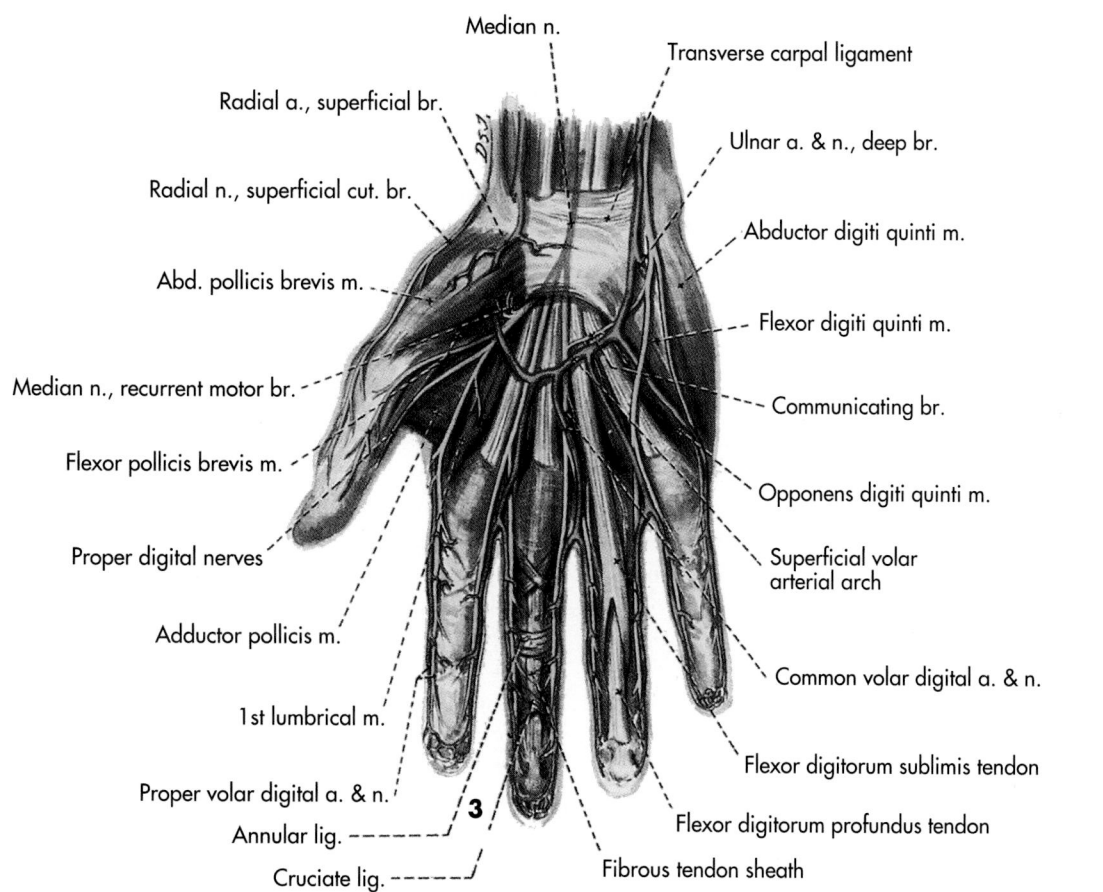

Median n.

Transverse carpal ligament

Radial a., superficial br.

Ulnar a. & n., deep br.

Radial n., superficial cut. br.

Abductor digiti quinti m.

Abd. pollicis brevis m.

Flexor digiti quinti m.

Median n., recurrent motor br.

Communicating br.

Flexor pollicis brevis m.

Opponens digiti quinti m.

Proper digital nerves

Superficial volar arterial arch

Adductor pollicis m.

Common volar digital a. & n.

1st lumbrical m.

Proper volar digital a. & n.

Flexor digitorum sublimis tendon

Annular lig.

Flexor digitorum profundus tendon

Cruciate lig.

Fibrous tendon sheath

3

THE UPPER EXTREMITY—PLATE 16

4. Deep muscular structures (Figs. 1 and 2)

a. ADDUCTOR POLLICIS—is seen on the radial side of the middle compartment, forming part of the floor of this area. It arises from the third metacarpal (transverse head) and from the carpal area (oblique head) and inserts into the base of the first phalanx. It is innervated by the deep ulnar nerve.

b. THREE VOLAR INTEROSSEI—make up the remainder of the deep muscles of the middle compartment. They arise from the second, fourth, and fifth metacarpal bones and insert on the extensor assembly. The first is inserted on the ulnar side of the index finger, the second on the radial side of the ring finger, and the third on the radial side of the little finger. These three muscles are innervated by the deep ulnar nerve. Their main function is adduction of the fingers with the middle finger as the axis. However, they also act in conjunction with the lumbricals and dorsal interossei as flexors of the metacarpophalangeal joints and extensors of the interphalangeal joints.

5. Deep neurovascular structures (see Figs. 1 and 2)

a. DEEP VOLAR ARCH—is formed by the radial artery and the deep branch of the ulnar artery. The radial artery enters the palm from the dorsum of the hand between the heads of the first dorsal interosseous muscle and then passes between the oblique and transverse heads of the adductor pollicis, where it joins the deep ulnar artery. Topographically, it lies two fingerbreadths distal to the rasceta. The rach gives rise to the following branches:

(1) *Princeps pollicis*—is actually a common digital branch to the thumb, dividing into two proper volar digitals. This artery may at times join the superficial ulnar artery to form the superficial volar arch.

(2) *Volar radial artery of index digit*—passes to the radial side of the index finger. It may in the absence of the superficial volar artery complete the superficial volar arch.

(3) *Volar metacarpals*—are three in number and descend in the second, third, and fourth interosseous spaces. They terminate by anastomosing with the common digitals of the superficial arch.

(4) *Carpal recurrent branches*—anastomose at the wrist with the volar radial and ulnar carpals to form the volar carpal network.

b. DEEP ULNAR NERVE—accompanies the deep volar arch through the middle compartment. It is described in more detail in the discussion of the hypothenar compartment.

Thenar compartment. (see Figs. 1 and 2)

1. Musculotendinous contents—three muscles form the eminence in this thenar compartment. They are all triangular in shape and are innervated by the recurrent branch of the median nerve.

a. ABDUCTOR POLLICIS BREVIS—arises from the volar surface of the transverse carpal ligament and greater multan-

gular and inserts on the base of the proximal phalanx of the thumb.

b. FLEXOR POLLICIS BREVIS—arises from the carpus and inserts on the ulnar side of the proximal phalanx.

c. OPPONENS POLLICIS—takes origin from the transverse carpal ligament and gains attachment to the radial side of the first metacarpal.

Two other muscles related to the thumb in this area are as follows:

d. ADDUCTOR POLLICIS—arises in the middle compartment from the third metacarpal and carpus and attaches to the proximal phalanx of the thumb on its ulnar side. This muscle is innervated by the deep ulnar nerve.

e. FLEXOR POLLICIS LONGUS TENDON—enters the hand deep to the transverse carpal ligament and enters the osteofibrous canal of the thumb, where it extends to the base of the distal phalanx. Its mucous tendon sheath is termed the *radial bursa* (see Fig. 1, Plate 18).

2. Neurovascular contents

a. RECURRENT BRANCH OF MEDIAN NERVE—is the motor nerve to this compartment. It arises from the lateral division of the medial nerve after the latter passes under the transverse carpal ligament. Topographically, its position may be located by flexing the ring finger to the thenar eminence.

b. PRINCEPS POLLICIS ARTERY (see Fig. 2).

Hypothenar compartment. (see Figs. 1 and 2)

1. Muscular contents—form the hypothenar eminence and are innervated by the deep ulnar nerve. The names of these muscles indicate their function.

a. ABDUCTOR DIGITI QUINTI—arises mainly from the pisiform bone and inserts into the ulnar side of the proximal phalanx of the little finger.

b. FLEXOR DIGITI QUINTA—takes origin from the hook of the hamate and transverse carpal ligament and gains attachment to the base of the proximal phalanx.

c. OPPONENS DIGITI QUINTI—has an origin similar to that of the flexor of the little finger. Its insertion is into the fifth metacarpal.

2. Neurovascular structures

a. ULNAR NERVE—enters the palm deep to the volar carpal but superficial to the transverse carpal ligament at the wrist. As it passes the radial side of the pisiform bone, it divides into superficial and deep branches. The *superficial ulnar nerve* is described on page 26. The *deep ulnar nerve* pierces the hypothenar compartment and continues into the middle component accompanying the deep volar arch. It innervates the hypothenar muscles, all the interossei, the two ulnar lumbricals, and the adductor pollicis.

b. ULNAR ARTERY—closely accompanies the ulnar nerve and also divides into superficial and deep branches. The *superficial ulnar artery* is considered on page 26, and the *deep ulnar artery* is discussed under the deep volar arch described previously.

PLATE 16

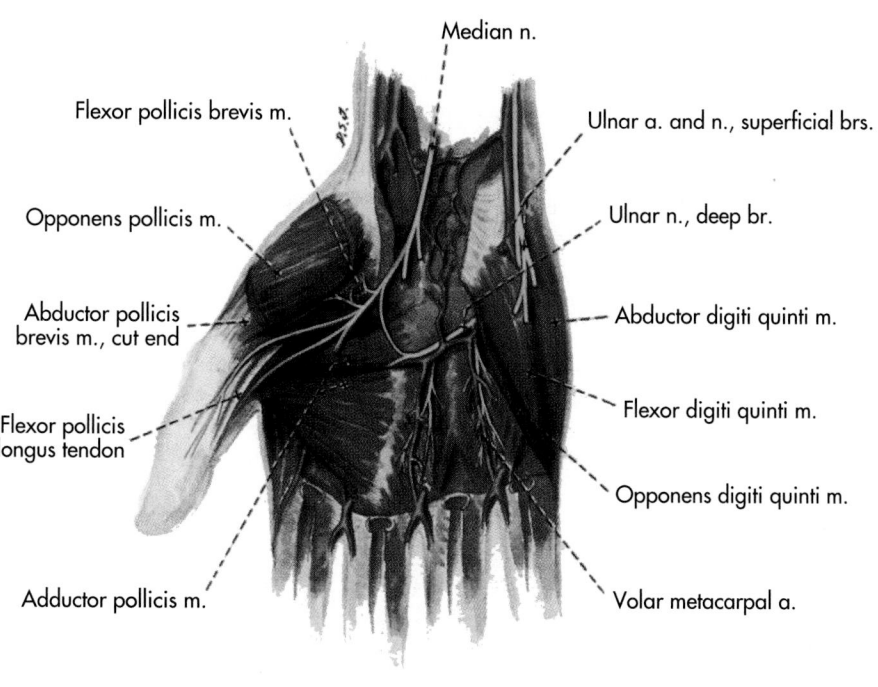

Median n.

Flexor pollicis brevis m.

Opponens pollicis m.

Abductor pollicis brevis m., cut end

Flexor pollicis longus tendon

Adductor pollicis m.

Ulnar a. and n., superficial brs.

Ulnar n., deep br.

Abductor digiti quinti m.

Flexor digiti quinti m.

Opponens digiti quinti m.

Volar metacarpal a.

1

Radial a., volar carpal br.

Radial a.

Volar carpal network

1st dorsal metacarpal a.

Princeps pollicis a.

Dorsal interosseous m.

Volar radial a. of index digit

Ulnar a., volar carpal br.

Ulnar n., deep br.

Carpal recurrent a.

Deep volar arch

Volar interosseous mm.

Common volar digital aa.

2

THE UPPER EXTREMITY—PLATE 17

The hand (dorsal surface) and wrist

Skin—the skin over the dorsal surface of the hand is so thin and freely movable that the underlying dorsal venous rete and extensor tendons are visible. The tendons of the thumb form an important topographic landmark: the *snuff-box* or *tabatière*. This is a triangular depression on the dorsal surface of the wrist bounded on the radial side by the tendons of the extensor pollicis brevis and abductor pollicis longus and on the ulnar side by the extensor pollicis longus. In the superficial fascia of this space is the lower portion of the cephalic vein, and in the depth, the radial artery.

Superficial fascia—in this plane are seen the vessels forming the dorsal venous rete and the superficial nerves.

1. DORSAL VENOUS RETE (Fig. 1)—arises from a longitudinal plexus of veins over the fingers that drain into the dorsal metacarpal veins. Communications between the lateral veins form the dorsal venous rete, which gives rise to the basilic and cephalic veins.

2. SUPERFICIAL NERVES (Figs. 1 and 2)—are derived from three sources: the dorsal ramus of the ulnar, the superficial branch of the radial, and the posterior antebrachial cutaneous nerve. Note that the dorsal surface of the distal portions of the index, middle, and radial half of the ring finger are innervated by the median nerve.

Extensor tendons (Fig. 3)—arise in the antebrachium and pass deep to the dorsal carpal ligament in synovial sheaths through specific osseofibrous canals. There are six such canals on the dorsum of the wrist. From radial to ulnar side, their contents are as follows:

1. Extensor pollicis brevis and abductor pollicis longus
2. Extensor carpi radialis longus and brevis
3. Extensor pollicis longus
4. Extensor digitorum communis and extensor indicis proprius
5. Extensor digiti quinti proprius
6. Extensor carpi ulnaris

Over the dorsal surface of the hand, the extensor tendons are joined by oblique tendinous bands (*juncturae tendinum*) and fascia, forming an aponeurotic extensor tendon sheet.

Dorsal subaponeurotic space (see Fig. 2, Plate 18)—is a loose connective tissue layer between the extensor tendon aponeurosis and the underlying interosseous muscles and bones.

Dorsal interosseous muscles (see Fig. 3)—four such muscles arising from adjacent sides of the metacarpal bones in each interspace. Each muscle inserts on the extensor assembly of the phalanges (Fig. 4). The first dorsal interosseous inserts on the radial side of the index finger; the fourth, on the ulnar side of the ring finger; and the second and third, on the radial and ulnar sides of the middle finger, respectively. These muscles act as abductors of the fingers and, in association with the lumbricals and volar interossei, as flexors of the metacarpophalangeal joint and extensors of the interphalangeal joints. They all are innervated by the deep ulnar nerve.

Dorsal metacarpal arteries (see Fig. 3)—the first dorsal metacarpal artery arises directly from the radial; the remaining three vessels arise from the *dorsal carpal rete*. The rete is formed by the dorsal carpal branches of the ulnar and radial arteries. The dorsal metacarpal arteries extend to the level of the metacarpophalangeal joints, where they divide into proper dorsal digital branches. At the base of the metacarpal bones, perforating branches anastomose with the branches of the deep palmar arch.

Extensor assembly—the extensor tendons of the second to fifth digit, as well as the tendons of the lubricals and interossei, insert onto the phalanges. This rather complex arrangement of fibers is illustrated in Fig. 4.

Volar aspect of the wrist (Fig. 5)

Because of the frequency of lacerations in the volar area of the wrist, knowledge of the relational anatomy of the volar surface of the wrist is important. Also of significance clinically is *carpal tunnel syndrome,* resulting from compression of the median nerve by chronic irritation and inflammation of the transverse carpal ligament.

Transverse carpal ligament—is a thick fibrous band extending from the pisiform and hook of the hamate on the ulnar side to the tubercle of the navicular and greater multangular on the radial side. The ligament splits at its radial attachment to form a separate compartment transversed by the flexor carpi radialis tendon and its sheath.

1. STRUCTURES SUPERFICIAL TO THE LIGAMENT (see Fig. 5, and Figs. 2 and 3, Plate 15)—include the following *palmaris longus tendon* in the midline, *palmar cutaneous branches of the median and ulnar nerves* on either side of the tendon, and *ulnar artery* and *nerve,* which lie in relation to the pisiform bone.

2. STRUCTURES DEEP TO THE LIGAMENT—lie in the *carpal tunnel* and, from radial to ulnar side, are as follows: *flexor pollicis longus* tendon with its mucous sheath (*radial bursa),* the *median nerve,* and the *flexor digitorum sublimis* and *profundus* tendons and their common mucous sheath (ulnar bursa).

The sublimis tendons of the middle and ring fingers are superficial in position, immediately deep to which are the sublimis tendons of the index and little fingers. The profundus tendons of all four fingers are aligned on the deepest level.

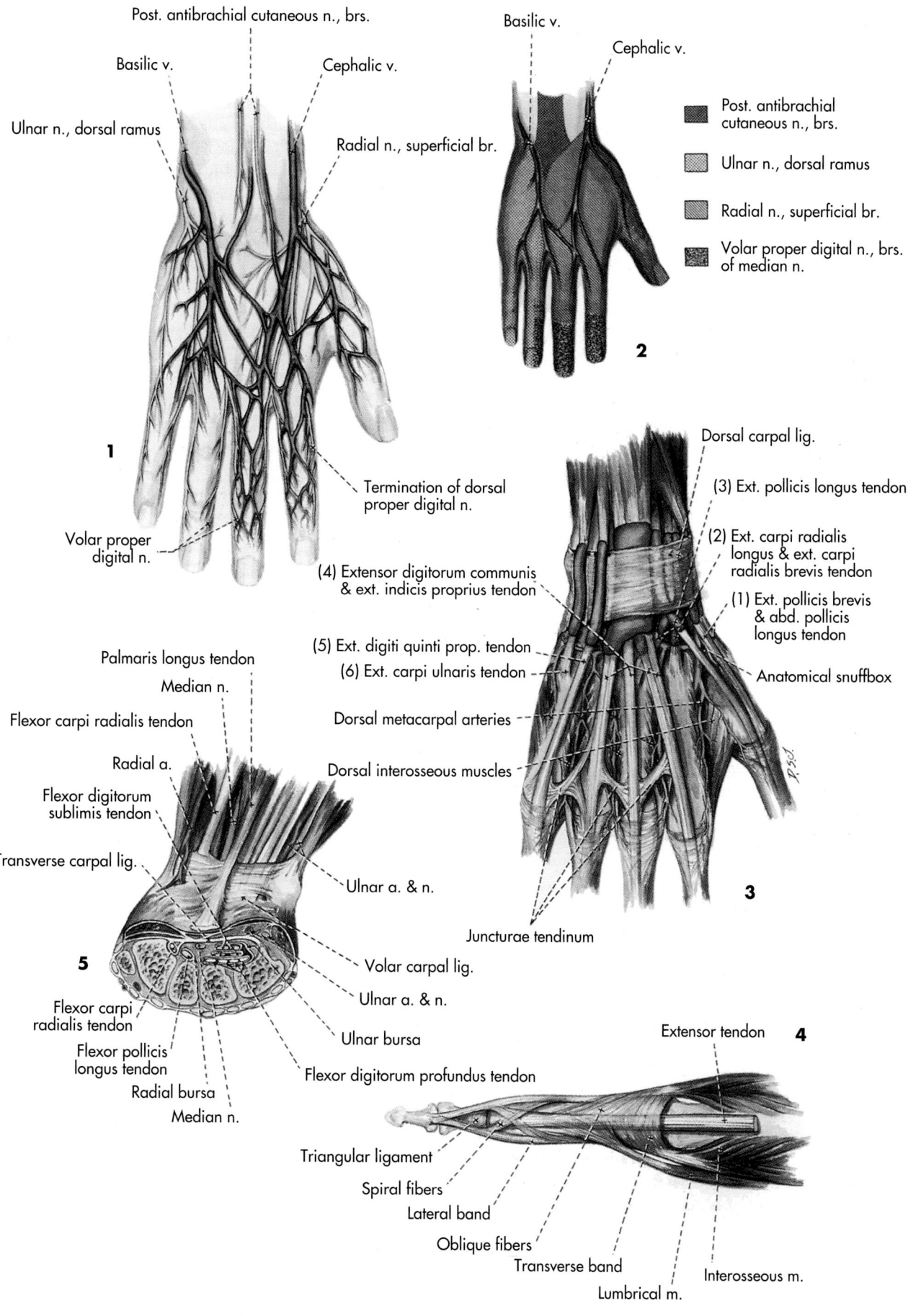

PLATE 17

1

Post. antibrachial cutaneous n., brs.

Basilic v.

Cephalic v.

Ulnar n., dorsal ramus

Radial n., superficial br.

Termination of dorsal proper digital n.

Volar proper digital n.

2

Basilic v.

Cephalic v.

Post. antibrachial cutaneous n., brs.

Ulnar n., dorsal ramus

Radial n., superficial br.

Volar proper digital n., brs. of median n.

3

Dorsal carpal lig.

(3) Ext. pollicis longus tendon

(2) Ext. carpi radialis longus & ext. carpi radialis brevis tendon

(1) Ext. pollicis brevis & abd. pollicis longus tendon

Anatomical snuffbox

(4) Extensor digitorum communis & ext. indicis proprius tendon

(5) Ext. digiti quinti prop. tendon

(6) Ext. carpi ulnaris tendon

Dorsal metacarpal arteries

Dorsal interosseous muscles

Juncturae tendinum

5

Palmaris longus tendon

Median n.

Flexor carpi radialis tendon

Radial a.

Flexor digitorum sublimis tendon

Transverse carpal lig.

Ulnar a. & n.

Volar carpal lig.

Ulnar a. & n.

Ulnar bursa

Flexor digitorum profundus tendon

Flexor carpi radialis tendon

Flexor pollicis longus tendon

Radial bursa

Median n.

4

Extensor tendon

Triangular ligament

Spiral fibers

Lateral band

Oblique fibers

Transverse band

Lumbrical m.

Interosseous m.

THE UPPER EXTREMITY—PLATE 18
The anatomy of hand infections

Only correct surgical care of deep infections in the hand can prevent serious destruction of tissue and permanent impairment of functions. Of particular importance are those infections located in the flexor synovial tendon sheaths and palmar fascial spaces. The latter are not spaces in the true sense of the word, but are fascial intervals that distend easily and limit the spread of pus or fluid. Infections of the tendon sheaths commonly spread to the fascial spaces and vice versa.

Mucous (synovial) tendon sheaths (Figs. 1 and 3) These sheaths are bursal protective elements that envelope the flexor tendons of the fingers.

1. Proper digital mucous tendon sheaths—extend from the neck of the metacarpal bones to the insertion of the long flexor tendons on the distal phalanx of the index, middle, and ring fingers. Like all mucous sheaths, they consist of parietal and visceral layers between which is found lubricating synovial fluid. Interrupted mesotendons of the sheath termed *vincula* (longus and brevis) transmit blood vessels to and from the tendon.

2. Radial bursa—is the mucous sheath of the flexor pollicis longus and extends from the insertion of the tendon on the distal phalanx of the thumb to a level in the forearm approximately 2.5 cm proximal to the transverse carpal ligament.

3. Ulnar bursa—is the common sheath that envelopes the tendons of the flexor digitorum sublimis and the flexor digitorum profundus, extending from the distal part of the forearm under the transverse carpal ligament to the middle of the palm, where it terminates along the tendon of the index, middle, and ring fingers, but on the ulnar side continues as the flexor digital sheath of the little finger. Often, there is a communication between the ulnar and radial bursae at the wrist, which accounts for the so-called horseshoe abscess.

Palmar fascial spaces. Between the flexor tendons of the fingers with their mucous sheaths and the accompanying lumbrical muscles anteriorly and the metacarpal bones with the interossei and the adductor pollicis muscles posteriorly, lie the thenar and midpalmar "spaces" (Figs. 1 and 2). They lie in the middle compartment of the palm separated by a fibrous partition at the third metacarpal (see Fig. 2). A third "space" of similar character and significance, the adductor space, exists behind the adductor pollicis muscle.

1. Thenar space (see Figs. 1 and 2)—is bounded by the flexor tendons of the index finger and the associated first lumbrical muscle on its volar side and the adductor pollicis muscle dorsally. It is limited on the radial side by the flexor

pollicis longus tendon and the radial bursa, and on the ulnar side by a firm anteroposterior septum extending from the fascia covering the flexor tendons to the third metacarpal bone. The proximal extension of the space is to the distal edge of the transverse carpal ligament and the distal limit at the line of the proximal transverse crease of the palm with an extension along the first lubrical muscle.

2. Midpalmar space (see Figs. 1 and 2)—has the same proximal and distal boundaries as the thenar space. Distally, however, it has extensions related to the second, third, and fourth lubrical muscles. Its volar boundary is the flexor tendons of the middle, ring, and little fingers and the associated lumbrical muscles. The fascia covering the anterior interosseous muscles and metacarpal bones form the dorsal limits. The space is limited on the ulnar side by the hypothenar muscles and fascia, and on the radial side by the same fascial septum extending to the third metacarpal as described previously.

3. Adductor space (Figs. 2 and 4)—is in continuity with the thenar space and lies between the adductor pollicis muscle and the first dorsal interosseous muscle. The two spaces communicate at the distal border of the adductor muscle.

Other fascial spaces. *Subcutaneous* and *subaponeurotic* spaces (see Fig. 2) are present on the dorsum of the hand. These are of much less importance than the palmar spaces.

Located in the forearm, but of importance because infection may reach it from the bursae in the deep palmar spaces, is the *retrotendinous space of Paroma*. It lies in the lower part of the anterior compartment of the forearm between the flexor pollicis longus and flexor digitorum profundus in front and the pronator quadratus behind.

Surgical incisions (see Fig. 3) Several incisions that may be used for drainage of closed-space infections of the hand are shown in Figs. 3 and 4. The proper digital sheaths may be opened as shown in Fig. 3, *A*. A lateral incision avoids transection of the flexion creases of the fingers. Incision for drainage of the radial bursa is shown in Fig. 3, *B*. The incision must not be extended too far into the palm for fear of injury to the recurrent branch of the median nerve. The ulnar bursa may be approached by any of three incisions, depending on the severity of the infection (Fig. 3, *C* through *E*).

The midpalmar space may be approached by an incision parallel to the distal palmar crease (Fig. 3, *F*) or through the web between the ring and middle fingers (Fig. 3, *G*). The thenar space may best be approached through an incision on the dorsal aspect of the web between the thumb and index fingers (see Fig. 4). Such an approach also permits drainage of the adductor space.

PLATE 18

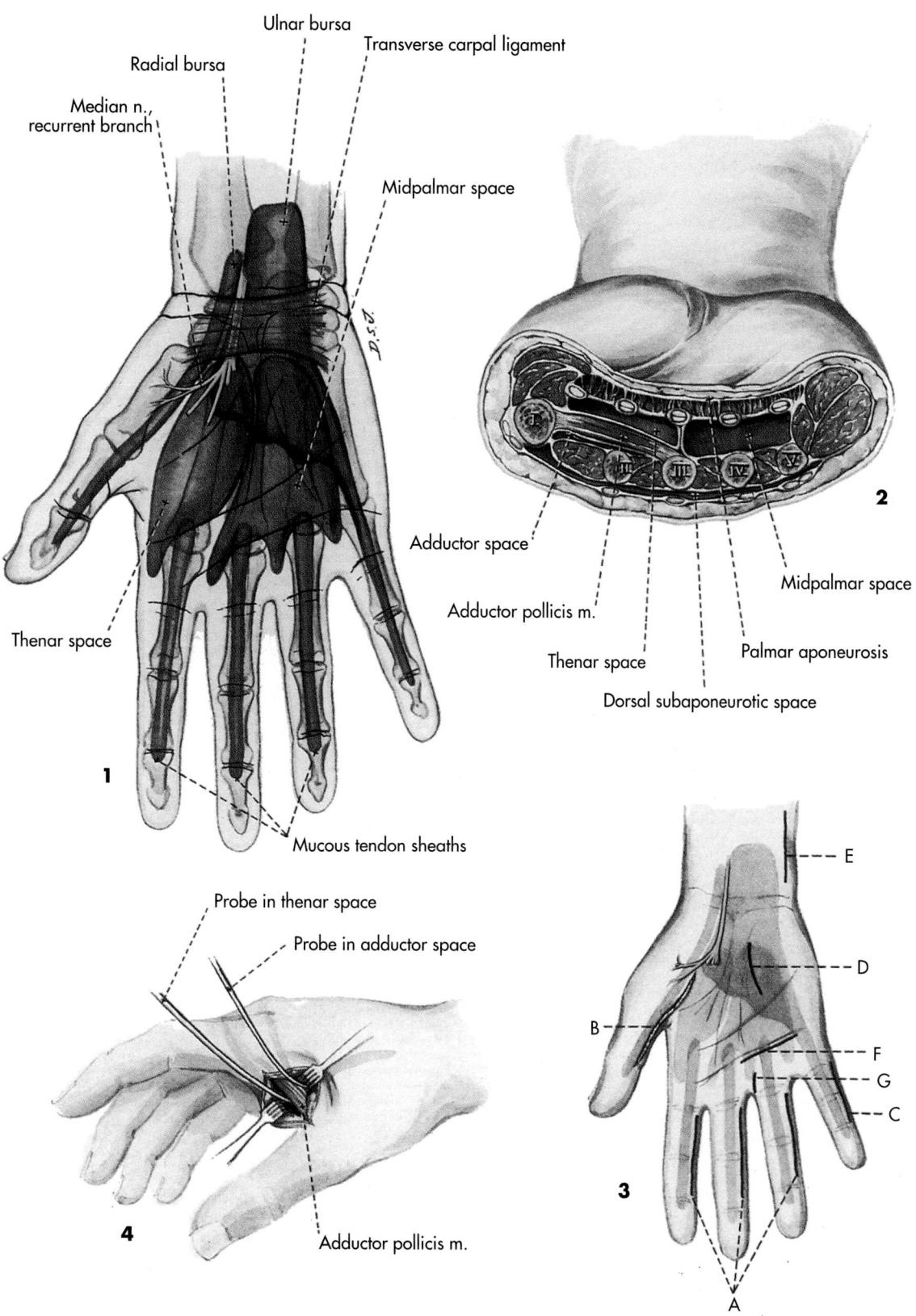

Ulnar bursa

Radial bursa

Transverse carpal ligament

Median n., recurrent branch

Midpalmar space

Thenar space

1

Mucous tendon sheaths

Adductor space

Adductor pollicis m.

Thenar space

Midpalmar space

Palmar aponeurosis

Dorsal subaponeurotic space

2

Probe in thenar space

Probe in adductor space

4

Adductor pollicis m.

E

D

B

F

G

C

3

A

THE UPPER EXTREMITY—PLATE 19
Major joints of the upper extremity

Although many bony articulations in the upper extremity are of clinical significance, only the three major joints are discussed here: the shoulder, elbow, and wrist joints. Each joint under consideration is a *diarthrodial joint*. This type of articulation has the following characteristics:

1. Each consists of two or more bones, each covered by articular hyaline cartilage.
2. The bones are united by a fibrous capsule continuous with the periosteum of the bone.
3. A synovial membrane lines the fibrous capsule and covers all portions of bone enclosed in the capsule and not covered with hyaline cartilage.

A generalization can be made in regard to the innervation of the joints: A joint is innervated by the same nerves that innervate the muscles that cross the joint. This is referred to as *Hilton's law.*

Shoulder joint. The shoulder joint is a diarthrodial joint of the enarthrodial (ball and socket) type. It is the most mobile of all the joints, permitting flexion, extension, abduction, adduction, medial and lateral rotation, and circumduction. Because of certain of its anatomic features, it is the most frequently dislocated in the body (page 42).

1. Bony parts (Figs. 1 and 2)—consist of the shallow, concave glenoid cavity of the scapula and the large convex head of the humerus, each covered by articular hyaline cartilage.

2. Articular capsule (Figs. 1 to 5)—is a lax fibrous layer uniting the bony parts. It is attached superiorly to the circumference of the glenoid cavity. The upper parts of the humeral attachment are on the anatomic neck, whereas the lower portion attaches to the shaft about 2 cm below the articular surface of the head (see Figs. 1 and 2). The looseness of the capsule is compensated in part by certain ligamentous reinforcements:

a. CORACOHUMERAL LIGAMENT (see Fig. 3)—is a broad band arising from the coracoid process and inserting into the greater tubercle of the humerus. This ligament strengthens the superior portion of the joint capsule.

b. GLENOHUMERAL LIGAMENTS (see Fig. 5)—are three ligamentous bands that reinforce the anterior portion of the capsular ligament. These bands can be distinguished by viewing the inner aspect of the capsule and are described as the *superior, middle,* and *inferior glenohumeral ligaments.* They arise from the rim of the glenoid cavity and insert on the humerus in relation to the lesser tubercle. Between the superior and middle band is seen an opening of varying size known as the *subscapular recess.*

c. GLENOID LABRIUM (see Fig. 5)—is a rim of dense fibrocartilage along the margin of the glenoid cavity. It deepens the cavity somewhat, thereby affording a better receptive area for the head of the humerus.

d. TRANSVERSE HUMERAL LIGAMENT (see Fig. 3)—extends between the lesser and greater tubercle and converts the intertubercular groove into a canal for passage of the tendon of the long head of the biceps.

3. Synovial membrane (Fig. 6)—lies deep to the articular capsule and attaches to the scapular and humeral articular margins. The synovial membrane has two constant extensions: one, as the *subscapular bursa* that extends through the subscapular recess described earlier; the second, as a prolongation inferiorly as the *synovial sheath of the long tendon of the biceps.* Sometimes, the synovial membrane of the joint extends through the posterior wall of the capsule as the *infraspinatus bursa.*

4. Musculotendinous relations (see Figs. 3 to 5)—are probably the most important anatomic feature of the shoulder joint because it depends on the muscular control for its integrity. Certain muscles are intimately related to the anterior, superior, and posterior surfaces of the capsule. The inferior aspect receives no musculotendinous reinforcement and constitutes the "weak area" of the articular capsule.

a. SUBSCAPULAR—reinforces the anterior portion of the capsule.

b. SUPRASPINATUS—is related to the superior aspect of the joint.

c. INFRASPINATUS AND TERES MINOR—strengthen the joint posteriorly.

d. LONG TENDON OF THE BICEPS—arises from the supraglenoid tuberosity and passes through the joint capsule surrounded by a tubular sheath derived from the synovial membrane. It performs a very important action in maintaining joint stability.

The subscapularis tendon in front and the supraspinatus, infraspinatus, and teres minor above and behind form what is known clinically as the *rotator cuff.*

5. Other relations—include bony, muscular, and neurovascular structures as well as bursae.

a. SUPERIORLY (see Fig. 3)—an osseofibrous arch, consisting of the *acromion process* and the *coracoacromial ligament,* protects the joint. Between this arch and the underlying capsule and supraspinatus tendon is the *subacromial bursa.*

b. ANTERIORLY (see Figs. 1 and 2, Plate 7)—the *axillary vessels* and terminal branches of the *brachial plexus* are separated from the joint by the subscapular muscle and bursa.

c. POSTERIORLY—overlapping the infraspinatus and teres minor muscles is the *deltoid muscle.* This muscle also is related to the superior, anterior, and lateral aspects of the joint, producing the rounded contour of the shoulder.

d. INFERIORLY (see Fig. 4)—the *axillary nerve* and *posterior humeral circumflex artery* and *vein* are closely related to the capsule. These vessels, along with the anterior humeral circumflex and transverse scapular vessels, supply and drain the shoulder joint. In this location, the *long head of the triceps* also may be seen.

PLATE 19

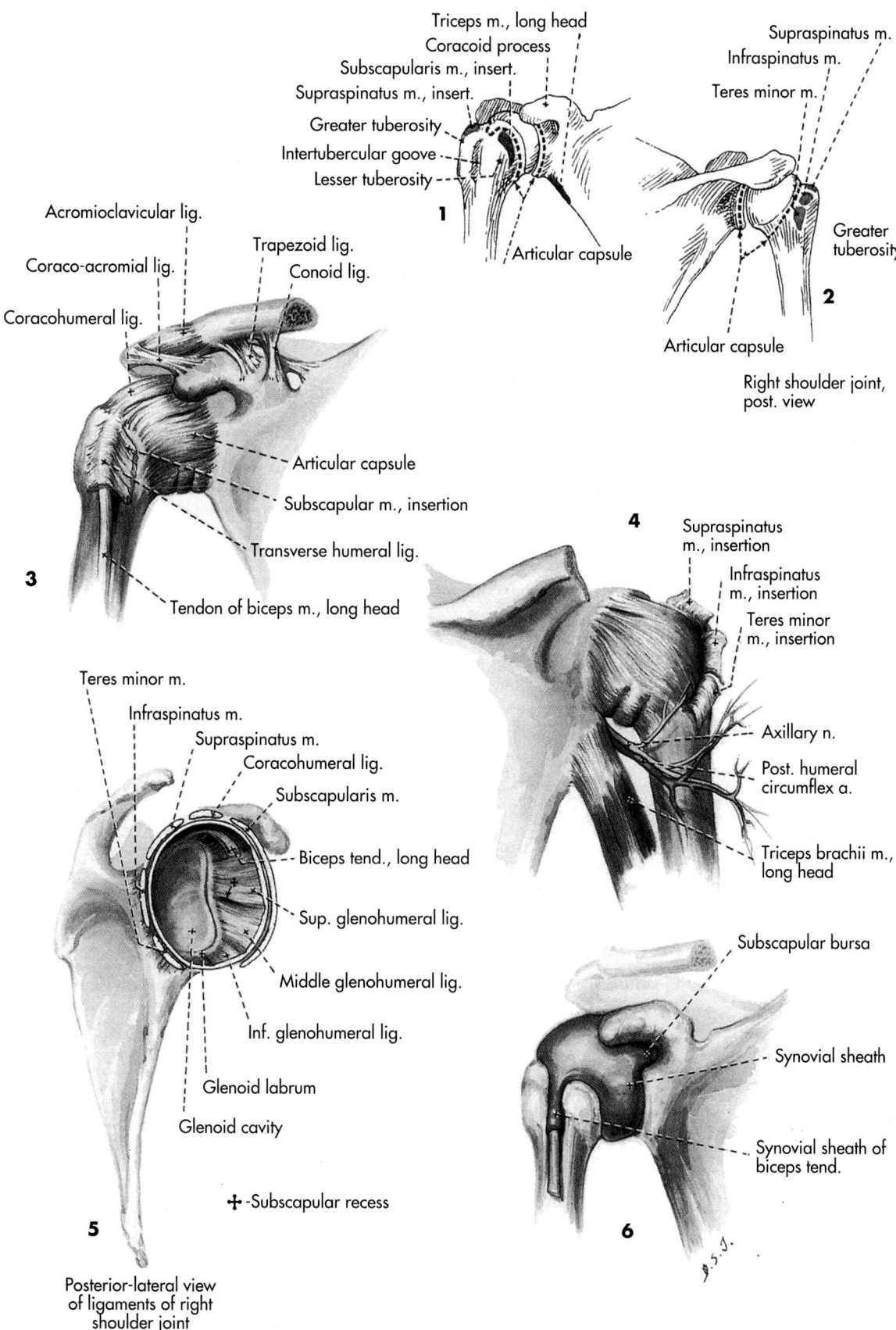

Triceps m., long head
Coracoid process
Subscapularis m., insert.
Supraspinatus m., insert.
Greater tuberosity
Intertubercular goove
Lesser tuberosity

Articular capsule

1

Supraspinatus m.
Infraspinatus m.
Teres minor m.

Greater tuberosity

2

Articular capsule

Right shoulder joint,
post. view

Acromioclavicular lig.
Coraco-acromial lig.
Coracohumeral lig.

Trapezoid lig.
Conoid lig.

Articular capsule

Subscapular m., insertion

Transverse humeral lig.

3

Tendon of biceps m., long head

4

Supraspinatus
m., insertion

Infraspinatus
m., insertion

Teres minor
m., insertion

Axillary n.

Post. humeral
circumflex a.

Triceps brachii m.,
long head

Teres minor m.
Infraspinatus m.
Supraspinatus m.
Coracohumeral lig.
Subscapularis m.

Biceps tend., long head

Sup. glenohumeral lig.

Middle glenohumeral lig.

Inf. glenohumeral lig.

Glenoid labrum

Glenoid cavity

✚-Subscapular recess

5

Posterior-lateral view
of ligaments of right
shoulder joint

Subscapular bursa

Synovial sheath

Synovial sheath of
biceps tend.

6

THE UPPER EXTREMITY—PLATE 20
Clinical considerations of the shoulder joint

The rotator cuff. Degenerative changes or rupture of fibers by trauma may produce significant lesions of an acute or chronic nature in the rotator cuff (page 40). *Calcific deposits* may develop in any of the tissues of the cuff (subscapularis, supraspinatus, and infraspinatus, and teres minor muscles), but in about half of the affected shoulders, it occurs as a single lesion in the supraspinatus portion of the cuff. The clinical term *bursitis* of the shoulder is usually a misnomer. Whereas calcium deposits may be present in the two bursae (the subacromial and subcoracoid) of the shoulder area to account for pain and limitation of motion of the joint, they usually are not in these bursae, but rather in the tissues of the rotator cuff.

Surgical approaches to the shoulder. Aspiration of the shoulder joint may be performed by inserting a needle just below the tip of the coracoid process and directing it posteriorly and slightly laterally.

Anterior approach (Figs. 1, 2, and 3)—is useful in exposing (1) the shoulder joint, (2) the long and short heads of the biceps, (3) the subscapularis muscle and tendon, (4) the glenoid fossa, and (5) the axillary surface of the scapula. Exposure of the latter two structures requires an osteotomy of the coracoid process. This incision is designed to protect the axillary nerve from injury. The position and course of the nerve must be constantly in the surgeon's mind. This approach through the deltopectoral cleft provides these two essentials: good exposure and protection of the axillary nerve. It may be extended superiorly (see Fig. 1, *dotted line*) for better access to the humeral head and inferiorly for the shaft of the humerus.

Posterior approach—by extension of the anterosuperomedial incision around the lateral and posterior margins of the acromion and the lateral part of the spine of the scapula, the posterior aspect of the shoulder joint may be exposed (Fig. 4, *dotted line*). However, exposure may be limited to the posterior aspect by an incision along the posterior margin of the deltoid (see Fig. 4).

Shoulder dislocations. The shoulder is the most frequently dislocated major joint in the body. Several anatomic freatures of the joint are responsible for this fact:

1. Its unprotected position, which makes it vulnerable to trauma
2. The extreme mobility of the joint, which is produced by the following:
   - The disparity in the size of the articular surface of the head of the humerus and the small, shallow glenoid fossa
   - The laxity of the joint capsule

Dislocating forces—a fall on the outstretched hand or on the elbow when the arm is adducted (Fig. 5), a direct blow on the shoulder, or violent muscle action alone may dislocate the shoulder.

Types of dislocation—the forces described previously also will determine in part the type of dislocation that will occur. Often, there is avulsion of the glenoid labrum, the fibrous capsule, and the glenohumeral ligaments from the anteroinferior aspect of the rim of the glenoid fossa, permitting displacement of the humeral head inferiorly (Fig. 6). Dislocations also may occur through a simple rent in the capsule or with an intact but stretched joint capsule.

1. SUBCORACOID (Fig. 7, *B*)—is the most common type. The head of the humerus lies below the coracoid process deep to the short head of the biceps and coracobrachialis muscles.

2. SUBGLENOID (Fig. 7, *C*)—is the second most common site for the head to lodge in dislocation. The subcoracoid and subglenoid types make up 98% of shoulder dislocations.

3. SUBCLAVICULAR (Fig. 7, *A*)—dislocation occurs if the dislocating force is great enough and properly directed. The head slides further anteriorly beneath the pectoralis minor and clavicle.

4. Subspinous type is a rare posterior displacement in which the humeral head passes backward to lie beneath the spine of the scapula.

Injuries to associated structures

1. To musculotendinous structures of the rotator cuff—is a common, if not constant and important, factor predisposing to recurrent dislocation. The injury usually involves tearing or stretching of the suprascapular and subscapularis muscles. The tendon of the long head of the biceps may be torn or dislocated.

2. To capsule—in addition to a tear in the inferior part of the capsule, other ligamentous reinforcements of the capsule may be disrupted. The most common injury is a detachment of the glenoid labrum (see Fig. 6) or disruption of the glenohumeral ligaments.

3. To bone—such as an associated fracture of the glenoid rim or neck of the scapula or the greater tuberosity of the humerus.

4. To nerves—in 5% of acute dislocations. Usually, it is temporary and involves only the ulnar nerve, but the radial, axillary, and median nerves may be damaged.

5. To vessels—contusion with thrombosis or laceration with severe hemorrhage occasionally may affect the axillary, subscapular, or posterior humeral circumflex arteries.

PLATE 20

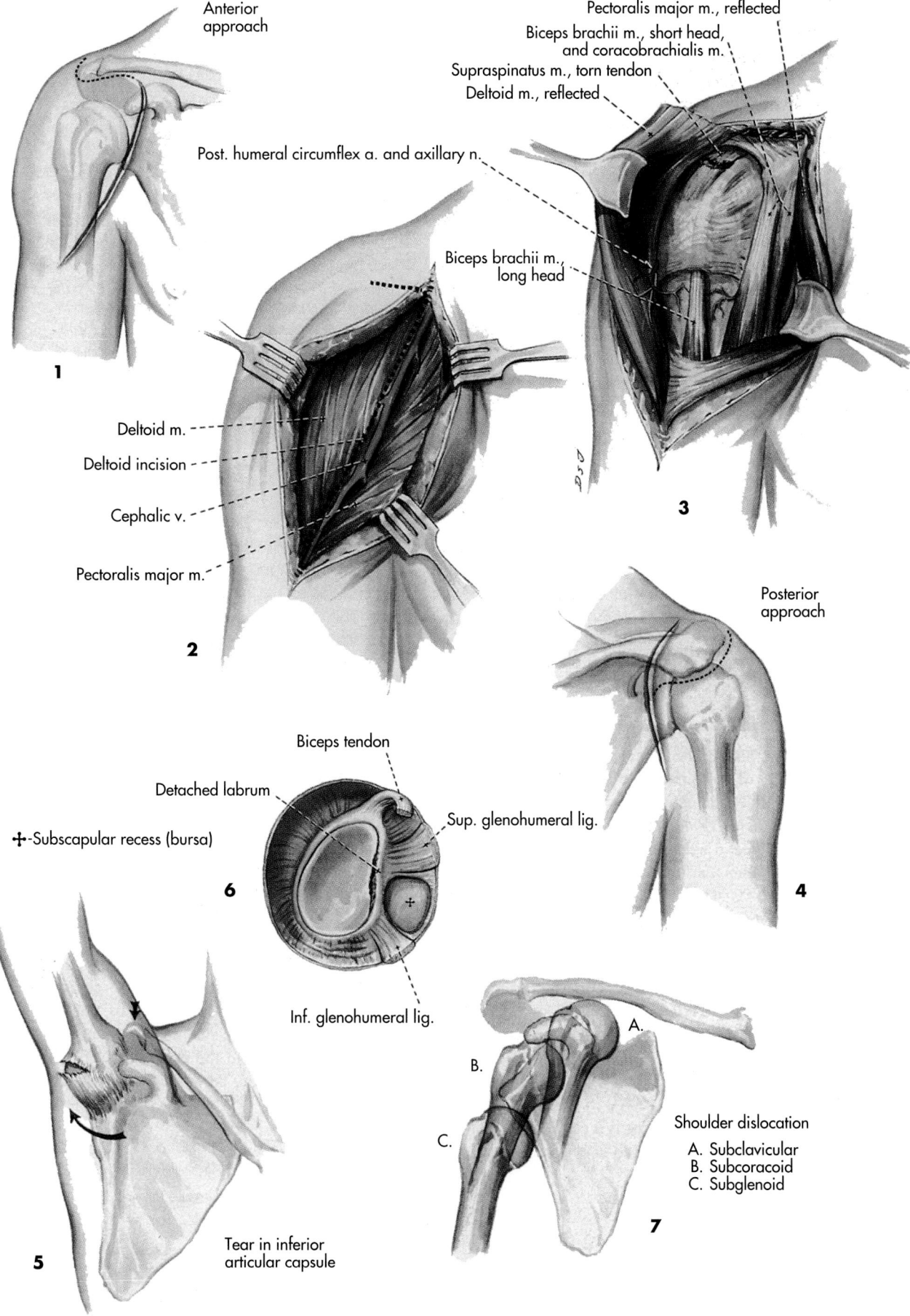

Anterior approach

Pectoralis major m., reflected

Biceps brachii m., short head, and coracobrachialis m.

Supraspinatus m., torn tendon

Deltoid m., reflected

Post. humeral circumflex a. and axillary n.

Biceps brachii m., long head

1

Deltoid m.

Deltoid incision

Cephalic v.

Pectoralis major m.

2

3

Posterior approach

Biceps tendon

Detached labrum

✝-Subscapular recess (bursa)

Sup. glenohumeral lig.

6

4

Inf. glenohumeral lig.

A.

B.

C.

Shoulder dislocation

A. Subclavicular
B. Subcoracoid
C. Subglenoid

7

Tear in inferior articular capsule

5

THE UPPER EXTREMITY—PLATE 21
Elbow joint

The elbow actually consists of three separate joints: the *humeroulnar, humeroradial,* and *proximal radioulnar joints.* They all are diarthrodial joints having a common synovial membrane. The humeral joints are the *ginglymus* (hinge-joint) type and are limited to extension and flexion. The radioulnar joint is classified as a *trochoidal type,* in which the articular surface of one bone is a disc that glides in a corresponding concave surface of the other bone, resulting in pronation and supination.

1. Bony parts (Figs. 1 and 2)—of the humeroulnar joint consist of the *trochlea of the humerus* and the *semilunar notch of the ulna.* The humeroradial joints join the *capitulum of the humerus* and the *fovea on the head of the radius.* The *medial part of the radial head* and the *radial notch of the ulna* make up the bony parts of the radioulnar articulation.

2. Articular capsule (see Figs. 1 and 2)—is attached to the anterior surface of the humerus on ridges extending from the medial and lateral epicondyles to a point above the *radial* and *coronoid fossae.* Below, it is attached to the articular margin of the coronoid process of the ulna and the neck of the radius *(anterior capsular ligament).* On the posterior surface of the humerus, it attaches to the margins of the olecranon fossa above and to the margins of the olecranon process of the ulna and neck of the radius below *(posterior capsular ligament).* This area is the weakest part of the joint, accounting for the fact that posterior dislocations are most frequent in occurrence. The capsule is reinforced by lateral and medial reinforcements.

a. ULNAR COLLATERAL LIGAMENT (Figs. 3 and 4)—is a triangular thickening in the capsule extending from the medial epicondyle of the humerus to the medial edge of the coronoid process of the ulna.

b. RADIAL COLLATERAL LIGAMENT (see Figs. 3 and 4)—extends from the lateral epicondyle and inserts into the neck of the radius and annular ligament.

c. ANNULAR LIGAMENT (see Figs. 3 and 4)—encircles the head of the radius, retaining it into the radial notch of the ulna.

3. Synovial membrane (Fig. 5)—extends from the margin of the articular surface of the humerus and lines the fossa of the humerus. It is reflected over the deep surface of the capsule and extends inferiorly as a pouch between the radial notch, annular ligament, and circumference of the head of the radius, the *sacciform recess.*

Wrist joint

Like the elbow joint, the wrist is a compound joint consisting of the *radiocarpal* and the *distal radioulnar joints.* The radiocarpal joint is a diarthrodial, *ellipsodial* type in which a convex surface is held in a concave surface. The actions of this joint are flexion, extension, abduction, adduction, and circumduction. The radioulnar is *trochoidal,* permitting pronation and supination.

1. Bony parts (Figs. 6 and 7)—of the radiocarpal joint consist on the proximal side of the concavity formed by the *articular surface of the radius* and the *articular disc* and the distal convex surface of the carpus, which is made up of the *navicular, lunate,* and *triquetral bones.* The radioulnar joint articulaton joins the *head of the ulna* with the *ulnar notch of the radius.*

2. Articular capsule (see Figs. 6 and 7)—extends from the anterior margin of the lower end of the radius and styloid process and the lower end of the ulna. The capsule attaches to the volar surface of the navicular, lunate, and triquetral carpal bones. The capsule is described as having four ligaments:

a. ANTERIOR RADIOCARPAL LIGAMENT (Fig. 8)—is attached to the styloid process and the anterior margin of the lower end of the radius and ulna above and the volar surface of the navicular, lunate, and triquetral below.

b. DORSAL RADIOCARPAL LIGAMENT (Fig. 9)—gains attachment to the dorsal end of the radius and its styloid process and the posterior margin of the articular disc. It passes downward to attach to the first row of carpal bones and the dorsal intercarpal ligament.

c. ULNAR COLLATERAL LIGAMENT (see Figs. 8 and 9)—extends from the styloid process of the ulnar and inserts by two divisions: one into the medial side of the triquetrum and the other to the pisiform and transverse carpal ligament.

d. RADIAL COLLATERAL LIGAMENT (see Figs. 8 and 9)—is attached to the styloid process of the radius above to the navicular below.

e. ARTICULAR DISK—is a fibrocartilaginous structure radiating from the radius to the base of the styloid process of the ulna. The disk enters into two distinct articulations, separating the distal radioulnar from the radiocarpal joints.

3. Synovial membranes (Fig. 10)—of the radiocarpal and the distal radioulnar joints are distinct from one another. The synovial membrane of the distal radioulnar joint is large and lax, extending between the articular surface of the ulna and the proximal surface of the articular disk and protruding between the radius and ulnar articular surfaces.

PLATE 21

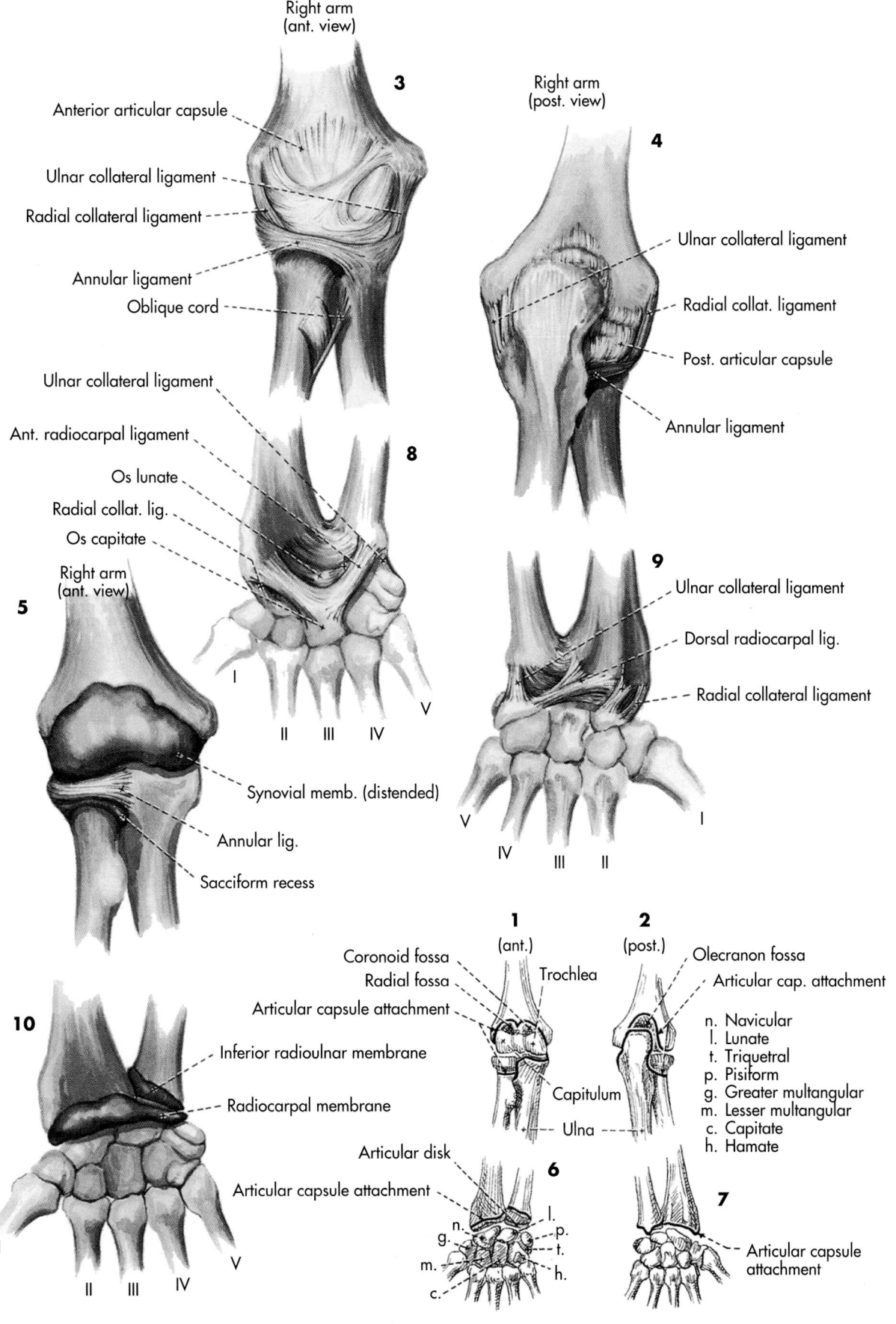

Right arm
(ant. view)

3

Anterior articular capsule

Ulnar collateral ligament

Radial collateral ligament

Annular ligament

Oblique cord

Right arm
(post. view)

4

Ulnar collateral ligament

Radial collat. ligament

Post. articular capsule

Annular ligament

Ulnar collateral ligament

Ant. radiocarpal ligament

Os lunate

Radial collat. lig.

Os capitate

Right arm
(ant. view)

5

8

I

V

II   III   IV

9

Ulnar collateral ligament

Dorsal radiocarpal lig.

Radial collateral ligament

V

I

IV

III   II

Synovial memb. (distended)

Annular lig.

Sacciform recess

10

Inferior radioulnar membrane

Radiocarpal membrane

I

V

II   III   IV

1
(ant.)

2
(post.)

Coronoid fossa

Radial fossa

Articular capsule attachment

Trochlea

Olecranon fossa

Articular cap. attachment

n. Navicular
l. Lunate
t. Triquetral
p. Pisiform
g. Greater multangular
m. Lesser multangular
c. Capitate
h. Hamate

Capitulum

Ulna

Articular disk

Articular capsule attachment

6

n.
g.
m.
c.

l.
p.
t.
h.

7

Articular capsule
attachment

THE UPPER EXTREMITY—PLATE 22
Clinical considerations of the elbow and wrist

Of particular clinical interest are the relations of certain muscles, nerves, and vessels that may be injured when the joints or the bones immediately about them are damaged. These same structures must be protected in the operative approach to the joints. Finally, as a result of pathologic changes in the joints, progressive lesions of clinical importance may affect these structures (e.g., delayed ulnar palsy, carpal tunnel syndrome).

1. Relation of the ulnar nerve to the medial epicondyle (Fig. 1)—is a posterior one. The nerve lies in a shallow groove secured and protected by an aponeurosis stretching between the epicondyle and the olecranon. It enters the forearm between the two heads of the flexor carpi ulnaris. In this superficial position behind the medial epicondyle, it is exposed to injury by a direct blow or by pressure. Its liability to damage in fractures of the medial epicondyle is apparent. Furthermore, because it is fixed in position by overlying strong fascia, progressive valgus deformity of the elbow, as may occur after ill-managed fractures of the capitellum, damages the nerve by stretching *(delayed ulnar palsy).* Release of the nerve and transplantation to a position in front of the medial epicondyle adds effective length to the nerve. This maneuver may be helpful in relieving delayed ulnar palsy or in accomplishing anastomosis of an ulnar nerve that has been divided at this level.

2. Relation of radial nerve to the lateral epicondyle and to the supinator muscle (Fig. 2)—the nerve lies on the front of the lateral epicondyle of the humerus in the interval between the brachioradialis and brachialis muscles. At this level, it divides into its two terminal branches: the superficial (sensory) and deep (motor). The *superficial ramus* passes distally deep to the brachioradialis. The *deep ramus* immediately turns posteriorly to reach the back of the forearm after passing around the lateral aspect of the radius, piercing the supinator muscle. Injuries to the radial nerve in fractures of the humerus already have been mentioned (page 22). It also may be injured by anterior dislocation of the head of the radius, and it is an important structure to be protected in the surgical approach to the elbow by the anterolateral route.

3. Anterolateral approach to the elbow—for open reduction of fractures of the radius and excision of tumors begins in the arm lateral to the biceps and extends distally along the anterior margin of the brachioradialis (Fig. 3). The deep fascia is then opened, and the radial nerve is brought into view on the front of the lateral epicondyle between the brachioradialis laterally and the biceps and brachialis muscles medially (see Fig. 2). Its superficial (sensory) and deep (motor) branches are identified (see previous discussion) and protected. The lateral antebrachial cutaneous nerve (branch of musculocutaneous) appears between the tendon of the biceps and the brachialis muscle and must be protected by retraction medially (see Fig. 2). With the hand supinated, the upper end of the radius is exposed and the joint is entered by an incision into the periosteum of the radius medial to the attachment of the supinator and lateral to the attachment of the pronator teres.

4. Exposure of ulnar nerve in region of the elbow joint through a posterior-medial incision (see Fig. 1)—an incision is centered over the groove between the medial epicondyle and the olecranon process. The nerve lies beneath the deep fascia in a groove in the triceps, just behind the medial intermuscular septum. The fascial roof bridging the interval between the epicondyle and the olecranon must be cut to expose and free the nerve as it enters the forearm between the two heads of the flexor carpi ulnaris. Branches of the nerve to this muscle must be preserved.

PLATE 22

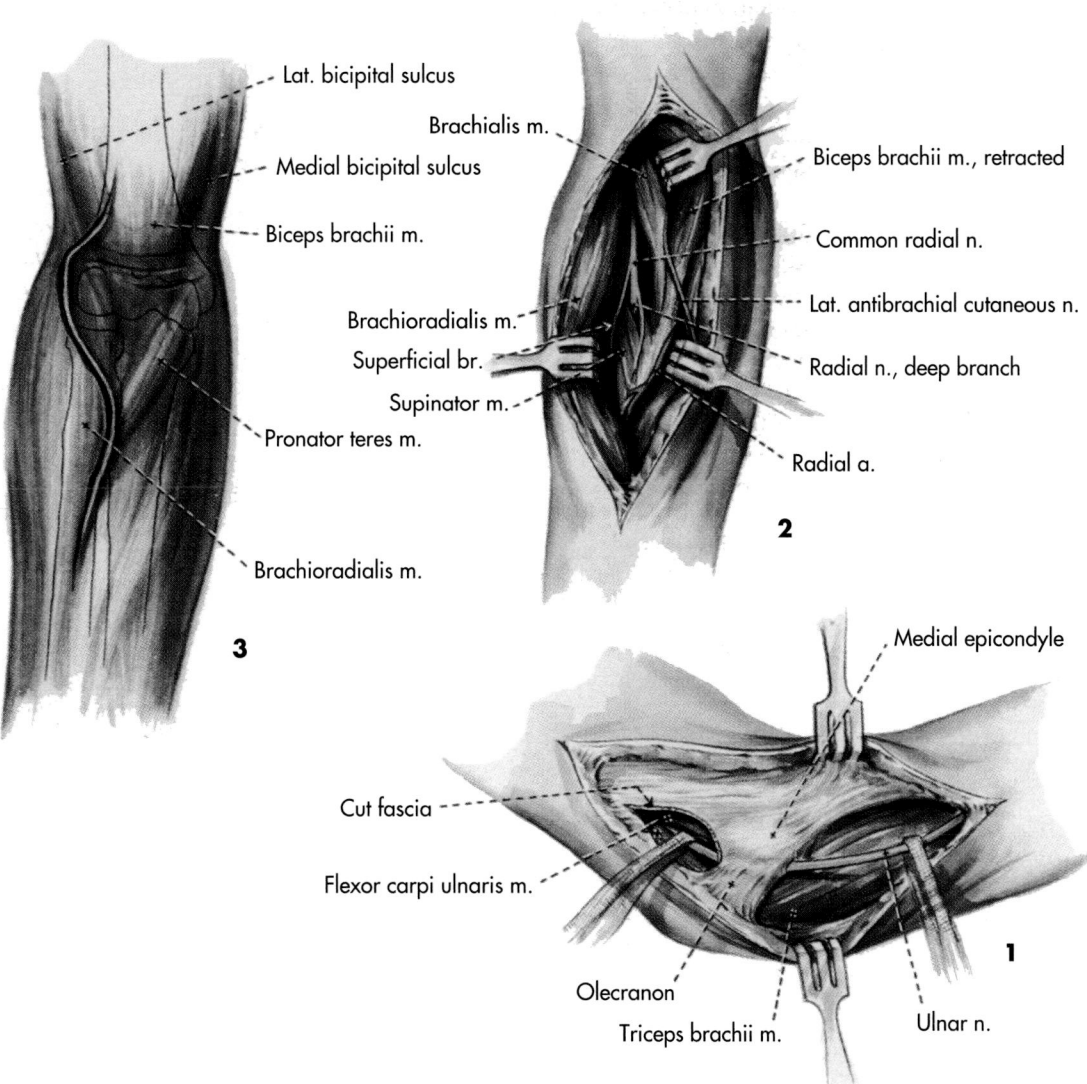

Lat. bicipital sulcus

Brachialis m.

Medial bicipital sulcus

Biceps brachii m.

Biceps brachii m., retracted

Common radial n.

Lat. antibrachial cutaneous n.

Brachioradialis m.

Superficial br.

Radial n., deep branch

Supinator m.

Pronator teres m.

Radial a.

Brachioradialis m.

2

3

Medial epicondyle

Cut fascia

Flexor carpi ulnaris m.

Olecranon

Triceps brachii m.

Ulnar n.

1

5. *Carpal tunnel syndrome or median neuritis at the wrist* (Fig. 4)—at the wrist, unyielding walls of a tunnel are formed by the carpal bones posteriorly and the strong transverse carpal ligament anteriorly that bridges the interval between the pisiform and hamate bones medially and the navicular and the greater multiangulum laterally. Through this closed space pass the flexor tendons with their mucous sheaths and the median nerve (see Fig. 5, Plate 17).

Any lesion that reduces the cross-sectional area of this tunnel may produce pressure on the median nerve. Distal to the *tunnel,* the median nerve furnishes sensory fibers to the radial three and a half fingers and motor fibers to the muscles of the thenar eminence. Pain and paresthesias, and weakness or paralysis with atrophy of the thenar muscles, are characteristic of the syndrome. A positive Tinel's sign (a tingling sensation in the distal end of the radial three fingers when percussion is made over the medial nerve at the wrist) and a delayed medial nerve conduction time are diagnostic of the syndrome.

Surgical decompression may be necessary. A longitudinal incision is made from the superior to the inferior border of the ligament medial to the median nerve, taking care to avoid its recurrent motor branch.

6. *Fracture of the navicular* (Fig. 5)—is a common carpal injury. The fracture occurs at the narrow "waist," producing two fragments. Normally, the navicular has a nutrient vessel entering the distal half and another entering the proximal half. Occasionally, both vessels go to the distal half, in which case fracture at the usual site deprives the proximal segment of its blood supply. Delayed union or nonunion may result. The latter may require excision of the proximal fragment. A characteristic clinical sign of the fracture is acute tenderness and swelling in the "anatomic snuffbox."

7. *Dislocation of the lunate* (Fig. 6)—is always anterior, and the bone comes to lie in the carpal tunnel. Impingement on the median nerve and flexor tendons produces symptoms as described under Carpal Tunnel Syndrome. There is also apparent shortening of the third metacarpal. Open reduction may be required.

PLATE 22–cont'd

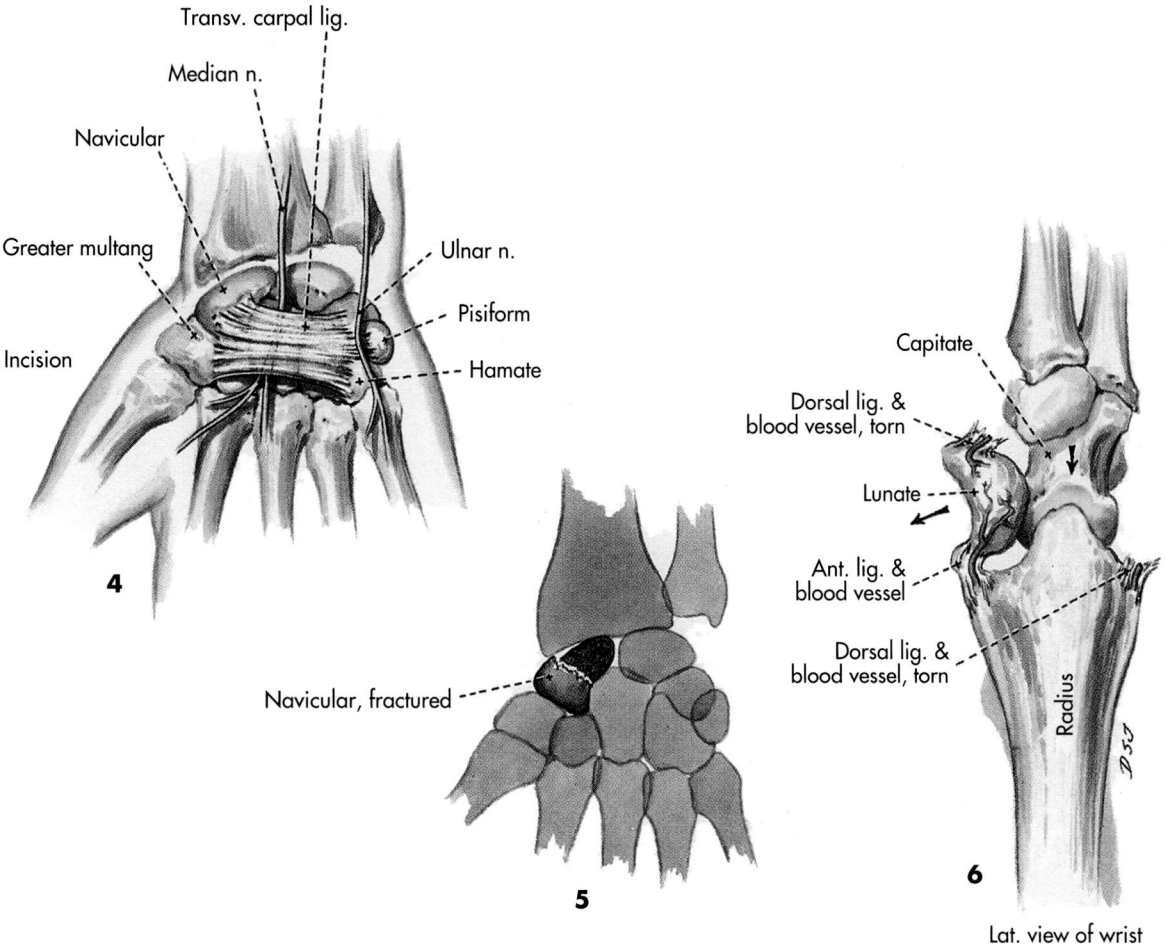

Transv. carpal lig.

Median n.

Navicular

Greater multang

Incision

Ulnar n.

Pisiform

Hamate

4

Navicular, fractured

5

Capitate

Dorsal lig. & blood vessel, torn

Lunate

Ant. lig. & blood vessel

Dorsal lig. & blood vessel, torn

Radius

6

Lat. view of wrist

Chapter 2

SURFACE ANATOMY
OF THE UPPER EXTREMITY

Neal E. Pratt

The purpose of this chapter is to present the surface anatomy of the upper extremity that is most relevant and useful to the clinician. The upper limb is presented regionally, starting proximally and proceeding distally. Each region is presented as a unit and organized in a similar manner so that the reader can follow the anatomy in a logical sequence. The specific regions are the posterior cervical triangle, shoulder, arm and elbow, forearm and wrist, and hand. In each region, the bony landmarks will be used as the basic references for most other structures.

Most of this chapter is devoted to the osteologic and muscular structures that are apparent through the skin. Because muscles are most readily palpable when they are active, the maneuvers necessary to produce specific muscle activity are included where appropriate. Nerve and vessel locations are included when they can be either palpated directly or specifically located relative to definitive landmarks. The names of structures appear in bold when their surface locations are described. Much of the information contained in this chapter is derived from multiple sources. As a result, specific references are not included in the text, but a variety of sources of additional information is included in a bibliography at the end of this chapter.

POSTERIOR CERVICAL TRIANGLE (Fig. 2-1)

The **posterior cervical triangle (posterior triangle of the neck)** is included because it houses the major neurovascular structures that supply the upper extremity and is the site of various clinical problems that can affect these structures and, potentially, the entire limb. The boundaries of this triangle are easily palpated and in most people can be identified visually. The base of the triangle is bony and formed by the **middle third** of the **clavicle;** the two sides are

muscular and formed by the posterior border of the **sternocleidomastoid** and the superior border of the **trapezius.** The borders of these muscles converge as they are followed superiorly toward the **mastoid process.** These boundaries can be accentuated by hunching the shoulder anteriorly and superiorly (trapezius) and rotating the head to the opposite side (sternocleidomastoid).

The **floor** of the triangle is muscular and palpable deep in the triangle. The **subclavian artery** and **proximal part** of the **brachial plexus** (roots and/or trunks) pass through this floor and are palpable in the anteromedial corner of the triangle (i.e., where the sternocleidomastoid muscle attaches to the clavicle). In the triangle, the **subclavian artery** is positioned medially and inferiorly; its pulse can be felt in the angle formed by the clavicle and sternocleidomastoid, just posterior to the clavicle where the artery passes superior to the first rib. The **superior trunk** of the brachial plexus is located approximately 2 to 3 cm superior to the clavicle at the posterior border of the sternocleidomastoid muscle. This structure feels like a strong cord or rope. Even though the **accessory nerve** is not palpable, its superficial course across the posterior triangle can be approximated because its course parallels a line between the ear lobe and the acromion process.

SHOULDER (Figs. 2-2 to 2-5)

The term *shoulder* is nonspecific because the areas and structures that can be included vary considerably. In this discussion, the "shoulder" includes the clavicle, the scapula, the proximal portion of the humerus, and all related articulations and soft tissues.

The **clavicle** is palpable throughout its length. In the midline, the **suprasternal (jugular) notch** is easily felt just

50

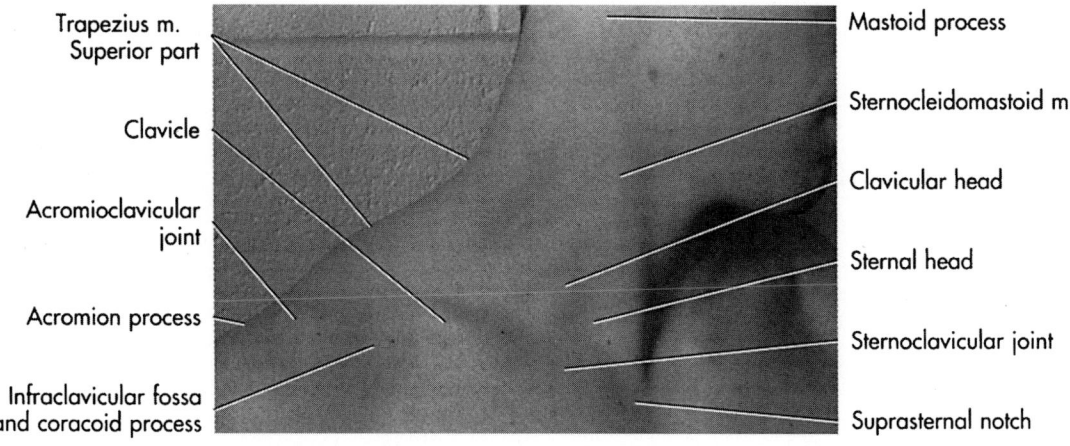

Trapezius m. Superior part

Clavicle

Acromioclavicular joint

Acromion process

Infraclavicular fossa and coracoid process

Mastoid process

Sternocleidomastoid m.

Clavicular head

Sternal head

Sternoclavicular joint

Suprasternal notch

Fig. 2-1. Anterolateral view of the right posterior cervical triangle. To accentuate the sternocleido-mastoid muscle, the head is rotated to the opposite side.

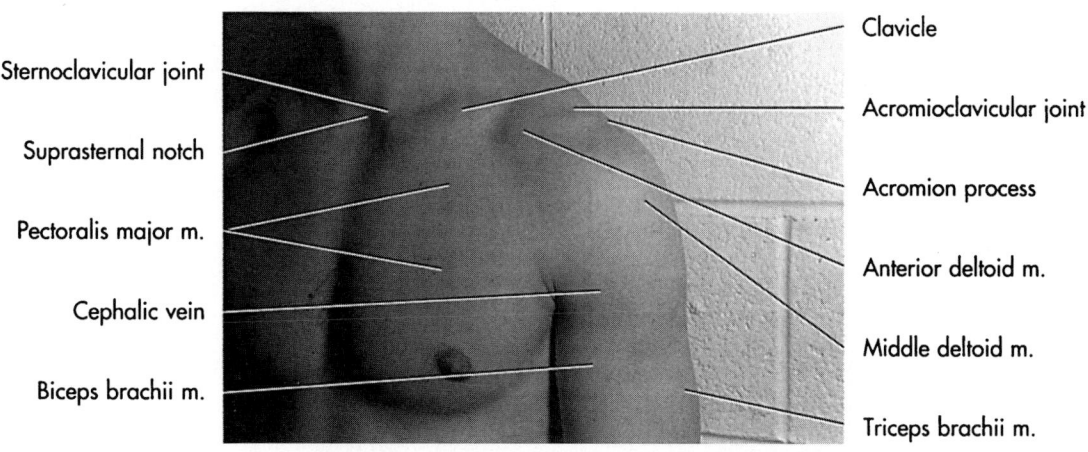

Sternoclavicular joint

Suprasternal notch

Pectoralis major m.

Cephalic vein

Biceps brachii m.

Clavicle

Acromioclavicular joint

Acromion process

Anterior deltoid m.

Middle deltoid m.

Triceps brachii m.

Fig. 2-2. Anterior view of the left shoulder, pectoral region, and proximal aspect of the arm.

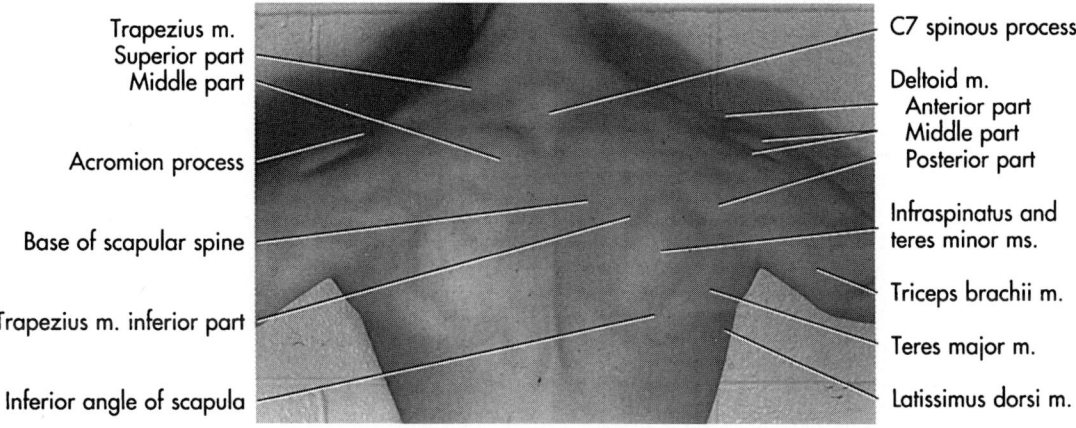

Trapezius m. Superior part Middle part

Acromion process

Base of scapular spine

Trapezius m. inferior part

Inferior angle of scapula

C7 spinous process

Deltoid m. Anterior part Middle part Posterior part

Infraspinatus and teres minor ms.

Triceps brachii m.

Teres major m.

Latissimus dorsi m.

Fig. 2-3. Posterior view of the cervical and thoracic portions of the back and the scapular regions. Horizontal abduction of the abducted upper limbs is resisted to reveal certain of the intrinsic and extrinsic muscles of the shoulder. Because the upper limbs are moderately abducted, the scapulae are rotated somewhat superiorly.

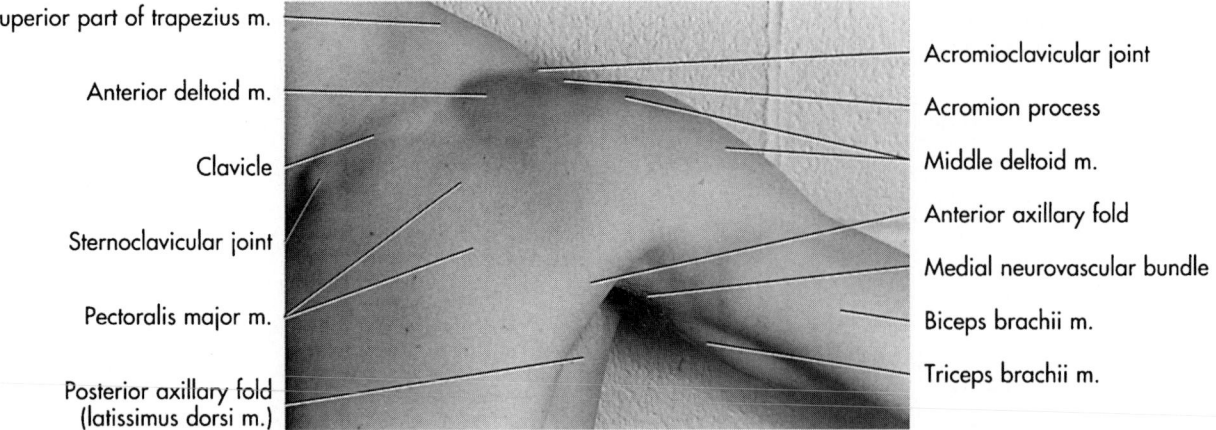

Superior part of trapezius m.

Anterior deltoid m.

Clavicle

Sternoclavicular joint

Pectoralis major m.

Posterior axillary fold
(latissimus dorsi m.)

Acromioclavicular joint

Acromion process

Middle deltoid m.

Anterior axillary fold

Medial neurovascular bundle

Biceps brachii m.

Triceps brachii m.

Fig. 2-4. Anterior and slightly inferior view of the shoulder and axillary region. The arm is moderately abducted to reveal both the anterior and posterior axillary folds and the medial neurovascular bundle.

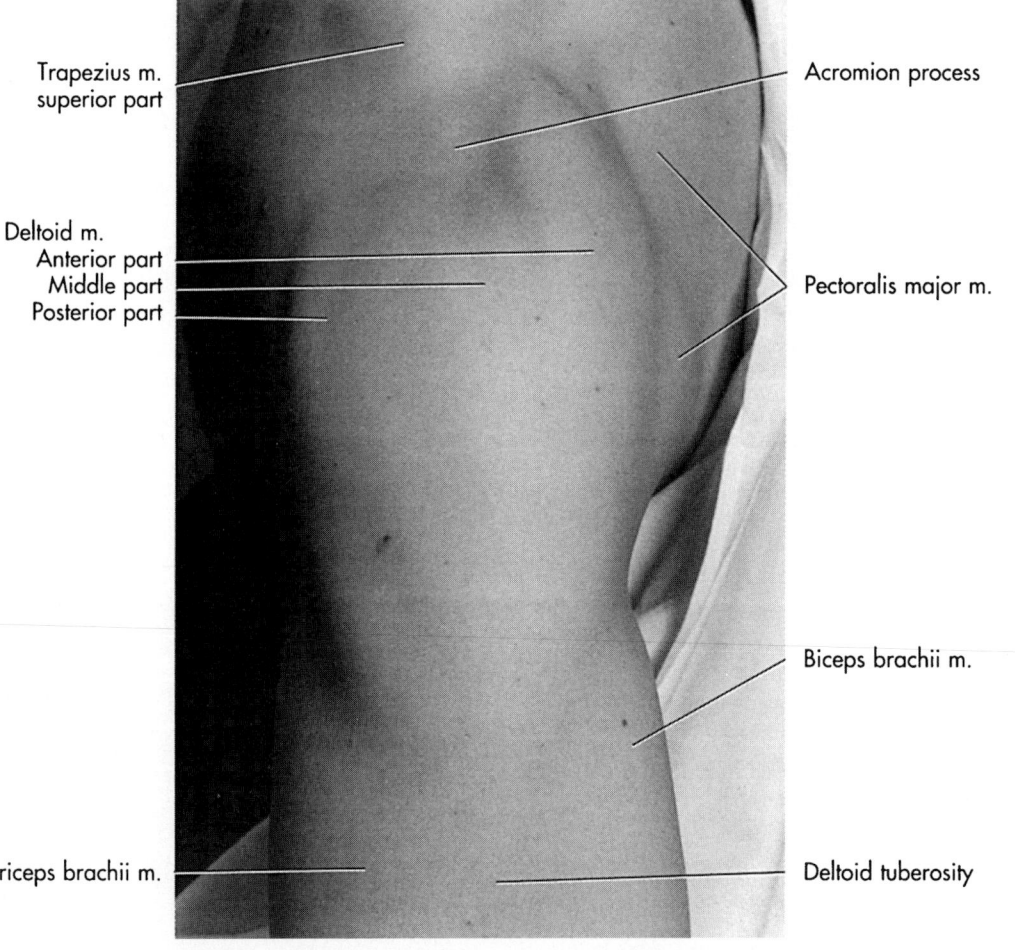

Trapezius m.
superior part

Deltoid m.
Anterior part
Middle part
Posterior part

Triceps brachii m.

Acromion process

Pectoralis major m.

Biceps brachii m.

Deltoid tuberosity

Fig. 2-5. Superolateral view of the shoulder.

superior to the manubrium of the sternum and between the medial ends of the clavicles. The **sternoclavicular joint** is located just lateral to the notch; its location can be verified by circumducting the arm and thereby moving the clavicle at the joint. From the joint, the shaft of the clavicle can be followed laterally; medially, it is anteriorly convex, and laterally, it is anteriorly concave. The clavicle ends laterally at the **acromioclavicular joint,** which is marked by either an elevation or a "step-off." The **infraclavicular fossa** is the depression inferior to the concavity of the clavicle; the **coracoid process** is palpable in the depths of that fossa.

The **acromion process** is the bony shelf just lateral to the acromioclavicular joint. The lateral border of this process ends abruptly and marks the most superior and lateral aspects of the **scapula.** The posterior aspect of the acromion continues medially and somewhat inferiorly as the **spine of the scapula.** The spine then ends medially, at its blunted **base,** at the **medial (vertebral) border** of the scapula. The base of the spine of the scapula typically is at the level of the spinous process of the third thoracic vertebra. From the base of the spine, the medial border of the scapula can be followed superiorly to the **superior angle** and inferiorly to the **inferior angle.** Most of the medial border is palpated through the trapezius muscle. From the inferior angle, the **lateral (axillary) border** can be followed superiorly to the glenoid fossa, which cannot be palpated.

Those aspects of the **proximal humerus** that can be palpated must be felt through the deltoid muscle around the edge of the acromion process. Because the head of the humerus articulates with the glenoid fossa of the scapula, it is positioned inferior to the acromion and therefore cannot be palpated. Even though the head of the humerus is not palpable, the tubercles surrounding it are. These are the **greater tubercle** laterally and posteriorly and the **lesser tubercle** anteriorly. These structures are separated by the **intertubercular groove,** which is positioned anterolaterally. The position of this groove can be verified by rotation of the humerus. The **deltoid tuberosity** is easily located on the lateral aspect of the shaft of the humerus, at about the midshaft level.

The muscles of the shoulder region can be classified as extrinsic and intrinsic. The **extrinsic muscles** interconnect the scapula, clavicle, or humerus with the axial skeleton and function to stabilize and move the shoulder girdle. Those that are palpable are the trapezius, pectoralis major, serratus anterior, and latissimus dorsi. The **trapezius** can be both visualized and palpated. The curvature of the neck between the head and the shoulder is formed by its superior part, and the middle and inferior parts extend laterally from the vertebral column and are superficial to most of the scapula. This muscle is prominent and easily palpable when the scapula is adducted. The **pectoralis major** forms the entire pectoral region, can be felt inferior to most of the clavicle, and forms the anterior axillary fold. It is active with horizontal adduction of the arm. The **latissimus dorsi** forms the most inferior part of the posterior axillary fold and can be palpated just lateral to the axillary border of the scapula, particularly when the arm is extended. The **serratus anterior** arises from the anterolateral aspects of most ribs and extends posteriorly and superiorly toward the vertebral border of the scapula. Because the muscle is largely deep to the scapula, only its anterior and inferior aspects can be felt. Forced scapular protraction (as during a push-up) makes these points of attachment easily identified. The **rhomboid major** and **minor** are located deep to the trapezius between

the scapula and vertebral column. Contraction of these muscles can be felt only when they are active and the trapezius is not, such as when the scapula rotates inferiorly (i.e., during resisted extension of the arm). The **levator scapulae** also is deep to the trapezius, specifically its superior part, as it extends from the superior angle of the scapula to the upper cervical vertebrae. Even though this muscle is ropelike in shape, as opposed to the broader trapezius, it can be difficult to distinguish from the trapezius because both muscles elevate the scapula.

The **intrinsic muscles** of the shoulder extend from the scapula or clavicle to the humerus and function to stabilize the glenohumeral joint and move the humerus. The largest of these is the **deltoid,** which forms the entire contour of the shoulder. Its three parts are easily palpable: the **middle part** with abduction of the arm, the **anterior part** with flexion, and the **posterior part** with extension. The **teres major** extends from the inferior aspect of the axillary border of the scapula to the anterior aspect of the proximal humerus; posteriorly, it is superior to the latissimus dorsi and forms part of the posterior axillary fold. Resisted medial rotation or extension of the humerus will make this stout muscle easily visible and palpable. Palpation of the **rotator cuff muscles** is difficult because they are covered (at least partially) by larger muscles, specifically the deltoid and trapezius. The tendons of all four muscles can be located through the deltoid, where they insert on the tubercles of the humerus. The **subscapularis** inserts anteriorly on the lesser tubercle, the **supraspinatus** superiorly on the greater tubercle, and both the **infraspinatus** and **teres minor** posteriorly on the greater tubercle. When external rotation of the humerus is resisted, portions of the muscle bellies of both the infraspinatus and the teres minor can be felt on the posterior aspect of the scapula in the interval between the deltoid and teres major.

The interval between the lateral aspect of the acromion process and the humerus, the **suprahumeral** or **subacromial space,** is important clinically because it is most often the site of pain associated with an impingement syndrome. The soft tissue structures in this interval and deep to the deltoid muscle are the **subacromial (subdeltoid) bursa,** the **tendon of the supraspinatus muscle,** and the superior aspect of the **glenohumeral joint capsule.** Even though each of these structures is palpable, each is palpated simultaneously with the others. As a result, distinguishing them is difficult. The **tendon of the long head of the biceps brachii muscle** also passes through this space. It is positioned somewhat anteriorly and is largely under the acromion, so it is palpable only in the intertubercular groove of the humerus.

Most **neurovascular structures** in the shoulder region are difficult to palpate because they are separated from the surface by a variety of other structures. However, the main **neurovascular bundle** that supplies the upper limb passes through the axilla, where it can be palpated with the arm moderately elevated. This bundle consists of the **axillary artery** and the **median, ulnar,** and **radial nerves.**

ARM AND ELBOW (Figs. 2-4, 2-6, and 2-7)

The bones of the arm and elbow region consist of the **distal half** of the **humerus** and **proximal aspects** of the **radius** and **ulna.** Because the humerus widens significantly at its distal end, the **medial** and **lateral humeral epicondyles** are easily palpable as the most pronounced medial and lateral prominences at the elbow. The soft tissue masses associated with these epicondyles are the **common tendons of origin** of the **superficial flexor** (medial) and **superficial extensor** (lateral) **muscles** of the forearm. From each of these epicondyles, the **supracondylar ridges** can be followed proximally for approximately 4 or 5 cm. Posteriorly, the **olecranon process** of the ulna forms the point of the elbow. From this process, the **shaft of the ulna** can be followed distally because it is subcutaneous throughout its length.

The location of the **elbow joint** can be determined both medially and laterally. The **lateral joint line** is marked by a depression distal to the lateral epicondyle between the capitulum and the **head of the radius;** the location of the radial head can be confirmed by supination and pronation of the forearm. Just distal to the radial head, the **radial neck** narrows to the shaft, which is deep to the lateral forearm musculature. The depression formed by the joint line is less distinct laterally than either anteriorly or posteriorly because of a thickening of the lateral aspect of the joint capsule—the **lateral (radial) collateral ligament.** The **medial joint line** of the elbow is less distinct because the medial epicondyle is prominent. In addition, the posterior and distal aspects of the epicondyle are commonly sensitive because of the presence of the **ulnar nerve.**

The **muscles of the arm** are separated into **anterior** and **posterior groups** by medial and lateral intermuscular septa. The **lateral septum** extends from the deltoid tuberosity to the lateral humeral epicondyle, and the location of the **medial septum** is marked by the medial neurovascular bundle, which continues from the axilla. Although there are three muscles in the anterior compartment, the **biceps brachii** is the most superficial; therefore its belly is readily palpable, particularly with resisted forearm flexion and supination. The **triceps brachii** occupies virtually the entire posterior compartment and is readily palpable throughout the posterior arm. Even its three heads can be identified (i.e., the **lateral head** proximally and laterally, the **long head**

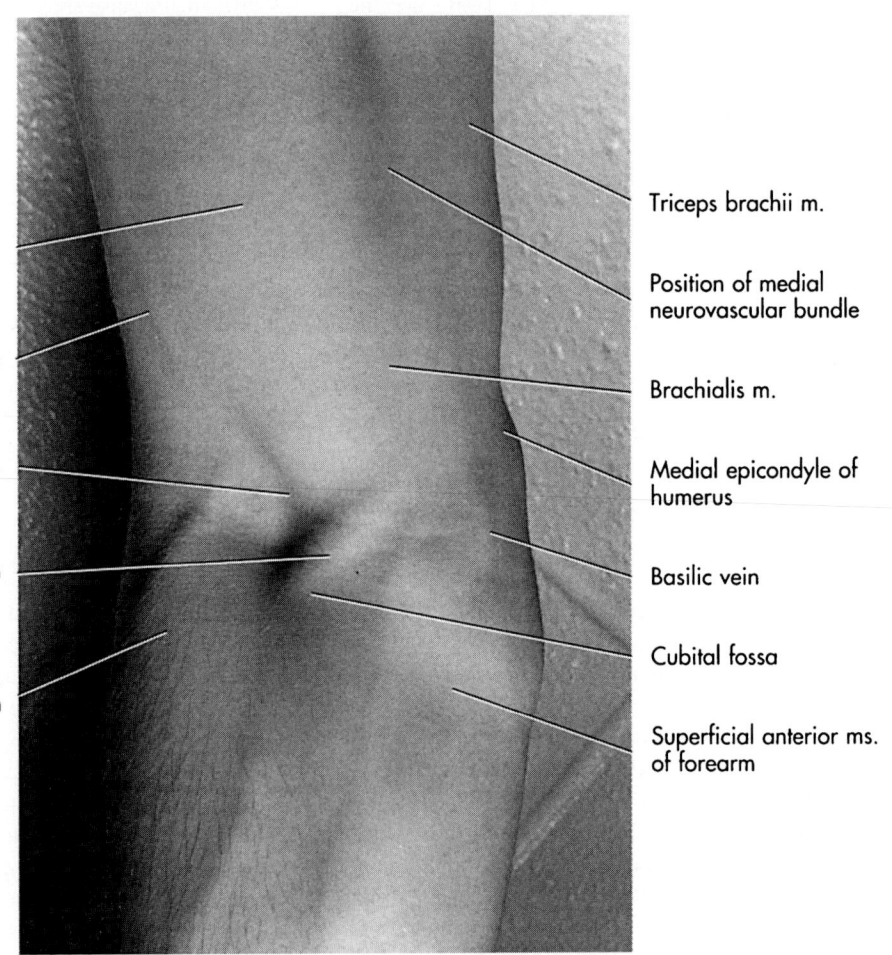

Biceps brachii m.

Cephalic vein

Tendon of biceps m.

Median cubital vein

Superficial posterior ms. of forearm

Triceps brachii m.

Position of medial neurovascular bundle

Brachialis m.

Medial epicondyle of humerus

Basilic vein

Cubital fossa

Superficial anterior ms. of forearm

Fig. 2-6. Anterior view of the elbow.

proximally and medially, and the **medial head** distally on either side of the triceps tendon).

The **muscles of the forearm** are separated into anterior and posterior groups even though their positions are not truly anterior and posterior. The **anterior muscles** are medial proximally and anterior distally; the **posterior muscles** are lateral proximally and posterior distally. Only a few of the forearm muscles can be palpated individually in the proximal forearm because they either have common tendons of origin or are deep to other structures. At the wrist, however, several of their tendons can be readily identified. Proximally and medially, the **pronator teres** can be palpated with resisted pronation; it feels like a distinct cord passing obliquely laterally from the medial epicondyle to the radius. It forms the medial boundary of the cubital fossa. Of the lateral muscles, the **brachioradialis** is most prominent. It is obvious when the forearm is flexed with the forearm midway between supination and pronation.

The **cubital fossa** is the triangular depression in front of

the elbow. Its medial and lateral borders are the pronator teres and brachioradialis muscles, respectively; its proximal border is a line between the humeral epicondyles. With the exception of the **ulnar nerve,** which enters the forearm by passing posterior to the medial epicondyle, the major neurovascular structures of the forearm and hand pass through this fossa. The **tendon of the biceps brachii** disappears into the center of the fossa. From this tendon, a fibrous band, the **bicipital aponeurosis (lacertus fibrosus),** passes medially to blend with the investing fascia of the forearm. The sharp proximal border of this aponeurosis can easily be identified when forearm flexion is resisted. The **brachial pulse** can be felt on the medial side of the biceps tendon, and the **median nerve** is between the tendon and the artery. Both the nerve and artery pass deep to the bicipital aponeurosis. The **median cubital vein** is superficial to the aponeurosis as it passes obliquely across the front of the elbow. This vein interconnects the major superficial veins of the upper limb (i.e., the **cephalic vein** laterally and the **basilic vein** medially).

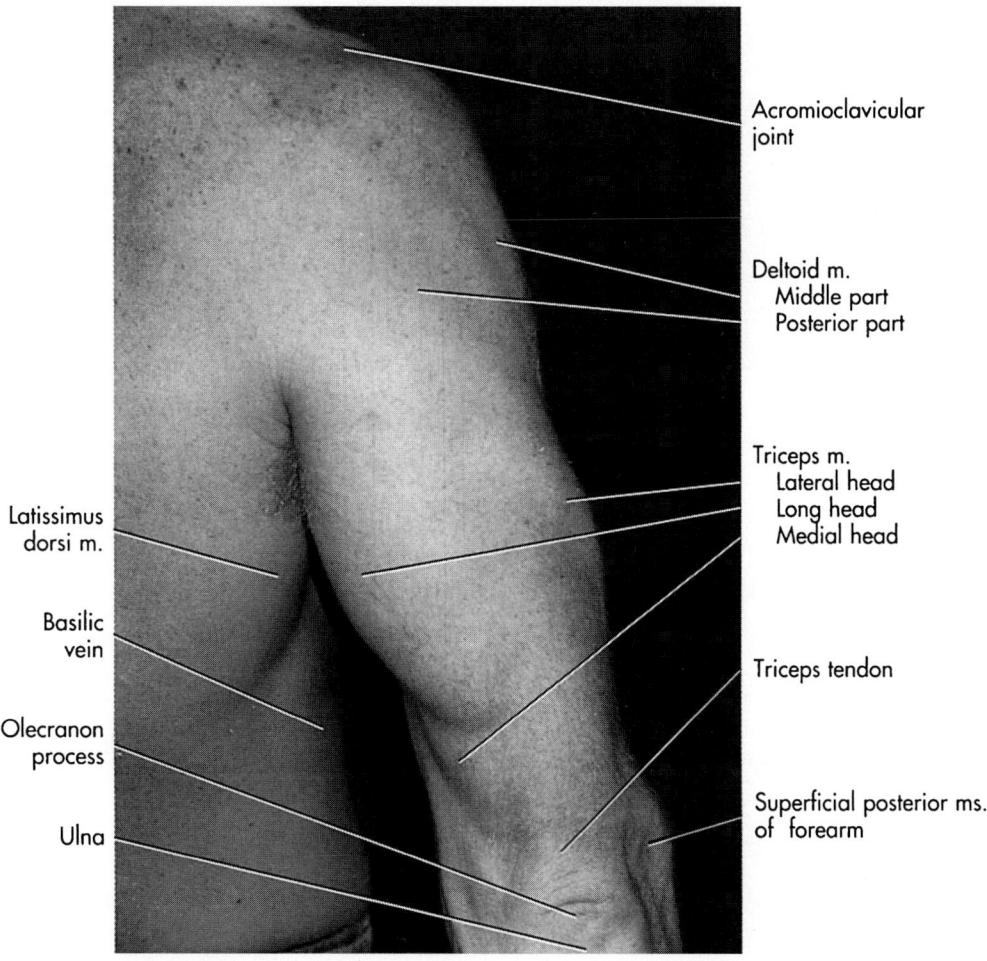

Fig. 2-7. Posterior view of the shoulder, arm, and elbow. Extension at the elbow is moderately resisted.

FOREARM AND WRIST (Figs. 2-8 to 2-12)

As mentioned, the **ulna** is palpable for its entire length, ending distally in the dorsomedially positioned **styloid process.** The **radius** cannot be palpated through most of the forearm, but at its distal end, it has two major landmarks. The most distal aspect of either forearm bone is the **styloid process of the radius,** which is easily felt on the lateral aspect of the wrist. The **dorsal radial (Lister's) tubercle** is the most apparent dorsal prominence. This tubercle is easy to locate when the thumb is extended because the tendon of the extensor pollicis longus makes a turn around the ulnar side of the tubercle.

Dorsally, the **distal end of the radius** forms a transverse ridge that marks the junction with the carpus or the **radiocarpal joint.** This ridge becomes more prominent when the hand is slightly flexed. Because the distal surface of the radius is concave (dorsal to palmar) and the dorsal aspect extends considerably more distally than the palmar aspect, the more proximal carpal bones are somewhat hidden

by this dorsal ridge of the radius when the hand is extended. With the hand in the neutral position or slightly flexed, a depression is apparent just distal to the radius approximately in line with the third ray. This depression marks the interval between the radius and base of the third metacarpal and contains the **lunate** proximally and **capitate** distally. The **scaphoid** forms the floor of the anatomic snuffbox. Palpation of this bone commonly produces moderate discomfort.

On the palmar side, the junction of the forearm and carpus along with the location of the carpal tunnel can be determined. The radiocarpal joint is located at the level of the **proximal palmar skin crease** of the wrist. The **distal skin crease** approximates the proximal border of the carpal tunnel. All four major bony attachments of the **transverse carpal ligament (deep flexor retinaculum)** can be identified. The **pisiform** is just distal to the distal carpal crease on the ulnar side. The **hamulus (hook)** of the **hamate** is slightly distal and lateral to the pisiform; it also is deeper than the pisiform, and its palpation may produce some discomfort

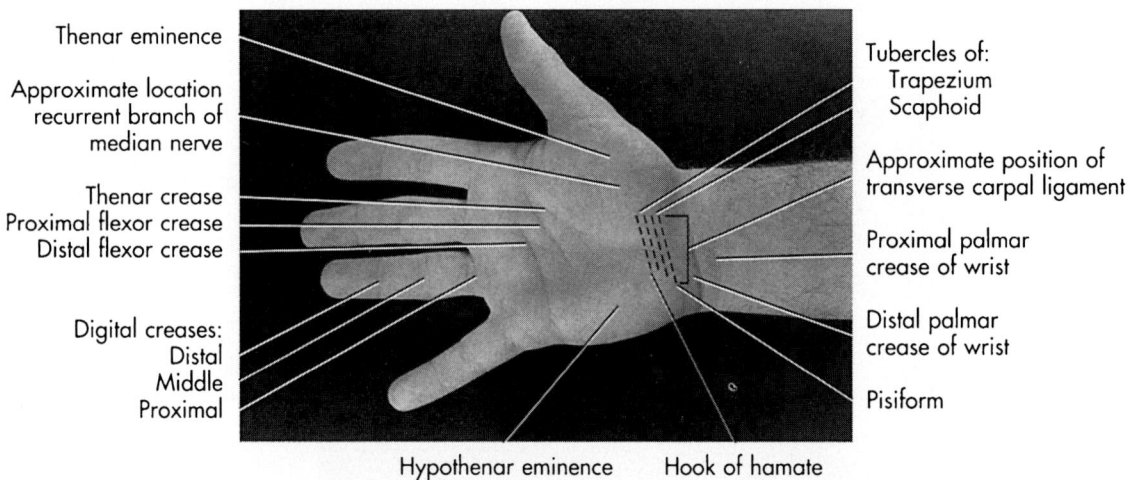

Thenar eminence

Approximate location
recurrent branch of
median nerve

Thenar crease
Proximal flexor crease
Distal flexor crease

Digital creases:
Distal
Middle
Proximal

Tubercles of:
Trapezium
Scaphoid

Approximate position of
transverse carpal ligament

Proximal palmar
crease of wrist

Distal palmar
crease of wrist

Pisiform

Hypothenar eminence   Hook of hamate

Fig. 2-8. Ventral or palmar view of the wrist and hand with the digits extended.

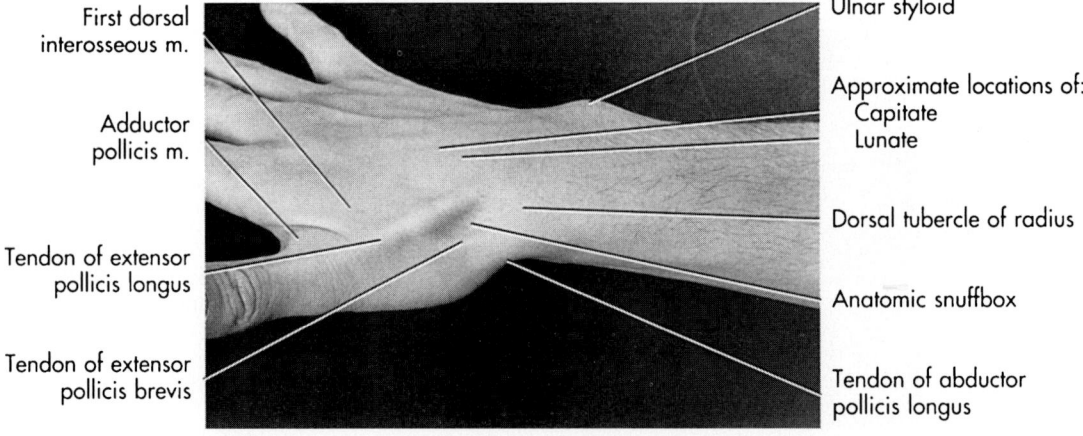

First dorsal
interosseous m.

Adductor
pollicis m.

Tendon of extensor
pollicis longus

Tendon of extensor
pollicis brevis

Ulnar styloid

Approximate locations of:
Capitate
Lunate

Dorsal tubercle of radius

Anatomic snuffbox

Tendon of abductor
pollicis longus

Fig. 2-9. Dorsomedial view of the distal aspect of the forearm, wrist, and hand, with the digits extended.

because of the proximity of the ulnar nerve. On the radial sides, the distal crease separates the **tubercles** of the **scaphoid** and **trapezium;** both tubercles are approximately in line with the tendon of the flexor carpi radialis.

On the **palmar aspect** of the **wrist** there are tendons of three muscles that are both constant and reliable landmarks.

The **tendon** of the **flexor carpi radialis** is large, crosses the wrist just lateral to the center, and is clearly visible when flexion of the hand is resisted. On the extreme ulnar side, the **tendon** of the **flexor carpi ulnaris** is directly in line with the pisiform. This tendon becomes more apparent with resisted flexion and ulnar deviation of the hand. The **tendons of the**

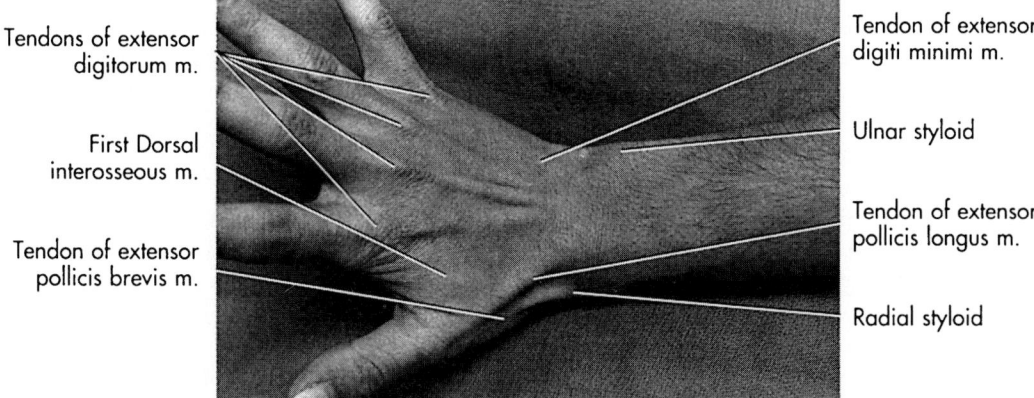

Fig. 2-10. Dorsal view of the distal aspect of the forearm, wrist, and hand, with the digits extended.

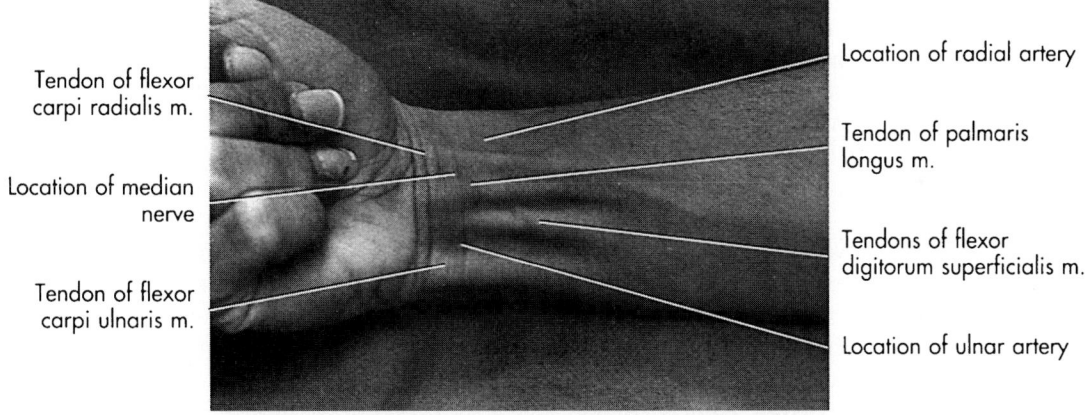

Fig. 2-11. Palmar view of the distal forearm, wrist, and hand. The fingers are flexed forcefully to reveal the tendons of certain forearm muscles.

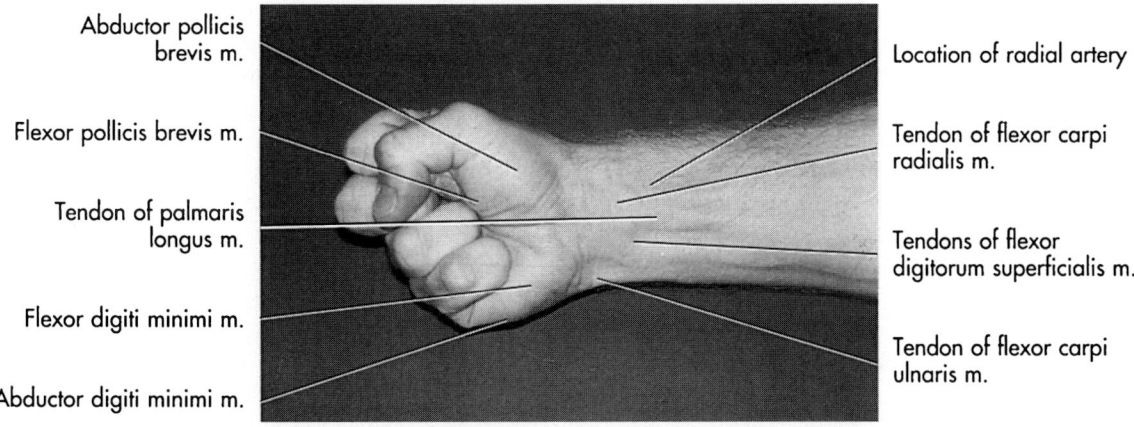

Fig. 2-12. Palmar view of the distal forearm, wrist, and hand. The hand is clenched into a strong fist.

flexor digitorum superficialis (sublimus) occupy the interval between the tendons of the flexor carpi radialis and flexor carpi ulnaris muscles. These tendons are arranged side-by-side and occupy most of the interval.

The **tendon of the palmaris longus,** which is present in approximately 85% of the population, is the most superficial tendon on the palmar aspect of the wrist. It is located on the ulnar side of the tendon of the flexor carpi radialis and superficial to the lateral tendon(s) of the flexor digitorum superficialis. The tendon of the palmaris longus becomes more prominent when the hand is slightly flexed and "cupped."

On the palmar wrist, the **median nerve** is in a deep position between the tendons of the flexor carpi radialis and the palmaris longus. When the palmaris longus is not present, the nerve is just ulnar to the tendon of the flexor carpi radialis. A very small branch of the median nerve, the **palmar branch,** arises from the radial side of the main trunk in the distal third of the forearm. This branch enters the hand superficially (not through the carpal tunnel) in line with the radial side of the median nerve or the radial side of the middle finger. In the distal forearm, the **ulnar nerve** and **artery** are deep to the flexor carpi ulnaris muscle. At the wrist, the nerve is deep to this tendon and the artery is just radial. The two structures then pass radial to the pisiform and ulnar to the hook of the hamate as they pass through Guyon's canal. Although the **radial artery** does not cross the palmar aspect of the wrist, its pulse is easily palpable 2 to 3 cm proximal to the wrist on the radial side of the tendon of the flexor carpi radialis.

The extensor tendons entering the hand cross both the radial and dorsal aspects of the wrist. The **tendons** of the **abductor pollicis longus** and **extensor pollicis brevis** typically occupy a common compartment as they cross the wrist. These two tendons are positioned superficial to the radial styloid as the most volar tendons on the radial aspect of the wrist. The **tendon** of the **extensor pollicis longus** muscle is apparent when the thumb is extended. This tendon crosses the wrist just ulnar to Lister's tubercle, then immediately turns radially as it passes toward the thumb. Along with the tendons of the abductor pollicis longus and extensor pollicis brevis, the tendon of the extensor pollicis longus forms the boundaries of the anatomic snuffbox. The **tendons** of the **extensor carpi radialis longus** and **brevis** muscles can be palpated just distal to the radius, in line with the index and middle fingers, respectively. Because both tendons are deep to other tendons, they are most apparent when extension of the hand is resisted while the fingers and thumb are relaxed. The **tendons** of the **extensor digitorum** are easily palpated after they are visualized; extension of the fingers makes them readily apparent. The most medial tendon is that of the **extensor carpi ulnaris.** It is in line with the ulnar styloid and bridges the indentation between that prominence and the base of the fifth metacarpal.

Other than the more deeply positioned radial artery, the neurovascular structures crossing the dorsal aspect of the wrist all are found in the subcutaneous tissue. The **radial artery** passes through the anatomic snuffbox, deep to all of the bordering tendons. **Superficial veins** contributing to both the **cephalic** and **basilic veins** usually can be observed on the lateral and medial aspects of the wrist, respectively. The **superficial radial nerve** crosses the dorsolateral aspect of the wrist. It usually can be palpated about midway between Lister's tubercle and the metacarpophalangeal joint of the thumb, where it crosses the tendon of the extensor pollicis longus muscle.

HAND (see Figs. 2-8 to 2-12)

Like the palmar wrist, the **palmar aspect of the hand** has skin creases that are consistently present and helpful in localizing deeper structures. There are three such creases on the palm, which usually appear to share a common point of origin at approximately the metacarpophalangeal joint of the index finger. The **distal volar flexor crease** extends across the palm from that point and marks the locations of the metacarpophalangeal joints. The **proximal volar flexor crease** is more oblique in position than the distal crease and ends at about the hypothenar eminence. The **thenar crease** outlines the border of the thenar eminence. The four fingers have three creases each. The **proximal digital crease** is located at the web space and the **middle** and **distal creases** are at the proximal and distal interphalangeal joints, respectively.

The approximate locations of the two arterial arches in the palm can be determined in the following manner. The **superficial palmar arterial arch** is at about the level of the proximal flexor crease in the center of the palm; this location also corresponds to the distal surface of the fully extended thumb. The **deep palmar arterial arch** is approximately the width of a finger proximal to the distal arch.

The nerves of the palm are the median and ulnar nerves. The main trunk of the **median nerve,** at the distal end of the carpal tunnel, is aligned with the middle finger. At that point, it separates into terminal branches. The **motor (recurrent, thenar) branch** recurs into the thenar musculature and is located midway between the first metacarpophalangeal joint and the pisiform. The **digital branches** of the median nerve pass toward the first, second, and third web spaces.

The **ulnar nerve,** after passing radial to the pisiform and ulnar to the hook of the hamate, bifurcates into **superficial** and **deep branches.** The superficial branch continues distally toward the fourth web space. Another branch, a proper digital nerve, passes toward the ulnar side of the little finger. The deep branch of the ulnar nerve passes deep and accompanies the deep arterial arch.

The **proper palmar digital nerves** and **arteries,** branches of both the median and ulnar nerves, provide the major nerve and arterial supplies to the digits. These nerves and vessels are located on both the ulnar and radial sides of the palmar aspects of the digits.

Only a small number of the **intrinsic muscles** of the hand can be palpated. In the most radial aspect of the thenar compartment, the **abductor pollicis brevis** is apparent when abduction of the thumb is resisted. With flexion of the thumb, the **flexor pollicis brevis** can be felt in the thenar compartment, in line with the flexor surface of the thumb. The **abductor digiti minimi** and **flexor digiti minimi** are apparent with abduction and flexion of the little finger, respectively. Two muscles can be distinguished in the first web space. Dorsally, the **first dorsal interosseous** is easily palpated with abduction of the index finger. In the palmar aspect of that web space, the distal aspect of the **adductor pollicis** is visible when thumb adduction is resisted.

BIBLIOGRAPHY

Backhouse KM, Hutchings RT: *Surface anatomy: clinical and applied,* Baltimore, 1986, Williams & Wilkins.

Basmajian JV: *Surface anatomy: an instructional manual,* ed 2, Baltimore, 1983, Williams & Wilkins.

Hamilton WJ, Simon G, Hamilton SGI: *Surface and radiological anatomy,* Baltimore, 1971, Williams & Wilkins.

Hoppenfeld S: *Physical examination of the spine and extremities,* New York, 1976, Appleton-Century-Crofts.

Lichtman DM: *The wrist and its disorders,* Philadelphia, 1988, WB Saunders.

Lockhart RD: *Living anatomy,* ed 6, London, 1963, Faber & Faber.

Morrey BF: *The elbow and its disorders,* Philadelphia, 1985, WB Saunders.

Spinner M: *Kaplan's functional and surgical anatomy of the hand,* ed 3, Philadelphia, 1984, JB Lippincott.

Tubiana R, Thomine JM, Mackin E: *Examination of the hand and upper limb,* Philadelphia, 1984, WB Saunders.

Watson MS: *Surgical disorders of the shoulder,* Edinburgh, 1991, Churchill Livingstone.

Chapter 3

ANATOMY AND KINESIOLOGY
OF THE HAND*

Robert A. Chase

The hand skeleton and associated ligaments constitute an architectural framework that allows the latitude of motion of the digits characteristic of human hand function. Some generalizations concerning allowable ranges of motion make up the patterns described by many observers through the centuries. The architectural units are divided into those functioning fixed and those with a sweep of motion in multiple planes. The mobile elements may be divided conveniently into three parts, each described in the following section and illustrated in a manner described by J. William Littler.[7,9-11,13,34]

THE FIXED UNIT OF THE HAND

The fixed unit of the hand (Fig. 3-1, *4*), consisting of metacarpals 2 and 3 and the distal row of carpals, has very limited motion at the intermetacarpal joints and the second and third carpometacarpal joints. The distal row of carpal bones forms a stable, unchanging, transverse arch. It is fixed by virtue of the tough intercarpal ligaments and the arch configuration of the carpal bones with the capitate as the keystone. The volar carpal ligament attaching to the hook of the hamate and the palmar ridges of the trapezium further prevents the collapse of the fixed transverse carpal arch. Articulating with the distal carpal row and projecting distally from it are the five metacarpals. The index and long finger metacarpals are fixed intimately to the distal carpal row, and together with it they form the fixed unit of the hand skeleton. This central fixed unit forms a supporting base for the remaining mobile units of the hand. The fixed unit projects distally from the wrist under the influence of the major wrist

extensors (extensor carpi radialis longus and extensor carpi radialis brevis) and the prime wrist flexor, the flexor carpi radialis. This central beam of the hand is then positioned for motion around it of the adaptive elements.

Mobile adaptive hand units

The adaptive units of the hand that move about the central I-beam consist of three elements, which are, in descending order of specialization, the thumb ray, the index finger, and the fourth and fifth rays together with the long finger.

The thumb ray. The thumb with its metacarpal and two phalanges (Fig. 3-1, *1*) has the greatest latitude and sweep of any of the digits. The metacarpotrapezial joint is a biconcave, saddle joint allowing a wide range of motion in many planes, because the joint capsule, although tough and unyielding, is loose enough to allow substantial movement. Five intrinsic muscles and four extrinsic muscles influence thumb positioning and activity.

The index finger. The index finger phalanges (Fig. 3-1, *2*) project from the fixed second metacarpal under the influence of three intrinsic and four extrinsic muscles. These muscles account for the relative independence of function of the index finger as compared with the long, ring, and little fingers. The interphalangeal joints move as hinge joints in flexion and extension, while the metacarpophalangeal (MP) joint has substantial medial and lateral range of motion (ROM) when the joint is in extension.

Long, ring, and little fingers together with the fourth and fifth metacarpals. This unit on the ulnar side of the hand functions as a stabilizing vise to grasp objects for manipulation by the thumb and index finger (Fig. 3-1, *3*). There is a ROM of approximately 30 degrees of flexion and extension at the fifth metacarpal hamate joint and approximately half this ROM at the fourth metacarpal hamate joint.

---

*From Flynn JE, Jupiter J: *Hand surgery,* ed 4, Baltimore, 1989, Williams & Wilkins.

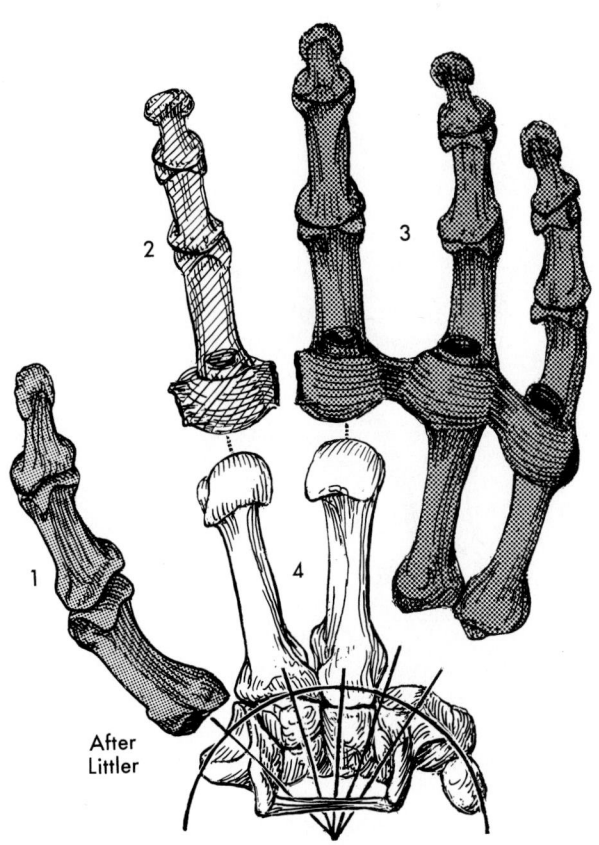

Fig. 3-1. The architectural components of the hand are divided into four separate units. Note the central fixed unit *(4)* and the mobile units *(1, 2,* and *3)*—see text. (After Littler, as shown in Chase RA: *Atlas of hand surgery,* Philadelphia, 1973, WB Saunders.)

This motion together with flexion capabilities at the MP joints and interphalangeal joints of the ulnar fingers allows adaptation of the part to work in concert with other hand units in powerful grasp. The units of the hand are illustrated after Littler (see Fig. 3-1): the fixed unit being designated number 4; the mobile first ray as number 1; the index digit with its independence as number 2; and the long, ring, and little fingers coupled with the fourth and fifth metacarpals as unit number 3.

Armed with an understanding of the degrees of motion in the various joints, one can understand the arch principles in hand architecture (Fig. 3-2). For example, the fixed transverse arch of the hand occurs at the level of the distal carpal row. It is fixed by virtue of the fitted arch of carpals with the capitate as the keystone and the tough intercarpal ligaments together with the flexor retinaculum or volar carpal ligament, which bridges between the extreme ends of the arch, taking attachment laterally on the hook of the hamate and pisiform and medially on the tubercle of the trapezium and tubercle of the scaphoid. At the level of the metacarpal heads, the arch becomes adaptive by virtue of the wide ROM of the first metacarpal at the metacarpotrapezial joint and the limited but definite ROM at the fourth and fifth carpometacarpal

joints. When the fixed transverse arch at the metacarpal heads is pulled into a half circle under the influence of the thenar and hypothenar muscles, the thumb is positioned to oppose the remaining digits as in pulp-to-pulp pinching. The fourth and fifth metacarpal heads are tethered to the central stable two metacarpals by the so-called intermetacarpal ligaments, which in fact attach to the volar plates of the MP joints. When the mobile metacarpal heads 1, 4, and 5 are pulled dorsally by the extrinsic extensor tendons with the thenar and hypothenar muscles relaxed, the transverse metacarpal arch is flattened or even reversed. Combined median and ulnar nerve palsy produce this picture.

The MP joints of each of the four fingers move medially and laterally with the joint in extension but lose this capability when the joint is flexed. The reinlike collateral ligaments are loose and redundant with the MP joints in extension and hyperextension, allowing maximum medial and lateral deviation. As the MP joint is flexed, the cam effect of the eccentrically placed ligaments and the epicondylar bowing of the collateral ligaments results in tightening and strict limitation of lateral mobility[33,46] (Fig. 3-3). Lateral mobility of the MP joints is stabilized somewhat by the interosseous muscles. The selected variable contraction of the interossei normally influences lateral motion to the extent allowed by the unyielding collateral ligaments. Should the collateral ligaments be destroyed or purposefully sacrificed, the interossei remain the sole source of lateral stability of the MP joints. Thus, when ulnar paralysis exists, caution must be exercised in MP joint capsulotomies because all lateral stability is lost and disastrous ulnar deviation may occur.[50]

The proximal interphalangeal (PIP) joints of the fingers act like hinge joints, because the medial and lateral collateral ligaments are radially fixed in a manner that allows no medial or lateral deviation of the joint in either flexion or extension. The PIP joints flex beyond the right angle to approximately 120 degrees. Generally, hyperextension is limited because of the ligamentous volar plate, an inseparable part of the joint capsule. A loose volar plate allows a variable amount of hyperextension beyond the usual 5 degrees. The distal interphalangeal (DIP) joints flex to about 90 degrees and usually extend to nearly 30 degrees of hyperextension.

FASCIA AND COMPARTMENTS OF THE HAND AND FOREARM

The deep fascia of the forearm invests the forearm musculature and divides it into flexor and extensor compartments separated by the interosseous membrane, the radius and ulna, and intermuscular septa. The anterior compartment is subdivided into three compartments, a deep and superficial compartment medially, and a lateral compartment containing the brachioradialis, extensor carpi radialis longus, and extensor carpi radialis brevis. The closed dorsal and ventral compartments are subject to compartment pressure syndromes when the deep fascia remains intact.

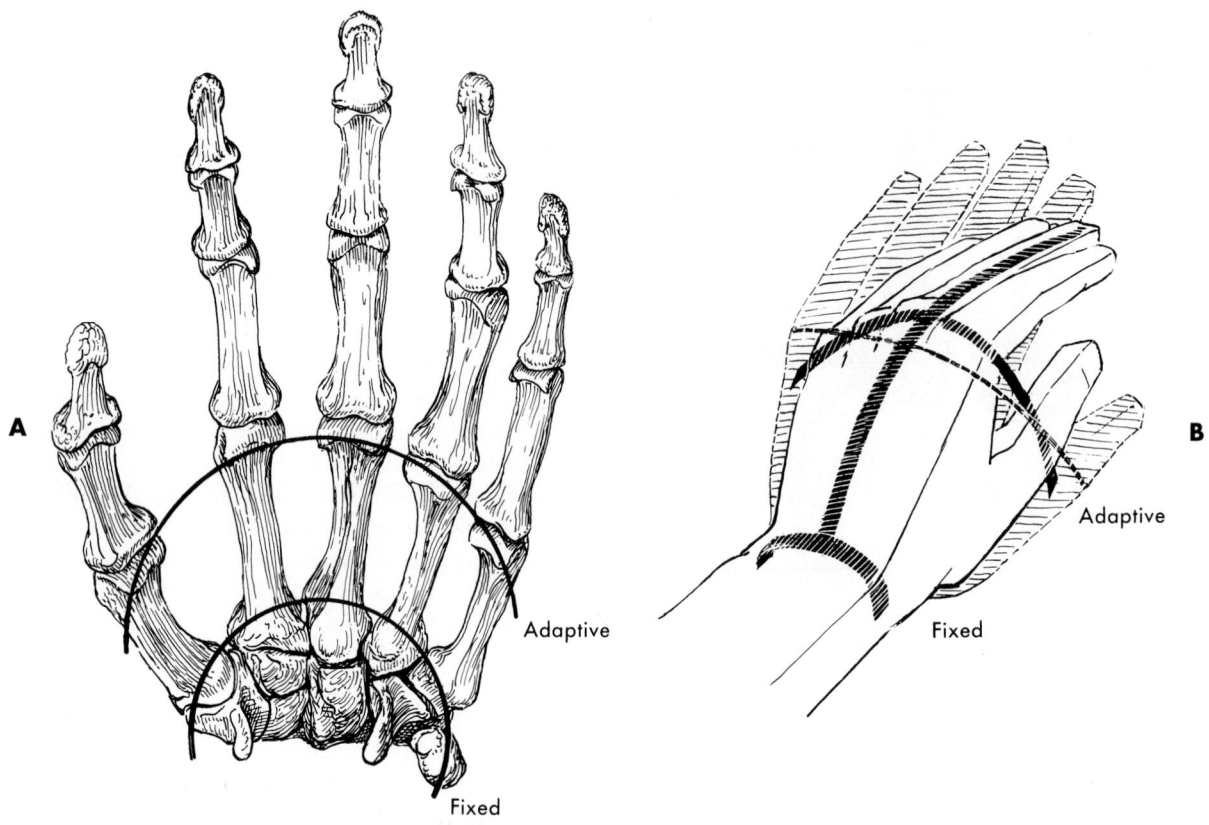

Fig. 3-2. A, The fixed and mobile transverse arches of the hand. **B,** Adaptive mobility at the level of the metacarpal heads, locus of the mobile transverse arch. This arch forms a semicircle with maximum action of the thenar and hypothenar positioning muscles. (From Jupiter JB: *Flynn's hand surgery,* ed 4, Philadelphia, 1991, Williams & Wilkins.)

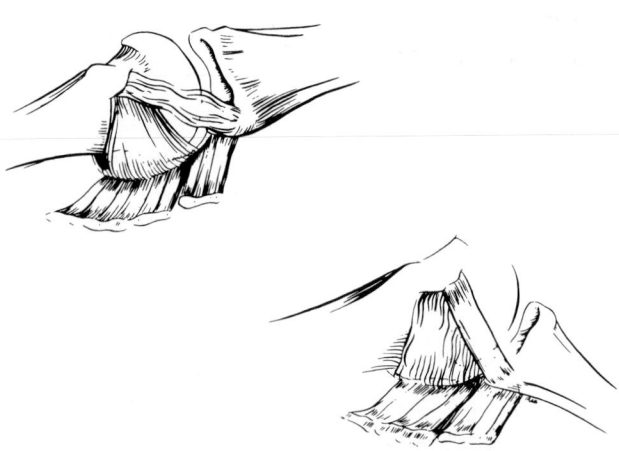

Fig. 3-3. Metacarpophalangeal joint collateral ligaments. With the joint extended, the metacarpophalangeal joint component of the collateral ligament is loose and the component from the metacarpal to the palmar plate is taut. Lateral movement is possible in extension. In flexion, the metacarpophalangeal joint collateral ligament is taut and the part attached to the palmar plate is loose. Thus no lateral movement is possible in metacarpophalangeal flexion. (From Jupiter JB: *Flynn's hand surgery,* ed 4, Philadelphia, 1991, Williams & Wilkins.)

In the hand, the fascia on the dorsum is quite different from that on the palm. Dorsally, the subcutaneous fascia is thin, loose, and areolar. The dorsal skin, therefore, is mobile and subject to avulsion injury and subcutaneous edema with swelling. A deep layer of fascia continuous with the extensor retinaculum at the wrist is present but thin. The extensor tendons are interlinked by membranous fascia that forms a distinct fascia layer.

The palmar fascia[4,20,35,36] is heavily fibrous and is arranged in longitudinal, transverse, oblique, and vertical fibers (Fig. 3-4). The longitudinally oriented fibers concentrate at the proximal origin from the palmaris longus at the wrist. If the palmaris longus is absent, which it is in about 15% to 20% of cases, the fascia terminates at the wrist crease. The fascia at the wrist level is separable from the underlying flexor retinaculum, the fibers of which are transverse in orientation in contrast to the longitudinal orientation of the palmar fascial fibers. From the proximal palm, the longitudinal fibers of the palmar fascia fan out, concentrating in flat bundles coursing toward each of the digits. These longitudinal fibers spread at the base of each digit and send minor fibers to the skin and the bulk of fibers distal into the fingers, where they attach to tissues making up

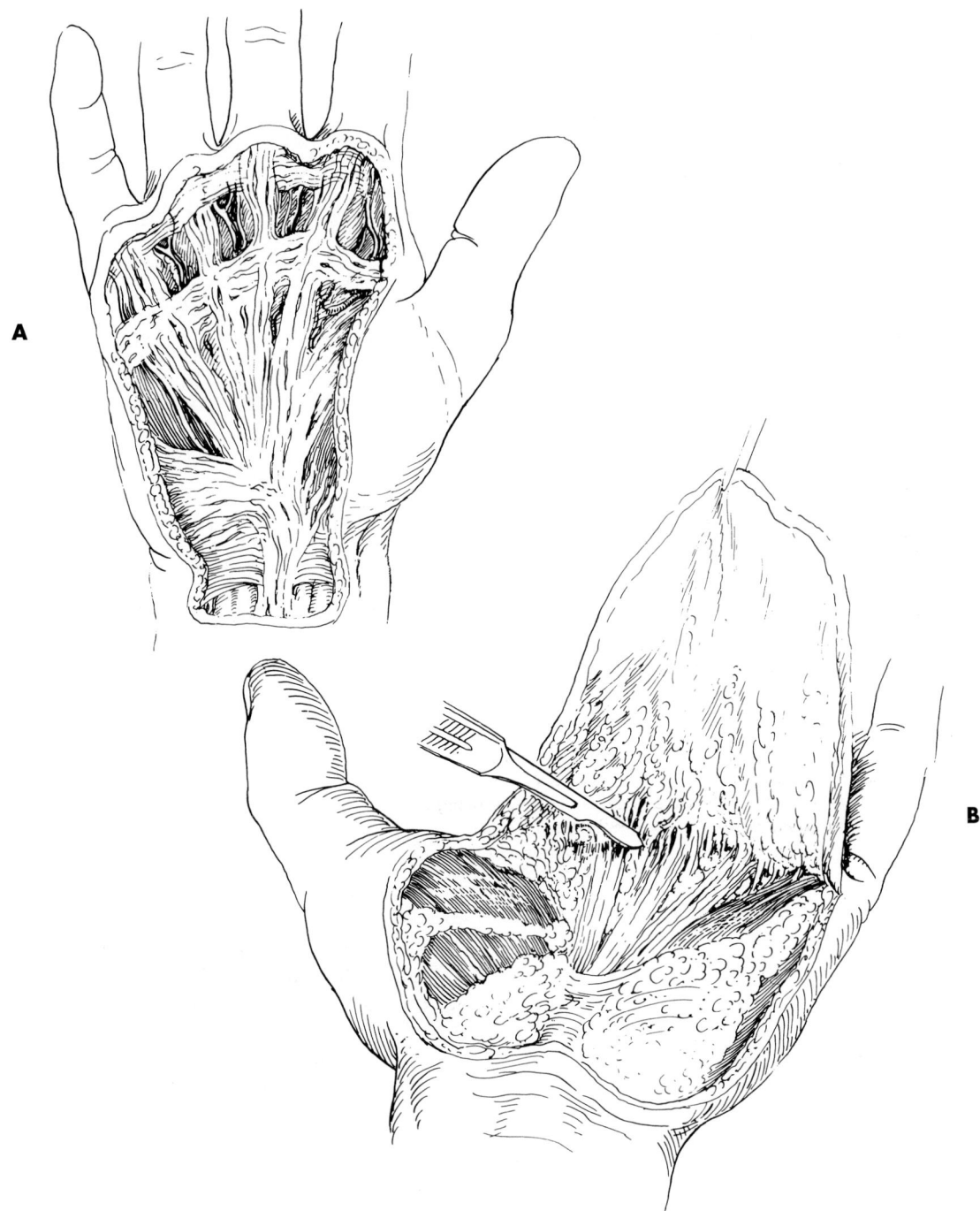

Fig. 3-4. The palmar fascia with its longitudinal, transverse, and vertical fibers. **A,** The longitudinal fibers originate in the palmaris longus (when present). Transverse fibers are concentrated in the distal palm supporting the web skin and in the midpalm are deep to the longitudinal fibers as the transverse palmar ligament. **B,** Vertical fibers extend superficially as multiple tiny tethering strands to stabilize the thick palmar skin. The deep vertical components concentrate in septa between the longitudinally oriented structures to the fingers. (From Chase RA: *Atlas of hand surgery,* Philadelphia, 1973, WB Saunders.)

the fibrous flexor sheath of the digits (Fig. 3-4, *A*). These fibers often extend well beyond the PIP joint and rarely as far as the DIP joint. There are some attachments of the fascia to the palmar plate and the intermetacarpal ligaments on each side of the flexor tendon sheath at the level of the MP joints.

A bundle of variable thickness courses toward the thumb. These fibers are sometimes difficult to identify and are customarily less concentrated and numerous than the fibrous bands to the four fingers. The thumb fibers blend into the deep fascia overlying the thenar muscles. On the ulnar

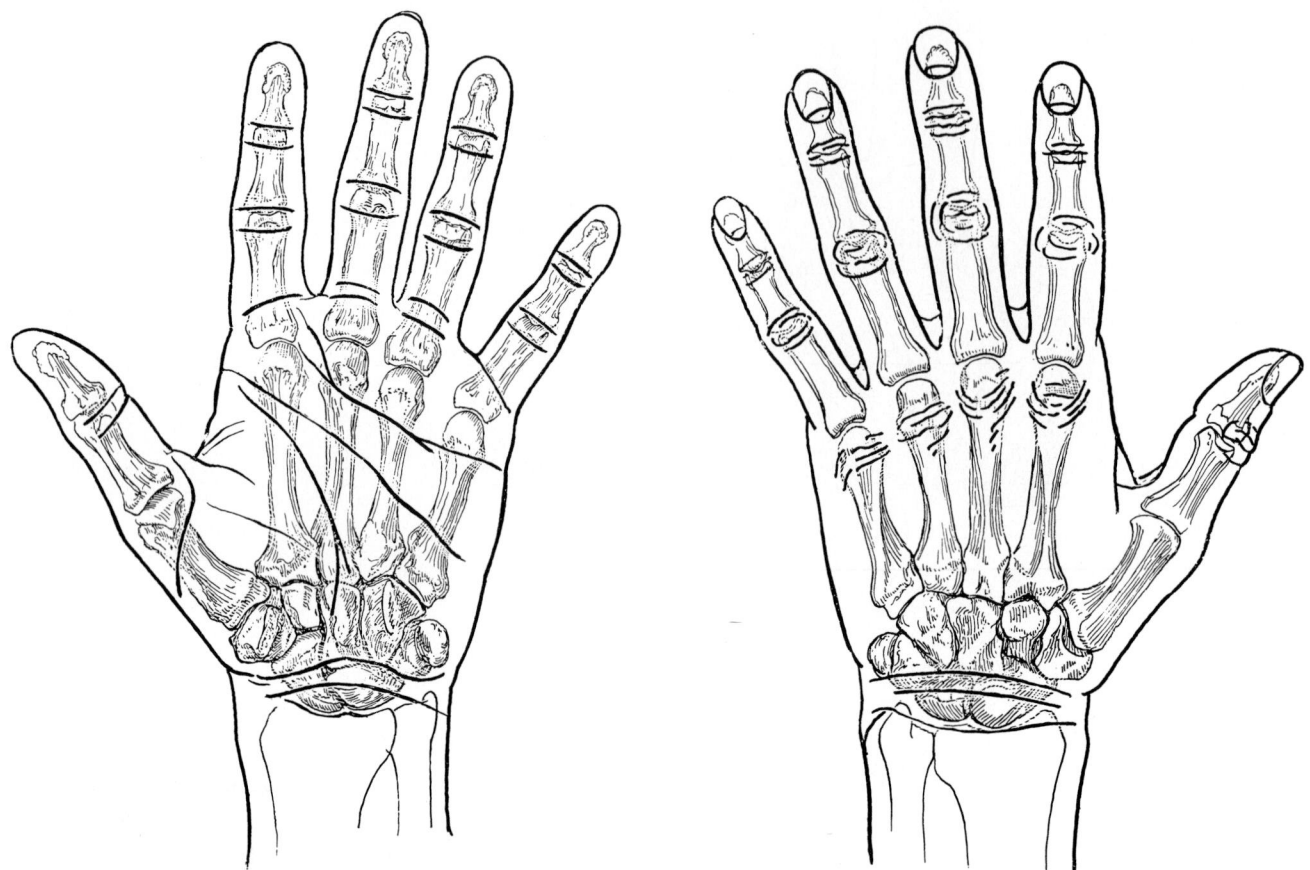

Fig. 3-5. Palmar and dorsal skin creases and their relationship to underlying joints. Note the fixed palmar creases resulting from skin fixation to the underlying palmar fascial plate by numerous vertical fibers. (From Jupiter JB: *Flynn's hand surgery,* ed 4, Philadelphia, 1991, Williams & Wilkins.)

extreme side of the longitudinal fibers, the fibers blend with the hypothenar fascia. The proximal portion of this ulnar border is the attachment site of the palmaris brevis muscle. Laterally, the muscle arises from hypothenar skin and fascia.

The transverse fibers of the palmar fascia are concentrated in the midpalm and the web spaces. The midpalmar transverse fibers lie deep to the longitudinal fibers, but they are inseparable from the deep vertical fibers that concentrate into the septa between the longitudinally oriented structures coursing to the digits. These transverse midpalmar fibers are called the transverse palmar ligament after the description by Skoog.[40] These transverse fibers form the roof of tunnels that act as palmar pulleys for the long flexors to the digits.

The vertical fibers of the palmar fascia, which lie superficial to the tough triangular membrane made up of the longitudinal and transverse fibers, consist of abundant vertical fibers attaching to the palm skin dermis (see Fig. 3-4, *B*). These fibers stabilize the palm skin and account for the palmar creases (Fig. 3-5). The vertical fibers on the deep side of the palmar fascial plate coalesce into a septa, forming compartments for the flexor tendons to each digit and

separate compartments for the neurovascular bundles and lumbrical muscles (see Fig. 3-4).

These eight compartments extend proximally to about the midpalm. Proximal to this, is a common central compartment. The medial and lateral marginal vertical septa extend more proximal than the seven intermediate septa, closing the central compartment laterally and medially. The presence of the adductor pollicis, which crosses the palmar aspect of the second metacarpal, results in the appearance of a major septum between the index flexor tendons and the neurovascular and lumbrical space to the third interspace. This thick septum attaches to the third metacarpal, dividing the palmar space into a thenar or adductor space and a midpalmar space (Fig. 3-6).[24]

At the level of the MP joint some of the longitudinal fibers extend down each side of the flexor tendon sheath as spiral bands passing superficial or deep to the proper digital artery and nerve. Occasionally, these bands extend dorsal to the neurovascular bundle at the base of the finger, then curl back around the bundle before crossing the PIP joint (Fig. 3-7). These spiral cords sometimes make dissection of the neurovascular bundle at this level in Dupuytren's contracture quite tedious.[35,36,43]

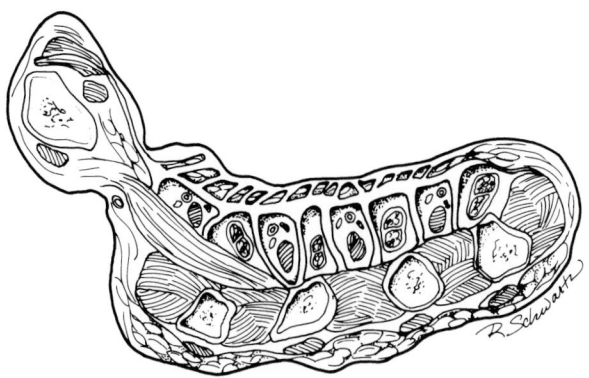

Fig. 3-6. Cross section at midpalm shows the white plaque of palmar fascia with vertical fibers extending upward to the dermis of the overlying skin. These tiny tethering strands stabilize the thick palmar skin. The deep vertical components of the fascia concentrate in septa between the longitudinally oriented structures to the fingers. Note the large fascial partition to the third metacarpal that separates the midpalmar space from the thenar space. (From Jupiter JB: *Flynn's hand surgery,* ed 4, Philadelphia, 1991, Williams & Wilkins.)

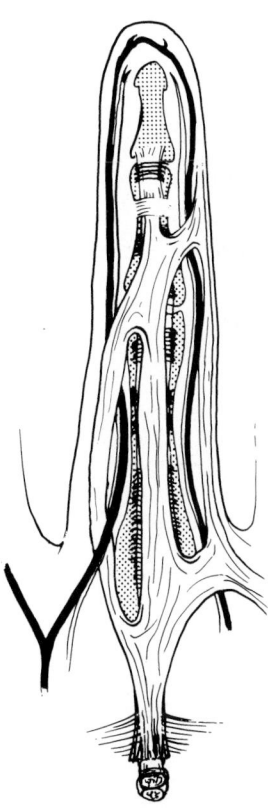

Fig. 3-7. Longitudinal fibers of the palmar fascia frequently extend down on each side of the flexor tendon sheath as spiral bands, often curling around the neurovascular bundles. (After McFarlane RM: Dupuytren's contracture. In Green DP: *Operative hand surgery,* New York, 1982, Churchill Livingstone.)

MUSCLES AND TENDONS
Extrinsic extensors

The extensor digitorum is a series of tendons with a common muscle belly (Fig. 3-8, *A*). The tendon itself enters into the central extensor of each of the fingers and terminates in its insertion into the middle phalanx at the central slip of the extensor mechanism. Its primary action in each finger is to extend the MP joint through the shroudlike fibers that pass around the proximal phalanx medially and laterally, just distal to the MP joint.

The interplay between the long extrinsic extensors and intrinsic muscles at the interphalangeal joint is the source of extension power to the phalanges of the fingers and thumb. The extrinsic extensors with muscle bellies in the forearm consist of a group of extensors, which work in unison with one another, and two independent long extensors, one for the index finger and another for the little finger (Fig. 3-8, *B* and *C*). Extrinsic extensors of the thumb consist of the extensor pollicis longus and the extensor pollicis brevis. The latter accompanies the abductor pollicis longus as one of the "outcropping" muscles emerging from beneath the long digital extensors and coursing superficial to the extensor carpi radialis longus and brevis to enter the first dorsal compartment at the wrist.[25]

On the dorsum of the hand, are intertendinous bridges between the separate tendons of the extensor digitorum. The extensor indicis is an independent long extensor to the index finger, and the extensor digiti minimi, usually represented by two separate tendons at the metacarpal level, acts as an independent extensor of the little finger. In each case, the independent extensor lies on the ulnar side of the extensor digitorum contribution to each of these two fingers. The extensor pollicis longus, like the independent extensors of the index and little fingers, has its own separate muscle belly, which lies deep to the extensor digitorum muscle bellies. Extensor pollicis longus inserts on the distal phalanx of the thumb and is the primary extensor of the interphalangeal joint, acting secondarily to extend the MP joint and the wrist (Fig. 3-9, *A*). The oblique muscles to the thumb, the tendons of which occupy the first dorsal fibrous compartment, consist of the tendons of the abductor pollicis longus and the extensor pollicis brevis. The extensor pollicis brevis insets on the proximal phalanx, acting primarily as an extensor of the MP joint (Fig. 3-9, *B*). The abductor pollicis longus inserts on the base of the first metacarpal, and it often sends tendon fibers to the proximal portion of the abductor pollicis brevis (Fig. 3-9, *C*). The abductor pollicis longus radially abducts the first metacarpal, but in bridging the wrist it, together with the extensor pollicis brevis, acts to aid in radial deviation of the wrist.

Extrinsic flexors

Three layers of muscles are in the flexor pronator group of the volar side of the forearm. The superficial group of muscles may be outlined by placing the hand on the palmar

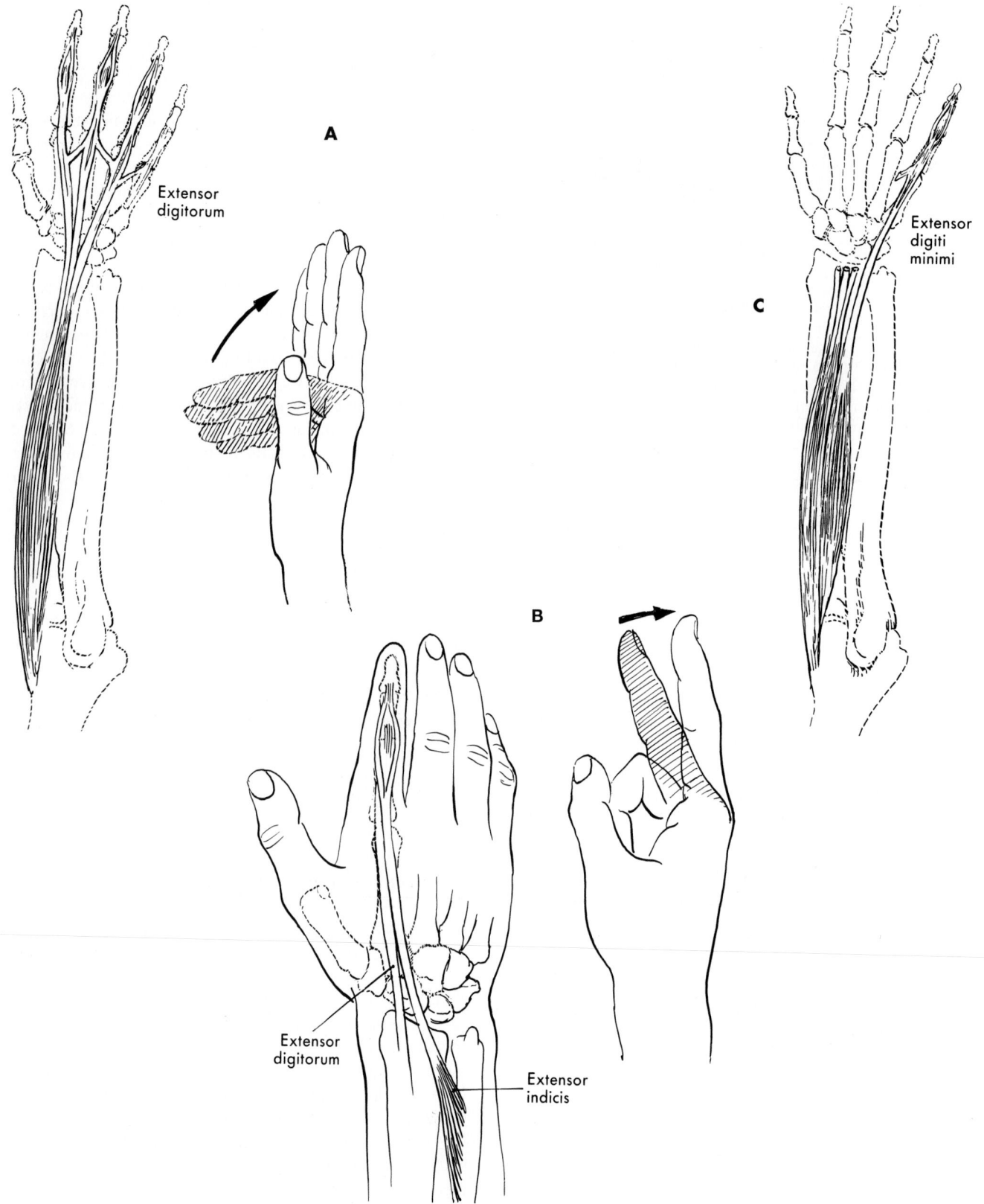

Fig. 3-8. A, Extensor digitorum has a common muscle belly and tendons extending to the four fingers. Note the intertendinous bridges at the level of the distal metacarpals. **B,** Extensor indicis to the index finger parallels the tendon to that finger from the extensor digitorum. **C,** Extensor digiti minimi allows independent extrinsic extension of the little finger. Tendons of the independent extensors of the index and little fingers lie on the ulnar side of the contribution to those fingers from the extensor digitorum. (From Chase RA: *Atlas of hand surgery,* Philadelphia, 1973, WB Saunders.)

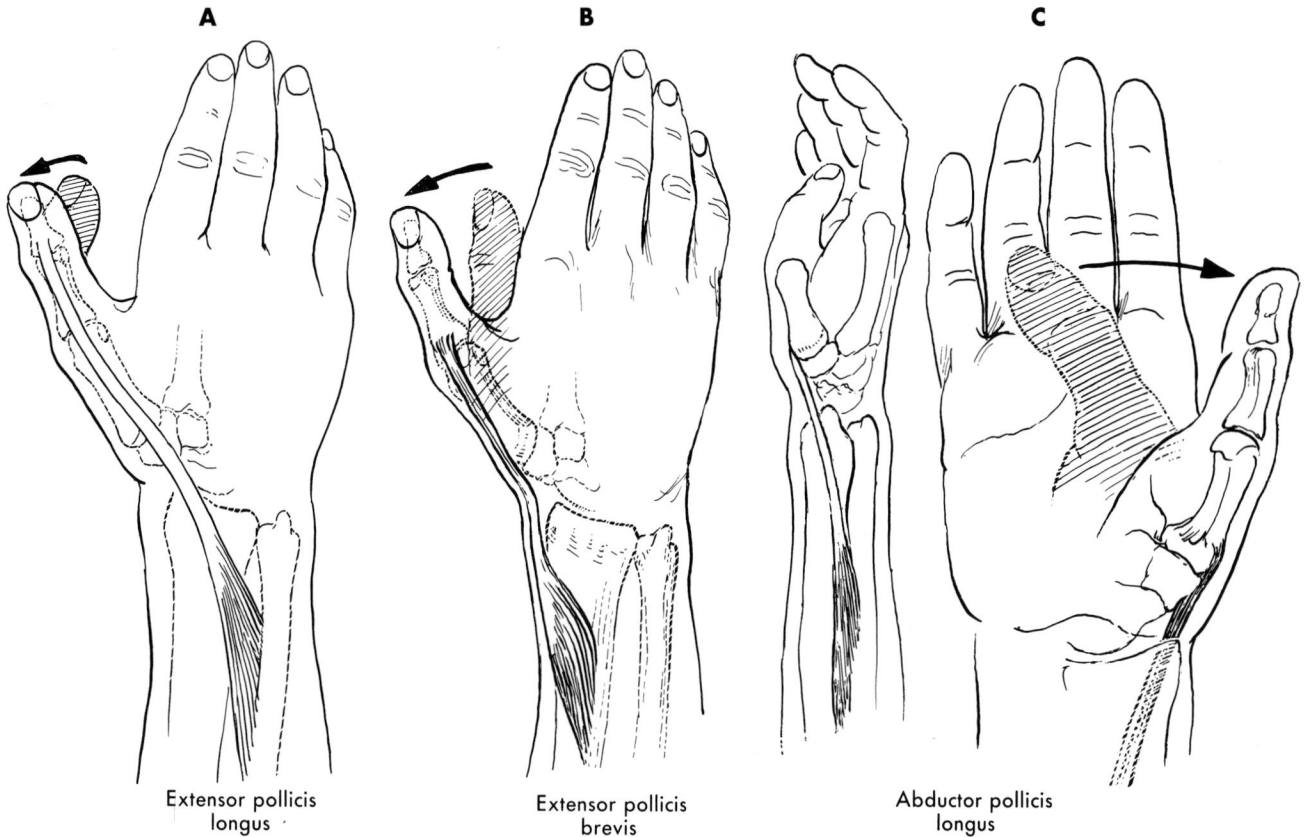

A   B   C
Extensor pollicis   Extensor pollicis   Abductor pollicis
longus   brevis   longus

Fig. 3-9. A, Extensor pollicis longus is the independent extensor of the distal phalanx of the thumb. **B,** Extensor pollicis brevis with attachment to the proximal phalanx extends to the metacarpophalangeal joint and aids in dorsal abduction of the thumb and radial deviation of the wrist. **C,** The abductor pollicis longus acts at the base of the first metacarpal to dorsally abduct the thumb and radially deviate the wrist. The extensor pollicis brevis and abductor pollicis longus, outcropping muscles to the thumb, occupy the first dorsal compartment at the wrist. (From Chase RA: *Atlas of hand surgery,* Philadelphia, 1973, WB Saunders.)

aspect of the opposite forearm with the thenar eminence at the medial epicondylar area and the ring finger along the ulnar border (Fig. 3-10). The thumb, index, long, and ring fingers then fall directly over the muscle tendon units, representing the superficial group of muscles on the flexor surface of the forearm. The thumb overlies the pronator teres; the index lies over the flexor carpi radialis; the long finger, over the palmaris longus; and the ring finger, over the flexor carpi ulnaris. The superficialis muscles make up the middle layer, and the deep layer consists of the flexor digitorum profundi, the flexor pollicis longus, and the pronator quadratus.

Each finger has a flexor digitorum profundus tendon inserting on the distal phalanx. The counterpart to the thumb is the flexor pollicis longus. The muscle bellies of the flexor profundi to the long, ring, and little fingers are often common and interdependent on the forearm, while the muscle belly of the flexor digitorum profundus to the index finger and the flexor pollicis longus each has a separate, identifiable independent muscle belly. Occasionally, there is some

interdependence between the flexor profundus to the index finger and the flexor pollicis longus. Each of the four fingers also has a flexor digitorum superficialis tendon, which lies superficial to the profundus tendon in the palm. As it passes into the finger, it flattens, then splits at the level of the proximal phalanx, and its two flat tails surround the profundus and decussate behind it to insert at the level of the middle phalanx (Fig. 3-11). The muscle bellies of the flexor digitorum superficialis tendons lie superficial on the palmar aspect of the forearm and are independent of one another. All of the extrinsic digital flexors pass through the carpal tunnel, where the flexor retinaculum acts as a major proximal pulley at the wrist.

THE RETINACULAR SYSTEM
Extensor retinaculum (Fig. 3-12)

The dorsal annular ligament of the wrist forms the roof over six separate extensor compartments at the level of the wrist. This dorsal transverse carpal ligament is essentially an area of thickening and specialization within the deep fascia

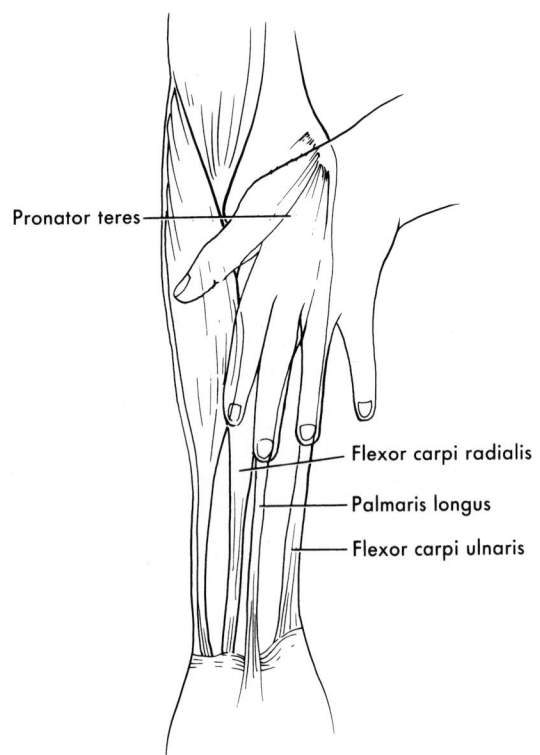

Fig. 3-10. The thumb, index, long, and ring fingers lie directly over the pronator teres, flexor carpi radialis, palmaris longus, and flexor carpi ulnaris if the contralateral hand is placed on the volar aspect of the forearm as shown. (After Henry AK: *Extensile exposure,* Baltimore, 1945, Williams & Wilkins.)

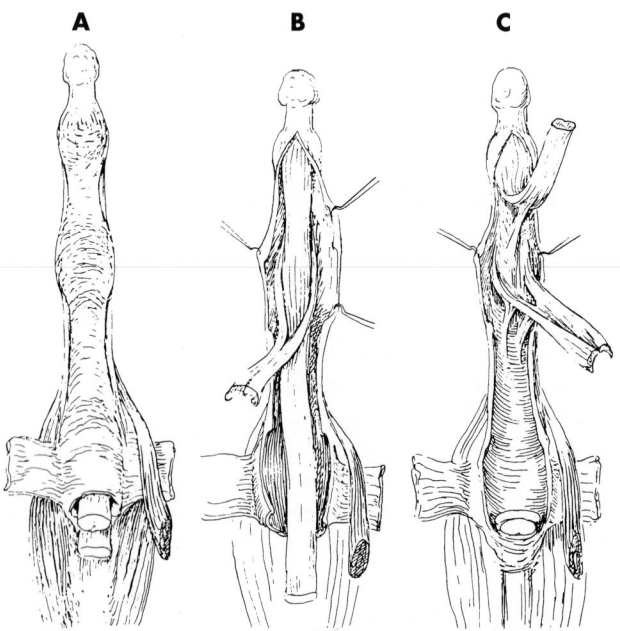

Fig. 3-11. A, Flexor tendons in the digit are surrounded by fibrous and synovial sheaths. **B,** The superficialis tendons split to allow the passage of the profundus tendon between its two tails to insert on the distal phalanx. **C,** The superficialis decussates behind the profundus tendon before inserting on the middle phalanx. (From Chase RA: *Atlas of hand surgery,* Philadelphia, 1973, WB Saunders.)

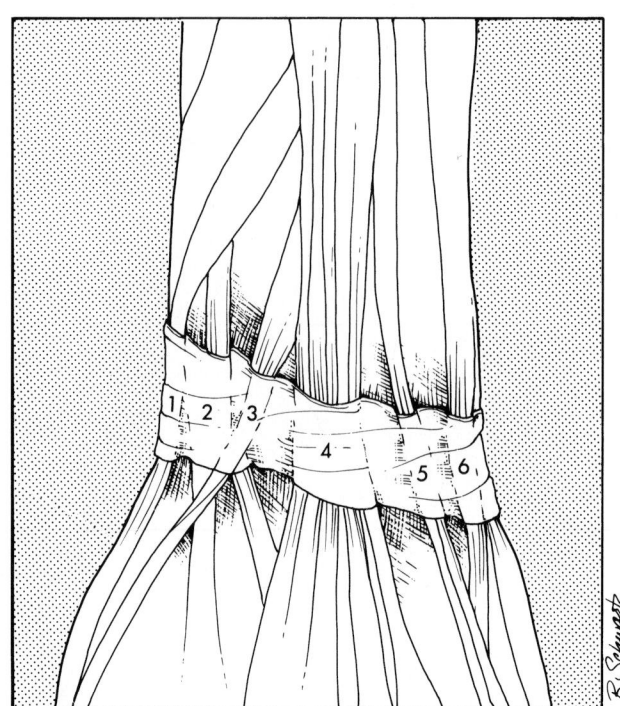

Fig. 3-12. The extensor retinaculum at the wrist forms a roof over the six extensor compartments. Each compartment has a synovial compartment that extends both proximally and distally to the retinaculum itself. (From Jupiter JB: *Flynn's hand surgery,* ed 4, Philadelphia, 1991, Williams & Wilkins.)

of the forearm and hand. The compartments are separated by vertical, longitudinal septa. The retinaculum itself is continuous across the dorsum of the tendons, then deep to the extensors, generating a floor for the compartments, particularly on the ulnar side of the hand.[45]

The first radial compartment may be subdivided into several compartments for the tendons of the abductor pollicis longus and the extensor pollicis brevis. The next compartment contains the two major wrist extensors, extensor carpi radialis longus and brevis. The third compartment forms a tunnel for the extensor pollicis longus just ulnar to Lister's tubercle. The fourth compartment houses the tendons of the extensor digitorum and the extensor indicis. The fifth compartment forms a pulley for the extensor digiti minimi. The sixth compartment houses the extensor carpi ulnaris.

The flexor retinacular system (Fig. 3-13, *A* and *C*)

Wrist pulley. The transverse carpal ligament forms a broad restraining pulley at the wrist level. It attaches on the radial side to the tubercle of the trapezium and scaphoid. On the ulnar side, it attaches to the hook of the hamate and the pisiform. The ligament confines the long flexor tendons and the median nerve within the carpal tunnel to prevent bowstringing of the long flexor tendons at the wrist.

Finger pulleys. (Fig. 3-13, *B* and *C*)[14,15,21,42] There are four or five discrete annular pulleys for the flexor tendons in

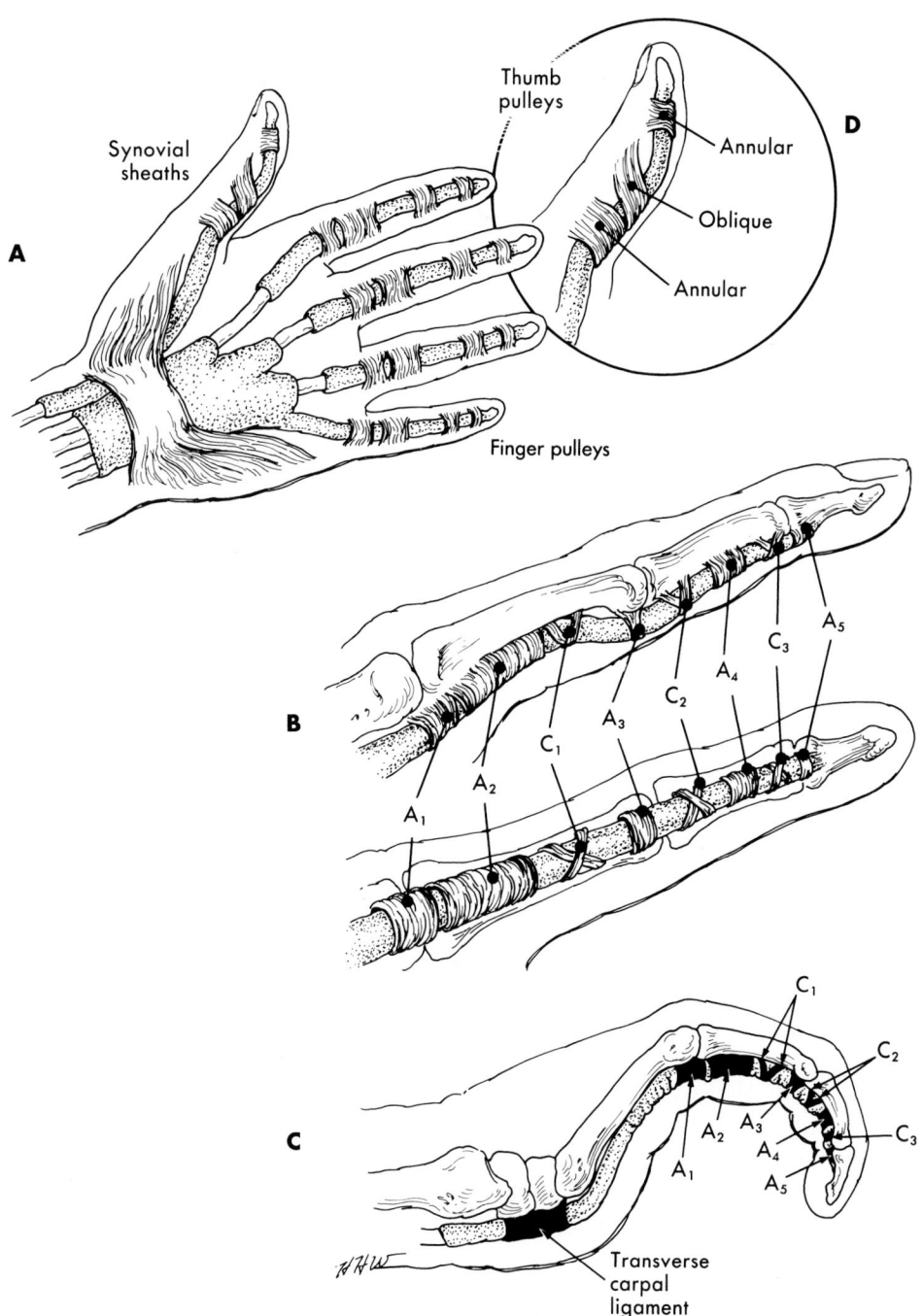

Fig. 3-13. **A,** Synovial and retinacular pulleys at the wrist and digit levels. **B,** The annular and cruciate pulleys within each of the fingers. **C,** The major retinacula occur where the longitudinal arches are adaptive at the wrist and within the digits. **D,** The thumb pulley. (From Chase RA: *Atlas of hand surgery,* vol 2, Philadelphia, 1984, WB Saunders.)

each finger. Between the annular pulleys one finds variable cruciate bands, which act as minor pulleys. The A_1 annular pulley begins 0.5 cm proximal to the MP joint and is anchored to the volar plate and the proximal phalanx. Immediately distal to it is the A_2 pulley, the largest of the annular pulleys, which extends about half the length of the proximal phalanx. The third annular pulley, A_3, lies over the PIP joint arising from its volar plate. The fourth annular

pulley is found over the middle one third of the middle phalanx, and a thickening of the sheath over the DIP joint is commonly designated as the fifth annular pulley, A_5. Between the A_2 and A_3 pulley,[5] between the A_3 and A_4 pulley,[5] and distal to the A_4 pulley, one commonly finds the more delicate cruciate ligaments, C_1, C_2, and C_3. The pulleys within the finger are placed to maintain the relationship of the flexor tendon to the long axis of each finger joint, and they prevent bowstringing of the tendon across the joints in flexion. The gaps between pulleys allow unrestrained flexion of the joints by allowing folding and pleating of the thin synovial sheath, which remains as the sole covering of the flexor tendons beneath the overlying finger fascia between the pulleys. Pulleys for the thumb consist of annular pulleys at the MP joints and an oblique pulley between (Fig. 3-13, *D*).

FLEXOR TENDON ZONES (FIG. 3-14)[7]

Based on the anatomy of the fibrous sheaths and the insertion of the flexor digitorum profundus and superficialis, the palmar aspect of the digits and hand are divided into specific zones.

Zone 1—Zone 1 is the area traversed by the flexor digitorum profundus distal to the insertion of the flexor digitorum superficialis on the middle phalanx.

Zone 2—Zone 2 extends from the proximal end of zone 1 to the proximal end of the digital fibrous sheath. It is subdivided into distal, middle, and proximal components.

   Distal—The distal portion extends from the insertion of the superficialis on the middle phalanx deep to the profundus to the proximal end of the A_3 pulley.

   Middle—The middle component extends from the insertion of the A_3 pulley to the distal end of A_2. The roof of the sheath in this zone consists only of synovial sheath and the C_1 cruciate ligament.

   Proximal—The proximal portion extends from the distal end of A_2 to the proximal end of A_1, a tunnel covered by the tough A_1 and A_2 pulley system.

Zone 3—Zone 3 is the area traversed by the flexor tendons in the palm and is free of fibrous pulleys. It extends, therefore, from the proximal end of the finger pulley system (A_1) to the distal end of the wrist retinaculum, the transverse carpal ligament.

Zone 4—Zone 4 is the carpal tunnel. It extends from the distal to the proximal borders of the transverse carpal ligament.

Zone 5—Zone 5 extends from the proximal border of the transverse carpal ligament to the musculotendinous junctions of the flexor tendon.

These tendon zones are particularly important to the hand surgeon treating tendon injuries. The management technique, postoperative rehabilitation, and prognosis vary according to the zone in which the flexor tendon injury occurs.

FUNCTION OF THE EXTRINSIC FLEXORS AND EXTENSORS[5]

In reviewing the function of muscles and their tendons, it is important to recall that a muscle-tendon unit affects every joint between its origin and insertion; that is, the flexor

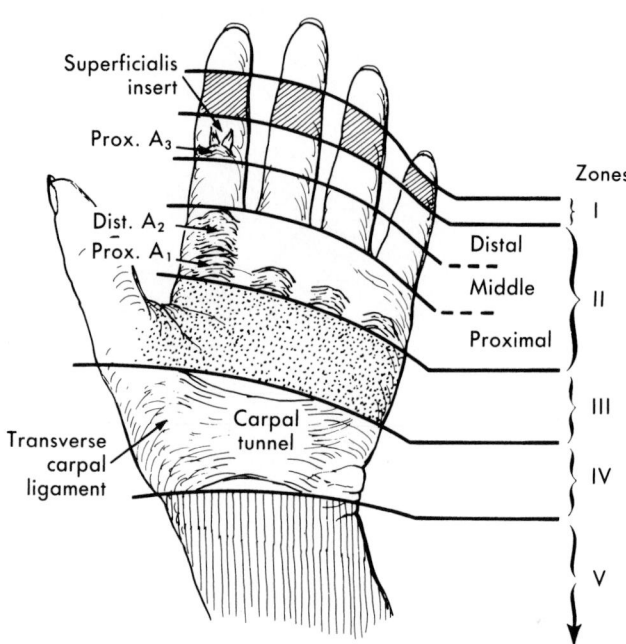

Fig. 3-14. Flexor tendon zones chosen for their relevance to flexor tendon injuries (see text). (From Chase RA: *Atlas of hand surgery,* vol 2, Philadelphia, 1984, WB Saunders.)

digitorum profundus crossing multiple joint linkages primarily flexes the DIP joint. However, secondarily, it flexes the PIP joint, followed by the MP joint, and, finally, the wrist. The complexity of its function multiplies when one considers the other antagonists and protagonists at each of the joints in the linkage of skeletal elements between the muscle's proximal and distal attachments. For example, flexion of the DIP and PIP joints by the profundus tendon is augmented by active extension of the MP joint by the long extensor tendon. Thus a principle is established that in a multiple linkage system, a tendon's function is, in fact, augmented at some joints by action of its antagonist at other joints in the system. It is certainly clear that wrist extensors that are antagonist to the profundus tendon at the wrist significantly augment profundus function at the MP and interphalangeal joints. This combination of wrist extension and finger flexion, in fact, is a synergistic function. The flexor digitorum profundus muscles that operate the ulnar three fingers are interdependent. Thus, if one restrains any of those three fingers in extension, function of the profundus tendon in the other two fingers is significantly diminished. This forms the basis for a test for superficialis tendon function. Muscle bellies of the flexor digitorum superficialis muscles are separate and independent. If one checkreins the func-

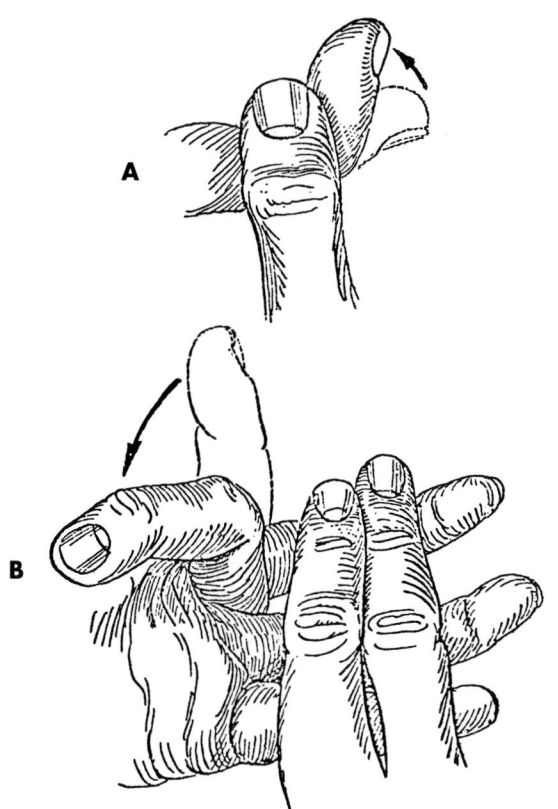

Fig. 3-15. A, The only flexor of the distal interphalangeal joint is flexor digitorum profundus. **B,** By checkreining the profundi, holding the fingers in extension, function of the superficialis muscle to the free finger may be tested. (From Chase RA: *Atlas of hand surgery,* vol 2, Philadelphia, 1984, WB Saunders.)

tion of the profundus tendons by holding the long finger or little finger in extension passively, the only effective flexor of the PIP joint is the superficialis tendon muscle unit. This is the basis for testing for superficialis function (Fig. 3-15).

The flexor pollicis longus is the only flexor of the interphalangeal joint of the thumb. Therefore testing for its function is simple. The extrinsic extensor muscles act primarily to extend the MP joints. Secondarily, they act as wrist extensors. Because of the nature of the extensor mechanism in the finger, if the MP joint is held passively in flexion, the long extensor tendon through its central slip and lateral bands acts to extend the interphalangeal joints. Thus, when the interossei and lumbricals act to flex or stabilize the MP joint, the long extensor mechanism will augment the extension of the interphalangeal joints. Absence of such intrinsic support of the MP joints in neutral position or flexion results in extension and hyperextension of the MP joints and in loss of influence of the extrinsic extensors at the interphalangeal joints, which are then at the mercy of the long flexors to the fingers. The result is the classic claw or intrinsic minus position.[48]

THE INTRINSIC MUSCLES OF THE HAND
Thenar muscles

The two and a half muscles lying lateral to the flexor pollicis longus on the palmar aspect of the thumb represent the median-innervated positioning muscles of that member. They are the abductor pollicis brevis, the opponens pollicis, and the superficial head of the flexor pollicis brevis. The abductor pollicis brevis originates from the fascia and flexor retinaculum on the palmar aspect of the wrist and extends to insert in part on the proximal phalanx and in part into the extensor mechanism of the thumb at and just beyond the MP joint. The fleshy opponens pollicis lies just deep to the abductor pollicis brevis and inserts all along the body of the metacarpal. The flexor pollicis brevis consists of two heads, one lateral to and one medial to the flexor pollicis longus. The lateral or superficial head regularly inserts into the proximal phalanx after surrounding the sesamoid at the radial side of the MP joint. The medial or deep head varies greatly in its insertion, inserting on the proximal phalanx sometimes through the sesamoid on the medial aspect of the MP joint, sometimes through the lateral sesamoid, and sometimes through both. The abductor pollicis muscle consists of transverse and oblique heads. It originates along the line of the palmar aspect of the third metacarpal and deep fascia of the hand. It inserts into the proximal phalanx by enshrouding the sesamoid on the ulnar side of the MP joint, often together with the deep head of the flexor pollicis brevis.

The hypothenar muscles are essentially mirror images of the thenar muscles except that there is no adductor. The muscles are abductor digiti minimi, flexor digiti minimi brevis, and opponens digiti minimi. The dorsal palmar interossei lie in the interosseous intervals taking origin from the opposing surfaces of the metacarpals. There are four dorsal interossei and three palmar. The interosseous tendons insert on the medial or lateral aspects of the proximal phalanx and have slips into the lateral band of the extensor mechanism. With the long finger as a central axis of the hand, the dorsal interossei are abductors, while the palmar interossei are adductors of the fingers. The lumbrical muscle has a moving site of origin from the profundus tendon or tendons in the palm of the hand. It extends palmar to the ligaments between the volar plates of the MP joints and inserts into the lateral band of the extensor mechanism. Diagrammatically, one sees that the relaxed lumbrical muscle is stretched by a separation of its origin and insertion as the finger is flexed by a pull on the profundus tendon. As the finger flexes, the extensor mechanism moves distally at the level of the interphalangeal joints, and thus the origin and insertion of the muscle are spread apart. If the muscle contracts, it produces flexion at the MP joint and extension at the PIP and DIP joints (Fig. 3-16).

The extensor mechanism in the finger[18,29-32,41,47]

There is a complex interdigitation of tendons of the extrinsic extensor mechanism and the intrinsic tendons

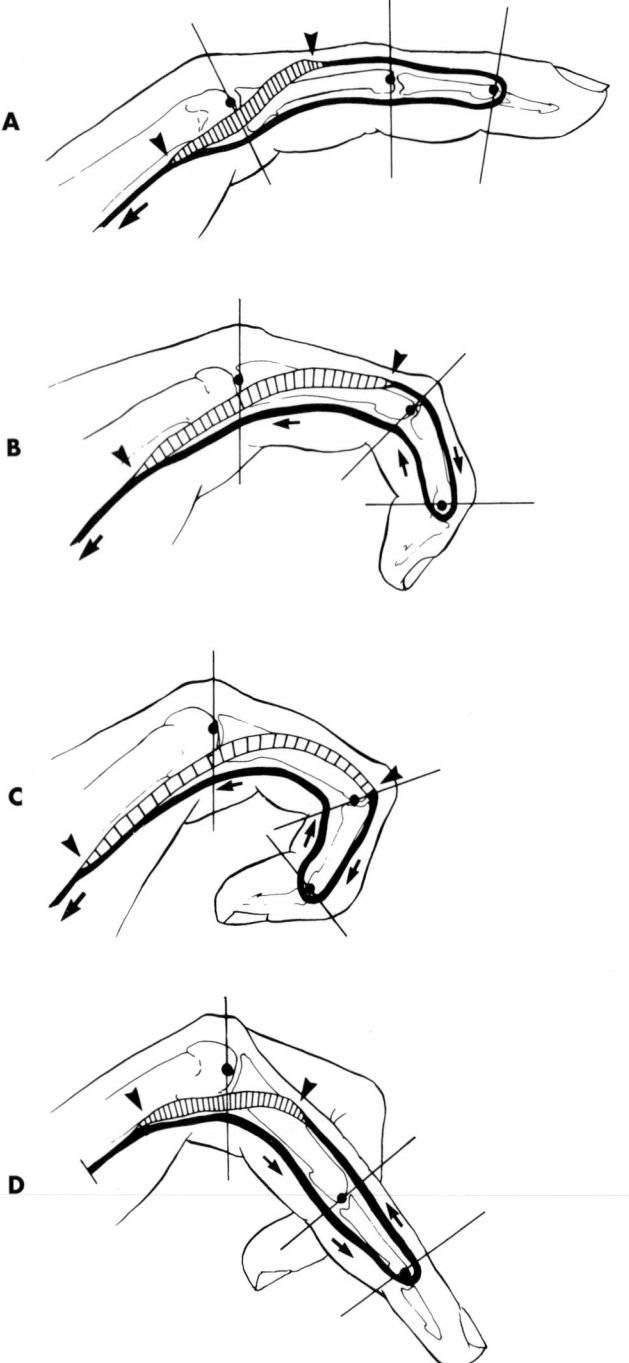

Fig. 3-16. The lumbrical muscle acts as a moderator band between the extensor and flexor mechanism in the finger. It has a moving origin from the profundus tendon and a moving insertion into the extensor mechanism through the lateral band. **A,** As the profundus tendon is pulled, the origin of the lumbrical moves proximal. **B,** Action of the profundus flexes the interphalangeal joints and moves the extensor mechanism distally, further separating the origin and insertion of the lumbrical. **C,** This becomes more exaggerated as the finger is pulled into flexion with the lumbrical relaxed. **D,** If the lumbrical muscle then contracts, its effect on the finger is to flex the metacarpophalangeal joint and extend the interphalangeal joints. This is the primary function of the lumbrical. (From Jupiter JB: *Flynn's hand surgery,* ed 4, Philadelphia, 1991, Williams & Wilkins.)

within the digit. The extrinsic extensor tendon is linked to shroud fibers at the level of the MP joint called the sagittal bands. It is through this sagittal band mechanism that the long extensors create extension at the MP joint as their primary function. The extensor, however, continues as a central slip inserting beyond the PIP joint into the middle phalanx. Before its insertion, it subdivides, giving off lateral slips, which join the lateral conjoint tendon or band through which the long extensor may influence the DIP joint. The tendinous extension of the interossei extends into the finger, forming a lateral tendon palmar to the joint axis of the MP joint. This extends distally, coursing dorsal to the PIP joint, where it is joined by the lateral slips of the common extensor mechanism. These lateral tendons of the interossei also give slips to the central slip for insertion into the proximal dorsal lip of the middle phalanx. The lumbrical muscle whose tendon lies just palmar to the intermetacarpal ligament extends as tendon to join the dorsal mechanism in passing dorsal to the axis of the PIP joint (see Fig. 3-16). In addition to these active structures, there is a passive oblique retinacular ligament, which inserts together with the distal insertion of the extensor mechanism on the distal phalanx. It therefore passes dorsal to the joint axis of the DIP joint, then obliquely palmar to take its origin from the fibrous tissues surrounding the flexor tendons just proximal to the PIP joint. It acts to extend the DIP joint when the PIP joint is extended.[8] The extensor mechanism is held centrally at the level of the PIP joint by the transverse retinacular ligaments.

The complex interplay of the extrinsic and intrinsic muscles within the finger allows wide variation of postures within the range allowed by the collateral ligaments and the capsular ligaments of the MP joint and the PIP and DIP joints.

BLOOD SUPPLY[1,12,37]

Arterial blood supply to the hand and forearm is furnished by branches from the brachial artery, including the superior and inferior ulnar collateral arteries and the profunda brachial artery, which contribute to the collateral anastomoses around the elbow. The terminal branches of the brachial artery, the radial and ulnar, are the major contributors of blood supply to the forearm and the hand. An early branch of the ulnar artery as it courses deep across the proximal forearm is the common interosseous artery, which gives rise to the anterior posterior interosseous arteries deep within the forearm. The radial and ulnar arteries continue through the forearm, contributing multiple muscular and osseous branches. At the wrist level, interarterial arches between the two major vessels furnish blood supply to the carpal bones. At the wrist level, the radial artery courses dorsally at the level of the radiocarpal joint to pass across the depression between the long and short extensors to the thumb, often referred to as the anatomic snuffbox. Before doing so, it generally gives off a superficial branch, which crosses the thenar eminence at various depths superficial to and deep within the thenar muscles to contribute to the superficial vascular arch. The branch crossing dorsally represents the major radial arterial contribution to the hand, particularly on its radial aspect. There are multiple variations in the nature of branching of the radial artery after it passes through the first web space between the second metacarpal and the first dorsal interosseous attachments to it. After giving off arterial branches to the thumb and index finger, it becomes the major contributor to the deep palmar vascular arch. The ulnar artery courses distally adjacent to the ulnar nerve lying just deep to the flexor carpi ulnaris. As it approaches the wrist, it contributes to the vascular arches at the wrist level, then turns superficial to lie just deep to the palmaris brevis muscles within Guyon's tunnel. After giving off a deep branch that anastomoses deep within the palm with the contribution to the deep vascular arch from the radial artery, the ulnar artery continues across the palm just deep to the palmar fascia as the superficial palmar arch. Arteries radiate distally from the superficial arch as common digital arteries that divide into proper digital arteries to the adjacent sides of the index, long, ring, and little fingers. Proper digital arteries arise from the superficial arch to the ulnar side of the little finger and from either the deep or superficial arch to the radial side of the index finger.

Blood supply to the thumb comes variably from the deep branch of the radial artery as a princeps pollicis or as branches directly from the deep arch. A discussion of the multiple variations of the blood supply within the hand is beyond the scope of this chapter, and the author suggests that a more complete review is available in the classic studies by Coleman and Anson[12] (1961) and the detailed studies by Murakami[37] (1969) and Adachi[1] (1928). Venous return from the hand is found both as classic venae comitantes from each of the arteries and the networks of veins that drain toward the dorsum of the fingers and hand into the cephalic and basilic venous systems. A detailed knowledge of vascular anatomy has become much more important with the advent of microvascular surgery with prospects for replantation and transfer of composite parts from one place to another.

NERVE SUPPLY[16,44,49]

Sensory nerve supply to the forearm and hand comes from the medial, lateral, and posterior antebrachial cutaneous nerves and the radial, ulnar, and median nerves within the hand. The radial aspect of the dorsum of the hand is innervated by the superficial sensory branch of the radial nerve. The dorsal branch of the ulnar nerve supplies the ulnar aspect of the dorsum of the hand and the palmar aspect of the little finger and ulnar half of the ring finger. The remaining portion of the palm, which includes the palmar aspect of the thumb, index, long, and half of the ring fingers, is supplied by the median nerve.

The median nerve

The median nerve enters the forearm lying adjacent to the brachial artery at the elbow and beneath the lacertus fibrosus or bicipital fascia. After giving off motor branches to the pronator teres muscle, the nerve passes between its deep and superficial heads. It gives off the anterior interosseous nerve in varying relationships to the pronator teres. The anterior interosseous nerve courses deep and distally along the interosseous membrane, giving motor branches to the flexor pollicis longus, and the flexor digitorum profundus to the index finger and to the pronator quadratus in which the nerve terminates. The main trunk of the median nerve passes through a second muscular arcade at the origins of the superficialis muscles of the forearm. It then lies on the deep surface of the superficialis muscles and tendons to the distal quarter of the forearm. In this position, it gives off motor branches to the flexor digitorum superficialis and the flexor carpi radialis. The nerve emerges to become superficial by coursing around the radial aspect of the superficialis tendons just above the wrist. It then becomes the most superficial structure within the carpal tunnel (Fig. 3-17, *A*). After passing through the carpal tunnel, the nerve arborizes into its sensory branches and the recurrent motor branch to the thenar muscles. The recurrent motor branch may come off at various levels, including a point within the carpal tunnel, where it may penetrate the volar carpal ligament to pass to the thenar muscles. The sensory nerves consist of a proper digital nerve to the thumb, which divides into a medial and lateral proper digital nerve, a proper digital nerve to the radial side of the index finger, and common digital nerves, which divide into proper digital nerves to the adjacent sides of the index, long, and ring fingers (Fig. 3-17, *B*). Tiny motor branches to the radial two lumbricals originate from the proper digital nerve to the radial side of the index finger and the common digital nerve to the adjacent sides of the index and long fingers.

Ulnar nerve

The ulnar nerve enters the forearm by passing through the cubital tunnel at the medial epicondylar groove of the humerus. It penetrates between the two heads of origin of the flexor carpi ulnaris. It lies on the deep side of that muscle throughout the forearm. It gives off motor branches to the flexor carpi ulnaris and the ulnar two or three flexor digitorum profundus muscles. At the wrist, the nerve courses superficial to enter the hand beneath the palmaris brevis muscle and fascia in Guyon's tunnel (Fig. 3-18), *A*). At this point, it gives off a deep motor branch and superficial branches, including a proper digital nerve to the ulnar side of the little finger and a common digital nerve to the adjacent sides of the little and ring fingers (Fig. 3-18, *B*). Other branches go to the palmaris brevis muscle and the abductor digiti minimi muscle. The deep motor branch of the ulnar nerve then passes through two more components of the ulnar tunnel at the wrist/hand level.[26] The first portion is that which lies between the hook of the hamate and the pisiform (called the *pisohamate tunnel*), and the second is a tunnel between the two heads of the opponens digiti minimi (called the *opponens tunnel*). The nerve then courses with the deep vascular arch and gives off tiny motor branches to the

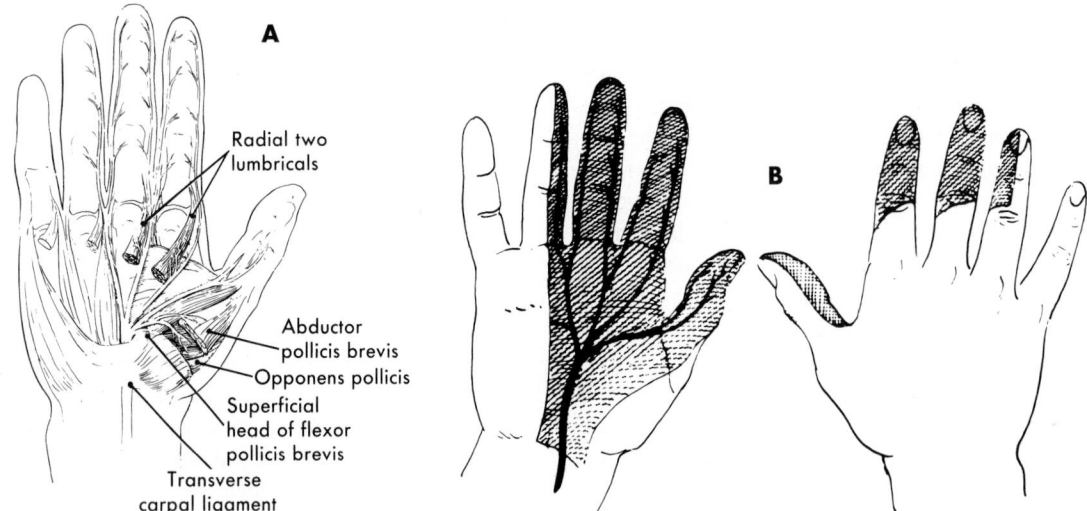

Fig. 3-17. A, The median nerve, the most superficial structure in the carpal tunnel, generally arborizes as it passes through the carpal tunnel into its terminal motor and sensory branches. The recurrent motor branches, which may actually pass through the flexor retinaculum rather than distal to it, generally innervate the two and a half thenar muscles on the radial side of the long flexor to the thumb, the abductor pollicis brevis, the opponens pollicis, and the superficial head of the flexor pollicis brevis. In addition, there are motor branches to the two radial lumbricals from the nerve branches coursing toward the index and long fingers. **B,** Sensory branches course to the thumb, index, and long fingers and to the radial side of the ring finger. The median nerve classically lends sensibility to the palmar aspect and the distal dorsum of the thumb, index, and long fingers and the radial one half of the ring finger. Intrinsic muscles radial to the flexor pollicis longus and the two radial lumbricals receive motor innervation from the median nerve. (From Chase RA: *Atlas of hand surgery,* vol 2, Philadelphia, 1984, WB Saunders.)

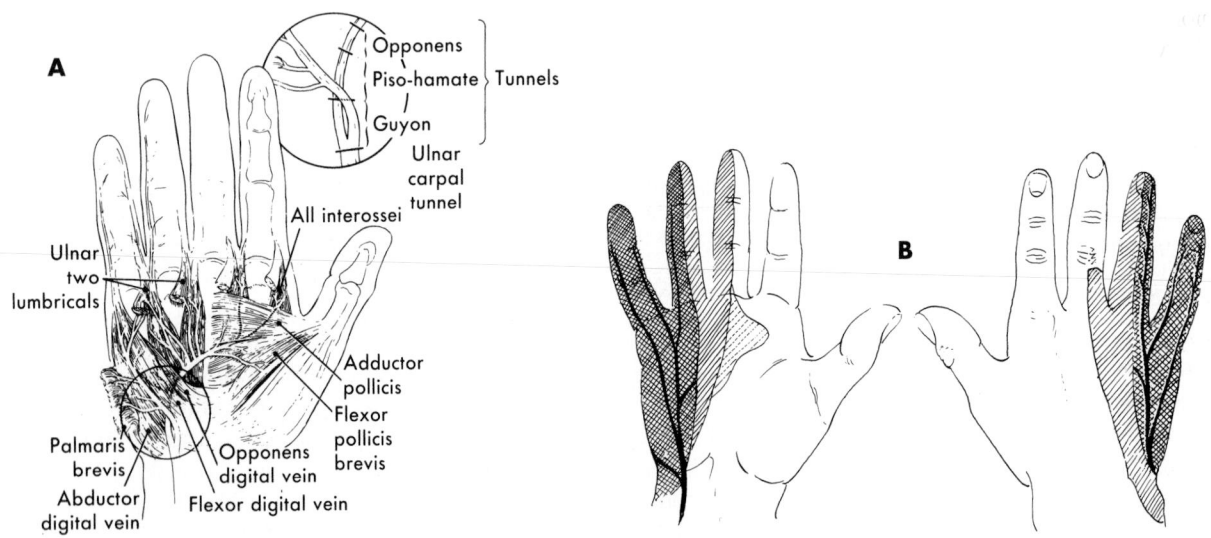

Fig. 3-18. A, The ulnar nerve arrives at the hand just medial to the flexor carpi ulnaris, where it becomes superficial coursing just beneath the palmaris brevis within Guyon's tunnel. The deep motor branch continues by coursing through the pisohamate tunnel and the opponens tunnel between the superficial and deep head of the opponens digiti minimi muscle. It courses across the deep palm in company with the deep vascular arch to give innervation to all of the interossei, the two ulnar lumbricals, the adductor pollicis, and generally the deep head of the flexor pollicis brevis. **B,** The superficial branch gives motor twigs to the palmaris brevis and the abductor digiti minimi before it continues to give sensory innervation to the little finger and ulnar side of the ring finger. (From Chase RA: *Atlas of hand surgery,* vol 2, Philadelphia, 1984, WB Saunders.)

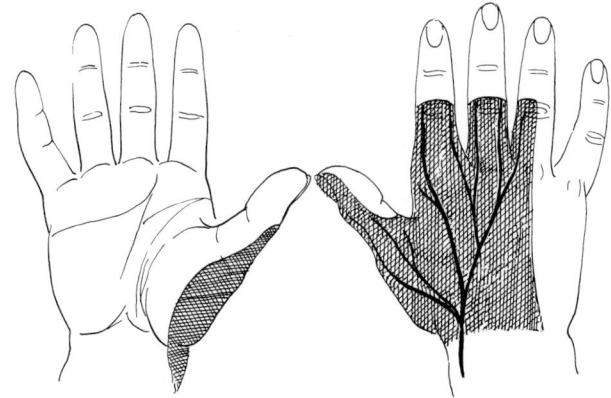

Fig. 3-19. The dorsal or sensory branch of the radial nerve courses over the radial dorsal aspect of the wrist to supply sensory innervation to the radial aspect of the dorsum of the hand and the proximal dorsal aspect of the thumb, index, and long fingers and variably the ring finger.

remaining hypothenar muscles, all of the interossei, the ulnar two lumbricals, the adductor pollicis, and the deep head of the flexor pollicis brevis. Variation in nerve supply to the intrinsic muscles between median and ulnar nerves occurs at the flexor pollicis brevis level.[49] The two heads of the muscle are often separately innervated by the median and ulnar nerve respectively, but often the superficial head may be innervated by the ulnar nerve or by both nerves.

Radial nerve

The radial nerve enters the forearm just deep to the brachioradiali muscle. It courses across the radial aspect of the elbow region close to the head of the radius, where it penetrates between the two heads of the supinator muscle at an arcade of fibers called the *Arcade of Frohse*. Before entering the arcade, the radial nerve gives motor branches to the brachioradialis, the flexor carpi, radialis longus and brevis, and a sensory branch that courses deep to the brachioradialis throughout the forearm to emerge as the dorsal sensory branch on the radial aspect of the dorsum of the hand (Fig. 3-19). The radial nerve passes through the Arcade of Frohse to become the posterior interosseous nerve. It innervates the supinator, and after passing between the two heads of the supinator, the nerve arborizes to give off motor branches to the extensor digitorum, the extensor carpi ulnaris, the extensor indicis, the extensor digiti minimi, the extensor pollicis longus, the extensor pollicis brevis, and the abductor pollicis longus.

HAND KINESIOLOGY—SOME PRINCIPLES[3,5,6]

Movements in the hand represent a complex series of muscular actions around multiple joint linkages. Muscle protagonists, antagonists, and modifiers all work in centrally controlled coordination based on movement commands voluntarily generated cerebrally, modified by reflex interactions at various levels in the central nervous system. A muscle rarely acts independently to create movement. For each muscle tendon unit, however, some principles apply:

1. A muscle tendon unit acts on every point between its origin and insertion (see Function of Extrinsic Flexors and Extensors).
2. Afferent fibers from stretch sensors within muscles serve as one arm of a reflex servo-mechanism to help control muscular contraction.
3. Reflexes may be conditioned through a complex learned reflexive response in such examples as those automatically demonstrated by complex movements done by conditioned athletes.
4. The arrangement of muscles and tendons in relationship to a specific joint determines their effect on joint action within the range allowed by the joint configuration and ligamentous limitations.
5. The forces on a joint by a muscle depend not only on muscle power but also on the combination of vectors affecting the joint at a given axis of motion.
6. The torque generated for rotary movement around a joint axis depends not only on the force generated by the muscle but also by the lever arm or perpendicular distance from the axis or center of rotation. This is popularly known as the moment arm.
7. The function of a muscle tendon unit that crosses several joints has its function augmented at any given joint by action of its antagonists at any or all other joints in the linkage. For example, the profundus flexors have their function at the MP and interphalangeal joints augmented by the wrist extensors, which are antagonists of the profundi at the wrist. This is the practical explanation of muscle synergism.

For an up-to-date, nicely presented, comprehensive discussion of upper limb kinesiology, see Brand.[5]

REFERENCES

1. Adachi B: *Das arterie system der Japaner,* vol 1, Maruzan, Kyoto, 1928.
2. Aubriot JH: The metacarpophalangeal joint of the thumb. In Tubiana R, editor: *The hand,* Philadelphia, 1985, WB Saunders.
3. Bell C: *The hand—its mechanism and vital endowments as evincing design,* London, 1834, The Pickering Press.
4. Bojsen-Moller F, Schmidt L: The palmar aponeurosis and the central spaces of the hand, *J Anat* 117:55, 1974.
5. Brand PW: *Clinical mechanics of the hand,* ed 2, St Louis, 1993, Mosby.
6. Bunnell S: *Surgery of the hand,* Philadelphia, 1944, JB Lippincott.
7. Chase RA: Surgical anatomy of the hand, *Surg Clin North Am* 44:1349, 1964.
8. Chase RA: Muscle tendon kinetics, *Am J Surg* 109:277, 1965.
9. Chase RA: *Atlas of hand surgery,* vol 1, Philadelphia, 1973, WB Saunders.
10. Chase RA: *Atlas of hand surgery,* vol 2, Philadelphia, 1984, WB Saunders.
11. Chase RA: Anatomy and examination of the hand. In May JW, Littler JW, editors: *Converse textbook of plastic surgery* (in preparation).
12. Coleman SS, Anson BJ: Arterial patterns in the hand based upon a study of 650 specimens, *Surg Gynecol Obstet* 113:408, 1961.

13. Dahhan P, Fischer L, Alliey Y: The trapeziometacarpal articulation, *Anatomia Clinica* 2:43, 1980.

14. Doyle JR, Blythe WF: *The finger flexor tendon sheath and pulleys: anatomy and reconstruction,* AAOS symposium on tendon surgery in the hand, St Louis, 1975, Mosby.

15. Doyle JR, Blythe WF: Anatomy of the flexor tendon sheath pulleys of the thumb, *J Hand Surg* 2:149, 1977.

16. Duchenne GBA: *Physiologie des Mouvements,* Paris, 1867, Bailliere (Translation by Kaplan EB, Philadelphia, 1959, JB Lippincott).

17. Eaton RG, Littler JW: A study of the basal joint of the thumb, *J Bone Joint Surg* 51A:661, 1969.

18. Eyler DL, Markee JE: The anatomy of the intrinsic musculature of the fingers, *J Bone Joint Surg* 36A:1, 1954.

19. Henry AK: *Extensile exposure,* Baltimore, 1945, Williams & Wilkins.

20. Hueston JT: *Dupuytren's contracture,* Baltimore, 1963, Williams & Wilkins.

21. Hunter JM, et al: The pulley system, *Proceedings of the American Society for Surgery of the Hand: orthopedic transactions,* 4:4, 1980.

22. Jones FW: *Principles of anatomy as seen in the hand,* Philadelphia, 1920, Blakistons' Son.

23. Joseph J: Further studies of the metacarpo-phalangeal and interphalangeal joints of the thumb, *J Anat* 85:221, 1951.

24. Kanavel AB: *Infections of the hand,* Philadelphia, 1925, Lea & Febiger.

25. Kaplan EB: *Functional and surgical anatomy of the hand,* Philadelphia, 1953, JB Lippincott.

26. Kim S: The ulnar tunnel at the wrist, Personal communication, 1986.

27. Kuczynski K: Carpometacarpal joint of the human thumb, *J Anat* 118:119, 1974.

28. Kuczynski K: The thumb and the saddle, *Hand* 7:120, 1975.

29. Landsmeer JMF: Anatomy of the dorsal aponeurosis of the human finger and its functional significance, *Anat Rec* 104:31, 1949.

30. Landsmeer JMF: Anatomical and functional investigations on the articulation of the human fingers, *Acta Anat* 25:1, 1955.

31. Landsmeer JMF: A report on the coordination of the interphalangeal joints of the human finger and its disturbances, *Acta Morphol Neerl Scand,* 2:59, 1958.

32. Landsmeer JMF: The coordination of finger-joint motion, *J Bone Joint Surg* 45A:1654, 1963.

33. Littler JW: Architectural principles of reconstructive hand surgery, *Surg Clin North Am* 31:463, 1951.

34. Littler JW: On the adaptability of man's hand (with reference to the equiangular curve), *Hand* 5:187, 1973.

35. McFarlane RM: Patterns of the diseased fascia in the fingers in Dupuytren's contracture, *Plast Reconstr Surg* 54:31, 1974.

36. McFarlane RM: Dupuytren's contracture. In Green DP: *Operative hand surgery,* New York, 1982, Churchill Livingstone.

37. Murakami T, Takaya K, Outi H: The origin, course and distribution of arteries to the thumb, with special reference to the so-called A. princeps pollicis, *Okajimas Folica Anatomica Japonica* 46:123, 1969.

38. Ou CJA: The biomechanics of the carpometacarpal joint of the thumb, doctoral dissertation, Department of Mechanical Engineering, Louisiana State University and Agricultural and Mechanical College. Ann Arbor, 1980,. University Microfilms International.

39. Pagalidis T, Kuczynski K, Lamb DW: Ligamentous stability of the base of the thumb, *Hand* 13:29, 1981.

40. Skoog T: The transverse elements of the palmar aponeurosis in Dupuytren's contracture, *Scand J Plast Reconstr Surg* 1:51, 1967.

41. Stack HG: A study of muscle function in the fingers, *Ann Royal Coll Surg Engl* 33:307, 1963.

42. Strauch B, Maura W: Digital flexor tendon sheath: an anatomic study, *J Hand Surg* 10A:785, 1985.

43. Strickland JW, Bassett RL: The isolated digital cord in Dupuytren's contracture: anatomy and clinical significance, *J Hand Surg* 10A:118, 1985.

44. Sunderland S: *Nerves and nerve injuries,* New York, 1978, Churchill Livingstone.

45. Taleisnik J, et al: Extensor retinaculum of the wrist, *J Hand Surg* 9A:495, 1984.

46. Tubiana R: *The hand,* vol 2, Philadelphia, 1985, WB Saunders.

47. Tubiana R, Valentine P: L'extension des doigts, *Rev Chir Orthop* 49:543, 1963.

48. White WL: Restoration of function and balance of the wrist and hand by tendon transfers, *Surg Clin North Am* 40:427, 1960.

49. Woodhall B, Beebe GW, editors: Peripheral nerve regeneration: a follow-up study of 3656 World War II injuries, *Veterans Administration Medical Monograph,* 1956.

50. Zancolli E: *Structural and dynamic bases of hand surgery,* Philadelphia, 1979, JB Lippincott.

Chapter 4

ANATOMY AND KINESIOLOGY OF THE WRIST

Richard A. Berger

The wrist is a unique joint interposed between the distal aspect of the forearm and the proximal aspect of the hand. There are common or shared elements to all three regions, which integrate from and function to maximize the mechanical effectiveness of the upper extremity. The wrist enables the hand to be placed in an infinite number of positions relative to the forearm and also enables the hand to be essentially locked to the forearm in those positions to transfer the forces generated by the powerful forearm muscles.

Although the wrist is truly a mechanical marvel when it is intact and functioning, loss of mechanical integrity of the wrist will inevitably cause substantial dysfunction of the hand and thus the entire upper extremity. It is vital that a thorough understanding of the wrist, including efforts in diagnosis, treatment, and rehabilitation, be acquired by all who treat the wrist. This chapter provides such a foundation by exploring the general architecture of the wrist, the bones, and joints that compose the wrists and the soft tissues that stabilize, innervate, and perfuse the wrist. In addition, an overview of the mechanics of the wrist, with a discussion of the motions of the wrist and its subparts and the force distribution across the wrist, is provided.

BONY ANATOMY

There are eight carpal bones, although many consider the pisiform to be a sesamoid bone within the tendon of the flexor carpi ulnaris (FCU), and thus not behaving as a true carpal bone. The bones are arranged into two rows (proximal and distal carpal row), each containing four bones. All eight carpal bones are interposed between the forearm bones and the metacarpals to form the complex called the *wrist joint.*

Distal radius and ulna

The distal surface of the radius articulates with the proximal carpal row through two articular fossae separated by a fibrocartilaginous prominence oriented in the sagittal plane called the *interfossal ridge* (Figs. 4-1 and 4-2). The scaphoid fossa is roughly triangular in shape and extends from the interfossal ridge to the tip of the radial styloid process. The lunate fossa is roughly quadrangular in shape and extends from the interfossal ridge to the sigmoid notch. On the dorsal cortex of the distal radius, immediately dorsal and proximal to the interfossal ridge, is a bony prominence called the *dorsal tubercle of the radius,* or *Lister's tubercle* (see Fig. 4-1). It serves as a divider between the second and third extensor compartments and functionally behaves as a trochlea for the tendon of extensor pollicis longus.

Under normal circumstances, the ulna does not articular directly with the carpus. Rather, a fibrocartilaginous wafer called the *triangular disc* is interposed between the ulnar head and the proximal carpal row (see Fig. 4-2). Even the ulnar styloid process is hidden from contact with the carpus by the ulnotriquetral (UT) ligament. The ulnar head is roughly cylindrical in shape, with a distal projection on its posterior border, called the *ulnar styloid process.* Approximately three fourths of the ulnar head is covered by articular cartilage, with the ulnar styloid process and the posterior one fourth as exposed bone or periosteum. A depression at the base of the ulnar styloid process, called the *fovea,* is typically not covered in articular cartilage.

Proximal carpal row bones

The proximal row consists of, from radial to ulnar, the scaphoid (navicular), lunate, triquetrum, and pisiform (Figs. 4-3 and 4-4). The scaphoid is shaped somewhat like

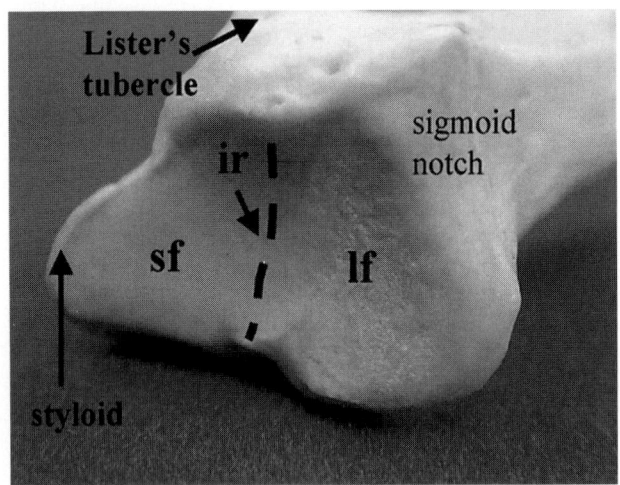

Fig. 4-1. Distal radius from a distal and ulnar perspective. *ir*, Interfossal ridge; *lf*, lunate fossa; *sf*, scaphoid fossa.

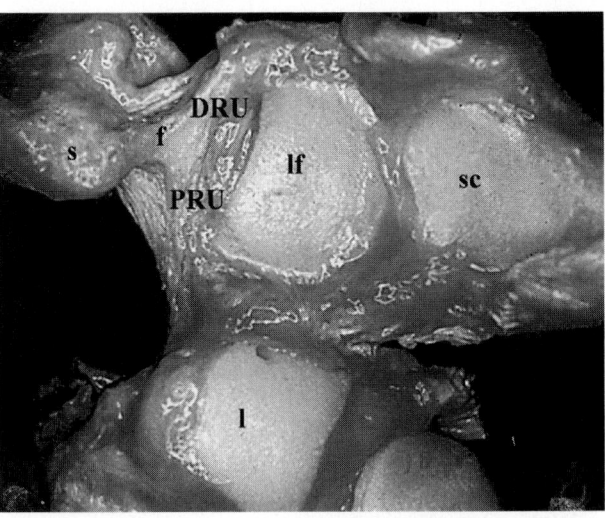

Fig. 4-2. Radiocarpal joint from a distal perspective, prepared by palmar-flexing the proximal carpal row. The triangular disc is seen between the distal radioulnar *(DRU)* and palmar radioulnar *(PRU)* ligaments. The interfossal ridge is seen between the scaphoid and lunate fossae. *f*, Foveal attachment of triangular fibrocartilage complex (TFCC); *L*, lunate; *lf*, lunate fossa of the distal radius; *s*, styloid attachment of TFCC; *sf*, scaphoid fossa.

Fig. 4-3. Wrist from palmar perspective. *Bones: C,* Capitate; *H,* hamate; *I,* first metacarpal; *L,* lunate; *P,* pisiform; *R,* radius; *S,* scaphoid; *Td,* trapezoid; *Tm,* trapezium; *U,* ulna; *V,* fifth metacarpal. *Ligaments: LRL,* Long radiolunate; *PCH,* palmar capitohamate; *PCT,* palmar trapezocapiate; *PLT,* palmar lunotriquetral; *RSC,* radioscaphocapitate; *SC,* scaphocapitate; *SRL,* short radiolunate; *STT,* scaphoid-trapezium-trapezoid; *TC,* triquetrocapitate; *TH,* triquetrohamate; *TT,* trapezium-trapezoid; *UL,* ulnolunate; *UT,* ulnotriquetral.

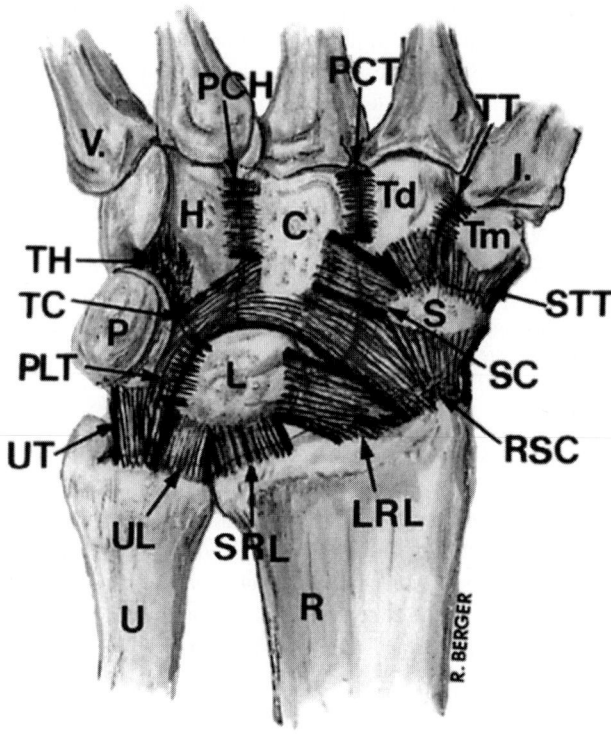

a kidney bean. The scaphoid is divided into three regions: the proximal pole, waist, and distal pole. The proximal pole has a convex articular surface that faces the scaphoid fossa and a flat articular surface that faces the lunate. The dorsal surface of the waist is marked by an oblique ridge that serves as an attachment plane for the dorsal joint capsule. The medial surface of the waist and distal surface of the proximal pole is concave and articulates with the capitate. The distal pole also articulates with the capitate medially, but distally it articulates with the trapezium and trapezoid. Otherwise, the distal pole is nearly completely covered with ligament attachments.

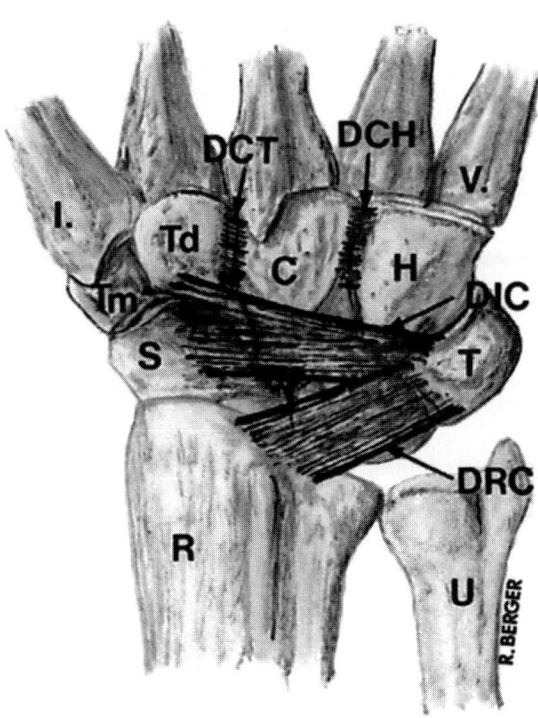

Fig. 4-4. Wrist from dorsal perspective. *Bones: C,* Capitate; *H,* hamate; *I,* first metacarpal; *R,* radius; *S,* scaphoid; *T,* triquetrum; *Td,* trapezoid; *Tm,* trapezium; *U,* ulna; *V,* fifth metacarpal. *Ligaments: DCH,* Dorsal capitohamate; *DCT,* dorsal trapezocapitate; *DIC,* dorsal intercarpal; *DRC,* dorsal radiocarpal.

The lunate is crescent-shaped in the sagittal plane, such that the proximal surface is convex and the distal surface concave, and it is somewhat wedge-shaped in the transverse plane. With the exception of ligament attachment planes on its dorsal and palmar surfaces, the lunate is otherwise covered with articular cartilage. It articulates with the scaphoid laterally, the radius and triangular fibrocartilage proximally, the triquetrum medially, and the capitate distally. In some individuals, the lunate has a separate fossa for articulation with the hamate, separated from the fossa for capitate articulation by a prominent ridge.

The triquetrum has a complex shape, with a flat articular surface on the palmar surface for articulation with the pisiform; a concave distal articular surface for articulation with the hamate; a flat lateral surface for articulation with the lunate; and three tubercles on the proximal, medial, and dorsal surfaces. The proximal tubercle is covered in cartilage for contact with the triangular disc, while the medial and dorsal tubercles serve as ligament attachment surfaces.

The pisiform, which means "pea-shaped," is oval in profile with a flat articular facet covering the distal half of the dorsal surface for articulation with the triquetrum. Otherwise, it is entirely enveloped within the tendon of FCU and serves as a proximal origin of the flexor digiti minimi muscle.

Distal carpal row bones

The distal carpal row consists of, from radial to ulnar, the trapezium, trapezoid, capitate, and hamate (see Figs. 4-3 and 4-4). The trapezium, historically referred to as the *greater multangular,* has three articular surfaces. The proximal surface is slightly concave and articulates with the distal pole of the scaphoid. The medial articular surface is flat and articulates with the trapezoid. The distal surface is saddle-shaped and articulates with the base of the first metacarpal. The remaining surfaces are nonarticular and serve as attachment areas for ligaments. The anterolateral edge of the trapezium forms an overhang, referred to as the *beak,* which is part of the fibro-osseous tunnel for the tendon of flexor carpi radialis (FCR).

The trapezoid, referred to historically as the *lesser multangular,* is a small bone with articular surfaces on the proximal, lateral, medial, and distal surfaces for articulation with the scaphoid, trapezium, capitate, and base of the second metacarpal, respectively. The palmar and dorsal surfaces serve as ligament insertion areas.

The capitate is the largest carpal bone and is divided into head, neck, and body regions. The head is almost entirely covered in articular cartilage and forms a proximally convex surface for articulation with the scaphoid and lunate. The neck is a narrowed region between the body and the head and is exposed to the midcarpal joint without ligament attachment. The body is nearly cuboid in shape with articular surfaces on its medial, lateral, and distal aspects for articulation with the trapezoid, hamate, and base of the third metacarpal, respectively. The large, flat palmar and dorsal surfaces serve as ligament attachment areas.

The hamate has a complex geometry, with a pole, body, and hamulus (hook). The pole is a conical proximally tapering projection that is nearly entirely covered in articular cartilage for articulation with the triquetrum, capitate, and variably the lunate. The body is relatively cuboid with medial and distal articulations for the capitate and fourth and fifth metacarpal bases, respectively. The dorsal and palmar surfaces serve as ligament attachment areas, except the most medial aspect of the body, where the hamulus arises. The hamulus forms a palmarly directed projection that curves slightly lateral at the palmar margin. This also serves as a broad area for ligament attachment.

JOINT ANATOMY

Before a discussion of the anatomy of the wrist can be pursued, it is important that a consensus of term definitions be reached. The terms *proximal* and *distal* are universally understood, but some confusion may exist regarding terms defining relationships in other planes. Although the terms *medial* and *lateral* are anatomically correct, they require a virtual positioning of the upper extremity in the classic anatomic position to be interpretable. Therefore the terms *radial* and *ulnar* have been introduced by clinicians to enable an instant understanding of orientation independent of upper extremity positioning, because the reference to these terms (the orientation of the radius and ulna) will not change significantly relative to the wrist. Likewise, the terms *anterior, volar,* and *palmar* all describe the front surface of the wrist, whereas *dorsal* and *posterior* describe the back surface of the wrist. Some may object to using the term *palmar* in reference to the wrist, but they should be reminded that the palmar, glabrous skin covers the anterior surface of the carpus; therefore it seems to have an acceptable use in the wrist.

Composed of eight carpal bones as the wrist proper, the wrist should be functionally considered as having a total of 15 bones. This is because of the proximal articulations with the radius and ulna and the distal articulations with the bases of the first through fifth metacarpals. The geometry of the wrist is complex, demonstrating a transverse arch created by the scaphoid and triquetrum/pisiform column proximally and the trapezium and hamate distally. In addition, the proximal carpal row demonstrates a substantial arch in the frontal plane.

From an anatomic standpoint, the carpal bones are divided into proximal and distal carpal rows, each consisting of four bones. This effectively divides the wrist joint spaces into radiocarpal and midcarpal spaces. Although mechanically linked to the distal radioulnar joint (DRUJ), the wrist is normally biologically separated from the DRIUJ joint space by the triangular fibrocartilage complex (TFCC).

Radiocarpal joint

The radiocarpal joint is formed by the articulation of confluent surfaces of the concave distal articular surface of the radius and the triangular fibrocartilage, with the convex proximal articular surfaces of the proximal carpal row bones.

Midcarpal joint

The midcarpal joint is formed by the mutually articulating surfaces of the proximal and distal carpal rows. Communications are found between the midcarpal joint and the interosseous joint clefts of the proximal and distal row bones, as well as to the second through fifth carpometacarpal joints. Under normal circumstances, the midcarpal joint is isolated from the pisotriquetral, radiocarpal, and first carpometacarpal joints by intervening membranes and ligaments. The geometry of the midcarpal joint is complex. Radially, the scaphoid-trapezium-trapezoid (STT) joint is composed of the slightly convex distal pole of the scaphoid articulating with the reciprocally concave proximal surfaces of the trapezium and trapezoid. Forming an analog to a "ball-and-socket joint" are the convex head of the capitate and the combined concave contiguous distal articulating surfaces of the scaphoid and the lunate. In 65% of normal adults, it has been found that the hamate articulates with a medial articular facet at the distal ulnar margin of the lunate, which is associated with a higher rate of cartilage eburnation of the proximal surface of the hamate. The triquetrohamate

region of the midcarpal joint is particularly complex, with the mutual articular surfaces having both concave and convex regions forming a helicoid-shaped articulation.

Interosseous joints: proximal row

The interosseous joints of the proximal row are relatively small and planar, allowing motion primarily in the flexion/extension plane between mutually articulating bones. The scapholunate (SL) joint has a smaller surface area than the lunotriquetral (LT) joint. Often, a fibrocartilaginous meniscus extending from the membranous region of the SL or LT interosseous ligaments will be interposed into the respective joint clefts.

Interosseous joints: distal row

The interosseous joints of the distal row are more complex geometrically and allow substantially less interosseous motion than those of the proximal row. The capitohamate joint is relatively planar, but the mutually articulating surfaces are only partially covered by articular cartilage. The distal and palmar region of the joint space is devoid of articular cartilage, being occupied by the deep capitohamate interosseous ligament. Similarly, the central region of the trapeziocapitate joint surface is interrupted by the deep trapeziocapitate interosseous ligament. The trapezium-trapezoid joint presents a small planar surface area with continuous articular surfaces.

LIGAMENT ANATOMY
Overview

The ligaments of the wrist have been described in a number of ways, leading to substantial confusion in the literature regarding various features of the carpal ligaments. Several general principles have been identified to help simplify the ligamentous architecture of the wrist. No ligaments of the wrist are truly extracapsular. Most can be anatomically classified as capsular ligaments with collagen fascicles clearly within the lamina of the joint capsule. The ligaments that are not entirely capsular, such as the interosseous ligaments between the bones within the carpal row, are intraarticular. This implies that they are not ensheathed in part by a fibrous capsular lamina. The wrist ligaments carry consistent histologic features, which are, to a degree, ligament specific. The majority of capsular ligaments are made up of longitudinally oriented laminated collagen fascicles surrounded by loosely organized perifascicular tissue, which are in turn surrounded by the epiligamentous sheath. This sheath is generally composed of the fibrous and synovial capsular lamina. The perifascicular tissue has numerous blood vessels and nerves aligned longitudinally with the collagen fascicles. The function of these nerves is currently not well understood. It has been hypothesized that these nerves are an integral part of a proprioceptive network, following the principals of Hilton's law of segmental innervation. The palmar capsular ligaments are more numerous than the dorsal, forming almost the entire palmar joint capsules of the radiocarpal and midcarpal joints. The palmar ligaments tend to converge toward the midline as they travel distally and have been described as forming an apex-distal V. The interosseous ligaments between the individual bones within a carpal row are generally short and transversely oriented and, with specific exceptions, cover the dorsal and palmar joint margins. Specific ligament groups are briefly described in the following sections and are divided into capsular and interosseous groups.

Distal radioulnar ligaments

Although a description of the DRUJ is beyond the scope of this chapter, a brief description of the anatomy of the palmar and dorsal radioulnar ligaments is required to understand the origin of the ulnocarpal ligaments. The dorsal and palmar DRUJ ligaments are believed to be major stabilizers of the DRUJ. These ligaments form the dorsal and palmar margins of the TFCC in the region between the sigmoid notch of the radius and the styloid process of the ulna (see Fig. 4-2). Attaching radially at the dorsal and palmar corners of the sigmoid notch, the ligaments converge ulnarly and pass in a cruciate manner such that the dorsal ligament attaches near the tip of the styloid process and the palmar ligament attaches near the base of the styloid process, in the region called the *fovea*. The palmar ligament has substantial connections to the carpus through the ulnolunate (UL), UT, and ulnocapitate (UC) ligaments. The dorsal ligament integrates with the sheath of extensor carpi ulnaris (ECU).

Palmar radiocarpal ligaments

The palmar radiocarpal ligaments arise from the palmar margin of the distal radius and course distally and ulnarly toward the scaphoid, lunate, and capitate (Figs. 4-3 and 4-5). Although the course of the fibers can be defined from an anterior view, the separate divisions of the palmar radiocarpal ligament are best appreciated from a dorsal view through the radiocarpal joint (see Fig. 4-5). The palmar radiocarpal ligament can be divided into four distinct regions. Beginning radially, the radioscaphocapitate (RSC) ligament originates from the radial styloid process, forms the radial wall of the radiocarpal joint, attaches to the scaphoid waist and distal pole, and passes palmar to the head of the capitate to interdigitate with fibers from the UC ligament. Very few fibers from the RSC ligament attach to the capitate. Just ulnar to the RSC ligament, the long radiolunate (LRL) ligament arises to pass palmar to the proximal pole of the scaphoid and the SL interosseous ligament to attach to the radial margin of the palmar horn of the lunate. The interligamentous sulcus separates the RSC and LRL ligaments throughout their courses. The LRL ligament has been called the *radioluno-triquetral ligament* historically, but the paucity of fibers continuing toward the triquetrum across the palmar horn of the lunate renders this name misleading. Ulnar to the origin

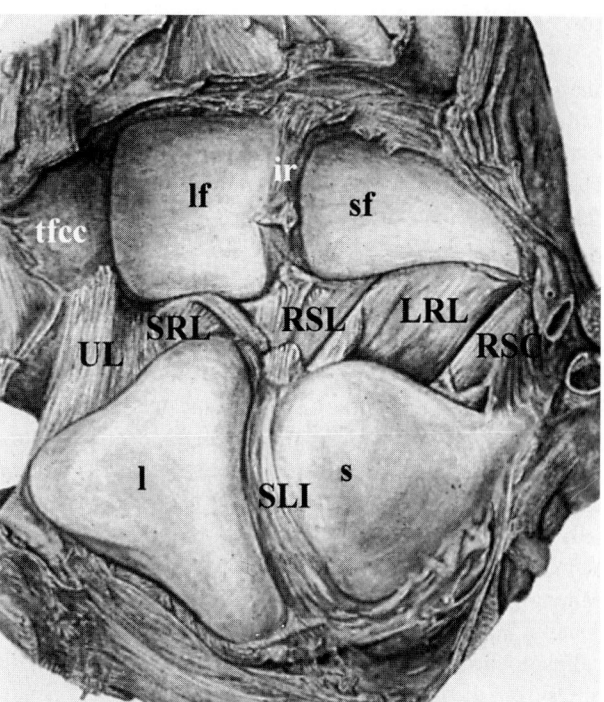

Fig. 4-5. Radiocarpal joint from distal perspective after palmar-flexing the proximal carpal row. *ir,* Interfossal ridge; *l,* lunate; *lf,* lunate fossa of distal radius; *LRL,* long radiolunate ligament; *RSC,* radioscaphocapitate ligament; *RSL,* radioscapholunate ligament; *s,* scaphoid; *sf,* scaphoid fossa of distal radius; *SLI,* scapholunate interosseous; *SRL,* short radiolunate ligament; *tfcc,* triangular fibrocartilage complex; *UL,* ulnolunate ligament.

of the LRL ligament, the radioscapholunate (RSL) "ligament" emerges into the radiocarpal joint space through the palmar capsule and merges with the SL interosseous ligament and the interfossal ridge of the distal radius. This structure resembles more of a "mesocapsule" than a true ligament, because it is made up of small-caliber blood vessels and nerves from the radial artery and anterior interosseous neurovascular bundle. Very little organized collagen is identified within this structure. The mechanical stabilizing effects of this structure have recently been shown to be minimal. The final palmar radiocarpal ligament, the short radiolunate (SRL) ligament, arises as a flat sheet of fibers from the palmar rim of the lunate fossa, just ulnar to the RSL ligament. It courses immediately distally to attach to the proximal and palmar margin of the lunate.

Dorsal radiocarpal ligament

The dorsal radiocarpal (DRC) ligament arises from the dorsal rim of the radius, essentially equally distributed on either side of Lister's tubercle (see Fig. 4-4). It courses obliquely distally and ulnarly toward the triquetrum, to which it attaches on the dorsal cortex. There are some deep attachments of the DRC ligament to the dorsal horn of the lunate. Loose connective and synovial tissue forms the capsular margins proximal and distal to the DRC ligament.

Ulnocarpal ligaments

The ulnocarpal ligament arises largely from the palmar margin of the TFCC, the palmar radioulnar ligament, and in a limited fashion, the head of the ulna. It courses obliquely distally toward the lunate, triquetrum, and capitate (Fig. 4-6). There are three divisions of the ulnocarpal ligament, designated by their distal bony insertions. The UL ligament is essentially continuous with the SRL ligament, forming a continuous palmar capsule between the TFCC and the lunate. Confluent with these fibers is the UT ligament, connecting the TFCC and the palmar rim of the triquetrum. In 60% to 70% of normal adults, a small orifice is found in the distal substance of the UT ligament, which leads to a communication between the radiocarpal and pisotriquetral joints. Just proximal and ulnar to the pisotriquetral orifice is the prestyloid recess, which is generally lined by synovial villi and variably communicates with the underlying ulnar styloid process. The UC ligament arises from the foveal and palmar region of the head of the ulna, where it courses distally, palmar to the UL and UT ligaments, and passes palmar to the head of the capitate, where it interdigitates with fibers from the RSC ligament to form an arcuate ligament to the head of the capitate. Few fibers from the UC ligament insert to the capitate.

Midcarpal ligaments

The midcarpal ligaments on the palmar surface of the carpus are true capsular ligaments, and as a rule, they are short and stout, connecting bones across a single joint space (see Figs. 4-3 and 4-6). Beginning radially, the STT ligament

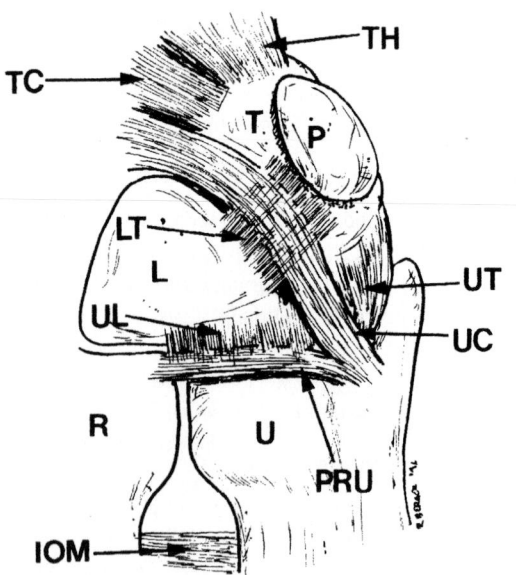

Fig. 4-6. Ulnocarpal and distal radioulnar joint complex from palmar perspective. *Bones: L,* Lunate; *P,* pisiform; *R,* radius; *T,* triquetrum; *U,* ulna. *Ligaments: LT,* Palmar lunotriquetral; *PRU,* palmar radioulnar; *TC,* triquetrocapitate; *TH,* triquetrohamate; *UC,* lunocapitate; *UL,* ulnolunate; *UT,* lunotriquetral.

forms the palmar capsule of the STT joint, connecting the distal pole of the scaphoid with the palmar surfaces of the trapezium and trapezoid. Although no clear divisions are noted, it forms an apex-proximal V shape. The scaphocapitate (SC) ligament is a thick ligament interposed between the STT and RSC ligaments, coursing from the palmar surface of the waist of the scaphoid to the palmar surface of the body of the capitate. There are no formal connections between the lunate and capitate, although the arcutate ligament (formed by the RSC and UC ligaments) has weak attachments to the palmar horn of the lunate. The triquetrocapitate (TC) ligament is analogous to the SC ligament. It is a thick ligament, passing from the palmar and distal margin of the triquetrum to the palmar surface of the body of the capitate. Immediately adjacent to the TC ligament, the triquetrohamate (TH) ligament forms the ulnar wall of the midcarpal joint and is augmented ulnarly by fibers from the TFCC. The dorsal intercarpal (DIC) ligament, originating from the dorsal cortex of the triquetrum, crosses the midcarpal joint obliquely to attach to the scaphoid, trapezoid, and capitate (see Fig. 4-4). The attachment of the DIC ligament to the triquetrum is confluent with the triquetral attachment of the DRC ligament. In addition, a proximal thickened region of the joint capsule, roughly parallel to the DRC ligament, extends from the waist of the scaphoid across the distal margin of the dorsal horn of the lunate to the triquetrum. This band, called the *dorsal scaphotriquetral ligament,* forms a "labrum," which encases the head of the capitate, analogous to the RSC and UC ligaments palmarly.

Proximal row interosseous ligaments

The SL and LT interosseous ligaments form the interconnections between the bones of the proximal carpal row and share several anatomic features. Each forms a barrier between the radiocarpal and midcarpal joints, connecting the dorsal, proximal, and palmar edges of the respective joint surfaces (see Fig. 4-5). This leaves the distal edges of the joints without ligamentous coverage. The dorsal and palmar regions of the SL and LT interosseous ligaments are typical of articular ligaments, composed of collagen fascicles with numerous blood vessels and nerves. However, the proximal regions are made up of fibrocartilage, devoid of vascularization and innervation and without identifiable collagen fascicles. The RSL ligament merges with the SL interosseous ligament near the junction of the palmar and proximal regions. The UC ligament passes directly palmar to the LT interosseous ligament with minimal interdigitation of fibers.

Distal row interosseous ligaments

The bones of the distal carpal row are rigidly connected by a complex system of interosseous ligaments (see Figs. 4-3 and 4-4). As is discussed later, these ligaments are largely responsible for transforming the four distal row bones into a single kinematic unit. The trapezium-trapezoid, trapeziocapitate, and capitohamate joints are each bridged by palmar and dorsal interosseous ligaments. These ligaments consist of transversely oriented collagen fascicles and are covered superficially by the fibrous capsular lamina, also consisting of transversely oriented fibers. This lamina gives the appearance of a continuous sheet of fibers spanning the entire palmar and dorsal surface of the distal row. Unique to the trapeziocapitate and capitohamate joints are the "deep" interosseous ligaments (Fig. 4-7). These ligaments are entirely intraarticular, spanning the respective joint spaces between voids in the articular surfaces. Both are true ligaments with dense, colinear collagen fascicles, but they are also heavily invested with nerve fibers. The deep trapeziocapitate interosseous ligament is located midway between the palmar and dorsal limits of the joint, obliquely oriented from palmar-ulnar to dorsal-radial, and each measures approximately 3 mm in diameter. The respective attachment sites of the trapezoid and capitate are angulated in the transverse plane to accommodate the orthogonal insertion of the ligament. The deep capitohamate interosseous ligament is found transversely oriented at the palmar and distal corner of the joint. It traverses the joint from quadrangular voids in the articular surfaces and measures approximately 5 × 5 mm in cross-sectional area.

TENDONS

The tendons that cross the wrist can be divided into two major groups: those that are responsible primarily for moving the wrist and those that cross the wrist in their path to the digits. Both groups impart some moment to the wrist, but obviously those that are primary wrist motors have a more substantial influence on motion of the wrist. The five primary wrist motors can be grouped as either radial or ulnar deviators and as either flexors or extensors.

The extensor carpi radialis longus (ECRL) and extensor carpi radialis brevis (ECRB) muscles are bipennate and originate from the lateral epicondyle of the humerus from a common tendon. Over the distal radius epiphysis, they are found in the second extensor compartment, from which they emerge to insert into the radial cortices of the bases of the second and third metacarpals, respectively. The ECRL imparts a greater moment for radial deviation than the ECRB, while the opposite relationship is found for wrist extension. Both the ECRL and the ECRB muscles are innervated by the radial nerve.

The ECU muscle is bipennate and originates largely from the proximal ulna and passes through the sixth extensor compartment. Within the sixth extensor compartment, the ECU tendon is contained within a fibro-osseous tunnel between the ulnar head and the ulnar styloid process. Distal to the extensor retinaculum, the ECU tendon inserts into the ulnar aspect of the base of the fifth metacarpal. The ECU muscle is innervated by the radial nerve.

The FCR muscle is bipennate and originates from the proximal radius and the interosseous membrane. The tendon of FCR enters a fibro-osseous tunnel formed by the distal pole of the scaphoid and the beak of the trapezium; it then angles dorsally to insert into the base of the second metacarpal. This fibro-osseous tunnel is separate from the carpal tunnel. The FCR muscle is innervated by the median nerve.

The FCU muscle is unipennate and originates from the medial epicondyle of the humerus and the proximal ulna. It is not constrained by a fibro-osseous tunnel, in distinction to the other primary wrist motors. It inserts into the pisiform and ultimately continues as the pisohamate ligament. The FCU muscle is innervated by the ulnar nerve.

VASCULAR ANATOMY
Extraosseous blood supply

The carpus receives its blood supply through branches from three dorsal and three palmar arches supplied by the radial, ulnar, anterior interosseous, and posterior interosseous arteries (Fig. 4-8). The three dorsal arches are named (proximal to distal) the *radiocarpal, intercarpal,* and *basal metacarpal transverse arches.* Anastomoses are often found between the arches, the radial and ulnar arteries, and the interosseous artery system. The palmar arches are named (proximal to distal) the *radiocarpal, intercarpal,* and *deep palmar arches.*

Intraosseous blood supply

All carpal bones, with the exception of the pisiform, receive their blood supply through dorsal and palmar entry sites and usually through more than one nutrient artery. Generally, a number of small-caliber penetrating vessels are found in addition to the major nutrient vessels. Intraosseous

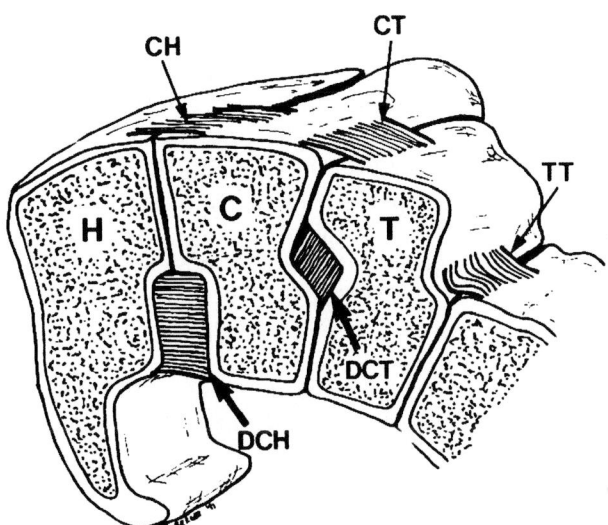

Fig. 4-7. Transverse section of the distal carpal row from distal and radial perspective. *C,* Capitate; *CH,* dorsal capitohamate ligament; *CT,* dorsal trapezocapitate ligament; *DCH,* deep capitohamate ligament; *DCT,* deep trapezocapitate ligament; *H,* hamate; *T,* trapezoid; *TT,* dorsal trapezium-trapezoid ligament.

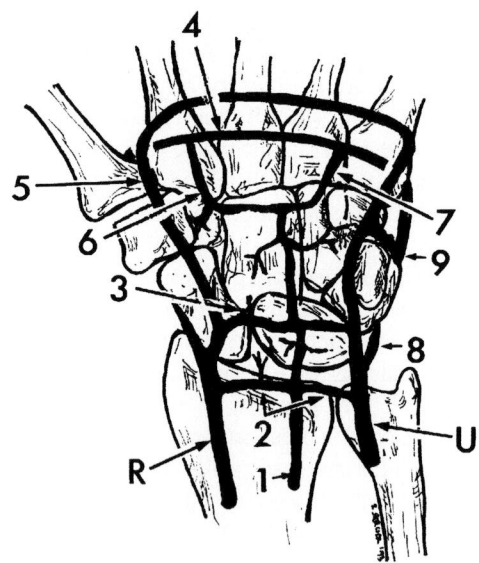

Fig. 4-8. Palmar extraosseous blood supply of the wrist. *1,* Anterior interosseous artery; *2-4,* transverse anastomotic arches; *5,* deep branch of radial artery; *6-9,* longitudinal anastomotic network. *R,* Radial artery; *U,* ulnar artery.

anastomoses can be found in three basic patterns. First, a direct anastomosis can occur between two large-diameter vessels within the bone. Second, anastomotic arcades may form with similar-sized vessels, often entering the bone from different areas. A final pattern, although rare, has been identified in which a diffuse arterial network virtually fills the bone.

Although the intraosseous vascular patterns of each carpal bone have been defined in detail, studies of the lunate, capitate, and scaphoid are particularly germane because of their predilection to the development of clinically important vascular problems. The lunate has only two surfaces available for vascular penetration: the dorsal and palmar. From the dorsal and palmar vascular plexuses, two to four penetrating vessels enter the lunate through each surface. Three consistent patterns of intraosseous vascularization have been identified, based on the pattern of anastomosis. When viewed in the sagittal plane, the anastomoses form either a Y, X, or an I pattern with arborization of small-caliber vessels stemming from the main branches. The proximal subchondral bone is consistently the least vascularized. The capitate is supplied by both the palmar and dorsal vascular plexuses; however, the palmar supply is more consistent and from larger-caliber vessels. Just distal to the neck of the capitate, vessels largely from the ulnar artery penetrate the palmar-ulnar cortex, while dorsal penetration occurs just distal to the midwaist level. The intraosseous vascularization pattern consists of proximally directed retrograde flow, with minimal anastomoses between dorsal and palmar vessels. When present, the dorsal vessels principally supply the head of the capitate, whereas the palmar vessels supply both the body and the head of the capitate. The scaphoid typically

receives its blood supply through three vessels originating from the radial artery: lateral-palmar, dorsal, and distal arterial branches. The lateral-palmar vessel is believed to be the principal blood supply of the scaphoid. All vessels penetrate the cortex of the scaphoid distal to the waist of the scaphoid, coursing in a retrograde fashion to supply the proximal pole. Although there have been reports of minor vascular penetrations directly into the proximal pole from the posterior interosseous artery, substantial risk for avascular necrosis of the proximal pole remains with displaced fractures through the waist of the scaphoid. Overall, it is thought that the remaining carpal bones generally have multiple nutrient vessels penetrating their cortices from more than one side, hence substantially reducing their risk of avascular necrosis.

KINEMATICS
Overview

Within 1 year after the announcement of the discovery of x rays, Bryce published a report of a roentgenographic investigation of the motions of the carpal bones. This marked a turning point for basic mechanical investigations of the wrist. The number of published biomechanical investigations of the wrist have increased almost exponentially over the past three decades. As such, a review of all mechanical analyses of the wrist is well beyond the scope of this chapter. Rather, a general overview of basic biomechanical considerations of the wrist is presented in the following categories: kinematics, kinetics, and material properties.

The global range of motion (ROM) of the wrist, measured clinically, is based on angular displacement of the hand about the "cardinal" axes of motion: palmar-flexion/dorsiflexion and radioulnar deviation. The conicoid motion generated by combining displacement involving all four directions of motion is called *circumduction*. A functional axis of motion has also been described as the *dart-throw axis,* which moves the wrist-hand unit from an extreme of dorsiflexion/radial deviation to an extreme of palmar-flexion/ulnar deviation. The magnitude of angular displacement in any direction varies greatly between individuals, but in "normal" individuals, it generally falls within the ranges of palmar-flexion (65 to 80 degrees), dorsiflexion (65 to 80 degrees), radial deviation (10 to 20 degrees), ulnar deviation (20 to 35 degrees), forearm pronation (80 degrees), and forearm supination (80 degrees).

Several attempts to define the "functional" ranges of wrist motion required for various tasks of daily living, as well as vocational and recreational activities, have been performed using axially aligned electrogoniometers fixed to the hand and forearm segments of volunteers. Although some variability between results was found, the vast majority of tested tasks could be accomplished with 40 degrees of dorsiflexion, 40 degrees of palmar-flexion, and 40 degrees of combined radial and ulnar deviation. The concept of a "center of rotation" of the wrist has been tested by a number

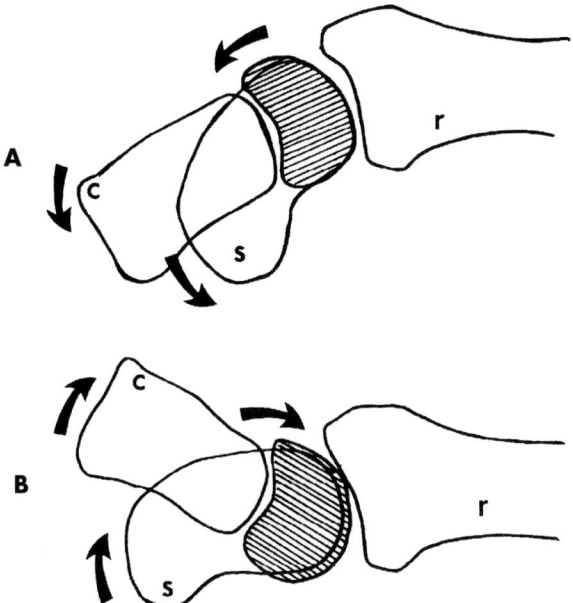

Fig. 4-9. Schematic of carpal bone motion during wrist palmar-flexion (**A**) and dorsiflexion (**B**). Note that all three bones essentially move in the same plane synchronously. *c,* Capitate; *r,* radius; *s,* scaphoid (lunate shown as shaded bone).

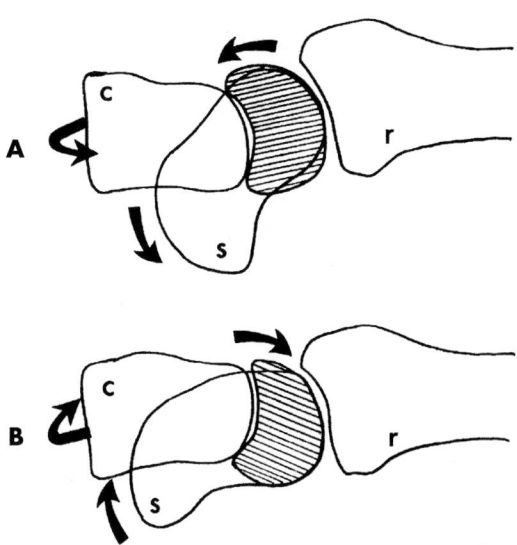

Fig. 4-10. Schematic of carpal bone motion during wrist radial deviation (**A**) and ulnar deviation (**B**). Note that the scaphoid and lunate primarily palmar-flex during radial deviation and dorsiflex during ulnar deviation. This behavior is called *conjunct rotation.* *c,* Capitate; *r,* radius; *s,* scaphoid (lunate shown as shaded bone).

of techniques and widely debated. It is generally agreed, however, that an approximation of an axis of flexion/extension motion of the hand unit on the forearm passes transversely through the head of the capitate, as does a separate orthogonal axis for radioulnar deviation. It must be remembered that the global motion of the wrist is a summation of the motions of the individual carpal bones through the intercarpal joints as well as the radiocarpal and midcarpal joints. Thus, although easier to understand, the concept of a center of rotation of the wrist is at best an approximation and of limited basic and clinical usefulness.

Individual carpal bone motion

The bones within each row display kinematic behaviors that are more similar than those observed between the two rows. Because the kinematic behaviors of the carpal bones are measurably different between palmar-flexion/dorsiflexion and radioulnar deviation, these two arcs of motion are considered separately (Figs. 4-9 and 4-10).

Palmar-flexion/dorsiflexion

The metacarpals are pulled through the range of palmar-flexion and dorsiflexion by the action of the extrinsic wrist motors attaching to their bases. The hand unit, made up of the metacarpals and phalanges, is securely associated with the distal carpal row through the articular interlocking and strong ligamentous connections of the second through fifth carpometacarpal joints. The trapezoid, capitate, and hamate undergo displacement with their respective metacarpals with

no significant deviation of direction or magnitude of motion (see Fig. 4-9). Because of the strong interosseous ligaments, the trapezium generally tracks with the trapezoid but remains under the influence of the mobile first metacarpal. The major direction of motion for this entire complex is palmar-flexion and dorsiflexion, with little deviation in radioulnar deviation and pronation/supination.

In general, the proximal row bones follow the direction of motion of the distal row bones during palmar-flexion/dorsiflexion of the wrist (see Fig. 4-9). However, the scaphoid, lunate, and triquetrum are not as tightly secured to the hand unit as are the distal row bones by virtue of the midcarpal joint. In addition, the interosseous ligaments between the proximal row bones allow substantial intercarpal motion. Thus there are measurable differences between the motions of the proximal and distal row bones, as well as between the individual bones of the proximal carpal row. This is most pronounced between the scaphoid and lunate. From the extreme of palmar-flexion to the extreme of dorsiflexion, the scaphoid undergoes substantially more angular displacement than the lunate, primarily in the plane of hand motion. There are measurable "out-of-plane" motions between the scaphoid and lunate as well because the scaphoid progressively supinates relative to the lunate as the wrist dorsiflexes. The effect of the differential direction and magnitude of displacement between the scaphoid and lunate is to create a relative separation between the palmar surfaces of the two bones as dorsiflexion is reached and a coaptation of the two surfaces as palmar-flexion is reached. The extremes of displacement are checked by the "twisting" of the fibers of the interosseous ligaments. Once this limit is reached, the scaphoid and lunate will move as a unit through the radiocarpal and midcarpal joints. Similar, although of lesser magnitude, behaviors occur through the LT joint. In all, the lunate experiences the least magnitude of rotation of all carpal bones during palmar-flexion and dorsiflexion. The radiocarpal and midcarpal joints contribute nearly equally to the range of dorsiflexion and palmar-flexion of the wrist when measured through the capitolunate/radiolunate joint column. In contrast, when measured through the radioscaphoid-STT joint column, more than two thirds of the ROM occurs through the radioscaphoid joint.

Radioulnar deviation

As with palmar-flexion and dorsiflexion, the bones of the distal row move essentially as a unit with themselves as well as with the second through fifth metacarpals during radial and ulnar deviation of the wrist (see Fig. 4-10). However, the proximal row bones display a remarkably different kinematic behavior. As a unit, the proximal carpal row displays a "reciprocating" motion with the distal row, such that the principal motion during wrist radial deviation is palmar-flexion (see Fig. 4-10). Conversely, during wrist ulnar deviation, the proximal carpal row dorsiflexes. In addition to the palmar-flexion/dorsiflexion activity of the proximal carpal row, a less pronounced motion occurs, resulting in ulnar displacement during wrist radial deviation and radial displacement during wrist ulnar deviation. Additional longitudinal axial displacements occur between the proximal carpal row bones, as they do during palmar-flexion and dorsiflexion. Although of substantially lower magnitude than the principal directions of rotation, these longitudinal axial displacements contribute to a relative separation between the palmar surfaces of the scaphoid and lunate in wrist ulnar deviation and a relative coaptation during wrist radial deviation, limited by the tautness of the SL interosseous ligament. Once maximum tension is achieved, the two bones will displace as a single unit. As with palmar-flexion and dorsiflexion, the lunate experiences the least magnitude of rotation of all carpal bones during radial and ulnar deviation. The magnitude of rotation through the midcarpal joint is approximately 1.5 times greater than the radiocarpal joint during radial and ulnar deviation.

KINETICS
Force analysis

Force analyses of the wrist have been attempted using a variety of methods, including the analytical methods of free-body diagrams and rigid-body spring models and experimental methods using force transducers, pressure-sensitive film, pressure transducers, and strain gauges. Because of the intrinsic geometric complexity of the wrist, the large number of carpal elements, the number of tissue interfaces that loads are applied to, and the large number of

positions that the wrist can assume, these analyses have been difficult and are riddled with assumptions. Thus relative changes and trends in forces brought about by the introduction of experimental variables are generally more useful than absolute values.

Normal joint forces

Experimental and analytical studies of force transmission across the wrist in the neutral position are in general agreement that approximately 80% of the force is transmitted across the radiocarpal joint and 20% across the ulnocarpal joint space (Fig. 4-11). This can be further compartmentalized into forces across the UL articulation (14%) and the UT articulation (8%). In the neutral position, one study reported that 78% of the longitudinal force across the wrist is transmitted through the radiocarpal articulation, with 46% transmitted by the radioscaphoid fossa and 32% by the lunate fossa. Forces across the midcarpal joint in a neutrally positioned joint have been estimated to be 31% through the STT joint, 19% through the SC joint, 29% through the lunocapitate joint, and 21% transmitted through the triquetrohamate joint. In general, it has been shown that forearm pronation increases ulnocarpal force transmission (up to 37% of total forces transmitted), with a corresponding decrease in radiocarpal force transmission. This has been theoretically linked to the relative distal prominence of the ulna that occurs in forearm pronation. The ulnocarpal force transmission increases to 28% of the total in ulnar deviation of the wrist, whereas radiocarpal forces increase to 87% of the total in radial deviation. Wrist palmar-flexion and dorsiflexion have only a modest effect on the relative forces transmitted through the radiocarpal and ulnocarpal joints.

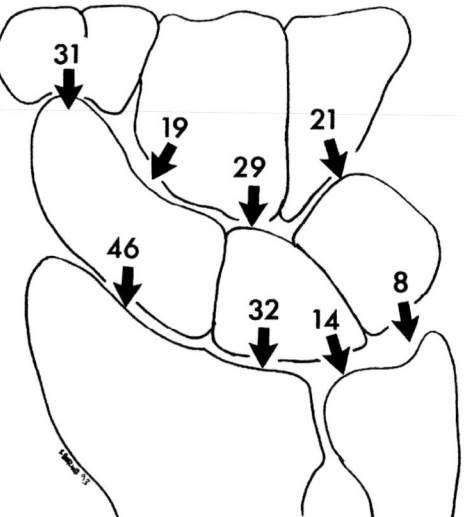

Fig. 4-11. Schematic of the wrist showing the approximate load percentages transmitted across the midcarpal joint and the percentages transmitted across the radiocarpal joint.

Normal joint contact area and pressure

With use of pressure-sensitive film placed in the radio-carpal joint space, three distinct areas of contact through the radiocarpal joint have been identified: radioscaphoid, radio-lunate, and UL. Overall, it has been determined that the actual area of contact of the scaphoid and lunate against the distal radius and TFCC are quite limited, regardless of joint position, averaging 20% of the entire available articular surface. The scaphoid contact area was greater than that of the lunate by an average factor of 1.5. The centroids of the contact areas shift with varying positions of the wrist, as do the areas of contact. For example, palmar-flexion of the scaphoid results in a dorsal and radial shift of the radio-scaphoid contact centroid and a progressive diminution of contact area. With externally applied loads, the peak articular pressures are low, ranging from 1.4 to 31.4 N/mm^2. The midcarpal joint has been difficult to evaluate using pressure-sensitive film because of its complex shape. It has been estimated that less than 40% of the available articular surface of the midcarpal joint is in actual contact at any one time. The relative contribution to the total contact of the STT, SC, lunocapitate, and triquetrohamate joints have been estimated to be 23%, 28%, 29%, and 20%, respectively. Thus it may be surmised that more than 50% of the midcarpal load is transmitted through the capitate across the scaphocapitate and lunocapitate joints.

BIBLIOGRAPHY

af Ekenstam FW: The distal radioulnar joint: an anatomical, experimental and clinical study with special reference to malunited fractures of the distal radius, *Abstracts of Uppsala Dissertations from the Faculty of Medicine* 505:1, 1984.

An K-N, Berger RA, Cooney WP, editors: *Biomechanics of the wrist joint,* New York, 1991, Springer-Verlag.

Berger RA: The anatomy and basic biomechanics of the wrist joint, *J Hand Ther* 84:93, 1996.

Berger RA: The ligaments of the wrist: a current overview of anatomy with considerations of their potential functions, *Hand Clin* 13:63, 1997.

Berger RA, Crowninshield RD, Flatt AE: The three-dimensional rotational behaviors of the carpal bones, *Clin Orthop* July:303, 1982.

Berger RA, Kauer JMG, Landsmeer JMF: The radioscapholunate ligament: a gross and histologic study of fetal and adult wrists, *J Bone Surg* 16A:350, 1991.

Berger RA, Landsmeer JMF: The palmar radiocarpal ligaments: a study of adult and fetal human wrist joints, *J Hand Surg* 1SA:847, 1990.

Bowers W: The distal radioulnar joint. In Green D, editor: *Operative hand surgery,* ed 3, New York, 1993, Churchill Livingstone.

Drewniany JJ, Palmer AK, Flatt AE: The scaphotrapezial ligament complex: an anatomic and biomechanical study, *J Hand Surg* 10A:492, 1985.

Gelberman RH, et a;: The arterial anatomy of the human carpus. Part I: the extraosseous vascularity, *J Hand Surg* 8:367, 1983.

Landsmeer JMF: *Atlas of anatomy of the hand,* New York, 1976, Churchill Livingstone.

Lange A, de Kauer JMG, Huiskes R: The kinematical behavior of the human wrist joint: a roentgenstereophotogrammetric analysis, *J Orthop Res* 3:56, 1985.

Lewis OJ: The development of the human wrist joint during the fetal period, *Anat Rec* 166:499, 1970.

Lewis OJ, Hamshire JR, Bucknill TM: The anatomy of the wrist joint, *J Anat* 106:539, 1970.

Mizuseki T, Ikuta Y: The dorsal carpal ligaments: their anatomy and function, *J Hand Surg* 14B:91, 1989.

Palmer AK, Warner FW: The triangular fibrocartilage complex of the wrist: anatomy and function, *J Hand Surg* 6:153, 1981.

Panais JS, et a;: The arterial anatomy of the human carpus. Part II. The intraosseous vascularity, *J Hand Surg* 8:375, 1983.

Ruby LK, et al: Relative motions of selected carpal bones: a kinematic analysis of the normal wrist, *J Hand Surg* 13A:1, 1988.

Schuind F, et al: The distal radioulnar ligament: a biomechanical study, *J Hand Surg* 16A:1106, 1991.

Seradge H, et al: Segmental motion of the proximal carpal row: their global effect on the wrist motion, *J Hand Surg* 15A:236, 1990.

Taleisnik J: The ligaments of the wrist, *J Hand Surg* 1:110, 1976.

Youm Y, et al: Kinematics of the wrist. I. An experimental study of radial-ulnar deviation and flexion-extension, *J Bone Joint Surg* 60A:423, 1978.

Chapter 5

ANATOMY AND KINESIOLOGY OF THE ELBOW

Stuart D. Patterson

The ability to bring the hand to one's mouth and perineum, in addition to placing the hand in space, is critically important to us as individuals. This motion, permitted by the elbow joint and the guiding neuromuscular system, allows us to perform our personal care and daily activities, which maintains our self-esteem and independence. While the shoulder allows us to place the hand on the surface of a hemisphere, it is the elbow that allows us to position the hand anywhere within that hemisphere (Fig. 5-1). As elbow motion is lost, the functional loss increases disproportionately. A 30-degree flexion contracture will result in a 28% functional loss, whereas a 60-degree flexion contracture will cause a 60% functional loss.[3,31]

Knowledge of the anatomic and biomechanical factors that contribute to the normal and pathologic function of the elbow joint is the foundation for successful treatment of our patients.

ANATOMY

The anatomy of the elbow joint is unique because of the proximity of three major peripheral nerves to the joint capsule (radial, ulnar, and median) and the presence of three major complex articulations within one joint capsule (ulnotrochlear, radiocapitellar, and proximal radioulnar). It is these characteristics, more so than any other, that has historically placed obstacles in the path of treatment. Extensive anatomic, kinematic, and biomechanical investigations of the elbow since the early 1980s, have significantly improved our knowledge. The joint is now viewed as being more forgiving as compared with the opinions and experiences of therapists and physicians 30 years ago.

The presence of the three articulations within the single synovial cavity of the elbow joint is a potentially compli-

cating situation. Infection or arthritis can affect all three, resulting in a loss of not only elbow flexion/extension but also forearm rotation. In addition, the functional linkage between the proximal and distal radioulnar joints has to be considered when dealing with conditions that may affect both, for example, a comminuted fracture of the radial head in association with an interosseous membrane disruption.

Despite the fact that we do not walk on our hands, the articular surfaces of the elbow joint are subjected to forces that equal or exceed those of the lower extremity joints. This is a consequence of long lever arms, which transmit high loads from the hand to the elbow. To overcome these forces, the elbow flexors and extensors generate large muscle tensions. This places large loads on the articular surfaces, which may exceed three times the body weight, as well as the soft tissue constraints.[1,2,31] These loads may compromise the outcome of elbow joint reconstruction, especially joint arthroplasty. An understanding of elbow anatomy and function will assist in formulating an appropriate management plan for patients.

Joint osteology and articulations

The elbow joint consists of the articulations between the humerus, radius, and ulna. The elbow is highly congruous and stable. The synovial cavity of the ulnotrochlear and radiocapitellar joints is continuous with the proximal radioulnar joint. The capitellum of the distal humerus is hemispherical, whereas the trochlea is shaped like a cotton reel, with a central trochlear groove and flared medial and lateral lips. The medial lip projects further distally than the lateral lip. Hyaline cartilage covers the anterior, inferior, and posterior articular surfaces of the trochlea, while only the anterior and inferior surfaces of the capitellum are covered (Fig. 5-2).

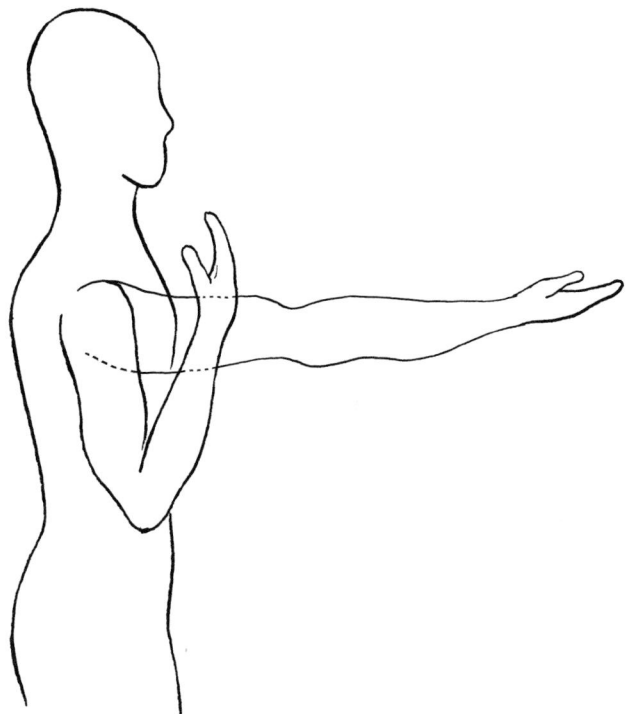

Fig. 5-1. Functional range of elbow motion. The elbow permits placement of the hand within the sphere circumscribed by the shoulder.

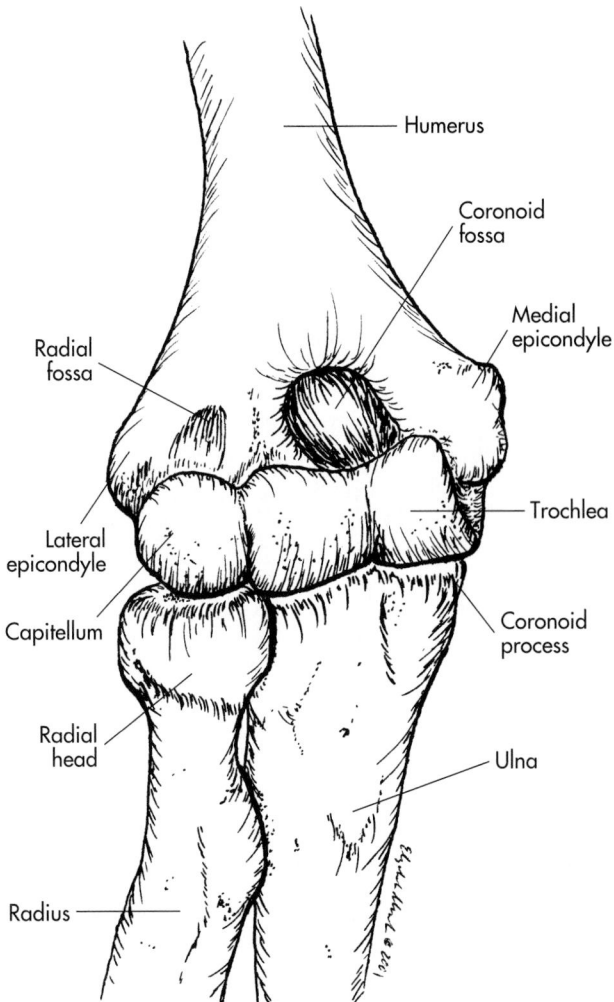

Fig. 5-2. Anterior elbow osseous anatomy.

Sagittal sections of the trochlea demonstrate that it has a slightly elliptical shape, which results in the olecranon and coronoid articular facets contacting the trochlea, but not the central area of the ulnar greater sigmoid notch.[1,2] Between the capitellum and trochlea is a shallow ridge, which articulates with the edge of the radial head through the full arc of flexion. The axis of rotation of the distal humerus lies at a 6- to 8-degree valgus tilt, relative to the long axis of the humerus.[22] This angulation contributes to the normal carrying angle of the elbow, which is a mean of 17.8 degrees in the adult population.[6] The axes of rotation of the capitellum and trochlea lie almost in a straight line, which facilitates reconstructive procedures on the elbow when replication of the axis is required (e.g., prosthetic arthroplasty, placement of dynamic external fixators).[1,22]

Anteriorly, there are fossae on the distal humerus to accommodate the tip of the coronoid (coronoid fossa) and radial head (radial fossa) in full flexion. Posteriorly, the olecranon fossa receives the tip of the olecranon in full extension. These fossae are necessary to allow full flexion and extension, respectively. Obliteration of these fossae as a result of malunion, heterotopic ossification, loose bodies, or osteoarthritic new bone formation will block motion (Fig. 5-3). The distal articular surface of the humerus is internally rotated 5 to 7 degrees, in 6 to 8 degrees valgus and flexed 30 to 45 degrees[16,21,22,31,34] (Fig. 5-4).

Supporting the articular surface of the distal humerus are the medial and lateral columns. The medial column includes the medial epicondyle, which gives origin to the flexor pronator muscles and the medial collateral ligament. The lateral epicondyle gives origin to the common extensor muscles and the lateral collateral ligament complex.

Articulating with the distal humerus are the ulna and radius. The proximal ulna is formed by the olecranon process, greater sigmoid or trochlear notch, and the coronoid process. The proximal ulna is angled on average 14 degrees varus to the shaft, with a range of 6 to 23 degrees.[1,2] When placing implants into the distal ulna, it is important to be aware of this to avoid perforating the ulna cortex. The greater sigmoid notch is concave with a central V-shaped ridge that articulates with the trochlear groove (Fig. 5-5). At the midportion of the greater sigmoid notch is a "bare spot" not covered by articular cartilage.[35] The olecranon process, into which the triceps inserts, serves as a secondary constraint to varus and valgus stress in full extension. Progressive loss of

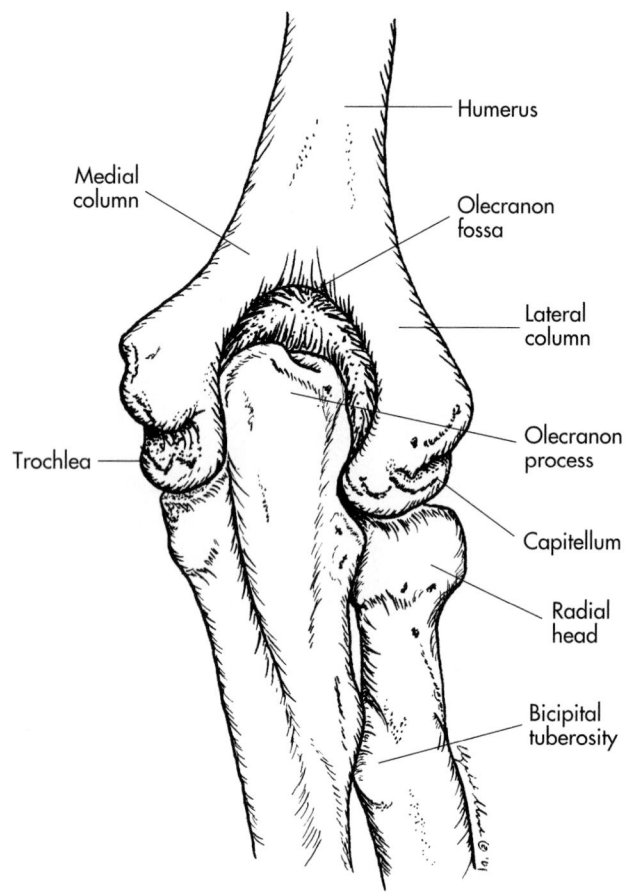

Fig. 5-3. Posterior elbow osseous anatomy.

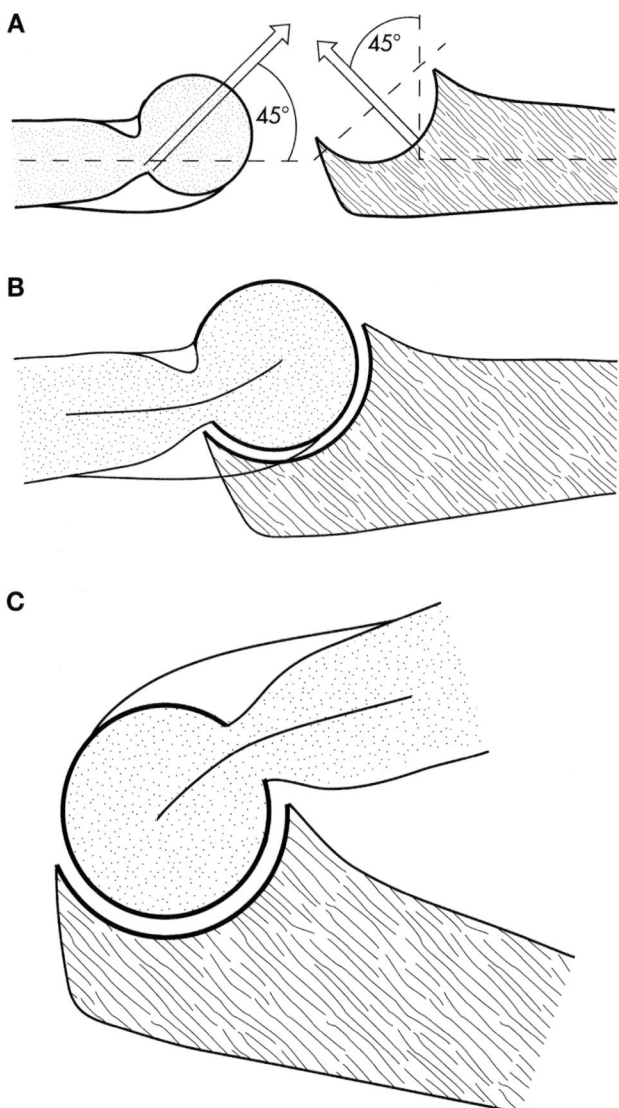

Fig. 5-4. Ulnohumeral joint alignment. **A,** Because of the 45-degree alignment of the capitellum and greater sigmoid notch of the ulna, the ulnohumeral joint has a theoretical range of motion from 0 to 180 degrees. **B,** Ulnohumeral joint alignment in full extension. **C,** Ulnohumeral joint alignment in full flexion.

the olecranon causes increasing instability of the ulno-humeral joint.[5] The coronoid process, which forms the anterior flare of the proximal ulna, acts as a major restraint to posterior instability of the elbow. The anterior joint capsule inserts, on average, 6.4 mm distal to the tip of the coronoid process.[7] Adjacent to the coronoid on the lateral aspect is the lesser sigmoid or radial notch, which articulates with the radial head. Distal to this is the supinator crest, into which the lateral ulnar collateral ligament inserts and from which the supinator muscle takes origin. Medial, and on average 18.4 mm dorsal to the tip of the coronoid process, is the sublime tubercle, into which the medial collateral ligament inserts and from which a portion of the flexor digitorum superficialis (FDS) originates.[7]

The proximal radioulnar joint permits rotation, translation, and axial motion (see Fig. 5-5). The radial head is oval, not round. The head of the radius has a concave surface, resembling a shallow dish; this surface articulates with the convex hemisphere of the capitellum. The beveled margins of the head articulate with the shallow ridge on the medial margin of the capitellum. The radius of curvature of the radial articular dish is larger than that of the capitellum, which permits translation of the head during forearm motion.

However, this lack of congruence also creates high contact pressures and probably accounts for the appearance of osteoarthritis at this articulation first.[1] Hyaline cartilage covers approximately 250 degrees of the margin of the radial head, which articulates with the lesser sigmoid notch of the ulna.[32] The 110-degree bare area on the radial head margin provides an area for the placement of internal fixation devices.[32] The radial head is set eccentrically on the radial neck, with an average offset of 4.2 ± 2.5 mm.[19] This creates a camshaft effect, with the center of the head moving away from the ulna in supination. There is no correlation between the radial head and neck diameter.[19] This has implications for prosthetic design.

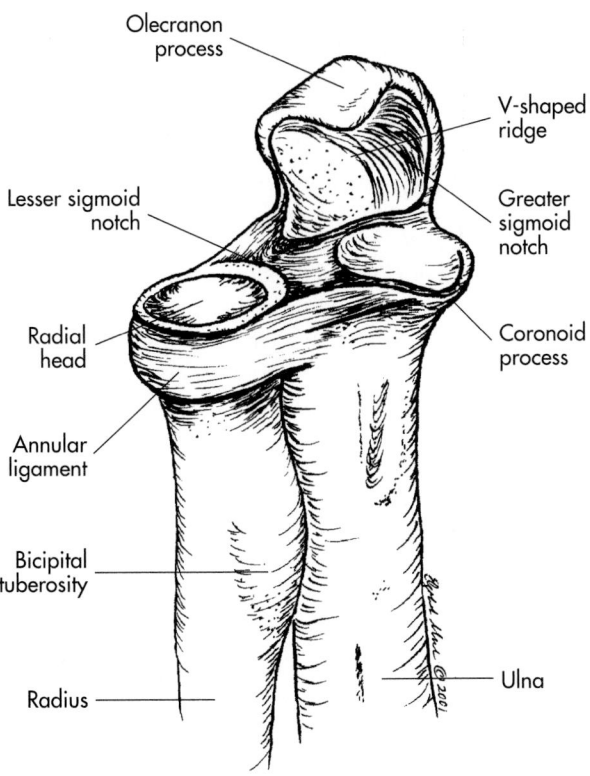

Fig. 5-5. Proximal radioulnar joint.

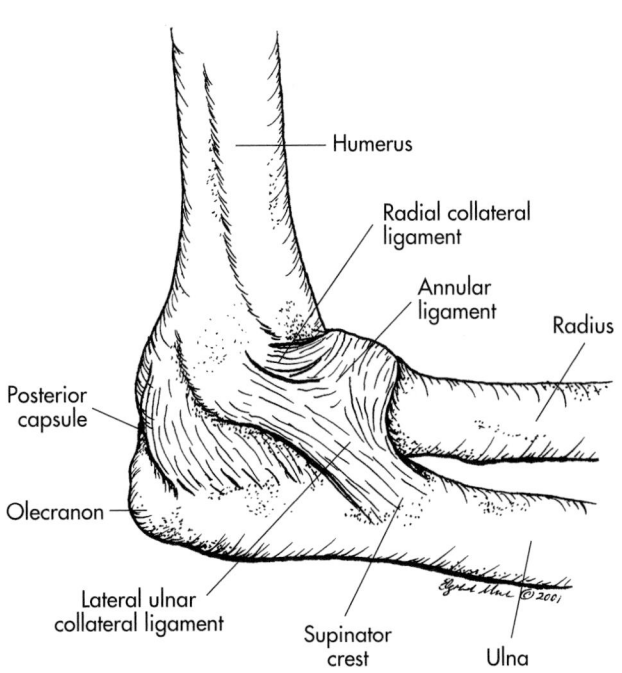

Fig. 5-6. Lateral elbow anatomy.

The bicipital or radial tuberosity serves as the insertion point for the biceps brachii tendon. The neck-shaft angle of the radius is, on average, 10 degrees, with the radial tuberosity sitting at the apex of the angle. Kapandji[16] has termed this angle the *supinator bend.* This angle permits the radius to rotate over the ulna in pronation and provides the biceps muscle with a crank to pull on. Distally, the natural radial bow results in the *pronator bend,* which provides another crank handle onto which the pronator teres inserts. These two bends lie on opposite sides of the forearm axis of rotation.[16]

During the management of radial shaft malunions, the radial tuberosity is a useful landmark to determine the rotation of the proximal radius relative to the distal radius on plain radiographs. Restoration of the radial bow is essential to preserve the normal range and power of forearm rotation.

Capsule, ligaments, and bursae

The elbow capsule attaches around the rims of the olecranon and coronoid fossae proximally, distally around the neck of the radius and distal to the tip of the coronoid.[35] At the distal edge of the annular ligament there is no discernible capsule. As a consequence, inflammatory synovium tends to extrude through this area and can infiltrate between the tissue planes, far into the midforearm.

The normal volume of the elbow joint is 25 ml.[22] In the

normal state, the capsule is extremely thin. However, after trauma, the capsule becomes markedly thickened, which may result in joint stiffness. The posterior and anterior joint capsule do not contribute to joint stability.[24] Lying posteriorly and anteriorly, between the capsule and synovium, are fat pads.[35] Joint effusions displace these away from the humerus and can be detected on radiographs, the so-called fat pad sign. Medially and laterally, the collateral ligament complexes develop from capsular thickenings.

The lateral collateral ligament complex consists of the radial collateral, annular, and lateral ulnar collateral ligaments[22,27] (Fig. 5-6). As a result of the recent interest in posterolateral rotatory instability of the elbow, the lateral collateral ligament complex has been extensively studied.[4,22,27,28,37]

The radial collateral ligament originates on the lateral epicondyle and merges with the annular ligament.

The annular ligament is a strong fibrocartilagenous band that encircles the radial head, stabilizing the proximal radius to the ulna.[20,35] It attaches to the anterior and posterior lips of the lesser sigmoid notch of the proximal ulna. It consists of three layers, formed by the inner joint capsule, intermediate radial fibers, and outer radial and lateral collateral ligament fibers.[20] Posteriorly, the annular ligament is wider and stronger. The inferior aspect of the annular ligament is continuous with the radius by virtue of a very tenuous membrane, which gives attachment to the synovium. This permits the radius to rotate relative to the ulna. With the radius in neutral rotation, the annular ligament is equally tensioned anteriorly and posteriorly. However, with full pronation, the posterior part of the annular ligament is tensioned. The opposite is true of full supination, when the anterior ligament is under tension.[20]

The quadrate ligament has been described as a thin structure lying on the inferior aspect of the annular ligament, between the radius and ulna.[35] However, the presence of this ligament is disputed.[20]

Posterior to the radial collateral ligament is the lateral ulnar collateral ligament. The ligament inserts on the lateral epicondyle and passes distally to insert onto the supinator crest, posterior to the radial head. This ligament is considered the primary constraint to posterolateral rotatory instability.[4,27,28] The lateral ulnar collateral ligament provides increasing stability to the elbow as it is flexed from full extension. Maximum stability is seen at 110 degrees. The corollary is true; that is, after disruption of this ligament, maximum laxity is seen at 110 degrees. During forced varus stress with the forearm supinated, the lateral collateral ligament is a primary stabilizer.[27,28] Reconstruction of the lateral collateral ligament restores stability.[37]

The medial collateral ligament insertion on the humerus is from the anteroinferior surface of the medial epicondyle.[26] It consists of anterior, posterior, and transverse bundles[12,13,22] (Fig. 5-7). The anterior bundle is the primary constraint to valgus instability.[4,22] This has been divided into anterior and posterior bands, with the anterior band being the more important stabilizer to valgus instability.[12] The greatest contribution to stability in valgus stress occurs between 60 and 90 degrees of flexion.[12] In full extension, the olecranon locks into the olecranon fossa and equal amounts of restraint

to valgus stress are contributed by the medial collateral ligament, articular surfaces, and joint capsule.[30] The medial collateral ligament is not isometric through flexion/extension. The most isometric portion of the anterior bundle is situated on the anterior and medial aspect. The anterior bundle is under tension throughout the flexion arc, whereas the posterior bundle is taut in flexion and loose in extension.[12,13] In patients undergoing a posterior elbow capsulectomy for loss of flexion, release of the posterior bundle may be required. Loss of the posterior bundle does not result in elbow instability.[13] The transverse bundle serves no significant purpose.

Bursae are found superficially over the olecranon process and deeply interposed between the biceps tendon and the bicipital tuberosity. The olecranon bursa first appears at the age of 7.[8] Inflammatory conditions such as gout or rheumatoid arthritis can affect the olecranon bursa. Most commonly, local repetitive trauma results in localized swelling. Bursae can also be found over the medial and lateral epicondyles.[9,22] The cubital or bicipitoradial bursa can also become inflamed and enlarged because of repetitive trauma or inflammatory conditions such as rheumatoid arthritis.[17] Other deeply placed bursae can be found between the capsule of the radiocapitellar joint and the deep surface of the extensor carpi radialis brevis (ECRB), and the olecranon process and triceps tendon.[22]

Muscles

The muscles of the elbow are divided into flexors, extensors, pronators, and supinators. Some muscles perform more than one activity, whereas others contract under specific conditions of load.

Surrounding the muscles of the arm is the deep investing fascia, which on the medial and lateral aspects, thickens to form the medial and lateral intermuscular septae, respectively. This divides the arm into anterior and posterior muscle compartments.[35]

The muscles have short lever arms because of their insertions close to the joint. This contrasts with the long lever arm of the hand and forearm. Consequently, the muscles need to generate large forces to overcome the biomechanical disadvantage. Therefore it is not surprising that the largest joint reaction forces occur in full extension.[1,2,4,31] Flexion and extension strength appears to be greatest between 60 and 90 degrees of flexion and neutral to full supination.[1,2,31] The greatest pronation and supination torques are generated when the forearm is fully supinated and pronated, respectively. This is due to the mechanical advantage provided by the tenodesis effect.[1]

The short lever arms of the elbow muscles have a kinematic advantage, in that a small amplitude contraction applied close to the joint axis of rotation will result in a large arc of motion for the distal extremity.[31]

The primary flexor of the elbow is the brachialis with the brachioradialis acting as the secondary flexor. Because of the

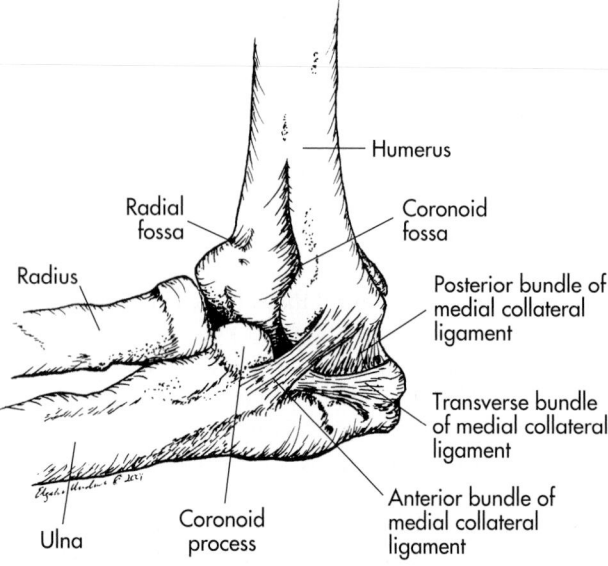

Fig. 5-7. Medial elbow anatomy.

insertion of the brachialis onto the ulna, the brachialis is active as an elbow flexor in any position of forearm rotation.[5a] Brachialis is innervated by the musculocutaneous nerve and brachioradialis by the radial nerve. The brachioradialis is always active in flexion, but more so when a load is applied.[1,2,5a] Brachioradialis also acts as a weak pronator and supinator when the forearm is in full resisted supination and pronation, respectively.[1,2]

Biceps brachii is the primary supinator of the forearm and a secondary flexor. The muscle has a long and short head, both of which are active during elbow flexion. In the supinated position, the biceps is usually active irrespective of the applied load. However, with the forearm fully pronated, the biceps is often inactive, even when a load is applied.[1,5a] Related to this finding is the observation that the biceps insertion on the radial tuberosity is closer to the elbow in pronation, compared with supination. This results in a 35% smaller moment arm. Therefore, for a given muscle force, this produces a reduced torque.[15] Similarly, the biceps is inhibited when the elbow is fully extended and recruited when a load is applied. The lacertus fibrosis is a sheet of strong fascia that arises from the medial border of the biceps tendon, which merges into the deep fascia on the medial aspect of the forearm.[35] The brachial artery and median nerve lie immediately beneath the lacertus fibrosis. Biceps brachii is innervated by the musculocutaneous nerve.

Triceps is the primary extensor of the elbow. It consists of the long, medial, and lateral heads; all are innervated by the radial nerve. The three heads are recruited sequentially, depending on the load applied to the extremity. The medial head is usually activated first, followed by the lateral and then the long. The medial head is always active, irrespective of the load applied.[5a] As the long head crosses the shoulder joint, it is suppressed when shoulder flexion is required.

The pronator teres acts primarily as a pronator of the forearm, but it is a secondary elbow flexor, especially when load is applied to the hand.[1,2,5a] When performing unresisted pronation, only the pronator quadratus contracts. However, with resisted pronation, the pronator teres is recruited.[5a] Elbow position does not affect the activity of the pronator teres.[5a] The pronator teres has a superficial and deep head between which passes the median nerve, which innervates both. The median nerve can be compressed where it passes beneath the fibrous arch that connects the two heads. The pronator teres inserts into the middle third of the radius.

The supinator muscle, innervated by the posterior interosseous nerve, is a secondary forearm supinator. Supinator acts alone when supination is unresisted, but with resistance, the biceps is recruited. It consists of a superficial and deep head, with the posterior interosseous nerve passing between the two heads, beneath the arcade of Frohse.[35] The deep head arises from the supinator crest of the ulna and the superficial head from the lateral humeral epicondyle. The two heads pass medially around the radius to insert between the anterior and posterior oblique lines of the radius.

Although the wrist extensors and flexors cross anterior to the axis of rotation of the elbow, their contribution to elbow flexion is small.[1]

The anconeus, innervated by the radial nerve, functions as both an extensor and possibly an abductor of the ulna. It appears to be active with most elbow motions and it has been proposed that it may act as an elbow stabilizer.[5a,22]

The anconeus epitrochlearis is a vestigial muscle found on the medial aspect of the elbow in 3% to 28% of the population.[25] It extends from the medial epicondyle of the distal humerus to the olecranon, superficial to the ulnar nerve. This may cause compression of the ulnar nerve.

Nerves

The major sensorimotor nerves that cross the elbow are the median, ulnar, and radial nerves. All of the motor nerves supply branches to the joint.[35] In addition, there are numerous cutaneous nerves that are important because of their propensity to lie in areas where skin incisions are made. To prevent significant injury to these nerves, knowledge of their relationships to surgical approaches is essential. Most reconstructive procedures on the elbow can be performed through a posterior midline skin incision, which avoids the major cutaneous nerves.[11]

The radial nerve, having passed posterior to the humerus in the spiral groove, wraps around the lateral margin of the humerus about 10 to 12 cm proximal to the lateral epicondyle. It then lies anterior to the humerus between the brachialis and brachioradialis, before passing deep to the brachioradialis, extensor carpi radialis longus, ECRB, and extensor digitorum communis. Beneath the brachioradialis, the radial nerve divides into the superficial radial nerve and posterior interosseous nerve.[35] The division is most commonly proximal to the radiocapitellar joint line.[35] The superficial branch continues distally beneath the brachioradialis, and the posterior interosseous nerve passes through the arcade of Frohse, between the superficial and deep heads of supinator, into the radial tunnel. The nerve is intramuscular in 98% of cases.[33] Before the nerve enters the radial tunnel, it innervates the ECRB and supinator.[35] After it exits the radial tunnel, branches of the posterior interosseous nerve supply the extensor muscles. The radial nerve may be compressed as it passes deep to the common extensors and through the radial tunnel. This may be due to anatomic variants (arcade of Frohse) or an abnormal pathologic condition (rheumatoid synovitis).

In the distal arm, the median nerve lies medial to the brachialis and brachial artery, along the medial intermuscular septum. Occasionally, a supracondylar process, 2 to 20 mm long, may be present 5 cm proximal to the medial epicondyle on the anteromedial humerus.[35] When this occurs, an associated ligament of Struthers passes from the supracondylar process to the medial epicondyle.[18] The median nerve and brachial artery may be compressed as they pass beneath the ligament.[18] The nerve passes into the forearm between the superficial and deep heads of pronator teres. The anterior interosseous nerve is given off at this point, which passes deep to the FDS.

The ulnar nerve lies on the medial aspect of the triceps and on the posterior aspect of the medial intermuscular septum (Fig. 5-8). It passes through the cubital tunnel, beneath the cubital tunnel retinaculum.[25] Articular branches are given to the joint at this level, before it passes between the humeral and ulnar heads of the flexor carpi ulnaris (FCU). The ulnar nerve can be compressed under the cubital tunnel retinaculum or the fascia between the two heads of FCU. With elbow flexion, there is stretching of the nerve over the medial epicondyle and narrowing of the cubital tunnel, with a decrease in cross-sectional area of the nerve[14] (Fig. 5-9).

The medial antebrachial cutaneous nerve lies on the anterior aspect of the medial intermuscular septum, dividing into two main branches above the medial epicondyle. The anterior branch passes down the median of the forearm, and the posterior branch crosses posteriorly over the medial epicondyle area. A direct medial approach to the elbow exposes this nerve to possible injury.[10]

The lateral antebrachial cutaneous nerve is the terminal branch of the musculocutaneous nerve.[35] It pierces the antebrachial fascia after passing across the anterolateral aspect of the elbow joint, where it lies on the lateral side of the biceps tendon. The nerve is at risk when surgery is undertaken on the biceps tendon. The posterior cutaneous nerve of the forearm, a branch of the radial nerve, lies on the posterolateral aspect of the arm and forearm.

Anatomic dissections of the midline of the elbow demonstrate a paucity of major cutaneous nerves.[11] This allows the surgeon to place a posterior longitudinal skin incision in the midline of the elbow, with a decreased risk of cutaneous nerve injury.[11]

Vascular

Anterior to the elbow lie the large subcutaneous veins. These veins drain into the lateral cephalic and medial basilic veins. The basilic vein lies deep to the superficial fascia in the distal arm, whereas the cephalic vein is superficial. Two large venae comitantes, or brachial veins, can be found adjacent to the brachial artery. No large veins are found on the posterior aspect of the elbow.[9,35]

The elbow has an excellent blood supply, with a profuse collateral vessel complex.[36] The brachial artery lies lateral to the median nerve in the cubital fossa. Within the fossa, at the level of the radial neck, it divides into the radial and ulnar arteries. The radial artery follows the medial edge of the biceps tendon, anterior to the supinator, before passing deep to the brachioradialis. The ulnar artery passes deep to the pronator teres.[35] Division of the brachial artery seldom results in an ischemic hand because of the collateral circulation. This collateral circulation is formed from the superior and inferior ulnar collateral arteries and radial and middle collateral arteries, which anastomose distally with the posterior and anterior ulnar recurrent arteries and radial and interosseous recurrent arteries respectively.[35,36]

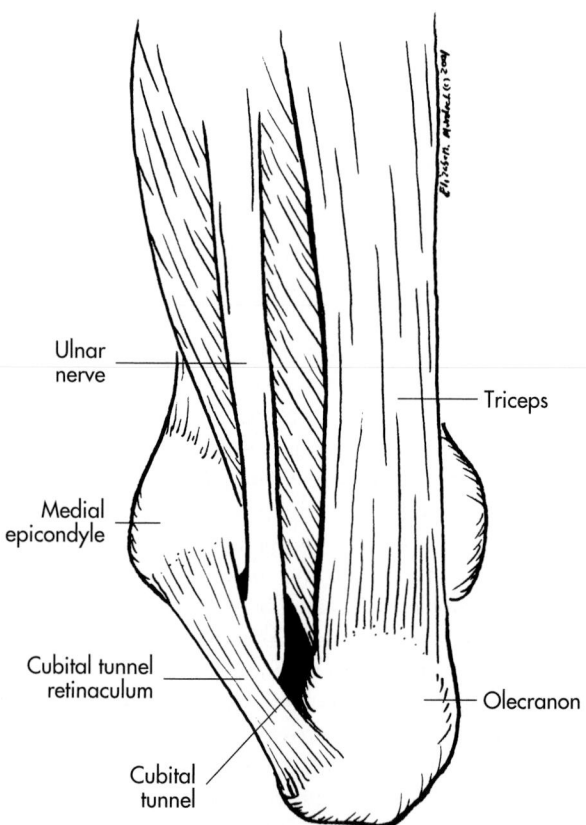

Fig. 5-9. Posterior cubital tunnel anatomy.

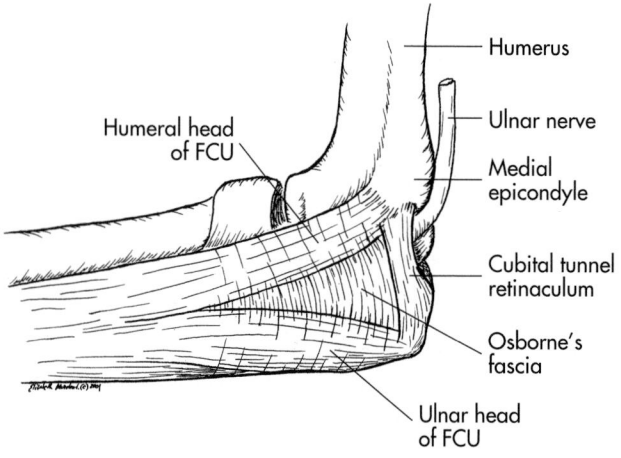

Fig. 5-8. Medial cubital tunnel anatomy. *FCU,* Flexor carpi ulnaris.

KINESIOLOGY

The study of joint movement is termed *kinesiology,* from the Greek words *kinein,* meaning "to move," and *logos,* meaning "to discourse."[29] Thus kinesiology combines the principles of anatomy, biomechanics, and physiology. The anatomic features of the elbow joint reviewed in the previous pages, along with the physiology of the connective tissues, determine the biomechanical factors that account for elbow motion.

In the anatomic position, the forearm is fully extended, maximally supinated, and adducted at the side. By convention, the 180-degree arc subtended by the humerus and ulna in the fully extended neutral position is measured as 0 degrees flexion (see Fig. 5-1). Additional extension is considered hyperextension. The elbow flexes from an average of 0 to 146 degrees.[1,23,30] Morrey and An[23] have demonstrated that most activities of daily living (ADLs) can be performed with a 100-degree arc of flexion between 30 and 130 degrees. Hyperextension occurs most commonly in skeletally immature females. This is limited by impingement of the olecranon process against the olecranon fossa. The anterior soft tissues interposed between the arm and forearm limit flexion (Fig. 5-4, *C*). Consequently, motion tends to be greater in children and those with thin extremities, compared with the elderly and those with obese or muscular extremities.

Forearm rotation occurs around an axis that passes through the capitellum, head of the radius, and distal ulna. The proximal and distal radioulnar joints act as a single functional unit with coaxial proximal and distal radioulnar joints. Kapandji[16] provides an excellent analogy to explain this important observation. Each radioulnar joint acts like the upper and lower hinges of a door. Malalignment of either hinge results in loss of normal rotation. Forearm rotation is measured with the elbow flexed to 90 degrees, the palm of the hand facing medially in the sagittal plane, and the extremity adducted at the side. Average pronation is 76 degrees, and supination is 81 degrees.[1,30] Morrey and An[23] have demonstrated that the majority of our ADLs can be performed with 50 degrees supination and 50 degrees pronation, for a total pronosupination arc of 100 degrees. In general, a loss of pronation is better tolerated than a loss of supination because of the compensatory motion of the shoulder. As we age, supination is lost.[1]

As the pronated radius supinates around the ulna, the ulna adducts and flexes.[16] The adduction-abduction or varus-valgus motion of the ulna occurs as a result of laxity of the collateral ligaments and averages 9 degrees.[1] This varus-valgus motion is also seen with elbow flexion/extension and averages 3 to 4 degrees.[1,4] Failure to recognize the mandatory varus-valgus movement of the ulna during the development of the totally constrained hinged elbow arthroplasties resulted in implant rapid loosening and failure. The current semiconstrained total elbow prostheses permit this motion through a "sloppy hinge."

Because of the oval shape of the radial head, as the forearm moves from pronation to supination, the radial head translates laterally. This moves the radial head center of rotation laterally about 2 mm.[16,30]

Pronation of the forearm results in proximal movement of the radius, whereas supination causes distal movement of the radius.[4]

SUMMARY

Elbow anatomy is the foundation on which we build our surgical approaches and operative interventions. Knowledge of elbow anatomy and kinesiology allows us to rehabilitate the elbow after trauma or surgery, enabling us to initiate early motion while ensuring joint stability.

REFERENCES

1. Amis AA: Biomechanics of the elbow. In Wallace WA, editor: *Joint replacement in the shoulder and elbow,* Oxford, 1998, Butterworth-Heinemann.
2. Amis AA: Biomechanics of the elbow. In Stanley D, Kay NRM, editors: *Surgery of the elbow: practical and scientific aspects,* London, 1998, Arnold.
3. An K-N, Morrey BF: Biomechanics: basic relevant concepts. Section I: basic science. In Morrey BF, Chao EYS, editors: *Joint replacement arthroplasty,* New York, 1991, Churchill Livingstone.
4. An K-N, Morrey BF: Biomechanics of the elbow. In Morrey BF, editor: *The elbow and its disorders,* Philadelphia, 2000, WB Saunders.
5. An K-N, Morrey BF, Chao EYS: The effect of partial removal of proximal ulna on elbow constraint, *Clin Orthop* 209:270, 1986.
5a. Basmajian JV: *Muscles alive,* ed 4, Baltimore, 1978, Williams & Wilkins.
6. Beals RK: The normal carrying angle of the elbow, *Clin Orthop* 119:194, 1976.
7. Cage DJN, et al: Soft tissue attachments of the ulnar coronoid process, *Clin Orthop* 320:154, 1995.
8. Chen J, et al: Development of the olecranon bursa: an anatomic cadaver study, *Acta Orthop Scand* 58:408, 1987.
9. De Boer P: Anatomy of the elbow. In Stanley D, Kay NRM, editors: *Surgery of the elbow,* London, 1998, Arnold.
10. Dellon AL, Mackinnon SE: Injury to the medial antebrachial cutaneous nerve during cubital tunnel surgery, *J Hand Surg* 10B:33, 1985.
11. Dowdy PA, et al: The midline posterior elbow incision, *J Bone Joint Surg* 77B:696, 1995.
12. Floris S, et al: The medial collateral ligament of the elbow joint: anatomy and kinematics, *J Shoulder Elbow Surg* 7:345, 1998.
13. Fuss FK: The ulnar collateral ligament of the human elbow joint: anatomy, function and biomechanics, *J Anat* 175:203, 1991.
14. Gelberman RH, et al: Changes in interstitial pressure and cross-sectional area of the cubital tunnel and of the ulnar nerve with flexion of the elbow, *J Bone Joint Surg* 80A:492, 1998.
15. Grabiner MD: The elbow and radioulnar joints. In Rasch PJ, editor: *Kinesiology and applied anatomy,* Philadelphia, 1989, Lea & Febiger.
16. Kapandji IA: *The physiology of the joints. Volume 1, Upper limb,* ed 2, New York, 1982, Churchill Livingstone.
17. Karanjia ND, Stiles PJ: Cubital bursitis, *J Bone Joint Surg* 70B:832, 1988.
18. Kessel L, Rang M: Supracondylar spur of the humerus, *J Bone Joint Surg* 48B:765, 1966.
19. King GJW, et al: An anthropometric study of the radial head: implications in the design of a prosthesis, *J Arthroplasty* 16:112, 2001.
20. Martin BF: The annular ligament of the superior radio-ulnar joint, *J Anat* 92:473, 1958.

21. Miyasaka KC: Anatomy of the elbow, *Orthop Clin North Am* 30:1, 1999.

22. Morrey BF: Anatomy of the elbow joint. In Morrey BF, editor: *The elbow and its disorders,* Philadelphia, 2000, WB Saunders.

23. Morrey BF, An K-N: Functional evaluation of the elbow. In Morrey BF, editor: *The elbow and its disorders,* Philadelphia, 2000, WB Saunders.

24. Nielsen KK, Olsen BS: No stabilizing effect of the elbow joint capsule: a kinematic study, *Acta Orthop Scand* 70:6, 1999.

25. O'Driscoll SW, et al: The cubital tunnel and ulnar neuropathy, *J Bone Joint Surg* 73B:613, 1991.

26. O'Driscoll SW, et al: Origin of the medial collateral ligament, *J Hand Surg* 17A:164, 1992.

27. Olsen BS, et al: Lateral collateral ligament of the elbow joint: anatomy and kinematics, *J Shoulder Elbow Surg* 5:103, 1996.

28. Olsen BS, et al: Kinematics of the lateral ligamentous constraints of the elbow joint, *J Shoulder Elbow Surg* 5:333, 1996.

29. Rasch PJ: The history of kinesiology. In Rasch PJ, editor: *Kinesiology and applied anatomy,* Philadelphia, 1989, Lea & Febiger.

30. Ries MD, Hurst LC, Dee R: Biomechanics of the elbow. In Dee R, editor: *Principles of orthopaedic practice,* New York, 1989, McGraw-Hill.

31. Simon SR, et al: Kinesiology. In Simon SR, editor: *Orthopaedic basic science,* Rosemont, 1994, American Academy of Orthopaedic Surgeons.

32. Smith GR, Hotchkiss RN: Radial head and neck fractures: anatomic guidelines for proper placement of internal fixation, *J Shoulder Elbow Surg* 5:113, 1996.

33. Tornetta P, et al: Anatomy of the posterior interosseous nerve in relation to fixation of the radial head, *Clin Orthop* 345:215, 1997.

34. Werner FW, An K-N: Biomechanics of the elbow and forearm, *Hand Clin* 10:357, 1994.

35. Williams PL, et al: *Gray's anatomy,* ed 38, Edinburgh, 1995, Churchill Livingstone.

36. Yamaguchi K, et al: The extraosseous and intraosseous arterial anatomy of the adult elbow, *J Bone Joint Surg* 79A:1653, 1997.

37. Zarzour ZDS, et al: Single strand reconstruction of the lateral ulnar collateral ligament restores posterolateral rotational stability to the elbow, *J Bone Joint Surg* 82B (suppl I):8, 2000.

Chapter 6

ANATOMY AND KINESIOLOGY OF THE SHOULDER

George P. Bogumill

The shoulder is the region of the body intervening between the upper limb proper and the trunk. It is composed of skeletal elements and the joints that connect them, as well as numerous muscles that serve to stabilize and to move the limb to place the hand in an advantageous position for the myriad functions unique to humans. The upper limb of humans is an organ for grasping and manipulating. The highly mobile joints and muscles that move them are able to so position and move the various parts of the limb that its terminal part, the hand, becomes the most effective tool in the animal kingdom.

SKELETON

The skeleton of the shoulder is composed primarily of three bones. The anteriorly situated clavicle and the posteriorly situated scapula constitute the shoulder girdle, to which is attached the humerus at the glenohumeral joint. The ribs, vertebrae, skull, and pelvis play a minor role in shoulder function by serving as sites of muscle attachments.

Clavicle

The clavicle (collar bone) is a short S-shaped bone that functions as a "tie-rod" connecting the axial skeleton to the upper limb (appendicular) skeleton. Although the rounded prominence on each end participates in synovial joints with sternum and acromion, motions are planar or adaptive and not as free as in true hinge joints. The S shape and mobile articulations on each end allow it to undergo complex rotation and elevation motions, facilitating adaptive changes in upper limb functional activity. The clavicle serves as an attachment site for a number of muscles that position and move the upper limb. It also protects the neurovascular bundle that passes from the neck into the arm. It is the most frequently fractured bone, especially in children. There is

normally a secondary ossification center medially, but none laterally. Injury to this lateral clavicle physis can mimic an acromioclavicular dislocation, and the diagnosis must be made clinically rather than by radiograph.

Scapula

The scapula (shoulder blade) is loosely attached to the posterior chest wall, ensheathed in muscle, and more or less "floating" in position depending on the muscle activity and function of the limb at any given time. The body of the scapula is a flattened blade of bone with a large ridge, the scapular spine, projecting from the posterior surface. This ridge begins at the medial border of the scapula and ends laterally as the large projecting acromion, overlying the humeral head and articulating with the clavicle. Extending anteriorly is the hook-shaped coracoid process. Laterally, the flat body expands into the glenoid, which articulates with the humerus. Numerous muscles arise from or insert onto the scapula and contribute to its infinitely varied movements.

Humerus

The humerus is the proximal lever arm of the upper limb, connecting the limb to the shoulder girdle through the glenoid. It is a large long bone whose rounded proximal end articulates with the glenoid surface of the scapula, although they do not fit well, in contradistinction to the ball and socket of the hip joint. The shaft of the humerus provides sites of attachment for prime shoulder movers as well as muscles that cross the elbow as prime movers of elbow, forearm, and even wrist and fingers.

JOINTS

The **shoulder "joint"** is actually composed of a series of articulations including the sternoclavicular, acromiocla-

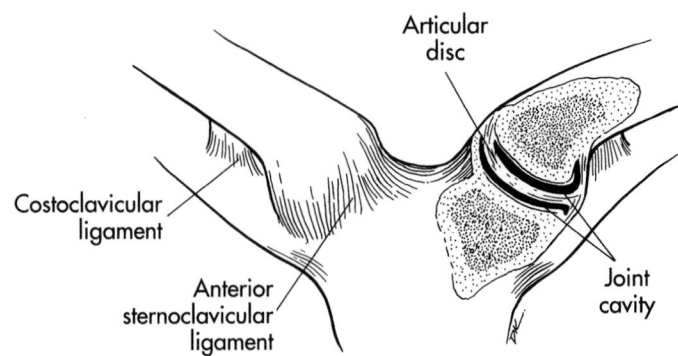

Fig. 6-1. Anatomy of sternoclavicular joint. Strong attachment of intraarticular disk to cranial portion of medial end of clavicle helps resist upward displacement of clavicle when weight is borne in hand and also helps cushion impacts directed medially along clavicle. (From Bogumill GP: Functional anatomy of the shoulder and elbow. In Pettrone FA, editor: *AAOS symposium on upper extremity injuries in athletes,* St Louis, 1986, Mosby.)

vicular, glenohumeral, and scapulothoracic joints. In addition, some clinicians consider the subacromial bursa a fifth "joint."

Sternoclavicular joint

The sternoclavicular joint is the only one that attaches the upper limb directly to the axial skeleton. The joint surfaces of the sternal manubrium and the clavicle are flat with a limited, mainly adaptive, range of motion. An articular disk allows increased freedom of motion while functioning as an intraarticular ligament (Fig. 6-1). With its strong attachment to the cranial aspect of the medial end of the clavicle, this articular disk tends to resist upward displacement when a weight is carried in the hand. It also serves to cushion compressive forces directed down the long axis of the clavicle in falls on the outer aspect of the shoulder. Stability also is provided by the anterior and posterior sternoclavicular ligaments, the configuration of the joint surfaces, and the costoclavicular ligament, which provides a strong ligamentous attachment medially to the first rib. The posterior sternoclavicular ligament is the strongest support of the joint and maintains the elevation of the *outer* end of the clavicle at rest. It also helps resist upward or backward displacement of the medial end of the clavicle.

Acromioclavicular joint

The acromioclavicular (AC) joint is a sliding (planar) joint with articular surfaces usually separated by a recognizable intraarticular disk, which varies from inconspicuous, to partial, to one that completely separates the AC joint into two compartments (Fig. 6-2, *A*). Occasionally the joint will have no synovial cavity but consist merely of a fibrous syndesmosis. Like the sternoclavicular joint, the AC joint is not a true hinge joint, but rather a sliding planar joint providing for adaptive motions. This joint is frequently injured in athletes, in part because it has a relatively weak, easily disrupted capsular ligament complex. Although the shape of the AC joint is quite variable (Fig. 6-2, *B* and *C*), the slope of the distal end of the clavicle often favors slippage of the acromion beneath the clavicle when an impact is placed on the outer aspect of the shoulder. More

important functionally, and of greater clinical significance in the athlete with a severe shoulder "separation," are the supporting conoid and trapezoid ligaments. These fibrous ligamentous structures originate from the cranial surface of the coracoid process and insert into the undersurface of the lateral clavicle, effecting control of clavicular displacement in a superior-inferior plane.

Glenohumeral joint

The glenohumeral joint has the greatest range of motion of any joint in the body. Unfortunately for some, such mobility is achieved at the expense of stability. Structurally, the humeral head's significantly larger surface area compared with the glenoid provides for a poor ball-and-socket joint (Fig. 6-3, *A* and *C*). Although the labrum broadens the articulating area (Fig. 6-3, *B* and *D*) and may significantly enhance the socket's depth by as much as 50%, the predominant role of joint stabilization is relegated to the surrounding soft tissue structures. These include the static restraints of the glenohumeral ligaments and the dynamic restraints of the rotator cuff. The glenohumeral ligaments arise from the humeral neck, attach along the glenoid rim, and blend with the joint capsule. There is often a defect in the capsule anteriorly that connects the joint cavity with the subscapularis bursa (Fig. 6-3, *B*). The laxity of the capsule is necessary, of course, for the large range of motion possible at this joint, but there is also a corresponding inability to provide stability. This helps explain why this joint is the most commonly dislocated joint in the body.

The dynamic restraints are the tendinous insertions of the rotator cuff, whose muscles are the subscapularis anteriorly, the supraspinatus superiorly, and the infraspinatus and teres minor posteriorly. Each of these provides fibrous insertion into the shoulder capsule; simultaneous activity of all of them serves to retain the humeral head in intimate contact with the glenoid. Muscular contraction of the rotator cuff produces force vectors whose orientation seats the humeral head within the glenoid, allowing other muscles, particularly deltoid, to then move the humerus.

There is some deepening of the glenohumeral joint socket by the coracoid process, the acromion, and the connecting

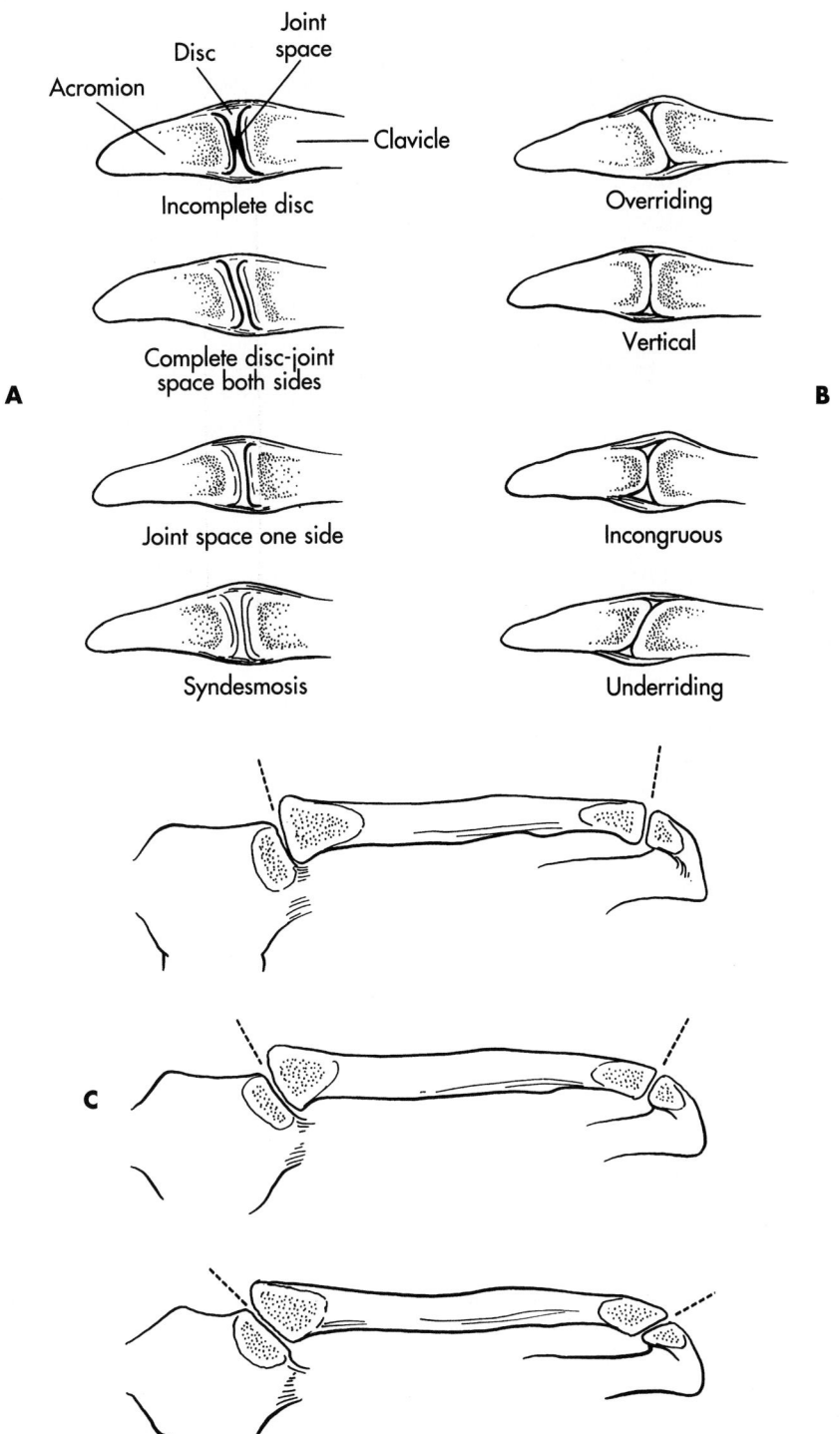

Fig. 6-2. Variations in acromioclavicular and sternoclavicular joints. **A,** Intraarticular disc in acromioclavicular joint is often incomplete, particularly in elderly. **B,** Varied configurations of clavicular alignment with acromion. **C,** Varied angles of ends of clavicle have bearing on ease of dislocation. (From Bogumill GP: Functional anatomy of the shoulder and elbow. In Pettrone FA, editor: *AAOS symposium on upper extremity injuries in athletes,* St Louis, 1986, Mosby.)

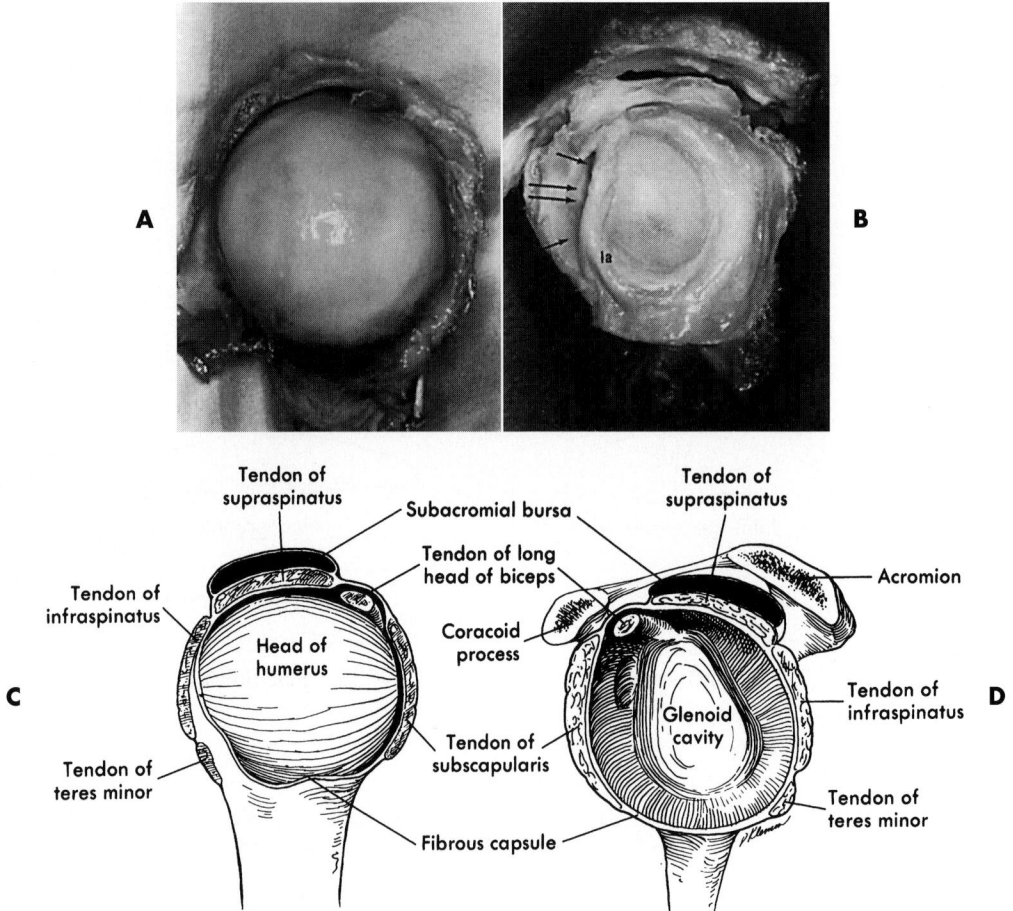

Fig. 6-3. Relationships of glenohumeral joint cavity, capsule, and bursae. **A** and **C,** Dissection and diagram of humeral head en face. **B** and **D,** Dissection and diagram of glenoid surface. *Arrows* indicate large subscapularis bursa. *1a,* Labrum.

coracoacromial ligament (Fig. 6-3, *B* and *C*). These structures are separated from the underlying supraspinatus tendon by a bursa (sometimes called the *subacromial joint* or *fifth joint*), which is often the site of inflammation and even dystrophic calcification. The bursa lies beneath both the acromion and deltoid and is a thin-walled potential space (Fig. 6-4, *C*) filled with synovial fluid that provides frictionless gliding between the supraspinatus tendon and the acromion. Because the tendon is blended with the superior joint capsule, it has an area covered with synovium on both surfaces (Fig. 6-4, *A* and *C*), and any blood supply to the tendon must enter it from the muscle belly on one side and the tendon insertion into the humerus on the other, leaving a relatively avascular "watershed" area in the tendon often subjected to "impingement" with abrasion caused by repetitive wear on the tendon. This problem may be aggravated by compression between the humeral head and acromion during muscular activity. This phenomenon may involve the infraspinatus tendon as well; the subscapularis and teres minor do not have the same problem, however, because they are not situated and moving between the acromion and humeral

head. The scapula must be rotated to tilt the glenoid upward to prevent the undersurface of the acromion and coracoacromial ligament from impeding overhead activities in throwing or racket sports. Pathologic involvement caused by primary bursal disease, overuse, or disease of the rotator cuff may lead to progressive inflammation, fibrosis, and obliteration of this space. Impingement of the rotator cuff, particularly with arm elevation in throwing athletes, is a common consequence.

The long head of the biceps is contained within the joint capsule; however, it is covered by synovium and thus is separated from direct contact with the joint fluid (Fig. 6-4, *B*). Its attachment to the supraglenoid tubercle helps it resist upward displacement of the humeral head. With its long intraarticular course, it obviously has to obtain its blood supply from its bony attachment, the musculotendinous junction, or both. Bicipital tendonitis with deterioration and fraying leading to painful inflammation often accompanies the impingement process and may be because of this tenuous relationship.

The subacromial (subdeltoid) bursa tends to be quite

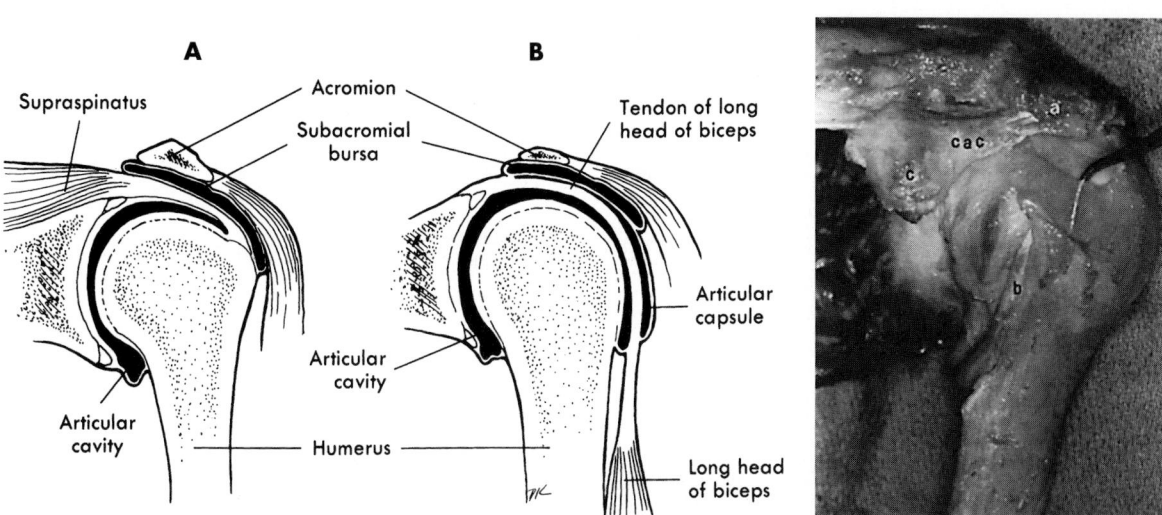

Fig. 6-4. Glenohumeral joint relationships with supraspinatus, long head of biceps, and subacromial (subdeltoid) bursae. **A,** Supraspinatus tendon is covered with synovium on both surfaces. **B,** Long head of biceps has intraarticular portion covered with layer of synovium. (Deltoid muscle is shown originating from acromion in **A** and **B** but is not marked.) **C,** Probe in well-defined subdeltoid portion of bursa. *a,* Acromion; *b,* long head of biceps; *c,* coracoid process; *cac,* coracoacromial ligament. (**A** and **B** from Bogumill GP: Functional anatomy of the shoulder and elbow. In Pettrone FA, editor: *AAOS symposium on upper extremity injuries in athletes,* St Louis, 1986, Mosby.)

large, and it extends laterally as one continuous space from under the acromion to lie deep to the deltoid muscle (Fig. 6-4, *C*). It facilitates motion of the shoulder and rotator cuff beneath the acromion and the coracoacromial ligament. It is more anterior than one would expect, and thus most of the painful impingements occur during flexion (anterior elevation) rather than during pure abduction (lateral elevation).

MUSCLES

Muscles and their functions can be described in several ways. For example, one can describe each muscle individually, listing its attachments, fiber direction, nerve supply, and function. This is the manner usually used for anatomic texts. However, it will better serve our purpose here to describe the various motions of the shoulder components and identify the muscles that take part in each motion. The reader soon will realize that many of the muscles can and do participate in more than one motion. For example, the pectoralis major is both a protractor and depressor of the shoulder girdle, as well as an adductor, internal rotator, flexor, and extensor of the arm; such varied functions of the pectoralis major, as well as other muscle groups, depend on the position of the humerus during the function attempted.

The large muscles attaching to the upper limb can be divided conveniently into an *extrinsic* group, which attach the limb girdle or the limb itself to the axial skeleton, and an *intrinsic* group, which go from the limb girdle to the limb.

Extrinsics

Muscles attaching from the thorax to the limb girdle are the subclavius, pectoralis minor, and serratus anterior. The large muscle attaching from the thorax to the humerus is the pectoralis major. Muscles attaching to the vertebrae and the limb girdle are the trapezius, levator scapulae, and rhomboideus major and minor. The single muscle connecting the vertebrae (and ilium) to the humerus is the latissimus dorsi.

Intrinsics

The deltoid is the only muscle running from clavicle to humerus, and it joins with numerous additional muscles going from scapula to humerus. These muscles are subscapularis, supraspinatus, infraspinatus, teres major and minor, and coracobrachialis. The long and short heads of the biceps go from scapula to radius, and the long head of the triceps attaches from scapula to ulna.

FUNCTIONAL MOVEMENT OF THE SHOULDER
Limb girdle

The sternoclavicular joint is the point of fixation of the upper limb to the axial skeleton. Because the length of the clavicle is finite and its medial end is spatially tied to the sternoclavicular joint, the clavicle functions as a spoke or radius of limb-girdle motion on this medially fixed point. We can change the position of this radius, but we cannot change its length. The scapulothoracic joint is not a true synovial

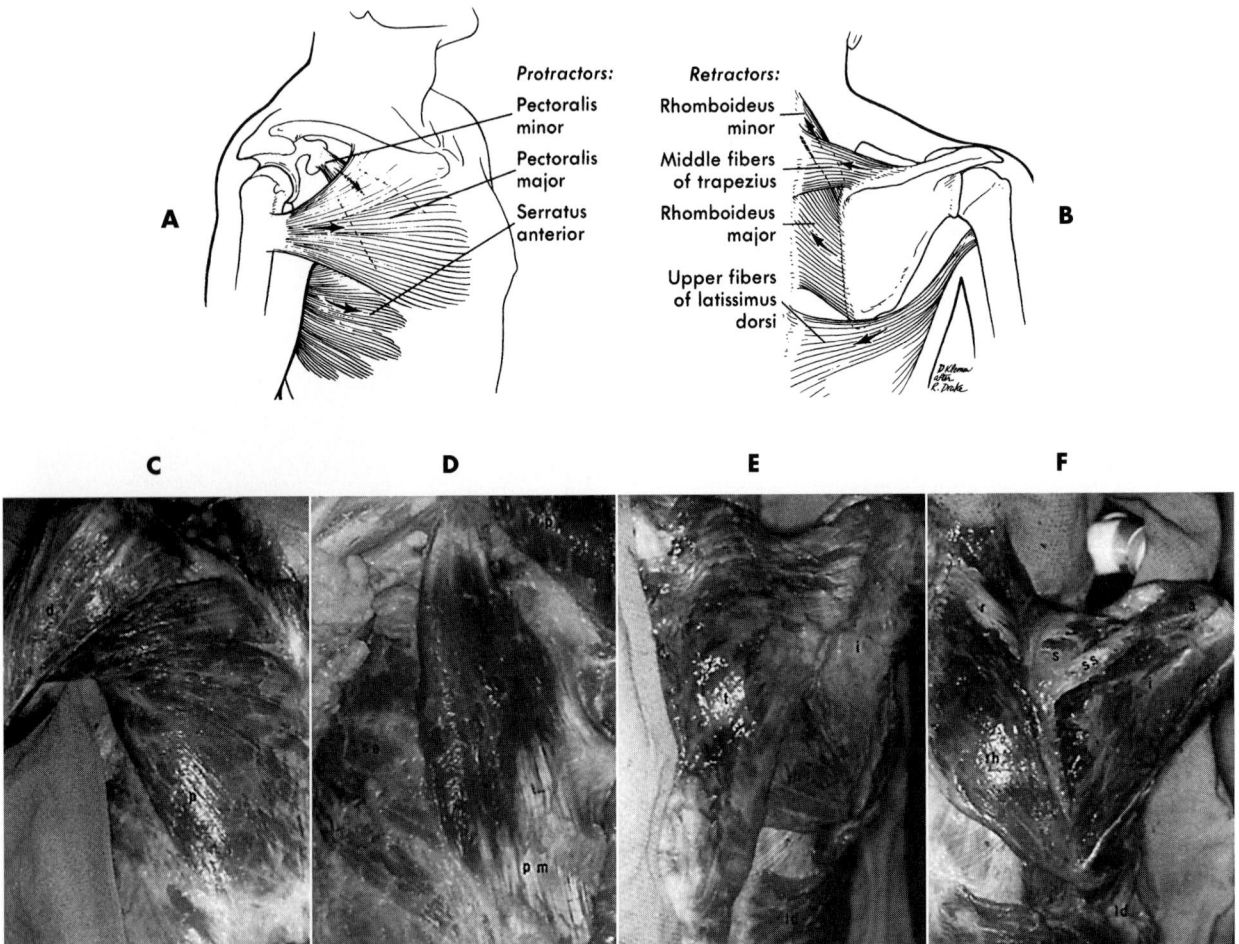

Fig. 6-5. Diagram and dissection of protractors and retractors of the shoulder girdle. **A** and **B,** Diagrams of anterior and posterior muscle groups. **C** and **D,** Dissection of the shoulder protractors. **E** and **F,** Dissection of shoulder retractors. *a,* Acromion; *d,* deltoid; *i,* infraspinatus; *ld,* latissimus dorsi; *p,* pectoralis major; *pm,* pectoralis minor; *r,* rhomboideus minor; *rh,* rhomboideus major; *s,* supraspinatus; *sa,* serratus anterior; *ss,* scapular spine; *t,* trapezius. (**A** and **B** from Bogumill GP: Functional anatomy of the shoulder and elbow. In Pettrone FA, editor: *AAOS symposium on upper extremity injuries in athletes,* St Louis, 1986, Mosby.)

joint, of course, but provides for rotation of the scapula "floating" on the chest wall. The radius of curvature of the chest wall is different from the functional radius of motion provided by the length of the clavicle. Thus the acromioclavicular joint, which has no prime movers, that is, no muscles crossing the joint to move it solely, has purely adaptive motions between the clavicle and scapula to compensate for the two different radii of motion.

Movements of the scapula are combined with the range of the glenohumeral joint to place the proximal limb segment, the humerus, in a functional position. Protraction, that is, "hunching" the shoulder forward as seen when boxers try to protect their chin, is done by the large, strong serratus anterior and pectoralis major and minor muscles (Fig. 6-5, *A, C,* and *D*). The muscles that retract the shoulder, that is, bring it posteriorly into the military "brace" position, are also large and strong and include the latissimus dorsi,

trapezius, and rhomboids (Fig. 6-5, *B, E,* and *F*). The elevators of the scapula are the levator scapulae; rhomboideus major and minor attaching to the medial border of the scapulae (Figs. 6-5, *F,* and 6-6); and the upper portion of the trapezius, which is the only elevator attaching to the outer end of the shoulder girdle (Figs. 6-5, *E,* and 6-6). With spinal accessory nerve injury and resultant paralysis of the trapezius, drooping of the outer aspect of the scapula is only partially compensated by the rhomboids and levator scapula medially, which are often painfully spastic from their overwork in trying to elevate the outer scapulae.

The serratus anterior, pectoralis minor, lower fibers of the pectoralis major, latissimus dorsi, and lower trapezius are depressors of the scapula (Fig. 6-7, *A, B,* and *C*), and are very important in lifting body weight from a chair or the floor when one presses downward on the hands. The latissimus dorsi is particularly important when using crutches.

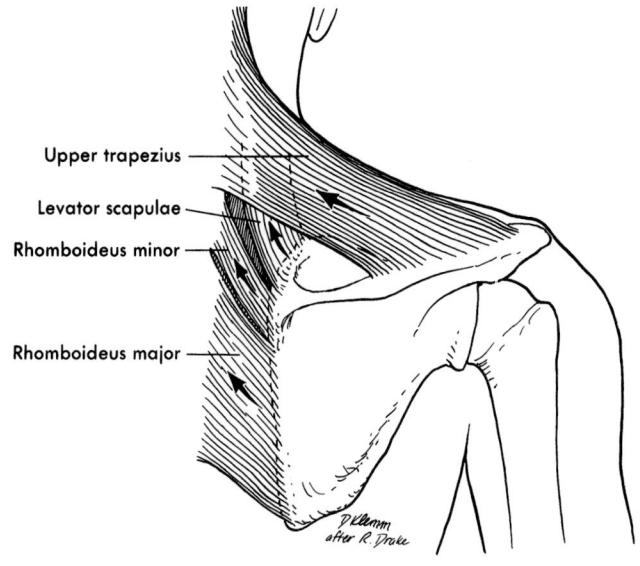

Fig. 6-6. Elevators of shoulder girdle ("shoulder shruggers"). (From Bogumill GP: Functional anatomy of the shoulder and elbow. In Pettrone FA, editor: *AAOS symposium on upper extremity injuries in athletes,* St Louis, 1986, Mosby.)

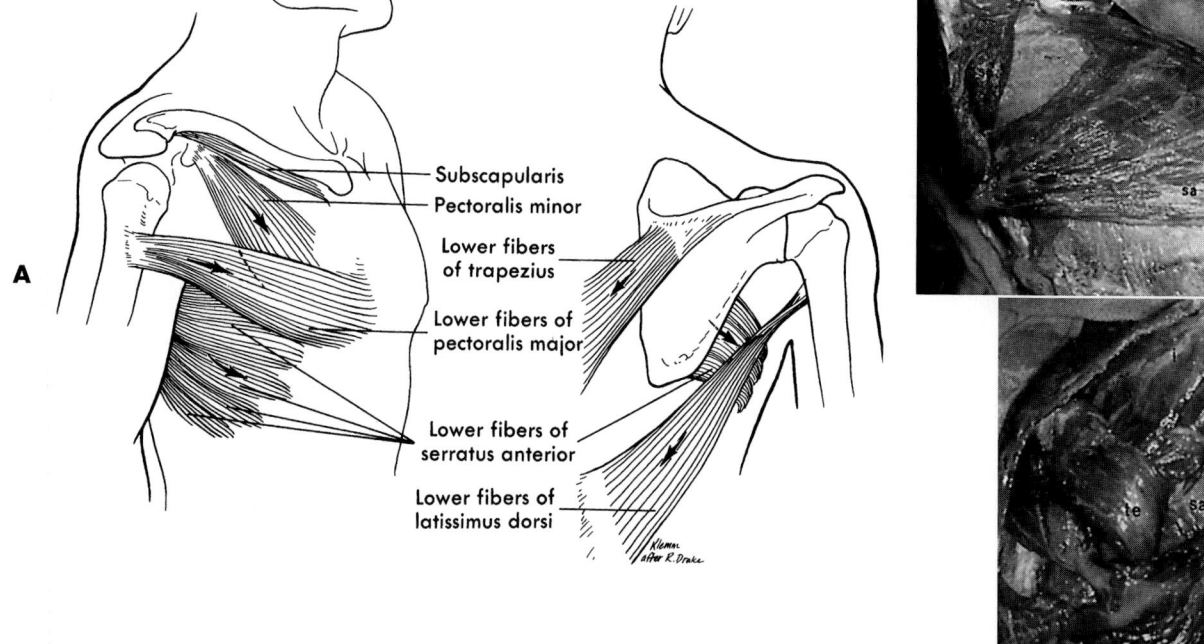

Fig. 6-7. Diagrams (**A**) and dissections (**B** and **C**) of shoulder girdle depressors. *i,* Infraspinatus; *ld,* latissimus dorsi; *sa,* serratus anterior; *sc,* subscapularis; *t,* trapezius; *te,* teres major (reflected); *tm,* teres minor. (**A** from Bogumill GP: Functional anatomy of the shoulder and elbow. In Pettrone FA, editor: *AAOS symposium on upper extremity injuries in athletes,* St Louis, 1986, Mosby.)

Rotation of the scapula is critical in effecting full normal range of motion of the glenohumeral joint. Upward rotation of the glenoid face is performed by upper and lower fibers of the trapezius and by the serratus anterior (Fig. 6-8). These two muscles are essential for successful use of the limb with a shoulder arthrodesis because upward rotation of the scapula then brings about elevation of the upper limb. Downward rotation of the glenoid surface of the scapula is produced by gravity and by the levator scapulae, rhomboids, latissimus dorsi, pectoralis minor, and lower fibers of the pectoralis major (Fig. 6-9) (see Table 6-1).

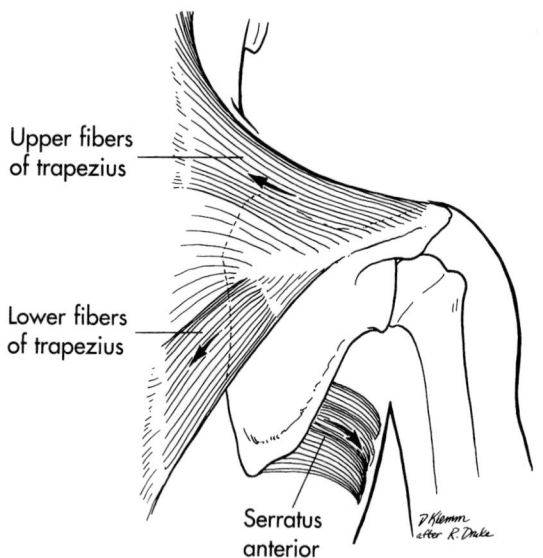

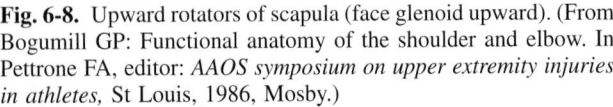

Fig. 6-8. Upward rotators of scapula (face glenoid upward). (From Bogumill GP: Functional anatomy of the shoulder and elbow. In Pettrone FA, editor: *AAOS symposium on upper extremity injuries in athletes,* St Louis, 1986, Mosby.)

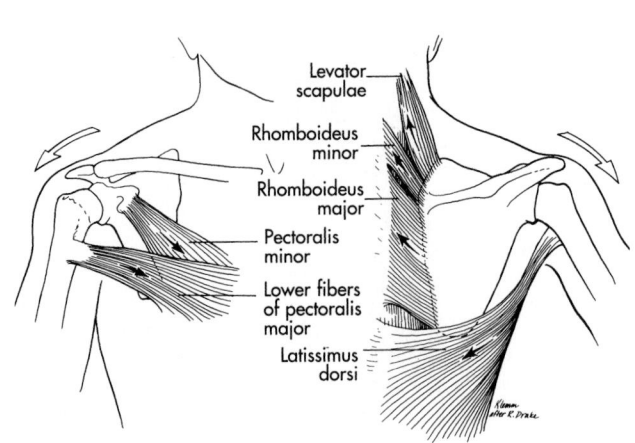

Fig. 6-9. Downward rotators of scapula (face glenoid downward). (From Bogumill GP: Functional anatomy of the shoulder and elbow. In Pettrone FA, editor: *AAOS symposium on upper extremity injuries in athletes,* St Louis, 1986, Mosby.)

Table 6-1. Muscles of the upper limb

Location	Muscle	Functional limb girdle movements	Functional glenohumeral motion
Extrinsic muscles of the upper limb (attach limb girdle or limb itself to the axial skeleton)			
Anterior (thorax to limb girdle)	Subclavius	Depress, stabilize clavicle	
Anterior (thorax to limb girdle)	Pectoralis minor	Protraction, depression, downward rotation	
Anterior (thorax to limb girdle)	Serratus anterior	Protraction, depression, upward rotation	
(Thorax to humerus)	Pectoralis major	Protraction, depression (lower fibers), downward rotation (lower fibers)	Flexion (clavicular head) Extension (sternocostal portion) Adduction, internal rotation
Posterior (vertebrae to limb girdle)	Trapezius	Retraction, elevation (upper portion), depression (lower portion), upward rotation (upper and lower portions)	
Posterior (vertebrae to limb girdle)	Levator scapulae	Elevation, downward rotation	
Posterior (vertebrae to limb girdle)	Rhomboid major	Retraction, elevation, downward rotation	
Posterior (vertebrae to limb girdle)	Rhomboid minor	Retraction, elevation, downward rotation	
(Vertebrae and ilium to humerus)	Latissimus dorsi	Retraction, depression, downward rotation	Extension, adduction, internal rotation
Intrinsic muscles of the upper limb (attach limb girdle to limb)			
Anterior (clavicle to humerus)	Deltoid		Flexion, adduction, internal rotation
Central	Deltoid		Abduction
Posterior	Deltoid		Adduction; external rotation
(Scapula to humerus)	Subscapularis		Internal rotation
(Scapula to humerus)	Supraspinatus		Abduction
(Scapula to humerus)	Infraspinatus		External rotation
(Scapula to humerus)	Teres major		Extension, adduction, internal rotation
(Scapula to humerus)	Teres minor		External rotation
(Scapula to humerus)	Coracobrachialis		Flexion, adduction
(Scapula to radius)	Long and short heads of biceps		Flexion
(Scapula to ulna)	Long head triceps		Extension

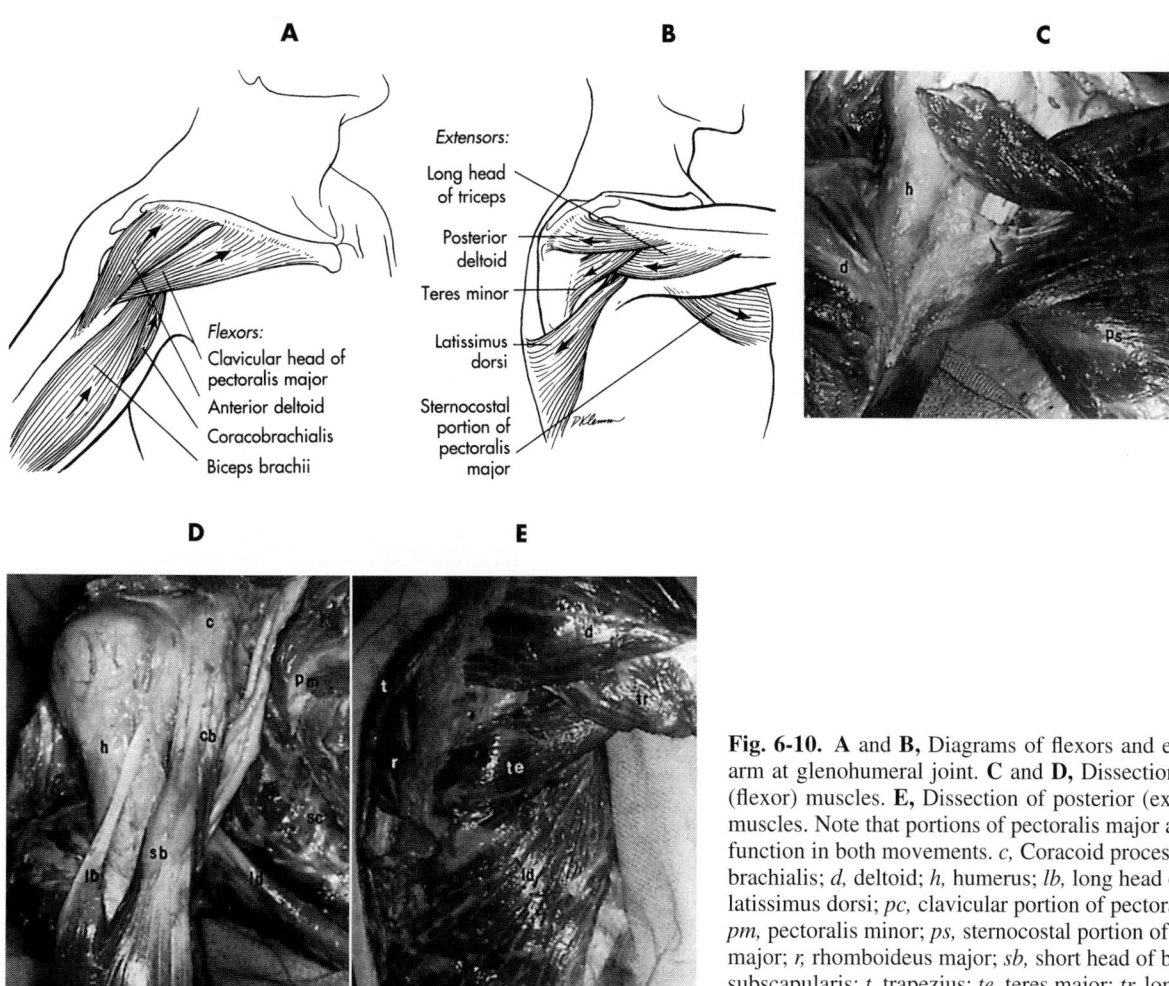

Fig. 6-10. A and **B,** Diagrams of flexors and extensors of arm at glenohumeral joint. **C** and **D,** Dissections of anterior (flexor) muscles. **E,** Dissection of posterior (extensor) muscles. Note that portions of pectoralis major and deltoid function in both movements. *c,* Coracoid process; *cb,* coracobrachialis; *d,* deltoid; *h,* humerus; *lb,* long head of biceps; *ld,* latissimus dorsi; *pc,* clavicular portion of pectoralis major; *pm,* pectoralis minor; *ps,* sternocostal portion of pectoralis major; *r,* rhomboideus major; *sb,* short head of biceps; *sc,* subscapularis; *t,* trapezius; *te,* teres major; *tr,* long head of triceps. (**A** and **B** from Bogumill GP: Functional anatomy of the shoulder and elbow. In Pettrone FA, editor: *AAOS symposium on upper extremity injuries in athletes,* St Louis, 1986, Mosby.)

Shoulder (glenohumeral) joint

The glenohumeral joint allows the greatest motion of any joint in the body, albeit at the expense of stability. It is difficult to define this motion because the glenoid faces forward 30 to 40 degrees; thus the motions in the planes of the body are not true motions in the planes of the joint. However, the motions are usually described in relation to the planes of the body. Thus there are motions in the sagittal and coronal planes as well as rotation about an axis down the shaft of the humerus regardless of the position of the humerus in space. In general, glenohumeral range of motion brings the arm slightly above horizontal, and the added scapulothoracic range of motion brings the arm vertical. Every individual has a distinct "scapulohumeral rhythm" that is approximately two thirds glenohumeral and one third scapulothoracic.

Flexion of the humerus is accomplished by the clavicular head of the pectoralis major, the anterior portion of the deltoid, the coracobrachialis, and the biceps brachii (Fig. 6-10, *A, C,* and *D*). Extension is accomplished by the triceps, teres major, latissimus dorsi, and posterior portion of the deltoid (Fig. 6-10, *B* and *E*). The sternocostal portion of the pectoralis major is also an extensor, as one can observe by placing one's hand on the edge of a table and pushing down while palpating the muscle because the sternocostal portion of the pectoralis major contracts. Conversely, the action of placing the hand beneath the edge of the table and lifting up causes contraction in the clavicular portion.

The abductors of the arm are primarily the supraspinatus and the central portion of the deltoid (Fig. 6-11). The adductors of the arm are large and numerous; they include the pectoralis major, anterior and posterior portions of the deltoid, coracobrachialis, teres major, and latissimus dorsi (Fig. 6-12). The relative strength of adductors over abductors helps explain why one cannot hold much weight with the arm

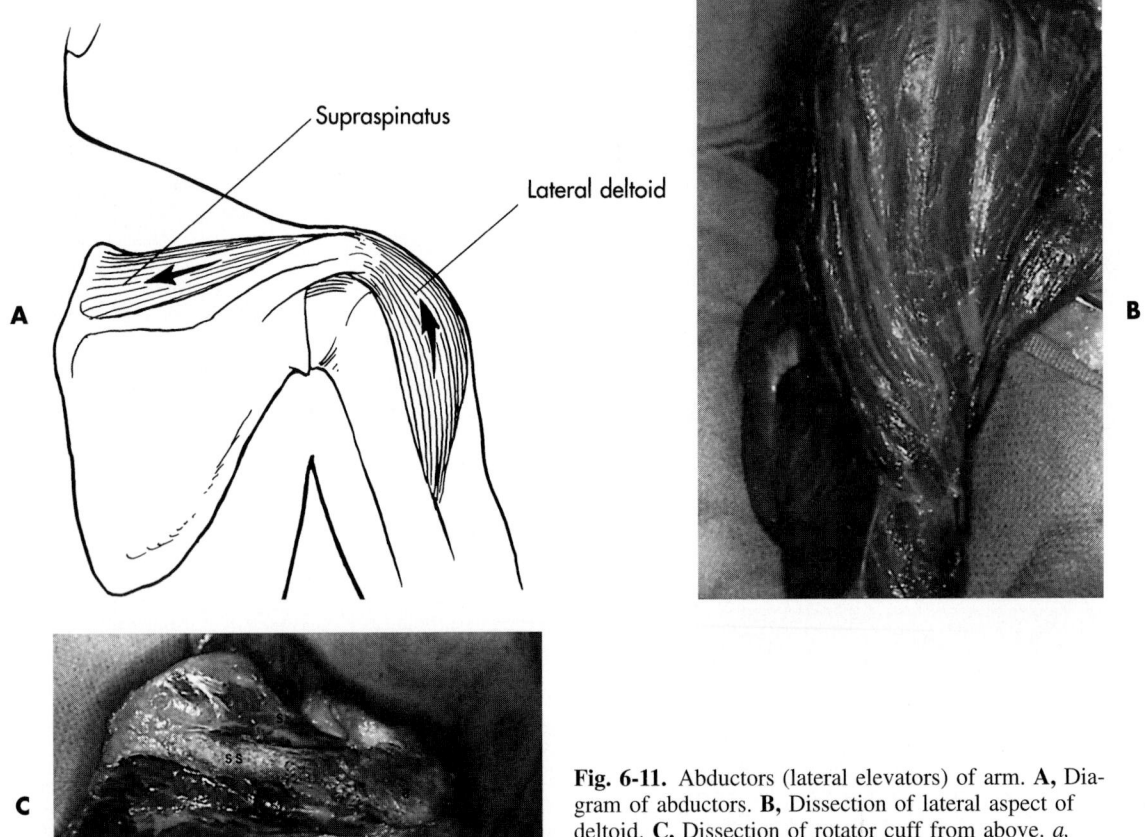

Fig. 6-11. Abductors (lateral elevators) of arm. **A,** Diagram of abductors. **B,** Dissection of lateral aspect of deltoid. **C,** Dissection of rotator cuff from above. *a,* Acromion; *i,* infraspinatus; *s,* supraspinatus; *ss,* spine of scapula. (**A** from Bogumill GP: Functional anatomy of the shoulder and elbow. In Pettrone FA, editor: *AAOS symposium on upper extremity injuries in athletes,* St Louis, 1986, Mosby.)

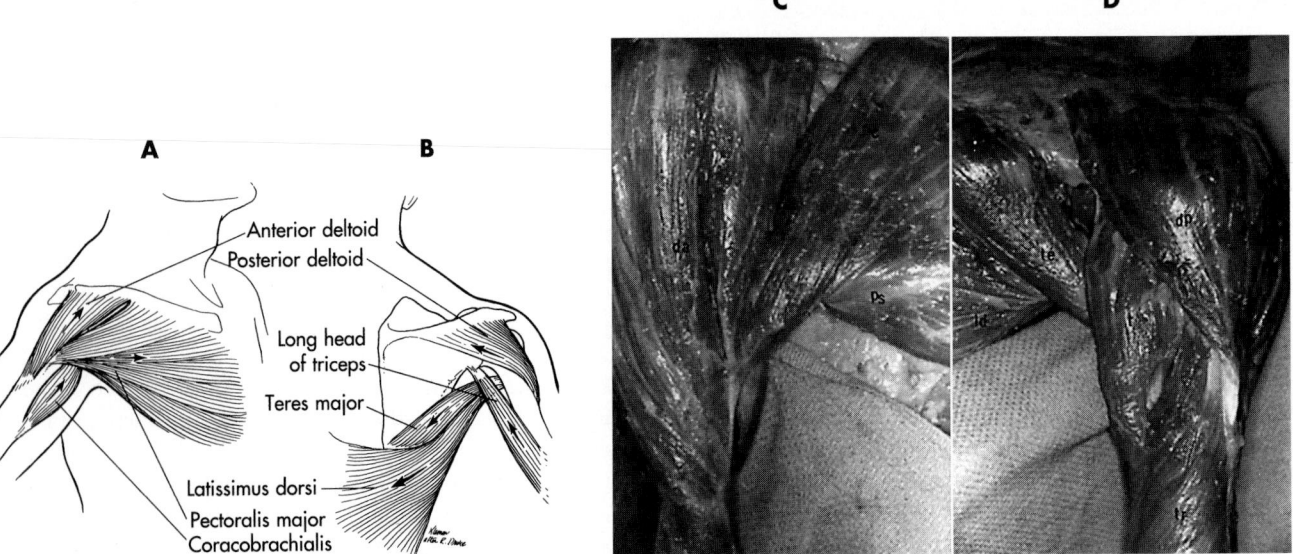

Fig. 6-12. A and **B,** Diagram of adductors of arm. **C,** Dissection of major anterior adductors. **D,** Dissection of major posterior adductors. *da,* Anterior deltoid; *dp,* posterior deltoid; *ld,* latissimus dorsi; *pc,* clavicular portion of pectoralis major; *ps,* sternoclavicular portion of pectoralis major; *t,* long head triceps; *te,* teres major; *tr,* lateral head of triceps. (**A** and **B** from Bogumill GP: Functional anatomy of the shoulder and elbow. In Pettrone FA, editor: *AAOS symposium on upper extremity injuries in athletes,* St Louis, 1986, Mosby.)

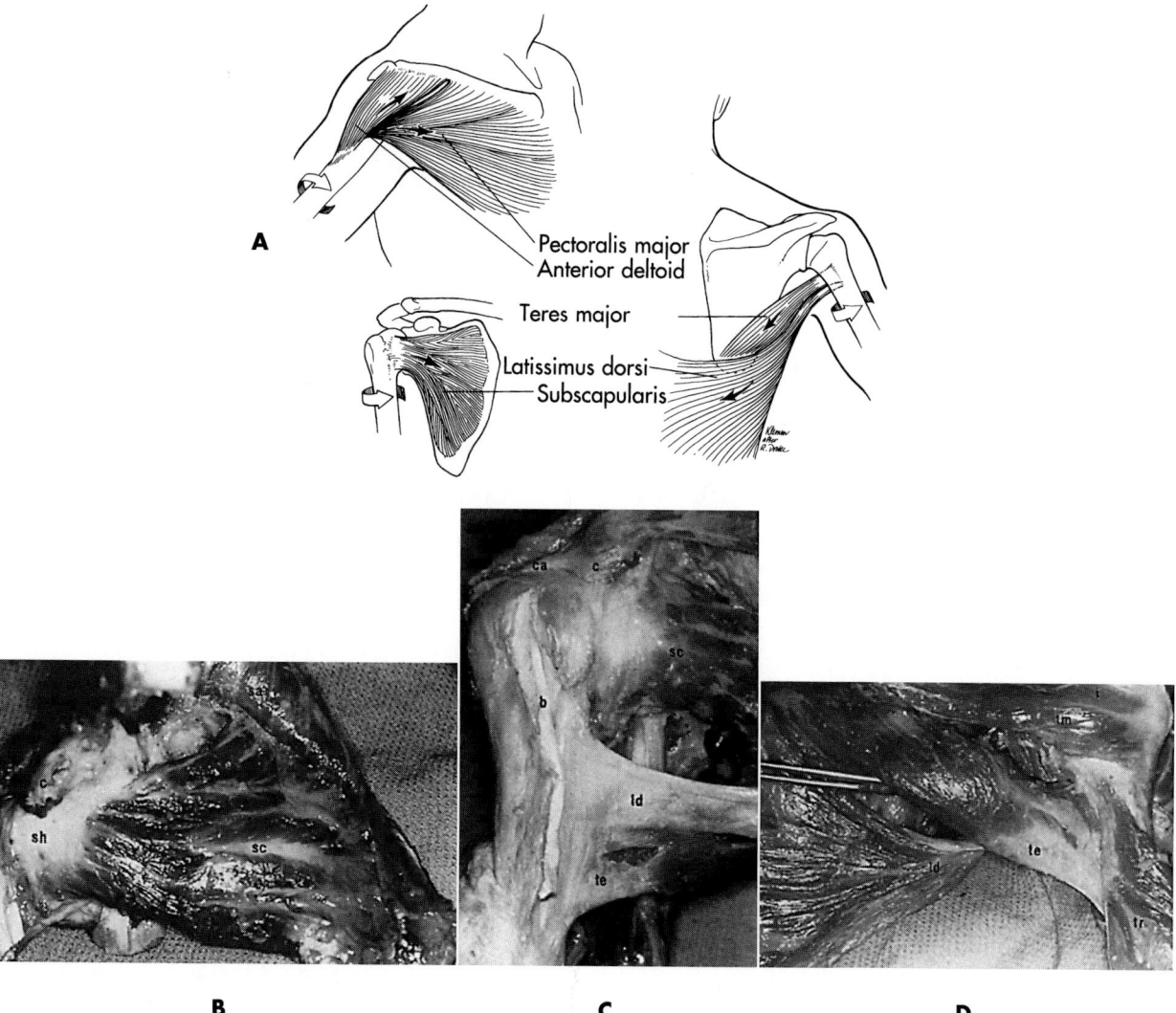

Fig. 6-13. Internal rotators of arm. **A,** Diagrams of anterior and posterior muscles that rotate humerus internally. **B,** Anterior dissection to illustrate insertion of subscapularis into anterior glenohumeral joint capsule. C, Insertion of latissimus dorsi and teres major onto anterior humeral shaft in bicipital groove. D, Posterior dissection of internal rotators. *c,* Coracoid process; *ld,* latissimus dorsi; *i,* infraspinatus; *sa,* serratus anterior; *sc* subscapularis; *sh,* shoulder joint capsule; *t,* long head of triceps origin from inferior glenoid tubercle (muscle belly has been removed to facilitate exposure); *te,* teres major; *tm,* teres minor. (**A** from Bogumill GP: Functional anatomy of the shoulder and elbow. In Pettrone FA, editor: *AAOS symposium on upper extremity injuries in athletes,* St Louis, 1986, Mosby.)

extended horizontally but can press downward with enough power to do the "iron cross" in gymnastics with the powerful adductor muscles.

A similar situation pertains to the rotators of the arm. The internal rotators are larger, stronger, and more numerous than external rotators (Fig. 6-13). Although the latissimus dorsi and teres major originate dorsally from the trunk, they attach to the anterior surface of the humerus (see Fig. 6-13, *C* and *D*) and are added to the pectoralis major, subscapularis, and anterior portion of the deltoid (see Figs. 6-10, *C* and *E,* 6-11,

B, and 6-13, *A* and *B*). The external rotators are much smaller and weaker and include the infraspinatus, teres minor, and posterior portion of the deltoid (Figs. 6-12, *D,* 6-14, *A* and *B,* and 6-15). The discrepancy between internal rotator-adductor power and external rotator-adductor strength is considered to have survival value in evolution; it helps the infant to hang onto its mother while she is fleeing from danger.

Muscular dysfunctions may be attributable to problems of the muscles, problems of the nerves to these muscles, and

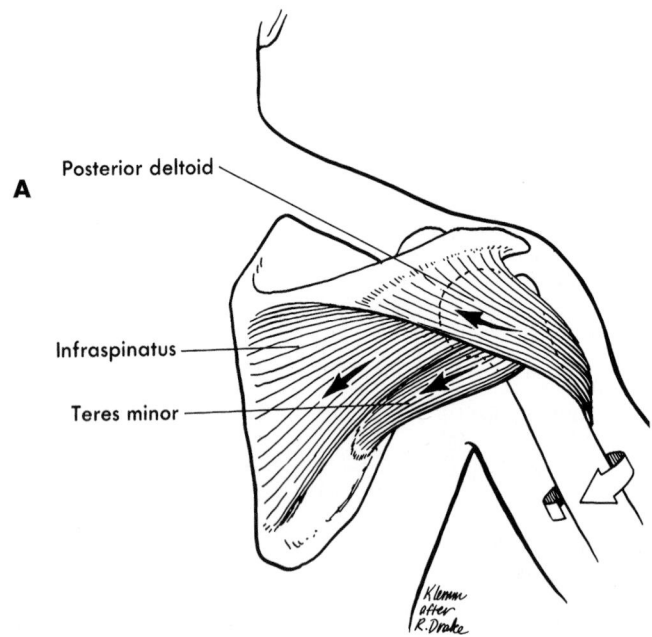

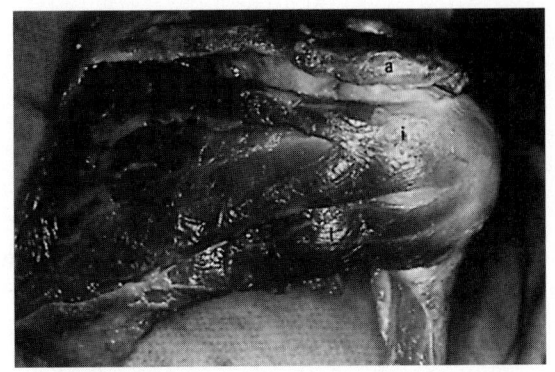

Fig. 6-14. External rotators of arm. **A,** Diagram of muscles that cause arm to rotate externally. **B,** Dissection of external rotators. Posterior deltoid has been removed for exposure of deeper muscles and capsule. *a,* Acromion; *i,* infraspinatus; *t,* teres minor; *ss,* spine of scapula. (**A** from Bogumill GP: Functional anatomy of the shoulder and elbow. In Pettrone FA, editor: *AAOS symposium on upper extremity injuries in athletes,* St Louis, 1986, Mosby.)

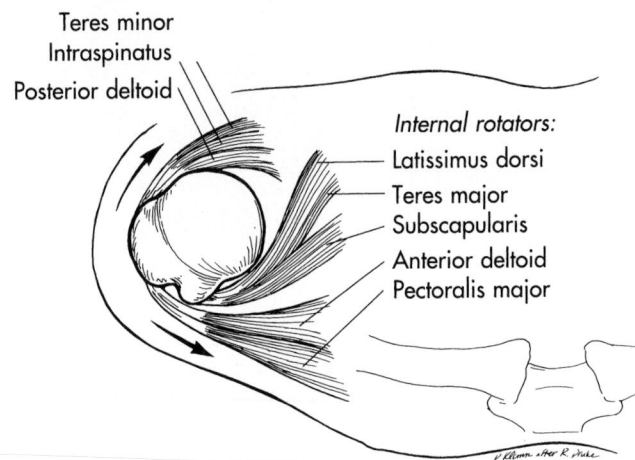

Fig. 6-15. Diagram from Fig. 6-14 of internal and external rotators of arm. (From Bogumill GP: Functional anatomy of the shoulder and elbow. In Pettrone FA, editor: *AAOS symposium on upper extremity injuries in athletes,* St Louis, 1986, Mosby.)

problems with the nerve roots supplying those nerves, as well as more proximally in the central nervous system. Diagnosis of a specific problem or site of a problem often is difficult. Patients quickly develop substitution patterns to replace a lost function. These patterns often can be very confusing to the examiner and require a great deal of therapy to overcome.

BIBLIOGRAPHY

Bogumill GP: Functional anatomy of the shoulder and elbow. In Pettrone FA, editor: *American Academy of Orthopaedic Surgery symposium on upper extremity injuries in athletes,* St Louis, 1986, Mosby.

Hollinshead WH: *Textbook of anatomy,* ed 3, Hagerstown, Md, 1974, Harper & Row.

Woodburne RT: *Essentials of human anatomy,* ed 5, New York, 1973, Oxford University Press.

Part II

EVALUATION

Chapter 7

UPPER QUARTER SCREEN

Philip McClure

Anatomically, the upper quarter includes the cervical spine, upper thoracic spine, and the upper extremity. Because the source of a patient's symptoms is often unclear, a screening examination can be helpful in providing an efficient mechanism to more precisely determine which region(s) may be contributing to the symptoms.[5] The upper quarter screening examination is designed to achieve two basic purposes: (1) to determine which anatomic region of the upper quarter is contributing to the patient's symptoms and therefore needs to be examined in greater detail and (2) to rule out gross sensory or motor neurologic deficits.

A screening examination is often unnecessary when the source of a patient's symptoms or dysfunction is very clear from the history such as postsurgical problems or cases in which the upper extremity has incurred some isolated traumatic injury. Cases for which the screening examination is most appropriate are those in which the diagnosis is unclear, or referred pain, typically emanating from more proximal structures, is a potential problem.

Referred pain can be defined simply as pain perceived in an area other than its source.[3] Although a complete discussion of referred pain is beyond the scope of this chapter, understanding some general characteristics of referred pain can be very helpful clinically. First, deeper, more proximal structures are most likely to refer pain. This is why the majority of the upper quarter screening examination focuses on the cervical spine and shoulder. These areas are known to be potential sources able to refer pain to multiple sites in the upper extremity.[1,2,8] However, it is rare that distal structures in the upper extremity refer pain proximally.

Referred pain also is typically described as a poorly localized, dull aching sensation. Therefore the patient who rubs the entire lateral aspect of the arm while describing a dull aching pain is more likely to have referred pain than a patient who, for example, complains of a sharp localized pain on the lateral aspect of the elbow.

While performing the examination, the chief goal is to reproduce the patient's chief complaint pain or symptom. Occasionally, patients will have mild restrictions in cervical range of motion (ROM) or complain of discomfort or pulling sensations during cervical spine testing. Painless restrictions in motion or symptoms that are not part of the patient's chief complaint should not be interpreted as positive tests but more likely represent normal variations.

Many variations exist on what is included in the screening examination; however, a suggested format is given in the form shown in Fig. 7-1. In general, the vigor and extent of the examination should be based on the patient's history. Also, tests or motions that are anticipated to most likely provoke symptoms should be saved for the end of the examination whenever possible to avoid clouding the remaining tests.

The screening examination includes inspection, progressively vigorous cervical spine testing, a systematic scan of the peripheral joints, myotome testing for motor weakness, sensory testing for diminished light touch sensation, reflex testing, and special tests related to neural tension and palpation of common entrapment sites.

INSPECTION

Inspection includes observation from the side as well as from anterior and posterior. Any asymmetry and gross postural abnormalities should be noted. Careful attention should be given to normal soft tissue contours to observe for muscle wasting in key areas such as the supraspinous and infraspinous fossae (rotator cuff atrophy), the upper trapezius, and deltoid musculature (Fig. 7-2, *A*). Anteriorly, the supraclavicular area should be inspected for any swelling (loss of normal concavity) that could represent the potential for an upper lung tumor (Fig. 7-2, *B*). An elevated shoulder girdle could represent guarding associated with a cervical spine or neural tension problem.

Patient Name:_____

Date:_____

Upper Quarter Screening Examination Form

Inspection:

❑ Forward Head Posture
❑ Asymmetry
❑ Muscle Atrophy
❑ Deformity

Cervical Spine (AROM + Passive overpressure)

	Pain	↓ROM
Flex	❑	❑
R Rot	❑	❑
L Rot	❑	❑
R SideBend	❑	❑
L SideBend	❑	❑
Ext	❑	❑

Distraction	❑
Compression	❑
L Spurling's	❑
R Spurling's	❑

Joint Scan (AROM + Passive overpressure)

	Pain	↓ROM
Shoulder Elev	❑	❑
Elb Flex (pron/sup)	❑	❑
Elb Ext (pron/sup)	❑	❑

Deep Tendon Reflexes

	Left	Right
Biceps	+1 2 3 4	+1 2 3 4
Brachioradialis	+1 2 3 4	+1 2 3 4
Triceps	+1 2 3 4	+1 2 3 4

Myotome Scan

	Weakness	Pain
Shdr Shrug (C2,3,4)	❑	❑
Shdr Abduct (C5)	❑	❑
Elbow Flex (C5-6)	❑	❑
Elbow Ext (C7)	❑	❑
Wrist Ext (C6)	❑	❑
Wrist Flex (C7)	❑	❑
Thumb Abd (C8)	❑	❑
Finger Abd/Add (T1)	❑	❑

Sensory Scan (light touch)

	Diminished
Supraclavicular (C4)	❑
Anterolat Arm (C5)	❑
Lat forearm/thumb (C6)	❑
Middle finger (C7)	❑
Ulnar hand (C8)	❑
Medial forearm (T1)	❑
Apex of axilla (T2)	❑

Neural Tension

	Symptoms
Shoulder abduct/ext rot	❑
+ elbow ext	
+ wrist/finger ext	

Palpation / Neural Compression

	Symptoms
Brachial Plexus	❑
Radial tunnel	❑
Cubital tunnel	❑
Carpal tunnel	❑

Fig. 7-1. Upper quarter screening form.

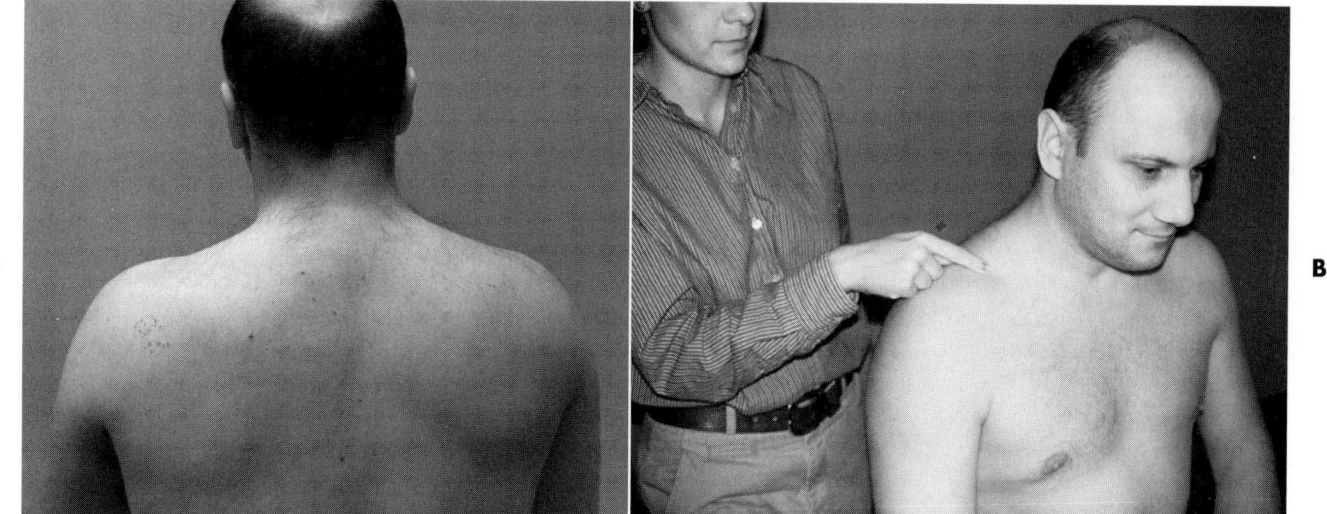

Fig. 7-2. A, Normal soft tissue contours for the upper trapezius, supraspinatus, and infraspinatus muscles. **B,** Normal concavity in supraclavicular area.

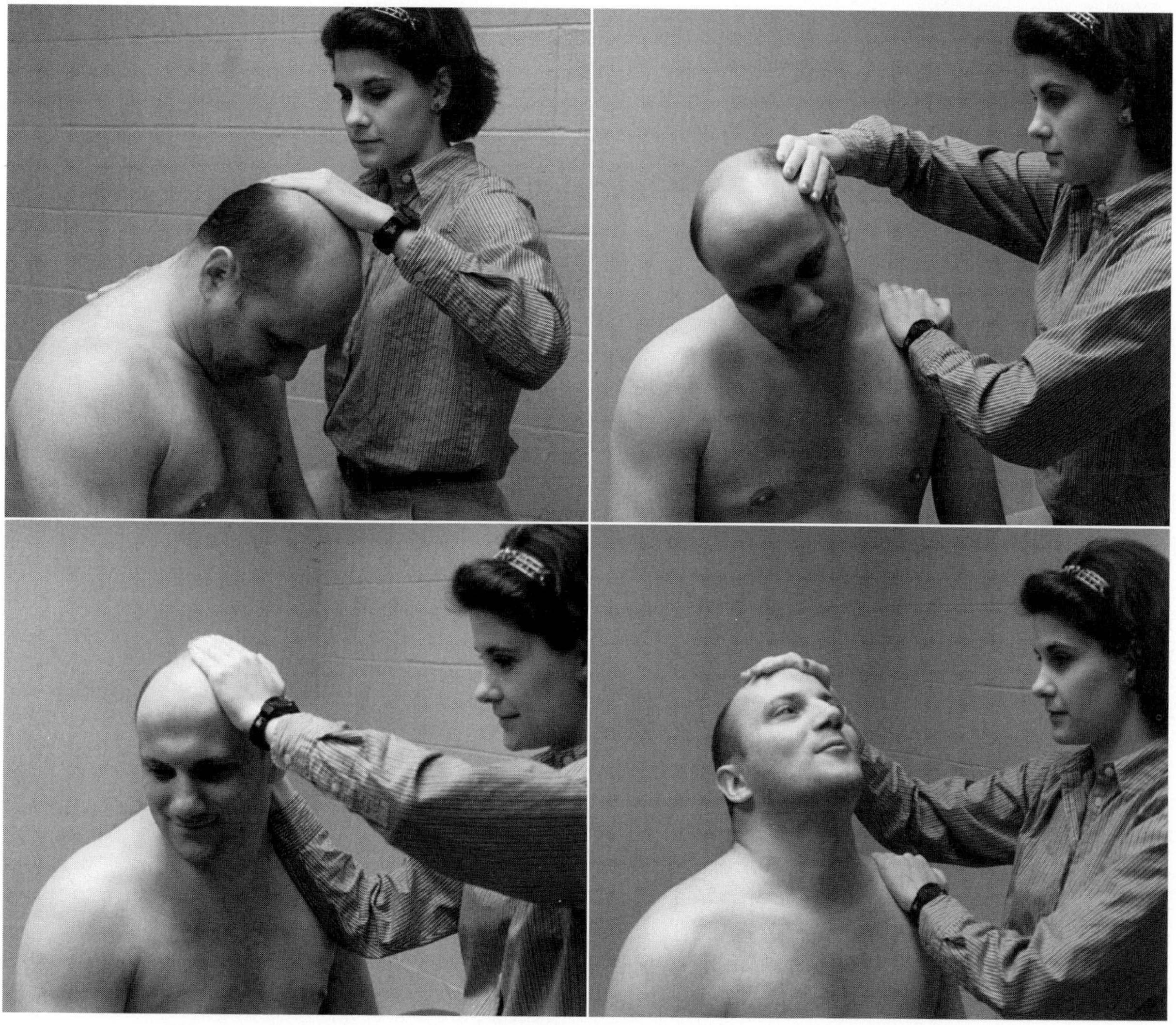

Fig. 7-3. Cervical range of motion testing. The patient first moves to the end-range actively. If no symptoms, passive over-pressure is added. **A,** Flexion. **B,** Side-bending. **C,** Rotation. **D,** Extension.

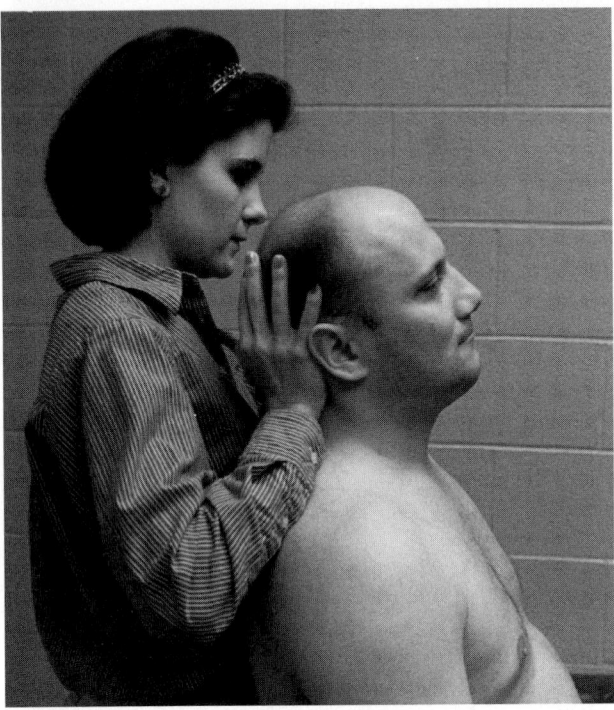

Fig. 7-4. Cervical distraction. The force is applied superiorly via the occiput. The patient must be completely relaxed, which is best achieved by asking him or her to lean back on the chair or on the examiner.

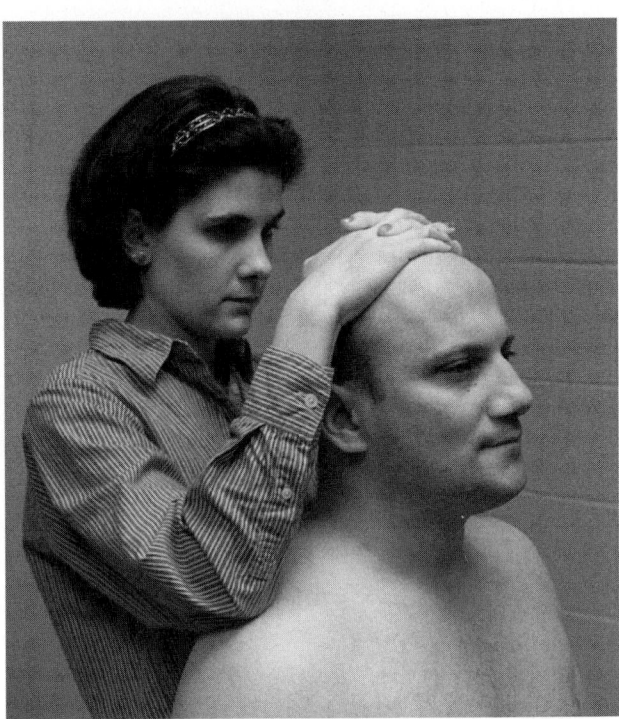

Fig. 7-5. Cervical compression. The force is applied inferiorly through the head. Care must be taken to avoid a forward head posture while applying this test.

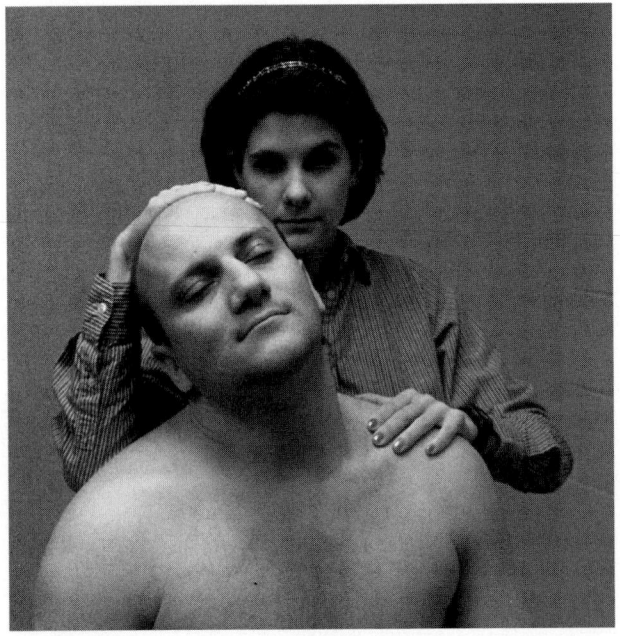

Fig. 7-6. Spurling's maneuver is performed by combining cervical extension, side-bending, and axial compression to the cervical spine.

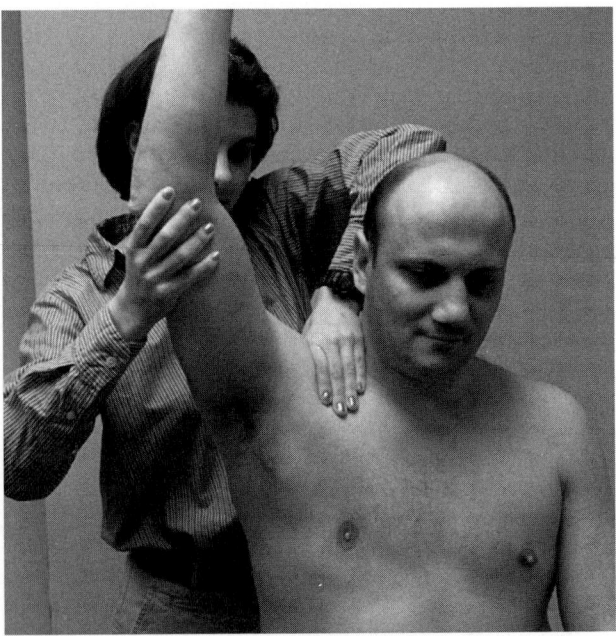

Fig. 7-7. Passive stress to the glenohumeral joint is accomplished by blocking upward scapular motion with one hand while passively elevating the arm.

CERVICAL SPINE

The cervical spine is probably the most common source of referred pain to the upper extremity. If the problem is from direct compression of a nerve root or spinal nerve, the symptoms will include either sensory disturbances or motor weakness.[2,4,10] More commonly, the cervical somatic tissues (ligaments, facet joints, disc, muscle) can refer pain to the upper extremity without direct neural compression.[2] In either case, the goal of the examination is to reproduce the chief complaint symptoms with ROM tests or special tests. ROM testing is done in each direction, first actively, then with passive overpressure applied at the end-range if the active motion was pain free (Fig. 7-3). Generally, cervical extension is the most provocative motion and should be performed last.

If standard motions do not provoke symptoms, cervical distraction, compression, and Spurling's tests are performed (Figs. 7-4 to 7-6). For cervical distraction (see Fig. 7-4), the patient must be relaxed, which is best accomplished by having them lean back slightly on the chair or directly on the examiner. For cervical compression (see Fig. 7-5), care must be taken to have the spine in a neutral position rather than a forward head posture while applying an axial compression force. The single most aggressive test to produce symptoms in the cervical spine is the Spurling's maneuver, which combines cervical extension and lateral bending along with axial compression (see Fig. 7-6). The basis for this test is that this position maximally narrows the intervertebral foramina on the side being tested.[6,7,9-11]

JOINT SCAN

Having tested the cervical spine, the joint scan is designed to quickly ascertain whether the shoulder or elbow joints may be a source of symptoms. The idea here is to take the glenohumeral and elbow joints through full passive motion and then apply overpressure. If no symptoms are produced, this is reasonable evidence that these joints are not the source of symptoms. For glenohumeral testing, the scapula must be blocked from gliding or rotating superiorly so the stress is focused on the glenohumeral joint (Fig. 7-7). Full elbow flexion and extension are combined with pronation and supination.

MYOTOME SCAN

During the myotome scan (Fig. 7-8), muscles that correspond to particular spinal segments are tested for the presence of weakness as listed in the form. The patient should be instructed to "hold, don't let me move you" while the examiner slowly increases the applied force in a controlled fashion. Because the primary goal here is to detect weakness associated with neurologic compromise, strength should be judged normal or diminished relative to the uninvolved side. If both sides are symptomatic, the examiner must use judgment based on past experience. The results

of manual muscle testing must be interpreted cautiously because the reliability of this technique is poor in muscles that are greater than a "fair" grade. If the strength of the muscle is questionable, *some* type of instrument (e.g., Nicholas Manual Muscle Tester, Lafayette Instruments, Lafayette, Indiana, or Microfet, Hoggan Health Industries, Draper, Utah) should be used to document muscle performance more precisely. Resistance that is initially strong but then is easily broken because of pain does not represent neurologic compromise but more likely some irritation of the muscle-tendon unit itself. Painless weakness is most suggestive of neurologic compromise or a complete tear within the muscle-tendon unit.

SENSORY SCAN

During the sensory scan (Fig. 7-9), dermatomes that correspond to particular spinal segments are tested for the presence of diminished sensitivity to light touch as listed in the form. A cotton ball or a brush of the examiner's fingertip may be used bilaterally while the patient is asked "Do these feel the same or different?" If the patient responds "different," the examiner asks "more or less?" The examiner should be careful not to lead the patient by saying something like "Does this feel less here?"

NEURAL TENSION

Specific tests for adverse neural tension within the upper quarter are discussed elsewhere in this text. A simple screening maneuver for the upper quarter is the combined active motions of full shoulder abduction in the frontal plane plus elbow, wrist, and finger extension (Fig. 7-10, page 118). Generally the elbow, wrist, and fingers are extended first, and shoulder abduction is the final motion. If the chief complaint symptoms are reproduced or shoulder abduction is appreciably reduced when combined with elbow, wrist, and finger extension, the possibility of adverse neural tension must be evaluated more fully.

PALPATION

If the history suggests the possibility of peripheral nerve entrapment, the more common sites of entrapment may be palpated in an effort to reproduce the symptoms (Fig. 7-11, page 118). These sites include the brachial plexus in the supraclavicular fossa, the posterior interosseous nerve in the radial tunnel as it pierces the supinator muscle, the ulnar nerve in the cubital tunnel, and the median nerve in the carpal tunnel.

DEEP TENDON REFLEXES

Reflex testing (Fig. 7-12, page 119) may be helpful in determining whether there is neurologic compromise; however, hyporeflexia is rather common so care must be taken to compare reflexes bilaterally.[4,5] Hyporeflexia represents lower motor neuron compromise, which may be at the nerve

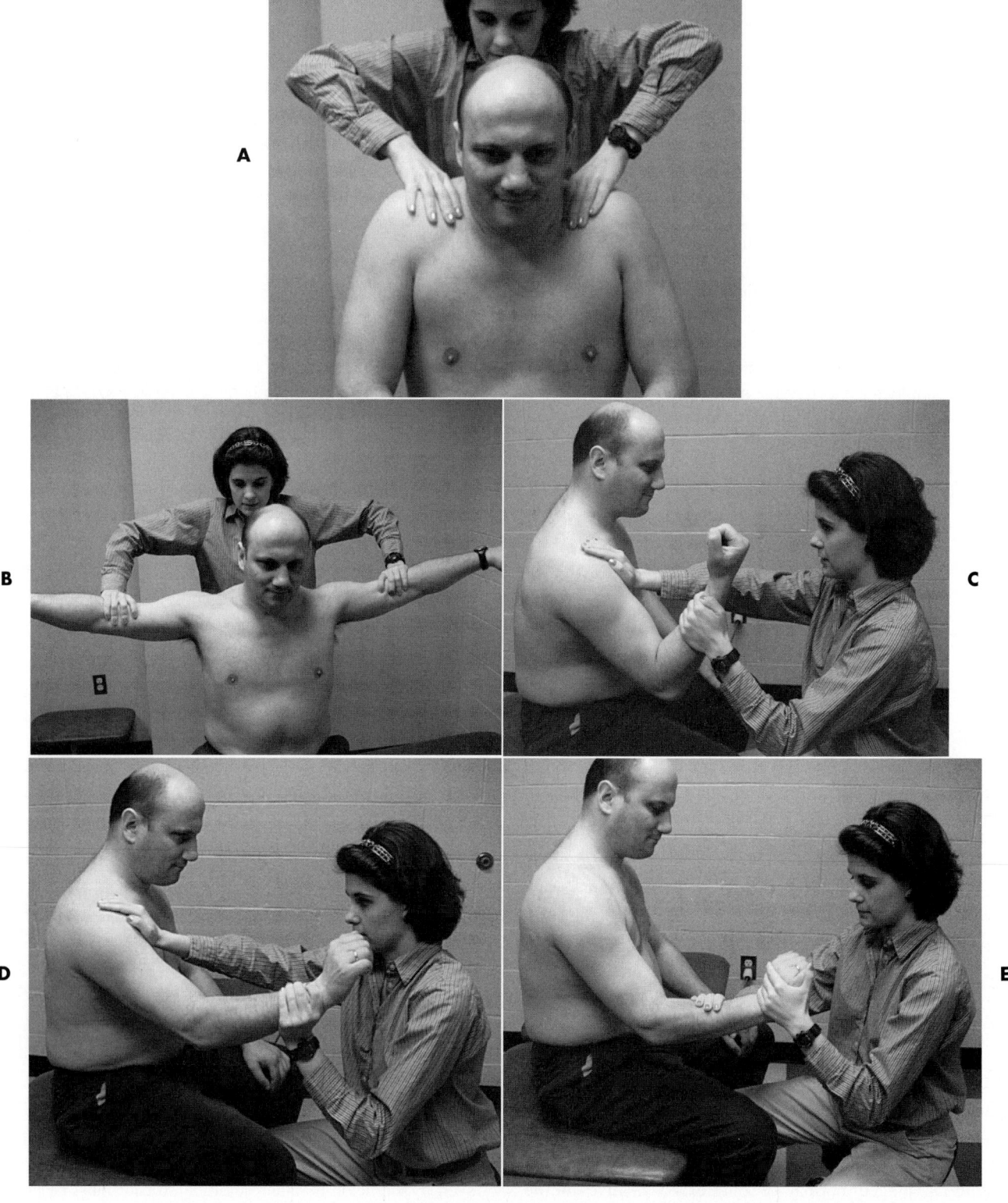

Fig. 7-8. Myotome scan. **A,** Shoulder shrug (C2-C4). **B,** Shoulder abduction (C5). **C,** Elbow flexion (C5-C6). **D,** Elbow extension (C7). **E,** Wrist extension (C6).

F G H I

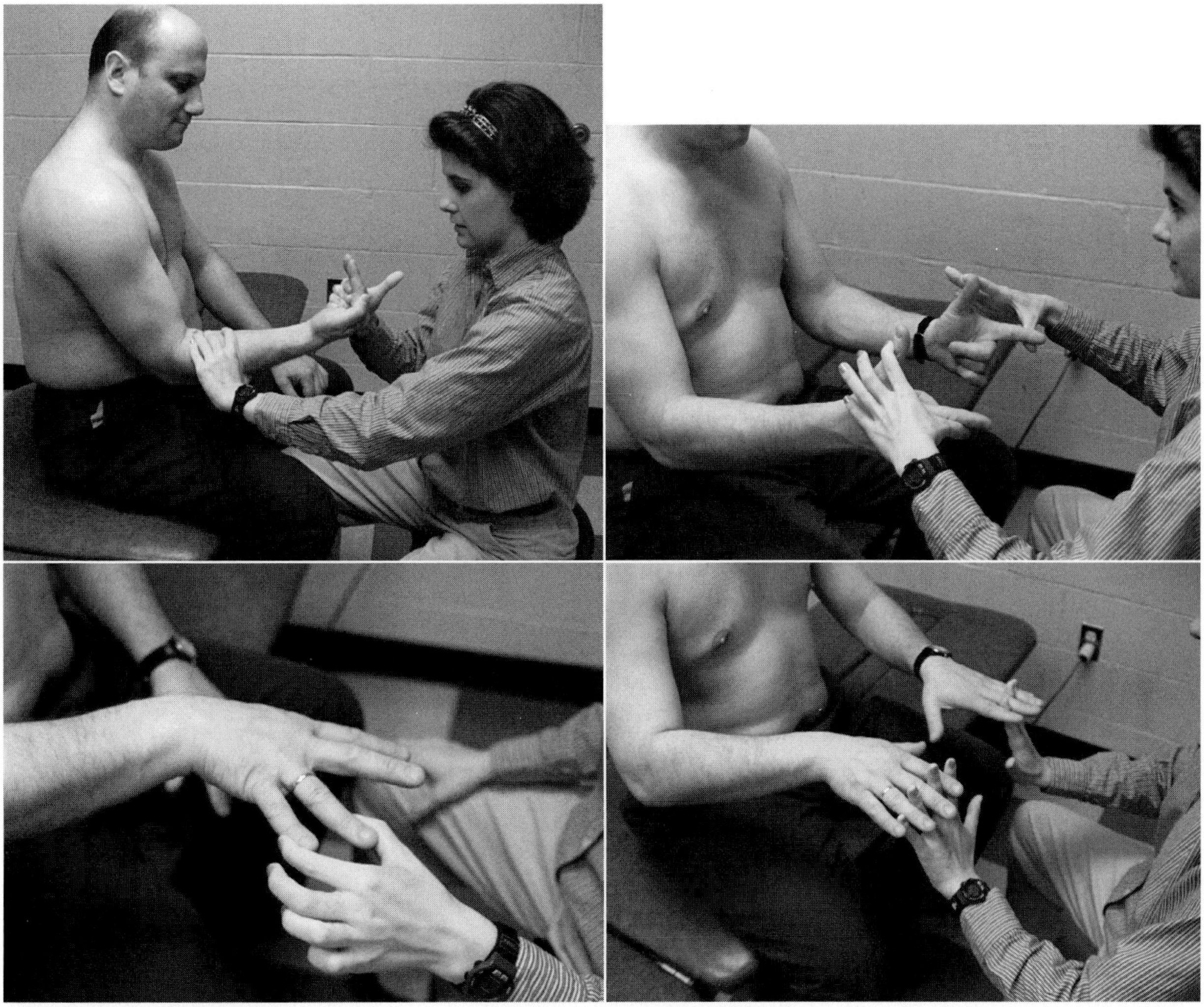

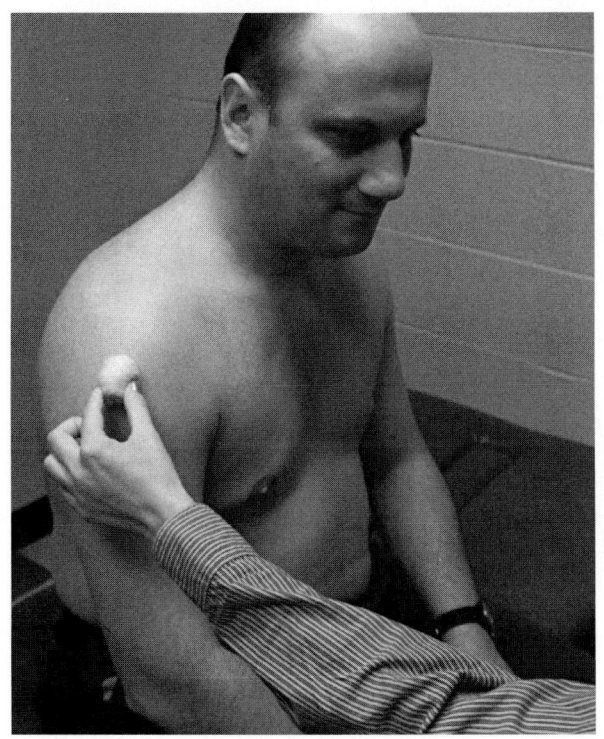

Fig. 7-8, cont'd **F,** Wrist flexion (C7). **G,** Thumb abduction (C8). **H,** Finger abduction. **I,** Adduction (T1).

Fig. 7-9. Sensory scan shown for C5 dermatome using a cotton ball.

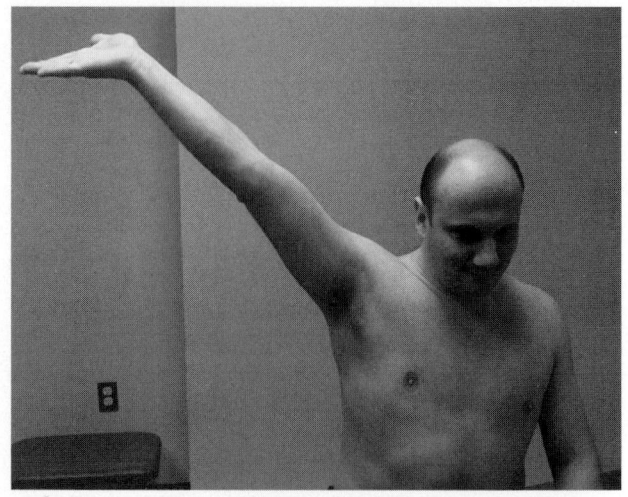

Fig. 7-10. Active test for neural tension. Elbow, wrist, and finger extension followed by shoulder abduction in the frontal plane.

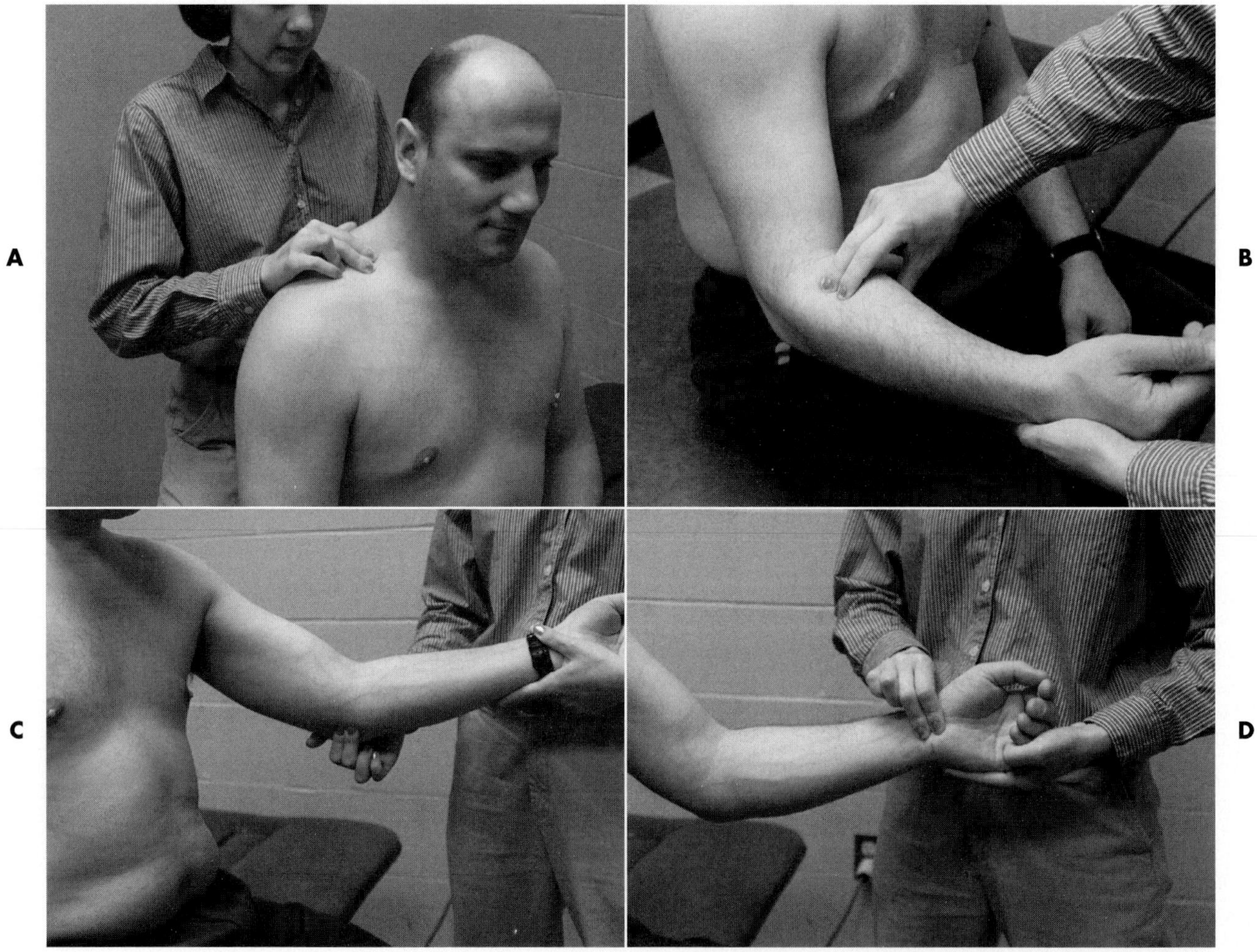

Fig. 7-11. Palpation of common entrapment points. **A,** Brachial plexus. **B,** Radial tunnel. **C,** Cubital tunnel. **D,** Carpal tunnel.

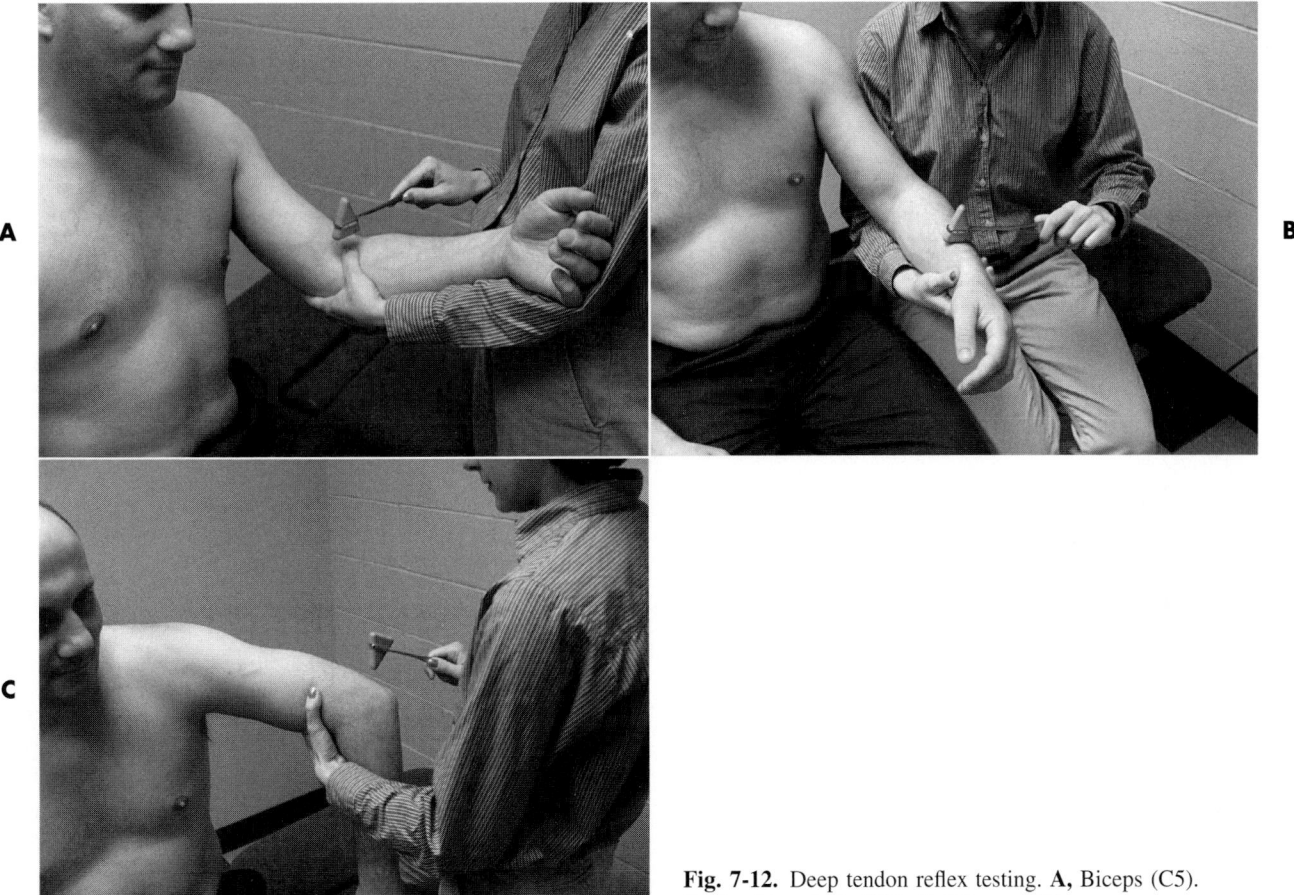

Fig. 7-12. Deep tendon reflex testing. **A,** Biceps (C5).
B, Brachioradialis (C6). **C,** Triceps (C7).

root, spinal nerve, or at a more distal level. If hyperreflexia is observed, upper motor neuron compromise should be suspected such as might occur with spinal stenosis in the cervical region.

SUMMARY

The upper quarter screening examination is designed to provide a quick (5 to 10 minutes) method of (1) determining the region(s) that should be examined in greater detail and (2) ruling out serious neurologic deficits. The screening is most useful in patients whose history suggests the possibility of cervical spine involvement, referred pain, or those for whom the source of symptoms is not clear.

REFERENCES

1. Bogduk N, Aprill C: On the nature of neck pain, discography and cervical zygapophysial joint blocks, *Pain* 54:213, 1993.
2. Bogduk N: Innervation and pain patterns of the cervical spine. In: Grant R, editor. *Physical therapy of the cervical and thoracic spine,* ed 2, New York, 1994, Churchill Livingstone.
3. Cyriax J: *Textbook of orthopedic medicine,* vol 1, *Diagnosis of soft tissue lesions,* ed 6, Baltimore, 1975, Williams & Wilkins.
4. Lestini WF, Wiesel SW: The pathogenesis of cervical spondylosis, *Clin Orthop* 239:69, 1989.
5. Magee David J: *Orthopedic physical assessment,* Philadelphia, 1992, WB Saunders.
6. Sandmark H, Nisell R: Validity of five common manual neck pain provoking tests, *Scand J Rehab Med* 27:131, 1995.
7. Spurling R, Coville W: Lateral rupture of the cervical intervertebral discs, *Surg Gynecol Obstet* 78:350, 1944.
8. Travell JG, Simons DG: *Myofascial pain and dysfunction: the trigger point manual,* Baltimore, 1983, Williams & Wilkins.
9. Viikari-Juntara E, Porras M, Laasonen EM: Validity of clinical tests in the diagnosis of root compression in cervical disc disease, *Spine* 14:253, 1989.
10. White A, Panjabi M: *Clinical biomechanics of the spine,* ed 2, Philadelphia, 1990, Lippincott.
11. Yoo JU, et al: Effect of cervical spine motion on the neuroforaminal dimensions of the human cervical spine, *Spine* 17:1131, 1992.

Chapter 8

CLINICAL EXAMINATION OF THE HAND

Pat L. Aulicino

Clinical examination of the hand is a basic skill that both the surgeon and the therapist should master. To master this skill, it is necessary to have an understanding of the functional anatomy of the hand. A thorough history, a systematic examination, and knowledge of disease processes that affect the hand will leave the examiner with few diagnostic dilemmas. Radiographs, computed tomographic (CT) scans, magnetic resonance imaging (MRI) scans, electrodiagnostics, and specialized laboratory tests are ancillary tools that only confirm a diagnosis that has been made on a clinical basis.

An organized approach and clear and concise records are of paramount importance. Either line drawings of the deformities or clinical photographs should be prepared for each new patient evaluated. Range of motion (ROM) of the affected parts should be recorded and dated in a table format. Any discrepancy between active and passive motion, if present, also should be noted. A good hand examination is useless if the results are not recorded accurately.

This chapter outlines one approach to examination of the hand. The most important points already have been made: perform a systematic, organized clinical examination and record the results accurately and clearly.

HISTORY

Before a patient's hand is examined, an accurate history must be taken. The patient's age, hand dominance, occupation, and avocations are elicited. If the patient has had an injury, the exact mechanism as well as the time and date of the injury and prior treatments are recorded. Prior surgical procedures, infections, medications, and therapy also are noted. After these background data are obtained, the patient is questioned specifically regarding the involved extremity.

Does he or she have pain? What is the character of the pain? When does it occur? Is it work related or constant? Does it occur at night or during the day? What relieves the pain, and what exacerbates it? What is the patient not able to do now that he could do before the injury? What does the patient desire from you? This last question is extremely important. The patient's reply will assist you in determining whether the patient has a realistic understanding of the true nature of the injury. Unrealistic expectations can never be fulfilled. They result in both an unhappy patient and an unhappy therapist and surgeon. During this interview, it is also important to assess the effect that the injury or disease process has on the patient's family, economic, and social life. Patients who have litigation pending or significant secondary gain are usually poorly motivated and are not optimal candidates for elective hand surgery. Successful hand surgery requires precise surgical techniques followed by expert hand therapy in conjunction with a well-motivated, compliant patient.

The patient's pertinent medical history is now obtained. Does he or she have rheumatoid arthritis or some other progressive collagen-vascular disease? Is the patient taking systemic steroids or some other medication? Does the patient have any other chronic systemic illness that would make him or her a poor surgical risk? The history is completed only after the surgeon or therapist has a complete understanding of the patient's problem and how this affects the patient physically, psychologically, and economically.

PHYSICAL EXAMINATION
General inspection

When examining a patient's upper extremity, one must be able to observe the shoulder, arm, forearm, and hand. Therefore the patient's entire upper extremity should be

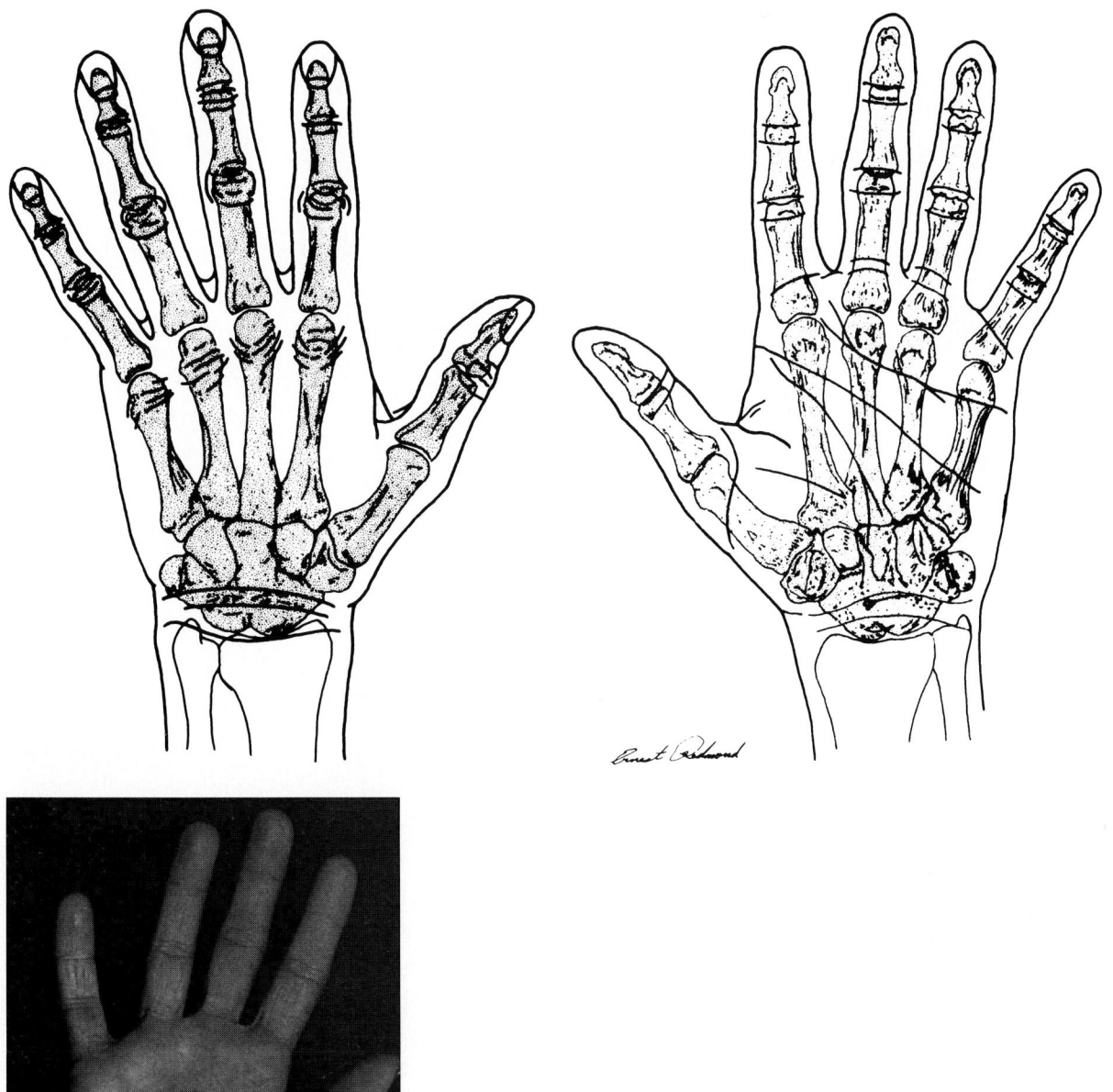

Fig. 8-1. Clinical photograph and diagrammatic illustrations of the relationship of the volar and dorsal skin creases to the underlying joints. The absence of a volar skin crease may indicate the presence of an underlying joint anomaly and thus the inability of the patient to flex that digit, as is seen in congenital symphalangism. The absence of both volar and dorsal skin creases is seen in conditions that cause edema, or as a result of the atrophic phase of a reflex sympathetic dystrophy. (Redrawn from Chase RA: *Atlas of hand surgery,* Philadelphia, 1973, WB Saunders.)

exposed. The gross appearance of the entire extremity is noted. Are the shoulder muscles atrophied? Does the patient have a normal-appearing upper extremity or is there a traumatic or congenital anomaly? Are there any scars? Are there numerous tattoos or needle marks? How does the patient carry this limb? Can he or she move the shoulder and arm without pain? Is the patient able to place his or her hand?

If the hand cannot be placed in a functional position, a brilliantly reconstructed hand is useless.

After the general appearance of the limb has been noted, attention is directed to the integument. The color, tone, and moisture of the skin are noted. Are the normal skin creases present (Fig. 8-1)? Is there any edema of the hand? Are the nails ridged, pitted, or deformed? Is there correct rotational

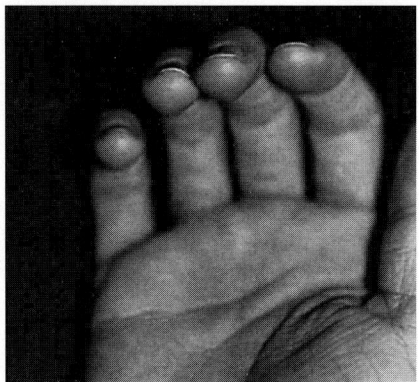

Fig. 8-2. Normal rotational alignment of nail plates.

alignment of the nail plates (Fig. 8-2)? Are there any obvious deformities of the hand? Do the thenar or hypothenar muscles appear atrophied? Are there any contractures? When the patient's injured extremity is being inspected, the uninjured extremity also should be inspected for comparison. The resting attitude of the hand is then noted. Normally, with the hand resting and the wrist in neutral, the fingers are progressively more flexed from the radial to the ulnar side of the hand. A loss of the normal resting attitude of the hand can indicate a tendon laceration, a contracture, or possibly a peripheral nerve injury (Fig. 8-3).

Part of the general inspection is noting how the patient treats the injured limb. Does he or she cradle the injured hand and stare at it as if it does not belong to him or her, or does the patient appear relatively unhampered by the injury? Bizarre posturing or overreaction may indicate deep-seated psychiatric problems. All observations are, of course, assiduously recorded.

Range of motion

The motion of the entire extremity should be measured and compared with that of the opposite side. As previously stated, discrepancies between active and passive motion should be noted. Fixed deformities also are noted.

The shoulder should be tested for forward flexion, extension, abduction, and internal and external rotation. Elbow extension and flexion and forearm supination and pronation also are measured and recorded. Wrist dorsiflexion, volar flexion, and ulnar and radial deviation are recorded. Thumb extension, flexion, opposition, and adduction; carpometacarpal (CMC) extension; and CMC abduction are recorded. A finger goniometer should be used to make each of these measurements.[36] If motion is lacking, the distance from the tip of the finger to the distal palmar crease (DPC) is measured. If the finger touches the palm but does not reach the crease, as in the profundus tendon disruption, this should be noted, and the distance from the tip of the finger to the DPC should be recorded; however, it should be stated that the finger did touch the palm but did not reach the DPC (Fig. 8-4).

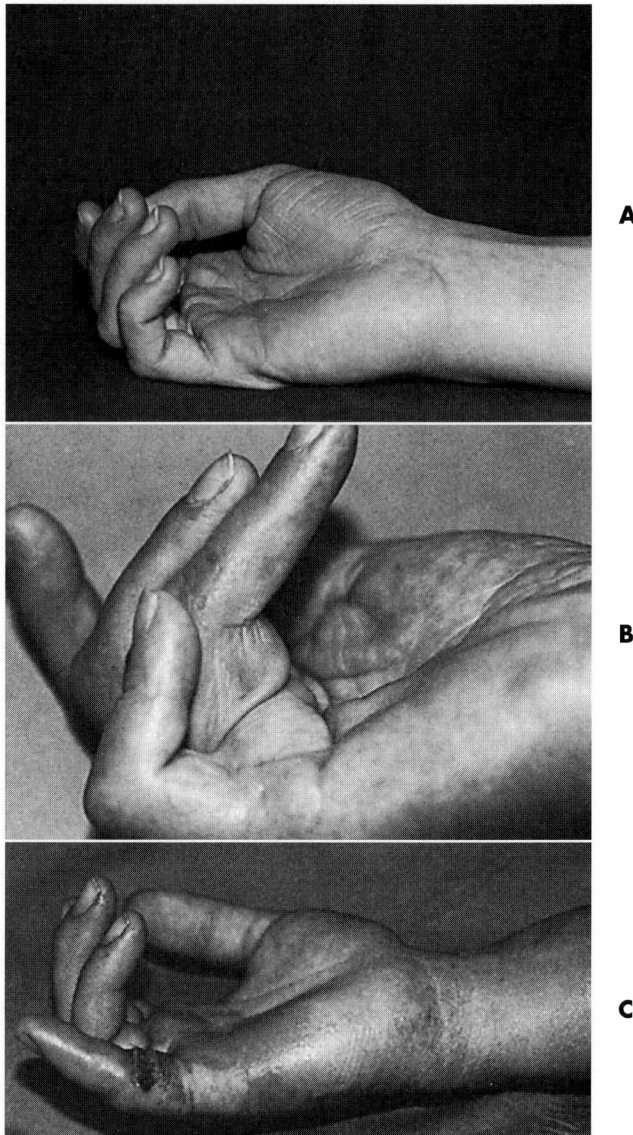

Fig. 8-3. A, Normal attitude of the hand in a resting position. Notice that the fingers are progressively more flexed from the radial aspect to the ulnar aspect of the hand. In **B,** this normal attitude is lost because of contractures of the digits as a result of Dupuytren's disease. **C,** Loss of the normal attitude as a result of a laceration of the flexor tendons to the fifth digit.

After all active and passive motions have been examined, the wrist is flexed and extended to see if the normal tenodesis effect is present. In an uninjured hand, when the wrist is flexed, the fingers and the thumb will extend, and as the wrist is extended, the fingers will assume an attitude of flexion and the thumb will oppose the fifth digit (Fig. 8-5). This is an automatic motion of the hand and does not require patient compliance. The alignment of the digits is then inspected. As stated, the nail plates all should be parallel to one another, and their alignment should be similar to that of the other hand. Each finger should point individually to the tuberosity

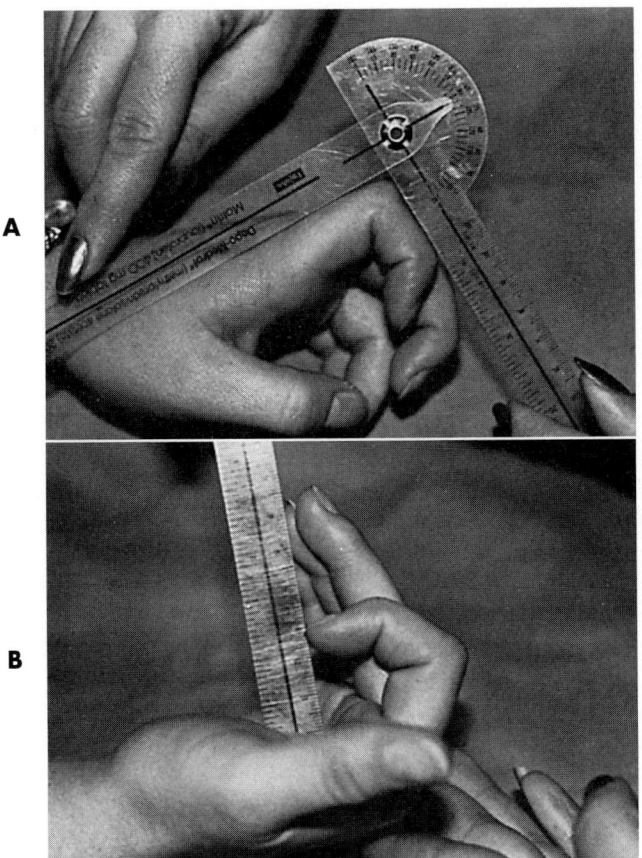

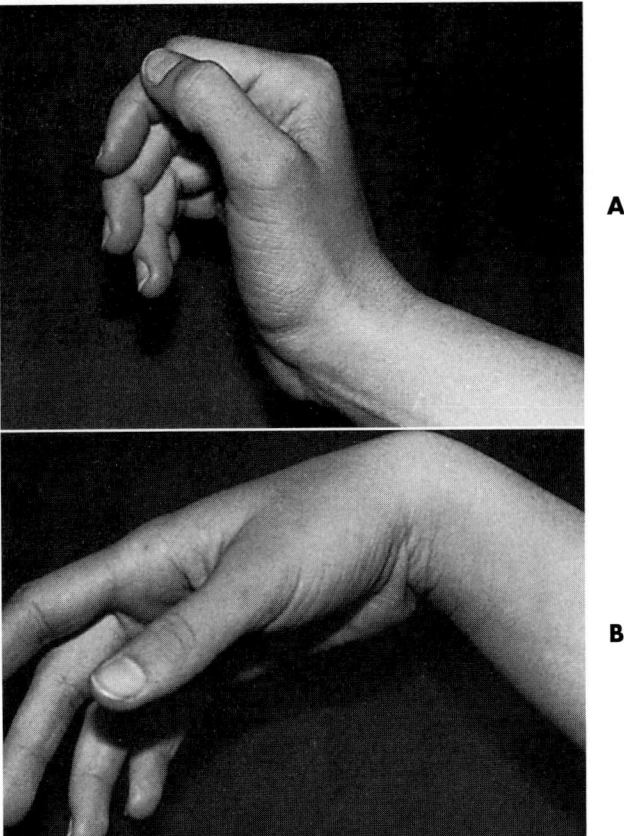

Fig. 8-4. A, A finger goniometer is used to measure the range of motion of the proximal interphalangeal joint of the index finger. **B,** A ruler is then used to measure the distance of the pulp of the finger from the distal palmar crease. Active and passive motions should be noted and recorded.

Fig. 8-5. Tenodesis of the hand. In an uninjured hand, on wrist dorsiflexion **(A)** the fingers and thumb will flex, and on flexion of the wrist **(B),** the thumb and fingers will extend. In the presence of a tendon laceration, contractures of the joints, or adhesions of the flexor or extensor systems, the normal tenodesis effect will be lost. This test can be performed actively by the patient or passively by the examiner.

of the scaphoid, and the longitudinal axis of all fingers when flexed should point in the direction of the scaphoid (Fig. 8-6).

Muscle testing

The hand is powered by intrinsic and extrinsic muscles. The extrinsic muscles have their origin in the forearm and the tendinous insertions in the hand. The extrinsic flexors are on the volar side of the forearm and flex the digits and the wrist. The extrinsic extensors originate on the dorsal aspect of the forearm and extend the fingers, thumb, and wrist. The intrinsic muscles originate and insert in the hand. These include the thenar and hypothenar muscles as well as the lumbricals and the interossei. The thenar and hypothenar muscles help position the thumb and the fifth finger and also aid in opposition of the thumb and in pinch. The interossei assist in abduction and adduction of the digits. The interossei flex the metacarpophalangeal (MP) joints and extend the interphalangeal (IP) joints. The function and testing of the intrinsic muscles is discussed later in this chapter.

Extrinsic muscle testing—the extrinsic flexors. As each specific extrinsic muscle-tendon unit is tested, its strength should be graded and recorded. Strength should be graded from 0 to 5, with 5 being normal. In grade 0, there is no evidence of contractility. In grade 1 (trace), there is slight evidence of contractility and no joint motion. In grade 2 (poor), there is complete ROM with gravity eliminated. In grade 3 (fair), there is complete ROM against gravity. In grade 4 (good), there is complete ROM against gravity with some resistance. In grade 5 (normal), there is complete ROM against gravity with full resistance.

The flexor pollicis longus (long flexor of the thumb) flexes the IP joint of the thumb. This muscle is tested by asking the patient to actively flex the last joint of his thumb (Fig. 8-7).

The flexor digitorum profundus of the fingers are then tested, in sequence, by having the patient flex the distal interphalangeal (DIP) joint of the finger being tested while the examiner holds the digit in full extension and blocks

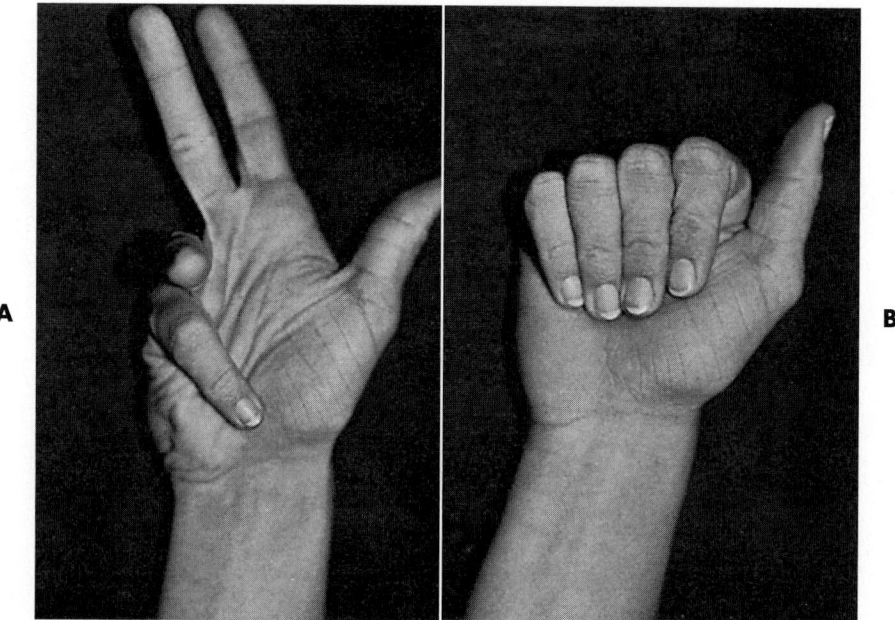

Fig. 8-6. A, On flexion the tip of the fifth finger will point directly to the tuberosity of the scaphoid, as will all the fingers when individually flexed. **B,** When all the digits are flexed simultaneously, the finger tips come together distal to the tuberosity, but the longitudinal axes of all fingers converge at an area proximal to the tuberosity of the scaphoid because of crowding of the adjacent digits. If there is a malunited fracture, the rotational alignment will be off and often there will be crossover of the digits.

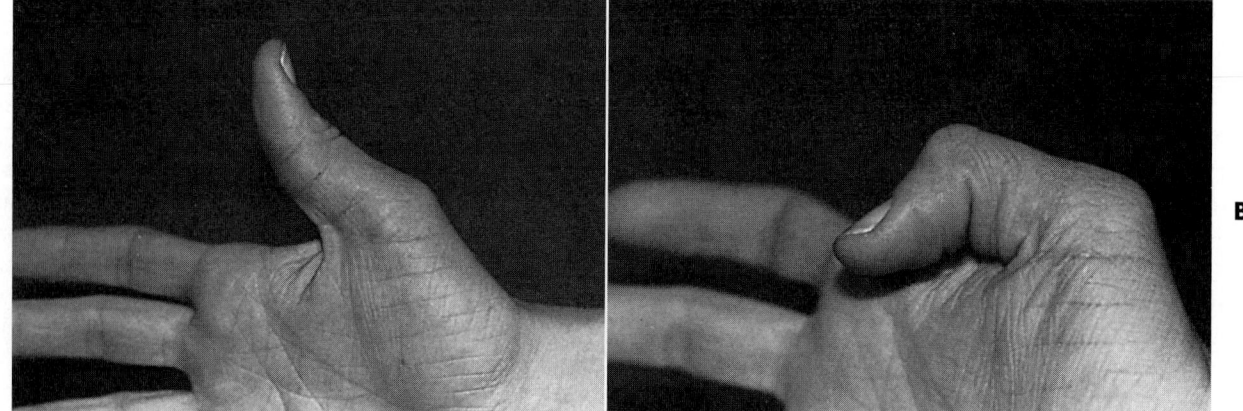

Fig. 8-7. Testing the flexor pollicis longus. **A,** With the thumb in a position of full extension at the interphalangeal joint, the patient is asked to actively flex this joint. **B,** The range of motion and grade of strength are recorded. It is also important to note whether the motion is obtained with or without blocking of the preceding joint by the examiner. This applies not only to testing the flexor pollicis longus but also to testing all other flexor systems because more power and motion can be obtained when blocking is used.

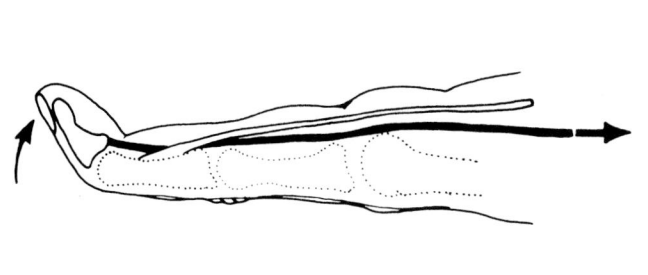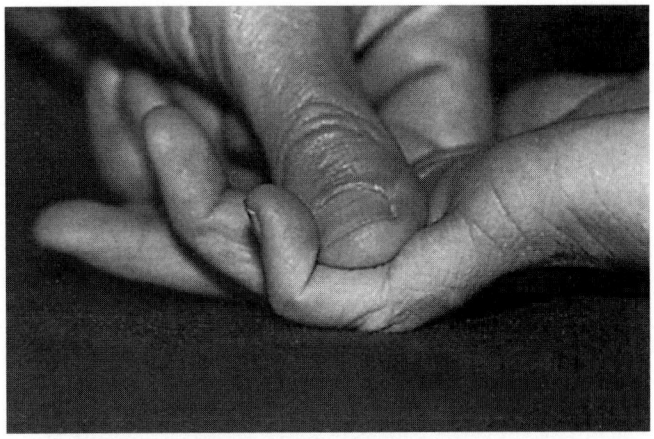

Fig. 8-8. Profundus test. The flexor digitorum profundus tendon flexes the distal interphalangeal joint. With the metacarpophalangeal joint and the proximal interphalangeal joint held in extension by the examiner, the patient is asked to flex the distal interphalangeal joint. (Redrawn from Hoppenfeld S: *Physical examination of the spine and extremities,* New York, 1976, Appleton-Century-Crofts.)

motion at the proximal interphalangeal (PIP) joint and the MP joint. During the testing of each profundus tendon, the other fingers are maintained in a slightly flexed position (Fig. 8-8).

The flexor digitorum superficialis of each finger is then tested. The examiner must hold the adjacent fingers in full extension. The PIP joint of the finger being tested is not blocked (Fig. 8-9). If the flexor system is functioning properly, the PIP will flex and the DIP joint will remain in extension. The fifth finger often has a deficient superficialis.[3] That is, it is not strong enough to flex the IP joint: on testing, the MP joint will flex and the DIP joint and the PIP joint will remain in extension. In the presence of a deficient superficialis tendon of the fifth digit, simultaneous testing of the fourth and fifth digits often reveals normal superficialis function of the fourth digit.

The flexors of the wrist can be tested by having the patient flex the wrist against resistance in a radial and then in an ulnar direction while the examiner palpates each tendon. The flexor carpi radialis (FCR) is palpated on the radial side of the wrist, and the flexor carpi ulnaris is palpated on the ulnar side of the wrist. The palmaris longus tendon can be palpated just ulnar to the FCR tendon.

Extrinsic muscle testing—the extensors. As previously stated, the extensors of the digits and the wrist originate on the dorsal aspect of the forearm and pass through six discrete retinacular compartments at the dorsum of the wrist before their insertions in the hand.

The first dorsal compartment contains the abductor pollicis longus (APL) and the extensor pollicis brevis (EPB) tendons. The APL usually has multiple tendon slips and inserts on the base of the first metacarpal and often has insertions on the trapezium. The EPB often runs in a separate compartment within the first dorsal compartment. The EPB and APL function in unison and are responsible for abduction of the first metacarpal and extension into the plane of the metacarpals. The EPB is also an extensor of the MP joint of the thumb. These musculotendinous units are tested by asking the patient to bring the thumb "out to the side and the back." Pain in the area of the first dorsal compartment and radial styloid is common and often a result of stenosing tenovaginitis of these tendons. This was first described by de Quervain in 1895 and now is a well-established clinical entity that bears his name. In 1930, Finkelstein stated that acute flexion of the thumb and deviation of the wrist in an ulnar direction would produce excruciating pain at the first dorsal compartment, near the radial styloid, in patients who had stenosing tenovaginitis. This examination is now universally known as *Finkelstein's test*[13] (Fig. 8-10). Failure to release the subcompartment of the EPB is a cause of persistent pain and a persistently positive Finkelstein's test after surgical release of the first dorsal compartment.

The extensor carpi radialis longus and brevis run in the second dorsal compartment. The longus inserts on the base of the second metacarpal and the brevis on the third. These are tested by asking the patient to make a tight fist and to strongly dorsiflex the wrist. The two tendons are then palpated by the examiner (Fig. 8-11).

The extensor pollicis longus (EPL) runs in the third dorsal compartment. This tendon both extends the IP joint of the thumb and adducts the first ray. The tendon passes sharply around Lister's tubercle and may rupture spontaneously after a Colles fracture or in rheumatoid arthritis.[38] Its function is tested by placing the patient's hand flat on the examining table and having him or her lift only the thumb off the table. The EPL can be visualized and palpated (Fig. 8-12).

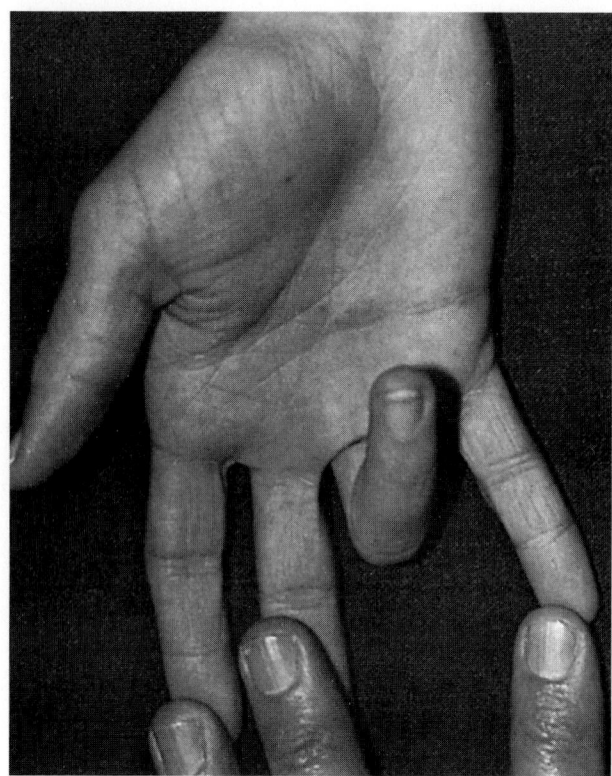

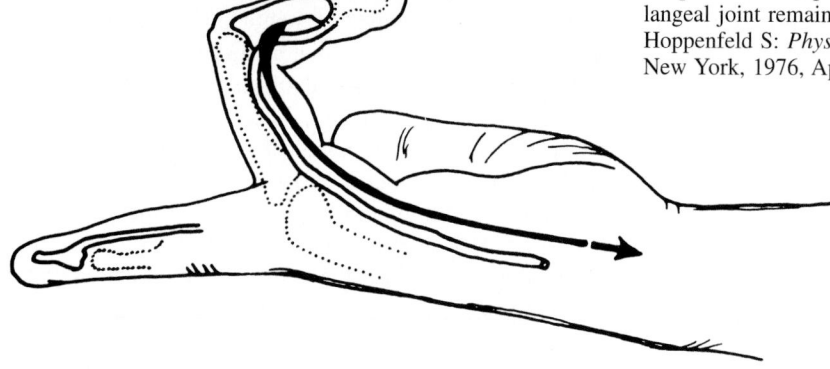

Fig. 8-9. Superficialis test. The flexor digitorum superficialis tendon flexes the proximal interphalangeal joint. The examiner must hold the adjacent fingers in full extension while asking the patient to flex the finger being tested. If the flexor system is functioning normally, the proximal interphalangeal joint will flex, while the distal interphalangeal joint remains in extension. (Redrawn by permission from Hoppenfeld S: *Physical examination of the spine and extremities,* New York, 1976, Appleton-Century-Crofts.)

The area of the wrist just distal to the radial styloid and bounded by the EPL ulnarly and the APL and EPB radially is known as the *anatomic snuffbox.* In this area runs the dorsal branch of the radial artery. A sensory branch of the radial nerve also passes over this area. The carpal scaphoid can be palpated in the base of the snuffbox. Tenderness in this area is suggestive of an acute scaphoid fracture or a painful scaphoid nonunion. However, strong pressure over this area will result in pain in the normal individual caused by pressure on the sensory radial nerve and dorsal branch of the radial artery.

The fourth dorsal compartment contains the extensor indicis proprius (EIP) and the extensor digitorum communis (EDC). These tendons are responsible for extension of the MP joints of the fingers. The EIP allows independent extension of the index MP joint. The EIP is tested by having the patient extend the index finger while the other fingers are flexed into a fist. The mass action of the EDC tendons is tested by having the patient extend the MP joints (Fig. 8-13). This test is performed with the IP joints flexed because the PIP joints are extended by the intrinsic muscles and not the long extensors of the hand. This may be a source of confusion to an uninitiated examiner. Patients with a high radial nerve palsy will still be able to extend the IP joints through the intrinsics.

The fifth dorsal compartment contains the extensor digiti

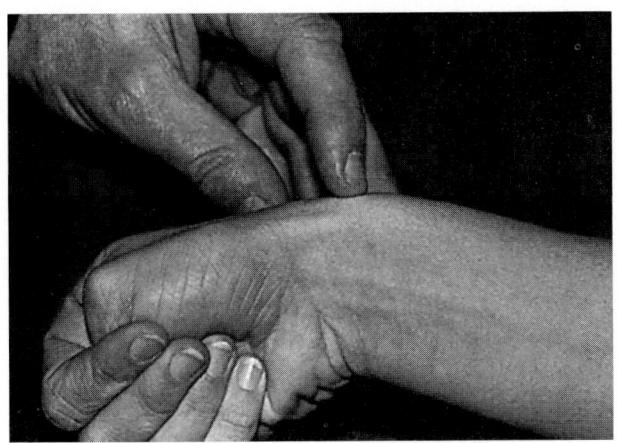

Fig. 8-10. Finkelstein's test for de Quervain's stenosing tenovaginitis of the first dorsal compartment. Acute flexion of the thumb and deviation of the wrist in an ulnar direction will produce excruciating pain at the first dorsal compartment, near the radial styloid, in patients who have this pathologic entity.

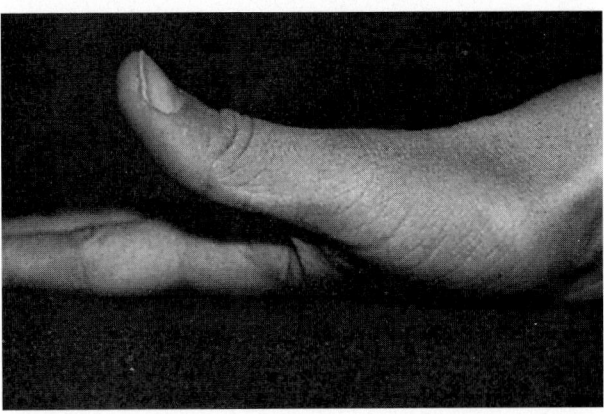

Fig. 8-12. The extensor pollicis longus tendon is tested by placing the patient's hand flat on the examining table and asking the patient to lift the thumb off the table. The extensor pollicis longus can then be visualized and palpated.

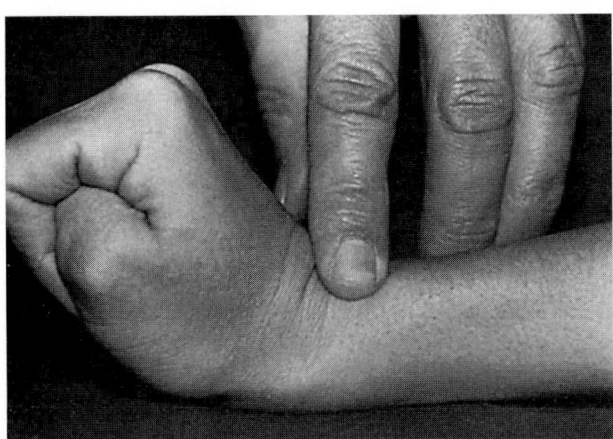

Fig. 8-11. On dorsiflexion of the wrist, the examiner can palpate the extensor carpi radialis longus, inserting on the base of the second metacarpal, and the extensor carpi radialis brevis, inserting on the base of the third metacarpal.

quinti (EDQ), which is responsible for independent extension of the MP joint of the little finger. It is tested by having the patient extend the fifth finger while the others are flexed. Because the EDQ and the EIP work independently of the communis tendons, most examiners test them simultaneously by having the patient extend the index and fifth fingers while the middle and ring fingers are flexed (Fig. 8-14).

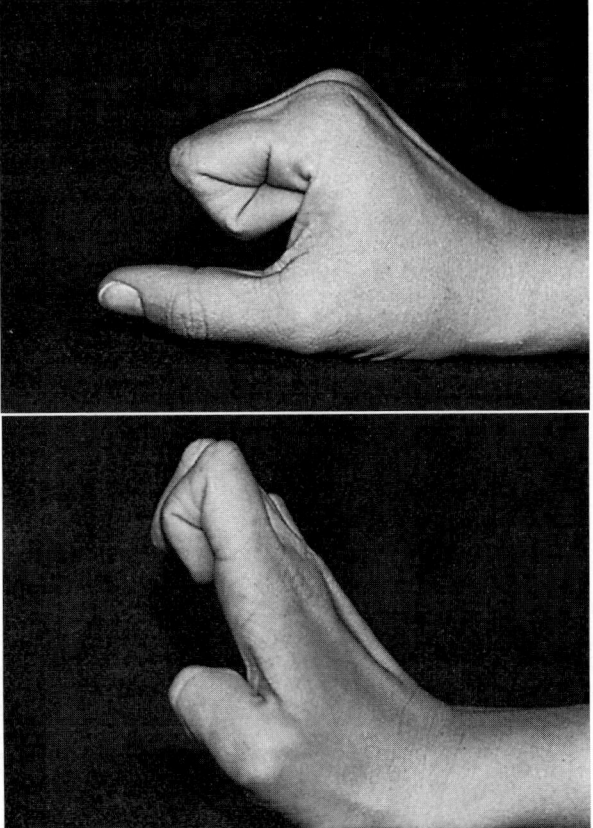

Fig. 8-13. The extensor digitorum communis tendons are tested by having the patient extend the metacarpophalangeal joints, with the proximal interphalangeal joints flexed.

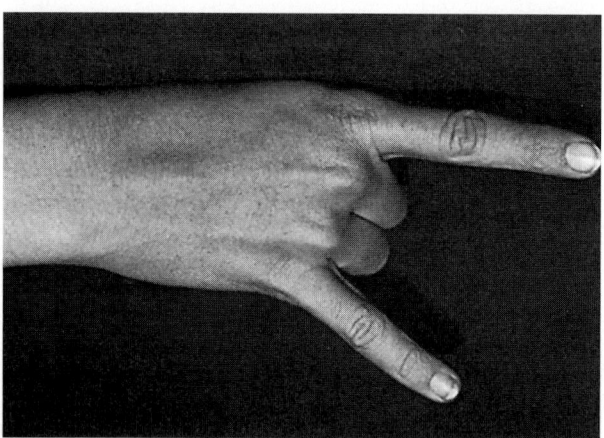

Fig. 8-14. The extensor digiti quinti and the extensor indicis proprius work independently of the communis tendons; they are tested by asking the patient to extend the index and fifth fingers while the middle and ring fingers are flexed.

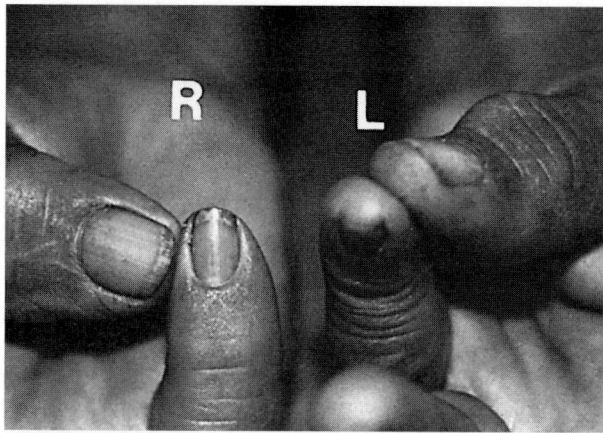

Fig. 8-16. Hands of a patient with a low median nerve palsy on the right side, resulting from a longstanding carpal tunnel syndrome. Notice that in attempted opposition, the nail plate is perpendicular to the plane of the metacarpals on the affected side *(R),* while the nail plate is parallel to the plane of the metacarpals on the normal side *(L).* Tip-to-tip pinch is impossible on the side with the loss of opposition.

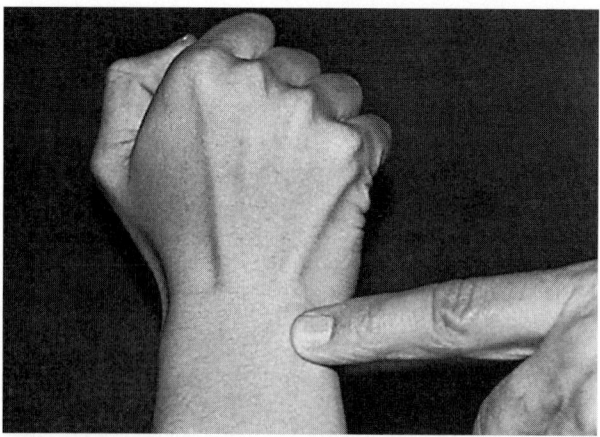

Fig. 8-15. The extensor carpi ulnaris can be visualized and palpated as it inserts on the base of the fifth metacarpal, while the patient dorsiflexes the wrist in an ulnar direction.

The sixth dorsal compartment contains the extensor carpi ulnaris, which inserts into the base of the fifth metacarpal and helps dorsiflex the wrist in an ulnar direction. This is tested by having the patient pull the hand dorsally and in an ulnar direction while the examiner palpates the tendon (Fig. 8-15).

Intrinsic muscle testing. The intrinsic musculature of the hand consists of the thenar and hypothenar muscles and the lumbricals and the interossei. All of these muscles originate and insert within the hand. There is a delicate balance between the intrinsic and extrinsic muscles, which is necessary for normal functioning of the hand.

The thenar muscles consist of the abductor pollicis brevis (APB), the flexor pollicis brevis, the opponens pollicis, and the adductor pollicis. These muscles position the thumb

and help perform the complex motions of opposition and adduction of the thumb.[28] Opposition, according to Bunnell, takes place in the intercarpal, CMC, and MP joints.[7] All three of these joints contribute to the angulatory and rotatory motions that produce true opposition. If one observes the thumb during opposition, it first abducts from the hand and then follows a semicircular path. The thumb pronates, and the proximal phalanx angulates radially on the first metacarpal. If the nail plate is observed, one can see that before beginning opposition, the thumbnail is perpendicular to the plane of the metacarpals. At the end of the opposition, the thumbnail is parallel to the plane of the metacarpals. During adduction, the thumb sweeps across the palm without following the semicircular path. The nail plate remains perpendicular to the plane of the metacarpals at all times. Because opposition is median-nerve innervated and adduction is usually ulnar-nerve innervated, one can easily see the difference between these two motions by comparing the hands of a patient with a longstanding low median nerve palsy on one side (Fig. 8-16).

Opposition is tested by having the patient touch the tip of the thumb to the tip of the little finger (Fig. 8-17). At the end of opposition, the thumbnail should be perpendicular to the nail of the little finger and parallel to the plane of the metacarpals.

The APB, which is the most radial and superficial of the thenar muscles, is usually the first to atrophy with severe median-nerve dysfunction, such as that resulting from a longstanding carpal tunnel syndrome. This muscle can be tested by having the patient abduct the thumb while the examiner palpates the muscle.

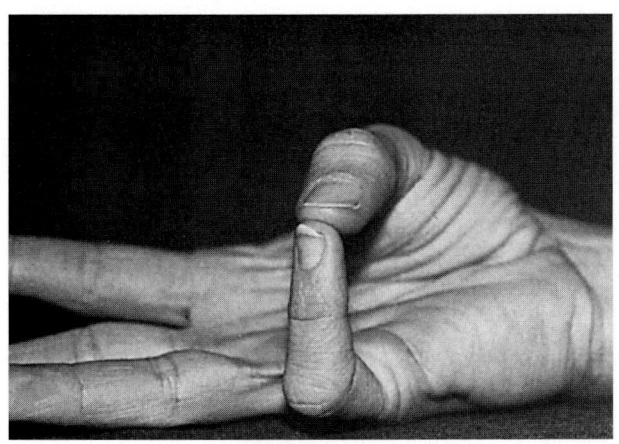

Fig. 8-17. Opposition of tip of thumb to tip of fifth digit. Notice tip-to-tip pinch and the relationship of the nail plate of the thumb to the plane of the metacarpals.

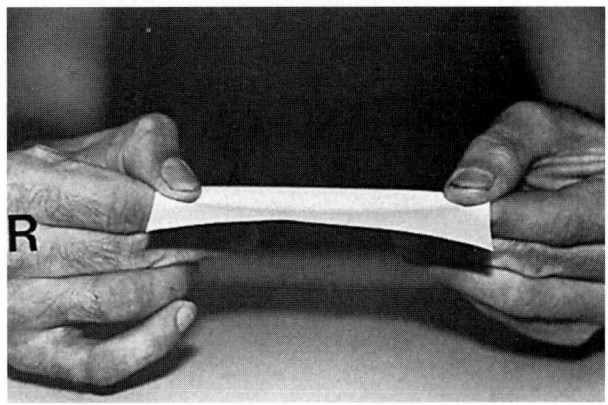

Fig. 8-18. Patient with low ulnar nerve palsy on the right. Weakness of pinch is demonstrated by Froment's and Jeanne's signs on the affected side *(R)*.

Thumb adduction is performed by the adductor pollicis, which is an ulnar-nerve innervated muscle. This muscle, in combination with the first dorsal interosseus, is necessary for strong pinch. The adductor stabilizes the thumb during pinch and also helps extend the IP joint of the thumb through its attachment into the dorsal apparatus. Thumb adduction can be tested by having the patient forcibly hold a piece of paper between his thumb and the radial side of the proximal phalanx of the index finger. When adduction is weak or nonfunctional, the IP joint of the thumb flexes during this maneuver; this is known as *Froment's sign* (1915).[26] *Froment's sign* is an indication of weak or absent adductor function. *Jeanne's sign* (1915) is hyperextension of the MP joint of the thumb during pinch[26] (Fig. 8-18).

The hypothenar muscles consist of the abductor digiti minimi, the flexor digiti minimi, and the opponens digiti minimi. The abductor and flexor aid in abduction of the fifth digit and in MP joint flexion of that digit. The deeper opponens digiti minimi aids in adduction and rotation of the fifth metacarpal during opposition of the thumb to the fifth finger. This helps cup the hand during grip and opposition. The hypothenar muscles are tested as one unit by having the patient abduct the little finger while the examiner palpates the muscle mass (Fig. 8-19).

The anatomy of the interossei is very complex, with much variation in their origins and insertions. There are seven interossei: four dorsal and three palmar. These muscles arise from the metacarpal shafts but have variable insertions. The palmar interossei almost always insert into the dorsal apparatus of the finger. The first dorsal interosseus almost always inserts into bone. The remaining dorsal interossei have varying insertions. (Refer to the work of Eyler and Markee for a more detailed description of the anatomy.[12]) The interossei are usually ulnar-nerve innervated, with a few exceptions.

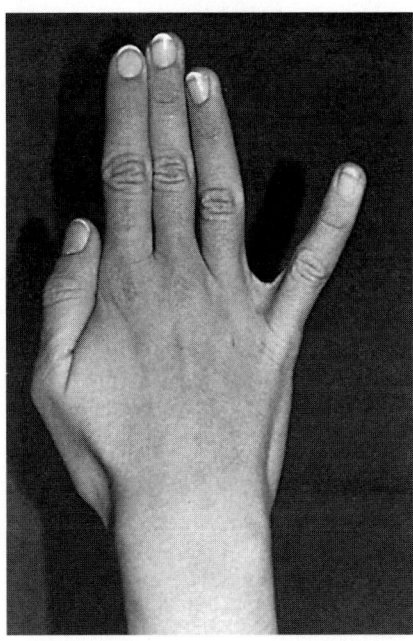

Fig. 8-19. Testing function of the hypothenar muscles by having patient abduct fifth digit.

There are four lumbricals, which originate on the radial side of the profundus tendons and usually insert on the dorsal apparatus. Occasionally, a few fibers insert into the base of the proximal phalanges. Because these muscles are a link between the extrinsic flexor and extrinsic extensor mechanisms, they act as a modulator between flexion and extension of the IP joints.[29]

The interossei are much stronger than the lumbricals; however, both muscle groups work in conjunction. All of

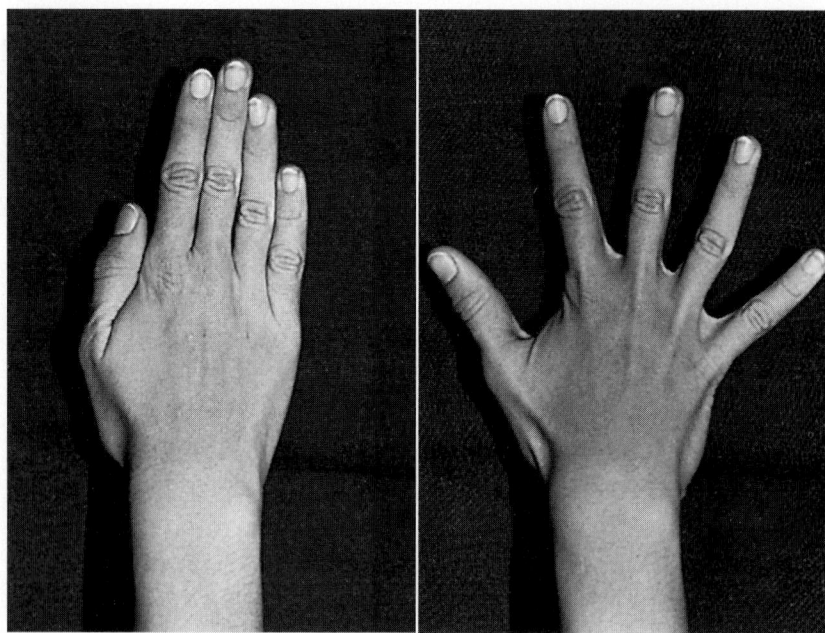

Fig. 8-20. Testing function of the interossei. With the hand flat on a table, the patient is asked to spread his or her fingers apart. Abduction and adduction are assessed from the relationship of the digits to the axis of the third metacarpal.

these muscle groups are of fundamental importance in extension of the IP joints and flexion of the MP joints. The interossei also abduct and adduct the fingers. The dorsal interossei are the primary abductors, and the volar interossei are the primary adductors of the fingers.

The preceding statements are an oversimplification of the anatomy and functional significance of the interossei and the lumbricals. The clinical examination of these two groups of muscles is, however, rather easy.

To test interossei function, one should ask the patient to spread his fingers apart. This is best done with the hand flat on the examining table to eliminate the action of the long extensors, which can simulate the function of the dorsal interossei (Fig. 8-20). To supplement this test, one can have the patient radially and ulnarly deviate the middle finger while it is flexed at the MP joint. This cannot be performed if the interossei are paralyzed; this test is known as *Egawa's sign* (1959).[26]

The first dorsal interosseus is a very strong radial abductor of the index finger and plays an important role in stabilizing that digit during pinch. It can be tested separately by having the patient strongly abduct the index finger in a radial direction while the examiner palpates the muscle belly (Fig. 8-21). The IP extension function of the lumbricals and interossei is tested by having the patient extend the PIP joints of the digits while the examiner holds the MP joints in flexion (Fig. 8-22).

If all of the interossei and lumbricals are functioning properly, the patient will be able to put his or her hand into the "intrinsic-plus position"; that is, the MP joints are flexed and the PIP joints are in full extension. J.I.P. James has recommended this as the position of immobilization for the injured hand.[18]

Injuries to the median or ulnar nerves, or both, or a crushing injury to the hand can result in paralysis or contractures of the intrinsic muscles. A hand without intrinsic function is known as the *intrinsic-minus hand*.[8,14] This hand will have lost the normal cupping of the hand. The arches of the hand will disappear, and there will be wasting of all intrinsic musculature (Fig. 8-23). There will be clawing of the fingers, as described by Duchenne in 1867.[26] The claw deformity is defined as hyperextension of the MP joints and flexion of the PIP and DIP joints (Fig. 8-24). This is the result of an imbalance between the intrinsic and extrinsic muscles of the hand.[48] The extrinsic extensors hyperextend the MP joints, and the extrinsic flexors flex the PIP and DIP joints. The flexion vector, induced by the intrinsics, across the MP joint is lost.[30] In time, the volar capsular-ligamentous structures will stretch out, and the claw deformity will increase in severity.[33]

Injury to the intrinsics, which can be caused by ischemia, crushing injuries, or other pathologic states (e.g., rheumatoid arthritis), can result in tightness of the intrinsic muscles. A test for intrinsic tightness was first described by Finochetto

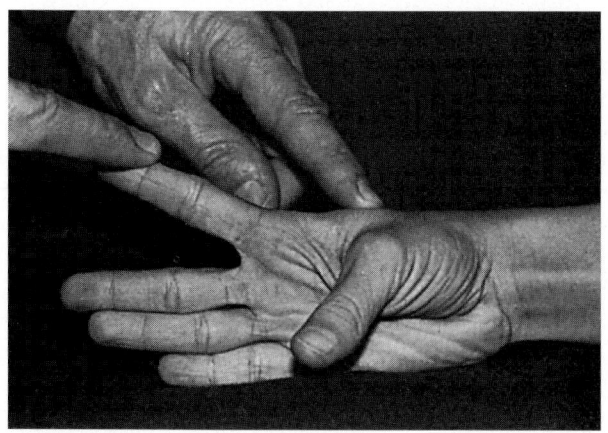

Fig. 8-21. On abduction of the patient's index finger, the examiner can palpate the first dorsal interosseus. This is the last muscle to receive innervation from the ulnar nerve.

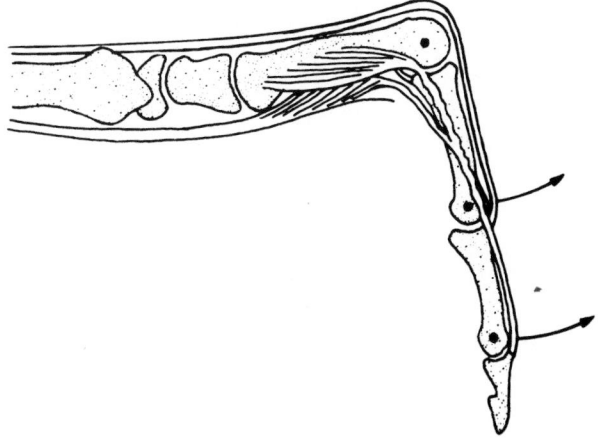

Fig. 8-22. The intrinsic muscles, by means of their attachment into the lateral bands and proximal phalanges, produce flexion of the metacarpophalangeal joints and extension of the proximal interphalangeal joints. The function of the lumbricals and interossei is tested by having the patient extend the proximal interphalangeal joints of the digits while the examiner holds the metacarpophalangeal joints in flexion. (Redrawn from Tubiana R: *The hand,* Philadelphia, 1973, WB Saunders.)

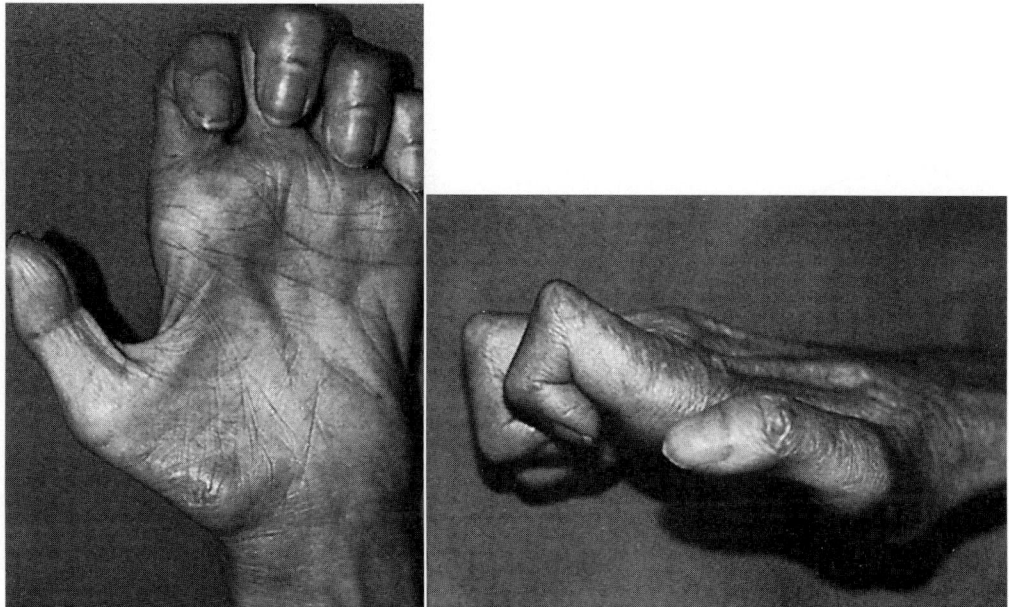

Fig. 8-23. Intrinsic-minus hand resulting from a longstanding low median and ulnar palsy. Notice loss of normal arches of the hand and wasting of all intrinsic musculature.

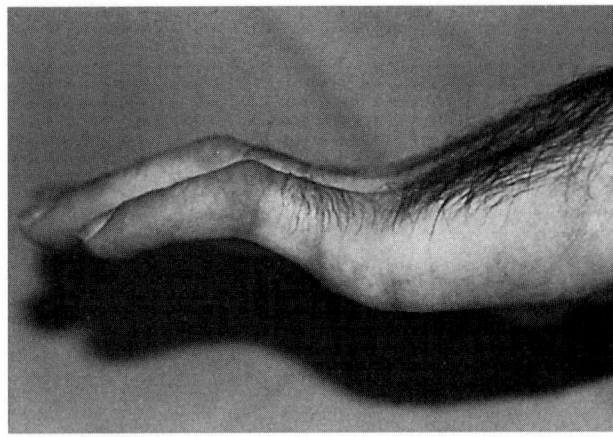

Fig. 8-24. Ulnar claw hand resulting from ulnar nerve laceration at the wrist. Notice hyperextension of the metacarpophalangeal joints and flexion of the proximal and distal interphalangeal joints because of an imbalance of the extrinsic flexor and extensor systems as a result of paralysis of the ulnar innervated intrinsic muscles.

in 1920.[55] Later, Bunnell and then Littler redescribed this test.[9] The intrinsic tightness test is performed by having the examiner hold the patient's MP joint in maximum extension (stretching the intrinsics) and then passively flexing the PIP joint. The MP joint is then held in flexion (relaxing the intrinsics), and the examiner passively flexes the PIP joint again. If the PIP joint can be passively flexed more when the MP joint is in flexion than when it is in extension, there is tightness of the intrinsic muscles[9,45,55] (Fig. 8-25). In patients with rheumatoid arthritis, intrinsic tightness is common and may result in a swan-neck deformity.[35] The swan neck is a result of the strong pull of the contracted intrinsics, through the lateral bands, which subsequently sublux dorsal to the axis of rotation of the PIP joint. The resultant deformity is one of hyperextension at the PIP joint and flexion at the DIP joint (Fig. 8-26). The boutonnière deformity also may occur in patients with rheumatoid arthritis.[34,54]

Occasionally, there is confusion as to the cause of limited PIP-joint motion. Is the condition a result of intrinsic

A

B

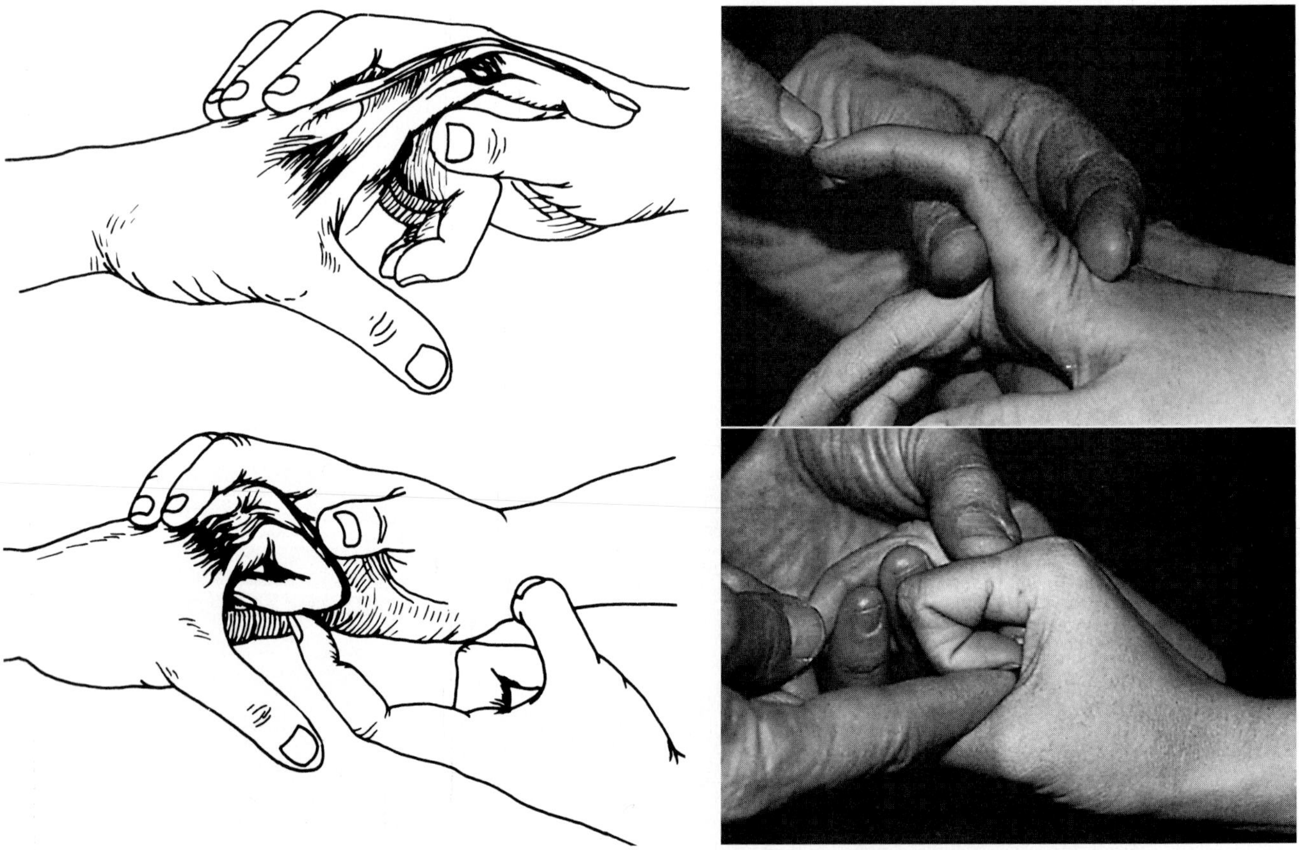

C

D

Fig. 8-25. Intrinsic tightness test. **A** and **B,** The intrinsics are put on stretch by the examiner, who then passively flexes the proximal interphalangeal joint. **C** and **D,** The intrinsics are then relaxed by flexing the metacarpophalangeal joint. If the proximal interphalangeal joint can be passively flexed more with the metacarpophalangeal joint in flexion than when it is in extension, the intrinsic muscles are tight. (Redrawn from Hoppenfeld S: *Physical examination of the spine and extremities,* New York, 1976, Appleton-Century-Crofts.)

tightness, of extrinsic tightness (e.g., scarring of the long extensors proximal to the PIP joint), or of the joint itself (i.e., collateral ligament tightness)? Three simple tests will clarify the situation. The intrinsic tightness tests help the examiner either rule out or identify intrinsic muscle problems. The extrinsic tightness test is just the opposite of the intrinsic test.

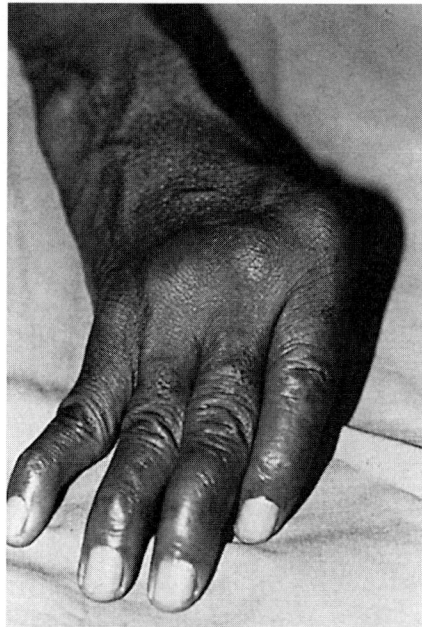

Fig. 8-26. Swan-neck deformity in a patient with rheumatoid arthritis. The swan-neck deformity is caused by intrinsic tightness, which causes the lateral bands to sublux dorsal to the axis of rotation of the proximal interphalangeal joint.

Again, the examiner holds the MP joint in maximum extension, passively flexes the PIP joint, and notes the amount of flexion. He or she then flexes the MP joint and passively flexes the PIP joint again. If extrinsic tightness (because the long extensors are scarred) is present, passive flexion of the PIP joint will be greater when the MP joint is held in extension than when it is held in flexion. Holding the MP joint in extension functionally lengthens the extrinsic extensor, whereas holding it in flexion relatively shortens it. If the motion of the PIP joint is unchanged regardless of the position of the MP joint, there is a joint contracture (Fig. 8-27).

OBLIQUE RETINACULAR LIGAMENT TEST

Occasionally, a patient exhibits a lack of active flexion at the DIP joint. This loss of active flexion may be caused by a joint contracture or a contracture of the oblique retinacular ligament.[22] The oblique retinacular ligament arises from the volar lateral ridge of the proximal phalanx and has a common origin with the distal A_2 and C_1 pulleys. It then traverses distally and dorsally to attach to the dorsal apparatus near the DIP joint (Fig. 8-28). As pointed out by Shrewsbury and Johnson, the tendon varies in its development and occurrence.[44] However, it is consistently made taut by flexion of the DIP joint. If this ligament is contracted, DIP motion will be limited. The oblique retinacular ligament tightness test is performed by passively flexing the DIP joint with the PIP joint in extension and then repeating this with the PIP joint in flexion. If there is greater motion when the PIP joint is flexed than when it is extended, there is a contracture of the ligament (Fig. 8-29). Equal loss of flexion indicates a joint contracture.

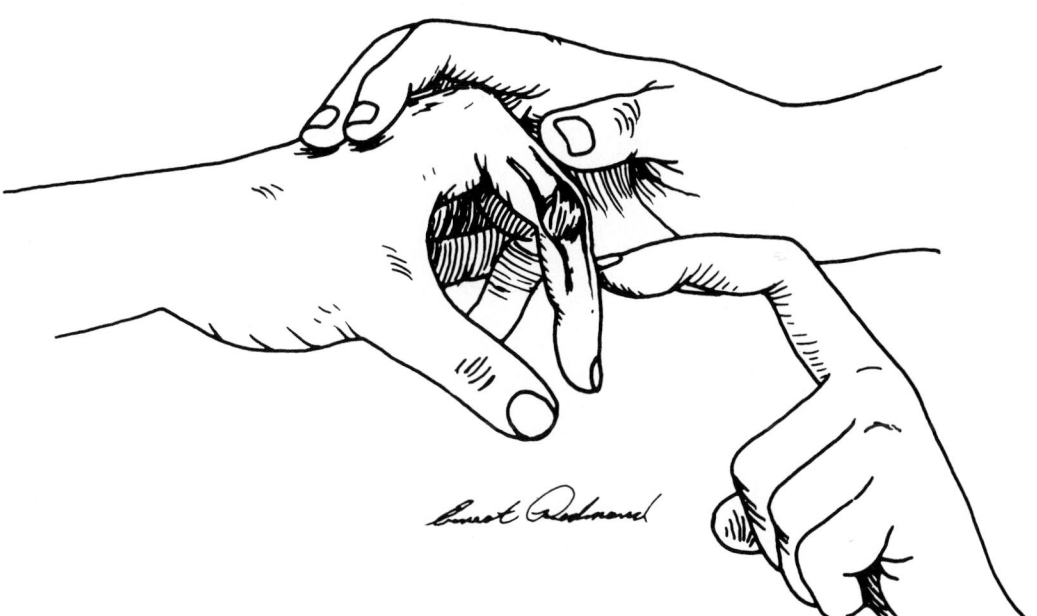

Fig. 8-27. Proximal interphalangeal joint contracture. Collateral ligament tightness will limit proximal phalangeal joint motion, regardless of the position of the metacarpophalangeal joint.

GRIP AND PINCH STRENGTH

The next step after evaluation of intrinsic and extrinsic musculature of the hand is determination of gross grip and pinch strength of the injured hand versus the noninjured hand. Several devices for objective measurement of grip strength are commercially available. The grip dynamometer (Fig. 8-30) with adjustable handle spacings provides an accurate evaluation of the force of grip.[4] This dynamometer has five adjustable spacings at 1, 1.5, 2, 2.5, and 3 inches. The patient is shown how to grasp the dynamometer and is requested to grasp it with his or her maximum force. The grip test position should be standardized. The forearm should be in neutral rotation and the elbow flexed 90 degrees. The shoulder should be adducted. The wrist should be between 0 and 30 degrees of extension and 0 and 15 degrees of ulnar deviation. The grip is measured at each of the five handle spacings. The right and left hands are tested alternately, and the force of each is recorded. The test is paced at a rate to eliminate fatigue. According to Bechtol, there is usually a 5% to 10% difference between the normal dominant hand and the normal nondominant hand.[4] Patients who use a less-than-maximal effort can be identified in two ways. First, if the test is repeated, a patient who applies less-than-maximal effort is usually not able to duplicate his or her previous performance. The discrepancy will be greater than 20% and sometimes as great as 100%.[4] Second, there is a normal bell curve of grip strength; the strength is greatest at the middle spacings and weakest at each end (e.g., level I, 20 pounds; level II, 25 pounds; level III, 35 pounds; level IV, 25 pounds; and level V, 20 pounds). A patient who applies less than maximal effort usually has a flat curve, with all values being approximately the same. If a patient has pain in the hand or forearm, of course the strength will be decreased. However, the bell curve pattern is usually still present (Fig. 8-31). Patients with an intrinsic-minus hand are an exception to this rule. Their grip will increase from level I to V because the extrinsic flexors are at a better mechanical advantage with the wider handle positions.

The rapid exchange grip (REG) test also may be used to detect submaximal effort. The REG test is administered with a dynamometer at the setting that achieves maximum grip during static testing. During testing, the physician holds the dynamometer in place. The patient is then instructed to maximally grip the dynamometer, alternating hands as

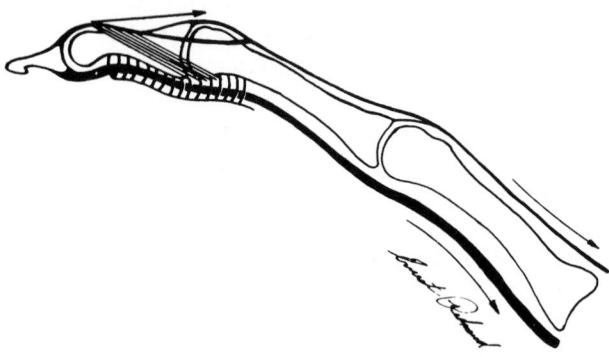

Fig. 8-28. Oblique retinacular ligament. (Redrawn from Tubiana R: *The hand,* Philadelphia, 1981, WB Saunders.)

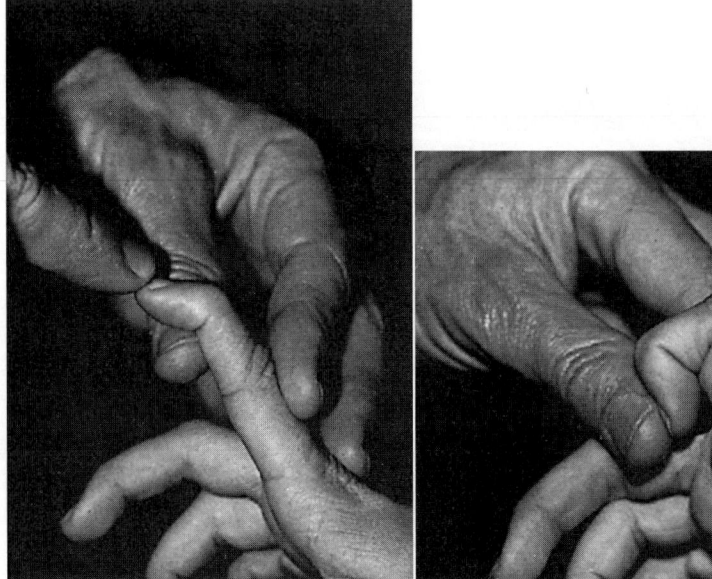

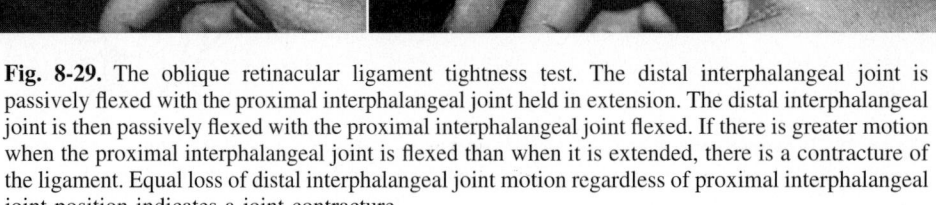

Fig. 8-29. The oblique retinacular ligament tightness test. The distal interphalangeal joint is passively flexed with the proximal interphalangeal joint held in extension. The distal interphalangeal joint is then passively flexed with the proximal interphalangeal joint flexed. If there is greater motion when the proximal interphalangeal joint is flexed than when it is extended, there is a contracture of the ligament. Equal loss of distal interphalangeal joint motion regardless of proximal interphalangeal joint position indicates a joint contracture.

rapidly as possible. Each hand grips the dynamometer 5 to 10 times. A positive REG test shows a significant increase in grip strength on the affected side as compared to static scores. A positive REG test in the presence of a flat curve on static testing suggests inconsistent effort by the patient.[16,49]

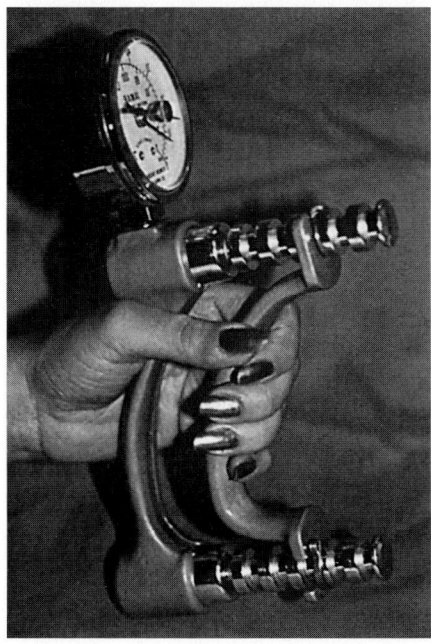

Fig. 8-30. Jamar grip dynamometer with five adjustable spacings. (Asimow Engineering Co, Los Angeles, Calif.)

There are three basic types of pinch: chuck, or three-fingered pinch; lateral, or key pinch; and tip pinch (Fig. 8-32). These can be tested with a pinch meter (Fig. 8-33). Many disease processes can affect pinch power: basilar arthritis of the thumb, ulnar nerve palsy, and anterior interosseus nerve palsy, to mention a few.

NERVE SUPPLY OF THE HAND—MOTOR AND SENSORY MOTOR

Three nerves provide motor and sensory function to the hand: the median, radial, and ulnar nerves (Fig. 8-34). The motor and sensory innervation of the hand also is subject to much variation, as pointed out by Rowntree.[41] However, we discuss the usual textbook innervation and ignore the variations.

The median, radial, and ulnar nerves are peripheral branches of the brachial plexus. The radial nerve is formed from the C6 and C7 nerve roots. The median nerve is formed by branches of the C7, C8, and T1 nerve roots. The terminal branches of the median, radial, and ulnar nerves are shown in Fig. 8-35. It is necessary to have a fundamental knowledge of the branches and their sequence of innervation to appropriately place the level of an injury or to follow the path of a regenerating nerve.

These three nerves enter the forearm through various muscle and fascial planes and have multiple potential sources of entrapment. Entrapment of these nerves results in classic clinical presentations, with loss of motor function and paresthesias in the distribution of each nerve.

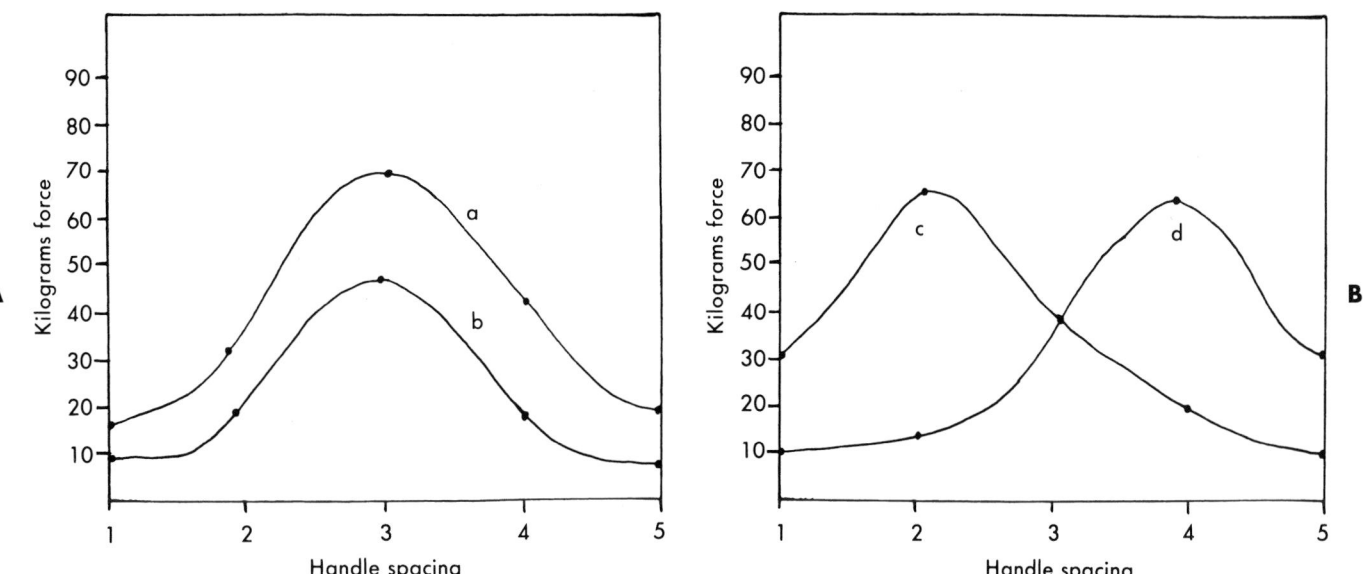

Fig. 8-31. A, The grip strengths of a patient's uninjured hand *(a)* and injured hand *(b)* are plotted. Despite the patient's decrease in grip strength because of injury, curve *b* maintains a bell-shaped pattern and parallels that of the normal hand. These curves are reproducible in repeated examinations, with minimal change in values. A great fluctuation in the size of the curve or absence of a bell-shaped pattern casts doubt on the patient's compliance with the examination and may indicate malingering. **B,** If the patient has an exceptionally large hand, the curve will shift to the right *(d);* with a very small hand, the curve will shift to the left *(c).* Notice, however, that the bell-shaped pattern is maintained despite the curve's shift in direction.

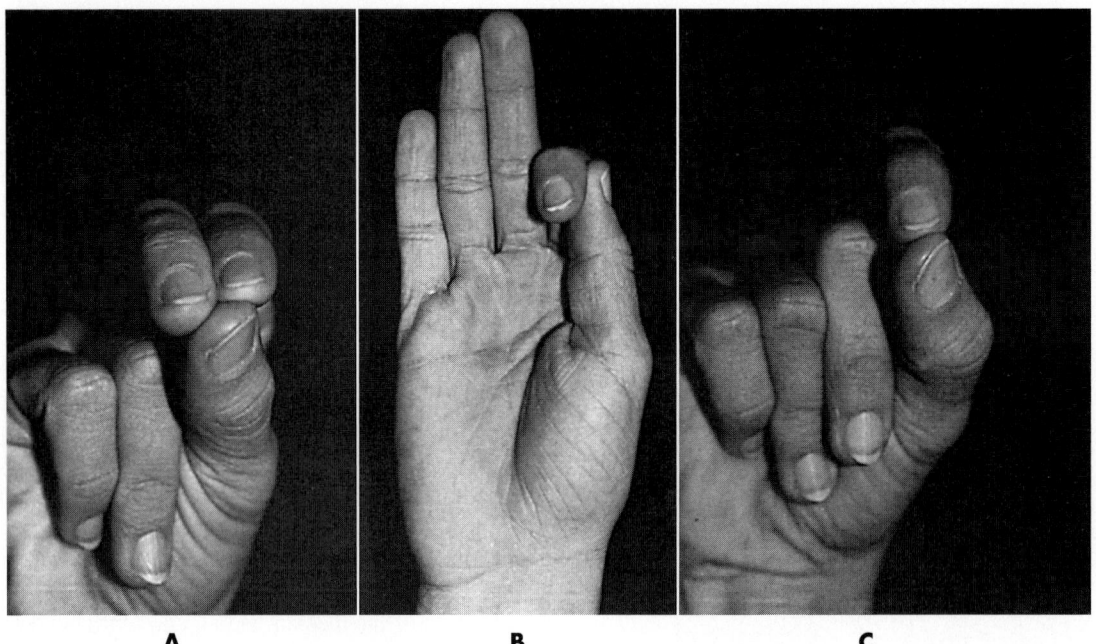

Fig. 8-32. A, Chuck, or three-fingered, pinch. **B,** Lateral, or key, pinch. **C,** Tip pinch.

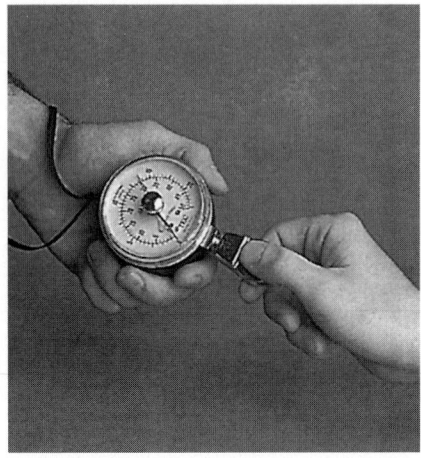

Fig. 8-33. Preston pinch gauge. (JA Preston Corp, Jackson, Mich.)

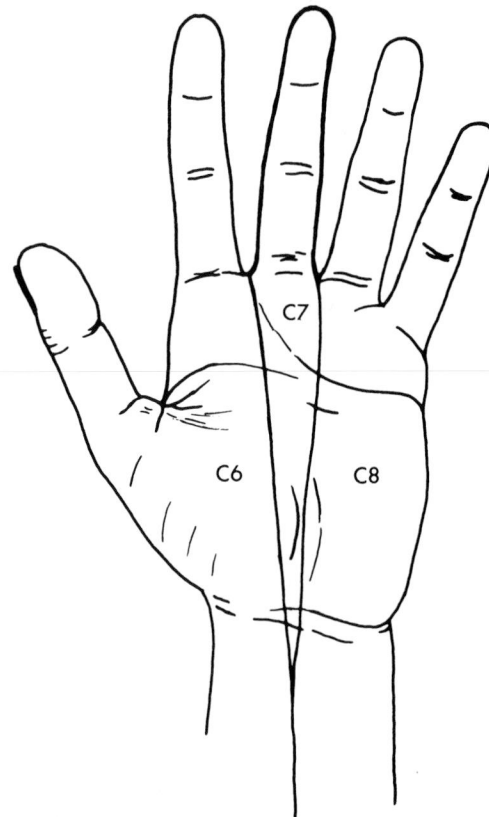

Fig. 8-34. Sensory dermatomes of the hand, by neurologic levels. (Redrawn from Hoppenfeld S: *Physical examination of the spine and extremities,* New York, 1976, Appleton-Century-Crofts.)

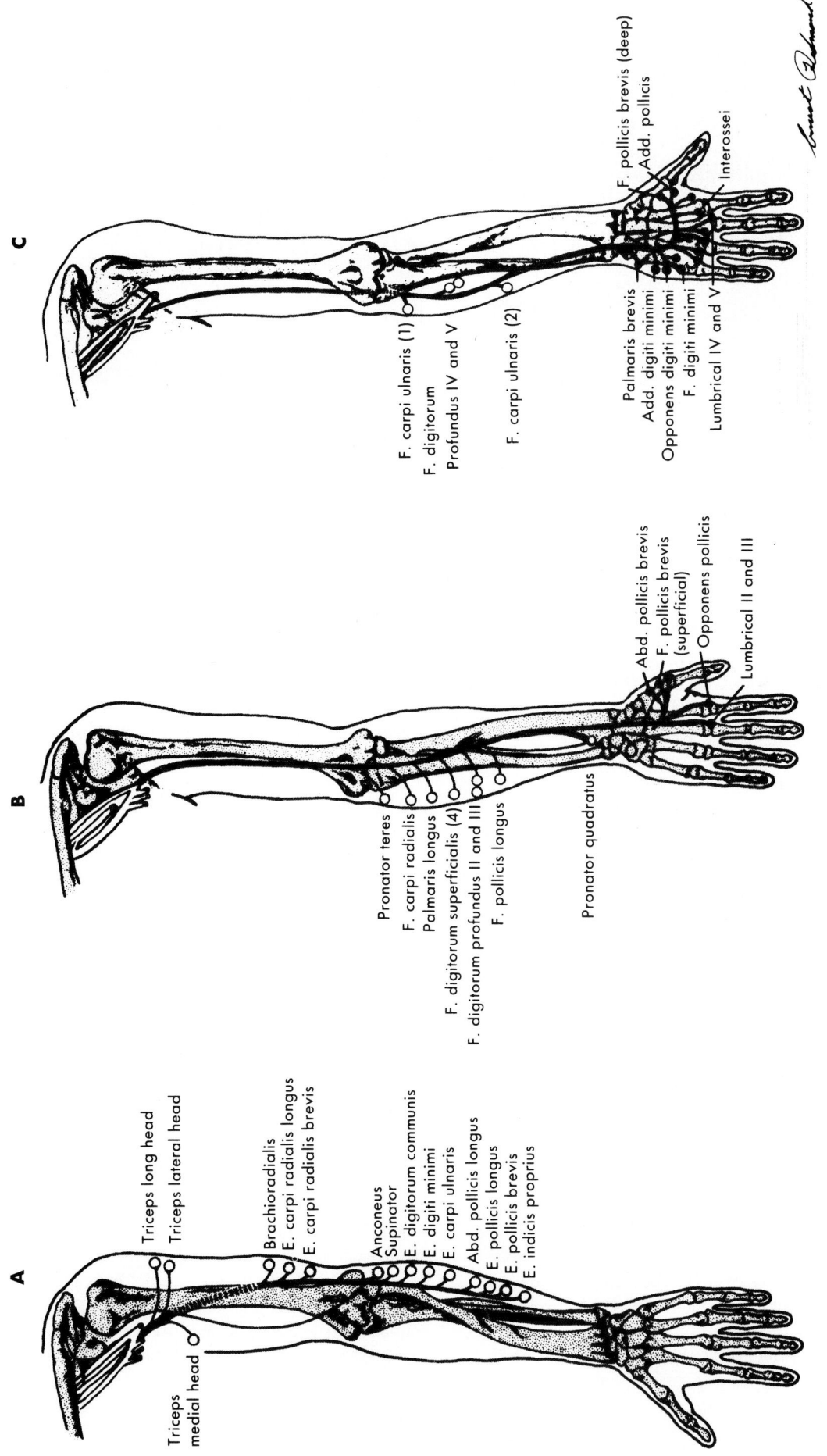

A
Triceps medial head
Triceps long head
Triceps lateral head
Brachioradialis
E. carpi radialis longus
E. carpi radialis brevis
Anconeus
Supinator
E. digitorum communis
E. digiti minimi
E. carpi ulnaris
Abd. pollicis longus
E. pollicis longus
E. pollicis brevis
E. indicis proprius

B
Pronator teres
F. carpi radialis
Palmaris longus
F. digitorum superficialis (4)
F. digitorum profundus II and III
F. pollicis longus
Pronator quadratus
Abd. pollicis brevis
F. pollicis brevis (superficial)
Opponens pollicis
Lumbrical II and III

C
F. carpi ulnaris (1)
F. digitorum
Profundus IV and V
F. carpi ulnaris (2)
Palmaris brevis
Add. digiti minimi
Opponens digiti minimi
F. digiti minimi
Lumbrical IV and V
F. pollicis brevis (deep)
Add. pollicis
Interossei

Fig. 8-35. Terminal branches of the radial (**A**), median (**B**), and ulnar (**C**) nerves. (Redrawn from American Society for Surgery of the Hand: *The hand, examination and diagnosis*, Aurora, Colo, 1978, The Society.)

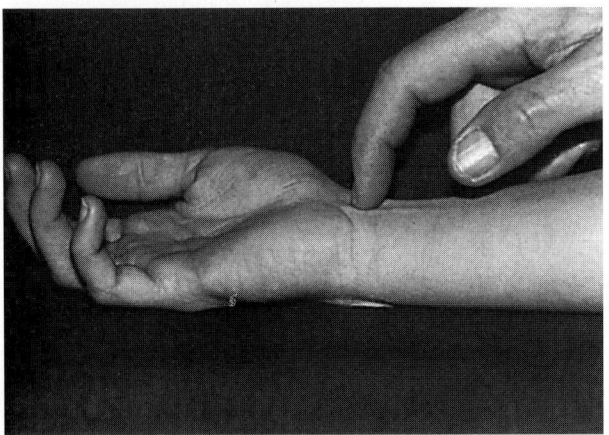

Fig. 8-36. Percussion of the median nerve at the wrist will elicit Tinel's sign in the presence of carpal tunnel syndrome.

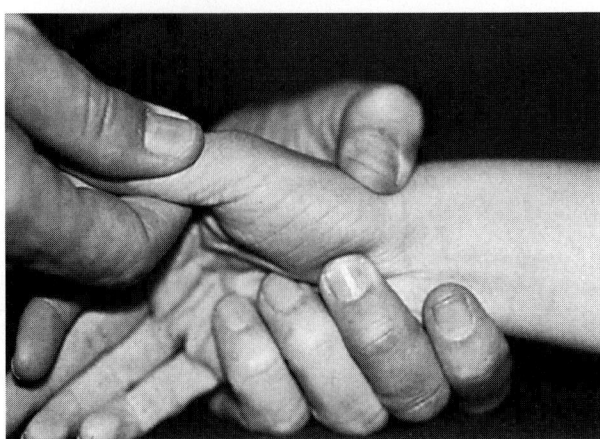

Fig. 8-37. The "grind test." Mild axial compression and gentle rotation of the thumb will elicit pain in the trapezial metacarpal joint if osteoarthritis is present.

The median nerve may be entrapped as it enters the forearm at the level of the pronator teres muscle, the lacertus fibrosus, or the superficialis arch.[15,19,47] As it enters the hand, it may be entrapped at the level of the carpal tunnel.[39] This common neuropathy has been termed *carpal tunnel syndrome* (CTS). Patients with CTS often complain of numbness in the thumb and the radial two and one-half fingers, as well as night pain, weakness of grip, and dropping of objects. With a longstanding compression, significant thenar atrophy and loss of thumb opposition are noted.[37,39,51]

Compression of the median nerve at the wrist was first described by Paget in 1854.[37] Several authors since then have reported this entity and have recommended division of the transverse carpal ligament. Phalen has most clearly defined this entity as a syndrome; in 1966, he reported his experience with 654 cases of CTS.[37] Phalen found that in a high percentage of cases, the wrist flexion test, now commonly known as *Phalen's test,* had a positive result and that Tinel's sign was present.

When performing Phalen's test, the patient holds his forearms vertically and allows both hands to drop into complete flexion at the wrist for approximately 1 minute. In this position, the median nerve is compressed between the transverse carpal ligament and the adjacent flexor tendons. This maneuver causes almost immediate aggravation of numbness and paresthesias in the fingers.

Percussion of the median nerve at the wrist produces paresthesias in the distribution of the nerve; this is known as *Tinel's sign* (Fig. 8-36). Tinel's sign is present not only in compressive neuropathies of nerves but also in partial and complete lacerations of nerves and in areas where neuromas have formed.[20,32,52]

The presence of thenar atrophy, paresthesias in the median nerve distribution, a positive Phalen's test, and Tinel's sign, in association with a history of night pain, is pathognomonic for a compressive neuropathy of the median nerve in the carpal tunnel.

The ulnar and radial nerves also are subject to compression as they enter the arm and hand. The ulnar nerve can be compressed near the medial intermuscular septum, near the cubital tunnel, or at the wrist (in Guyon's canal).[17,21,43,53] The radial nerve is subject to compression at the radial tunnel and as it passes between the two heads of the supinator muscle in an area known as the arcade of Frohse, or it can be compressed superficially at the wrist.* As with compression of the median nerve, patients will complain of paresthesias in the sensory distribution of the irritated nerve and may have a positive Tinel's sign. In longstanding or severe acute compressive neuropathies, there will be atrophy or even paralysis of the muscles innervated distal to the area of compression. If one is aware of the sequence of innervation of each nerve and performs a good manual motor examination, it is usually not hard to make a diagnosis of a nerve entrapment.

Patients with CTS, especially postmenopausal women, may have pain at the base of the thumb, which may be thought to be caused by a compressive neuropathy. In this particular patient population, osteoarthritis of the metacarpal trapezial joint is common. The diagnosis can be made by performing the "grind test" and of course by radiographic examination. The grind test (Fig. 8-37) is performed by manipulating the patient's thumb with mild axial compression and gentle rotation. This maneuver will induce pain in the metacarpal trapezial joint if degenerative joint disease is present. Often, CTS and metacarpal trapezial arthritis will coexist, and it is sometimes difficult to identify the pain-causing lesion. The test performed for CTS and the grind test will help clarify the situation.[50]

*References 6, 24, 25, 40, 42, 46.

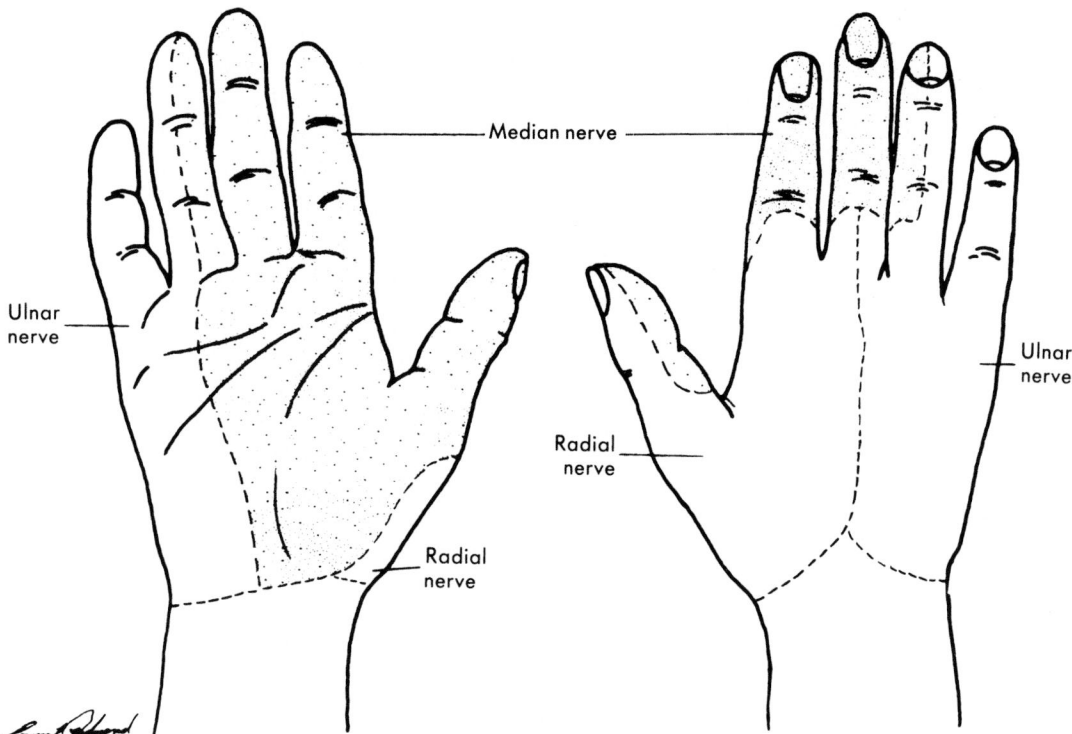

Fig. 8-38. Sensory distribution of the median, radial, and ulnar nerves in the hand. (Redrawn from Weeks PM, Wray RC: *Management of acute hand injuries: a biological approach,* St Louis, 1973, Mosby.)

CUTANEOUS SENSIBILITY

Normal sensibility is a prerequisite to normal hand function. A patient with a median nerve injury has essentially a "blind hand" and is greatly disabled, even if all motor function is present. The assessment of sensibility is therefore an integral and important part of the examination of the hand.

The distribution of sensory nerves is subject to as much variation as the distribution of the motor branches.[41] The classic distribution of the median, ulnar, and radial nerves is shown in Fig. 8-38.

There are many ways to assess sensibility, including von Frey filaments, Moberg's pickup test, Seddon's coin test, the moving two-point discrimination test described by Dellon, and Weber's two-point discrimination test.[5,11,23,31] Each test has its supporters and detractors. Other chapters in this book address sensibility testing and sensory reeducation in detail.

From a practical standpoint, an adequate sensibility examination can be performed by using the two-point discrimination test and by careful examination of the patient's skin. Skin that has been deinnervated has lost its autonomic input and sudomotor function (i.e., it does not sweat). The finger pulp becomes atrophic, smooth, and dry, with relative loss of dermal ridges. Deinnervated skin will not wrinkle when placed in warm water (the "wrinkle test").[31] Tinel's sign will be present at the site of a nerve injury (Fig. 8-39).

The two-point discrimination test is performed with a paper clip that has been bent into a caliper. With the patient's eyes closed and his or her hand cradled in the examiner's, the examiner gently places the caliper on the skin in a longitudinal direction, that is, on either the ulnar or the radial side of the digit. The ends of the paper clip must touch the skin lightly, just to the point of blanching. The ends should be smooth and not barbed. The patient is then asked whether he feels one point or two. Gradually the points are brought closer together and reapplied until the patient feels only one point. Normal two-point discrimination at a fingertip is 5 mm or less (Fig. 8-40). Although this is not the most sensitive of tests and the result does not correlate with function of the hand, it is an adequate screening test and is much less time consuming than the more involved tests described.

VASCULARITY OF THE HAND

The vascular supply of the hand is usually extensive; however, it should be evaluated carefully before any surgery of the hand. The primary blood supply to the hand is through the radial and ulnar arteries. In some individuals, the dominant blood supply to the hand can be from one artery. The ulnar artery gives rise to the superficial palmar arch, and the radial artery gives rise to the deep arch. These arches usually have extensive anastomoses.[10,27] The superficial palmar arch gives rise to four common digital arteries, which

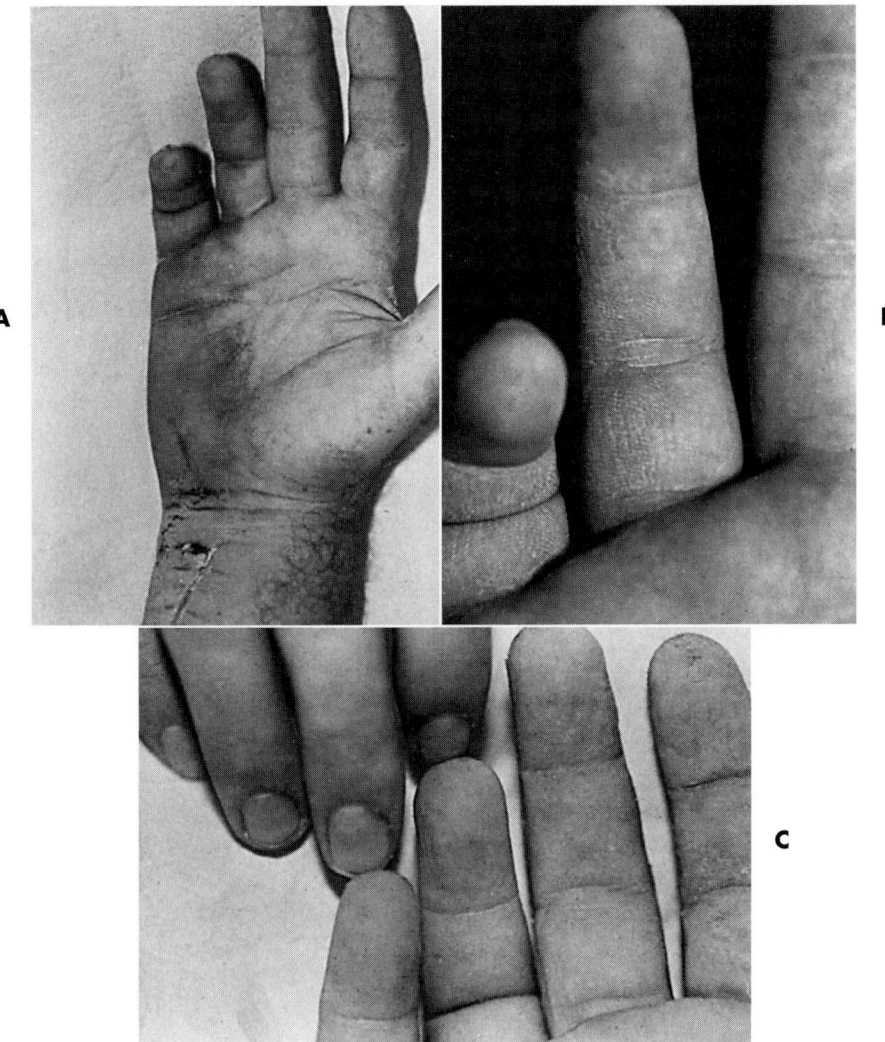

Fig. 8-39. Photographs illustrating loss of autonomic function after a peripheral nerve injury. **A,** The injury level to the ulnar nerve at the wrist is seen. The accumulated dry skin after the first postoperative dressing change can be seen in the classic ulnar nerve distribution. **B,** Closer view of the dry skin, which indicates a loss of sudomotor function. Notice how the fourth ray is split. **C,** Positive result of "wrinkle test" in same patient.

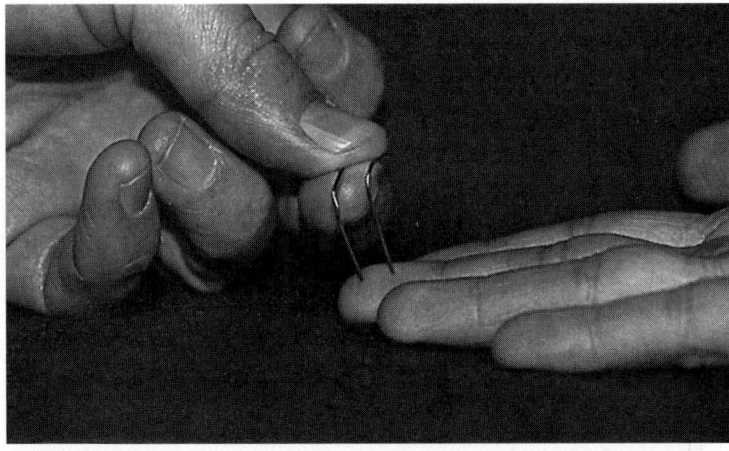

Fig. 8-40. Two-point discrimination test using a bent paper clip.

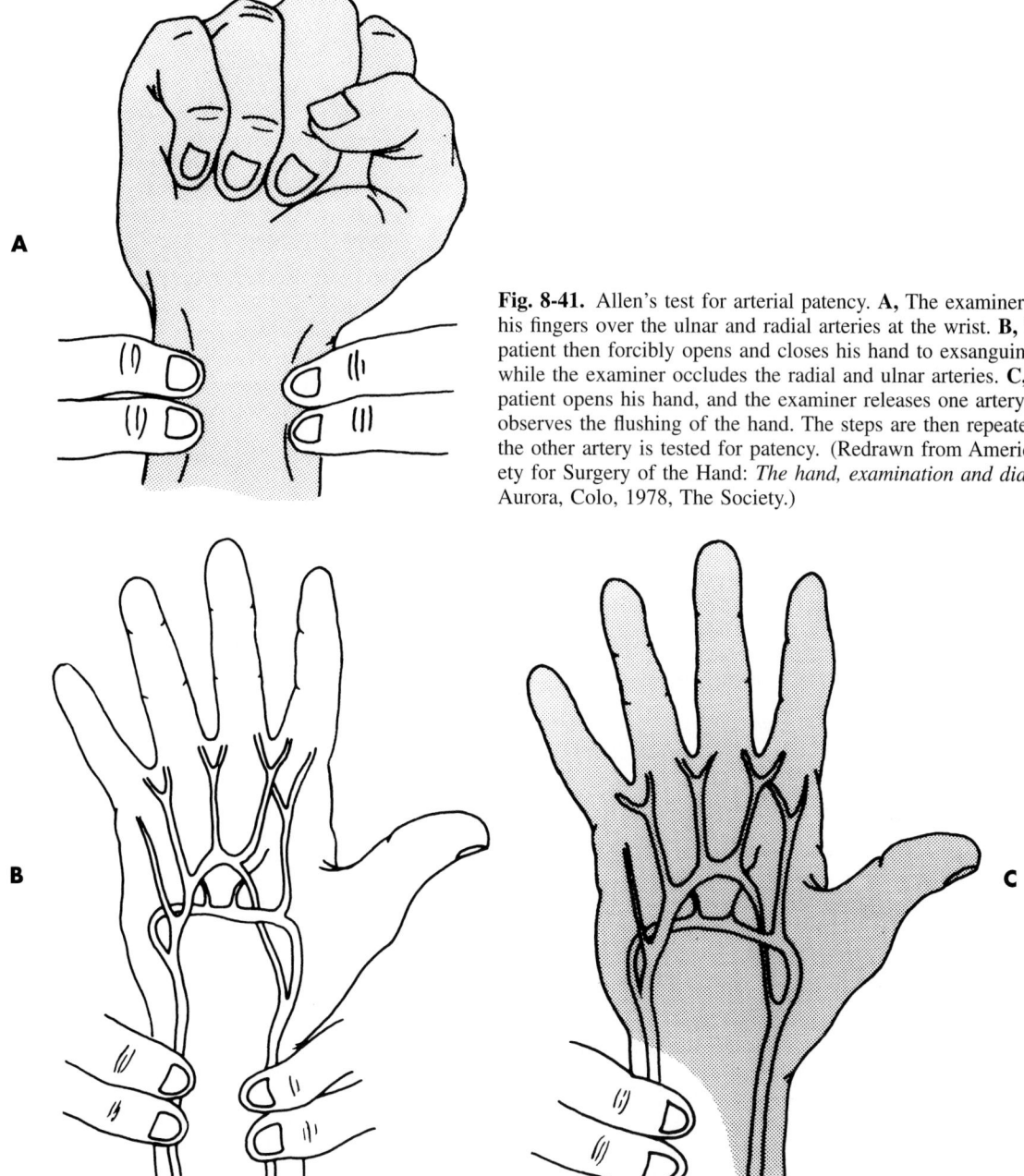

Fig. 8-41. Allen's test for arterial patency. **A,** The examiner places his fingers over the ulnar and radial arteries at the wrist. **B,** The patient then forcibly opens and closes his hand to exsanguinate it while the examiner occludes the radial and ulnar arteries. **C,** Next the patient opens his hand, and the examiner releases one artery and observes the flushing of the hand. The steps are then repeated, and the other artery is tested for patency. (Redrawn from American Society for Surgery of the Hand: *The hand, examination and diagnosis,* Aurora, Colo, 1978, The Society.)

then branch to form the proper digital arteries. The superficial arch may supply blood to the thumb, or the thumb may be completely vascularized by a branch of the radial artery known as the princeps pollicis artery. To assess blood supply to the hand, one should check the color of the hand (pale, red, or cyanotic), digital capillary reflux, and the radial and ulnar pulses at the wrist, and perform Allen's test. In 1929, Allen described a simple clinical test to determine the patency of the radial and ulnar arteries in thromboangiitis obliterans.[1] This test is performed by having the patient open and close his or her hand to exsanguinate it while the

examiner occludes the radial and ulnar arteries at the wrist with digital pressure. The patient then opens the hand, which will be white and blanched. The examiner then releases either the ulnar or the radial artery and watches for revascularization of the hand. If the hand does not flush, the artery is occluded. This test is then repeated with the opposite artery (Fig. 8-41).

A modification of Allen's test can be performed on a single digit.[2] The steps are the same as just outlined, except that the examiner occludes and releases the radial and ulnar digital arteries.

CONCLUSION

In this chapter, we have presented an organized approach to clinical examination of the hand. The books and articles listed at the end of this chapter provide more detailed descriptions of the tests and clinical entities that have been presented here. Clinical examination is an art that improves with practice and experience.

ACKNOWLEDGMENTS

We thank Cynthia DuPuy for her assistance in preparation of the illustrations and Mavis Stinus for her secretarial assistance in the preparation of this chapter.

REFERENCES

1. Allen E: Thromboangiitis obliterans: methods of diagnosis of chronic occlusive arterial lesions distal to the wrist with illustrative cases, *Am J Med Sci* 178:237, 1929.
2. Ashbell T, Kutz J, Kleinert H: The digital Allen test, *Plast Reconstr Surg* 39:311, 1967.
3. Baker D, et al: The little finger superficialis: clinical investigation of its anatomical and functional shortcomings, *J Hand Surg* 6:374, 1981.
4. Bechtol C: Grip test: the use of a dynamometer with adjustable handle spacings, *J Bone Joint Surg* 36A:820, 1954.
5. Bowden R, Napier J: The assessment of hand function after peripheral nerve injuries, *J Bone Joint Surg* 43B:481, 1961.
6. Braidwood A: Superficial radial neuropathy, *J Bone Joint Surg* 57B:380, 1975.
7. Bunnell S: Opposition of the thumb, *J Bone Joint Surg* 20:269, 1938.
8. Bunnell S: Surgery of the intrinsic muscles of the hand other than those producing opposition of the thumb, *J Bone Joint Surg* 24:1, 1942.
9. Bunnell S: Ischaemic contracture, local, in the hand, *J Bone Joint Surg* 35A:88, 1953.
10. Coleman S, Anson B: Arterial patterns in the hand based upon a study of 650 specimens, *Surg Gynecol Obstet* 113:408, 1961.
11. Dellon A: The moving two-point discrimination test: clinical evaluation of the quickly adapting fiber-receptor system, *J Hand Surg* 3:474, 1978.
12. Eyler D, Markee J: The anatomy and function of the intrinsic musculature of the fingers, *J Bone Joint Surg* 36A:1, 1954.
13. Finkelstein H: Stenosing tenovaginitis at the radial styloid process, *J Bone Joint Surg* 12:509, 1930.
14. Harris C, Riordan D: Intrinsic contracture in the hand and its surgical treatment, *J Bone Joint Surg* 36A:10, 1954.
15. Hartz C, et al: The pronator teres syndrome: compressive neuropathy of the median nerve, *J Bone Joint Surg* 63A:885, 1981.
16. Hildreth D, et al: Detection of submaximal effort by use of the rapid exchange grip test, *J Hand Surg* 14A:742, 1989.
17. Hunt JR: Occupation neuritis of the deep palmar branch of the ulnar nerve: a well-defined clinical type of professional palsy of the hand, *J Nerv Ment Dis* 35:673, 1908.
18. James JIP: The assessment and management of the injured hand, *Hand* 2:97, 1970.
19. Johnson RK, Spinner M, Shrewsbury MM: Median nerve entrapment syndrome in the proximal forearm, *J Hand Surg* 4:48, 1979.
20. Kaplan E: Translation of J. Tinel's "Four millement" paper. In Spinner M, editor: *Injuries to the major branches of peripheral nerves of the forearm*, ed 2, Philadelphia, 1978, WB Saunders.
21. Kleinert H, Hayes J: The ulnar tunnel syndrome, *Plast Reconstr Surg* 47:21, 1971.
22. Landsmeer JMF: The anatomy of the dorsal aponeurosis of the human finger and its functional significance, *Anat Rec* 104:31, 1949.
23. Levin S, Pearsall G, Ruderman R: Von Frey's method of measuring pressure sensibility in the hand: an engineering analysis of the Weinstein-Semmes pressure aesthesiometer, *J Hand Surg* 3:211, 1978.
24. Linscheid R: Injuries to radial nerve at the wrist, *Arch Surg* 91:942, 1965.
25. Lister GD, Belsole RB, Kleinert HE: The radial tunnel syndrome, *J Hand Surg* 4:52, 1979.
26. Mannerfelt L: Studies on the hand in ulnar nerve paralysis: a clinical-experimental investigation in normal and anomalous innervation, *Acta Orthop Scan* 87(suppl):1, 1966.
27. Markee J, Wray J: Circulation of the hand: injection-corrosion studies, *J Bone Joint Surg* 41A:673, 1959.
28. McFarlane R: Observations on the functional anatomy of the intrinsic muscles of the thumb, *J Bone Joint Surg* 44A:1073, 1962.
29. Mehta H, Gardner W: A study of lumbrical muscles in the human hand, *Am J Anat* 109:227, 1961.
30. Mickes J, Reswick J, Hager DL: The mechanism of the intrinsic-minus finger: a biomechanical study, *J Hand Surg* 3:333, 1978.
31. Moberg E: Objective methods for determining the functional value of sensibility in the hand, *J Bone Joint Surg* 40B:454, 1958.
32. Moldaver J: Tinel's sign: its characteristics and significance, *J Bone Joint Surg* 60A:412, 1978.
33. Mulder J, Landsmeer J: The mechanism of the claw finger, *J Bone Joint Surg* 50B:664, 1968.
34. Nalebuff E, Millender L: Surgical treatment of the boutonniere deformity in rheumatoid arthritis, *Orthop Clin North Am* 6:753, 1975.
35. Nalebuff E, Millender L: Surgical treatment of the swan-neck deformity in rheumatoid arthritis, *Orthop Clin North Am* 6:733, 1975.
36. Noer H, Pratt D: A goniometer designed for the hand, *J Bone Joint Surg* 40A:1154, 1958.
37. Phalen G: The carpal tunnel syndrome: seventeen years' experience in diagnosis and treatment of 654 hands, *J Bone Joint Surg* 48A:211, 1966.
38. Riddell D: Spontaneous rupture of the extensor pollicis longus: the results of tendon transfer, *J Bone Joint Surg* 45B:506, 1963.
39. Robbins H: Anatomical study of the median nerve in the carpal tunnel and etiologies of the carpal tunnel syndrome, *J Bone Joint Surg* 45A:953, 1963.
40. Roles N, Maudsley R: Radial tunnel syndrome: resistant tennis elbow as a nerve entrapment, *J Bone Joint Surg* 54B:499, 1972.
41. Rowntree T: Anomalous innervation of the hand muscles, *J Bone Joint Surg* 31B:505, 1949.
42. Shaw J, Sakellarides H: Radial nerve paralysis associated with fractures of the humerus: a review of forty-five cases, *J Bone Joint Surg* 49A:899, 1967.
43. Shea J, McClain E: Ulnar nerve compression syndromes at and below the wrist, *J Bone Joint Surg* 51A:1095, 1969.
44. Shrewsbury M, Johnson R: A systematic study of the oblique retinacular ligament of the human finger: its structure and function, *J Hand Surg* 2:194, 1977.
45. Smith R: Non-ischemic contractures of the intrinsic muscles of the hand, *J Bone Joint Surg* 53A:1313, 1971.
46. Spinner M: The arcade of Frohse and its relationship to posterior interosseous nerve paralysis, *J Bone Joint Surg* 50B:809, 1968.
47. Spinner M: The anterior interosseous nerve syndrome with special attention to its variations, *J Bone Joint Surg* 52A:84, 1970.
48. Srinivasan H: Clinical features of paralytic claw fingers, *J Bone Joint Surg* 61A:1060, 1063, 1979.
49. Stokes H, et al: Identification of low-effort patients through dynamometer, *J Hand Surg* 20A:1047, 1995.
50. Swanson A: Disabling arthritis at the base of the thumb: treatment by resection of the trapezium and flexible (silicon) implant arthroplasty, *J Bone Joint Surg* 54A:456, 1972.
51. Tanzer R: The carpal tunnel syndrome: a clinical and anatomical study, *J Bone Joint Surg* 41A:626, 1959.
52. Tinel J: Le signe du "fourmillement" dans les lesions des nerfs peripheriques, *Press Med* 47:388, October 1915.
53. Uriburu I, Morchio F, Marin J: Compression syndrome of the deep motor branch of the ulnar nerve (Piso-Hamate hiatus syndrome), *J Bone Joint Surg* 58A:145, 1976.
54. Vaughn-Jackson O: Rheumatoid hand deformities considered in the light of tendon imbalance, *J Bone Joint Surg* 44B:764, 1962.
55. Zancolli E: *Structural and dynamic basis of hand surgery*, Philadelphia, 1968, JB Lippincott.

Chapter 9

DIAGNOSTIC IMAGING
OF THE UPPER EXTREMITY

John S. Taras
Mark E. Schweitzer

The diagnosis of upper extremity disorders relies on information obtained in the history, physical examination, and views of the region acquired through one or more imaging techniques. Plain radiography provides adequate visualization of most problems and, for that reason, is a standard part of the initial evaluation. Excellent depiction of fractures, fracture alignment, site of fracture healing, dislocation, soft tissue calcification, foreign bodies, and bony detail can be obtained by this readily available, cost-effective, and noninvasive means. In certain cases, the problem cannot be properly assessed by routine measures; thus other imaging modalities must be used to provide further diagnostic information. In this chapter, radiography and advanced imaging techniques are discussed in relation to the diagnosis of hand disorders.

RADIOGRAPHY
Routine studies

Routine studies of the hand consist of posteroanterior (PA), lateral, and oblique views, which are evaluated for bone density, bony lesions, fractures and dislocations, integrity of the articular surfaces and joint spaces, and irregularities of the soft tissue (Fig. 9-1).[9]

Bone density, which is evaluated grossly, may be normal, less than normal (osteopenia), or greater than normal (osteosclerotic). Osteopenia is most often encountered in the elderly and is known as *senile osteoporosis* when associated with advanced age. Osteosclerosis occurs in conditions such as avascular necrosis (Fig. 9-2), fracture healing, and metabolic bone disease.[11] Plain films may reveal discrete or diffuse bone lesions, including primary or metastatic bone tumors, infection, and metabolic bone disease (Fig. 9-3). The

cortical integrity is carefully inspected for evidence of acute fracture (Fig. 9-4) and the joint alignment evaluated for subluxation or dislocation.[10] Abnormalities of the articular surface and cartilage joint space also are documented. Narrowing of the cartilage space and/or erosive changes may indicate arthritis, resulting from degeneration, inflammation, infection, or trauma (Figs. 9-5 and 9-6).[4] Finally, the soft tissue shadows are evaluated for irregularities. Any evidence of calcification (Fig. 9-7), foreign bodies (Fig. 9-8),[22] or soft tissue masses must be correlated with the clinical findings.

Special views

If the history and physical examination indicate a localized problem, a coned-down view of the area can be obtained. This approach is especially useful for isolated disease of the carpal bones because fractures and abnormalities in this region often cannot be seen on plain views (Fig. 9-9). Special positioning and maneuvers also are used to allow more complete visualization of a suspected pathologic condition. For example, stress views may demonstrate joint malalignments that are not evident on routine films. Tears of the ulnar collateral ligament of the thumb metacarpophalangeal (MP) joint are a case in point because these can become apparent by applying a force to this joint in radial deviation (Fig. 9-10).[5] A special maneuver is often needed to demonstrate damage to the scapholunate ligament complex. This complex is important in stabilizing the scaphoid and preventing rotatory subluxation. When it is injured, the scapholunate interval may appear completely normal on a routine view, but it widens when a compression load is applied by clenching the fist in supination (Fig. 9-11). Special views also are useful in demonstrating the bony

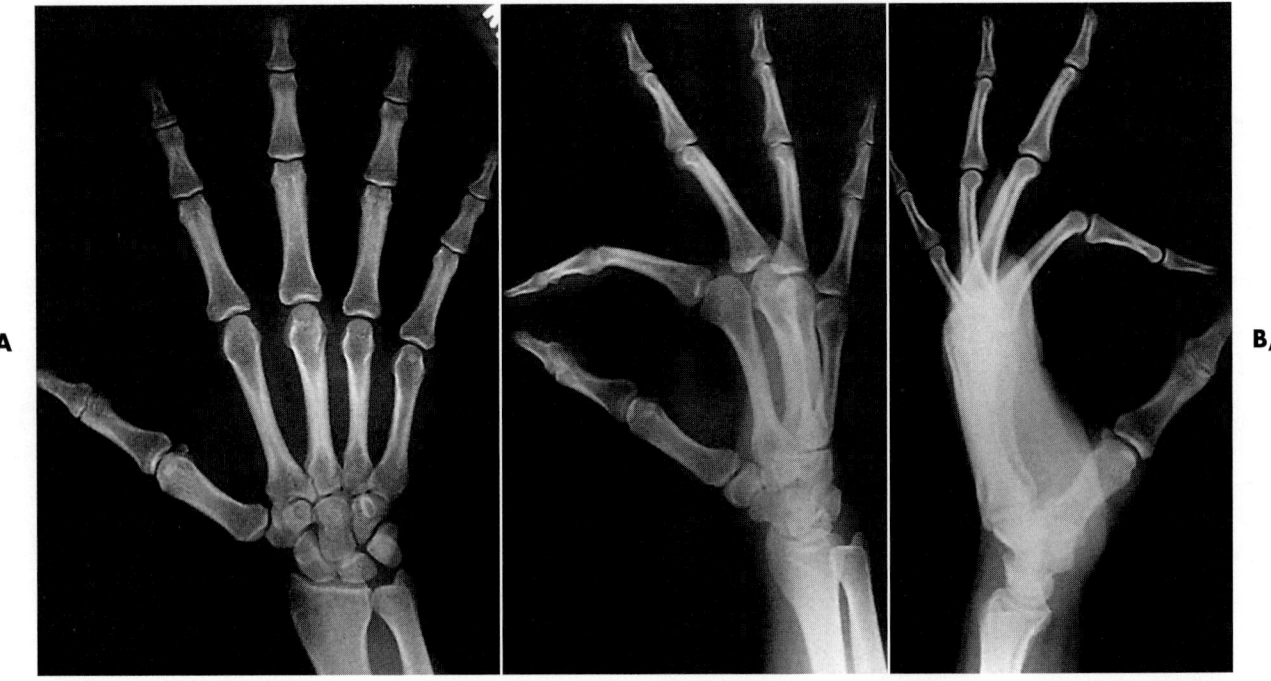

Fig. 9-1. Routine views of the hand. **A,** Posteroanterior. **B,** Oblique. **C,** Lateral.

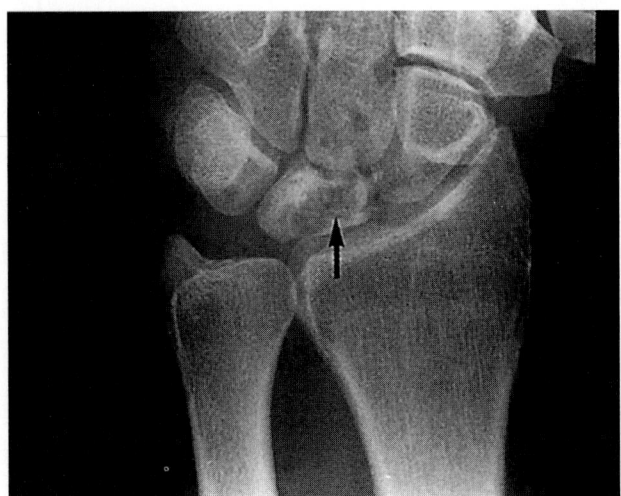

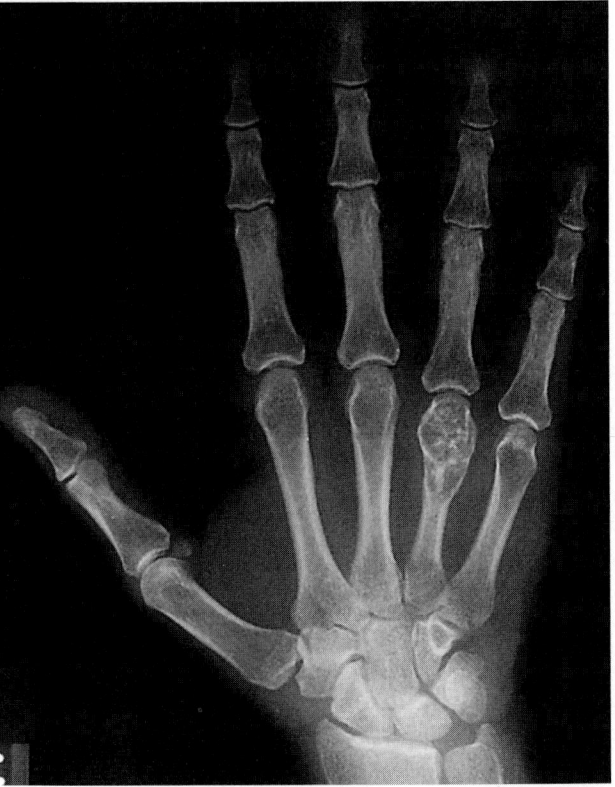

Fig. 9-2. Avascular necrosis of the lunate, or Kienbock disease. Coned-down posteroanterior views of the wrist demonstrate two manifestations of avascular necrosis: bony sclerosis, seen in the ulnar aspect of the lunate, and osteopenia, seen in the radial side of the lunate *(straight arrow)*. The latter is due to increased blood flow as the bone attempts to heal.

Fig. 9-3. An enchondroma is demonstrated in this posteroanterior view. Note the decreased bone density of the fourth metacarpal head and shaft, which also are increased in size. Within the area of decreased bone density are stippled calcifications—a classic finding in this type of lesion.

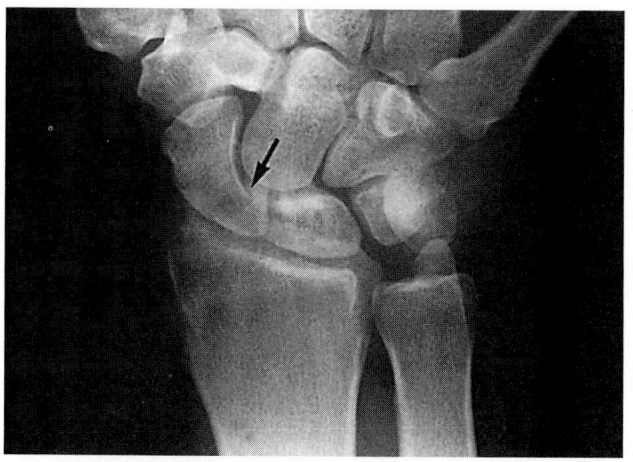

Fig. 9-4. This posteroanterior view of the wrist shows a fracture of the proximal third of the scaphoid *(arrow)* with an associated cyst.

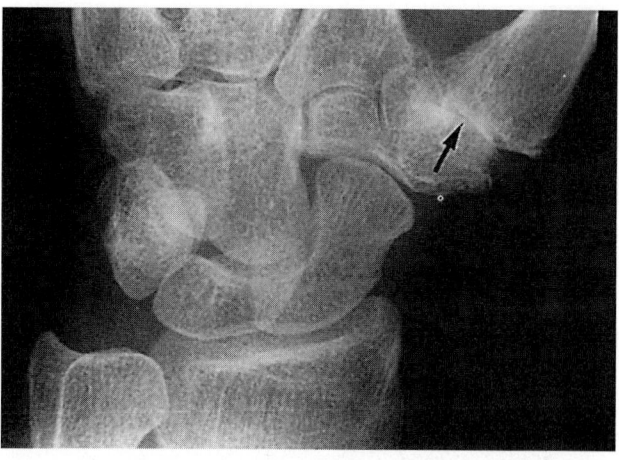

Fig. 9-6. Osteoarthritis. Oblique view of the wrist showing decreased height of the articular cartilage at the first metacarpal joint *(arrow)*. The disease also has resulted in increased bone density on both sides of the joint.

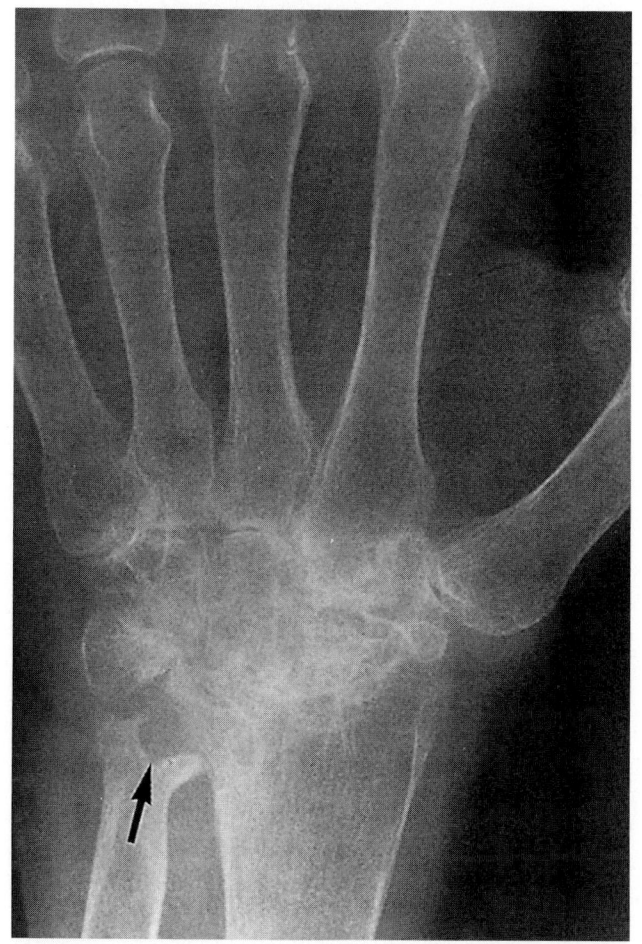

Fig. 9-5. Posteroanterior views of the wrist demonstrating the hallmarks of rheumatoid arthritis: osteopenia, which may be the earliest sign of the disease (compare with normal bone density in Fig. 9-1, *A*), loss of articular cartilage, and erosions. In this patient, erosion is evident at the ulnar styloid *(arrow)*.

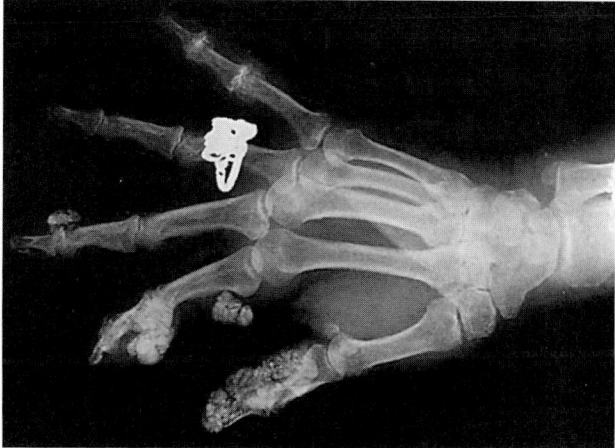

Fig. 9-7. Oblique view of the hand demonstrating extensive calcification in the soft tissues of the digits.

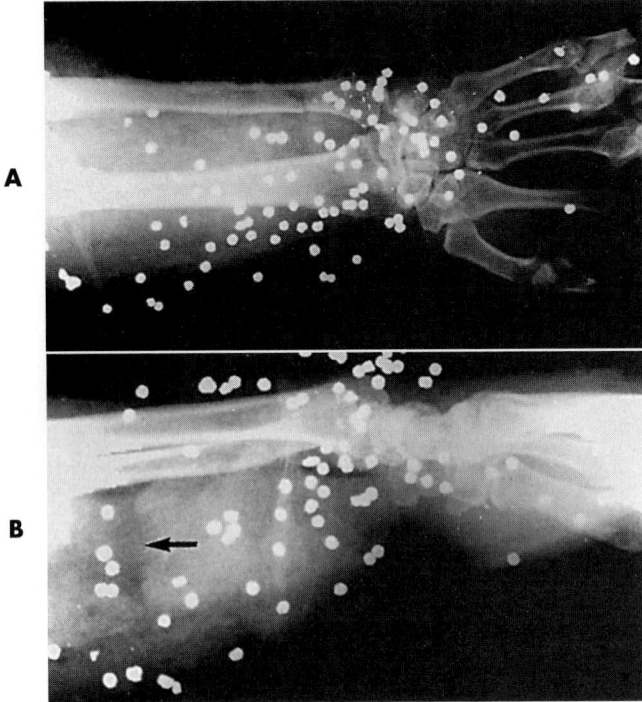

Fig. 9-8. Posteroanterior (**A**) and lateral (**B**) views of the wrist and distal forearm showing multiple shotgun pellets. Note the air in the soft tissues (areas of lucency *[arrow]*) caused by the penetrating trauma.

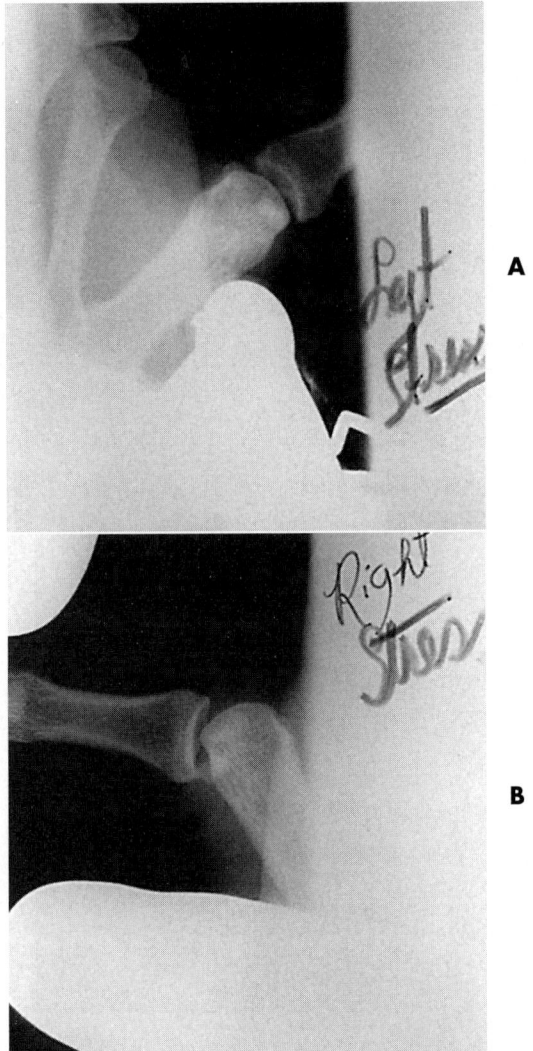

Fig. 9-10. Thumb dislocation. **A,** This patient's left thumb appears normal under radial stress. **B,** The right thumb, which had a disruption of the ulnar collateral ligament, shows subluxation of the first metacarpophalangeal joint when subjected to the same stress.

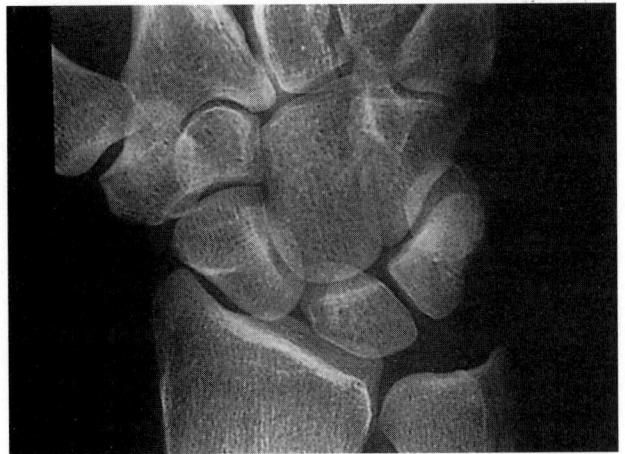

Fig. 9-9. Coned-down posteroanterior views of the wrist provide greater bony detail and are useful when wrist pathology is suspected.

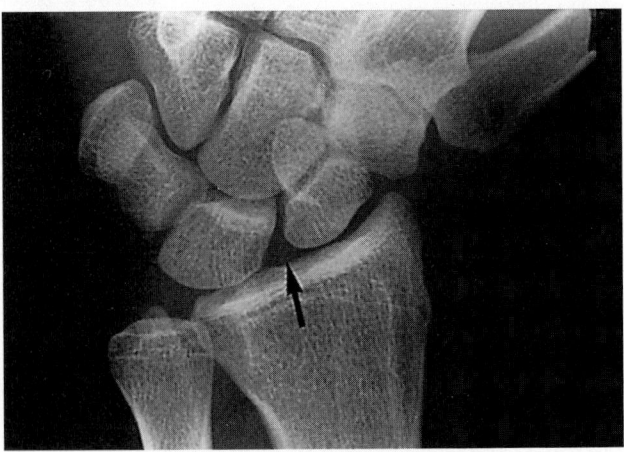

Fig. 9-11. When this patient clenched the fist in supination, subluxation of the scaphoid *(arrow)* occurred.

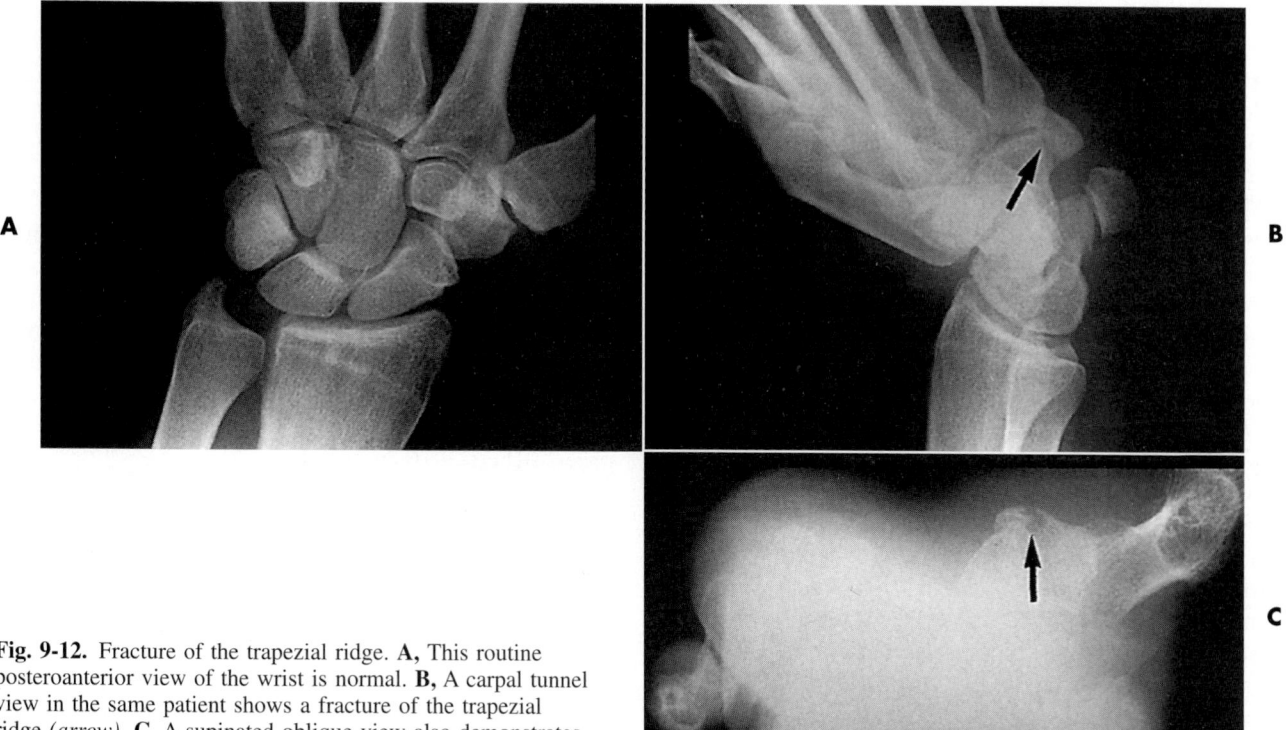

Fig. 9-12. Fracture of the trapezial ridge. **A,** This routine posteroanterior view of the wrist is normal. **B,** A carpal tunnel view in the same patient shows a fracture of the trapezial ridge *(arrow).* **C,** A supinated oblique view also demonstrates this type of fracture *(arrow).*

Fig. 9-13. Carpal tunnel view showing a fracture of the hook of the hamate *(arrow).*

Table 9-1. Imaging techniques used in diagnosing hand disorders: invasiveness and cost

Technique	Cost	Invasiveness
Plain radiography	+	0
Plain tomography	++	0
Computed tomography	+++	0
Bone scintigraphy	++	+
Magnetic resonance imaging	+++	0
Wrist arthography	++	++
Arteriography	+++	++++

+, $50-$300; ++, $400-$900; +++, >$1000.

anatomy of the carpal tunnel and certain fractures, such as those of the trapezial ridge (Fig. 9-12) and hook of the hamate (Fig. 9-13).

Advanced imaging techniques

When a diagnosis cannot be made on the basis of the routine clinical examination and plain radiographs, more advanced imaging techniques can be used to visualize the bone and soft tissue anatomy more completely. The decision to use another technique must consider the invasiveness and cost of the procedure (Table 9-1) as well as its specificity.

Plain tomography

Plain tomography is capable of visualizing healing bone and fracture nonunion better than routine radiographs, especially in cases involving the scaphoid and hook of the

hamate. This examination is noninvasive and relatively inexpensive, and although it may have limited availability in outpatient clinics, it is available in most hospitals. The technologist must know how to correctly position the patient and be familiar with the special equipment used. The bony detail revealed on plain tomograms is obscured by cast material, so the cast must be removed before the examination.

Computed tomography

Computed tomography (CT) is useful in evaluating complex fractures and bony lesions, providing superior detail of cortical invasion, marrow abnormalities, and matrix calcification.[3,5,25] It, too, is noninvasive but has a great advantage over plain tomography because it can image through cast material. CT enhances soft tissue contrast, so it is of great value in diagnosing soft tissue masses. It also provides excellent depiction of subluxations and dislocations of the distal radioulnar joint.[15] With the advent of spiral and multislice CT, thin 1-mm slices provide sagittal and coronal reconstruction identical to direct imaging.

Bone scintigraphy

Bone scintigraphy involves the intravenous injection of ^{99m}Tc-labeled monodiphosphonate (MDP), which is preferentially taken up by bone. Flow images are generated after 60 seconds, and a nuclear medicine angiogram is obtained. Delayed images are generated after 3 hours. Areas of abnormal blood flow and bone turnover can be detected on the scan, making it useful in the evaluation of infection, avascular necrosis of the lunate, tumors, and reflex sympathetic dystrophy. It also is used to screen patients who have unexplained wrist pain (Fig. 9-14).[18]

The examination is minimally invasive and moderately expensive. The poor anatomic resolution of the scan is the primary drawback of this modality. The test also is nonspecific, so the results must be carefully correlated with the clinical findings to be properly interpreted.

Arteriography

Arteriography is the most specific means of evaluating vascular anatomy and pathology; it is used to evaluate aneurysms, traumatic vessel injuries, and tumor vascularity (Fig. 9-15).[27] The examination is performed by threading a catheter into the brachial artery using a femoral approach, injecting contrast material, and then taking multiple radiographs. The procedure is often painful, even with the use of new nonionic contrast material. The contrast medium may cause arterial spasm, although this can be controlled with the use of vasodilators. Anaphylaxis is another potential complication when iodinated contrast material is used, but severe episodes are rare, occurring in only 1 of 40,000 cases. Magnetic resonance (MR) and CT angiography can replace conventional angiography for large vessel disease.

Magnetic resonance angiography

MR angiography can easily demonstrate vascular abnormalities such as arterial thrombosis and arteriovenous fistulas, and it also can help identify abnormal vasculature within soft tissue tumors.[26] Eventually, this technique may be capable of providing detailed images of vessels as small as the digital arteries. MR angiography is noninvasive because it does not require the use of intravenous contrast material (Figs. 9-16 and 9-17).

Arthrography

Arthrography is used to evaluate the integrity of the carpal ligaments and triangular fibrocartilage (Fig. 9-18). The examination involves injecting dye into the radiocarpal, radioulnar, and midcarpal compartments, so it must be performed carefully.[9] Communication of dye between the compartments of the wrist can be caused by a clinically unimportant perforation and does not necessarily indicate pathology.[28] Thus the test results must be correlated with the clinical examination and interpreted with a great deal of caution. The examination is invasive but can be administered with minimal discomfort to the patient. Arthrography is currently used as a complement to magnetic resonance imaging (MRI).

Cineradiography

Continuous radiographic imaging of the wrist in motion is a useful method of evaluating dynamic carpal instability.

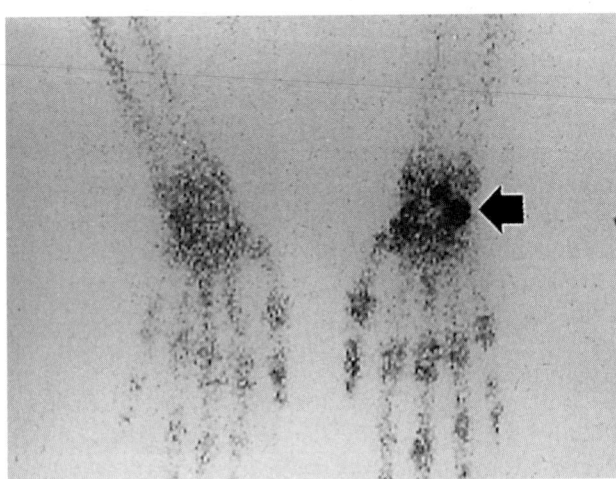

Fig. 9-14. This bone scan demonstrates increased uptake in the right lunate, the right pisiform/triquetral area, and the first carpal metacarpal joint *(arrow)*. Such findings are nonspecific. Avascular necrosis of the lunate was demonstrated on other imaging studies.

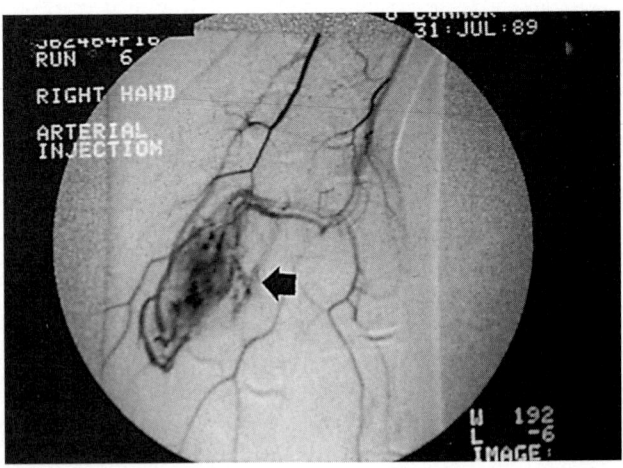

Fig. 9-15. Contrast arteriogram of the wrist showing a hemangioma *(arrow)* in the ulnar aspect of the palm.

This noninvasive and inexpensive technique is the diagnostic imaging procedure of choice for determining and documenting the presence of dynamic rotatory subluxation of the scaphoid.[19]

Magnetic resonance imaging

MRI not only provides excellent detail of soft tissue structures but also is completely noninvasive and involves no ionizing radiation. Among its minor drawbacks are its contraindications in patients with pacemakers, cochlear implants, and/or ferromagnetic aneurysm clips. In addition, the examination is performed with the patient lying in a narrow cylinder within the bore of a magnet—a closed space that may cause some individuals to become claustrophobic.

(In the event of such anxiety, the patient may be administered intravenous benzodiazepam, provided that the patient also can be monitored properly during sedation.) Evaluating a suspected pathology with MRI involves the optimization of many parameters; for this reason, close communication between the orthopedist and radiologist is absolutely essential.

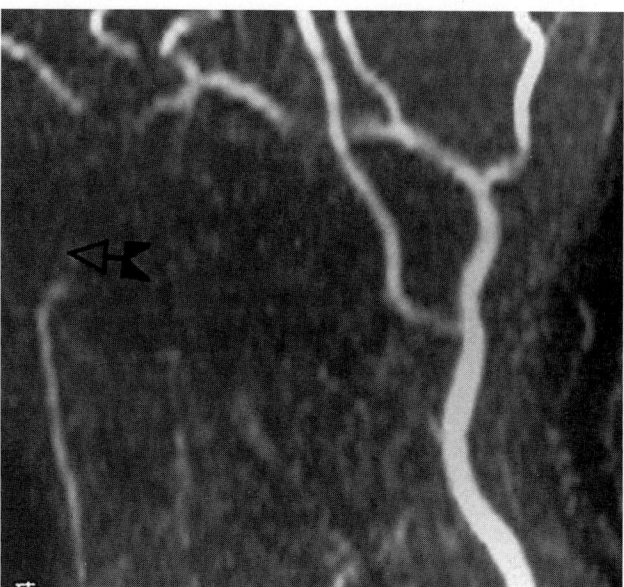

Fig. 9-17. Magnetic resonance (MR) angiogram demonstrating ulnar artery thrombosis *(left)*. (Compare with normal MR angiogram in Fig. 9-16.)

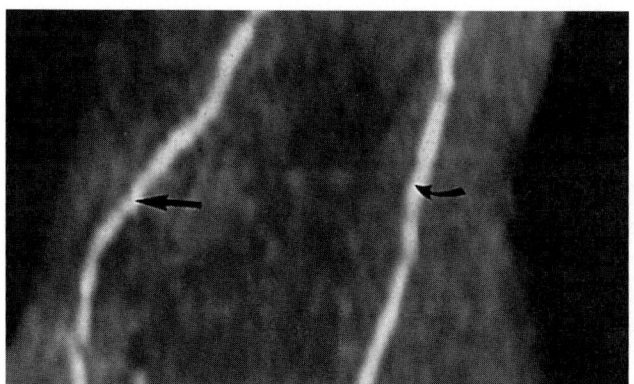

Fig. 9-16. Magnetic resonance angiogram of a normal radial *(curved arrow)* and ulnar *(straight arrow)* artery.

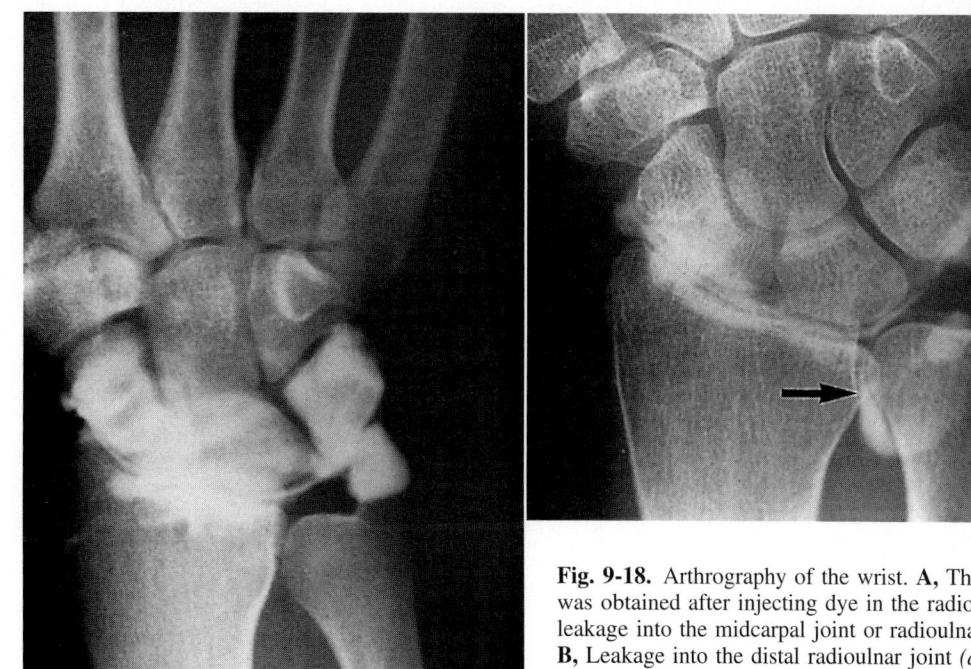

Fig. 9-18. Arthrography of the wrist. **A,** This normal arthrogram was obtained after injecting dye in the radiocarpal joint. No leakage into the midcarpal joint or radioulnar joint is seen. **B,** Leakage into the distal radioulnar joint *(arrow)* is evident in this patient. Clinical correlation is needed to accurately interpret this finding.

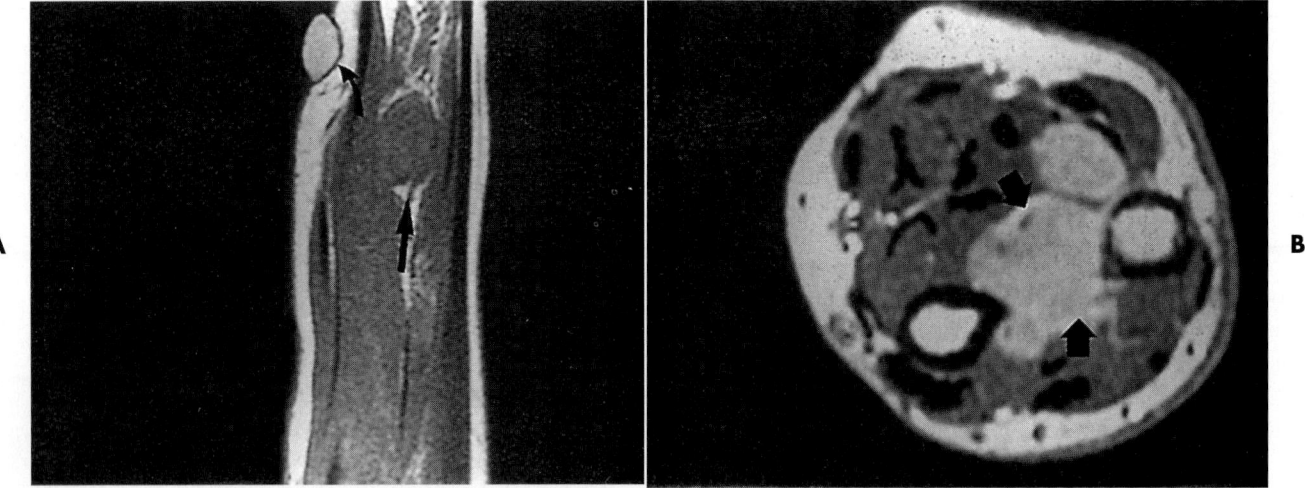

Fig. 9-19. Synovial sarcoma. **A,** Sagittal magnetic resonance image showing a soft tissue mass *(arrow)*. The white object *(curved arrow)* is a marker (raw almond) placed over the palpable mass *(straight arrow)*. **B,** Axial magnetic resonance image obtained after contrast enhancement demonstrates the mass again *(arrows)* and shows that the neurovascular bundle is encased by tumor.

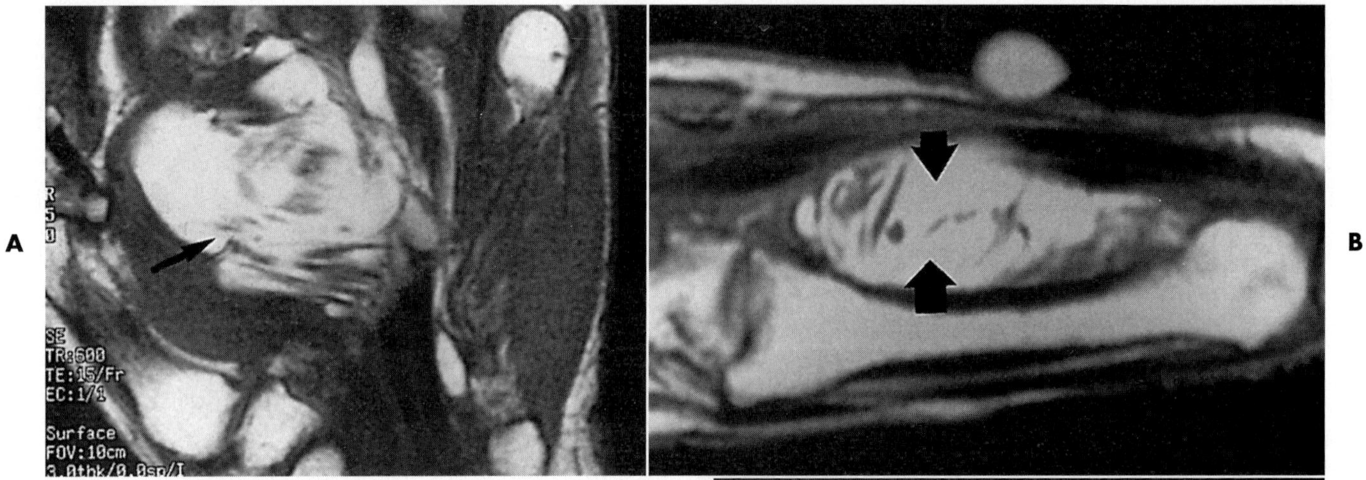

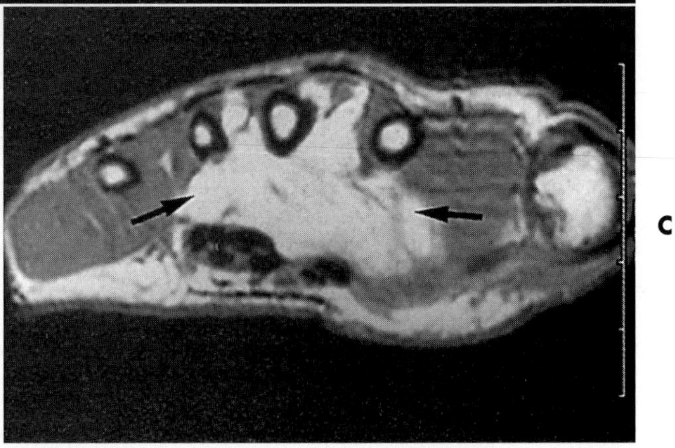

Fig. 9-20. Infiltrating lipoma of the palm. Magnetic resonance images of the sagittal **(A)**, coronal **(B)**, and axial **(C)** planes show the extent of the lesion *(arrows)*.

MRI is of great value in defining soft tissue abnormalities (Figs. 9-19 to 9-21). In the evaluation of tumors, it cannot provide a specific diagnosis, but it can define the size of the lesion and the extent of involvement of marrow and neurovascular structures (Fig. 9-22).[1] Other soft tissue abnor-

malities diagnosed more easily by MRI include ganglions, ligament tears, and cartilage abnormalities (Fig. 9-23).[2,30] Hypertrophy of the dorsal capsule can cause dorsal wrist pain and progress to the formation of a ganglion that may not be palpable. Patients with dorsal wrist pain of unknown

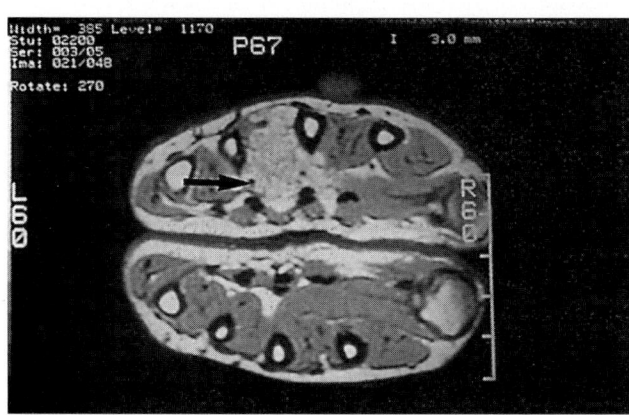

Fig. 9-21. Hemangioma. Axial magnetic resonance images through the palm show a mass between the third and fourth metacarpals *(arrow)*. Magnetic resonance imaging is capable of depicting the extent of a soft tissue mass but cannot provide a specific pathologic diagnosis. A contrast arteriogram of this hand is shown in Fig. 9-15.

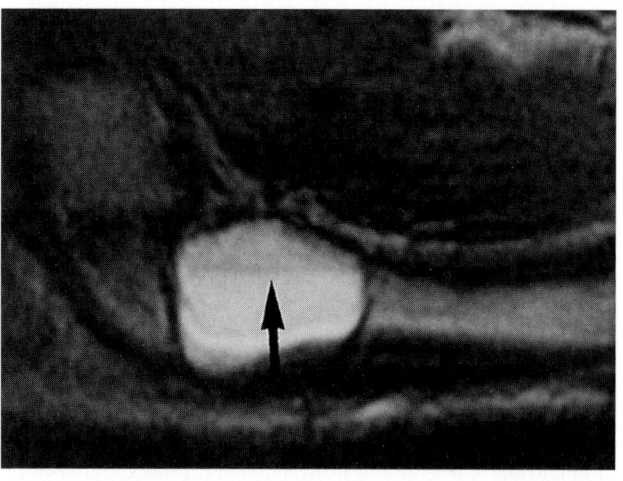

Fig. 9-22. Aneurysmal bone cyst. This magnetic resonance image reveals an abnormality at the base of the second metacarpal. The fluid-filled level *(arrow)* is a typical finding in such cases.

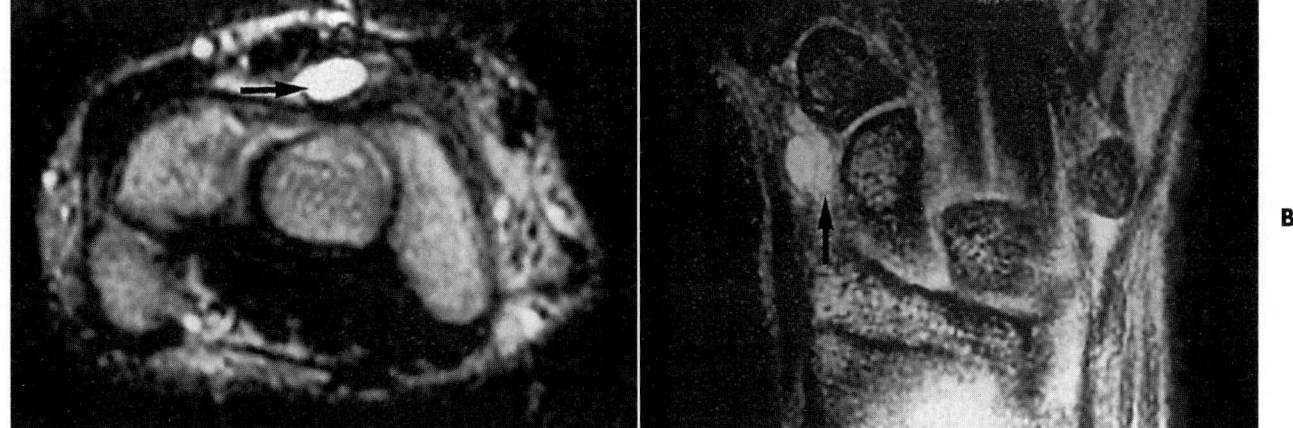

Fig. 9-23. Ganglion. **A,** This axial magnetic resonance image demonstrates a dorsal mass *(arrow)* that was not palpable on clinical examination. **B,** Coronal magnetic resonance image in another patient showing a mass in the abductor canal *(arrow).*

origin are therefore candidates for evaluation by MRI. MRI is especially helpful in diagnosing tears of the scapholunate and lunotriquetral ligaments, particularly when dissociation of the scapholunate is not evident on plain films.[20] Excellent depiction of the triangular fibrocartilage can be achieved with MRI, but the image must be interpreted carefully; thinning of the disc occurs in many patients, but a tear of this structure is not diagnosed unless an avulsion from the ulnar or radial insertion can be observed.[7,8,14]

Evaluation of the wrist has traditionally been performed with plain film radiography. More recently, CT has been used, especially for the evaluation of subtle fractures, and

MRI is becoming a more frequently used tool to evaluate internal derangements of the wrist. An internal derangement is any abnormality of a joint that is visible when the joint is examined by arthroscopy or arthrotomy. High-resolution MRI images and small field of views are commonly used to image this small and complex joint. The triangular fibrocartilage, ligaments and tendons, synovium and cartilage, and carpal tunnel are commonly evaluated.

There are three compartments of the wrist: the distal radioulnar, radiocarpal, and midcarpal joints. Normally, no communication is seen between these compartments. However, communication does exist between the midcarpal and common carpometacarpal compartments. There is also normal communication between the triquetral-pisiform and either the midcarpal or radiocarpal compartments. Any other communications imply an internal derangement. The prestyloid and triquetral-pisiform are the most commonly visualized recesses of the wrist.

A small amount of fluid in the radiocarpal joint is normal. Only a minimal amount of fluid should normally be seen in the midcarpal joint, except for the triquetral-pisiform recess. Fluid should not be visible in the common carpometacarpal compartment. Fluid in the distal radioulnar joint (DRUJ) is always abnormal. This may be painful and is often associated with triangular fibrocartilage (TFC) tears. DRUJ fluid is less commonly associated with arthritis.

The tendon sheaths of the wrist may normally contain a small amount of synovial fluid; however, fluid should not be visible in any of the extensor tendon sheaths. If a moderate amount of tendon sheath fluid is visible by MRI, it should be described as abnormal. Fluid in multiple sheaths should raise the possibility of an inflammatory arthropathy. Synovitis of the flexor tendons demonstrates complex fluid and synovial proliferation, which on MRI appears as gray signal that is hypointense to joint fluid on T_2-weighted images. This is significantly enhanced with contrast administration.

There are no true bursae in the wrist. Acquired or adventitial bursa may be seen deep or superficial to the carpal tunnel flexor tendons, adjacent to the ulna styloid, or adjacent to the bases of the first or fifth metacarpals.

Some problems are most efficiently diagnosed by using the available clinical information to direct the imaging workup. The anatomic structures involved determine the modalities used. Examples of this approach are outlined on the following sections.

Extensor tendons

The extensor tendons are contained in six dorsal compartments numbered from the radial (I) to ulnar (VI) sides of the wrist. Lister's tubercle separates compartments II and III. Extensor disorders outside of compartments I or VI are rare; thus fluid in multiple compartments usually represents synovitis and is often a marker for an inflammatory arthritis such as rheumatoid.

More commonly, the tendons of compartment I abductor pollicis longus and extensor pollicis brevis are affected with stenosing tenosynovitis. This disorder is termed *de Quervain's syndrome* and is related to overuse. It is more common in women and also may occur as a complication of pregnancy. Patients typically present with pain radiating from the radial styloid to the thumb and proximally into the forearm. Pain is increased with passive movement of the thumb and swelling/tenderness over the first dorsal compartment of the wrist. This disorder usually is diagnosed clinically. On MRI fluid within the tendon sheath is increased, and the tendons themselves, which may show increased intrasubstance signal, are enlarged. On coronal images, there is focal obliteration of the adjacent subcutaneous fat and intense synovial enhancement following gadolinium administration. This stenosing tenosynovitis is analogous to adhesive capsulitis in the shoulder.

Compartment VI contains the extensor carpi ulnaris (ECU) tendon, which is another common site for disorders such as synovitis or tenosynovitis. ECU subluxation may occur, which can lead to synovitis and/or intrasubstance tears; thus dynamic imaging may be performed to confirm the diagnosis. It should be recognized that artifactual increased signal within the ECU is commonly seen, which may represent subclinical degeneration or normal fascicular anatomy.

Ligaments

The ligamentous anatomy of the wrist is complex because of the stabilization required for the numerous carpal bones and extensive range and axes of motion in this joint. The intrinsic carpal ligaments connect the carpal bones to each other, while the extrinsic ligaments connect the carpus to both the radius and ulna and to the metacarpals. The extrinsic ligaments are more important for overall carpal stability and have a complex nomenclature. In general, tears of the extrinsic ligaments are less common and more difficult to diagnose than intrinsic ligament tears. Ligaments can be injured by trauma or by inflammatory processes such as rheumatoid arthritis.

The two main intrinsic ligaments of the wrist are the scapholunate (SL) and lunatotriquetral (LT) ligaments. SL ligament tears may be spontaneous, secondary to a fall on an outstretched hand, or associated with the subtypes of carpal instability. LT ligament tears also can be spontaneous or posttraumatic. LT tears are not uncommonly associated with instability patterns of the wrist and also have a high association with TFC tears.

Mechanically, both the SL and LT ligaments are divided into three portions: dorsal, volar, and central. The central or membranous portion is thin, whereas the dorsal and volar portions are thicker with individual fascicles usually visible. The membranous aspect is the easiest to visualize on MR and is the portion most commonly perforated. Membranous tears can cause pain but are biomechanically unimportant. The dorsal and volar aspects of these ligaments are more important to the mechanical stability of the carpus; however, these are the most difficult portions to reliably evaluate for abnormalities. Consequently, secondary signs of dorsal or volar ligamentous injury are important to note. Normally, joint fluid should go up to, but not extend through, these ligaments. Fluid violating the intercarpal intervals is the most reliable secondary sign of a tear. This also can be used to evaluate for central tears. The failure of fluid to normally enter the scapholunate and lunatotriquetral interspaces is a sign of chronic ligament tear with scarring.

The carpal ligaments are best visualized on thin section 3D-gradient recalled MR sequences in the coronal and axial planes. They appear as signal voids bridging the carpal bones. Ligament strains can be diagnosed if there is abnormal signal and/or attenuation of the structure. Discontinuity, complete absence, and increased intercarpal distances are findings compatible with ligament tears. The best finding for an intrinsic tear is fluid violating the space extending from the radiocarpal to the midcarpal joints. Normally, the ends of the lunate, scaphoid, and triquetrum should appear smoothly rounded. The presence of osteophytes is abnormal and often is caused by biomechanically incompetent ligaments, usually resulting from partial dorsal or volar aspect tears. The presence of marrow edema, subchondral sclerosis, or other signs of focal articular disease should suggest ligament dysfunction. Focal offset of two adjacent carpal bones and the lack of the normal articular parallelism also are signs suggestive of ligament dysfunction. Remember that perforation of the SL or LT ligaments occurs with aging; thus, in a patient older than 35 to 40 years of age, a tear should be diagnosed only if the ligament is morphologically abnormal.

Carpal instability

The three most commonly imaged instability patterns are rotatory subluxation of the scaphoid (associated with radioscaphocapitate and SL ligament tears), volar intercalated segmental instability (VISI), and dorsal intercalated segmental instability (DISI). Rotatory subluxation and DISI are usually traumatic and present in young adulthood. VISI, although usually degenerative or traumatic, has an association with rheumatoid arthritis.

The diagnosis of many patterns of carpal instability can be established by routine radiographic findings. The lateral projection is useful in evaluating both DISI and VISI. In DISI, the lunate is flexed dorsally, with the scaphoid displaced vertically. The angle of intersection between the main longitudinal axis (along the radius, scaphoid, lunate, capitate, and third metacarpal) and the long axis of the scaphoid is greater than 60 degrees where it should normally be 30 to 60 degrees. The radioscapholunate ligament should be evaluated for tear. This injury is typically degenerative in origin and is thought to be the sequela of trauma to the outstretched hand in a young adult.

In VISI, the lunate is flexed toward the palm, and the angle between the two longitudinal axes is less than 30 degrees. Note that this finding may be normal if bilateral and in a young female patient. VISI is less common than DISI overall. Most cases are thought to be degenerative in origin, although there is an association with rheumatoid arthritis.

Carpal fusion

Carpal fusion or coalition is clinically important because it places the patient at a somewhat higher risk for carpal instability and secondary SL ligament tears. There are three types of carpal fusion:

1. Congenital: Isolated fusions involve bones of the same carpal row, whereas syndrome-related fusions may affect bones in different rows (both proximal and distal). LT and capitate-hamate are the most common types of isolated fusion, although fusion may occur in almost any combination. LT fusion may be asymptomatic, but widening of the scapholunate interosseous space may be seen radiographically. Partial fusions may be associated with pain and cystic changes in the adjacent bones. Massive carpal fusion, which affects both carpal rows, is associated with congenital syndromes/chromosomal anomalies (e.g., Turner's, Holt-Oram, Ellis von Creveldt).
2. Surgical/posttraumatic.
3. Inflammatory: Pericapitate fusions are seen in adult Still's disease.

Triangular fibrocartilage complex

The most common internal derangement of the wrist involves the TFC. The triangular fibrocartilage complex (TFCC) consists of the triangular fibrocartilage, the meniscal homologue, the ulnolunate and ulnotriquetral (volar ulnocarpal) ligaments, and the extensor carpi ulnaris tendon. The TFC is a biconcave fibrocartilage band that normally appears dark on all imaging sequences and is surrounded by higher signal synovial fluid or hyaline cartilage. Its function is similar to that of the menisci in the knee. The TFC arises from the ulnar aspect of the distal radius and extends to the junction between the ulnar head and styloid process, adjacent to the meniscal homologue. The meniscal homologue at the ulnar edge of the TFC is made up of fibrofatty tissue that appears as high signal on T_1 and proton-density images in contrast to the low signal TFC. Many authorities currently believe that the homologue is not a fibrofatty structure, but rather fat interposed between the extrinsic ligaments at the ulnar aspect of the wrist. The meniscal homologue should never appear similar to fluid on T_2 images.

The TFC is best demonstrated on coronal images, especially on thin-section 3D-gradient echo sequences. A suspected tear of the TFC is a common indication for MR evaluation of the wrist. These tears are divided into degenerative and traumatic types. Degenerative tears are much more common and are often termed *central tears*. These occur in the thinnest portion of the TFC, which is central but slightly eccentric toward the radial aspect of this structure. Traumatic tears occur after a discrete injury and usually are located at the ulnar or radial side of the TFC. Traumatic tears tend to be perpendicular to the long axis of the TFC and are associated with fluid in the DRUJ and, to a lesser degree, with excessive fluid in the radiocarpal joint. TFCC tears can be partial or full thickness. Ulnar-sided tears may be in the region of the meniscal homologue. It is these traumatic TFC tears that are most easily missed on MRI. High-signal intensity in this region on T_2-weighted sequences is the most reliable finding. Any fluid at the periphery of the TFCC on T_2-weighted images that is not in the prestyloid recess or ECU tendon sheath should be described as a peripheral tear. TFCC tears are typically associated with LT, and less frequently, SL ligament tears.

Although the TFC is usually low in signal on all pulse sequences, increased internal signal may sometimes be seen on GRE or T_1-weighted images. This represents degeneration of the TFC and not a true tear. This degenerative signal is globular, is hypointense to cartilage, and does not extend to both sides of the TFC. Another diagnostic pitfall is the line of high-signal hyaline cartilage seen at the insertion of the TFC onto the radius, which can be mistaken for a tear. True radial sided tears are rare. They usually are caused by acute trauma and consist of a radial avulsion of the TFC with increased signal intensity on T_2 images. Tears should be seen on at least two pulse sequences.

Ulnar variance

Ulnar variance refers to the relationship between the distal ulna and radius, excluding their respective styloid processes. Normally, the articular surfaces of these bones are aligned. Changes in the length of the ulna relative to that of the radius will alter the compressive forces across the wrist. In positive ulnar variance, the ulna is longer than the adjacent articular aspect of the radius, while with negative variance the ulna is shorter. Any variance greater than 2.5 mm is biomechanically significant. Ulnar variance may be difficult to accurately assess on MRI, other than to describe the relationship between the ulna and the sigmoid sulcus of the radius. Negative ulnar variance is weakly associated with Kienbock disease. Positive ulnar variance is associated with degenerative type TFC tears due to mechanical erosion.

Positive ulna variance can eventually lead to impaction of the lunate by the ulna through a chronic TFC tear. This is known as *ulnalunato abutment syndrome*. This also may affect the triquetral bone of the carpus. On MRI, abutment is manifested by cartilage loss of the lunate with resultant marrow edema and eventual subchondral sclerosis. Cartilage defects are best seen on high-resolution images, whereas the sclerosis is seen as low signal on T_1- and T_2-weighted sequences. Gradient echo sequences often accentuate this dark signal. The best markers for abutment are subchondral cysts, usually at the proximal and ulnar aspects of the lunate and distal ulna. Ultimately, chronic abutment may result in osteonecrosis of the lunate. Of note, TFC tears do not need to be present in the setting of abutment.

Distal radioulnar joint disorders

There are four types of problems affecting the DRUJ: incongruity, instability, impaction, and isolated tears of the TFC.[16] The presence or absence of each can be confirmed by using the various imaging techniques in a logical sequence.

Joint incongruity is evaluated on plain PA radiographs, which can demonstrate irregularity, sclerosis, spurs, and erosions of the articular surface of the sigmoid notch of the radius and ulnar head (Fig. 9-24). Instability is caused by a deficiency of the fibrocartilaginous support structure of the

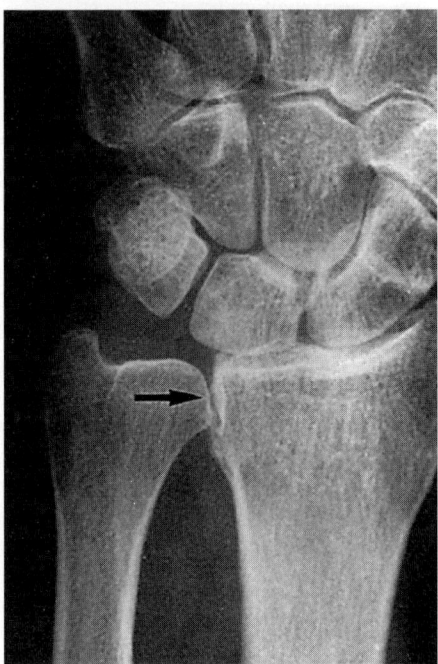

Fig. 9-24. Incongruity of the distal radioulnar joint. Narrowing of the normal cartilage space *(arrow)* demonstrates loss of the articular cartilage.

DRUJ, and this problem can be determined on the basis of the clinical examination. Plain radiographs taken with the patient properly positioned will confirm the diagnosis if subluxation or dislocation of the ulnar head within the sigmoid notch of the radius is shown (Fig. 9-25). CT or MRI also can confirm the subluxation or dislocation by demonstrating the orientation of the DRUJ in the axial plane.[15]

Impaction of the DRUJ is caused by a length discrepancy between the radius and ulna. If the ulna is too long, it impacts or abuts on the carpus during rotation (Fig. 9-26). Positive ulnar variance may be demonstrated on plain radiographs, especially if the fist is clenched in pronation. Isolated tears of the TFC disc may cause pain without instability. This condition can be diagnosed on the basis of the clinical examination and confirmed with MRI (Fig. 9-27).

Avascular necrosis

Avascular necrosis (AVN) is common in the wrist. It may be the result of overuse, occur spontaneously, or be secondary to local trauma or systemic disease. Examples of systemic processes that can lead to AVN include steroid usage and systemic lupus erythematosus (SLE).

An example of AVN related to overuse occurs in the lunate and is termed *Kienbock disease*. Repetitive microtrauma is thought to be the major cause, although it may occur after a single major traumatic event. The dominant extremity is usually affected, and young males are more commonly affected than females. The blood supply to the

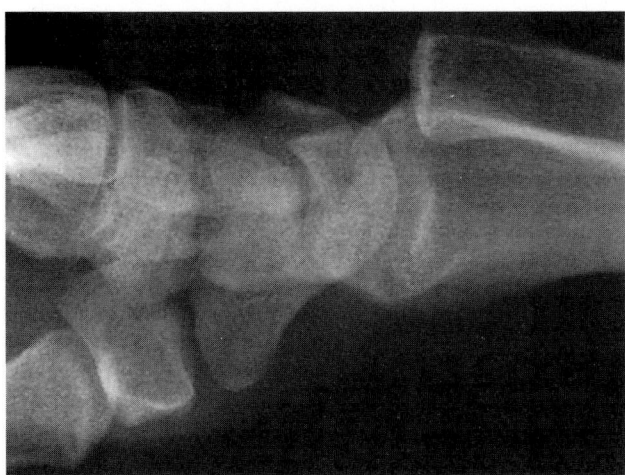

Fig. 9-25. Lateral view of the wrist showing dorsal subluxation of the ulna after trauma.

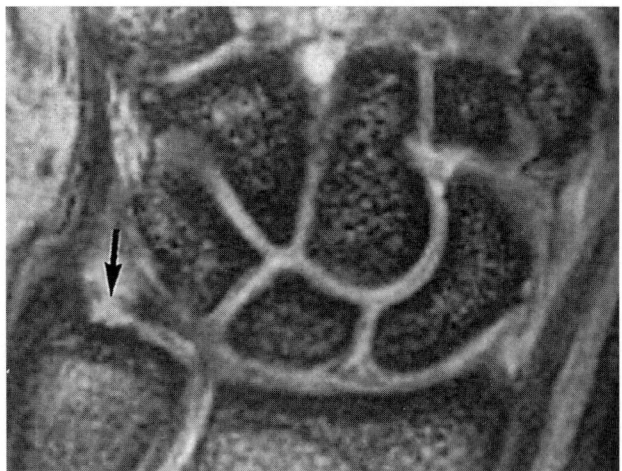

Fig. 9-27. Coronal magnetic resonance image showing an avulsion of the triangular fibrocartilage complex from its attachment to the ulna *(arrow).*

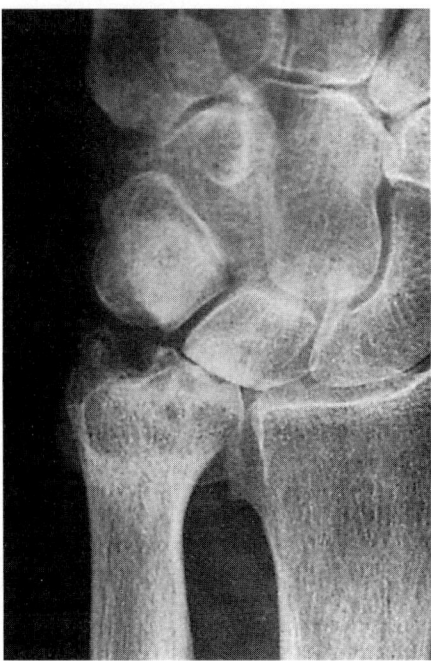

Fig. 9-26. Positive ulnar variance of the distal radioulnar joint seen in this posteroanterior view has resulted in impaction of the ulna into the lunate. The sclerosis indicates a chronic bone reaction to this trauma. Loss of the articular cartilage also is evident.

lunate is tenuous because most of this bone is covered with hyaline cartilage. The proximal aspect of the lunate is most vulnerable to injury, and if AVN involves only one part of the bone, it affects the radial side. Kienbock disease also is associated with negative ulnar variance. The MR staging of Kienbock disease (modified from plain film staging) is as follows:

Stage 1: normal contour of the lunate, with a radiolucent or radiodense line representing the compression fracture; fracture is seen as a zone of decreased T_1 signal

Stage 2: resorption of bone along the fracture line
Stage 3: all of the changes of stages 1 and 2, plus sclerosis of the bone; necrotic bone has variably decreased T_1 signal
Stage 4: fragmentation or flattening of the lunate
Stage 5: secondary osteoarthritis of the radiocarpal and intercarpal joints; fragmentation and decreased T_1 signal of the lunate combined with osteophyte formation, subchondral sclerosis, and/or edema involving the adjacent articular surfaces; often an associated joint effusion

Because of its anatomic specificity, MRI is capable of demonstrating marrow abnormalities caused by AVN, and it can reveal these changes earlier than is possible with bone scintigraphy (Fig. 9-28).[17,21,23,24,30] Bone islands have a similar appearance on MR images, so the results must be correlated with plain films. The imaging findings of Kienbock disease show marrow replacement, best assessed on the T_1-weighted images as decreased signal.[17,21,23,24,30] The T_2 appearance varies somewhat but usually shows increased signal. As with all cases of AVN in the wrist, the classic "double-line" sign is rarely seen. The surrounding soft tissues are usually normal, and a joint effusion is variably present.

Posttraumatic AVN may be seen in any carpal bone; however, it is most common in the scaphoid. This is due to its blood supply because the proximal pole is fed from the terminal branches of the artery passing through the middle segment of the scaphoid. A scaphoid waist fracture may disrupt this supply, and in up to 60% of cases, AVN may result. The risk of AVN increases as fracture becomes more proximal. Fractures that have a visible step-off also have a higher risk of AVN. On MRI, the proximal pole of the fractured navicular may show decreased bone marrow signal on T_1 images. The contour of the cortex may become

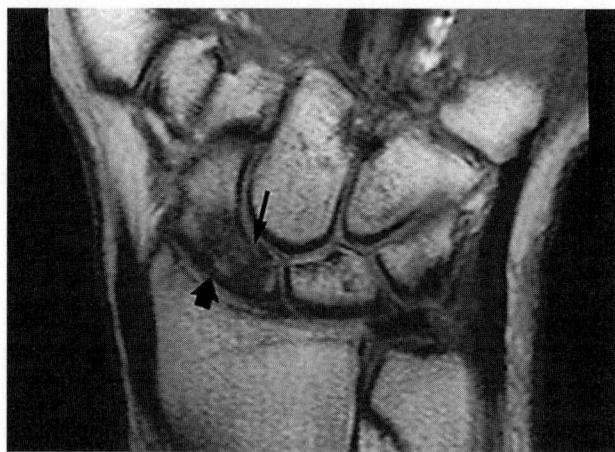

Fig. 9-28. Magnetic resonance image demonstrating a scaphoid fracture (disruption in the black cortical line at the *thin arrow*). The marrow of the scaphoid is relatively darker *(thick arrow),* indicating edema from the fracture.

indistinct and irregular subsequent to collapse. MRI also can show reactive changes in the distal fracture fragment, with AVN rarely occurring here. Again, the "double-line" sign on T_2 images is rarely seen. An acutely "negative" MR for scaphoid AVN is unreliable because false-negative results can occur up to 1 to 2 months.

Spontaneous or idiopathic AVN occurring in the scaphoid is termed *Preiser's disease.* Preiser's disease demonstrates complete marrow replacement on T_1-weighted images, with typical edema on T_2-weighted images. Associated ligamentous injury is uncommon, as is collapse. The capitate bone is the third most common carpal bone to undergo AVN, but this occurs rarely, and when it does, is usually spontaneous in origin.

Carpal tunnel syndrome

The carpal tunnel is bounded by the concave volar surface of the carpus in continuity with the flexor retinaculum, which extends from the trapezium to the hook of the hamate. It consists of the eight flexor digitorum tendons (flexor digitorum superficialis [FDS] and flexor digitorum profundus [FDP]), the flexor pollicis longus tendon, and the median nerve.

Carpal tunnel syndrome (CTS) is a common overuse syndrome characterized by pain, paresthesias, and weakness in the distribution of the median nerve. It is bilateral in 50% of cases and associated with repetitive mechanical activity, such as typing. Other causes of CTS include tenosynovitis, rheumatoid arthritis, amyloidosis, infection, mass (intrinsic or extrinsic), pregnancy, or developmental anomalies. Diagnosis is usually made clinically and confirmed with electromyography (EMG) examinations.

MRI plays a limited role in the evaluation of carpal tunnel disease. By and large, the diagnosis of this problem should be reached clinically, but MRI may be used occasionally if

the symptoms derive from a soft tissue mass or an infection within the carpal tunnel.[12,13] Indications for wrist MRI include atypical symptoms, a lack of EMG findings, high clinical suspicion for mass, young patient age (possible congenital anomalies), and recurrent symptoms in postoperative patients.

On MRI, the flexor retinaculum is normally taut to minimally convex, the median nerve is of uniform size (4×2 mm) and ovoid in shape with signal isointense to muscle, and the flexor tendons are not distinguishable from one another on T_2-weighted sequences. MR findings of CTS include volar bowing of the flexor retinaculum, synovitis of the tendon sheaths within the carpal tunnel, focal enlargement of the median nerve at the level of the pisiform, and increased signal of the nerve itself. The median nerve may alternatively appear flattened. Note that these findings are nonspecific in the absence of symptoms. High signal within the median nerve is the least reliable sign and is often seen in asymptomatic individuals. Mild bowing of the flexor retinaculum may be physiologic; thus CTS should not be suggested unless this finding is marked. Masses rarely cause CTS, but the search for masses must be diligent. Ganglion cysts, lipomas extending from the thenar or hypothenar eminences, or focal amyloid deposition may be causative lesions. A dedicated extremity MRI may be a cost-effective way to make this diagnosis.

In postoperative patients, it is important to check for incomplete lysis of the flexor retinaculum. Although the retinaculum may have been completely severed at surgery, it may regrow and appear intact. Assessment for recurrent or residual masses or recurrent synovitis also should be performed. Postoperatively, the flexor tendons will migrate volarly and the median nerve will usually regain normal size and signal.

Ulnar nerve compression

Compression of the ulnar nerve also may occur at the wrist, resulting in tingling and pain along the hypothenar region, ulnar side of the fourth and fifth fingers. The ulnar nerve, along with the ulnar artery and vein, travels within Guyon's canal. This space lies superficial to the retinaculum of the carpal tunnel, adjacent to the hook of the hamate. Processes that affect or extend into this space may cause the characteristic symptoms.

Ulnar neuropathy (Guyon's canal)

Guyon's canal is formed on the medial side by the pisiform and flexor carpi ulnaris and on the lateral side by the hook of the hamate. The splitting of the flexor retinaculum forms the roof of Guyon's canal. Within the canal lies the ulnar nerve, ulnar artery, and vena comitans.[29] Pain in the ulnar aspect of the palm may be caused by a pathologic condition in the canal and may involve the hook of the hamate, pisiform, ulnar artery or vein, or ulnar nerve. A tumor such as a lipoma or ganglion that extends into or arises within the canal also may cause symptoms by compressing any of these structures.

Fractures involving the hamate or pisiform may be difficult to visualize on plain films and are best evaluated on a carpal tunnel view or CT scan. An anteroposterior oblique view also should be obtained to evaluate the possibility of pisotriquetral arthritis. Pisotriquetral arthritis may be idiopathic or the result of a fracture. MRI is the best option for evaluating vascular and other soft tissue structures. Routine MRI and MR angiography can definitively establish vessel patency noninvasively.

As with CTS, MRI may reveal masses, most commonly ganglion cysts and/or inflammatory changes within Guyon's canal. Compression of the ulnar nerve most commonly results from fibrous bands, which may not be visualized on MRI. Beware of looped ulnar vessels, which may mimic ganglia in this region.

Arthritis

Several types of arthritis affect the wrist, including osteoarthritis (OA), rheumatoid arthritis (RA), crystal deposition diseases (most notably gout and calcium pyrophosphate deposition disease) and hemochromatosis. The presence of cysts and the specific distribution of disease can be helpful in differentiating the various types of arthritis.

Because the wrist is a non–weight-bearing joint, osteoarthritis is usually secondary to other processes such as prior trauma, inflammatory arthritides (RA), or infection. The radial distribution of OA is well recognized, with changes usually confined to the first carpometacarpal joint and the trapezioscaphoid space of the midcarpal joint. Clinical symptoms include pain, restricted movement, and instability. Increasing radial subluxation of the metacarpal base, narrowing of the interosseous space, sclerosis and cystic change of the subchondral bone, and osteophytosis is seen radiographically. Changes of osteoarthritis on MRI are characterized by joint space loss, subchondral cyst or geode formation, and bony production manifested by subchondral sclerosis and osteophyte formation.

Focal arthritis also may occur secondary to a type II lunate or in the scapholunate advanced collapse (SLAC) wrist. OA at the base of the first metacarpal often demonstrates marked proliferative change, with large osteophyte production and synovial cysts that can sometimes mimic masses on MRI. This form of OA also can mimic a subluxation because the osteophytes may appear to displace the base of the first metacarpal radially. OA about the scaphoid is common and is usually not related to instability. However, this type of OA can be the sequelae of a ligament tear or instability, particularly if the arthritis is focal. Usually, this focal type of arthritis occurs as the result of an SL or LT ligament tear.

The SLAC wrist may occur as a complication in patients with long standing SL ligament tears and secondary widening of the SL interval. There is proximal migration of the capitate, leading to focal arthritis at the capitoscaphoid and capitolunate joints. On MRI, the SLAC wrist demonstrates cartilage loss and subtle marrow edema at the distal central SL joint and the proximal capitate. The SLAC wrist may lead to CTS because of the shortening of the carpal tunnel with an infolding of the median nerve.

The last subtype of OA occurs in patients with a type II lunate. In this variant, an extra facet of the lunate articulates with the hamate. This is a common finding, occurring in approximately half of affected individuals. Accelerated cartilage loss with underlying marrow edema may be seen as the sequelae of the type II lunate. Frank osteoarthritis may appear at the lunatohamate junction. The edema from the cartilage loss in this entity may mimic AVN or stress fractures of the hamate.

The next most common type of arthritis to affect the wrist is RA. RA has certain characteristic sites of involvement in the wrist, including the ulna styloid (secondary to extensor carpi ulnaris synovitis) and the first and second MP joints. The cartilage loss in RA presents as diffuse, symmetric joint space loss in contrast to the focal changes seen in OA. Joint effusions are common, with marked synovial proliferation (pannus) often seen. This pannus mimics fluid on T_2-weighted images but may also demonstrate low signal secondary to ferritin deposition. The number and size of erosions, as well as the volume of pannus, are good markers for rheumatoid activity. These findings may be used to assess the effectiveness of medical intervention in this disease.

Calcium pyrophosphate deposition disease (CPPD) often affects the wrist. Usually, calcification is seen in the TFC, but it also may affect the SL and LT ligaments. Capsular calcification also can occur, but this type of calcification is usually senile or related to hyperparathyroidism caused by renal failure. On MR, it may be difficult to see the calcifications of CPPD. This is because the TFC is normally low in signal intensity; therefore the signal void of calcification does not show up against it. Occasionally, the calcifications may appear bright, particularly on intermediate-weighted images. Calcifications may mimic either a TFC, SL, or LT ligament tear because of the artifactual junction between the low signal calcification and the higher signal of a degenerated, but not torn, ligament.

The urate crystal deposition of gout tends to be low in signal on T_1- and T_2-weighted images. Sharply marginated erosions usually are seen, and there is often pancarpal involvement with variably sized lesions of high signal on T_2-weighted images. Diseases with similar signal characteristics include amyloidosis, synovial chondromatosis, and pigmented villonodular synovitis (PVNS). All of these entities also show variable, but often significant, susceptibility artifact. Of note, some types of productive osteoarthritis can occasionally have a peculiar appearance, which may mimic gout or PVNS. Last, the arthritis resulting from silicone implants also can have a similar appearance to this group of disorders.

Fracture

Most displaced wrist fractures can be adequately assessed by plain film. Frontal and lateral views are routine projections, with radiographs obtained during radial and ulnar deviation helpful in the evaluation of the carpal bones. In addition to evaluation for carpal fracture, the orientation of the carpal rows and the intercarpal relationships is important in the assessment of carpal instability. Fractures of the scaphoid are most common, with classification and prognosis for healing or complications based on the location of the fracture line. Isolated fractures of the triquetrum (dorsal surface), lunate, and hamate are less common but also are seen.

MR plays a role in the evaluation of occult fractures. The most commonly suspected occult fracture of the wrist involves the scaphoid. In this clinical setting, advanced imaging is often required because scaphoid fractures are difficult to visualize on routine radiographs. In the past, CT, routine tomography, or more frequently, scintigraphy had been used to evaluate occult fractures, but even in cases with negative CT or tomographs, patients often were treated as if a true fracture were present, if the clinical suspicion was high enough. Treatment was withdrawn if follow-up radiographs remained negative.

More recently, MRI has become the test of choice to evaluate for the presence of a scaphoid fracture. In patients in whom scaphoid fractures are clinically suspected, MRI can clearly demonstrate the abnormality, which appears as a dark, linear fracture line on T_1-weighted images. It also has the advantage of showing other associated occult fractures, usually involving the triquetrum or distal radius. The MR protocol should include coronal T_1 and short inversion recovery (STIR) images. If the STIR images are negative, a fracture can be confidently excluded. Many patients with suspected scaphoid fractures have only soft tissue injuries, including collateral ligament tears, peripheral TFCC tears, radial TFCC avulsions, and SL or LT ligament tears.

Occult fractures may occur elsewhere in the wrist, but they are much less common and have infrequent complications. Triquetral fractures are the second most common carpal fracture, but they rarely require advanced imaging for diagnosis. The third most common carpal bone fracture involves the hamate. Hamate fractures usually occur either dorsally or involve the hook, with both areas often difficult to visualize radiographically. Thin-section axial CT images through this area may be required to diagnose a fracture. On MRI, hook of the hamate fractures are best evaluated on axial images, and they are clinically important because of the proximity to Guyon's canal and the possibility of ulnar nerve impingement. Even though lunate fractures are rare, AVN is a common complication (similar to the scaphoid). Some

cases of Kienbock disease likely result from this posttraumatic scenario. Occasionally, cysts in the lunate may mimic fractures.

Bone bruises are intimately related to occult fractures, and differentiating the two by MRI alone can be difficult. Bone bruises should be diffuse, have little articular or cortical extension, and show no obvious fracture line. In the wrist, however, occult fractures may be present with these findings alone. Bone bruises, although they may be symptomatic, heal spontaneously in 8 to 10 weeks without treatment and have no known sequelae. Occult fractures, on the other hand, are true fractures and may go on to nonunion and the other typical complications. It is our philosophy that in the hand and wrist, abnormalities seen on both T_1 and STIR (or fat-suppressed T_2 images) represent true fractures. Those injuries with abnormalities on STIR sequences only should be termed *bone bruises*.

Lunate fractures, proximal capitate fractures, and hook of hamate fractures may occur because of stress injuries. However, stress fractures are much less common in the upper extremity than the lower extremity. The differentiation of an acute traumatic fracture from a stress fracture is made on the basis of time. An acute traumatic fracture occurs at one specific episode of time, while a stress fracture has no discrete episode leading to it. In general, stress fractures are more common in the lower extremities, but they can occur in the wrist especially in active sports participants. Before a stress fracture occurs, there is the normal physiologic response of the bone to attempt to remodel (Wolff's Law). This remodeling might be visible on MRI as subtle areas of marrow edema. The stress response may be painful and can show uptake of moderate intensity on bone scintigraphy. The stress response can be thought of as a bone bruise, which can be a self-limited condition that heals spontaneously once the causative activity is stopped. If this activity continues, a fatigue-type stress fracture may result. This occurs in normal bones undergoing abnormal stresses. In older individuals, insufficiency-type fractures may occur when injury is due to normal stresses applied to abnormal underlying bone (usually as a result of osteoporosis).

Nonunion

Nonunion or delayed union occurs when a fracture does not heal within the first 6 months following the injury. *Delayed union* refers to complete healing occurring after a significant time interval, while healing never occurs in nonunion. Systemic diseases such as alcoholism, pancreatitis, cirrhosis, and malnutrition all contribute to delayed union. Nonunion is usually related to the type and location of the fracture and whether it was immobilized adequately or not. In particular, scaphoid fractures have a relatively high incidence of nonunion. Scaphoid nonunion may be fibrous, cartilaginous, or synovial (pseudoarthrosis).

A fibrous nonunion demonstrates low signal on T_1- and T_2-weighted images. Because this appearance is similar to the MR characteristics of some united fractures, only the presence of motion on physical examination can definitely define nonunion. Evaluation with thin section CT may be a helpful adjunct in evaluating for subtle bony bridging. Motion at a site of nonunion is indirectly visible on MRI as high T_2 signal about the fracture. This perifractural edema is either a sign of healing or abnormal motion, and distinguishing between the two can be difficult. In small bones, this edema is more likely secondary to pathologic motion. Cartilaginous nonunion shows intermediate T_1- and T_2-weighted signal and also can demonstrate motion/edema around the fracture line. If synovial fluid is present in the fracture line after 6 months, this represents a pseudoarthrosis or synovial nonunion. This is the only type of nonunion that is surgically treated. To diagnose a pseudoarthrosis on MR, the fluid at the fracture site should be differentiated from the perifractural edema of healing by using heavily T_2-weighted images. The granulation tissue of normal fracture healing will fade on these long TE (time to echo) images.

Masses

The most common mass in the wrist is a ganglion. Occasionally, these can extend intraosseously, typically into the lunate. Ganglia are often signs of an internal derangement and may be a cause of pain if occult. The second most common wrist mass is a lipoma, characteristically located in the thenar or hypothenar eminence. Within the hand, tendon sheath fibromas and giant cell tumors of the tendon sheath may occur. Distally, masses may occur in the tuft of the digits. These include glomus tumors, foreign body granulomas, paronychia, or felons.

Dorsal wrist pain

Dorsal wrist pain may be caused by pathology in the extensor tendon compartment, dorsal wrist capsule, or bony structures.

Bony structures. Evaluation of the bony structures begins with routine plain views. If the bone density is increased, advanced Kienbock disease is a possibility; otherwise, early avascular necrosis of the lunate must be ruled out. Bone scintigraphy is then performed and, in Kienbock disease, may show decreased uptake within the first 48 hours and 10 increased uptake as the bone repairs. Bone scintigraphy is nonspecific, however, and will demonstrate increased uptake wherever bone turnover is increased, such as in joints with synovitis. It also provides poor anatomic resolution and does not effectively distinguish between the joint space and the bone. MRI provides far greater resolution than bone scintigraphy in the evaluation of avascular necrosis. It also can reveal pathology of the bone vascularity earlier than any other imaging techniques (Fig. 9-29).

Dorsal capsule. Hypertrophy of the synovium of the dorsal capsule may be clinically indistinguishable from other causes of dorsal wrist pain, but MRI can provide a definitive diagnosis because of its excellent resolution of soft tissue structures (Fig. 9-30).

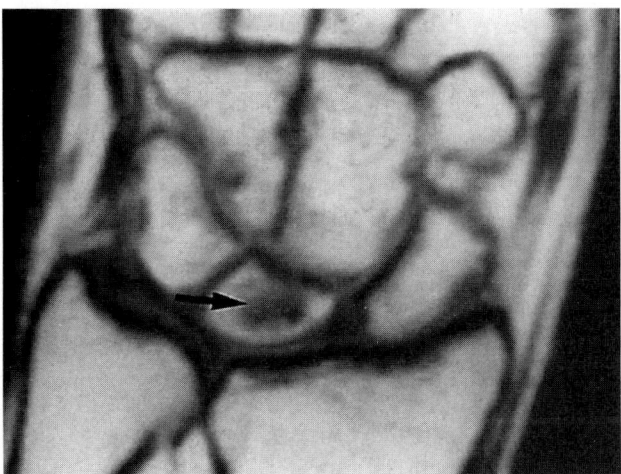

Fig. 9-29. Avascular necrosis of the lunate *(arrow).* Coronal magnetic resonance image shows a dark area in the marrow. The corresponding nuclear medicine scan is seen in Fig. 9-14.

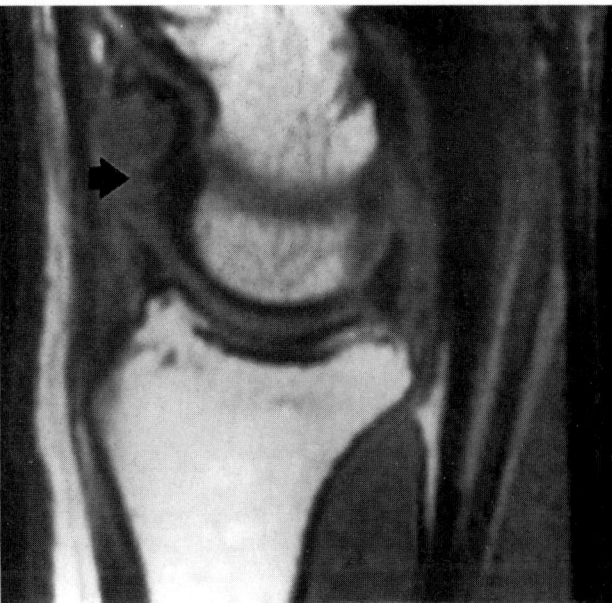

Fig. 9-30. This patient's dorsal wrist pain was caused by hypertrophy of the dorsal capsule *(arrow),* seen in this sagittal magnetic resonance imaging (MRI) scan. MRI is useful in distinguishing this condition from avascular necrosis of the lunate.

REFERENCES

1. Binkovitz LA, Berquist TH, McLeod RA: Masses of the hand and wrist: detection and characterization with MR imaging, *AJR Am J Roentgenol* 154:323, 1990.
2. Binkovitz LA, et al: Magnetic resonance imaging of the wrist: normal cross-sectional imaging and selected abnormal cases, *Radiographics* 8:1171, 1988.
3. Brondelt RP, et al: Wrist: coronal and transaxial CT scanning, *Radiology* 163:149, 1987.
4. Buckwalter KA, Swan JS, Braunstein EM: Evaluation of joint disease in the adult hand and wrist, *Hand Clin* 7:135, 1991.
5. Cone RO, et al: Computed tomography of the normal radioulnar joint, *Invest Radiol* 18:541, 1983.
6. Campbells CS: Gamekeeper's thumb, *J Bone Joint Surg* 37B:148, 1955.
7. Certolini E, et al: MR evaluation of triangular fibrocartilage complex tears in the wrist, *J Comput Assist Tomgr* 14:963, 1990.
8. Golimbu CN, et al: Tears of the TFCC of the wrist: MR imaging, *Radiology* 173:731, 1989.
9. Linn MR, Mann FA, Gilula LA: Imaging the symptomatic wrist, *Orthop Clin* 21:515, 1990.
10. Manaster BJ: Cortical efficacy of triple injection arthrography, *Radiology* 178:267, 1991.
11. Mann FA, Wilson AJ, Gilula LA: Radiographic evaluation of the wrist: what does the hand surgeon need to know? *Radiology* 184:15, 1992.
12. Meena HE: Radiologic study of endosteal, intracortical, and periosteal surfaces of the hand bones in metabolic bone disease, *Hand Clin* 7:37, 1991.
13. Mesgarzadeh M, et al: Carpal tunnel: MR imaging. Part I. Normal anatomy, *Radiology* 171:743, 1989.
14. Mesgarzadeh M, et al: Carpal tunnel: MR imaging. Part II. Carpal tunnel syndrome, *Radiology* 171:749, 1989.
15. Metz VM, Schratter M, Dock WI: Age associated changes of the triangular fibrocartilage: evaluation of the diagnostic performance of MR imaging, *Radiology* 184:217, 1992.
16. Mino DE, Palmer AK, Levinsohn EM: Role of radiography and computerized tomography in the diagnosis of the subluxation and dislocation of the distal radioulnar joint, *J Hand Surg* 8:23, 1983.
17. Nathan R, Schneider LH: Classification of distal radioulnar joint disorders, *Hand Clin* 7:239, 1991.
18. Perlik PC, Guilford WB: Magnetic resonance imaging to assess vascularity of scaphoid nonunion, *J Hand Surg* 16A:479, 1991.
19. Pin PG, et al: Role of radionuclide imaging in the evaluation of wrist pain, *J Hand Surg* 13A:810, 1988.
20. Protas JM, Jackson WR: Evaluating carpal instabilities with fluoroscopy, *AJR Am J Roentgenol* 135:137, 1980.
21. Reicher MA, Kellerhouse L: *Carpal instability in MRI of the wrist and hand,* New York, 1990, Raven Press.
22. Reinus WR, et al: Carpal avascular necrosis MR imaging, *Radiology* 160:689, 1986.
23. Russell RC, et al: Detection of foreign bodies in the hand, *J Hand Surg* 16A(1):2, 1991.
24. Schweitzer ME, et al: Chronic wrist pain: spin-echo and short tau inversion recovery MR imaging and conventional and MR arthrography, *Radiology* 182:205, 1992.
25. Sowa DT, et al: Application of magnetic resonance imaging to ischemic necrosis of the lunate, *J Hand Surg* 14A:1008, 1989.
26. Stewart NR, Gilula LA: CT of the wrist: a tailored approach, *Radiology* 183:13, 1992.
27. Swan JS, et al: Preoperative evaluation of giant cell tumors of the radius with MR angiography, *J Hand Surg* 18A:499, 1993.
28. Vogelzang RL: Arteriography of the hand and wrist, *Hand Clin* 7:63, 1991.
29. Wilson AJ, Gilula LA, Mann FA: Unidirectional joint communications in wrist arthrography: an evaluation of 250 cases, *AJR Am J Roentgenol* 157:105, 1991.
30. Zeiss J, Jakum C, Khimji T: Ulnar tunnel at the wrist (Guyon's canal): normal MR anatomy and variants, *AJR Am J Roentgenol* 158:1081, 1992.

Chapter 10

CLINICAL INTERPRETATION OF NERVE CONDUCTION STUDIES AND ELECTROMYOGRAPHY OF THE UPPER EXTREMITY

Glenn A. Mackin

Nerve conduction studies (NCS) and electromyography (EMG) rank second in importance only to careful history and neurologic examination for accurate and localizing diagnosis of nerve entrapments and disorders of the peripheral nervous system (PNS). Unlike batteries of clinical tests designed for specific nerve entrapments such as carpal tunnel syndrome (CTS),[8,20] well-designed NCS and EMG provide not only *objective,* localizing, prognostically important data about the suspected lesion but also indispensable PNS context about concurrent mononeuropathies, polyneuropathy, myopathy or other neuromuscular disorders. Neurophysiologists should provide prompt, understandable, "bottom line" answers that define PNS *lesion and context* in terms of the referral question. The optimal neurophysiologist is a physician, fellowship trained and board certified in electrodiagnostic medicine, adept in sophisticated examination and neuromuscular pattern recognition, and flexible enough to consistently perform studies tailored to each patient.[5] This chapter develops a practical framework for referring physicians and hand therapists to use for clinically correlating results and judging the quality of NCS and EMG reports.

Clinicians seek pragmatic answers that will help their patients. Is CTS or another entrapment present? How severe is it? What is the precise localization? Are there atypical features or concurrent disorders such as radiculopathy or polyneuropathy? Do the neurophysiologic findings explain the patient's symptoms and signs, or are they at least consistent with them? Do they indicate additional or unsuspected diagnoses, or reveal a need for radiologic or other testing? Do the study design and results support the final interpretation logically and scientifically? Numerous textbooks, reviews, and courses are available with background information on neurophysiologic theory and techniques. Patients are best served when referring clinicians and neurophysiologists communicate on the basis of mutually understood interpretative principles, including what NCS and EMG actually test, their limitations, and timing considerations that are crucial to meaningful conclusions. The purpose of this chapter is to elucidate that conceptual framework.

NERVE CONDUCTION STUDIES
General principles

NCS are generally more important in diagnosing nerve entrapments and injuries, but needle EMG is necessary to most studies for the complementary information it provides. Both tests measure electrical potentials generated by nerves and muscles. In sensory and motor NCS, a square-wave stimulus in milliamps (mA) is delivered, usually percutaneously, at test points along the nerve causing it to depolarize. The patient feels an instantaneous shock but not the wave of induced depolarization as it travels up and down the nerve. NCS measure voltage potential differences between two electrodes, the first recording over a nerve or muscle at an informative site away from the stimulation point, the second a "neutral" reference. Recording electrodes are arranged for

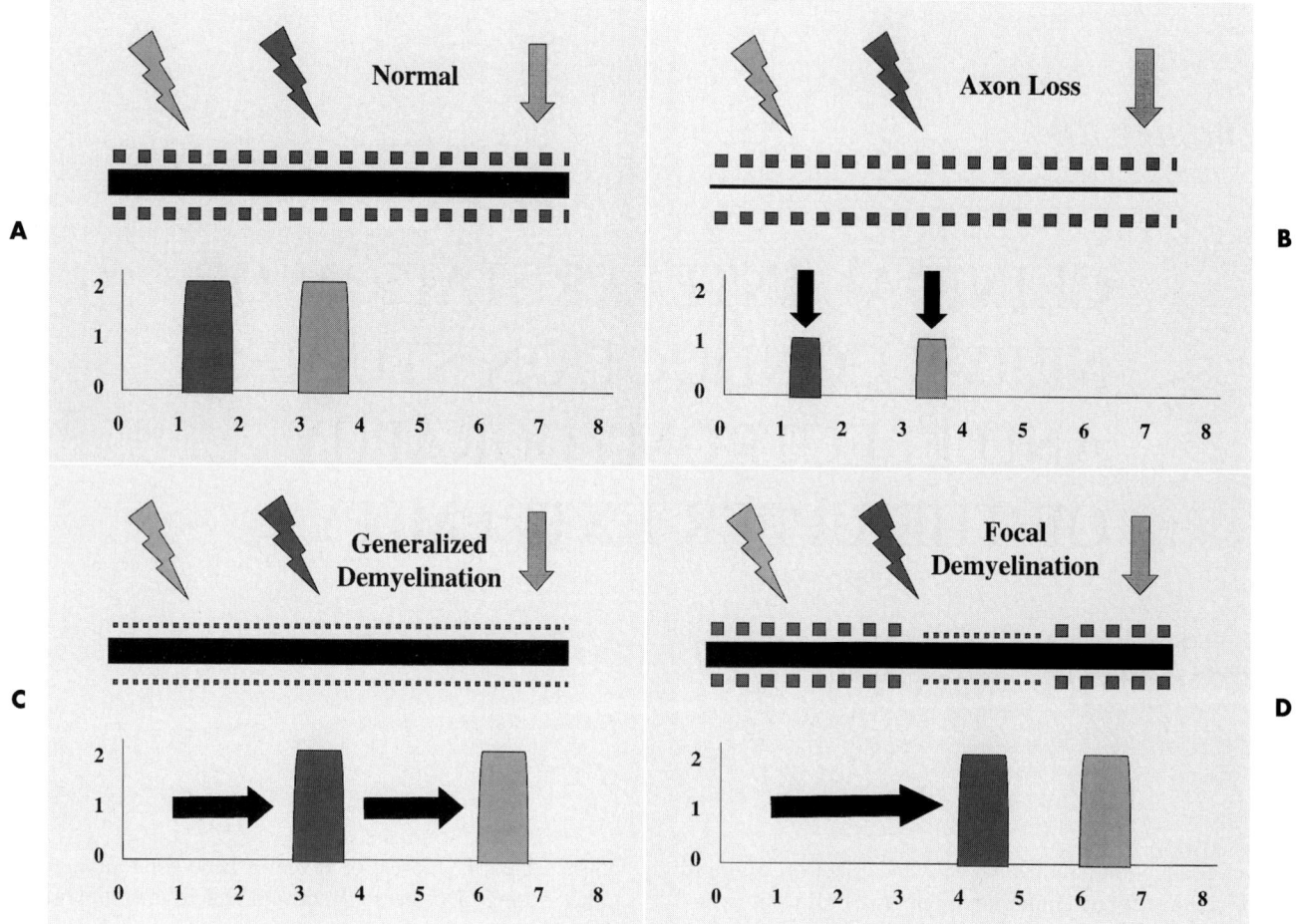

Fig. 10-1. Schematic peripheral nerves illustrate "nerve conduction study (NCS) templates" in text. In all nerves, the *black horizontal bar* reflects the proportion of large sensory or motor axons, and *blue dotted lines* reflect myelin on large sensory and motor fibers, available for testing. The *gray down arrow* indicates the recording electrodes placed distally over a named sensory nerve, or over the motor point and reference site for a motor NCS. The *blue "lightning bolt"* reflects the more distal point of stimulation along the nerve tested, and the *blue rectangle* reflects the recorded waveform amplitude, area, and morphology as a function of time. The *red "lightning bolt"* and *rectangle,* respectively, reflect the more proximal point of stimulation and recorded waveform. Arbitrary numbers on the *y*-axis for amplitude and *x*-axis for time of the recorded response are provided to facilitate visual comparison between normal and the different nerve injury patterns. **A,** Normal nerve. **B,** Axon loss (AL). **C,** Generalized demyelinating synchronous slowing (SS), as in Charcot-Marie Tooth polyneuropathy, Type 1. **D,** Focal, distal, demyelinating synchronous slowing (SS), as in carpal tunnel syndrome.

sensory NCS over the nerve, and for motor NCS mostly over compact superficial muscles. NCS parameters include *amplitude* (μV for sensory, mV for motor), *distal latency* (DL, in msec) from the most distal point of stimulation, and *conduction velocity* (CV, in m/sec) calculated in nerve segments demarcated by the selected stimulation points. Although caveats after nerve injury are discussed, as a rule of thumb, the *size* (amplitude or area) of the NCS response is proportional to the quantity of measurable axons, while the *speed* (CV, DL) may provide information about the integrity of myelin over the nerve segment tested.

Templates for interpretation of nerve conduction studies

The primary objectives of NCS are to localize the nerve lesion, characterize it as predominantly caused by axon loss (AL) or demyelination, determine severity and prognosis, facilitate surgical planning when appropriate,[2] and monitor the pace of nerve regeneration.[3]

In normal nerve, the DL, amplitudes, and segmental CV are normal (Fig. 10-1, *A*, and Plate 25, *A*). With loss of large sensory or motor axons (AL), the amplitude of proximal and distal responses are reduced and CV may be normal or

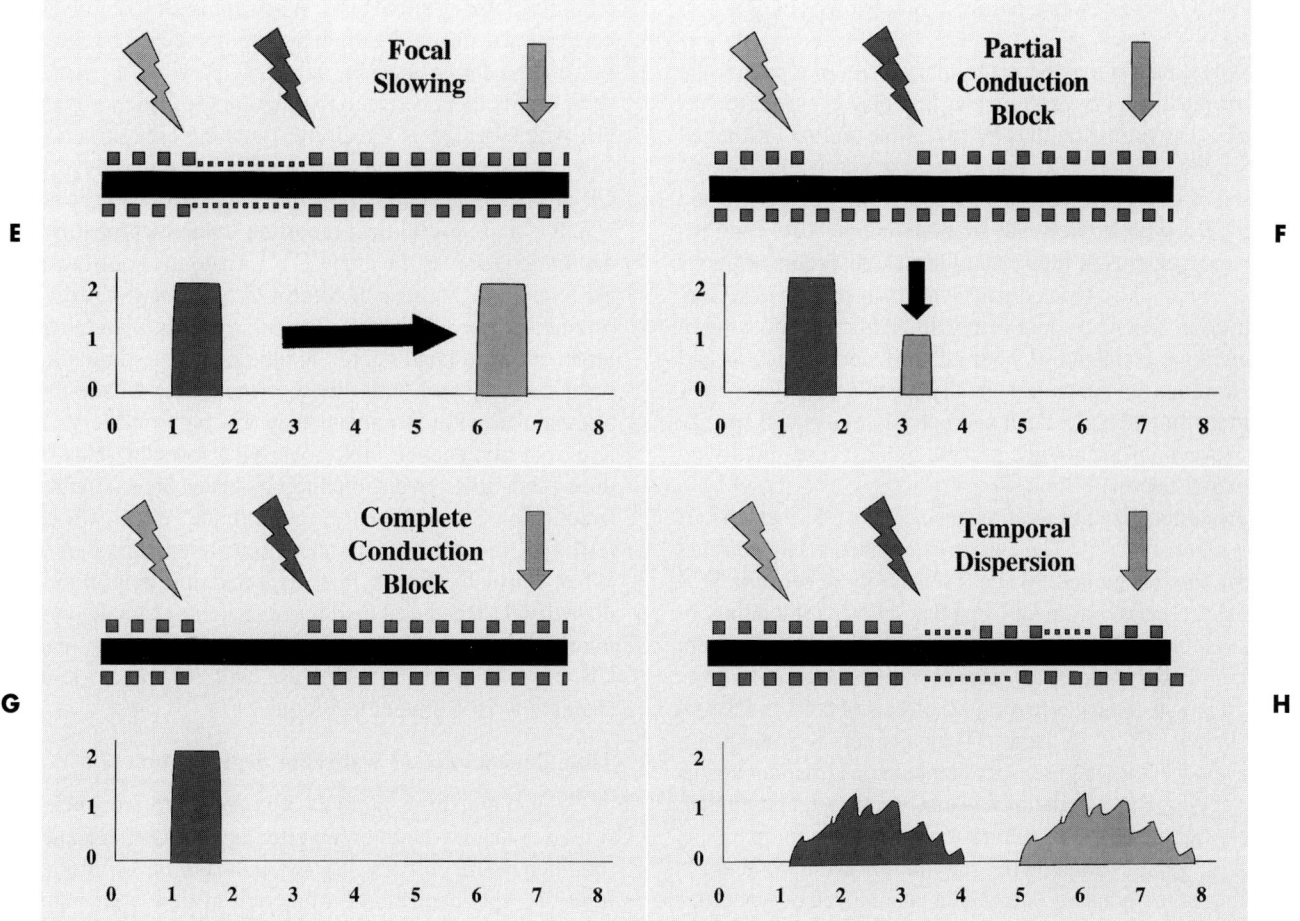

Fig. 10-1, cont'd E, Focal, proximal, demyelinating synchronous slowing (SS), as in ulnar neuropathy across the elbow. **F,** Focal, partial, demyelinating conduction block (CB), shown proximally as in ulnar neuropathy at elbow. **G,** Focal, complete, demyelinating CB, proximally. **H,** Temporal dispersion (TD), as in Guillain-Barré syndrome, chronic inflammatory demyelinating polyneuropathy, and some entrapments.

mildly slowed, although not more than 20% below the lower limit of normal (Fig. 10-1, *B,* and Plate 25, *B*). Clinical examples include focal mononeuropathies and most poly-neuropathies. Demyelinating patterns include significant *synchronous slowing* (SS) diffusely or focally (Fig. 10-1, *C* to *E,* and Plate 25, *C* to *E*); *conduction block* (CB) or "neurapraxia," which may be partial or complete (Fig. 10-1, *F* and *G,* and Plate 25, *F* and *G*), in which the proximally elicited response is smaller than distal; and *temporal disper-sion* (TD) in which proximal response has significantly lon-ger duration and an often irregular shape (Fig. 10-1, *H,* and Plate 25, *H*). Clinical examples of demyelination include SS across wrist in CTS and across elbow in ulnar neuropathy, CB at or near the elbow in some ulnar neuropathies and radial nerve compression at spiral groove, and TD in ac-quired demyelinating polyneuropathies such as Guillain-Barré syndrome (GBS) and chronic inflammatory demyelin-ating polyneuropathy (CIDP).[1,5,12]

Conduction slowing, demyelination, and remyelination

NCS patterns suggesting primary demyelination in-clude significant SS, TD, and CB that meet published criteria.[8] All are seen in acquired neuropathies, but only SS is seen in hereditary polyneuropathies such as the demy-elinating form of Charcot-Marie-Tooth disease. Primary demyelinating range slowing is not necessarily seen in a nerve segment with TD, unless SS also is present among the conducting fibers. As a rule of thumb, when amplitudes are normal or nearly so, slowing suggests primary demyelina-tion when DL (or long latency motor "F waves" to and from the spinal cord) is prolonged 30% above the upper limit of normal, or CV is reduced 30% or more below the lower limit of normal. CB and AL are more likely to correlate with symptoms than SS or TD, especially when motor axons are involved. SS and TD may be asymptomatic, although mild degrees of both may be seen with AL of large myelinated axons over long nerve segments. Muscles supplied by nerves showing TD are not weak, unless significant AL or CB is also present.

Demyelination may be the primary result of a pathologic process such as nerve entrapment that may progress to AL. Primary demyelination may be reversible and AL mitigated or avoided, if the focal entrapment is surgically decompressed or if an acquired generalized GBS or CIDP is treated effectively with appropriate immunotherapy. By contrast, other mechanisms of injury and intrinsic disorders of axons cause primary AL, which disrupts the axon-myelin interface, resulting in secondary loss of myelin. Although most nerve lesions have elements of both AL and demyelination and NCS findings are not pathologically specific as nerve biopsy, clinicians should expect that neurophysiologists will specify the *predominant* pathologic process in most cases involving disordered nerves.

Precise localization requires *focal SS or CB over a short nerve segment.*[15,16,19] The classic example is CTS, in which current practice guidelines stress sensitivity of sensory NCS over short nerve segments (median nerve stimulating in palm, recording proximal to wrist), and recent literature favors *internal comparison studies* between adjacent nerves over identical distances to mitigate effects of cold on DL and CV (below 32° C in hand). Typical internal comparison studies in CTS include sensory comparisons (median versus ulnar nerve palm to wrist or wrist to ring finger, and median versus radial wrist to thumb) and motor comparisons (median versus ulnar wrist to lumbrical-interosseus).[17] Slowing in many nerves suggests a generalized polyneuropathy, making it difficult to be sure that any focal slowing seen is sufficiently disproportionate to attribute to superimposed entrapment (e.g., CTS in diabetic polyneuropathy). Focal slowing may confirm demyelination (or fail to meet criteria) and may occur in a symptomatic or asymptomatic location (e.g., ulnar slowing across the elbow). Focal slowing demonstrable across multiple points of entrapment, common and uncommon, symptomatic or not, suggests autosomal-dominant "hereditary neuropathy with liability to pressure palsies" (HNPP), for which a gene test is available.

Conduction block is present when the amplitude and area of the wave obtained by stimulating proximal to the lesion is at least 20% less (ideally 50% less) than the wave obtained by stimulating distal to it, provided duration of the proximally elicited response does not exceed the distally elicited one by more than 15%. *Temporal dispersion* is present when the duration of the former exceeds the latter by more than 15%, irrespective of the amplitude change. Like the velocity criteria for demyelination, these rules apply only when amplitudes are near normal. Larger amplitude drops are required proximally when assessing CB in the presence of low distal amplitudes. Given that motor responses are orders of magnitude larger than sensory, it is technically easier to show CB in the former.

Reliable neurophysiologists rigorously exclude technical errors before diagnosing CB (and minimal abnormalities) to minimize false-positive tests. When apparent CB is observed between two standard stimulation points separated by a long nerve segment, it may be useful, if possible, to stimulate short segments in between to pinpoint the lesion. For example, with ulnar CB at the elbow, "inching" the stimulator in 1 to 2 cm steps along the nerve course may precisely localize CB at the humeroulnar aponeurosis or retrocondylar space, which is more useful than reporting "ulnar neuropathy with neurapraxia across the elbow."[6,11] Anatomic considerations are important because a Martin-Gruber anastomosis may resemble ulnar CB in the forearm, yielding a significantly larger ulnar-to-hand motor amplitude after stimulating at wrist as compared with elbow.[7] Attempting to stimulate a segment of nerve percutaneously too far from nerve itself (e.g., obesity, edema, bulky overlying muscles) may introduce technical errors including inadequate stimulation (mimicking CB) and the "virtual cathode" effect (CV errors resulting from uncertainty about actual depolarization site). When unusually distal CB is suspected, it is helpful to stimulate distal to the usual distalmost site. For example, without midpalmar sensory stimulation recording fingers, median CB 2 cm distal to wrist crease will resemble AL using standard wrist-to-finger technique.

Time dependence of wallerian degeneration

To distinguish AL and CB, it is crucial to recognize that wallerian degeneration (WD) after axonotmesis is an active, time-dependent process. The key indicator of AL after nerve injury is what happens as a function of time after injury to the wave amplitude elicited distal to the lesion as compared with the wave amplitude elicited proximal to it.

Immediately after nerve injury before WD has taken place, the distal amplitude is normal and the proximal is reduced or absent, reflecting conduction failure and resembling the CB pattern (see Fig. 10-1, *F* and *G*). If pure demyelinating CB is present, axon continuity is preserved through lesion and a CB pattern persists until remyelination occurs. If pure AL is present, the distal stump undergoes WD, the distal amplitude declines to approximate the low proximal amplitude, resulting in an AL pattern (see Fig. 10-1, *B*). Although the time course of WD is similar for motor and sensory axons, it takes 3 to 4 days to observe a decline in distal motor amplitudes after AL lesions versus 10 to 12 days in distal sensory amplitudes. The difference is explained by neuromuscular junctions (NMJs) in the motor unit between stimulated nerve and depolarizing muscle. Axonotmesis disrupts axonal trophic support of muscle mediated by the slow axon transport system, and NMJs fail before WD affects amplitudes. WD is a stump length–dependent process, seen sooner in lesions near muscle.

When NCS are performed immediately after nerve injury, they may make a unique contribution to the evaluation, if some conduction across the lesion is seen, proving *at least partial continuity* that is not clinically evident. Although an immediate NCS provides a baseline for future studies, it cannot define the status of *nonconducting* axons in lesion, whether caused by AL, CB, or both. In general, the amount serially determined amplitudes decline from baseline in an injured nerve is reasonably proportional to the amount of AL.

Sensory nerve conduction studies, injury, and regeneration

Sensory nerve action potential (SNAP) is a summation of normally synchronous waves of depolarization traveling in large sensory axons as they pass recording electrode. Large sensory axons carry electrical impulses to the spinal cord that the brain interprets as vibration, proprioception, two-point discrimination, touch, and complex cortical perceptions. Conventional sensory NCS do not record these encoded impulses, resulting perceptions, or depolarization of *small* axons (c-nociceptors). Nor does SNAP count the sensory axons. (Separate quantitative sensory tests [QST] are available to measure and follow vibratory thresholds in large axons and temperature perception and pain thresholds in small axons.)

Because peripheral axons are living structures supported by sensory neurons in dorsal root ganglia (DRG) located in or near spinal neural foramina, a recordable SNAP confirms the continuity of large DRG neurons with their peripheral processes. In the arms, the "peripheral" or *postganglionic* process of DRG cells traverses brachial plexus and peripheral nerves. The "central" or *postganglionic* process, which SNAP does not test, traverses spinal roots to enter the spinal cord. A reduced or absent SNAP amplitude indicates postganglionic AL at or distal to the DRG and is therefore not localizing. An absent SNAP means there has been total loss of large DRG cells (sensory neuronopathy) or peripheral processes (peripheral neuropathy). An abnormally low SNAP amplitude indicates a partial loss of large DRG cells or their peripheral processes, provided adequate (supramaximal) stimulation has been delivered. A normal SNAP amplitude indicates the presence of "enough" large sensory axons, defined by formal normative studies. A low-normal SNAP amplitude in a symptomatic dermatome or nerve distribution calls for side-to-side comparison because a twofold or greater asymmetry is abnormal.

SNAPs are fraught with potential technical and interpretive pitfalls. First, with side-to-side comparisons, both sides may be affected (e.g., CTS). Second, although SNAP amplitudes usually are more affected than motor after WD has occurred, testing in the 5- to 9-day window after postganglionic AL is confusing because the reduced CMAP but not SNAP amplitude falsely suggests a preganglionic lesion. Third, a postganglionic lesion (e.g., plexopathy) does not exclude a concurrent preganglionic lesion (e.g., radiculopathy), especially when the injury may involve both (e.g., traction injury to arm). Finally, when neurophysiologists approach nerve segments with undue clinical expectation of a specific lesion, they may uncritically accept a reduced or absent *sensory* response as confirmatory. Common examples include absent ulnar sensory response stimulating wrist recording from small finger in *suspected* ulnar neuropathy at elbow, and absent median sensory response stimulating wrist recording from middle finger in *suspected* CTS. The most circumspect interpretation of these isolated findings, respectively, is a partial AL lesion at or distal to the C8 and C7 DRGs in either brachial plexus or individual peripheral nerves. Particularly in the case of ulnar neuropathy, for which there are many potential sites of axonotmesis from axilla to palmar branch, the burden of localization shifts to *motor* NCS and EMG.

Clinicians approach sensory symptoms thinking of the cutaneous distributions of spinal roots (dermatomes) and peripheral nerves. To understand what SNAP actually tests, it is crucial to recognize that dermatomal symptoms can arise from preganglionic axons, postganglionic axons, or both. For example, there is clinical overlap of cutaneous numbness and tingling between C6 radiculopathies and upper trunk brachial plexopathies. With preganglionic C6 radiculopathies, postganglionic C6 axons are intact, so SNAPs are normal when recorded in the C6 dermatome, however numb the skin (e.g., median nerve recording thumb, or superficial radial nerve). With an upper trunk plexopathy, sensory symptoms on the radial forearm or thumb could correspond with SNAP amplitudes that are absent, reduced in absolute terms, low-normal but less than half contralaterally, or *normal* if symptoms arise from irritation of large C6 postganglionic processes without AL or selective injury to c-nociceptor axons in the C6 dermatome.

Sensory nerve injuries recover through remyelination (weeks to months) or regeneration of cut axons (1 inch/month or 1 to 2 mm/day). If sensory amplitudes are reduced, it means either that one cannot stimulate and record distal to the point of actual partial or CB or that the nerve is not there. As CB lesions remyelinate or large axons regenerate, SNAP amplitudes increase. However, sensory (and motor) axon sprouts may not reach their targets because of misdirection, scarring, neuroma formation, or regeneration failure.

Motor nerve conduction studies, injury, and regeneration

Interpretation of compound muscle action potentials (CMAP) uses similar principles and "templates" as for SNAPs, but several differences should be recognized.

Even though both test living peripheral nerve systems, the proximal anatomy of the "motor unit" differs from the large DRG and peripheral process sensory system. First, the different locations of lower motor neurons (LMNs) and sensory DRG neurons are electrodiagnostically important. LMNs (anterior horn cells) are located in the spinal cord ventral horn, *proximal to both spinal roots and sensory neurons* located in the DRG at or near the intervertebral foramina. SNAPs do not reflect sensory root disease in cervical radiculopathies. For both motor NCS and needle

EMG studies, the living "motor unit" tested neurophysiologically consists of LMNs, motor root and axons, NMJ, muscle membrane, and myofibers. Significant motor AL at the LMN or root level may be reflected in motor NCS results (see Fig. 10-1, *B,* and Plate 25, *B*) and abnormal EMG. Because muscles are supplied by more than one motor root, acute AL in a one motor root must be severe to reduce CMAP amplitudes recorded distally in the limb, although side-to-side CMAP comparisons may be informative. Second, given the rather different locations of anterior horn cell (AHC) and DRG, abnormalities in CMAP or EMG together with normal SNAP from the same spinal segment define a *preganglionic* lesion. Although neurophysiologic interpretations should pass the test of reasonableness, CMAP, EMG, and SNAP findings that align to suggest a preganglionic versus a postganglionic lesion should be taken quite seriously and not ignored when they do not fit the clinical expectation. When clinical and neurophysiologic localization appear to disagree, the neurophysiologist has a responsibility to consider the timing of the study relative to WD, additional testing (side-to-side, specialized, and serial), unexpected concurrent lesions, and neuromuscular diagnoses. Occasional patients with painless thenar atrophy referred for CTS are found to have clinically subtle widespread motor denervation consistent with motor neuron disease.

Although the rates of WD and axon regeneration are similar for sensory and motor axons, the distal anatomy of the "motor unit" and recording site for CMAP relative to it differ significantly from the sensory system as reflected in SNAP. First, unlike the SNAP, which amounts to a "snapshot" of a traveling wave of depolarization passing under the recording electrodes over a named nerve, the CMAP represents the potential difference between a recording electrode on a muscle's "motor point" and a reference electrode off the muscle. Although most reduced CMAPs recorded in patients with hand problems are caused by AL or demyelination related to focal mononeuropathies, it is important to recall that the motor unit reflected in CMAP tests more structures than individual nerves. Thus reduced or absent CMAP may reflect disorders of LMNs, roots (compressive and infiltrative), polyneuropathies, NMJ, muscle membranes, and muscles themselves. Second, reinnervation after motor AL may show increasing CMAP amplitudes and areas (but often different morphologies) by two distinct mechanisms. Unlike sensory reinnervation, which proceeds only by distal *regeneration* of cut nonbranching axons, motor reinnervation reflected in CMAP proceeds through distally branching motor axons by two mechanisms. After partial AL, motor axons in continuity with muscle may undergo *collateral sprouting* by 3 to 6 months to resupply isolated muscle fibers. Transected axons may *regenerate* at similar rates as sensory axons to grow back into muscle, provided they are not blocked or diverted from their target. Muscle fibers remain receptive to motor sprout ingrowth for a finite time, a year or possibly more, depending on age and

investigational treatments to prolong receptivity. Because the CMAP measures the end organ where the SNAP does not and because there are two mechanisms of motor reinnervation, a "normal" CMAP amplitude in the acute phase after injury and chronic phase after reinnervation has different implications regarding the rough quantity of axons supplying muscle. EMG is more informative on that point.[13]

ELECTROMYOGRAPHY

It is beyond the scope of this chapter to discuss the enormous value of EMG in neuromuscular diagnosis. In the evaluation of focal mononeuropathies, EMG plays an indispensable role by identifying unsuspected or concurrent PNS lesions, demonstrating partial motor continuity that might be clinically inapparent immediately after nerve injury, providing insight into the acuity of motor denervation and extent of chronic denervation, and the pace of motor regeneration to muscle. Well-designed and skillfully performed EMG studies provide such crucial information complementary to NCS data that test requisitions that to stipulate "NCS only" invites an incomplete evaluation in most instances.

In standard EMG, a sterile concentric or monopolar needle electrode is inserted into a muscle to record electrical activity on needle insertion, spontaneous activity in the resting muscle, and motor unit potentials (MUP) with voluntary contraction.

Insertional activity in the resting muscle on needle insertion is often overinterpreted but, when marked, reflects muscle membrane irritability a few days before spontaneous activity appears or an underlying disorder of membrane or muscle proper.

Spontaneous activity in the resting muscle includes *fibrillations and positive sharp waves,* which reflect "acute" AL in denervating disorders and muscle fragmentation or necrosis in myopathic disorders. Fibrillations and positive sharp waves are seen in neuropathic disorders when the EMG needle tip is near viable muscle fibers disconnected from axons and appears in an axon stump-length dependent pattern. In acutely denervated muscles with short stumps, such as cervical paraspinals after radiculopathies and nerve transactions near muscle, these discharges may appear within 7 to 10 days. In most evaluations, however, the muscle of interest is well distal to the site of injury, such as an ulnar innervated intrinsic hand muscle after acute AL at elbow. In such instances, fibrillations and positive sharp waves appear after WD has occurred and therefore require 3 to 4 weeks to appear. They persist until "silenced" by muscle reinnervation by either collateral sprouting or regeneration or muscle fibrosis when isolated too long from axon trophic support. Fasciculations are spontaneous discharges in resting muscle that reflect motor unit irritability anywhere from the LMN to muscle and may be seen in motor neuron diseases, radiculopathies, mononeuropathies, polyneuropathies, and myopathies.

Voluntary activity generates an "interference pattern" on the EMG screen and reflects ideally graded patient effort from minimal contraction to full. Analysis includes MUP amplitude, duration and morphology (generally larger and more polyphasic after reinnervation), and firing patterns. MUP recruitment analysis assesses the firing rates of individual MUPs relative to the number of MUPs firing. In normal muscle, no MUP should fire excessively fast, and as increasing graded force is required, more MUPs are recruited to fire. In denervating processes, recruitment is reduced and a reduced number of MUPs are seen firing at excessive rates. It is important to recognize that immediately after focal nerve injury, before WD has taken place and emergence of fibrillations and positive waves demonstrates the presence of some AL, recruitment is reduced in affected muscles whether the lesion includes AL, CB, or both. Neurophysiologists should provide a semiquantitative severity estimate for recruitment abnormalities because these, taken together with NCS abnormalities, assist in decision making for surgical repair.

"Positive" sensory symptoms and test sensitivity

Patients with nerve problems seek help for *negative* symptoms indicating a lack of sensory or motor function or *positive* symptoms indicating an excess or ectopic function. Negative sensory symptoms include numbness and perceived deadness, whereas positive sensory symptoms include tingling and burning. Negative motor symptoms include weakness, whereas positive motor symptoms include fasciculations and cramps. Negative sensory and motor symptoms from PNS correlate well with NCS and EMG abnormalities. Likewise, positive motor symptoms and signs often correlate with specific discharges on resting EMG and abnormalities on motor NCS or EMG during muscle contraction.

By contrast, positive sensory symptoms are elusive and sometimes frustrating for referring clinicians and neurophysiologists alike.[21] The SNAP correlate of *tingling* from large sensory axons may be a normal study, a nonlocalizing AL pattern, or localizing demyelinating SS, CB, or TD if recorded over a suspect short nerve segment. The SNAP correlate of *burning* from small sensory axons may be a normal study, unless there are relevant associated NCS abnormalities. The words "this study provides neurophysiologic *evidence* of" should precede lists of conclusions because, strictly speaking, a normal study does not "rule out" a PNS basis for positive sensory symptoms. It is crucial to recall the tradeoff between the sensitivity and specificity of diagnostic tests in general[9] and the sensitivity and specificity of electrophysiologic tests for particular entrapments. In CTS, 10% to 15% of patients with "classic" sensory symptoms have normal NCS, a state of affairs sometimes criticized as unacceptable "false-negatives." Some clinicians have responded by devising clinical test batteries for specific entrapments with sensitivities said to

rival NCS, although the definitions of "classic" and electrophysiologically abnormal are critical. Some neurophysiologists respond by performing multiple sensitive NCS tests to detect any abnormality whatsoever or emphasize borderline results. Such strategies risk unacceptably high false-positive rates, particularly for entrapments such as CTS and ulnar neuropathy for which NCS are very sensitive. (For entrapments such as superficial radial neuropathy for which NCS are less sensitive, appropriate caveats to guide the clinician should be made.)

The approach recommended herein recognizes the dearth of solid natural history studies of very mild clinical entrapments, the illusion of the perfectly sensitive and specific test,[18] and the strengths of properly performed electrophysiologic consultation (objectivity, context, prognosis). It is important that electrophysiologists remind referring clinicians that conventional sensory NCS do not test small sensory axons or DRG central processes that, when irritated, may underlie paresthesias from named nerves, myofascial structures, and/or sensory roots. However, normal results in suspected entrapments for which NCS are highly sensitive (e.g., CTS, ulnar) provide reassurance that significant AL is absent and conservative vigilance is justified.

CONCLUSION: QUALITY ASSURANCE AND PATIENT AND CLINICIAN SATISFACTION

Published neurophysiologic guidelines delineate professional, technical, and *ethical* standards for physicians providing electrodiagnostic consultation.[10] Although clinicians look first for responsive "bottom line" results on NCS and EMG reports and may lack the experience to evaluate study design, certain reliability markers should be readily apparent on the face of each report.

Hallmarks of *careful studies tailored to the patient* include occasional departures from routine to confirm borderline abnormalities, circumspect interpretation of minor abnormalities, routine adjectives that estimate severity of NCS[4] and EMG findings, "fit" between referral issues and anatomic scope of study, substantive clinical correlations, and interpretations that sometimes suggest alternative diagnoses based on independent study. *External indicators of technical quality on reports* include specification of the predominant pathologic process in neuropathic cases, reported NCS normal values and temperature measures, "internal comparison" studies, side-to-side NCS comparisons for borderline results (especially in brachial plexopathies), repetition and verification of difficult subtests, actual NCS waveforms included with the report, and patient satisfaction.

The importance of patient satisfaction with reassuring manner and thoroughness of the neurophysiologist cannot be overemphasized, given discomfort inherent in NCS and EMG and the necessity of patient cooperation and relaxation for optimal results. Optimal neurophysiologic consultation is a process that calls for excellent communication not only between patient and neurophysiologist during the study but also between neurophysiologist and referring clinician before and after the study.

REFERENCES

1. Aminoff MJ: *Electrodiagnosis in clinical neurology,* ed 3, New York, 1992, Churchill Livingstone.
2. Arle JE, Zager EL: Surgical treatment of common entrapment neuropathies of the upper extremities, *Muscle Nerve* 23:1160, 2000.
3. Berry H: Traumatic peripheral nerve lesions. In Brown WF, Bolton CF, editors: *Clinical electromyography,* ed 2, Boston, 1993, Butterworth-Heinemann.
4. Bland JDP: A neurophysiological grading scale for carpal tunnel syndrome, *Muscle Nerve* 23:1280, 2000.
5. Brown WF, Bolton CF, editors: *Clinical electromyography,* ed 2, Boston, 1993, Butterworth-Heinemann.
6. Campbell WW: The value of inching techniques in the diagnosis of focal nerve lesions: inching is a useful technique, *Muscle Nerve* 21:1554, 1998.
7. Campbell WW, et al: Variations in anatomy of the ulnar nerve at the cubital tunnel: pitfalls in the diagnosis of ulnar neuropathy at the elbow, *Muscle Nerve* 14:733, 1991.
8. Consensus Criteria for the Diagnosis of Partial Conduction Block, AAEM guidelines in electrodiagnostic medicine, *Muscle Nerve* 22(suppl 8):S225, 1999.
9. Eisen A, et al: Receiver operating characteristic curve analysis in the prediction of carpal tunnel syndrome: a model for reporting electrophysiologic data, *Muscle Nerve* 16:787, 1993.
10. The Electrodiagnostic Medicine Consultation, AAEM guidelines in electrodiagnostic medicine, *Muscle Nerve* 22(suppl 8):S73 1999.
11. Kimura J: *Electrodiagnosis in diseases of nerve and muscle: principles and practice,* ed 2, Philadelphia, 1989, FA Davis.
12. Kincaid JC: AAEE Minimonograph #31: the electrodiagnosis of ulnar neuropathy at the elbow, *Muscle Nerve* 11:1005, 1988.
13. Mackin GA: Electrophysiologic testing of injured and regenerating nerves. In Hunter JM, Schneider LH, Mackin EJ, editors: *Tendon and nerve surgery in the hand: a third decade,* St Louis, 1997, Mosby.
14. Massy-Westrop N, Grimmer K, Bain G: A systematic review of the clinical diagnostic tests for carpal tunnel syndrome, *J Hand Surg* 25A:120, 2000.
15. Practice Parameter for Electrodiagnostic Studies in Carpal Tunnel Syndrome, AAEM guidelines in electrodiagnostic medicine, *Muscle Nerve* 22(suppl 8):S139, 1999.
16. Practice Parameter for Electrodiagnostic Studies in Ulnar Neuropathy at the Elbow, AAEM guidelines in electrodiagnostic medicine, *Muscle Nerve* 22(suppl 8):S169, 1999.
17. Preston DC, Logigian EL: Lumbrical and interossei recording in carpal tunnel syndrome, *Muscle Nerve* 15:1253, 1992.
18. Rosenbaum R: Editorial: Carpal tunnel syndrome and the myth of El Dorado, *Muscle Nerve* 22:1165, 1999.
19. Stevens JC: AAEM Minimonograph # 26: the electrodiagnosis of carpal tunnel syndrome, *Muscle Nerve* 20:1377, 1997.
20. Szabo RM, et al: The value of diagnostic testing in carpal tunnel syndrome, *J Hand Surg* 24A:704, 1999.
21. You H, et al: Relationships between clinical symptom severity scales and nerve conduction measures in carpal tunnel syndrome, *Muscle Nerve* 22:497, 1999.

Chapter 11

RANGE-OF-MOTION MEASUREMENT OF THE HAND

Catherine A. Cambridge-Keeling

Rarely, if ever, is assessment of hand function discussed without some reference to the range of motion (ROM) of the involved extremity. According to Cantrell and Fisher, "A considerable bulk of the medical, rheumatological and surgical literature on the hands has concentrated on ROM of the fingers as a primary source of data on the success or failure of many of our forms of treatment."[9] In each edition of *Rehabilitation of the Hand: Surgery and Therapy,* chapters on evaluation have included ROM as an essential component.[2,3,12,32] Swanson[31] and Swanson et al.[32] relied significantly on limitation of motion in assessing impairment of the hand. The American Society of Hand Therapists' *Clinical Assessment Recommendations* gave ROM prominence.[10,13] Likewise, the American Society for Surgery of the Hand's, *The Hand: Examination and Diagnosis* gives considerable emphasis to joint motion measurements.[18] This is because many clinicians consider ROM to be a measurable definable entity. Norms for joint motion have been recorded in *Joint Motion: Method of Measuring and Recording,* allowing the examiner to compare readily the involved joint with the patient's own uninvolved contralateral joint or established values.[24]

Is ROM really reliable as an assessment tool? Does it meet the criteria of being objective, measurable, and unbiased? Is the use of a goniometer necessary, or are estimated motion measurements as reliable? If a motion-measuring device is used, what is the most objective type? Is it a standard manual goniometer based on a protractor with one fixed arm and one movable arm, an inclinometer, which measures the absolute orientation of a line in a vertical plane, or one of the many electrogoniometers being produced for specific computer systems or research projects? Are the measurements taken by the various types of commercially available and custom-made devices interchangeable? In addition, does dorsal or lateral positioning change the measurement? Many such questions arise when health professionals who evaluate and treat patients with hand injuries discuss the role of ROM. One must answer these questions to determine the role of ROM in the battery of assessment tools available to help evaluate the injured hand. The goal of this chapter is to address some of the questions about ROM and discuss some of the more common methods used to determine ROM in the hand and wrist.

REVIEW OF THE LITERATURE
Range of motion—examiner estimation versus use of a goniometer

Little information can be found in the literature comparing the accuracy of joint motion measured with and without a goniometer. In *Joint Motion: Method of Measuring and Recording,* the use of a goniometer is left to the surgeon's discretion.[24] In a study by Low,[26] 50 examiners were asked to estimate the angle of first the author's left elbow in full flexion and then his wrist in full extension. They then measured the angles with a standard goniometer. No instruction was given to the examiners regarding methodology. The mean error in estimating elbow flexion was 9.3 degrees, compared with a 5-degree mean error in measured flexion. The mean estimated error for wrist extension was 12.8 degrees, with the measured mean error being 7.8 degrees.[26] The author did not note the statistical significance of the greater error when estimated values were compared with measured values. He did conclude that a goniometer was more reliable than estimated motion values. A study by Watkins et al.[33] comparing visual estimates of passive knee ROM indicated greater intratester error for visual estimation compared with goniometer measurements, but the reliability was greater than expected by the researchers. No statistical analysis was completed to determine the level of significance of the variances. Further research is needed before any firm conclusions can be reached, but the indication from this starting point is that reliability is improved by use of a goniometer.

What is the reliability of ROM measurements made with a standard goniometer? An early study by Hellebrandt et al.[19] found that a skilled observer varied 3 degrees or less in 70% of his or her measurements and 7 degrees or less in 95% of measurements when 780 paired observations were compared. The eight physical therapist subjects used were found to be within 7 degrees or less of their first measurements in duplicate trials in 62% to 72% of their observations. Statistical comparisons showed the average therapist to be reliable in duplicating measurements made by a highly skilled observer.[19] Hamilton and Lachenbruch[17] also found a statistically significant level of reliability among investigators measuring the joint motion of the metacarpophalangeal (MP), the proximal interphalangeal (PIP), and distal interphalangeal (DIP) joints of the hand. Boone et al.[4] compared four testers' measurements taken at the shoulder, elbow, wrist, hip, knee, and foot. They found reliability was greater for the three upper extremity measurements than for the lower extremity measurements. Their upper extremity–motions intratester reliability compared favorably with the earlier work by Hellebrandt et al.[19]

Significance of goniometric placement and design

Hamilton and Lachenbruch[17] investigated three types of goniometers: a 180-degree finger goniometer for dorsal placement, a 360-degree universal goniometer for lateral placement, and a pendulum type of goniometer that is placed dorsally on the digit. Statistical analysis indicated equal reliability among all three goniometers. The authors discussed factors such as edema and deformity that would influence the choice of instrument and may make one type more reliable than another given such complications.[17] Armstrong et al.[1] used a universal goniometer and an NK computerized goniometer to measure the flexion and extension of the elbow. They found that the intrarater reliability for the same instrument was high but that the two instruments gave significantly differing results. Marshall et al.[27] also found poor concurrent validity in the ROM measurements taken with a manual goniometer compared with the electrogoniometer they used. The findings of poor interchangeability between the manual and computerized goniometers in the Armstrong and Marshall studies were not consistent with the results of work presented by Brown et al.[1,8,27] Their research on the validity and reliability of the Dexter Hand Evaluation found concurrent validity when measuring the Dexter goniometer against the standard finger goniometer, as well as high intrarater and interrater reliability.[8] The different results found in these three studies point out the danger in comparing measurements made by different instruments that have not been studied for concur-

rent validity. As new joint measuring devices become available, they should not be considered interchangeable until proven to be so.

Lateral and dorsal goniometer placement at the elbow was studied by Grohmann[16] using a noninjured elbow that was positioned in a stabilizing device. No statistical difference was found in the measurements made by either lateral or dorsal placement of the goniometer.[16,17] However, LaStayo and Wheeler[25] concluded that the results of ulnar, radial, and volar/dorsal placement of the goniometer when measuring passive range of motion (PROM) of the wrist were statistically different from each other. Therefore consistency of measurement technique is necessary. Also, of the three techniques, the volar/dorsal placement gave the greatest intertester and intratester reliability. Until further research examines the other joints of the upper extremity, choice of lateral or dorsal placement should be based on the experience of the tester and considerations of the injury, such as edema, dressings, and deformity.

Intratester error compared with intertester error

The studies surveyed for this chapter were in agreement that the margin of error was greater when more than one tester measured the ROM on the same patient.* Specialty experience with hands or a definite protocol to follow improved intertester reliability.[1,20] In the Horger study,[20] in which no set protocol was followed, interrater reliability was considered excellent among specialized therapists (employed in hand clinics) compared with nonspeciality therapists when wrist motions were measured. In the Armstrong study in which both experienced hand therapists and inexperienced therapists used a standard goniometer and an NK computerized goniometer following a set protocol, the intratester reliability was high for both instruments. The authors postulated that the similarities of the intratester variations between therapists resulted from the uniformity of the methods used to measure the joint motion.[1] LaStayo and Wheeler[25] concluded that when the three techniques they studied for measuring wrist motion were used interchangeably, the results were not consistent. They stated not only were the motion results more reliable when the same technique was used but also the volar/dorsal technique was the most reliable of the techniques studied.[25]

Active, active-assisted, and passive range-of-motion measurements

The motion that is recorded at a joint may be active, active-assisted, or passive (Box 11-1). According to Hurt,[22] "There are two primary purposes in measuring joint motion: to determine the degree of joint motion which can be accomplished by the active contraction of the governing muscle, and to determine the freedom existing at a joint by

*References 1, 4, 17, 25, 26, and 33.

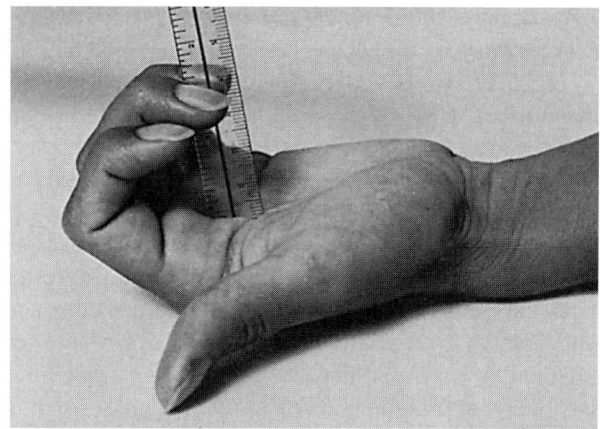

Fig. 11-1. Measuring from pulp of distal phalanx to distal palmar crease gives an easily understood value indicating the limitation of total finger flexion.

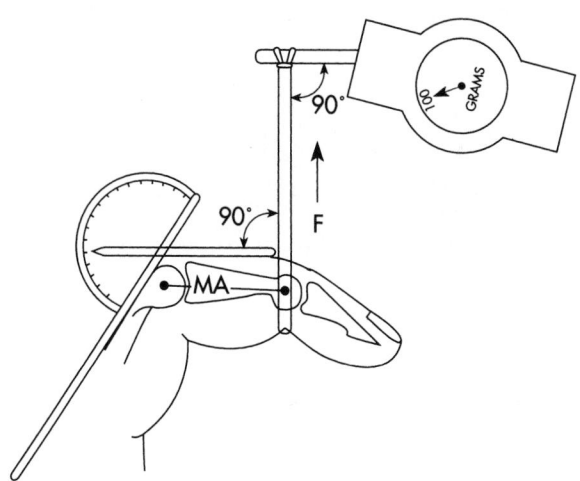

Fig. 11-2. Torque is applied to extend the proximal interphalangeal joint at right angles in the middle segment of the finger. Torque 5 force 3 moment arm. (Moment arm 5 perpendicular distance from the joint axis.) (From Breger-Lee D, Bell-Krotoski J, Brandsma JW: *J Hand Ther* 3:7, 1990.)

measuring the range through which it can be moved when all the muscles are relaxed.'' Unless active motion is contraindicated, the patient is first instructed in active motion to determine available range when the joint is powered by its own musculature.[22] When the patient has full active joint excursion, passive motion values need not be taken, because a joint that has full active range also will have full passive range. However, if the patient cannot actively move through the full range, active-assisted and/or passive motion measurements become necessary to gain an accurate picture of a joint's movement.[5,22,29] Active-assisted motion allows for stabilization of a segment to improve the mechanical advantage of the muscles that move the joint being measured. An example given by Brand[5] is the stabilization of the MP joint in extension to give greater mechanical advantage to the interphalangeal (IP) joint flexors at the more distal joints.

Accurate measurement of active and active-assisted ROM depends on patient compliance and the tester's skill. PROM measurements might be considered more objective because patient compliance is no longer a factor,[5] but according to Goodwin,[15] "Sufficient evidence is available to suggest that PROM is more difficult to measure reliably than active." Multiple authors have noted the difficulty in controlling, quantifying, and reproducing the force applied to a joint when measuring PROM.[5-7,17]

Total active motion, total passive motion, and fingertip to distal palmar crease measurements

Total active motion (TAM) or total passive motion (TPM) values and composite finger flexion to distal palmar crease (DPC) measurements allow one number to represent the total motion capacity for a single finger (see Box 11-1). Total active and passive motion sums facilitate statistical analysis of ROM progression or regression for an entire finger because only one numerical value per finger is involved. A single number may be helpful in plotting generalized trends of change in a finger's motion but is not specific to any particular joint.[10]

The difference between TAM and TPM is in the force causing the movement. Because the fisted position is used to measure both total active and total passive range of

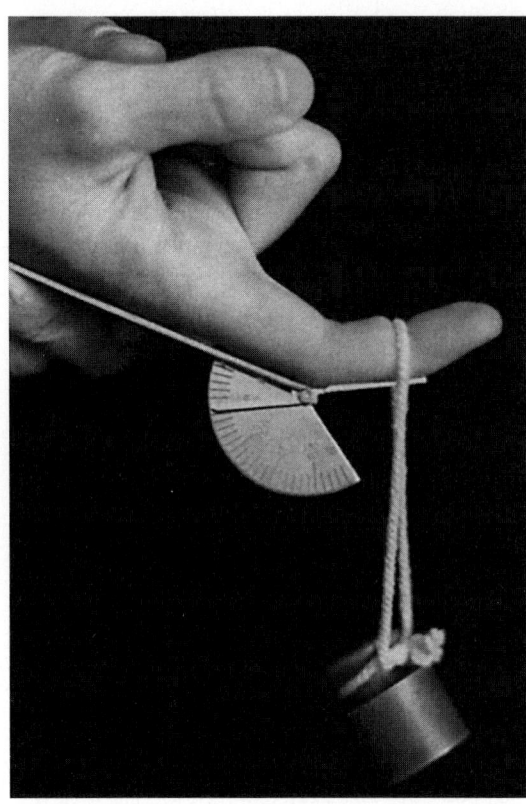

Fig. 11-3. A simple way to obtain a torque-angle measurement is to position a hand so that a hanging weight of, for example, 250 g, is pulling at right angles to a segment of a finger and at a finger crease. Alternatively, the weight may hang over a pulley wheel so that the string is horizontal and the hand is more easily positioned. (From Brand P, Hollister A, editors: *Clinical mechanics of the hand,* ed 2, St Louis, 1993, Mosby.)

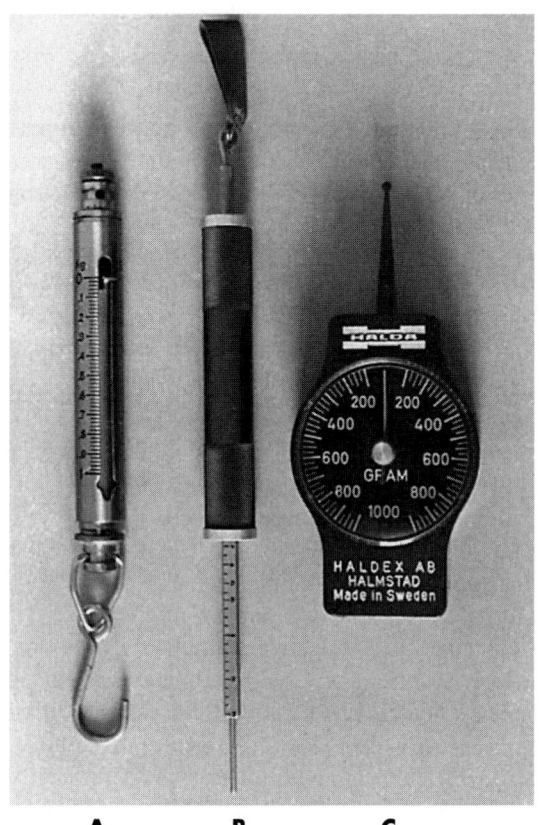

Fig. 11-4. We have used many different devices for applying torque to joints. **A,** A simple spring scale, from a hardware store, used by sport fishermen for weighing their catch. It is calibrated in grams to 1 kg. **B,** A push-pull device to which, at one end *(top),* a sling may be attached for measuring pull while a pencil eraser (not shown) is used to cap the other end so that the narrow metal end (used sometimes a dolorimeter) does not cause harm when used to push a digit into flexion. **C,** A Haldex lever device in which the dial records the force needed at the end of the lever to displace it. We attach a string sling to the end and pull at right angles to the lever. We also use the end of the lever to push. In either case, the reading of the dial is recorded. (**B** and **C** available from Fred Sammons, Inc., Box 32, Brookfield, Ill; from Brand P, Hollister A, editors: *Clinical mechanics of the hand,* ed 2, St Louis, 1993, Mosby.)

motion, a total (active or passive) motion measurement may not correlate with the sum of individual joint motion measurements.

Another useful measurement technique records the distance from the finger pulp to the DPC when the patient attempts to make a fist.[13] This measurement gives an approximation of the total digital motion in flexion and is more comprehensible to many patients than motion measured in degrees. Centimeters or inches can be used to record the distance, with zero indicating full flexion to the DPC (Fig. 11-1).

Torque-angle range of motion

As mentioned in the section on PROM, the difficulty in measuring the force applied during the measurement of PROM makes the reliability of sequential PROM measurements questionable. Torque-angle range of motion (TROM) uses a constant measured force to passively move a joint through its PROM. TROM has been advocated by Brand as a clinically feasible method of objectively measuring PROM.[5] Brand's methods have been used by several

authors[6,7,14] and may improve the reliability of ROM measurements.[7]

Both Brand[5] and Breger-Lee et al.[6] describe the torque-angle measurement in a clinical setting using a Haldex gauge to measure the force applied (Fig. 11-2). Brand also describes using a known weight (Fig. 11-3), a spring scale, or a push-pull device calibrated in grams up to 1 kg (Fig. 11-4) to measure force. In a preliminary study, Breger-Lee et al.[7] questioned whether TROM would produce a more reliable measurement of passive motion. They used forces of 200 g, 400 g, 600 g, and 800 g to measure ROM of a small number of PIP and DIP joints. The researchers noted higher and more consistent correlations as force levels were increased, especially at the 800-g level.

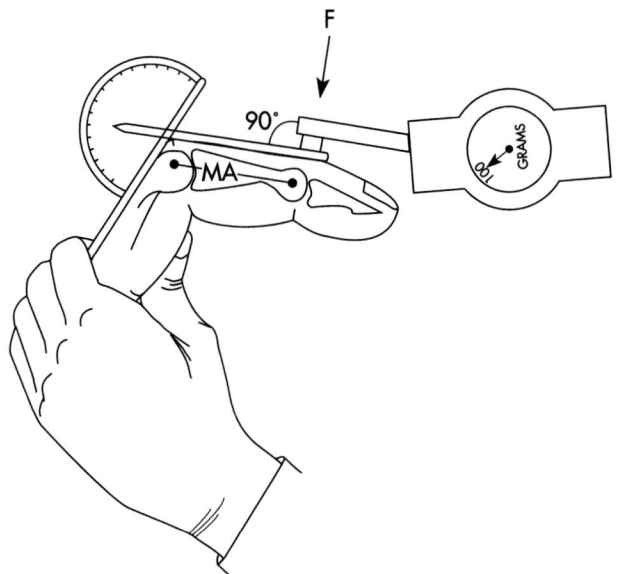

Fig. 11-5. To apply flexion force, a pusher such as the eraser end of a pencil or a small, narrow, flat piece of foam may be attached to the tip of the lever arm of the measurement gauge. The force applied must be perpendicular to the moment arm, applied to the dorsum of the phalanx opposite the joint crease. (From Breger-Lee D, Bell-Krotoski J, Brandsma JW: *J Hand Ther* 3:7, 1990.)

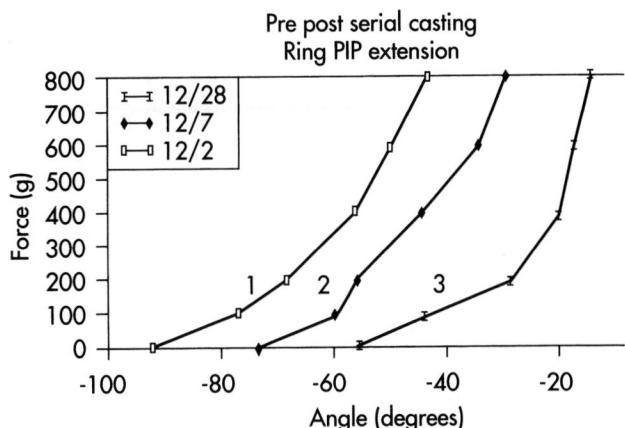

Fig. 11-7. Case example of a patient who underwent plaster of paris casting to the proximal interphalangeal *(PIP)* of the ring finger. This represents torque-angle range of motion (TROM) of PIP extension. From left to right, *1,* the curve created before casting was initiated to increase PIP extension. The gentle slope indicates that the joint has some mobility. *2,* TROM 1 week after casting to ring finger. Improvement is noted, with a slope indicating more casting may be beneficial. *3,* TROM after 3 weeks of casting. Note that the steep curve indicates a plateau is reached in ability to remodel the joint. If the curve continues to be steep in the next week, we would consider discontinuing the casting. (From Breger-Lee D, Bell-Krotoski J, Brandsma JW: *J Hand Ther* 3:7, 1990.)

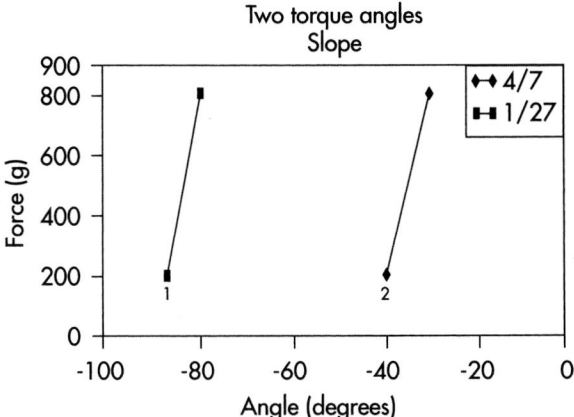

Fig. 11-6. A slope created by two torque angles is depicted with applied loads of 200 g and 800 g of force (tension), *1,* before, and, *2,* after casting. From left to right, note the improved ROM of the patient's PIP extension gained from serial PIP casting:

   1/27/88 200 g, 293 degrees; 800 g, 280 degrees
   4/7/88 200 g, 243 degrees; 800 g, 234 degrees

(From Breger-Lee D, Bell-Krotoski J, Brandsma JW: *J Hand Ther* 3:7, 1990.)

The study also found that intrarater reliability was higher than interrater reliability, a finding common with many standard goniometric studies.[7]

The technique described by Brand[5] and Breger-Lee et al.[6] for measuring TROM requires a finger goniometer, a Haldex orthotic-pinch gauge, a thick loop of string, and an eraser end of a pencil. The finger goniometer is placed dorsally over the joint to be measured, and the Haldex gauge with the loop for measuring extension force is placed at the flexion crease of the joint distal to the joint being measured (see Fig. 11-2). The torque must remain constant for subsequent trials to be comparable. For the torque to remain constant, the force (as measured by the Haldex gauge) and the moment arm (the perpendicular distance from the joint axis to the applied force) must remain constant. Torque = force × moment arm. As the force is being applied in a dorsal direction, the TROM is into extension. An anatomic landmark such as a flexor or extensor crease can be used to keep the moment arm constant. For TROM flexion measurement, a pushing force such as a pencil eraser attached to the end of the Haldex gauge is suggested (Fig. 11-5).[6]

TROM for the same joint can be demonstrated on a graph representing the changing motion at a given joint with increasing torque.[5,7,14] If only two different loads are used, a slope is created (Fig. 11-6). If more than two torque angles are plotted using three or more loads with a constant moment arm, a TROM curve can be plotted. Brand[5] and others note that the slope of the torque angle curve gives information regarding the potential for joint motion improvement with appropriate therapy intervention. The gentler the angle of the slope, the greater the potential for improvement (Fig. 11-7).

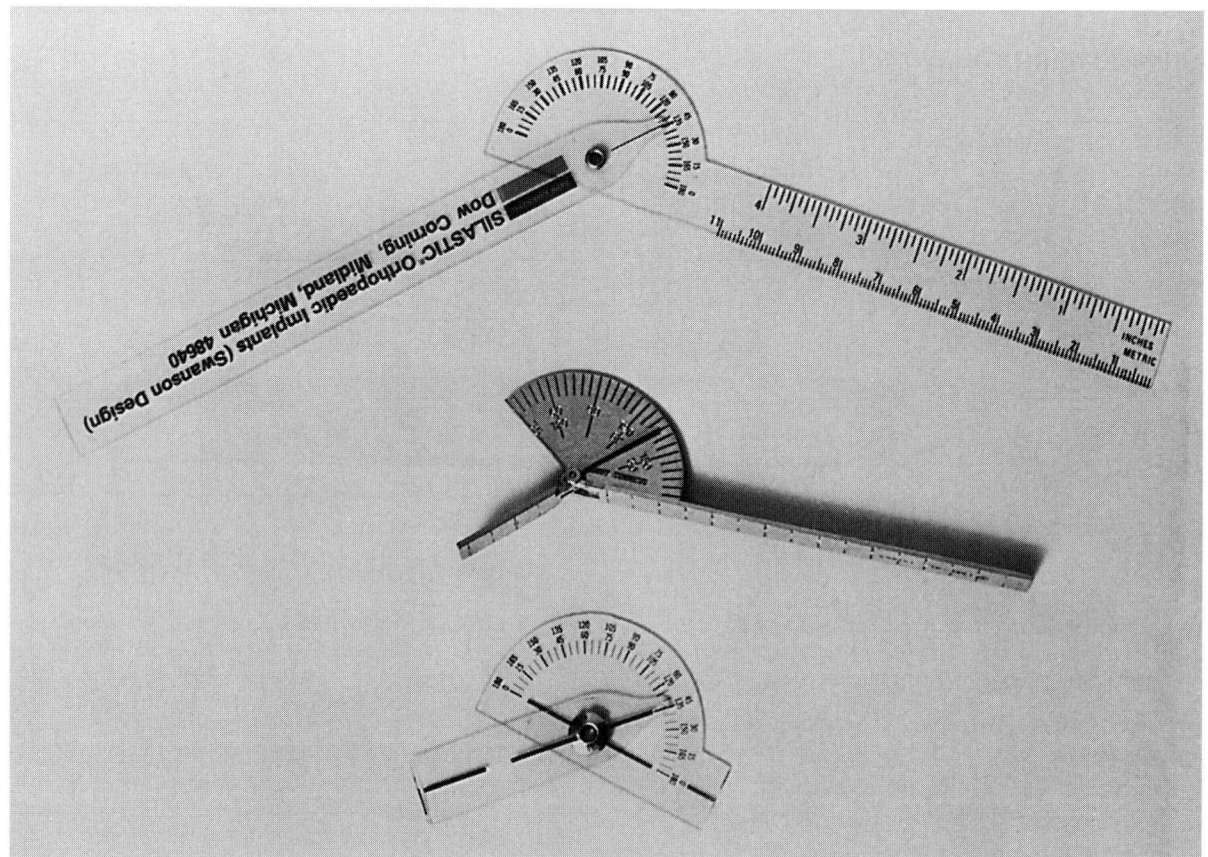

Fig. 11-8. Goniometer size and design should be appropriate for size of joint being measured and the technique being used.

Sequential plotting of TROM curves or TROM slopes over multiple treatment sessions will indicate improvement or lack thereof in therapy.[5-7,14]

TECHNIQUES FOR MEASURING RANGE OF MOTION OF WRIST AND HAND USING A GONIOMETER
General considerations for all joints

The patient should be as comfortable as possible without sacrificing joint positioning or musculotendinous dynamics. To facilitate cooperation, the patient must have clear understanding of the motion he or she is to perform during AROM. The patient also should know that the movement is to take place only in the assigned joints so as to avoid substitution motions.[21,28] During PROM, the patient should be as relaxed as possible, avoiding the problem of tensing muscles around the joint being measured. The force exerted on a joint during passive motion should be minimal and consistent from one test to another. Swanson[32] suggests that a force of 0.5 kg applied to the middle of the adjacent distal phalanx is adequate for evaluation of passive motion. Brand[5] and others[6,7] suggest TROM as previously described.

Goniometer size and placement. Goniometers are manufactured in a variety of forms and sizes. The size of the goniometer should be appropriate for the joint being measured. The wrist and forearm motions are adequately measured with a standard 14.5-cm-length arm.[11] The finger joints are more easily measured by use of a commercially available finger goniometer made for dorsal alignment or by shortening the arms of a small goniometer. Such an adapted goniometer is suitable for lateral or dorsal measurements of the finger joints (Fig. 11-8).

When a lateral measurement is being made, the goniometer must be placed so that the arms are parallel to the long axis of the adjacent bones forming the joint. The fulcrum should be as close to the axis of motion of the joint as possible[11,22] (Fig. 11-9). When a goniometer is placed dorsally on a digit, the fulcrum should be centered over the joint, with the arm lying dorsally along the long axis of the adjacent bones (Fig. 11-10).

In the case of a multiarticular joint complex such as the wrist, an anatomic landmark often is used for an approximate axis of motion. In the wrist, the styloid process of the radius laterally (Fig. 11-11) and the capitate dorsally and volarly are such landmarks (Fig. 11-12).

Goodwins's study,[15] discussed earlier, suggests that the interchangeable use of different types of goniometers in a clinical setting is inadvisable. As more types of goniometers

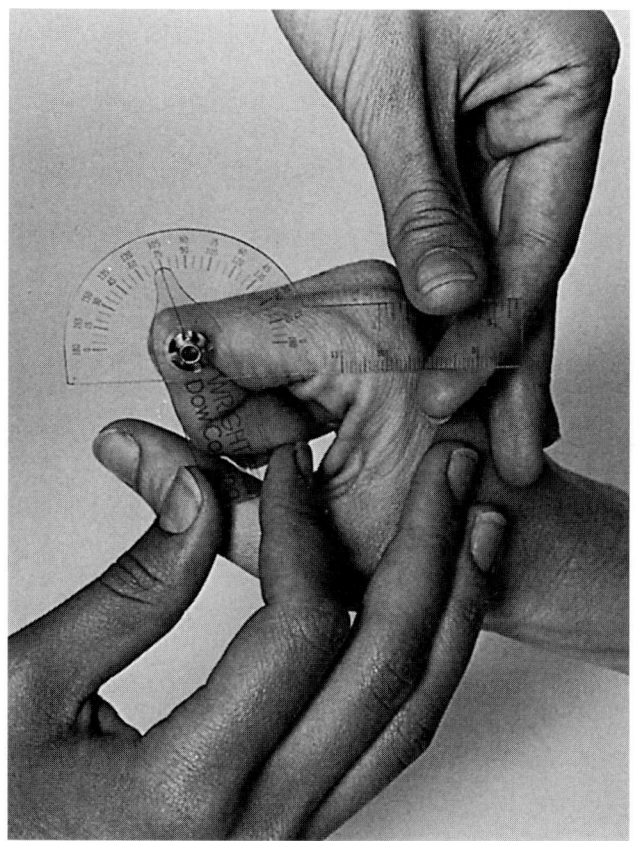

Fig. 11-9. Lateral placement of goniometer with shortened arms is suitable for finger joint measurements.

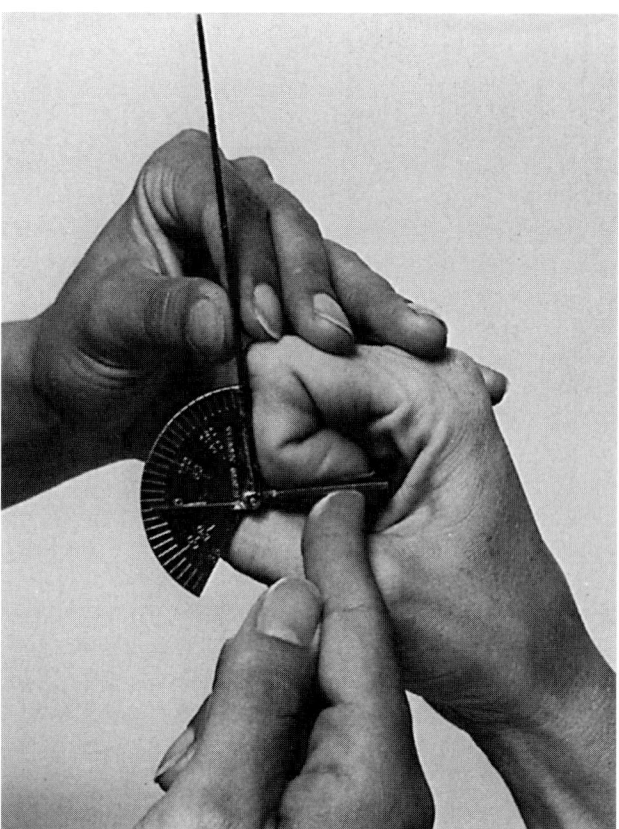

Fig. 11-10. Slight metacarpophalangeal extension allows full excursion of goniometer without interference by touching palm.

become available, using a specific device will become more important. The danger of comparing measurements generated by the multiple types of manual and/or electric goniometers, without evidence that the various systems give corresponding results, is great. Invalid comparisons not only would affect the outcome of research data, but also could do a major disservice to a patient.[1,27]

Limiting the effect of positioning on range-of-motion values

Hurt[21] states that "the resting length of a two joint muscle is insufficient to allow full motion in the direction away from itself simultaneously in both joints over which it passes" (Fig. 11-13). However, full motion is normally available at either joint with relaxation of the other.[21] The extrinsic finger flexors and extensors cross one or more finger joints and the wrist as well. In the case of the flexor digitorum superficialis, extensor digitorum communis, and the flexor pollicis longus, just distal to their origins, the elbow is crossed as well. To avoid having a resting length insufficiency interfere with ROM readings, the wrist should be neutral when digital motion measurements are being taken. Furthermore, to limit the influence of forearm positioning on wrist and finger measurements, the forearm should be pronated[13] (Fig.

11-14). Radial and/or ulnar deviation of the wrist while measuring wrist flexion and extension should be avoided because these motions have influence on the excursion of the wrist flexor and extensor tendons according to work done by Marshall et al.[27]

Recording range-of-motion measurements

Experts disagree about how ROM measurements should be recorded so that other professionals can accurately interpret the results. Several authors cited here comment on the importance of clearly defining a motion as being within the realm of normal flexion and extension or as an abnormal movement, such as hyperextension, but exact guidelines for unequivocal interpretation are not given. The American Academy of Orthopaedic Surgeons and the American Society for Surgery of the Hand recommend a system of notation in which all motions are measured from 0 degrees (neutral) starting position.[18,24] Flexion measurements are recorded as positive (+) numbers; extension and hyperextension beyond the 0-degree starting position are recorded as negative (−) numbers. Thus 15/110 passive motion of the PIP joint indicates a 15-degree flexion contracture and full passive flexion. Similarly, −15/110 indicates 15 degrees hyperextension and full passive flexion. Written statements

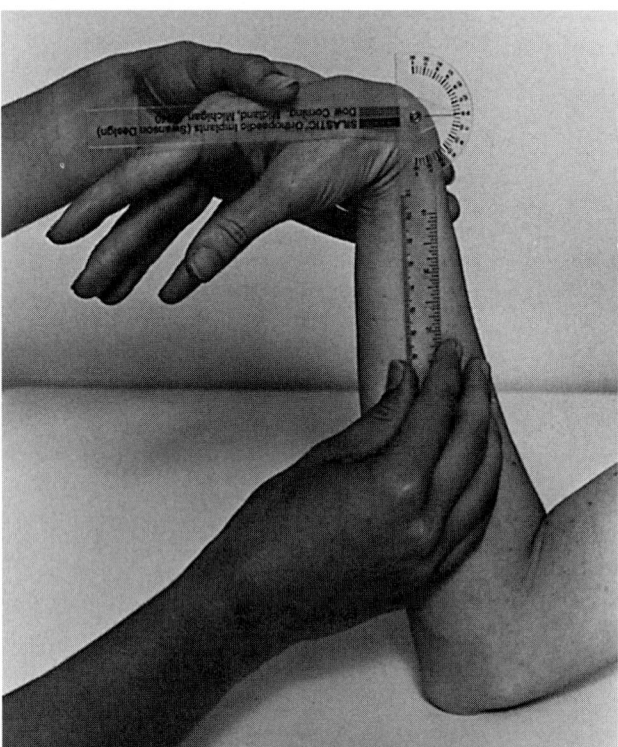

Fig. 11-11. Lateral measurement on radial aspect of wrist is preferred because of stability of second carpometacarpal joint.

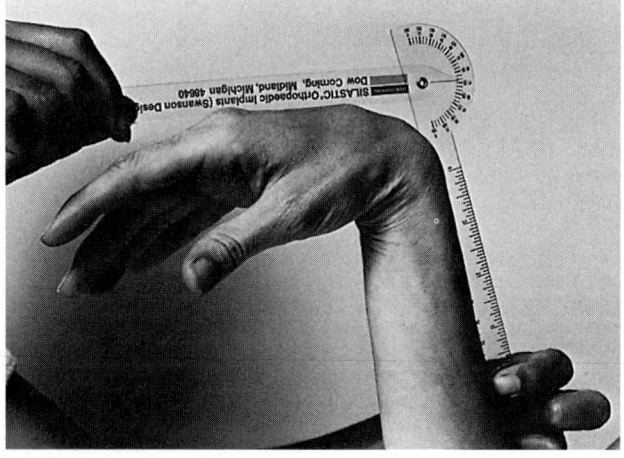

Fig. 11-12. The third carpometacarpal joint is stable and allows the metacarpal to be used for alignment of the dorsally placed goniometer.

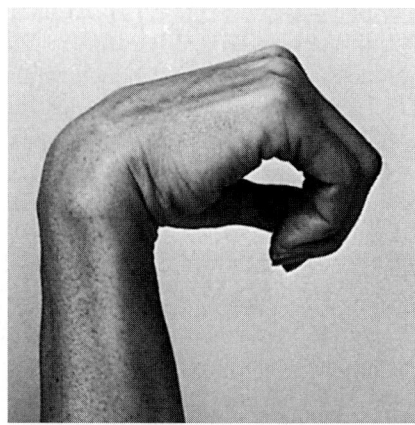

Fig. 11-13. Because of elongation of the extrinsic finger extensors over the fully flexed wrist, the remaining available excursion is inadequate to allow for full finger flexion.

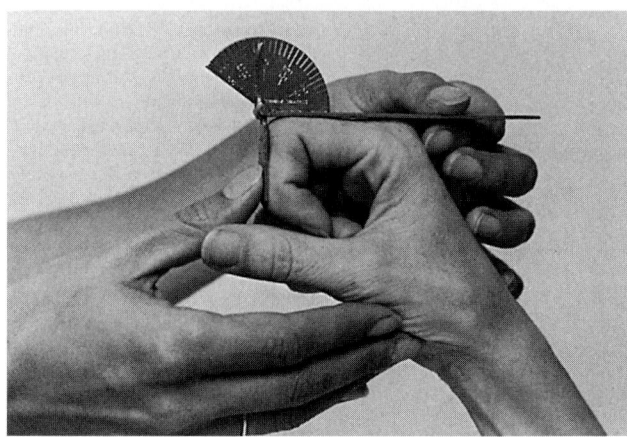

Fig. 11-14. Taking digital motion measurements with wrist in neutral and forearm in pronation eliminates possible effects of normal tendon-excursion limitation on range-of-motion measurements.

can be used to indicate rotation and alignment deformities.[32] The American Society of Hand Therapists endorses the American Medical Society's method of using plus (+) to indicate joint hyperextension, and minus (−) to indicate the inability to fully extend a joint (extension lag). Using this notation system, −15/110 indicates 15-degree extension lag and 110 degrees of flexion.[10]

Because of the lack of uniformity in recording motion measurements, a statement must accompany ROM records explaining the notation system and the type of goniometer used. Otherwise, accurate data could be inaccurately interpreted.

METHODS FOR MEASURING JOINT MOTION
Pronation and supination of the foreman

Measuring rotational movements at the radioulnar joints is difficult because of the long axis of movement and the lack of stable anatomic lever arms with which to align the goniometer. The method used by Downer incorporates the salient points of other techniques and does not require special equipment other than a standard goniometer.[11,21,28]

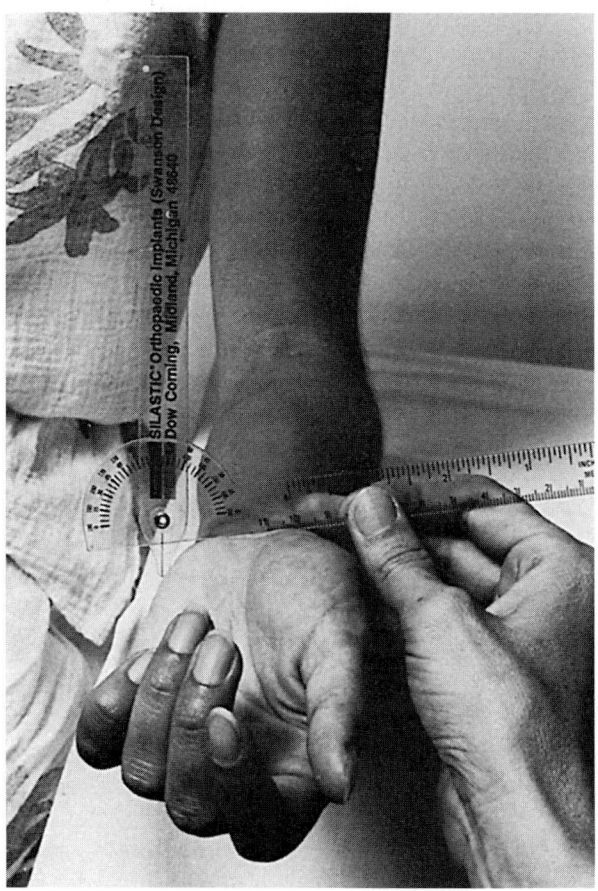

Fig. 11-15. Abduction of shoulder or extension of elbow allows substitution of shoulder movement for true supination or pronation.

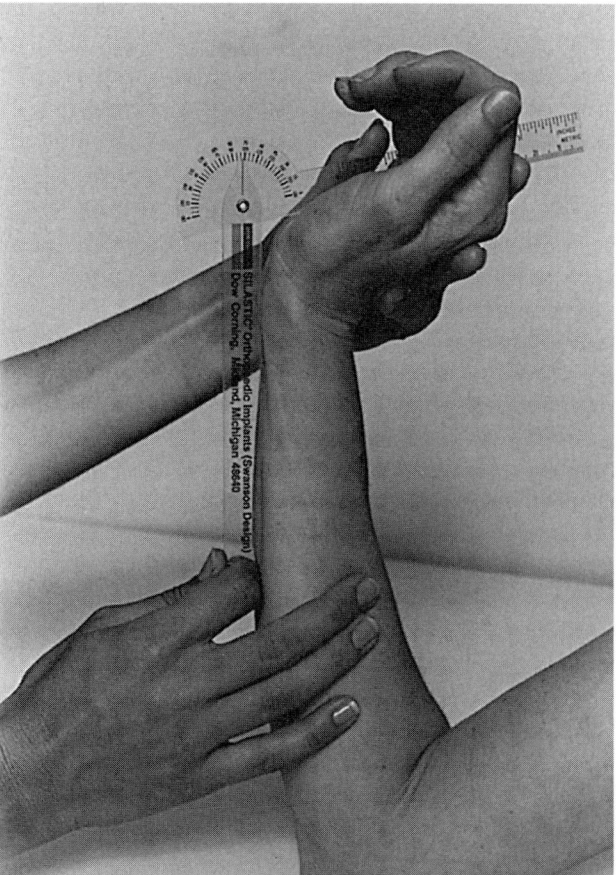

Fig. 11-16. Movable arm of goniometer will be over third metacarpal bridging palmar arc.

The patient may be sitting or standing, but the elbow must be flexed to 90 degrees with the arm close to the side of the body. The arm position is important to avoid substitution movements of the shoulder.[11,23] The forearm should be in midposition with the palm vertical in relation to the floor. This position is defined as 0 degrees.[24]

For measurements of supination, the patient rotates the hand and forearm to its maximum palm-up position without extending the elbow or abducting the upper arm. The stationary arm of the goniometer is aligned with the humerus or held perpendicular to the floor.[11] The movable arm is placed on edge across the volar aspect of the wrist at the level of the ulnar styloid. The axis of the goniometer is just medial to the ulnar styloid (Fig. 11-15). Normal ROM in supination is 0 to between 80 and 90 degrees. The starting position for pronation is the same as for supination. The patient rotates the hand and forearm into the maximum palm-down position. The stationary arm again is aligned with the humerus or perpendicular to the floor. The only change is the position of the movable arm, which is now on the dorsum of the wrist at the level of the styloid processes.[28] Normal motion is from 0 to between 80 and 90 degrees.[24]

Motion at the wrist

The wrist motions usually measured are flexion, extension, and radial and ulnar deviation. Wrist circumduction cannot be measured adequately.[24]

Flexion. Wrist flexion can be measured with the goniometer placed dorsally on the wrist[13,33] or laterally along the radial border of the forearm and second metacarpal.[23,29] Placement of the goniometer along the ulnar border of the wrist and the fifth metacarpal also has been suggested.[11,29] However, the mobility of the carpometacarpal (CMC) joints of the fourth and fifth metacarpals could skew the measurements of wrist flexion when an ulnar placement is used.[13] For measurement of wrist flexion (volar flexion) on the radial aspect of the forearm, the elbow is flexed and the forearm and wrist are placed in neutral for the starting position. The wrist is then flexed, and the stationary arm of the goniometer is aligned with the radius while the movable arm is aligned with the second metacarpal.[23] The axis of motion of the goniometer is approximately at the level of the radial styloid (see Fig. 11-11). Wrist flexion (volar flexion), with the goniometer placed dorsally, requires the elbow to be flexed and the forearm in neutral with the wrist in neutral as the starting position. The wrist is flexed with the fingers relaxed.

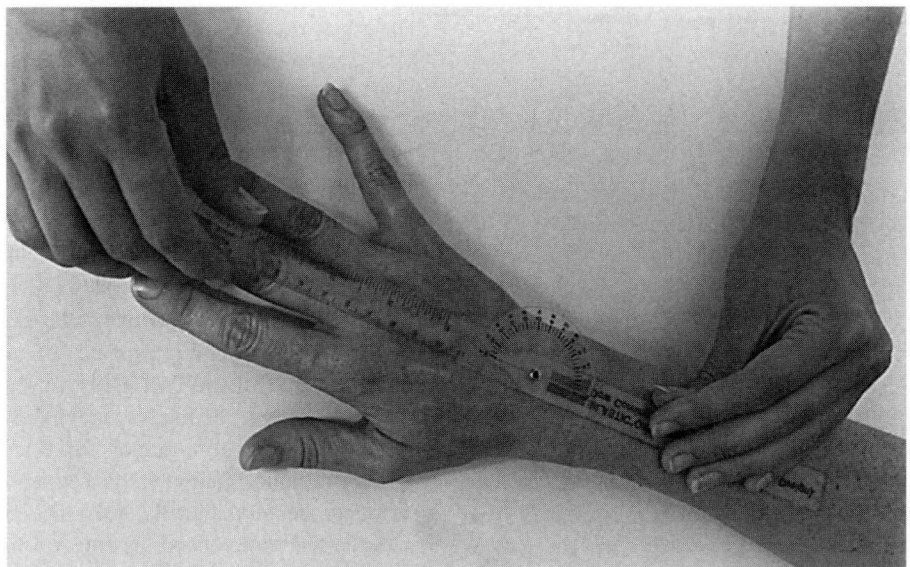

Fig. 11-17. Starting position for measurement of radial and ulnar deviation requires wrist to be in neutral in both planes of motion—flexion-extension and radial and ulnar deviation.

The stationary arm of the goniometer is aligned with the long axis of the forearm while the movable arm is aligned with the third metacarpal.[13] The fulcrum of the goniometer is approximately at the level of the capitate (see Fig. 11-12). According to *Joint Motion: Method of Measuring and Recording,* the normal arc of motion for wrist flexion is 0 to 80 degrees.[24]

Extension. To measure wrist extension (dorsiflexion) using the lateral placement, the wrist is extended with the fingers allowed to flex passively.[23] The normal arc of motion is 0 to 70 degrees.[24] For measurement of wrist extension with the goniometer volarly placed, the starting position of the arm is the same as for wrist flexion. However, goniometer placement is different. After the wrist is extended, the stationary arm is aligned with the long axis of the forearm on the volar surface and the movable arm is aligned with the volar surface of the third metacarpal.[13] The fingers should be relaxed (Fig. 11-16).

Radial and ulnar deviation. The starting positions for taking measurements of radial and ulnar deviation are the same. The forearm is in pronation, and the goniometer is placed dorsally.[13] The zero position is with the wrist in neutral.[24] The stationary arm is aligned in midposition along the forearm. The capitate and lateral epicondyle of the elbow can be used as reference points for the stationary arm, and the movable arm is placed along the third metacarpal (Fig. 11-17). In both radial and ulnar deviation, wrist flexion and extension must be avoided. The wrist is angled toward the thumb for radial deviation or angled toward the fifth finger for ulnar deviation.[11,13,29] The normal range of radial deviation is 0 to 20 degrees, and for ulnar deviation, 0 to 30 degrees.[24]

Motion of the fingers

The wrist and forearm should be in neutral to allow full tendon excursion of the long finger flexors and extensors when one is measuring the motion of the MP, PIP, and DIP joints.[13] This is true for both active and passive motion studies. Unless otherwise noted, AROM values for flexion are taken with all three joints of each finger actively flexed to their maximum. For the measurement of extension, all three joints are actively extended to their maximum. Simultaneous flexion or extension of the finger joints during measurement gives the examiner a better picture of the musculotendinous limitations affecting active motion of the joints. Passive motion is measured on a joint-by-joint basis, with the adjacent joint or joints in neutral so that the musculotendinous effects are minimized and only the excursion of the joint is being measured.[22]

Metacarpophalangeal joint flexion and extension. MP motion can be measured laterally or dorsally. The landmarks used for lateral measurements of joint flexion and extension are the same. For lateral placement of the goniometer on the index or middle fingers, the stationary arm is aligned with the lateral longitudinal axis of the second metacarpal. The moving arm is aligned with the lateral longitudinal axis of the proximal phalanx (Fig. 11-18). In the case of the middle finger, this requires the examiner to have the index MP joint slightly extended so that the middle finger can be clearly sighted (Fig. 11-19). The ring and little fingers are measured from the ulnar border of the hand with the same techniques.

Dorsal placement of the goniometer to measure MP joint flexion and extension is the same for both. The stationary arm is placed over the dorsum of the metacarpal, the fulcrum is superior to the joint axis, and the movable arm is placed

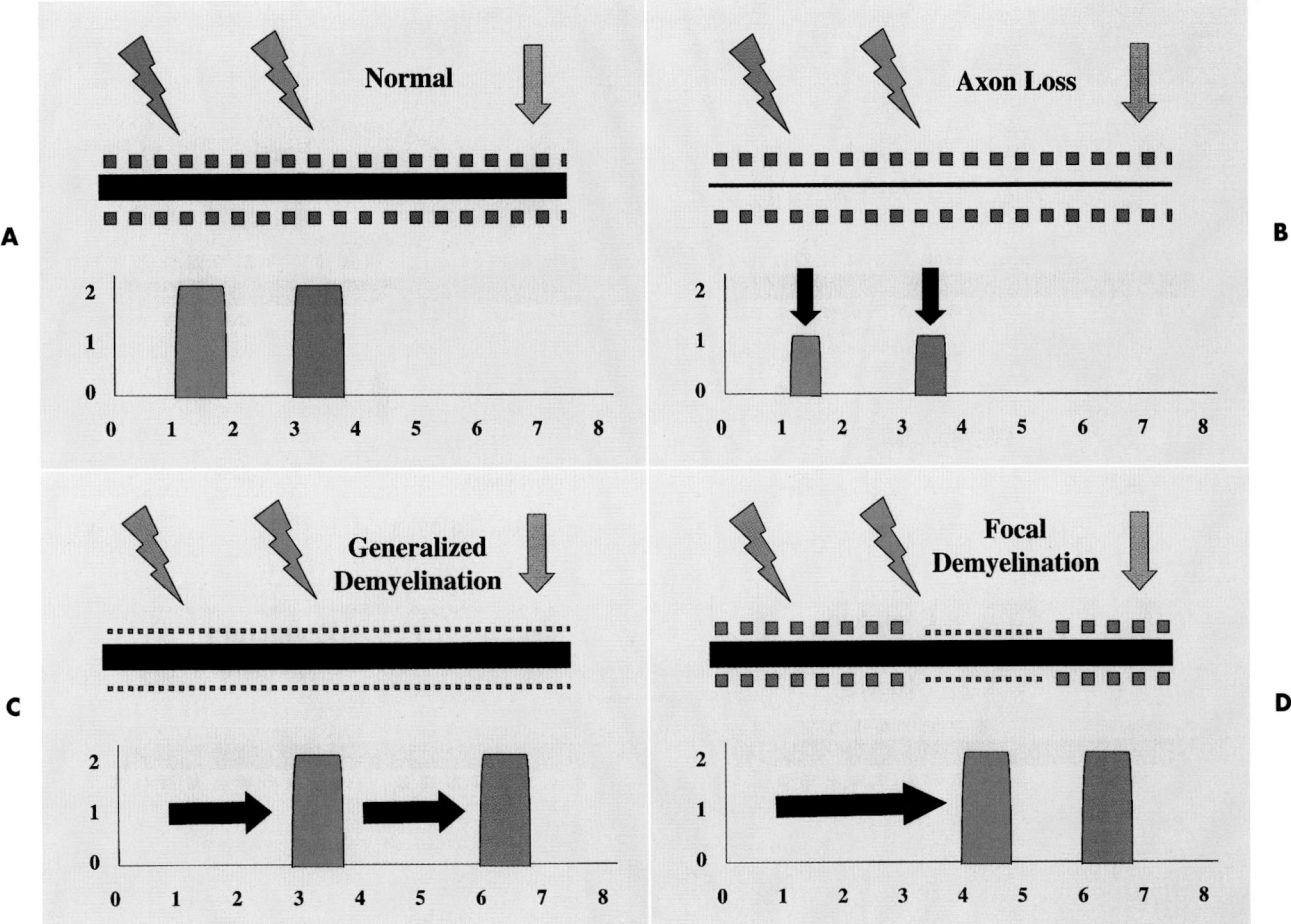

Plate 23. Schematic peripheral nerves illustrate "nerve conduction study (NCS) templates" in text. In all nerves, the *black horizontal bar* reflects the proportion of large sensory or motor axons, and *blue dotted lines* reflect myelin on large sensory and motor fibers, available for testing. The *gray down arrow* indicates the recording electrodes placed distally over a named sensory nerve, or over the motor point and reference site for a motor NCS. The *blue "lightning bolt"* reflects the more distal point of stimulation along the nerve tested, and the *blue rectangle* reflects the recorded waveform amplitude, area, and morphology as a function of time. The *red "lightning bolt"* and *rectangle,* respectively, reflect the more proximal point of stimulation and recorded waveform. Arbitrary numbers on the *y*-axis for amplitude and *x*-axis for time of the recorded response are provided to facilitate visual comparison between normal and the different nerve injury patterns. **A,** Normal nerve. **B,** Axon loss (AL). **C,** Generalized demyelinating synchronous slowing (SS), as in Charcot-Marie Tooth polyneuropathy, Type 1. **D,** Focal, distal, demyelinating synchronous slowing (SS), as in carpal tunnel syndrome.

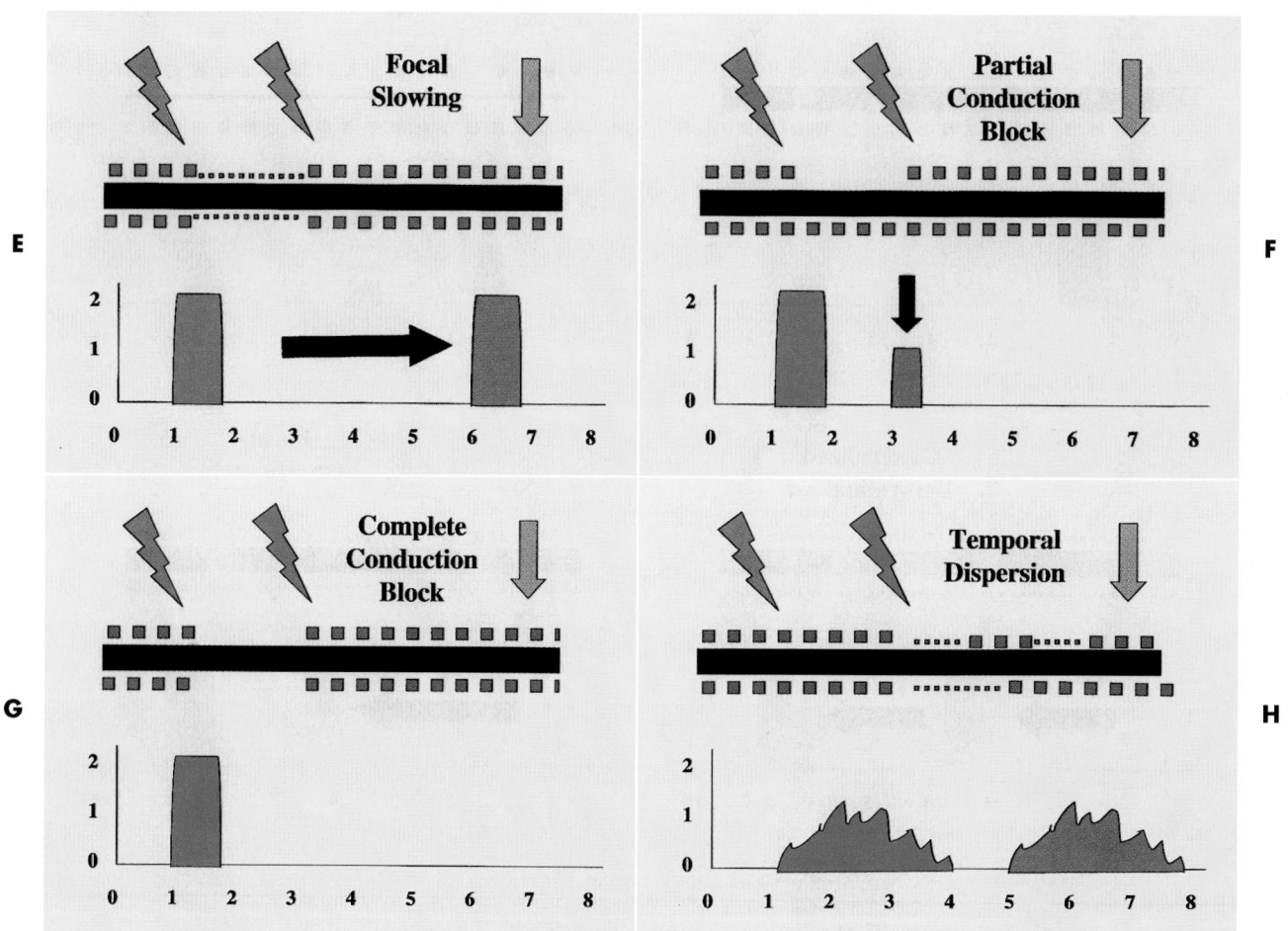

Plate 23, cont'd E, Focal, proximal, demyelinating synchronous slowing (SS), as in ulnar neuropathy across the elbow. **F,** Focal, partial, demyelinating conduction block (CB), shown proximally as in ulnar neuropathy at elbow. **G,** Focal, complete, demyelinating CB, proximally. **H,** Temporal dispersion (TD), as in Guillain-Barré syndrome, chronic inflammatory demyelinating polyneuropathy, and some entrapments.

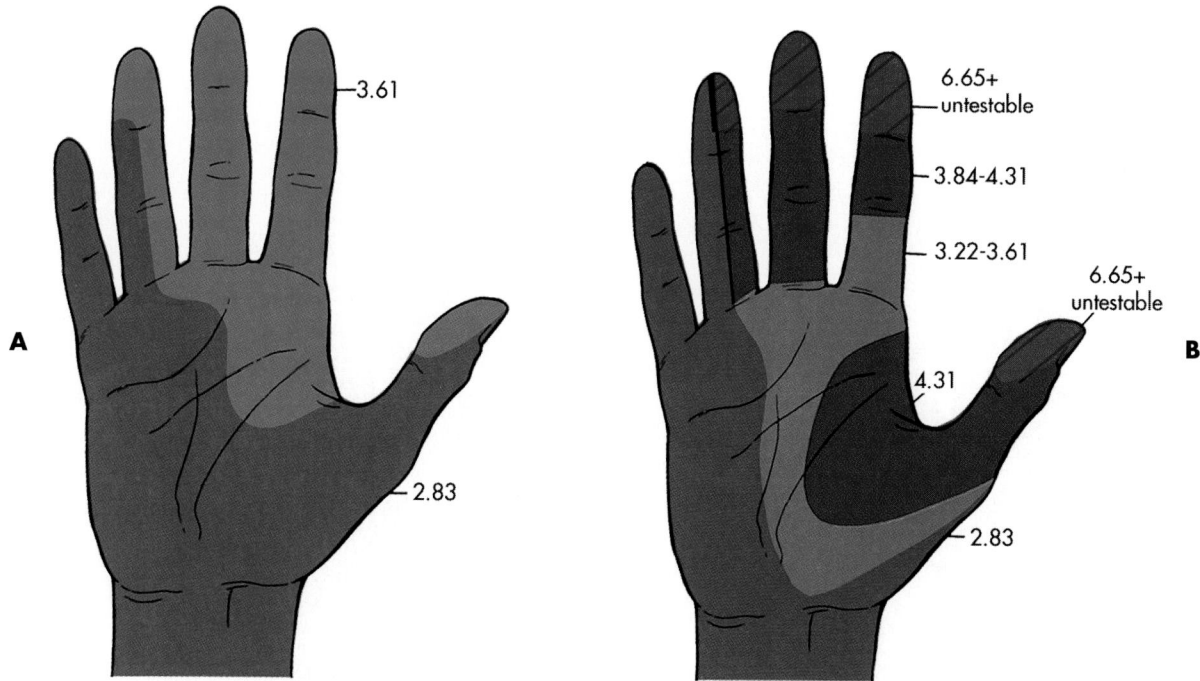

Plate 24. A, Monofilament mapping showing a median nerve compression as measured in a woman with a history of numbness for 2 years and no corrective intervention. **B,** Same patient as measured 4 months later. Touch-pressure recognition has become worse from diminished light touch to untestable with monofiaments.

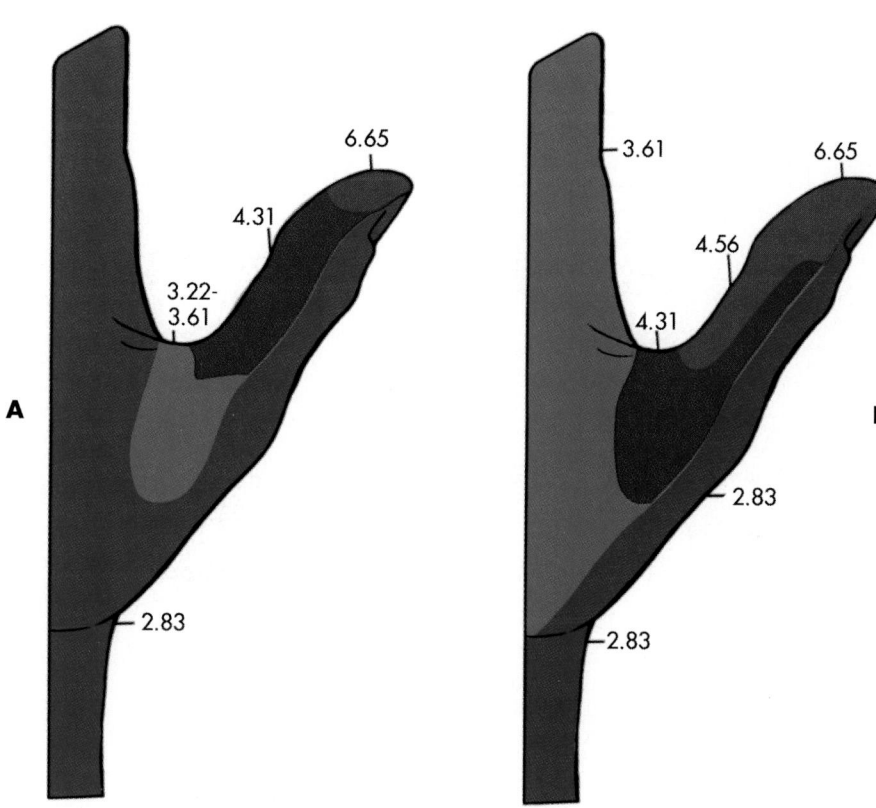

Plate 25. A, Two years after incomplete amputation of right thumb. Digital nerves were not resutured. Small centimeter pedicle of dorsal skin was intact. **B,** Same patient after injection of lidocaine around median nerve to determine whether innervation was radial nerve or median. Notice that although the volar thumb sensation was downgraded, it and the palmar area of the median nerve did not become asensory. This finding brings into question the blocking of the contralateral nerve in testing. Such blocks may be incomplete and lead to false conclusions.

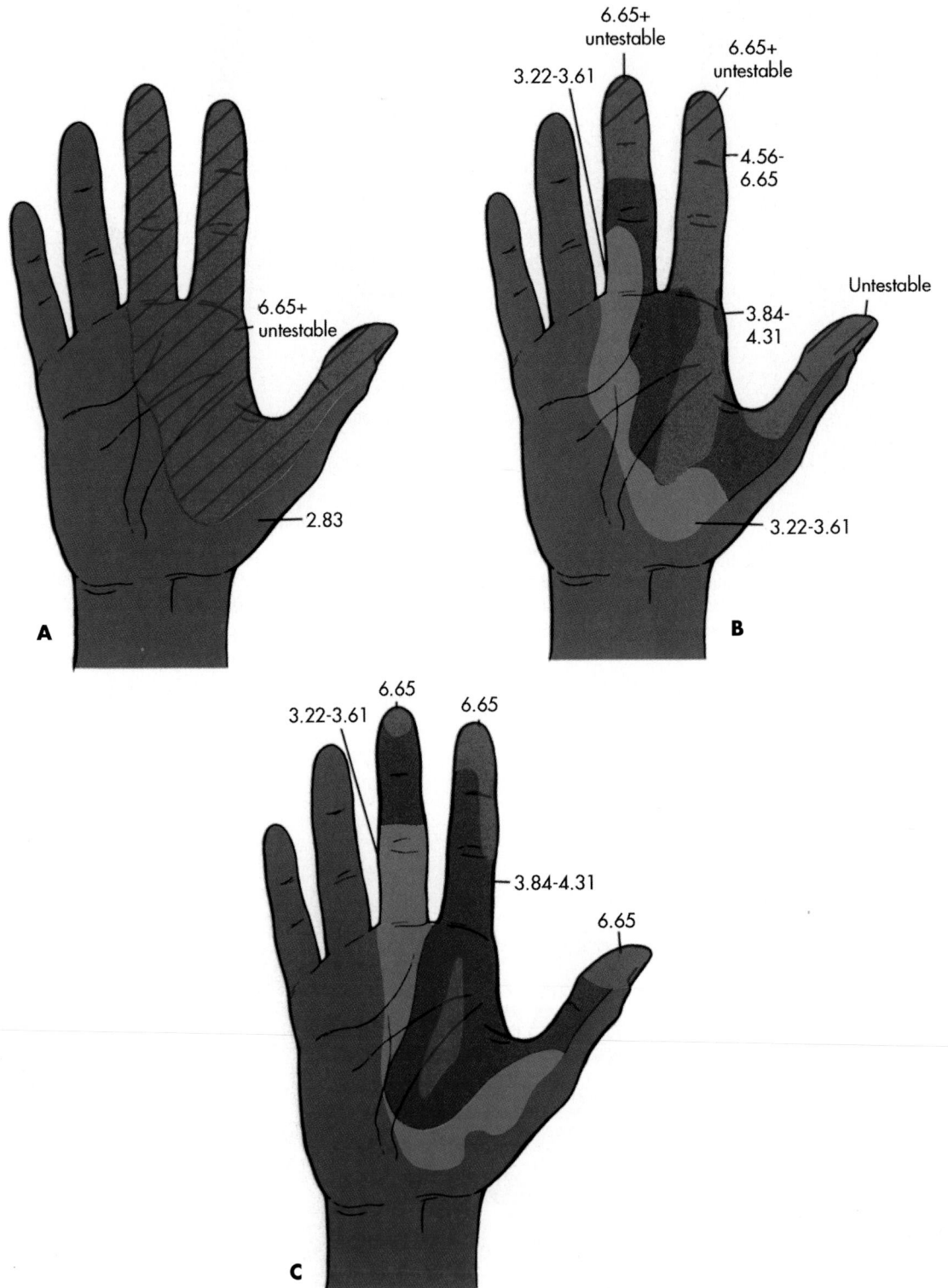

Plate 26. A, Monofilament mapping showing a median nerve laceration before surgery. Two-point untestable. **B,** Same patient 3 months after surgery. Two-point untestable. **C,** Same patient 7 months after surgery. Two-point untestable, fingertips now testable with monofilaments.

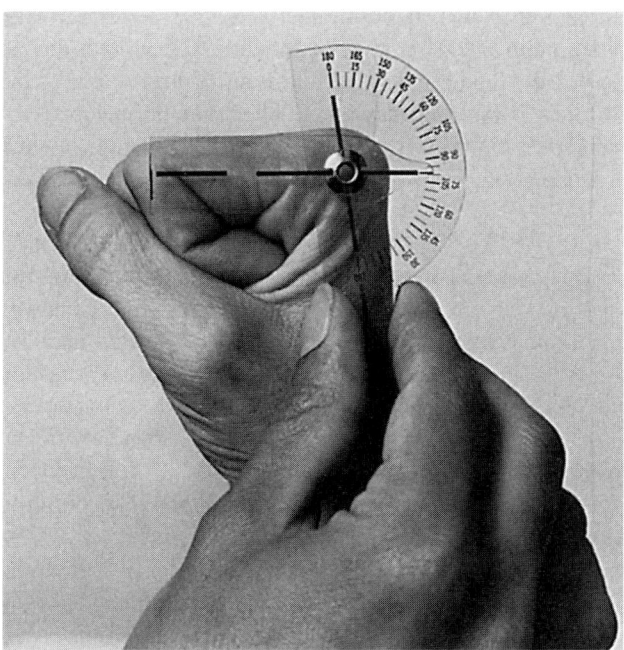

Fig. 11-18. Thumb should be held in abduction or adduction and slight extension when one is laterally measuring metacarpophalangeal joint motion of index finger so as not to block full metacarpophalangeal flexion of index finger.

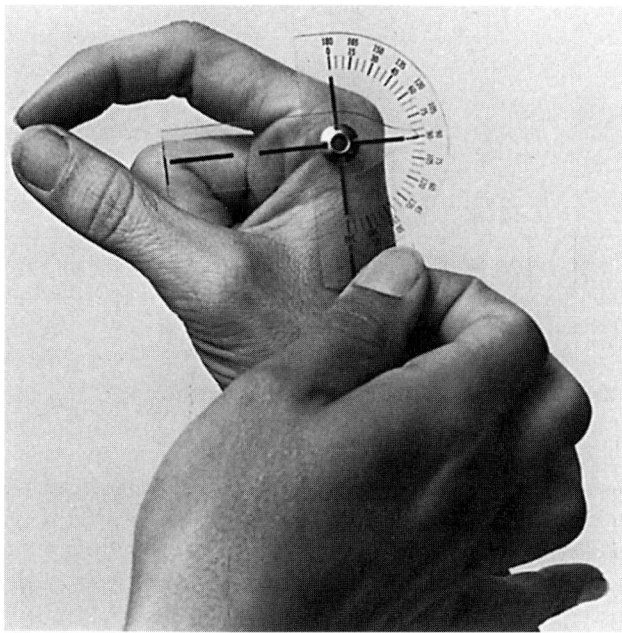

Fig. 11-19. Movable phalanx must be sighted as clearly as possible for an accurate measurement.

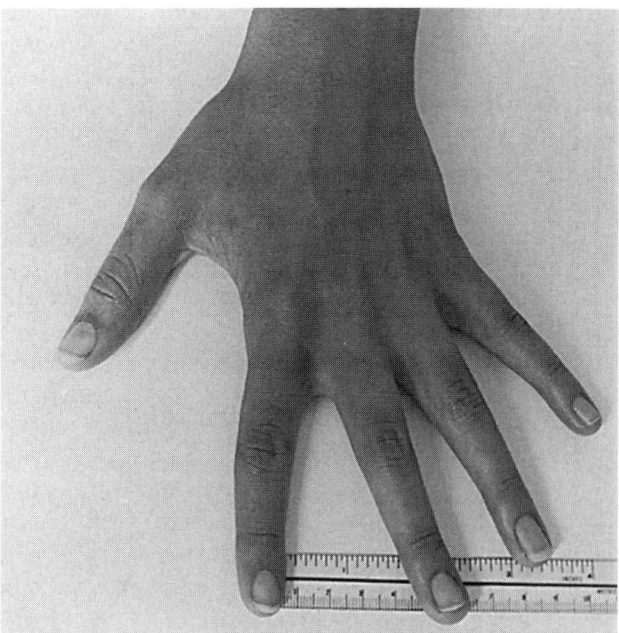

Fig. 11-20. Measuring distance between midpulps of adjacent maximally abducted fingers allows for comparisons of abduction to help in evaluation of treatment effectiveness.

over the dorsum of the adjacent phalanx.[13,23] The arc of motion usually evaluated when one is measuring MP joint motion is 0 to 90 degrees, but hyperextension of up to 45 degrees also is normal.[24]

Metacarpophalangeal joint abduction and adduction. *Joint Motion: Method of Measuring* does not give norms for finger abduction and adduction. It suggests measuring the distance from finger tip to finger tip in inches or centimeters. These measurements can be used for pretreatment and posttreatment comparisons only[24] (Fig. 11-20).

Proximal and distal interphalangeal joint flexion and extension. Because the techniques used for measurement of joint motion at the PIP and DIP joints are very similar, they are described together here. The use of a commercially available finger goniometer for dorsal placement (see Fig. 11-10) or a small goniometer in which the arms have been shortened for dorsal or lateral placement (see Fig. 11-9) helps with the measurement of the finger joints.

For lateral measurements, the stationary arm is placed along the long axis of the proximal phalanx and the moving arm is placed along the long axis of the adjacent distal phalanx. The fulcrum approximates the axis of motion of the joint[30] (see Fig. 11-18). The MP joints may have to be extended slightly when one is measuring the DIP flexion to allow the goniometer to clear the palm during full active flexion. When one is measuring extension of the PIP and DIP joints, the same goniometer placement is used along the lateral long axis if the adjacent phalangeal joints have been extended.

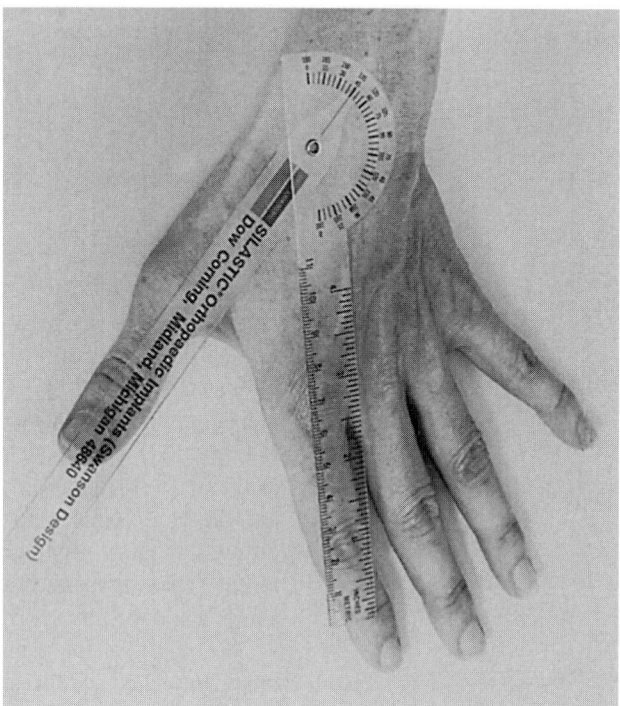

Fig. 11-21. Measurement of thumb extension is done with thumb in plane of palm.

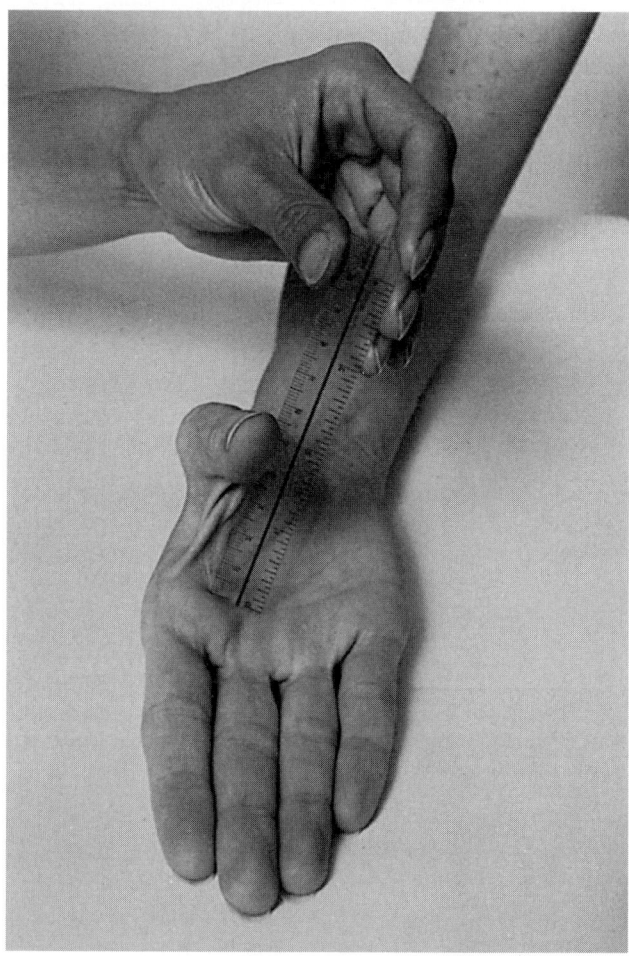

Fig. 11-22. Thumb abduction is measured in a plane perpendicular to palm.

Dorsal measurements of PIP and DIP flexion are made by placing the stationary arm on the dorsal long axis of the proximal phalanx and the movable arm on the dorsum of the adjacent distal phalanx.[11,23] The examiner should keep the goniometer in as complete contact with the dorsal finger surface as possible to avoid errors in measurement[30] (see Fig. 11-10). As with lateral placement, slight MP extension may be necessary for measurement of DIP flexion if total active flexion is complete or nearly so (see Fig. 11-10). The placement of the arms of the goniometer remains the same when one measures the extension of the PIP and DIP joints, except that the joints are in maximum extension.[24] The ROM of the PIP joints is 0 to 110 degrees, and that of the DIP joints is 0 to 60 or 70 degrees.[24]

Thumb motions. The thumb's movement pattern is the most complex of all the digits because of its highly mobile CMC joint. Flexion describes the movement across the palm that terminates with the tip of the thumb at the base of the fifth finger. It involves flexion of the CMC, MP, and IP joints for full excursion. Extension of the thumb involves the same joints in a movement away from the second metacarpal, again in the plane of the palm.[24]

Thumb flexion and extension can be measured with a goniometer placed laterally or dorsally along the appropriate adjacent bones. CMC joint flexion requires the stationary arm to be aligned with the lateral or dorsal long axis of the radius with the movable arm aligned with the first metacar-

pal. The approximate axis of motion is level with the anatomic snuffbox. Flexion of the CMC joint is 15 degrees.[24] CMC extension can be measured with the stationary arm aligned with the second metacarpal and the movable arm aligned over the first metacarpal (Fig. 11-21). MP and IP flexion and extension can be measured with the same lateral or dorsal technique appropriate for the index finger MP and PIP joints. Thumb MP joint motion is 0 to 50 degrees, and IP joint motion is 0 to 80 degrees.[24] The IP joint of the thumb has varying degrees of hypertension and should be compared with the contralateral thumb if a pathologic condition is suspected.

Thumb abduction and adduction occur in a plane perpendicular to the palm and normally involve only movement of the CMC joint. Norms for abduction have not been established by the American Academy of Orthopaedic Surgeons, but the measurement can be compared with that of the contralateral hand. *Adduction* is defined as the thumb in line with the radius lying immediately beside the second metacarpal, whereas *abduction* is the angle that occurs as the

CONCLUSION

The research done on assessment of the reliability of measuring joint motion indicates that use of the same goniometer by the same tester using the same method for measuring serial motion increases reliability. When the same tester is not available, the use of the same type of goniometer and method of measurement may help improve reliability. Documentation of the methods used and of the type of goniometer is important. With the rapid development of computerized evaluation programs for the clinical setting as well as custom-made goniometers for research projects, the potential for differences and errors in measurement is expanding. Only after the reliability and validity of the computerized goniometer has been established and the concurrent validity between the manual and computerized goniometer has been determined can manual and computerized goniometric measurements be compared.

The methods for measuring joint motion presented in this chapter are for the evaluation of hands without major deformities that cause excessive joint deviations, subluxations, and dislocations, such as advanced rheumatoid arthritis. Refer to the chapters in this text on arthritis for more detailed information on the evaluation of the arthritic hand.

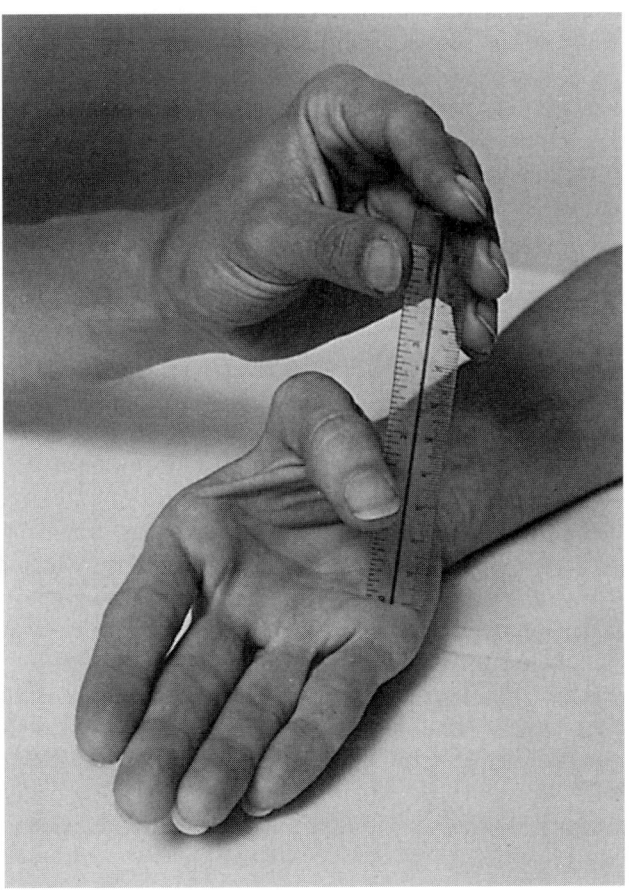

Fig. 11-23. During opposition, thumb must move out of plane of palm while approaching fifth finger.

thumb moves perpendicularly away from the plane of the palm.[24] This angle can be measured in degrees with a goniometer. The stationary arm is aligned with the lateral aspect of the second metacarpal, and the moving arm is placed dorsally along the long axis of the first metacarpal.[23] An alternative method is to measure in inches or centimeters the distance from the DPC of the index finger to the pulp or IP crease of the thumb[24] (Fig. 11-22). Other methods of measurement, using special measuring devices such as dental calipers, have been suggested in the hand literature and may be helpful in some circumstances.

Thumb opposition is a composite motion comprising abduction, rotation, and flexion. Opposition is usually measured in inches or centimeters between the thumb tip and the tip or base of the fifth finger[24] (Fig. 11-23). For true opposition and not just thumb flexion, the thumb must move out and away from the plane of the palm with the thumbnail approximately parallel to the plane of the palm.

REFERENCES

1. Armstrong AD, et al: Reliability of range of motion measurement in the elbow and forearm, *J Shoulder Elbow Surg* 7:573, 1998.
2. Aulicino PL: Clinical examination of the hand. In Hunter JM, Mackin EJ, Callahan AD, editors: *Rehabilitation of the hand: surgery and therapy,* ed 4, St Louis, 1995, Mosby.
3. Bell-Krotoski J, Breger D, Beach R: Application of biomechanics for evaluation of the hand. In Hunter JM, Mackin EJ, Callahan AD, editors: *Rehabilitation of the hand: surgery and therapy,* ed 4, St Louis, 1995, Mosby.
4. Boone DC, et al: Reliability of goniometric measurements, *Phys Ther* 58:1355, 1978.
5. Brand P: Methods of clinical measurement in the hand. In Brand PW, Hollister A, editors: *Clinical mechanics of the hand,* ed 2, St Louis, 1993, Mosby.
6. Breger-Lee D, Bell-Krotoski J, Brandsma J: Torque range of motion in the hand clinic, *J Hand Ther* 3:7, 1990.
7. Breger-Lee D, et al: Reliability of torque range of motion: a preliminary study, *J Hand Ther* 6:29, 1993.
8. Brown A, et al: Validity and reliability of the Dexter hand evaluation and therapy system in hand injured patients, *J Hand Ther* 1:37, 2000.
9. Cantrell T, Fisher T: The small joints of the hand, *Clin Rheum Dis* 8:545, 1982.
10. Clapper MP, Wolf SL: Comparison of the reliability of the orthoranger and standard goniometer for assessing active lower extremity range of motion, *Phys Ther* 68:214, 1988.
11. *Clinical assessment recommendations,* ed 2, Chicago, 1992, American Society of Hand Therapists.
12. Downer A: *Goniometry: measurement of joint range of motion,* Columbus, 1982, Ohio State University Press (unpublished).
13. Fess EE: Documentation: essential elements of an upper extremity assessment battery. In Hunter JM, Mackin EJ, Callahan AD, editors: *Rehabilitation of the hand: surgery and therapy,* ed 4, St Louis, 1995, Mosby.
14. Fess EE, Moran CA: *Clinical assessment recommendations,* 1981, American Society of Hand Therapists.

15. Goodwin J, et al: Clinical methods of goniometry: a comparative study, *Disabil Rehab* 1:10, 1992.
16. Grohmann JEL: Comparison of two methods of goniometry, *Phys Ther* 63:922, 1993.
17. Hamilton GF, Lachenbruch PA: The reliability of goniometry in assessing finger joint angle, *Phys Ther* 49:465, 1969.
18. *The hand: examination and diagnosis,* Aurora, Colo, 1978, American Society for Surgery of the Hand.
19. Hellebrandt FA, Duvall EN, Moore ML: The measurement of joint motion. Part III. Reliability of goniometry, *Phys Ther Rev* 29:302, 1949.
20. Horger MM: The reliability of goniometric measurements of active and passive wrist motions, *Am J Occup Ther* 44:342, 1990.
21. Hurt SP: Considerations in muscle function and their application to disability evaluation and treatment: joint measurement. Part I, *Am J Occup Ther* 1:69, 1947.
22. Hurt SP: Considerations in muscle function and their application to disability evaluation and treatment: joint measurement. Part I, *Am J Occup Ther* 1:209, 1947.
23. Hurt SP: Considerations in muscle function and their application to disability evaluation and treatment: joint measurement. Part II, *Am J Occup Ther* 1:281, 1947.
24. *Joint motion: method of measuring and recording,* Chicago, 1965, American Academy of Orthopaedic Surgeons.
25. LaStayo PC, Wheeler DL: Reliability of passive wrist flexion and extension goniometric measurements: a multicenter study, *Phys Ther* 74:162, 1994.
26. Low JL: The reliability of joint measurement, *Physiotherapy* 62:227, 1976.
27. Marshall MM, Mozrall JR, Shealy JE: The effects of complex wrist and forearm posture on wrist range of motion, *Human Factors* 41:205, 1999.
28. Moore ML: The measurement of joint motion. Part I. Introductory review of the Literature, *Phys Ther Rev* 29:195, 1949.
29. Moore ML: The measurement of joint motion. Part II. The technic of goniometry, *Phys Ther Rev* 29:256, 1949.
30. Perry JF, Bevin AG: Evaluation procedures for patients with hand injuries, *Phys Ther* 54:593, 1974.
31. Swanson AB: *Flexible implant resection arthroplasty in the hand and extremities,* St Louis, 1973, Mosby.
32. Swanson AB, Goran-Hagert C, Swanson G: Evaluation of impairment of hand function. In Hunter JM, Mackin EJ, Callahan AD, editors: *Rehabilitation of the hand: surgery and therapy,* ed 4, St Louis, 1995, Mosby.
33. Watkins M, et al: Reliability of goniometric measurement and visual estimates of knee range of motion obtained in a clinical setting, *Phys Ther* 71:98, 1991.

Chapter 12

EDEMA: THERAPIST'S MANAGEMENT

June P. Villeco
Evelyn J. Mackin
James M. Hunter

Persistent edema presents a constant challenge to hand surgeons and hand therapists. If unresolved, it will delay healing and can result in pain and stiffness, thereby compromising functional results. This chapter addresses the development and treatment of local edema with intact (although overwhelmed) venous, arterial, and lymphatic systems. The physiology and treatment of lymphedema are discussed separately in Chapters 53 and 54.

EDEMA DEFINED

Edema is the accumulation of excessive fluid in the intercellular spaces.[18,19] The process of controlling fluid accumulation involves a variety of factors that influence capillary filtration and lymph drainage. This process is affected by both vascular and nonvascular processes.

All cells are bathed in extracellular fluid. This fluid can be divided into two main components: the interstitial fluid and the blood plasma.[18,19] The interstitial fluid is outside of the closed vascular system.[15] Blood plasma is the fluid noncellular part of blood in which red blood cells, white blood cells, and platelets are suspended to collectively form total blood volume.[18,19] This circulating blood tissue fills the vascular system and is circulated through the heart, arteries, capillaries, and veins.

The arterial system brings oxygen and nutrients to the cells, whereas the venous system is responsible for waste and carbon dioxide removal. The exchange of nutrients and cellular waste between the tissues and the circulating blood takes place at the level of the capillaries, primarily through diffusion and filtration. The capillary wall consists of a single layer of highly permeable endothelial cells and is surrounded by a basement membrane. The diameter of the capillary is just large enough for red blood cells and other blood cells to pass through[15,18,19] Blood enters the capillaries through arterioles and metarterioles and exits through venules. It is rare that any single functional cell is more than 20 to 30 microns away from a capillary.[18,19]

Oxygen and glucose are in higher concentration in the bloodstream than in the interstitial fluid and diffuse into the interstitial fluid, whereas carbon dioxide diffuses in the opposite direction.[15,19] Proteins are too large to diffuse easily through the capillary membrane and primarily flow linearly along the capillary.[18] However, small amounts of proteins leak out of the blood capillaries into the interstitium, where they accumulate in the interstitial fluid.[18,19] The lymphatic system is responsible for returning proteins that have accumulated in the interstitial spaces back into the venous system until the system is back in balance. Lymph is fluid collected from tissues; it flows via lymphatic vessels through the lymph nodes and drains into the venous system.[15,18,19] Fig. 12-1 illustrates the exchange process between substances in the interstitial fluid spaces with blood and lymphatic capillaries.

The spaces between cells are collectively called the *interstitium.* The fluid between cells (or interstitial fluid) is derived by filtration from the capillaries. There is a constant exchange of fluid between the intercellular tissue spaces and the blood plasma across the capillary membrane. Fluid in the interstitium is trapped by proteoglycan filaments, which cause the fluid to have the characteristics of a gel.[18,19] This "tissue gel" contains almost the same constituents as plasma, except for proteins, because proteins do not filter out

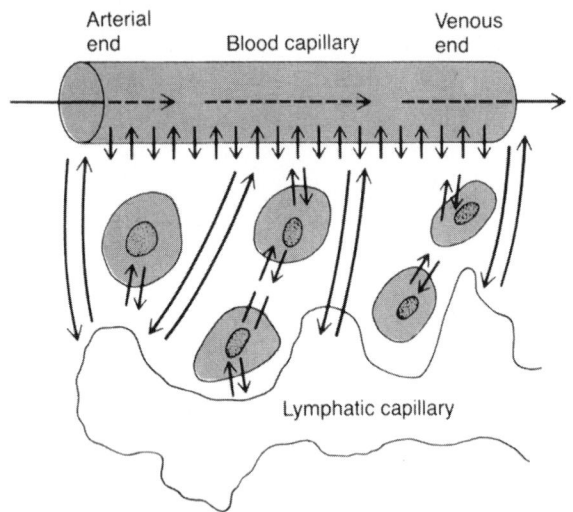

Fig. 12-1. Diffusion of fluid molecules and dissolved substances between the capillary and interstitial fluid spaces. (From Guyton AC, Hall JE: *Textbook of medical physiology,* ed 9, Philadelphia, 1996, WB Saunders.)

of the capillaries easily. Water molecules, electrolytes, nutrients, and cellular waste *diffuse* through the interstitium rapidly, although fluid *flows* very poorly in the tissue gel.[18,19] Generally, there is only a very slight amount of fluid that is free from these proteoglycan filaments and not trapped in the tissue gel. In normal tissues, the "free" fluid is usually much less than 1%. When tissues start to develop edema, the gel can swell from 30% to 50% to accommodate the increased volume of interstitial free fluid.[18,19] After this point, the gel can not accommodate additional fluid, and the amount of free fluid increases. The amount of the free fluid may expand to equal more than half of the interstitial fluid,[18,19] and the interstitial fluid volume can increase to several hundred percent above normal in seriously edematous tissues.[19] Pitting edema is made up of large amounts of free fluid in the tissues that can be displaced briefly by pressure, leaving a pit that slowly fills with fluid flowing back from the surrounding tissues.[19] Fig. 12-2 illustrates this effect in a woman who has pitting edema in her hand. When fluid in the interstitium becomes clotted with fibrinogen, preventing it from moving freely, or when tissue cells rather than the interstitium swell, brawny edema results.[19] Brawny edema is firm to the touch.

Lymphedema refers to the specific type of edema caused by accumulation of protein-rich fluid in the extracellular space of skin and subcutaneous tissue, which results from obstruction of superficial extremity lymphatics.[11] Although most edemas are caused by increased capillary filtration, which overwhelms lymph drainage, lymphedema represents failure of the lymphatic system to drain lymph from a defined region, usually a limb.[29] The lymphatics are responsible for draining excess fluid as well as cells, proteins, lipids, microorganisms, and debris from tissues. The main function of the lymphatic system is to return large molecules, such as

proteins, to the blood. The lymphatic system influences the volume of interstitial fluid and the interstitial fluid pressure as it compensates to balance the rate of protein and fluid leakage from the blood capillaries. The pathophysiology and treatment of lymphedema are discussed in greater depth in Chapters 53 and 54.

NET CAPILLARY FILTRATION AND EFFECT ON EDEMA

Net filtration of fluid across the capillary membrane is determined by the balance between the forces that tend to force fluid outward into the interstitial spaces (filtration) and the forces that move fluid inward (resorption). Normally, the filtration pressures slightly exceed the reabsorption pressures, and the lymphatics balance the system by pulling excess fluid and proteins out of the interstitial spaces and returning them to the blood.[18,19]

Substances are transferred between the plasma and interstitial fluid primarily by diffusion through the capillary membrane. This diffusion provides continual mixing between the interstitial fluid and the plasma.[18,19] Lipid-soluble substances such as oxygen and carbon dioxide can diffuse directly through the cell membranes. Lipid-insoluble substances, such as chloride ions, sodium ions, and glucose, as well as water, diffuse through capillary pores or periodic intercellular clefts that connect the interior of the capillary with the exterior. These clefts or slit pores are about 20 times the diameter of a water molecule but slightly less than the diameters of plasma proteins such as an albumin molecule. The net rate of diffusion depends on the concentration difference between the two sides of the capillary membrane.

Minute vesicles are also located on the surface of the endothelial cells.[15,18,19] These vesicles transport plasma and extracellular fluid through the capillary wall by imbibing small amounts and then moving slowly through the endothelial cells, releasing the contents to the outer surface.[15,18,19]

Fluid exchange depends on the properties of the capillary walls and the pressures acting across the capillary membrane. Capillary permeability is selective and is affected by pressures and relative concentrations on either side of the membrane and on the integrity of the membrane itself.[36] Capillary permeability is increased following external injury, operative trauma, and burns.[43]

The primary four pressures that influence net capillary filtration are the capillary (hydrostatic) pressure, the interstitial fluid (hydrostatic) pressure, the plasma colloid osmotic pressure, and the interstitial fluid colloid osmotic pressure. The *capillary pressure* is the blood pressure in the capillaries that tends to move fluid from the capillary outward through the membrane at any given point.[18,19,36,43] This pressure is greater at the arterial end than at the venous end of the capillary, resulting in fluid filtering out at the arterial end and being reabsorbed at the venous end of the blood capillaries.

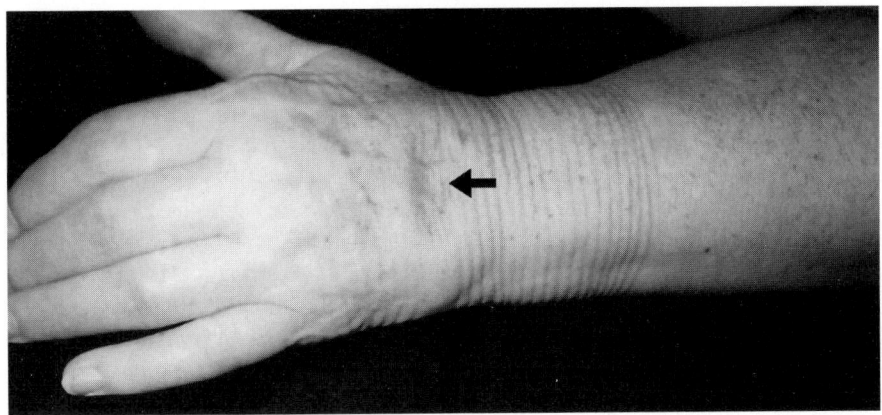

Fig. 12-2. Patient with pitting edema of the hand.
Note the "pit" left by the therapist's thumb *(arrow).*

The *interstitial fluid pressure* tends to force fluid inward through the capillary membrane when it is positive but outward when it is negative. This can be subdivided into the pressure of the fluid within the gel (integral pressure) and the free fluid pressure. There is a slight pressure difference between these pressures caused by the osmotic pressure of the gel. When acute edema develops, the free fluid portion swells. Normally, in loose tissue, interstitial free fluid pressure is slightly less than atmospheric pressure and exerts a suction force, drawing fluid out of the capillaries.[18,19] The direct cause of edema is positive pressure in the interstitial fluid spaces.[19]

Colloid osmotic or *oncotic pressures* are the pressures created by dissolved proteins, causing osmosis of fluid. The plasma colloid osmotic pressure draws fluid inward through the membrane, whereas the interstitial fluid colloid osmotic pressure draws fluid outward through the membrane. The concentration of protein in the plasma is generally two to three times that of the interstitial fluid. Approximately 75% of the plasma colloid osmotic pressure results from albumin. The plasma colloid osmotic pressure is important in preventing loss of fluid volume from the blood into the interstitial spaces.

The capillary pressure, *negative* interstitial free fluid pressure, and interstitial fluid colloid osmotic pressure all tend to force fluid outward, whereas the plasma colloid osmotic pressure causes osmosis of fluid inward. The balance of pressure between these four forces is called the *net capillary filtration pressure.* There is usually a higher outward force (filtration pressure) at the arterial end of the capillary because of the higher capillary pressure at this end, and a higher inward force, or reabsorption pressure, is seen at the venous end. About nine tenths of what is filtered out at the arterial end of the capillary is reabsorbed back in at the venous end, with the remaining fluid going through the lymph vessels.[18,19] When the net filtration pressure rises excessively, too much fluid is moved outward into the interstitial spaces for the lymphatics to manage and *extracellular edema* results.

Abnormal leakage of fluid from the capillaries into the extracellular (interstitial) spaces can be caused by increased capillary pressure (as with arteriolar dilation, venular constriction, increased venous pressure, failure of venous pumps, or lack of active muscular activity), decreased plasma proteins (as with loss of proteins from denuded skin areas in burns and wounds), increased capillary permeability (as results from release of histamine and related substances, from kinins such as bradykinin, or from bacterial infections), or blockage of lymph return.[15,18,19] All of these will result in an increased volume of interstitial fluid with subsequent expansion of the extracellular fluid of volume.[18,19]

Widespread edema may be caused by heart failure, loss of proteins in the urine or decreased ability to produce proteins, and excessive kidney retention of salt and water.[15,18,19]

Trauma can cause venous obstruction or arteriolar dilation and thus result in increased capillary pressure and a higher net filtration pressure.[36] The capillary filtration pressure will also be elevated by local or general heating that causes arterial dilation. Burns not only decrease plasma proteins (as discussed earlier) but also lead to increased capillary permeability and may allow fluid to spill into the tissues as a result of damage to the integrity of the capillary endothelium or enlarged capillary pores.[36] Release of histamine and bradykinin is part of an initial inflammatory response and will increase capillary permeability and blood flow, allowing large quantities of fluid and protein, including fibrinogen, to leak into the tissue. This in turn will cause increased interstitial fluid to accumulate.[19]

Intracellular edema can occur in conditions in which the metabolic systems of tissues are depressed or lack adequate nutrition to the cells, and it may occur in inflamed tissue areas as cell membranes increase their permeability to sodium and other ions, with subsequent osmosis of water into the cells.[18,19]

EDEMA AND RESPONSE TO INJURY

In the hand, afferent blood flow occurs on the volar surface and is controlled by arterial blood pressure. The major portion of the return blood flow takes place on the dorsal surface through the lymphatic and venous systems. The return systems require active movement of the hand to compress and produce retrograde venous and lymphatic flow by joint movement and compression of the fascial compartments. The dynamics of return flow are further augmented by motion of the elbow and shoulder.[28]

In the *normal* extremity, mild edema of the hand may be produced in a few hours by immobilizing the upper extremity with the hand in a dependent position, such as in a sling. Edema produces bloating of the skin on the dorsum of the hand, which results in flattening of the hand and loss of the longitudinal and transverse arches.[20]

EDEMA AND STAGES OF WOUND HEALING

The nature and treatment of edema differ for the three stages of wound healing. The stages are described here and consist of the inflammatory phase, which usually lasts the first 3 to 5 days; the fibroplastic or proliferative phase, which may last 2 to 6 weeks depending on the nature and degree of injury; and the maturation or remodeling phase, which may last from 6 months to 2 years.[14,37]

Edema is the first and most obvious reaction of the hand to injury. Most wounds have an excess of fluid content early in the healing process. Release of histamine and bradykinin increases capillary permeability and is part of a normal acute inflammatory reaction that occurs in response to tissue injury from a variety of causes, including trauma, heat, chemicals, and bacteria. Edema in the early phase of wound healing is liquid, soft, and easy to mobilize and reduce. At this stage, the excess fluid, called *transudate,* consists mainly of water and dissolved electrolytes.[27] This type of edema should not alarm the therapist as long as the principles of compression, elevation, use of cold, and active motion are observed to minimize pooling of blood in injured areas.[25,32] However, excessive edema can inhibit wound healing by decreasing arterial, venous, and lymphatic flow.[44]

The primary function of the inflammatory phase is to wall off the injured area, dispose of injury byproducts through phagocytosis, and prepare for the fibroplastic repair phase. Chemical mediators initially cause vasoconstriction, followed by vasodilation. Increased cell permeability allows passage of fluid and white blood cells through cell walls to form plasma.[32] Leukocytes and other phagocytic cells accumulate at the site of injury to clean up the debris, and fibrogen is converted to fibrin. Key to treatment in the inflammatory phase of wound healing is pain control and a balance between gentle active range of motion (AROM) in an elevated position and rest of the involved structures.

Excessive exercise in this phase can delay clot formation and increase inflammation.[32] Heat is also contraindicated in the inflammatory stage because it will cause further vasodilation and increase membrane permeability, capillary infiltration, and arterial blood flow, which will result in additional edema.

Fibroplasia begins as early as 3 to 5 days after injury and lasts from 2 to 6 weeks, depending on the extent of the wound.[14,37] During the fibroplastic or repair stage of wound healing, repair of the injured tissue is initiated. Fibroplasia is characterized by increased capillary growth, increased fibroblasts, and new collagen synthesis. Clinically, scar production is heightened, and the wound begins to gain tensile strength.

Edema that persists into the fibroplasia phase is of particular concern to the surgeon and therapist. This edema is likely to become an ongoing problem unless early intervention is applied. The edema fluid becomes more viscous from the elevated protein content, and the excess fluid is called *exudate.*[27] The protein-rich fluid or exudate associated with edema causes fibrosis and thickening of the tissues, with subsequent shortening of structures such as ligaments and tendons. As fibrin is deposited between the structures of the hand, organized adhesions result between structures such as tendon and their sheaths, joint capsules, synovial membranes, and fascial layers.[9,36] Structures will continue to swell, thicken, and shorten, and eventually will be replaced by dense fibrous tissue.[25,46] The greater the edema and the longer it persists, the more extensive the scarring and the resultant pain, adhesions, disfigurement, and disability. All tissues—vessels, nerves, joints, and intrinsic muscles—become involved in a state of reduced nutrition and inelasticity. The combination of persistent edema with immobilization and poor positioning ultimately results in a stiff hand and must be circumvented.

If the lymphatic system becomes blocked or metabolites are allowed to accumulate in the interstitial spaces, colloid osmotic pressure is increased by the relative increase in concentration of proteins, again resulting in a higher capillary net filtration pressure. The coagulating effect of tissue exudates causes the interstitial and lymphatic fluid to clot, preventing the fluid from being expulsed by pressure and resulting in brawny edema in the spaces surrounding the injured cells.[19] Brawny or nonpitting edema can also be caused by swelling of the tissues cells from trauma, disease, or inadequate nutrition.[19]

The final phase of healing is called the *maturation* or *remodeling phase;* it is initiated as fibroplasia subsides. In this stage, tissue remodeling and realignment are achieved by placing tensile stresses on collagen fibers. At this point, persistent, stagnant edema may have led to fibrosis with elevated protein content. Chronic edema will result in stretching of the tissue spaces, necessitating long-term use of continuous compressive garments to prevent recurrence of any gains made in edema reduction. If allowed to progress to the maturation phase, edema will become hard, thick, and brawny as the result of connective tissue infiltration and fibrosis. In the worst scenario, edema compromises arterial flow, causing anoxia and impaired metabolic circulation and cellular nutrition, and necrosis of tissues may ensue.

PREVENTION OF EDEMA

The prevention and treatment of edema are of paramount importance during all phases of management of the injured hand.[20] Measures need to be taken before edema is visible because interstitial fluid volume will increase 30% above normal before detection.[19] According to Brand and Thompson,[6] as much as 50 ml of edema may accumulate in the hand without being noticed "by a busy therapist dealing with a succession of patients." Elevation and compressive bandaging, in addition to use of cold, are helpful techniques for preventing posttraumatic edema.

After surgery or trauma, the extremity should be positioned above the heart as much of the time as possible. If the hand must be immobilized, when possible, it should be positioned in the intrinsic-plus position of flexed metacarpophalangeal (MP) joints (to 70 degrees) and extended interphalangeal (IP) joints to prevent shortening of the MP joint collateral ligaments and IP volar plates because a first web space contracture limiting spread of the thumb can be very disabling. The wrist should be positioned in neutral or slight extension. The first web space also needs to be maintained via thumb abduction and extension. This is particularly true with burn patients, whose wounds will contract as they heal. If the intrinsic-plus position is not feasible, the patient's hand should be positioned in the best approximation and the splint adjusted when feasible.

Dressings after injury or surgery should be bulky and firm, with the fingers separated. Light gauze fluff can be used between fingers and in the palm. Bandaging should be applied uniformly and with even pressure from distal to proximal, using a spiral or figure-of-eight technique. Splints should support the hand and wrist to offer comfortable immobilization, and they should be padded carefully to avoid pressure at bony prominences or over the dorsal venous system.

Cold application may be helpful in limiting edema formation by producing vasoconstriction and reducing metabolic rate and arteriolar blood flow, reducing membrane permeability and capillary infiltration, and providing a counterirritant to pain. However, careful attention to vascular status must be provided when cold packs are used because excessive cooling may result in tissue ischemia and damage. Cold is contraindicated in the presence of arterial compromise or repair. Cold is especially helpful during the initial inflammatory phase and should be used in combination with other principles of edema management, such as elevation and compression. The use of cold modalities will be helpful if properly used and cold packs are arranged so that their weight is not carried on the hand.

Edema in its early stages is reversible. If edema can be controlled early, subsequent scar formation is minimized in comparison with the scar that forms if edema is prolonged and brawny. Postoperative efforts are directed toward minimizing edema and promoting uncomplicated wound healing. Patient education is vital. Beginning with the initial treatment in the hospital or clinic, the patient must be made aware of the factors that can exacerbate or alleviate edema.

ASSESSMENT OF EDEMA

As discussed previously, a significant amount of edema may accumulate in a hand without visible detection.[6] For this reason, the ability to establish and measure changes in edema with standardized and reliable procedures is critical for the effective management of edema.

The volumeter is a standardized tool that allows the therapist to measure hand edema by measuring the amount of water the limb displaces.[5,45] Patients are assessed, if possible, on their initial visit and thereafter checked routinely before and after exercise or use of a modality for changes in hand size from edema. Brand and Thompson[6] recommend the regular use of a volumeter for every postoperative hand.

The concept of the volumeter to measure swelling by water displacement was designed by Dr. Paul Brand and Helen Wood, O.T.R., at the United States Public Health Service Hospital in Louisiana. Waylett-Rendall and Seibly[45] have shown that the volumeter is reliable within ± 10 ml (1%) if successive measures are performed by the same examiner. A subsequent study done by King[23] assessed the effect of water temperature on hand volume during volumetric measurement. Although there was a significant difference in volumes using extreme temperatures (41° versus 113° F), it was found that the use of "cool" (68° F) versus "tepid" (95° F) water does not appear to alter hand volume readings significantly enough to be of concern.[23]

The difference in volume of dominant versus nondominant hands was studied by Van Velze et al.[42] for 263 male laborers. They concluded that, on average, the left nondominant hand was 3.43% smaller (16.9 ml) than the right dominant hand for male laborers.[42]

The effect of exercise of the asymptomatic hand on volumetric and sensory status has been studied by McGough and Surwasky.[26] Their results on 20 subjects suggest that exercise influences volumetric measurements. Specifically, females in the study demonstrated a 3.6% increase in volumetrics immediately after exercise, with a decline in volume at 10 minutes after exercise to 2.4%.[26] The males in the study demonstrated a 5.2% volume increase immediately after exercise, with a decline in volume at 10 minutes after exercise to 5%. McGough and Surwasky[26] encourage further statistical investigation on a larger scale of the role of hand dominance, gender, and age on hand volume.

It is important to follow the standardized procedure for the volumeter and to standardize alternative techniques as

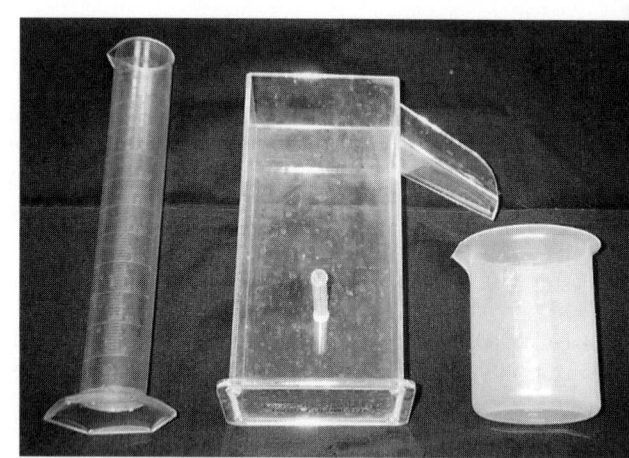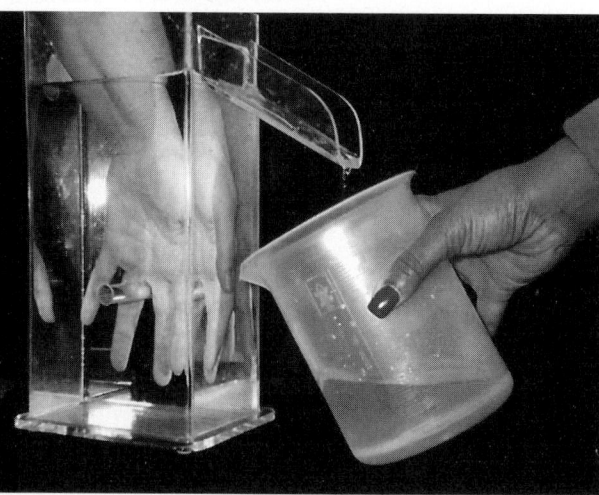

A

B

Fig. 12-3. A, The volumeter, beaker, and graduated cylinder used to collect and measure the amount of water displaced by edematous hand. **B,** The hand placed in pronation inside the volumeter, with the ring and middle fingers straddling the rod and the web space in contact with the bar.

much as possible. Fig. 12-3, *A,* shows the components of the volumetric kit, which includes the volumeter, the 800-ml collection beaker, and the 500-ml graduated cylinder. Fig. 12-3, *B,* shows a patient's hand positioned in the volumeter. Instructions for the standardized procedure to use with the commercially available volumeters accompany each volumeter purchased from equipment companies. The volumeter should be placed on the same level surface for each use. Specific instructions for measurement are as follow[5,21,30,36]:

1. Fill the volumeter with tepid (room temperature) water until water overflows into the beaker. Discard the overflow, and reposition the beaker beneath the volumeter's spout for collection.
2. Remove all jewelry from both upper extremities of the patient.
3. Position the patient with the thumb facing the spout and the forearm in pronation (the palm facing the patient). Any variations from this position should be documented so that future measures can be taken in the same position.
4. While the patient is standing, have him or her slowly immerse the hand into the volumeter until the fingers firmly straddle the rod between the ring and middle fingers and the web space is in contact with the bar. The hand needs to be kept as vertical as possible, avoiding contact with the sides of the volumeter. Water will overflow into the beaker. Maintain this position until water stops spilling from the spout.
5. Pour the water from the beaker into the graduated cylinder and record the volume displaced. If the overflow is greater then 500 ml, it will be necessary to pour the contents from the overflow beaker into the graduated cylinder twice and add the sums together.

When volumetric measures cannot be taken, circumferential measurements of the hand and forearm are an option. Measurements are taken with a tape measure before and after treatment. When only one or two digits are involved, circumferential measurement is more useful because the edema in an individual joint or digit may not be detected by the volumeter. To allow more valid comparison of sequential measurements, anatomic landmarks are used as reference points for placement of the tape.

Edema will fluctuate daily with changes in diet, activity level, water retention, temperature, and time of day. Therefore it is important to measure both the involved and uninvolved extremity for comparison.

TECHNIQUES FOR REDUCTION OF EDEMA

The specific techniques used to promote resolution of edema and their effectiveness vary depending on whether the edema is in the inflammatory, fibroplastic, or maturation phase of wound healing.

Treatment in the inflammatory stage was described earlier and consists primarily of use of cold, compression, elevation, and active motion.

Treatment of edema in the fibroplasia phase should stress AROM and tendon gliding exercises to prevent the development of adhesions, splinting to maintain and increase range of motion (ROM), use of pressure to apply stress to influence collagen fibers via massage, compression garments, and vibration in an effort to soften forming scar and minimize adhesions between developing scar and surrounding tissues.[22] Intermittent compression can be used to facilitate removal of byproducts from the area. Although heat is generally contraindicated with edema, it may be helpful in the fibroblastic repair phase to precondition tight structures, influence extensibility of connective tissues, increase circulation, and provide pain relief before ROM exercises, as long as edema is mild. If heat is used, the extremity needs to be elevated during and monitored before and after heating to assess any increase in swelling that would contraindicate that modality. Moist hot packs, paraffin, and fluidotherapy are all are able to provide superficial heat *in combination with elevation.* Heat is contraindicated in patients who have vascular insufficiency. Massage and active exercise should follow application of heat.

Brawny edema is difficult to influence. In this stage, techniques that increase tissue hydrostatic pressure, such as compressive garments and massage, are indicated. Intermittent compression protocols require longer durations and use of compression garments to prevent recurrence of edema. Developing adhesions and ROM restrictions are more firmly established and difficult to influence because collagen formation and reabsorption slow during the maturation phase. Splinting used to influence tissue remodeling should be applied with low load and for a long duration.

A combination of approaches can be used to treat edema. The following specific approaches are discussed in more detail in the following sections: (1) elevation, (2) active motion, (3) massage, (4) intermittent compression, (5) continuous passive motion (CPM), (6) compressive bandages, (7) string wrapping, and (8) electrical modalities (high volt, NMES).

Elevation

Elevation uses gravity to enhance venous and lymphatic flow out of traumatized areas. Elevation is especially helpful when initiated immediately after surgery. For elevation to be effective, a gentle decline from distal to proximal with the entire limb slightly above the level of the heart should be achieved. In other words, the hand should be slightly higher than wrist, the wrist should be slightly higher than the elbow, and the elbow should be positioned slightly higher than the shoulder. Pillows or wedge supports can be used to position the extremity appropriately at a table or in bed. If arterial systems are compromised or if elevation causes ischemia of the extremity, the level of elevation will need to be altered. When arterial occlusion is diagnosed, the arm should be lowered below the heart. When venous occlusion is diagnosed, the extremity should be elevated.[39]

Precautions must be observed for the replanted arm, hand, or digit. In this case, excessive elevation is to be avoided because it can stress the arterial system. Elevation for the transplanted limb should be at the level of the heart and modified according to the patient's arterial and venous status.[8] Healthy replanted digits are warm and pink. Arterial occlusion may be indicated by a cool, pale digit, whereas venous insufficiency is associated with a dusky hue in the replanted part. The therapist should instruct the patient to make sure that the elbow is not kept in a flexed position because this may create an obstruction to venous drainage.

A sudden increase in edema or an alteration in color or temperature should be reported immediately to the surgeon.[25]

In addition to facilitating venous and lymphatic outflow from the limbs, elevation decreases the hydrostatic pressure in the blood vessels, which in turn decreases the capillary filtration pressure at the arterial end.[43] As discussed previously, hydrostatic pressure occurs in the vascular system because of the weight of blood in the vessels.[15] Peripheral venous and arterial pressures are influenced by gravity. The pressure in any vessel held below heart level is increased by gravity, and the pressure in any vessel held above the level or the heart is decreased by gravity.[15] When the hand is lower than the heart, the intravascular pressure is increased, in turn increasing the capillary filtration pressure.[43] Consequently, interstitial fluid will accumulate in the dependent hand. In contrast, keeping the limb above the level of the heart decreases the intravascular pressure and decreases the capillary filtration pressure.[15]

Active motion

Active exercises create muscle pumping, soft tissue movement, and compression of veins and lymphatic vessels, all of which are helpful in edema control.[3,8,16,38] Strong muscular contractions assist in venous and lymphatic drainage.[38] Active motion prevents stagnation of tissue fluids that can result from lack of use.

Schuind and Burny[35] state that the postcapillary blood pressure facilitating venous return is less than 15 mm Hg, whereas the hydrostatic pressure opposing venous return from the dependent hand is approximately 35 mm Hg. Active movement is required to produce venous return.[35] There are also data supporting the benefits of exercise in enhancing lymph flow and improving resorption.[7,29] However, Mortimer[29] cautions that when treating lymphedema patients, exercise must be neither excessive nor isometric because the resulting increased blood flow will increase the lymph load.

AROM and tendon gliding exercises also help prevent adhesions from developing, especially after surgery. All joints that are not required to be immobilized should be able to move freely in the cast or splint and taken through their full ROM.[2] The therapist should alert the surgeon when a cast inadvertently restricts full motion at uninvolved joints. In particular, casts that are not intended to restrict MP joint motion should be cut back to the level of the distal palmar crease to allow full motion at these joints.

It is important to include the more proximal joints in an ROM program. These joints will become stiff if not taken through their ROM, and active pumping of the proximal muscles will help clear any proximal edema, thus allowing more efficient drainage of distal edema. An effective exercise that incorporates elevation and active motion of the digits and shoulders is to have the patient elevate both arms over the head and make firm fists at least 25 repetitions each hour.[2,25]

Massage

Techniques for massage include retrograde massage, effleurage, and stroking to produce a mild pressure gradient, acting to remove edema from the limb.[7] These techniques may also aid in the removal of lymphatic fluid. Manual massage can increase lymphatic flow, affect intramuscular adhesions, and mobilize tissue fluid.[43] The continuous compression of massage may decrease local interstitial fluid content.[44] Manual edema mobilization, a technique that provides gentle stimulation of the lymphatics to facilitate flow of excessive tissue fluid and protein from an edematous area, is discussed in depth in Chapter 53.

Intermittent compression

Intermittent compression has been shown to be an effective tool for reducing edema, although there is controversy as to the treatment protocols with regard to pressure, duration, and frequency.* The intermittent pressure works by increasing tissue hydrostatic pressure and acceleration of the lymphatic and venous flow via massage.[43] This in turn drives lymphatic fluid back into the venous system. To be effective, the pump pressure must be greater than the 25-mm Hg[18] mean capillary pressure and should not exceed the diastolic blood pressure of the patient. Treatment duration generally ranges between 30 minutes and 2 hours for the patient with acute edema. Separate protocols for pressure and duration exist for the patient with an impaired lymphatic system. For example, Leduc et al.[24] advise that pneumatic compression not exceed 40 mm Hg in these patients. With both populations, the limb should be elevated during treatment, with intermittent compression. The compression/release ratio is usually 3:1 or 4:1.[9] Interestingly, Leduc et al.[24] cite studies that did not demonstrate uptake of proteins by the lymphatic system with compression pumping.

The amount of pressure must be adjusted according to each patient's diagnosis and condition. Acute conditions, such as fractures, begin with a low amount of pressure and are supervised carefully by the therapist. An edematous crushed hand may be placed in the pneumatic appliance as early as the first day after the trauma or surgery. The presence of open wounds does not prohibit intermittent pressure as long as sterile dressings are used. Felt pads can be positioned around pins to prevent pressure on them. More chronic edema will require higher pressures and longer treatment times.

Intermittent compression may be helpful in decreasing edema during the inflammatory phase by facilitating the lymphatic system's ability to reabsorb byproducts and by assisting in the removal of byproducts during the fibroplasia phase.[32]

A number of different models of pneumatic pumps provide compression, including single-chamber and multi-chamber pumps. A multichamber sequential pressure sleeve inflates from distal to proximal and is theoretically more effective at returning fluid to the lymphatics by preventing back flow. One concern with the single-chamber unit is that it may merely redistribute fluid into areas of low hydrostatic pressure and spread the edema over a larger area.[1]

Intermittent compression is contraindicated in patients with infection, deep vein thrombosis, or vascular compromise, or with any patient who has a medical condition such as congestive heart failure, cardiac or renal insufficiency, or pulmonary edema, who may not be able to safely handle the additional fluid load into their circulatory system.

Continuous passive motion

CPM is another method available for the therapist to consider using to reduce hand edema in postoperative patients, especially patients who have undergone surgical release procedures such as tenolysis or capsulectomy. This group of patients may be predisposed to the development of adhesions and hand stiffness. Hand CPM units include parameters that may be set by the therapist to control the specific ROM desired and velocity of movement. Many units include an MP joint block to isolate IP joint motion. CPM is most effective during the early phases of wound healing and early scar formation. CPM in the pain-free range of motion allows for improved gliding, nutrition of tissues, and scar lengthening.[22] CPM may also have a role with patients who have an impaired ability to actively use their hand, such as patients who have hemiplegia secondary to a cerebrovascular accident.[16] Passive ROM will maintain joint mobility in the specified range and can improve lymphatic flow.

Compressive bandages

Various compressive dressings are available commercially. These include Tubigrip stockinet, tubular elastic bandage, finger sleeves, Tubigrip pressure garments, biforme pressure gloves, and Isotoner gloves, among others.[38] Ace wrapping or a self-adherent wrap such as Coban can also be used to provide compression. As with any bandaging, the extremity should be wrapped from distal to proximal to assist with lymphatic and venous drainage, and a spiral or figure-of-eight technique (not circular) should be used.

In the acute stage of wound healing, compression limits the amount of space available for swelling to accumulate.[32] Compression may decrease fibroblast synthesis of collagen by decreasing the blood flow and causing local hypoxia,[44] which is especially important in the fibroplasia phase. Pressure may mechanically force fluid out of the tissue.[44] In the later stages of wound healing, compression maintains

*References 1, 7, 17, 33, 38, 44.

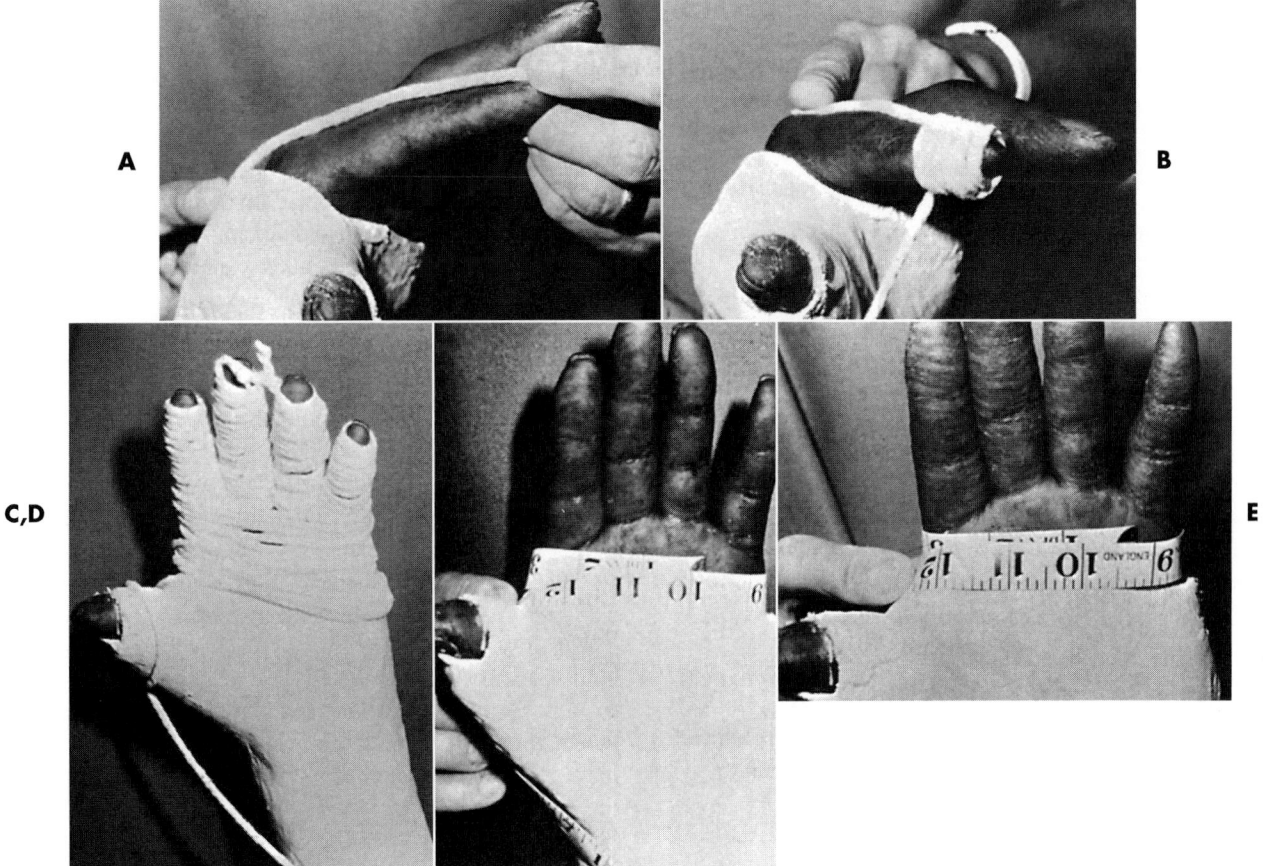

Fig. 12-4. A, String wrapping may be started while the patient is in cast to begin reduction of edema. **B,** Starting at the distal end of the index finger, the cord is wrapped closely and firmly around the finger. **C,** The patient's hand is placed in elevation. The cord remains on the hand for 5 minutes. String wrapping is followed by active fist-making. **D** and **E,** Circumferential measurements taken before and after string wrapping with retrograde massage indicated a decrease in edema.

gains made in edema reduction by reducing capillary filtration. Compressive garments help reinforce tissue hydrostatic pressure and facilitate venous and lymphatic flow. The use of compressive garments or wrapping is especially important with brawny (fibrotic) edema and should always be used following pneumatic pumping to maintain reductions in edema. Compressive garments are contraindicated for patients with arterial compromise, new skin grafts, or unhealed burn wounds.

All forms of external compression need to be monitored by the patient to make sure that capillary flow is not restricted. The patient who is using compression wrapping at home must be instructed to observe for any signs of compromised circulation, such as changes in color, coldness, or numbness in the fingertips.

Self-adherent wrap is an effective way to provide constant, light compression of the digit or hand. A 1-inch tape can be used to wrap the digit. Care must be taken not to apply tension while wrapping because this can restrict circulation. Self-adherent wrap maintains compression while allowing unrestricted motion, and it will not prevent the patient from carrying out the exercise program. With a reliable patient, this offers excellent support and compression to the edematous digit or hand.

String wrapping

String wrapping has been advocated as an easy, inexpensive, and effective means to decrease edema[13] (Fig. 12-4). For this technique, a soft cord is used and is wrapped closely and firmly around the finger, proceeding distally to proximally, with the hand in elevation. After 5 minutes, the cord is removed, and the patient is instructed to make a fist 10 times. The protocol suggested by Flowers[13] includes repeating this treatment three times a day until return flow circulation is restored adequately.

In a study done by Flowers,[13] massage and string wrapping were found to be equally effective in the reduction of edema, whereas a combined approach (using retrograde massage while the string was in place) was found to be more effective than either technique used alone.

Electrical modalities

High-volt pulsed direct current (HVPC) has been hypothesized to decrease edema by reducing microvascular permeability to plasma proteins.[3,4,31,34,40] It is hypothesized that the current reduces edema by repelling negatively charged proteins in the edematous interstitial spaces.[31,40] It is suggested that when the negative polarity of HVPC repels negatively charged cells and protein, a fluid shift occurs.[31] High volt includes intensities greater than 100 volts.

The effect of HVPC in reducing edema has been assessed in experiments with frogs following impact injury and hyperflexion injury.[3,4,41] In these studies, continuous cathodal HVPC was administered at 120 Hz and at voltages 10% lower than those needed to evoke muscle contraction. Significant differences between treated and untreated limbs were evident after the first 30-minute treatment ($p < .01$). Edema formation was curbed for between 4 and 7.5 hours following a single 30-minute administration and gains maintained for 17 hours following the final administration of a series of four 30-minute sessions.[3,4,41] The amplitude used in these studies was set below the threshold required to elicit a muscle contraction in order to separate out the effect of active muscle contraction on edema reduction.

Stralka et al.[40] conducted a study on the use of HVPC in reducing chronic hand edema. In this study, the HVPC was incorporated into a wrist splint. Subjects received twenty 30-minute sessions at the work site over a 35-day period. Posttreatment evaluation showed significant decreases for hand edema and pain, as well as statistically significant decreases in the amount of stimulation required to stimulate the median nerve.

Chu et al.[10] studied the effect of direct current on wound edema after full-thickness burn injury in rats and found that direct electric current had a beneficial effect in reducing wound edema after burn injury. Immediate and continuous application of −40, −4, or +40 µA direct current was applied through silver-nylon dressings. At least 8 hours of treatment was required to achieve a sustained maximum effect. In this study, polarity was also studied. Neither reversal of electrode polarity nor change in current density had any significant effect on the results of treatment.

Griffin et al.[17] compared the effectiveness of a single treatment HVPC, intermittent pneumatic compression, and placebo-HVPC. Differences between the HVPC and placebo-HVPC group approached .036 but did not reach statistical significance ($p = .04$). Reduction in hand edema was significant for the intermittent pneumatic compression group compared with the placebo-HVPC group, at the $p = .01$ level.

Although electrical stimulation may be helpful in decreasing edema in any of the three stages of wound healing, it has been suggested that intensities that produce muscle contractions should be avoided in the inflammatory phase because they may increase clotting time.[32]

Faghri[12] studied the effects of neuromuscular stimulation (NMS)-induced muscle contraction and elevation on hand edema in flaccid cerebrovascular accident patients. He concluded that NMS was more effective for reduction of edema than elevation alone. He suggests that NMS may provide an effective alternative for patients who are unable to effectively use active motion for edema reduction.

All patients who are candidates for electrical modalities must be cleared medically before initiating this type of therapy. The use of electrical modalities is contraindicated in patients who have a pacemaker, cardiac arrhythmias, seizures, myocardial disease, or any other condition that may be adversely affected by current.

SUMMARY

The best treatment of edema is to prevent and minimize occurrence through the use of atraumatic surgical techniques, appropriate postoperative dressings and positioning, judicious and monitored use of cold, comfortable elevation, and early motion when possible. If edema persists, various approaches may be considered and should be used in combination whenever helpful to enhance arterial systems, venous return, and lymphatic flow. Control of edema is essential to optimize the benefits of therapy and, ultimately, hand function.

REFERENCES

1. Ause-Ellias KL, et al: The effect of mechanical compression on chronic hand edema after burn injury: a preliminary report, *J Burn Care Rehabil* 15:29, 1994.
2. Beasley RW: Vascular injuries. In Beasley RW, editor: *Hand injuries,* Philadelphia, 1981, WB Saunders.
3. Bettany JA, Fish DR, Mendel FC: Influence of high voltage pulsed direct current on edema formation following impact injury, *Phys Ther* 70:219, 1990.
4. Bettany JA, Fish DR, Mendel FC: The effect of high voltage pulsed direct current on edema formation following hyperflexion injury, *Arch Phys Med Rehabil* 71:677, 1990.
5. Brand PW: Methods of clinical measurement of the hand. In Brand PW, Hollister A, editors: *Clinical mechanics of the hand,* ed 2, St Louis, 1993, Mosby.
6. Brand PW, Thompson DE: Mechanical resistance. In Brand PW, Hollister A, editors: *Clinical mechanics of the hand,* ed 2, St Louis, 1993, Mosby.
7. Brennan MJ, Miller LT: Overview of treatment options and review of the current role and use of compression garments, intermittent pumps, and exercise management of lymphedema, *Cancer* 15:83(12 suppl Am):2812, 1998.
8. Buncke HJ, et al: Surgical and rehabilitative aspects of replantation and revascularization of the hand. In Hunter JM, Schneider LH, Mackin EJ, Callahan AD, editors: *Rehabilitation of the hand: surgery and therapy,* ed 4, St Louis, 1995, Mosby.
9. Bunnell S: Bunnell's *surgery of the hand,* Philadelphia, 1970, JB Lippincott.
10. Chu CS, et al: Direct current reduces wound edema after full-thickness burn injury in rats, *J Trauma* 40:738, 1996.
11. Daane S, Poltoratszy P, Rockwell WB: Postmastectomy lymphedema management: evaluation of the complex decongestive therapy technique, *Ann Plast Surg* 40:128, 1998.

12. Faghri PD: The effects of neuromuscular stimulation-induced muscle contraction versus elevation on hand edema in CVA patients, *J Hand Ther* 10:29, 1997.

13. Flowers K: String wrapping versus massage for reducing digital volume, *J Hand Surg* 10A:583, 1985.

14. Flowers KR: Edema: differential management based on the stages of wound healing. In Hunter JM, Schneider LH, Mackin EJ, Callahan AD, editors: *Rehabilitation of the hand: surgery and therapy,* ed 4, St Louis, 1995, Mosby.

15. Ganong WF: The general & cellular basis of medical physiology. In Ganong WF, editor: *Review of medical physiology,* ed 20, Stamford, Conn, 2001, Appleton & Lange.

16. Giudice ML: Effects of Continuous passive motion and elevation on hand edema, *Am J Occup Ther* 44:914, 1990.

17. Griffin JW, et al: Reduction of chronic posttraumatic hand edema: a comparison of high voltage pulsed current, intermittent pneumatic compression and placebo treatments, *Phys Ther* 70:279, 1990.

18. Guyton AC: Capillary fluid exchange, interstitial fluid dynamics, and lymph flow. In Guyton AC, Hall JE, editors: *Human physiology and mechanism of disease,* ed 6, Philadelphia, 1997, WB Sanders.

19. Guyton AC, Hall JE: *Textbook of medical physiology,* ed 10, Philadelphia, 2000, WB Saunders.

20. Hunter JM: Salvage of the burned hand, *Surg Clin North Am* 47:1060, 1967.

21. Jaffe R, Farney-Mokris S: Edema. In Casanova JS, editor: *Clinical assessment recommendations,* ed 2, Chicago, 1992, ASHT.

22. King JW: Traumatic injuries of the hand. In Stanley BG, Tribuzi SM, editors: *Concepts in hand rehabilitation,* Philadelphia, 1992, FA Davis.

23. King TI II: The effect of water temperature on hand volume during volumetric measurement using the water displacement method, *J Hand Ther* 6:202, 1993.

24. Leduc O, et al: The physical treatment of upper limb edema, *Cancer* 15(12 suppl Am):2835, 1998.

25. Mackin EJ: Prevention of complications in hand therapy. In *Complications of hand surgery, hand clinics,* 2:429, 1986.

26. McGough CE, Surwasky ML: Effect of exercise on volumetric and sensory status of the asymptomatic hand, *J Hand Ther* 4:177, 1991.

27. Michlovitch SL: *Thermal agents in rehabilitation,* ed 3, Philadelphia, 1996, FA Davis.

28. Moberg E: Shoulder-hand finger syndrome, *Surg Clin North Am,* 40:365, 1960.

29. Mortimer PS: Therapy approaches for lymphedema, *Angiology* 48:87, 1997.

30. NC Medical: Hand volumeter for measuring edema by fluid displacement, Directions for use (instruction sheet, not dated).

31. Newton R: High-voltage pulsed current: theoretical bases and clinical application. In Nelson RM, Currier DP, editors: *Clinical electrotherapy,* ed 2, Norwalk, Conn, 1991, Appleton & Lange.

32. Prentice WE: Guidelines for using therapeutic modalities in rehabilitation. In Prentice WE, editor: *Therapeutic modalities in sports medicine,* ed 3, St Louis, 1994, Mosby.

33. Ramesh M, et al: Effectiveness of the A-V impulse hand pump, *J Bone Joint Surg* 81B:229, 1999.

34. Reed BV: Effect of high voltage pulsed electronical stimulation on microvascular permeability to plasma proteins, a possible mechanism in minimizing edema, *Phys Ther* 68:491, 1988.

35. Schuind F, Burny F: Can algodystrophy be prevented after hand surgery? *Hand Clin* 13:455, 1997.

36. Schultz-Johnson K: *Volumetrics: a literature review,* Santa Monica, Calif, 1988, Upper Extremity Technology.

37. Smith KL: Wound healing. In Hunter JM, Schneider LH, Mackin EJ, Callahan AD, editors: *Rehabilitation of the hand: surgery and therapy,* ed 4, St Louis, 1995, Mosby.

38. Sorenson MK: The edematous hand, *Phys Ther* 69:1059, 1989.

39. Steichen JB, Idler RS: Surgical aspects of replantation and revascularization. In Hunter JM, Schneider LH, Mackin EJ, Callahan AD, editors, *Rehabilitation of the hand: surgery and therapy,* ed 3, St Louis, 1990, Mosby.

40. Stralka SW, Jackson JA, Lewis AR: A randomized clinical trial of high voltage pulsed, direct current built into a Wrist Splint, *AAOHN J.* 46:233, 1998.

41. Taylor K, e al: Effect of a single 30-minute treatment of high voltage pulsed current on edema formation in frog hind limbs, *Phys Ther* 72:63, 1992.

42. Van Velze CA, et al: The difference in volume of dominant and nondominant hand, *J Hand Ther* 4:6 1991.

43. Vasudevan SV, Melvin JL: Upper extremity edema control: rationale of the techniques, *Am J Occup Ther* 33:520, 1979.

44. Walsh M, Muntzer E: Wound management. In Stanley BG, Tribuzi SM, editors: *Concepts in hand rehabilitation,* Philadelphia, 1992, FA Davis.

45. Waylet-Rendall J, Seibly D: A study of the accuracy of a commercially available volumeter, *J Hand Ther* 4:10, 1991.

46. Weeks P, Wray RC: Management of the stiff hand. In Weeks PM, editor: *Management of acute hand injuries,* St Louis, 1978, Mosby.

Chapter 13

SENSIBILITY TESTING WITH THE SEMMES-WEINSTEIN MONOFILAMENTS

Judith A. Bell-Krotoski

The Semmes-Weinstein monofilament form of testing provides information that is not duplicated by any other test, adds insight into the physiology of the peripheral nerve system, and quantifies abnormality.[59] When calibrated correctly, it is one of the few, if not the only, sensibility measurement instruments that approaches requirements for an objective test.[2,3,8,72,75] This chapter is a summary of what is fact or fiction, what is known and not known regarding monofilament testing, and what is necessary in technique to produce an accurate measurement of sensibility.

The first edition of *Rehabilitation of the Hand* was intended to record technique for education in hand therapy as correlated with surgery. In this fifth edition, it is rewarding to be able to reference excellent studies that have been done with the monofilaments in various applications that advance our knowledge base for patient treatment.[29,33-35,39,58,61,65,75]

MYTHS AND TRUTHS

Many fascinating studies of cutaneous sensibility have been executed since the age of Aristotle.* Each offers insight into the many facets of sensory function and what has and has not been attempted in its measurement. All articles list a bibliography of referenced information sources. By reading these references and the studies they in turn reference, one comes into direct contact with the original sources of information. It is often surprising to find that one's personal interpretation of the original study is quite different

from the interpretation of the study by another author. Serious researchers need to obtain original reports that often are more comprehensive and important to understanding than later reviews. A review of only the last 10 years can be misleading.

Neurophysiologists are still trying to isolate the components of "normal" sensibility, and much is yet unknown.[19,21,35] Quite naturally, the neurophysiologist is interested in "normal" sensory function, and his or her test requirements are adjusted accordingly for normal detection thresholds.[41,49,51] The clinician is interested in abnormal thresholds as they compare with normal and needs a test that can clearly define when a subject has dropped off from a normal baseline.* Abnormal thresholds are referenced against normal detection threshold values so that degrees of loss can be determined accurately and monitored for improvement or worsening with treatment.[52,60,62,63]

Simplicity

The monofilament test is simple to perform accurately. It provides an absolute numerical and pictorial record for serial measurements of the same patient, or across patients, for comparison with treatment. The monofilaments can be used in a 10-minute screen at predetermined sites, for limited mapping such as a specific digital nerve area, or for a full mapping to show clearly the relative relationship of an abnormal nerve versus other areas of response. The test's versatility is one of its strengths.

*References 9, 18, 20, 37, 59, 69, 71.

*References 24, 28, 43, 44, 49, 51.

Application

The monofilament test, described in this chapter as used in the hand and upper extremity, has great value in providing similar screening and mapping all over the body.* Even on the face, where sensitivities far exceed that of the hand, areas of abnormality can be accurately mapped. Only in the plantar area of the foot, which often has degrees of callus, is some allowance needed in the interpretation of higher detection thresholds.

Sensitivity

Semmes et al[59] and Weinstein[73,75] used the lightest monofilaments in the test for discrimination of detection areas with normal subjects. For test comparison within normal subjects, different scales of interpretation than those presented here (i.e., between men and women, left and right hands, age groups, and so on) are needed to address finite differences found within normal subjects.[27,66] However, the intent of the monofilament test in evaluating clinical subjects is to identify abnormal subjects and when patients first fall off from a normal baseline (for both males and females).[29] To identify abnormal subjects from those who fall "within normal limits," one scale of interpretation has been determined based on known threshold detection values and patient "functional discrimination and recognition."[1,3,70,77] This interpretation scale, described in this chapter, is used for the hand, arm, shoulder, and rest of the body.

Instrument reliability

An instrument has to be shown to have instrument reliability before it can be considered valid and used in clinical studies. The repeatability of an instrument is related to its validity. If an instrument is shown not to be repeatable (i.e., in its strength of application), then its validity is nonexistent. One cannot use human performance alone to prove reliability of an instrument that measures in units defined by the National Institute of Standards and Technology (NIST).

The monofilaments clearly have been shown to be accurate and repeatable as an instrument if calibrated correctly, and they have the unique ability to dampen the vibration of the examiner's hand that occurs with hand-applied devices that do not control for this vibration.[4,7,11]

It is true that some closeness in force of application is produced by the monofilaments in the long kit and occasions may occur when forces overlap. This simply means that not all the monofilaments available for testing need to be used. For the sake of time, it is more expedient to use those monofilaments determined most critical for identification of "normal versus abnormal" and changes in "functional discrimination and recognition." This is why certain monofilaments are specifically selected for the mini-kit, and in most cases, these are all that is needed for screen-ing or full mapping of sensibility. The forces of application of the monofilaments in the minikit never overlap; thus the minikit is actually more sensitive as an instrument than the long kit. The long kit does include additional monofilaments needed for testing within normal subjects. In normative studies, inclusion of the lighter above-threshold monofilaments is critical for accurate measurement.

That the monofilaments have instrument reliability if calibrated correctly does not mean there is no room for improvement. The Weinstein Enhanced Sensory Test (WEST) was developed as an improved instrument.[72] Following review and discussion regarding the minikit filaments and a prototype set that placed the minikit monofilaments in one holder, Weinstein, one of the original authors of the Semmes-Weinstein monofilament test, added nonslip coating and a rounded tip, less fragile handle and certified the monofilament force of application. Because the changes in the WEST monofilaments are potentially different enough in stimulus to affect threshold detection, exact comparisons cannot yet be drawn between the WEST and the original Semmes-Weinstein. Although the instruments are very close in stimulus, additional clinical testing in patients will direct whether interpretation scales need be adjusted for the WEST.

Other versions of the Semmes-Weinstein monofilaments have been designed.[6,14,42] Most of these keep the original 90-degree angle of the filament to the rod and 38-mm length of the monofilament and include monofilaments of standard diameter. In particular, instrument versions in other handles have been made available for overseas testing in countries where cost is often a deciding factor in the availability of instruments and equipment. The application technique has been found to be important in ensuring accuracy of any form of the Semmes-Weinstein monofilament test.[7,11,67]

Validity

When calibrated and applied correctly, the monofilaments are a valid test for testing sensibility detection thresholds. Studies have clearly demonstrated their ability to accurately detect the clinical condition intended.* Used in standard protocols, the monofilament test is being used to compare patient data in multicenter studies and is providing information regarding peripheral nerve changes with treatment not previously available with less sensitive and uncontrolled instruments.[39,65]

Normative studies

Normative studies were originally conducted by Semmes and Weinstein.[59,73,75] Weinstein has published extensively on the monofilaments over a 50-year period. More recent normative studies have been made and are available for reference, but these only confirm the original normative thresholds defined by Weinstein with current instruments.[8a]

*References 12, 31, 54, 56, 57, 68, 71.

*References 12, 26, 30, 38, 40, 47.

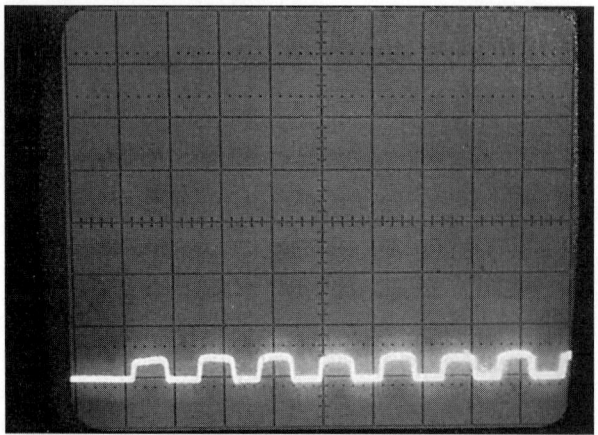

Fig. 13-1. Oscilloscope screen showing force on repeat application of the 2.83 (marking number) "within normal limits" Semmes-Weinstein monofilament (250 mg/division). The instrument applications force is repeatable within a small range if the lengths and diameters of the monofilament are correct.

Newer instruments need review and clinical trials as well as comparison with results from currently available touch-detection threshold instruments.

Calibration

The force of application the monofilaments produce is related to their diameter size and length. Monofilaments, sized according to their diameter, if of the same length, will be repeatable in force of application within a very small range, usually within milligrams[4,7] (Fig. 13-1). By comparison, peripheral nerves that are clinically acute and changing increase or decrease in their threshold detection by several grams, and changes in nerve function and the improvement or worsening direction of change are detected and documented quite easily. Very small changes in force of application would not be expected to significantly affect threshold of detection. However, testing should be as controlled and repeatable as possible if results are to be considered reliable. Clinicians either need to request calibration information on test kits they use or measure the calibration, particularly for reports on patient studies.

Unfortunately, the readily available top-loading balances can be inaccurate for measurement of monofilament force of application because the scales depend on a spring mechanism for measurement.[4,7] Because the monofilament is elastic (one of its desired physical properties), it is opposed by the spring mechanism, and the balance readout is variable. If a top-loading instrument such as a Metlar is all that is available for measurement, some estimate of its force of application can be made. However, these should not be used to adjust the application force of a given filament because the result may be to make changes that make the instrument out of standard with other instruments used for

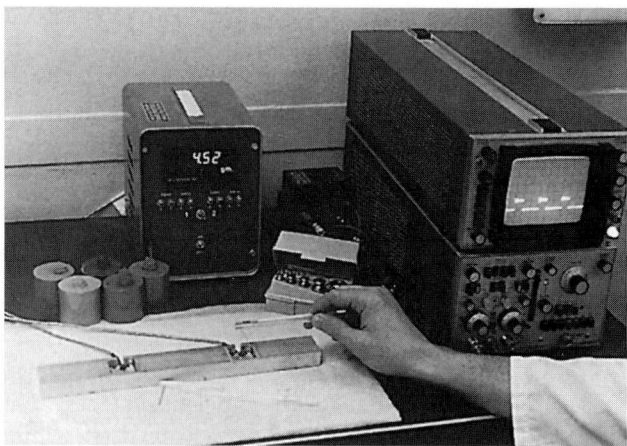

Fig. 13-2. Sensory instrument measurement system.

patient comparison. If measured on a top-loading balance-type scale, a monofilament should not be hand applied, but rather should be mounted in a test tube holder and brought down to where it bends in contact with the scale for a reading. The scale should be allowed to accommodate for the elasticity of the monofilament. This can be reasonably accomplished by waiting a few seconds and then taking the measurement at the same point in time for each measurement.

Accurate measurement of the dynamic force of the monofilaments requires instrumentation that can measure their force dynamics exactly. Special instrumentation was created for this purpose in earlier measurements. Bell and Buford developed measurement instrumentation sensitive enough to measure the dynamic force of application of the monofilaments[4,7,10,11] (Fig. 13-2). The signature of a monofilament repeatedly applied can be measured and examined for spikes in force, vibration of the tester's hand, or subthreshold application. In more recent sensory instrument testing, researchers have developed an instrument measuring system using commercially available force transducers and a custom program to measure the force output (developed in Labview, National Instruments, Austin, Texas). Newer measurement systems include a direct reading into a computer program for analysis.

Test selection

It is not uncommon to find that in the area of sensibility testing, authors and clinicians champion one or more methods of sensibility testing.[14,16,17,23,52] Often, this is based on tradition, on what seems to be most popular, or on opinion that has been raised about a particular test. Sensory function is complicated, and depending on the question, one may need more than one test to obtain an adequate picture of abnormality.

One real criticism of most instruments for measuring sensibility is their lack of control on applied stimulus, which the monofilaments do have by virtue of their elastic property and ability to accommodate some of the normal and variable vibration of the examiner's hand (which often exceeds the resolution for normal touch detection threshold). The elasticity of the monofilament and its bending at a specific force means the force it can apply is limited. Without this elasticity, any application by any probe instrument far exceeds the resolution of normal touch detection threshold and widely varies from a few milligrams in one application to over several grams or several hundred grams in another. This is because there is no limit on the force and no control on variables such as vibration.

Computerized instruments

Several computerized instruments that can reproduce part of the monofilament touch-threshold stimulus available range have been developed, and some of these are becoming commercially available.[14,17,32,42] It should be recognized that computerized instruments have the same limitations as handheld instruments if their stimulus is hand applied. The best of the computerized instruments is designed to automatically apply and control the stimulus and has a built-in limit on how much force is applied.[34,41] In instruments that still depend on a hand application of the stimulus, some improved control is possible with the accompanying direct feedback of measured force (or pressure) output, but in measurements in our laboratory, it was impossible for any instrument to have sufficient control on force of application if the testing probe was hand applied.

In addition, force measurement systems must be carefully examined for sensitivity. It is rare that one is accurate to less than 1 g. In fact, testing of strain gauges reported in literature to be accurate for less than 1 g found they often were not. The measurement system needs to be shown not to just average or electronically filter and smooth signals because averaging can hide peaks of higher force and the hand-applied vibration to which the patient would most certainly respond. It is common for computerized instruments to filter and average signals; some filtering of external "noise" such as the frequency produced by lights in a measurement area is even required. Instruments reported to be accurate need to have their forces and range of forces measured, and these measurements need to be available along with instrument specifications for any instrument sold for clinical testing of patients.

One of the biggest criticisms of the computerized instruments for threshold detection is that they have yet to produce, in one stimulus probe of a single diameter, the full range of application forces available in the Semmes-Weinstein monofilament set.[20,21] Interestingly, proponents of computerized instruments argue that the computerized stimulus is better because it does not change for area.[17] The area would change if the stimulus was designed to measure greater levels of sensory loss as needed to define "loss of protective sensation." Computerized instruments are primarily designed to assess light touch thresholds and do not yet offer a test to determine "protective sensation" threshold. Certainly, when it comes to sensory abnormality and function discrimination or recognition, whether or not protective sensation is present is a defining factor needed for patient treatment because it determines if the patient is still relatively safe with sharp or hot objects, or conversely, in danger of wounds and amputations from complications of burns and injuries that could be incurred through use of everyday objects.[1,20,52,70]

Undoubtedly, computerized instruments with sufficient control and range eventually will be available and add to our understanding of sensibility and abnormality. They also may help us define and adjust what is needed for an optimal touch-threshold test and have more application in research laboratories than in clinical settings. Once optimal stimulus and control are defined, the real challenge is to make this a readily available practical instrument at a reasonable cost so that it can be widely used for patient testing. To this end, the monofilaments have so far remained a valuable test with relative control and practicality and may eventually be found to be as accurate in needed sensitivity and accuracy and more desirable for practicality and portability than a more expensive computerized battery-dependent instrument.

Because of the large differences in sensibility testing instruments and techniques, practitioners wanting to develop an objective sensibility testing technique cannot escape the need to critique references and instruments for their merits and limitations. An instrument is not accurate or inaccurate just because it is said to be so; rigorous studies and measurements have to be conducted and published. Clinicians should treat as fact only what can be clearly proven as fact; all else should be treated as conjecture and opinion. In this way, advances in sensibility testing can be made that will help put to rest some of the myths perpetuated in testing and prevent a very good test like the Semmes-Weinstein monofilament test from not being used just because it is not recommended by some experienced examiners who champion another form of testing.

Comparison trials

Most research that criticizes monofilaments does so without actual direct comparison to the monofilament test in terms of results. Studies that do compare another instrument to the monofilament testing are not always done in a protocol that would stand up to requirements for a fair comparison and also ignore unique aspects of the monofilament test. One must be wary of instrument studies that use only two examiners, particularly those that use the study to support their conclusion for another form of testing.[55] It is easy to find agreement between two examiners, whereas the addition of a third examiner can adversely change the level of interrater reliability. To determine the relative control and validity of another instrument with the monofilaments, a comparison study requires a valid protocol with direct comparison instrument stimulus. Confirmation of results by independent examiners is preferable before judgments are made regarding the relative validity or usefulness of one test versus another.

End-organ specificity

Attempts have been made to divide clinical testing instruments into those that test slowly versus quickly adapting end organs, referencing the monofilaments as only testing slowly adapting fibers.[15,53] However, in any given skin area of 10 mm^2, there are close to 3000 sensory end organs.[25,64] Given the stimulus variability in application force of most instruments used for testing sensibility it would seem impossible to selectively stimulate slowly versus quickly adapting fibers.

Although in a laboratory situation some end organs can be shown to be rapidly adapting in response to a stimulus and other end organs to be slowly adapting, such laboratory testing requires highly sophisticated instrumentation and measures end organ response under extreme control and artificial circumstances. Any clinical sensibility testing instrument would have to be much more controlled before it could possibly duplicate the testing of a controlled laboratory setting. In addition, neurophysiologists tell us that still other nerve fibers respond in between the quickly or slowly adapting and possibly act as moderators of the other two types. Still to be determined is their role in response to a stimulus and how all the nerve fibers are interpreted at the central cortex level; certainly instruments with variable application force cannot accomplish this.

The application force frequency of the monofilaments has been examined in a laboratory setting with and without strict control. The findings suggest that they cannot, even with the best of control, stimulate only one fiber population (slowly or rapidly adapting fibers).[7,11] The monofilaments were applied to a strain gauge that could measure both the frequency of their application signal and their force of application (Fig. 13-3). Frequency signals were detected throughout the available frequency spectrum at both low and high frequency. End organs are known to respond at certain defined levels of low or high frequencies. All instruments tested produced low and high frequency signals of sufficient strength to stimulate all end organs. It makes sense clinically that both rapidly and slowly adapting end organs are stimulated in the monofilament test, in that a patient will respond quickly with initial application of the stimulus. A slow enough monofilament application that does not appear to excite the rapidly adapting end organs is harder for a patient to perceive.

Thus arguments that the monofilament test should not be used because it stimulates only the slowly adapting end

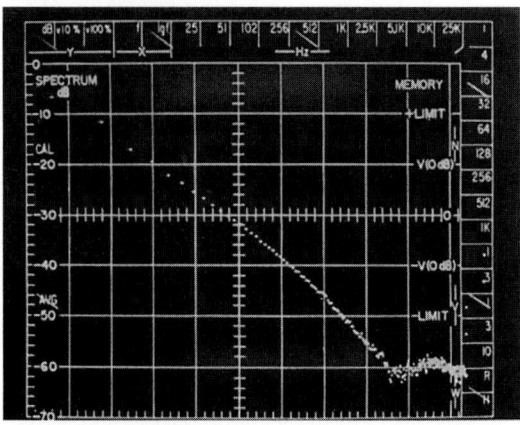

Fig. 13-3. On an expanded scale is shown the force spectral content of a 4.17 (marking number) Semmes-Weinstein monofilament applied 16 times and averaged. The horizontal axis spans 1 to 512 Hz (cycles per second). The vertical axis is in decibels referenced to 5 g (OdB) on the left (at 100 Hz the signal is 50 dB below 5 g, which is 15.8 mg). The energy from the instrument application occurs throughout a broad frequency spectrum (both low and high) sufficient enough to stimulate both slowly and rapidly adapting end organs.

organs are without merit. However, regardless of whether the monofilament test measures slowly or rapidly adapting end organs, what is most important is that it is clinically reliable as an instrument and valid in identifying the abnormal condition it is intended to measure.

Force versus pressure

Monofilaments have been reported in "force" values to understand relative differences in their weight (applied to the skin during application). Force is easier to understand in ordinal rank than pressure. Pressure is force divided by area. Because pressure values can change by changing the area measured, they can be misleading. Both pressure and force are units of measurement and do not change the stimulus applied, only the way it is reported. However, at least two areas of variability exist in accurate reporting of pressure measurements of the monofilament as applied to the skin:

1. When a monofilament is bent against the skin, the full area of the monofilament tip does not always come into full contact with the skin, but rather with a crescent-shaped edge. For an accurate calculation of the pressure applied with a filament of a particular force, one would have to calculate the area of the crescent-shaped edge that comes in contact with the skin and divide this into the force. This is not practical if even possible.
2. The area of application of a monofilament applied to the skin can and does change with clinical situations. Soft pliable skin may fully accommodate the whole area of the filament tip, whereas hard, inelastic skin that occurs with callus and scar may not. The area of

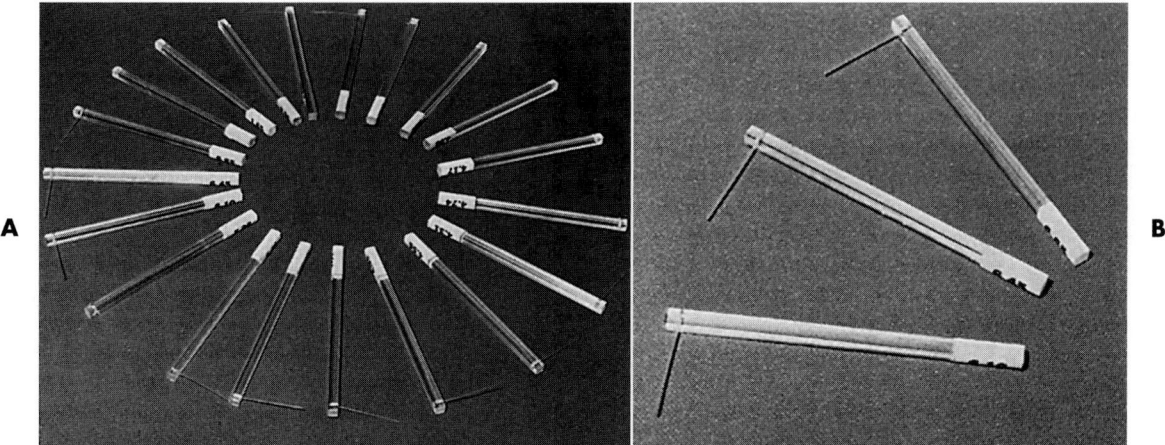

Fig. 13-4. A, Semmes-Weinstein Anesthesiometer monofilament testing set. **B,** Close-up view of filaments.

Table 13-1. Interpretation scale for monofilaments

		Filament markings*	Calculated force (g)
Green	Normal	1.65-**2.83**	0.0045-0.068
Blue	Diminished light touch	3.22-**3.61**	0.166-0.408
Purple	Diminished protective sensation	3.84-**4.31**	0.697-2.06
Red	Loss of protective sensation	**4.56-6.65**	3.63-447
Red-lined	Untestable	>6.65	>447

Force data from Semmes J, Weinstein S: *Somatosensory changes after penetrating brain wounds in man,* Cambridge, Mass, 1960, Harvard University Press.
*Minikit monofilaments are in bold.[59] Descriptive levels based on other scales of interpretation and collapse of data from 200 patient tests.[1,70]

a given sized monofilament is constant. It is no more accurate to report the monofilament application in pressure than it is to report it in force, and it is less accurate to report the stimulus in pressure because of the possibilities for inaccuracy induced by variable contact. The monofilaments are reported in force along with their area for each size monofilament. Their relative pressure can be calculated simply by dividing the force by the area.

Full spectrum

The monofilament test is capable of measuring a range of responses, for example, from "within normal limits" to "diminished light touch," to "diminished protective sensation" to "loss of protective sensation" and detection of any residual sensibility that may still be responsive to treatment.

Instrument specifications

Although the marking numbers of the monofilaments are related to a log scale of the force, they are used primarily as index numbers for ordering and for identification of filaments included in sets. Conversion tables specify the relative force for interpretation (Fig. 13-4, Table 13-1).

Cost

Monofilaments are relatively inexpensive and can be made available to national and international treatment programs for standard measurement and comparison. However, one should keep in mind that realities of the business side of medicine may cause financial considerations to drive opinion more than the accuracy and practical value of the instrument. So long as clinicians continue to buy inaccurate instruments, they will continue to be sold and their accuracy potentially exaggerated. As the demand for monofilaments grows, more and more companies will make them available. Clinicians need to critically evaluate instruments they use, ask for measurement specifications, and return inaccurate instruments for replacement.

Nerve conduction velocity

Tests of nerve conduction velocity are recommended along with the Semmes-Weinstein monofilament test where available.[23] Nerve conduction tests depend greatly on examiner technique and other variables. The test can vary according to the time of day, temperature of the extremity, size of the electrodes, placement of the electrodes, and individual testing instrument. Used with other tests of sensibility, the test can be of great help in determining the

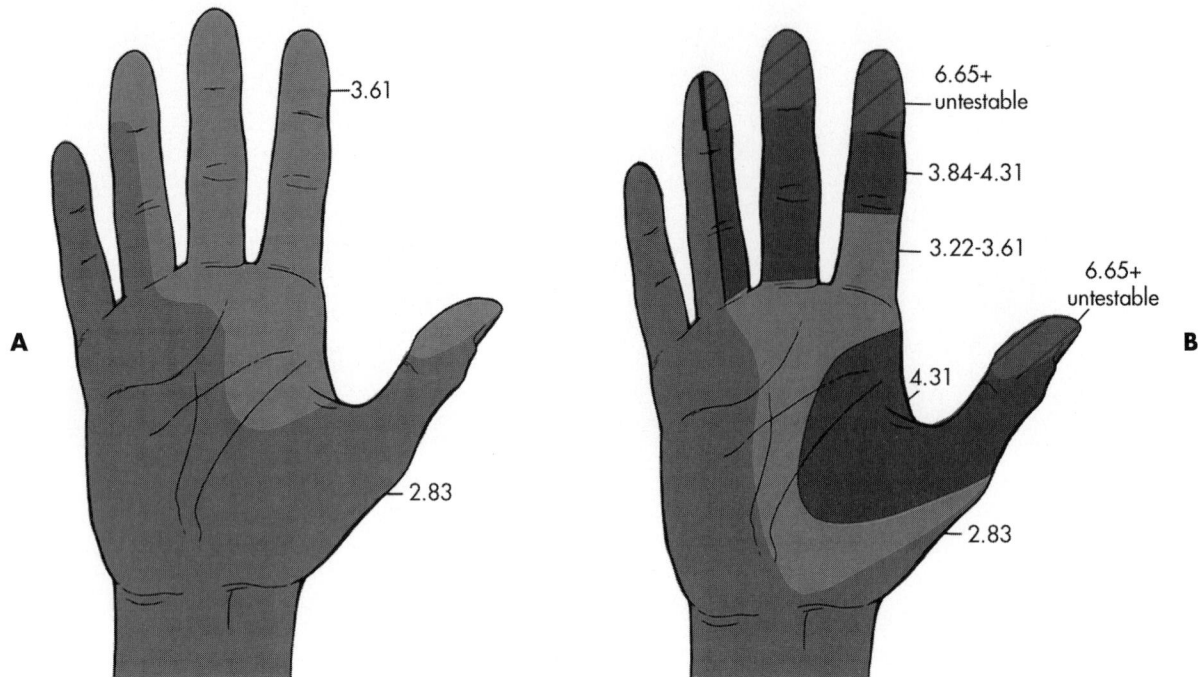

Fig. 13-5. A, Monofilament mapping showing a median nerve compression as measured in a woman with a history of numbness for 2 years and no corrective intervention. **B,** Same patient as measured 4 months later. Touch-pressure recognition has become worse from diminished light touch to untestable with monofilaments.

location of nerve injury and in numerically quantifying and documenting nerve problems. It is important to realize that the test in no way can determine what a patient does and does not feel. Attempts to directly correlate nerve conduction with diminished functional cutaneous sensation have been largely unsuccessful. Both nerve conduction tests and cutaneous sensibility tests appear to be needed to adequately clinically classify and monitor peripheral nerve function. Usually, the tests will correlate for evidence of involvement or noninvolvement of a nerve. However, exceptions are found. I have found cases in which nerve conduction was "absent" when some Semmes-Weinstein monofilaments could still be felt. In less frequent instances, cases have been seen in which the monofilaments have been "within normal limits" and a nerve shows a "slowed" nerve conduction response.

ADVANTAGES OF MONOFILAMENT TESTING

Advantages of monofilament testing include that the filaments bend when the peak-force threshold has been achieved and that a relatively consistent force is continued by the filaments until they are either removed from the skin contact or are severely curved. When they are severely curved, the force on the skin is less than the desired threshold. In addition to controlling the force of application, the filament design attempts to control the velocity of application. If applied too quickly, the filament force will

exceed the desired threshold. Otherwise, the bending of the filament minimizes the vibration of the examiner's hand.

A minikit set containing a normal threshold filament and the heaviest filament for each functional level was developed in 1977. This kit greatly reduces testing time. The instrument can be used for screening at selected sites or full mapping.

Color coding of the filament force produces a mapping that provides the examiner with differential thresholds of touch in areas of normal or relatively normal sensibility and areas of diminution. If the application technique is consistent, the mappings produced can be serially compared for changes in neural status. The mappings can be predictors of the rate of neural return or diminution. They can be predictors as well of the quality of neural return, or severity of diminution (Figs. 13-5 to 13-7 and Plates 24 to 26). Attempts to correlate increasing or decreasing touch thresholds with levels of patient function appear superior to that associated with many other forms of testing. Used in combination with other clinical tests of sensory function, particularly a test of sensory nerve conduction, the monofilament test can lead to the resolution of patient problems not resolved by other forms of testing and can clarify other test results. The monofilaments are increasingly used by neurophysiologists in studies to determine end-organ response. Like the other tests of sensibility, they could be made more objective through careful consideration of their physical properties.

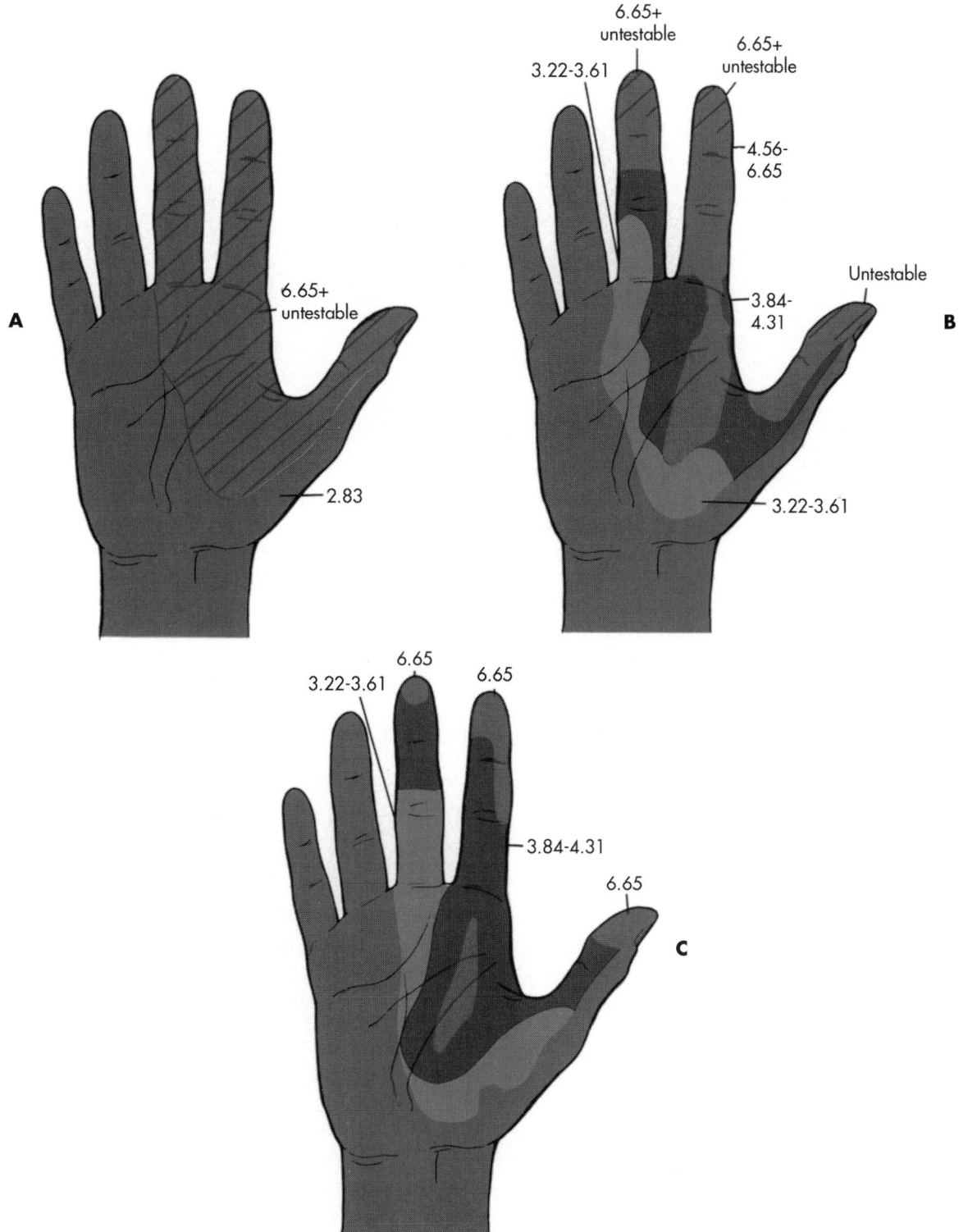

Fig. 13-6. A, Monofilament mapping showing a median nerve laceration before surgery. Two-point untestable. **B,** Same patient 3 months after surgery. Two-point untestable. **C,** Same patient 7 months after surgery. Two-point untestable, fingertips now testable with monofilaments.

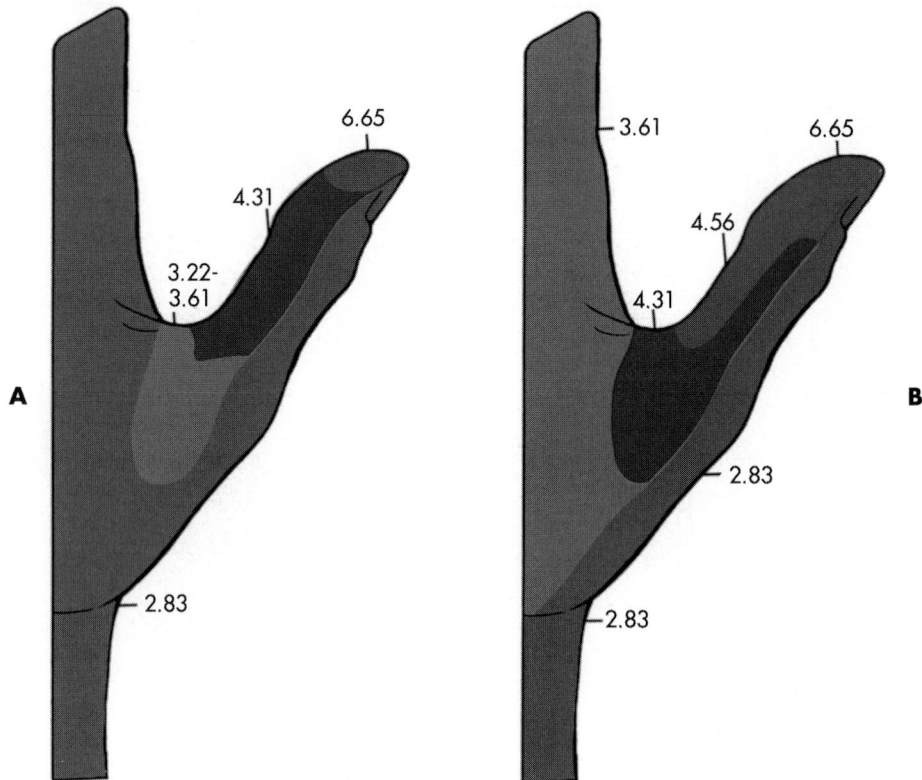

Fig. 13-7. A, Two years after incomplete amputation of right thumb. Digital nerves were not resutured. Small centimeter pedicle of dorsal skin was intact. **B,** Same patient after injection of lidocaine around median nerve to determine whether innervation was radial nerve or median. Notice that although the volar thumb sensation was downgraded, it and the palmar area of the median nerve did not become asensory. This finding brings into question the blocking of the contralateral nerve in testing. Such blocks may be incomplete and lead to false conclusions.

CURRENT SEMMES-WEINSTEIN DESIGN

Although von Frey[69] was the inventor of the monofilament form of testing, the currently available testing sets are not identical to the test instrument he described. Von Frey was interested in normal physiology, and the hairs did not provide the full spectrum of forces needed for measuring levels of functional loss, as do the Semmes-Weinstein monofilaments.

The current testing instrument was developed by Semmes and Weinstein and is described in their book *Somatosensory Changes After Penetrating Brain Wounds in Man.*[25,59] Semmes and Weinstein desired a measure that would be applicable over a wider range of intensities than von Frey's and one that would provide a progressive force scale. The investigators attempted to show that with their filaments, which increase in diameter to exert increased forces, the common logarithm of the force increases in an approximately linear fashion with the ordinal rank of the filaments. The force increments between filaments are not equal.

Semmes et al[59] and Weinstein,[74] using the monofilaments, established a threshold below which stimuli are never (or rarely) perceived and above which they are always (or nearly always) perceived. In their studies of 20 normal

subjects, each with two hands, they found the left hand only slightly more sensitive than the right, with only the left thumb reaching a significant level of difference. The left hand exhibited a more pronounced gradient of sensitivity between parts (thumb and palm) than the right hand, in which there was *no* significant difference in parts (thumb and palm). Thus, even if the monofilaments were ordered with equal force increments between filaments, there are few clear lines, if any, in threshold differences between fingers, thumbs, and palms for adjustments in the testing scales. Testing scales then cannot be arbitrarily altered for fingers, thumb, and palm areas without invalidation of data from areas altered.

I recommend that the examiner use one scale consistently and allow for slight diminutions in sensibility in areas of the skin believed to be slightly less sensitive in touch pressure thresholds, such as callused skin. An example would be with testing of the plantar surface of the foot. One would not be concerned if this surface reflects a diminished light touch, because one knows the keratin layer of the plantar cutaneous skin to be relatively thick. However, one would be concerned if the plantar surface reflected a diminished protective sensation because even with callus, the normal patient will have "protective sensation." It is emphasized that variations in normal cutaneous sensitivity thresholds can be measured in milligrams. The force range of the monofilaments is from 4.5 mg, the lightest, to 447 g, the heaviest (Weinstein's original calculation) measuring rudimentary residual sensibility.[59,73]

Although the early investigators using the filaments did succeed in standardizing the filaments with normal subjects and referenced the filaments of increasing and decreasing forces to "normal" thresholds, the filaments were not standardized to functional levels of diminution in the manner they are utilized today. Their greatest value at present is their sensitivity, which allows testing of normal versus abnormal thresholds of sensibility and answers the question, "Is potential sensibility normal or not?" After an area of normal sensibility has been established, the other filaments of increasing forces can be referenced to this area of normal sensibility to establish a light touch–deep pressure differential in sensory areas, as between the ulnar and median nerves of the right and left hands.

INTERPRETATION SCALE

The credit for equating increasing levels of forces required by the monofilaments to levels of diminution in sensory function goes to Kilulu von Prince.[70] Von Prince began grouping the filaments into levels that could be equated with expected levels of function on the part of the patient. Von Prince was greatly influenced by the work of Napier[48] and Moberg.[45] Concurrently with studies being done by Semmes in sensory losses arising from central origin in determining normal thresholds, von Prince began to investigate the residual function of patients who had received a multiple variety of peripheral nerve injuries from war wounds. Von Prince realized that although some patients would have injuries similar to those of other patients, there was a considerable difference in the level of function of the patients. For example, of two patients who could not tell a difference in testing between one and two points, one could feel a match that would burn his finger and the other could not. Thus she perceived that there must be a protective level of sensation that was not measured by the other test. Of two patients who would have a response to a pinprick, one would have the ability to discriminate textures and one would not. Thus she perceived that there must be a light touch level of sensation that would be equated with the patient's ability to discriminate textures.

Von Prince may have been one of the earliest hand therapists. She was considered radical in ideas at the time she developed her concepts of sensory testing. She broke with what was then tradition for therapists in the armed services to develop a common base of training. Considering the development of testing to measure the level of function of peripheral nerve injuries so important, she requested 6 months in which to investigate this area and develop testing scales.

In her early scales, von Prince attempted to equate levels of diminished sensory function with levels of two-point discrimination testing. This was a logical assumption, because the Weber[71] two-point discrimination test was frequently used in practice. This would be changed in later scales when it would be found that although there appears to be a relationship between diminishing levels of two-point discrimination and increasing levels of force required by the monofilaments, the two tests cannot be directly equated.[1,77]

Omer in particular realized the value of von Prince's work and was instrumental in ensuring that other investigators would continue her work when von Prince was sent to other assignments. He published a paper with Werner in 1970[78] that would add to the "classic" publications in sensibility testing. The testing scale of von Prince was changed in the article by Werner and Omer to omit two-point discrimination as a consideration in the filament testing and to treat it as a separate test.

Werner and Omer, who were concerned with point localization of a touch stimulus, developed two interpretation scales, one for point localization and one for area localization. They also described a level of diminished epicritic sensation (diminished light touch).

The interpretation scales of von Prince and Werner and Omer were used frequently and additional variations developed for sensory testing in the ensuing years.

The current interpretation scale was developed in 1976 based on previous scales and patient performance on function tests (Table 13-2). This scale was used by the author and reviewed in more than 200 tests of patients with nerve compression and lacerations from 1976 to 1978. Later it was discovered to be identical to that of the "area-localization" scale described by Werner and Omer. If their level of diminished light touch is further divided into two levels and the full range of filaments are included, this comparison can be seen.[3,78] (Werner and Omer chose to leave out a few filaments.) The chances that two independent investigators would settle on the same interpretation scale for clinical use are small unless there are indeed differences in the patient's level of sensory function—that is, light touch and protective sensation—that are measurable at specific forces in a spectrum from light touch to deep pressure.

An area localization scale was chosen over scales for point localization because nerves after laceration often have referred touch, and the maturation of referred touch after nerve injuries in our measurements improved independently of light touch–deep pressure thresholds.

James M. Hunter, at the Philadelphia Hand Center, realized the value of the filament mapping in producing information on the patient's neural status that was not forthcoming from other sensory examinations. He encouraged this form of testing with his surgical patients, many of whom came to him with longstanding unresolved peripheral nerve problems.

Table 13-2. Rod markings versus calculated force in gram increments from filament to filament

Rod markings (Log 10 force, 0.1 mg)	Calculated force (g)*		
	Force between filaments		Force between filaments
Loss of protective sensation*			
6.65†			
6.45	165.5	{ 447.0	
6.10		{ 281.5 }	154.5
5.88	52	{ 127.0 }	
5.46		{ 75.00 }	46
5.18	14	{ 29.00 }	
5.07		{ 15.00 }	3.3
4.94	3.05	{ 11.70 }	
4.74		{ 8.650 }	3.15
4.56†	1.868	{ 5.500 }	
		{ 3.632 }	
Diminished protective sensation			1.57
4.31†		{ 2.052 }	
4.17	0.568	{ 1.494 }	
4.08		{ 1.194 }	0.3746
3.84	0.4972	{ 0.6958 }	
Diminished light touch			0.2886
3.61†		{ 0.4082 }	
3.22	0.2422	{ 0.1660 }	
Normal			0.0983
2.83†		{ 0.0677 }	
2.44	0.0402	{ 0.0275 }	
2.36		{ 0.0230 }	0.0045
1.65	0.0185	{ 0.0045 }	

*Scale is linear but does not occur at regular force increments.
†Minikit monofilaments (monofilaments used in short version of test).

The monofilaments are being used to map sensibility diminutions and losses in patients with Hansen's disease. These patients can have diminution or loss of feeling in one of three ways—through end-organ invasion by bacilli, nerve trunk invasion by bacilli, or nerve compression secondary to swelling. The involvement of peripheral nerves can mimic a peripheral nerve lesion or compression from other causes. The filaments are being used as a sensitive monitor of early changes in sensory status in these patients, who can have reversal or improvement of their neural damage through timely use of steroids and other medications.

Detection threshold

In contrast with point localization and two-point discrimination, normal detection threshold for touch pressure is not widely variable over the entire body.[74] This makes mapping of the peripheral nerve system possible. The 2.83 SW filament (marking number), detected over most of the body, serves as a cut-off reference for normal versus abnormal peripheral nerve function, and the heavier filaments quantify levels of abnormality and loss.

Although suitable for use on most of the body, in particular the upper extremity, the 2.83 filament is supra-threshold for the face, and subthreshold for contact areas of the foot. The detection thresholds were originally tested by Weinstein, and mapping of abnormal peripheral nerve function was based on his and other work. Although the filament forces have varied slightly in subsequent testing, there is little change in detection thresholds with newer instruments compared with his original results. The same relative relationship of threshold detection with newer instruments is confirmed in a recent study by Bell-Krotoski and others, in which six examiners used both the Gillis W. Long Hansen's Disease Center (GWLHDC) minikit filaments and North Coast Medical (NCM) long kit filaments in a study of 131 subjects (262 hands, 520 tests; 182 feet, 364 tests).[8a] The study, using the test protocol described in this chapter, found no significant difference in threshold testing with the GWLHDC or NCM 2.83 filaments. The results show the percentage affirmative response from testing with the GWLHDC 2.83 SW filament (measured 62 mg mean application force) (Fig. 13-8).

A normal person will not feel the 2.83 filament 100% of the time, but a normal person will feel the filament the majority of times it is applied. It is possible to have 100% detection on the hand with heavier filaments, but this would

Threshold Detection - 2.83 S-W Filament
(62 mg)

Upper Extremity

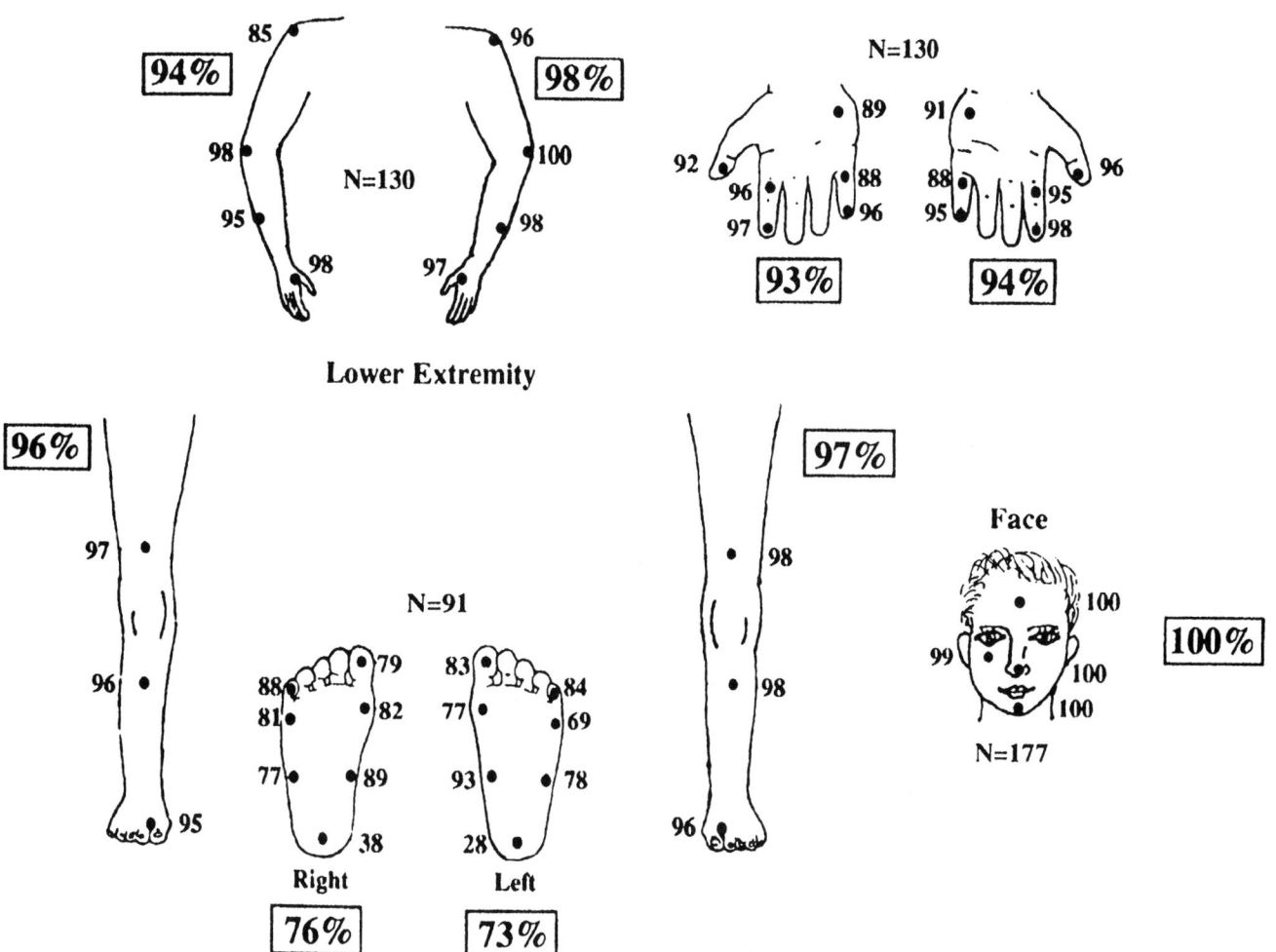

Fig. 13-8. Normal threshold touch-pressure detection.

lose test sensitivity (i.e., include many subjects as normal who should feel the 2.83 filament).[8] Detection levels actually can be set at different sensitivities, but the optimum is the greatest detection with the fewest false positives. Detection on the face for the 2.83 filament is 100%. This indicates the 2.83 filament is suprathreshold—not sensitive enough to test the face, and a lighter filament is felt by most subjects. The detection on the contact areas of the foot is less than 80%. These areas then would need a heavier filament to rule out abnormality. (The 3.61 filament was found to be a better predictor of normal at these sites.)

There is an even more important reason that the 2.83 filament has been selected as the cut-off filament for "normal detection." The 2.83 filament is detected in broad areas inconsistent with specific peripheral nerve innervation, but

the next heavier filaments single out specific areas that are frequently found to upgrade or worsen on subsequent testing. More proximal parts of the upper extremity can be tested, and large areas can be screened for closer examination. This has been found true even for the face and contact surface of the foot, where peripheral nerves are now being frequently mapped (if an area of the foot not responding to the 2.83 filament is only consistent with the plantar contact area, there is little reason for concern; if including other areas and specific nerve distributions, there is good reason to consider it abnormal).

Some believe even lighter filaments should be used as cut-off filaments for normal. Most of these are examiners of carpal tunnel and other entrapment syndromes where the earliest detection of change is sought for early intervention.

If a patient scores "within normal limits" to the 2.83 filament, it is possible to obtain a differential in nerve areas in some patients, for instance, between the ulnar and median nerve with lighter filaments. It is difficult, however, to establish that differences at these sensitive levels are in fact abnormal.

The establishment of a detection level is most important on initial patient testing. On subsequent testing, the previous test serves as a baseline for comparison to establish the direction of change, if any. Peripheral nerves frequently change in status if abnormal, and determination of the direction of change with treatment is one of the biggest advantages of using the filament test. Small and large changes in nerve function and areas consistent with specific nerves can be easily detected and recorded.

PATIENT TESTING TECHNIQUE

Testing with the monofilaments begins with filaments in the normal threshold level and progresses to filaments of increasing pressure until touch is identified by the patient. The filaments 1.65 to 4.08 are applied three times to the same spot, with one response out of three considered an affirmative response. This was found necessary in measurements of the filament forces.[2] One touch may not reach the required threshold of these light filaments, but one out of three almost certainly reaches intended threshold. All the filaments are applied in a perpendicular fashion in 1 to 1.5 seconds, continued in pressure in 1 to 1.5 seconds, and lifted in 1 to 1.5 seconds. The filaments 1.65 to 6.45 should bend to exert the specific pressure. The 6.65 filament has been found most repeatable if applied just to bending. If we are careful to differentiate a false-positive response from a true detection, we may stimulate each site three to five times to ensure it is not felt. Filaments should be applied a minimum of three times, *with one response out of three taken as an affirmative response.* All sensibility testing is performed with careful attention to the normal distribution of the sensory nerves and common variations. A detailed history is taken from the patient and charted as an aid in close examination of the nerve distribution of suspected involvement and the screening of other areas. Unless a higher lesion is suspected from the history, it is often necessary to examine only the hands with the filaments, although *it is possible to test the entire body with the filaments.*

As nerve return progresses proximally to distally except for cases such as syringomyelia and localized partial lesions, the fingertip in the median and ulnar nerve distributions will be the first area to lose sensibility and the last area for return of sensibility. Testing of the fingertips can serve as a limited monitor of corresponding nerve status.

It is more accurate for the same examiners to repeat successive evaluation, but because this is not always possible, the testing can be repeated by other examiners using the same technique.[4] Testing by other examiners is possible when a double-blind situation is desired for studies.

What is mandatory is a quiet testing area; unfortunately, this makes the use of the filaments questionable in an open clinic. It is sometimes very difficult for the patient to attend the filaments in a diminished sensory area. As one patient described the problem, it is like asking him to read a technical journal when he does not recognize all the words. Any sound is distracting, and sounds such as people walking by or typing can make it impossible for some patients to feel filaments they may feel in a quiet area. To ensure an accurate examination, it is most critical for the examiner to be certain the patient can attend and is attending to the filaments.

The testing technique described is in contrast to that of other authors who have required area and point localization when testing with the monofilaments. In area localization, after being touched, the patient responds by indicating the *area* that was touched. In point localization, the patient responds by covering the *point* touched with a wooden dowel within a centimeter. Normal point localization varies widely in the extremity and body, and testing by the latter method is more time consuming and is sometimes confusing to patients who have referred touch.[1,72] It is believed that point localization may reflect the cognitive ability of a patient to adapt to new sensory pathways more than the actual level of return of the nerve and its response to touch. If what we are actually attempting to test is threshold of touch, it is believed that it can be more simply and aptly measured by having the patient respond to stimulation by the monofilament by saying the word *touch.* An argument to this effect is that under nerve retraining we can effect an improvement in a patient's point localization and discrimination of sensory input, but few examiners would believe we are actually effecting a change in the physiologic status of the nerve. Point localization is tested in the sensory evaluation but is treated as a tactile discrimination requiring cortical participation. It can be tested quickly, and a note made of the direction and distance in centimeters into another point, area, or finger where the touch is referred.

Consistent colors from cool to warm are used to correspond with the diminishing sensibility levels. These allow a quickly read, consistent, easily comparable mapping of sensibility.

Procedure for mapping

The procedure is the same for the long or minikit except more monofilaments are used in the long.

1. Draw a probe (a Boley gauge) across the area to be tested in a radial-to-ulnar and proximal-to-distal manner. Ask the patient to describe where and if his or her feeling changes. *Do not ask for numbness because the patient's interpretation of numbness varies*

    Draw the area described as "different" with an ink pen (Fig. 13-9). The examination is easier if the patient can identify the gross area of involvement as

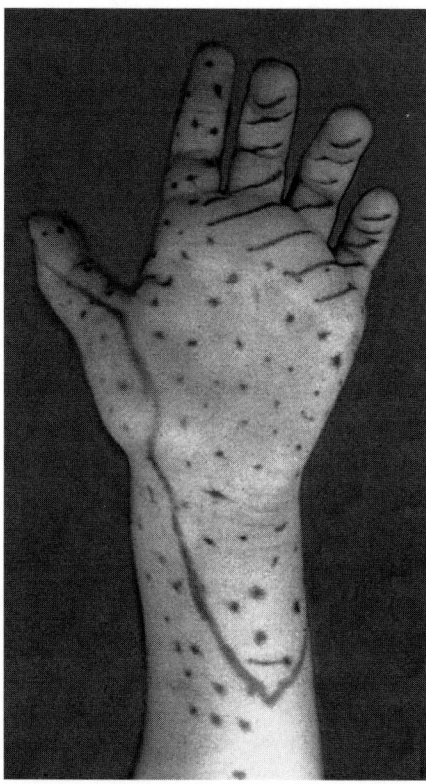

Fig. 13-9. Peripheral nerve mapping in a young male patient a few weeks after an axonotmesis injury of the peripheral nerves following a car accident. Each filament was applied three times to each site tested, with one response out of three accepted as an affirmative. The proximal areas (outside line drawn) is used for differential reference (tests within normal limits using 2.83 marking number Semmes-Weinstein monofilament). The areas distal to the line progressively decreases in threshold detection, requiring heavier filament forces for threshold detection toward the fingertips. The ulnar nerve–innervated fingers on this measurement have no response. This patient was followed with repeat testing for returning nerve function and had a normal response in all hand areas within a 1-year period.

a reference; if the patient cannot, proceed the same way on testing but allow more testing time.

2. Establish an area of *normal sensibility* as a reference. Familiarize the patient with the filament to be used and demonstrate it in the proximal area believed to be normal. Then, with the patient's eyes occluded, demonstrate the filament until the patient can easily identify the filament on the low side of normal (2.83).

 This reference of normal is extremely important because the examiner returns to it frequently to establish a differential between it and a site the patient does not feel. Guessing is eliminated if a patient responds at the reference site but not the site tested.

 Test the involved hand (volar surface) by applying the same filament (2.83) to the fingertips first and working proximally. Dot the spots correctly identified with a *green* felt-tip pen. (Explain to the patient that the second touch he feels is a marking of the pen.) In

general, the patient is tested distally to proximally, but a consistent pattern is not used to avoid patient anticipation of the area to be touched. When all the area on the volar surface of the hand that can be identified as within normal limits is marked in green, proceed to the dorsum of the hand and test in the same fashion. Because the sensibility on the dorsum of the hand is not always as well defined as the volar surface, it is easier to establish areas of decreased sensibility on the volar surface first. *Now the gross areas of normal and decreased sensibility have been defined.*

3. Return to the volar surface of the hand. Proceed to the filaments within the level of *diminished light touch* (see Table 13-1) but change the color of the marking pen for this level to *blue*. Test as above in the unidentified areas remaining, working again first on the volar surface and then on the dorsum.

4. If areas remain unidentified, proceed to the filaments in the *diminished protective sensation level (purple)* and then *loss of protective sensation level (red)* and continue testing until all the areas have been identified.

5. Record the colors and filament numbers on the report form to produce a sensory mapping. (Color and mark hands on form.) Note any variations and unusual responses, especially delayed responses. Delayed responses (more than 3 seconds) are considered abnormal. Note the presence and direction of referred touch with arrows. Note and draw on the form any unusual appearances on the hands, including sweat patterns, blisters, dry or shiny skin, calluses, cuts, blanching of the skin, and so on.

Hand screen

 A hand screen examination with minikit filaments has been developed to reduce testing time and allow monitoring of patients over time with treatment (Fig. 13-10, *A*). The minikit filaments represent the cut-off forces for each functional level of sensibility—normal, diminished light touch, diminished protective sensation, and loss of protective sensation.[6] Two filaments are included for the loss of protective sensation level. For returning nerve function, the heaviest of these (marking number 6.65) is important to signal rudimentary deep-pressure sensation. The lightest of these is important to define loss of protective sensation versus diminished protective sensation (marking number 4.56).[1] Sites for median nerve monitoring are the tip of the thumb, index, and proximal index. (The radial base of the palm is specifically avoided to eliminate variation from the recurrent branch of the median nerve.) Sites for the ulnar nerve are the distal little finger, proximal phalanx, and ulnar base of the palm. The site for the radial nerve is the dorsal aspect of the thumb apex (web space). More data points can be included if desired, but these represent the minimum critical consistent data points for monitoring the peripheral nerves (Fig. 13-10, *B*).

Program Name:		HAND SCREEN RECORD	Initial F/U __ __	Date:
Patient's Name *(Last, First, Middle)*:			Date of Birth:	SS No.	ID No:
Patient's File No.	Medications:			Date Diagnosis:	Date Onset:

Section I. SENSORY TESTING: Use first filament (A) at site indicated *(apply three times)*: If no response, use next heavier filament to determine level of loss.

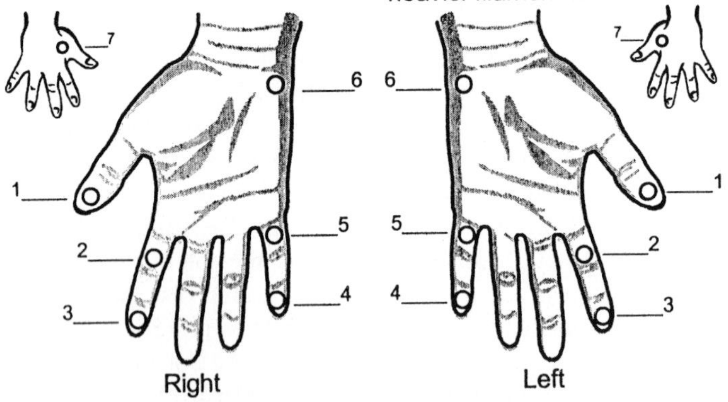

Right   Left

Filament	Force, gms	Interpretation	(Grade Pts.)
A Green (2.83)	0.05	Normal	(5)
B Blue (3.61)	0.20	Residual Texture	(4)
C Purple (4.31)	2.00	Residual Protective Sensation	(3)
D Red (4.56)	4.00	Loss of Protective Sensation	(2)
E Orange (6.65)	300.00	Residual Deep Pressure	(1)

Section II. SKIN INSPECTION: Draw and label *(above)*: **W** - Wound, **C** - Callus, **S** - Swelling, **R** - Redness, **D** - Dryness, **T** - Temperature, **M** - Missing, **J** - Contracture, **O** - Other

Section III. MUSCLE TESTING: Mark *(below)*: **S** = Strong, **W** = Weak, **P** = Paralysis *(or Grade 5 to 0)*

(Ulnar Nerve)   (Median Nerve)   (Radial Nerve)

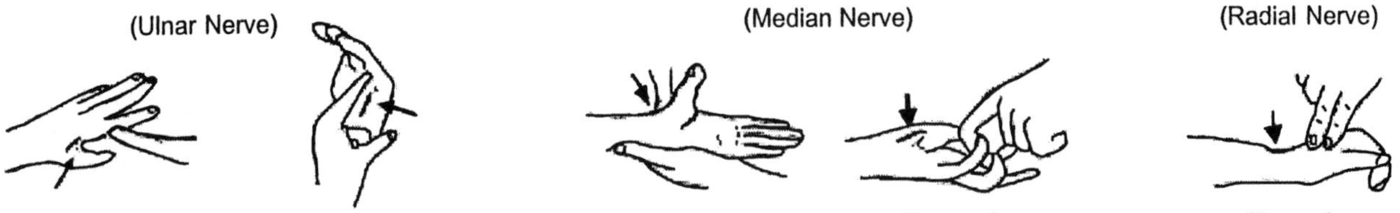

R__ L__   R__ L__   R__ L__   R__ L__   R__ L__

1) Index finger Abduction (FDI) 2) Little Finger MP Joint Flex. (L) 3) Thumb Abduction Out of Palm (APB) 4) Thumb to Little Finger (OP) 5) Radial Wrist Extension (ECR)

Section IV. PERIPHERAL NERVE RISK: Mark: **U** = Ulnar, **M** = Median, **R** = Radial, (or **UM**)

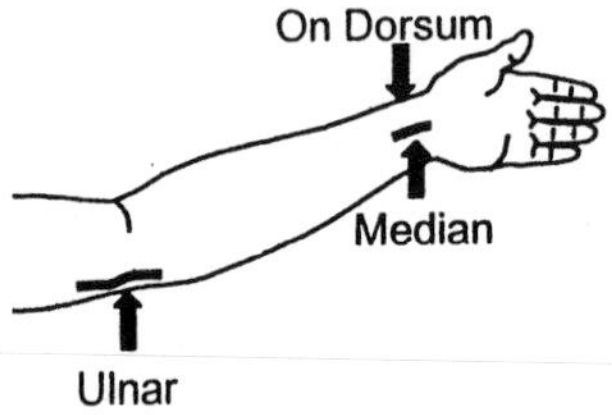

Radial Cutaneous On Dorsum
Median
Ulnar

1) Enlarged or swollen nerve   R ___   L ___
2) Tender / painful on stretch or compression   R ___   L ___
3) Sensory change in the last 12 months   R ___   L ___
4) Muscle change in the last 12 months   R ___   L ___

High Risk *(acute or changing nerve)* Yes ___ No ___
(refer to physician / therapist)

Section V. DEFORMITY RISK: *(Check if present)*

1) Loss of Protective Sensation   R ___ L ___   4) Injuries *(wounds, blisters, etc.)* R ___ L ___
2) Clawed but Mobile Hand   R ___ L ___   5) Contracted or Stiff Joints   R ___ L ___
3) Fingertip Absorption (Mild___ Severe___) R ___ L ___   6) Wrist Drop *(radial nerve)*   R ___ L ___

High Risk *(any of the above)*:   Yes ___ No ___
(refer for appropriate treatment)

Has there been a **change in the hand since last exam**?   Yes __ No __

Examined by:_____

NHDP FORM 130
HAND SCREEN RECORD

Fig. 13-10. A, Hand screen form used for initial evaluation.

Program Name:	**PERIPHERAL NERVE MONITORING**			
Patient's Name *(Last, First, Middle)*:		Date of Birth:	SS No:	ID No:
Patient's File No.	Other Diagnoses:		Date Diagnosis:	Date Onset:

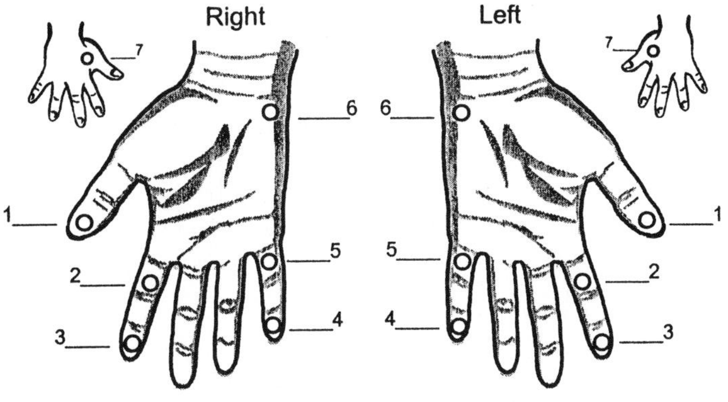

Right   Left

1 FDI ___   4 OP ___
2 L ___   5 ECR ___
3 APB ___

1) Enlarged Nerve ___
2) Tender Nerve ___
3) Sensory Change ___
4) Muscle Change ___

1) Protective Loss ___
2) Clawed/MobileJts ___
3) Absorption:
   Mild ___ Severe ___
4) Injuries ___
5) Contracted/Stiff Jts ___
6) Wrist Drop ___

1 FDI ___   4 OP ___
2 L ___   5 ECR ___
3 APB ___

1) Enlarged Nerve ___
2) Tender Nerve ___
3) Sensory Change ___
4) Muscle Change ___

1) Protective Loss ___
2) Clawed/MobileJts ___
3) Absorption:
   Mild ___ Severe ___
4) Injuries ___
5) Contracted/Stiff Jts ___
6) Wrist Drop ___

Comment: _____ Date: _____

Medication: _____ Examined by: _____

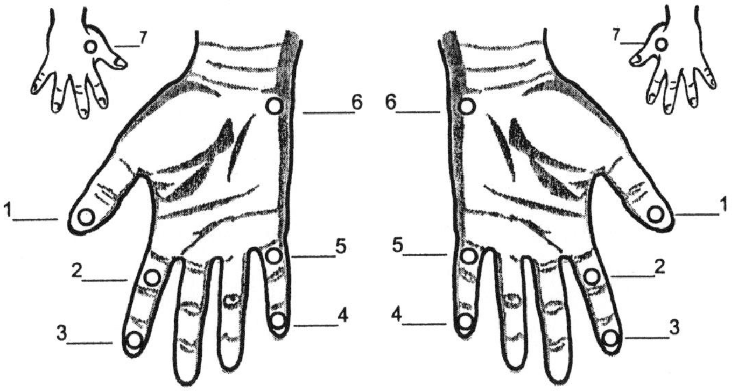

1 FDI ___   4 OP ___
2 L ___   5 ECR ___
3 APB ___

1) Enlarged Nerve ___
2) Tender Nerve ___
3) Sensory Change ___
4) Muscle Change ___

1) Protective Loss ___
2) Clawed/MobileJts ___
3) Absorption:
   Mild ___ Severe ___
4) Injuries ___
5) Contracted/Stiff Jts ___
6) Wrist Drop ___

1 FDI ___   4 OP ___
2 L ___   5 ECR ___
3 APB ___

1) Enlarged Nerve ___
2) Tender Nerve ___
3) Sensory Change ___
4) Muscle Change ___

1) Protective Loss ___
2) Clawed/MobileJts ___
3) Absorption:
   Mild ___ Severe ___
4) Injuries ___
5) Contracted/Stiff Jts ___
6) Wrist Drop ___

Comment: _____ Date: _____

Medication: _____ Examined by: _____

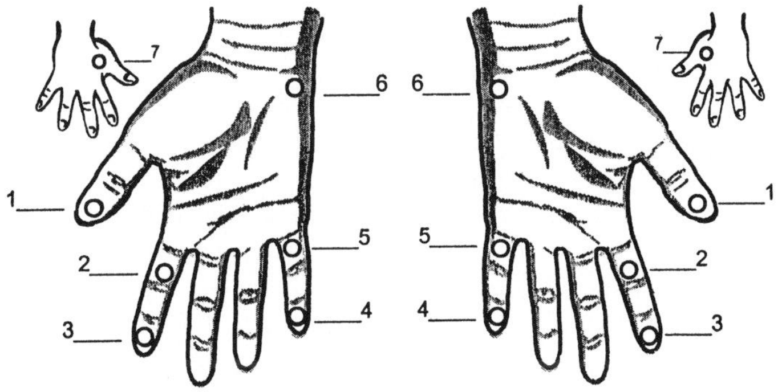

1 FDI ___   4 OP ___
2 L ___   5 ECR ___
3 APB ___

1) Enlarged Nerve ___
2) Tender Nerve ___
3) Sensory Change ___
4) Muscle Change ___

1) Protective Loss ___
2) Clawed/MobileJts ___
3) Absorption:
   Mild ___ Severe ___
4) Injuries ___
5) Contracted/Stiff Jts ___
6) Wrist Drop ___

1 FDI ___   4 OP ___
2 L ___   5 ECR ___
3 APB ___

1) Enlarged Nerve ___
2) Tender Nerve ___
3) Sensory Change ___
4) Muscle Change ___

1) Protective Loss ___
2) Clawed/MobileJts ___
3) Absorption:
   Mild ___ Severe ___
4) Injuries ___
5) Contracted/Stiff Jts ___
6) Wrist Drop ___

Comment: _____ Date: _____

Medication: _____ Examined by: _____

NHDP FORM 131
PERIPHERAL NERVE MONITORING

Fig. 13-10, cont'd B, Peripheral nerve monitoring form; same information as hand screen form but allows several evaluations on one page for easy comparison.

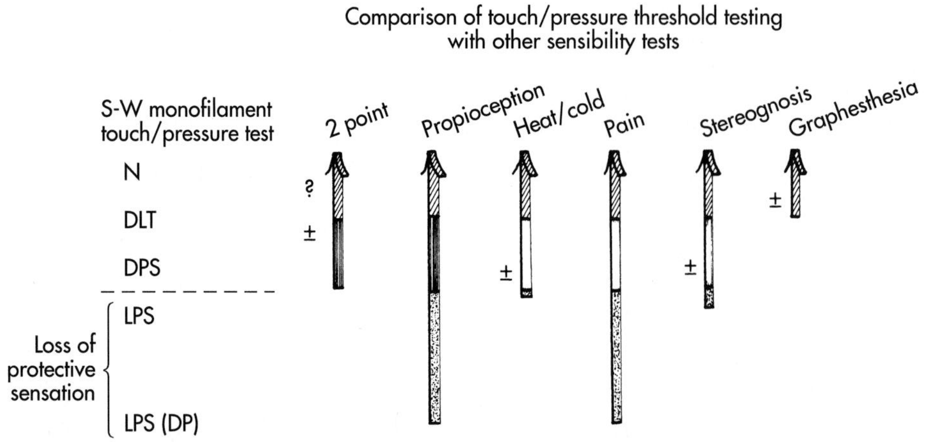

Comparison of touch/pressure threshold testing
with other sensibility tests

Fig. 13-11. Results of comparison review of 150 cases, 200 tests of patients with nerve compressions or lacerations, and other tests given in a 1976 to 1978 test battery. Semmes-Weinstein monofilament functional levels (*N*, normal; *DLT*, diminished light touch; *DPS*, diminished protective sensation; *LPS*, loss of protective sensation; *DP*, deep pressure) can be read vertically. The relationship of the monofilament levels to other sensibility tests can be read horizontally. Although the tests did in general correlate with respect to involvement or noninvolvement, no direct correlation could be made in level results from two-point discrimination testing and monofilament testing. Several cases with nerve compressions measured two-point discrimination within normal limits (3 to 5 mm or 6 mm at fingertips), whereas light touch–deep pressure thresholds were decreased to as low as the diminished protective sensation level. In four patients, two-point discrimination testing was abnormal, whereas monofilament light touch–deep pressure testing was within normal limits (two old burns, one cerebrovascular accident, and one partial thumb amputation).

Data are digitized for computer analysis by giving each filament a weighted score: green, 2.83 equals 5; blue, 3.61 equals 4; purple, 4.31 equals 3; red, 4.56 equals 2; red-orange, 6.65 equals 1; no response equals zero. Scores can be totaled for each nerve and overall. A normal hand then would have a score of 15 for the median nerve, 15 for the radial nerve, and 5 for the radial, for a total of 35 points.

INTERPRETATION AND RELATIONSHIP TO FUNCTION

The interpretation of monofilament force levels was based on a review of 150 cases and 200 tests of patients with peripheral nerve problems at the Philadelphia Hand Center, Ltd, Philadelphia, from 1976 to 1978. Subsequent discussion of the data with von Prince and experience in use of the interpretation in patients with peripheral nerve problems over the last 23 years has continued to support the relationship of force thresholds to functional sensibility. Comparisons were made between the Semmes-Weinstein monofilaments and other tests of sensibility routinely given to patients as a test battery. The results are summarized in Fig. 13-11.

Normal touch is a recognition of light touch, and therefore deep pressure, that is, within normal limits. This level is the most significant of all levels because it allows the examiner to distinguish between areas of normal sensibility and areas of sensory diminution.

Diminished light touch is diminished recognition of light touch. If a patient has diminished light touch, provided that the patient's motor status and cognitive abilities are in play, he or she has fair use of the hand; graphesthesia and stereognosis are both close to normal and adaptable; he or she has good temperature appreciation and definitely has good protective sensation; he or she most often will have fair to good two-point discrimination; and the patient may not even realize he or she has had a sensory loss.

Diminished protective sensation is just that. If a patient has diminished protective sensation, he or she will have diminished use of the hands, difficulty manipulating some objects, and a tendency to drop some objects; in addition, the patient may complain of weakness of his or her hand, but the patient will have an appreciation of the pain and temperature that should help keep him or her from injury, and the patient will have some manipulative skill. Sensory reeducation can begin at this level. It is possible for a patient to have a gross appreciation of two-point discrimination at this level (7 to 10 mm).

Loss of protective sensation is again what it says. If a patient has loss of protective sensation he or she will have little use of the hand; a diminished, if not absent, temperature appreciation; an inability to manipulate objects outside his or her line of vision; a tendency to injure himself or herself easily; and it may even be dangerous for the patient to be around machinery. The patient will, however, be able to feel a pinprick and have *deep pressure sensation,* which does not make him or her totally asensory. Instructions on protective care are helpful to prevent injury.

If a patient is *untestable,* he or she may or may not feel a pinprick but will have no other discrimination of levels of feeling. If a patient feels a pinprick in an area otherwise untestable, it is important to note this during the mapping. Instructions on protective care of the hand are mandatory at this level to prevent the normally occurring problems associated with the asensory hand.

Further interpretation of the effect the decrease or loss of sensibility has on patient function depends on the area and extent of loss and whether musculature is diminished.

FUTURE CONSIDERATIONS

A few cases of suspected nerve compression have been found in which all the testing of neural status described is within normal limits, and a patient history is the only indicative finding. A review of the literature quickly shows similar cases. It is suspected that in these cases the patient is not always being tested at the time of the symptoms. The patient comes in for testing after he or she has slept late, had a good breakfast, and had a more quietly paced and lighter-duty morning than the normal routine, but in reality the patient complains of problems only after heavy-duty work of a few hours' duration. Hunter has termed this condition *transient stress neuropathy* and has referred patients for testing before and after activities and positions that reproduce their symptoms.[28]

SUMMARY

The recognition of threshold levels of light touch–deep pressure is invaluable in peripheral nerve evaluation. Mappings of such thresholds enable the examiner to "see" what is otherwise invisible. Handheld instruments without sufficient control on application are not repeatable and valid in clinical testings. Computerized test instruments are becoming available and will help test longstanding physiologic concepts.[14,21,22,32,49] Not only will it be possible to eliminate uncontrolled variables of handheld tests, but also computer-driven instruments will make it possible to test with a full range of controlled graduated stimuli to determine optimal test stimuli. After optimal stimuli are determined, results could improve handheld tests. Even the computerized instruments must meet the sensitivity or repeatability requirements for objective testing and will have to be validated in controlled clinical studies.

Accurate, repeatable, and valid color-coded hand screening or mapping of the peripheral nerves is made possible by the Semmes-Weinstein monofilaments. Data from consistent tests can be numerically quantified and compared among measurements, with treatment, and among patient groups. The instrument is portable, practical, and available for clinical testing of patients with peripheral nerve disease or injury.

ACKNOWLEDGMENTS

I gratefully acknowledge Bill Buford, Bioengineer formerly at the Paul W. Brand Research Laboratory, Gillis W. Long Hansen's Disease Center, Carville, Louisiana, for his help in reviewing the monofilament calculations in developing instrument measurements and collaborating on sensibility test design. Also acknowledged is the help of Lillian Brewder, M.Ed., for statistical consultation.

REFERENCES

1. Bell JA: Sensibility evaluation. In Hunter J, et al, editors: *Rehabilitation of the hand,* St Louis, 1978, Mosby.
2. Bell JA, Buford W: Comparison of forces and interpretation scales as used with the von Frey Aesthesiometer. Paper presented at Hand Surgery Correlated with Hand Therapy meeting, Philadelphia, 1978.
3. Bell JA, Buford WL Jr: Assessment of levels of cutaneous sensibility. Presented at the sixteenth annual meeting of the United States Public Health Professional Association, Houston, 1979.
4. Bell JA, Tomancik E: Repeatability of testing with Semmes-Weinstein monofilaments, *J Hand Surg* 12A:155, 1987.
5. Bell-Krotoski J: A study of peripheral nerve involvement underlying physical disability of the hand in Hansen's disease, *J Hand Ther* 5:3, 1993.
6. Bell-Krotoski J: "Pocket filaments" and specifications for the Semmes-Weinstein monofilaments, *J Hand Ther* 3:1, 26, 1993.
7. Bell-Krotoski J, Buford W Jr: The force/time relationship of clinically used sensory testing instruments, *J Hand Ther* 1:76, 1988.
8. Bell-Krotoski J, Weinstein S, Weinstein C: Testing sensibility, including touch-pressure, two-point discrimination, point localization, and vibration, *J Hand Ther* 6:2, 1993.
8a. Bell-Krotoski JA, et al: Threshold detection and Semmes-Weinstein monofilaments: a comparative study, *J Hand Ther* 8:155, 1995.
9. Boring EG: *Sensation and perception in the history of experimental psychology,* New York, 1942, Appleton-Century-Crofts.
10. Brand PW: Symposium, Assessment of cutaneous sensibility. Comments of chairman. National Hansen's Disease Center, Carville, La, 1980.
11. Buford WL, Bell JA: Dynamic properties of hand held tactile assessment stimuli. Proceedings of the thirty-fourth annual conference of Engineering in Medicine and Biology, 23:307, 1981.
12. Chochinov RH, Onyot LE, Moorehouse JA: Sensory perception thresholds in patients with juvenile diabetes and their close relatives, *N Engl J Med* 286:1233, 1969.
13. Curtis RM: Sensory reeducation after peripheral nerve injury. In Fredricks S, Brody GS, editors: *Symposium on the neurologic aspects of plastic surgery,* vol 17, St Louis, 1978, Mosby.
14. Dellon AL: The moving two-point discrimination test: clinical evaluation of the quickly adapting fiber/receptor system, *J Hand Surg* 3:474, 1978.
15. Dellon AL: The sensational contributions of Erik Moberg, *J Hand Surg [Br]* 15:14, 1990.
16. Dellon AL, Mackinnon SE, Crosby PM: Reliability of two-point discrimination measurements, *J Hand Surg* 12A:5, 1987.
17. Dellon ES, Mourey R, Dellon AL: Human pressure perception values for constant and moving one- and two-point discrimination, *Plast Reconstr Surg* 90:1, 112, 1992.
18. Demichells F, et al: Biomedical instrumentation for the measurements of skin sensitivity, *Trans Biomed Eng BMR* 26:326, 1979.
19. Dyck PJ: Quantitation of cutaneous sensation in man. In Dyck PJ, Thomas PK, editors: *Peripheral neuropathy,* Philadelphia, 1975, WB Saunders.
20. Dyck PJ: Assessment of cutaneous sensibility. Symposium presented at National Hansen's Disease Center, Carville, La, 1980.
21. Dyck PJ, et al: Clinical vs quantitative evaluation of cutaneous sensation, *Arch Neurol* 33:651, 1976.

22. Dyck PJ, et al: *Peripheral neuropathy,* ed 3, Philadelphia, 1993, WB Saunders.

23. Gelberman RH, et al: Sensibility testing in peripheral nerve compression syndromes: an experimental study in humans, *J Bone Joint Surg* 65A:632, 1983.

24. Gelberman RH, et al: Results of treatment of severe carpal tunnel syndrome without internal neurolysis of the median nerve, *J Bone Joint Surg* 69:896, 1987.

25. Greenspan JD, LaMotte RH: Cutaneous mechanoreceptors of the hand: experimental studies and their implications for clinical testing of tactile sensation, *J Hand Ther* 6:2, 75, 1993.

26. Grimaund JF, et al: How to detect neuropathy in Leprosy, *Rev Neurol (Paris)* 150:785, 1994.

27. Hage JJ, et al: Difference in sensibility between the dominant and nondominant index finger as tested using the Semmes-Weinstein monofilament pressure aesthesiometer, *J Hand Surg* 20:227, 1995.

28. Hunter JM, Read RL, Gray R: Carpal tunnel neuropathy caused by injury: reconstruction of the transverse carpal ligament for the complex carpal tunnel syndromes, *J Hand Ther* 6:2, 1993.

29. Imai HT, et al: Interpretation of cutaneous pressure thresholds (Semmes-Weinstein monofilament measurement) following median nerve repair and sensory reeducation in the adult, *Microsurgery* 10:142, 1989.

30. Jamison DG: Sensitivity testing as a means of differentiating the various forms of leprosy found in Nigeria, *Int J Lepr* 39:504, 1972.

31. Jeng CJ, et al: Sensory thresholds of normal human feet, *Foot Ankle Int* 21:501, 2000.

32. Jimenez S, et al: A study of sensory recovery following carpal tunnel release, *J Hand Ther* 6:2, 124, 1993.

33. Kets CM, et al: Reference values for touch sensibility thresholds in healthy Nepalese volunteers, *Lepr Rev* 67:28, 1966.

34. Koris MR, et al: Carpal tunnel syndrome: evaluation of a quantitative provocational diagnostic test, *Clin Orthop* 251:157, 1990.

35. Kuipers M, Schreuders T: The predictive value of sensation testing in the development of neuropathic ulceration on the hands of leprosy patients, *Lepr Rev* 65:253, 1994.

36. LaMotte RH: Assessment of cutaneous sensibility, sensory discrimination and neural correlation. Symposium presented at National Hansen's Disease Center, Carville, La, 1980.

37. LaMotte RH, Mountcastle VB: Capacities of humans and monkeys to discriminate between vibratory stimuli of different frequency and amplitude: a correlation between neural events and psychophysical measurements, *J Neurophysiol* 38:539, 1979.

38. LaMotte RH, Srinivasan MA: Tactile discrimination of shape: responses of quickly adapting mechanoreceptive afferents to a step stroked across the monkey fingerpad, *J Neurosci* 8:1672, 1987.

39. Lehman LF, et al: The development of the Semmes-Weinstein monofilaments in Brazil, *J Hand Ther* 6:290, 1993.

40. Looft FJ, Williams WJ: One-line receptive field mapping of cutaneous receptors, *Trans Biomed Eng BME* 26:350, 1979.

41. Lundborg G, et al: Digital Vibrogram: a new diagnostic tool for sensory testing in compression neuropathy, *J Hand Surg* 11A:5, 1986.

42. Lundborg GB, et al: Artificial sensibility based on the use of piezoresistive sensors. Preliminary observations, *J Hand Surg [Br]* 23:620, 1998.

43. MacDermid JC, et al: Decision making in detecting abnormal Semmes-Weinstein monofilament thresholds in carpal tunnel syndrome, *J Hand Ther* 7:158, 1994.

44. Millesi H, Renderer D: A method of training and testing sensibility of the fingertips, from the Department of Plastic and Reconstructive Surgery, Surgical University Clinic of Vienna and Ludwig-Boltzmann, Institute for Experimental Plastic Surgery, Vienna, Austria, 1978.

45. Moberg E: Objective methods of determining the functional value of sensibility of the hand, *J Bone Joint Surg* 40B:454, 1958.

46. Mountcastle VB: *Medical physiology,* ed 12, vol 2, St Louis, 1968, Mosby.

47. Naafs B, Dagne T: Sensory testing: a sensitive method in the follow-up of nerve involvement, *Int J Lepr* 45:364, 1978.

48. Napier JR: *Hands,* New York, 1980, Pantheon Press.

49. Novak CB, et al: Evaluation of hand sensibility with single and double latex gloves, *Plast Reconstr Surg* 103:128, 1999.

50. O'Brien PC, Dyck PJ, Kosanke JL: *A computer evaluation of quantitative algorithms for measuring detection thresholds of cutaneous sensation clinical applications,* Boston, 1989, Butterworths.

51. Omer GE Jr: Median nerve compression at the wrist, *Hand Clin* 8:317, 1992.

52. Omer GE, Bell-Krotoski JA: Sensibility testing. In Omer GE, et al, editors: *Management of peripheral nerve problems* ed 2, Philadelphia, 1998, WB Saunders.

53. Paul RL, Merzesich M, Goodman H: Representations of slowly and rapidly adapting mechanoreceptors of the hand in Broadman's areas 3 and 1 of *Macaca mulatta, Brain Res* 36:239, 1972.

54. Pham HD, et al: Screening techniques to identify people at high risk for diabetic foot ulceration: a prospective multicenter trial, *Diabetes Care* 23:606, 2000.

55. Poppen NK: Sensibility evaluation following peripheral nerve suture: critical assessment of the von Frey, two-point discrimination, and ridge tests. In Jewett DL, McCarroll HK Jr, editors: *Symposium on nerve repair: its clinical and experimental basis,* St Louis, 1979, Mosby.

56. Premkumar RE, et al: Quantitative assessment of facial sensation in leprosy, *Int J Lepr Other Mycrobat Dis* 66:384, 1998.

57. Rosen BL: Recovery of sensory and motor function after nerve repair: a rational for evaluation, *J Hand Ther* 9:315, 1996.

58. Rosen BL, et al: Assessment of functional outcome after nerve repair in a longitudinal cohort, *Scand J Plast Reconst Surg Hand Surg* 43:71, 2000.

59. Semmes J, et al: *Somatosensory changes after penetrating brain wounds in man,* Cambridge, Mass, 1960, Harvard University Press.

60. Szabo RM, et al: Sensibility testing in patients with carpal tunnel syndrome, *J Bone Joint Surg* 66:60, 1984.

61. Tadjalli HE, et al: Importance of crossover innervation in digital nerve repair demonstrated by nerve isolation technique, *Ann Plast Surg* 35:32, 1995.

62. Tajima T, Imai H: Results of median nerve repair in children, *Microsurgery* 10:145, 1989.

63. Trumble TE, et al: Seural nerve grafting for lower extremity nerve injuries, *J Orthop Trauma* 9:158, 1995.

64. Vallbo AB, Johansson RS: The tactile sensory innervation of the glabrous skin of the human hand. In Gordon G, editor: *Active touch,* Oxford, England, 1978, Pergamon Press.

65. van Breckel WH, et al: Functional sensibility of the hand in leprosy patients, *Lepr Rev* 68:25, 1997.

66. van Turnhout AA, Hage JJ: Lack of difference in sensibility between the dominant and non-dominant hands as tested with Semmes-Weinstein monofilaments, *J Hand Surg [Br]* 22:768, 1997.

67. van Vliet DC, et al: Duration of contact time alters cutaneous pressure threshold measurements, *Ann Plast Surg* 31:335, 1993.

68. Voerman VF, et al: Normal values for sensory thresholds in the cervical dermatomes: a critical note on the use of Semmes-Weinstein monofilaments, *Am J Phys Med Rehabil* 78:24, 1999.

69. Von Frey M: Zur Physiologie der Juckempfindung, *Arch Neurol Physiol* 7:142, 1922.

70. von Prince K, Butler B: Measuring sensory function of the hand in peripheral nerve injuries, *Am J Occup Ther* 21:385, 1967.

71. Weber EH: Ueber den Tastsinn, *Muller Archiv* 61:152, 1935.

72. Weber EH: Data cited by Sherrington CS, in *Shafer's textbook of physiology,* Edinburgh, 1900, Young J Pentland.

73. Weinstein S: Intensive and extensive aspects of tactile sensitivity as a function of body part, sex, and laterality. In Kenshalo DR, editor: *The skin senses,* Springfield, Ill, 1968, Charles C Thomas.
74. Weinstein S: Fifty years of somatosensory research from the Semmes-Weinstein monofilaments to the Weinstein enhanced sensory test, *J Hand Ther* 6:1, 11, 1993.
75. Weinstein S: Tactile sensitivity of the phalanges, *Percept Motor Skills* 14:351, 1962.
76. Weise MD, et al: Lower extremity sensibility testing in patients with herniated lumbar intervertebral discs, *J Bone Joint Surg* 68:1219, 1985.
77. Werner G, Mountcastle VB: Neural activity in mechanoreceptive cutaneous afferents: stimulus-response relations, Weber functions and information transmission, *J Neurophysiol* 28:359, 1965.
78. Werner JL, Omer GE: Evaluating cutaneous pressure sensation of the hand, *Am J Occup Ther* 24:5, 1970.

Chapter 14

SENSIBILITY ASSESSMENT FOR NERVE LESIONS-IN-CONTINUITY AND NERVE LACERATIONS

Anne D. Callahan

The challenges inherent in sensibility assessment of the upper extremity have increased in recent years. In the past, it seemed the majority of patients referred for evaluation had diagnoses of median nerve compression at the wrist or nerve lacerations at the wrist. The latter 1980s and 1990s saw a shift in referral population toward nerve lesions in continuity at all segments of upper extremity nerves. Schwartzman[72] states that brachial plexus traction injuries are "common, overlooked, and often misdiagnosed." Whitenack et al.[87] and Hunter et al.[44,45] attribute the increasing incidence of high-level traction neuropathies to several factors, including high-speed vehicular trauma, falls on the outstretched arm, extensive computer use, repetitive assembly work (especially lateral abduction or overhead lifting), women in the workplace performing heavy work that exceeds their physical capacity, and poor posture.

With these trends in referral population in mind, the therapist must have a working knowledge of the sensory patterns of the upper extremity nerves at all levels, from roots to distal cutaneous branches. In addition, the evaluating therapist must approach sensibility assessment of nerve lesions in continuity differently than for nerve lacerations. The purpose of this chapter is to discuss prerequisites for sensibility assessment and current clinical techniques for assessment of nerve lesions in continuity and nerve lacerations.

PREREQUISITES FOR ASSESSMENT

Meaningful sensibility assessment requires adequate history, good clinical skills in assessment of sympathetic function, and appropriate test selection and administration. However, before the therapist ever meets the patient, certain prerequisites of knowledge are essential to clinical competence in sensibility assessment. These knowledge domains are nerve pathways and areas of cutaneous supply, knowledge of the effects of nerve injury, and control of test variables. These prerequisites are discussed before proceeding to the actual components of clinical assessment (Table 14-1).

Prerequisite: knowledge of nerve pathways and cutaneous supply

The region of skin that the therapist assesses for sensibility will depend on the cutaneous distribution of the affected nerve segment. Therefore the therapist must be familiar with upper extremity nerve pathways from spinal roots to distal cutaneous branches. In addition, the therapist must be aware of the location of sensory signs and symptoms resulting from lesions at different sites along the nerve pathways (Table 14-2). In some cases, clinicians may use certain provocative positions or maneuvers to duplicate the patient's symptoms; some examples are listed in Table 14-2.

Roots of the brachial plexus. Operative words in anatomic descriptions of the brachial plexus are "usually,

214

Table 14-1. Prerequisites and components of sensibility assessment

Prerequisites of sensibility assessment	Components of sensibility assessment
Knowledge of nerve pathways	Referral and history
Knowledge of effects of nerve injury	Assessment of sympathetic function
Pathomechanics and degrees of injury	Mapping the area of dysfunction
Patterns of sensibility loss and recovery	Test selection and administration
Control of test variables	Sensibility evaluation battery
Environment-related variables	Nerve lesions in continuity
Patient-related variables	Divided nerves (postoperative)
Instrument-related variables	
Method-related variables	
Examiner-related variables	

Table 14-2. Location of sensory signs and symptoms of upper extremity nerve lesions in continuity*

Nerve segment	Location of sensory signs and symptoms	Provocative tests and maneuvers
Roots	Segmental distribution; focal signs in part of the nerve root distribution	Spurling's maneuvers[72]
Trunks	Segmental distribution	
Upper trunk	Pain in C2 distribution of cranium; pain across trapezial ridge; pain radiating down the medial scapular border to its tip[72]	Arms placed over the head and adjacent to the ears[72] Deep pressure to supraclavicular fossa[72]
Lower trunk	Dull ache and paresthesias in IV and V and medial forearm[72]	Elevated arm stress test (EAST)[70] Hunter test[87]
Cords	Cutaneous nerve distribution	
Lateral cord	Paresthesias of I, II, and radial half of III. (If there is concomitant median nerve injury, the tip of II will be subjectively more insensitive to pinprick than either I or tip of III.)[72]	EAST[70] Hyperabduction with internal rotation[72] Deep pressure to infraclavicular fossa (under lateral clavicle)[72]
Medial cord	Medial aspect of upper arm and forearm; ulnar half of III, IV, and V have decreased sensitivity to pinprick[72]	Deep pressure to supraclavicular fossa[72]
Posterior cord	Paresthesias with minimal sensory loss from dorsal area of the forearm, I and II[72]	
Peripheral nerves		
Superficial radial nerve	Dorsal web space between I and II (autonomous supply)	Hyperpronation of forearm[52]
Ulnar nerve palmar digital branches	Distal ulnar pulp V (autonomous supply)	
Median nerve terminal branches	Distal radial pulp II (autonomous supply)	Thenar muscle abduction test[44] Hyperextension wrist and finger test[44] Tethered median nerve stress test

*Also listed is a sampling of provocative tests and maneuvers. *Note:* Contrary points of view exist regarding the specificity of certain of these maneuvers.†
†16, 17, 51, 66, 69, 70, 72, 89, 90.

generally, mainly, and most often"; variations are common. The roots of the brachial plexus, C5, C6, C7, C8, and T1 anterior primary rami exit the spinal cord at the intervertebral foramina. (Branches from C4 and T2 ventral rami also may contribute.) C5, C6, and C7 nerve roots give rise to the long thoracic nerve close to the intervertebral foramina; it innervates serratus anterior. The dorsal scapular nerve arises mainly from the C5 nerve root and provides variable

innervation to levator scapulae and full innervation to the rhomboids (Fig. 14-1).[41]

There is considerable innervation overlap between the sensory fibers of adjacent spinal nerves at the periphery.[31] Sunderland[77] has represented the sensory dermatomes "without reference to variations or the zones of overlap of adjacent spinal nerves" (Fig. 14-2). Despite variations in dermatome charts, one can confidently use these reference points when assessing segmental innervation: C5 supplies the outer aspect of the shoulder tip, C6 supplies the thumb, C7 (longest cervical spinous process) supplies the middle finger (the longest finger), C8 the little finger, and the T3 dermatome lies in the axilla.[10] Division of a single nerve root generally does not result in anesthesia in its dermatomal area because of the innervation overlap between cutaneous branches at the periphery. However, irritation of a nerve root does result in focal pain, paresthesia, dysesthesia, and altered sensation, often in only a part of the nerve root distribution[77,88] (see Table 14-2).

According to Schwartzman,[72] Spurling's (foraminal compression) test (see Chapter 7) may help differentiate nerve root from plexus injury; it also may be positive with brachial plexus injury but usually not to the same degree.

Trunks. The roots combine to form the upper, middle, and lower trunks at the level of the scalene muscles. Fibers from C5 and C6 combine to form the upper trunk. The

middle trunk is a continuation of C7 fibers. C8 and T1 fibers combine to form the lower trunk. These trunks are located mainly in the supraclavicular fossa. Two nerves come off the upper trunk: the subclavian nerve to the subclavian muscle and the suprascapular nerve. The latter nerve passes through the suprascapular foramen to the supraspinatus and infraspinatus muscles[41] (Fig. 14-3). According to Backhouse,[3] the upper portion of the plexus is much more vulnerable to traction, compression, and direct trauma than the lower portion. The lower roots and trunk are more susceptible to trauma related to adjacent anatomic structures.

Schwartzman[72] has described the sensory and motor effects of traction injuries to the upper and lower trunks of the brachial plexus. He states that no single test is diagnostic of brachial plexus traction injury or thoracic outlet syndrome at this time, but some maneuvers are helpful in localizing the site of injury (see Table 14-2).

Divisions. Each of the three trunks divides into an anterior and posterior division. The divisions lie deep to the middle third of the clavicle and extend distally to the lateral border of the first rib (Fig. 14-4). Fibers in the anterior divisions innervate the anterior aspect of the upper extremity; fibers in the posterior divisions innervate the posterior aspect.

Cords. The divisions unite to form the lateral, posterior, and medial cords, named for their position relative to the axillary artery. The cords lie below the clavicle behind the pectoralis minor tendon in the axilla. The posterior divisions from all three trunks combine to form the posterior cord. The anterior divisions from the upper and middle trunks form the lateral cord; the anterior division of the lower trunk forms the medial cord (frequently with a contribution from the middle trunk)[41] (Fig. 14-5).

Similar to the upper and lower trunks, the lateral and medial cords are vulnerable to compromise by traction and epineural fixation to surrounding tissues (see Table 14-2).

Nerves. The *lateral cord* gives rise to three nerves[41] (Fig. 14-6):

1. The lateral pectoral nerve, which branches off from the proximal portion of the cord and provides partial innervation to pectoralis major
2. The musculocutaneous nerve (motor to coracobrachi-

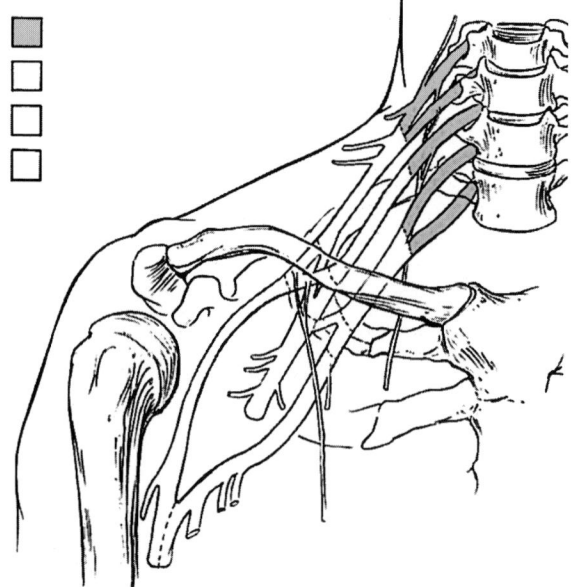

Fig. 14-1. Roots of the brachial plexus. Note the long thoracic and dorsal scapular nerves arising from the roots. (From Callahan AD: Nerve injuries in the upper extremity. In Malick MH, Kasch MC, editors: *Manual on management of specific hand problems,* Pittsburgh, 1984, AREN.)

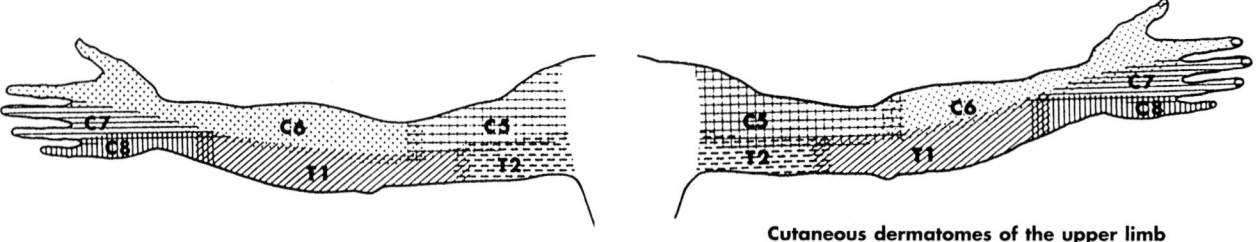

Cutaneous dermatomes of the upper limb

Fig. 14-2. Cutaneous dermatomes of the upper limb. (From Sunderland S: *Nerves and nerve injuries,* ed 2, New York, 1978, Churchill Livingstone.)

alis, biceps, and brachialis; sensory via the lateral cutaneous nerve of the forearm, to the lateral forearm on both its dorsal and volar surfaces)

3. The lateral head of the median nerve (motor to all median innervated muscles except the intrinsics)

The *posterior cord* gives rise to five nerves[41] (Fig. 14-7):

1. Upper subscapular nerve innervates subscapularis.
2. Lower subscapular nerve innervates teres major and provides a branch to subscapularis.
3. Thoracodorsal nerve (also called the *middle subscapular nerve*) motors latissimus dorsi.
4. Axillary nerve innervates the deltoid and teres minor muscles and a small area of skin overlying the lower part of the deltoid muscle.
5. Radial nerve motors the extensors of the elbow, wrist, and digits.

The cutaneous branches of the radial nerve are as follows:

1. Lower lateral cutaneous nerve of the arm supplies lower lateral aspect of the arm.
2. Posterior cutaneous nerve of the arm supplies central posterior aspect of the arm.
3. Posterior cutaneous nerve of the forearm supplies the central posterior aspect of the forearm.
4. Terminal sensory branches supply the dorsal aspect of I, II, and (radial half of) III to the level of the proximal interphalangeal joints.

There is considerable overlap with other cutaneous nerves in each of these areas.

The *medial cord* gives rise to five nerves[41] (Fig. 14-8):

1. Medial pectoral nerve branches off proximally and provides partial innervation to pectoralis major and full innervation to pectoralis minor.
2. Medial brachial cutaneous nerve supplies the medial aspect of the arm on its dorsal and volar surfaces.
3. Medial antebrachial cutaneous nerve of the forearm supplies the medial aspect of the forearm on its dorsal and volar surfaces.
4. Ulnar nerve motors the ulnar wrist flexors, ulnar digital flexors, and ulnar intrinsics in the hand. It

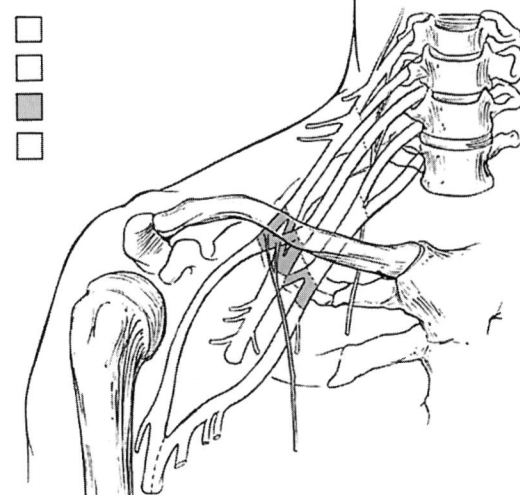

Fig. 14-4. Anterior and posterior divisions of the brachial plexus. (From Callahan AD: Nerve injuries in the upper extremity. In Malick MH, Kasch MC, editors: *Manual on management of specific hand problems,* Pittsburgh, 1984, AREN.)

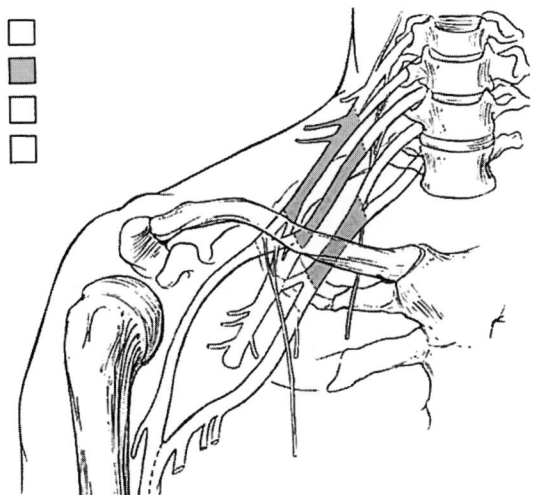

Fig. 14-3. The nerve roots of the brachial plexus combine to form the upper, middle, and lower trunks at the level of the scalene muscles. Note the subclavian and suprascapular nerves arising from the upper trunk. (From Callahan AD: Nerve injuries in the upper extremity. In Malick MH, Kasch MC, editors: *Manual on management of specific hand problems,* Pittsburgh, 1984, AREN.)

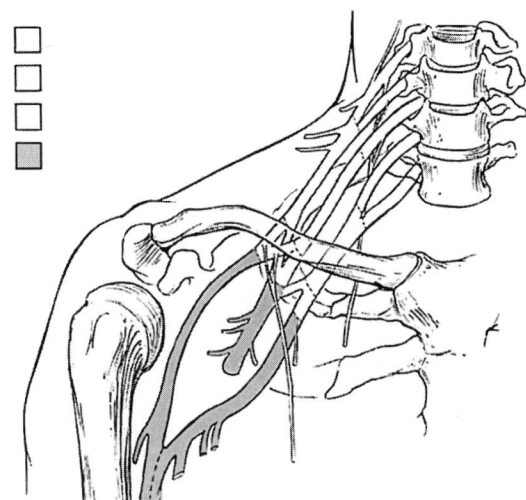

Fig. 14-5. Below the clavicle, the divisions unite to form the lateral, posterior, and medial cords of the brachial plexus.[65] (From Callahan AD: Nerve injuries in the upper extremity. In Malick MH, Kasch MC, editors: *Manual on management of specific hand problems,* Pittsburgh, 1984, AREN.)

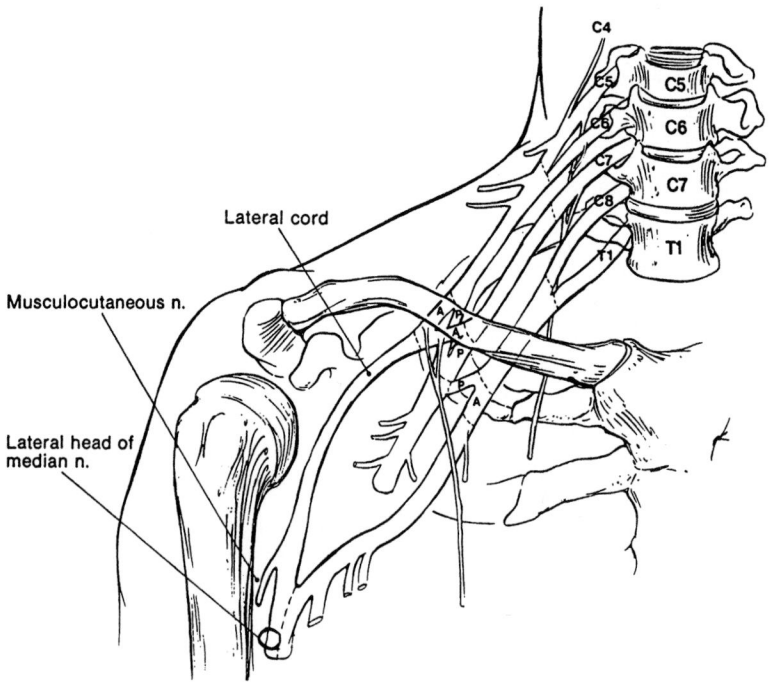

Fig. 14-6. The lateral cord gives rise to three nerves: lateral pectoral nerve, musculocutaneous nerve, and the lateral head of the median nerve.[65] (From Callahan AD: Nerve injuries in the upper extremity. In Malick MH, Kasch MC, editors: *Manual on management of specific hand problems,* Pittsburgh, 1984, AREN.)

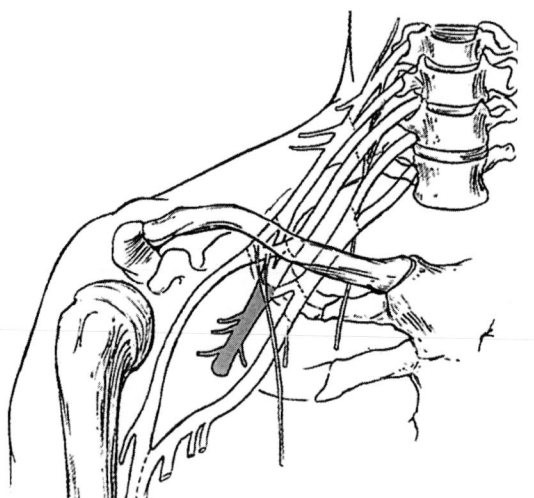

Fig. 14-7. The posterior cord gives rise to five nerves: upper subscapular nerve, lower subscapular nerve, thoracodorsal nerve, axillary nerve, and the radial nerve.[65] (From Callahan AD: Nerve injuries in the upper extremity. In Malick MH, Kasch MC, editors: *Manual on management of specific hand problems,* Pittsburgh, 1984, AREN.)

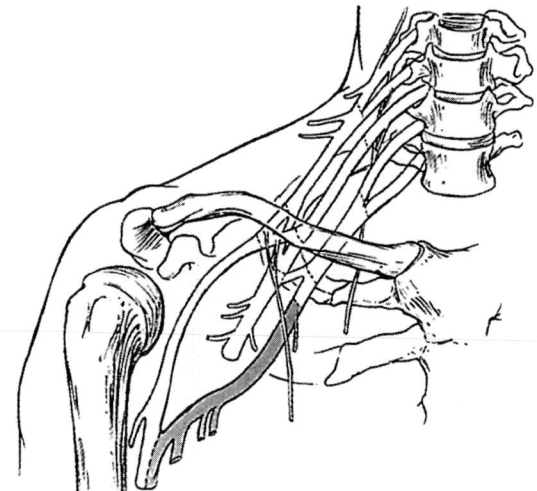

Fig. 14-8. The medial cord gives rise to five nerves: medial pectoral nerve, medial brachial cutaneous nerve, medial antebrachial cutaneous nerve, ulnar nerve, and the medial head of the median nerve.[65] (From Callahan AD: Nerve injuries in the upper extremity. In Malick MH, Kasch MC, editors: *Manual on management of specific hand problems,* Pittsburgh, 1984, AREN.)

provides cutaneous innervation to the skin overlying the ulnar half of IV and all of V.

5. Medial head of the median nerve innervates the median intrinsic muscles in the hand and the skin overlying I, II, III, and radial half of IV on the volar surface and distal to the proximal interphalangeal joints on the dorsal surface.[41]

Box 14-1 lists common sites for nerve lesions in continuity caused by compression, entrapment, or traction.

Prerequisite: knowledge of the effects of nerve injury

Pathomechanics and degrees of injury. Agents of nerve injury are mechanical, thermal, chemical, or ischemic. Trauma results in a nerve lesion in continuity (i.e., compression, constriction, entrapment, or traction) or a divided nerve in which continuity is disrupted and the ends retract (i.e., laceration). Gilliat[36] has noted distinctions between compression, constriction, and entrapment, and defined them as indicated in Table 14-3.

The prognosis for recovery of nerve function depends on which nerve structures are damaged (i.e., axons, endoneurium, perineurium, or epineurium) and the degree of severity. Sunderland[77] describes five degrees of severity of nerve injury, ranging from axonal conduction block in a first-degree injury to transection of the nerve in a fifth-degree injury. His classification is described in detail in Chapter 32.

Sunderland's first-degree injury corresponds to Seddon's "neuropraxia."[73,74] Sunderland[77] observed that *third-degree injury* often occurs in entrapment lesions; in these cases, recovery is spontaneous but incomplete because regenerating axons may be prevented by scar from re-entering their original endoneurial tubes. *Fourth-degree injury* results in much more scarring and internal disorganization than lower levels of injury because the strong perineurial sheath that surrounds fiber bundles is disrupted. There may be some hardly useful spontaneous recovery; therefore surgical intervention is essential if functional recovery is to occur. Even so, residual deficits are to be expected because of internal scarring and faulty regeneration and reinnervation. In *fifth-degree injury,* the entire nerve trunk is transected. As in level four injury, surgical repair is necessary; residual sensory and motor deficits are to be expected. Third-, fourth-, and fifth-degree injuries are the most commonly referred for sensibility assessment.

Patterns of sensibility loss and recovery. When the injury is above the clavicle, affecting the roots and/or trunks, the motor and sensory deficits are segmental in nature. If the injury is below the clavicle, the cords and/or the nerves to which they give rise are affected. The motor and sensory deficits then follow the distribution of the affected peripheral nerves.[41] Because of the overlap between adjacent cutaneous nerves, the area of sensory deficit in a peripheral nerve lesion may be limited to a small region of autonomous supply (see Table 14-2).

Nerve lesions in continuity

Pattern of loss as detected by conventional test instruments.* Sensory fibers are more susceptible to early compression than motor fibers, and the large myelinated (touch) fibers are more susceptible than the small thinly myelinated (pain) or unmyelinated (burning pain, hot, cold) fibers. A specific pattern of sensory loss in nerve compression, specifically carpal tunnel syndrome (CTS), has been demonstrated by the work of Dellon,[21] Lundborg et al.,[50] Gelberman et al.,[32,33] and Szabo et al.[79,80]

Dellon[21] studied a group of 45 patients with 61 compressed nerves, using vibration (256- and 30-cps tuning forks), static and moving two-point discrimination, electrodiagnostic studies, Tinel's sign, and Phalen's sign. Among these seven tests, he found that diminished vibratory perception was the earliest detectable clinical abnormality in compression syndromes of insidious onset.

Lundborg et al.[50] studied the effects of controlled acute external compression to the median nerves of 16 volunteer subjects. They compared motor nerve conduction, sensory nerve conduction, and two-point discrimination findings at three different levels of compression. Among these three tests, the researchers found a decrease in sensory potential amplitude to be the first detectable abnormality. In several cases, even when sensory potential amplitude was severely reduced, two-point discrimination tested within normal limits.

In another study using the same model of controlled compression on 12 volunteer subjects, Gelberman et al.[33] compared findings from the following tests: vibration (256 cps), Semmes-Weinstein Pressure Aesthesiometer (monofilament test), static two-point discrimination, and moving two-point discrimination. They also monitored sensory and motor nerve conduction, subjective findings, and muscle strength. Their results follow:

1. A decrease in sensory amplitude was the earliest electrodiagnostic indication of impaired nerve function.
2. A high correlation was present between the Semmes-Weinstein monofilament test, vibratory testing, and sensory amplitude.
3. Changes in static and moving two-point discrimination consistently occurred together and occurred significantly later than abnormalities on the threshold test (i.e., Semmes-Weinstein and vibration tests).
4. Regarding the two threshold tests, they noted a problem with the quantitation of vibratory stimulus

---

*In this chapter, tests or instruments referred to as "conventional" denote handheld instruments as opposed to computer-assisted test instruments.

Box 14-1 Common sites for sensory nerve lesions in continuity

Within the scalene triangle

- The roots or trunks of the brachial plexus and the subclavian artery are vulnerable to potential mechanical pressure from the borders of the triangle or from other structures. The lower trunk and the subclavian artery are the most susceptible. Their locations adjacent to the first rib or perhaps their arching courses across the first rib make them susceptible to tension exerted by the dependent limb.
- Potential hazards are as follows:
    Hypertrophied scalene muscles
    Sharp fibrous bands associated with the scalene attachments to the first rib
    Developmental variations
    Presence of a cervical rib (the most clearly documented cause and effect)
    Presence of a scalene minimus muscle
    Faulty posture

Lateral to the scalene triangle

- As it exits the posterior triangle of the neck, the brachial plexus passes between the clavicle and first rib. Clavicle depression or rib cage elevation reduces the bony interval, especially medially, and can compress the nerve trunks or axillary vessels.
- More laterally, the neurovascular bundle passes inferior to the coracoid process and posterior to the pectoralis minor. During extreme excursions of the upper limb, especially abduction and external rotation, the brachial plexus is stretched around the coracoid process where it is thought to be vulnerable to stretching.

Musculocutaneous nerve

- This nerve is vulnerable where its terminal branch, the lateral antebrachial cutaneous nerve, pierces investing fascia in the distal arm lateral to biceps and becomes superficial. Here, external compression, such as the strap of a heavy handbag, can injure the nerve.

Radial nerve

In the arm:

- In the axilla, it is vulnerable to the fibrous tendinous edges of latissimus dorsi and the long head of triceps as it passes through the angle between them. It also is vulnerable to an external compressive force such as an axillary crutch.
- In the spiral groove, it is vulnerable to lacerations by sharp bony edges of midshaft humeral fractures.
- Posterior and then inferior to the deltoid tuberosity, it is vulnerable because it is superficial.
- It also is vulnerable where it pierces the lateral intermuscular septum to enter the anterior compartment in the distal lateral arm.

In the forearm and hand:

- The radial nerve crosses the anterolateral aspect of the elbow to enter the forearm. At or about the level of the elbow, the

nerve splits into its *superficial (cutaneous) and deep (posterior interosseous) branches.*

The superficial radial nerve is vulnerable to laceration throughout its course in the hand because it is superficial. It also is vulnerable to compression by external weight.

Median nerve

In the arm:

- The median nerve descends in the neurovascular bundle (median nerve, ulnar nerve, and brachial artery) that passes through the arm at the junction of the investing fascia and the medial intermuscular septum. It is vulnerable to compression by aneurysm within this bundle.

In the forearm, the median nerve is vulnerable:

- At the sharp proximal edge of the bicipital aponeurosis
- By supracondylar fracture or elbow dislocation
- Where it passes between the two heads of pronator teres
- At the proximal border of flexor digitorum superficialis (the "sublimus bridge"). The anterior interosseous nerve branches off distal to the sublimus bridge. The median nerve is vulnerable to compression at pronator or the sublimus bridge. There is no sensory defect.

In the hand:

- The most ventral structure passing through the carpal tunnel, the median nerve is subject to compression within the tunnel.
- The palmar cutaneous branch of the median nerve arises proximal to the wrist and passes superficially to the carpal tunnel; it is spared in carpal tunnel syndrome.

Ulnar nerve

In the arm:

- Within the neurovascular bundle the nerve is vulnerable to compression by aneurysm.
- At the midarm level, it enters the posterior compartment by passing through a fibrous opening where it is subject to entrapment.
- In the posterior compartment, it occupies a groove in the medial head of the triceps brachii muscle (the arcade of Struthers), where it is firmly anchored and has little padding between it and the bone. Here, it is vulnerable to external compression such as from a tourniquet or the hard edge of an operating table.

In the forearm:

- The ulnar nerve enters the forearm by passing posterior to the medial epicondyle in the cubital tunnel. Here it is vulnerable to major and mild trauma.

In the hand:

- The nerve passes through Guyon's canal. It gives off its superficial and deep branches, which are vulnerable to compression.
- The dorsal cutaneous branch of the ulnar nerve arises deep to flexor carpi ulnaris, approximately 5 to 7 cm proximal to the wrist and passes to the dorsum of the hand, sparing the dorsal ulnar innervated skin when the ulnar nerve proper is injured at the wrist.

The information in this box, which has been adapted for boxed format with permission, is compiled from and closely paraphrases text from Pratt NE: *Clinical musculoskeletal anatomy,* Philadelphia, 1991, Lippincott.

Table 14-3. Types of nerve lesions in continuity

Compression	Sustained pressure is applied to a localized region of nerve, either through the skin or internally (e.g., from a hematoma adjacent to the nerve). There is a pressure differential between one part of the nerve and another.[36]
Constriction	A reduction in nerve diameter caused by adjacent tissues.[36]
Entrapment	Constriction or mechanical distortion by a fibrous band or within a fibrous or fibroosseous tunnel.[36]
Traction	Stretching of neural tissue. This condition may coexist with compression, constriction, or entrapment.

and response using the tuning fork, and they described the Semmes-Weinstein monofilament test as the most accurate quantitative test in their model of acute compression.

In the next study in the series, Szabo, Gelberman, and Dimick[79] evaluated 20 patients with idiopathic CTS. All patients had objective abnormalities in median nerve conduction at the wrist level. Sensibility tests were administered before and after surgery. The researchers used a fixed-frequency (120 Hz), variable-amplitude vibrometer (Bio-Thesiometer), and a 256-cps tuning fork to test vibration. The other tests were Semmes-Weinstein Pressure Aesthesiometer, two-point discrimination, Phalen's test, Tinel's test, and the tourniquet test. Their study confirmed that the threshold tests (i.e., vibrometry and Semmes-Weinstein monofilaments) are more sensitive than two-point discrimination in assessing sensibility in chronic compression neuropathies.

In the next study, Szabo et al.[80] returned to the model of controlled acute compression in 12 volunteer subjects. Because of the previously noted problem with quantitation of the tuning fork, they sought to compare findings from the vibrometer with findings from the 256-cps tuning fork, Semmes-Weinstein Pressure Aesthesiometer, static and moving two-point discrimination, and electrodiagnostic tests. They used the same vibrometer (Bio-Thesiometer) as in the previously cited study. They found that vibrometer abnormalities were the earliest clinical findings and had a high correlation with the less quantifiable tuning fork and slightly less sensitive Semmes-Weinstein Pressure Aesthesiometer. All three threshold tests were significantly more sensitive than two-point discrimination ($p = .01$). They concluded that the vibrometer has significant potential as a clinical and research instrument in nerve compression syndromes.

To summarize, the conclusions to be drawn from these studies of acute and chronic compression neuropathies using conventional test instruments, are the following:

1. The earliest objective finding is decreased sensory amplitude in electrodiagnostic testing.
2. The threshold tests, vibration and Semmes-Weinstein pressure test, are the most sensitive indicators of clinical abnormality in compression neuropathies.
3. A vibrometer offers the advantage of quantification over a tuning fork.
4. Abnormalities in moving and static two-point discrimination are late findings in compression neuropathy.

Pattern of loss as detected by the Pressure-Specified-Sensory-Device. In his recent text, Dellon[23] describes a test instrument that he helped develop, the Pressure-Specified-Sensory-Device, which became available in 1989. Dellon reports that it detects a different sequence of sensory loss in chronic nerve compression than the previously cited studies. The instrument is designed to measure four submodalities of touch threshold: cutaneous pressure threshold for one-point static and for one-point moving touch, the pressure threshold for distinguishing one from two static points, and the distance threshold for distinguishing one from two points. In a study of 125 CTS and 71 cubital tunnel syndrome patients, Dellon and Keller[24] found the following:

1. The first parameter to become abnormal with chronic nerve compression was the *pressure threshold for static two-point discrimination.* (This result occurred while the distance for discriminating one from two points remained normal, that is, 3 to 4 mm.)
2. Often, when the pressure threshold for distinguishing one from two static points was already abnormal, the pressure threshold for one-point testing (static or moving) tested normal.

These clinical findings are specific to this instrument. The same order of abnormal thresholds was found in a separate study of patients with tarsal tunnel syndrome and compression of the peroneal nerve at the fibular head. Dellon's conclusion is that given a sensitive enough test instrument, the earliest change that can be detected in chronic nerve compression is the pressure required to distinguish one from two static points touching the skin. He states that for evaluation or screening of chronic nerve compression, just the static touch thresholds (one point and two point) need to be measured.

Intermittent symptoms. Some patients with nerve lesions in continuity complain of sensory symptoms brought on or intensified by certain positions or activities. At rest, they may test normal on both electromyography and clinical sensibility tests. These patients are candidates for "stress testing" in which the affected extremity is subjected to positions or activities selected to provoke sensory symptoms. The patients are tested at rest and after stress. Results of prestress and poststress testing are compared for indications of transient stress neuropathy.

Bell noted the use of sensory stress testing at the Philadelphia Hand Center in 1978.[4] Stress electromyography has been a formal part of the testing protocol there since 1982.[67] Recent reports have confirmed the clinical usefulness of stress testing in patients with transient symptoms of neuropathy.[12,48,78]

Pattern of recovery. The degree of recovery depends on the severity of compression. Mild compression can undergo spontaneous recovery if the initiating cause is removed. Moderate to severe cases that require surgical intervention might respond in one of several ways, including immediate full recovery; gradual full recovery; a period of postoperative hypersensitivity and nerve irritability followed by gradual full recovery; and partial recovery, with or without accompanying hypersensitivity and nerve irritability. Gelberman et al.[32,33] have classified CTS into four stages (early, intermediate, advanced, and acute) and have described the response to treatment of patients in each category.

Divided nerves

Pattern of loss. Immediately after denervation, the autonomous area of nerve supply is anesthetic. Overlapping areas of supply with neighboring cutaneous nerves are hypesthetic. Therefore careful testing should elicit a borderline transition area between the zones of normal and absent sensibility. The transition area is smaller for touch sensibility than for pain sensibility.[73]

During the early weeks after denervation, some ingrowth of nerve supply from normal nerves occurs along the borders of the anesthetic area, thereby causing apparent shrinkage of the anesthetic zone. The exact mechanism for initiation of this phenomenon is not known.[73,77]

Pattern of recovery. The rate of regeneration of sensory fibers in humans generally falls within an average range of 1 to 2 mm per day, with wider ranges reported by some investigators[73,77] An initial recovery rate of 3 mm per day is not unusual, with slowing of the rate over time. Factors affecting the rate of regeneration within an individual include the nature and level of the lesion and the age of the patient.[84]

Pain elicited by pinch is a very early sign of sensory recovery and may precede a positive Tinel's sign.[77] Tenderness to pressure and to pinprick precede sensitivity to moving touch, which precedes light touch and discriminative touch.[14,74,77] At first, perceptions are poorly localized and may radiate proximally or distally. Accurate localization is among the last sensory functions to recover.[82]

Prerequisite: control of test variables

Many variables contribute to the subjective nature of sensibility testing. Ideally, sensory instruments should meet stringent tests of reliability and validity. Although efforts are being made to achieve that goal,* none of our conventional instruments yet meets all seven requirements of standardized tests noted by Fess.[29] These requirements are (1) reliability, (2) validity, (3) administrative instructions, (4) equipment criteria, (5) norms, (6) instructions for interpretation, and often, (7) a bibliography. Note that Dellon[23] states that the Pressure-Specified-Sensory-Device meets all of the criteria of the consensus reports of the American Diabetes Association and the American Peripheral Neuropathy Association for quantitative sensory testing. In a clinical setting, skilled evaluators attempt to control as much as possible for the variables discussed in the following sections.

Environment-related variables. Background noise is distracting to the patient and the tester. A test administered in a noisy environment is not the same as one administered in a quiet environment. All testing should be done in a quiet room. The examiner must be alert for sound made by a testing instrument before or during the application of a stimulus, which will cue the patient to a change in stimulus. Similarly, the sound of a starched lab coat sleeve as the examiner moves about will cue the patient to the arrival of a stimulus. These extraneous noises must be eliminated from the sensibility examination.

Patient-related variables. Patient-related variables have to do with patient attitude, level of concentration, and possibly anxiety level (see Chapter 122 for helpful guidelines on evaluating elderly patients in whom inattention might be a problem). Each patient brings his or her own agenda to a sensibility test. Some will want to test well; others will not. Some are suggestible and may imagine a stimulus when there is none; others admit a sensation only if they are absolutely positive they felt it.

Normal callused skin has a higher sensory threshold than normal uncallused skin in the hand because a given stimulus will deform callused skin less than soft, supple skin. Therefore areas of callosity should be noted so that test results can be more validly assessed. Because sensitivity varies within the normal population, the uninvolved hand is usually the best control in the determination of sensibility dysfunction.

Instrument-related variables. Instrument-related variables include quality control in the manufacturing of instruments and variations in the same instrument over time.[49] Instruments that can be calibrated should be calibrated regularly. Dellon[23] notes that the National Institute of Standards and Technology (NIST) defines measurements, for example, for grams. If a testing device can be calibrated to meet NIST's standards, the device is said to be traceable; the Pressure-Specified-Sensory-Device is a traceable instrument.

The examiner should be aware of the idiosyncrasies of each instrument that he or she uses. For example, some

---

*References 4, 7, 8, 15, 27, 40, 43, 46.

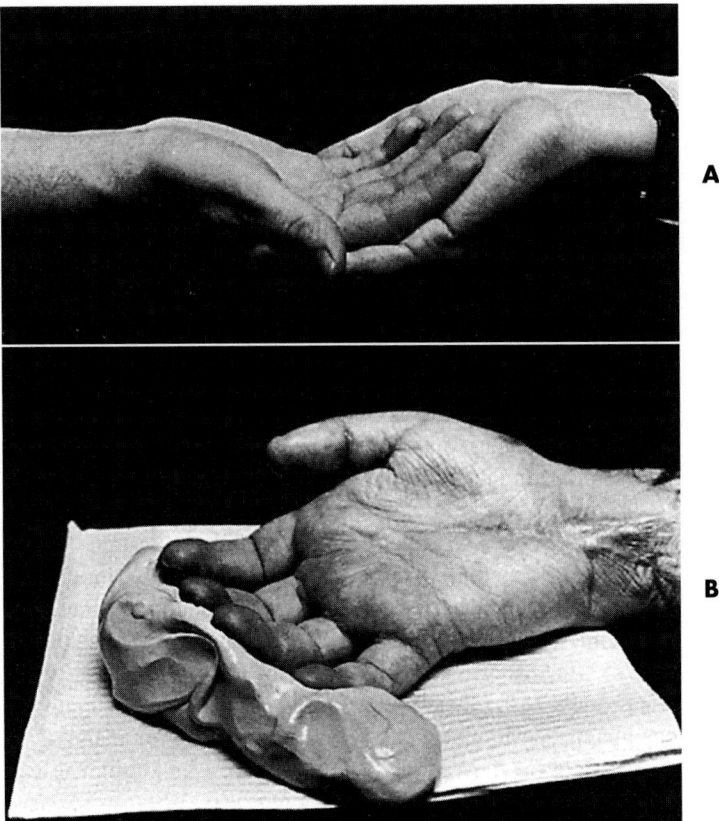

Fig. 14-9. Hand to be tested should be fully supported in examiner's hand (**A**) or fully supported in putty or a similar medium (**B**).

two-point discrimination instruments are heavier than others; the examiner must be careful not to exert a heavier pressure when testing with a heavier instrument.

Greenspan and LaMotte[37] note that in laboratory studies of sensitivity, the experimenter controls either the amount of force that is applied to the skin or the amount of skin indentation (displacement) induced by the instrument. The clinical evaluator should be able to do the same with his instruments. Regardless of which of the two variables are controlled, the evaluator also must be able to control or at least measure various temporal factors, such as the rate and duration of the stimulus. Each of these variables can influence the measurement of threshold sensitivity.[37]

Method-related variables. The same test instrument in two different examiners' hands can produce different results because of differences in the methods of administration. For example, one examiner may use more pressure than the other or may stimulate with a moving instead of a constant touch. Control of method-related variables can be assisted by the following:

1. Provide standard instructions to the patient before each test.

2. Use a standard method of supporting the hand during threshold testing and certain functional tests. Brand[11] has recommended that the hand be fully supported in the examiner's hand so that inadvertent stretch of tissues and movement of joints can be avoided (Fig. 14-9, *A*). He has further suggested that a better method of support would be to rest the hand in putty or a similar medium that would provide full support (Fig. 14-9, *B*). Use of such a medium would have the advantage of eliminating transmission of random vibration in the supporting hand to the hand being tested.[8,11]

3. Parameters of stimulus application must remain the same within a test and between tests. Important parameters include speed of stimulus application, which is known to affect perception,[38] the amount of pressure exerted on the skin, and whether the stimulus is moving or constant.

4. Vary the time interval between applications of the stimulus and the spacing of stimuli so that the patient cannot anticipate the timing or location of the next stimulus.[37]

5. Carefully document the results for better comparison between successive tests.

Bell and Buford[8] demonstrated that when a stimulus is applied with a handheld instrument, the examiner is unable to control for force of application. In part, this is caused by vibration of the hand holding the instrument. An exception is the Semmes-Weinstein Pressure Aesthesiometer. Bell and Tomancik[5] showed that if the lengths and diameters of the filaments are correct, the application forces they produce are repeatable within a predictable range.

Examiner-related variables. Experience, attention to detail, and concern for adherence to methods of administration will affect test results, as will the examiner's level of concentration and fatigue. To minimize the effect of the former variables, the same examiner should perform successive tests on a given patient.

COMPONENTS OF SENSIBILITY ASSESSMENT

Armed with a knowledge of nerve pathways and the effects of injury on sensory function, and prepared to control for as many variables as current instruments and techniques allow, the therapist is prepared to begin the sensibility evaluation.

A thorough assessment includes the following: a careful history, examination of sympathetic function, appropriate selection of tests, administration of the tests in a standard manner so that as many testing variables as possible can be minimized and follow-up evaluation can be reliably compared, and knowledgeable interpretation of information gathered.

REFERRAL AND HISTORY
Candidates for evaluation

Patients may be referred for sensibility evaluation for any of the following reasons: (1) to aid in diagnosis, (2) to aid in serial follow-up after nerve repair, (3) to aid in impairment assessment in compensation cases, and (4) to determine the need or readiness for sensory reeducation.

Obtaining the history

A careful history, based on medical chart information and skillful interviewing of the patient, will provide the examiner with information that cannot be gained by any specific clinical test. Such information will aid in shortening the time required for testing and will help determine the prognosis for recovery.

A history should include name, age, sex, dominance, and occupation. Age influences prognosis for recovery. Occupation and whether the dominant or nondominant extremity was injured will help in estimating degree of sensibility recovery required for functional use of the extremity in work and leisure activities.

The date, nature, and level of injury also should be recorded. The time elapsed since the date of injury or repair helps in proper assessment of Tinel's sign and in better interpretation of the presence or absence of sympathetic function. The nature of the injury (e.g., laceration, crush, traction, compression) will influence the amount of scarring that occurs, in turn influencing the quality of regeneration. Prognosis for recovery of distal sensory function partially depends on the level of the injury; injuries at or proximal to the wrist level rarely result in good functional sensation in the adult.[25,56,59]

The medical chart often documents a patient's involvement in litigation. This is important information for the examiner because litigation might influence the level of cooperation of the patient. The best candidate for sensibility evaluation is one who has nothing to gain by abnormal test results.

Skillful interviewing is important. Questions should be phrased in such a way as to avoid leading the patient. Thus an appropriately worded initial question would be, "Please tell me what problems you have in this hand." The patient will then tend to rank his or her nerve-related complaints without artificial emphasis on sensory disturbances. For example, a patient with CTS may not describe any sensory-related problems, limiting the complaint to a weakness in grip strength. In this case, one could expect that the patient would probably test with normal or only slightly diminished sensibility. On the other hand, if the patient states, "It feels like there is a veil on my fingertips when I try to pick up something," he or she could be expected to test with slight to moderate loss of sensibility. Terms such as *numbness, dead, asleep,* and *pins and needles* may refer to hypesthesia, anesthesia, or paresthesia, depending on the patient, and should be clarified.

After the patient has described his or her dysfunction in his or her own words, the examiner can ask more leading questions to elicit greater detail about the current status of sensibility. Such questioning will help the nonsophisticated or nonobservant patient articulate his or her problems. The examiner will want to know if sensibility is improving, getting worse, or staying the same. Are symptoms aggravated by certain positions or activities or temperatures (i.e., cold intolerance)? Are they relieved by certain positions or motions (e.g., "shaking of the arm")? Does the sensibility deficit affect performance of activities of daily living (ADLs)?

At this time in the examination, it is convenient to assess briefly motor function, including grip and pinch strength and, in selected cases, individual muscle strength because motor function will affect performance on certain sensibility tests that may be used. The patient's performance during these motor tests can suggest to the examiner the patient's general level of cooperation, as evidenced by the shape of his or her strength curve on the Jamar dynamometer (see Chapter 8) and exertion of maximal effort during muscle testing.

Table 14-4. Sympathetic changes after nerve injury

Sympathetic function		Early changes	Late changes
Vasomotor	Skin color	Rosy	Mottled or cyanotic
	Skin temperature	Warm	Cool
Sudomotor	Sweat	Dry skin	Dry or overly moist
Pilomotor	Gooseflesh response	Absent	Absent
Trophic	Skin texture	Soft; smooth	Smooth; nonelastic
	Soft-tissue atrophy	Slight	More pronounced, especially in finger pulps
	Nail changes	Blemishes	Curved in longitudinal and horizontal planes; "talonlike"
	Hair growth	May fall out or become longer and finer	May fall out or become longer and finer
	Rate of healing	Slowed	Slowed

ASSESSMENT OF SYMPATHETIC FUNCTION IN THE HAND

Sympathetic fibers subserve vasomotor (*vas,* Latin "vessel"), sudomotor (*sudor,* Latin "sweat"), and pilomotor (*pilus,* Latin "hair") functions in the extremity. After nerve injury, the area of loss of sympathetic function closely corresponds to the area of loss of sensory function because the cutaneous sympathetic fibers follow essentially the same pathway to the periphery as the cutaneous sensory fibers.[77] The actual autonomous area of sympathetic function may be smaller than the corresponding autonomous area of cutaneous sensory function because there is more overlap between sympathetic fibers of different nerves than between sensory fibers.[41] The combination of sympathetic and sensory dysfunction results in characteristic trophic (*trophe,* Greek "nourishment") changes in all tissues of the involved area.[77] Examination of the sympathetic function and trophic changes in the hand (Table 14-4) provides definite information on the nutritional state of the part and suggestive information on sensory function in the part.

The correlation between presence of sympathetic function and sensibility is greatest immediately after nerve laceration and in long-term cases in which little or no regeneration has occurred. However, if the original injury were partial or the nerve undergoes incomplete regeneration, sympathetic function may return without significant return of sensation.[60,62,76,77]

Vasomotor changes

Vasomotor function is reflected in skin temperature, color, edema, and cold intolerance. For 2 to 3 weeks after complete denervation, or longer in some incomplete lesions, the skin feels warm to the touch because of vasodilation secondary to paralysis of the vasoconstrictors.[74] This warm phase is gradually superseded, for reasons not completely understood, by a phase in which the skin feels cool to the touch. According to Richards,[68] normal warmth of the skin does not occur until there is a high degree of sensory recovery.

Skin temperature is quickly assessed by use of the dorsum of the examiner's hand to compare the involved cutaneous area with the contralateral normal area. The dorsum is used because it is rich in temperature receptors and is less likely than the warm, moist volar skin to result in a false reading.

During the warm phase, the skin is flushed or rosy. During the cold phase, it is usually mottled (a combination of pallor and cyanosis) or, in severe cases, reddish blue from stasis.[14] Color is assessed by visual comparison with the uninvolved hand.

Edema may occur as a result of decreased circulatory function and is more likely after brachial plexus injuries than distal injuries.[74]

During the cold phase, the patient may complain of cold intolerance. The skin temperature is abnormally influenced by environmental temperature, particularly cold, and when exposed to cold, the part becomes cold and rewarms slowly.[77] There may be mild to severe pain that is relieved when the extremity is warmed or the pain may last several hours after exposure. Cold intolerance may extend beyond the denervated part to include the entire hand and will recover only as reinnervation restores normal circulation.[74,77]

McCabe et al.[53] developed a seven-item patient-answered questionnaire to measure the severity of cold sensitivity in the hand and to grade potential exposure of the hands to cold in the workplace (Fig. 14-10). They established high test-retest reliability and demonstrated construct validity.

The questionnaire was used later in a prospective cohort study[18] of 123 patients with acute hand and forearm injuries over a period of 11 months after injury. A subset of 25 patients with more severe symptoms at 11 months was reassessed at 3 years. The results indicated that the severity of cold sensitivity increased from the time of injury until 3 months after injury and then remained constant until the assessment at 11 months after injury. The more severely symptomatic patients who answered the questionnaire again at 3 years after the injury had reduced severity of symptoms (67% of the 11-month level scores) as measured by this

A

1. How much does cold bother your injured hand while holding a glass of ice water?

2. How much does cold bother your injured hand when you get out of a hot shower or hot bathtub with the air at room temperature?

3. How much does cold bother your injured hand holding a frozen package from the freezer?

4. How much does cold bother your injured hand when you wash in cold water?

← —————— 100 mm —————— →

not at all   mild   moderate   severe   extreme

B

1. How much of your work requires manipulation of objects with your hands at temperature near or below freezing?

2. At work, how much time are you required to be working either outside in the cold or in a refrigerated environment?

3. How much do you do with the temperature at or near freezing when you are not able to wear warm gloves or mittens?

never   rarely   occasionally   usually   all the time

Fig. 14-10. The Cold Sensitivity Severity Scale (**A**) and the Potential Work Exposure Scale (**B**) developed by McCabe et al.[53] to measure cold sensitivity. Subjects responded to each item by placing an "X" on a 100-mm line with indicators at 25-mm intervals and underlying descriptors. The distance in mm from the beginning of the line to the X is the score for that item. Scores are summed for a total score for cold sensitivity severity and for potential work exposure. (From reference 53.)

scale. (For a more detailed discussion of cold intolerance see Chapter 91.)

Sudomotor changes

Lack of sweating occurs in the autonomous area of the sympathetic fibers immediately after denervation. Abnormally increased sweating, such that beads of sweat are clearly visible, may occur after partial nerve injury, especially when the nerve is irritated and pain is present, or during regeneration of a lacerated nerve.[41]

The presence of sweating does not imply the return of sensory function.[50,60,62] However, the absence of sweating in a recent nerve laceration or in a long-term injury does strongly correlate with a lack of discriminative sensation.[30,55]

Pilomotor changes

Absence of the "gooseflesh" response occurs when there is complete interruption of sympathetic supply to an area.[41] This phenomenon is not included in a routine sensibility evaluation.

Trophic changes

Interruption of normal nerve supply results in interruption of the normal nutritive process of the tissues, thereby causing some atrophy of all tissues from skin to bone.[14] Decreased nutrition is evident in skin texture, the soft tissue of the finger pulps, nail changes, hair growth, increased susceptibility to injury, and slowed healing.

Trophic changes are reversible as regeneration occurs. Persistent changes are associated with failure of regeneration or chronic irritation of a partial nerve lesion. Some nerves carry more sympathetic fibers than others; thus median nerve lesions result in more trophic changes (particularly noticeable in the index finger) than ulnar nerve lesions, which result in more changes than the radial nerve. Trophic changes are more pronounced in causalgic states and in brachial plexus lesions than in simple nerve lacerations.[14,77]

Skin texture. Early on, the skin is thin and smooth, almost "velvety" because atrophy of the epidermis has caused the papillary ridges and finger creases to become less distinct. In long-term cases, the skin becomes shiny, smooth, and inelastic.[77] Examination is by visual observation and by palpation.

Atrophy of finger pulps. The generalized atrophy that follows denervation is most obvious in the pulps of the fingers, which may take on a tapered appearance. In fact, the entire digit may appear noticeably smaller than its corresponding digit on the other hand. This change occurs with long-term denervation because of irreparable injury or failure of regeneration; therefore it is not generally observed to reverse itself.[77]

Nail changes. Changes within the first few months include striations, ridges and similar blemishes, slowed growth, and increased hardness.[77] Later, in response to atrophy of the soft tissue of the digits, the nails conform to the shape of the atrophied pulp. They become smaller than the corresponding nail on the opposite hand and curve in the longitudinal and horizontal planes. They may become talonlike in appearance. The lunula is diminished or absent (Fig. 14-11). Severe nail changes are signs of long-term denervation and therefore are not likely to improve with time.[77]

Hair growth. Hair loss may occur in the region of denervation or may become longer and finer.[14] Occasionally, it demonstrates increased growth, termed *hypertrichosis,* which is most often noted on the forearm in radial nerve and median nerve injuries and occasionally in injuries of the brachial plexus.[41] Seddon[74] states that the apparent increase

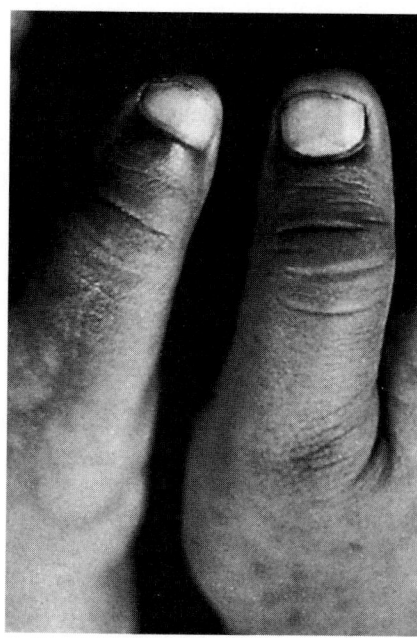

Fig. 14-11. Thumbnail changes in a case of chronic median nerve denervation. Notice that the nail on the left is smaller than the one on the right and has no visible lunula. The thumb has atrophied, and the nail has curved to conform to tapered tip.

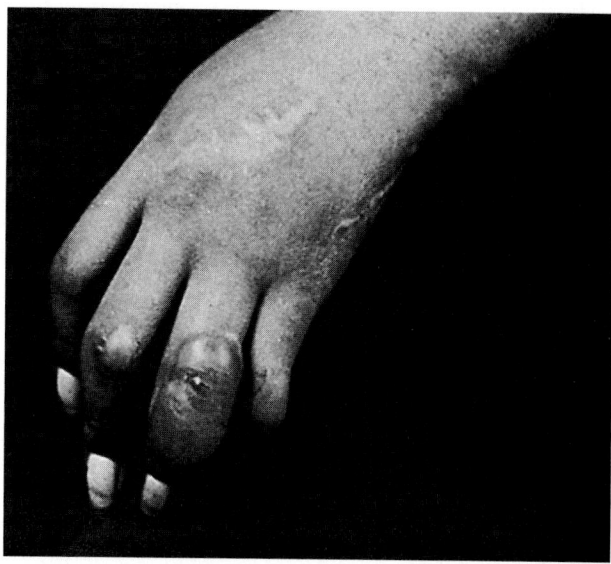

Fig. 14-12. This hand with median and ulnar nerve injury was allowed to rest against a hot radiator, resulting in second-degree burns, to ulnar three digits.

in growth of hair on the forearm is often attributable to atrophy of the denervated part. In causalgia, there is loss of hair where the skin is atrophic and shiny.[77]

Susceptibility to injury and slowed healing. Atrophy of the epidermis and underlying tissue causes the skin to become more delicate and therefore more susceptible to injury from noxious stimuli, including pressure, temperature, and sharp objects. This is clearly exemplified during the pinprick test when atrophic skin is penetrated by a sharp pin and responds with a minute spot of blood, whereas normal skin on the same extremity does not. Healing takes longer than in normal skin because of decreased nutrition and vascularity, a condition that reverses itself as reinnervation occurs.[77] The patient who does not compensate for increased susceptibility to injury will often present with blisters and ulcers on the denervated skin (Fig. 14-12), whereas the presence of "wear" marks[54] such as dirt stains and calluses, indicates functional use of the hand and is a sign of useful sensibility. Absence of "wear" marks on skin that has undergone reinnervation and has adequate motor function while other parts of the same hand demonstrate them indicates lack of use and useful sensibility of the unmarked parts (Fig. 14-13).

A thorough history and examination of the hand will clue the experienced examiner to the status of sensibility in the hand. However, the details of sensory dysfunction and the progress of regeneration can be determined only through the administration of specific clinical tests designed to assess sensibility.

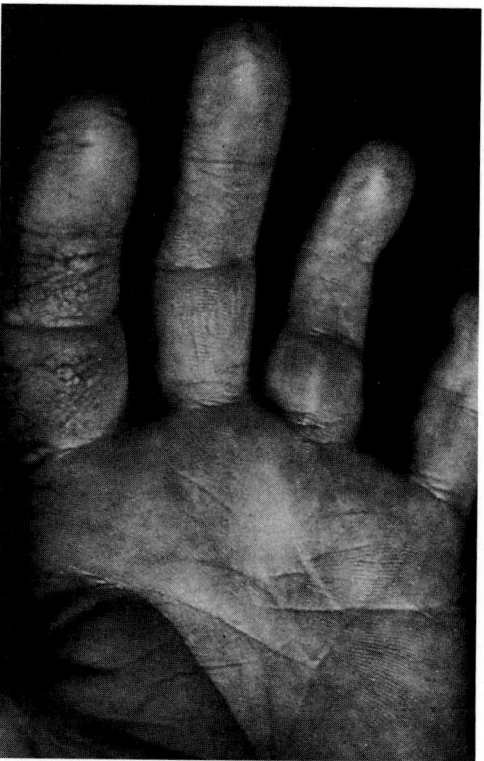

Fig. 14-13. "Wear marks" on the hand of a mechanic indicate that index finger is used for functional activities, but ulnar three digits, which had sustained digital nerve injury 1 year previously are not. Testing revealed presence of light touch but poor discriminative sensation in involved digits.

MAPPING THE AREA OF SENSORY DYSFUNCTION

Assessment of sensibility is faster and more precise when one maps out the area of sensibility dysfunction before the administration of specific tests. This can be done in two ways.

Mapping by examiner

The examiner draws a probe, such as the blunt end of a pen, lightly over the skin, starting from an area of normal sensibility and proceeding to the area of suspected abnormal sensibility. The patient, whose vision is occluded, is asked to immediately say "now" when the sensation produced by the probe is suddenly "different." Using a felt-tip pen, the examiner marks the skin at the spot where the patient said "now" and then proceeds to approach the area of dysfunction from another starting point. The area is thus approached from all directions—proximal, distal, radial, and ulnar—until all boundaries are marked (Fig. 14-14).

Note that in early or mild nerve lesions in continuity, mapping may not produce an identifiable area of dysfunction, thereby indicating that light-touch perception has not been affected to a degree detectable by this technique. This is a good prognostic sign for resolution of sensory symptoms by conservative or surgical intervention. Note also that in later stages of regeneration after nerve repair, mapping may not produce an identifiable area of light-touch dysfunction. This condition can be interpreted as excellent recovery of light touch.

Mapping by patient

Some examiners prefer to have the patient map the area of dysfunction. With vision unoccluded, the patient draws

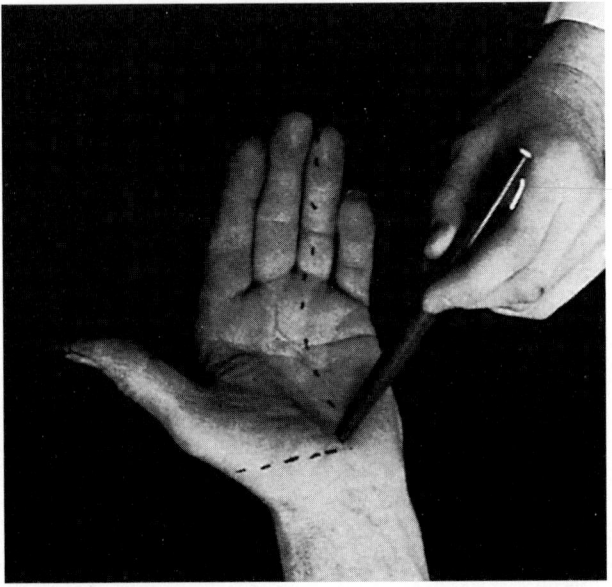

Fig. 14-14. Mapping area of dysfunction helps make subsequent testing faster and more accurate.

the probe across his or skin as described previously and marks on the skin where the sensation produced by the probe suddenly feels different. This method may allow for a more precise mapping.

With either method of mapping, the probe should be drawn fairly slowly across the skin with a light touch so that no drag is produced. Each time the probe passes over the same path, a reliable patient will say "now" at the same location. Progress in reinnervation will be reflected in a progressively diminishing "map" size over time. The results of mapping should be transferred to an outline of the hand or photographed to provide a permanent record.

TEST SELECTION AND ADMINISTRATION
Categories of sensibility tests

Our current sensibility tests can be divided into four categories: threshold tests, functional tests, objective tests, and provocative or stress tests.

Threshold tests. Threshold tests seek to determine the minimum stimulus (within the limitations of the test instrument) that can be perceived by the subject. They measure sensory impairment. Threshold tests include those for the four classic cutaneous functions (pain, heat, cold, and touch-pressure) and for vibration.[18]

The Semmes-Weinstein pressure aesthesiometer[4,75,83,86] and the Automated Tactile Tester (ATT)[40,43,46] are examples of threshold test instruments for one-touch pressure threshold. The latter instrument is a computer-controlled device used to test low- and high-frequency vibration, pinprick, warmth, and two-point discrimination, as well as light touch.

Dellon's Pressure-Specified-Sensory-Device is another computer-assisted device useful for measuring pressure threshold for static and moving one-point touch, the distance threshold for detection of two points, and the pressure threshold for detection of two points. Traditionally, two-point discrimination testing has been thought of as a functional test[54] (described in the following discussion) or a test of innervation density.[22] Because of the ability of his instrument to test for two-point discrimination *pressure* threshold, Dellon[23] now categorizes two-point discrimination as a threshold measurement test. He explains that innervation density is a necessary but not sufficient determinant of two-point discrimination; stimulus intensity is another component.

Functional tests. Functional tests assess the usefulness of the sensibility and address the issue of disability caused by sensory impairment. For example, is sensibility present on a gross level only, or on a fine discriminative level? Is it useful for fine-prehension tasks? Is it sufficient for daily activities and work tasks in which vision is occluded during manipulation of objects? It is these qualities that Moberg termed *tactile gnosis*. These tests are considered integrative tests because they require a higher level of sensory processing than the threshold tests do.

Functional tests include classic static two-point discrimination and moving two-point discrimination (i.e., as tested with conventional handheld instruments), touch localization, Moberg pickup test and its variations, and other tests of tactile gnosis.[13,64,71] Some of these require active manipulation of an object rather than simply passive recognition of a stimulus. The requirement for active manipulation is based on recognition that touch is an active, exploratory process of the hand, not merely a passive receptive sense, and therefore touch can be more accurately assessed if the hand is permitted to actively explore and "scan" the object presented.[34] Note the converse: Requiring active manipulation when there is a motor defect can result in *under*estimation of sensory function.

Other tests of function include ADL assessment, job simulation, and assessment of cold intolerance.

Objective tests. Objective tests include the Ninhydrin sweat test and other tests of sudomotor function, nerve conduction studies, and the wrinkle test.[61] These are termed *objective* because they require only passive cooperation of the patient and not his or her subjective interpretation of a stimulus. They do not directly correlate with functional sensation after nerve repair.[1,60,62,76] However, the sudomotor and wrinkle tests can be useful in obtaining information about the function of a nerve in children and suspected malingerers, and nerve conduction tests provide useful information about conduction parameters in a nerve (see Chapter 10).

Provocative tests and stress tests. Stress tests are designed to elicit or increase latent sensory symptoms. A patient is tested under normal "at rest" conditions and after subjecting the affected part to stress.* Stress tests can be useful in those patients whose history indicates intermittent symptoms or symptoms brought on by particular activities or positions. The particular stress test chosen might be a provocative position (e.g., maximal wrist flexion and extension for CTS), maneuver (see Table 14-2), or work-simulation activity. A study by Gillenson et al.[35] supports the use of Semmes-Weinstein monofilaments for stress testing. They measured touch threshold with the monofilaments in normal subjects with the wrist in neutral, maximal active flexion, and maximal active extension. They found no change in threshold caused by wrist position. They concluded that if a change in sensation is found when the wrist is positioned in a provocative posture, of either flexion or extension, the result may suggest the presence of a pathologic condition.

Administration of specific tests

Determination and interpretation of Tinel's sign. Tinel's sign[81] is assessed by gentle percussion from distal to proximal along the nerve trunk. The most distal point at which the patient experiences a tingling sensation that radiates distally in the cutaneous distribution of the nerve is the point of positive Tinel's sign. This sign is said to represent the advancing terminations of the regenerating sensory axons. Progress in regeneration can be documented by recording the level of Tinel's sign in successive examinations, using an anatomic landmark as a point of reference. For nerve lesions in continuity, a positive Tinel's sign helps localize the site of injury.

Seddon[74] states that a positive sign can occur in the presence of a partial, unrepaired nerve lesion, thereby falsely indicating regeneration. He credits Henderson[42] with making the sign more informative by his repeated observations on 400 cases of nerve injury in prisoner-of-war hospitals in World War II. Seddon[74] states:

Henderson found that Tinel's sign became important about 4 months after the time of injury. If it was strongly positive at the level of the lesion but persistently absent below, spontaneous regeneration could not be expected. If the sign was strongly positive at the site of damage and also appeared weakly distal to it, the quality of regeneration would be poor. But a strongly positive sign at the level of the lesion that gradually faded as the response moved peripherally and became stronger in the distal part of the nerve indicated that satisfactory regeneration was in progress.

One must always assess the meaning of Tinel's sign in the context of other information gathered about sensory function. The sign may be absent where too much muscle lies over the nerve to allow adequate percussion of it.[74]

Threshold tests. Details on administration of proprietary computer assisted tests, such as the Automated Tactile Tester,[43] The Case IV System,[28] and the Pressure-Specified-Sensory-Device, is beyond the scope of this chapter. The reader is referred to the original authors and to Dellon[23] for a review of these systems. Discussion in this chapter focuses on administration of conventional threshold tests.

Conventional threshold tests of pain and touch-pressure are useful for monitoring return of sensibility in the early months after nerve laceration. Threshold tests of vibration and touch-pressure are used to assess early changes in sensibility caused by nerve compression.[21,33,79,80]

A goal in threshold testing is to record information in a way that allows for more reliable comparison with follow-up reports. When testing for pain, temperature, or touch-pressure, one can make testing more systematic and documentation more accurate by use of a worksheet that has a grid superimposed on an outline of the hand (Fig. 14-15). The grid is divided into zones, whose longitudinal lines parallel the rays of the hand and whose horizontal lines correspond to the flexion creases of the digits and palm. This grid was devised by von Prince[83] for use in her studies of light-touch dysfunction in nerve-injured patients in the 1960s, but the grid is useful for other tests as well. During testing, the examiner visualizes the grid on the patient's hand and applies the test stimulus to a particular zone. Correct and incorrect responses are recorded in the corresponding zone on the worksheet. A different worksheet can be used for each

*References 3, 6, 12, 45, 48, 67, 68.

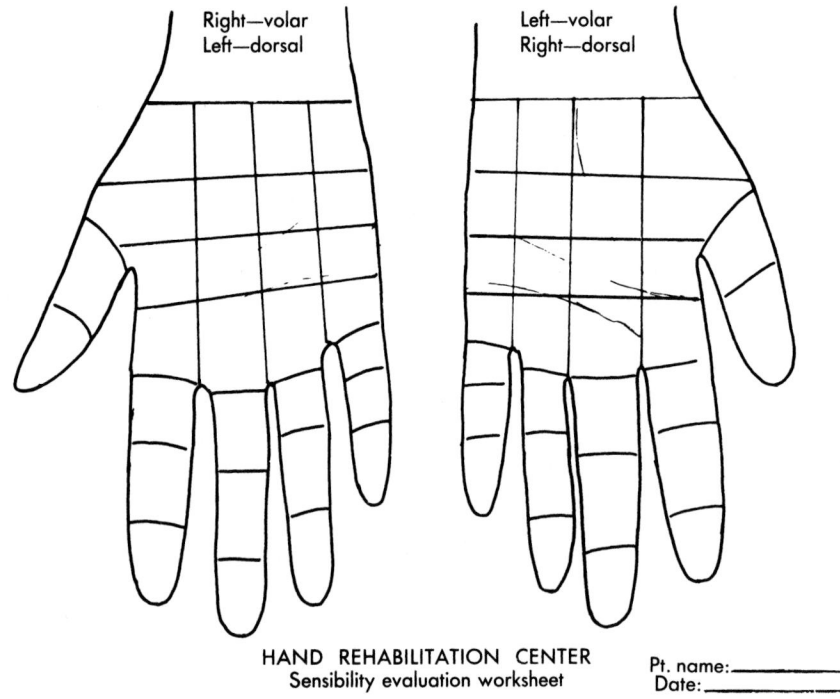

Right—volar
Left—dorsal

Left—volar
Right—dorsal

HAND REHABILITATION CENTER
Sensibility evaluation worksheet

Pt. name:_____
Date: _____

Fig. 14-15. Grid worksheet is recommended during threshold testing to make testing and documentation more systematic.

test, and the worksheets can be filed for permanent records or the information on the worksheet can be transferred to a more formal report. The use of this grid is explored in the following description of methodology for the threshold tests.

During all threshold tests, the hand is fully supported in the examiner's hand or in putty (see Fig. 14-9). Vision is occluded by use of a blindfold, by the patient simply closing his or her eyes, or by a screen. The last method is ideal because it allows test instruments and recording sheets to be hidden from view even between tests when vision might not otherwise be occluded.

Pinprick. Protective sensation is the ability to perceive painful or potentially harmful stimuli on the skin and in the subcutaneous tissue. Heat, cold, deep pressure, low-grade repetitive pressure, and superficial pain are examples of such stimuli. Of these, the most commonly tested and the one regarded as the best test of protective sensation is superficial pain tested with a safety pin. It is not sufficient simply to require the patient to say "now" when touched with the sharp end of the pin because the patient may respond simply to pressure of the stimulus and not sharpness of the stimulus. A more accurate assessment of protective sensation requires that the patient discriminate between the sharp and dull sides of the pin.

When testing with a pin, the examiner should keep in mind that during nerve regeneration, a period of hypersensitivity to pinprick will occur. In the area of hyperanalgesia, the response to pinprick will be hyperacute, that is,

abnormally unpleasant. For patient comfort, testing should proceed in such a way that the number of applications of the stimulus in one "zone" of the hand is minimized.

The amount of pressure necessary to elicit correct responses on the uninvolved hand is used as a guide for pressure to be used on the involved hand. The examiner alternates randomly between the sharp and dull sides of the pin, being sure that each "zone" has been stimulated at least once by each end of the pin so that true discrimination within an area has been ascertained. The entire area of dysfunction, as determined previously by mapping, is tested.

Results within a zone are scored as follows: correct response to both sharp and dull, intact protective sensation; incorrect response to both sharp and dull, absent protective sensation; hyperalgesic; or pressure awareness only.

Sunderland[77] notes that the perception of pinprick ranges along a hierarchy that includes absence of awareness, pressure sensation without distinguishing between sharp and dull, hyperanalgesia with radiation, sharp sensation with some radiation and gross localization, sensation of sharpness with or without slight stinging or radiation and fair localization, and finally, normal perception. Seddon[74] likewise grades the response to pinprick along several parameters.[74]

Moberg[56] and Dellon,[22] among others, have stated that they do not test for pinprick because of the discomfort involved to the patient and because the information gained does not correlate directly with functional sensation. However, one can argue for testing pinprick after nerve laceration

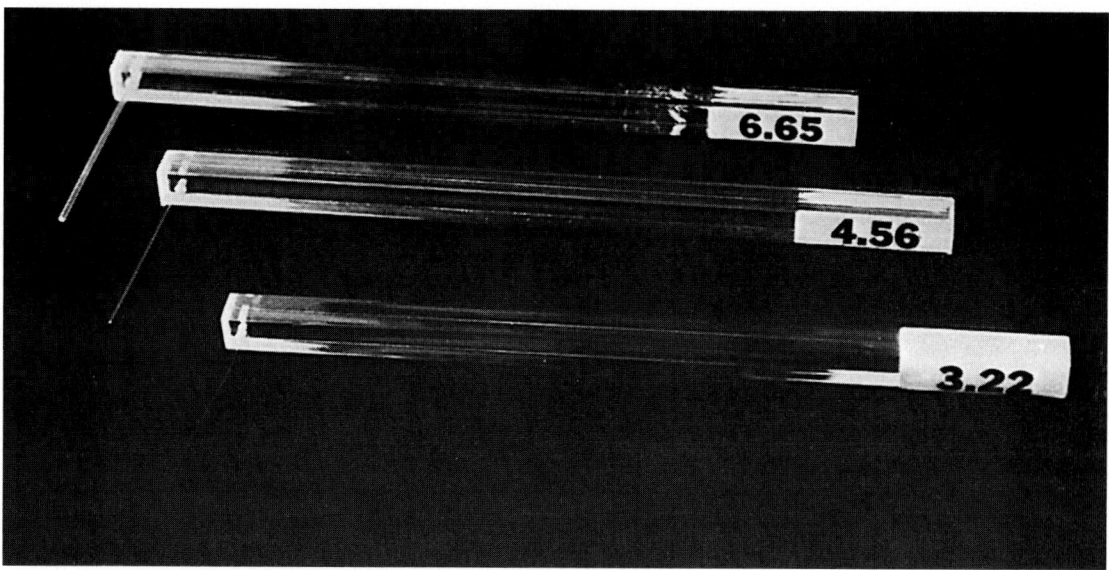

Fig. 14-16. Each probe consists of a nylon monofilament attached to a Lucite rod.

if other indications of sensibility return are absent. In these instances, it becomes important to know if this parameter of protective sensation is intact.

Temperature. Test tubes or metal cylinders filled with hot and cold fluids have been used for clinical testing of temperature perception. Because of the difficulties in controlling test conditions within a test and between tests and the lack of direct correlation with functional sensation, many clinicians do not test for temperature discrimination.[22,55,74,77] Some satisfy themselves with testing simply for the perception of hot and cold on a gross level; others do not test for temperature at all, preferring to allow the presence of pinprick perception to be sufficient evidence of protective sensation.

Touch-pressure. Light touch and deep pressure sensibility are considered to represent two ends of a continuum of cutaneous sensibility, with light touch being perceived by receptors in the superficial skin layers and pressure being perceived by receptors in the subcutaneous and deeper tissue.[77] Pressure sensibility is a form of protective sensation because it warns of deep pressure or of low-grade repetitive pressure, which might result in injury to the skin. Light touch sensibility is a necessary component of fine discrimination.

In 1960, Semmes and Weinstein[75] developed a graded light-touch testing instrument for use in a study of somatosensory changes in brain-injured adults. This instrument, the Semmes-Weinstein Pressure Aesthesiometer (North Coast Medical, Campbell, California) is a kit of 20 probes, each probe consisting of a nylon monofilament attached to a Lucite rod (Fig. 14-16). Each probe is marked with a number ranging from 1.65 to 6.65 that represents the logarithm of 10 times the force in tenths of milligrams (log 10 force 0.1 mg) required to bow the monofilament when it is

applied perpendicular to the skin.[85] Thus, correctly applied, the finest monofilament, labeled 1.65, produces a pressure of 1.5 g/mm^2, and the thickest filament, 6.65, produces a pressure of 439 g/mm^2.[26,84]

In 1967, von Prince[83] introduced this instrument into the therapy clinic for use in testing touch-pressure sensibility in the nerve-injured hand. Her pioneering efforts were taken up by Werner and Omer[86] and Bell.[4] The methods of administration and interpretation of this test are described in detail in Chapter 13.

The latest modifications of the instrument are a minikit of five specially selected monofilaments from the full set[6,9] and the Weinstein Enhanced Sensory Test (WEST) (Connecticut Bioinstruments Inc., Danbury, Connecticut).[84] The latter instrument includes modifications designed to increase ease of portability, to increase speed of testing, to increase resistance to damage, to reduce tip slippage on the skin, and to provide consistent pressures on the skin. These instruments are described fully by Bell-Krotoski in Chapter 13.

Vibration. Bell-Krotoski has noted that tests of vibration with handheld instruments are particularly prone to lack of control because of variations in force of stimulus and the manner in which the stimulus is applied. Moreover, although decreased vibration sense is an early finding in compression neuropathy, a correlation of decreased vibration with decreased tactile function (be it touch-pressure, protective sensation, or discriminative sensation) has yet to be established.[7,8,9] The tuning fork, vibrometer, and Automated Tactile Tester (ATT),[40,43,46] three clinical instruments currently used for testing vibration, vary in the amount of stimulus control they afford the tester.

Tuning fork. According to the methods of Dellon,[22] testing with a 256-cps tuning fork in nerve compression syndromes is done as follows. The tuning fork is first struck against a surface, and then one of the prong ends is applied tangential to the surface being tested. (Bell and Buford[8] found that force amplitude is more controllable when the base of the tuning fork is applied.) The examiner attempts to control intensity of amplitude by trying to maintain the same striking force with each application of the tuning fork. The fingertips of the thumb and index fingers are the test sites in median nerve compression, and the tip of the small finger is the test site in ulnar nerve compression. The patient closes his or her eyes during the test. The vibrating tuning fork is applied to the test site and to two control sites: the contralateral fingertip and an ipsilateral noninvolved fingertip. After each paired stimulation to a test site and control site, the patient is asked, "How did they feel different?" Responses such as "didn't feel anything," "softer," "louder," "quieter," and others are recorded as "abnormal" perception. Dellon also requires that the vibration be localized to rule out perception by a neighboring nerve or distant receptors.

Vibrometer. The vibrometer (Bio-Thesiometer) consists of a handheld, variable-amplitude, fixed-frequency vibrator and a voltage meter (which measures increasing voltage as vibration amplitude is increased). Instructions for operation and administration accompany the instrument. The stimulus is first demonstrated to the patient on an uninvolved area of the hand, starting at an amplitude below threshold and continuing up to and past threshold. The patient is instructed to close his or her eyes during the test and to say "now" as soon as the first sensation of vibration is felt. The examiner supports the finger being tested and applies the stimulus through a button-shaped vibrating head held against the finger. The suspected involved fingertips are tested, as well as ipsilateral and contralateral fingertips.

The threshold level is recorded in volts from the voltage meter. This reading can be converted to absolute amplitude (measured in microns) through a calibration table furnished with the instrument. Although the vibrometer has limitations in common with other handheld testing instruments[7] (see Chapter 13), it provides a more quantitative assessment of vibration than the tuning fork and allows for more reliable comparison of preoperative and postoperative thresholds.

Automated tactile tester. The ATT[43] is a computer-controlled device able to vary the intensity of the stimulus at low and high frequencies of vibration. The instrument also controls the rate and duration of the stimulus. These are definite improvements over handheld instruments in stimulus control. Initial normative[43] and clinical trials[40,46] have been carried out and indicate that the ATT is a sensitive and reliable tool for the diagnosis of compressive peripheral neuropathy. Dellon discusses in more detail the limitations of current electronic vibrometers in his text.[23]

Functional tests

The quality of fine discriminative sensation determines the usefulness of sensibility in daily activities. Therefore selection of tests and interpretation of results must be done carefully before one declares that a patient has normal discriminative sensibility.

Static two-point discrimination. Two-point discrimination is the classic test of functional sensibility because it is generally acknowledged to relate to the ability to use the hand for fine tasks.[23,54,60] (However, Dellon[22] has summarized several studies that refute this correlation.) Moberg[54] observed that 6 mm of two-point discrimination is required for winding a watch, 6 to 8 mm for sewing, and 12 mm for handling precision tools, and that above 15 mm gross tool

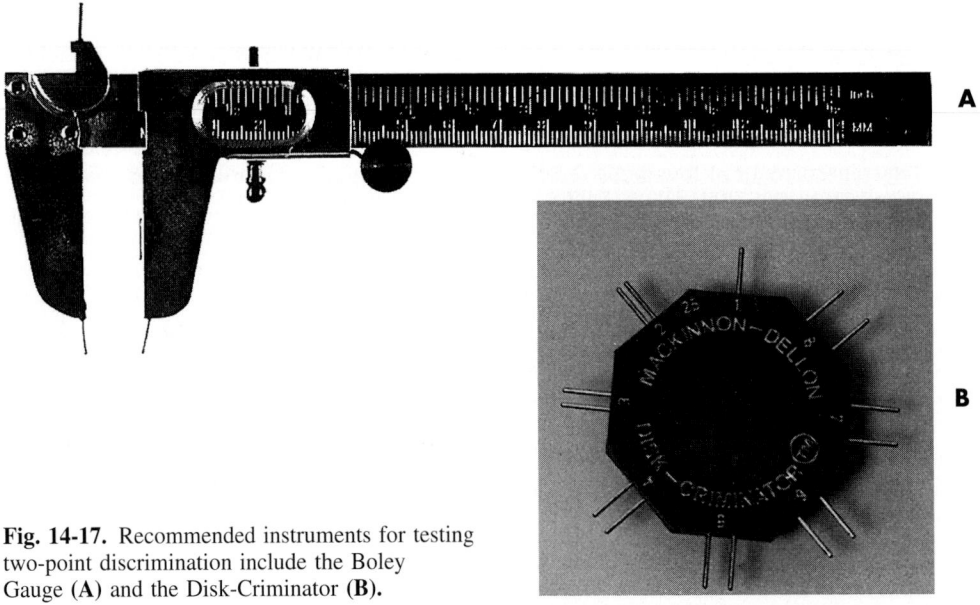

Fig. 14-17. Recommended instruments for testing two-point discrimination include the Boley Gauge (**A**) and the Disk-Criminator (**B**).

handling may be possible, but only with decreased speed and skill.

The test instrument should be light and have blunt testing ends. The Disk-Criminator (Disk-Criminator, P.O. Box 16392, Baltimore, Maryland)[19] and the Boley Gauge (Boley Gauge, Research Designs, Inc., Houston, Texas) are two such instruments (Fig. 14-17).

During the test, the patient's hand should be fully supported. Vision is occluded. Only the fingertips need be tested because the fingertips are the most important in active exploration and tactile scanning of an object. Testing is begun with 5 mm of distance between the two points. One or two points are applied lightly to the fingertip in a random sequence in a longitudinal orientation to avoid crossover from overlapping digital nerves. A common error is to apply too much pressure. Because it is light-touch discrimination that is being tested and because the patient is to be compared with the normal population, the pressure applied should be very light and stop just at the point of blanching.[11] Seven of ten responses must be accurate for scoring. If the responses are inaccurate, the distance between the ends is increased by increments of 1, 2, or 5 mm, depending on the suspected severity of the dysfunction, until the required accurate responses are elicited. Testing is stopped at 15 mm (or less, if the pulp is not of sufficient length) if responses are inaccurate at that level. Interpretation of scores is based on the guidelines set by the American Society for Surgery of the Hand[2] (Table 14-5).

Localization of touch. None of the tests described thus far have required localization of a stimulus. Localization represents a more integrated level of perception than simple recognition of a stimulus; therefore it should be tested as a separate function. The ability to localize was found by Weinstein[84] in a study of 48 normal adults to have a high correlation with two-point discrimination (.92), while neither two-point discrimination nor localization was found to have a high correlation with light-touch threshold (.17 and .28, respectively). Because of its high correlation with two-point discrimination, localization is considered a test of functional sensation.

Localization is most appropriate for testing after nerve repair because the poor localization that typically occurs after repair can seriously limit function. The stimulus used is the finest diameter Semmes-Weinstein monofilament that can be perceived throughout the area of dysfunction. Localization is tested over the entire area of dysfunction with this single filament.

Table 14-5. Two-point discrimination norms

Normal:	<6 mm
Fair:	6-10 mm
Poor:	11-15 mm
Protective:	One point perceived
Anesthetic:	No points perceived

The grid is useful for recording the results of this test.[86] With the patient's vision occluded and the hand fully supported, the selected monofilament is applied to the center of a zone. (Similarly, moving-touch localization can be tested by applying a moving-touch stimulus along the longitudinal midline of a selected zone.) Patients are instructed to open their eyes each time they feel a touch and point to the exact spot touched. Patients' responses will be more accurate if they use their vision to help localize than if they attempt to localize with their eyes closed.[39] If the stimulus is correctly localized, a dot is marked in the corresponding zone on the worksheet. If the stimulus is incorrectly localized, an arrow is drawn on the worksheet from the site of stimulation to the site of referral (Fig. 14-18). Each zone is stimulated only once. The resulting data on the worksheet are used as the permanent record. The worksheet gives the examiner and the patient a graphic representation of the quality of localization and points out patterns of referral that might be amenable to sensory reeducation. With improvement in localization over time, the localization worksheets should demonstrate fewer and shorter arrows.

The preceding method of mapping localization provides a quick screen and "impression" of localization, but results are not objectively measured. In a preliminary study, Nakada[57] provided a method to more objectively document and score errors in both constant and moving-touch

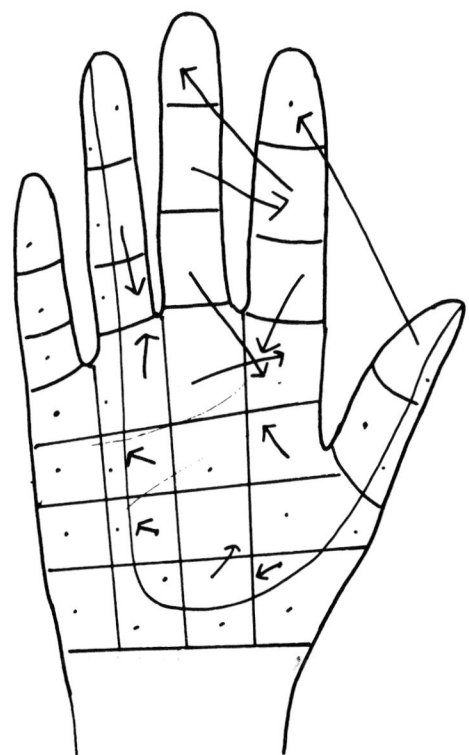

Fig. 14-18. Mapping of localization. *Dot,* Stimulus that was accurately perceived; *arrow,* referred stimulus; *arrowhead,* points to which stimulus was referred.

localization. In her method, the grid is drawn on the hand, the Semmes-Weinstein monofilament marked 4.17 is used to apply the stimulus, and errors in localization are measured with a vernier caliper. Although this method is more time-consuming, it does offer greater consistency in results and a better baseline for evaluating progress in localization.

Moving two-point discrimination. The rationale for this test, devised by Dellon,[19,20] is that because fingertip sensibility is highly dependent on motion, the stimulus for discrimination testing should be moving. As when testing static two-point discrimination, the test instrument for moving two-point discrimination should be light and have blunt testing ends. In accordance with the methods described by Dellon,[19] testing is begun with the instrument set at an 8-mm distance between the two points. The instrument is moved proximally to distally on the fingertip parallel to the long axis of the finger, with the testing ends side by side. The pressure used is just light enough so that the subject can appreciate the stimulus. Once the patient is inaccurate or hesitant in responding, he or she is required to respond accurately to 7 of 10 stimuli before the distance is narrowed. Testing is stopped at 2 mm, which represents normal moving two-point discrimination.

Dellon has reported that moving two-point discrimination always returns earlier than two-point discrimination after nerve laceration and approaches normal 2 to 6 months before two-point discrimination reaches normal. Therefore he advocates this test as a more valid assessment of discrimination and as an earlier means of assessing return of discrimination than the classic two-point test.

Moberg pickup test. The Moberg pickup test[54,55] requires motor participation and is most appropriate for median or combined medioulnar lesions. An assortment of everyday objects, the number and nature of which are determined by the examiner, is placed on a table in front of the patient, who is instructed to pick them up one at a time, as fast as possible, and place them into a box using his or her involved hand (Fig. 14-19, *A*). The examiner times the patient and notes which digits are used for prehension. The patient repeats the task with the uninvolved hand. Finally, the patient is asked to pick up objects again, but this time with the eyes closed. Again, time required and manner of prehension are noted. When locating and picking up objects with vision occluded, the patient will tend not to use sensory surfaces that have poor sensibility (Fig. 14-19, *B*).

Norms have not been established for this test. Its value lies in the observations that can be made during the brief time it requires to administer. Taking into account motor deficits, the best comparison for the involved hand is the performance by the uninvolved hand. The test can be made more difficult by requiring the patient to identify the objects as he or she picks them up.

Ng et al.[58] have proposed a standard protocol for administering the pickup test. Using a standard set of test items, instructions, and test layout, they found that hand dominance and gender had significant effects on test performance. Their study was limited by lack of establishing intrarater reliability, too small of a sample to establish interrater reliability, and limited subject age range (majority between 20 and 39 years old). However, these limitations could be overcome and the authors' conclusion that administering the test with a standard protocol may be clinically sound is supported by their preliminary findings.

Dellon modification of Moberg pickup test. Dellon modified the pickup test by standardizing the items used and requiring identification of them. He chose objects of similar material to avoid giving cues by texture or temperature and objects graded to require increasing ability to discriminate (Fig. 14-20).[22]

In cases in which the ulnar nerve is not involved, the ulnar digits are taped to the palm. The patient is timed while picking up the objects and placing them into a box. If the motor deficit is judged too severe during this sighted part of the test, the test is discontinued. If the deficit is not too severe, vision is occluded and the examiner places one item at a time into the median three digits for patient identification. The time required for identification is recorded; no more than 30 seconds is permitted per object. Each object is presented twice.

Dellon's recording of response time for object identification is a useful modification of the test. A recent study by King[47] draws attention to the clinical importance of response time in object identification and texture discrimination. King correlated the results of Semmes-Weinstein monofilament testing in CTS patients with their response times for texture and object recognition. She found a significant association between level of touch perceived and time required to identify the test items. Further confirmation of this association is needed, but the study successfully draws attention to the need to factor in response times in our tests of tactile gnosis.

Objective tests

Two objective tests, the Ninhydrin sweat test and the wrinkle test, are described in the following sections because of their occasional usefulness in testing, especially for children and suspected malingerers. As stated previously, they can give suggestive evidence of sensory function early after nerve laceration and in long-term cases in which regeneration has failed, but they do not correlate directly with the presence or absence of sensibility during regeneration.[62,63,77]

Ninhydrin sweat test. Methods of administration have been described by several authors,[30,54,62,63,76] but those described by Perry[62] and Phelps[63] are the easiest to follow because they make use of commercially available Ninhydrin developer and fixer. The essentials of their techniques are subsequently presented.

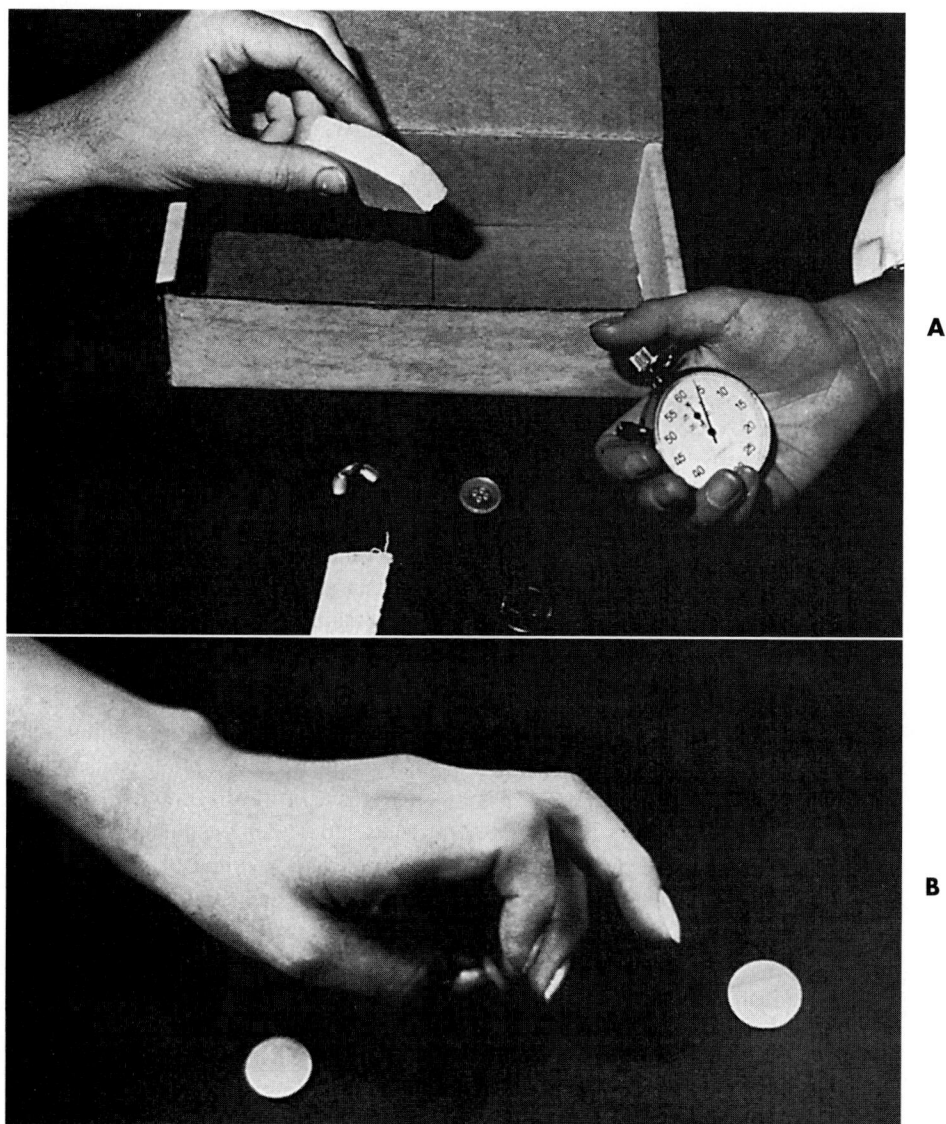

Fig. 14-19. A, Moberg pickup test. **B,** When locating and picking up objects with vision occluded, patient will tend not to use sensory surfaces that have poor sensibility.

The patient's hand is cleansed thoroughly with soap and warm water; rinsed thoroughly; and then wiped with ether, alcohol, or acetone. Perry recommends a 5-minute waiting period to allow the normal sweating process to ensue, whereas Phelps requires a 20- to 30-minute period to elapse before proceeding with the test. During the waiting period, the patient's fingertips must not come into contact with any surface.

At the end of the waiting period, the fingertips are pressed with a moderate amount of pressure against a good quality bond paper (e.g., no. 20) that has previously been untouched. The fingertips are traced with a pencil and held in place for 15 seconds. During this time the examiner must be careful not to touch any part of the paper and the patient's fingertips must not slide on the paper to avoid contamination of the results.

The paper is then sprayed with ninhydrin spray reagent (N-0507) (Sigma Chemical Company, St. Louis, Missouri) and allowed to dry for 24 hours or heated in an oven for 5 to 10 minutes at 200° F (93° C). During the development period, the ninhydrin stains purple the amino acids and lower peptide components of sweat that have penetrated the paper. After development, the prints are sprayed with ninhydrin fixer reagent (N-0757) (Sigma Chemical Company, St. Louis, Missouri) for a permanent record of the results.

According to Perry, a good normal print is one in which dots representing discrete sweat gland orifices can be clearly

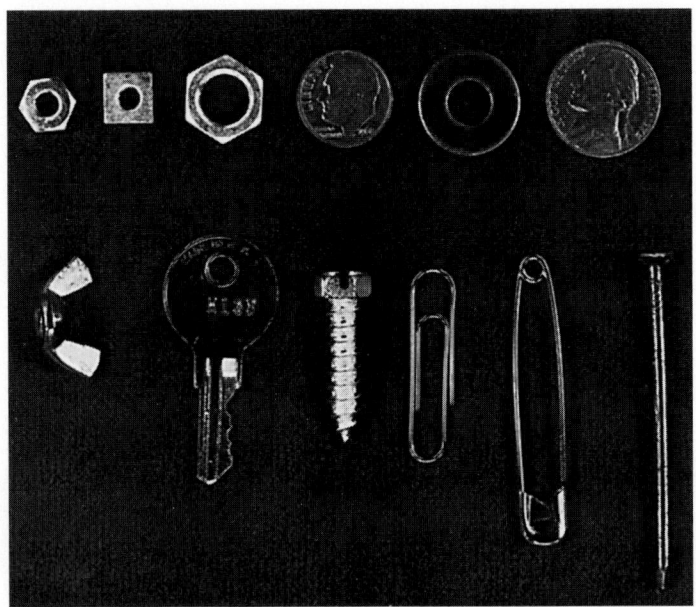

Fig. 14-20. Items used in Dellon modification of Moberg pickup test.

visualized. A blank print indicates that no sweating has occurred. A smudged print may represent a finger that moved during testing, or hyperhidrosis that has stained beyond its boundaries and may be masking an area of anhidrosis.[62]

Moberg has scored ninhydrin test results on a scale of 0 to 3, with 0 representing absent sweating and 3 representing normal sweating.[56]

Wrinkle test. The wrinkle test was described by O'Riain[61] in 1973. He observed that a denervated hand placed in warm water (40° C; 104° F) for 30 minutes does not wrinkle in the denervated area as normal skin does. He associated this phenomenon with an absence of sensory function and the return of wrinkling with a return of sensory function.

In a study of 41 nerve-injured patients, using the same finger-wrinkling method, Phelps[63] found that only after recent complete laceration did an absence of finger wrinkling always correlate with an absence of sensibility. In patients with nerve compression, the presence of wrinkling does not indicate intact sensibility. Therefore the wrinkle test appears to be of most use after recent nerve laceration, particularly in children and others unable or unwilling to cooperate with a sensibility examination.

Phelps noted that the results of finger wrinkling are difficult to document, even photographically. She used the same 0 to 3 scoring system to rate the amount of wrinkling that Moberg used for scoring the ninhydrin test.

Provocative tests and stress tests

There is not a standard stress test to document sensibility dysfunction in patients whose symptoms are intermittent or aggravated by activity. Stress tests can be positional[48,67] (e.g., wrist flexion or extension at end range for 1 minute) or dynamic[12,67] (e.g., putty squeeze for 5 minutes or work/ activity induced).

RECOMMENDATIONS FOR SENSIBILITY EVALUATION BATTERY

Because no single test can adequately assess the complex function of sensibility, evaluation is best approached by a battery of tests. Presented here are recommendations for test selection for nerve lesions in continuity and for nerve lacerations (postoperative). Test selection will be influenced by time available for testing, examiner familiarity with a particular test and instrument, and age and concentration level of the patient. In all cases, however, the selected battery must be administered in a manner designed to minimize variables, and the results must be interpreted knowledgeably.

Nerve lesions in continuity

Recommended components of a sensibility battery are as follows:

- History
- Tinel's test at the suspected compression site(s) (*Note:* A negative test does not rule out compression at that site.)
- With limb positioned at rest:
  Nerve conduction testing to detect early decrease in sensory nerve potential amplitude
  Vibratory testing to detect early sensory changes
  Semmes-Weinstein monofilament testing to detect early changes in touch-pressure threshold (If NCV, vibration, and touch-pressure tests are abnormal, test static and moving two-point discrimination to detect advanced sensory changes.)

- For patients who complain of intermittent symptoms or symptoms aggravated by particular position or activities:

    Subject the affected part to positional and/or dynamic stress.

    Follow stress with NCV, vibration, and/or touch-pressure threshold tests.

Nerve lacerations—postoperative

Recommended components of a sensibility battery are as follows:

- History
- Examination of the hand for evidence of sympathetic dysfunction and administration of Cold Sensitivity Severity Scale[53]
- Tinel's test to determine distal progression of regenerating axons
- Serial mapping to demarcate area of touch-pressure dysfunction
- Semmes-Weinstein monofilament testing to assess level of touch-pressure return (In areas of the hand that are unresponsive to the thickest diameter filaments, consider the pinprick test to evaluate protective sensation.)

If there is return of touch to the fingertips, static and moving two-point discrimination tests on the fingertips and touch localization tested on the entire area of dysfunction will provide information on the level of functional return.

The Moberg pickup test and Dellon modification of the pickup test integrate motor and sensory function and are administered quickly. Either is appropriate for median or combined medioulnar nerve dysfunction. Inspection of the hand for "wear marks" and the patient's reported functional use of the hand in ADLs will provide further evidence of functional sensibility.

For those suspected of malingering, the Semmes-Weinstein Pressure Aesthesiometer can be especially useful in documenting inconsistencies in responses. For the child, the wrinkle test, possibly the ninhydrin sweat test, and the Moberg pickup test may provide the information desired regarding function.

SUMMARY

A thorough and accurate sensibility evaluation requires that the therapist have a sound knowledge of nerve pathways, the effects of nerve injury, current instruments, and methods of controlling test variables. The assessment battery includes a careful history, skillful interviewing of the patient, examination of sympathetic function in the hand, and appropriate test selection and administration. The careful examiner who critiques his or her methods and who listens to his or her patients will learn from each patient and become a skilled examiner. The skilled examiner will accept the challenge of evaluating sensibility as an always interesting and at times fascinating task.

REFERENCES

1. Almquist E, Eeg-Olofsson O: Sensory nerve conduction velocity and two-point discrimination in sutured nerves, *J Bone Joint Surg* 52A:791, 1970.
2. American Society for Surgery of the Hand: *The hand: examination and diagnosis,* Aurora, Colo, 1978, The Society.
3. Backhouse KM: Nerve supply in the arm and hand. In Tubiana R, editor: *The hand,* vol 1 Philadelphia, 1991, WB Saunders.
4. Bell JA: Sensibility evaluation. In Hunter JM, et al, editors: *Rehabilitation of the hand,* St Louis, 1978, Mosby.
5. Bell J, Tomancik E: Repeatability of testing with Semmes-Weinstein monofilaments, *J Hand Surg* 12A:155, 1987.
6. Bell-Krotoski JA: Light touch-deep pressure testing using Semmes-Weinstein monofilaments. In Hunter JM, et al, editors: *Rehabilitation of the hand,* ed 3, St Louis, 1989, Mosby.
7. Bell-Krotoski J: Advances in sensibility evaluation, *Hand Clin* 7:527, 1991.
8. Bell-Krotoski JA, Buford WL: The force/time relationship of clinically used sensory testing instruments, *J Hand Ther* 1:76, 1988.
9. Bell-Krotoski J, Weinstein S, Weinstein C: Testing sensibility, including touch-pressure, two-point discrimination, point-localization, and vibration, *J Hand Ther* 6:114, 1993.
10. Bickerstaff ER, Spillane JA: *Neurological examination in clinical practice,* ed 5, Oxford, 1989, Blackwell.
11. Brand PW: Functional manifestations of sensory loss. Presented at symposium, Assessment of levels of cutaneous sensibility, US Public Health Service Hospital, Carville, La, Sept 1980.
12. Braun RM, Davidson K, Doehr S: Provocative-testing in the diagnosis of carpal tunnel syndrome, *J Hand Surg* 14A:195, 1989.
13. Brunelli SG: Gnostic rings for assessment of tactile gnosis, *Am Soc Surg Hand Newslett* no 53, 1981.
14. Bunnell S: *Surgery of the hand,* ed 5, revised by Boyes JH, Philadelphia, 1970, JB Lippincott.
15. Clark WC: Pain sensitivity and the report of pain: an introduction to sensory decision theory, *Anesthesiology* 40:272, 1974.
16. Campbell JN, Naff NJ, Dellon AL: Thoracic outlet syndrome: neurosurgical perspective, *Neurosurg Clin North Am* 2:227, 1991.
17. Costigan DA, Wilbourn AJ: The elevated arm stress test: specificity in the diagnosis of thoracic outlet syndrome, *Neurology* 35(suppl):74, 1985 (poster abstract).
18. Craigen M, et al: Patient and injury characteristics in the development of cold sensitivity of the hand: a prospective cohort study, *J Hand Surg* 24:8, 1999.
19. Dellon AL: The moving two-point discrimination test: clinical evaluation of the quickly-adapting fiber/receptor system, *J Hand Surg* 3:474, 1978.
20. Dellon AL: The paper clip: light hardware to evaluate sensibility in the hand, *Contemp Orthop* 1:39, 1979.
21. Dellon AL: Clinical use of vibratory stimuli to evaluate peripheral nerve injury and compression neuropathy, *Plast Reconstr Surg* 65:466, 1980.
22. Dellon AL: *Evaluation of sensibility and reeducation of sensation in the hand,* Baltimore, 1981, Williams & Wilkins.
23. Dellon AL: *Somatosensory testing and rehabilitation,* Baltimore, 2000, The Institute for Peripheral Nerve Surgery.
24. Dellon AL, Keller K: Cutaneous pressure threshold measurement in carpal and cubital tunnel syndrome, *Ann Plast Surg* 38:493, 1997.
25. Dellon AL, Curtis RM, Edgerton MT: Reeducation of sensation in the hand after nerve injury and repair, *Plast Recosntr Surg* 53:297, 1974.
26. Dellon AL, Mackinnon SE, Brandt KE: The markings of Semmes-Weinstein nylon monofilaments, *J Hand Surg* 18A:756, 1993.

27. Dellon ES, Mourey R, Dellon AL: Human pressure perception values for constant and moving one- and two-point discrimination, *J Plast Reconstr Surg* 90:112, 1992.
28. Dyck PJ, et al: Introduction of automated systems to evaluate touch-pressure, vibration, and thermal cutaneous sensation in man, *Ann Neurol* 4:502, 1978.
29. Fess E: The need for reliability and validity in hand assessment instruments, *J Hand Surg* 11A:621, 1986.
30. Flynn JE, Flynn WF: Median and ulnar nerve injuries: a long range study with evaluation of the Ninhydrin test, sensory and motor return, *Ann Surg* 156:1002, 1962.
31. Foerster O: The dermatomes in man, *Brain* 56:1, 1933
32. Gelberman RH, et al: Carpal tunnel syndrome: scientific basis for clinical care, *Orthop Clin North Am* 19:115, 1988.
33. Gelberman RH, et al: Sensibility testing in peripheral-nerve compression syndromes, *J Bone Joint Surg* 65A:632, 1983.
34. Gibson J: Observations on active touch, *Psychol Rev* 69:477, 1962.
35. Gillenson SP, et al: The effect of wrist position on testing light touch sensation using the Semmes-Weinstein Pressure Aesthesiometer: a preliminary study, *J Hand Ther* 11:27, 1998.
36. Gilliat RW, Harrison MJG: Nerve compression and entrapment. In Asbury AK, Gilliat RW, editors: *Peripheral nerve disorders,* London, 1984, Butterworths.
37. Greenspan JD, La Motte RH: Cutaneous mechanoreceptors of the hand: experimental studies and their implications for clinical testing of tactile sensation, *J Hand Ther* 6:75, 1993.
38. Grindley GC: The variation of sensory thresholds with the rate of application of the stimulus, *Br J Psychol* 27:86, 1936.
39. Halnan CRE, Wright GH: Tactile localization, *Brain* 83:677, 1960.
40. Hardy M, et al: Evaluation of nerve compression with the Automated Tactile Tester, *J Hand Surg* 17:838, 1992.
41. Haymaker W, Woodhall B: *Peripheral nerve injuries: principles of diagnosis,* ed 2, Philadelphia, 1953, WB Saunders.
42. Henderson WR: Clinical assessment of peripheral nerve injuries: Tinel's test, *Lancet* 2:801, 1948.
43. Horch K, et al: An automated tactile tester for evaluation of cutaneous sensibility, *J Hand Surg* 17A:829, 1992.
44. Hunter JM: Recurrent carpal tunnel syndrome, epineural fibrous fixation, and traction neuropathy, *Hand Clin* 7:491, 1991.
45. Hunter JM, Read RL, Gray R: Carpal tunnel neuropathy caused by injury: reconstruction of the transverse carpal ligament for the complex carpal tunnel syndromes, *J Hand Ther* 6:145, 1993.
46. Jimenez S, et al: A study of sensory recovery following carpal tunnel release, *J Hand Ther* 6:124, 1993.
47. King PM: Sensory function assessment: a pilot comparison study of touch pressure threshold with texture and tactile discrimination, *J Hand Ther* 10:24, 1997.
48. Koris M, et al: Carpal tunnel syndrome: evaluation of a quantitative provocational diagnostic test, *Clin Ortho Rel Res* 251:157, 1990.
49. Levin S, Pearsall G, Ruderman RJ: Von Frey's method of measuring pressure sensibility in the hand: an engineering analysis of the Weinstein-Semmes Pressure Aesthesiometer, *J Hand Surg* 3:211, 1978.
50. Lundborg G, et al: Median nerve compression in the carpal tunnel: functional response to experimentally induced controlled pressure, *J Hand Surg* 7:252, 1982.
51. Luoma A, Nelems B: Thoracic outlet syndrome: thoracic surgery perspective, *Neurosurg Clin North Am* 2:187, 1991.
52. MacKinnon SE, Dellon AL: Two-point discrimination tester, *J Hand Surg* 10A:906, 1985.
53. McCabe SJ, Mizgala C, Glickman L: The measurement of cold sensitivity of the hand, *J Hand Surg* 16A: 1037, 1991.
54. Moberg E: Objective methods for determining the functional value of sensibility in the hand, *J Bone Joint Surg* 40B:454, 1958.
55. Moberg E: Criticism and study of methods for examining sensibility in the hand, *Neurology* 12:8, 1962.
56. Moberg E: Nerve repair in hand surgery: an analysis, *Surg Clin North Am* 48:985, 1968.
57. Nakada M: Localization of a constant-touch and moving touch stimulus in the hand: a preliminary study, *J Hand Ther* 6:23, 1993.
58. Ng CL, Ho DD, Chow SP: The Moberg Pickup Test: results of testing with a standard protocol, *J Hand Ther* 12:309, 1999
59. Omer GE: Sensation and sensibility in the upper extremity, *Clin Orthop Rel Res* 104:30, 1974.
60. Onne L: Recovery of sensibility and sudomotor activity in the hand after nerve suture, *Acta Chir Scand* 300(suppl):1, 1962.
61. O'Riain S: New and simple test of nerve function in the hand, *Br Med J* 22:615, 1973.
62. Perry JF, et al: Protective sensation in the hand and its correlation to the Ninhydrin sweat test following nerve laceration, *Am J Phys Med* 53:113, 1974.
63. Phelps P, Walker E: Comparison of the finger wrinkling test results to established sensory tests in peripheral nerve injury, *Am J Occup Ther* 31:9, 1977.
64. Poppen NK: Clinical evaluation of the von Frey and two-point discrimination tests and correlation with a dynamic test of sensibility. In Jewett DL, McCarroll HK, editors: *Symposium on nerve repair: its clinical and experimental basis,* St Louis, 1979, Mosby.
65. Pratt NE: *Clinical musculoskeletal anatomy,* Philadelphia, 1991, JB Lippincott.
66. Quintner JL: A study of upper limb pain and paraesthesias following neck injury in motor vehicle accidents: assessment of the brachial plexus tension test of Elvey, *Br J Rheumatol* 28:528, 1989.
67. Read R: Stress testing in nerve compression, *Hand Clin* 7:521, 1991.
68. Richards RL: Vasomotor and nutritional disturbances following injuries to peripheral nerves. In Seddon HJ, editor: *Peripheral nerve injuries,* London, 1954, Her Majesty's Stationery Office.
69. Roos DB: Thoracic outlet and carpal tunnel syndromes. In Rutherford RB, editor: *Vascular surgery,* Philadelphia, 1984, WB Saunders.
70. Roos DB: The thoracic outlet syndrome is underrated, *Arch Neurol* 47:328, 1990.
71. Rosen B, Lundborg G: A new tactile gnosis instrument in sensibility testing, *J Hand Ther* 11:251, 1998
72. Schwartzman RJ: Brachial plexus traction injuries, *Hand Clin* 7:547, 1991.
73. Seddon HJ, editor: *Peripheral nerve injuries,* London, 1954, Her Majesty's Printing Office.
74. Seddon HJ: *Surgical disorders of the peripheral nerves,* ed 2, New York, 1975, Churchill Livingstone.
75. Semmes J, et al: *Somatosensory changes after penetrating brain wounds in man,* Cambridge, Mass, 1960, Harvard University Press.
76. Stromberg WB, et al: Injury of the median and ulnar nerves: one hundred and fifty cases with an evaluation of Moberg's Ninhydrin test, *J Bone Joint Surg* 43A:717, 1961.
77. Sunderland S: *Nerves and nerve injuries,* ed 2, New York, 1978, Churchill Livingstone.
78. Szabo R, Chidgey L: Stress carpal tunnel pressures in patients with carpal tunnel syndrome and normal patients, *J Hand Surg* 14A:624, 1989.
79. Szabo RM, Gelberman RH, Dimick MP: Sensibility testing in patients with carpal tunnel syndrome, *J Bone Joint Surg* 66A:60, 1984.
80. Szabo RM, et al: Vibratory sensory testing in acute peripheral nerve compression, *J Hand Surg* 98A:104, 1984.
81. Tinel J: The "tingling" sign in peripheral nerve lesions (translated by Emanual B. Kaplan). In Spinner M: *Injuries to the major branches of peripheral nerves of the forearm,* ed 2, Philadelphia, 1978, WB Saunders.
82. Trotter W, Davies HM: Experimental studies in the innervation of the skin, *J Physiol* 38:134, 1909.
83. Von Prince K, Butler B: Measuring sensory function of the hand in peripheral nerve injuries, *Am J Occup Ther* 21:385, 1967.

84. Weinstein S: Intensive and extensive aspects of tactile sensitivity as a function of body part, sex and laterality. In Kenshalo DR, editor: *The skin senses,* Springfield, Ill, 1968, Charles C Thomas.

85. Weinstein S: Fifty years of somatosensory research: from the Semmes-Weinstein monofilaments to the Weinstein enhanced sensory test, *J Hand Ther* 6:11, 1993.

86. Werner JL, Omer GE: Evaluating cutaneous pressure sensation of the hand, *Am J Occup Ther* 24:347, 1970.

87. Whitenack SJ, et al: Thoracic outlet syndrome complex: diagnosis and treatment. In Hunter JM, et al, editors: *Rehabilitation of the hand,* ed 3, St Louis, 1990, Mosby.

88. Wienir MA: Limb radicular pain and sensory disturbances. In Wienir MA, editor: *Spine: state of the art reviews,* Philadelphia, 1988, Hanley & Belfus.

89. Wilbourn AJ, Porter JM: Thoracic outlet syndromes. In Weiner MA, editor: *Spine: state of the art reviews,* Philadelphia, 1988, Hanley & Belfus.

90. Wilbourn AJ: Thoracic outlet syndromes: a plea for conservatism, *Neurosurg Clin North Am* 2:235, 1991.

Chapter 15

BIOMECHANICS AND EVALUATION OF THE HAND*

Judith A. Bell-Krotoski
Donna E. Breger-Stanton

MEASUREMENTS MUST BE PRECISE AND REPEATABLE

Objective measures are efficient measures that justify case referral, show efficacy of treatment, and help substantiate practice. They help eliminate guesswork and ensure that clinical treatment is focused on what works.† The need for the application of biomechanical terms and principles in patient treatment is increasing, as is the need for assurance that measurement techniques are objective. The engineer, skilled in requirements for objective measurement as well as for the use of objective measurement instruments, adds insight and depth to the understanding of hand function and evaluation.[66] Dr. Paul Brand envisioned a biomedical engineer as a regular member of the surgical/therapy team, promoted this concept, and demonstrated the value of the engineer on the team in the rehabilitation research laboratory he established in Carville, Louisiana.‡ Basic principles of soft tissue mechanics, hand mechanics, and materials mechanics ensuing from this program, which interrelated rehabilitation research with therapy clinical practice, are included in this chapter.§ The direct application of engineering terms and principles rewards the clinician with records that are objective, repeatable, and comparable.

*The authors thank Robert Beach, M.A., P.T., for his contributions to this chapter in previous editions.
†References 16, 18, 36, 45, 57, 64.
‡Paul W. Brand Research Laboratory, U.S. Public Health Service, Gillis Long Hansen's Disease Center, Carville, Louisiana; relocated to National Hansen's Disease Programs, Summit Medical, Baton Rouge, Louisiana. Web site: bhpc.hrsa.gov/nhdp.
§References 1, 7, 11, 18, 30, 33, 41, 72.

MECHANICS OF FORCE AND PRESSURE ON SKIN

In consideration of the mechanics of pressure from splinting, traction, and measurement of forces used in therapy treatment, of first concern is the force, or *pressure* (force per unit area), applied to the skin and other soft tissue. There are limits to how much *stress* the skin can tolerate before its integrity is compromised (stress occurs in the skin when a force is applied). Some stress on and within skin tissue is usual and is needed to maintain normal healthy tissue. Skin that does not receive enough stress becomes thin and shiny and tears easily; however, too much stress can be harmful, and repetitive stress can be harmful even at low levels.

The safe and effective limits of stress on skin and the soft tissue reaction to stress are important in patient treatment. One may question how to determine what force can be both safe and maximally effective. Knowledge of materials and soft tissue mechanics, with direct measurement of force applied to the skin and soft tissue, can help determine optimum force for treatment. Brand[15] points out that every pressure sore results from excessive mechanical force. With this understanding, the mechanical environment can be modified and controlled so that problems from too much stress can be prevented. Living skin and soft tissue can be injured or destroyed by mechanical force in at least four ways. These four ways are associated with (1) degree, (2) duration, (3) repetition, and (4) direction.

Degree and duration of stress

Low stress can be damaging to tissue if it is of long duration, and it can result in ischemic necrosis. The effect of continuous, low force under constricting circumferential bandages, straps, or areas of splint contact can be seen. Capillary flow in the skin will be obstructed with very little pressure—from 30 to 50 mm Hg.[37] To prevent ischemic necrosis, it is necessary to control either the degree of pressure, the duration of pressure, or both.[15,71] By pressing a clear piece of glass on the skin and observing the results, one can appreciate how little pressure it takes to blanch the skin and shut down capillary flow. The same blanching can occur under a splint, strap, or cuff but go unseen.

In its usual state, the skin uses pain as a protective mechanism against sustained low-pressure ischemia (i.e., pressure that is not immediately uncomfortable but is strong enough to cause some decrease in capillary flow and eventual ischemia). The skin was not designed to sustain constant low pressure that causes ischemia. At some point before actual tissue damage occurs, an ischemic area begins to become uncomfortable. The reaction of the individual is to move and redistribute the pressure. This is why some patients do tolerate ill-fitted splints. Before they get an ulcer from ischemia, they must first have some other factor that overrides the usual protective response, such as generalized or specific muscle weakness, sensory impairment, or sedation. However, when a patient expresses discomfort from a splint, there may be areas of ischemic pressure, which the patient cannot explain.

High stress (i.e., stress sufficiently high to tear and destroy tissue) can destroy tissue in a short period (injury resulting from trauma). Human skin can resist stresses of 100 kg/cm^2 according to Yamada.[79] High stress may be as high as 1000 times the amount of pressure that causes ischemia. High stress can result from a force impact against the skin from any object. The smaller the object or its edge, the greater the stress produced. A prick of a pin or needle is an injury of great stress because the force is concentrated on the small area of the tip.

Repetition of stress

Low or moderate stress can be damaging to tissue if it is repetitive. At first the stress, if low, may be acceptable and harmless for a number of repetitions. If this is followed by continuous repetitive *moderate stress,* it will eventually result in tissue damage and an inflammatory response.[12,43] The inflammation will occur before necrosis unless the tissue gets mechanically torn apart (pulverized, where vascular tissue and skin cells are torn apart before an inflammation response can occur).

Repetitive stress is more damaging than normal (direct) stress at higher levels. The effect that repetitive stress adds to normal stress can be seen on the fingertip of a patient undergoing rubber band traction if the patient continually flexes the finger against the cuff and rubber band. A seemingly moderate force at some point can eventually become inflammatory. It is necessary to reduce traction force if repetitive use is required of the finger in a splint or if the

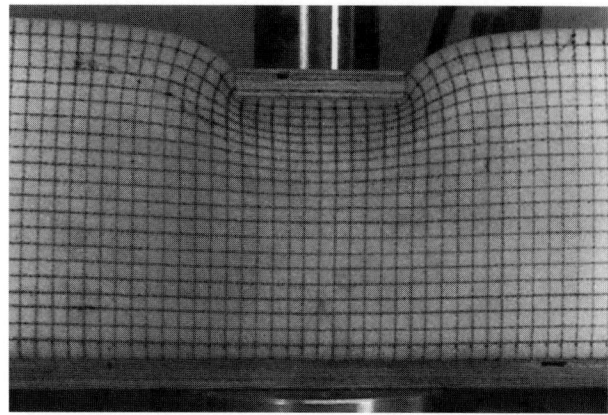

Fig. 15-1. Shear force. Shear force that is tangential is more damaging than normal force that is direct. As a piston and block compress a foam model, note the twisting and angulation of squares at edge of the block, compared with the compressed rectangular "cells" underneath. (Photograph by David E. Thompson, Ph.D.)

skin has become sensitized. In animal models, histologic changes following repetitive stress were seen microscopically before there was actual breakdown of skin; thus potential damage can occur even before it is easily observed.

Skin that receives mild repetitive stress over time can react by forming callus and becoming tougher. This reaction in normal living tissue helps prevent further tissue damage. However, even with mild callus, skin can be injured if it receives cumulative or excessive stress in an area. Also of note, excessive callus can actually contribute to underlying tissue damage from its relative hardness, tendency to crack, and lack of flexibility.

Direction of stress

Studies have shown that the most damaging type of stress to the skin is not *normal stress* (i.e., perpendicular to the surface), but rather is shear (i.e., produced by lateral force).[16,71] This type of stress occurs where edges of objects, such as splints, come into contact with the skin and have a force component parallel to or tangent to the surface. *Shear stress* has a rotational effect on the skin cells and can tear and deform skin cells (Fig. 15-1). Seemingly low shear can be damaging and can easily cause damage before the injury is perceived. The blister that forms in the palm of the hand from a screwdriver handle results from the twisting of the handle as it grabs the skin and tears it from other soft tissue. The shearing force separates the outer skin layers, making the blister, which fills with fluid. The skin can absorb relatively high direct impact, but does not so readily accommodate shear stress.

PHYSICAL AND MECHANICAL PROPERTIES OF SKIN

The skin and its associated soft tissue's inherent physical properties make it an ideal covering for the structural mechanics of the skeletal system. The skin's plastic

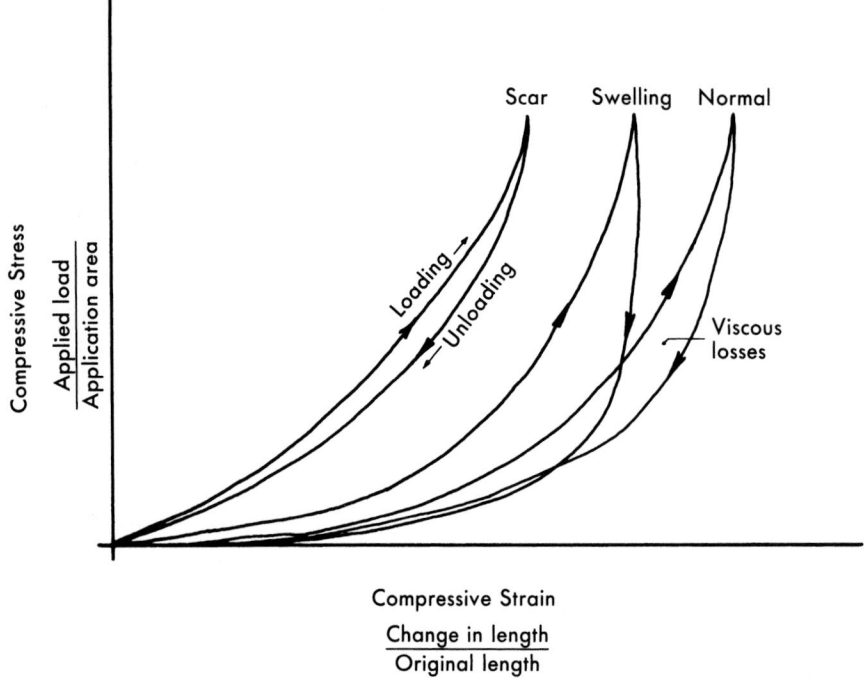

Fig. 15-2. Stress/strain measurement showing viscoelastic properties of skin and soft tissue under various conditions. Minimal force on normal tissue results in significant strain until the "elastic limit" is reached. Scar tissue builds up stress rapidly, producing increasing strain and a steeper curve. Swelling increases the viscous content of tissue, producing a steeper curve and greater distance between loading and unloading. (Researched by William Buford, B.M.E., Ph.D., and David E. Thompson, Ph.D.)

characteristics allow it to mold and reshape to various surfaces, thus allowing the patient to grip objects without slipping. The skin absorbs impact, cushions, and expands to meet the limits of joint range of motion (ROM), returning to a normal resting position on release of tension. Engineers call these characteristics *plasticity* (degree of moldability) and *viscoelasticity* (degree of viscosity and elasticity).[71] The plastic and viscoelastic properties of the skin enable it to resist breaking down under stress in usual situations.

The effect that force has on skin and soft tissue varies according to the condition of the tissue. Tissue that has changed in quality by disuse or as a result of injury has lost some of its ability to sustain stress and to absorb impact. The condition of skin must be considered carefully along with mechanical measures when judgments are made regarding "safe" amounts of force the skin can sustain. Skin quality affects the onset of ischemic necrosis. Tissue that is tense and more rigid from edema will more quickly develop ischemic necrosis, as will inflamed tissue. Skin overlying stiff joints lacks the joint movement that redistributes pressure (Fig. 15-2).

Thermography measurement (i.e., measurement of temperature) monitors patient reaction to stress and tolerance to stress. By using thermography in soft tissue studies, Brand[17,18] demonstrated the cumulative effects of stress. He found that if the baseline skin temperature is measured, and

a subject receives stress on the skin for a given period, the time it takes for skin temperature and redness to return to normal can be observed and documented. On the second day of the same activity, the skin has become sensitized. It takes less time for the skin temperature to be elevated and redness to reoccur, and a longer time for them to return to the baseline initial measurement[15,18] (Fig. 15-3).

A healing wound or injury will have an elevated temperature compared with other tissue.[13,17,52] By establishing a baseline temperature measurement in cases of injury, subsequent increases or decreases in temperature can be recognized and used to help guide treatment. For instance, if an injured joint has a several-degree elevation in temperature in the hours or day after being exercised in therapy, indications are that it was exercised too much. If repeated measurement shows only a degree or two temperature increase in the hours or day after being exercised in therapy, the exercise level is shown to be "within tissue tolerance" and could possibly be increased, speeding up recovery.

Infections result in the greatest change in skin temperature. A delta T (i.e., change in temperature) can sometimes be as high as 7° C in an infected area compared with uninfected areas. Any skin or joint area with a large increase in temperature is suspect for infection, and the area should be examined closely for any additional signs of infection, hyperemia, puncture wounds, drainage, foul odor, pus,

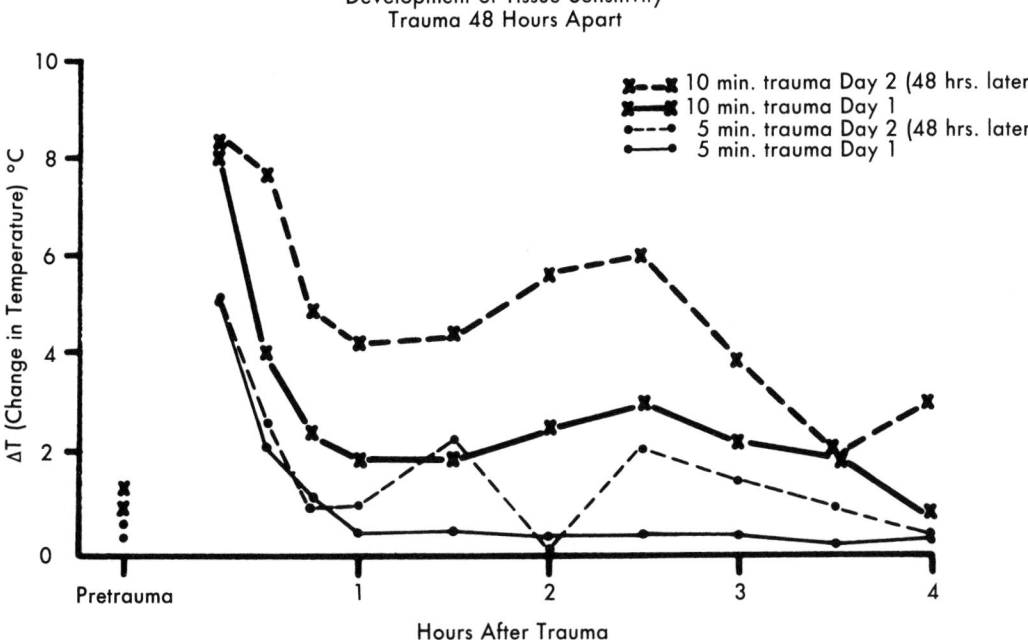

Fig. 15-3. Tissue reaction from repetitive force. Note the temperature elevation that occurred with repetitive force of two durations and sensitivity that had developed by day 2. The result of repetitive stress on tissue can be long-lasting and continue for several weeks. (From Brand PW, Sabin TD, Burke JP: Sensory denervation: a study of its cause and its prevention in leprosy and of management of insensitive limbs. Final Report, Carville, Louisiana, US Public Health Service Hospital, SRS Project No. RC-40-M, June 30, 1970.)

discoloration, and necrosis. However, not all temperature elevation is bad. The temperature elevation of the infected wound indicates that activity to heal the wound is occurring.

In chronic ulcers the initial inflammatory stage of healing has subsided and the wound may actually be cool in comparison with other skin areas. Absence of temperature elevation in the wound signals that the infection is chronic or that the tissue has little blood supply with little healing activity. To help the wound heal, it sometimes is necessary to abrade lightly an unhealing wound with a piece of sterile gauze to create a mild inflammatory process to promote healing. (Abrading a wound should be performed only with the concurrence of a physician and when the wound looks clean and the granulation bed looks good, but epithelialization is not progressing.)

Laboratory strength testing of skin shows its viscoelastic characteristics.[74,79] When a tensile elongation or compression load is applied to the skin (as in measurement with standard materials testing equipment), initially there is a gradual increase of stress in the skin. Within a given range, the skin has a capacity for elastic deformation; it can be elongated or compressed and then return to normal resting length without injury or deformity when the elongation or compression load is discontinued. With increasing pressure, stress in the skin increases. At a certain point, stress in the skin begins to occur rapidly (as it begins to approach the limits of its accommodation), and if the load is continued, the skin becomes tense and begins to fatigue (break down). Beyond a certain point, the skin will undergo *plastic deformation* or creep (i.e., permanent deformity and inability to return to normal resting length). If the compression load is further increased, the skin will eventually rupture.

The *stress* (load force per unit area) versus *strain* (change in length) of the skin as it is subjected to increasing load can be plotted on a *stress/strain curve* (graph of stress versus strain) (see Fig. 15-2). The slope of the stress/strain curve reveals the *modulus of elasticity* of what is being measured and is important in analysis of the viscoelastic properties of tissue. Analysis of the *elastic* properties of tissues tells how different tissues respond to elongation or *compression*.[16,18,41,42] The elastic modulus of bone or tendon is high (the curve is steep and almost vertical) when compared with that of skin, which is much more elastic (lower, more relaxed curve). All tissues have their own elastic modulus that is relative to the degree of their elasticity. Yamada[79] measured and published the relative elasticity of every tissue in an animal model, providing an understanding of the relative elasticity of various tissues.

The increased *viscous* fluid volume that accompanies swollen tissue mechanically changes normal soft tissue that is plastic (flexible and compliant) and elastic (returning to resting position) (see Fig. 15-2). Edema limits longitudinal movement of collagen fibers by reorienting them in a transverse direction, and it limits the tissue's ability to be compliant. These changes decrease skin and joint ROM, are directly related to the amount of fluid volume in the tissues, and can be reduced or eliminated in direct relationship to a corresponding reduction in the fluid volume. A hand with swollen tissue will not have a normal ROM as long as there is edema in and under the skin. Permanent deformity of the tissue, or *remodeling,* does not occur unless swelling is prolonged or excessive. Measurement of hand volume allows edema to be quantified and compared (see Hand volume measurement, page 256).[18]

Healthy joints and tendons have minimal friction, but swollen skin, joints, and tendons have an increase in friction relative to the amount of increased fluid. This friction inhibits ROM. Intercellular swelling (i.e., intercellular increase in fluid volume) can change the apparent elastic modulus of the skin and soft tissue. The increased tension in the tissue has the effect of making tissue more impacted and rigid, thus producing a steeper stress versus strain curve.

Scar tissue dramatically changes the ability of the skin to serve as a cushion for deeper structures and to elongate and contract for joint ROM (see Fig. 15-2). Scar tissue does not react like normal tissue. The more scar that develops in tissue, the more the tissue's normal inherent plastic and viscoelastic properties change. Scar tissue is more rigid and less elastic; thus it has a much steeper stress/strain curve in comparison with normal healthy tissue. Scarred tissue is more vulnerable to injury from areas of stress concentration and reduced compliance. Scar limits joint ROM of skin by reduced capacity for excursion with load from force of muscles and excursion of tendons.

Clinical measurement of joint ROM can reveal changes in the skin and soft tissue's viscoelastic characteristics and document clinical conditions. For accurate measurement, it is necessary to use a consistent tension or strain on the joint being measured (see Torque range-of-motion measurement page 252).[18]

MECHANICS OF SOFT TISSUE REMODELING

Skin and soft tissue with reduced tension will remodel into deformity. With reduced tension from limited joint positioning, joint deformity, or muscle loss, skin and other soft tissues remodel and lose tissue cells. Even ligaments and blood vessels lose cells and thus the ability to elongate to previous lengths, resulting in contracture. Contracture usually occurs on the volar surface of fingers, wrists, and elbows, where tissue more often undergoes long periods of decreased tension and limited elongation from disease or injury. Dorsal skin overlying joint flexion contractures typically lengthens and becomes redundant as a result of sustained elongation tension (Fig. 15-4). These changes occur regardless of the underlying cause of the joint restriction because they result from the change in the forces acting on the skin and soft tissue.[18]

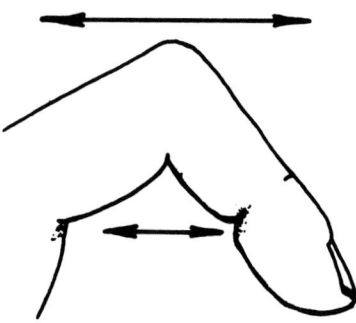

Fig. 15-4. Skin and soft tissue remodeling with interphalangeal joint contracture. Tissue is lost on volar surface, where stress is less, and grows on dorsal surface, where stress is greater. This process can be reversed if stress is made to be greater on the dorsal surface and less on the volar.

The skin and joint tissues can remodel and grow new tissue by static positioning at the limits of their elongation. Skin that is fully elongated to its elastic limit will have a low increase in tension. Living tissue responds to a low increase in *tension* by growing new cells until tension is reduced back to the tissue's original physiologic resting state. The skin may then be elongated further to its new elastic limit, which is longer. The remodeling process can be repeated as long as progressive gain is seen. Brand[18] conceived, described, and applied the technique of serial casting for *tissue remodeling.* With use of this technique on small or large joints or over several joints for muscle/tendon unit tightness, gradual remodeling of the connective tissue has been shown to occur when the tissue is held at the end of its elastic limit for 1 or 2 days. For optimal remodeling to occur, tension must be continuous or almost continuous, or at least frequent. Any interruption of tension may slow the process. Dynamic traction does not usually work as effectively as serial casting for skin and soft tissue contractures because it is difficult to design a dynamic splint that fits well enough to apply a continuous low-tension traction.[58] Pressure garments for scar prevention and remodeling in burn patients are other methods using the principle of controlled tension for tissue remodeling.

Stretch of tissue occurs when tissues are taken beyond their elastic limit and results in rupture of cellular material. Tissue remodeling does not include stretch. Treatment of contracture should be done with no or minimal actual "stretch" of skin and soft tissue, only a gentle elongation within the skin's elastic limit. Cellular rupture releases protein material that will create scar and further increase inelasticity. Remodeling cannot occur in an hour's treatment. Improvement in joint ROM measured in therapy sessions in a short period of time arises from fluid shifts, or tissue rupture, and may even decrease in subsequent hours or days if treatment has been too aggressive and caused actual tissue damage. It takes time for skin to grow, just as it took time for the tissue to develop contracture.

MOVEMENT, STRESS, AND WOUNDS

The effect of movement can be detrimental to wound healing because of the stress placed on new, fragile tissue. Progressive mobilization of injured tissue and careful assessment of the tissue's response are indicated whether a wound is the result of trauma or is controlled, as with elective surgery. For progressive return to movement, immobilization restraints should be weaned away, not just removed after a period of restricted movement. During a period of restoration of movement and function, hand volume and temperature elevations signal overuse. Monitors of wound color, temperature, and volume help determine the stress on wounds and the direction of improvement or worsening. Serial tracings of area and extent of wounds can be used along with photographs for the record. The edges of the wound and the extent of contraction or expansion can be recorded by their tracing on clear plastic.

Movement and mechanical stress can be particularly damaging to infected tissue. When tendons and joints move through their normal ROM, blood and other tissue fluids are forced into motion. The effect of movement on infected tissue, particularly impacted tissue, can be to drive the infection deeper into other tissue areas, thereby increasing the area of infection and delaying healing. Moving any hand in the initial stages of infection may extend the course of treatment needed. Often, it is better to completely immobilize an infected part (one joint higher than the infection) for a few days and allow it to localize, and then allow gentle ROM when it is safer for the tissues.

For patients without pain, the normal mechanism by which the injured hand is functionally splinted and protected is lost.[20] It is not uncommon to see patients with insensitive extremities with infections extending into the axillae. The effect of mechanical irritation is well demonstrated when these patients with insensitive hands are immobilized (in functional positions). Erythema quickly subsides and the wounds become localized.

INTERFACE OF SOFT TISSUE WITH MATERIALS

Materials used for splinting have degrees of plastic and viscoelastic properties.[18,27,65,73] Selection of materials based on their inherent mechanical properties can be used to an advantage in patient treatment.[9,25,26] The splint is therefore designed for the patient, rather than the patient being fitted to the splint.

Rigid splints

Some materials are rigid and nonconforming in comparison with other materials. Splints and casts traditionally have been made of rigid materials and can be designed to minimize stress. An optimal material for padding the interface of hard material with skin is one that simulates the plastic and viscoelastic properties of skin. In our Rehabilitation Research Laboratory, it has been found that Spenco elastic (i.e., cloth-covered microcellular rubber [AliMed,

Inc., Dedham, Massachusetts]) most nearly simulated the elastic quality of normal human skin. This material has been used with success for years in shoe insoles as an interface between skin and hard, rigid materials, particularly for patients with insensitivity, and is a material available for use in hand splinting. Other materials are also available for use as padding. One wants to select a material that holds up under repeated use, that does not allow the fingers to come in direct contact when pinched, and that will allow lateral sliding of the fingers to help eliminate shear.

Soft splints

Soft splints have some pliability and are supportive along certain planes of movement but flexible in others. Soft splints made with semirigid materials have become required in sports medicine because of the physical contact nature of games and potential injury to others from rigid splints. They should not be so tight or compliant that they produce vascular compromise, and they should conform well enough to minimize shear stress on repetitive movement. Soft splints are particularly helpful in the treatment of children and patients with insensitivity who are much more vulnerable to injury from hard, rigid materials. Soft materials can be combined and laminated to each other to provide more stability and contact cushioning. Many materials are available for soft splints, including Aliplast, Plastazote, and Spenco elastic. Elastic adhesive wrap and paper tape can be combined with rigid substructures such as plaster, but care must be taken to prevent vascular compromise.

Bandages

Bandages can create varying amounts of pressure on the skin and underlying tissue. Circular bandages generally are wrapped in a figure-of-eight fashion rather than in a repeated circular manner to avoid inadvertent band-type constrictive areas of tissue (vascular and lymphatic). Circular pressure can be uneven because one point of the wrap may be pulled tighter than another, thereby concentrating pressure in one area, or resulting in a tourniquet. A nonexpandable bandage material (i.e., material not cut on a bias or with little, if any, elasticity) will apply more pressure than bias-cut material or elastic materials that permit some expansion if swelling occurs.

Elastic materials

Every layer of an elastic wrap mechanically carries its elastic pressure. Elastic bandages should be used with particular care regarding the amount of tension with which they are wrapped, even with the first wrap. In the second wrap, the pressure under the bandage is doubled, with the third wrap the pressure is tripled, and so forth.[18] Movement of the hand in the bandage further concentrates pressure, particularly over prominent areas. For example, the circumference of a wrist is larger when the wrist is extended rather than neutral; therefore, if wrapped in neutral, pressure under

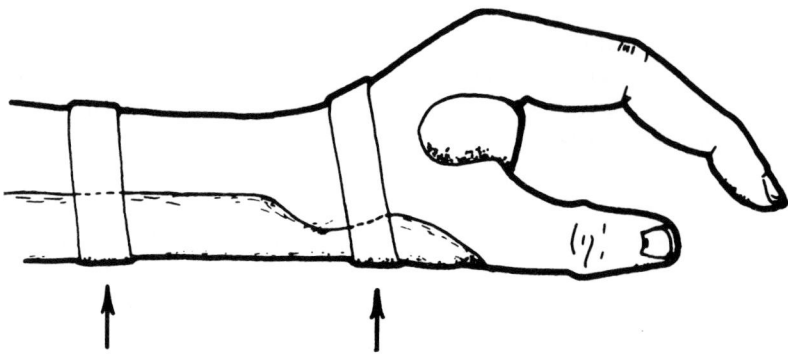

Fig. 15-5. Splints should be molded to conform to the hand and forearm's curved surfaces and to lift straps away from the sides of fingers and hands where straps can cause high concentration of pressure. Splint with molded support around edges allows straps to apply more dorsal force over a broader area to anchor the hand and prevent a tourniquet effect, enabling a better vascular return.

the bandage will be greater when the wrist is extended.[6] Direct pressure is increased where bending of joints creates folds in the material. Self-adhesive elastic bandages carry more risk than do nonadhesive bandages because gliding of the individual wraps is less likely if swelling occurs. Patients might also apply the material incorrectly. Self-adhesive elastic bandages such as Coban (Minnesota Mining and Manufacturing Company [3M], North Coast Medical Inc., Morgan Hill, California) should be used only with caution when a patient has reduced sensibility.

SPLINT MECHANICS

Localized pressure from splinting occurs when contact force on the skin is concentrated at any small area, such as over a bony prominence or over any area with a small radius. If an elastic bandage is wrapped around the hand, the areas of greatest pressure are at the curved lateral sides of the index and little fingers, as well as over the dorsum of joints, where the bones and tendons are prominent. Damage from direct pressure created by the elastic bandage is likely at any point that the anatomic area for pressure concentration is small. Normal direct or shear stress should be kept to a minimum in splinting by spreading out contact force over a broad area and avoiding small or concentrated areas.

Hyperemia and the length of time hyperemia persists after pressure is removed (longer than 15 minutes) indicate inflammation from pressure. Persistent hyperemia, swelling, and heat are cardinal signs that the tissue is becoming damaged. Objective monitors of elevated temperature and swelling help quantify skin response to stress.

Patients without sensitivity or with loss of protective sensation are particularly vulnerable to injury from pressure. The examiner should use other treatment methods and completely avoid traction in these patients, or monitor traction aggressively for signs of persistent redness or blisters, heat, or swelling. Patients with nerve injuries and degrees of insensitivity have been found to develop skin changes of scar, decreased vascularity, and tissue absorption

from repetitive stress even when the skin has not been broken.[18]

Mechanics of straps

Splint straps can cause localized pressure as they course around fingers and the sides of the hand, and can adversely affect vascular flow. The splint should be designed to lift the straps away from the sides of the hand and fingers rather than anchor to and conform around the sides of the hand and fingers (Fig. 15-5). The aim is to anchor the hand by anterior-posterior pressure over a broader area of the hand, thus reducing the pressure. The rigid part of the splint can be made to curve around the sides of the hand and fingers. Straps that are too flexible may be too compressive, thus adding to vascular ischemia. Leather makes a good strap or cuff because it usually is semirigid. Shear is likely if movement occurs under the straps, casts, or splints, and it adds to injury from direct stress over a bony prominence or over any area with a small radius. Shear stress is produced anywhere high force is concentrated, such as at splint holes or edges. Broadening the area of contact reduces the stress.

To understand the ischemic pressure effect that straps or cuffs have on fingers, Brand[16,18] suggests wrapping clear plastic cuffs around three fingers. To simulate the various forces of traction, fishing weights can be applied to the cuffs; the first to just short of blanching, the second to mottled blanching, and the third to full blanching. The time it takes for each to become uncomfortable should be noted. One would not think of wearing either of the cuffs that cause blanching for any extended period. However, this is exactly what is sometimes asked of patients undergoing traction splinting. One must splint to tissue tolerance where sustained low stress will not cause sustained skin blanching—not just splint to patient tolerance.

Mechanics of padding

Padding can effectively help reduce shear, but it adds bulk and can add to normal direct pressure. Padding of edges and contact surfaces where shear is likely to occur can help reduce shear, but often, a splint is better remolded or otherwise readjusted to fit rather than being padded, unless the padding is molded into the design of the splint. Straps with foam or other padding can also increase conformation so well that vascular supply is compromised. If a "dough-nut" is made to relieve a skin area, the skin can be injured by shear stress caused at the inner edge of the hole. Rounding the edges of a splint or a doughnut area can help prevent injury by increasing the contact area, which spreads force over a larger area. Shear is critical to avoid in patients with loss of protective sensation.

Traction and dynamic assists

Dynamic assists are the power behind mobilization splints, but tissue damage and ineffective treatment may occur with incorrect traction. The objective in using dynamic traction is to aid the patient in reaching full rehabilitative potential from treatment without additional inflammation, scarring, and deformity of skin.

The skin and underlying soft tissue are the limiting factors in determining the maximum amount of force that can be used to mobilize a stiff joint by dynamic traction. Tendon and bone can usually withstand additional torque in most cases. Greater force for traction of joints could be used if the skin under the traction could safely sustain higher force. Traction is adjusted to skin tissue tolerance for this reason, and traction is relaxed or discontinued if evidence of inflammatory response is seen, then continued with a reduced force after obvious signs of inflammation have subsided. It is better to start traction with a low force and to gradually increase the force over a few days rather than to have to back off after tissue injury. Further injury may be prevented by having both the patient and examiner look for early stages of traumatic inflammation, and adjusting traction accordingly.

Mechanics of cuffs

A traction cuff (sling) that is either too flexible or too rigid can cause injury (Fig. 15-6, *A*). A cuff made of very flexible material can bend and conform so much that it causes high shear at the sides of the finger and at edges where it contacts the finger. Highly flexible material may conform so closely that vascular compromise occurs under a cuff's arc of contact. A cuff that is too rigid also can be injurious (edge pressure more than triple) because it tilts when the direction of traction is angulated.

Patient compliance with traction splinting is increased by attention to materials and design of cuffs. Actual pressure necrosis from splinting is likely only in patients with insensitive hands. Patients with sensitivity will generally remove cuffs if they become uncomfortable. Leather, which is flexible while being firm enough to reduce shear at the sides and edges of the contract arc, makes a good material for a traction cuff because it simulates normal skin. The loop of the cuff should not be too shallow because this increases

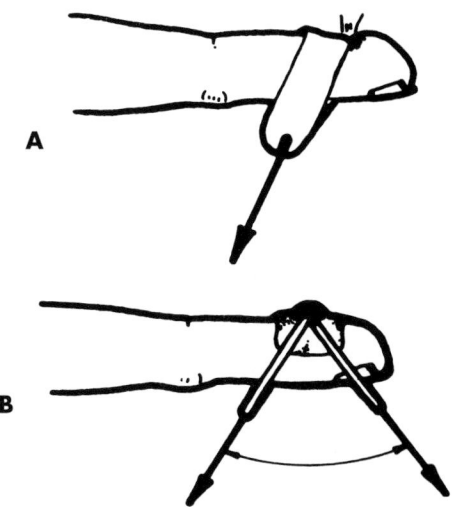

Fig. 15-6. A, Shear at edge of traction cuffs can result in injury to tissue. **B,** Brand suggests anchoring rigid cuffs at middle position to minimize rotation of the cuff on the finger with finger movement and changes in angle of traction.

the lateral side contact stress. A loop length extending at least 2 to 2.5 cm beyond the finger is desirable. Thin cuffs should be avoided. The cuff should be as wide as is possible to distribute pressure over as wide an area as possible (no less than 1 cm wide). If the cuff (area in which the force is applied to the skin) is wider, more traction force is possible. If a thin cuff is used, less traction force may be necessary. There is no "safe" amount of force against the skin per se because the quality of skin and soft tissue dictates the maximum that can be applied without damage. The skin needs to be examined for areas of sustained redness an hour after traction has been applied and again the next day.

Brand[18] has suggested an inexpensive rigid cuff design that spreads pressure over a larger area without causing edge shear. This cuff consists of a plaster shell of two to three layers molded in an arc around the finger. When the plaster is formed and hardened, a loop of thread can be added to the center back of the plaster cuff. (The thread loop is used for traction.) The cuff does not tilt against the finger, but rather moves with the finger. The rigid cuff also serves to lift the thread away and to eliminate shear stress at the lateral sides of the finger. Plaster is preferred because it conforms well and will stick to the skin, eliminating shear, but thermoplastic material can also be used in the same design (Fig. 15-6, *B*).

Mechanics of outriggers

Both low-profile and high-profile traction splint designs have advantages and disadvantages. Low-profile outriggers can be used effectively if well designed and adjusted. They can be more cosmetic but do not necessarily offer any mechanical advantage (and sometimes have less), and they usually require more frequent adjustment to create and maintain desired traction. A high-profile splint is often more efficient, and sometimes—if traction is indicated—is optimal. A high-profile outrigger can provide the distance necessary for extension and recovery of the bands in a direct line of pull. Any angulation in the direction of pull, as is introduced in a low-profile design, can create drag. Clinicians debate the advantage of one design over another, but both high- and low-profile splints have their place, and the design that best fits the patient's needs should be used.

Drag is a biomechanical term encompassing both frictional and tissue restraint, such as is seen in adhesions. It is any factor within the limb that tends to prevent or hinder the free motion of a joint. In the case of dynamic assists, the effect of external drag can be seen when the rubber band or nylon thread is moving around an outrigger, with *friction* being caused by the actual materials used. Friction can cause a band or nylon thread around the bar to move like a ratchet in slips and starts. The result is additional and unwanted force that can directly affect the skin and cause ischemic pressure. Ratchetlike movement from friction is seen when rubber bands or nylon thread passes over an outrigger that is made from thermoplastic materials or when hook Velcro is used to provide retainers to hold thread in place.

In a study by Chow et al.,[35] the varying traction systems of splints were compared against one another, including the standard rubber band traction, a single strand of rubber band used with and without a palmar pulley, a single-core elastic band, and variations thereof. The results were significant. In this study of 28 subjects, the system of a palmar pulley, a single-core–coated elastic band, and a spring wire lever arm was consistently the most mechanically and functionally efficient system compared with the other traction systems. The rubber band traction without a pulley required the greatest effort to extend the distal interphalangeal (DIP) and proximal interphalangeal (PIP) joints. It is desirable to use a free and frictionless bar. It is even better to use a wheel pulley or smooth steel bar, both of which are available as prefabricated splint accessories.

Mechanics of reaction bars

Reaction bars, which are used to stabilize parts of fingers and joints for traction to be applied to other joints, are common components of splinting. Pressure problems occur with the use of reaction bars because, for every gram of force exerted by the rubber band traction, there is at least twice as much force pushing down on the reaction bar.[18] The *lumbrical bar* is one of the most common reaction bar stabilizers and is also one of the most frequent areas for splint pressure problems. In a system in which there is tension, such as in dynamic splinting, any movement is toward the tension. If a joint is stiff, the rubber band will pull or tilt the whole finger toward the outrigger. For example, in a dorsal splint with a proximal phalanx block built into the body of the splint, the metacarpophalangeal (MP) joints will move away from the inside surface of the splint. The MP

joints have to be secured in the splint so that they will not angulate volarly with traction. A molded pad that fits the palmar arch can help anchor the MP joints securely. To further disburse pressure on the dorsum of the fingers, the surface of a reaction bar can be curved to fit the shape of the fingers. The bar can be made as wide as possible and semirigid padding added. If the hand fits into the splint well, more force for traction is possible than if the splint is ill fitted and creates dorsal pressure.

Static or dynamic splints

Insight into the biomechanics of soft tissue and of hand functions makes it necessary to redefine the concept of static versus dynamic splints—there is no static splint.[2,18] A so-called static splint is not at all static in its function—it is an *immobilization splint*. A splint that immobilizes one joint dynamically affects the action at another joint. Immobilization of the DIP joint of a finger transfers the flexion force of the flexor digitorum profundus (FDP) more proximally to the PIP joint, thus increasing the flexion force acting at the PIP joint (see Fig. 114-15).

Calculated and purposeful dynamic transfer of force can help in the treatment of stiff joints. For example, when a joint such as the PIP is injured, the other joints with the least resistance to glide will be the first to move. The injured and perhaps swollen PIP joint will be the least likely to move and thus is in danger of becoming stiff. If the DIP joint is casted, the flexion force at the DIP joint is transferred more proximally to the PIP joint and can help overcome resistance caused by injury and restore flexion ROM.

When tendon repairs are functioning primarily at the distal joints, casting or splinting the distal joints with removable casts will encourage normal ROM at the more proximal joints. Conversely, casting of the more proximal joints will transfer power of motion force to the more distal joints. This is what happens when a therapist blocks the more proximal joints to concentrate movement at the distal joints. For instance, after a boutonnière repair, the interphalangeal (IP) joint that most easily moves in flexion is the PIP joint. This is, in fact, dangerous to the repair at the level of the dorsum of the PIP joint because the repair can be given too much tension too early. By casting the PIP joint, the therapist dynamically decreases its flexion and shifts the flexion power of the FDP, which normally flexes two joints to the DIP joint (see Fig. 114-16).

A stiff or fused joint acts as an internal splint, and the force that was acting on that joint is transferred to other joints. The normally balanced biomechanics of the flexors and extensors is disrupted. Without realizing the dynamic transfer of force that occurs with splinting, the surgeon or therapist can be causing undesirable results. Often, the results of joint fusions are not satisfactory, but it is not always understood why. Fusions of the IP joints of the fingers often result over time in progressive flexion contractures at the DIP joints. The flexion force of PIP joint flexor muscles is transferred to MP and DIP joints, and at the DIP joint flexion force is unopposed by the extensors that were disrupted during surgery. Thus a mechanical imbalance has been created at surgery. Fusion of a joint affects the biomechanics of the thumb even more than of the fingers because the thumb has more rotational forces. The effect of this transfer in force needs to be evaluated over time because the remodeling that takes place in other joints may not be apparent for the first few months, or even in a year, and the examiner can think no problem was created.

MEASUREMENT OF FORCE AND PRESSURE ON SKIN

Patients with intrinsic muscle weakness and other muscle imbalances will demonstrate increased and abnormal concentration of force on the fingertips rather than even pressure distribution throughout a normal contact area. Repeat measurements after tendon-rebalancing surgery or casting for contracture can demonstrate an increase in area of contact and a more uniform pressure distribution. Excessively high force occurs particularly on the fingertips of patients with loss of sensitivity and lack of pressure feedback.

Pressure transducers

A pressure *transducer* can be used to provide measurement of relative magnitude and concentration of pressure under materials or from objects when the hand is used.[56] These can be placed under bandages or used in a glove system in which they are attached to a recording device or computer. Most commercially available transducers are subject to some variability depending on where the pressure is on their surface and they should be used under the same conditions and in the same position. Pressure transducers need to be as thin as possible or incorporated as a part of the material tested so their bulk does not add pressure (Fig. 15-7).

Pressure prints

Gloves impregnated with pressure-sensitive capsules have been used to demonstrate relative differences in pressure with tools and objects. These gloves consist of open-cell polyurethane foam with a cotton outer cover impregnated with dye-filled microcapsules. Staining occurs as the weakly acidic bromophenol solution contacts the alkaline powder (used as an activator) that is dusted over the inner surface of the glove. The microcapsules are broken by a single application of a large force (60 pounds per square inch [psi]) or by repetition of smaller forces (20 to 30 psi). Differential staining provides mapping of the location and distribution of stress[17] (Fig. 15-8).

Weighted cylinders

Contact areas during grip can be measured by counting the number of phalanges that come into contact with a 1-, 2-, or 3-inch cylinder. The measurement is even more useful

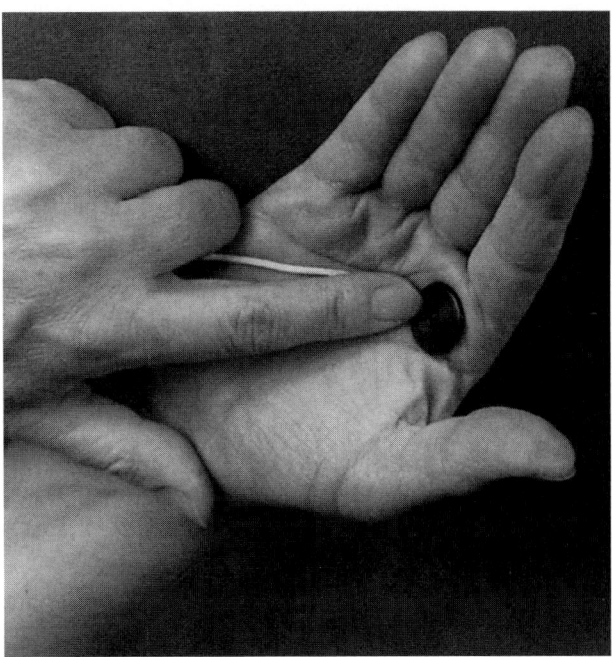

Fig. 15-7. Pressure transducer. Small pressure transducers can be useful aids in determining the amount and area of pressure concentration under splints, straps, and bandages.

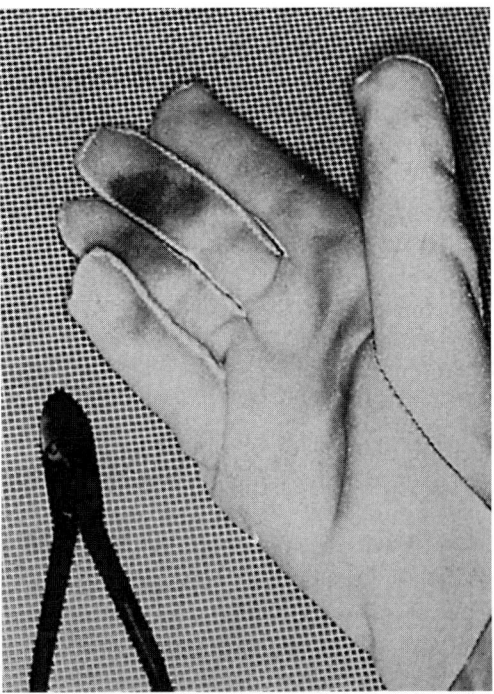

Fig. 15-8. Microcapsule staining of glove in areas of high-pressure concentration from a hand tool. Inking of a tool can similarly demonstrate on a glove areas of contact pressure and concentration of pressure in a small area that can cause hand injury.

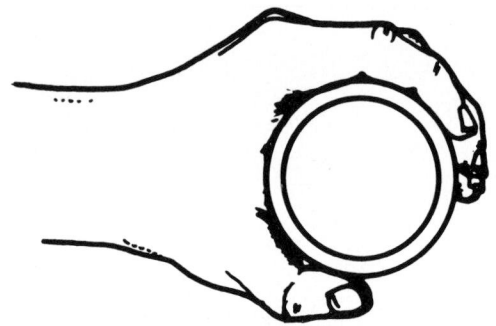

Fig. 15-9. Weighted cylinders of graduated sizes enable contact area of fingers during grasp to be evaluated. Intrinsically imbalanced hands will be unable to contact the cylinder with a normal, broad, palmar contact area.

when the cylinders are of progressive weights. Weighted cylinders are particularly helpful in the evaluation of changes in grasp and pinch with increasing load. In patients with muscle imbalances of the hand, it often can be demonstrated that a light pinch or grasp may appear normal until the fingers are loaded with a weight and then collapse on sustained positioning. This evaluation is helpful because it is not enough for a patient's fingers simply to work in selective positions. What happens to the fingers when loaded with weight is the real test of how fingers function, and rebalancing in reconstructive surgery is needed (Fig. 15-9).

Inked cylinders

Cylinders for grasp can be inked and covered with paper. The ink transfers to the paper on contact of the hand, and the paper is saved as a record. A Harris mat, originally designed to measure contact pressure on the sole of the foot, has been added to a cylinder covered with paper. The mat contains a grid of squares with ridges of various sizes and heights. The more pressure exerted against the pad, the more details the grid will show on the print.[53,59]

MEASUREMENT OF SPLINT FORCES

Measurement of *force* used in splinting is not limited to the laboratory but should be a part of everyday patient treatment. Measurements can be quick and repeatable and do not necessarily add greatly to the time for clinical treatment beyond records that are needed to document and substantiate treatment.[16,18,30,47,61]

Measurement of pressure under cuffs

The pressure that cuffs produce on the skin can be measured with an orthotic gauge, which measures the force of traction and the area of contact from the cuff. Pressure is the force divided by the unit area of contact. It has been suggested that as a rule, traction force on the skin by typical traction cuffs should not exceed 300 g.[46] A 300-g traction force for a semirigid leather cuff that is 2 cm wide and contacts a 2-cm length of skin thus provides a 4-cm^2 contact area, which does not exceed 75 g/cm^2 (or 0.025 psi, 13 mm Hg).[18,30] This is a guideline for an estimate of traction. If the same cuff was only 1.5 cm wide, pressure on the skin would be higher; thus the traction force might need to be reduced to accommodate the thinner cuff (300 divided by 3 cm^2 = 100 g/cm^2).

Measurement of rubber band traction

Rubber bands, like soft tissue and other splinting materials, have viscoelastic properties. The elastic restraint component is the tension that is seen in the rubber band. The tension of rubber bands is determined by their length and thickness. Short, thick bands produce high forces, and long, thin bands produce relatively low forces (Fig. 15-10). A relationship exists between the elongation and tension of a given rubber band. When there is a change in length of the rubber band, there is a relative change in the tension it produces. A graph of this tension is called a *length/tension curve*. Each band of a different length and width will have its own tension-producing capacity.[18,25,26] Limited excursion will limit joint ROM. In general, short bands produce a large amount of tension with a limited excursion. Length/tension measurements suggest the use of longer bands that are not too thick (1 to 3 mm) and that have a more desirable length/tension ratio for traction splinting.

Fess[44] found that a given size and quality of rubber band can have a fairly predictable force spectrum. Rubber bands tested by Buford[32] were found to demonstrate as much as 200 g of tension difference between bands of the same batch. Variations in the size of bands in the same batch accounted for much of the variation in force. The rubber bands tested were size 33, which is a commonly used rubber band size for splinting. Therefore, for consistent traction, it is important to pick bands of the same relative size and tension even within a given batch. Mildenberger et al.[61] published a valuable systematic approach to selection of rubber band traction.

Another physical property of rubber bands is their *hysteresis*—the change that occurs in the bands with loading and unloading. The tension (elastic restraint component) during loading (stretching) is more than the tension that occurs during unloading. This adds to the variable force of the stretched rubber band at any given length of the band. The hysteresis is variable, depending on the size, material, and age of the band. Bands age quickly and *fatigue* easily, increasing their hysteresis.

Breger-Lee and Buford[26] found that rubber bands of various lengths and thicknesses exhibited *creep* over time when subjected to a constant load for 3 weeks. The shortest, thickest bands exhibited the least creep. Fess[44] tested tension of rubber bands chosen by experienced and inexperienced therapists, and found therapists with experience in dynamic splinting were much more likely to select bands of appropriate length and tension than inexperienced therapists and students, who often selected too much tension. These studies emphasize that it is safer to initially use bands of less

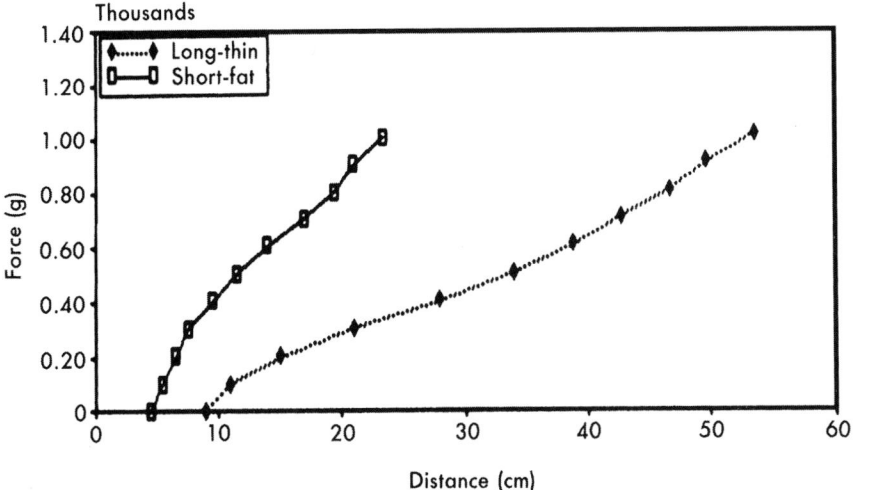

Fig. 15-10. Stress/strain curve of rubber bands. Each band of a different length and width will have its own stress/strain curve that can be measured.

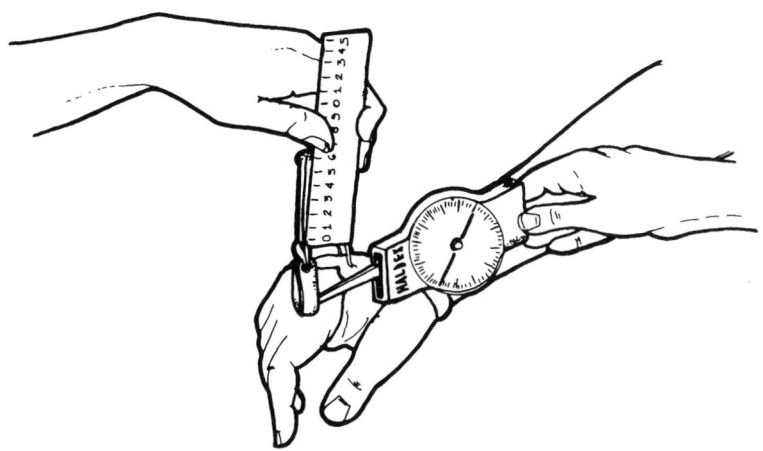

Fig. 15-11. Rubber band traction measurement. Rubber band traction is measured in place, on the splint, in the same position and distance force will be applied. (Researched by William Buford, B.M.E., Ph.D.)

tension (in the range of 300 g) and to check band tension and skin tolerance frequently. There is no way to adequately guess the force, but through routine measurement the therapist can enhance his or her estimation of forces required.

Rubber bands of the same size will vary in length and tension, and thus vary in the force applied to the skin for joint movement. Rubber bands of the same tension for replacement traction can be identified by the length they hang with a weight. Rubber bands hang from a post in the clinic that has been mounted on a board. One standard repeatable weight is used to hang on the bands (e.g., 300 g).[26]

Rubber band force is measured directly on the splint in the direction and for the length the traction will be applied. While the traction cuff is on the patient in a resting position, the length of the band is measured with a standard ruler, from the band's attachment point on the splint to its attachment point on the traction cuff. The cuff and rubber band unit only is removed. Using the ruler as the guide for length, the clinician extends the cuff with the rubber band for the same length and in the same direction as it was when on the patient (with the tip of the arm of a Haldex or other measurement gauge used to extend and hold the cuff (Be OK Sammons, Inc., Bessell Healthcare Co., Brookfield, Illinois). The resultant force is read (Fig. 15-11).

The maximum force that will be exerted on the fingers at extremes of ROM can be similarly calculated with the aforementioned technique. The patient extends or flexes the finger undergoing traction in the splint, and the cuff is removed but extended to the same position and in the same direction with the Haldex gauge. The bands are measured at the longest length at which they will exert pressure against

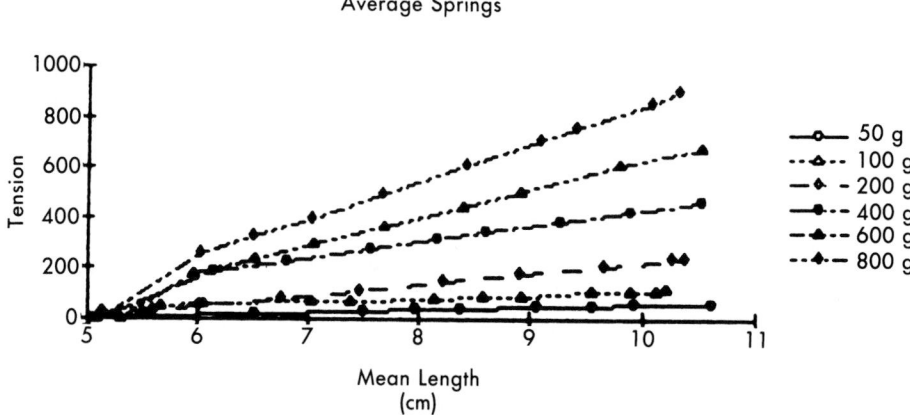

Fig. 15-12. Spring traction measurement. Springs of progressive lengths and forces can be selected and progressively increased in specific increments of force/tension. (From Robertson, et al: *J Hand Ther* 1:110, 1988.)

the skin and at the shortest length at which they will apply pressure when the patient fully extends or flexes the splinted joint or finger. Higher forces may be acceptable at extremes of joint motion (full extension or full flexion) if they are intermittent and do not cause damage from repetitive stress. The amount of safe force will also vary according to the amount of wearing time and other variables. Patient compliance is a consideration. In general, the more the patient understands that long periods of mild force are desirable for optimal correction, the more compliant he or she is in using the splint for long periods.

Measurement of springs

Springs are more durable than rubber bands, their shelf life is excellent, and they provide a consistent and controlled force. The use of graded springs can be an improvement over rubber bands. The length/tension measurements of springs are often available through manufacturers. A wide range of spring forces suitable for splinting are available commercially. Springs need to be measured in the position they will be used on the patient with the same technique as for rubber bands.

Springs in the SCOMAC Low Profile Outrigger Kit developed by Rouzaud and Allieu (available through North Coast Medical, San Jose, California; Smith, Nephew, and Rolyan, Germantown, Wisconsin; and Wise, Ali Medical Corp., Dedham, Massachusetts) are color-coded for specific force, and range from 50 to 2000 g. In an independent study, Roberson et al.[65] tested the SCOMAC springs for their length-tension relationships, creep, hysteresis, and fatigue. The springs were consistent in length/tension measurements among those studied and with the forces specified by the manufacturer. No creep (deformity-causing changes in force) was found in the tested springs, indicating reliability of the force exerted at a given length after a given amount of time. Little hysteresis was found (the springs provided a controlled, repeatable force at each length, whether the

spring was stretching or contracting). With repeated elongation, they maintained their original length/tension measurements and did not break or bend (Fig. 15-12).

TORQUE RANGE-OF-MOTION MEASUREMENTS

Careful clinical measurements of joint ROM provide significant insight into the cause and treatment of joint problems. Almost all stiffness is caused by ligaments, capsules, skin, or scar.[18,67,78] Measurements can help determine the type of therapy to recommend, whether conservative treatment may be a waste of time, or whether surgery is indicated.[23,24] Measurements are used to monitor changes as a result of pathologic conditions and to evaluate effectiveness of treatment modalities or the rebalancing of muscle power on joints introduced by tendon transfers.

Two approaches can be taken when measuring a joint angle: (1) to estimate the joint axis and align the arms of a goniometer along the side of the bony shafts or (2) to measure the angle above the joint. There is no clear way to locate the axis of the joint being measured. However, it does not matter how far above or below the joint the axis of the goniometer is placed; the axis alignment is accurate as long as the goniometer arms are aligned along the bony shafts (unless there is excessive swelling or bony misalignment).

Passive ROM measurement either along the side or over the joint has been the traditional method for evaluation of the joint mobility. The actual joint angle measured depends on the position of the other joints and the amount of torque placed on the joint. Without consistent positioning or consistent torque, measurements are inaccurate.

The need for more objective measurements of joint angles led Brand[18] to introduce the torque ROM concept for measurements of the hand as "windows into the mechanics of the joint." In addition to being accurate, this method can be used to more specifically differentiate joint stiffness that is caused by adhesions around tendons from that which is caused by stiffness around joints (Fig. 15-13).

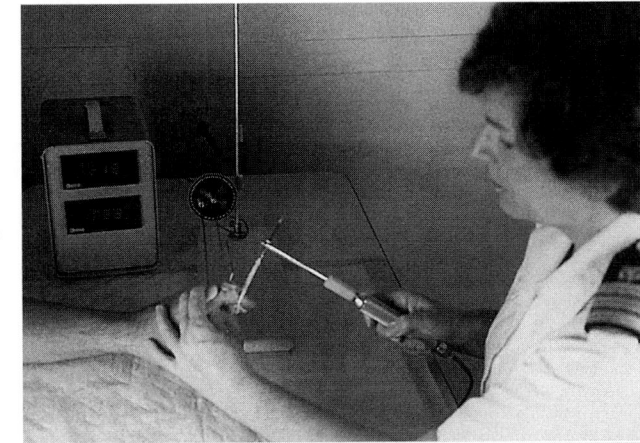

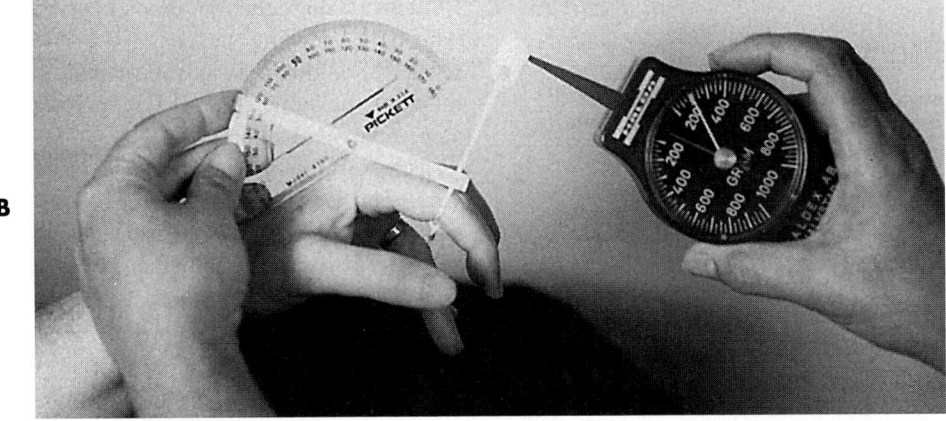

Fig. 15-13. Instrument technique for measuring torque range of motion. **A,** Original prototype strain gauge. **B,** Haldex strain gauge and goniometer adaptation for clinic measurements. (Research by Paul W. Brand Research Laboratory, Carville, La.)

Torque is what occurs at the joint as the force is applied at a given distance from the joint axis. Torque at the joint is the force multiplied by the distance the force is applied. In a technique described by Beach and Bell,[5] the distance is kept the same for repeat measurements to simplify the procedure and to allow the examiners to be concerned only about the force that is applied. The actual torque will be higher the farther the measurement is made from the joint. The loop for traction is placed at the same distance for measurement, usually at the more distal joint crease. If desired, a water-soluble ink can be used to mark for distance of measurement.

The clinical reliability of torque ROM measurements has been examined to determine the intrarater and interrater reliability of the method.[29] Although the intrarater reliability is more consistent than interrater reliability, the tests moderately correlated with each other overall. A consistent force and position of the other, more proximal joints can make a tremendous difference in resultant joint-angle measurement. The joint angle increases with increased force, and is often different if the wrist is placed in flexion or extension.

Instrument specifications

Engineers in the Rehabilitation Research Laboratory have developed several prototype measurement instruments to control the force applied to the joint for torque ROM measurement.[21] Buford[30] developed a cantilever, beam-type force transducer with digital readout for use in the clinic, and newer models are still being developed (Fig. 15-13, *A*). A computerized torque ROM device has been designed by the NK Biotechnical Corporation (Minneapolis, Minnesota). Other models will become available as the technique is more widely used. However, expensive instrumentation is not needed in the clinic; torque ROM measurements can be performed using a standard goniometer, a strain gauge, and a finger loop (cuff).

Measurement procedure

An orthotic gauge, Haldex or similar, is used with a 2-inch loop of string attached to the most distal part of the device arm. A ⅛-inch string is used for the loop, which provides traction against the measurement arm of the gauge. The distance from the joint axis that the gauge string combination is to be applied for traction is measured and recorded.

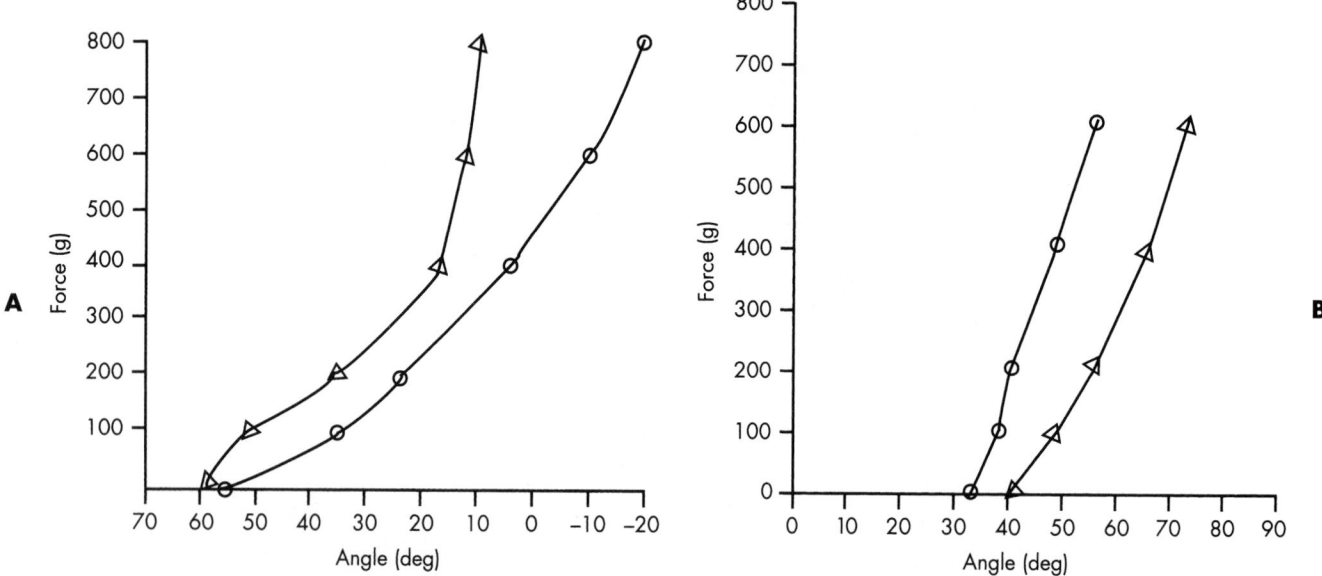

Fig. 15-14. A, Normal torque-angle curves for (1) proximal interphalangeal *(PIP)* joint and (2) metacarpophalangeal joint extension. (Note similarities in slope with earlier stress/strain curve of normal tissue.) **B,** Abnormal torque-angle curves for PIP joint flexion before and after paraffin treatment. (Note shift to the right in second measurement and more relaxed curve.)

Traction is applied to the desired force (as read on the gauge), and the resultant angle is recorded (Fig. 15-13, *B*).

A voice recorder is helpful to record the resultant joint-angle measurements of the different forces applied (and leaves the hands free for measurement). The position of the proximal joints must be consistent for repeatable measurement. A universal (reusable) cock-up splint can be made to stabilize the wrist position in degrees of flexion, neutral, or extension during measurements. This splint is made as with any cock-up splint, but with thenar cutouts on both sides so that it can fit the right or left.

For measurement of the PIP joint in extension, the crease of the DIP joint is used for the loop, moving the PIP joint into extension. The gauge measures the G force applied. A finger goniometer is placed over the dorsum of the finger to read the ROM. The traction must be maintained at right angles to the segment distal to the joint measured.

To measure PIP flexion, the arm of an orthotic gauge is applied to the finger using a pencil eraser tip (eraser has been attached to measurement arm of the gauge for this purpose). The dorsum of the middle phalanx opposite the finger distal flexion crease is used to determine a repeatable distance through which the force is applied. The direction of application of force must be at right angles to the segment of the digit that is to move. The position of the MP joints and the wrist should be noted and maintained constant.

Torque angle

ROM measurements are immediately more objective if one standard force (e.g., 300 g) is used to measure every joint. *Torque angle* refers to the resultant angle measurement at a specific force applied at a given distance from the joint.

Torque-angle measurements

Useful information about the mechanical quality (elasticity or inelasticity) of the joint tissues may be obtained by making a succession of torque-angle measurements at different levels of force (at the same distance from the axis). Torque-angle measurements refer to a sequence of incremental force and resultant changes in joint angle. The forces may be applied at from 100 to 800 g, but the maximum amount of safe force varies according to the size of the hand and the pathologic condition. With small, fragile hands, the force should not exceed 300 to 600 g. The greatest changes in angle will be produced with the lower levels of force (100 to 400 g), with higher forces producing little change; thus higher force beyond 400 g is not always needed for measurement). Brand recommends the use of four forces, another variation uses only two (e.g., 200 and 600 g of force).[5,18,24,28] Arthritic joints or joints with instability should not be measured with more force than that necessary to gently straighten the joint (100 to 200 g). (It takes approximately 100 g to completely straighten a finger to 180 degrees extension.)

Torque-angle curves

A torque-angle curve is the line plot produced by successive torque-angle measurements of a joint. A graph is made by recording measurement force on the vertical axis and angle on the horizontal axis. A normal torque-angle

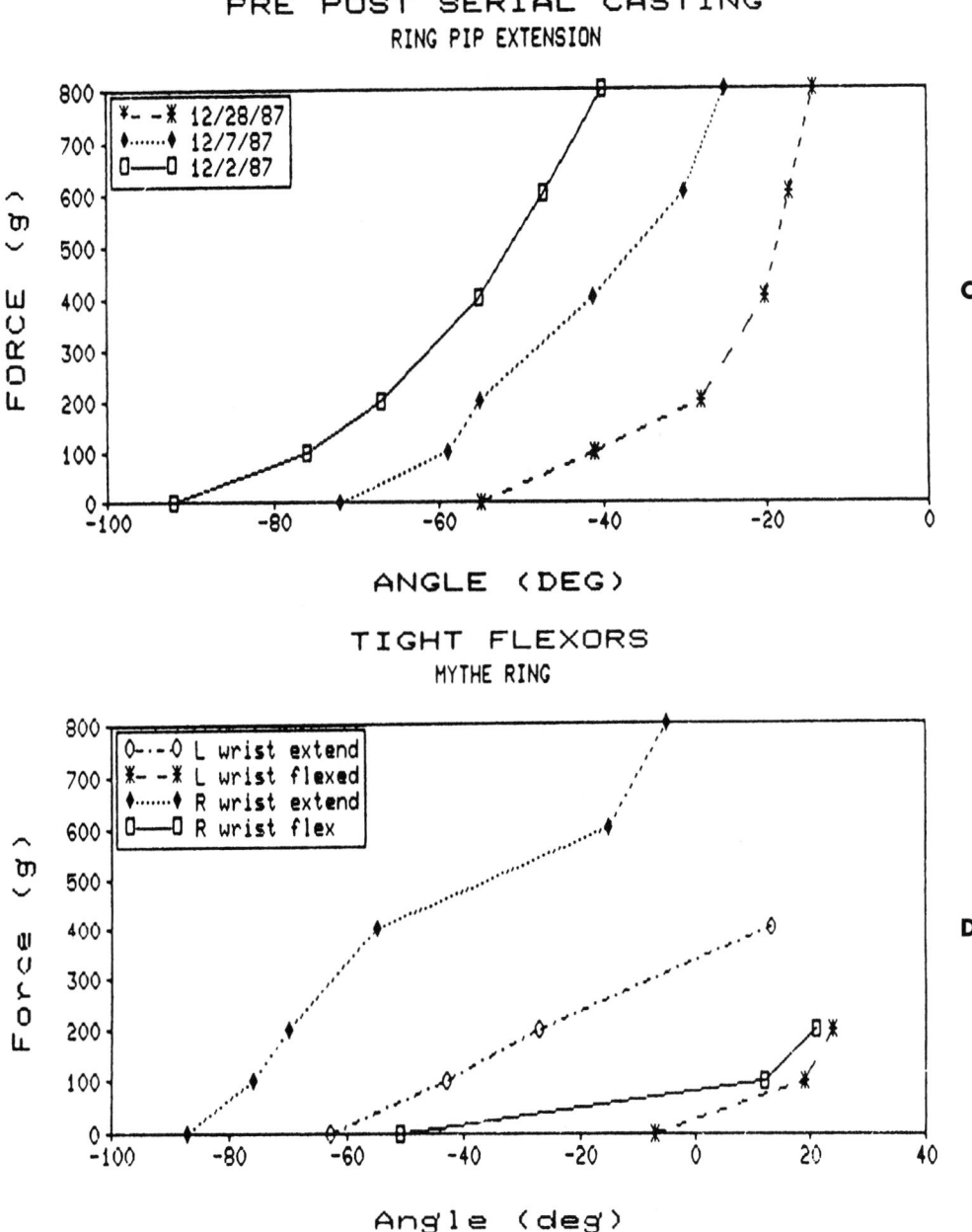

Fig. 15-14, cont'd. **C,** Torque-angle curve measurements precasting and postcasting for extension. (From Breger-Lee DE, Bell Krotoski JA, Brandsma JW: *J Hand Ther* 3:12, 1990.) **D,** Torque-angle curves from flexor muscle tendon unit tightness. (From Breger-Lee DE, Bell Krotoski JA, Brandsma JW: *J Hand Ther* 3:12, 1990.)

curve shows that the joint has a soft end-feel (springiness).[49] A normal torque-angle curve for the PIP joint and the MP joint is shown in Fig. 15-14, *A,* and Fig. 15-14, *B,* shows an abnormal torque-angle curve for a proximal interphalangeal joint before and after its shift toward normal with treatment. The viscoelasticity of the joint's restraining tissue is revealed in the curve. A normal curve begins in a soft slope that changes quickly with increased gram load. A fixed, con-

tracted joint comes to an abrupt halt in slope and has a steep curve with increasing *load.*

Torque-angle curves can document and show improvement with and the efficacy of treatment, as well as help identify optimum treatment technique.[22,28,50] Fig. 15-14, *C,* shows the improvements in measurement of a ring PIP joint with treatment by casting for remodeling (see Chapter 114). In Fig. 15-14, *D,* measurements show tightness of the sublimis muscle tendon unit in the left hand compared with the right when a ring finger IP joint is measured with the wrist flexed and extended.

Optimally, repeat measurements are taken at the same time of day and with the hand in the same relative position. The viscosity of normal joints changes with elevation or dependent positioning and time of day. This change is even more dramatic after hand injury and disease, and the amount of fluid can change the torque-angle curve. Arthritic patients who have morning stiffness have an increase in viscosity.[78]

HAND VOLUME MEASUREMENT

Brand[14,18] invented the hand volumeter (Volumeters Unlimited, Idyllwild, California) to objectively measure edema, to monitor edema, and to help direct treatment[4] (see Hand volume measurement procedure, page 188). Independent authors have reported on the reliability of hand volume measurements.[38,39,69,77] After surgery, swelling can persist into the period of remobilization. If the edema during return to function is from inactivity or dependent positioning, there will be a hand volume change in a short period after elevation of the extremity. This type of edema responds to movement, massage, and compressive treatment to the hand. In patients with inflammatory edema from infection or overuse, hand volume will not show a change in a short period, and treatment indicated is rest or at least a decrease in activity. Exercise, if allowed, is initially limited to that necessary to maintain joint and tendon gliding. Hand volume measurements can be particularly helpful in following patients with arthritic hands who can have fluid volume changes with time of day and with treatment. Volume measurements help determine whether medications, night splinting, or splinting during activities have an effect of reducing fluid volume of the hand.

Waylett and Seibly[77] studied the average deviation accuracy of the Brand-designed volumeter and reported 10 ml or less of measurement variation with one examiner, and 10- to 15-ml variation between examiners. A hand could have a fluid change in distinct areas, such as from palm to fingers, and still maintain the same volume. Circumferential measurements of the hand and fingers with a tape is a useful adjunct to volume measurement (note the exact location of measurement).

TEMPERATURE ASSESSMENT

A prolonged elevation in skin temperature from too much stress can be accurately measured.[12,13,18,52] Any exercise of the hand will result in some temperature elevation but should be of short duration. The examiner can learn to discern changes in temperature with measurement. A hand that has swelling from disuse will be cool by comparison with normal. Temperature differentials are more important than the absolute temperature. One area of skin is compared with other areas on the same hand or with the same site on the other hand. The skin temperature can vary, particularly from the dorsal to volar surfaces of the hand, but the difference often is only 1° C; thus a difference more than this is suspect.

Thermography, or infrared heat photography, has been used in research for several years.[14] Even in black and white, an isotherm picture mapping is produced from hot to cool, and hot spots can easily be recognized. In color, temperature changes by color for each degree. Warm colors are red, orange, and white, and cooler colors are green, blue, and purple. Although mappings are highly valuable to clinical treatment, equipment costs have made instruments impractical. Thermography instruments are now available at less cost (Ircon, Inc., Niles, Illinois; Teletherm Infrared Thermal Image Corp., Dunedin, Florida). These use a camera to take an infrared photograph of the hand that can directly read into a computer. Temperature mappings can be stored and compared with serial maps and among patients. If a hand has been warmed in a glove or has been exercised a lot, it

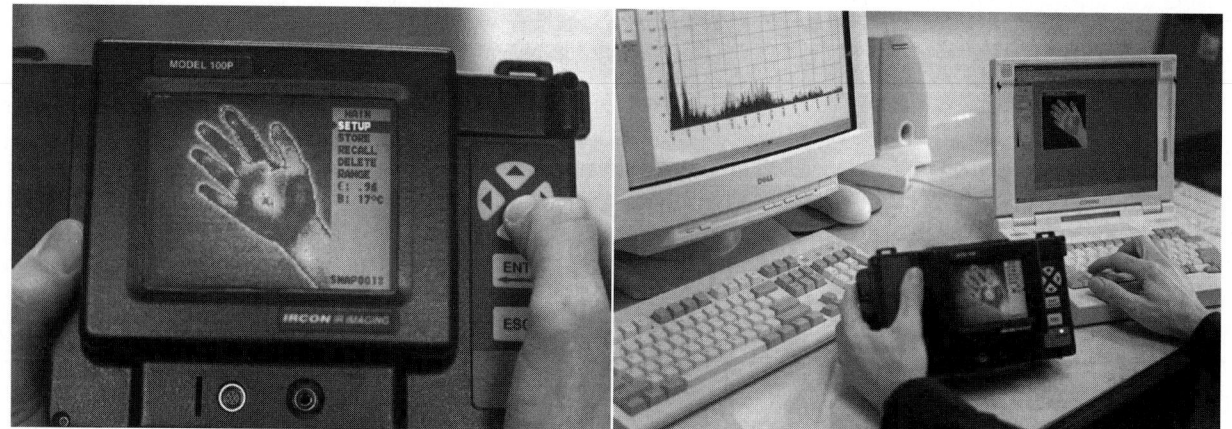

Fig. 15-15. A, Currently available thermography equipment. A camera (Ircon) records the temperature mapping and reads directly into a portable or desktop computer for record and analysis. **B,** Close-up of the temperature mapping on the camera, which can be in black and white or color. (Courtesy Ircon, Inc., Niles, Ill.)

may be necessary to cool the extremity for approximately 5 minutes before measurement (Fig. 15-15).

Surface skin thermometers are inexpensive but unfortunately take time to register and are not practical. Handheld radiometer instruments for measuring absolute skin temperature at one site are relatively inexpensive and are readily available (Mikron Infrared Thermometer, Mikron Instrument Co., Inc., Midland Park, New Jersey; Model KM 900, Probe KS, Measurements, Inc., New Orleans, Louisiana). Battery-operated temperature probe instruments provide accurate measurement and site comparison, but not easy mapping.

STRENGTH MEASUREMENT

Strength of a muscle is the tension a muscle can develop and is related to the cross-sectional area of its fibers and its excursion.[19] *Excursion* is the distance through which the strength can be used and is related to work capacity of the muscle itself.[34] Strength of a muscle provided at a given joint depends on how far it is from the joint axis and on the number of joints it is crossing. The distance that the muscle or tendon is from the axis in part determines the usable external strength of an individual, which is not the same as the strength or tension produced by the muscle.

Grip strength measurements are used as a collective measure of a patient's overall strength or weakness. Although populations vary in mean grip strength, grip strength can be measured in absolute values on an instrument such as the Jamar dynamometer.[46,60] The Jamar dynamometer has been shown to be a sensitive and repeatable test instrument when calibrated correctly and used in a procedure that is in itself repeatable.[46] It is most useful when the patient can be used as his or her own control, such as in comparing

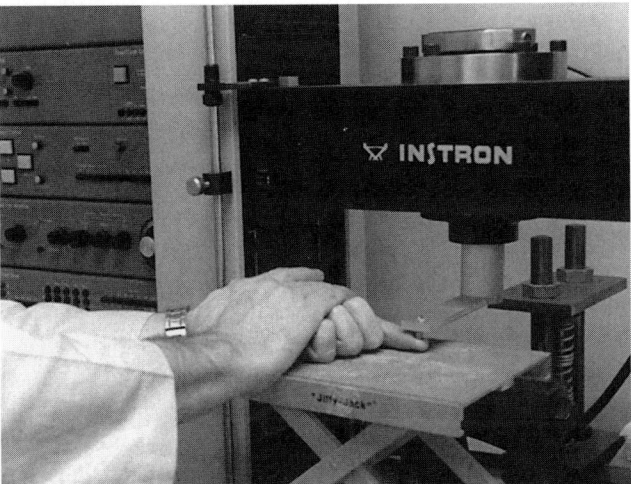

Fig. 15-16. Instron materials measurement instrument. Laboratory testing of materials can measure their viscoelastic properties and allow comparison of materials used for padding and splinting. With adaptation the instrument can be used for measuring individual finger strength or for stress testing.

right and left hands and when comparing baseline measurements with subsequent measurements.

Grip strength measurement with current instruments cannot be individualized to different muscles or fingers. Experimental instruments have been explored. A gyroscopic grip strength dynamometer with force transducers for each finger was designed experimentally at the National Institutes of Health by a therapist formerly associated with the authors' laboratory during its early years.[68] The Instron Materials Testing Instrument (Model II 22, Instron Instruments and Systems, Houston, Texas) used for studies of viscoelastic properties of materials can be adapted experimentally to test strength of individual muscles or fingers (Fig. 15-16). This instrument is essentially a large-scale stress/strain gauge that can be connected to an instrument with a calibrated graph readout. The flexion strength of a ring finger before and after a sublimis transfer, and radial wrist extensors for intrinsic replacement procedures, have been tested in this fashion. Testing is position dependent, and requires identical positioning for repeat testing.

Similar individual finger testing can be performed in the clinic with strain gauges, such as the Haldex orthotic gauge. The gauge can be mounted, and positioning devices can be made to ensure repeatable positioning. For example, weak radial wrist extension can be measured to find the exact load it can resist before it can no longer extend beyond neutral. On subsequent measurement, progressive improvement or weakness can be measured. Brand[18,19] emphasizes that endurance is as important as initial strength. He suggests the use of a metronome with selected gram weights, which are measured. The examiner counts the number of possible contractions through a full ROM with a given weight.

Electromyography numerically grades muscle strength and endurance. Validity of this testing depends on the experience and interpretation of the examiner. An integrating monitor can remove some subjectivity. The amplitude of the signal is considered more important than the wave form for strength (the abnormal wave forms are the basis for noting pathologic conditions). A weak strength of signal (amplitude) indicates weak muscle fiber–contraction activity. The duration, or continued muscle activity over time, is important in measurement because some muscles will show a good amount of contraction activity but drop off quickly.

Relative strength of muscles versus excursion

Individual strength measurement is variable in different populations; thus average muscle performance values are meaningful only for limited groups of similar individuals. There are numerous grip strength studies and there is question regarding what norms should be used for different patients. Brand,[19] like Bunnell in describing muscle balance and imbalance, considers the relative strength to be more important than absolute strength. He has found the relative muscle strength in most normal individual forearms and hands to be fairly constant and published this information

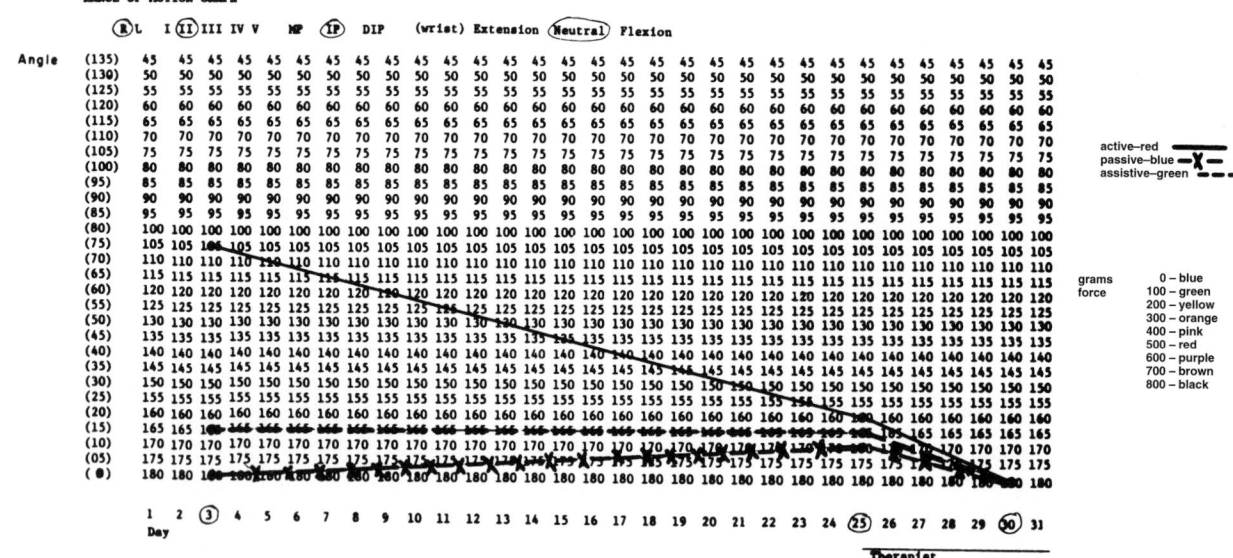

Fig. 15-17. Simplified measurement graph. By listing the possible range of data in rows and columns, a predesigned graph can be created. Serial measurements can be marked on the graph for comparison with previous measurements, whether or not a computer is available. Use of exact numbers can possibly eliminate errors that are possible with data point–type entry.

with Beach and Thompson in a review of 15 cadaver specimens. The study did not measure muscle strength in cadavers but implied strength or relative tension based on a cross-sectional area.

Brand et al.[19] found that the fiber lengths of the muscles are about equal when the muscles are displayed with the fibers aligned and that all fibers reach from the tendon of origin to the tendon of insertion. This is important because it means the fiber masses and lengths can be measured to determine the relative strengths of the muscles. Elftman,[40] after the work of Blix, previously demonstrated the relationship between fiber length, tension, and excursion.

The fiber length of a muscle is proportional to its potential excursion. Muscles with short fibers do not move far, whereas muscles with long fibers have long excursions. Muscles with short fibers and with large mass will be powerful muscles, but for short distances. Muscles with long fibers but with small mass will move relatively long distances, but with relatively little strength. Some muscles have many short fibers but potentially have the same relative volume; thus they have the same total work capacity as muscles with long fibers with less volume. A relative muscle-mass table was developed for all of the muscles of the hand and forearm. Each muscle has its own *mass fraction,* that is, the individual muscle mass percentage of total muscle mass of all muscles of the hand and forearm.

The cross-sectional area of all fibers is proportional to the maximum tension or tension-producing capacity of the muscles. A relative muscle-tension table was developed for all of the muscles of the forearm and hand. Each muscle has its own *tension fraction,* or individual muscle percentage of total cross-sectional areas for muscles of the hand and

forearm. The table contains highly valuable information for surgeons and therapists comparing strength and excursion of muscles used for tendon transfers.[14,19]

MEASUREMENT GRAPHS

Graphs allow measurements to be compared over time and among patients, and they reveal trends and associations that are not as easy to understand in statistical data alone.[16] Graphs of patient performance are easy for the professional and patient to understand as well as the employer and referral service. As with the simple temperature graph found in every hospital record, it is easy to see when a measurement goes above or below certain thresholds. The peaks on graphs can be associated with improvement in treatment and the valleys with regression, and vice versa. With computers, graphs are being used more frequently for displaying clinical measurements. Computerized data entry programs such as Excel now allow data to be directly entered into spread sheets that automatically convert to graphs. Data entered can be analyzed by the program or through compatible programs such as statistical analysis system.

The most helpful clinical graphs show the complete measurement range possible and a normal baseline. Deviation in measurement can then be quickly noted. Computers also make it possible for the clinician to easily design his or her own graphs. A simplified design for easy recording can be made by simply grouping in rows and columns the pertinent numerical data and range[8] (Fig. 15-17). For example, for IP joint measurement, a graph needs a range in joint-angle degrees from 0 degrees flexion through degrees of hyperextension. Measurements should then be noted directly on the form whether or not a computer is available.

INSTRUMENT TESTING

Many commonly used clinical measurement instruments can be found to fall short of the requirements for valid instruments.[30,45] Information presented in this chapter underlines the need for valid objective instruments. To describe and analyze clinical problems accurately, one must record data in terms other than subjective and have educated experience. There is no substitute for hands-on experience and educated intuition, and a clinician with the best of measurement and treatment techniques still needs to exercise good judgment. However, experience is enhanced and misconception is eliminated through reliable assessment of patient performance with sensitive and repeatable measures. How else can patient data be compared with normal subjects and with expected improvement? New knowledge and the most effective and efficient treatment can be found only with sensitive and accurate measurement.

Particularly with managed care and more limited time for treatment, examiners need to be aware of the shortcomings of ineffective measurements and instruments. The following are some routine questions when using any instrument or technique: (1) How sensitive is the instrument? (2) Is it calibrated and accurate? (3) Is it valid for what is being measured? (4) Is it quantifiable in repeatable increments for monitoring? and (5) Is it technique dependent?

There is a great difference between an instrument that has become *standard* or recommended in traditional practice and one that has been *standardized* through accepted clinical trials.[45,46] One of the greatest criticisms of tests for measurement of sensibility, for instance, is the variation in application induced by test instruments being handheld without control on force of application.[10] The examiner should at least be aware of what could be subjective in a measurement, and rely most heavily on instruments that have been found to be as controlled as possible given the limits of what is possible.

Unfortunately, there appears to be a renewed trend for products to be marketed through word-of-mouth "testimony." As a selling technique, it has been said and included in product promotional material that an instrument has been tested and is used at a recognized clinic. This type of promotion places even more burden on clinics to use reliable instruments, but on follow-up of supposed "testing," this amounts to therapists trying a device and liking it, but with no real investigative comparison study. Testimony and use does not identify valid instruments and can perpetuate the acceptance of ineffective instruments.

When clinicians accept as reliable only valid and objective instruments and devices that have been shown to be effective, not only will more improved instruments become available, but some of the ineffective ones will be recognized and eliminated. When clinicians check the calibration of instruments and return those that are out of calibration, manufacturers will be more exacting and more concerned about design specifications. All claims of validity and reliability should be backed not only by literature and expert references, but by hard studies, and at best independent or multicenter studies confirming similar findings. Newer instruments and devices are often still in development and often need continued testing and improvements for clinical application to be practical and valid.

Equally, one must not assume that an instrument is reliable and valid just because it is computerized. Computerized instruments still have to meet standards for reliable instruments. For instance, the measurements cannot be subject to fluctuations in power, life of batteries, and drive mechanisms that lack sensitivity or are not accurate. Signal filtering can eliminate application and technique variation in recorded and reported results, and should be examined specifically. A handheld instrument that is sensitive and repeatable within requirements for testing may be the most desirable in many situations for cost and practicality.

INTERACTIVE SURGICAL WORKSTATION PROJECT

Computer models of the hand are advancing both knowledge of hand biomechanics and teaching of biomechanics. A degree in biomechanics should not be necessary to learn what is needed for optimal patient treatment.[3,16,54,70] Computers help serve as a database in which knowledge of hand biomechanics is stored and can be accessed in examples or interactive learning sets for those needing specific information and techniques.[63,75,76] Models aid understanding of measurement and normal hand function that can be adjusted to simulate abnormal clinical situations. For example, in a normal hand, the full extension of the fingers by the extrinsic muscles is made possible through stabilization of the fingers by the intrinsic finger flexors. If the intrinsic muscles are lost, as happens with ulnar and median nerve paralysis, the extensor digitorum communis (EDC) can no longer fully extend the fingers. This can be demonstrated on a fresh cadaver section for students or can be simulated in a computer program designed to quickly show the biomechanical results of an intrinsic paralysis (Fig. 15-18).

One day an interactive workstation will be available for students and clinicians to accelerate quick understanding and knowledge of hand biomechanics resulting from injury and disease.[2,15,33,48] By changing the normal balance of muscles in and around joints of a computer model, the resultant imbalance can be recreated on the screen. A surgeon can key in critical elements specific to a patient, and propose surgical transfers using preprogrammed data of patient-relative muscle strength and excursion. The therapist can design splints for biomechanically imbalanced hands, learn what is needed for correction, and directly see results of new designs. An interactive work-station is being developed and programmed to include data from objective clinical measurements of hand biomechanics.[1,21,31,51,55,62,75,76]

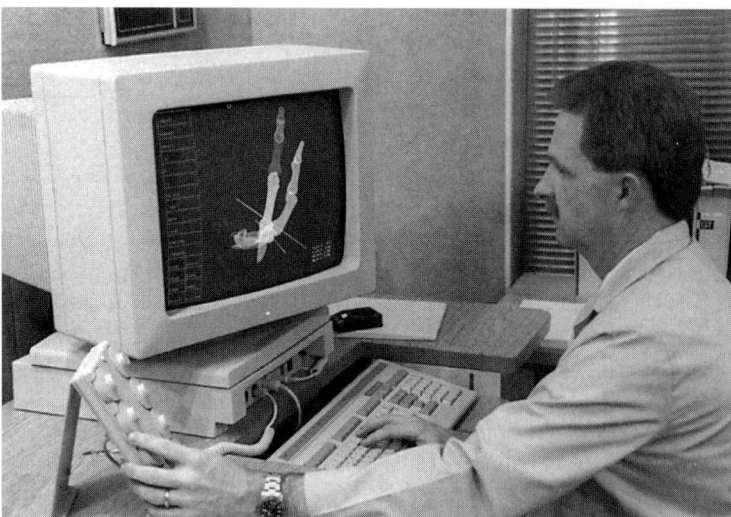

Fig. 15-18. Interactive surgical workstation. Computer modeling of the hand in an educational workstation has been a long-term project of the Paul W. Brand Research Laboratory. This includes years of data from soft tissue studies and actual cadaver measurements. The workstation will allow accelerated education in biomechanics of the hand and splints through examples, as well as simulation of various clinical conditions such as muscle mechanics before and after tendon transfer surgery.

COMPUTERIZED MEASUREMENT SYSTEMS

Computerized measurement systems* are exciting in the possibilities they offer in patient measurement and documentation, which in the past have been limited by bulky filing systems and time-absorbing documentation. Computer patient workstations have attachments that can be used for measurements such as grip and ROM and the measurements are entered directly into a database. Direct-reading instruments reduce the possibility of examiner error and facilitate multiple measurement and performance analyses of the same patient or groups of patients. Computer-driven systems allow controlled measurements that can be interactively adjusted according to patient response. Subject to proven accuracy, the increasing use of computers in clinics enhances the ability to generate quick and accurate reports and to show progress.

SUMMARY

Understanding the biomechanics of the hand and requirements for objective measurement can add new knowledge to hand therapy and surgery. Measurement techniques need to be performed by clinicians who are sensitive and attentive to biomechanical principles. With an understanding of soft tissue mechanics, the clinician can design splints to eliminate, minimize, or shift pressure to a larger area to prevent ischemia; can provide safe and effective correction of clinical conditions; and can improve the design of objects the hand must use. Advances in treatment depend on objective measurements and subsequent clinical research integrated with clinical treatment.

DEFINITION OF TERMS

Compression force loading that acts in opposite directions to push materials together

Creep continued and progressive deformation of soft tissue resulting from constant loading over an extended time (as opposed to remodeling of tissue, which involves growth of tissue)

Elasticity the property by which a material returns to its original form after deformation

Elastic deformation a deformation that is reversible when loading is released

Fatigue failure of material under loading

Force the direct or indirect action of one body on another

Friction tangential force acting between two structures in contact that opposes motion or impending motion (static friction if the structures are at rest, kinetic friction if the structures are in relative motion)

Length-tension curve variation in length with graphed variation in tension (force loading in opposite directions)

Load force or stress applied to a structure

Modulus of elasticity slope of the curve in the elastic region produced by graphing a ratio of stress versus strain: stiff materials have higher elastic modulus than soft materials

*DataGlove, Hand Evaluation System, Greenleaf Medical, Palo Alto, California; Automated Tactile Tester, Topical Testing, Inc, Salt Lake City, Utah; Cedaron DEXTER Physician Work Station, Davis, California; Key Assessment Station, Key Functional Assessments, Minneapolis, Minnesota; EXOS, Exos, Inc., Burlington, Massachusetts; Henley Evaluation System, Sugarland, Texas; Tracker Comprehensive Hand and Upper Extremity Evaluation, Salt Lake City, Utah; Biometrics Ltd., EVAL Computerized Hand and Upper Extremity Evaluation System, Ladysmith, Virginia.

Normal stress direct or perpendicular stress that occurs in soft tissue

Plastic deformation a strain in a material that is not recoverable when loading is released

Plasticity the property by which a material retains its form after deformation; a plastic material that is moldable

Pressure force per unit area acting on a structure from a load

Shear stress angular stress that occurs tangentially in soft tissue

Strain change in length of a structure under loading

Stress tensile or compressive force per unit area within a structure in response to an externally applied load

Stress-strain curve graph of variation in strain output (length or angle) with variation in stress (force per unit area)

Tangential force force that occurs at angles to the surface of tissue and has lateral and rotational components that produce shear

Tension force loading acting in opposite directions that tends to pull an object apart

Tissue remodeling growth and relaxation of tissue held under low constant tension, thereby returning to its homeostatic resting state

Transducer a device that converts one form of energy to another such as pressure to electrical energy, where it can be measured and quantified

Torque force times distance from the center of the joint axis

ACKNOWLEDGMENTS

We acknowledge with appreciation the critique and assistance of William Buford, M.E., Ph.D., former Chief, Paul W. Brand Research Laboratory; and David E. Thompson, Ph.D., former Professor of Electrical Engineering, Louisiana State University.

REFERENCES

1. Agee M, Brand W, Thompson E: The moment arms of the carpometacarpal joint of the thumb: their laboratory determinations and clinical application. Proceedings of the 37th annual meeting of the American Society for Surgery of the Hand, New Orleans, January, 1982.
2. American Society of Hand Therapists: *Splint classification system,* Chicago, 1992, The Society.
3. An KN, Chao EY, Cooney WP: Normative model of human hand for biomechanical analysis, *J Biomech* 12:775, 1979.
4. Beach RB: Measurement of extremity volume by water displacement, *Phys Ther* 57:28, 1977.
5. Beach RB, Bell JA: Torque range-of-motion curve: an objective method for passive joint range-of-motion measurement. Proceedings of the 5th annual meeting of the American Society of Hand Therapists, *J Hand Surg* 7:308, 1982.
6. Beach RB, Bell JA: Ace, Coban, and bias stockinette: pressures resulting from their use. Proceedings of the 6th annual meeting of the American Society of Hand Therapists, *J Hand Surg* 8:627, 1983.
7. Beach RB, Thompson DE: Selected soft-tissue research: an overview from Carville, *Phys Ther* 59:30, 1979.
8. Bell JA: Simplified measurement graphs: a new approach. Proceedings of the 6th annual meeting of the American Society of Hand Therapists, *J Hand Surg* 8:626, 1983.
9. Bell JA: Plaster casting for the remodeling of soft tissue. In Fess EE, Phillips CA, editors: *Hand splinting: principles and methods,* ed 2, St Louis, 1987, Mosby.
10. Bell Krotoski JA, Buford WL: The force/time relationship of clinically used sensory testing instruments, *J Hand Ther* 1:76, 1988.
11. Bell Krotoski JA, et al: Biomechanics of the hand, *J Hand Ther,* Special Edition, 8, 1995.
12. Bergtholdt HT, Brand PW: Thermography: an aid in the management of insensitive feet and stumps, *Arch Phys Med Rehabil* 56:205, 1975.
13. Blakeney AB, Bergtholdt HT, Wood HL: Injury splinting and temperature assessment of the insensitive hand. Proceedings of the 12th annual professional meeting of the Commissioned Officers Association of the U.S. Public Health Service, San Francisco, April, 1977.
14. Brand PW: Evaluation of the hand and its function, *Orthop Clin North Am* 4:1127, 1973.
15. Brand PW: Pathomechanics of pressure ulceration. In Brody GS, Fredericks S, American Society of Plastic and Reconstructive Surgeons, editors: Symposium on the neurological aspects of plastic surgery, vol 17, St Louis, 1978, Mosby.
16. Brand PW: Mechanics of dynamic splinting. In Boswich JA, editor: *Current concepts in hand surgery,* Philadelphia, 1983, Lea & Febiger.
17. Brand PW, Ebner JD: A pain substitute, pressure assessment in the insensitive limb, *Am J Occup Ther,* 51A:109, 1969.
18. Brand PW, Hollister A: *Clinical mechanics of the hand,* ed 3, St Louis, 1993, Mosby.
19. Brand PW, Beach RB, Thompson DE: Relative tension and potential excursion of muscles in the forearm and hand, *J Hand Surg* 6:209, 1981.
20. Brand PW, Sabin TD, Burke JF: *Sensory denervation: a study of its cause and its prevention in leprosy and of management of insensitive limbs.* Final Report, Carville, LA U.S. Public Health Services Hospital, SRS Project No. RC-40-M, August, 1966 through June, 1970.
21. Brand PW, Thompson DE, Micks JE: *The biomechanics of the interphalangeal joint: the proximal interphalangeal joint,* London, 1987, Churchill & Livingstone.
22. Brandsma JW: Preoperative and postoperative evaluation of the hand with intrinsic paralysis. Proceedings of the International Conference on Biomechanics and Clinical Kinesiology of Hand and Foot, Indian Institute of Technology, Madras, India, December 16-18, 1985.
23. Brandsma JW, Brand PW: Quantification and analysis of joint stiffness. Proceedings of the International Conference on Biomechanics and Clinical Kinesiology of Hand and Foot, Indian Institute of Technology, Madras, India, December, 1985.
24. Breger DE: Torque ROM: quantification of joint stiffness. Proceedings of the 22nd annual professional meeting of the Commissioned Officers Association of the U.S. Public Health Service, November, 1987.
25. Breger DE: Biomechanics of splinting. Proceedings of the 11th annual meeting of the American Society of Hand Therapists, San Antonio, September, 1987.
26. Breger-Lee DE, Buford WL: Update in splinting materials and methods: frontiers in hand rehabilitation, *Hand Clin* 7:3, 1991.
27. Breger-Lee DE, Buford WL: Properties of thermoplastic splinting materials, *J Hand Ther* 5:4, 1992.
28. Breger-Lee DE, Bell Krotoski J, Brandsma JW: Torque range of motion in the hand clinic, *J Hand Ther* 3:1, 1990.
29. Breger-Lee D, et al: Reliability of torque range of motion: a preliminary study, *J Hand Ther* 6:29, 1993.
30. Buford WL: Clinical evaluation of orthotic devices. Proceedings of the 13th annual professional meeting of the Commissioned Officers Association of the U.S. Public Health Service, March, 1978.
31. Buford WL: An interactive three-dimensional simulation of the kinematics of the human thumb, doctoral dissertation, Baton Rouge, 1984, Louisiana State University.
32. Buford WL, Bell JA: Working analysis of dynamic splinting. Proceedings of the 14th annual professional meeting of the Commissioned Officers Association of the U.S. Public Health Service, Phoenix, April, 1979.
33. Buford WL, Thompson DE: A system for three-dimensional interactive simulation of hand biomechanics, *IEEE Trans Biomed Eng* 34:444, 1987.
34. Chao EY, et al: *Biomechanics of the hand.* New Jersey, 1989, World Scientific.
35. Chow SP, et al: A splint for controlled active motion after flexor tendon repair, *J Hand Surg* 25:645, 1990.

36. Cromwell L, Weibell J, Pfeiffer EA, editors: *Biomedical instrumentation and measurements,* ed 2, Englewood Cliffs, NJ, 1980, Prentice Hall.

37. Daly CH, et al: The effect of pressure loading on the blood flow rate in human skin. In Kennedi RM, et al, editors: *Bed sore biomechanics,* New York, 1976, Macmillan Press.

38. DeVore GL, Hamilton GF: Volume measuring of the severely injured hand, *Am J Occup Ther* 22:16, 1968.

39. Eccles MV: Hand volumetrics, *Br J Phys Med* 19:5, 1956.

40. Elftman H: Biomechanics of muscle, *J Bone Joint Surg* 48A:363, 1966.

41. Evans RB, Thompson DE: An analysis of factors that support early active short arc motion of the repaired central slip, *J Hand Ther* 5:4, 1992.

42. Evans RB, Thompson DE: The application of force to healing tendons, *J Hand Ther* 6:4, 1994.

43. Fernie G: Instrumentation in studies of the effects of pressure on soft tissue. In Brand PW, Mooney V, editors: Proceedings of the Workshop on Effects of Pressure on Human Tissue, Carville, LA, March, 1977.

44. Fess EE: Rubber-band traction: physical properties, splint design, and identification of force magnitude. Proceedings of the 7th annual meeting of the American Society of Hand Therapists, *J Hand Surg* 9A:610, 1984.

45. Fess EE: The need for reliability and validity in hand assessment instruments, *J Hand Surg* 11:621, 1986.

46. Fess EE: A method for checking Jamar dynamometer calibration, *J Hand Ther* 1:28, 1987.

47. Fess EE, Phillips C, editors: Principles of using dynamic assists for mobilization. In *Hand splinting: principles and methods,* ed 2, St Louis, 1987, Mosby.

48. Flatt AE, Fischer GW: Biomechanical factors in the replacement of rheumatoid joints, *Ann Rheum Dis* 28:36, 1969.

49. Flowers KR, LaStayo P: The effect of total end range time on improving passive range-of-motion, *J Hand Ther* 7:150, 1994.

50. Flowers KR, Pheasant SD: The use of torque angle curves in the assessment of digital joint stiffness, *J Hand Ther* 1:69, 1988.

51. Giurintano DJ, et al: The five-link manipulator thumb model, *Med Eng Phys* 17:297, 1995.

52. Goiler H, Lewis DW, McLaughlin RE: Thermographic studies of human skin subjected to localized pressure, *Am J Roentgenol Radium Ther Nucl Med* 113:749, 1971.

53. Harris JR, Brand PW: Patterns of disintegration of tarsus in anaesthetic foot, *J Bone Joint Surg* 48B:4, 1966.

54. Hazelton FT, et al: The influence of wrist position on the force produced by the finger flexors, *J Biomech* 8:301, 1975.

55. Hollister AM, et al: The axes of rotation of the metacarpophalangeal and the interphalangeal joints of the thumb, *Clin Orthop Rel Res* 320:188, 1995.

56. Horner RL, Kenyon PB, Hackencamp T: The role of high-tech systems in hand rehabilitation. Science and Industry Exhibit. Proceedings of the 48th annual meeting of the American Society for Surgery of the Hand, Kansas City, Mo, September 29-October 2, 1993.

57. Johnston MV, Keith RA, Hinderer SR: Measurement standards for interdisciplinary medical rehabilitation, *Arch Phys Med Rehabil* 73:S3, 1992.

58. Kolumban SL: The role of static and dynamic splints: physiotherapy techniques and time in straightening contracted interphalangeal joints, *Lepr India* 41:323, 1969.

59. Kumar RP, Brandsma JW: A method to determine pressure distribution of the hand, *Lepr Rev* 57:39, 1986.

60. Mathiowetz V, et al: Reliability and validity of grip and pinch strength evaluations, *J Hand Surg* 9A:222, 1984.

61. Mildenberger LA, Amadio PC, An KN: Dynamic splinting.: systematic approach to the selection of elastic traction, *Arch Phys Med Rehabil* 67:241, 1986.

62. Myers LM, et al: Interactive segmentation of three-dimensional anatomical data for musculoskeletal modeling. *Proceedings of the 9th annual meeting of the National Computer Graphics Association* III:143, 1988.

63. Odesanya O, Waggenspack WN, Thompson DE: Construction of biological surface models from cross-sections, *IEEE Trans Biomed Eng* 40:329, 1993.

64. Roberson L, Giurintano DJ: Objective measurement of joint stiffness, *J Hand Ther* 8:163, 1995.

65. Roberson L, et al: Analysis of the physical properties of SCOMAC springs and their potential for use in dynamic splinting, *J Hand Ther* 1:110, 1988.

66. Rodgers MM, Cavanaugh PR: Glossary of biomechanical terms, concepts, *J Phys Ther* 64:1886, 1984.

67. Salter RB, et al: The biological effect of continuous passive motion on the healing of full-thickness defects in articular cartilage: an experimental investigation in the rabbit, *J Bone Joint Surg* 62A:1232, 1980.

68. Schneiderwind W: A new method for simultaneously evaluating individual finger function during power grip, master's thesis, Boston, 1972, Boston University.

69. Schultz-Johnson KS: *Volumetrics: a literature review.* Santa Monica, Calif, Upper Extremity Technology, 1988.

70. Swanson AB: Pathomechanics of deformities in hand and wrist. In Brand PW, Mooney V, editors: *Flexible implant resection arthroplasty in the hand and extremities,* St Louis, 1973, Mosby.

71. Thompson DE: Mechanical principles. In Fess EE, Phillips CA, editors: *Hand splinting: principles and methods,* ed 2, St Louis, 1987, Mosby.

72. Thompson DE, Giurintano DJ: A kinematic model of the flexor tendons of the hand, J Biomech *22:327, 1989.*

73. Thompson DE, Hussen HM: Characteristics of orthotic materials by mechanical impedance method. Proceedings of the 30th annual ACEMB, Los Angeles, 1977.

74. Thompson DE, Hussein HM, Perritt R: Point impedance characterization of soft tissue in vivo. Proceedings of the Second International Symposium for Bioengineering of the Skin, Cardiff, Wales, 1979.

75. Thompson DE, et al: Simulating hand surgery: a work in progress, *SOMA* 2:6, 1987.

76. Thompson DE, et al: A hand biomechanics workstation. Proceedings of the ACM/SIGGRAPH Conference, Atlanta, Ga, August, 1988.

77. Waylett J, Seibly D: A study to determine the average deviation accuracy of a commercially available volumeter, *J Hand Surg* 6:3, 1981.

78. Wright V, Johns R: Quantitative and qualitative analysis of joint stiffness in normal subjects and in patients with connective tissue diseases, *Ann Rheum Dis* 20:36, 1961.

79. Yamada H, Evans FG: Strength of biological materials, Baltimore, 1970, Williams & Wilkins.

Chapter 16

DOCUMENTATION: ESSENTIAL ELEMENTS OF AN UPPER EXTREMITY ASSESSMENT BATTERY

Elaine Ewing Fess*

"I often say that when you can measure what you are speaking about and express it in numbers, you know something about it; but, when you cannot measure it in numbers your knowledge is of a meagre and unsatisfactory kind; it may be the beginning of knowledge but [you] have scarcely in your thought advanced to the stage of science whatever the matter may be."

—Lord Kelvin

Objective measurements provide a foundation for hand rehabilitation efforts by delineating baseline pathologic conditions from which patient progress and treatment methods may be assessed. A thorough and unbiased assessment procedure furnishes information that helps predict rehabilitation potential, provides data with which subsequent measurements may be compared, and allows medical specialists to plan and evaluate treatment programs and techniques. Conclusions gained from evaluation procedures guide treatment priorities, motivate staff and patients, and define functional capacity at the termination of treatment. Assessment through analysis and integration of data also serves as the vehicle for professional communication, eventually influencing the body of knowledge of the profession.

The quality of assessment information depends on the objectivity, sophistication, predictability, sensitivity, selectivity, and accuracy of the tools used to gather data. It is of utmost importance to choose assessment instruments wisely. Dependable, precise tools allow clinicians to reach conclu-

sions that are minimally skewed by extraneous factors or biases, thus diminishing chances of subjective error and facilitating more accurate understanding. Instruments that measure diffusely produce nonspecific results. Conversely, instruments with proven accuracy of measurement yield precise and selective data.

The manner in which assessment tools are used is also critical. Deviations in recommended equipment, procedure, or sequence invalidate test results. A cardinal rule of assessment is that instruments must not be used as therapy practice tools for patients. Information obtained from tools that have been used in patient training is radically skewed, rendering it invalid and meaningless. Testing equipment also should not be substituted or altered from the original equipment on which reliability and validity statements were based, and test procedure and sequence must not vary from that described in administration instructions. Patient fatigue, physiologic adaptation, test difficulty, and length of test time also may influence results. Clinically, this means that sensory testing is done before assessing grip or pinch; rest periods are provided appropriately; and if possible, more difficult procedures are not scheduled early in testing

*The author receives no compensation in any form from products discussed in this chapter.

sessions. Good assessment technique should reflect both test protocol and instrumentation requirements.

Communication is the underlying rationale for requiring good assessment procedures. The acquisition and transmission of knowledge, both of which are fundamental to patient treatment and professional growth, are enhanced through development and use of a common professional language based on strict criteria for assessment instrument selection. The use of "home-brewed," evaluation tools that are unreliable and unvalidated is never appropriate because their baseless data may misdirect or delay therapy intervention. The purposes of this chapter are to (1) define measurement terminology and criteria, (2) identify factors that influence the development of an upper extremity battery, and (3) review current upper extremity assessment instruments in relation to accepted measurement criteria. It is not within the scope of this chapter to recommend specific test instruments. Instead readers are encouraged to triage the instruments used in their practices according to accepted instrument selection criteria,[74] keeping those that best meet the criteria and discarding those that do not.

ASSESSMENT TERMINOLOGY AND CRITERIA

Standardized tests, the most sophisticated assessment tools, are statistically proven to be reliable and valid, indicating (1) that they measure consistently within their testing unit, between like instruments, between examiners, and from trial-to-trial, and (2) that they measure what they were designed to measure. "Reliability deals with whether a measurement consistently reflects something, whereas validity deals with how the measurement is used."[69-71,159] The few truly standardized tests available in hand rehabilitation are limited to instruments that evaluate hand coordination, dexterity, and work tolerance, and unfortunately, not all of these tools meet all of the requirements of standardization. The remaining hand/upper extremity assessment tools fall at varying levels along the reliability and validity continuums according to how closely their inherent properties match measurement criteria.

As consumers, medical specialists must require that all assessment tools have appropriate documentation of reliability and validity. "Data regarding reliability [and validity] should be available and should not be taken at face value alone; just because a manufacturer states reliability studies have been done, or a paper concludes an instrument is reliable, does not mean the instrument or testing protocol meets the requirements for scientific design."[20] *Purchasing and using assessment tools that do not meet fundamental measurement criteria limits potential at all levels, from individual patients to the scope of the profession.*

Standardized tests must have all of the following elements: (1) Statistical proof* of reliability; (2) statistical

proof* of validity; (3) a statement defining the purpose/intent of the test; (4) detailed equipment criteria; (5) specific administration, scoring, and interpretation instructions; and (6) normative data, drawn from a large population sample, that is divided, with statistically suitable numbers of subjects in each category, according to appropriate variables such as hand dominance, age, sex, and occupation. A bibliography of related literature also may be included. Although many instruments are touted as "standardized," most lack even the fundamental elements of statistical reliability and validity, relying instead on normative statements such as means or averages. Instruments without statistical reliability and validity have no basis for justifying either their consistency of measurement or their capability to measure the entity for which they were designed. Because relatively few evaluation tools fully meet standardization criteria, instrument selection must be predicated on satisfying as many of the listed requisites as possible.[67]

Through interpretation, standardized tests provide information that may be used to predict how a patient may perform in normal daily tasks. For example, if a patient achieves "x" score on a standardized test, it may be predicted that the patient would perform at an equivalent of the "75th percentile of normal assembly line workers." Standardized tests allow deduction of anticipated achievement based on narrower performance parameters as defined by the test.

In contrast, observational tests assess performance through comparison of subsequent test trials and are limited to like-item-to-like-item comparisons. Observational tests are often scored according to how patients perform specific test items, that is, independently, independently with equipment, needs assistance, and so on. "The patient is able to pick up a full 12-ounce beer can with his injured hand without assistance." Progress is based on the fact that he could not do this 3 weeks ago. However, this information cannot be used to predict whether the patient will be able to dress himself or herself or run a given machine at work. Assumptions beyond the test item trial-to-trial performance comparisons are invalid and irrelevant. Observational tests may be included in an upper assessment battery so long as they are used appropriately.

COMPUTERIZED EVALUATION EQUIPMENT

Computerized assessment tools must meet the same measurement criteria as noncomputerized instruments. Unfortunately, both patients and medical personnel tend to assume that computer-based equipment is more trustworthy than its noncomputerized counterparts. This assumption is erroneous. In hand rehabilitation, some of the most commonly used noncomputerized evaluation tools have been or are being studied for instrument reliability and validity (the

*Correlation statistics or another appropriate measure of instrument reliability.

*Correlation statistics or another appropriate measure of instrument validity.

two most fundamental instrumentation criteria). However, at the time of this writing, none of the computerized hand evaluation instruments have been statistically proven to have intrainstrument and interinstrument reliability, via comparison to National Institute of Standards and Technology (NIST) criteria. Some have "human performance" reliability statements, but these are based on the fatally flawed premise that human normative performance is equivalent to mechanized NIST calibration criteria.[72,73,75] Who would accept the accuracy of a watch that had been "calibrated" by timing 20 "normal" individuals in a 20-yard dash? Human performance is not an acceptable criterion for defining the reliability, that is, the calibration, of mechanical devices such as those used in upper extremity rehabilitation clinics.

Furthermore, one cannot assume that a computerized version of an instrument is reliable and valid because its noncomputerized counterpart has established reliability. For example, although some computerized dynamometers have identical external components to those of their manual counterparts, internally they have been "gutted" and no longer function on a hydraulic system. Reliability and validity statements for the manual dynamometer are not applicable to the "gutted" computer version. Even if both dynamometers were hydraulic, separate reliability and validity data would be required for the computerized instrument.

Because of its inherent complexity, it is often difficult to determine instrument reliability of computerized test equipment without the assistance of qualified engineers and computer experts. Compounding the problem, stringent federal regulation often does not apply to "therapy devices." Without sophisticated technical assistance, medical specialists and their patients have no way of knowing the true accuracy of the data produced by computerized therapy equipment.

DEVELOPMENT OF AN ASSESSMENT BATTERY

An assessment battery must be reflective of the environment in which it is used. Types of patients, expectations and use of data, and physical setting should be considered to ensure that the selected group of tests meets the unique needs of the practice. Age, diagnosis, intelligence, socioeconomic background, language, and other patient population variables are important in selecting evaluation tools. Tests requiring high levels of cooperation may not be appropriate for a practice dealing primarily with children, mentally retarded individuals, or persons with limited language skills. The intent for gathering information is also important when creating an assessment battery. Requirements are often more stringent for research evaluation equipment than for instruments used in daily clinical testing. Staff qualifications, fiscal criteria, and state and federal regulations also influence selection of tests in an assessment battery.

Specific considerations

An assessment battery should address the full spectrum of upper extremity performance, including physiologic status, motion, sensibility, and function. In addition, it should define a patient's medical history, vocational and avocational information, and relevant administrative data that allow subsequent intervention to be tailored to the specific needs of patients. Specialized tests such as an upper extremity prosthetic check-out and a splint evaluation are also invaluable.

Because there is no single universal upper extremity assessment instrument, clinicians must rely on a variety of tools to measure the various parameters of hand condition and performance. A minimum of one instrument per area should be selected to measure each of the five basic domains: physiologic status, motion, sensibility, function, and patient satisfaction. Although this minimum-requirement five-instrument assessment battery is sufficient for cursory evaluation, practices specializing in hand/upper extremity dysfunction routinely include several instruments specific to each domain, generating gradation and verification of information.

The American Society for Surgery of the Hand (ASSH)[7] and the American Society of Hand Therapists (ASHT)[3,4] have established guidelines for clinical assessment of the hand and upper extremity. These guidelines are meaningful in defining the quality of professional communication and understanding of hand/upper extremity dysfunction. It is important that those responsible for developing evaluation protocols seriously consider these guidelines and generate assessment batteries that reflect the recommendations of these two professional organizations.

TIMING AND USE OF ASSESSMENT TESTS

Not all patients who are evaluated need to be given all of the tests within an assessment battery. Hand specialists routinely use a few quick tests to check hand function initially, adding more sophisticated testing procedures as dictated by the patient's condition. For example, if a patient tests normal with the Semmes-Weinstein monofilaments, other sensibility tests can be eliminated in most cases. To conserve time and decrease frustration, tests within each domain should be scheduled according to type of information provided and degree of difficulty, beginning with an easy, dependable test that supplies basic data and working toward the more esoteric instruments.

Initial and final evaluations usually are comprehensive in scope, and intervening evaluations are less formal, concentrating on assessing progress in specific areas according to the problems exhibited by the patient. Frequency of reevaluation sessions depends on the patient, progress demonstrated, and the nature of the test itself. Range of motion (ROM) may be measured several times during a therapy session for an early postoperative tenolysis patient. However, grip strength measurements for this patient may not be appropriate because of wound healing and tensile strength limitations until 7 to 8 weeks postoperatively, and then strength measurements, because of the time required to effect change, are not measured as often as ROM.

Recording of assessment data also varies with the situation. For the early tenolysis patient, unless significant problems are encountered requiring frequent documentation to demonstrate lack of cooperation or other mitigating issues, only one set of ROM measurements are recorded per day, although multiple readings are taken. As change occurs less rapidly, motion values may be recorded two or three times a week, eventually decreasing to once every 2 weeks, once a month, and so on. Change in status is documented through objective measurements at appropriate intervals.

HISTORY AND PHYSICAL STATUS

In addition to recording the patient's condition, the initial history should contain information about how and when the injury occurred, including time and place. Documentation of changes in vocational, avocational, and daily living skills (DLS) is important, as is close observation of the patient's spontaneous use of the extremity before, during, and after the evaluation session. When identifying the source of pain, obtaining the patient's subjective assessment of its perceived intensity and its impact on his or life, helps provide insight into the patient's attitude and ability to cope with the situation.

Obtaining a history is not only amassing of facts, it is also an opportunity to begin building a foundation of trust and communication between patient and examiner. Genuine concern and an unhurried manner facilitate discussion, yielding cooperation and understanding as the patient participates in his or her rehabilitation process.

Examination

The detail in which the examination is accomplished, and by whom, depends on the clinical setting and on the division of duties between surgeons and therapists. Regardless of who is responsible for conducting the formal intake evaluation, patients are assessed for general condition and configuration of the extremity, including skin and soft tissue; skeletal stability; articular motion and integrity; tendon continuity and glide; neurovascular status; isolated muscle function, sensibility, and vessel patency; and finally, general function, coordination, and dexterity.

The combination of clinical examination and precise measurement allows examiners to identify and make judgments regarding patient rehabilitative potential and need for therapeutic intervention. Assessment instruments delimit problems through numerical data, quantifying and adding definition to knowledge and understanding. Without measurement, perceptions are diffuse and unclear.

CURRENT HAND/UPPER EXTREMITY ASSESSMENT INSTRUMENTS

Assessment instruments may be divided into groups according to five basic domains: extremity condition, motion, sensibility, function, and patient satisfaction. (1) Condition involves the neurovascular system as it pertains to tissue

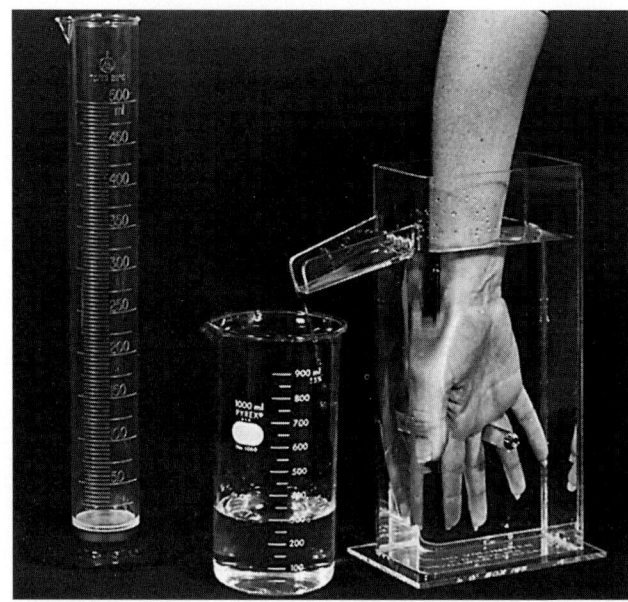

Fig. 16-1. Volumeter accuracy has been shown to be within 10 ml when used according to instructions.

viability; nutrition; vessel patency; and arterial, venous, and lymphatic flow. Noninvasive monitoring of extremity volume, skin color, and temperature, and arterial pulses provides important information about the status of skin and subcutaneous tissue and neurovascular function. (2) Measurement of motion depends on muscle-tendon continuity, contractile and gliding capacity, neuromuscular function, and volitional control. Goniometric measurements and isolated muscle strength testing are commonly used methods for evaluating upper extremity motion. (3) Relying on neural continuity, impulse transmission, receptor acuity, and cortical perception, sensibility assessment may be divided into sudomotor or sympathetic response and the ability to detect, discriminate, quantify, and identify stimuli.[110] (4) Reflecting the integration of all systems, hand function is evaluated through measurements of grip and pinch; coordination and dexterity; and vocational, avocational, and DLS activities. (5) Patient satisfaction tests assess patients' endorsement/ approval of the therapeutic intervention they received.

Condition assessment instruments

Based on Archimedes' principle of water displacement, the *volumeter*, as designed by Brand,[35] measures composite extremity mass (Fig. 16-1). Available in a range of sizes, volumeters monitor physiologic changes within the extremity as evidenced by changes in hand/extremity size, provided immersion of the extremity in water is not contraindicated. Although volumeter measurements are crucial for monitoring the inflammatory stage of wound healing, they also may be used to assess atrophy. Volumeter measurements are accurate to within 10 ml when used according to manufacturer specifications.[194] Variables that reduce accuracy include use of an aerated faucet for tank filling, extremity motion post immersion, inconsistent pressure on the stop rod, and inconsistent placement of the volumeter for successive measurements. Measurements from both extremities are recorded initially with successive measurements of the symptomatic extremity recorded at appropriate intervals.

When volumeter assessment is contraindicated, *circumferential* or *external diameter measurements,* using a flexible tape measure or external millimeter caliper, may be used to assess extremity size. Although less exact and inclusive in scope, accuracy of these tools is improved with consistent placement[163] and tension of the tape or caliper on the extremity. Suspension of a 10- to 20-g weight from the end of the tape measure allows consistent tension from trial to trial, and caliper measurements are more appropriate for monitoring smaller diameters as with digital joints or segments. Serial measurements are recorded (Fig. 16-2) at appropriate intervals as dictated by patient progress.

Directly related to digital vessel patency, skin temperature is a valuable indicator of tissue viability. Used to monitor the status of early postoperative revascularized hands or digits, cutaneous temperature gauges are placed on three areas, on a revascularized digit, on a normal adjacent or corresponding digit, and on the dressing, to monitor the relative temperature differences in the reattached digit, a matching digit, and room temperature. It is important to report any decrease in temperature in the revascularized segment, with critical temperature being 30° C, with lower readings indicating possible vascular compromise. Normal digital temperature ranges between 30° and 35° C.

Doppler scanners are used to map arterial flow through audible ultrasonic response to arterial pulsing. Although inconsistencies continue to plague attempts to quantify Doppler readings, to date these scanners are accepted as important noninvasive assessment tools.

Motion assessment instruments

Goniometric evaluation of the upper extremity is essential to monitoring articular motion and musculotendinous function (Fig. 16-3). Passive range-of-motion (PROM) measurements reflect the ability of a joint to be moved through its normal arc of motion, with limitations indicative of problems within the joint or capsular structures surrounding the joint. Active range-of-motion (AROM) measurements reflect the muscle-tendon unit's ability to effect motion of the osseous kinetic chain. Limitations in AROM may be caused by lack of tendon continuity; adhesions; tendon sheath constriction; tendon inflammation; tendon subluxation, dislocation, or bowstringing; or tendon attenuation. With diminished PROM, AROM may seem impaired, although tendon amplitude and muscular contraction are normal. Conversely, normal PROM may seem limited when tendon gliding is reduced. Because AROM cannot

exceed the passive capacity of joint motion, it is essential that both AROM and PROM are assessed and recorded (Fig. 16-4). It is also important to analyze carefully the cause of limited motion to properly direct therapeutic intervention.

Proven more precise than visual estimates,[92,115] goniometric measurements are accurate, provided standard procedures are followed.[61,90,96,119,158-160] Accuracy of goniometric measurements differs according to joint complexity,[86,92,115] between PROM and AROM measurements,[10,31,191] between same and multiple examiners,[34,90,115] and according to patient diagnosis.[13,90] For both intraexaminer and interexaminer reliability, repeated measures under controlled conditions allow variance of 4 degrees[124] and for intraexaminer measurements, a difference of 3 to 4 degrees indicates change in upper extremity joint status.[34] Although further study is needed to address the validity of using a fixed-axis device to assess joints with nonfixed axes of motion that are influenced by articular glide and rotation,[161] most clinicians accept the assumption of rotation around a central point axis when assessing joint motion. Normative data for goniometric measurements are available.[1,7] Multiaxis goniometers, video recordings, and fiber optics may be the equipment of the future.[37,119,171,199]

An adjunct to individual joint measurement, *composite digital motion,* is computed as total active motion (TAM) and total passive motion (TPM).[7] TAM is the sum of simultaneous (full fist) active flexion measurements of the metacarpal, and proximal and distal interphalangeal joints of a digit, minus the simultaneous (full finger extension) active extension deficits of the same three joints. TPM is computed in a similar manner except that passive measurements are used. TAM and TPM each are expressed as single numerical values, reflecting both flexion and extension capacity of a single digit and providing a composite assessment of single digit function (Fig. 16-5).

Torque range of motion (TQROM), as described by Brand, applies a series of increasing forces to a stiff joint to quantify measurement of PROM. When translated into torque-angle curves, the composite mechanical qualities of the restraining tissues are visualized, allowing better understanding of the pathologic condition involved (Fig. 16-6). With good repeatability, TQROM provides a quantifiable method of predicting and monitoring stiff joint response to therapy intervention.

Manual muscle testing (MMT) appraises isolated muscle strength (Fig. 16-7). MMT is used to evaluate nerve lesions, monitor nerve regeneration, and assess preoperative potential of tendon transfers. Although criteria for grading muscle strength have improved, portions of the test are subject to examiner interpretation. To increase interrater reliability, it is important to have a common method of conducting and interpreting manual muscle examinations. Various grading systems exist, but the two most commonly used are Seddon's[163] numerical system (from 0 to 5) and the method recommended by the Committee on After-Effects, National

VOLUMETER MEASUREMENTS

	DATE:	DATE:	DATE:	DATE:	DATE:	DATE:
800 ml.						
700 ml.						
600 ml.						
500 ml.						
400 ml.						
300 ml.						
200 ml.						

NORMAL VOLUME (opposite hand):_____

CIRCUMFERENCE / DIAMETER:*

BICEPS**					
FOREARM**					
DPC					
DIGIT (_____)					

NORMAL MEASUREMENT (opposite hand): _____

	BICEPS:	FOREARM:	DPC:	DIGIT:	

* circle method used

** 10 cm. above/below medial epicondyle of humerus

NAME:

NUMBER:

HAND:

Fig. 16-2. Recording of volumetric data on a graph facilitates explanations of progress for patients and medical personnel.

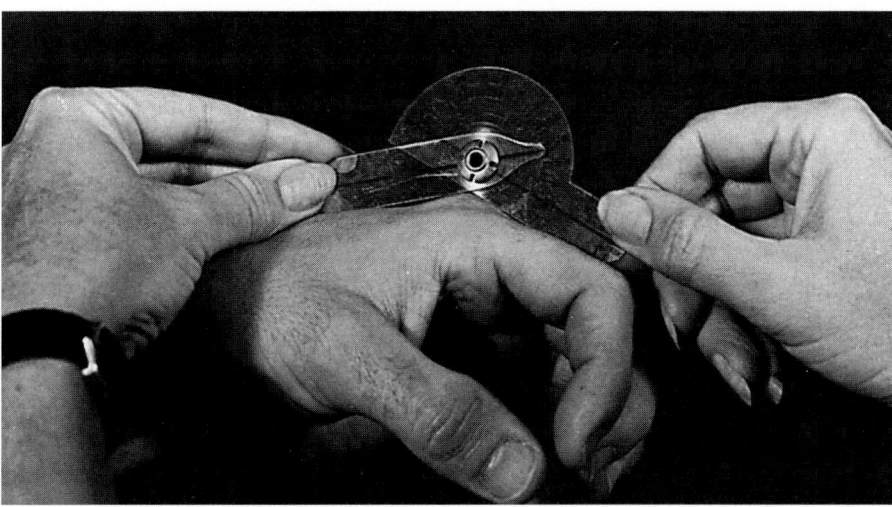

Fig. 16-3. A shortened goniometer facilitates range-of-motion measurements on the small joints of the hand.

Foundation for Infantile Paralysis[103] using "zero," "trace," "poor," "fair," "good," and "normal." The latter is further refined by a plus-minus system, determining half-ranges. Fluctuations of muscle tone and altered reflex activity make MMT of little value in upper motor neuron lesions such as cerebral palsy or cerebrovascular accidents.

Sensibility assessment instruments

When assessing sensibility, it is important to use a technique of recording that is accurate, that allows quick understanding by others, and in an age of computerization, that is readily adaptable to computerization to facilitate follow-up. Color helps define areas of diminished and impaired sensibility (see color plates that accompany Chapter 13). Also, using area identification coordinates (Fig. 16-8) speeds communication and data transfer. The "numbers" illustrated in Fig. 16-8 are area coordinates of the palm of the hand, with the first number in each two-digit sequence representing ray longitudinal position; that is, the thumb is 1, the index finger is 2, and the small finger is 5. The second number in the two-digit sequence represents transverse position of an area; that is, 1 equals the distal phalanx area, 2 the middle phalanx, 3 the proximal phalanx, and so on. When combined, the two digits allow immediate identification of a specific area; that is, area 21 is the index distal phalanx, 31 is the long distal phalanx, 53 is the small finger proximal phalanx, and area 54 is the field distal to the distal palmar crease over the fifth ray. The "numbers" illustrated are not true integers. Instead, they are single-digit coordinates that, when combined, allow accurate definition of the areas of the palm. Each area may be further divided into radial and ulnar and proximal and distal. Area 11RP is the distal phalanx of the thumb, radial proximal side (quadrant); area 32UD is the ulnar (U), distal aspect (D) of the long (3) middle phalanx (2). Accurate recording is critical to good assessment technique.

Sympathetic response tests are applicable to patients with complete nerve disruption and who are within 6 months of initial injury. Volitional participation is required for motor, sensibility, and dexterity testing, but the problem is compounded in assessing sensibility because the stimulus, when received, is also interpreted by the patient, resulting in test information that is vulnerable to bias. Although most patients are cooperative, occasions arise when dealing with children, patients with language problems, or patients whose motives may be suspect, in which a test that relies on sudomotor or sympathetic response may be helpful. These tests should not be relied on as the primary sensibility test in an assessment battery.

The ninhydrin test identifies areas of disturbance of sweat secretion after peripheral nerve disruption. Denervated skin does not produce a sweat reaction because of involvement of sympathetic fibers in the distribution area of the injured peripheral nerve. Ninhydrin spray, a colorimetric agent, turns purple when it reacts with small concentrations of sweat. Unfortunately, sympathetic return after a peripheral nerve injury is variable, and on long-term follow-up, sudomotor response does not correlate with sensibility return.[140]

The wrinkle test[141] is based on a similar concept of sympathetic fiber involvement in peripheral nerve injuries, in that denervated palmar skin, as opposed to normal skin, does not wrinkle when soaked in warm water. As with sweating, palmar wrinkling has diminishing correlation to sensory function as the postinjury time increases, and it has no correlation to sensory capacity in nerve compression injuries.[146]

Detection of a punctate stimulus is the most simple level of function in the hierarchy of sensibility capacity of the hand/upper extremity, requiring ability to distinguish a single-point stimulus from normally occurring atmospheric

UPPER EXTREMITY ASSESSMENT BATTERY

RANGE OF MOTION

HAND

A

DATE: _____	THUMB	CHANGE +/-	INDEX	CHANGE +/-	LONG	CHANGE +/-	RING	CHANGE +/-	SMALL	CHANGE +/-
MP	( ) ( )		( ) ( )		( ) ( )		( ) ( )		( ) ( )	
PIP	IP ( ) ( )		( ) ( )		( ) ( )		( ) ( )		( ) ( )	
DIP	CMC ( ) ( )		( ) ( )		( ) ( )		( ) ( )		( ) ( )	
TAM (TPM)	( ) ( )		( ) ( )		( ) ( )		( ) ( )		( ) ( )	

DATE: _____	THUMB	CHANGE +/-	INDEX	CHANGE +/-	LONG	CHANGE +/-	RING	CHANGE +/-	SMALL	CHANGE +/-
MP	( ) ( )		( ) ( )		( ) ( )		( ) ( )		( ) ( )	
PIP	IP ( ) ( )		( ) ( )		( ) ( )		( ) ( )		( ) ( )	
DIP	CMC ( ) ( )		( ) ( )		( ) ( )		( ) ( )		( ) ( )	
TAM (TPM)	( ) ( )		( ) ( )		( ) ( )		( ) ( )		( ) ( )	

DATE: _____	THUMB	CHANGE +/-	INDEX	CHANGE +/-	LONG	CHANGE +/-	RING	CHANGE +/-	SMALL	CHANGE +/-
MP	( ) ( )		( ) ( )		( ) ( )		( ) ( )		( ) ( )	
PIP	IP ( ) ( )		( ) ( )		( ) ( )		( ) ( )		( ) ( )	
DIP	CMC ( ) ( )		( ) ( )		( ) ( )		( ) ( )		( ) ( )	
TAM (TPM)	( ) ( )		( ) ( )		( ) ( )		( ) ( )		( ) ( )	

KEY:

Active: extension/flexion

Passive: (extension/flexion)

Thumb CMC: adduction/abduction

Change: record in red

Name: _____

Number: _____

Hand: _____

Fig. 16-4. Active and passive range-of-motion (ROM) and total motion values should be recorded at appropriate intervals. Improvements or losses in motion may be expressed as plus or minus the amount of change, such as 115 or 25. **A,** ROM for the hand. **B,** ROM for the wrist, forearm, elbow, and shoulder.

UPPER EXTREMITY ASSESSMENT BATTERY

RANGE OF MOTION

WRIST, FOREARM, ELBOW, SHOULDER

		DATE:___		DATE:___		DATE:___	
			CHANGE +/−		CHANGE +/−		CHANGE +/−
W R I S T	EXTENSION	( )( )		( )( )		( )( )	
	FLEXION	( )( )		( )( )		( )( )	
	RADIAL DEVIATION	( )( )		( )( )		( )( )	
	ULNAR DEVIATION	( )( )		( )( )		( )( )	
F O R E A R M / **E L B O W**	SUPINATION	( )( )		( )( )		( )( )	
	PRONATION	( )( )		( )( )		( )( )	
	EXTENSION	( )( )		( )( )		( )( )	
	FLEXION	( )( )		( )( )		( )( )	
S H O U L D E R	EXTENSION	( )( )		( )( )		( )( )	
	FLEXION	( )( )		( )( )		( )( )	
	ABDUCTION	( )( )		( )( )		( )( )	
	INTERNAL ROTATION	( )( )		( )( )		( )( )	
	EXTERNAL ROTATION	( )( )		( )( )		( )( )	

B

KEY:
  Active: #°
  Passive: (#°)
  Change: Record in red

Name:___
Number:___
Extremity:___

Fig. 16-4 cont'd. For legend see page 270.

DATE: 6-1-02	THUMB	CHANGE +/−	INDEX	CHANGE +/−	LONG	CHANGE +/−	RING	CHANGE +/−	SMALL	CHANGE +/−
MP	( ) ( )		10/30 ( ) ( )		( ) ( )		( ) ( )		( ) ( )	
PIP	IP ( ) ( )		30/45 ( ) ( )		( ) ( )		( ) ( )		( ) ( )	
DIP	CMC ( ) ( )		0/75 ( ) ( )		( ) ( )		( ) ( )		( ) ( )	
TAM (TPM)	( ) ( )		110 ( ) ( )		( ) ( )		( ) ( )		( ) ( )	

Fig. 16-5. Total motion provides a single numerical value for composite digital motion: summation of digit flexion (30 + 45 + 75 = 150); summation of digit-extension deficits (10 + 30 + 0 = 40); flexion sum minus extension deficit sum (150 − 40 = 110); total active motion of digit equals 110 degrees.

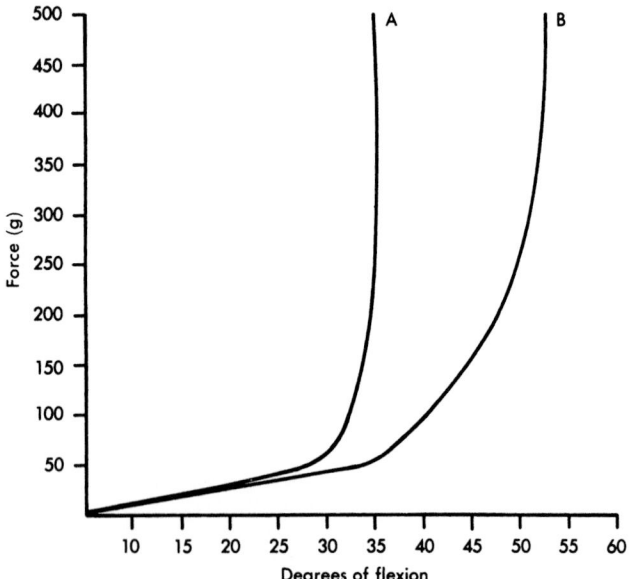

Fig. 16-6. This torque-angle, range-of-motion graph reveals that the long finger proximal interphalangeal joint, *B,* has more passive "give" than that of the index finger, *A,* indicating that the long finger may respond more readily to splinting and exercise programs. (From Fess EE and Philips CA: *Hand splinting: principles and methods,* ed 2, St Louis, 1987, Mosby.)

background stimuli. Normal touch force threshold using Semmes-Weinstein monofilaments is approximately 4.86 g/mm² (pressure).[20,26] As testing devices, the monofilaments are uniquely important to clinicians and researchers alike in that they control the amount of force applied (Fig. 16-9). These filaments consistently produce repeatable forces within a predictable range from set to set and from examiner to examiner, provided their lengths and diameters are correct.[22,24,25] Clinical validity of the monofilaments is documented for assessment and monitoring peripheral nerve disruption, compression, and regeneration[2]; prediction and monitoring peripheral neuropathic diseases and their complications; and for prediction of function.[78,88,108,109,139,142,143,156,157,176,177,182,186,190,197]

An experience related by Weinstein[196] regarding collaborative work with a neurosurgeon provides important insight into face validity of the monofilaments and the inherent difference between sensibility detection and discrimination levels. During craniotomies on conscious patients, Weinstein tested sensibility using two tests: the monofilaments and two-point discrimination. As weak electrical stimulation was applied to the cortical areas representing the hands, normal threshold values remained constant bilaterally for the monofilament test. In contrast, ability to perceive two points from one point even at large distances was abolished in the hand associated with the stimulated side, while the hand associated with the nonstimulated cortex area retained normal two-point discrimination, indicating a major differ-

ence between the two tests. Neurologically, detection is more fundamental than discrimination, which requires cortical integrity. Interestingly, this concept may be obliquely substantiated by rat model research in which neurophysiologists use the monofilaments to test extremity acuity of their animal subjects.[17,63,152]

Duration of contact time, speed of filament application, soaking the hand before testing, and sites tested alter monofilament test results.[118,125,126,188,189] It is imperative that consistent procedures be used with monofilament assessment of sensibility.[128] In addition, it has been shown that use of the monofilaments in combination with wrist flexion provocative testing provides more accurate and sensitive results when testing for median-nerve compression.[107]

The monofilaments are available in the original 20-filament set and in a 5-filament mini set. Supplying a no-overlap range of reproducible stimuli from normal to absent light touch, the 5-filament set is quick and easy to use in the clinic. Normative data for the filaments are available.[26,56,84,130,187] A touch-force assessment instrument should produce stimuli that measure lighter than normal threshold. The 20-filament kit has two filaments that are lighter than the normal 2.83 filament, satisfying this requisite. The WEST 5-filament set has specialized tip geometry to decrease slippage upon contact and is certified for calibration accuracy.[196]

The Dellon-Curtis evaluation has four categories, assessing moving touch, constant touch, flutter (30-cps tuning fork), and vibration (256-cps tuning fork).[51] Controversy exists concerning this test, with some neurophysiologists and neurologists questioning use of vibration because of lack of stimulus specificity to evaluate nerve status in a confined space such as the hand.[60,110] Bell-Krotoski and Buford[22] found that applied force produced by either size tuning fork is uncontrolled, and oscillation is influenced by random vibration of the examiner's hand, strike force, and how long oscillation persists. In addition, they report that force amplitude of a tuning fork is more uncontrolled with side application than tip application. Physicists note that use of a tuning fork in attitudes other than perpendicular to the surface of application changes the vibratory stimulus to a compression stimulus and may elicit a pain response.[129] Force control is also absent for both the moving and constant touch portions of the test. Lack of control of stimulus force and disputed recovery of sequence[193] as originally described raises reliability and validity questions.

Product development in the area of sensibility testing is rapidly changing, and most experts now acknowledge that control of stimulus force is a fundamental concept. One area in which force control has not been associated with stimulus application is that of vibrometry. Although several variations of vibrometers currently are available, for most vibrometers the issue of control of stimulus force continues to be absent, making their reliability questionable.

MANUAL MUSCLE TEST

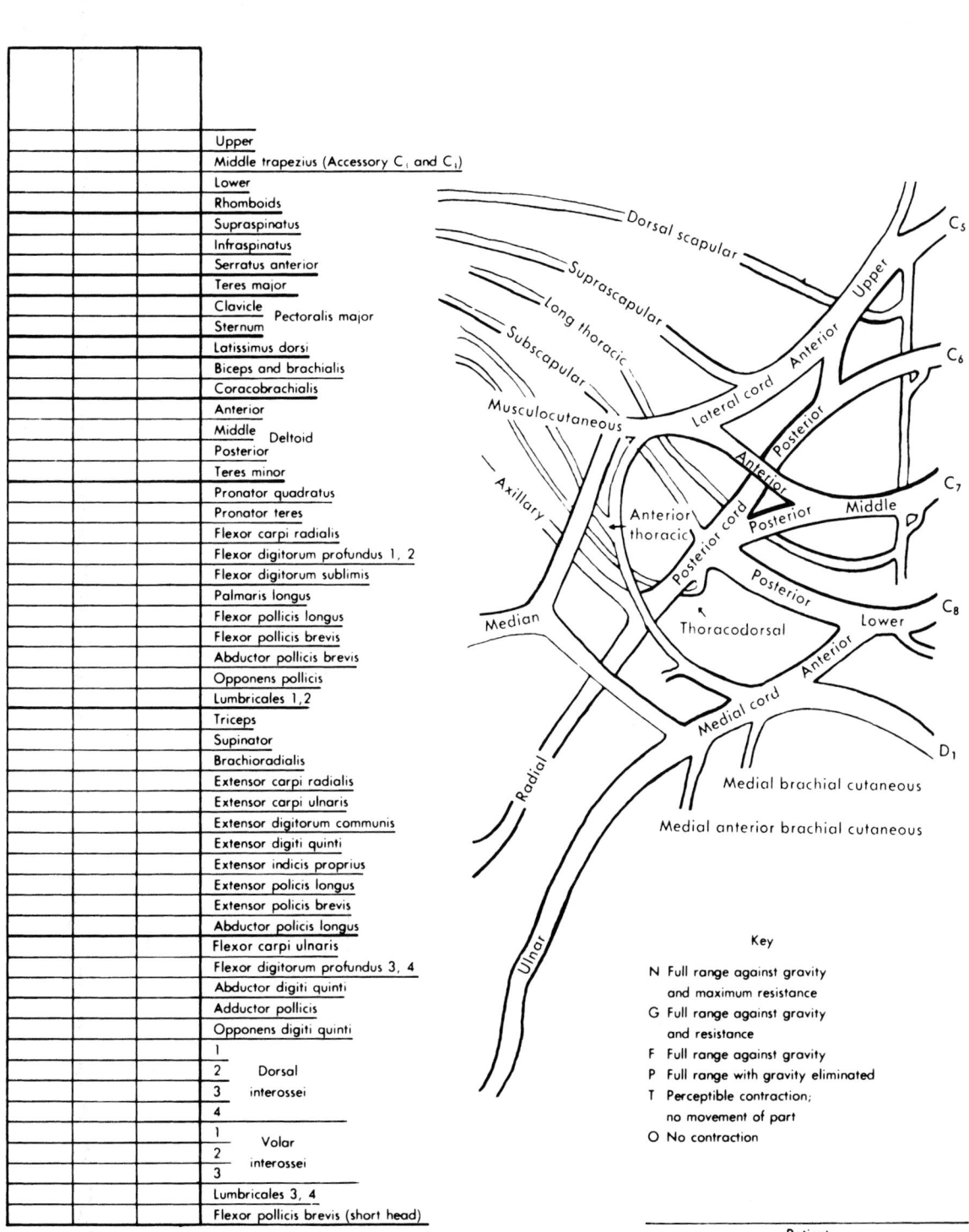

			Upper
			Middle trapezius (Accessory C₁ and C₁)
			Lower
			Rhomboids
			Supraspinatus
			Infraspinatus
			Serratus anterior
			Teres major
			Clavicle / Pectoralis major
			Sternum
			Latissimus dorsi
			Biceps and brachialis
			Coracobrachialis
			Anterior
			Middle / Deltoid
			Posterior
			Teres minor
			Pronator quadratus
			Pronator teres
			Flexor carpi radialis
			Flexor digitorum profundus 1, 2
			Flexor digitorum sublimis
			Palmaris longus
			Flexor pollicis longus
			Flexor pollicis brevis
			Abductor pollicis brevis
			Opponens pollicis
			Lumbricales 1,2
			Triceps
			Supinator
			Brachioradialis
			Extensor carpi radialis
			Extensor carpi ulnaris
			Extensor digitorum communis
			Extensor digiti quinti
			Extensor indicis proprius
			Extensor policis longus
			Extensor policis brevis
			Abductor policis longus
			Flexor carpi ulnaris
			Flexor digitorum profundus 3, 4
			Abductor digiti quinti
			Adductor pollicis
			Opponens digiti quinti
			1
			2 / Dorsal
			3 / interossei
			4
			1
			2 / Volar
			3 / interossei
			Lumbricales 3, 4
			Flexor pollicis brevis (short head)

Date   Nerve-muscle examination   Brachial plexus

Key

N Full range against gravity
  and maximum resistance
G Full range against gravity
  and resistance
F Full range against gravity
P Full range with gravity eliminated
T Perceptible contraction;
  no movement of part
O No contraction

Patient

Fig. 16-7. Basic concept of this manual muscle test was inspired by a form designed by Dr. Lorraine F. Lake, Ph.D., Assistant Professor of Physical Therapy and Anatomy and Associate Director of Irene Walter Johnson Institute of Rehabilitation Medicine. Washington University School of Medicine, St. Louis, Mo.

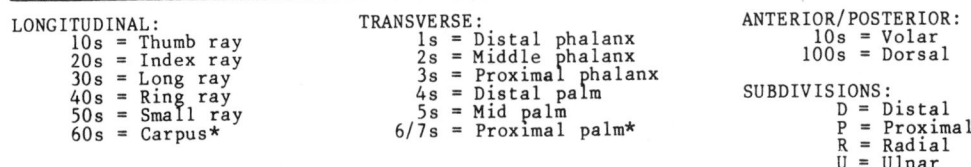

UPPER EXTREMITY ASSESSMENT BATTERY

SENSORY EVALUATION:
COMPUTER KEY

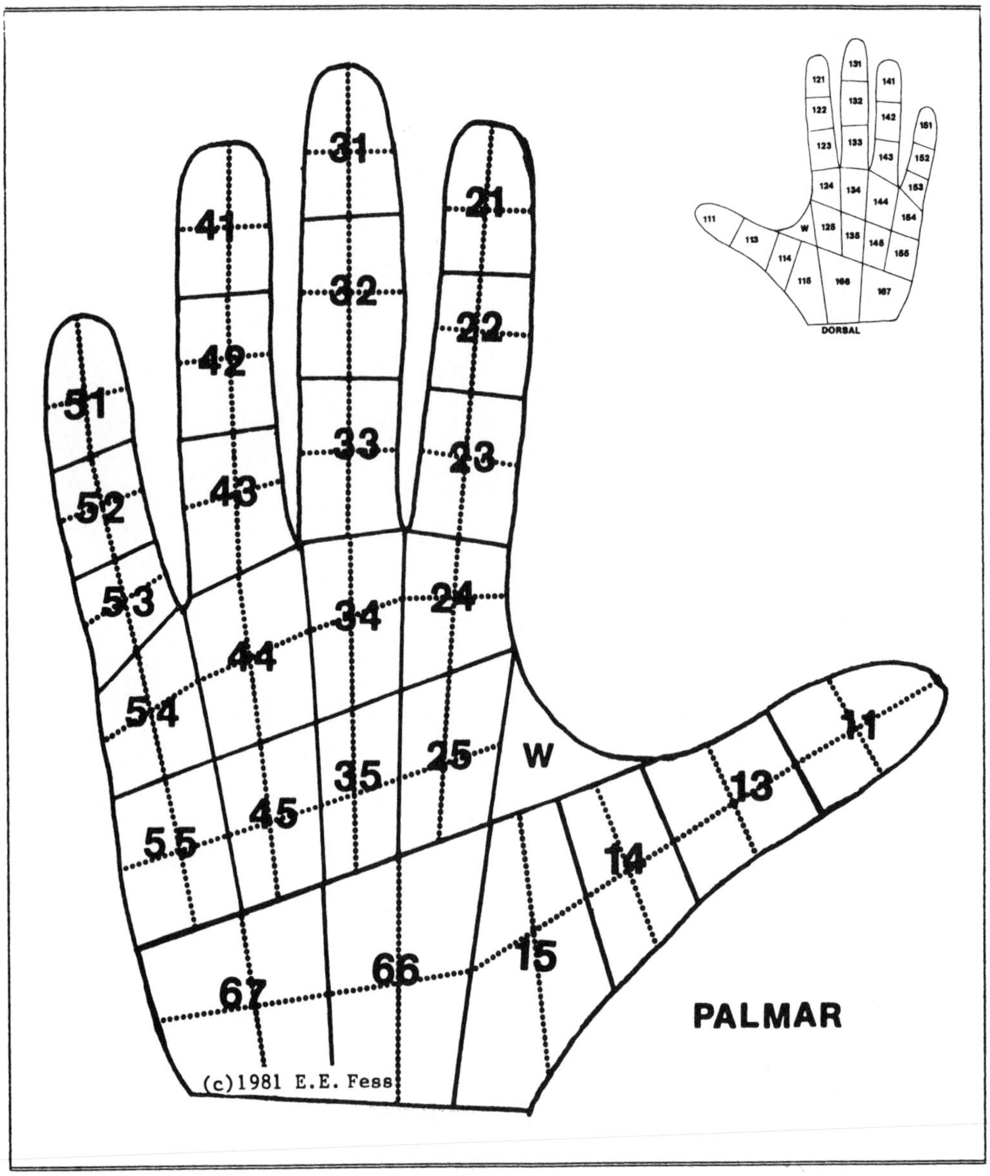

LONGITUDINAL:
    10s = Thumb ray
    20s = Index ray
    30s = Long ray
    40s = Ring ray
    50s = Small ray
    60s = Carpus*

TRANSVERSE:
    1s = Distal phalanx
    2s = Middle phalanx
    3s = Proximal phalanx
    4s = Distal palm
    5s = Mid palm
    6/7s = Proximal palm*

ANTERIOR/POSTERIOR:
    10s = Volar
    100s = Dorsal

SUBDIVISIONS:
    D = Distal
    P = Proximal
    R = Radial
    U = Ulnar

* Modification suggested by J. Bell, 1982.

Fig. 16-8. Coordinates identify specific areas of the palm. The first numbers in the two-digit code represents the longitudinal ray and the second number is the transverse location.

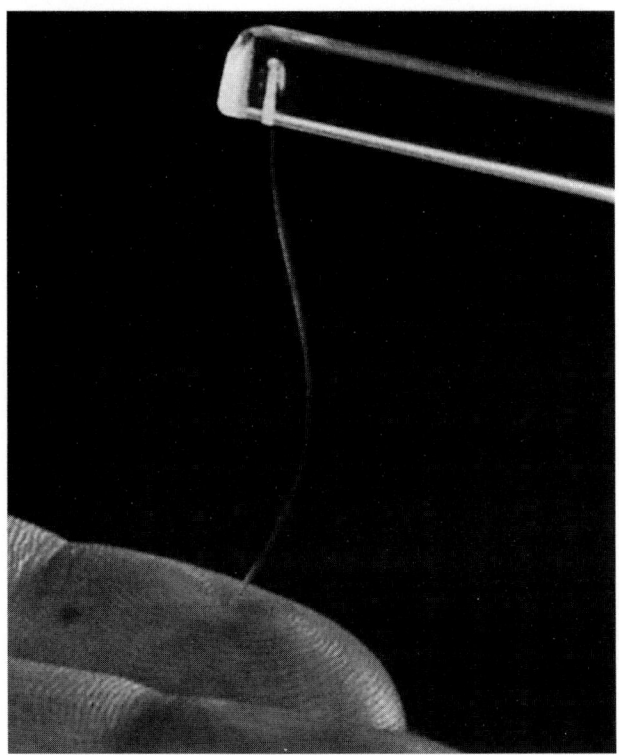

Fig. 16-9. The monofilament collapses when a given force, dependent on filament diameter and length, is reached, controlling the magnitude of the applied touch-pressure.

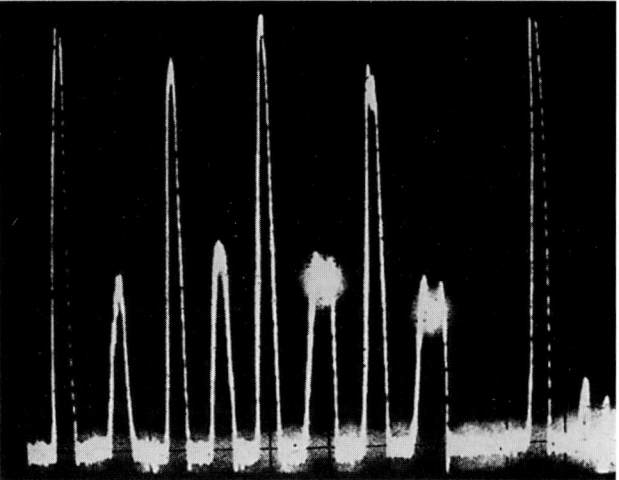

Fig. 16-10. Monitoring the applied force between one and two points, a transducer and oscilloscope graphically show the discrepancies in the amount of force applied between one and two points in a two-point discrimination test by an experienced hand specialist using skin deformation and lack of blanching as the clinical criteria. (Courtesy Judith A. Bell and W. Buford, Carville, La.)

Discrimination is the second level in the sensibility assessment continuum. The ability to perceive one stimulus from a second, different stimulus, involves the capacity to detect each stimulus separately and to differentiate between them. Discrimination requires finer reception acuity and more judgment by the patient than does detection, the first level on the continuum.[196]

Two-point discrimination[7,195] is the most commonly used method of assessing sensibility of the hand. In giving this test, disagreement exists as to whether it is preferable to begin the test with a large or small distance between the two points, and the number of correct responses required varies slightly among examiners. Moving two-point discrimination[52] adds the variable of motion to the test.

The two-point discrimination test has some instrumentation problems. Bell-Krotoski and Buford[21,22] found that even among experienced hand surgeons and therapists, differences between the amount of force applied to the one point and that applied to two points easily exceeded the resolution or sensitivity threshold for normal sensibility (Fig. 16-10). Lack of force consistency is amplified with the introduction of motion in the moving two-point test. Directly influenced by cutaneous topography, applied forces were found to be 400 times the sensitivity of normal cutaneous receptors. They also discovered that because of the varying pressures applied, interrater reliability was poor, perhaps explaining the lack of agreement in reporting and the multiplicity of current clinical sensibility assessment tools.

In contrast, Dellon et al.[53] reported high interrater reliability using standard testing methods and a commercially available two-point discriminator instrument. However, this study involved only two examiners. More study is needed with multiple examiners in different conditions before conclusive statements may be made regarding reliability. Even more important, before examiner reliability is addressed, instrument reliability first must be documented in the laboratory.

In 1995, Tassler and Dellon[179] reported validity of a new computerized sensibility testing tool, the pressure-specified sensory device (PSSD). In clinical comparisons to electro-diagnostic testing (EDT) in nerve entrapment patients, they found this handheld instrument with metal probe tips connected via force transducer to a computer, to have high sensitivity but low specificity. Although several published clinical studies using the PSSD exist,[14,54,185] instrument reliability studies for the PSSD were not found. A prerequisite for all mechanical device validity studies, intrainstrument and interinstrument reliability must first be established through independent laboratory analysis using NIST criteria. Once this is done, independent intrarater and interrater reliability needs to be defined. One study reported that PSSD results were "highly operator dependent and difficult to reproduce" but encouraged further investigation of the device.[82] Although the PSSD eventually may be found to be a useful instrument for testing sensibility, currently much more information is needed in terms of instrumentation criteria.

The Ridge device* introduces the important concept of control of amount of tissue displacement rather than control of applied force. Sensibility instruments should control either the force or the displacement variable, and although most aesthesiometer designs involve force application, the ridge device is unique because of its displacement design. Consisting of a rectangular piece of plastic, from the center of which a narrow ridge gradually rises to a height of 1.5 mm, the ridge device is believed to be useful in identifying patients whose two-point discrimination is between 8 and 12 mm. Instrumentation problems with the ridge device include reliability and validity issues. More intelligent patients have higher scores and the device tends to "bounce" across the skin as it is pulled. In addition, lack of measurement specificity relating to the amount of tissue deformation is problematic, in that the ridge rises without interruption, decreasing accuracy and rater reliability.

Quantification is the third level of sensory capacity. This level involves organizing tactile stimuli according to degree. A patient may be asked to rank in order several alternatives according to roughness, irregularity, thickness, or weightiness. *Identification,* the final and most complicated sensibility level, is the ability to identify objects. At this time, no standardized tests are available for these two categories, although their concepts are commonly used in sensory reeducation treatment programs. Some observational, function-based, sensibility tests such as the Moberg picking-up test and the coin test are adapted to test identification by eliminating sight cues, but none of these have reliability or validity, and they lack even simple equipment standards.

The major problem in assessing sensibility is cortical modification of thresholds. With the exception of sudomotor tests, all of the sensibility evaluation instruments currently available have the potential for producing subjective information. Another variable is callous formation or the hardness of the cutaneous surface (Fig. 16-11). Keratin layers alter the amount of force transferred to sensory receptors by increasing the area of force application. Therefore occupation is a factor in assessment of sensibility. Furthermore, studies indicate that specific receptors cannot be isolated with current unrefined assessment instruments.[22,60]

Sensibility assessment instrumentation is in an early developmental phase. Representing a final, high priority, frontier generation of instruments that better evaluate sensibility of the upper extremity will influence significantly the scope and direction of the profession in the next several decades. The inherent properties of instruments, current and future, must be analyzed and triaged in terms of statistical reliability and validity. To progress, we must first be able to measure. To measure, we must look carefully at our tools. (Refer to Chapters 13 and 14 for specific test protocols.)

*Although clinical use of the Ridge device has decreased, it is included in this chapter because of its unique tissue displacement design.

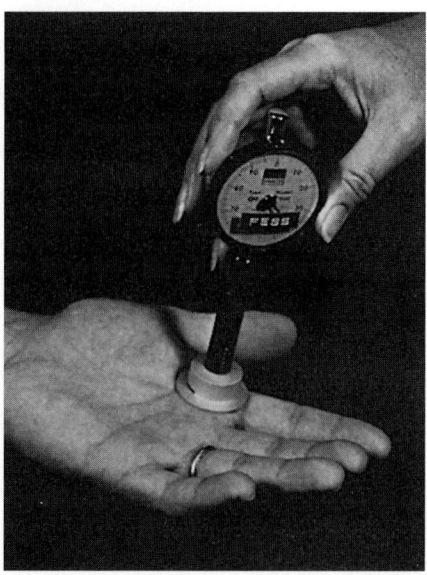

Fig. 16-11. A search for an instrument that will measure skin hardness involves instrumentation studies for reliability and validity.

Function assessment instruments

Handedness is an essential component of upper extremity function. Traditionally, the patient self-report (SR) is the most common method of defining hand preference in the upper extremity rehabilitation arena. Although hand preference tests with established reliability and validity have been used by psychologists to delineate cortical dominance for several decades,[127,169] knowledge of these tests by surgeons and therapists is relatively limited. Recent studies show that the Waterloo Handedness Questionnaire (WHQ),[144,169,178] a 32-item function-based survey with high reliability and validity, more accurately and more extensively defines hand dominance than does the patient self-report.[105,117] The WHQ is inexpensive, simple and fast to administer, and easy to score; in addition, patients respond positively to it, welcoming its user-friendly format and explicitness of individualized results. Better definition of handedness is important to clinicians and researchers alike, in that it improves treatment focus and outcomes on a day-to-day basis, and through more precise research studies, it eventually enhances the professional body of knowledge.

Grip assessment is most often measured with a commercially available hydraulic Jamar dynamometer (Fig. 16-12), although other dynamometer designs are available.[15,77,112,114,192] Developed by Bechtol[19] and recommended by professional societies,[5,7,106] the Jamar dynamometer has been shown to be a reliable test instrument,[68] provided calibration is maintained and standard positioning of test subjects is followed.* In an ongoing instrument reliability study, of 190 used Jamar and Jamar design

*References 111, 120, 138, 153, 154, 168, 173.

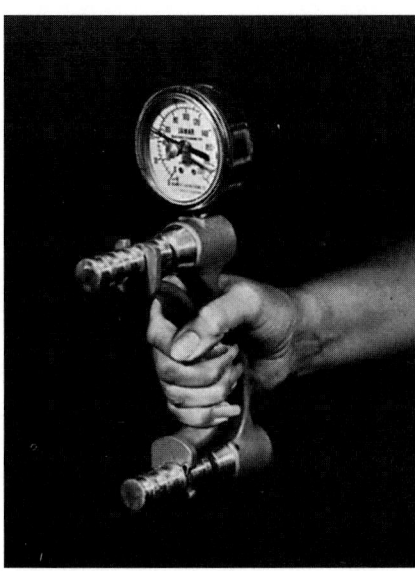

Fig. 16-12. The Jamar dynamometer provides reliable and accurate measurement of grip strength.

dynamometers evaluated by the author, 51% passed the requisite +.9994 correlation criterion when compared to NIST test weights. Of these (.9994 and above), 27% needed minor faceplate adjustments to align their read-out means with the mean readings of the standardized test weights. Of 30 brand new dynamometers, 80% met the correlation criterion of +.9994. Interestingly, two Jamar dynamometers were tested multiple times over more than 8 years with less than .0004 change in correlation, indicating that these instruments do maintain their calibration if carefully used and stored.[66]

Test procedure is important. In 1978 and 1983, the ASSH recommended that the second handle position be used in determining grip strength and that the average of three trials be recorded.[6,7] Of importance is the concept that grip changes according to size of object grasped. Normal adult grip values for the five consecutive handle positions, when plotted on a graph, consistently create a bell-shaped curve, with the first position (smallest) being the least advantageous for strong grip, followed by the fifth and forth positions; strongest grip values occur at the third and second handle positions.[19,134] If inconsistent handle positions are used to assess patient progress, normal alterations in grip scores may be erroneously interpreted as advances or declines in progress. Fatigue is not an issue for the three-trial test procedure but may become a factor when recording grip strengths using all five handle positions (total of 15 trials with 3 trials at each position).[150] A 4-minute rest period between handle positions helps control potential fatigue effect.[200] Percent of maximal voluntary contraction (MVC) required is also important in understanding normal grip strength and fatigue.[94] For example, it is possible to sustain

isometric contraction at 10% MVC for 65 minutes without signs of muscle fatigue.[98] Although Young[200] reported no significant difference in grip scores between morning and night, his data collection times were confined in comparison to those of other investigators who recommend that time of day should be consistent from trial-to-trial.[19,65]

Better definition of handedness directly influences grip strength. Using the WHQ, Lui and Fess found a consistent polarization pattern with greater differences between dominant and nondominant grip strengths in normal subjects with WHQ classifications of predominantly left or right preference versus those who were ambidextrous or with slight left or right preferences. This polarization pattern was especially apparent in the second Jamar handle position.[116]

Norms for grip strength are available,[87,89,121,122] but several of these studies involve altered Jamar dynamometers or other types of dynamometers.[132,133,135,162] Independent studies refute the often cited 10% rule (for normal subjects dominant hand strength is 10% greater than nondominant hand), with reports finding that the minor hand has a range of equal to or stronger than the major hand in up to 31% of the normal population.[145,162,174] The "10% rule" also is not substantiated when the WHQ is used to define handedness.[116] Grip has been reported to correlate with height, weight, and age[16,19,162]; socioeconomic variables such as participation in specific sports or occupations also influence normal grip.[49,50] Grip strength lower than normal is predictive of deterioration and disability in elderly populations.[33,48,79,147,149,175]

Although grip strength often is used clinically to determine sincerity of voluntary effort, validity of its use in identifying submaximal effort is controversial, with studies supporting* and refuting its appropriateness.[12,64,85,136,184] Niebuhr and Marion[137] recommend use of surface EMG in conjunction with grip testing to more accurately determine sincerity of effort. The rapid exchange grip test,[91,97] a popular test for insincere effort, has been shown to have problems with procedure and reliability[180]; even with a carefully standardized administration protocol, its validity is disputed because of low sensitivity and specificity.[166]

The Jamar's capacity as an evaluation instrument, the effects of protocol, and the ramification of its use have been analyzed by many investigators over the years with mixed, and sometimes conflicting, results. Confusion largely results from the fact that most studies reported have relied on nonexistent, incomplete, or inappropriate methods for checking instrument accuracy of the dynamometers used in data collection. A second and more recent development is the ability to better define handedness using the WHQ. Scientific inquiry is both ongoing and progressive as new information is available. Although past studies provide a springboard and

*References 42, 80, 81, 131, 164, 172.

direction, it is important to understand that all grip strength studies need to be reevaluated using carefully calibrated instruments and in context of the more accurate definition of handedness provided by the WHQ.

Other grip strength assessment tools need to be selected according to stringent instrumentation criteria including longitudinal effects of use and time. Although spring-load instruments or rubber bulb/bladder instruments may demonstrate good instrument reliability when compared with corresponding NIST criteria, both categories of instruments exhibit deterioration with time and/or use, rendering them inaccurate as assessment tools.

Pinch strength is measured with a commercially available pinchometer. Reliability of pinchometers needs investigation. Generally speaking, hydraulic pinch instruments are more accurate than spring-loaded. A commonly used pinchometer in the shape of an elongated C with a plunger dial on top is, mechanically speaking, a single large spring, in that its two ends are compressed toward each other, against the counter force of the single center C spring. This design has inherent problems in terms of instrument reliability.[57]

Three types of pinch are usually assessed: (1) prehension of the thumb pulp to the lateral aspect of the index middle phalanx (key, lateral, or pulp-to-side), (2) pulp of the thumb to pulps of the index and long fingers (three-jaw chuck, three-point chuck), and (3) thumb tip to the tip of the index finger (tip-to-tip). Lateral is the strongest of the three types of pinch, followed by three-jaw chuck. Tip-to-tip is a positioning pinch used in activities requiring fine coordination rather than power. As with grip measurements, the mean of three trials is recorded, and comparisons are made with the opposite hand. Better definition of handedness via the WHQ will impart improved understanding of the relative value of dominant and nondominant pinch strength. Cassanova and Grunert[40] describe an excellent method of classifying pinch patterns based on anatomic areas of contact. In an extensive literature review, they found more than 300 distinct terms for prehension. Their method of classification avoids colloquial usage and eliminates confusion when describing pinch function.

Standardized tests for assessing *manual dexterity* and *coordination* are available in several levels of difficulty, allowing selection of instruments that best suit the needs/abilities of individual patients. As noted, when using a standardized test instrument, it is imperative not to deviate from the method, equipment, and sequencing described in the test instructions. Test calibration, reliability, and validity are determined using very specific items and techniques, and any change in stipulated pattern renders resultant data invalid and meaningless. Using a standardized test as a teaching/training device in therapy also excludes its use as an assessment instrument because of skewing data.

Of the tests available, the Jebsen-Taylor hand function test[95] requires the least amount of extremity coordination and is inexpensive to assemble and easy to administer and score. The Jebsen consists of seven subtests: (1) writing, (2) card turning, (3) picking up small objects, (4) simulated feeding, (5) stacking, (6) picking up large lightweight objects, and (7) picking up large heavy objects. Originally developed for use with rheumatoid arthritic patients,[95,165] the Jebsen has been used to assess aging adults,[83] hemiplegic persons,[167] children,[181] and wrist immobilization,[39] among others. Jebsen norms are categorized according to maximum time, hand dominance, age, and gender.[170] Rider and Lindon[155] report a statistically significant difference in times with substitution of plastic checkers for the original wooden ones, and a trend of faster times with use of larger paper clips than originally described, invalidating the test. Equipment for standardized tests cannot be substituted/altered from that of the original test unless the test is restandardized completely with the new equipment. Capacity to measure gross coordination makes this test an excellent instrument to assess individuals whose severity of involvement precludes use of many other coordination tests that often require very fine prehension patterns.

Based on placing blocks into spaces on a board, the Minnesota Rate of Manipulation Tests (MRMT) include five activities: (1) placing, (2) turning, (3) displacing, (4) one-hand turning and placing, and (5) two-hand turning and placing. Originally designed for testing personnel for jobs requiring arm-hand dexterity, the MRMT is another excellent example of a test that measures gross coordination and dexterity, making it applicable to many of the needs encountered in hand/upper extremity rehabilitation. Norms for this instrument are based on more than 11,000 subjects. Unfortunately, some of the commercially available versions of the MRMT are made of plastic. Reliability, validity, and normative data were established on the original wooden version of the test and are not applicable to the newer plastic design. Essentially, the plastic MRMT is an unknown, needing reliability, validity, and normative investigation before it may be used as a testing instrument.

Requiring prehension of small pins, washers, and collars, the Purdue Pegboard Test[183] evaluates finer coordination than the two previous dexterity tests. Subcategories for the Purdue are (1) right hand; (2) left hand; (3) both hands; (4) right, left, and both; and (5) assembly. Normative data are presented in categories based on gender and job type: male and female applicants for general factory work, female applicants for electronics production work, male utility service workers, and so on. Normative data also are available for 14- to 19-year-olds,[123] and for those ages 60 and older[55] Reddon et al.[151] found a learning curve for some subtests when the Purdue was given five times at weekly intervals, reinforcing the concept that standardized tests should not be used as training devices for patients.

In terms of psychomotor taxonomy, all of the previously described tests assess activities that are classified as skilled movements. Evaluating compound adaptive skills, the

Crawford Small Parts Dexterity Test adds another dimension to hand function assessment by introducing tools into the test protocol. Increasing the level of difficulty, this test requires subjects to control implements in addition to their hands/fingers. The Crawford involves use of tweezers and a screwdriver to assemble pins, collars, and small screws on the test board. It relates to activities requiring very fine coordination, such as engraving, watch/clock making, office machine assembly, and other intricate skills. The O'Connor[93] test also requires use of tool manipulation to place small pegs on a board.

Other hand-coordination and dexterity testing instruments are available. They should be evaluated carefully in terms of the criteria for standardization outlined earlier in this chapter to ensure that they have been proved to measure appropriately and accurately.

Work hardening tests span a wide range in terms of meeting instrumentation criteria, with many falling into the category of specific item/task longitudinal tests designed specifically to meet the needs of an individual patient. On the sophisticated end of the continuum, the Valpar Work Sample consists of 19 work samples that meet all the criteria for a standardized test, and the individual tests may be used alone or in multiple groupings depending on patient requirements. With the exception of the Valpar Work Samples, many "work hardening" tests are not standardized.

The Baltimore Therapeutic Equipment (BTE) Work Simulator uses static and dynamic modes to produce resistance to an array of tools and handles that are inserted into a common exercise head. Although the basic concept of this machine is innovative and the static mode has been shown to be accurate with high reliability correlation coefficients, the dynamic mode has problems producing consistent resistance. Dynamic mode resistance has been found seriously variable both within and between machines, making the Work Simulator inappropriate for assessment when consistent resistance is required.[41,45,58] Because of the fluctuating and unpredictable dynamic mode resistance changes that are not accurately reflected by the computer printout, caution should be used in allowing patients with acute injuries, geriatric patients, pediatric patients, patients with inflammatory problems such as rheumatoid arthritis, patients with unstable vascular systems, and/or patients with impaired sensibility to exercise on this machine. Volumetric measurements may be helpful in identifying patients whose inflammatory response to working on the Work Simulator dynamic mode may be increasing. Interestingly, a review of reliability studies involving the Work Simulator identifies a pattern that is all too often found with mechanical rehabilitation devices, in that multiple studies were conducted and reported using human performance to establish its reliability as an assessment instrument.* Human performance is not an appropriate indicator of accuracy/calibration for mechanical

*References 11, 29, 47, 62, 104, 148, 198.

devices. Later, when consistency of resistance of the dynamic mode was evaluated according to NIST standards, reliability/accuracy was found to be lacking. A second-generation "work simulator," the Primus, is currently on the market, along with similar machines from other companies. At the time of this writing, no NIST-based reliability information is available for any of these additional machines, including the Primus.[38,46,59,99]

Traditionally, the extent to which DLS are assessed has depended on the type of clientele treated by the rehabilitation center. Facilities oriented toward treatment of trauma injury patients required less extensive DLS evaluation and training than a center specializing in arthritis patients. However, with increased emphasis on patient satisfaction reporting, it has become apparent that more extensive DLS evaluation is needed to identify specific factors that are individual and distinct to each patient. The Flinn Performance Screening Tool (FPST)[76] is important because it is, and continues to be, tested for reliability, and it allows patients to work independently of the evaluator in deciding what tasks they can and cannot perform. The FPST consists of two volumes of more than 300 laminated daily activity photographs that have been tested and retested for specificity and sensitivity of task. Volume One assesses self-care tasks and Volume Two evaluates home/outside activities and work activities. This test represents a major step toward defining function in a scientific manner.

Assessment of a patient's potential to return to work is based on a combination of standardized and observational tests, knowledge of the specific work situation, insight into the patient's motivational and psychologic references, and understanding of the complexities of normal and disabled hands/upper extremities in general. Although its importance has been acknowledged in the past, vocational assessment of the patient with an upper extremity injury is now given a higher priority in most of the major hand rehabilitation centers throughout the country. Treatment no longer ends with achievement of skeletal stability, wound healing, and a plateau of motion and sensibility. This shift in emphasis has been the result, in large part, of the contributions of the Philadelphia Hand Center.

Patient satisfaction assessment instruments

Testing of *patient satisfaction* has become an integral part of rehabilitation endeavors.[8,18] Just as other test instruments must meet instrumentation criteria, so too must patient satisfaction assessment tools,[30,32,36] which are often in the form of patient-completed questionnaires. Current symptom/satisfaction tools used in evaluating patients with upper extremity injury or dysfunction include the Medical Outcomes Study 36-Item Health Survey (SF-36), the Upper Extremities Disabilities of Arm, Shoulder, and Hand (DASH),[9] the Michigan Hand Outcomes Questionnaire (MHQ),[43,44] and the Severity of Symptoms and Functional Status in Carpal Tunnel Syndrome questionnaire.[27,28,100-102,113]

CONCLUSION

Evaluation with instruments that measure accurately allows physicians and therapists to correctly identify hand/upper extremity disease and dysfunction, assess the effects of treatment, and realistically apprise patients of their progress. Accurate assessment data also permit analysis of treatment modalities for effectiveness, provide a foundation for professional communication through research, and eventually influence the scope and direction of the profession as a whole. Because of their relationship to the kind of information obtained, assessment tools cannot be chosen irresponsibly. The choice of tools directly influences the quality of individual treatment and the quality of understanding between hand specialists. Criteria exist for identifying instruments on which we can depend to measure accurately when used by different evaluators and from session to session. Unless the results of a "home-brewed" test are statistically analyzed, the test is tried on large numbers of normal subjects, and the results are analyzed again, it is naive to assume that such a test provides meaningful information. Current tools may be better understood by checking their reliability and validity levels with bioengineering technology,[23] and statisticians may be of assistance in devising protocols that will lead to more refined and accurate information. We as hand specialists have a responsibility to our patients and to our colleagues to continue to critique the instruments we use in terms of instrumentation criteria. Without assessment, we cannot treat, we cannot communicate, and we cannot progress.

REFERENCES

1. American Academy of Orthopedic Surgeons (AAOS): *Joint motion: method of measuring and recording,* Chicago, 1965, The Academy.
2. American Medical Association (AMA): The upper extremities. In Cocchiarella L, Andersson G, editors: *Guides to the evaluation of permanent impairment,* Chicago, 2000, AMA Press.
3. American Society of Hand Therapists (ASHT): American Society of Hand Therapists clinical assessment recommendations. In Fess EE, Moran C, editors: *American Society of Hand Therapists clinical assessment recommendations,* Garner, 1981, The Society.
4. American Society of Hand Therapists (ASHT): *American Society of Hand Therapists clinical assessment recommendations,* Chicago, 1992, The Society.
5. American Society of Hand Therapists (ASHT): *American Society of Hand Therapists splint classification system,* Chicago 1992, The Society.
6. American Society for Surgery of the Hand (ASSH): *The hand: examination and diagnosis,* Aurora, Colo, 1978, The Society.
7. American Society for Surgery of the Hand (ASSH): *The hand: examination and diagnosis,* New York, 1983, Churchill Livingstone.
8. Amadio PC: Outcomes research and the hand surgeon, *J Hand Surg* 19A:351, 1994 (editorial).
9. Amadio PC: Outcomes assessment in hand surgery: what's new? *Clin Plast Surg* 24:191, 1997.
10. Amis A, Miller J: The elbow, *Clin Rheum Dis* 8:571, 1983.
11. Anderson PA, et al: Normative study of grip and wrist flexion strength employing a BTE Work Simulator, *J Hand Surg* 15A:420, 1990.
12. Ashford RF, Nagelburg S, Adkins R: Sensitivity of the Jamar Dynamometer in detecting submaximal grip effort, *J Hand Surg* 21A:402, 1996.
13. Ashton B, Pickles B, Roll J: Reliability of goniometric measurements of hip motion in spastic cerebral palsy, *Dev Med Child Neurol* 20:87, 1978.
14. Aszmann OC, Dellon AL: Relationship between cutaneous pressure threshold and two-point discrimination, *J Reconstr Microsurg* 14:417, 1998.
15. Aveque C, et al: The evaluation of the Artem grip in its function assessment, *Ann Chir Main Memb Super* 13:334, 1994.
16. Backous DD, Farrow JA, Friedl KE: Assessment of pubertal maturity in boys, using height and grip strength, *J Adolesc Health Care* 11:497, 1990.
17. Barbay S, et al: Sensitivity of neurons in somatosensory cortex (S1) to cutaneous stimulation of the hindlimb immediately following a sciatic nerve crush, *Somatosens Mot Res* 16:103, 1999.
18. Barr JT: The outcomes movement and health status measures, *J Allied Health* 24:13, 1995.
19. Bechtol C: Grip test: use of a dynamometer with adjustable handle spacing, *J Bone Joint Surg* 36A:820, 1954.
20. Bell-Krotoski J: Advances in sensibility evaluation, *Hand Clin* 7:527, 1991.
21. Bell-Krotoski J, Buford W: The force/time relationship of clinically used sensory testing instruments, *J Hand Ther* 1:76, 1988.
22. Bell-Krotoski JA, Buford WL Jr: The force/time relationship of clinically used sensory testing instruments, *J Hand Ther* 10:297, 1997.
23. Bell-Krotoski JA, Fess EE: Biomechanics: the forces of change and the basis for all that we do, *J Hand Ther* 8:63, 1995.
24. Bell-Krotoski J, Tomancik E: The repeatability of testing with Semmes-Weinstein monofilaments, *J Hand Surg* 12A:155, 1987.
25. Bell-Krotoski J, Weinstein S, Weinstein C: Testing sensibility, including touch-pressure, two-point discrimination, point localization, and vibration, *J Hand Ther* 6:114, 1993.
26. Bell-Krotoski JA, et al: Threshold detection and Semmes-Weinstein monofilaments, *J Hand Ther* 8:155, 1995.
27. Bessette L, et al: Patients' preferences and their relationship with satisfaction following carpal tunnel release, *J Hand Surg* 22A:613, 1997.
28. Bessette L, et al: Prognostic value of a hand symptom diagram in surgery for carpal tunnel syndrome, *J Rheumatol* 24:726, 1997.
29. Bhambhani Y, Esmail S, Brintnell S: The Baltimore Therapeutic Equipment work simulator: biomechanical and physiological norms for three attachments in healthy men, *Am J Occup Ther* 48:19, 1994.
30. Bieliauskas LA, et al: Use of the odds ratio to translate neuropsychological test scores into real-world outcomes: from statistical significance to clinical significance, *J Clin Exp Neuropsychol* 19:889, 1997.
31. Bird H, Stowe J: The wrist, *Clin Rheum Dis* 8:559, 1982.
32. Blevins L, McDonald CJ: Fisher's Exact Test: an easy-to-use statistical test for comparing outcomes, *MD Comput* 2:15, 1985.
33. Bohannon RW: Hand-grip dynamometry provides a valid indication of upper extremity strength impairment in home care patients, *J Hand Ther* 11:258, 1998.
34. Boone D: Reliability of goniometric measurements, *Phys Ther* 58:1355, 1978.
35. Brand PW: *Hand volumeter instruction sheet,* Carville, La, 1977, US Public Health Services Hospital 1977.
36. Bridge PD, Sawilowsky SS: Increasing physicians' awareness of the impact of statistics on research outcomes: comparative power of the t-test and Wilcoxon Rank-Sum test in small samples applied research, *J Clin Epidemiol* 52:229, 1999.
37. Brosseau L, et al: Intratester and intertester reliability and criterion validity of the parallelogram and universal goniometers for active knee flexion in healthy subjects, *Physiother Res Int* 2:150, 1997.
38. Capodaglio P, et al: Work capacity of the upper limbs after mastectomy, *G Ital Med Lav Ergon* 19:172, 1997.
39. Carlson JD, Trombly CA: The effect of wrist immobilization on performance of the Jebsen Hand Function Test, *Am J Occup Ther* 37:167, 1983.

40. Casanova J, Grunert B: Adult prehension: patterns and nomenclature for pinches, *J Hand Ther* 2:231, 1989.
41. Cetinok EM, Renfro RR, Coleman EF: A pilot study of the reliability of the dynamic mode of one BTE Work Simulator, *J Hand Ther* 8:199, 1995.
42. Chengalur SN, et al: Assessing sincerity of effort in maximal grip strength tests, *Am J Phys Med Rehabil* 69:148, 1990.
43. Chung KC, et al: Reliability and validity testing of the Michigan Hand Outcomes Questionnaire, *J Hand Surg* 23A:575, 1998.
44. Chung KC, et al: The Michigan Hand Outcomes Questionnaire (MHQ): assessment of responsiveness to clinical change, *Ann Plast Surg* 42:619, 1999.
45. Coleman EF, et al: Reliability of the manual dynamic mode of the Baltimore Therapeutic Equipment Work Simulator, *J Hand Ther* 9:223, 1996.
46. Cooke C, et al: Relationship of performance on the ERGOS work simulator to illness behavior in a workers' compensation population with low back versus limb injury, *J Occup Med* 36:757, 1994.
47. Curtis RM, Engalitcheff J Jr: A work simulator for rehabilitating the upper extremity-preliminary report, *J Hand Surg* 6A:499, 1981.
48. Davies CW, Jones DM, Shearer JR: Hand grip: a simple test for morbidity after fracture of the neck of femur, *J R Soc Med* 77:833, 1984.
49. De AK, et al: Respiratory performance and grip strength tests on the basketball players of inter-university competition, *Indian J Physiol Pharmacol* 24:305, 1980.
50. De AK, et al: Respiratory performance and grip strength tests in Indian school bodys of different socio-economic status, *Br J Sports Med* 14:145, 1980.
51. Dellon A, Curtis R, Edgerton M: Reeducation of sensation in the hand after nerve injury and repair, *Plast Reconst Surg* 3:297, 1974.
52. Dellon AL: The moving two-point discrimination test: clinical evaluation of the quickly adapting fiber/receptor system, *J Hand Surg* 3A:474, 1978.
53. Dellon AL, Mackinnon SE, Crosby PM: Reliability of two-point discrimination measurements, *J Hand Surg* 12A:693, 1987.
54. Dellon ES, et al: The relationships between skin hardness, pressure perception and two-point discrimination in the fingertip, *J Hand Surg* 20B:44, 1995.
55. Desrosiers J, et al: Normative data for grip strength of elderly men and women, *Am J Occup Ther* 49:637, 1995.
56. Desrosiers J, et al: Hand sensibility of healthy older people, *J Am Geriatr Soc* 44:974, 1996.
57. Dunipace K: Personal communication, 1990.
58. Dunipace KR: Reliability of the BTE work simulator dynamic mode, *J Hand Ther* 8:42, 1995 (letter).
59. Dusik LA, et al: Concurrent validity of the ERGOS work simulator versus conventional functional capacity evaluation techniques in a workers' compensation population, *J Occup Med* 35:759, 1993.
60. Dyck P, et al: Clinical vs quantitative evaluation of cutaneous sensation, *Arch Neurol* 33:651, 1976.
61. Ekstrand J, et al: Lower extremity goniometric measurements: a study to determine their reliability, *Arch Phys Med Rehab* 63:171, 1982.
62. Esmail S, Bhambhani Y, Brintnell S: Gender differences in work performance on the Baltimore Therapeutic Equipment work simulator, *Am J Occup Ther* 49:405, 1995.
63. Esser MJ, Sawynok J: Acute amitriptyline in a rat model of neuropathic pain: differential symptom and route effects, *Pain* 80:643, 1999.
64. Fairfax AH, Balnave R, Adams RD: Variability of grip strength during isometric contraction, *Ergonomics* 38:1819, 1995.
65. Ferraz MB, et al: The effect of elbow flexion and time of assessment on the measurement of grip strength in rheumatoid arthritis, *J Hand Surg* 17A:1099, 1992.
66. Fess E: Instrument reliability of new and used Jamar and Jamar design dynamometers (ongoing study).
67. Fess EE: Editorial: The need for reliability and validity in hand assessment instruments, *J Hand Surg* 11A:621, 1986.
68. Fess EE: A method of checking Jamar dynamometer reliability, *J Hand Ther* 1:28, 1987.
69. Fess EE: Letter to the editor: response—reliability and validity, *J Hand Ther* 1:219, 1988.
70. Fess EE: Research for the clinician: using research terminology correctly—reliability, *J Hand Ther* 1:109, 1988.
71. Fess EE: Research for the clinician: using research terminology correctly—validity, *J Hand Ther* 1:148, 1988.
72. Fess EE: Research for the clinician: why trial-to-trial reliability is not enough, *J Hand Ther* 7:28, 1994.
73. Fess EE: Research for the clinician: how to avoid being misled by statements of average, *J Hand Ther* 7:193, 1994.
74. Fess EE: Guidelines for evaluating assessment instruments, *J Hand Ther* 8:144, 1995.
75. Fess EE: Research for the clinician: human performance—an appropriate measure of instrument reliability? *J Hand Ther* 10:46, 1997.
76. Flinn S, Ventura D: *The Flinn performance screening tool,* Cleveland, 1997, Functional Visions.
77. Fraser A, et al: Predicting 'normal' grip strength for rheumatoid arthritis patients, *Rheumatology* (Oxford) 38:521, 1999.
78. Gelberman RH, et al: Sensibility testing in peripheral-nerve compression syndromes: an experimental study in humans, *J Bone Joint Surg* 65A:632, 1983.
79. Giampaoli S, et al: Hand-grip strength predicts incident disability in non-disabled older men, *Age Ageing* 28:283, 1999.
80. Gilbert JC, Knowlton RG: Simple method to determine sincerity of effort during a maximal isometric test of grip strength, *Am J Phys Med* 62:135, 1983.
81. Goldman S, Cahalan TD, An KN: The injured upper extremity and the JAMAR five-handle position grip test, *Am J Phys Med Rehabil* 70:306, 1991.
82. Grime PD: A pilot study to determine the potential application of the pressure specified sensory device in the maxillofacial region, *Br J Oral Maxillofac Surg* 34:500, 1996.
83. Hackel ME, et al: Changes in hand function in the aging adult as determined by the Jebsen Test of Hand Function, *Phys Ther* 72:373, 1992.
84. Hage JJ, van der Steen LP, de Groot PJ: Difference in sensibility between the dominant and nondominant index finger as tested using the Semmes-Weinstein monofilaments pressure aesthesiometer, *J Hand Surg* 20A:227, 1995.
85. Hamilton A, Balnave R, Adams R: Grip strength testing reliability, *J Hand Ther* 7:163, 1994.
86. Hamilton G: Reliability of goniometers in assessing finger joint angle, *Phys Ther* 49:465, 1969.
87. Hanten WP, et al: Maximum grip strength in normal subjects from 20 to 64 years of age, *J Hand Ther* 12:193, 1999.
88. Hargens AR, et al: Effects of local compression on peroneal nerve function in humans, *J Orthop Res* 11:818, 1993.
89. Harkonen R, Piirtomaa M, Alaranta H: Grip strength and hand position of the dynamometer in 204 Finnish adults, *J Hand Surg* 18B:129, 1993.
90. Harris S, Smith L, Krukowski L: Goniometric reliability for a child with spastic quadriplegia, *J Pediatr Orthopaed* 5:348, 1985.
91. Hildreth D, et al: Detection of submaximal effort by use of the rapid exchange grip, *J Hand Surg* 14A:742, 1989.
92. Hillenbrandt F, Duval E, Moore M: The measurement of joint motion: III reliability of goniometry, *Phys Ther Rev* 29:302, 1949.
93. Hines M, O'Connor J: A measure of finger dexterity, *Personnel J* 4:379, 1926.

94. Jaskolska A, Jaskolski A: The influence of intermittent fatigue exercise on early and late phases of relaxation from maximal voluntary contraction, *Can J Appl Physiol* 22:573, 1997.

95. Jebsen RH, et al: An objective and standardized test of hand function, *Arch Phys Med Rehabil* 50:311, 1969.

96. Jeng SF, et al: Reliability of a clinical kinematic assessment of the sit-to-stand movement, *Phys Ther* 70:511, 1990.

97. Joughin K, et al: An evaluation of rapid exchange and simultaneous grip tests, *J Hand Surg* 18A:245, 1993.

98. Kahn JF, Favriou F, Jouanin JC et al: Influence of posture and training on the endurance time of a low-level isometric contraction, *Ergonomics* 40:1231, 1997.

99. Kaiser H, Kersting M, Schian HM: Value of the ERGOS work simulator as a component of functional capacity assessment in disability evaluation, *Rehabilitation (Stuttg)* 39:175, 2000.

100. Katz JN, et al: Symptoms, functional status, and neuromuscular impairment following carpal tunnel release, *J Hand Surg* 20A:549, 1995.

101. Katz JN, et al: Workers' compensation recipients with carpal tunnel syndrome: the validity of self-reported health measures, *Am J Public Health* 86:52, 1996.

102. Katz JN, et al: Maine Carpal Tunnel Study: outcomes of operative and nonoperative therapy for carpal tunnel syndrome in a community-based cohort [published erratum appears in *J Hand Surg* 24A:201], *J Hand Surg* 23A:697, 1998.

103. Kendall H, Kendall F, Wadsworth G: *Muscle testing and function,* ed 4, Baltimore 1993, Williams & Wilkins.

104. Kennedy LE, Bhambhani YN: The Baltimore Therapeutic Equipment Work Simulator: reliability and validity at three work intensities, *Arch Phys Med Rehabil* 72:511, 1991.

105. Kersten K, et al: *A correlational study between self-reported hand preference and results of the Waterloo Handedness Questionnaire, Occupational Therapy,* New York, 1995, Columbia University 1995.

106. Kirkpatrick J: Evaluation of grip loss: a factor of permanent partial disability in California, *Industrial Med Surg* 26:285, 1957.

107. Koris M, et al: Carpal tunnel syndrome: evaluation of a quantitative provocational diagnostic test, *Clin Orthop* 1990:157, 1990.

108. Kuipers M, Schreuders T: The predictive value of sensation testing in the development of neuropathic ulceration on the hands of leprosy patients, *Lepr Rev* 65:253, 1994.

109. Kumar S, et al: Semmes-Weinstein monofilaments: a simple, effective and inexpensive screening device for identifying diabetic patients at risk of foot ulceration, *Diabetes Res Clin Pract* 13:63, 1991.

110. LaMotte R: Testing sensibility. Symposium: assessment of levels of cutaneous sensibility, United States Public Health Service Hospital, Carville, La, 1980.

111. LaStayo P, Chidgey L, Miller G: Quantification of the relationship between dynamic grip strength and forearm rotation: a preliminary study, *Ann Plast Surg* 35:191, 1995.

112. LaStayo P, Hartzel J: Dynamic versus static grip strength: how grip strength changes when the wrist is moved, and why dynamic grip strength may be a more functional measurement, *J Hand Ther* 12:212, 1999.

113. Levine DW, et al: A self-administered questionnaire for the assessment of severity of symptoms and functional status in carpal tunnel syndrome, *J Bone Joint Surg* 75A:1585, 1993.

114. Lindahl OA, et al: Grip strength of the human hand—measurements on normal subjects with a new hand strength analysis system (Hastras), *J Med Eng Technol* 18:101, 1994.

115. Low JL: The reliability of joint measurement, *Physiotherapy* 62:227, 1976.

116. Lui P, Fess EE: Comparison of dominant and nondominant grip strength: the critical role of the Waterloo Handedness Questionnaire (submitted for publication).

117. Lui P, Fess EE: Establishing hand dominance: self-report versus the Waterloo Handedness Questionnaire (submitted for publication).

118. MacDermid JC, Kramer JF, Roth JH: Decision making in detecting abnormal Semmes-Weinstein monofilament thresholds in carpal tunnel syndrome, *J Hand Ther* 7:158, 1994.

119. MacDermid JC, et al: Intratester and intertester reliability of goniometric measurement of passive lateral shoulder rotation, *J Hand Ther* 12:187, 1999.

120. Mathiowetz V, Rennells C, Donahoe L: Effect of elbow position on grip and key pinch strength, *J Hand Surg* 10A:694, 1985.

121. Mathiowetz V, Wiemer DM, Federman SM: Grip and pinch strength: norms for 6- to 19-year-olds, *Am J Occup Ther* 40:705, 1986.

122. Mathiowetz V, et al: Grip and pinch strength: normative data for adults, *Arch Phys Med Rehabil* 66:69, 1985.

123. Mathiowetz V, et al: The Purdue Pegboard: norms for 14- to 19-year-olds, *Am J Occup Ther* 40:174, 1986.

124. Mayerson NH, Milano RA: Goniometric measurement reliability in physical medicine, *Arch Phys Med Rehabil* 65:92, 1984.

125. McAuley DM, Ewing PA, Devasundaram JK: Effect of hand soaking on sensory testing, *Int J Lepr Other Mycobact Dis* 61:16, 1993.

126. McGill M, et al: Possible sources of discrepancies in the use of the Semmes-Weinstein monofilament. Impact on prevalence of insensate foot and workload requirements, *Diabetes Care* 22:598, 1999.

127. McMeekan E, Lishman W: Retest reliabilities and interrelationship of the Annett hand preference questionnaire and the Edinburgh handedness inventory, *Br J Psychol* 66:53, 1975.

128. Mielke K, et al: Hand sensibility measures used by therapists, *Ann Plast Surg* 36:292, 1996.

129. Mitchell E: Symposium: assessment of levels of cutaneous sensibility, United States Public Health Service Hospital, Carville, La 1980.

130. Mitchell PD, Mitchell TN: The age-dependent deterioration in light touch sensation on the plantar aspect of the foot in a rural community in India: implications when screening for sensory impairment (in process citation), *Lepr Rev* 71:169, 2000.

131. Mitterhauser MD, et al: Detection of submaximal effort with computer-assisted grip strength measurements, *J Occup Environ Med* 39:1220, 1997.

132. Montoye HJ, Lamphiear DE: Grip and arm strength in males and females, age 10 to 69, *Res Q* 48:109, 1977.

133. Montpetit RR, Montoye HJ, Laeding L: Grip strength of school children, Saginaw, Michigan, 1899 and 1964, *Res Q* 38:231, 1967.

134. Murray J: Presidential address, *J Hand Surg* 7:543, 1982.

135. Newman DG, et al: Norms for hand grip strength, *Arch Dis Child* 59:453, 1984.

136. Niebuhr BR, Marion R: Voluntary control of submaximal grip strength, *Am J Phys Med Rehabil* 69:96, 1990.

137. Niebuhr BR, Marion R, Hasson SM: Electromyographic analysis of effort in grip strength assessment, *Electromyogr Clin Neurophysiol* 33:149, 1993.

138. O'Driscoll S, Horii, E: The relationship between wrist position, grasp size, and grip strength, *J Hand Surg* 17A:169, 1992.

139. Omer GE Jr: Median nerve compression at the wrist, *Hand Clin* 8:317, 1992.

140. Onne L: Recovery of sensibility and sudomotor activity in the hand after severe injury, *Acta Chir Scand (Suppl)* 1:300, 1962.

141. O'Rain S: New and simple test for nerve function in the hand, *Br Med J* 3:615, 1973.

142. Palumbo CF, Szabo RM, Olmsted SL: The effects of hypothyroidism and thyroid replacement on the development of carpal tunnel syndrome (in process citation), *J Hand Surg* 25A:734, 2000.

143. Peeters GG, Aufdemkampe G, Oostendorp RA: Sensibility testing in patients with a lumbosacral radicular syndrome, *J Manipulative Physiol Ther* 21:81, 1998.

144. Peters M, Murphy K: Cluster analysis reveals at least three, and possibly five distinct handedness groups, *Neuropsychologia* 30:373, 1992.

145. Petersen P, et al: Grip strength and hand dominance: challenging the 10% rule, *Am J Occup Ther* 43:444, 1989.

146. Phelps P, Walker E: Comparison of the finer wrinkling test results to established sensory tests in peripheral nerve injury, *Am J Occup Ther* 31:565, 1977.

147. Phillips P: Grip strength, mental performance and nutritional status as indicators of mortality risk among female geriatric patients, *Age Ageing* 15:53, 1986.

148. Powell DM, et al: Computer analysis of the performance of the BTE Work Simulator, *J Burn Care Rehabil* 12:250, 1991.

149. Rantanen T, et al: Midlife hand grip strength as a predictor of old age disability, *JAMA* 281:558, 1999.

150. Reddon JR, et al: Hand dynamometer: effects of trials and sessions, *Percept Mot Skills* 61:1195, 1985.

151. Reddon JR, et al: Purdue Pegboard: test-retest estimates, *Percept Mot Skills* 66:503, 1988.

152. Ren K: An improved method for assessing mechanical allodynia in the rat, *Physiol Behav* 67:711, 1999.

153. Richards LG: Posture effects on grip strength, *Arch Phys Med Rehabil* 78:1154, 1997.

154. Richards LG, Olson B, Palmiter-Thomas P: How forearm position affects grip strength, *Am J Occup Ther* 50:133, 1996.

155. Rider B, Linden C: Comparison of standardized and non-standardized administration of the Jebsen Hand Function Test, *J Hand Ther* 1:121, 1988.

156. Rosen B: Recovery of sensory and motor function after nerve repair. A rationale for evaluation, *J Hand Ther* 9:315, 1996.

157. Rosen B, Dahlin LB, Lundborg G: Assessment of functional outcome after nerve repair in a longitudinal cohort, *Scand J Plast Reconstr Surg Hand Surg* 34:71, 2000.

158. Rothstein J, Miller P, Roetiger R: Goniometric reliability in a clinical setting: elbow and knee measurements, *Phys Ther* 63:1611, 1983.

159. Rothstein JM: Measurement and clinical practice: theory and application. In Rothstein JM: *Measurement in physical therapy: clinics in physical therapy,* New York, 1985, Churchill Livingstone.

160. Sabari JS, et al: Goniometric assessment of shoulder range of motion: comparison of testing in supine and sitting positions, *Arch Phys Med Rehabil* 79:647, 1998.

161. Schmidt G: Biomechanical analysis of knee flexion and extension, *J Biomech* 6:79, 1973.

162. Schmidt R, Toews, J: Grip strength as measured by the Jamar dynamometer, *Arch Phys Med Rehab* June:321, 1970.

163. Seddon H: *Surgical disorders of the peripheral nerves,* ed 2, New York 1973, Churchill Livingstone.

164. Seki T, Ohtsuki T: Influence of simultaneous bilateral exertion on muscle strength during voluntary submaximal isometric contraction, *Ergonomics* 33:1131, 1990.

165. Sharma S, Schumacher HR Jr, McLellan AT: Evaluation of the Jebsen hand function test for use in patients with rheumatoid arthritis [corrected] [published erratum appears in *Arthritis Care Res* 7:109, 1994], *Arthritis Care Res* 7:16, 1994.

166. Shectman O, Taylor C: The use of the rapid exchange grip test in detecting sincerity of effort, part I: administration, *J Hand Ther* 13:195, 2000.

167. Spaulding SJ, et al: Jebsen Hand Function Test: performance of the uninvolved hand in hemiplegia and of right-handed, right and left hemiplegic persons, *Arch Phys Med Rehabil* 69:419, 1988.

168. Spijkerman DC, et al: Standardization of grip strength measurements. Effects on repeatability and peak force, *Scand J Rehabil Med* 23:203, 1991.

169. Steenhuis RE, et al: Reliability of hand preference items and factors, *J Clin Exp Neuropsychol* 12:921, 1990.

170. Stern EB: Stability of the Jebsen-Taylor Hand Function Test across three test sessions, *Am J Occup Ther* 46:647, 1992.

171. Stillman B, McMeeken J: A video-based version of the pendulum test: technique and normal response, *Arch Phys Med Rehabil* 76:166, 1995.

172. Stokes H, et al: Identification of low-effort patients through dynamometry, *J Hand Surg* 20A:1047, 1995.

173. Su CY, et al: Grip strength: relationship to shoulder position in normal subjects, *Kao Hsiung I Hsueh Ko Hsueh Tsa Chih* 9:385, 1993.

174. Su CY, et al: Performance of normal Chinese adults on grip strength test: a preliminary study, *Kao Hsiung I Hsueh Ko Hsueh Tsa Chih* 10:145, 1994.

175. Sunderland A, et al: Arm function after stroke. An evaluation of grip strength as a measure of recovery and a prognostic indicator, *J Neurol Neurosurg Psychiatry* 52:1267, 1989.

176. Szabo RM, Gelberman RH, Dimick MP: Sensibility testing in patients with carpal tunnel syndrome, *J Bone Joint Surg* 66A:60, 1984.

177. Tairych GV, et al: Normal cutaneous sensibility of the breast, *Plast Reconstr Surg* 102:701, 1998.

178. Tan U: Normal distribution of hand preference and its bimodality, *Int J Neurosci* 68:61, 1993.

179. Tassler PL, Dellon AL: Correlation of measurements of pressure perception using the pressure-specified sensory device with electro-diagnostic testing, *J Occup Environ Med* 37:862, 1995.

180. Taylor C, Shechtman O: The use of the rapid exchange grip test in detecting sincerity of effort, part I: administration of the test, *J Hand Ther* 13:195, 2000.

181. Taylor N, Sand PL, Jebsen RH: Evaluation of hand function in children, *Arch Phys Med Rehabil* 54:129, 1973.

182. Temple CL, Hurst LN: Reduction mammaplasty improves breast sensibility, *Plast Reconstr Surg* 104:72, 1999.

183. Tiffin J, Asher E: The Purdue Pegboard: norms and studies of reliability and validity, *J Appl Psychol* 32:234, 1948.

184. Tredgett M, Pimble LJ, Davis TR: The detection of feigned hand weakness using the five position grip strength test, *J Hand Surg* 24B:426, 1999.

185. Trott SA, et al: Sensory changes after traditional and ultrasound-assisted liposuction using computer-assisted analysis, *Plast Reconstr Surg* 103:2016, 1999.

186. van Brakel WH, et al: Functional sensibility of the hand in leprosy patients, *Lepr Rev* 68:25, 1997.

187. Van Turnhout AA, et al: Lack of difference in sensibility between the dominant and non-dominant hands as tested with Semmes-Weinstein monofilaments, *J Hand Surg* 22B:768, 1997.

188. van Vliet D, Novak CB, Mackinnon SE: Duration of contact time alters cutaneous pressure threshold measurements, *Ann Plast Surg* 31:335, 1993.

189. Voerman VF, van Egmond J, Crul BJ: Normal values for sensory thresholds in the cervical dermatomes: a critical note on the use of Semmes-Weinstein monofilaments, *Am J Phys Med Rehabil* 78:24, 1999.

190. Voerman VF, van Egmond J, Crul BJ: Elevated detection thresholds for mechanical stimuli in chronic pain patients: support for a central mechanism, *Arch Phys Med Rehabil* 81:430, 2000.

191. Wagner C: Determination of the rotary flexibility of the elbow joint, *Eur J Appl Physiol* 37:47, 1977.

192. Walamies M, Turjanmaa V: Assessment of the reproducibility of strength and endurance handgrip parameters using a digital analyser, *Eur J Appl Physiol* 67:83, 1993.

193. Waylett-Rendall J: Sequence of sensory recovery: a retrospective study, *J Hand Ther* 2:245, 1989.

194. Waylett-Rendal J, Seibly D: A study of the accuracy of a commercially available volumeter, *J Hand Ther* 4:10, 1991.

195. Webber E: Data cited by Sherringron CS: *Shafer's textbook of physiology,* Edinburgh, 1900, Young J Pentland.

196. Weinstein S: Fifty years of somatosensory research: from the Semmes-Weinstein monofilaments to the Weinstein Enhanced Sensory Test, *J Hand Ther* 6:11, discussion 50, 1993.

197. Weise MD, et al: Lower-extremity sensibility testing in patients with herniated lumbar intervertebral discs, *J Bone Joint Surg* 67A:1219, 1985.

198. Wilke NA, et al: Baltimore Therapeutic Equipment work simulator: energy expenditure of work activities in cardiac patients, *Arch Phys Med Rehabil* 74:419, 1993.

199. Wise S, et al: Evaluation of a fiber optic glove for semi-automated goniometric measurements, *J Rehabil Res Dev* 27:411, 1990.

200. Young VL, et al: Fluctuation in grip and pinch strength among normal subjects, *J Hand Surg* 14A:125, 1989.

Chapter 17

OUTCOME MEASUREMENT
IN THE UPPER EXTREMITY

Joy C. MacDermid

WHAT IS AN OUTCOME MEASURE?

An outcome measure is any measurement of a patient's health status that can change. Health status can change as a result of time, treatment, or disease.

The World Health Organization has characterized health status by considering the effect of disease at various levels.[83] These levels have been characterized as impairment, disability, and handicap. Revision of the terminology has been proposed to emphasize the capability rather than the deficit, although the original terminology continues to be widely used. Although the "impairment" label remains unchanged, "disability" has been referred to as "activity" and "handicap" as "participation." Pathology affects the biologic level but can be manifested as an inability to perform tasks and fulfill normal societal roles. Thus the effect of pathology is mitigated by a variety of personal, psychologic, social, and societal factors.[17,35,41,83] Outcome instruments may measure this effect at different levels.

Impairment is the loss or abnormality of psychologic, physiologic, or anatomic structure or function.[83] Examples of impairments that hand therapists typically measure include hand size, appearance, strength, range of motion (ROM), volume, sensory threshold, and pain. Methods and interpretation for measuring impairments of the hand are the traditional focus of hand therapy and are detailed in many of the chapters in this book discussing evaluation.

Disability is the restriction or lack of ability to perform an activity in a manner or within a range that is considered normal.[83] Tests that measure disability by assessing performance of specific tasks includes tests such as the TEMPA,[24] Jebson Test of Hand Function,[39] Purdue Pegboard,[72] Minnesota Rate of Manipulation Test,[43] and other functional tests in which the patient is observed performing the specific task being evaluated. Disability can also be measured by

scoring the patient's ratings from questionnaires that ask about his or her ability to perform a specific task.

Handicap is a disadvantage for a given individual, resulting from impairment or a disability that limits or prevents the fulfilment of a role that is normal for that individual.[83] By definition, it depends on a variety of personal, psychosocial, societal, and cultural factors. Thus *handicap* is often defined by an individual person using health status questionnaires. Questionnaires that assess quality of life, satisfaction, or ability to perform an individual's usual role are measuring aspects of a handicap. Indicators of return-to-work status also reflect one aspect of a person's handicap.

A standardized outcome measure is one that has specific properties: It is published; there are detailed instructions on how to administer, score, and interpret the test; it has a defined purpose; it was designed for a specific population; and there are published data indicating acceptable reliability and validity.[21] Standardization in clinical measurement is essential to ensure that outcome measures are capable of providing valid information about a patient's health status.

HOW CAN CLINICIANS USE OUTCOME MEASURES?

Three evaluative procedures can be performed with outcome scores: evaluation of change over time, discrimination between groups of patients, and prediction of future status.[21,33,47]

Evaluation of change over time is the most common clinical purpose for measuring health status. Therapists need to know whether treatments are causing a change. Furthermore, therapists need to demonstrate to others that their treatment has resulted in a clinically important change. When designing a treatment plan, therapists determine which impairments are contributing to the disability and handicap and design a treatment program to minimize the extent of impairment and disability. When a treatment is designed to minimize a specific impairment, evaluation before and after is required to determine whether the impairment has been affected by the treatments selected. For example, if a therapist evaluates a tendon repair and decides that the tendon is not gliding, active range of motion (AROM) is appropriate to measure. Treatment for this patient would include a variety of interventions that are expected to improve tendon glide. The efficacy of these interventions would be determined by reevaluating the impairment in AROM.

Increasingly, therapists are using outcome measures to determine how their treatments affect disabilities and handicaps. If the impairments we treat are important and if we can make clinically significant changes in them, the treatment effect should be measurable not just at the impairment level but also at the disability and handicap level. Thus the patient who is treated because his or her tendon glide is impaired should experience improvements in ability to perform specific tasks such as gripping a handle (disability) and in quality of life. These effects should be measured on standardized outcome instruments.

When evaluation over time is being done on groups of patients, programs can be evaluated, subgroups who benefit most can be identified, quality improvement programs can be evaluated, or clinical research can be conducted. Outcome measures that are responsive (i.e., able to measure change over time) are essential to the evaluation of treatment effects resulting from hand therapy.

Discrimination between groups is required when the purpose is to discern cutoff points on a rating scale that can be used to identify certain outcomes.[33] Which patients have maintained sympathetic pain syndrome, which are able to return to work, and which require a nursing home? These are the types of questions that require a discriminative analysis. Although most therapists do not perform this type of analysis as part of their practice, they do read these types of research studies so that they can improve their skill in treatment planning and goal setting.

Finally, outcome measures can be used to predict future outcomes. What will be the final strength 1 year after a fracture? What is the final active motion of a distal interphalangeal (DIP) joint after a profundus repair? Who will return to work? Who will require surgery for median nerve compression? Can we predict preoperatively who will develop maintained sympathetic pain syndrome? These are prediction questions that might interest clinicians. Prediction analyses use scores on rating scales at some preliminary stage to predict future scores or outcomes.

Outcome measures have specific measurement properties that determine how well they function to evaluate change, discriminate, or predict. To a certain extent, these measurement properties can be competing; therefore an instrument designed for one type of analysis may not be suited to other types of analysis.[33] For example, AROM may be used to evaluate a change in tendon glide over time, but does AROM at baseline predict final AROM or ability to return to work? Does AROM at 8 weeks discriminate between patients who are capable of returning to work and those who are not? Although we have some evidence in our clinical literature on the evaluative aspects of AROM as an outcome measure, we really do not have much evidence on its predictive or discriminative properties. To truly understand clinical measurement, we need to understand important measurement properties of the measures we select and how these properties relate to different purposes and different clinical situations.

WHAT ARE THE IMPORTANT MEASUREMENT PROPERTIES OF OUTCOME MEASURES?

The three measurement properties fundamental to how a tool can be used are reliability, validity, and responsiveness.[21]

Reliability is the consistency or repeatability of a measurement. Reliability is fundamental to other measurement properties because without stability, the utility of any measure is compromised. However, high reliability, in itself, does not ensure that other measurement properties are also acceptable. Therefore both reliability and validity of outcome measures should be documented before clinicians use them to make decisions.

Measurements can be repeated by the same therapist (intrarater), by different therapists (interrater), or on different occasions (test-retest). Generally, intrarater reliability is higher than other forms of reliability analysis because the measurement error attributable to differences between testers and occasions is not considered. However, for evaluating patients over time, it is important to know that a measure remains constant over time if the patient remains stable (i.e., test-retest reliability). When we expect to share our measurements with others through clinical assessment notes, progress reports, or research studies, it is important that we present results that another therapist would attain if he or she performed the measurement (i.e., interrater reliability).

Standardized methods are important to attain reliability. It has been demonstrated that certain clinical measures such as ROM can be performed reliably by both novice and experienced therapists when a standardized method is used.[5] For this reason, detailed descriptions of how tests are performed should be documented in research studies and taught by hand therapy educators. Therapists should ensure that any measurement delegated to support personnel is one that can be performed reliably by a nontherapist with proper training in the correct procedure. Evidence for decisions about who should perform measurements and how the measurements should be performed is published in reliability studies. Differences in how tests are performed on different test occasions or by testers contributes to greater measurement error and thus makes it more difficult to assess when a true clinical change has occurred.

Reliability can be assessed using different statistics. Basic understanding of these statistics is important for clinicians because it helps them understand how to use published reliability studies to improve clinical expertise. Correlation coefficients are ratios of variance that approximate one when the relationship is perfect and disintegrate to zero when the measurements are not related to each other.[62] The intraclass correlation coefficient (ICC) is the format used when measurements are taken within the same class (i.e., repeated measurements).[25,68] The ICC is one of the most common statistics in reliability literature. Because these statistics are a ratio, they tend to be compared against benchmarks of what is acceptable reliability. Various benchmarks have been posed. Fleiss suggested that <.40 indicated poor reliability, that 0.40 to 0.75 was moderate, and that >.75 was excellent.[30] The problem with comparing a study result against a benchmark is that it portrays reliability as a pass/fail situation. However, measurement error occurs with every measurement. Statistics like the standard error of measurement (SEM) or mean error allow therapists to view measurement error in more quantitative terms.[13-16,36] For example, it has been shown that ROM measurements of elbow flexion and extension vary 3 to 5 degrees on average for the same tester and 5 to 8 degrees for different testers.[5] It is advisable for reliability studies to examine measurement error both in absolute quantity (SEM, mean error) and relative to group variability (ICC) so that the reader understands how the measurement is likely to perform when used for either individual patients or groups.

Quantifying the amount of error that occurs with specific types of clinical measures helps clinicians know whether observed changes are likely to indicate a treatment effect or not. When the change observed in a particular patient is greater than that which could be anticipated to occur because of measurement error, the clinician can say with confidence that the patient has changed. For this reason, outcome measures that are used to measure change in individual patients should have a high reliability (ICC > .75). Furthermore, therapists should incorporate techniques to minimize measurement error into their clinical practice. Taking the average of multiple measurements, standardized test protocols, training of testers, and regular calibration of instruments are steps used to reduce error in clinical measurement.

Validity is the extent to which the measure accurately portrays the aspect of health status that it was intended to describe. It can be thought of as the "trueness" of the measure.[21] Validity is difficult to ascertain in many cases because the true answer is often unknown. Furthermore, a measure may be valid for one purpose but not for other purposes. For example, a general health instrument may be a valid indication of overall health but may not be valid when assessing change in upper extremity function after certain hand injuries. Therefore validity needs to be assessed by a

variety of methods and in various situations. Validity is the cumulative evidence provided to support the use of outcome instruments in specific situations to perform specific analytic functions. For this reason, various forms of validity are recognized.

Content validity is the extent to which a measure represents an adequate sampling of the content. This can be ensured in the development of patient questionnaires by using survey and data analysis methods to determine which items are contained in a questionnaire.[32,47] It can be determined for developed questionnaires through consensus reviews or expert panels. For example, we would expect a carpal tunnel instrument to include questions about classic symptoms of carpal tunnel syndrome (CTS), such as numbness, tingling, and waking at night.[51]

Construct validity is the extent to which scores obtained agree with theories underlying the content. Testing constructs derived from the theoretical underpinnings of an instrument requires that relationships be investigated. Does the instrument relate to other instruments the way in which one would expect? Do groups expected to be different turn out to be different on the outcome measure evaluated (discriminant validity)? For example, do people with more severe fractures score more poorly? Do patients in a nursing home have lower scores than patients living independently?

Validity is an important aspect of clinical measurement and deserves increased attention by clinical researchers. Validity studies provide evidence as to whether an instrument can be used to make certain types of clinical decisions.

Clinicians are often tempted to devise their own instruments or modify existing instruments to make something that is directly applicable to their clinical situation. Although this may improve the validity of the modified scale to serve their specific purpose, the onus is on developers to prove that new or modified instruments are both reliable and valid.

WHAT DO I NEED TO KNOW BEFORE USING OUTCOME TOOLS?

It is important to select the right instrument for the purpose required and to ensure that the instrument is used correctly in any clinical evaluation. Numerous methods and measures have been developed for clinical evaluation. A literature search may uncover instruments that are related to your specific needs. Because development of an instrument is a time-consuming process, a thorough search of the literature for a measure that meets your clinical evaluation needs is advisable. Then literature on the measurement properties of potentially useful instruments should be reviewed to determine which ones have acceptable measurement properties.

Once a measure with acceptable measurement properties has been identified, the clinician needs to investigate issues of practicality. Some patient questionnaires require permission from the authors and/or payment before being used. The time required to complete the test, language requirements, cost, data analysis requirements, and training requirements must be determined. Consideration of all of these factors is required before clinicians can determine which instrument is most appropriate for their clinical practice.

Standards for the use of measures have been described in 1991 by the American Physical Therapy Association's Task Force in their *Standards for Tests and Measurements in Physical Therapy.*[4] Other sources of information on standardization are the Advisory Group on Measurement Standards of the American Congress of Rehabilitation Medicine and a variety of publications that focus on outcome measures.[42] The general standards for use of measures discussed here are also addressed elsewhere.[4,21,42]

Users of measures should know the technical aspects of the instrument; that is, they should have documentation of the scoring, interpretation, reliability, and validity of the instrument. Some instruments, such as the Disability of the Arm, Shoulder and Hand (DASH)[75] or the Patient-Rated Wrist Evaluation (PRWE),[52] can be easily scored by the therapist at the time of evaluation. Others have more complicated scoring algorithms, such as Short-Form 36 (SF-36).[77,79]

When using an instrument, one should be certain that one has a valid basis to do so. Is the measure appropriate for the population on which it will be applied? Is it able to measure the amount of change expected or a clinically important change in status? Is it the "right" measure for the patient characteristics that are of clinical interest?

Clinicians also should know and reveal to others the importance of specific measures in the decision-making process. For example, when evaluating whether a patient is benefitting from a home transcutaneous electrical nerve stimulation (TENS) unit, one might assess both a pain scale and a quality-of-life scale. The therapist should be able to state, before treatment, that the purpose of the TENS unit is to decrease pain and increase quality of life. If concrete changes in these two outcomes can be documented with use of TENS, its continued use can be justified. If the outcome measures do not indicate that these changes have occurred, TENS is discontinued.

Measures should be used by the individuals who have the necessary training, experience, and or professional qualifications. Certain types of evaluations tend to fall in the domain of specific professionals. For example, certain psychometric evaluations are performed only by licensed psychologists. There are some aspects of hand evaluation that require the expertise of a trained hand therapist. However, a number of outcomes can be evaluated by other professionals or even support staff. One purpose of reliability studies is to define what level of training and experience is required to administer a measure. Some assessments may not be technically demanding, and thus both inexperienced and experienced testers may achieve highly reliable results. For example, elbow flexion and extension and forearm rotation have been shown to be reliably measured when the

tester is either an experienced orthopedic surgeon, an experienced hand therapist, or an inexperienced physical therapist.[5] Some physical assessments may require greater technical skill. For example, passive movement characteristics of the shoulder have been measured reliably when the tester is an experienced manual therapist.[19]

Therapists should make themselves aware of the training procedures required to properly administer a test and ensure that they are adhered to. One problem in many tests within the realm of hand therapy is that the detail on how to perform the test and/or train personnel to perform the test is incomplete. Dexterity tests such as the Jebson Hand Function Test are widely used to assess patient outcomes. However, the detail on how the test is performed is insufficient, resulting in variations in how different clinicians perform the test. Therapists can find details about how to perform a test in a manual or reliability studies. When the details of how to perform a test are incomplete, it is the tester's responsibility to investigate where more detailed instructions may be found and to document the specific methodology used.

In addition, therapists should know what normative data or comparative data were collected for the measures that they use. For example, when commenting on a patient's strength, it is advisable to compare the patient's injured hand with the best estimate of that particular patient's normal strength (i.e., his or her uninjured side) and to also compare that patient's strength against scores considered normal for patients of a similar size, age, and sex. Thus conclusions about the extent of strength recovered during rehabilitation or ability to perform strength-based tasks are made on the basis of quantified data. When outcomes are health status questionnaires like the SF-36, normative data and data for pathologic conditions are available for comparison.[79] When more specific instruments like the DASH, Patient-rated wrist evaluation, or a CTS questionnaire are used, comparative data may be less accessible. Few of these instruments have published normative data, and it is often assumed that the absence of pain and disability is normal. However, with aging, pain and disability become more prevalent and may be considered more "normal"; thus we do not know the true normal score for many disability questionnaires. In these types of patient questionnaires, we should compare our data against the long-term results of similar patients in published case series.

Use of comparative data requires that we understand which patient characteristics are expected to influence the outcome. For example, therapists should have access to normative data for hand strength. A number of factors are known to be important predictors of hand strength, including hand size, age, sex, and body size. Clinicians should have tables or equations that will take these predictors into consideration when assessing whether a particular patient's hand strength is abnormal. With respect to patient questionnaires, it is important to have comparative data of specific pathologic conditions at various stages of recovery so that comparisons can be made as to the severity of any given score. Therapists also should consider the cost benefit aspects of any measure to which they expose a patient. Is there any risk? For example, when testing a patient's maximal strength, is there any risk of injury such as tendon rupture, muscle strain, or fracture displacement? When asking patients to complete questionnaires, one must consider that the patient's time has value and that unless the questions are meaningful, you might be wasting the patient's time. The therapist must be convinced that the outcome evaluation has the potential to provide the patient benefit. This benefit may be better treatment, an appropriate disability pension, a correct diagnosis, or appropriate job restrictions.

Therapists should know the proper environmental conditions and equipment requirements for completing the outcome evaluation. For example, evaluation of sensory thresholds requires specific equipment and environmental conditions. The patient must be positioned properly, and the surroundings must be quiet if an accurate measurement is to be achieved. Instruments must be sensitive to small increments in pressure and must be calibrated to ensure that they remain consistent over time. Environment can also affect questionnaires. Patients may feel uneasy about expressing dissatisfaction to their doctor or therapist, but they can be more frank when an independent assessor administers the questions.

When tests are used to diagnose or classify patients, the therapist should be aware of the sensitivity, specificity, and pretest probability of the tests. Clinical diagnostic tests such as provocative testing provide insight into the probability of a diagnosis but should be interpreted considering the potential for measurement error.

HOW DO I FIND OUTCOME MEASURES THAT ARE SUITABLE FOR ME?

The first step in identifying an appropriate instrument is to decide which clinical characteristics are most relevant to your patient population. Outcome measures can be found by searching the literature and textbooks. By searching the topic area that pertains to your clinical practice, you should locate instruments relevant to your clinical population. Sometimes, the instrument will be published and thus readily available; other times, you may need to contact authors to obtain it. Before using any instrument, you should ensure that you have proper and updated forms or equipment and are aware of the proper scoring of the instrument. The *Journal of Hand Therapy* and reference lists at the end of chapters in this text are good sources of articles that document reliable and valid methods of measuring both impairment and disability as they relate to hand therapy.

A number of scales that combine measures of impairments, such as ROM and strength, have been devised, with ability to perform specific tasks—usually evaluated by the clinician. Example of such scales are the Mayo Performance Index (MEPI)[61] and the Constant-Murley score.[22] Scores from these scales are often rated as excellent, good, fair, or poor so that the number of each type of result can be reported in case series or outcome studies. Clinicians should be aware that these scales have limitations. The subjective categories are not meaningful because they have not been validated, are not consistent between scales, and are not reliable.[73] These scales tend to be developed according to observer opinion rather than by a systematic method. Items included and their weighting are arbitrary. The reliability and validity of these scales tends to be poorly addressed. Furthermore, because the disabilities are recorded by the observer, not the patient, a potential for bias exists. Considering these limitations, it seems advisable for therapists to measure impairments separate from measures of disability and to report raw scores rather than subjective ratings for outcomes.

Patient rating scales allow patients to self-report the extent of difficulty they are experiencing. Table 17-1 describes patient rating scales that can be used to measure disability in the upper extremity.

When introducing a new impairment or disability measure into your clinical practice, you must ensure that it is used as designed by the developers. Sometimes, because of the space limitations in scientific journals, the methodology description for tests has been abbreviated and the detail is insufficient to allow replication. In these cases, the user is obligated to contact the authors of the new methodology to provide more precise instructions.

HOW DO I ADMINISTER THE OUTCOME MEASURE TO MEASURE CHANGE IN MY PATIENTS?

When using outcome tools to assess change in individual patients, a number of practical details must be considered. Who will administer the questionnaire? Some therapists like to introduce the questionnaire to their patients as a way to facilitate their subjective evaluation of them. Other therapists prefer the questionnaire to be administered by an independent person to minimize the opportunity for bias. My personal preference is to have an independent person provide the questionnaire and provide assistance with completing it only to the extent required.

The way in which the questionnaire is administered may depend on the patient's capacity. The effect of illiteracy is grossly underestimated. When patients ask a spouse or family member to fill out forms, refuse to cooperate, or ask to take questionnaires home, illiteracy may be the underlying reason. Others may try to mask their illiteracy by completing the forms, but their answers will be nonsensical. By offering to read questions to patients in a circumspect way, one can allow these patients the opportunity to convey their opinions on their status without insulting their dignity.

It is important to have a plan of how often outcome instruments will be administered. A baseline and final status

Text continued on p. 294

Table 17-1. Patient rating scales for outcome evaluation in the upper extremity

Measure	Purpose	Format	Reliability	Validity	Responsiveness
Visual Analogue Scales (VAS)— Pain[18,26,27,40,50,80]	To measure quantity of pain	10-cm line—in a variety of formats; requires careful instruction; score is distance from zero (no pain) to end (worst pain imaginable)	Can vary, but high test-retest has been demonstrated[26,67]	High correlation between VAS and numeric pain rating scale,[27] finger dynamometer,[80] and a verbal description of pain[80]	Able to detect 21 levels of just noticeable differences[50]; some believe that it is less sensitive to change in acute pain than in chronic pain[18]
Numeric Rating Scales (NRS)—Pain	To measure quantity of pain	0-10 scale for pain administered verbally or on paper; typically 0 = no pain and 10 = worst pain imaginable	Not specifically reported but high when used as a subscale in other measures[54]	High correlation with VAS,[27] finger dynamometer,[80] and other outcome measures	High in distal radius fractures as subscale[56]
Sickness Impact Profile (SIP)[10-12]	Health status across demographic and cultural groups	136 items that are divided into two dimensions (physical and psychosocial) and 12 categories	Internal consistency test-retest and interrater reliability (interview) are all high	Construct, concurrent validity, reported[11]; has not been widely used for upper extremity	Responsive in low back pain[25]
(Medical Outcomes) Short-Form SF-36[77,79]	Health status across demographic and cultural groups	36 items; 8 subscales (physical function, physical role, vitality, bodily pain, general health, social function, emotional role, and mental health and vitality); two summary component scales are calculated (physical and mental), which standardize the patient's score to the U.S. population norms	Has been reported to be high[77,79]	Numerous validity studies and normative data abundant[77,79]; instrument well supported by Medical Outcomes Trust; may be preferable to sickness impact profile[70]; authors suggest that for upper extremity it should be combined with a more specific instrument[8,9]	Less responsive than the DASH or patient-rated wrist evaluation in evaluating wrist fractures[56]
(Medical Outcomes) Short-Form SF-12[78]	Health status across demographic and cultural groups	12 items; two summary component scales are calculated (physical and mental), which standardize the patient's score to the U.S. population norms	Has been reported to be high[77,79]	Numerous validity studies and normative data abundant[77,79]; instrument well supported by Medical Outcomes Trust; may be preferable to Sickness Impact Profile[70]	Summary scores less responsive than the DASH or patient-rated wrist evaluation in evaluating wrist fractures[55]

Instrument	Purpose	Description	Reliability	Validity	Responsiveness
Musculoskeletal Function Assessment (MFA)[28,29,57,58,71]	Health status instrument for use with a broad range of musculoskeletal disorders; to complement SF-36	100 items; subscales include self-care, sleep/rest, hand/fine motor, mobility, housework, employment/work, leisure/recreation, family relationships, cognition/thinking, emotional adjustment	High[71]	Appropriate correlations with other instruments and other clinical measures[29,58,71]; normative and comparison data reported[28]	Moderate to large effect sizes reported
Disability, Arm, Shoulder and Hand (DASH)[9,26,37,54,74,75]	Upper-extremity disability	30 items rated 1-5; majority of questions assess upper extremity function	Can be high[9,75]	Construct validity has been demonstrated[9,38,75]	More responsive than generic measures for patients with upper extremity pathology[56,75]; shown to be reliable, valid, and responsive for a variety of upper extremity problems,[9] for ulnar-sided wrist problems,[38] and for distal radius fractures[56]
Upper Extremity Function Scale (UEFS)[64]	To measure impact of upper-extremity disorders on function	8 items scored 0-10	Internal consistency high	Excellent convergent and discriminative validity when compared with measures of symptom severity[64]	More responsive than grip and pinch in CTS[64]
Shoulder Pain and Disability Index (SPADI)[8,34,66,81]	Shoulder pain and disability	Pain and disability scored as 50% each; items scored on a visual or numeric analog scale; 5 pain questions, 8 function; a numeric (0-10) version has been shown to be highly correlated with VAS version[81]	High internal consistency and moderate test-retest[59]	Construct and criterion validity have been evaluated[59,81]	Discriminated with high likelihood between patients who were better or worse[81]
Shoulder Rating Questionnaire[49]	Severity of symptoms and functional status of the shoulder	21 questions in total, including 1 global rating on a VAS and 18 questions in a likert format—4 pain, 5 ADL, 3 recreation, 4 work, 1 satisfaction	High internal consistency and test-retest reliability[49]	Moderate to high validity coefficients compared with arthritis impact measurement scales[49]	Responsive[49]
Western Ontario Rotator Cuff WORC[2]	Quality of life in patients with rotator cuff pathology	21 questions on visual analog scales; sections on physical symptoms, sports/recreation, work, lifestyle, and emotions	High	Moderate correlation with strength and ROM in patients with rotator cuff[31]	Manuscript in progress; presented but not published

Continued

Table 17-1. Patient rating scales for outcome evaluation in the upper extremity—cont'd

Measure	Purpose	Format	Reliability	Validity	Responsiveness
Western Ontario Instability Index WOSI[45]	Quality of life in patients with shoulder instability	21 questions on visual analog scales; sections on physical symptoms, sports/recreation, work, lifestyle, and emotions	High[45]	Correlated appropriately with other instruments[45]	More responsive than 5 other instruments (DASH, ASES, UCLA, Constant score and Rowe Rating)[45]
Shoulder Arthritis Questionnaire (publication in process by above authors)[46]	Quality of life in patients with shoulder osteoarthritis	19 questions on visual analog scales; sections on physical symptoms, sports/recreation, work, lifestyle, and emotions	Not published	Not published yet; same format as previously published shoulder scales[2,45]	Not published
American Shoulder and Elbow Surgeons (ASES) Patient Form[65]	Patient-rated pain and disability for a wide variety of shoulder problems	1 pain question (VAS); 10 function questions (0-3)	Shown to have high reliability and internal consistency[60]	Construct, content, and discriminative validity demonstrated[60]	Not published
Shoulder Pain Score[82]	For assessing pain in patients with shoulder pathology	7 questions; 5 on a 4-point Likert scale and 1 VAS for global rating of pain	Not published	Factor analysis used to determine that question addresses two factors considered passive and active situations by authors[82]	Not published
Constant Shoulder Score (patient component)[22]	Used for a variety of shoulder problems, including instability	Pain rated 0-4; function (work, recreation, sleep position of arm work)	Not published		Not published
Shoulder Disability Questionnaire[76]	Functional disability in patients with shoulder disorders	16 yes/no questions on pain, related disability	Not published		Responsive in 349 primary care patients with shoulder disorders[76]
Subjective Shoulder Rating Scale[48]	To briefly measure subjective shoulder complaints	Multiple-choice questions; 1 pain, 1 motion, 1 stability, and 1 activity	Not published	Highly correlated to Constant-Murley score but much faster to complete[48]	Not published
Simple Shoulder Test[59]		Yes/no responses; 2 pain, 7 function, 3 motion questions		Discriminant in patients with rotator cuff pathology[31]	
American Shoulder and Elbow Surgeons (ASES) Elbow Form[44]	To measure pain, disability, and patient satisfaction in patients with elbow pathology	Patient rating scales for pain ranked 0-10 for 5 pain items, 0-3 for 12 function items, and 0-10 for 1 satisfaction question	High[53]	Appropriate (high) correlation with patient-rated elbow evaluation[53]	Not published
Patient Rated Elbow Evaluation (PREE)[53]	To measure pain and disability in patients with elbow pathology	5 pain questions scored 0-10; 15 function questions scored 0-10	High[53]	Appropriate (high) correlation with ASES elbow form[53]	Not published

Instrument	Purpose	Items	Reliability	Validity	Responsiveness
Patient-Rated Ulnar Nerve Evaluation	For patients with symptoms of ulnar nerve compression	Pain, sensory/motor scale, and function subscales	Not published	Not published; format similar to previous questionnaires by same author[53]	Not published
Forearm Rating Scale[63]	To measure pain and disability in patients with lateral epicondylitis	Items scores 0-10; 5 pain items; 6 specific function tasks; 4 items on usual ability in personal care, work, household work, and recreation	Excellent test-retest reliability[63]	Not published	Not published
Patient-Rated Wrist Evaluation[52,54,56]	To measure pain and disability in patients with wrist pathology	Items scores 0-10; 5 pain items; 6 specific function tasks; 4 items on usual ability in personal care, work, household work, and recreation	High test-retest[52,54]	Content based on expert survey/patient interviews construct and criterion validity evaluated[52,54]	More responsive than DASH or SF-36 for wrist fractures[56]
(Carpal Tunnel) Symptom Severity Scale and Functional Scale[51]	To measure severity of symptoms in patients with carpal tunnel syndrome; to measure functional problems in patients with carpal tunnel syndrome	5 point Likert score questions in 2 subscales; symptom severity scale has 11 items; function subscale has 8 items	High in original format and a modified Swedish version[7,51]	Symptom severity scales differentiated between patients with CTS and without CTS[6]; a modified version added 2 items on palmar pain, 8 items on satisfaction, and 4 items on patient opinions on satisfaction with surgery; this scale was translated into Swedish and shown to be valid[7]	More responsive than generic measures or impairment scores[3]; responsive in Swedish version[7]
Alderson-McGall Hand Function Questionnaire[1]	To measure hand function in patients with CTS	Items rated 1-7	High internal consistency in pilot data (17 carpal tunnel patients)		
Michigan Hand Questionnaire[20]	Health domains in patients with hand disorders	37 items: domains overall hand function, activities of daily living, pain, work performance, aesthetics, and patient satisfaction	Substantial test-retest reliability[20]	Factor analysis supported subscales; appropriate correlations between subscales and with SF-12; discriminant validity demonstrated[20]	
Patient Specific[69]	To measure severity of problems in patients self-selected items	Patients select up to 5 items and rank difficulty 0-10			Preliminary results reported suggest appropriate responsiveness

ADL, Activities of daily living; *CTS,* carpal tunnel syndrome; *ROM,* range of motion.

evaluation are the minimum requirements to determine the effect of treatment. However, when instruments are used throughout a treatment program, they can be used to assess the course of recovery. In this case, they must be applied at intervals over which important clinical change is expected to occur. Instruments should generally not be reapplied within the same week because patients can be anticipated to be relatively stable within this time frame. Overly frequent application of instruments may allow patients to remember their previous responses and contaminate the validity of your evaluation process.

Some forms of clinical evaluation (i.e., research, program evaluation, quality improvement, and marketing research) may require that a postdischarge evaluation be performed. This evaluation is generally considered a final outcome. It should be performed when surgical and rehabilitation efforts have been maximized and a patient has resumed normal activity. Long-term follow-up can also be performed to gauge deterioration in patients with chronic disease or to gauge the effects of long-term complications.

HOW DO I ANALYZE THE EFFECT OF MY TREATMENT ON OUTCOME?

Treatment effects are the change in score from baseline evaluation. For individual patients, this information is descriptive. When measuring changes in impairment or disability scores for individual patients, the emphasis should be on whether this represents a clinically important change and whether patients have reached a "normal" score. When analyzing group data for research or program evaluation, an analysis that takes into consideration the repeated nature of the measurement is indicated. Where only a baseline evaluation and final evaluation are performed, a simple paired t-test is sufficient. When multiple time frames have been measured, a repeated-measures analysis of variance is required to detect change over time. More complicated statistical analyses can be used to adjust for important predictors of outcome.

WHAT ARE IMPORTANT PREDICTORS OF OUTCOME?

When measuring outcome and describing it to others, it is important to know and document important predictors of outcome. Unfortunately, we are at a preliminary stage in our understanding of how impairment translates into disability and handicap. Understanding this relationship is important in providing an accurate prognosis for patients, determining who will benefit from treatment, and designing treatment programs that focus on the critical components of the disability and handicap. The traditional predictors that are documented with all clinical phenomena are age and sex.

Severity of injury is an important consideration in evaluating outcome. Therapists need to understand how severity of injury affects prognosis and treatment response. For ex-

ample, it has been suggested that conservative management is most effective for mild CTS. Our outcome data on distal radius fractures suggest that patients with more severe fractures (i.e., those with more radial shortening) will experience more pain and disability in their long-term outcome.[55] On the other hand, patients with severe limitation at a baseline assessment have the most "room for improvement" and may experience the greatest change in raw scores.

Patient characteristics can also be powerful predictors of outcome. Further research is required to fully understand which patient characteristics affect outcome in upper extremity conditions. When patient characteristics and injury characteristics present at baseline evaluation of distal radius fractures are evaluated, the most important predictor of the extent of pain and disability at 6 months after fractures was the potential for secondary gain (i.e., legal or worker's compensation).[55] Level of education was also shown to be predictive of outcome. Educational level may relate to a number of other factors, such as ability to modify job demands, ability to acquire less demanding employment, ability to understand home programs, and compliance.

CONCLUSIONS

Hand therapists assess their patients to determine how pathology of the upper limb has caused impairment, disability, and handicap. They formulate treatment plans to mitigate these problems and assess the treatment program effectiveness by using standardized outcome evaluations. The foundations of hand therapy rest on standardized outcome measures used to improve our ability to diagnose patients, assess change in patient status, predict future outcomes, conduct clinical research, and institute continuous quality improvement.

REFERENCES

1. Alderson M, McGall D: The Alderson-McGall hand function questionnaire for patients with carpal tunnel syndrome: a pilot evaluation of a future outcome measure, *J Hand Ther* 12:313, 1999.
2. Alvarez C, et al: *The development and evaluation of a disease specific quality of life measurement tool for rotator cuff disease.* Annual Meeting Book of Abstracts, New Orleans, 1998, American Academy of Orthopaedic Surgeons.
3. Amadio PC, et al: Outcome assessment for carpal tunnel surgery: the relative responsiveness of generic, arthritis-specific, disease-specific, and physical examination measures, *J Hand Surg Am* 21:338, 1996.
4. American Physical Therapy Association's Task Force on Standards for Measurements in Physical Therapy: Standards for tests and measurements in physical therapy, *Phys Ther* 71:589, 2000.
5. Armstrong AD, et al: Reliability of range-of-motion measurement in the elbow and forearm, *J Shoulder Elbow Surg* 7:573, 1998.
6. Atroshi I, Breidenbach WC, McCabe SJ: Assessment of the carpal tunnel outcome instrument in patients with nerve-compression symptoms, *J Hand Surg* 22A:222, 1997.
7. Atroshi I, Johnsson R, Sprinchorn A: Self-administered outcome instrument in carpal tunnel syndrome: reliability, validity and responsiveness evaluated in 102 patients, *Acta Orthop Scand* 69:82, 1998.
8. Beaton DE, Richards RR: Measuring function of the shoulder: a cross-sectional study of five questionnaires, *J Bone Joint Surg Am* 78A:882, 1996.

9. Beaton DE, et al: Measuring the whole or parts? Validity, reliability and responsiveness of the DASH outcome measure in different regions of the upper extremity, *J Hand Ther* 14:128, 2001.

10. Bergner M, et al: The sickness impact profile: conceptual formulation and methodology for the development of a health status measure, *Int J Health Serv* 6:393, 1976.

11. Bergner M, et al: The sickness impact profile: validation of a health measure, *Med Care* 14:57, 1976.

12. Bergner M, et al: The sickness impact profile: development and final revision of a health status measure, *Med Care* 19:787, 1981.

13. Bland JM, Altman DG: Statistical methods for assessing agreement between two methods of clinical measurement, *Lancet* 1:307, 1986.

14. Bland JM, Altman DG: Statistical methods for assessing agreement between measurements, *Biochem Clin* 11:399, 1987.

15. Bland JM, Altman DG: A note on the use of the intraclass correlation coefficient in the evaluation of agreement between two methods of measurement, *Comput Biol Med* 20:337, 1990.

16. Bland JM, Altman DG: This week's citation classic: comparing methods of measurement, *Curr Contents* 40:8, 1992.

17. Brandsma JW, Heerkens YF, van Ravensberg CD: Impairments and disabilities in hand therapy: the necessity of a uniform terminology for communication and research purposes, *J Hand Ther* 6:252, 1993.

18. Carlsson AM: Assessment of chronic pain part 1: aspects of reliability and validity of the visual analogue scale, *Pain* 16:87, 1983.

19. Chesworth BM, et al: Movement diagram and "end-feel" reliability when measuring passive lateral rotation of the shoulder in patients with shoulder pathology, *Phys Ther* 78:593, 1998.

20. Chung KC, et al: Reliability and validity testing of the Michigan Hand Outcomes Questionnaire, *J Hand Surg Am* 23:575, 1998.

21. Cole B, Finch E, Gowland C: Physical outcome measures, Toronto, 1993, Canadian Physiotherapy Association.

22. Constant CR, Murley AHG: A clinical method of functional assessment of the shoulder, *Clin Orthop* 214:160, 1987.

23. Davis AM, et al: Measuring disability of the upper extremity: a rationale supporting the use of a regional outcome measure, *J Hand Ther* 12:269, 1999.

24. Desrosiers J, et al: Development and reliability of an upper extremity function test for the elderly: the TEMPA, *Can J Occup Ther* 60:9, 1993.

25. Deyo RA, Diehr P, Patrick DL: Reproducibility and responsiveness of health status measures: statistics and strategies for evaluation, *Control Clin Trials* 12:142S, 1991.

26. Dixon JS, Bird HA: Reproducibility along a 10cm vertical visual analogue scale, *Ann Rheum Dis* 40:87, 1981.

27. Downie WW, Leatham PA, Rhind VM: Studies with pain rating scales, *Ann Rheum Dis* 37:378, 1978.

28. Engelberg R, et al: Musculoskeletal Function Assessment instrument: criterion and construct validity, *J Orthop Res* 14:182, 1996.

29. Engelberg R, et al: Musculoskeletal function assessment: reference values for patient and non-patient samples, *J Orthop Res* 17:101, 1999.

30. Fleiss JL: Reliability of measurement. In Fleiss JL, editor: *The design and analysis of clinical experiments,* Toronto, 1986, John Wiley & Son.

31. Getahun T, MacDermid JC, Patterson SD: Concurrent validity of patient rating scales in assessment of outcome after rotator cuff repair, *J Musculoskel Res* 4:119, 2000.

32. Guyatt G, Feeny D, Patrick D: Issues in quality-of-life measurement in clinical trials, *Control Clin Trials* 12:81S, 1991.

33. Guyatt GH, Feeny DH, Patrick DL: Measuring health-related quality of life, *Ann Intern Med* 118:622, 1993.

34. Heald SL, Riddle DL, Lamb RL: The shoulder pain and disability index: the construct validity and responsiveness of a region specific disability measure, *Phys Ther* 77:1079, 1997.

35. Heekens YF, et al: Impairments and disabilities: the difference—proposal for adjustment of the international classification of impairments, disabilities and handicaps, *Phys Ther* 74:430, 1994.

36. Hove LM, et al: Fractures of the distal radius in a Norwegian city, *Scand J Plast Reconstr Surg Hand Surg* 29:263, 1995.

37. Hudak PL, Amadio PC, Bombardier C, The Upper Extremity Collaborative Group: Development of an upper extremity outcome measure: the Dash (disabilities of the arm, shoulder and head [sic]). *Am J Ind Med* 29:602, 1996.

38. Jain R, Hudak PL, Bowen CVA: The validity of health status measures in patients with ulnar wrist disorders, *J Hand Ther* 14:147, 2001.

39. Jebson RH, et al: An objective and standardized test of hand function, *Arch Phys Med Rehabil* 50:311, 1969.

40. Jensen MP, Karoly P, Braver S: The measurement of clinical pain intensity: a comparison of six methods, *Pain* 27:117, 1986.

41. Jette AM: Physical disablement concepts for physical therapy research and practice, *Phys Ther* 74:380, 1994.

42. Johnston MV, Keith RA, Hinderer SR: Measurement standards for interdisciplinary medical rehabilitation, *Arch Phys Med Rehabil* 73:S3, 2000.

43. Jurgenson CE: Extension of the Minnesota Rate of Manipulation Test, *J Appl Psych* 27:164, 1943.

44. King GJW, et al: A standardized method for assessment of elbow function, *J Should Elbow Surg* 8:351, 1999.

45. Kirkley A, et al: The development and evaluation of a disease-specific quality of life measurement tool for shoulder instability: the Western Ontario Shoulder Instability Index (WOSI), *Am J Sports Med* 26:764, 1998.

46. Kirkley A, et al: *Shoulder arthritis questionnaire,* Orlando, 2000, American Society of Elbow and Shoulder Surgeons Specialty Day.

47. Kirshner B, Guyatt G: A methodological framework for assessing health indices, *J Chronic Dis* 38:27, 1985.

48. Kohn D, Geyer M: The subjective shoulder rating system, *Arch Orthop Trauma Surg* 116:324, 1997.

49. L'Insalata JC, et al: A self-administered questionnaire for assessment of symptoms and function of the shoulder (see comments). *J Bone Joint Surg* 79A:738, 1997.

50. Langley GB, Sheppeard H: The visual analogue scale: its use in pain measurement, *Rheumatol Int* 4:145, 1985.

51. Levine DW, et al: A self-administered questionnaire for assessment of severity of symptoms and functional status in carpal tunnel syndrome, *J Bone Joint Surg Am* 75A:1585, 1993.

52. MacDermid JC: Development of a scale for patient rating of wrist pain and disability, *J Hand Ther* 9:178, 1996.

53. MacDermid JC: Reliability and validity of the patient rated elbow evaluation compared to the ASES Elbow Form, DASH and SF-36, *J Hand Ther* 14:105, 2001.

54. MacDermid JC, et al: Patient rating of wrist pain and disability: a reliable and valid measurement tool, *J Orthop Trauma* 12:577, 1998.

55. MacDermid DC, et al: Baseline predictors of pain and disability six-months after a distal radius fracture. In MacDermid JC, editor: *Baseline predictors of pain and disability six-months following distal radius fracture,* London, Ontario, 1999, University of Western Ontario.

56. MacDermid JC, et al: Responsiveness of the Sf-36, DASH, patient rated wrist evaluation and physical impairments in evaluating recovery after a distal radius fracture, *J Hand Surg Am* 25A:330, 2000.

57. Martin DP, et al: Development of a musculoskeletal extremity health status instrument: the Musculoskeletal Function Assessment instrument, *J Orthop Res* 14:173, 1996.

58. Martin DP, et al: Comparison of the Musculoskeletal Function Assessment questionnaire with the Short Form-36, the Western Ontario and McMaster Universities Osteoarthritis Index, and the Sickness Impact Profile health-status measures, *J Bone Joint Surg Am* 79:1323, 1997.

59. Matsen FA, et al: Evaluating the shoulder. In *Practical evaluation and management of the shoulder,* Philadelphia, 1994, WB Saunders.

60. Michener LA, McClure PW, Sennett BJ: American Shoulder and Elbow Surgeons standardized shoulder assessment form: reliability, validity and responsiveness, *J Orthop Sports Phys Ther* 30:A-30, 2000.

61. Morrey BF, An KN, Chao EYS: Functional evaluation of the elbow. In Morrey BF, editor: *The elbow and its disorders,* Philadelphia, 2000, WB Saunders.

62. Norman GR, Streiner DL: *Biostatistics: the bare essentials,* St Louis, 1994, Mosby.

63. Overend TJ, et al: Reliability of a patient-rated forearm evaluation questionnaire for patients with lateral epicondylitis, *J Hand Ther* 12:31, 1999.

64. Pransky G, et al: Measuring functional outcomes in work-related upper extremity disorders: development and validation of the Upper Extremity Function Scale, *J Occup Environ Med* 39:1195, 1997.

65. Richards RR, et al: A standardized method for the assessment of shoulder function, *J Shoulder Elbow Surg* 3:347, 1994.

66. Roach KE, et al: Development of a shoulder pain and disability index, *Arth Care Res* 4:143, 1991.

67. Scott J, Huskisson EC: Vertical or horizontal visual analogue scales, *Ann Rheum Dis* 38:560, 1979.

68. Shrout PE, Fleiss JL: Intraclass correlations: uses in assessing rater reliability, *Psychol Bull* 86:420, 1979.

69. Stratford P, et al: Assessing disability and change of individual patients: a report of a patient specific measure, *Physiother Can* 47:258, 1995.

70. Stucki G, et al: The Short Form-36 is preferable to the SIP as a generic health status measure in patients undergoing elective total hip arthroplasty, *Arthritis Care Res* 8:174, 1995.

71. Swiontkowski MF, et al: Short musculoskeletal function assessment questionnaire: validity, reliability, and responsiveness, *J Bone Joint Surg* 81A:1245, 1999.

72. Tiffin J, Asher EJ: The Purdue Pegboard: norms and studies of reliability and validity, *J Appl Psych* 32:234, 1948.

73. Turchin DC, Beaton DE, Richards RR: Validity of observer-based aggregate scoring systems as descriptors of elbow pain, function and disability, *J Bone Joint Surg Am* 80A:154, 1998.

74. Upper Extremity Collaborative Group: Measuring disability and symptoms of the upper limb: a validation study of the DASH questionnaire, *Arthritis Rheum* 39:S112, 1996.

75. Upper Extremity Collaborative Group: *The Dash Outcome Measure: user's manual,* 1999, Institute for Work and Health.

76. van der Windt DA, et al: The responsiveness of the Shoulder Disability Questionnaire, *Ann Rheum Dis* 57:82, 1998.

77. Ware JE, Kosinski M, Keller SD: *SF-36 physical and mental health summary scales: a user's manual,* Boston, 1994, The Health Institute, New England Medical Center.

78. Ware JE, Kosinski M, Keller S: *SF-12: how to score the SF-12 Physical and Menyat Summary Scales,* Boston, 2000, The Health Institute, New England Medical Centre.

79. Ware JE, et al: *SF-36 health survey manual and interpretation guide,* Boston, 1993, The Health Institute, New England Medical Center.

80. Wilkie D, et al: Cancer pain intensity measurement: concurrent validity of three tools—finger dynamometer, pain intensity number scale, visual analogue scale, *Hospice J* 6:1, 1990.

81. Williams JWJ, Holleman DRJ, Dimel DL: Measuring shoulder function with the Shoulder Pain and Disability Index, *J Rheumatol* 22:727, 1995.

82. Winters JC, et al: A shoulder pain score: a comprehensive questionnaire for assessing pain in patients with shoulder complaints, *Scand J Rehabil Med* 28:163, 1996.

83. World Health Organization: *International Classification of Impairments, Disabilities and Handicaps: a manual of classification relating to the consequences of disease,* Geneva, 1980, World Health Organization.

Chapter 18

IMPAIRMENT EVALUATION

Lawrence H. Schneider

In the United States, disorders of the upper extremities are widespread and cause associated disability and great expense.[27] Injuries and arthritic conditions are the most common disorders of the upper extremity, and musculoskeletal problems involving the upper and lower extremity and the spine are the most common cause of work-related disability.[14] As documented by Kelsey et al.,[17] approximately 18 million acute upper extremity injuries occur per year, and at any given time, approximately 31 million people have arthritis, many with upper extremity involvement. Twenty-four million visits are made to physicians' offices each year for upper extremity problems, at a cost of almost $19 billion in 1995. These statistics illustrate the current significance of these problems.

HISTORY OF IMPAIRMENT EVALUATION

The need for impairment and disability evaluation was brought forth with the development of entitlement programs and worker's compensation awards (private or public programs for the disabled).[22] Evidence indicates that some of these systems existed in ancient times, and in the Middle Ages, merchant and craft guilds organized to protect their members.[6,22]

Many guides developed in Europe in the nineteenth century.[18] These showed great variability in assigning value to the same impairment because of a lack of established standards. Rating was a conglomerate of many factors, and the physician was in a weak position to defend his or her opinion because of a lack of definitive standards. In 1927, Kessler[18] proposed that medical decisions be based on measurable factors. McBride[23,24] then developed a complex system of medical measurements in disability evaluation. The first rating system for the American orthopedic surgeon, authored by McBride,[24] was published in 1936 and focused on worker's compensation laws. It was an attempt to standardize ratings on a more scientific basis. Unfortunately,

problems remained because of the degree of subjectivity involved. Slocum and Pratt[30] offered a schedule based on function, which when reviewed today appears rudimentary. In response to the problem of impairment evaluation, the American Medical Association (AMA) appointed a Committee on Medical Rating of Physical Impairment in September of 1956 that was authorized to establish guides for a rating system. Drs. Kessler and McBride served as consultants on this committee. The first of these Guides was published as a special edition of the *Journal of the American Medical Association* on February 15, 1958[1]; it covered the upper and lower extremities and the back in three sections. The upper extremity section, "a unit of the whole man" was divided into four sections: hand, wrist, elbow, and shoulder. The hand was further subdivided into the five digits and the digits into their respective joints.[1] Impairments were then rated based on loss of motion or ankylosis at the joints or secondary to amputation of a part as assigned by the committee and given on a provided chart. A functional value was derived for the deficit and then applied from the digit to the hand and the hand to the upper extremity and from there onto the whole person.

An attempt to give guidelines for standardization of evaluations done by the orthopedic surgeons also was developed and published in 1962 by the American Academy of Orthopedic Surgeons (AAOS) Committee on Disability Evaluation chaired by Dr. McBride.[3] This 30-page pamphlet was intended to standardize orthopedic evaluations. Despite the use of the term *disability* in the committee's name, this paper makes it clear that a disability rating is an administrative not a medical responsibility. This effort was soon superseded by the AMA Guides.

In 1970, Kessler[18] pushed for more objectively obtained measurements. He stressed loss of function over anatomic loss. Extensive interplay was involved in trying to work out the multiple problems he encountered.[18]

Subsequent to the first attempt in 1958, the AMA Committee's scope was broadened, and from 1958 to 1970 it published 13 separate "Guides to the Evaluation of Permanent Impairment" in the *Journal of the American Medical Association.* A second edition of these guides was published as separate chapters in a single volume in 1971 entitled "Guides to the Evaluation of Permanent Impairment." These AMA Guides, now in a fourth edition (June 1993)[2] (with updates), are an "attempt to estimate the severity of human impairments based on accepted medical standards."[1] The concept here is that a loss of function could be translated to a percentage loss of the whole person. Although the Guides are needed, the complexity of issues in impairment evaluation makes them imperfect.[29] This is recognized by most experts, including the framers, who are cautious in their choice of language, stating, "this is an attempt to standardize these evaluation proceedings."[1] Frequent updates in response to inconsistencies will gradually further improve their utility. The section of the Guides devoted to the upper extremity was updated and developed by Dr. Alfred Swanson et al.,[32,34] and we are indebted for their work in this difficult area.[28] They also have provided the section on impairment evaluation in prior editions of this text. This chapter does not attempt to serve as a substitute for the AMA Guides, but rather serves to help the reader in the application of the Guides, pointing out the pitfalls and adding some opinionated views on their use.

THE IMPAIRMENT EVALUATION

When is an impairment evaluation indicated? Impairment evaluation is not undertaken early, but rather is done after the patient's condition has stabilized for some time. Impairment, to be evaluated, must be permanent; that is, the patient's condition should be stabilized and unlikely to change either with time or further treatment.[7,8] When performing a rating examination, the rating physician should understand the use of the terms *impairment* and *disability.*

Impairment versus disability

Impairment is a deviation from normal in a body part and its functioning. It marks the degree to which an individual's capacity to carry out daily activities has been diminished. Impairment can be determined and thus is a medical decision made with the use of the Guides after a thorough review of the medical history and a medical examination conducted in combination with appropriate laboratory tests and diagnostic procedures. Physical impairment involves an anatomic or physiologic loss that interferes with the subject's ability to perform a certain function. After evaluation an impairment rating can be assigned. This impairment rating can then be used to determine *disability,* which is a decrease in, or the loss of, the capacity of the individual to meet personal, social, or occupational demands, or activities that the individual cannot accomplish because of the impairment.

Many people with an impairment but with adaptation do not have a disability. An example would be an elevator operator or a surgeon[9] who loses an index finger; although each has a 20% impairment of the hand, he or she has no disability.

It was originally intended that the medically determined impairment rating would be taken to a legal entity, such as a worker's compensation board or some other administrative body, that would then award the disability rating, but today it appears that these organizations more frequently rely on examining physicians to make the disability determination. This is in spite of the Guides telling us that impairment percentages derived according to Guides criteria should not be used to make direct estimates of disabilities. These impairment examinations are being performed by physicians who specialize in occupational medicine or disability rating and specialists who, in some states, take a course and then are certified to perform such evaluations. Again, an impaired person is not necessarily disabled, and all impairments do not result in the same degree of disability in all cases. The impairment rating is a medical determination and directly related to the medical status of the individual, whereas disability can be determined only within the context of the personal, social, or occupational demands that the individual is unable to meet as a result of the impairment.[22] Ideally, impairment evaluation should provide only one element of the disability rating.

The medical evaluation

The medical evaluation is based on clinical findings in a physical examination after a detailed history. The examiner must recognize that the examinee is heavily invested in the result of the examination, which consequently is often adversarial in nature. Despite this, the examiner should always present a neutral demeanor. The complaints and findings should be reasonably relatable to the nature of the injury or condition. The examiner should be cognizant of the difficulties in this evaluation and search for objective findings that will correlate with the subjective symptoms. Psychologic overlay, symptom magnification, and suspected malingering should be noted and attention called to them in the final report with terms that point out such inconsistencies. These issues should not be confronted at the time of the examination, with the examiner maintaining an impartial attitude. On subjective testing, the experienced and sophisticated examinee will present findings that may invalidate the meaning of a particular test.

Medical history. The examination should be preceded by a review of the available records, which the examiner should *insist* be made available. A detailed history of present illness is then taken along with the current complaints and the examinee's reported functional difficulties. In trauma, it is useful to understand the details of the injuring situation. This information may help the examiner judge whether the incident is likely to have led to the current complaints. The history of treatment is developed along with the patient's perceived response to that treatment.

Health history may be significant in that certain medical conditions will predispose to and/or explain certain conditions or symptoms. Prior trauma should be elucidated along with its possible relation to present symptoms. Knowledge of current medications and treatment will bring out any concurrent problems. The use of inappropriate medications should be known. For example, the use of narcotics in a less than major problem greatly influences that patient's response and reporting of pain symptoms. In my experience, many of these patients who are on inappropriate narcotics for long periods would ideally benefit from withdrawal of their medication as part of their treatment and before their evaluation. A patient's social history may indicate a healthy or unhealthy lifestyle and reveal issues that may be adding undue stress to his or her life. A work history often reveals much about the patient. A physically heavy job may explain their symptoms. Other jobs, in which the worker perceives mental stress, can explain symptoms, the origin of which are otherwise obscure. Diffuse, poorly localized symptoms; vague chronic pain; intolerance of treatment; worsening with every treatment modality; excessive drug use; and poor compliance in treatment all should be noted in gaining an overall picture of the patient.

Physical examination. The physical examination should include the usual elements of a complete physical. Needed instruments include a goniometer, a Jamar dynamometer, a pinch gauge, tape measure, a reflex hammer, and a device that allows measurement of two-point discrimination. A current copy of the Guides is necessary to complete the report generated by the evaluation procedures.

The appearance of the upper extremity is noted, including obvious deformities, amputations, scars, masses, atrophy of muscles or finger pulps, trophic changes, skin discoloration, or sweat pattern abnormalities. The extremity, especially the hand, is palpated to determine temperature and sweat pattern. Range of motion (ROM) is measured at all joints in the involved area. A sensory evaluation is carried out. All data are recorded on the multitude of forms and outlines available for this purpose. Appropriate imaging studies and neurodiagnostic testing, when indicated, can be critical. All of this is put together in a comprehensive report.

It is good discipline to conclude the physical examination with a usable diagnosis that is consistent with the current ICD-9 code. This diagnosis should be responsive to the findings and considered very carefully because it can, to a great degree, become a label that, if inaccurate, is difficult to eradicate. At times a clear-cut diagnosis cannot be made. The use of the nonjudgmental diagnostic code 729.5 for "pain—upper extremity" is an excellent tool when the diagnosis is not confirmable. It is useful in an examinee without recognizable objective justification for his or her pain and is superior to assigning arbitrary terms such as "fibromyalgia

syndrome, cumulative trauma disease, or chronic pain syndrome."[15,16] Much confusion is created when patients, reporting wrist pain, are labeled as having "tendonitis" or "tenosynovitis" when, in fact, these easily confirmable inflammatory conditions are not truly present.[36] The use of the 729.5 code then serves to point out the lack of an objective or rational explanation for the symptoms and avoids a confirmatory label that will confuse the issues. In such cases, the examiner should give the reasons for the offered opinion in the discussion section of the report. After the examination, the history and measurements and the subsequent diagnosis are then used with the Guides to estimate the impairment, which should be backed by the rationale that went into the awarding of the rating.

Using the Guides for evaluation of upper extremity impairment[2]

Chapter 1 of the Guides deals with general information, definitions, and how to apply the information derived through the Guides. The upper extremity is covered in the section on the musculoskeletal system, Chapter 3 sections 3.1a an 3.1o, and is relatively straightforward. In the upper extremity, impairment is based on amputation, ankylosis, or restricted motion of joints, and nerve problems with sensory and/or motor ramifications. All of these are relatively straightforward and, with proper use of the Guides, easily ratable. Other issues that are more difficult to assess include weakness, pain, reflex sympathetic dystrophy, and so-called cumulative trauma disease. These are addressed in the Guides, as are conditions such as strength, vascular disorders, wrist instabilities, arthritis, and joint subluxation or dislocation. Most of these latter conditions should, in large part, be evaluated and rated through the use of primary criteria (i.e., amputation, ankylosing or restricted joint motion, nerve problems).[2] When this is not possible, the Guides have sections of other conditions that can be helpful to the rater.

When applying the material in the Guides, the upper extremity is covered as follows:

1. Amputation of a part, 3.1b
2. Nerve damage with sensory loss, 3.1c
3. Ankylosis or restricted motion of joints of the hand, 3.1f and 3.1g
4. Loss of motion to the wrist shoulder and elbow, 3.1h, 3.1i , and 3.1j
5. Impairment due to peripheral nerve disorders, 3.1k
6. Impairment due to vascular disorders, 3.1l
7. Impairment due to other disorders of the upper extremity, 3.1m

Although nerve problems and vascular deficits in the upper extremity are covered in Chapter 3, we also may need to refer to Chapter 4 on the nervous system and Chapter 6 on the cardiovascular system. Chapter 14, which covers mental and behavioral disorders, and Chapter 15, on pain, also may need to be referenced. When pain is a factor, the percentage of impairment awarded in the various sections makes allowance for the pain that may accompany the primary impairing condition.

Each section of the Guides includes a discussion of measurement techniques; tables of relative impairment due to restriction of motion, ankylosis, and amputations; and methods for combining and relating various impairments.[1]

Limitations of the Guides

In this section, I discuss the relevant sections of the Guides and offer my advice and comments on the strengths and weaknesses of each. There are however, some obvious overall limitations, that should be noted first. These include the following:

1. Age-related changes are difficult to separate from those related to an injury, but an attempt should be made to do so.
2. Some measurements lack reliability and validity.
3. Many of the clinical tests are subjective.
4. Psychosocial factors can greatly affect the examinee's presentation. Psychogenic overlay, symptom magnification, and malingering may make it difficult to obtain an accurate estimate of impairment.
5. It is not possible to rate pain in a meaningful manner, especially with conditions such as reflex sympathetic dystrophy, arthritis, wrist conditions and incomplete nerve recovery, which may be unresolved.

These limitations are not the fault of the Guides. These problems may never be totally resolvable. This was recognized by Swanson and colleagues,[34] who clearly warned us that there would be patients whose "complaints are not justified by objective findings or whose responses to testing are not felt to be justified by the diagnosis or the nature of the condition or whose response to testing varies widely from time to time." They went on to say that such patients should put the examiner on guard.

Unfortunately, many of the standardized and provocative tests done on a physical examination are by their nature subjective, that is, under the control of the examinee. This includes such time-honored tests as Tinel's sign or Phalen's test for carpal tunnel syndrome. Most of the clinical tests for patients who present with upper extremity pain attributed to thoracic outlet syndrome or brachial plexopathy when anatomic neuromuscular objective signs are not present, particularly are not completely reliable in the impairment evaluation setting. Many patients have had multiple examinations and become sophisticated enough to learn to supply the expected answers. The evaluation in those cases will test the ingenuity of the examiner. The Guides, which represent a noble effort in a difficult area, require frequent reevaluation and updating, which fortunately is continuing. They are justifiably widely used.

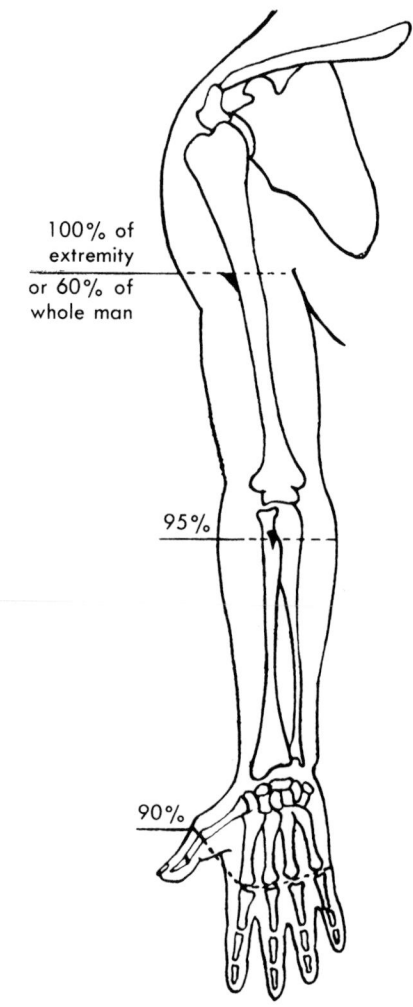

100% of extremity or 60% of whole man

95%

90%

Fig. 18-1. Impairment of the upper extremity from amputation at various levels. (From *The guides to the evaluation of permanent impairment,* ed 4, Chicago, 1993, American Medical Association.)

Relevant sections of the Guides

The following is a commentary concerning relevant sections of the Guides, including a discussion of strengths and weaknesses.

Amputation. Standard percentage values have been assigned to the various amputation levels in the upper extremity. When these percentages are learned, it is a relatively simple matter to assign impairment to the extremity resulting from amputation. Impairment of the entire upper extremity is equivalent to 60% of the whole person; therefore total amputation, or 100% loss of the limb, would be evaluated as a 60% impairment of the whole person. Amputation of the upper extremity from the level of the biceps insertion to the level proximal to the metacarpophalangeal (MP) joints is equivalent to a 95% loss of the upper extremity or 57% of the whole person (Fig. 18-1). Amputation at the MP joints is rated as a 90% loss of the upper extremity. In regard to the hand, individual digits have been assigned values in relation to the whole hand: The thumb is evaluated as 40%, index and

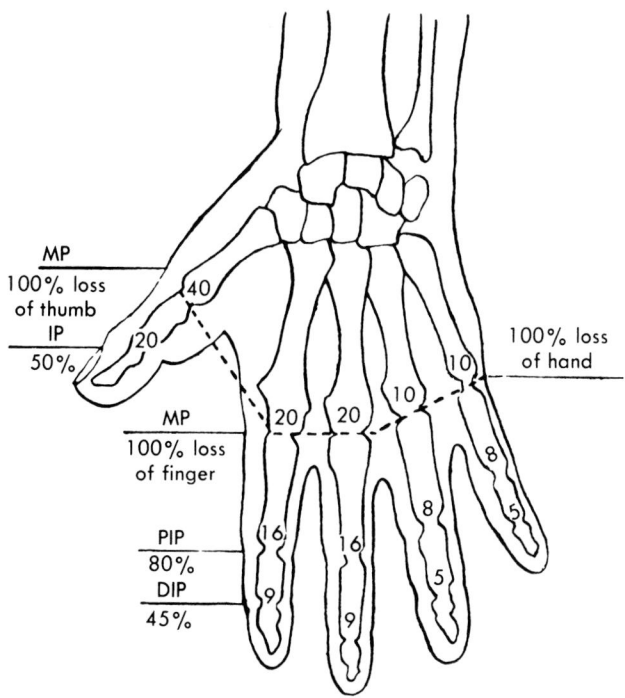

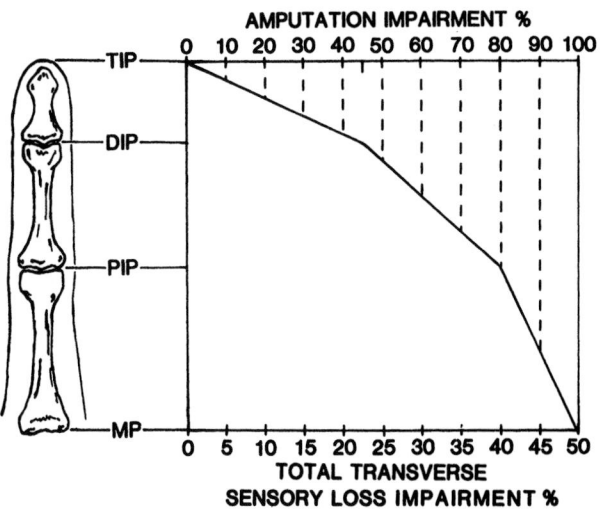

Fig. 18-3. Finger impairment from amputation at various lengths *(top scale)* and total transverse sensory loss *(bottom scale)*. Total transverse sensory loss impairments correspond to 50% of amputation impairments. *DIP,* Distal interphalangeal; *MP,* metacarpophalangeal; *PIP,* proximal interphalangeal; *TIP,* tip of finger. (From *The guides to the evaluation of permanent impairment,* ed 4, Chicago, 1993, American Medical Association.)

Fig. 18-2. Impairment of the digits and of the hand for amputations at various levels. *DIP,* Distal interphalangeal; *IP,* interphalangeal; *MP,* metacarpophalangeal; *PIP,* proximal interphalangeal. (From *The guides to the evaluation of permanent impairment,* ed 4, Chicago, 1993, American Medical Association.)

long fingers 20% each, and ring and little fingers 10% each (Fig. 18-2).

In turn, each portion of an amputated digit is given a value in relation to the entire digit. Amputation of the digit at the MP joint is equal to a 100% loss of that digit; amputation at the proximal interphalangeal (PIP) level is 80% loss of the digit, and distal interphalangeal (DIP) amputation is equal to a 45% loss of the digit (see Fig. 18-2). Awards for amputations at intervals between the joints are adjusted proportionally. If all fingers and thumb are amputated at the MP joints, it is equivalent to 100% loss of the hand, which is equal to 90% of the upper extremity or 54% of the whole person. Learning these simple rules helps keep the relative values for amputation in perspective (Fig. 18-3). The total impairment awarded for a nonamputated finger with, for example, restricted motion and/or nerve damage should not exceed that given for amputation of that finger. Knowing the value of each finger in amputation sets a boundary for estimating impairment for other less definitive injuries.

Range of motion. Diminished ROM of the joints of the upper extremity is a measurable factor used in the evaluation of loss of function.[11] The arc of motion (angular measurement) of the finger joints, for example, is represented by two numbers, one at the extreme of extension and the other the extreme of flexion. Therefore each joint is assigned a numerator and a denominator. Obtaining these measurements (14 in all just for the thumb and fingers) is

cumbersome and time-consuming, but no better method is available.[21] The use of glove-embedded sensors or an electronic goniometer may help gather this data in the future. For now, a simple goniometer is used. ROM measurements are rounded off to the nearest 10 degrees. The goniometer, as placed over the dorsum of the finger joints, is not perfect. Swelling or deformity of the finger skews the measurement. The examiner and the Guides should recognize that this technique for measurement is somewhat of a compromise and that for the measurement to be truly accurate, it would have to be obtained via longitudinal lines drawn through the midaxis of the adjacent phalanges at the joints. The ROM can be better estimated by placing a goniometer lateral to the joint or using a straight edge as a reference point against the phalanx proximal to that particular joint (Fig. 18-4). Although use of the goniometer is required, an experienced examiner often can reproduce the measurements using an estimate obtained with a straight edge alongside the joint. If a patient demonstrates active motion that is short of the expected, in view of the history, examination findings, and radiograph studies, then the examiner should try to find out whether maximum effort is being exercised. The examinee's active ROM should be consistent with the pathologic signs and the medical evidence. The examiner is essentially forced to accept the offered active motion but when concerned about compliance can try gentle passive motion to check on the validity of the motion demonstrated. One must not unduly push the patient or cause discomfort, but when there are obvious discrepancies, the data may have to be discarded or labeled as inconsistent. The examiner may have the patient "warm up" and try again later in the examination.

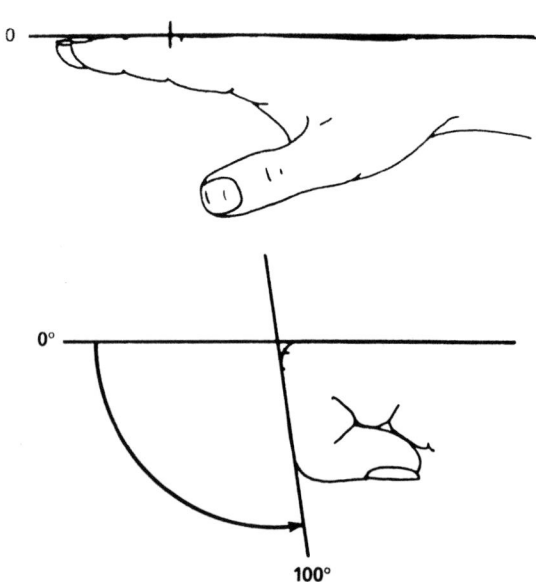

Fig. 18-4. Neutral position *(top)* and flexion *(bottom)* of finger, proximal interphalangeal joint. (From *The guides to the evaluation of permanent impairment,* ed 4, Chicago, 1993, American Medical Association.)

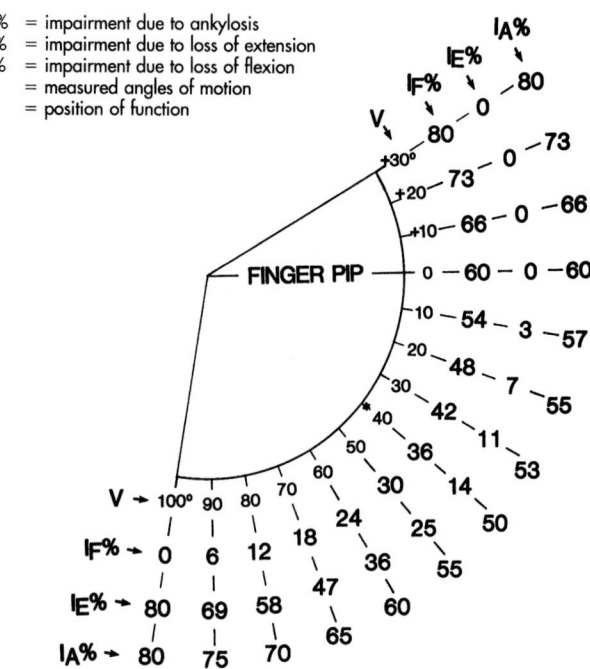

Fig. 18-5. Finger impairments resulting from abnormal motions at the proximal interphalangeal; *(PIP)* joint. (From *The guides to the evaluation of permanent impairment,* ed 4, Chicago, 1993, American Medical Association.)

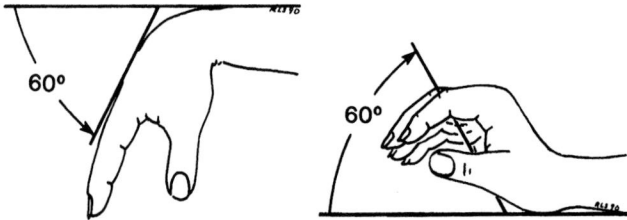

Fig. 18-6. Wrist flexion *(left)* and extension *(right).* (From *The guides to the evaluation of permanent impairment,* ed 4, Chicago, 1993, American Medical Association.)

Some advise rescheduling the examination for another day, but this is rarely practical.

Tables provided in the Guides relate deficiencies in joint motion in all the joints in the upper extremity from the shoulder to the interphalangeal (IP) joints to specific percentages of impairment (Fig. 18-5). The finger motion impairment values of the MP, PIP, and DIP joints are then combined to get the impairment for the finger, which can then be used to find the impairment as it relates to the hand, upper extremity, and then to the whole person. When multiple fingers are involved, one must determine the impairment of each digit and its relationship to the hand. These values are then added to determine the loss of function of the hand. This total is then combined with loss of function attributed to, for example, ankylosis or restriction of motion of the wrist as derived from the Guides (Figs. 18-6 and 18-7).

In general, if there is a question of abnormal motion, one can compare the ROM in question to the contralateral unimpaired joint for comparison. This is generally reliable, except in the thumb, where ROM is not as consistent bilaterally.

Impairment caused by peripheral nerve disorders

Sensory deficits. The Guides tell us that any sensory loss or deficit that contributes to permanent impairment must be unequivocal and permanent.[2] It must be remembered that there is no perfect, objective test for determination of sensory loss, and the examiner depends on the examinee's input. Sudomotor function is an objective reflection of sensory integrity, but except for the clinical observation of a sweat pattern, it is not a practical test for everyday use. The Ninhydrin test[25] has not been widely used but can occasionally be useful in cases that have no other solution. Neurodiagnostic testing is helpful to document the presence or absence of nerve deficiency. For sensory evaluation, the Guides recommend using two-point discrimination testing and, in particular, moving two-point discrimination, which is said to be more accurate, especially in the recovering nerve.[12] In the hand, when two-point discrimination exceeds 15 mm, the area is said to be totally deficient in sensation or to have a 100% sensory impairment. Six-millimeter two-point discrimination and below is regarded as normal sensibility. Percentage impairment of the finger is then assigned as indicated in Fig. 18-8). Confirmatory findings in significant sensory deficit are loss of sudomotor function manifested by dryness of the finger pulps, which also may

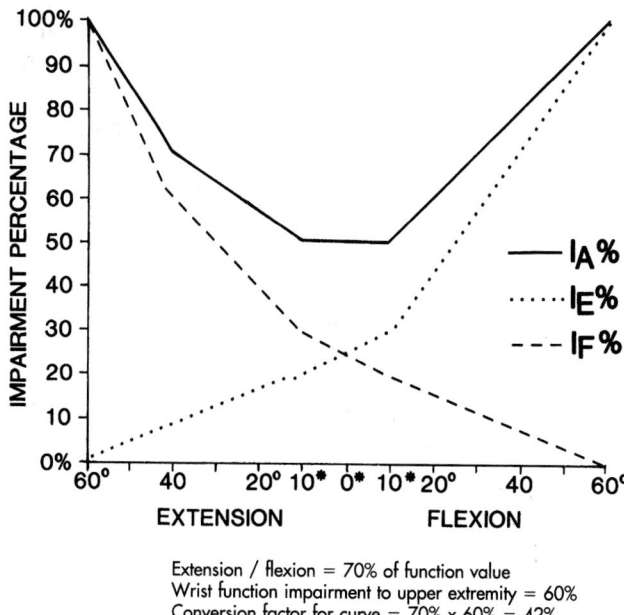

Extension / flexion = 70% of function value
Wrist function impairment to upper extremity = 60%
Conversion factor for curve = 70% x 60% = 42%

Fig. 18-7. Impairment curves for ankylosis *(IA%)*, loss of extension *(IE%)*, and loss of flexion *(IF%)* of the wrist. (From *The guides to the evaluation of permanent impairment,* ed 4, Chicago, 1993, American Medical Association.)

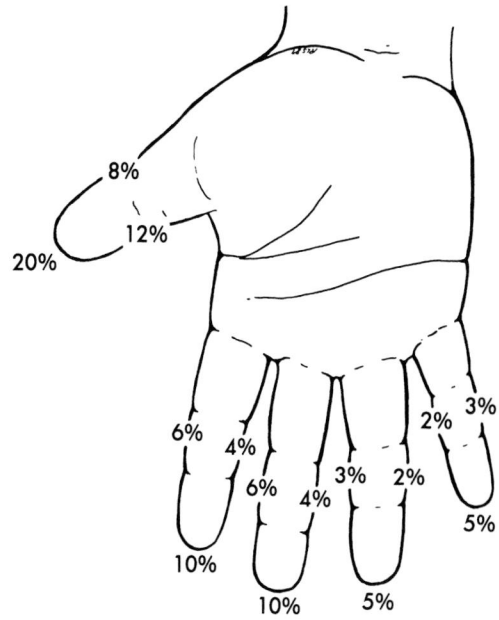

Fig. 18-8. Impairment of hand resulting from total transverse sensory loss of digits (numbers at tips of digits) and longitudinal sensory loss of radial and ulnar sides of the digits (numbers at sides of digits). (From *The guides to the evaluation of permanent impairment,* ed 4, Chicago, 1993, American Medical Association.)

be atrophic. Because the two-point discrimination test, when done correctly, is a complex undertaking requiring an experienced and patient examiner, in critical issues the use of a certified hand therapist with training and experience is advised for this examination.[5] In most instances when I evaluate sensation, I have used the modality of light touch to evaluate for sensory function, comparing the sensation reported in the area in question with that of an area of agreed-upon normality. I do not advocate the use of the pin to test for sensory function and have not used it for many years because I have found that when a nerve is completely nonfunctional, the examinee is left with bloody pinholes in that nerve's distribution. Alternatively, when the nerve is intact the examination can become very unpleasant for the examinee. Neither is a happy situation. The sensory picture obtained should concur with anatomy and correlate with the patient's history and other findings. To calculate the loss resulting from sensory loss in the fingers, the examiner can refer to Table 18-1).

Motor deficits. In cases of total denervation of a muscle, the problem is relatively simple to rate, but in cases of weakness or partial paralysis, detailed muscle testing may be required. This necessitates a knowledgeable examiner skilled in this examination. A standardized rating system, adapted by the Guides, for rating muscle power applies a rating of 5 for a full range of active motion against full resistance and at the other end of the scale, 0 for complete paralysis.

In relation to nerve problems, the framers of the Guides agreed upon certain guidelines. There is also an established maximum value to be assigned as a result of any particular nerve dysfunction. For example, a completely nonfunctional median nerve injured in the proximal forearm, which will have complete sensory and motor implications, is given a 65% impairment of the upper extremity. The ulnar nerve at a similar level is equivalent to a 50% impairment of the upper extremity. With the application of these guidelines, the examiner has a reference to aid in rating nerve impairment in the upper extremity. Similarly, each digital nerve, which is a purely sensory nerve, has been assigned a value (see Fig. 18-8).

It is noted that the evaluator is instructed not to use impairment values from more than one section because this overlap will lead to a too high impairment rating. When multiple areas of impairment are involved because of injury to the peripheral nerves, they are combined using the combined values chart.

Pain. Evaluation of chronic pain in impairment examination is a difficult problem. Besides being addressed in several areas of the Guides, an entire chapter[20] is devoted to this symptom. Chapter 15 provides an excellent discussion of pain entities and refers the reader to appropriate areas of the Guides when chronic pain is the presenting symptom. In general, pain should be explainable by some underlying and definable problem. A percentage impairment can then be given based on that estimated for the primary problem

Table 18-1. Relationship of impairment of the upper extremity to impairment of the whole person

% Impairment of		% Impairment of		% Impairment of	
Upper extremity	Whole person	Upper extremity	Whole person	Upper extremity	Whole person
0 = 0		35 = 21		70 = 42	
1 = 1		36 = 22		71 = 43	
2 = 1		37 = 22		72 = 43	
3 = 2		38 = 23		73 = 44	
4 = 2		39 = 23		74 = 44	
5 = 3		40 = 24		75 = 45	
6 = 4		41 = 25		76 = 46	
7 = 4		42 = 25		77 = 46	
8 = 5		43 = 26		78 = 47	
9 = 5		44 = 26		79 = 47	
10 = 6		45 = 27		80 = 48	
11 = 7		46 = 28		81 = 49	
12 = 7		47 = 28		82 = 49	
13 = 8		48 = 29		83 = 50	
14 = 8		49 = 29		84 = 50	
15 = 9		50 = 30		85 = 51	
16 = 10		51 = 31		86 = 52	
17 = 10		52 = 31		87 = 52	
18 = 11		53 = 32		88 = 53	
19 = 11		54 = 32		89 = 53	
20 = 12		55 = 33		90 = 54	
21 = 13		56 = 34		91 = 55	
22 = 13		57 = 34		92 = 55	
23 = 14		58 = 35		93 = 56	
24 = 14		59 = 35		94 = 56	
25 = 15		60 = 36		95 = 57	
26 = 16		61 = 37		96 = 58	
27 = 16		62 = 37		97 = 58	
28 = 17		63 = 38		98 = 59	
29 = 17		64 = 38		99 = 59	
30 = 18		65 = 39		100 = 60	
31 = 19		66 = 40			
32 = 19		67 = 40			
33 = 20		68 = 41			
34 = 20		69 = 41			

From Swanson AB, de Groot Swanson G: Principles and methods of impairment evaluation in the hand and upper extremity. In *Guides to the evaluation of permanent impairment*, ed 4, Chicago, 1993, American Medical Association.

causing the symptom. Pain is otherwise not easily ratable. I have found self-reporting pain scales worthless in the setting of an impairment evaluation when the patient has a great investment in the final rating. With many warnings and precautions, the Guides tell us that chronic pain, in the absence of objectively validated conditions, should be evaluated on a multidisciplinary basis by physicians with a special interest and background in pain medicine. This is not always a practical solution. We also are asked to rate the effects of the pain on the patient's ability to carry out daily activities. A pain-intensity grid is provided[2] that is a self-reporting evaluation of the patient's pain. Although no examiner can feel the patient's pain, this self-reporting scale is not a satisfactory answer to the issue of pain rating. There is no immediate solution to this problem, and I recommend rating pain in the context of the underlying medical problem. This is recognized by the framers of the Guides who have given us the various tables applicable to permanent impairments and are said to have included allowances for the pain that may occur with those impairments. The rater is given considerable leeway to override the system when in his or her judgment there is a cause to do so.[2,32] Nowhere are the limitations of impairment evaluation better illustrated than when rating those complaining of chronic pain.

Reflex sympathetic dystrophy. Reflex sympathetic dystrophy (RSD), now referred to as *complex regional pain syndrome* (CRPS), has been divided into two types: type 1, traditional RSD, and type 2, RSD with a recognizable peripheral nerve abnormality. Type 2 is what was referred to as *causalgia* in the older literature.[20] The presence of pain is primary, but it is further associated with swelling, stiffness, and discoloration in this diagnosis according to the Guides.[2] I would add trophic changes and sweat pattern abnormalities to the list of findings necessary to make this diagnosis. The diagnosis may be verified by or supported with a three-phase nucleotide scan or by the response to a successful stellate ganglion block. It is recommended that the examiner not label a patient reporting chronic pain as having CRPS without the indicated findings. Because impairment evaluation is a late procedure in an injury or illness, the impairment examiner may not see the acute stage of CRPS but should recognize the late ravages of the condition which may present with joint restriction and ongoing peripheral nerve problems. It is important not to use the diagnosis casually but only when a strong history and clinical picture demands because this diagnosis carries many legal implications with it. It is recommended that in late RSD the impairment rating be based on the following:

1. Loss of motion at each involved joint
2. Sensory deficit in the involved peripheral nerve territory
3. Motor deficit if present due to an involved nerve

The impairment ratings for these findings can then be combined using the combined values chart.

Although pain is an absolute requirement for a CRPS diagnosis, impairment resulting from CRPS is not assessed using the Guides' Chapter 15 on pain. Ensalata[13] presents an excellent discussion of the difficulties in the evaluation of these conditions and brings to our attention the great amount of work that needs to be done in this area.

Impairment caused by other disorders of the upper extremities. Several derangements are covered in the Guides that were not mentioned elsewhere, and they may need inclusion in a final impairment determination. This gives the rater a lot of leeway when evaluation finds such conditions as joint crepitation, joint swelling, digit rotational deformity, digit lateral deviation, subluxation or dislocation, joint instability, arthroplasty, and trigger finger. Tables are provided to assign the various impairment ratings to be applied. These conditions should, for the most part, be covered by underlying anatomic and physiologic findings, and impairment therefore is estimated using other more primary criteria such as restriction in ROM. We are told to avoid duplicate rating and that this section is to be used only when other criteria have not sufficed to cover the impairment.

In the case of carpal instability, ratings given are based on x-ray measurements (which may be a source of error) and the presence of arthritic changes. These x-ray criteria are to be used only when all other wrist factors are normal. I believe that in such cases impairment ratings are better arrived at on the basis of clinical findings with emphasis on restriction of ROM. It is noted that there are variations in the measurements used in the evaluation of these problems, and this area of impairment rating needs the work of experienced hand surgeons to give the impairments assigned more validity. This is discussed in an article[10] that points out the problems in these evaluations.

Grip testing. One of the parameters on which hand function is based is the evaluation of grip strength in the hand.[4,19] Quantification of grip strength is said to be measurable and repeatable by the use of the Jamar dynamometer.[4] Unfortunately, the subjectivity of this evaluation when used under impairment evaluation conditions greatly reduces the value as a reliably measurable parameter. Swanson[33] tells us that many factors determine the strength of grip, including age, handedness, pain, finger amputations, and restricted motion among others. Not the least is the compliance of the patient in the test and his or her willingness to put effort into the examination. When obvious deficiencies are present, they may be used to determine a percentage of impairment. In my opinion, it is rarely valid to register the loss of strength as a factor in the evaluation in the absence of confirmatory deficiencies. Despite this, I always measure the grip strength on an evaluation to gain additional information about the patient.

When grip testing is carried out, some standard techniques are applicable.[31,34] The examinee is seated with the arm carried at the side of the trunk and the elbow flexed at 90 degrees. Grip testing is generally done using the Jamar dynamometer at the second and third handle positions. In weak arthritic hands, one can use a blood pressure cuff inflated to 50 mm Hg, and the change in pressure with grip is recorded as strength.[33] Also suggested are two methods that help detect those who are not exerting their maximal strength on grip testing:

1. Testing at all five handle positions of the Jamar dynamometer and plotting the measurements should show a bell curve rather than a flat line.[33]

2. Using rapid exchange gripping, that is, using one hand and then the other for at least 5 repetitions, helps show those who are not compliant because they will exert much higher levels than on the routine tests, and when they realize this, their performance will drop precipitously.[32]

Although it has been my observation that many people are stronger by approximately 10% on their dominant side, Swanson et al.,[34] in their study of unimpaired subjects found a remarkable bilateral similarity of strength in a wide range of subjects; however, manual workers were usually stronger on their dominant side.

Pinch strength is also measurable using a pinch gauge. Key pinch is usually used, but again, is also of little value as a measurement in adversarial situations. In this test the non-compliant individual is able to directly view the measurements on the gauge and may consciously or subconsciously adjust his or her pinch pressure.

Overall I agree that when there is suspicion or evidence that the subject is exerting less than maximal effort during grip testing, the measurements become invalid for impairment evaluations. This is supported by Swanson et al.[34] who do not assign a large role to grip and pinch values in an evaluation system based on anatomic impairment.

Functional capacity evaluation

One of the weaknesses of impairment and subsequent disability evaluation is the lack of ability to look at the functional capacities of the examinee—the ability to actually perform work. The entities we are able to measure may not correlate with the ability to perform a function.[26,28,34] Today the difference between impairment and disability rating seems to be blurring, and examining physicians are frequently called upon to fill out work evaluation certificates.[22] These forms may be for general work restrictions or for specific jobs, our knowledge of which may be rudimentary. Even with expertise in impairment evaluation we are at a disadvantage.[26] The ability to perform work is directly related to the physical capacities of a person, but in addition, philosophic and psychologic issues are involved. The ability and desire to perform work has multitudes of determinants both conscious and subconscious. Illness behavior can pervade the evaluation. The use of a functional capacities evaluation performed by an upper extremity therapist trained in the administration of these studies would be of great assistance to the physician doing an impairment evaluation.

Functional capacity evaluation (FCE) can be subdivided into physical capacity evaluation and work capacity evaluation.[35] Physical capacity evaluation examines isolated parts of the body or functional units. Work capacity evaluations assess performance involving several functional units.

These studies essentially were designed to assist the worker getting back to work after an injury but also could be of value in a permanent impairment situation. These evaluations are especially pertinent because the Americans with Disability Act prohibits exclusion of qualified persons with disabilities from employment,[28] and some mechanism is needed to evaluate the worker with a permanent impairment. The FCE can assist in the determination and validity of occupational disability. On the negative side is the fact that the examination is not standardized and there is a need for better validity testing if it is to have real value. The evaluator needs to be trained and skilled to make these evaluations pertinent. I have seen situations in which the findings were in great excess to the objective impairment, thereby creating great confusion. Although their value in cases with difficult patients is questionable,[28] I believe these evaluations could have great value in the process and would hope that better validity standards would make them even more useful.

Combining impairments

When there is more than one impairing factor to be considered in a part, then the Guides want us to combine them before converting to the next unit. To combine impairments in the upper extremity, the rater must first determine the impairments of each region (hand, wrist, elbow, and shoulder joints), if multiple regions are impaired. Combining is done using the combined values chart at the back of the Guides. When multiple areas within a unit contribute to impairment (e.g., in a finger), these impairments, such as restriction of motion and sensory loss, are combined before conversion to impairment of the hand. In the case of digit and hand impairments, convert to impairment of the upper extremity before regional impairments can be combined. After combining, the impairment can then be converted to whole body impairment using the appropriate table (see Table 18-1).

Rule: When there are several impairments of a unit, they must be combined before going to the next unit. It must be remembered that one should not assign an impairment value that exceeds that for amputation of that part.

SUMMARY

When an impairment evaluation is performed, the extremity is examined and deficits are noted, including amputation, nerve impairments, and decrease in ROM. Other criteria that may be associated with impairment also are credited from the appropriate charts in the Guides. In the case of deficiencies of function resulting from digital problems, the individual digital impairments are converted to impairment of the hand, which is then converted to impairment percentage of the upper extremity. If other areas of the upper extremity, such as at the wrist, elbow, or shoulder, are involved, these are calculated and combined and related to the whole person. If both upper extremities are involved, the whole person impairment percentage for each is established and then combined.

It should be noted that the final percentages represent an estimate rather than a precise determination and are rounded off to the nearest 0% or 5% value.

Results should be consistent with the results of previous clinical studies and the pertinent examination. One must appreciate that there are controversies and contradictions within the Guides. Their framers acknowledge that imperfections in the rating procedure are unavoidable. The Guides allow that they cannot always provide complete and definitive answers,[2] but considerable leeway is given to the rater in difficult areas. This may be in the form of "severity modifiers" or in impairments that are not clearly covered by the primary measurable areas.

As I see it, the main problem in these evaluations exists in areas that use self-reporting in the awarding of a rating. In these examinations, the patient is heavily invested in the outcome and decisions made by the rating physician. This may lead to what has been called "symptom exaggeration." This is not to say that the examinee is necessarily malingering, that is, making an outright conscious attempt to deceive, but he or she may be influenced by subconscious emotional overlay. It is my impression that the actual percentage of people malingering is probably low, but this must be considered as a factor in those cases that are not explainable in reasonable terms. The problem is that many of the presentations are not objectively measurable, and there is little hope in the system that impairment can be measured accurately in those persons who may have other motives.

REFERENCES

1. AMA Committee on Medical Rating of Physical Impairment: A guide to the evaluation of permanent impairment of the extremities and back, *JAMA* Special Edition Feb 15, 1958.
2. *AMA Guide to the evaluation of permanent impairment,* ed 4, Chicago, 1993, American Medical Association, 3rd printing, August 1995.
3. American Academy of Orthopedic Surgeons: *Manual for orthopaedic surgeons in evaluating permanent physical impairment,* Committee on Disability Evaluation, Chicago, 1962, AAOS.
4. Bechtold CO: Grip test. The use of a dynometer with adjustable handle spacings, *J Bone Joint Surg* 36A:820, 1954.
5. Bell J: Sensibility testing. In Hunter JM, et al., editors: *Rehabilitation of the hand,* ed 3, St Louis, 1990, Mosby.
6. Bertelsen A, Capener N: Fingersex and King Canute, *J Bone Joint Surg* 42B:390, 1960.
7. Blair SJ, Swanson AB, Swanson GD: Evaluation of impairment of hand and upper extremity, *AAOS Instr Course Lect* 38:73, 1989.
8. Blair SJ, et al: Evaluation of impairment of the upper extremity, *Clin Orthop* 221:42, 1987.
9. Brown PW: Less than ten: surgeons with amputated fingers, *J Hand Surg* 7A:31, 1982.
10. Cohen M: Instability of the wrist, *The Guides Newsletter* March/April, 1998.
11. Cambridge CA: Range-of-motion measurements of the hand. In Hunter JM, et al, editors: *Rehabilitation of the hand,* ed 3, St Louis, 1990, Mosby.
12. Dellon AL, Kallman CH: Evaluation of functional sensation in the hand, *J Hand Surg* 8:865, 1983.
13. Ensalata LH: The challenge of evaluating RSD impairment and disability (Part II), *AMA Guides Newsletter,* Jan/Feb, 1998.

14. Frymoyer JW, Mooney V: Current concepts review. Occupational orthopaedics, *J Bone Joint Surg* 68A:469, 1986.
15. Hadler N: Occupational illness: the issue of causality, *J Occup Med* 26:587, 1984.
16. Hadler NM: Cumulative trauma disorders: an iatrogenic concept, *J Occup Med* 32:38, 1990.
17. Kelsey J, et al: *Upper extremity disorders: frequency impact and cost,* New York, 1997, Churchill Livingstone.
18. Kessler HH: *Disability-determination and evaluation,* Philadelphia, 1970, Lea & Febiger.
19. Kirkpatrick EJ: Evaluation of grip loss, *California Medicine* 85:314, 1956.
20. Koman AI, Smith BP, Smith TL: Reflex sympathy dystrophy (Complex Regional Pain Syndrome). In Mackin EJ, et al., editors: *Rehabilitation of the hand and upper extremity,* ed 5, St Louis, 2001, Mosby.
21. Litchman HM, Paslay PR: Determination of finger-motion impairment by linear measurement, *J Bone Joint Surg* 56A:85, 1974.
22. Luck JV, Florence DW: A brief history and comparative analysis of disability systems and impairment rating guides, *Orthop Clin North Am* 19:839, 1988.
23. McBride ED: *Disability evaluation and principles of treatment of compensable injuries,* ed 6, Philadelphia, 1963, JB Lippincott.
24. McBride ED: Concept of disability (the classic), *Clin Orthop* 221:3, 1987.
25. Moberg E: Objective methods for determining the functional value of sensibility in the hand, *J Bone Joint Surg* 40B:454, 1958.
26. Mooney V: Impairment, disability and handicap, *Clin Orthop Rel Res* 221:14, 1987.
27. Praemer A, Furner S, Risce DP: *Musculoskeletal conditions in the United States,* Rosemont, Ill, 1999, American Academy Orthopedic Surgeons.
28. Pransky G: Functional capacity evaluations and disability, *AMA Guides Newsletter* March/April, 1998.
29. Rondellini RD, Katz RT: *Impairment rating and disability evaluation,* Philadelphia, 2000, WB Saunders.
30. Slocum DB, Pratt DR: Disability evaluation for the hand, *J Bone Joint Surg* 28:491, 1946.
31. Stokes HM: The seriously injured hand: weakness of grip, *J Occup Med* 25:683, 1983.
32. Swanson AB, Goran-Hagert C, Swanson G DeG: Evaluation of impairment in the upper extremity, *J Hand Surg* 12A:896, 1987.
33. Swanson AB, Matev IB, de Groot G: The strength of the hand, *Bull Prosthet Res* Fall;145, 1970.
34. Swanson AB, Swanson G DeG, Goren-Hagbert, C: Evaluation of impairment of hand function. In Hunter JM, et al, editors: *Rehabilitation of the hand, surgery and therapy,* ed 4, St Louis, 1995, Mosby.
35. Velozo CA: Work evaluations: critique of the state of the art of functional assessment of work, *Am J Occup Ther* 47:203, 1993.
36. Weiland AJ: Editorial-repetitive strain injuries and cumulative trauma disorders, *J Hand Surg* 21A:337, 1996.

Part **III**

WOUND MANAGEMENT

Chapter 19

WOUND CLASSIFICATION AND MANAGEMENT

Roslyn B. Evans
John A. McAuliffe

WOUND CLASSIFICATION AND MANAGEMENT: THE SURGEON'S PERSPECTIVE

The surgeon usually begins and sets the tone for the process of wound management because he or she generally is responsible for the first encounter with the wound. This is obviously true of elective surgical wounds, in which case the surgeon has designed, executed, and repaired the wound under ideal, controlled, and aseptic circumstances. In the case of the traumatic open wound, it is the surgeon who makes the decision regarding the need for operative treatment in the simplest cases and determines the timing and extent of surgical intervention for more complex injuries involving multiple tissues.

Throughout the process of wound care, we must always treat the patient and not simply the injured hand.[29] Care of the wounded hand may assume secondary or lesser importance in the multiply injured patient. We must be able to stage and temporize our treatment in such cases, while leaving available all possible options for delayed, but still state-of-the-art, reconstruction and rehabilitation. In cases of isolated upper extremity injury, we must remember that the patient's personality, vocation, and avocation may demand significant alteration in the treatment plan from what we may otherwise consider ideal.[28] We must avoid the temptation to allow technology to overcome reason as much in surgery of the hand as in any other medical endeavor. Our ability to perform a given procedure is not a necessary or sufficient medical indication.

Elective wounds

Although surgeons may vary in their recommendations for the care of incisions, there is little controversy regarding the treatment of these wounds. We rely on the fact that surgical wounds generally heal rapidly by first intention, and this expectation usually is realized. However, we must not neglect to consider those factors that may adversely affect this expected outcome. Preoperative assessment of immunologic, metabolic, and vascular compromise is mandatory[156] and usually can be accomplished with a thorough history and physical examination. Basic laboratory evaluation also may be helpful in the assessment of metabolic or nutritional factors that may negatively affect the process of wound healing,[98,109] particularly in the elderly or debilitated patient. The anticipation and prevention of wound healing complications are far superior to the treatment of such complications and generally result in an improved functional outcome.

The placement of surgical incisions so as to avoid scar contracture and dysfunction is of critical importance in surgery of the hand.[1] Even well-accepted surgical exposures can sometimes be altered to the potential benefit of both the wound and the patient. For example, although technically more demanding, anterior capsulectomy to relieve flexion contracture of the elbow is best performed via a lateral approach.[150] This skin incision placed in the midaxial line will be under no tension as the underlying joint is moved. Therapy will not have to be suspended or postponed because of fears of dehiscence of the more conventional and very tight anterior wound. Placing incisions in lines of limited tension also decreases pain with motion.

Similarly, selected proximal phalanx fractures are best approached by a midaxial incision in the digit, accompanied by careful retraction of the intact dorsal hood mechanism. This exposure may serve to minimize the scarring and subsequent loss of motion associated with the more traditional dorsal tendon-splitting technique.

From this discussion, we see that the focus of our attempts to influence the healing wound is the minimization of scar that restricts motion. To this end, control of wound hematoma is another variable over which the surgeon must attempt to exert maximal control. I (JAM) strongly advocate that the tourniquet be deflated and hemostasis be achieved before wound closure. Postoperative edema also must be aggressively prevented with appropriate dressings and strict elevation. Hematoma and edema are the harbingers of deep scar that will unnecessarily complicate and delay rehabilitation.

The surgeon and therapist must be aware that they have not completed their tasks until the scar has matured and remodeled. The critical details of scar management are discussed elsewhere in this chapter and text.

We all aspire to achieve uneventful wound healing, so that our attention may be more appropriately focused on the timetable for healing and rehabilitation of the deeper tissues that have been repaired or reconstructed. Strict attention to detail and basic principles helps ensure that healing of the wound does not interfere with the other priorities of patient management.

Traumatic wounds

Although much can be learned from the masters of the subject,[29,36] the judgment of the individual surgeon often remains the most significant determinant of success in healing of the traumatic wound. There is some potential predictive advantage to categorization of these wounds[88,198]; however, attempting to apply these schemes to any given wound may prove difficult. Despite the available guidelines, "each hand, each wound, and each damaged structure must be individually assessed,"[29] also taking into account the capabilities and experience of the individual surgeon.

Certain basic tenets apply in the care of all traumatic wounds, regardless of their magnitude. A thorough history is critical to the complete appreciation of the severity of the wound. Certain mechanisms of injury may prompt grave concern for a small and innocuous-appearing violation of the skin. Classic examples include the punctate wound that accompanies high-pressure injection injury and the tiny laceration on the dorsum of a hand that has contacted the tooth of an adversary. The environment in which the injury occurred may signal the need for more aggressive treatment, as may a significant delay in caring for the wound. A history of a crush component to the wounding mechanism indicates that the zone of injury may extend far beyond the obvious skin defect.

Inquiry regarding the status of tetanus prophylaxis and appropriate supplementation of active immunization or provision of passive immunization for those previously unvaccinated are mandatory.[10]

Physical examination must be performed before the use of any type of anesthetic agent to accurately assess neurologic function. It is not necessary to probe the wound; documentation of deep injury can be obtained by careful examination of the distal extremity. Vascular examination must be performed with a high index of suspicion based on proximity of the wound to known arterial anatomy. In certain individuals, significant collateral circulation can exist despite laceration of both digital arteries or both major arteries at the wrist. The location of the wound in these cases should prompt emergent exploration without delay. The possibility of compartment syndrome in the hand, as well as the forearm, always must be considered. The elevation of compartment pressures to critical levels may not occur for several hours after injury, and this diagnosis may not be apparent at the time of initial presentation.

The classification of wounds into tidy and untidy categories provides a fairly intuitive framework in which to consider surgical treatment.[170] A sharp laceration that divides flexor tendons and a digital nerve represents a tidy wound that can be successfully treated with immediate repair and closure by a competent surgeon. The hand crushed beneath the tire of a tractor with complex dorsal and volar lacerations containing imbedded soil clearly represents an untidy wound that would prove disastrous if closed primarily. Both of these wounds are contaminated. They differ in the degree of contamination and the presence and amount of nonviable tissue; these are the variables we must consider most carefully when judging a wound. In these cases, it is usually best to overestimate the severity of the wound and err on the side of conservatism in its treatment. The first priority in care of the wound that might be considered untidy is the wound itself.[33] Without control of the wound, repair or reconstruction of deeper structures, whether performed early or late, is doomed to failure.

One of the major controversies in care of the wounded hand is the advisability of primary wound closure.[33,107,132,214] Recent military surgical experience has clearly demonstrated the safety and efficacy of delayed primary closure. There is no proven advantage to repair on the day of injury and no evidence suggesting a disadvantage to delayed closure within the first week.[107,132] Delayed closure allows for somewhat less aggressive initial debridement, which can be critical in the hand, where many vital structures lie in close proximity. Delayed closure also permits a second-look debridement before one passes final judgment. Wounds in the hand can safely be left open. Certainly, a wound that is prematurely closed and becomes frankly infected is far worse than one that has not been closed.[26] Wound closure is an elective procedure that should be performed only when the surgeon feels entirely confident in its outcome.[35,64]

Certain wounds may never be closed and are allowed to heal by secondary intention. This may be true in cases of

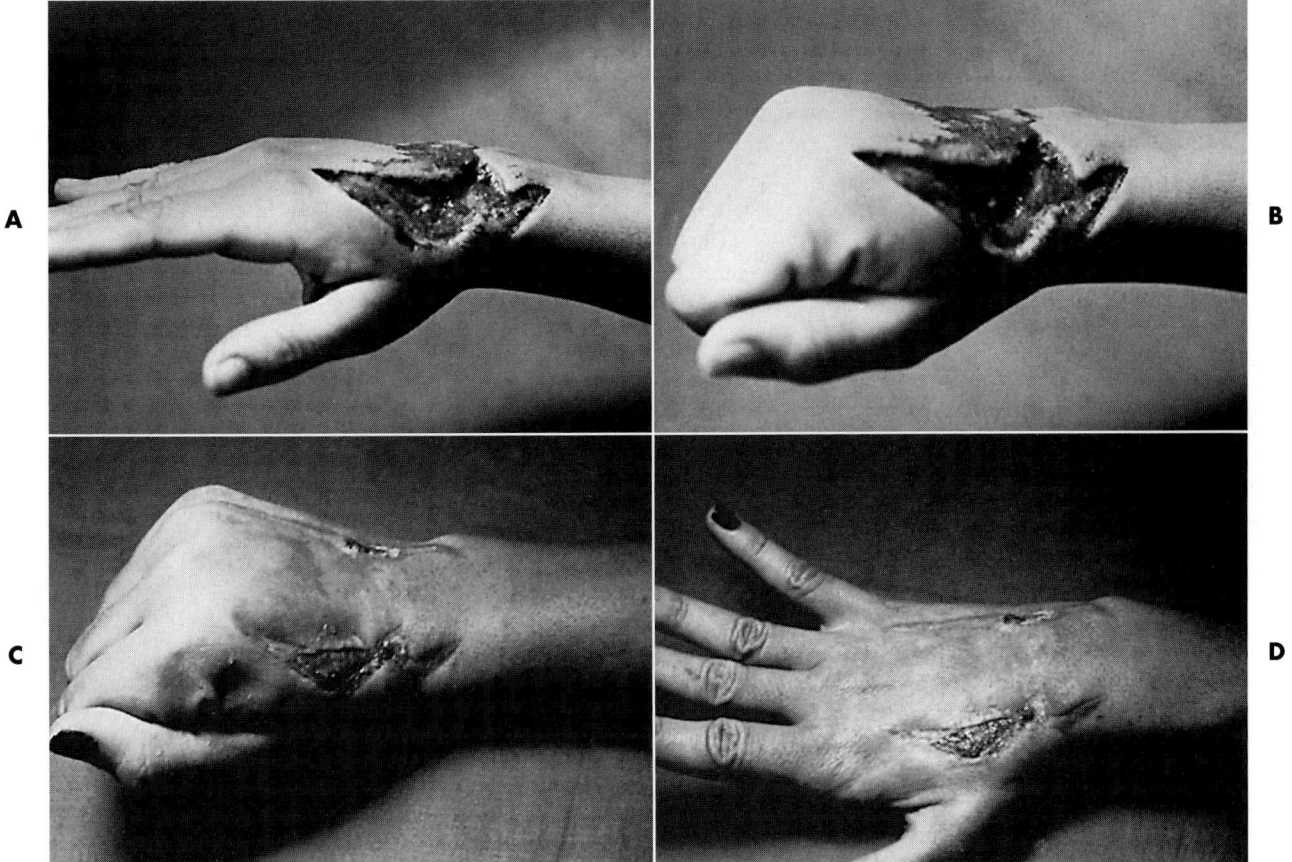

Fig. 19-1. A and **B,** Subcutaneous dorsal infection treated by debridement and early motion. **C** and **D,** Healing progresses while the patient actively exercises the hand. (From Burkhalter WE: Wound classification and management. In Hunter JM, et al, editors: *Rehabilitation of the hand,* ed 3, St Louis, 1990, Mosby.)

frank infection (Fig. 19-1) or for other wounds, such as fingertip injuries, in which the benefits of wound contraction afforded by secondary intention healing may serve to significantly decrease the size of the scar.[43] Throughout this process, restoration of motion and function of the injured part remains a far greater priority than closure of the wound.[33]

Repair of associated injuries to deeper structures usually can be conducted at the time of delayed primary wound closure. Even if the more complex reconstruction of deeper tissues is delayed further, there is significant advantage to performing fracture fixation at this time. Control of the wound may be more readily obtained in the presence of skeletal stability, and early motion can be initiated.[35,78,106]

Wound closure usually can be accomplished by simple suture or the use of split-thickness skin graft (STSG). Provisional wound closure with STSG may be preferable in certain complex, untidy wounds. Early rehabilitation then can be instituted and motion recovered, leaving more definitive coverage procedures for a later date.[35] In some cases, the skin defect may overlie vital deeper tissues that

will not accept split graft. Several studies have advocated early flap coverage in this instance,[37,84] provided that the surgeon is certain of the character of the deeper aspects of the wound at the time this is performed.

One of the most challenging decisions in the care of complex wounds is often whether salvage of the injured part is feasible or advisable.[195] Amputation never should be considered lightly, if only based on the consideration of potential complications.[26,154] We must not, however, allow function of the entire hand to be sacrificed while attempting salvage of a marginal digit or struggle for months to maintain a dysvascular insensate hand that is of far less functional value than an appropriate prosthesis would be. Mature surgical judgment is required in these instances. If amputation is to be performed, we must consider the salvage of viable portions of the deleted part to aid in the repair of the residual hand or limb.[39]

Surgical treatment of the open wound must be performed in the appropriate setting, just as is the case for elective surgery. There is no place for hurried exploration in the emergency department. Adequate anesthesia, proper light-

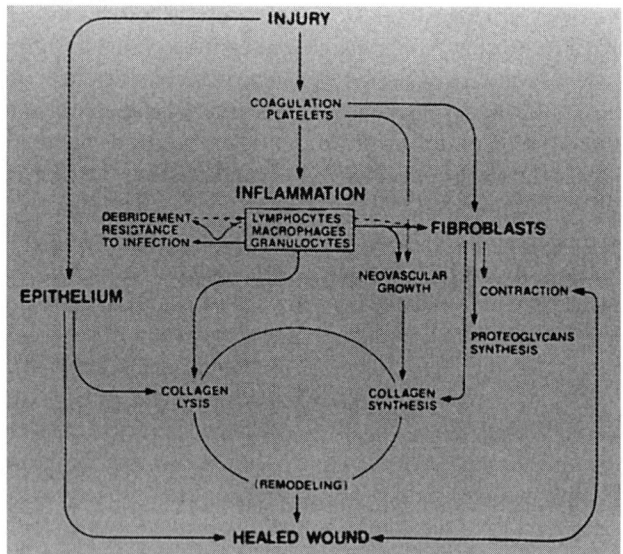

Fig. 19-2. Schematic concept of wound healing. (From Hunt TK, et al, editors: *Soft and hard tissue repair,* New York, 1984, Praeger, an imprint of Greenwood Publishing Group, Westport, Conn.)

ing, tourniquet control, magnification, and the availability of instruments to complete whatever repair is deemed necessary, are all prerequisites. Care of the open wound is a constantly challenging process; we should not choose to handicap ourselves in its performance.

WOUND EVALUATION AND TREATMENT: THE THERAPIST'S PERSPECTIVE

Knowledge of wound biology and the physiology of tissue repair is the basis of clinical decision making in the treatment of the simple, complex, or multilayered wound.

Wound healing is a cellular event. Each phase of wound healing is characterized by changes in cellularity as different cell types, primarily neutrophils, monocytes, macrophages, fibroblasts, and endothelial cells, migrate into and out of the wound bed[42,52,58,71,126] (Fig. 19-2). This cellular activity, initiated by tissue and platelet disruption, is regulated by a complex interaction of biochemical exchanges that orchestrate the events of phagocytosis, neovascularization, and biosynthesis of reparative collagen.[52,67,71,76,87,100,126,141,165]

The dramatic changes in wound healing activity usually are divided into three overlapping stages.* In the first stage of repair, the inflammatory or exudative stage, the neutrophil and macrophage are responsible for clearing the wound of debris to set the stage for subsequent repair.[15,201,208] The macrophage is the most important regulatory cell in the inflammatory stage because it is critical to bactericidal control and is chemotactic to the fibroblast.[24,87,118,165,200] Secretory products of the macrophage, such as interleukin-1 (IL-1), can enhance fibroblast proliferation and collagen synthesis.[187] The macrophage also may be important in

the normal process of angiogenesis, the formation of new blood vessels in granulation tissue.[114,201,210] A nonmitogenic chemoattractant for endothelial cells, possibly derived from macrophages, has been isolated from wound fluid.[14]

The migration of epithelial cells, the process known as *epithelialization,* is initiated within hours of injury, sealing the cleanly incised and sutured wound within 6 to 48 hours.[193] Epithelial cell movement is stimulated by an apparent loss of cellular contact that occurs with wounding and is stimulated by the process of contact guidance.[193] This cellular migration is terminated when advancing cells meet like advancing cells by the phenomenon known as *contact inhibition.*[183] Epidermal cells will migrate toward the area of cell deficit, following the predictable pattern of mobilization, migration, mitosis, and cellular differentiation.[183] The cells maintain their numbers by mitosis, both in fixed basal cells away from the wound edges, and in migrating cells, with the net result being a resurfacing of the wound and thickening of the new epithelial layer.[178,193] This reepithelialization process is influenced and possibly directed by a bath of cytokines arising from cells in the wound environment and in distant tissues.[193]

In the second stage of healing, the fibroblastic or reparative stage, the fibroblast will begin the process of collagen synthesis.[55,149] The fibroblast, signaled by the macrophage, platelet-derived growth factor (PDGF), or other mononuclear cells, initially secretes the elements of ground substance, protein polysaccharides, and various glycoproteins, and at approximately the fourth to fifth day after wounding, collagen synthesis begins.[87,133,141,178]

The myofibroblast, a highly specialized form of fibroblast, is thought to be responsible for the phenomenon of wound contraction.[185] This contractile fibroblast has the characteristics of both the smooth muscle cell and the fibroblast and is found in open granulating wounds, whereas fibroblasts are found in closed incised wounds.[185] The role of the myofibroblast and the mechanism of contraction are still controversial. Researchers have suggested that the histologic existence of myofibroblasts is related to a transitional state of fibroblasts in granulation tissue, wherein they prepare to migrate from a healed wound.[185]

Endothelial cells form the new blood vessels in granulation tissue, which provide oxygen and nutrients to the wound site.[77] These nutrients are necessary for the synthesis, deposition, and organization of the extracellular matrix.[200] Angiogenesis is thought to be directed chemically by growth factors and macrophage-secreted angiogenic peptides.[14,29,101,119,200,201,210]

The third stage of wound healing is characterized by the maturation and remodeling of scar tissue or extracellular matrix manufactured during the second or reparative stage.[145,165,183]

Several excellent texts and articles are available that provide a more detailed review of current research on all aspects of wound healing.[42,75,85,116,134,184]

---

*References 41, 58, 102, 116, 165, 183, 208, 217.

Understanding the normal cellular activity of wound repair and regeneration is critical to accurate wound assessment, which in turn determines successful wound treatment. The key issue in wound management is understanding the physiologic effect of our actions, be they debridement, cleansing, disinfection, dressing, or the use of modalities or motion, on the natural response of wound healing. These treatments all contribute, either positively or negatively, to that cellular response.

Applied basic science: what's new?

Recent advances in the bioregulation of normal wound repair may suggest new modalities to hasten healing in the simple wound and to stimulate healing in the nonhealing wound.* Much of this new research defines the role of peptides, IL-1, growth factors, and wound fluids in wound metabolism† and supports the concept of maintaining a moist wound environment in the noninfected wound as a means of facilitating biochemical and cellular activity.‡ The deleterious effects of desiccation, mechanical trauma, and some topical treatments have been studied in terms of their inhibition of normal cellular function, and the results should alter some currently popular, but unscientific, wound management techniques.[22,68,90,110,160,163,179]

The concept of tissue engineering has been the focus of much study in the past decade. Woo et al.[219] define *tissue engineering* as the manipulation of biochemical and cellular mediators to effect protein synthesis and to improve tissue remodeling. They make the point that this aspect of wound manipulation is in the early stages of research. The new biologic therapies being developed from this basic science research use the application of growth factors to both cutaneous wounds and fibrous structures and use gene transfer techniques and cell therapy to alter wound healing. This new technology will most likely alter future treatment techniques,[21,32,152,219] but these new techniques do not have much clinical application for the hand clinician as of this writing. Buckwalter and Grodzinsky[32] remind us that even though tissue engineering promises to facilitate bone and fibrous tissue healing in the future, to date, none has proven to be as effective as the mechanical loading of healing tissues with controlled stress.

Products that interact with biologic tissues (the application of topically applied growth factors, and biologic dressing impregnated with growth factors) flood the marketplace, and although they also will alter clinical management,[120,188] some researchers warn that we have not yet met with appropriate use of this new technology,[177] and that "a serious lack of knowledge exists with clinicians who use the clinical application of topically applied solutes in wounds."[46] Several articles are suggested to help the reader

gain perspective regarding clinical application of this new technology.[19,21,32,120,177,188,219]

For the most part, management of the upper extremity cutaneous wound by the hand surgeon or hand therapist is not an issue. The cleanly incised and sutured wound epithelializes within 6 to 48 hours,[193] and the noninfected wound allowed to heal by secondary intention is expected to contract at a predictable pace.[165,185] The normal phases of wound healing usually proceed without difficulty when the wound is managed with careful debridement of nonviable tissue, physiologic repair, and routine wound care with cleansing and dressing.[175] The hand clinician will in most cases focus attention on the schedules for healing, immobilization, and mobilization for the deeper injured and repaired tissues. However, with complications of infection or dehiscence, and healing altered by malnutrition, irradiation, medication, immunosuppression, or a poor local blood supply, wound management becomes more of an issue and the significance of scientific clinical management becomes more apparent.* Depressed healing associated with vasculitis, venostasis, diabetes, immunosuppression, and burn care has inspired much of the work produced by multidisciplinary specialties that has produced the new clinical treatments with biologic dressings, oxygen therapy, and growth factors.[116,117,125] Cancer research has had a significant effect on the body of wound healing knowledge, providing the early analysis of peptide growth factors.[101,141] As previously noted, manipulation of the microenvironment of the wound and enhancement of cellular activity through the use of growth factors are still in the early experimental stages but predictably will alter clinical management of repaired tendon, nerve, and the complex wound.† The integration of biotechnology and the biochemical aspects of wound research may have tremendous relevance to our specialty because many of these new treatments claim to regulate cellular activity, speed epithelialization and contraction, and decrease inflammation.‡ The application of a more scientific approach to wound healing may alter scar deposition and speed healing, decreasing the associated factors of morbidity—delayed healing, pain, excess fibrosis, longer treatment time, and increased expense. Treatment that may be helpful but not critical for the uncomplicated wound may be obligatory for the complex wound.

The next section addresses clinical decision making in wound evaluation and the effects of therapeutic management techniques on the cellular events in the different stages of wound healing.

Wound assessment: a traditional approach

Traditional wound assessment is well described in the literature.‡ Wounds are evaluated in terms of risk factors for

---

*References 19, 21, 32, 83, 87, 99, 119, 177, 188, 219.
†References 53, 54, 63, 87, 166, 173, 207.
‡References 13, 17, 62, 71, 72, 119, 186, 200, 203, 206, 211, 213.

*References 6, 16, 18, 31, 118, 128, 146, 148, 153, 175, 178.
†References 11, 40, 45, 74, 79, 82, 151, 167, 173, 219.
‡References 4, 5, 7-9, 29, 55, 192, 206, 207, 211.

altered healing, the presence or absence of infection, physical location, size, appearance, and the stage of wound healing. Wound edema, presence of hematoma, vascular perfusion, and the status of the deeper tissues are noted. The rate of healing in relation to the date of injury or surgery and the duration of previous treatment or chronicity of the wound are important factors in treatment planning.

Assessment of infection includes a review of risk factors for the individual case, visual inspection, and tissue cultures.[34,191,205] Before surgery or medical management, the surgeon will have established the factors that are predictive of susceptibility to infection or an altered rate of healing. As discussed previously, this information determines timing of technique for wound closure or surgical management. Risk factors are determined based on an accurate history, including information concerning the mechanism of injury, the environment in which the injury occurred, the patient's medical and immunosuppressive state, systemic or local nutritional status, and previous medical treatment with medication or radiation.* These risk factors should be known to the hand therapist and the surgeon because the therapist in most cases will be monitoring the wound more intensively than the surgeon. Patients at high risk for infection may need to be seen more often than those who will predictably experience benign wound healing.

Visual inspection will help determine whether a wound is healing with a normal inflammatory response or, if in fact, it has become infected. The cardinal signs of inflammation, redness, swelling, pain, and heat, accompany the biochemical and fluid aspects of the early inflammatory stage of wound healing and are not to be confused with infection.[165,208] The therapist should understand that purulence does not always represent the presence of infection.[176,178] If the inflammatory response is exaggerated or if the drainage is purulent, then bacterial counts must be obtained to determine the level of wound contamination.[135]

Clinical measurements of wound sepsis are determined by wound culture. The U.S. Institute of Surgical Research defines wound sepsis caused by bacterial overgrowth as bacterial counts exceeding 10^5 organisms per gram of tissue.[72,177] Traumatic wounds with multiple layers of injury to skin, muscle, and bone are difficult to evaluate because the colony count may be variable at each level (Burkhalter WE, personal communication, 1990).

One must understand that wound healing in the clinical situation will occur in the presence of bacteria; it is the quantity of and not the mere presence of bacteria that creates alterations in the reparative process.[178] Acceptable levels of endogenous, nonpathogenic microflora, as opposed to frank infection, will determine the rate of wound healing and may actually stimulate tissue repair.[47] Favorable microflora in the wound bed may stimulate epidermal cell migration and healing.[121,122] Wound fluid monocyte and macrophage

*References 6, 15, 16, 18, 34, 47, 61, 62, 146, 148, 153, 175.

counts have been found to be markedly elevated, and collagen deposition increased, in wounds inoculated with 10^2 organisms.[122] Lower bacterial counts or well-controlled infection have been found to enhance chemotactic and bactericidal activity.[178]

However, in the presence of significant infection (greater than 10^5 organisms per gram of tissue), impaired leukocyte function, decreased chemotaxis, impaired cellular migration, epithelialization, and intracellular killing are noted.[139,178] Superficial infection may damage new epithelium through the release of neutrophil proteases,[163] and bacterial counts greater than 10^5, may retard wound contraction.[178] Infected wounds are affected adversely by the formation of thicker connective tissue and excessive angiogenesis, which is associated with prolific scar formation.[31,55,101,122,178] Robson,[178] in a review of studies on the effect of bacterial count on fibroplasia, found the results to be inconsistent, but noted that collagen and hydroxyproline contents were consistently higher in infected wounds.

Thus infection control is important not only to the rate of healing but also to the management of scar, which ultimately can interfere with tissue gliding and excursion for tendon, nerve, ligament, joint, and skin.

The wound healing by primary intention is usually simple to evaluate and treat. Attention in these cases is usually directed to protection of the deeper structures, the status of suture or staples, tension at the suture line, quality or quantity of drainage, and viability of the tissue. These wounds are described in terms of periwound edema, inflammation, infection, wound tension, viability, and rate of epithelialization.

If the wound closed by primary intention develops complications and dehisces, it becomes a wound healing by secondary intention.[34] Wounds left to heal by secondary intention, or the chronic or infected wound, pose more complex questions and require more clinical problem-solving and decision-making skills of the health care practitioner.

The following section attempts to simplify decision making and treatment planning for the hand therapist who may be confused by the many issues surrounding the management of the complex wound.

Wound assessment: the three-color concept

Marion Laboratories introduced a universal classification system for open wounds in the late 1980s that simplifies wound description and wound treatment. Their approach uses a "three-color concept" to describe wound status. Wounds are described as red, yellow, black, or a combination of two or three colors. The clinical application of this classification system is described by Cuzzel[49,50,194] in several articles. The following color descriptions for evaluation and treatment are summaries of her articles. Clinical decision making as it relates to therapeutic management by debridement, cleansing, disinfecting, and dress-

Table 19-1. Simplifying clinical decision-making for open wounds

	Black wound	Yellow wound	Red wound
Description	Covered with thick necrotic tissue or eschar	Generating exudate, looks creamy, contains pus, debris, and viscous surface exudate	Uninfected, properly healing with definite borders, may be pink or beefy red, granulated tissue and neovascularization
Cellular activity	1. Autolysis, collagenase activity 2. Defense, phagocytosis 3. Macrophage cell	1. Immune response, defense 2. Phagocytosis 3. Macrophage cell	1. Endothelial cells—Angiogenesis 2. Fibroblast cells—collagen and ground substance 3. Myofibroblast—wound contraction
Débridement	1. Surgical, preferred 2. Mechanical, whirlpool, dressings 3. Chemical, enzymatic digestion	Separate wound debris with aggressive scrubs, irrigation, or whirlpool	N/A—avoid any tissue trauma or stripping of new cells
Cleansing	1. Whirlpool 2. Irrigation 3. Soap and water scrubs	1. Use no antiseptics 2. Soap and water 3. Surfactant-soaked sponge 4. Polaxmer 188, Pluronic F-68	1. No antiseptics 2. Ringer's lactate 3. Sterile saline, sterile water
Topical treatment	Topical antimicrobials with low WBC or cellulitis	1. Topical antimicrobials to control bacterial contamination 2. Silver sulfadiazine, bactroban, neomycin, polymixin B, neosporin	1. N/A for simple wounds 2. Vitamin A for patients on steroids 3. Antimicrobials for immunosuppressed
Dressing	1. Wet-to-dry for necrotic tissue 2. Proteolytic enzyme to débride 3. Synthetic dressing, autolysis 4. Dress to soften eschar	1. Wet-to-dry—wide mesh to absorb drainage 2. Wet-to-wet—saturated with medicants 3. Hydrocolloid or semipermeable foam dressings, hydrogels	1. Occlusive or semiocclusive dressings; semipermeable films 2. Protect wound fluids and prevent dessication
Desired goal	1. Remove debris and mechanical obstruction to allow epithelialization, collagen deposition to proceed 2. Evolve to clean, red wound	1. Light débridement without disrupting new cells 2. Exudate absorption 3. Bacterial control 4. Evolve to red wound	1. Protect new cells 2. Keep wound moist and clean to speed healing 3. Promote epithelialization, granulation tissue formation, angiogenesis, wound contraction

From Evans RB: *Hand Clin* 7:418, 1991.
N/A, Not applicable; *WBC,* white blood cell.

ing is reviewed in a brief synopsis as it relates to wound color[42,50,67,179] (Table 19-1).

The red wound. The red wound is uninfected, healing according to a predictable schedule, and characterized by definite borders, granulation tissue, and apparent revascularization (Fig. 19-3 and Plate 27). The fibroblast, myofibroblast, endothelial, and epithelial cells are active in this wound, orchestrating the events of epithelialization, angiogenesis, and collagen synthesis. Skin-donor sites or surgical wounds healing by secondary intention, as in the case of an open Dupuytren's release, are examples of red wounds often seen in the hand clinic. Superficial wounds and acute partial or second-degree burns are classified as red wounds if they are uniformly pink in appearance.

Tissue oxygenation determines the color of the wound. A chronic red wound has pale pink to beefy red granulation tissue and usually is in the late stages of repair. Red wounds closing by secondary intention fill with granulation tissue from the edge of the wound to the center, closing by contraction and epithelialization, or they may be closed by grafting at the appropriate time.

Cellular activity in the clean red wound must be protected and facilitated by the appropriate therapy. Therapeutic goals are to protect the local wound environment, maintain

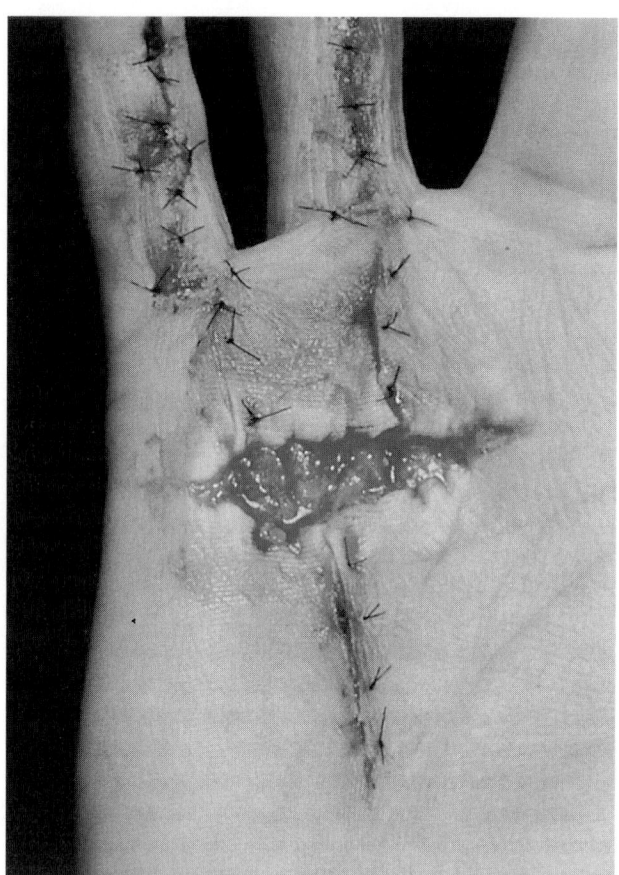

Fig. 19-3. A red wound in a Dupuytren's fasciectomy 3 days after surgery. The wound in the palm is beefy red, without infection, with epithelial, endothelial myofibroblast, and fibroblast cellular activity taking place. Note that the digital wounds are already epithelized.

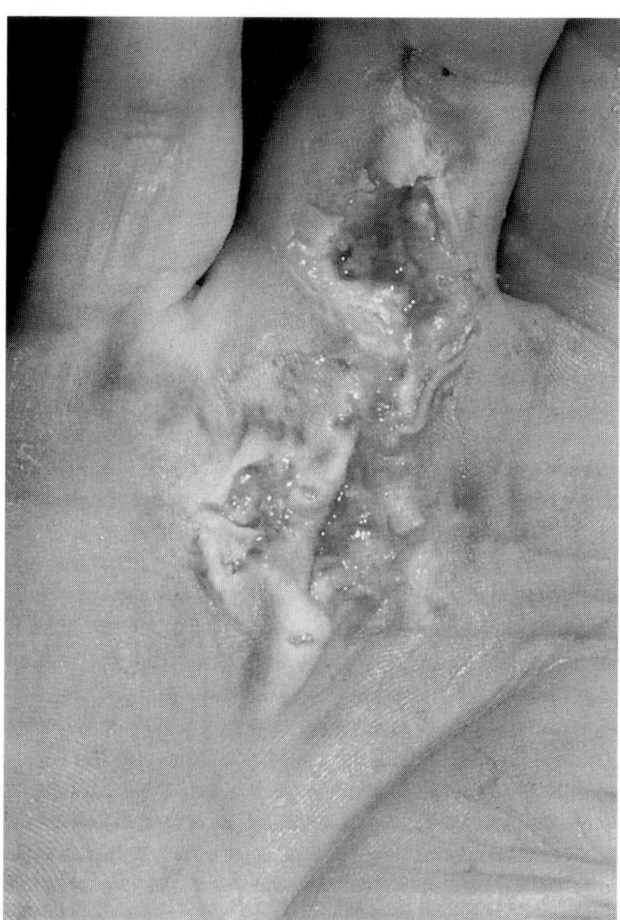

Fig. 19-4. A yellow wound infected with *Pseudomonas* in a postsurgical Dupuytren's fasciectomy closed by primary intention with subsequent dehiscence. Although some of the green color is from skin pencil, the wound is yellow-green with a distinctive odor. Cellular activity is dominated by the macrophage, which is stimulated by bacteria and inflammation. (From Evans RB: *Hand Clin* 7:419, 1991.)

humidity, protect the wound fluids from desiccation, and protect the newly forming granulation tissue and epithelial cells. These wounds should be cleansed with lactated Ringer's solution or for home care with a nondetergent, mild pump soap such as Ivory or Dove. The soap should be applied to the periwound area only and rinsed with running water. Antiseptics should not be used on the red wound. Topical treatment may include an antibiotic ointment if the patient is at high risk for developing infection. The newly forming cells should be protected from noxious mechanical forces (tapes, dry dressings, wet-to-dry dressings, whirlpool agitation, and wound scrubbing). Occlusive or semiocclusive dressings, which are described in the following section, may be used to protect the local wound environment and wound humidity.

The yellow wound. The yellow wound may range in color from a creamy ivory to a canary yellow. Colonization with *Pseudomonas* gives the wound a yellow-green appear-

ance and a distinctive odor. The yellow wound is draining, purulent, and characterized by slough that is liquid or semiliquid in texture; it contains pus, yellow fibrous debris, or viscous surface exudate (Fig. 19-4 and Plate 23). The generating exudate may promote bacterial growth. Cellular activity is dominated by the macrophage, which is stimulated by the presence of bacteria and inflammation. The macrophage functions to clear the tissue of debris and to remove pathogenic organisms; thus it is critical to bactericidal control and phagocytosis.[200]

Epithelialization and wound contraction, activity controlled by the epithelial cells and myofibroblasts, may be occurring at the pink wound margins but, in general, are delayed until infection or excessive inflammation are under control.

The goal of treatment in the case of the yellow wound is to facilitate cellular activity so that it can evolve into a red wound. Continual cleansing, removal of nonviable tissue, and absorption of excess drainage are important to decrease the workload of the macrophage.[217] These wounds may be washed with soap and water aggressively, irrigated with a water pick[204] or syringe, or treated with sterile whirlpools to separate surface debris and necrotic tissue. Topical antiseptics are cytotoxic and depress leukocyte function, thus depleting the body's natural defense mechanism.[48,61,62,72,180] If bacterial proliferation requires control, an antibiotic such as Silvadene or Bactroban, and not a topical antiseptic, should be used in the wound.[182,191] Wet-to-dry dressings should be placed over only the wound because their application to the periwound area may cause skin maceration. Wet-to-dry dressings should be used with care because their removal may disturb new cells that are forming at the edge of the wound in addition to necrotic tissue. Dressings to absorb excess exudate while maintaining a moist environment, such as semipermeable foams, hydrocolloids, or hydrogels, may be used in the noninfected wound.[72]

The black wound. The black wound ranges in color from dark brown to gray-black; it is covered with eschar or thick necrotic tissue (Fig. 19-5 and Plate 29). Cellular activity represents several stages of wound repair that may be occurring simultaneously. The macrophage is working to clear the area of bacteria and debris and to signal fibroblasts to the area. The fibroblast and endothelial cells are beginning to synthesize collagen and new vessels as the debris is removed. This cellular activity is facilitated by the removal of the eschar surgically, mechanically, or enzymatically, in an effort to decrease the workload of the macrophage and to allow for unimpeded cellular migration. Eschar impedes cellular migration and proliferation by acting as a mechanical block and provides a medium in which bacteria can proliferate.

Debridement is the therapeutic goal for the black wound. Meticulous and timely debridement decreases the risk of infection and hastens healing by facilitating normal cellular response. These wounds may be debrided surgically, mechanically, or with proteolytic enzymes[49,72,191] such as Travase or Elase. Before mechanical debridement, the tissue may be softened as it is cleansed with scrubs or whirlpool to loosen dead tissue from the viable wound bed.

Topical antibiotics may soften eschar and decrease bacterial count. These wounds should be dressed to protect the wound environment, soften eschar, and facilitate autolysis. Synthetic dressings may facilitate autolysis by protecting wound fluids that contain the white cells responsible for phagocytosis.

Wound management: the therapist's role

The therapist can contribute to the wound healing process by using management techniques that protect wound fluids, help prevent or control infection, minimize adverse mechanical influences, and control the collagen maturation process. Physical agents may facilitate cellular movement associated with increased blood flow, epithelialization, and macrophage

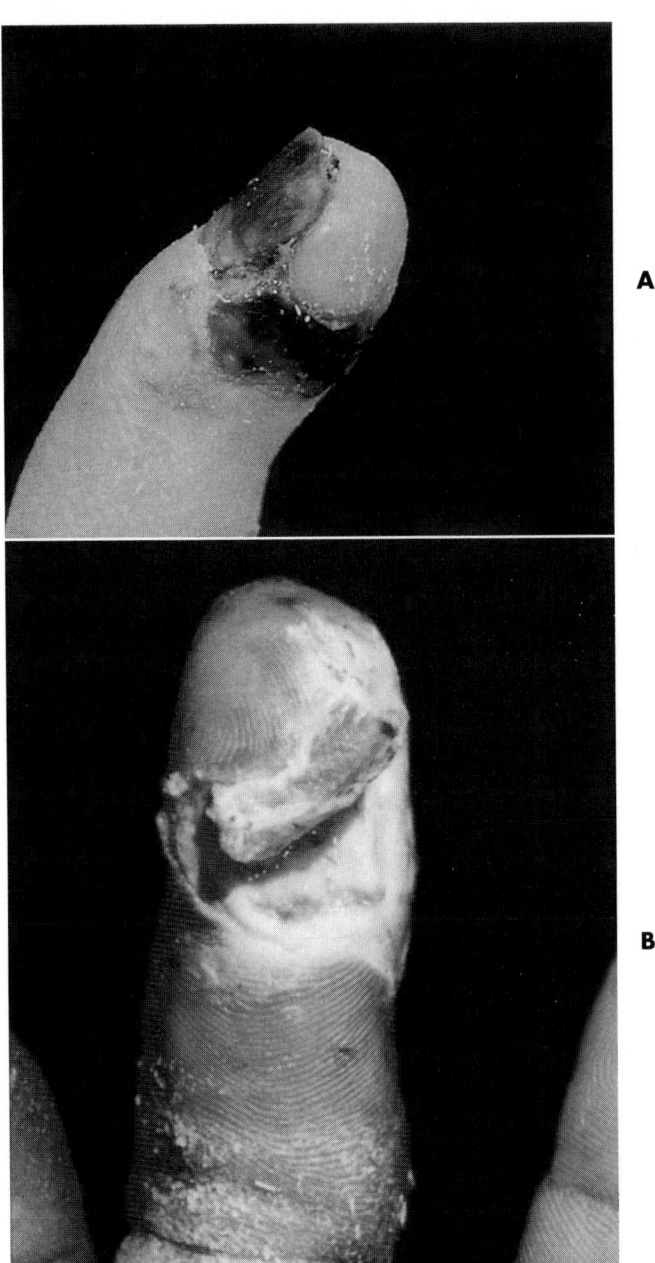

Fig. 19-5. A, A black wound on the fingertip that required mechanical debridement in therapy after whirlpool. The macrophage is working to clean the area of bacterial and debris. The fibroblast and endothelial cells will begin to synthesize collagen and new vessels as the debris is removed. **B,** A failed fingertip skin graft seen as a black and yellow wound with red at its periphery. The black portion was mechanically debrided, the yellow portion gently scrubbed, and the red portion protected. (From Evans RB: *Hand Clin* 7:420, 1991.)

or fibroblast activity and may have a role in the stimulation of growth factors.

Protecting wound fluids. The positive role of humidity in wound resurfacing, first reported more than four decades ago,[96,215,216] has been recognized as one of the most important factors in wound healing by several researchers.* Wound fluids contain certain growth factors, including somatomedins, interleukin-4, and other cytokines, that interact with the host tissue, promote cellular activity, and contribute to wound metabolism.† Polypeptide growth factors are proteins that are mitogens and chemoattractants, serving to recruit leukocytes and fibroblasts to the wounded tissue.[87,141] IL-1, a secretory product of the macrophage, has been demonstrated to enhance fibroblast activity and collagen synthesis.[187] Somatomedins are anabolic hormones that affect cell replication, protein and glycogen synthesis, and nutrient transport.[192]

This cellular infiltrate is thought to guide the reparative process and to determine the final result after injury.[71] The tissue fluids that accumulate in a wound create a favorable environment for angiogenesis and granulation tissue formation on which epithelialization can occur.[17,58,69,72,100,118,208,216]

An accelerated rate of healing in moist wounds is supported by histologic evaluation of full-thickness wounds in porcine skin.[58] Neutrophils and macrophages decreased in number more rapidly under moist conditions, and the proliferative phase cells (fibroblasts and endothelial cells) increased more rapidly. Progression to the remodeling phase and advanced angiogenesis was noted in moist as compared with dry wounds.[58]

Dessication. In an unprotected wound, evaporation occurs within hours of tissue disruption, allowing wound fluids to escape the wound bed.[72] An open wound exposed to air for 2 to 3 hours will become necrotic to a depth of 0.2 to 0.3 mm.[216] The desiccated dermis or scab impedes epithelial cell migration and acts as a mechanical barrier, creating a dell or depression in the wound as the epidermal cells are required to migrate from the wound margins deep beneath the dried tissue.[215] This process is minimized in a wound that is occluded and not allowed to dessicate.[7]

Human skin has measurable transcutaneous electrical potential differences that are decreased with wounding.[44,66,69] Dehydration of wound tissue may decrease the lateral electrical gradient thought to control epidermal cell migration.[72,73,108]

Exposed wounds tend to be more inflamed and necrotic than occluded wounds.[217] In later stages, the dermis of exposed wounds is more fibroblastic, fibrotic, and scarred.[217]

Occlusion is a term that refers to the ability of a wound dressing to allow the transfer of water vapor and gases from a wound surface to the atmosphere.[217] The concept of sequestering wound fluids in the noninfected open wound for the purpose of enhancing cellular activity or facilitating autolytic debridement with occlusive or semiocclusive dressings has led to the development of many environmental dressings.[8,13,56,59,69,72,97,99,111,123,143,168,206]

These microenvironmental dressings may be categorized as films, foams, hydrocolloids, hydrogels, and calcium alginates.* Although there are substantial differences in these dressings, they are similar in that they maintain wound humidity (are impermeable to water but not always water vapor), may permit exchange of gases, reduce pain, reduce mechanical trauma associated with dressing removal, and absorb exudate in some cases.[72] The properties and indications for the dressings are summarized as an introduction (Table 19-2), and several excellent review articles are recommended for more detailed study.[13,46,69,72,131,152,188,189,211,217]

Preventing and controlling infection. The therapist can contribute to infection control by using the appropriate therapeutic techniques to maintain a clean wound bed free of necrotic tissue or excess drainage, by protecting the wound from its external environment with the proper dressings and by instructing the patient concerning home wound care.

Cleansing. Cleanly incised and sutured wounds may be washed with a mild soap and running water as early as 24 hours after surgery.[157] I (RBE) generally rinse the sutured wound with saline until it is epithelialized at about 48 hours, and then briefly wash the periwound area and suture line with soap and water. The red wound may be rinsed with lactated Ringer's solution, which is more biologically compatible with the wound environment than saline. Some wound therapists currently believe that the pH of saline is too acidic for wound care. The red wound should not be scrubbed because this mechanical trauma could disrupt newly forming epithelium and vessels.[212] The yellow and black wound may be scrubbed with a mild soap and water. Dove or Ivory are recommended for home care (Crossland M, personal communication, 1990), or Pluronic F-68 or Poloxamer 188, nontoxic surfactants, can be used when more vigorous cleansing is needed.[62,179] A high-porosity sponge (90 ppi) may be used for mechanical scrubs because it is minimally abrasive and thus imposes less tissue damage.[62] The object of wound cleansing is to separate soil, particle, and debris from the wound but not to create cellular destruction. Hydraulic irrigation with a water pick or whirlpool are indicated only for yellow and black wounds to loosen debris from the wound bed.[182,203]

Cleansing solutions such as Hibiclens, hexachlorophene, and povidone-iodine or Betadine may be used on intact skin before surgery on the periwound area, but if applied to the wound itself, are cytotoxic and will invite infection by destroying macrophages.[18,23,61,90,179]

---

*References 4, 5, 7-9, 59, 97, 99, 123, 152, 158, 168, 211, 217.
†References 14, 17, 71, 87, 141, 155, 171, 192, 200, 208.

*References 13, 56, 64, 72, 97, 105, 123, 131, 137, 189, 203, 213, 217.

Table 19-2. Properties, indications, and precautions for microenvironmental dressings*

	Semipermeable film	Semipermeable foam	Semipermeable hydrogel	Hydrocolloid
Commercial name	Bioclusive Blisterfilm Ensure-It Omniderm Oproflex Opsite Polyskin Tegaderm Uniflex	Coraderm Lyofoam Lyofoam C Primaderm Synthaderm	Geliperm Intrasite Scherisorb Spenco Secondskin Vigilon	Biofilm Comfeel ulcus Demiflex Duoderm Granuflex Intact J&J Ulcer Dressing Restore
Indications	Clean, minimally exudative wound; red wound, sutured wounds, donor graft sites (split-thickness grafts), superficial burns, IV site dressing, superficial ulcers	Yellow wound, moderate to high exudate, skin ulcers, odiferous cancers, venous ulcers when combined with stockings or pressure dressings	Donor sites, superficial operation sites, chronic damage to epithelium, yellow exudating wounds; may apply over topical antimicrobials	Yellow wounds, friction blisters, postoperative dermabrasions, decubitus ulcers, venous stasis ulcers, cutaneous ulcers
Characteristics	Semiocclusive, occlusive, nonabsorbent, transparent, thin, adhesive, resistant to shear, low friction, does not control temperature, permeable to O_2 gas and water, impermeable to water and bacteria	Hydrophilic properties on wound side, hydrophobic on other side; limited absorbent capacity; permeable to water vapor and gas; polyurethane foams with a heat- and pressure-modified wound contact surface	Three-dimensional hydrophilic polymers that interact with aqueous solutions, swell and maintain water in their structure; insoluble in water; conform to wound surface; permeable to water vapor and gas, impermeable to water; tape required for fixation	Combine benefits of occlusion and absorbency; absorbs moderate to high exudate: expands into wound as exudate is absorbed to provide wound support; vision occluded; atraumatic removal; outer layer impermeable to gas, water, bacteria
Function	Mimics skin performance protects from pathogens, decreases pain, maintains wound humidity, enhances healing by protecting wound fluids; protects from pressure, shear, friction	Maintains wound humidity, absorbs excess exudate, maintains warmth, decreases pain, cushions wound while averting "strikethrough"	Maintains wound humidity; facilitates autolytic debridement; absorbs excess exudate; allows evaporation without compromising humidity; removes toxic components from wound; maintains warmth; decreases pain	Absorbs exudate to form a gel that swells; applies firm pressure to the floor of a deep ulcer; autolytic debridement maintains wound humidity; maintains warmth; removes toxic compounds; decreases wound site
Precautions	Only for uninfected, red wounds; apply to dry periwound area; frame wound by 2 in; break-in seal allows microbes to enter wound from dressing margins	Visual monitoring occluded; low adherence, must tape	Permeable to bacteria; for moderate exudate; dehydrates easily; nonadhesive	Vision occluded; do not use on hairy surfaces

*Disclaimer/contraindications: All environmental dressings must be used in accordance with product information, which provides guidelines for indications, application, and contraindications. Some contraindications are wounds ulcerated into the muscle, tendon, bone; third-degree burns edge-to-edge eschar; wounds associated with osteomyelitis and active vasculitis, ischemic ulcers, and infected wounds. These products are all-inclusive and are not necessarily endorsed by the author or publisher but are provided as a source for further study.

Several authors have studied the adverse effects of povidone-iodine.[18,23,62,179] Aronoff[12] has demonstrated that long-term povidone-iodine topical application may result in systemic absorption with resulting negative effects. Wound epithelialization and early tensile strength are affected negatively by 1% povidone-iodine solution. Researchers have reported that this solution must be diluted to 0.001% concentration to be nontoxic to human fibroblasts.[130] At this strength, the solution is still bactericidal to *Staphylococcus aureus*. However, Rodeheaver[179] has demonstrated that cleansing with povidone-iodine offers no advantage over cleansing with saline solution. He found the same level of viable bacteria in wounds contaminated with *S. aureus* when treated with either saline or povidone-iodine. Both hexachlorophene and povidone-iodine scrubs have been found to instantaneously lyse white blood cells that are critical to wound defense,[179] and povidone-iodine damages red blood cells, resulting in significant hemolysis.[30] Feedar and Kloth[72] urge that povidone-iodine solution in whirlpools and on gauze dressings be reconsidered, and other authors[62,179,202] recommend cessation of this practice altogether.

Although we all have observed wound healing in the presence of these cleansing agents, it may be that the wounds we have treated could have responded more quickly, decreasing time, discomfort, and expense, had we more carefully protected the wound fluids and cellular environment.

Disinfecting. Many wound specialists have condemned the practice of decontaminating a wound after cleansing with topical antiseptics. The often-quoted adage that "the only solution that should be placed in a wound is one that can safely be poured in the physician's eye" is supported by most wound therapists.[22] Rodeheaver[182] has demonstrated that all antiseptic agents are cytotoxic and their only mechanism of action is to destroy cell walls. Almost four decades ago he reviewed commonly used antiseptics and found iodine, chlorhexidine, peroxide, boric acid, alcohols, hexachlorophene, formaldehyde, hypochlorite, acetic acid, silver nitrate, merthiolate, gentian violet, permanganate, and aluminum salts to be cytotoxic.[182]

Hydrogen peroxide (H_2O_2), which has little bactericidal action, is perhaps misused as often as povidone-iodine. Hydrogen peroxide is appropriately used on a crusted wound, or to cleanse periwound skin, but should not be used after crust separation, on new granulation tissue, or on closed wounds.[72]

Researchers have suggested that topical antibiotics are the only antimicrobial agents that are nontoxic and beneficial to wound cellular activity.[182] Bactroban is a broad-spectrum antimicrobial recommended for its bactericidal capacity, which is greater than that of other topical antimicrobials. Neosporin ointment has a wide spectrum of bactericidal activity, including most gram-positive and gram-negative bacteria found in both human and porcine skin.[72] Zinc bacitracin, which is one of the three antibacterial com-

ponents of Neosporin, was found to increase epidermal healing by 25% when compared with controls.[72] Contaminated blister wounds treated with a triple antibiotic of neomycin, polymyxin B, and bacitracin ointment demonstrated lower bacterial counts and faster healing when compared with similar wounds treated with only protection or antiseptics.[129] One percent Silvadene cream acts on a wide range of gram-negative and gram-positive bacteria as well as fungi. It has been used to prevent infection in burn wounds[95] and to salvage some or all parts of questionable flaps.[191] Silvadene treatment has been reported to reduce bacterial counts in wounds contaminated with less than 10^5 bacteria in 100% of the cases tested.[179] Silvadene also has been found to speed epithelialization in experimental animal studies.[179]

With each dressing change, the wound should be cleansed thoroughly of these ointments, and surface coagulum should be gently removed so that the fresh application of the topical antibiotic will gain contact with the wound bed.[60, 61] By using only antibiotic ointments and avoiding the use of cytotoxic antiseptics, bacterial count is controlled and macrophage function, so critical to wound defense, is protected. These ointments may speed epithelialization by keeping the wound moist, thereby preventing crust formation and desiccation, which serve as mechanical barriers to cell migration.

Debridement. Necrotic tissue promotes bacterial growth and, by mechanical impedance, interferes with epithelial cell migration.[62] Removal of this necrotic tissue by meticulous debridement may be the most critical aspect of care to prevent infection in the acute wound and in the management of the contaminated or chronic wound.[62,94]

Debridement can be accomplished mechanically, enzymatically, or biologically through the normal phagocytic activity of white blood cells (autolysis).[72] Mechanical debridement by the surgeon is a critical component of both primary and chronic care. The therapist can remove small areas of black or gray eschar or debris from combination yellow and black wounds with fine forceps and sharp scissors. The necrotic debris should be separated from the wound edges, working toward the center, to facilitate the process of wound contraction. The yellow wound can be gently debrided with a small bone curette, but care must be taken not to fracture new capillaries at the wound edges. Before mechanical debridement, the wound may be cleansed and softened in a clear water whirlpool. A scab may serve as a biologic dressing and left in place on a superficial wound, but if drainage occurs from beneath the scab, it is mandatory that it be debrided.[191]

Enzymatic debridement with topical enzymes such as Travase or Elase may be used to hasten separation of eschars, scabs, or fibrinous coagulum.[72,191] Collagenase debridement products Biozyme C and Santyl may hydrolyze undenatured collagen or facilitate debridement of difficult necrotic tissue.[72] Feedar and Kloth[72] categorize these topical en-

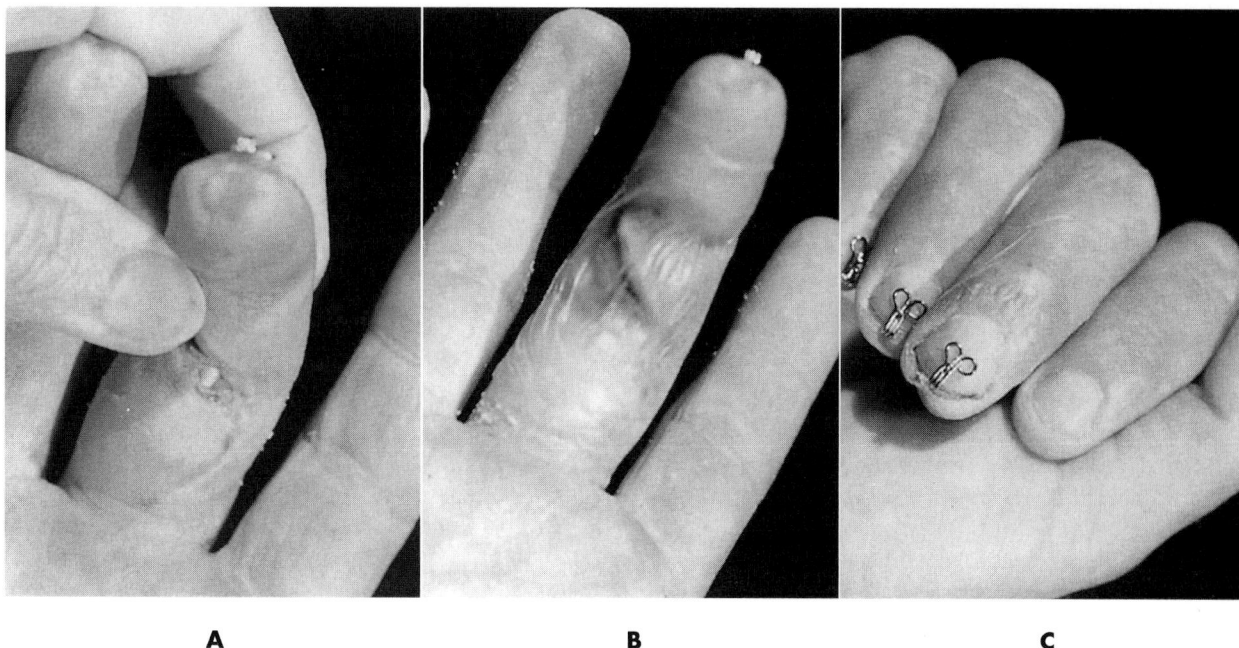

Fig. 19-6. A, Exposed repaired flexor tendon at 3 weeks after surgery. **B,** A Tegaderm dressing sequestered wound fluids and protected the exposed tendon until the wound was revised. **C,** The thin Tegaderm dressing offered minimal impedance to active flexion exercise, which was critical to maintaining tendon glide while the tendon was exposed.

zymes as selective, that is, working on only necrotic tissue, and their claim is supported by others who have demonstrated that these enzymes spare viable tissue.[92,220] Although these proteolytic enzymes may depress leukocyte phagocytosis, they do not significantly interfere with wound healing.[180] Hydrocolloid, alginate, or hydrogel dressings can be used to achieve natural autolytic cleansing.[189]

Autolytic debridement or biologic debridement is considered the most selective type of debridement because this process relies on the body's natural defense system.[72] The noted importance of this natural phagocytic activity has led to the concept of sequestering wound fluids to facilitate macrophage debridement and has led to the development of synthetic dressings that enhance autolytic debridement.[72,189]

Selective debridement by careful mechanical debridement, proteolytic enzymes, or autolytic debridement facilitates positive cellular response and is indicated for the yellow or black wound. Nonselective debridement, or that which indiscriminately removes both viable and nonviable tissue from the wound, may disturb new epithelial cells and granulation tissue and should be used with discretion. Nonselective debridement includes wet-to-dry, wet-to-wet, and dry-to-dry dressings, whirlpool therapy, vigorous scrubs, Dakin's solution, or hydrogen peroxide solutions.[72]

Dressing to prevent or control infection. The act of covering a wound is an attempt to reproduce the barrier function of epithelium.[217] The primary dressing, or that which is placed in direct contact with the wound, provides a barrier to the external environment and functions to prevent infection. Nonadherent, nonabsorbent contact layers such as Adaptic, Xeroform, Aquaphor, or Transite may help prevent desiccation and adhesion of the secondary dressing to the wound. These nonadherent contact layers are used postsurgically before the wound is sealed or epithelialized or can be used on a clean, red wound. The red wound can be protected from its environment with nonabsorbent film dressings such as Tegaderm, Opsite, or Bioclusive (see Table 19-1). These dressings are impermeable to water and provide all the benefits of moist wound healing previously described. I (RBE) have successfully used Tegaderm to protect the humidity of exposed tendon in the digit. This film allows complete motion, adheres with an airtight seal to the periwound area, and prevents tendon desiccation until the wound is closed by secondary intention or surgical means (Fig. 19-6 and Plate 30). These dressings provide a physiologic solution to a difficult problem, but they are not appropriate for infected wounds. Biolex wound gel (Bard Patient Care) with mesh dressings is another new product that provides a moist, acidic environment to maintain humidity for an exposed tendon.

When excess drainage or infection is present, dressing changes should be performed as often as demanded by the accumulation of debris and fluid and the overload of absorbent materials.[217] The absorption of exudate into a dressing reduces the work requirement of the macrophage for phagocytosis and autolytic debridement and also removes a potential substrate for microbial growth.[217] The accumulation of wound fluid to the point of flooding will cause maceration and bacterial overgrowth. Therefore an absorbent dressing should imbibe exudate, but not allow fluid accumulation to the level of the most superficial dressing layer ("strikethrough").[217] If "strikethrough" does occur, a channel is created that will allow microorganisms to enter the wound from the external environment.[217] The absorbent dressing should match the requirement of the wound. The acute, noninfected wound will exude maximally at 24 hours after surgery and may have as its secondary layer sterile absorbent woven or nonwoven gauze products that usually are made of cotton or rayon.[217]

Yellow, noninfected, exuding wounds may be dressed with some of the newer microenvironmental dressings that function to absorb fluid without "strikethrough," encourage autolytic debridement, and maintain body temperature[6,69,123,217] (see Table 19-2). Hydrocolloid and hydrogel dressings are those that combine the benefits of occlusion and absorption and are most often used for chronic yellow wounds.[56,137,213,217] Alginates absorb exudate, facilitate moist wound healing, and can be used to obtain hemostasis in an oozing wound.[105,123,203] Excess exudate also may be absorbed with hydrophilic products.[72] Yellow wounds should be irrigated of the yellow-brown gelatinous mass that remains on the wound after dressing removal when hydrocolloids are used.[217] The yellow wound also may be dressed with a wide meshed 4 × 4 dressing changed every 4 to 6 hours to absorb purulent drainage, or with a wet dressing saturated with saline or topical medicants. If topical medicants are used, they should not be allowed to dry out because this would increase the concentration of the medication, possibly rendering it cytotoxic.[191]

Open wounds with dead space should be lightly packed with a fine mesh strip gauze (e.g., Nu Gauze) to keep the superficial portions of the wound open while the deeper layers contract. Tight packing should be avoided because it could retard drainage and create tissue ischemia. A fine mesh (44/36) gauze prevents epithelial growth into the weave.[191]

Minimizing mechanical influences. Mechanical influences that affect healing include wound edema, hematoma, tension at the wound site or incision line, foreign bodies, crust or necrotic tissue, iatrogenic manipulation, and overly aggressive debridement.

Edema. Swelling is a normal occurrence in the inflammatory stage of wound healing, but its control decreases the inflammatory response, which in turn decreases fibrosis.[208] The edematous wound environment contributes to sustaining and perpetuating a chronic inflammatory state associated with excessive scarring.[72] Gross edema in the periwound area decreases vascularization by altering hydrostatic capillary pressure; decreased oxygen and nutrient supply subsequently decrease the proliferation of granulation tissue.[101,117,125] Therapeutic management of edema

includes elevation techniques, controlled motion when possible, and application of a bulky dressing during the inflammatory stage. Single Coban wraps control edema in digital wounds. The application of stress to injured tissues with manual exercise should be applied judiciously in all phases of wound healing. Exercise that is painful or increases swelling increases inflammation and should be avoided.

Hematoma. Hematoma formation compromises the repair process. The space-occupying blood coagulum decreases perfusion capability, may cause graft separation or wound dehiscence, and increases the workload of the phagocytic cells.[86] The increased inflammatory response associated with hematoma increases fibrosis and scar. Hematoma also serves as a perfect culture medium for bacteria and increases the risk for infection.

Correct surgical management with proper hemostasis before closure, adequate approximation of tissue defects, and drains where deemed necessary may prevent hematoma. The postoperative bulky dressing should be used for 24 to 48 hours with most surgical wounds about the hand or wrist and continued with each dressing change for as long as the first 5 to 7 days after surgery for surgeries in the vascular forearm, such as tumor excision or release of the median or radial nerves at this level.

Large mesh grafts, such as those that would provide coverage for the dorsum of the hand, can be dressed with 4 × 4 wide mesh gauze dressings, wet with saline, to provide a continuous wicking action for exudate and to reduce fluid viscosity. These dressings serve to protect the graft from hematoma and excess accumulation of exudate, which should cause graft separation. These dressings must be kept wet, because allowing them to dry out would cause adherence and disturb the graft tissue during removal. This regimen is carried out in a hospital environment with 24-hour elevation.[35a]

Dressings that function to maintain the configuration of a wound or to ensure graft contact to the wound, such as a bolus, should be made of cotton instead of synthetic materials, which compress and lose their shape.[190]

Negative-pressure dressings have recently been described as a technique for preventing hematoma formation or serum collection postoperatively as an alternative to protecting skin grafting with bolstered dressings.[20,112] The technique, termed *vacuum-assisted closure* (VAC), uses negative pressure to eliminate fluid collections, to increase oxygen tension, and to decrease contamination. The treatment consists of insertion of sterile sponge into the wound bed connected to the negative pressure device by a suction hose. The device as described by Blackburn operated at a negative pressure of 125 mm Hg with a 5-minute on, 2-minute off cycle.[20] VAC has been used in the treatment of degloving injuries,[142] for the coverage of radial forearm free flap donor-site complications,[86] and for closure of chronic wounds [93]

Decreasing wound site tension. Wound site tension may reduce the rate of repair, compromise tensile strength, and increase the final width of the scar.[25,183,196] Excessive tension at the wound site may cause necrosis by jeopardizing local blood supply.[1,69] Sutures that are tied too tightly may need to be released; tension on an incision line may be relieved with wound tapes, pressure dressings, or splints that limit motion and stress.[22,172,181]

Physical agents. Physical agents offer the therapist additional options in wound management. The use of physical agents and their effect on cellular function is yet another expanding frontier in the area of wound manipulation, but a detailed discussion is beyond the scope of this chapter. Several sources are suggested for further study on the application of exogenously applied electrical stimulation,* the effects of ultrasound (US) on the various connective tissues,† and the use of heat and cold as an adjunct to wound treatment.[91,127,144]

Definitive research is lacking for clinical application of these modalities.[81] A number of review articles are available to offer perspective to the clinician.[21,91,99,124,159]

A few important studies are mentioned to emphasize the point that with all applied modalities, as with other wound management techniques, the therapist should have an understanding of the physiologic response of the tissues to the treatment applied.

Electrical stimulation. Therapeutic doses of electrical current have been shown to augment healing in chronic wounds in human subjects and induced wounds in animal models.[73] Studies of cell cultures have shown that electrical fields can influence migrating, proliferative, and functional capacity of cells involved in the healing process, and that growth factors may be stimulated by electrical current.[73] One clinical study has demonstrated the beneficial effect of pulsed electrical stimulation on the healing of stage II, III, and IV chronic dermal ulcers, with treatment times that do not exceed 60 minutes per day, 5 to 7 days per week,[73] substantially less than the 20 to 42 hours of electrical stimulation per week recommended in earlier studies.[38] In vitro electrical stimulation has been shown to stimulate local growth factor activity, affecting human dermal fibroblasts and leading to greater collagen synthesis.[70]

Isolated epidermal cells, cell clusters, and cell sheets have demonstrated galvanotaxis (electrotaxis) in migrating toward the cathode in in vitro studies.[44,66] Macrophages have been shown to migrate toward the anode,[164] whereas neutrophils have been observed to migrate toward both the anode and cathode.[147]

Researchers have demonstrated that dermal fibroblasts in culture, stimulated with pulsed current at 100 pulses per second (pps) and 100 v, had increases in the expression of

*References 21, 70, 73, 81, 99, 114, 115, 124, 189.
†References 57, 80, 89, 99, 138, 159, 197, 199, 209.

receptors for transforming growth factor-β that were six times greater than those of control fibroblasts.[70] A negative effect has been demonstrated on tendon healing. The effect of pulsed electromagnetic fields (PEMF) stimulation on early flexor tendon healing in a chicken model (using a similar stimulus to that used clinically) caused a decrease in tensile strength and an increase in peritendinous adhesions.[174]

Ultrasound. The effect of low-intensity US on the healing strength of 24 repaired rabbit Achilles tendons was studied.[65] The tendons were excised after nine treatments and compared with non-US tendons. The US group demonstrated a significant increase in tensile strength, tensile stress, and energy absorption capacity. These findings suggest that high-intensity US is not necessary to augment the healing strength of tendons, but that low-intensity US may enhance the healing process of surgically repaired Achilles tendons.[65]

A study that describes the influence of US administered at different postoperative intervals on several aspects of healing in the surgically repaired zone II flexor tendon in 76 white leghorn chickens has indicated that use during the early stages of wound healing increases range of motion, decreases scar formation, and shows no adverse effect on strength.[104]

The effect of US on the healing human tendon has not yet been established, and US is not yet ready for clinical application. However, experimental studies suggest that positive effects are found with sonication limited to the very earliest stages of healing, and negative results when sonication is continued for several weeks.[65] Clinical guidelines in regard to timing, duration, and intensity of application have not yet been established, but these parameters evidently must be matched to specific cellular activity to maximize the effectiveness of this modality.

The effect of US on bone repair has been investigated recently. It has been demonstrated that low intensity US can accelerate the healing of fresh fractures.[89,209] Some preliminary evidence suggests its usefulness in treatment of delayed healing and nonunions as well.[89,138] A single case study credits low-intensity ultrasound with union of an ununited hook of the hamate fracture.[80]

Nussbaum[159] provides a nice review of studies on ultrasound that will be of clinical interest to the hand clinician.

Scar management. Scar management should be addressed from the first wounding day. Judicious planning of surgical procedures, full-thickness skin grafting where necessary, and infection control are immediate concerns.[185] Control of the variables that could lead to infection, an exaggerated inflammatory state, or a dehydrated wound, will help minimize fibrosis and hypertrophic scarring.[217]

Adhesion control in the case of the deeper tissues is discussed in other chapters on rehabilitation of the tendon, ligament, and joint. The negative biochemical and biomechanical changes in immobilized connective tissue studied both experimentally and clinically have been defined in many articles (see also Chapter 31) and are not reiterated here, except to point out that some controlled motion for these deeper tissues should be applied where possible with respect to the tensile strength of the repair to maintain tissue homeostasis and to promote a more organized deposition of collagen at the wound site.[218] Motion in the inflammatory stage biochemically stimulates cellular response.[11,32,218] Early passive motion has been correlated to an increased fibronectin (FN) concentration in the adult canine tendon; by 7 days after repair, controlled motion flexor tendons had FN concentrations two times that of immobilized tendons.[11] Fibroblast chemotaxis and adherence to the substrate in the days after injury and repair appear to be directly related to FN concentration.[82] Motion during the reparative stages will biomechanically affect tissue glide for tendon and ligament and nutrient transport for cartilage. Tissue engineering promises to alter the management of healing connective tissue in the future,[219] but at this writing, none of these new experimental techniques have been as effective as the application of controlled load to healing tendon and ligament.[32]

Techniques for the management of cutaneous scars—pressure garments, elastomeres, silicone gel sheeting, and the use of paper tape— are well known to the hand therapist (see Chapter 90).[77,158,161,162,172,186,196,221]

Hypertrophic scars are found most commonly in areas of high tension and movement as with the flexor surfaces of the extremities.[196] Applying tension to suture lines with aggressive splinting and exercise can contribute to hypertrophic scarring on these surfaces and functional limitation. An example of commonly misapplied force by the hand therapist is the postoperative Dupuytren's case. These cases as with others fare better with tension eliminated with splinting and careful exercise technique.

Topical silicone gel sheeting (SGS) is a relatively new technique used to prevent, control, and reduce hypertrophic scar (HS) formation.[196] Clinically, it decreases scar redness and elevation of the scar area, and patients seem to have fewer complaints of itching and painful sensations.[113]

The mechanism of action of the SGS is unknown.[113,196] Pressure exerted by the SGS applied to the scar with paper tape is negligible (less than 3 mm Hg).[169] Temperature and differences in oxygen transmission have been excluded. The gel is occlusive with a water vapor rate lower than that of skin (4.5 versus 8.5 g/m²/hr).[162] However, other polyurethane films do not have the same effect on HS. Researchers postulate that because the scar surface does not become wet or macerated with prolonged wear, the SGS may promote hydration of the scar, but changes in scar water content have not been directly measured. Researchers also postulate that the reduction in water vapor loss may decrease capillary

activity, thereby reducing collagen deposition and scar hypertrophy.[51] There is no histologic or scanning electron microscopic evidence of silicone absorption, but a chemical effect has not been excluded. Several clinical studies have demonstrated the clinical benefits of SGS in minimizing HS in surgical scars and keloid scars with at least 12 hours of treatment daily over periods of up to 6 months.[3]

SGS also has been found to prevent development of these scars and is effective as a wound dressing. In a controlled analysis of fresh surgical incisions, SGS was found to significantly inhibit the formation of HS when used at least 12 hours daily for 2 months.[113] They have been used with postoperative punch grafting to prevent cobblestoning, graft dislocation, and to provide sterile atmosphere for the grafts,[2] and as a method of treating painful fingertip injuries in children.[161]

Paper tape applied longitudinally along an incision line as soon as epithelialization takes place prevents wound site tension and clinically appears to minimize scarring. This technique has been studied recently,[158,172,186] with one researcher finding that it is even more effective than SGS.[158] Reiffel applied paper tape longitudinally along susceptible wounds and found that hypertrophic scarring was prevented.[172] He hypothesized that the tape worked by preventing longitudinal stretching of the incision line. He also proposed that SGS was effective in scar management because it prevents tension at the incision line not because of compression forces.[172]

SUMMARY

The wound healing process is subject to manipulation and facilitation by the clinician. The importance of a physiologic approach to the management of both the simple and complex wound may prove to speed the processes of epithelialization and contraction and help control collagen deposition. The importance of careful attention to this aspect of our discipline cannot be overemphasized.

REFERENCES

1. Adamson JE, Fleury AF: Incisions in the hand and wrist. In Green DP, editor: *Operative hand surgery*, ed 2, vol 3, New York, 1988, Churchill Livingstone.
2. Agarwal US, et al: Silicone gel sheet dressings for prevention of post-minigraft cobblestoning in vitiligo, *Dermatol Surg* 25:102, 1999.
3. Ahn ST, Monafo WW, Mustoe TA: Topical silicone gel for the prevention and treatment of hypertrophic scar, *Arch Surg* 126:499, 1991.
4. Alper JC, Tibbetts LL, Sarazen AA: The in vitro response of fibroblasts to the fluid which accumulates under a vapor permeable membrane, *J Invest Dermatol* 84:513, 1985.
5. Alper JC, et al: Moist wound healing under a vapor permeable membrane, *J Am Acad Dermatol* 8:347, 1983.
6. Altemeier W: The significance of infection in trauma, *Bull Am Coll Surg* 57:7, 1972.
7. Alvarez O: Moist environment in healing-matching dressing to wound, *Wounds* 2:59, 1989.

8. Alvarez OM, Hefton JM: Healing wounds: occlusion or exposure, *Infect Surg* 173, 1984.
9. Alvarez OM, Mertz PA, Eaglstein WH: The effect of occlusive dressings on collagen synthesis and reepithelialization in superficial wounds, *J Surg Res* 35:142, 1983.
10. American College of Surgeons Committee on Trauma: *Early care of the injured patient,* ed 2, Philadelphia, 1976, WB Saunders.
11. Amiel D, et al: Fibronectin in healing flexor tendons subjected to immobilization and early controlled passive motion, *Matrix* II:184, 1991.
12. Aronoff GR, et al: Increased serum iodide concentration from iodide absorption through wounds treated topically with povidone-iodine, *Am J Med Sci* 297:173, 1980.
13. Aubock J: Synthetic dressings, *Curr Probl Dermatol* 27:26, 1999.
14. Banda MJ, et al: Isolation of a nonmitogenic angiogenesis factor from wound fluid, *Proc Natl Acad Sci USA* 79:7773, 1983.
15. Barbul A: Immune aspects of wound repair, *Clin Plast Surg* 17:433, 1990.
16. Barbul A: Role of the immune system. In Cohen IK, Diegelman RF, Lindblad WJ, editors: *Wound healing: biochemical and clinical aspects,* Philadelphia, 1992, WB Saunders.
17. Barbul A, et al: Growth factors and other aspects of wound healing; biological and clinical implications. In Barbul A, et al: *Progress in clinical and biological research,* vol 266, New York, 1988, Alan R Liss.
18. Becker GD: Identification and management of the patient at high risk for wound infection, *Head Neck Surg* 8:205, 1986.
19. Bello YM, Phillips TJ: Recent advances in wound healing, *JAMA* 283:716, 2000.
20. Blackburn JH II, et al: Negative-pressure dressings as a bolster for skin grafts, *Ann Plast Surg* 40:453, 1998.
21. Braddock M, Campbell CJ, Zuder D: Current therapies for wound healing: electrical stimulation, biological therapeutics, and the potential for gene therapy, *Int J Dermatol* 38:808, 1999.
22. Branemark PI, et al: Local tissue effects of wound disinfectants, *Acta Scand* 357(suppl):166, 1966.
23. Brennan SS, Leaper DJ: The effect of antiseptics on the healing wound: a study using the rabbit ear chamber, *Br J Surg* 72:780, 1985.
24. Browder W, et al: Effect of enhanced macrophage function on early wound healing, *Surgery* 104:224, 1988.
25. Brown GL, et al: Enhancement of wound healing by topical treatment with epidermal growth factor, *N Engl J Med* 321:76, 1989.
26. Brown PW: Open wounds of the hand. In Tubiana R, editor: *The hand,* vol 2, Philadelphia, 1985, WB Saunders.
27. Brown PW: Complications following amputation of parts of the hand. In Boswick JA, editor: *Complications in hand surgery,* Philadelphia, 1986, WB Saunders.
28. Brown PW: The role of motivation in recovery of the hand. In Kasdan, editor: *Occupational hand and upper extremity injuries and disease,* Philadelphia, 1991, Hanley & Belfus.
29. Brown PW: Open injuries of the hand. In Green DP, editor: *Operative hand surgery,* ed 3 New York, 1993, Churchill Livingstone.
30. Bryant CA, et al: Search for a non-toxic surgical scrub solution for periorbital laceration, *Ann Emerg Med* 13:317, 1984.
31. Bucknall TE: The effect of local infection upon wound healing: an experimental study, *Br J Surg* 67:851, 1980.
32. Buckwalter JA, Grodzinsky AJ: Loading of healing bones, fibrous tissue, and muscle: implications for orthopaedic practice, *J Am Acad Orthop Surg* 7:291, 1999.
33. Burkhalter WE: Experiences with delayed primary closure of war wounds of the hand in Viet Nam, *J Bone Joint Surg* 50A:45, 1968.
34. Burkhalter WE: Care of war injuries of the hand and upper extremity: report of the war injury committee, *J Hand Surg* 8:810, 1983.
35. Burkhalter WE: Mutilating injuries of the hand, *Hand Clin* 2:45, 1986.
36. Burkhalter WE: Wound classification and management. In Hunter JM, et al, editors: *Rehabilitation of the hand,* ed 3, St Louis, 1990, Mosby.
37. Byrd HS, Cierny G, Tebbets JB: The management of open tibial fractures with associated soft tissue loss, *Plast Reconstr Surg* 68:73, 1981.
38. Carley P, Wainapel S: Electrotherapy for acceleration of wound healing: low intensity direct current, *Arch Phys Med Rehabil* 66:443, 1985.
39. Chase RA: The damaged index digit, *J Bone Joint Surg* 50A:1152, 1968.
40. Clark RAF: Cutaneous tissue repair: basic biologic considerations I, *J Am Acad Dermatol* 13:701, 1985.
41. Clark RAF, et al: Platelet isoforms of platelet derived growth factor stimulate fibroblasts to contract collagen lattices, *J Clin Invest* 84:1036, 1989.
42. Cohen IK, Diegelmann RE, Lindblad WJ: *Wound healing. Biomechanical and clinical aspects,* Philadelphia, 1992, WB Saunders.
43. Conolly WB: Spontaneous healing and wound contraction of soft tissue wounds of the hand, *Hand* 6:26, 1974.
44. Cooper NS, Schliwa M: Electrical and ionic control of tissue cell locomotion in a DC electrical field, *J Neurosci Res* 13:223, 1985.
45. Cordeiro PG, et al: Acidic fibroblast growth factor enhances peripheral nerve regeneration in vivo, *Plast Reconstr Surg* 83:1013, 1989.
46. Cross SE, Roberts MS: Defining a model to predict the distribution of topically applied growth factors and other solutes in excisional full-thickness wounds, *J Invest Dermatol* 112:36, 1999.
47. Cruse PJE, Foord R: The epidemiology of wound infection, *Surg North Am* 66:27, 1980.
48. Custer J, et al: Studies in the management of the contaminated wound. An assessment of the effectiveness of pHisoHex and Betadine surgical scrub solutions, *Am J Surg* 121:572, 1971.
49. Cuzzell J: The new red, yellow, black color code, *Am J Nurs* 10:1342, 1988.
50. Cuzzell J: Wound care forum: tell it like it is: a realistic approach to wound documentation, *Am J Nurs* 86:600, 1986.
51. Davey RB, Wallis KA, Bowering K: Adhesive contact media: an update on graft fixation and burn scar management, *Burns* 17:313, 1991.
52. Davidson JM: Wound repair, *J Hand Ther* 11:80, 1998.
53. Devel TF, Senior KM, Chang D: Platelet factor 4 is chemotactic for neutrophils and monocytes, *Proc Natl Acad Sci USA* 78:4584, 1981.
54. Devel TF, et al: Chemotaxis of monocytes and neutrophils to platelet-derived growth factor, *J Clin Invest* 69:1046, 1982.
55. Diegleman RR, Lindblad WJ: Cellular sources of fibrotic collagen, *Fundam Appl Toxicol* 5:219, 1985.
56. Draye JP, Delaney B, Van de Voorde: In vitro and in vivo biocompatibility of dextran dialdehyde cross-linked gelatin Hydroget films, *Biomaterials* 19:1677, 1998.
57. Dyson M: Role of ultrasound in wound healing. In Kloth LC, McCulloch JM, Feedar JA, editors: *Wound healing: alternatives in management,* Philadelphia, 1990, FA Davis.
58. Dyson M, et al: Comparison of the effects of moist and dry conditions on dermal repair, *J Invest Dermatol* 91:434, 1988.
59. Eaglstein WH: Experiences with biosynthetic dressings, *J Am Acad Dermatol* 12:434, 1985.
60. Edlich RF, et al: Studies in the management of contaminated wounds: VI. The therapeutic value of gentle scrubbing in prolonging the limited period of effectiveness of antibiotics in contaminated wounds, *Am J Surg* 121:668, 1971.
61. Edlich RF, et al: Technical factors in wound management. In Hunt TK, Dunphy JE, editors: *Fundamentals of wound management,* New York, 1979, Appleton-Century-Crofts.
62. Edlich RF, et al: Principles of emergency wound management, *Ann Emerg Med* 17:1284, 1988.

63. Eisinger M, et al: Wound healing by epidermal derived factors: experimental and preliminary clinical studies. In Barbul A, et al, editors: *Growth factors and other aspects of wound healing, biological and clinical implications,* New York, 1987, Alan R Liss.

64. Elton RC, Bouzard WC: Gunshot and fragment wounds of the metacarpus, *South Med J* 68:833, 1975.

65. Enwemeka CS, Rodriguez O, Mendoza S: The biomechanical effects of low intensity ultrasound on healing, *Ultrasound Med Biol* 16:807, 1990.

66. Erickson CA, Nuccitelli R: Embryonic fibroblast motility and orientation can be influenced by physiological electrical fields, *J Cell Biol* 98:296, 1984.

67. Evans RB: An update on wound management, *Hand Clin* 7:409, 1991.

68. Faddis D, Daniel D, Boyer J: Tissue toxicity of antiseptic solutions. A study of rabbit articular and periarticular tissues, *J Trauma* 17:845, 1977.

69. Falanga V: Occlusive wound dressings: why, when, which? *Arch Dermatol* 124:872, 1988.

70. Falanga V, Bourguignon GL, Bourguignon LYN: Electrical stimulation increases the expression of fibroblast receptors for transforming growth factor-beta, abstracted, *J Invest Dermatol* 88:488, 1987.

71. Falcone PA, Caldwell MP: Wound metabolism, *Clin Plast Surg* 17:443, 1990.

72. Feedar JA, Kloth LC: Conservative management of chronic wounds. In Kloth LC, McCulloch JM, Feedar JA, editors: *Wound healing: alternatives in management,* Philadelphia, 1990, FA Davis.

73. Feedar JA, Kloth LC, Gentzkow GD: Chronic dermal ulcer healing enhanced with monophasic pulsed electrical stimulation, *Phys Ther* 71:639, 1991.

74. Fernandez E, Pallini R, Mercanti D: Effects of topically administered nerve growth factor on axonal regeneration in peripheral nerve autografts implanted in the spinal cord of rats, Neurosurgery 26:37, 1990.

75. Ferraro MC, Lauckhardt KHP, special edition editors: Tissue repair, *J Hand Ther* 11, 1198.

76. Folkman J, Klagsbrun M: Angiogenesis factors, *Science* 235:442, 1987.

77. Forrester JC, et al: Wolff's law in relation to the healing skin wound, *J Trauma* 10:770, 1970.

78. Freeland AE, Jabaley ME, Hughes JL: *Stable fixation of the hand and wrist,* New York, 1986, Springer-Verlag.

79. Frykman GK: The quest for better recovery from peripheral nerve injury: current status of nerve regeneration research, *J Hand Ther* 6:83, 1993.

80. Fujioka H, et al: Treatment of ununited fracture of the hook of hamate by low-intensity pulsed ultrasound: a case report, *J Hand Surg* 25A:77, 2000.

81. Gardner SE, Frantz RA, Schmidt FL: Effect of electrical stimulation on chronic wound healing: a meta-analysis *Wound Repair Regen* 7:495, 1999.

82. Gelberman RH, et al: Fibroblast chemotaxis after repair, *J Hand Surg* 16A:686, 1991.

83. Gibson T, Kenedi RM: Biomechanical properties of skin, *Surg Clin North Am* 47:279, 1967.

84. Godina M, Lister G: Early microsurgical reconstruction of complex trauma of the extremities, *Plast Reconstr Surg* 78:285, 1986.

85. Granick MS, Long CD, Ramassastry SS, editors. Wound healing: state of the art, *Clin Plast Surg* 25, 1998.

86. Greer SE et al: The use of subatmospheric pressure dressing for the coverage of radial forearm free flap donor-site exposed tendon complications, *Ann Plast Surg* 43:551, 1999.

87. Grotendorst GR: Chemoattractants and growth factors. In Cohen IK, Diegelman RF, Linblad WJ, editors: *Wound healing,* Philadelphia, 1992, WB Saunders.

88. Gustilo RB, Anderson JT: Prevention of infection in the treatment of one thousand and twenty-five open fractures of long bones, *J Bone Joint Surg* 58A:453, 1976.

89. Hadjiargyrou M, et al: Enhancement of fracture healing by low intensity ultrasound, *Clin Orthop* Oct (suppl):8216, 1998.

90. Hamed LM, et al: Hibiclens keratitis, *Am J Ophthalmol* 184:50, 1987.

91. Hardy M, Woodall W: Therapeutic effects of heat, cold, and stretch on connective tissue, *J Hand Ther* 11:148, 1998.

92. Harmel RP, Vane DP, King DR: Burn care in children: special considerations, *Clin Plast Surg* 13:95, 1986.

93. Hartnett JM: Use of vacuum-assisted wound closure in three chronic wounds, *J Wound Ostomy Continence Nurs* 25:281, 1998.

94. Haury B, et al: Débridement: an essential component of traumatic wound care, *Am J Surg* 135:238, 1978.

95. Hermans RP: Topical treatment of serious infections with special reference to the use of a mixture of silver sulfadiazine and cerium nitrate: two clinical studies, *Burns* 2:59, 1984.

96. Hinman CD, Maibach H: Effect of air exposure and occlusion on experimental human skin wounds, *Nature* 200:377, 1963.

97. Hom DB, et al: Choosing the optimal dressing for irradiated tissue wounds, *Otolaryngol Head Neck Surg* 121:591, 1999.

98. Hopf HW, Hunt TK: Wound repair and nutrition. In Esterhai JL, Gristina AG, Poss R, editors: *Musculoskeletal infection,* Park Ridge, Ill, 1992, American Academy of Orthopaedic Surgeons.

99. Houghton PE, Campbell KE: Choosing an adjunctive therapy for the treatment of chronic wounds, *Ostomy Wound Manage* 45:43, 1999.

100. Hunt TK, Hussain Z: Wound microenvironment. In Cohen IK, Diegelman RF, Lindblad WJ, editors: *Wound healing: biochemical and clinical aspects,* Philadelphia, 1992, WB Saunders.

101. Hunt TK, LaVan FB: Enhancement of wound healing by growth factors, *N Engl J Med* 321:111, 1989.

102. Hunt TK, et al: Cellular control of repair. In Hunt TK, et al, editors: *Soft and hard tissue repair: biological and clinical aspects,* New York, 1984, Praeger.

103. Hunt TK, et al: Studies on inflammation in wound healing: angiogenesis and collagen synthesis stimulated in vivo by resident and activated wound macrophages, *Surgery* 96:48, 1984.

104. Huys S, et al: The effects of ultrasound on flexor tendon healing in the chicken limb, *J Hand Surg* 20B:809, 1995.

105. Ichioka S et al: An experimental comparison of hydrocolloid and alginate dressings, and the effect of calcium ions on the behavior of alginate gel, *Scand J Plast Reconstr Surg Hand Surg* 32:311, 1998.

106. Jabaley ME, Freeland AE: Rigid internal fixation in the hand: 104 cases, *Plast Reconstr Surg* 77:288, 1986.

107. Jabaley ME, Peterson HD: Early treatment of war wounds of the hand and forearm in Vietnam, *Ann Surg* 177:167, 1973.

108. Jaffe LF, Vanable JW: Electrical fields and wound healing, *Clin Dermatol* 2:34, 1984.

109. Jensen JE, et al: Nutrition in orthopaedic surgery, *J Bone Joint Surg* 64A:1263, 1982.

110. Johnson AR, White AC, McAnalley: Comparison of common topical agents for wound treatment: cytotoxicity for human fibroblasts in culture, *Wounds* 1:186, 1989.

111. Kahanovich S, et al: The best of wound cover methods, *Q Med Rev* 1:236, 1986.

112. Kalailieff D: Vacuum-assisted closure: wound care technology for the new millennium, *Perspectives* 22:28, 1998.

113. Katz BE: Silastic gel sheeting is found to be effective in scar therapy, *Cosm Derm* June:1, 1992.

114. Kloth LC, Feedar JA: Acceleration of wound healing with high voltage, monophasic, pulsed current, *Phys Ther* 68:503, 1988.

115. Kloth LC, Feedar JA: Electrical stimulation in tissue repair. In Kloth LC, McCulloch JM, Feedar JA, editors: *Wound healing: alternatives in management,* Philadelphia, 1990, FA Davis.

116. Kloth LC, McCulloch JM, Feedar JA: *Wound healing: alternatives in management,* Philadelphia, 1990, FA Davis.

117. Knighton DR, et al: Oxygen tension regulates the expression of angiogenesis factor by macrophages, *Science* 221:1283, 1983.

118. Knighton DR, et al: Classification and treatment of chronic non-healing wounds, *Ann Surg* 204:322, 1986.

119. Knighton DR, et al: The use of topically applied platelet growth factors in chronic non-healing wounds: a review, *Wounds* 71, 1989.

120. Kunimoto BT: Growth factors in wound healing: the next great innovation? *Ostomy Wound Manage* 45:56, 1999.

121. Laato M, Lehtonen OP, Niinikoski J: Granulation tissue formation in experimental wounds inoculated with *Staphylococcus aureus, Acta Chir Scand* 151:313, 1985.

122. Laato M, et al: Inflammatory reaction and blood flow in experimental wounds, inoculated with *Staphylococcus aureus, Eur Surg Res* 20:33, 1988.

123. Ladin DA: Understanding dressings, *Clin Plast Surg* 25:433, 1998.

124. Lampe KE: Electrotherapy in tissue repair, *J Hand Ther* 11:131, 1998.

125. LaVan FB, Hunt TK: Oxygen and wound healing, *Clin Plast Surg* 17:463, 1990.

126. Lawrence WT: Physiology of the acute wound, *Clin Plast Surg* 25:321, 1998.

127. Lehmann JF, DeLateur BJ: Therapeutic heat. In Lehmann JF, editor: *Therapeutic heat and cold,* ed 4, Baltimore, 1990, Williams & Wilkins.

128. Levenson SM, Demetriou AA: Metabolic factors. In Cohen IK, Diegelman RF, Linblad WJ, editors: *Wound healing, biochemical and clinical aspects,* Philadelphia, 1992, WB Saunders.

129. Leyden JJ, Bartelt NM: Comparison of topical antibiotic ointments, a wound protectant, and antiseptics for the treatment of human blister wounds contaminated with staphylococcus aureus, *Fam Pract* 24:601, 1987.

130. Lineaweaver W: Topical antimicrobial toxicity, *Arch Surg* 120:267, 1985.

131. Lyall PW, Sinclair SW: Australian survey of split skin donor site dressings, *Aust N Z J Surg* 70:114, 2000.

132. Lowry KF, Curtis GM: Delayed suture in the management of wounds, *Am J Surg* 80:280, 1950.

133. Madden JW, Peacock EE: Studies on the biology of collagen during wound healing. I. Rate of collagen synthesis and deposition in cutaneous wounds of the rat, *Surgery* 64:288, 1968.

134. Mani R, et al, editors: *Chronic wound healing: clinical measurements and basic science,* Philadelphia, 1999, WB Saunders.

135. Mann RS: Hand infections, *Hand Clin* 5:4,1989.

136. Martin GR, Peacock EE: Current perspectives in wound healing. In Cohen IK, Diegelman RF, Linblad WJ, editors: *Wound healing: biochemical and clinical aspects,* Philadelphia, 1992, WB Saunders.

137. Matzen S, Peschardt A, Alsbjorn B: A new amorphous hydrocolloid for the treatment of pressure sores: a randomized controlled study, *Scand J Plast Reconstr Hand Surg* 33:13, 1999.

138. Mayr E, Rankel V, Ruter A: Ultrasound: an alternative healing method for nonunions? *Arch Orthop Trauma Surg* 120:1, 2000.

139. McCall CE, et al: Functional characteristics of human toxic neutrophils, *J Infect Dis* 124:68, 1971.

140. McCulloch JM, Kloth LC: Evaluation of patients with open wounds. In Kloth LC, McCulloch JM, Feedar JA, editors: *Wound healing: alternatives in management,* Philadelphia, 1990, FA Davis.

141. McGrath MH: Peptide growth factors and wound healing, *Clin Plast Surg* 17:421, 1990.

142. Meara JG, et al: Vacuum-assisted closure in the treatment of degloving injuries, *Ann Plast Surg* 42:589, 1999.

143. Mertz PM, Eaglstein WH: The effect of a semiocclusive dressing on the microbial population in superficial wounds, *Arch Surg* 119:287, 1984.

144. Michlovitz SL: *Thermal agents in rehabilitation,* Philadelphia, 1990, FA Davis.

145. Mignatti P, Welgus HG, Rifkin DB: Role of degradative enzymes in wound healing. In Clark RAF, Henson PM, editors: *The molecular and cell biology of wound repair,* New York, 1988, Plenum Press.

146. Miller SH, Rudolph R: Healing in the irradiated wound, *Clin Plast Surg* 17:503, 1990.

147. Monguio J: Uber die polar wirkung des galvanischen stromes auf leukozyten, *Z Biol* 93:553, 1933.

148. Morain WD, Colen LB: Wound healing in diabetes mellitus, *Clin Plast Surg* 17:493, 1990.

149. Morgan CJ, Pledger J: Fibroblast proliferation. In Cohen IK, Diegelman RF, Lindblad WJ, editors: *Wound healing: biochemical and clinical aspects,* Philadelphia, 1992, WB Saunders.

150. Morrey BF: Anterior capsular release for flexion contracture. In Morrey BF, editor: *The elbow-master techniques in orthopaedic surgery,* New York, 1994, Raven Press.

151. Morris J, et al: Platelet derived growth factor enhances healing in a rabbit deep flexor tendon model, unpublished research, 1992.

152. Morykwas MJ, Argenta LC: Nonsurgical modalities to enhance healing and care of soft tissue wounds, *J South Orthop Assoc* 6:279, 1997.

153. Mulder CD: Factors complicating wound repair. In Kloth LC, McCulloch JM, Feedar JA, editors: *Wound healing: alternatives in management,* Philadelphia, 1990, FA Davis.

154. Murray JF, Carman W, MacKenzie JK: Transmetacarpal amputation of the index finger: a clinical assessment of hand strength and complications, *J Hand Surg* 2:471, 1977.

155. Nemeth AJ, Hebda PA, Eaglstein WH: Stimulating effect of human wound fluid on epidermal outgrowth from porcine skin explant cultures, abstracted, *J Invest Dermatol* 86:497, 1986.

156. Nerlich ML, Tscherne H: Biology of soft tissue injuries. In Browner BD, et al, editors: *Skeletal trauma,* Philadelphia, 1992, WB Saunders.

157. Noe JM, Keller M: Can stitches get wet? *Plast Reconstr Surg* 81:82, 1988.

158. Niessen FB, et al: The use of silicone sheeting (Sil-K) and silicone occlusive gel (Epiderm) in the prevention of hypertrophic scar formation, *Plast Reconstr Surg* 102:1962, 1998.

159. Nussbaum E: The influence of ultrasound on healing tissues, *J Hand Ther* 11:140, 1998.

160. Oberg MS: Do not put hydrogen peroxide or povidone iodine into wounds! *Am J Dis Child* 141:27, 1987.

161. O'Donovan DA, Mehdi SY, Eadie PA: The role of Mepitel silicone net dressings in the management of fingertip injuries in children, *J Hand Surg* 24B:727, 1999.

162. Ohmori S: Effectiveness of silastic sheet coverage in the treatment of scar keloid, *Aesthetic Plast Surg* 12:95,1988.

163. Orgil D, Deming RH: Current concepts and approaches to wound healing, *Crit Care Med* 16:899, 1989.

164. Orida N, Feldman JD: Directional protrusive pseudopodia activity and motility in macrophage induced by extracellular electric fields, *Cell Motil* 2:243, 1982.

165. Peacock EE: *Wound repair,* ed 3, Philadelphia, 1984, WB Saunders.

166. Pessa ME, Bland KL, Copeland EM III: Growth factors and determinants of wound repair, *J Surg Res* 42:207, 1987.

167. Pierce CF, et al: Role of platelet derived growth factor in wound healing, *J Cell Biochem* 45:319, 1991.

168. Pirone LA, et al: Wound healing under occlusion and non-occlusion in partial thickness wounds in swine, *Wounds* 2:74, 1990.

169. Quinn KJ: Silicone gel in scar treatment, *Burns* 13:933, 1987.

170. Rank BK, Wakefield AR: *Surgery of repair as applied to hand injuries,* ed 2, Edinburgh, 1979, E & S Livingstone.

171. Rappolee DA, et al: Wound macrophages express TGF (alpha) and other growth factors in vivo: analysis by an RNA phenotyping, *Science* 241:708, 1988.
172. Reiffel RS: Prevention of hypertrophic scars by long term paper tape application, *Plast Reconstr Surg* 96:1715, 1995.
173. Rich KM, et al: Nerve growth factor enhances regeneration through silicone chambers, *Exp Neurol* 105:162, 1989.
174. Robotti E, et al: The effect of pulsed electromagnetic fields on flexor tendon healing in chickens, *J Hand Surg* 2424B:56, 1999.
175. Robson MC: Disturbances of wound healing, *Ann Emerg Med* 17:219, 1988.
176. Robson MC, Heggars JP: Quantitative bacteriology and inflammatory mediators in soft tissue. In Hunt TK et al, editors: *Soft and hard tissue repair: biological and clinical aspects,* New York, 1984, Praeger.
177. Robson MC, Mustoe TA, Hunt TK: The future of recombinant growth factors in wound healing, *Am J Surg* 176(2A suppl):808, 1998.
178. Robson MC, Stenberg BD, Heggers JP: Wound healing alterations caused by infection, *Clin Plast Surg* 17:485, 1990.
179. Rodeheaver G: Controversies in topical wound management, *Ostomy Wound Management* 20:59, 1988.
180. Rodeheaver G: Side-effects of topical proteolytic enzyme treatment, *Surg Gynecol Obstet* 148:562, 1979.
181. Rodeheaver GT, Spengler MD, Edlich RF: Performance of new wound closure tapes, *J Emerg Med* 5:451, 1987.
182. Rodeheaver GT, et al: Mechanical cleansing of contaminated wounds with a surfactant, *Am J Surg* 129:241, 1975.
183. Rohrich RJ: The biology of wound healing. Techniques of wound closure, abnormal scars, envenomation, *Selected Readings in Plastic Surgery* 5:1, 1988.
184. Rudolph R, Miller SH: Wound healing, *Clin Plast Surg* 17:457, 1990.
185. Rudolph R, VandeBerg J, Ehrlich HP: Wound contracture. In Cohen IK, Diegelman RE, Lindblad WJ, editors: *Wound healing: biochemical and clinical aspects,* Philadelphia, 1992, WB Saunders.
186. Sawada Y, Urushidate S, Nibei Y: Hydration and occlusive treatment of a sutured wound, *Ann Plast Surg* 41:508, 1998.
187. Schmidt JA, et al: Interleukin-1, a potential regulator of fibroblast proliferation, *J Immunol* 128:2177, 1982.
188. Sefton MV, Woodhouse KA: Tissue engineering, *J Cutan Med Surg* 1(suppl):18, 1998.
189. Senet P, Meaume S: Decubitus sores in geriatric medicine. Local and general treatment of pressure sores in the aged, *Presse Med* 28:1840, 1999.
190. Singer PI, Moore JH, Byron PM: Management of skin grafts and flaps. In Hunter JM, et al, editors: *Rehabilitation of the hand,* ed 3, St Louis, 1990, Mosby.
191. Smith KL: Wound care for the hand patient. In Hunter JM, et al, editors: *Rehabilitation of the hand,* ed 3, St Louis, 1990, Mosby.
192. Spencer EM, Skover G, Hunt TK: Somatomedins: do they play a pivotal role in wound healing? In Barbul A, et al, editors: *Growth factors and other aspects of wound healing: biological and clinical implications,* New York, 1988, Alan R Liss.
193. Stenn KS, Malhotra R: Epithelialization. In Cohen IK, Diegelman RE, Lindblad WJ, editors: *Wound healing: biochemical and clinical aspects,* Philadelphia, 1992, WB Saunders.
194. Stotts N, Cuzzell J: Toward a universal standard for wound assessment and therapy. Seminar proceedings from the American Association of Critical Care Nurses Teaching Institute, Kansas City, Mo, 1988, Marion Laboratories.
195. Strickland JW: A rationale for digital salvage. In Strickland JW, Steichen JB, editors: *Difficult problems in hand surgery,* St, Louis, 1982, Mosby.
196. Su CW, et al: The problem scar, *Clin Plast Surg* 25:451, 1998.
197. Sun JS, et al: Bone defect healing enhanced by ultrasound stimulation: an in vitro tissue culture model, *J Biomed Mater Res* 46:253, 1999.
198. Swanson TV, Szabo RM, Anderson DD: Open hand fractures: prognosis and classification, *J Hand Surg* 16-A:101, 1991.
199. Taskan I, et al: A Comparative study of the effect of ultrasound and electrostimulation on wound healing in rats, *Plast Reconstr Surg* 100:966, 1997.
200. Ten Dijke P, Iwata KK: Growth factors for wound healing, *Bio/Technology* 7:793, 1989.
201. Thakral KK, Goodson WH, Hunt TK: Stimulation of wound blood vessel growth by wound macrophages, *J Surg Res* 26:430, 1979.
202. Thomas C: Nursing alert—wound healing halted with the use of povidone-iodine, *Ostomy Wound Management* 18:30, 1988.
203. Timmons J: Alginates and hydrofibre dressings, *Prof Nurse* 14:501, 1999.
204. Trelstad A, Osmundson D: Water pick: wound cleansing alternative, *Plast Surg Nurs* 9:117, 1989.
205. Trott A: Mechanisms of surface soft tissue trauma, *Ann Emerg Med* 17:1279, 1988.
206. Varghese MC, et al: Local environment of chronic wounds under synthetic dressings, *Arch Dermatol* 122:52, 1986.
207. Wahl LM, Wahl SM: Inflammation. In Cohen IK, Diegelman RF, Lindblad WJ, editors: *Wound healing: biochemical and clinical aspects,* Philadelphia, 1992, WB Saunders.
208. Wahl SM, Allen JB: T-lymphocyte dependent mechanisms of fibrosis. In Barbul A, et al, editor: *Growth factors and other aspects of wound healing: biological and clinical implications,* New York, 1988, Alan R Liss.
209. Warden SJ, et al: Acceleration of fresh fracture repair using the sonic accelerated fracture healing system (SAFHS): a review, *Calcif Tissue Int* 66:157, 2000.
210. Whalen GF, Zetter BR: Angiogenesis. In Cohen IK, Diegelman RF, Lindblad WJ, editors: *Wound healing: biochemical and clinical aspects,* Philadelphia, 1992, WB Saunders.
211. Wheeland RG: The newer surgical dressings and wound healing, *Dermatol Clin* 5:393, 1987.
212. Wheeler CB, et al: Side effects of high pressure irrigation, *Surg Gynecol Obstet* 234:775, 1976.
213. Williams C: Hydrocoll: a "new breed" of hydrocolloid wound dressing, *Br J Nurs* 7:1337, 1998.
214. Wilson H: Secondary suture of war wounds, *Ann Surg* 121:152, 1945.
215. Winter GD: The formation of the scab and the rate of epithelialization of superficial wounds in the skin of the young domestic pig, *Nature* 193:293, 1962.
216. Winter GD: Effect of air drying and dressings on the surface of wound, *Nature* 197:91, 1963.
217. Wiseman DM, et al: Wound dressings: design and use. In Cohen IK, Diegelman RF, Lindblad WJ, editors: *Wound healing: biochemical and clinical aspects,* Philadelphia, 1992, WB Saunders.
218. Woo SL-Y, Buckwalter JA, editors: *Injury and repair of the musculoskeletal soft tissues,* Park Ridge, Ill, 1988, American Academy of Orthopaedic Surgeons.
219. Woo SL-Y, et al: Tissue engineering of ligament and tendon healing, *Clin Orthop* 367 (suppl):8312, 1999.
220. Zawack BE: The effect of Travase on heat injured skin, *Surgery* 77:132, 1975.
221. Zukin DD: New wound closure tapes, *J Emerg Med* 5:553, 1987 (editorial).

Chapter 20

CARE OF THE HAND WOUND

Kevin L. Smith
James L. Price, Jr.

Wound care has, since the beginning of time, figured prominently in daily life, religion, and ritual. People have treated wounds with potions and poisons, with nostrums and hokums, and with substances as far ranging as wine, honey, ashes, animal excrement, boiling oil, and salves of earthworms in turpentine added to puppies boiled in oil of lilies.[9] With so many products on today's market, there is understandable confusion in the choice of the most appropriate dressing regimen. Because there are so many different kinds of wounds, each with specific requirements for dressings, there is probably no one best wound dressing or technique.

Wound management is often an emotional issue, guided more by experience than science. As long as the dressing material or technique does not harm the wound, healing will occur (given conditions such as sufficient time, adequate state of nutrition, and lack of disease). The purpose of this chapter is to provide an overview of wound management and dressing techniques based on sound biologic principles. The patient with a posttraumatic or postoperative hand wound presents problems that are unique to hand surgery. For most wounds, an optimal environment for healing usually requires immobilization, but total immobility can run counter to the successful maintenance of gliding surfaces. The goals of conservative debridement, wound immobilization, and aggressive therapy are often difficult to balance in the presence of an unstable wound. Although the decision to institute therapy is made with the surgeon, it is necessary for the therapist to be able to diagnose and appropriately treat wounds ranging from clean to dirty.

WOUND HEALING

Wound healing is a coordinated dynamic event involving cell multiplication and active migration. Cells are stimulated to increase intracellular synthetic activity and produce substrate for extracellular biochemical events. The entire sequence of events of wound healing is geared to produce new collagenous tissue to replace that which was destroyed. With application of the proper dressings, the process of wound healing can be facilitated. Whether a wound is incised or excised and regardless of the amount of tissue lost, all wounds progress through the same phases of wound healing.

Phase 1: inflammation

The inflammatory phase is the immediate vascular and cellular response to wounding that clears the wound of devitalized tissue, debris, and foreign materials. This cleansing effect is mediated by (1) dilution through vascular dilation and subsequent edema, (2) chemical neutralization with the release of proteolytic and collagenolytic enzymes, (3) the precipitation of toxins, and (4) a cellular response leading to the phagocytosis of debris and invading bacteria by polymorphonuclear leukocytes and macrophages. Damage to blood vessels exposes subendothelial collagen, which stimulates platelet adherence. Platelet agglutination initiates the coagulation sequence, and a clot is formed within the injured vessels. Then, leucocytes and macrophages enter the extravascular space by diapedesis and begin their cleansing activity.

Within a clean wound (i.e., little debris), there is little work to be done and the inflammatory phase is usually over in 5 days. Conversely, a dirty wound with considerable debris requires a longer inflammatory phase to clean up the debris, resulting in a delay in the fibroplastic phase of wound healing. A prolonged inflammatory phase also can result from severe tissue trauma at the time of injury, rough tissue handling during surgery, overly aggressive therapy, or inappropriate damaging dressings. If the inflammatory phase is affected by steroid administration or chronic debilitation—factors that decrease both the quality and quantity of cellular participation—wound healing is prolonged.[9,21,30]

Phase 2: fibroplasia

The fibroplastic or proliferative phase of repair lasts from 2 to 6 weeks, depending on the extent of the wound. This phase, beginning 3 to 5 days after sustaining the wound, consists of fibroblast proliferation, accompanied by endothelial budding, yielding new capillary growth. On a framework of fibrin and fibronectin, the fibroblasts lay down collagen, on which the fragile capillary buds grow, and together they form granulation tissue. During this period, immobilization helps prevent collagen-fiber disruption and facilitates the increase in tensile strength of the wound.[30,38]

It is the granulation tissue bed on which epithelial cells migrate in a centripetal fashion, thereby resurfacing the wound with immature "scar" epithelium. This newly formed epithelium is characterized by lack of dense attachment to an underlying dermis, causing it to be thin and fragile.[30] Traumatic handling during therapy or pressure points from dressings or splints should be avoided because they can lead to blistering and deepithelialization.

There is an increase of tensile strength during this phase that parallels the increase in collagen content for about 3 weeks. The collagen accumulation then reaches a plateau in which collagen synthesis becomes balanced by collagen degradation. When this plateau is reached, tensile strength is approximately 15% of normal and continues to increase linearly for at least 3 months.[22] Epithelialization occurs during this time, independent of, but usually in concert with, contraction. Peacock defines *contraction* as "an active process which attempts to close a wound in which a loss of tissue has occurred."[30] *Contracture,* on the other hand, refers to a result that may or may not be caused by contraction. Skin wounds contract by the stretching of surrounding skin to close the defect and not by the production of new skin. Contraction proceeds even after epithelial coverage is achieved, but to a lesser degree. The only way to effectively reduce wound contraction is to obtain wound closure (e.g., by skin graft) and maintain appropriate splinting regimens.[5,21] If coverage is inadequate and splinting is ignored, contracture can reach unreconstructable degrees (Fig. 20-1). When one is attempting to avoid contraction by skin grafting, the thickness of the graft is important. Split-grafted wounds contract 25% more than full-thickness skin-grafted wounds.[33] It is the dermis that

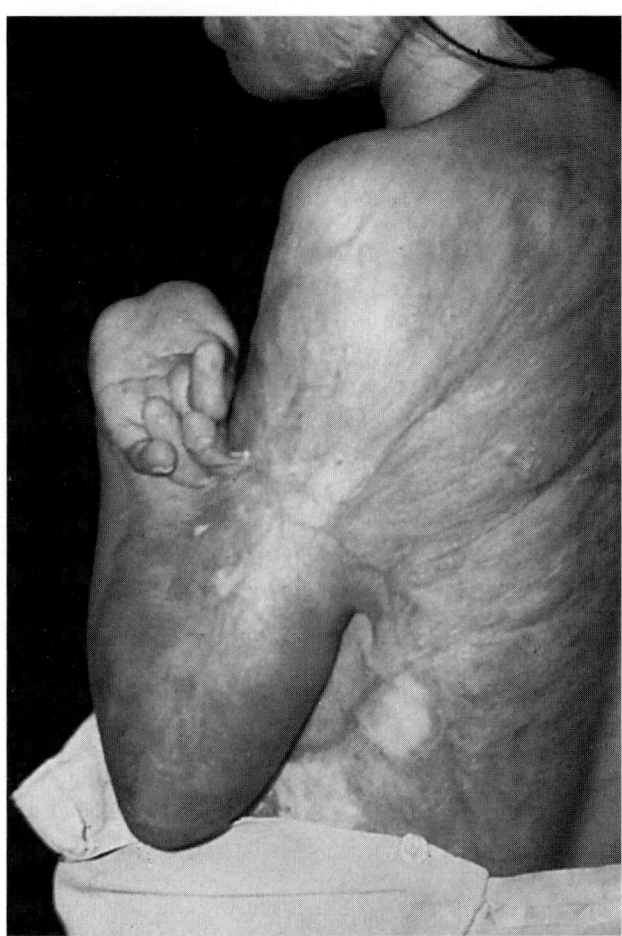

Fig. 20-1. An example of end-stage wound contracture caused by allowing a burn wound to heal without treatment by wound contraction and secondary epithelialization.

plays the key role in reduction of wound contraction.[4] Recent studies have shown that Biobrane—a synthetic, temporary, polypeptide-coated, nylon-silicone fabric—when applied to an open wound, inhibits contraction as well. The mechanism for this is not elucidated.[11] A synthetic dermal substitute (collagen/glycosaminoglycan/silastic), Integra, may also serve to limit wound contraction by providing dermal architecture below thin split grafts.[20]

Phase 3: maturation

The last phase of wound healing is the maturation, or remodeling, phase, which begins as the fibroblastic activity decreases. This phase may last for years. During this phase, the amount of collagen decreases and the wound becomes stronger.[22] Tensile strength progressively increases, with approximately 50% of normal tensile strength regained by 6 weeks.[38] Early, new scar is red, raised, thick, and rigid, but given time, scar maturation proceeds and the scar softens and becomes more pliable and thin. Scar never reaches normal skin tensile strength. Therefore, when subjected to transverse stress, scars tend to widen over time.

SURGICALLY CLOSED WOUNDS

In a surgically closed wound with minimal debris, reepithelialization seals the wound by 48 hours.[21] The basal layer of the epithelial cells at each margin of the wound multiply and migrate to close the defect over a "bridge" provided by accurate dermal approximation. These wounds are not usually problems for the patient, therapist, or surgeon. Barring the formation of an abscess or marginal tissue necrosis necessitating debridement in a surgically closed wound, minimal dressings are required. For the first 24 hours after surgery, light gauze dressing moistened with saline serves to absorb wound exudate by capillarity. This leads to a clean wound that is free of crust.[3] On the morning of the first postoperative day, this light dressing can be removed and the wound safely washed with mild soap and water without causing increased wound complications.[29] A light dressing of bland antibiotic ointment, such as Neosporin or Polysporin, can be applied to the wound with or without light gauze dressing. This will allow better fit of a splint and greater potential for range of motion to facilitate hand therapy if it is to be started this early. Tensile strength is provided initially by the sutures, safely allowing early therapy (as directed by the specifics of the wound).

THE OPEN WOUND

When a patient presents with an open wound, the evaluation of surface tissue viability is all-important. The wound should be completely undressed, and the presence of necrotic debris, drainage, odor, eschar, or protein coagulum should be noted. The color of the surrounding skin and the presence or absence of granulation tissue in the wound should be appreciated. The warmth of the tissue should be assessed. The sensibility of the tissues should be determined (providing nerve damage has not occurred) because its presence implies viable tissue. Assessment of vascularity should be made by the observation of direct dermal or wound bed bleeding and the "blanch and blush" of capillary refill. The latter can be a deceptive sign, and a comparison should be made with normal tissue. Too-rapid capillary refill implies venous congestion and that the viability of the tissues may be in jeopardy. Dangerous venous congestion is further indicated by an increased tissue turgor or a peau d'orange appearance. A sound foundation in anatomy is necessary to know what adjacent tissues risk exposure and further injury. This knowledge will guide the aggressiveness with which the wound will be treated.

Debridement

Wound healing will not progress in the presence of active infection or excessive necrotic debris. Any open wound needs to be kept meticulously free of dead material and exudate to facilitate healing. A "natural dressing," such as a scab, which is made of dried blood and protein coagulum, or an eschar, which is a thick covering of denatured collagen, is protective and can be left in place and the wounds treated by this "exposure" method (when the eschar or scab does not interfere with range of motion). Healing progresses as the epithelium migrates from the wound margin, aided by the elaboration of collagenases. As the eschar or scab is elevated, it can be trimmed. This method is suitable as long as there is no drainage or purulent liquefaction below the eschar. If this occurs, debridement is mandatory.

When eschar or necrotic debris must be removed, it requires mechanical debridement using fine forceps and sharp scissors or a knife. Hydrotherapy or wet dressings can soften this debris and ease its removal. Debridement is not generally painful to the patient because only the nonviable tissue is excised. When the wound is filled with numerous small patches of necrotic debris, mechanical debridement with forceps and scissors can be tedious. In this case, frequent wet dressings, by adherence to the debris and wick action, can effectively remove these smaller fragments (Fig. 20-2).

In the hand wound, it is not uncommon to see tendons exposed. An exception to the rule of aggressive debridement of nonviable tissue exists when tendons are considered. Even though a tendon may be devitalized by the loss of its peritenon, if it is protected and not allowed to dessicate, the stability of the collagen matrix remains and this devitalized tendon can serve in much the same manner as a tendon graft. If the wound is treated and closed with the devitalized tendon placed beneath adequate skin and soft tissue, the tendon ultimately will be cellularized and retain the potential for good function.[30]

Separation of eschars, scabs, or fibrinous coagulum can be hastened by commercially available proteolytic enzyme ointments such as Travase (Flint Pharmaceuticals—bacillus subtilis protease) or Elase (Parke-Davis Pharmaceuticals—fibrinolysin and deoxyribonuclease). These are indicated for short-term use to hydrolyze the protein-rich fibrinous coagulum found on many draining wounds. Although these enzymes may interfere with leukocyte phagocytosis, they do not appear to interfere with wound healing.[32] Some have even suggested that these enzymes spare viable tissue.[12,42] The authors suggest that these enzyme preparations should be used sparingly and only after the evaluation of the character of the wound debris before each use. These preparations are sometimes painful on application and can cause a burning sensation. Their action seems to be facilitated by their application under an occlusive dressing.

Bacteria and wound infection

The presence of bacteria can be demonstrated in any open wound, and sterilization of the wound can be achieved only by closure, not with drugs or dressings. The factors that determine clinical infection are the number of bacteria, their virulence, and host resistance. Resistance relates to systemic factors as well as local factors, such as amounts of wound debris, foreign body, and compromised tissue. Quantitative tissue culture, the bacterial count per gram of sampled tissue,

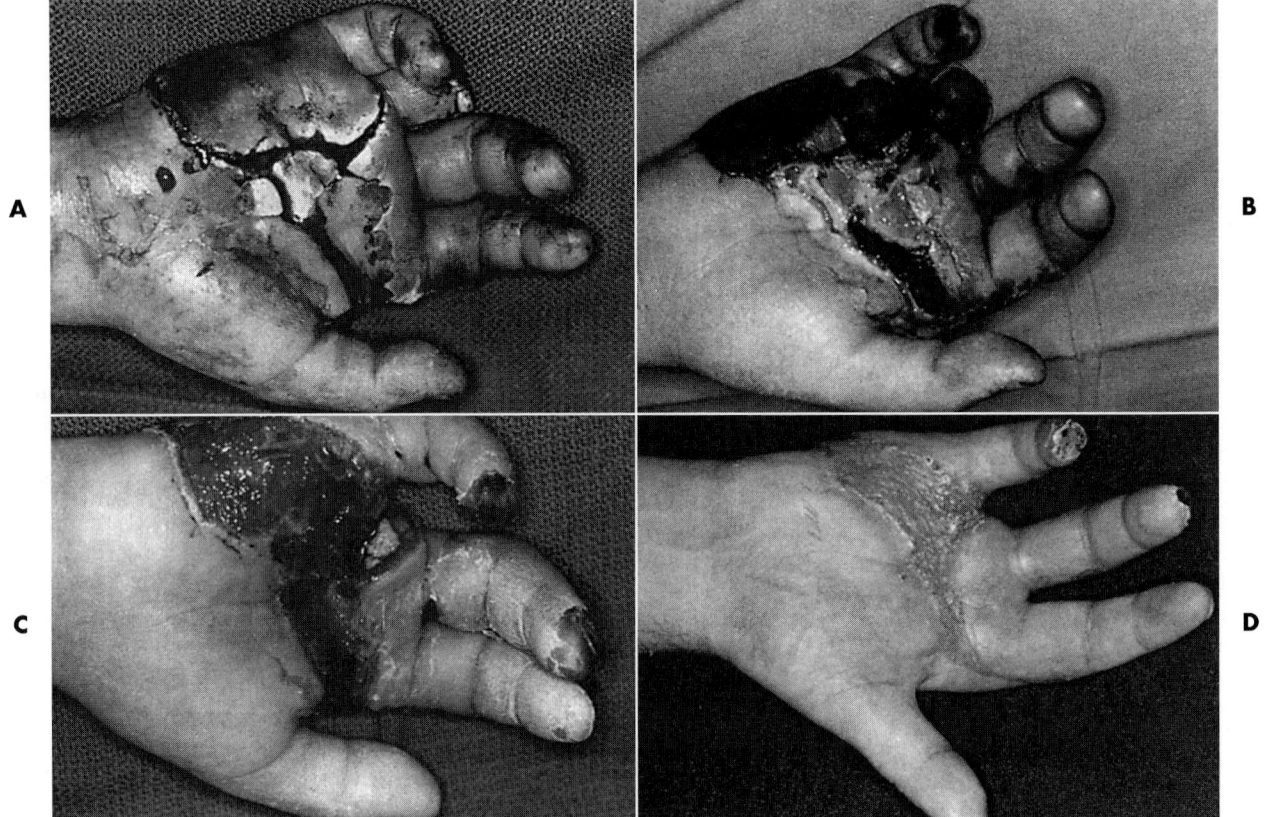

Fig. 20-2. A, Printing press crush with extensive soft tissue injury before the first debridement.
B, Five days later, "second-look" debridement necessitates a fourth ray amputation. **C,** After 10 days
of wet dressings allowing aggressive hand therapy, the granulating bed of the wound and marginal
epithelial migration denotes readiness for closure with skin graft. **D,** Six weeks after injury, the
wounds are healed with skin graft. Hand therapy was suspended only during the initial 5 days after
skin grafting.

is necessary to differentiate between colonization and
infection.

A wound is considered clinically infected if the concentration of bacteria is greater than $10^5/g$. If closure is
attempted with bacterial counts greater than 10^5, it is likely
to fail, especially if the organism is *Staphylococcus* or
Pseudomonas. Most organisms can be reduced in number by
adequate debridement and an effective dressing regimen.
Occasionally, the topical application of antimicrobial or
antiseptic agents is useful. The exception to this is
β-hemolytic streptococcus, which produces the wound
lysins streptokinase and streptodornase. This organism must
be eliminated before wound closure, and fortunately *Streptococcus* is very sensitive to systemic penicillin.[26,39]

WOUND DRESSING
Functions of a dressing

When a dressing is prescribed for a patient, many factors
should be taken into account, including the patient, the
wound, and the goals of treatment. A dressing should fulfill

basic criteria and can be adjusted to meet the specific needs
of each patient (Box 20-1). The ideal dressing should be
designed to protect the wound from the external environment, isolating it from trauma, exogenous bacteria, and
temperature changes. A supportive dressing immobilizes the
wound. Motion, by disruption of immature fibrin scaffolding
and capillary budding, increases inflammation, which ultimately increases scarring and extends the wound healing
process.[3] Splinting also becomes an integral part of wound
immobilization and support. The dressing for the hand
should be designed to immobilize the wound and provide
protective positioning in whatever position is dictated by the
injury. This dressing should also be nonrestrictive to allow
motion in the noninjured portions of the hand.

The ideal dressing can control the microenvironment of
the wound. Healing proceeds best in a moist environment.[6]
A drying wound will extend tissue damage, and the resultant
denatured collagen and dessicated protein coagulum will
create an impermeable scab, which will retard epithelialization. The epithelialization will be forced to proceed at a

deeper level at the junction of the live tissue with the dead tissue. A moist environment also allows gaseous exchange, which is necessary to maintain Po_2 and pH at optimal levels.[36] By the hydrostatic characteristics of the dressings, the level of moisture can be controlled. Too wet of an environment will cause maceration and possibly enhance bacterial proliferation.[28] Too dry of an environment will encourage further tissue loss caused by dessication.

The ideal dressing provides comfort during its application and removal and when it is in place. It also provides the psychologic purpose of reminding the patient that he or she has a wound and reporting the same to the people he or she contacts. A dressing also serves to cover, aesthetically, a highly visible wound to decrease associated anxiety. An expertly applied dressing also can increase the confidence a patient has in those providing care. Most important, the dressing should do no harm to the wound and should not impede the healing process.

Special wounds and dressing requirements

After the nature of a wound is assessed, the dressing is prescribed accordingly. A dressing may need to be absorptive for use on the secreting or draining wound. It may be designed to debride the wound, apply topical medicaments, or both. It may be adherent or nonadherent or wet or dry. The dressing may be designed to be compressive to help minimize scar volume.[10,28]

As a wound progresses through the healing process, the method of dressing should change according to the requirements of the wound. One dressing style will not be sufficient for the entire healing phase.

The dirty or infected wound

The dirty or infected wound (Fig. 20-3) is first treated by adequate surgical debridement. Then dressings are applied with the intention of hastening further removal of necrotic debris or drainage. Historically, dry dressings have been prescribed. A dry dressing of wide mesh gauze (standard 4×4s) is absorptive and serves to remove the transudate or exudate from the wound. In addition, this dressing will adhere to loose necrotic debris, which is then removed with the dressing. The frequency of dressing changes is determined by the amount of drainage and debris, and changes are performed before the dressing is saturated. The usual interval of dressing change is about every 4 to 6 hours. Disadvantages of the dry (dry-to-dry) dressings are many and probably outweigh any advantages of this dressing technique. The dressings are painful, and they cause dessication of the superficial layers of the open wound. Debridement is indiscriminate, and fragile fibroblasts and epithelial cells from the healing wound are likely to be removed with any necrotic debris. For these reasons, dry dressings have largely been abandoned for the open wound because dressing techniques should not replace surgical debridement, especially in the hand wound, where debridement must be very precise. Dry dressings are still appropriate for the surgically closed wound when protection of a suture line is indicated.

Wet dressings can be used and are an effective means of softening adherent crusts and debris. The wet wide mesh gauze has greater capillarity than dry dressings[27] and can enhance the removal of wound drainage. There is less adherence of the dressing to the wound, and consequently, less pain is caused with its removal; however, this affords relatively less debriding action than dry dressings. A moist physiologic environment provided by a wet dressing encourages reepithelialization,[40] and the topical application of gentle heat or cold over the dressing is better transmitted to the wound. These dressings should be changed every 2 to 4 hours and can be kept wet with a variety of solutions, the best being lactated Ringer's solution warmed to body temperature. The wet dressing also can be saturated with topical medicaments to provide bacteriostatic or bactericidal action.[28]

Although wet dressings provide a moist physiologic environment for healing, bacteria can flourish in this situation, complicating healing. In addition, the constantly wet dressing may macerate intact skin and thus effect an unwanted keratolytic action.

Topical medicaments in the wet dressing

A decided advantage of the wet dressing technique is the ability to apply topical antibiotics or nonspecific antimicrobial solutions directly to the wound surface. Most solutions in use today are efficacious bacteriocidal agents, but recent studies have shown that most have significant cytotoxic properties in commonly used concentrations.[16-18,37]

These solutions should be applied at least every 4 hours to keep the dressing wet. If the wound has little exudate and the dressing remains clean, the dressing need not be changed

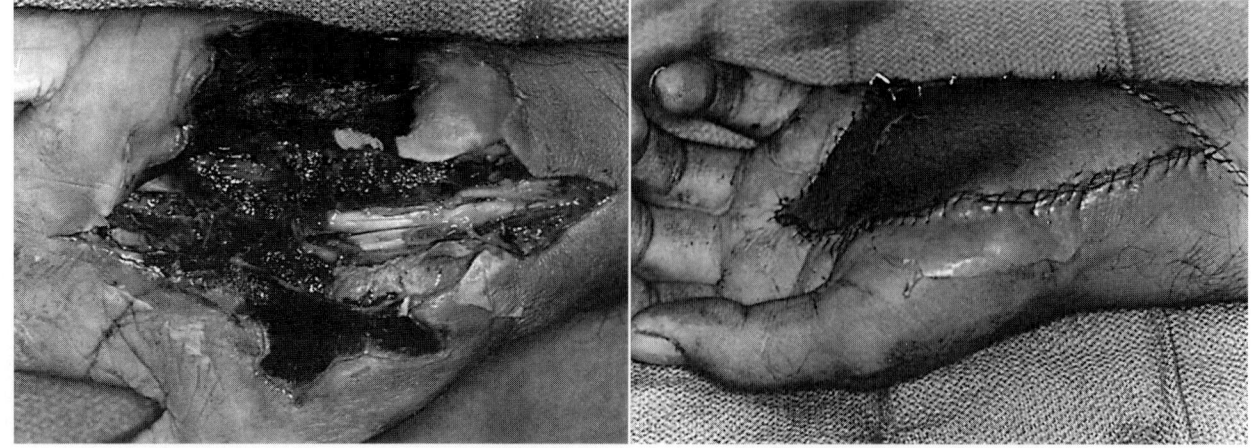

Fig. 20-3. A, This 33-year-old immunosuppressed diabetic renal transplant patient developed a necrotizing fasciitis of the left palm. After several staged debridements and wet dressings to prevent dessication, the wound is ready for definitive debridement and microvascular flap closure. **B,** Closure is obtained by free transfer of a neurotized lateral arm flap to allow healing by first intention.

each time it is moistened. Care must be taken to avoid the drying of these dressings because evaporation can yield medicament concentrations that are toxic. Occlusive overwraps, such as Saran Wrap, can be helpful to prevent evaporation.

The choice of topical antibiotics should be governed by specific wound cultures, and antibiotics, which are rarely given systemically, should be used to reduce the risk of compromising further parenteral therapy. Preference should be given to those drugs that have been shown to be effective, such as neomycin, kanamycin, cephaloridine, and bacitracin (penicillin, ampicillin, and cephalothin are possibly effective). These drugs should be used in concentrations two to four times the minimum inhibitory concentration (MIC).[31,35]

Nonspecific antimicrobials such as 1% povidone-iodine (Betadine), 0.5% sodium hypochlorite (Dakin's solution), 0.25% acetic acid, and 3% hydrogen peroxide, all can be toxic to some degree at full strength. Of these, there was no bactericidal concentration of acetic acid, hydrogen peroxide, or sodium hypochlorite that was not cytotoxic.[16,18] Therefore it is recommended that these solutions be abandoned for dressing care. Although 1% povidone-iodine did not appear to disturb the normal wound healing process,[37] fibroblast toxicity was apparent until dilutions of 0.001% (1:1000), a level at which bactericidal activity was maintained.[18]

The wet-to-dry dressing

A combination of these two dressing techniques is the commonly used "wet-to-dry" dressing. The same wide mesh gauze is placed on the dirty wound and is applied wet. The dressing is then allowed to dry. The wick action pulls necrotic material, exudate, or transudate into the gauze, which is removed with the gauze during dressing changes every 4 to 6 hours. Unfortunately, the debridement is indiscriminate, and healthy granulation and immature epi-

thelium are removed with the dressing, causing pain, bleeding, and damage to the wound.[28] This technique is perhaps the most widely used dressing technique, and although it is effective in debriding a dirty wound, it is not surpassed by careful surgical debridement and a wet dressing regimen and should be avoided.

Wound packing

Packing of a wound is indicated when the wound has significant dead space and the superficial portions of the wound need to be kept open while the deeper recesses are allowed to contract. The packing must be in contact with all wound edges, and the wound cavity should not be packed too tightly. Tight packing will retard drainage, create tissue ischemia, and cause the wound to behave in a fashion similar to the abscess that created it. Many materials can be used in wound packing, the most common being wide mesh gauze, such as 4 × 4s or Kling, or fine mesh strip gauze commercially available as Nugauze. Rarely, however, does a hand wound require packing, and generally, the aforementioned dressings will suffice.

Use of topical creams and ointments

Aside from simple suture line care, there are a few special instances in which topical creams—primarily silver sulfadiazine—have been useful. Generally, the cream is placed on the wound directly and then covered with gauze wraps to hold it in place. For burns of the hand, the wounds are coated with silver sulfadiazine and the hand is then placed within an appropriately sized plastic bag (10 × 18 inches) (Fig. 20-4). Motion is then encouraged, and hand therapy is instituted immediately. The patient is encouraged to manage his or her own activities of daily living and is kept out of any protective splinting during times of exercise, meals, and hygiene. The hand is fitted for proper splints

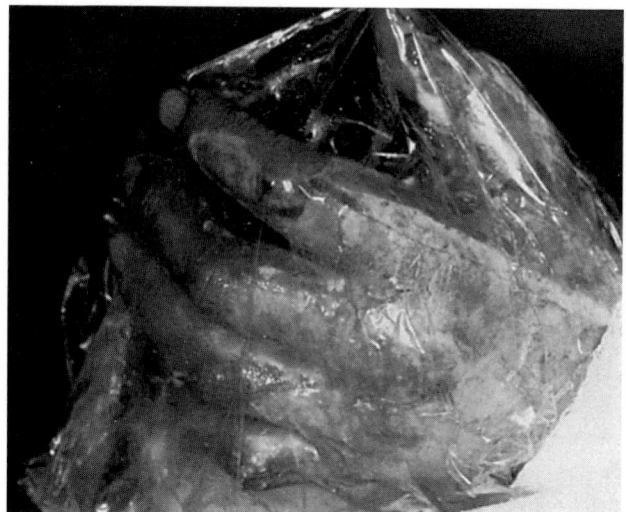

Fig. 20-4. This acutely burned hand has been placed in a plastic bag dressing with silver sulfadiazine after initial debridement and escharotomy. This allows close application of the protective positional splint and also allows the hand to be used for daily life skills. The dressing is comfortable and does not interfere with hand therapy.

while in the plastic bag "dressing," thereby allowing closer fit without the interference of bulky dressings.[2,34] Of interest, commercially available plastic bags are sterile as a result of the manufacturing process and require no further preparation off the shelf.[24,34]

Topical silver sulfadiazine also has been used in attempts to salvage some or all portions of "questionable" flaps (Fig. 20-5). Treatment of the compromised margin of the flaps with topical antibacterial creams applied under dry gauze twice daily reduced the depth of tissue loss and consequently increased the surviving length of experimental flaps. This dressing regimen seemed to improve survival by the prevention of dessication and not by the inherent augmentation of vascularity. Although bacterial counts were three logarithms higher in flaps treated with only inactive vehicles, there was no appreciable difference in survival between flaps treated with topical antibiotic and those not.[25] We continue to use Silvadene dressings as a last resort for compromised flaps, under the assumption that a three-logarithm decrease in bacterial load may decrease potential wound complications associated with flap failure.

The clean open wound

The distinguishing feature of a clean open wound is that it demonstrates a uniform presence of flat, healthy granulation tissue with evidence of epithelial proliferation and migration at the wound margin (Fig. 20-6). A wound such as this requires a dressing different from that of the dirty or infected wound. This dressing should most of all be nonadherent and designed to maintain a moist environment for healing (Fig. 20-7).

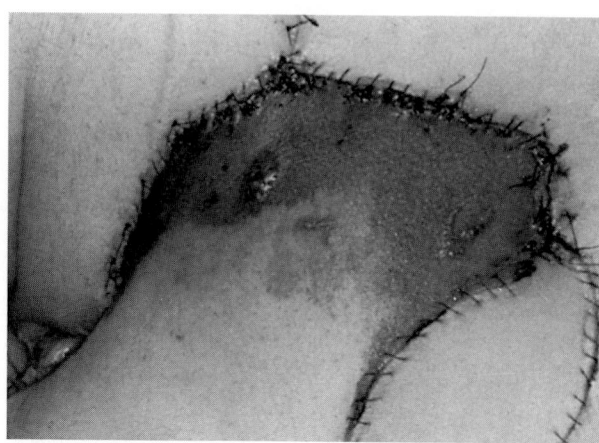

Fig. 20-5. Pedicle flap clearly showing ischemic changes in its distal margin with a clear line of demarcation marked by deep blue coloration and early epidermolysis. Just proximal to the line of demarcation, venous congestion with too-brisk capillary refill and slow bleeding can be seen. Experience has shown that a flap such as this can be partially salvaged by the application of topical dressings (silver sulfadiazine). Experiments have shown that this is likely to be because of the dressing being occlusive.[25]

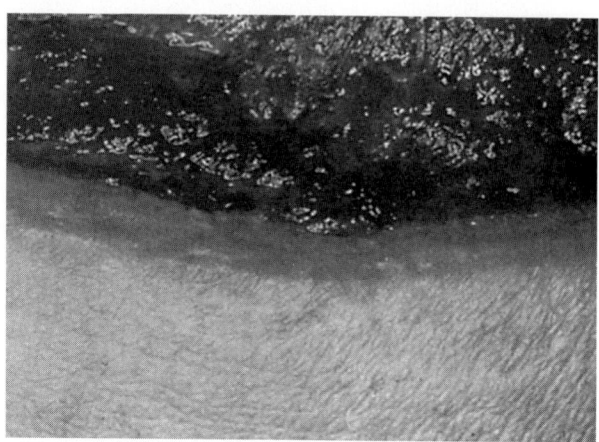

Fig. 20-6. Clean, open wound revealing a uniform bed of granulation tissue with an advancing epithelial margin at the skin-wound junction.

The dressing for the clean wound starts with a contact layer. This layer determines how the dressing will interact with the wound. The contact layer must be sterile; it must contact all surfaces of the wound by conforming to its contours; and there must be no gaps to allow collections of serum, blood, or pus to form. The nonadherent contact layer should be of gauze mesh sufficiently fine to prevent the growth of granulations within the interstices but open enough to allow drainage to pass through into the overlying absorbent layer of the dressing.

The choice of a nonadherent contact layer is dictated by the character of the wound drainage. If the wound has little

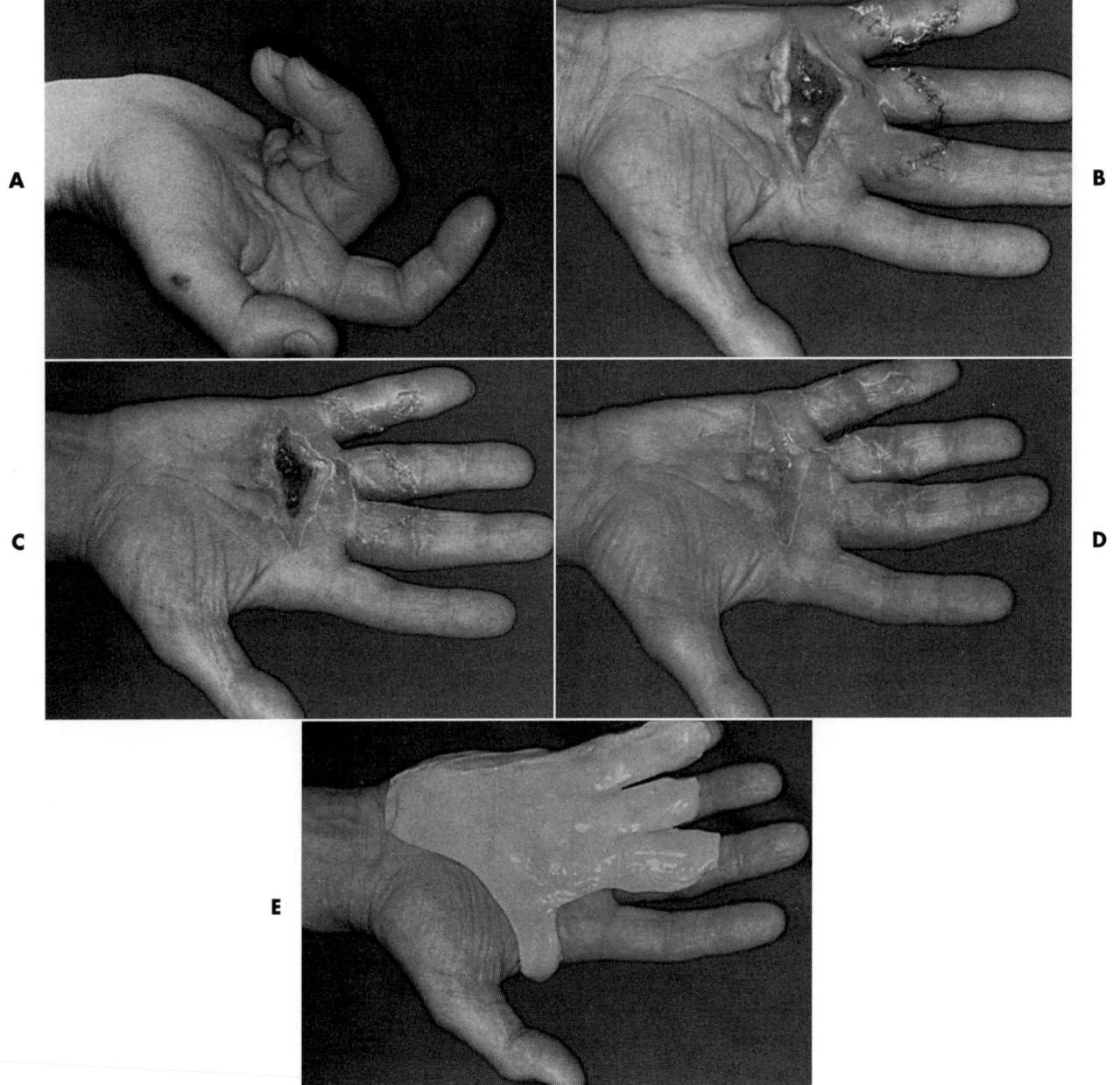

Fig. 20-7. A, A 67-year-old patient with Dupuytren's contracture. **B,** Three days after release using open technique. **C,** This clean open wound is managed with Xeroform, fluff gauze, and Kling wraps with range-of-motion therapy four times daily and continuous splinting in extension. **D,** Twenty-two days after surgery, the wound is closed and splinting is reduced to nighttime only in extension. **E,** Compression is applied to the wound and is directed by using silastic 382 medical grade Elastomer (Dow Corning Corp., Midland, Mich.) with continued extension splinting at night.

or no drainage, this layer need only be nonadherent. If moderate drainage exists, the contact layer must allow the passage of some of the fluid into the overlying absorptive dressing. Most medicated dressings are made by impregnating fine mesh rayon or cotton gauze, and common examples are Vaseline gauze, Xeroform, Xeroflo, and Adaptic. Other nonadherent dressings combine a permeable or perforated polymeric film, which allows immediate strikethrough and

an absorptive intermediate layer. Examples of these products are Telfa, Exudry, and Dermasel. Of these, Xeroform and Vaseline gauze tend to allow less drainage and can lead to wound maceration in a heavily draining wound.

The central or intermediate layer in the dressing for a clean wound is absorptive to the degree necessary for the wound. This layer is also protective and supportive. It is commonly "fluffed" gauze, mechanics waste, cotton, or

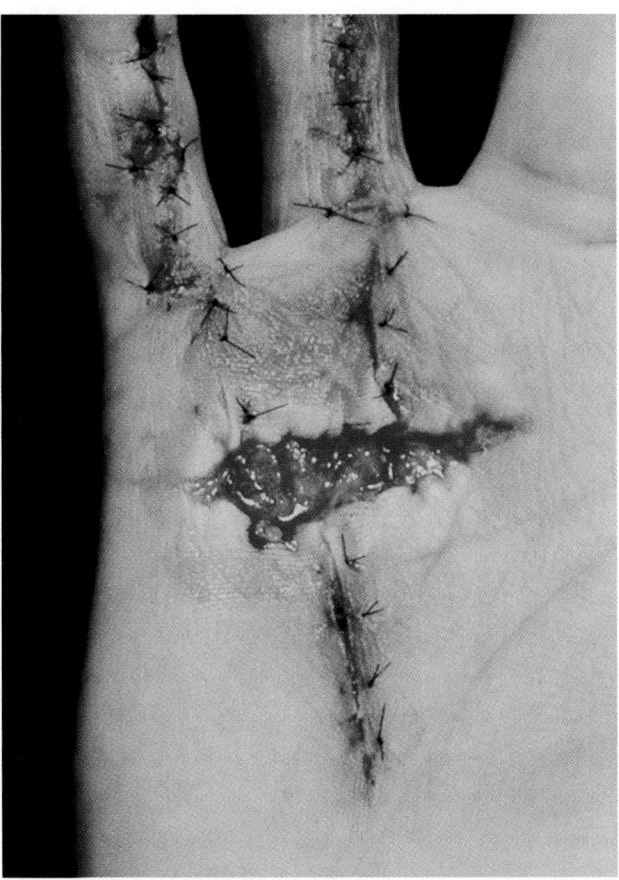

Plate 27. A red wound in a Dupuytren's fasciectomy 3 days after surgery. The wound in the palm is beefy red, without infection, with epithelial, endothelial myofibroblast, and fibroblast cellular activity taking place. Note that the digital wounds are already epithelized.

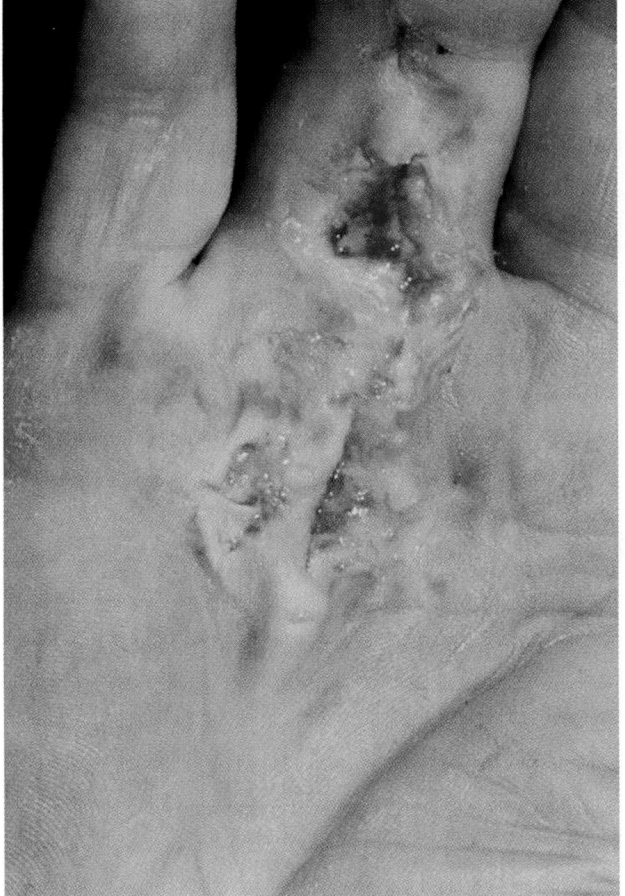

Plate 28. A yellow wound infected with *Pseudomonas* in a postsurgical Dupuytren's fasciectomy closed by primary intention with subsequent dehiscence. Although some of the green color is from skin pencil, the wound is yellow-green with a distinctive odor. Cellular activity is dominated by the macrophage, which is stimulated by bacteria and inflammation. (From Evans RB: *Hand Clin* 7:419, 1991.)

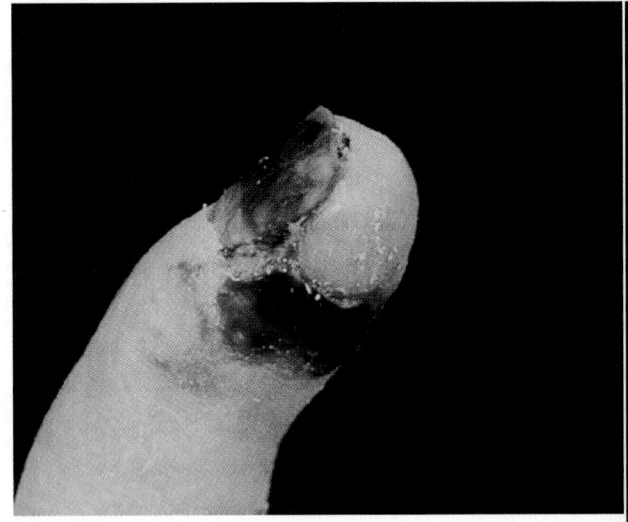

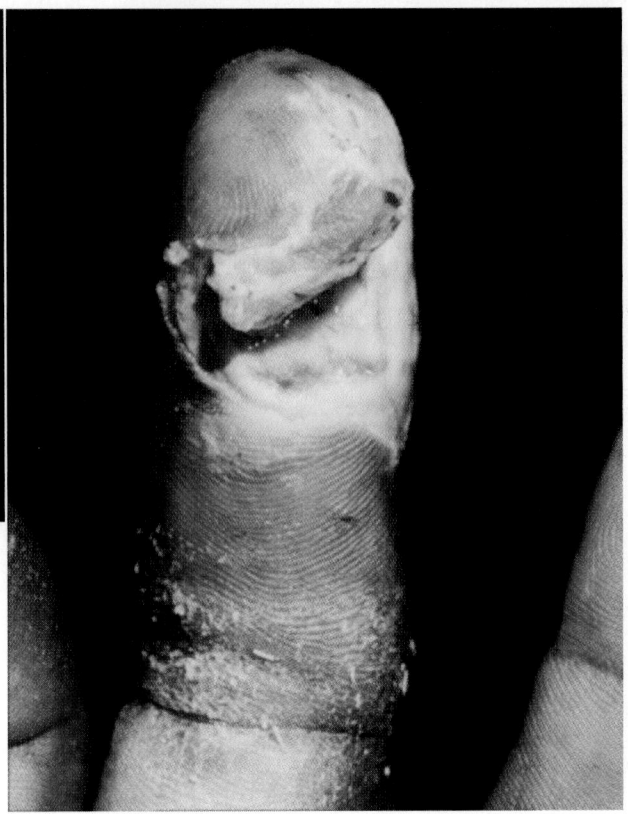

Plate 29. A, A black wound on the fingertip that required mechanical debridement in therapy after whirlpool. The macrophage is working to clean the area of bacterial and debris. The fibroblast and endothelial cells will begin to synthesize collagen and new vessels as the debris is removed. **B,** A failed fingertip skin graft seen as a black and yellow wound with red at its periphery. The black portion was mechanically debrided, the yellow portion gently scrubbed, and the red portion protected. (From Evans RB: *Hand Clin* 7:420, 1991.)

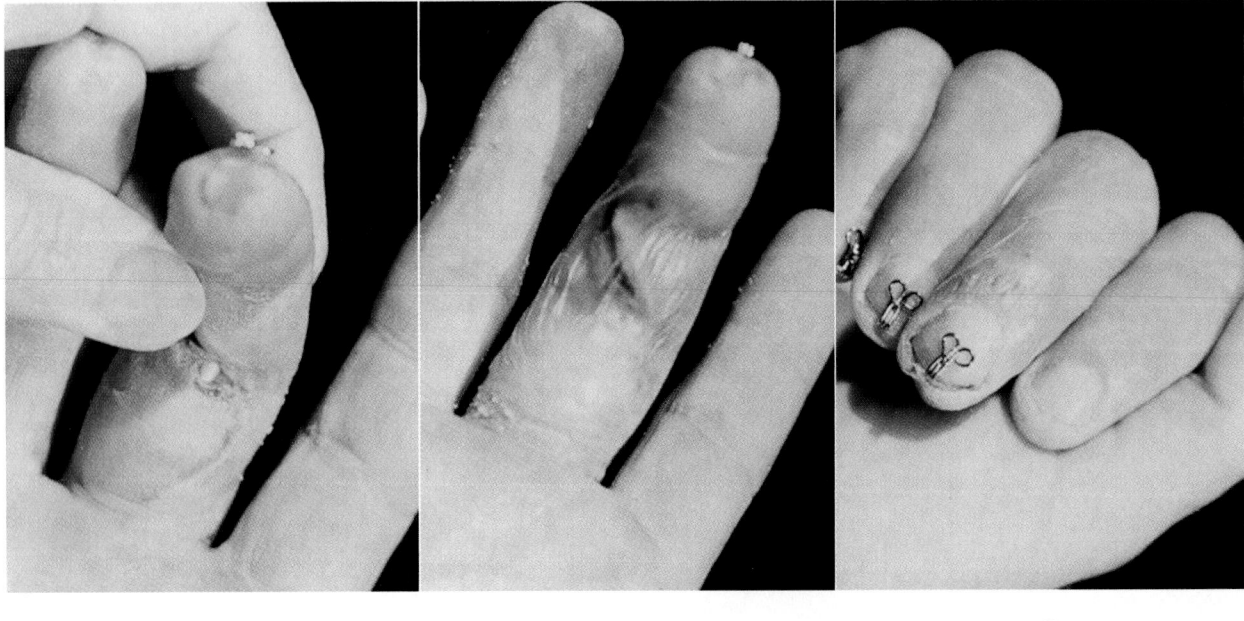

A   B   C

Plate 30. A, Exposed repaired flexor tendon at 3 weeks after surgery. **B,** A Tegaderm dressing sequestered wound fluids and protected the exposed tendon until the wound was revised. **C,** The thin Tegaderm dressing offered minimal impedance to active flexion exercise, which was critical to maintaining tendon glide while the tendon was exposed.

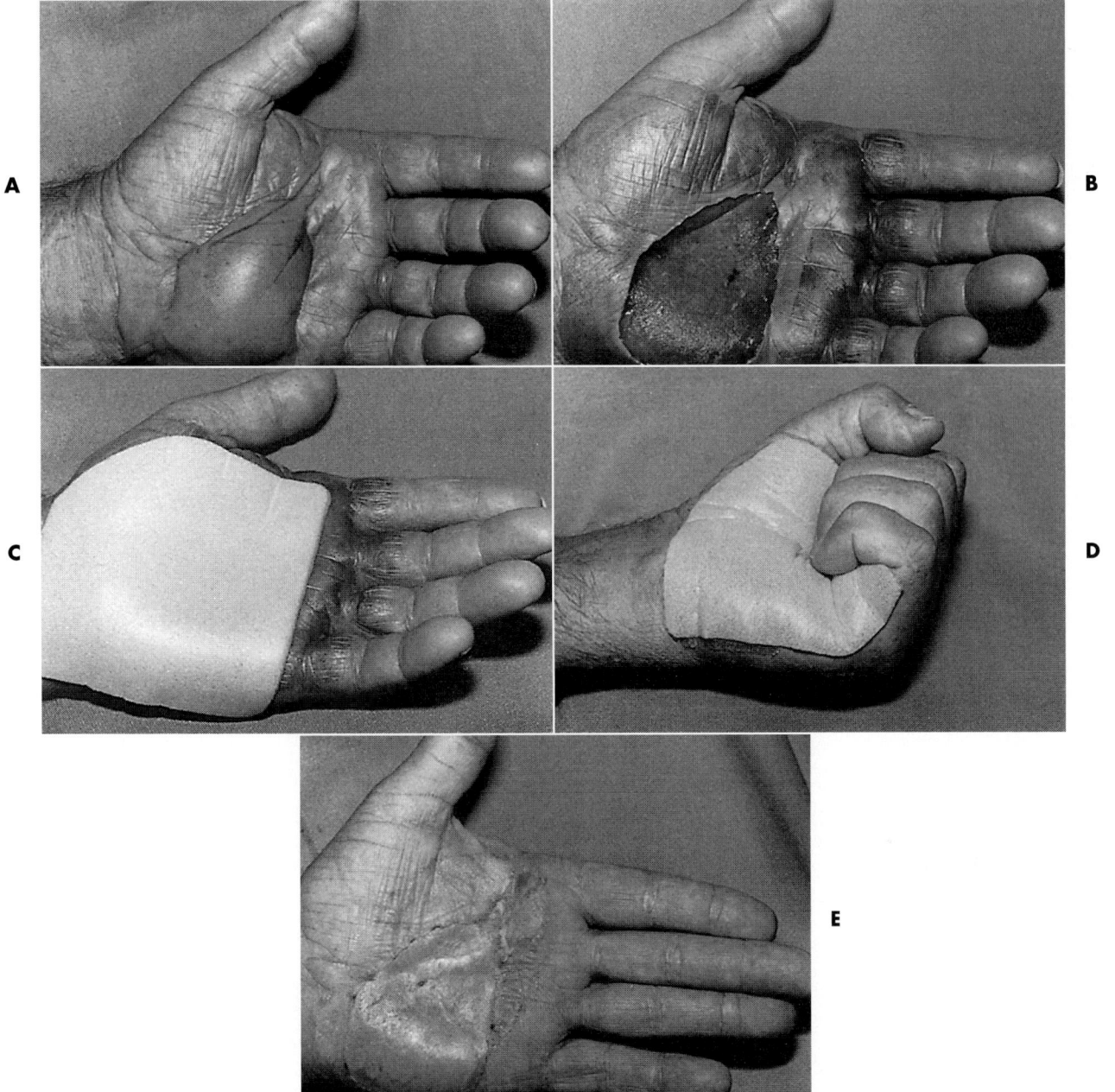

Fig. 20-8. A, This 29-year-old fireman sustained a partial-thickness palmar burn and presented with a large palmar blister. **B,** The blister is debrided. **C,** A hydrocolloid dressing (Duoderm) is applied. **D,** A pain-free wound and thin dressing allow full range of motion. **E,** Two weeks after every-3-day dressing changes, the burn is healed.

Dacron batting. This is changed as often as is necessary before saturation. Improved wicking is achieved if the material (most commonly, wide mesh gauze 4 × 4s) is applied moist. Antimicrobials can effectively be used in this layer.

The final layer of a dressing for the clean wound binds the dressing and holds it in place. This layer may incorporate a rigid splint or may be elastic. In either case, it stabilizes the dressing and the underlying wound. If therapy is to be done

while the hand dressing is in place, it is necessary to determine how much shear the dressing creates at the wound surface. If there is shear, therapy should be done only when the dressing is off or sufficiently reduced.

Occlusive dressings for the clean open hand wound

Over the last decade, occlusive dressings have left the realm of pressure sore therapy and skin-graft-donor-site dressing, and their use has expanded to include wounds that are difficult to dress, such as those of the hand. Occlusive hydrocolloid dressings (HCDs) such as Duoderm and Cutinova Hydro interact with the wound surface by creating a microenvironment in which leukocytes, macrophages, and endogenous proteolytic enzymes can function and facilitate the wound healing process. The wound contact surface is an exudative slurry that can be malodorous and resemble infected pus, but it is, in fact, this slurry that facilitates "physiologic debridement" and a favorable environment for reepithelialization. The greatest advantages of occlusive dressings are that they speed reepithelialization in acute wounds, promote the formation of granulation tissue in chronic wounds, and provide reduction in wound pain. In experimental studies, epithelialization was increased as much as 40% (in the knife-wounded pig), and dermal fibroblasts appeared in the wound more quickly, enhancing the granulation tissue formation.[1,6] HCD also may enhance wound healing by their more efficient prevention of dessication.[19]

An often-stated concern about wounds treated with an occlusive regimen is that they appear to be more likely to become infected. Although bacteria are more numerous in wounds covered with occlusive dressings, the bacteria mostly comprise the skin's normal flora, to the exclusion of pathogens, and are not found clinically to interfere with the wound healing process.[7] Efficient functioning of the host defense mechanism was credited with an overall infection rate of 2.6% under occlusive dressings, as compared with a rate of 7.1% under conventional dressings.[6,8,13] However, it is inappropriate to use occlusive dressings in wounds that are clinically grossly contaminated or that have been shown to be colonized with anaerobic organisms.[23]

Ideally, occlusive hydrocolloid dressings are best applied to flat surfaces. HCDs, relatively thin dressings even in the thickest forms, provide little interference with finger range of motion when used on the palmar surface of the hand (Fig. 20-8). Also, their ease of application and adherence make them ideal dressings for fingertip burns (Fig. 20-9) and partial fingertip amputations (Fig. 20-10). In these cases, the occlusive dressing can be supported with an overwrap of Coban for added stability. HCDs are also available in "thin" forms, which are useful in dressing across joints and still allowing motion. HCDs are also useful in dressing the skin avulsion wounds so common in the aged and steroid-dependent patients. In all cases, the HCD is usually left in place until the underlying slurry begins to drain from the edge—from 3 to 6 days.

Biobrane dressings for clean hand wounds

The use of Biobrane as a contact layer dressing also has been helpful, especially in burn wounds to the hand. Biobrane acts as a semipermeable "pseudoepithelium" and allows gas exchange at the wound surface. It is a very thin

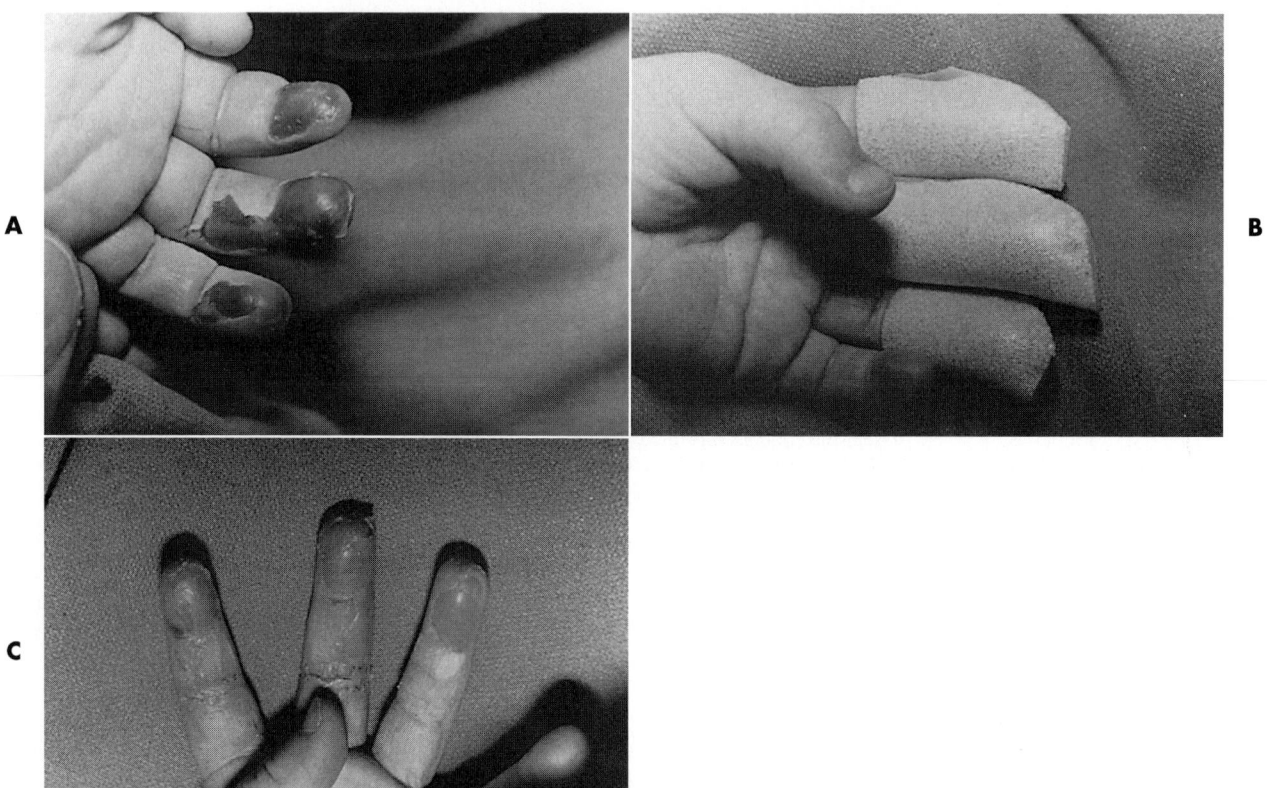

Fig. 20-9. **A,** This 2-year-old girl sustained partial-thickness burns to her fingertips. **B,** Duoderm dressings applied every 3 to 4 days. **C,** The healed burns 7 days after injury.

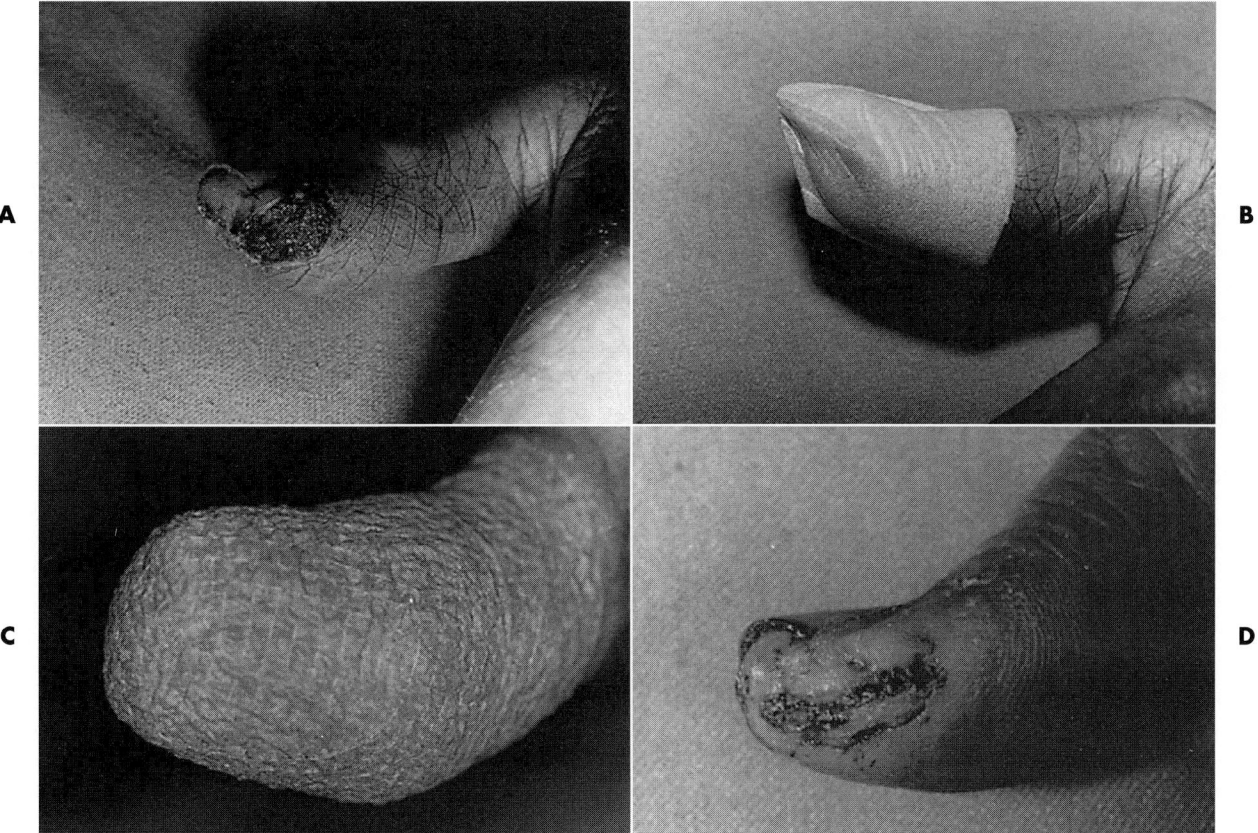

Fig. 20-10. A, A partial fingertip amputation from a saw injury (no exposed bone). **B,** Duoderm dressing over wound. **C,** The hydrocolloid dressing is supported by Coban to allow work. **D,** The nearly healed wound 3 weeks after injury (no time lost from work).

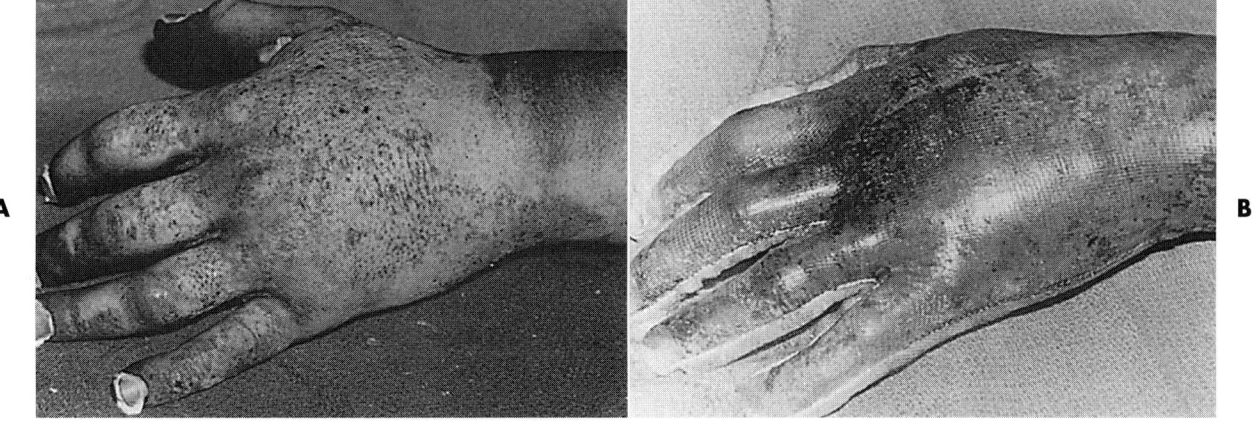

Fig. 20-11. A, This 62-year-old patient sustained deep partial-thickness and full-thickness burns over the dorsum of her hand and forearm. **B,** After initial tangential excision, a Biobrane glove is placed on the hand. Wet dressings are then placed over the Biobrane (until it becomes adherent), and the patient is splinted as necessary. Therapy can proceed while the hand is undressed down to the Biobrane.

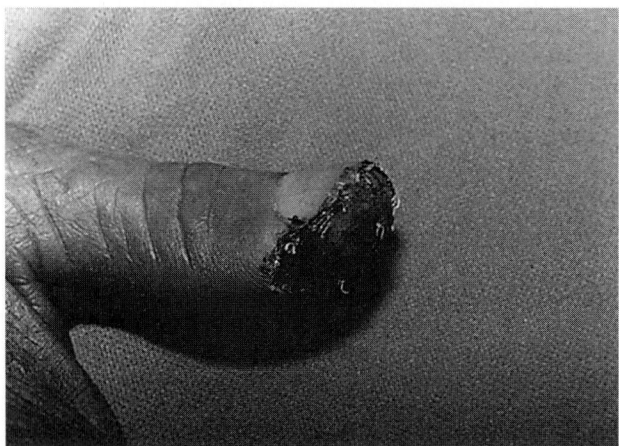

Fig. 20-12. This 42-year-old patient sustained a full-thickness skin loss in a planer injury (no exposed bone). Biobrane is applied to the wound and sutured with absorbable suture to the margins. Wet dressings are applied until the Biobrane is adherent, then only protective dry dressing is indicated. The wound is then allowed to reepithelialize, and the Biobrane is sloughed as this occurs. Patients are generally rendered pain free with this dressing technique.

membrane of silicone mechanically bonded on one side to a flexible nylon fabric, which is then linked covalently to porcine collagenous peptides. The structural and chemical properties of the Biobrane allow binding of wound fibrin, which adheres the fabric to the wound bed until cell ingrowth occurs, tightly binding the mesh to the wound. Evaporative water loss from the wound is decreased 90%, and because of the tight adherence of the Biobrane to the wound surface, there is significant pain relief and minimal bacterial proliferation.[14] Biobrane must adhere to the wound surface to be effective; therefore care must be taken to prevent the accumulation of fluids under the material. Most of the complications associated with Biobrane, such as infection, delayed epithelialization, and pain, are directly related to fluid collections.[41]

For burns, Biobrane can be applied as a glove or in isolated patches sutured to the margins of the wound. Until the Biobrane adheres to the wound bed, wet overdressings should be applied three or four times per day. They are useful to wick the exudate from beneath the sheet and can be used to deliver topical antibiotics if necessary. Between dressing changes, gentle range-of-motion exercise is encouraged. When the Biobrane is adherent, no overdressing is necessary and patients may be allowed to gently shower (Fig. 20-11).

In a partial-thickness wound that is expected to reepithelialize, the Biobrane can be left in place and the edges trimmed as they lift off the healing skin surface. Biobrane also facilitates the preparation of the wound bed for grafting by protecting fragile granulation tissue. The Biobrane is then removed and the wound grafted in one stage. Biobrane also has shown great utility for patients who have sustained partial fingertip amputations and for whom it is elected to

allow wound healing by secondary intent. Often, the Biobrane dressing with a light Coban protective wrap renders the patient sufficiently pain free to allow early return to work (Fig. 20-12).

SUMMARY

This chapter has summarized basic dressing principles and has described dressings useful in many types of wounds. The injured hand presents unique problems to the surgeon and therapist that are different from wound problems in other areas of the body. Optimal care requires a coordinated effort among the surgeon, therapist, and patient to yield a maximally functioning hand with a healed wound. After initial assessment of the patient with an open hand wound, the surgeon will either close the wound or apply the first dressing. For a severely injured hand, the patient often must be returned to the operating room for a "second look" to assess the viability of compromised tissues left during the initial conservative debridement. The patient is then referred to the hand therapist, who makes the decision regarding appropriate dressing in conjunction with the surgeon. If the wound is open and in need of debridement, wet dressings are prescribed. When the wound is sufficiently debrided by surgery or these dressings, the dressing is advanced to the three-layer nonadherent clean wound dressing or an occlusive hydrocolloid or Biobrane dressing. This is maintained until healing is completed by secondary intention or until the wound is closed by skin graft, flap, or delayed primary techniques. As long as the wound is maintained stable during the entire period that the hand is dressed, therapy can proceed and will not delay wound healing.

The open wound therefore should not cause a delay in therapy, and wound dressing is an important part of the care of the patient from injury to complete rehabilitation.

REFERENCES

1. Alvarez OM, Mertz PM, Eaglestein WH: The effect of occlusive dressings on collagen synthesis and re-epithelialization in superficial wounds, *J Surg Res* 35:142, 1983.
2. Beasley RW: *Hand injuries,* Philadelphia, 1981, WB Saunders.
3. Brody GS: Dressings, splints and casts. In Goldwyn RM, editor: *The unfavorable result in plastic surgery: avoidance and treatment,* ed 2, vol 1, Boston, 1984, Little, Brown.
4. Brown D, Garner W, Young VL: Skin grafting: dermal components in inhibition of wound contraction, *South Med J* 83:789, 1990.
5. Donoff RB, Grillo HC: The effects of skin grafting on healing open wounds in rabbits, *J Surg Res* 19:163, 1975.
6. Eaglestein WH: The effect of occlusive dressings on collagen synthesis and reepithelialization in superficial wounds. In Ryan TJ, editor: *An environment for healing: the role of occlusion,* London, 1984, Royal Society of Medicine.
7. Eaglestein WH, Mertz PM, Falanga V: Occlusive dressings, *Am Fam Physician* 35:211, 1987.
8. Eriksson G: Bacterial growth in venous leg ulcers: its clinical significance in the healing process. In Ryan TJ, editor: *An environment for healing: the role of occlusion,* London, 1984, Royal Society of Medicine.

9. Falcone PA, Caldwell MD: Wound metabolism, *Clin Plast Surg* 17:443, 1990.
10. Finley JM: *Practical wound management: a manual of dressings,* Chicago, 1981, Yearbook Medical.
11. Frank DH, Bonaldi LC: Inhibition of wound contraction: comparison of full-thickness skin grafts, Biobrane, and aspartate membranes, *Ann Plast Surg* 14:103, 1985.
12. Harmel RP, Vane DP, King DR: Burn care in children: special considerations, *Clin Plast Surg* 13:95, 1986.
13. Hutchinson JJ: Prevalence of wound infection under occlusive dressings: a collective survey of reported research, *Wounds* 1:123, 1989.
14. Klein RL, Rothman BF, Marshall R: Biobrane: a useful adjunct in therapy of outpatient burns, *J Pediatr Surg* 19:846, 1984.
15. Knight B: The history of wound treatment. In Westaby S, editor: *Wound care,* London, 1985, William Heinemann Medical Books.
16. Kozol RA, Gillies C, Elgebaly SA: Effects of sodium hypochlorite (Dakin's solution) on cells of the wound module, *Arch Surg* 123:420, 1988.
17. Lineweaver W, et al: Antimicrobial toxicity, *Arch Surg* 120:267, 1985.
18. Lineweaver W, et al: Cellular and bacterial toxicities of topical antimicrobials, *Plast Reconstr Surg* 75:394, 1985.
19. Linsky CB, Rovee DT, Dow T: Effects of dressings on wound inflammation and scar tissue. In Hildick-Smith G, editor: *The surgical wound,* Philadelphia, 1981, Lea & Febiger.
20. Machens HG, Berger AC, Mailaender P: Bioartificial skin, *Cells Tissues Organs* 167:88, 2000.
21. Madden JW: Wound healing: biological and clinical features. In Sabiston DC Jr, editor: *Davis-Christopher textbook of surgery: the biological basis of modern surgical practice,* Philadelphia, 1977, WB Saunders.
22. Madden JW, Peacock EE: Studies on the biology of collagen during wound healing. III. Dynamic metabolism of scar collagen and remodeling of dermal wounds, *Ann Surg* 174:511, 1971.
23. Marshall DA, Mertz PM, Eaglestein WH: Occlusive dressings: does dressing type influence the growth of common bacterial pathogens? *Arch Surg* 125:1136, 1990.
24. Matthews DC: unpublished observations, 1982.
25. McGrath MH: How topical dressings salvage "questionable" flaps: experimental study, *Plast Reconstr Surg* 67:653, 1981.
26. McKinney P, Cunningham BL: *Handbook of plastic surgery,* Baltimore, 1981, Williams & Wilkins.
27. Noe JM, Kalish S: The mechanisms of capillarity in surgical dressings, *Surg Gynecol Obstet* 143:454, 1976.
28. Noe JM, Kalish S: Dressing materials and their selection. In Rudolph R, Noe JM, editors: *Chronic problem wounds,* Boston, 1983, Little, Brown.
29. Noe JM, Keller M: Can stitches get wet? *Plast Reconstr Surg* 81:82, 1988.
30. Peacock EE Jr: *Wound repair,* ed 3, Philadelphia, 1984, WB Saunders.
31. Polk HC, Finn MP: Chemoprophylaxis and immunoprophylaxis in surgical wound infection. In Simmons RL, Howard RJ, editors: *Surgical infectious disease,* New York, 1982, Appleton-Century-Crofts.
32. Rodeheaver G, et al: Side-effects of topical proteolytic enzyme treatment, *Surg Gynecol Obstet* 148:562, 1979.
33. Sawhey CP, Monga HL: Wound contraction in rabbits and the effectiveness of skin grafts in preventing it, *Br J Plast Surg* 23:318, 1970.
34. Slater RM, Hughes NC: A simplified method of treating burns of the hands, *Br J Plast Surg* 24:396, 1971.
35. Tobin GR: The compromised bed technique: an improved method for skin grafting problem wounds, *Surg Clin North Am* 64:653, 1984.
36. Turner TD: Which dressing and why? In Westaby S, editor: *Wound care,* London, 1985, William Heinemann Medical Books.
37. Viljanto J: Disinfection of surgical wounds without inhibition of normal wound healing, *Arch Surg* 115:253, 1980.
38. Westaby S: Fundamentals of wound healing. In Westaby S, editor: *Wound care,* London, 1985, William Heinemann Medical Books.
39. Westaby S, White S: Wound infection. In Westaby S, editor: *Wound care,* London, 1985, William Heinemann Medical Books.
40. Wheeland RG: The newer surgical dressings and wound healing, *Dermatol Clin* 5:393, 1987.
41. Yang J-Y, Tsai Y-C, Noordhoff MS: Clinical comparison of commercially available Biobrane preparations, *Burns* 15:197, 1989.
42. Zawacki BE: The effect of Travase on heat injured skin, *Surgery* 77:132, 1975.

Chapter 21

MANAGEMENT OF SKIN GRAFTS AND FLAPS

L. Scott Levin
Gregory J. Moorman
Lior Heller

Reconstructive surgery of the upper extremity has developed significantly over the last three decades. Microsurgical techniques, a variety of new flaps, and the increasing use of functional free tissue transfer have greatly enhanced the armamentarium of reconstructive surgical concepts and procedures.[13] At the same time, the continuing sophistication of postoperative wound management has created an optimal environment for wound healing, rehabilitation, and overall recovery. Reconstructive surgery has evolved from the practice of simply providing soft tissue coverage for traumatic defects, to a complex algorithmic process of wound management involving thorough clinical assessment, evaluation of individual functional and social needs of the patient, creation and implementation of a surgical plan, and meticulous postoperative management. The algorithmic approach offers a reconstructive ladder for the evaluation and treatment of wounds ranging from acute traumatic injuries to various chronic conditions, including osteomyelitis, nonhealing wounds, and defects following tumor resection.[23] This ladder directs the reconstructive surgeon to the indicated reconstructive surgical approach, based on the extent and severity of the wound, the functional needs of the patient, and the availability of required tissue elements. The initial goal of the reconstructive surgeon is the reconstitution of the soft tissue envelope, providing a well-vascularized, healthy environment to facilitate localized healing. With successful recovery and healing, the reconstructive surgeon can attain his or her ultimate goal: to optimize rehabilitation based on individual needs and thus maximize functional restoration, providing the patient with the opportunity for rapid social reintegration and the overall improvement of their quality,

productive recovery. This chapter discusses an algorithmic approach to reconstruction of the hand and upper extremity, providing examples of excellent reconstructive options for complex surgical problems, ranging from skin grafts, to local tissue flaps, to advanced free tissue transfer. Management strategies to facilitate localized healing and optimize functional rehabilitation and recovery are outlined.

PATIENT EVALUATION

The first step in developing a reconstructive strategy is the assessment of the patient. The surgeon must recognize the clinical reconstructive needs of the patient, based on the severity of a traumatic injury, the extent of a chronic wound, or the tumor mass requiring resection. Important considerations include age, significant medical conditions, preinjury functional status, occupation, dominance of the extremity involved, psychosocial considerations, and individual patient motivation and compliance. In patients with acute traumatic injuries of the upper extremity, a thorough clinical evaluation is necessary to first rule out the presence of other significant life-threatening injuries. Once a patient's overall condition is known to be stable, the clinician may proceed with further assessment of the extremities. Evaluation of the hand and upper extremity involves a systematic approach to the extremity as a functional organ.[13] Complete examination includes gross visual inspection, evaluation of limb perfusion, assessment of passive and active motion, and a review of neurologic function. Imaging studies such as radiographs, ultrasonography, computed tomography scanning, magnetic resonance imaging, and/or angiography are incorporated as indicated to further establish the extent of soft tissue, bone, and vascular involvement. Once the clinical needs of the patient have been clearly established, an algorithmic surgical management strategy can then be created to optimize the reconstruction, postoperative management, and the overall functional rehabilitation of the patient, based on those individual needs.

MANAGEMENT STRATEGY

A reconstructive management strategy is created based on the evaluation of an injury or wound and the individual needs of the patient. The complexity of the surgical reconstruction is directed by the severity and extent of the wound, the viability of the remaining tissues, and the exposure of underlying vital structures. The first step in surgical wound management is exploration, irrigation, and meticulous debridement. Adequate debridement of all non-viable tissues is required to establish a healthy environment for healing and to decrease the risk of potential infection. Underlying injuries to vital structures of function must be identified and repaired. Neurovascular injuries need to be repaired either primarily or with the use of conduits as indicated. Fractures must be recognized, irrigated, and debrided appropriately, and then they must be stabilized with internal or external fixation. Tendon injuries should be repaired primarily, if possible, or prepared for more extensive future reconstruction as a staged procedure. Following repair of these underlying vital structures, soft tissue coverage becomes the primary consideration. Soft tissue reconstruction options include primary closure, delayed primary closure, healing by secondary intention, skin grafts, local tissue transfer, free tissue transfer, or any combination of these.

Primary wound closure

Primary wound closure simply involves reapproximating the wound edges. This is accomplished with the use of sutures, staples, tapes, or skin glue, as a single or multilayered repair. Delayed primary closure suggests a delay in the repair, such as waiting to allow associated edema to resolve enough to facilitate primary closure, or to allow future reassessment of the soft tissue viability before closure considerations.

Healing by secondary intention

Healing by secondary intention refers to leaving a wound open and allowing it to heal spontaneously through contraction and epithelialization. In the hand and upper extremity, healing by secondary intention can be successfully used with acceptable results in small wounds, such as fingertip injuries involving less than a 1-cm defect, without exposed underlying bone. Healing of larger hand and upper extremity wounds by secondary intention, however, can result in significant scar formation and contracture, with subsequent limitations in range of motion (ROM) and function.

Skin grafts

A skin graft is a harvested segment of epidermis and dermis that has been elevated and separated completely from its blood supply. The first reported transfer of skin was credited to Reverdin in 1870,[19] but skin grafting did not become common until the invention of the dermatome by Padget[28] during the time of World War II. The dermatome simplified the method of elevating a skin graft, providing a reliable instrument to harvest a skin graft of a desired size and depth, consistently. The dermatome remains the primary tool used today for harvesting skin grafts. With the increased use of skin grafts, it was recognized that their early use for wound coverage could retard the extent of wound contracture, thus limiting deformity and functional disability.[10]

Skin grafts can either be full thickness or split thickness. A full-thickness skin graft refers to harvesting a segment of skin, including the epidermis and entire dermis. A full-thickness skin graft resembles normal skin more closely, including texture, color, and potential for hair growth. A full-thickness skin graft demonstrates the greatest amount of primary contracture, but the least amount of secondary wound contracture. That is, after the harvest of a full-thickness skin graft, it quickly contracts and appears much smaller because of the elasticity of the tissues. However, when that full-thickness skin graft is applied to a wound defect early, it maintains its size, and can completely stop the contracture of the wound. Full-thickness skin grafting does have limitations. There is a slightly greater risk of nonadherence of the graft, and donor site availability must be considered before full-thickness skin harvest. A full-thickness skin graft donor site must be amenable to primary closure, or the created donor defect may require an additional split-thickness skin graft for coverage.

A split-thickness skin graft is a partial-thickness skin graft consisting of the entire epidermis and a portion of the dermis. Partial-thickness skin grafts can be harvested at varying depths and are classified according to the thickness of dermis included: thin split-thickness grafts, intermediate- or medium-thickness grafts, or thick split-thickness skin grafts. Compared with a full-thickness graft, a split-thickness skin graft demonstrates less primary contracture following harvest, but greater secondary contracture of the grafted wound. A thin split-thickness skin graft produces the least primary contracture because of the decreased elastic tissues, but it produces the greatest secondary wound contracture. A thick split-thickness graft can decrease the rate of wound contracture, but it will not retard it completely as a full-thickness graft can.

A split-thickness skin graft can be either meshed or unmeshed. Split-thickness grafts are typically meshed at ratios of 1:1 to 3:1, with the ratio selected dependent on the size of the defect needed to be grafted and the skin available for grafting. Meshing of the harvested skin graft facilitates expansion of the graft for coverage of more extensive wound defects. A split-thickness skin graft also may be left unmeshed and used to cover a wound as a sheet graft. A sheet graft avoids the meshed-pattern scarring associated with meshed skin grafts, thus resulting in a more cosmetic appearance.

Skin grafts may be secured to the margins of the wound with sutures, staples, tape, or skin glue. At this point, the wound dressing and the postoperative management take precedence. The postoperative wound care can greatly influence the survival of the transferred skin graft. Various potential postoperative complications can lead to the demise of a skin graft. The best method to avoid failure is prevention by meticulous postoperative management. The number one reason for failure of a skin graft is hematoma. A hematoma can form beneath the graft, preventing adherence and promoting graft loss. Prevention includes meticulous perioperative hemostasis and appropriate postoperative dressings. Dressings over a skin graft must provide lubrication to prevent desiccation, appropriate compression to eliminate the potential space between the skin graft and the wound bed, and local immobilization to prevent shearing of the graft. An appropriate dressing promotes imbibition, inosculation, adherence, and success of the skin graft. A lubricating gauze such as Adaptic, Xeroform, or Xeroflo initially is placed directly over the skin graft, followed by layered moist cotton balls, cotton sheets, or gauze, saturated in a solution such as Bunnells', or mineral oil. Bunnells' solution, consisting of benzalkonium chloride, acetic acid, and glycerin, is the lubricating liquid we prefer. A convex wound may only require a simple dressing under which compression will occur naturally because of the projection of the convex surface of the wound. A concave wound often requires a tie-over dressing, also called a *bolster* or *stent,* to compress the skin graft against the surface of the wound defect. This is accomplished with the use of sutures, staples, or a circumferential dressing, to secure the bolster dressing over the skin graft, facilitating graft adherence and healing.

Graft survival also is enhanced by strict local immobilization. This is achieved by splinting the appropriate associated joint(s), at the level of the digits, wrist, or elbow, to maintain a constant protective position and decrease the risk of shearing of the graft.

Postoperative follow-up and management. The dressing over an upper extremity skin graft typically is removed in 4 to 7 days, and the wound is reevaluated. By this time, the skin graft should be adherent to the wound bed, but meticulous wound care is still required to preserve the reconstruction. It remains important to maintain a moist/lubricated environment to prevent the persistent risk of desiccation of the skin graft and facilitate complete healing. This is accomplished with either continued wet-to-dry dressing changes or the application of a lubricating agent such as an antibacterial ointment, bacitracin or an equivalent. Once complete epithelialization of the skin graft is recognized, the use of the lubricating ointments and dressings can be discontinued and a simple moisturizing cream started.

The continued serial application of a moisturizing cream, such as Eucerin or the equivalent, in combination with gentle massage, can facilitate progressive contoured scar maturation with flattening of the grafted surface and improve the overall cosmetic results. Once adherence of the skin graft is recognized, and as long as there are no significant underlying injuries, rehabilitation of the upper extremity can be initiated and aggressively advanced. Neurovascular, tendon, and bone injuries will influence the rehabilitation plan, with timing directed by the individual extent of their involvement.

Management of the skin graft donor site. We prefer to simply cover the harvested split-thickness skin graft donor site with an op-site, a transparent, adherent dressing, and allow spontaneous reepithelialization of the donor bed. Reepithelialization of the graft donor site typically occurs in approximately 1 week. If fluid collects beneath the dressing, it is simply drained with a needle and the dressing patched with an additional op-site, or the entire dressing is changed. Following complete reepithelialization of the donor site, dressings are discontinued and the healing bed can be treated for dryness as needed, using a moisturizing lotion such as Eucerin or an equivalent.

Local tissue transfer. Earlier in this chapter, we noted that skin grafts are not appropriate for all wounds. For traumatic defects of the upper extremity involving soft tissue loss, with associated exposure of underlying vital structures, such as blood vessels, nerves, tendons devoid of paratenon, bones devoid of periosteum, or wounds with insufficient vascularity to support a skin graft, a more complex reconstructive approach must be used. The surgeon's initial consideration in this situation is the next step in the algorithmic approach to reconstruction of the upper extremity, that is, use of a local tissue flap. Local tissue transfer refers to the dissection, elevation, and transfer of skin, combined with a varied amount of underlying tissue, potentially including subcutaneous tissue, fascia, muscle, nerve, tendon, and/or bone. The composition of the tissue harvested and used is determined by the type and extent of tissue loss. During the elevation of a local tissue flap, the local blood supply supporting the flap is preserved. This undivided portion of the flap containing the vascularity required for flap survival, is labeled the pedicle. A local tissue flap can close a local tissue defect, establishing a well-vascularized, healthy environment to potentiate healing of the associated underlying injuries. Local tissue flaps are labeled according to the layers of tissue used, the pattern of the blood supply, and the type of mobilization required.

Skin flaps. Using a local skin flap for reconstruction of an upper extremity defect refers to rotating adjacent skin and subcutaneous tissue into a wound to supply coverage and closure. A skin flap design is based on the local vascular anatomy of the skin. A random pattern flap is a local skin flap that has no specific arterial-venous system.[26] An axial pattern flap is a single pedicle skin flap with an anatomically established arterial-venous system along its longitudinal axis.[26] An island flap is an axial pattern flap in which the skin bridge has been separated, leaving only the vascular pedicle intact at the base.[11] Skin flaps are also classified by mobilization techniques, rotational versus advancement. Rotation flaps are skin flaps that rotate around a fixed point to reach a wound defect (Fig. 21-1). An advancement flap is a skin flap that advances from the donor site to the recipient wound bed in a straight line, without any rotation (Fig. 21-2). Numerous accounts of local flaps are well described in the literature; local flaps are traditionally valuable and versatile options in the reconstruction of many upper extremity defects at all levels: the fingers, hands, forearm, and upper arm.

Digital reconstruction. Our fingers are the tools we use to reach out and engage our environment. Whether at work or at play, our fingers are always in front of us and subsequently are injured often. Fingertip injuries involving a surface area of less than 1 cm, without exposed bone or vital structures, can simply be allowed to close by secondary intention. Moist dressings can be applied until the wound has reepithelialized. In fingertip injuries involving a surface area defect greater than 1 cm, or digital defects with exposed underlying vital structures, a reconstructive procedure is indicated. The reconstructive goal is to provide wound closure and restore functional sensibility to the finger. As

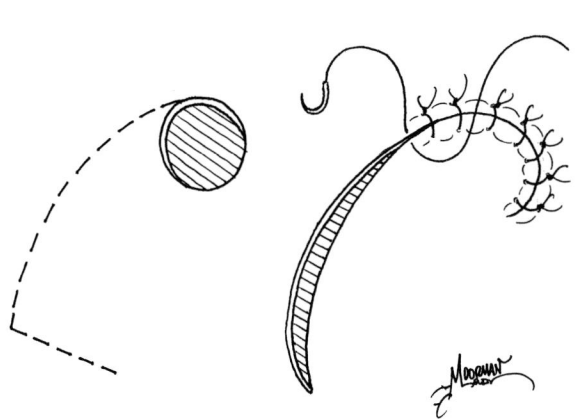

Fig. 21-1. Rotation flap. The flap is designed to rotate around a fixed point to reach a wound defect.

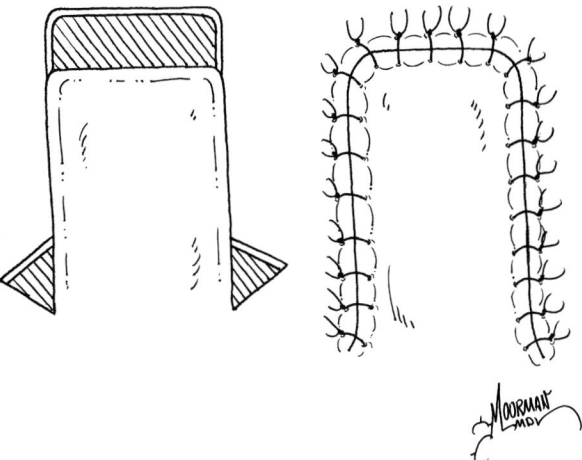

Fig. 21-2. Advancement flap. The flap is designed to advance from the donor site to the recipient wound bed in a straight line, without any rotation.

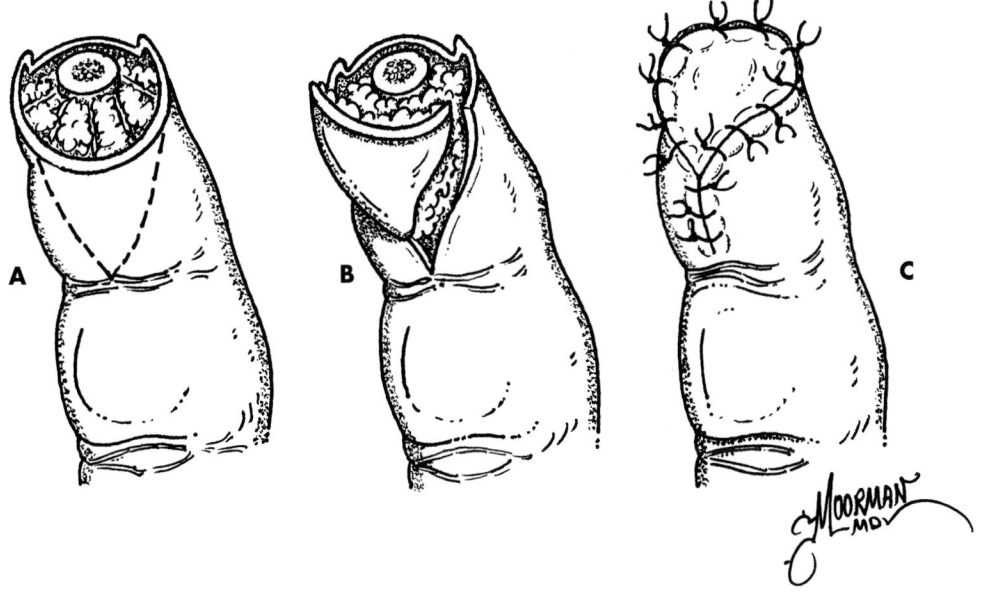

Fig. 21-3. V-Y advancement flap. **A,** Fingertip injury with planned V-shaped volar incision. **B,** Elevation of volar flap. **C,** Distal advancement of volar flap and closure in a Y-pattern.

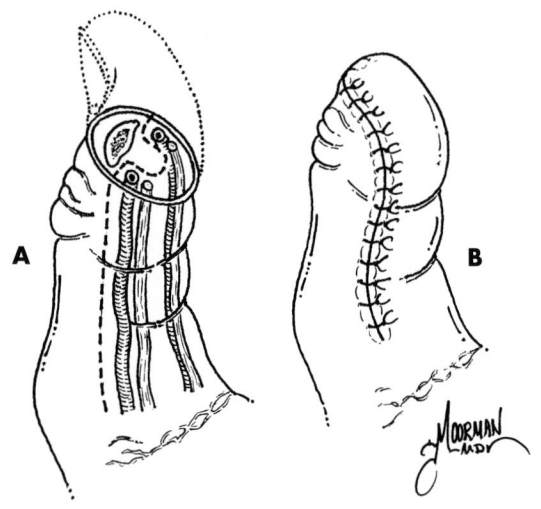

Fig. 21-4. Moberg flap. **A,** Distal thumb amputation with planned midlateral incisions. The neurovascular bundles are preserved and advanced with the volar flap. **B,** Advancement of the volar flap and suture closure.

noted before, many well-described local skin flap procedures are illustrated in the reconstructive literature. The selection of a particular surgical procedure is individualized to the patient, based primarily on the size and the location of the wound defect.

V-Y advancement flap.[12] The volar V-Y (Atasoy, Tanquilli-Leali)[2,32] or lateral V-Y (Geissendorfer, Kutler)[12,22] advancement flaps are skin flaps indicated for small fingertip injuries. These flaps offer a reconstructive dimension of 1 to 1.5 cm. Following appropriate debridement of the injured tissues, the volar V-Y flap is created by making a triangular skin incision(s) just below the defect. The subcutaneous tissue is preserved, and the fibrous septa from the pulp to the periosteum is released. The dissected V-shaped flap is then advanced distally to cover the defect, and subsequently closed in a Y-pattern with surgical sutures (Fig. 21-3). The flap is covered with a nonadherent lubricating gauze and protected with a bulky dressing. Sutures are typically removed in 2 weeks, and early motion is initiated.

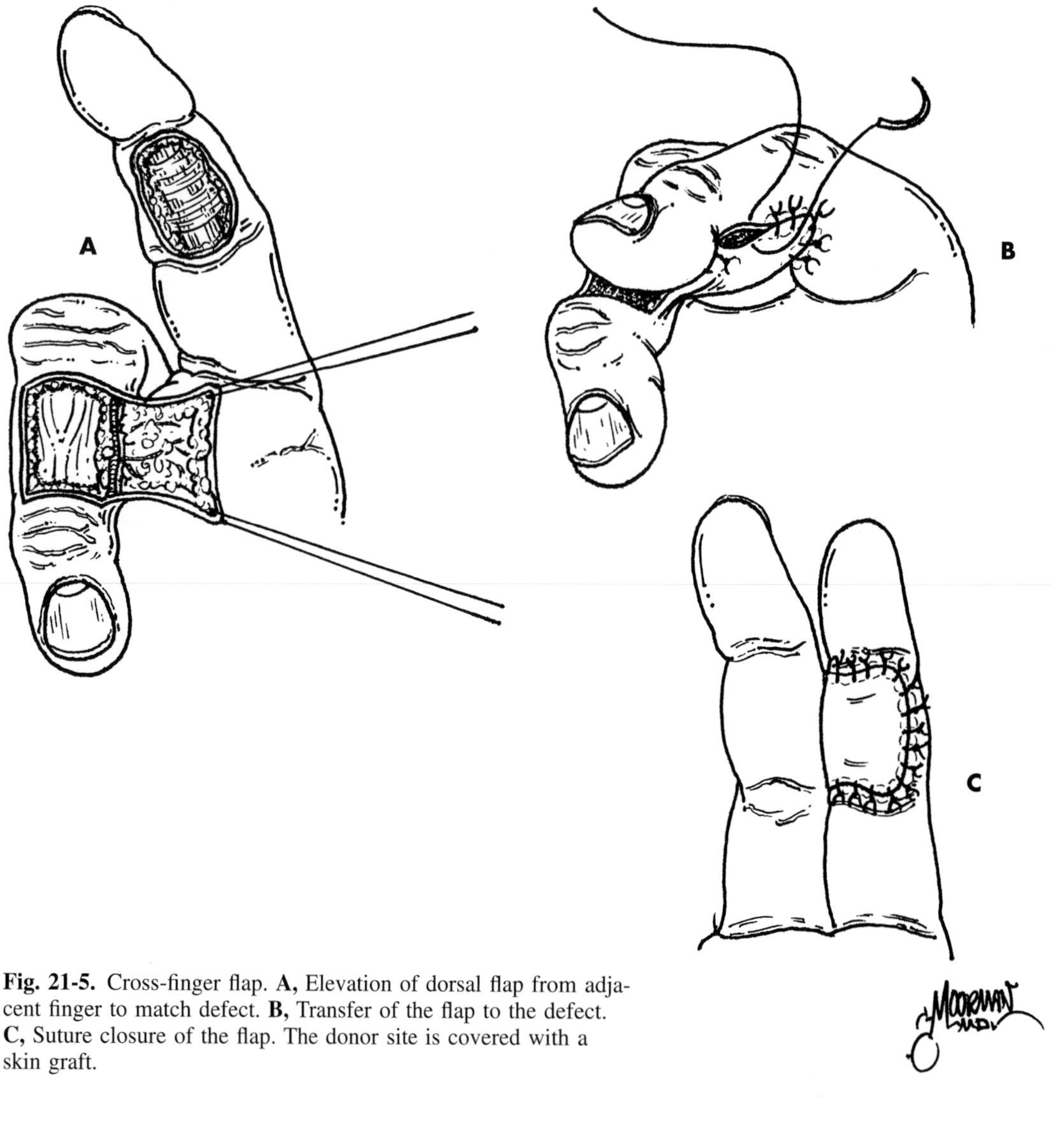

Fig. 21-5. Cross-finger flap. **A,** Elevation of dorsal flap from adjacent finger to match defect. **B,** Transfer of the flap to the defect. **C,** Suture closure of the flap. The donor site is covered with a skin graft.

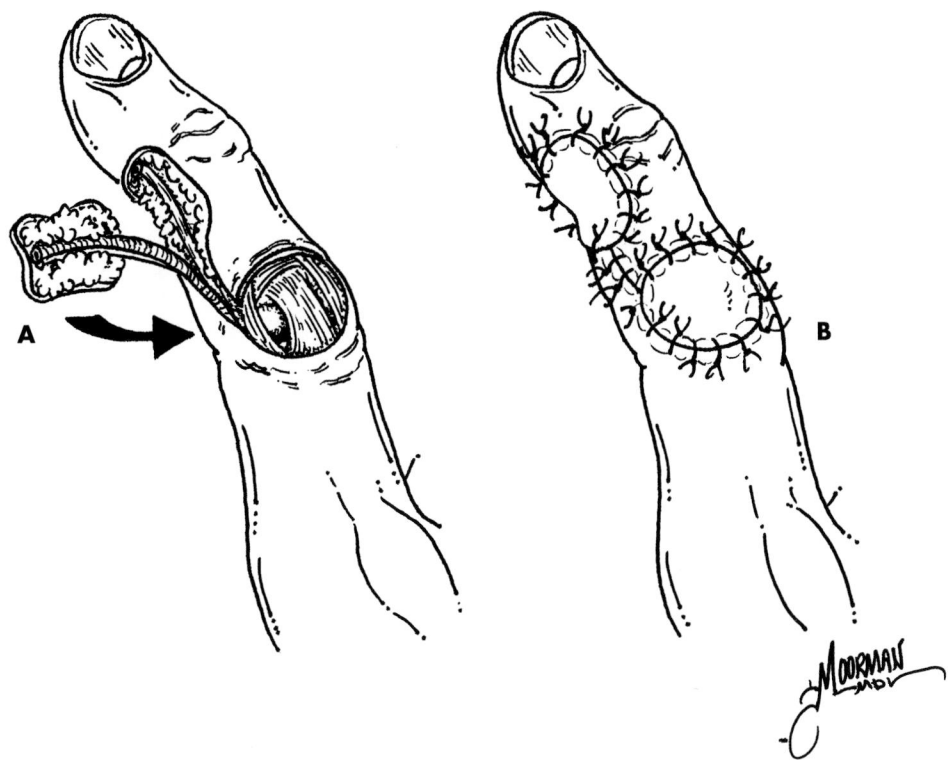

Fig. 21-6. Digital island flap. **A,** Dissection and elevation of skin flap based on the proper digital artery and vein, designed to cover the illustrated defect over the dorsal surface of the proximal interphalangeal joint. **B,** Rotation of the island flap to cover the defect and closure of the donor site with a skin graft.

Volar advancement Moberg flap. Defects of the pulp of the thumb or other digital defects that are too large for coverage with a V-Y advancement flap, may be approached with a Moberg flap.[27]

Moberg volar advancement flap may be advanced a distance of 1.5 to 2.0 cm and used to cover a traumatic defect involving the entire volar surface of the thumb or another digit. The Moberg flap is created by making midlateral incisions below the fingertip defect. The neurovascular bundles are preserved, and the created volar flap is then advanced to cover the defect (Fig. 21-4). This is a reliable sensate flap that restores sensibility to the pulp. The flap is dressed with a nonadherent lubricating gauze, followed by the application of a protective dressing and splint.

Cross-finger flaps. A conventional cross-finger flap uses an elevated skin flap from the dorsal aspect of one finger to cover an open volar or tip wound with exposed tendon or bone of an adjacent finger.[9] The donor site is then covered with a skin graft (Fig. 21-5). A reverse cross-finger flap involves dissecting an additional adipofascial flap beneath the skin flap, which is then used to cover a dorsal wound defect of an adjacent finger.[1] The skin flap is then reinset over the donor defect and a skin graft is placed over the transferred adipofascial flap. Each of these flaps can cover a digital defect up to 2 cm. The skin grafts are then supported

with a bolster dressing, and the fingers are splinted or pinned to protect the created flaps. The patient returns in 2 weeks for separation and insetting of the flap. Hand therapy is initiated early to maintain optimal ROM and function.

Digital island flaps. Digital island flaps are excellent reconstructive tools to cover either distal or proximal digital defects up to 2.5 cm, overlying exposed joints or tendons (Fig. 21-6). A skin flap is created in a pattern indicated by the local defect and then harvested based on the proper digital artery and vein.[21] The associated proper digital nerve can be included to add sensibility to the reconstructed flap, or preserved in its natural anatomic state. The pedicle flap is then transferred distally or proximally to the digital defect and secured with permanent sutures. The donor site is reconstructed with a small full-thickness skin graft.

Muscle, musculocutaneous, and fasciocutaneous flaps. Muscle, musculocutaneous, and fasciocutaneous flaps are more complex reconstructive tools available for surgical coverage of local wound defects of the upper extremity. Reconstruction proximal to the fingers typically involves more extensive injuries with larger soft tissue defects requiring more elaborate reconstruction. Vital structures, such as tendons, blood vessels, nerves, and bone are often exposed, requiring appropriate healthy soft tissue coverage to optimize healing of the underlying injuries. Muscle,

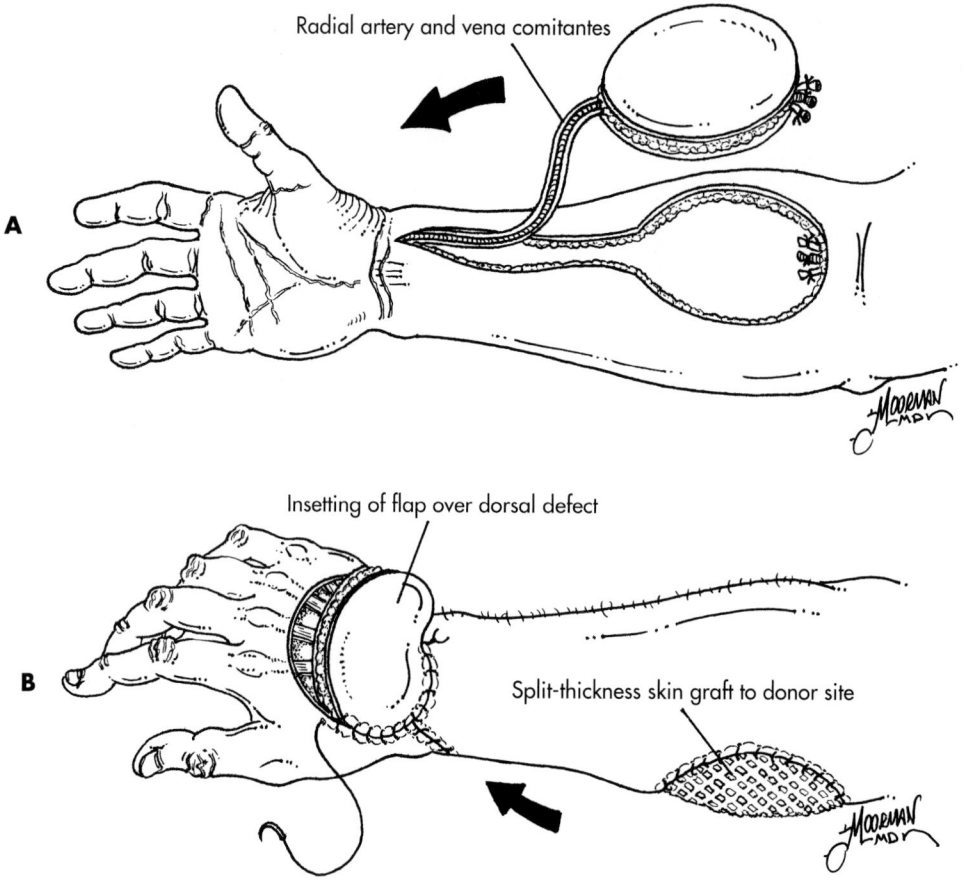

Radial artery and vena comitantes

A

Insetting of flap over dorsal defect

B

Split-thickness skin graft to donor site

Fig. 21-7. Radial forearm flap. **A,** Elevation of the fasciocutaneous flap based on the radial artery and veins, designed to cover a wound defect on the dorsum of the hand. **B,** Rotation of the flap distally and suture closure. Coverage of the donor site with a skin graft.

musculocutaneous, and fasciocutaneous flaps, either harvested and used as local flaps or as free tissue transfers, can provide sufficient healthy tissue bulk to fill large wound defects. These soft tissue flaps are based on defined vascular anatomy with associated versatility and reliability.[31] The upper extremity offers several excellent choices for local tissue transfer reconstruction of amenable wound defects.

Radial forearm flap. The radial forearm flap is a fasciocutaneous flap harvested from the volar forearm, based on the radial artery and concomitant veins[30] (Fig. 21-7). This flap offers the reconstructive surgeon an excellent option for coverage of defects requiring thin, pliable tissue. The radial forearm flap can be raised on its pedicle and rotated locally, either proximally, based on antegrade flow, or distally, based on retrograde flow. This flap also may be harvested as a free flap, and/or combined with a strip of palmaris longus or brachialis for associated tendon reconstruction, a portion of the radius for bony reconstruction,[8] or the lateral antebrachial cutaneous nerve to establish an innervated flap. The disadvantages of this procedure are the sacrifice of a major forearm artery, and the unsightly donor harvest site, which requires a skin graft for coverage.

Posterior interosseus flap. The posterior interosseous flap is a fasciocutaneous flap that can be used as a reverse pedicled local tissue transfer based on the posterior interosseous artery, to cover distal defects of the wrist, dorsal hand, and first web space. A reconstructive dimension of 8 × 15 cm may be elevated and rotated, but any skin island greater then 4 cm wide will require a skin graft for closure of the donor site. This flap is dissected and harvested from the dorsal forearm, rotated distally, and secured into the defect with surgical sutures. The flap is protected with sterile dressings and immobilization.

Lateral arm flap. The lateral arm flap is an excellent flap for reconstruction of upper extremity soft tissue defects. This flap can be used as a local pedicled flap, based on antegrade or reverse flow, or as a free flap. The lateral arm flap represents an innervated cutaneous flap with a reconstructive dimension of 15 × 18 cm. It may be harvested as an osteocutaneous flap with a portion of the humerus and may include a fasciocutaneous forearm extension, or a tendon strip from the triceps, depending on the individual needs for reconstruction.[18] The lateral arm flap may be rotated on its pedicle to cover large defects either proximally around

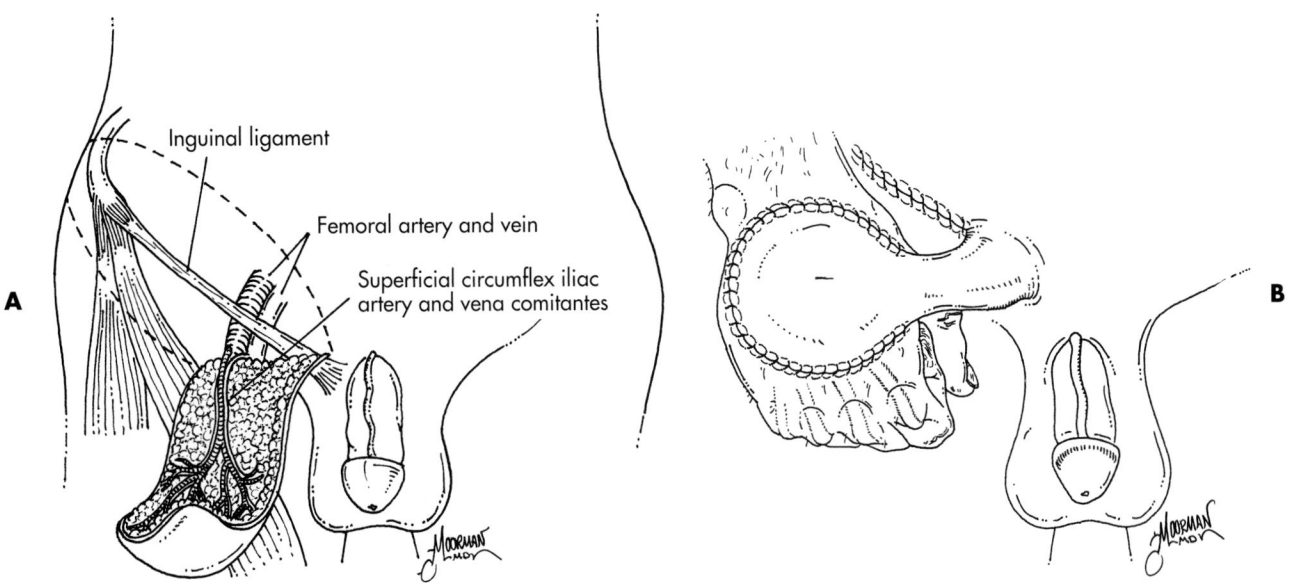

Fig. 21-8. Groin flap. **A,** Elevation of the groin flap. **B,** Contouring the flap as a tube for coverage of a complex degloving hand injury.

the shoulder or distally around the elbow. As a free flap, the lateral arm flap may be further used for coverage of defects involving the dorsum of the hand or the first web space.

Groin flap. The groin flap is an axial pattern flap that provides a reliable surgical option for reconstruction of distal upper extremity injuries. This flap is elevated as a pedicle flap based on the superficial circumflex iliac artery and concomitant veins, and then used to cover either hand or forearm defects[26] (Fig. 21-8). The donor defect may close primarily, or it may require a skin graft for coverage. Once the flap is secured to the defect, the upper extremity must be immobilized to eliminate tension on the vascular pedicle. Immobilization of the flap may be achieved with circumferential dressings, tape, or supportive splints, and carefully maintained as an outpatient. The patient then returns in 2 to 3 weeks for surgical division of the vascular pedicle and final contouring and insetting of the flap. Before division of the flap, gentle ROM of the uninvolved digits should be performed.

Parascapular and scapular flaps. The parascapular and scapular flaps are cutaneous flaps based on a branch of the circumflex scapular artery[33] (Fig. 21-9). Each of these flaps has a reconstructive dimension of about 10×25 cm. A parascapular or scapular flap can be rotated locally and used as a pedicled flap for coverage of shoulder or proximal, posterior arm defects. These flaps can be harvested and transplanted as free flaps for coverage of both forearm and dorsal hand defects.[4] Parascapular and scapular flaps also provide the reconstructive surgeon the opportunity to incorporate additional fascial extensions to provide gliding surfaces for associated tendon repairs, if necessary, or include a portion of scapular bone for reconstruction of segmental forearm defects.

Latissimus dorsi flap. The latissimus dorsi flap is an excellent reconstruction option for the coverage of large surface area defects. This flap may be harvested as a muscle or musculocutaneous flap and used as a pedicled tissue transfer to cover significant local defects of the shoulder and upper arm, or as a free flap to cover extensive distal upper extremity wounds. As a free tissue transfer, the latissimus dorsi flap is harvested based on the thoracodorsal artery and concomitant vein[3] and contoured to fit the defect. The thoracodorsal vessels are anastomosed to prepared recipient vessels out of the zone of injury, followed by insetting of the flap to cover the defect. This flap has an incredible reconstructive dimension of about 20×35 cm, depending on the size of the individual.

Postoperative management of local tissue flaps. At the time of the operation, the local tissue flap is protected with a sterile dressing and a supportive splint at the appropriate joint level. A window is cut out of the dressing over the created flap to allow direct visualization of the reconstruction. This allows meticulous clinical observation of the local tissue flap vascularity, which is monitored by color and capillary refill. Lack of color or delayed capillary refill may represent lack of blood flow within the flap, whereas discoloration or rapid capillary refill suggests flap congestion. Each of these clinical findings suggests potential flap failure and the need for continued meticulous clinical monitoring, with a low threshold for surgical reexploration and revision. Postoperatively, the reconstructed upper extremity is elevated on a couple of pillows or a prefabricated foam wedge commercially designed for limb elevation. Elevation is of utmost importance to prevent upper extremity swelling and the associated potential risk of increased flap congestion. Upon discharge home, elevation

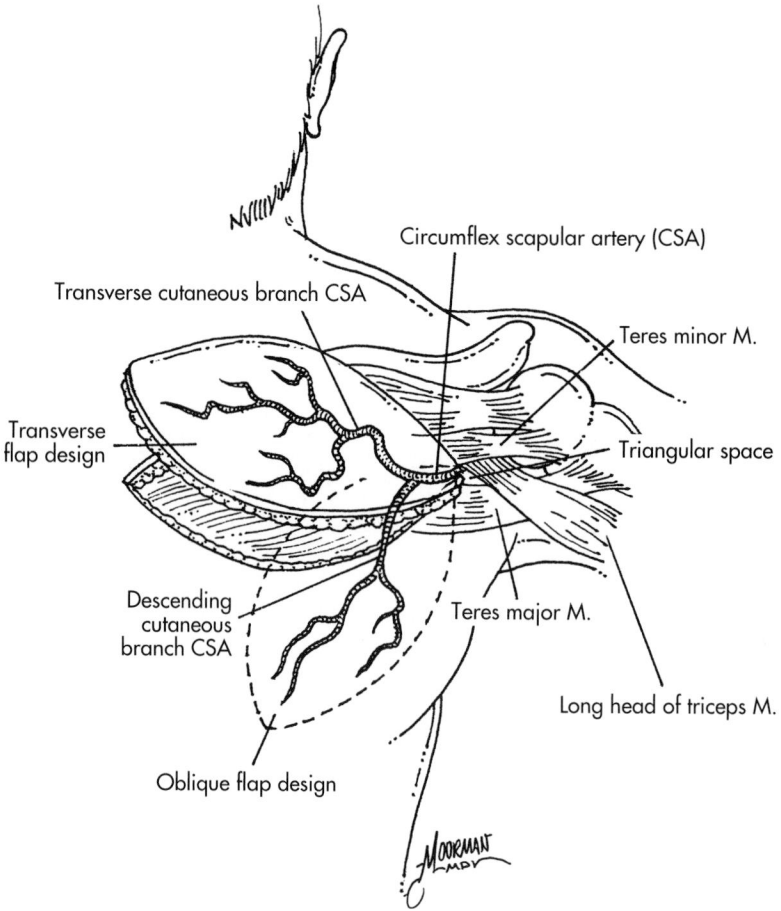

Fig. 21-9. Surgical anatomy of the scapular flap.

is continued and splints are left intact to maintain support and protection, facilitating complete healing of the local tissue reconstruction.

The patient or a home health care agency monitors operative drains at home, where output is measured and recorded over 24-hour periods. The drains are removed at clinic follow-up when the reported output falls below our set minimum of 30 ml for a 24-hour period. Sutures and/or staples are removed 2 weeks postoperatively, and an early rehabilitation protocol is instituted to facilitate progressive functional restoration and overall recovery. As noted earlier, the intensity and timing of the postoperative rehabilitation therapy depend on the extent and specific nature of the underlying structural injuries.

Free tissue transfer

Reconstruction of an upper extremity wound defect using a local tissue flap is not always feasible. Local tissue transfer may be limited because of the wound location or regional donor site deficiencies. A vascular pedicle may not be long enough to reach a particular defect, or the defect may be too large to cover completely with local tissue. In these instances, the reconstructive surgeon looks to our final rung in the reconstructive ladder, free tissue transfer.

Autologous free tissue transfer refers to the transplant of tissue from one location of the body to another. This is achieved by using an operating microscope and meticulous techniques of microsurgery to perform small vessel anastomoses between the pedicle of the transferred free tissue flap and the prepared local recipient vessels.

Microsurgery for extremity reconstruction began more than three decades ago with the introduction of the operating microscope for anastomoses of blood vessels, described by Jacobson.[17] The operating microscope was first used to repair injured digital arteries, which began the age of digital replantation in the 1960s.[6,20] In the 1970s, the use of the microscope was expanded to microsurgical composite free tissue transplantation.[29] Composite free tissue transplantation describes the harvesting and transfer of a composite (or collection) of tissues, including muscle, fascia, skin and subcutaneous tissue, nerve, tendon, bone, or any combination of these. The vascular inflow and outflow of the harvested free tissue flap is preserved for anastomosis with the local blood supply. Efforts of the modern microsurgeon have expanded from just providing soft tissue bulk for coverage of a wound defect to the ultimate reconstructive goal of full functional restoration.[15]

Free tissue transfer continues to play an increasingly vital

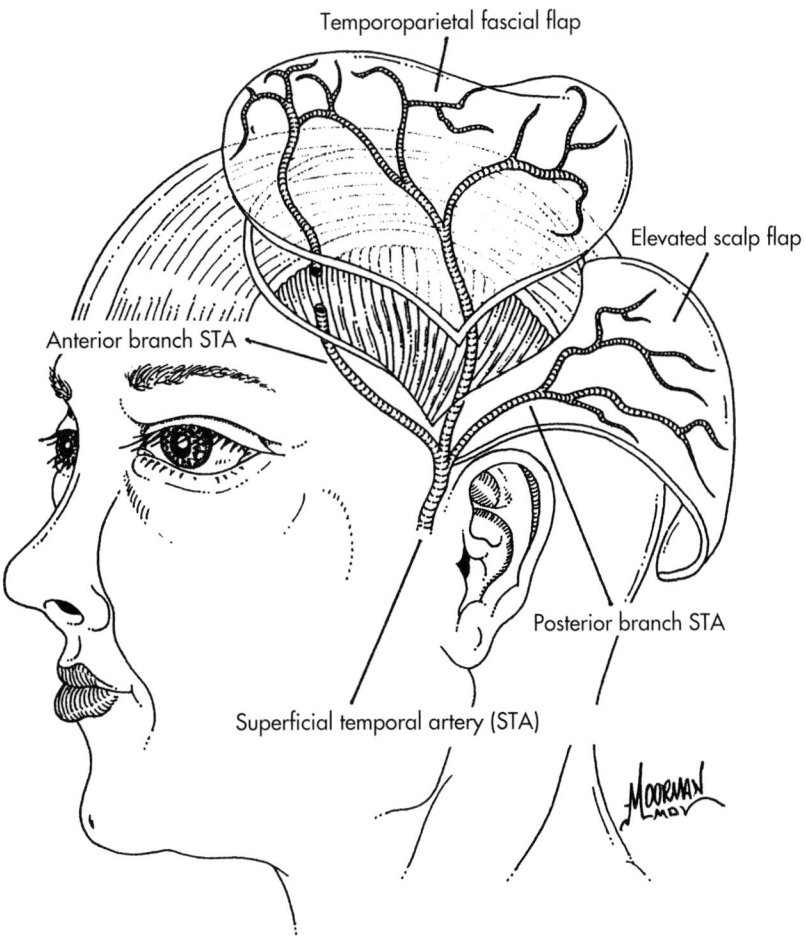

Temporoparietal fascial flap

Elevated scalp flap

Anterior branch STA

Posterior branch STA

Superficial temporal artery (STA)

Fig. 21-10. Anatomy of the temporoparietal fascial flap.

role in the reconstruction of upper extremity complex wounds. Free tissue flaps, dissected as muscle, musculocutaneous, or fasciocutaneous flaps, can be harvested out of the zone of injury and transferred to a distant extensive wound, providing healthy tissue for coverage and optimizing the healing potential.

Free tissue transplantation offers many advantages, primarily including early mobilization and rehabilitation. Free flaps also offer the possibility of using composite free tissue transplantation, as a single-stage procedure, even in the acute emergency setting.[24] Free flaps may include a combination of tissues that can be harvested and transferred as a single unit, including vessels, nerves, tendons, muscle, skin, and bone. These flaps can be tailored specifically to fit a particular wound defect, with associated improved cosmesis. In addition, free muscle flaps can provide potential restoration of specific upper extremity motor function and/or sensibility.[25] In Volkmann's contracture of the forearm, flexion of the fingers is lost due to the ischemic injury associated with a local traumatic event. In this instance, a gracilis muscle may be harvested with its motor nerve and transferred as an innervated free muscle flap to restore finger flexion. Similarly, an innervated latissimus dorsi free muscle

flap may be used to restore elbow flexion in individuals lacking elbow function secondary to traumatic injury or congenital anomaly. A cutaneous sensory nerve also may be preserved with a harvested free musculocutaneous flap and used to create a neurosensory flap, potentially restoring sensibility to a particular area. In free tissue reconstruction of the upper extremity, the ultimate feat of functional restoration is the replantation of amputated digits or the transfer of entire toes to the hand. In summary, a free flap offers contoured soft tissue coverage, provides a healthy wound environment to facilitate healing, offers functional reconstruction, and allows early mobilization and rehabilitation to optimize the potential for full recovery.

There are multiple excellent free flaps described for reconstruction of upper extremity wound defects, each individually indicated by the location and extent of the particular wound. Several of these flaps, which can be used for either local tissue transfer or as free flaps for upper extremity reconstruction, were discussed earlier in this chapter, including the radial forearm flap, lateral arm flap, parascapular and scapular flaps, and the latissimus dorsi flap. Other reconstructive options using free tissue transfer are described in the following sections.

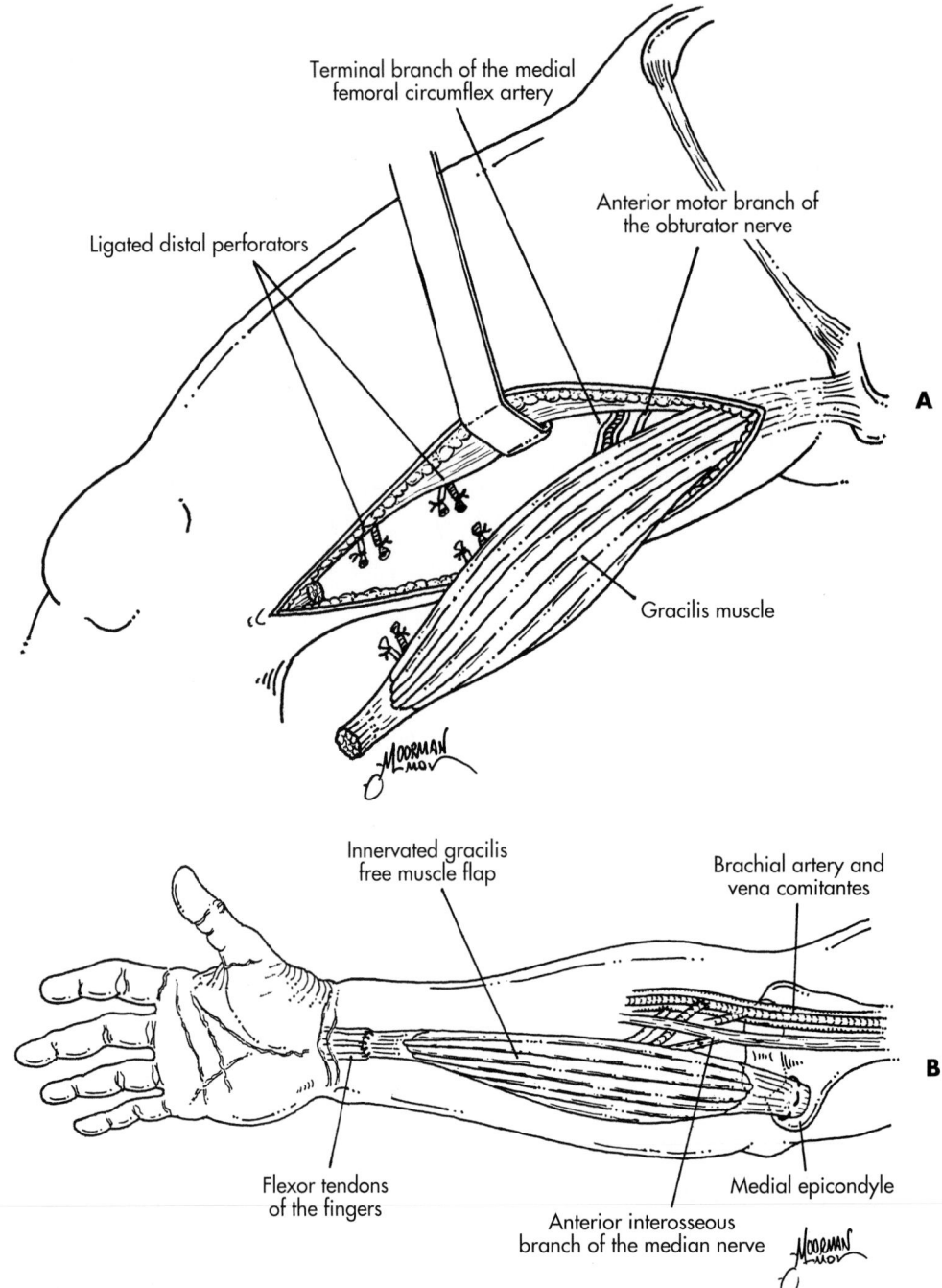

Terminal branch of the medial
femoral circumflex artery

Anterior motor branch of
the obturator nerve

Ligated distal perforators

Gracilis muscle

Innervated gracilis
free muscle flap

Brachial artery and
vena comitantes

Flexor tendons
of the fingers

Anterior interosseous
branch of the median nerve

Medial epicondyle

Fig. 21-11. A, Elevation of a gracilis muscle flap. **B,** Transfer of the gracilis as an innervated free muscle flap to restore flexor function to the upper extremity.

Serratus muscle/fascial flap. The serratus flap is harvested as a muscular or fascial flap with or without a skin island, based on the serratus vascular arcade. This flap has a reconstructive dimension of about 10 × 18 cm, and provides the reconstructive surgeon with another versatile option for repair of upper extremity defects requiring thin pliable tissue or gliding tissues for associated tendon

reconstructions. Vascularized ribs may be harvested with this flap, for additional bony reconstruction.

Temporoparietal fascial flap. The temporoparietal fascial flap consists of thin, supple fascia, harvested as a free flap, based on the superficial temporal artery and vein[5,7] (Fig. 21-10). This flap has a reconstructive dimension of 8 × 15 cm and is often used for defects of the dorsal hand, palm, and digits. The temporoparietal fascial flap conforms nicely to the contour of a wound surface but requires the addition of a skin graft for completion of the surface coverage. Appropriate dressings are required for maintenance of a moist environment to facilitate skin graft survival and healing.

Gracilis flap. The gracilis flap can be harvested as a muscle or musculocutaneous flap and transplanted to the upper extremity as a free tissue transfer. This flap is based on the terminal branch of the medial femoral circumflex artery and concomitant veins[14] and can be used to cover defects up to 6 × 25 cm. The gracilis muscle also can be harvested with a motor branch of the obturator nerve and used as an innervated free muscle flap to restore flexor function to the upper extremity[16] (Fig. 21-11).

Fibular flap. The fibular flap involves the harvest of bone, with or without a skin paddle and/or muscle, for reconstruction of segmental defects of the shoulder, humerus, radius, ulna, or wrist, and associated soft tissue loss. This flap is based on the peroneal artery and veins and can include a segment of fibula up to 26 cm.[34] The proximal and distal 6 cm of the fibula are preserved to maintain stability of the extremity. A skin island with a reconstructive dimension of 8 × 15 cm may be included, based on septal perforators from the peroneal vascular pedicle. The donor site may or may not require a skin graft for closure, depending on the size of the skin paddle harvested.

Postoperative management of free flaps

Following free tissue transfer, the free flap is protected with sterile dressings and a supportive splint. When the wound is dressed and the splint is molded, great care is taken to avoid any pressure on the vascular pedicle. A window in the dressing is created over the reconstruction to allow meticulous postoperative clinical observation. We prefer to monitor free flaps with the aid of a laser Doppler.[17] A laser Doppler probe is secured to the flap surface with either suture or a double-sided adhesive. The laser Doppler projects a numerical value from a Doppler signal, representing the vascular flow within the flap. An elevated, stable value corresponds to a viable, stable free flap. Dropping numerical values may suggest vascular compromise and impending failure of the free flap, unless addressed expeditiously in the operating room. The most reliable method of accurate free flap monitoring remains meticulous clinical observation.

Most patients are treated with Dextran 40 postoperatively for 4 days, followed by the initiation of aspirin, each for their antiplatelet effects. The laser Doppler is typically removed on postoperative day 4. Without complication, our patients are typically discharged the next day, postoperative day 5. At the time of discharge, splint immobilization of the upper extremity is maintained for continued support and protection and patients are instructed to continue strict upper extremity elevation. Operative drains are removed from the reconstruction and donor sites when the drain output subsides to a minimum, typically under 30 ml for a 24-hour period. Sutures and staples are left intact for 2 weeks and then removed in the clinic. Depending on the underlying injuries to vital structures, such as tendons or bone, early rehabilitation, including occupational therapy and social reintegration, can now be initiated.

CONCLUSION

Reconstructive surgery of the upper extremity has continued to make progressive and significant clinical advances. These impressive advances have been facilitated by the continual addition and use of new flaps and the increasing use of functional free tissue transfer, with improved microsurgical techniques, postoperative management, and intensive rehabilitation. We have successfully incorporated an algorithmic approach to reconstruction of the upper extremity. We have established this reconstructive ladder for the evaluation and treatment of upper extremity wounds and defects, directing the surgeon to the indicated reconstructive surgical options, based on the extent and severity of the wounds, the functional needs of the patient, and the availability of required tissue elements. The reconstructive options, surgical techniques, and postoperative pearls, illustrated and described in this chapter, are used daily in our practice and offered as excellent reconstructive management strategies to facilitate localized healing and optimize each individual patient's functional rehabilitation and overall recovery.

REFERENCES

1. Atasoy E: Reversed cross-finger subcutaneous flap, *J Hand Surg* 7:481, 1982.
2. Atasoy E, et al: Reconstruction of the amputated finger tip with a triangular volar flap: a new surgical procedure, *J Bone Joint Surg* 52A:921, 1970.
3. Bartlett SP, May JW Jr, Yaremchuk MJ: The latissimus dorsi muscle: a fresh cadaver study of the primary neurovascular pedicle, *Plast Reconstr Surg* 67:631, 1981.
4. Barwick WJ, Goodkind DJ, Serafin D: The free scapular flap, *Plast Reconstr Surg* 69:779, 1982.
5. Brent B, et al: Experiences with the temporoparietal fascial free flap, *Plast Reconstr Surg* 76:177, 1985.
6. Buncke CM, Schultz WB: Experimental digital amputation and replantation, *Plast Reconstr Surg* 36:62, 1965.
7. Chowdary RP, Chernofsky MA, Okunski WJ: Free temporoparietal flap in burn reconstruction, *Ann Plast Surg* 25:169, 1990.
8. Cormack GC, Duncan MJ, Lamberty BG: The blood supply of the bone component of the compound osteo-cutaneous radial artery forearm flap: an anatomical study, *Br J Plast Surg* 39:173, 1986.
9. Cronin TD: The cross-finger flap: a new method of repair, *Am Surg* 17:419, 1951.
10. Fisher JC: Skin grafting. In Georgiade GS, Reifkohl R, Levin LS, editors: *Plastic maxillofacial and reconstructive surgery*, ed 3, Baltimore, 1997, Williams & Wilkins.
11. Fisher J, Gingrass MK: Basic principles of skin flaps. In Georgiade GS, Reifkohl R, Levin LS, editors: *Plastic maxillofacial and reconstructive surgery*, ed 3, Baltimore, 1997, Williams & Wilkins.
12. Geissendorffer H: Beitrag zur Fingerkuppenplastik (Thoughts on fingertip plasty—first description of a lateral V-Y flap), *Zbl Chir* 70:1107, 1943.

13. Germann G, Sherman R, Levin LS: *Decision-making in reconstructive surgery: upper extremity,* New York, 2000, Springer.

14. Giordano PA, Abbes M, Pequignot JP: Gracilis blood supply: anatomical and clinical re-evaluation, *Br J Plast Surg* 43:266, 1990.

15. Godina M: Early microsurgical reconstruction of complex trauma of the extremities, *Plast Reconstr Surg* 78:285, 1986.

16. Hari K: Microvascular free flaps for skin coverage: indications and selection of donor sites, *Clin Plast Surg* 10:37, 1983.

17. Jacobson JH: Microsurgery and anastomosis of small vessels, *Surg Forum* 243, 1960.

18. Katsaos JM, et al: The lateral upper arm flap: anatomy and clinical applications, *Ann Plast Surg* 12:489, 1984.

19. Klasen HJ: *History of free skin grafting,* Heidelberg, 1981, Springer-Verlag.

20. Kleinert HE, Kasden M, Romero JL: Small blood vessel anastomosis for salvage of severely injured upper extremity, *J Bone Joint Surg* 45A:788, 1963.

21. Kojima T, et al: Reverse vascular pedicle digital island flap, *Br J Plast Surg* 43:290, 1990.

22. Kutler W: A new method for fingertip amputation, *JAMA* 133:29, 1947.

23. Levin LS: The reconstructive ladder: an orthoplastic approach, *Orthoped Clin North Am* 24:393, 1993.

24. Lister G, Shecker L: Emergency free flaps to the upper extremities, *J Hand Surg* 13A:22, 1988.

25. Manktelow RT, McKee NH: Free muscle transplantation to provide active finger motion, *J Hand Surg* 3:416, 1978.

26. McGregor IA, Jackson IT: The groin flap, *Br J Plast Surg* 25:3, 1972.

27. Moberg E: Aspects of sensation in reconstruction of the upper limb, *J Bone Joint Surg* 46A:17, 1964.

28. Padget EC: Skin grafting in severe burns, *Am J Surg* 43:626, 1939.

29. Serafin D, Buncke HJ: *Microvascular composite tissue transplantation,* St Louis, 1979, Mosby.

30. Solitar D, Tanner NS: The radial forearm flap in the management of soft tissue injuries of the hand, *Br J Plast Surg* 37:19, 1984.

31. Taylor GI, Palmer JH: The vascular territories (angiosomes) of the body: experimental study and clinical applications, *Br J Plast Surg* 40:113, 1987.

32. Tranquilli-Leali LE: Ricostruzione dellapice delle falangi ungeali mediante autoplastica volare peduncolata per scorrimento (Reconstruction of the fingertip by a medial volar flap), *Infort Traum Lavoro* 1:186, 1935.

33. Urbanic JR, et al: The vascularized cutaneous scapular flap, *Plast Reconstr Surg* 69:772, 1982.

34. Wei FC, et al: Fibular osteoseptocutaneous flap: anatomical study and clinical applications, *Plast Reconstr Surg* 78:191, 1986.

Part IV

INFECTIONS

Chapter 22

COMMON INFECTIONS IN THE HAND

Ross Nathan
John S. Taras

Although infections have declined in incidence since the advent of antibiotics, they remain among the most disabling of any condition affecting the hand.[3,4] Infection in this part of the body holds great potential for damage, which is why patients often require prolonged hospitalization and rehabilitation. In most cases, the infection begins with a minor penetrating trauma or small open wound.* Its character and progression are determined by its specific location within the specialized tissues of this extremity,[25] so treatment can vary to a considerable degree. The key to minimizing the incidence and severity of hand infections is the prompt administration of appropriate treatment for even the most minor injuries.

GENERAL CONSIDERATIONS

Injuries that break the skin barrier nearly always create a wound contaminated by bacteria. Whether the microorganisms multiply and establish an infection, however, is determined by the virulence of the microorganisms and the host's immune response.[32] Poor arterial blood supply, venous congestion,[36] the presence of necrotic or damaged tissue,[12,32] and the presence of foreign bodies are all local wound factors that increase the likelihood of infection. The patient's resistance can be compromised by certain systemic conditions, the most common of which is diabetes mellitus.[12,29,34] Others include acquired immunodeficiency syndrome,[13] Raynaud's disease, agranulocytosis and related disorders, severe chronic illness, immunosuppressive therapy, and chronic drug abuse.

*References 3, 4, 22, 23, 32, 36.

Although almost any type of microorganism can cause a hand infection, most cases involve *Staphylococcus aureus* (50% to 80%)[26] and ß-hemolytic streptococci (15%).[16,22] The next most common pathogens are *Aerobacter aerogenes* (10%), *Enterococcus* (10%), and *Escherichia coli* (5%).[22] Infections secondary to penetrating trauma usually involve a single species, but those associated with bites and intravenous drug use are polymicrobic in over 50% of cases.[16,24,43]

ANATOMY

A detailed understanding of the hand's specialized anatomy is crucial to determining the location and character of the infection, predicting its likely path, and optimizing surgical drainage without injuring vital structures or extending the infection to uninvolved tissues.[19] The skin, subcutaneous tissue, tendon sheaths, and joint spaces are some of the specialized structures in the hand, and their anatomy is covered elsewhere in this text. The fascial spaces and lymphatics are other important components of the hand's anatomy and merit a brief review here.

The hand contains five fascial spaces in which pus can accumulate: (1) dorsal subcutaneous, (2) dorsal subaponeurotic, (3) hypothenar, (4) thenar, and (5) midpalmar.[19] Other spaces that provide an optimal environment for the rapid growth of microorganisms are the flexor tendon sheaths and the joint spaces, which contain synovial fluid and are lined with a specialized layer of synovial tissue. Infections within the synovial spaces are among the most devastating of all hand disorders.

The lymphatics of the hand can be classified into two types according to their origin and location. The superficial lymphatics arise in the skin and course through the subcutaneous tissue, and the deep lymphatics arise in deeper tissue and follow the blood vessels.[29] The lymph vessels in the fingers follow the digital arteries and are most abundant on the volar surface. From this point, the channels flow dorsally in the interdigital spaces along the medial and lateral borders of the hand[42] and then travel proximally up the dorsal surface.[29] (This anatomy explains why a primary infection in the palmar surface can initially present with dorsal swelling.[19,20,29,38])

DIAGNOSIS

The routine evaluation of a patient with a suspected hand infection consists of a general medical history,[34] physical examination, and standard radiographs. Laboratory and microbiologic studies, including a culture of a specimen from the involved site, may aid the diagnosis of more serious infections and direct antimicrobial therapy.

The history usually discloses a trivial injury that received inappropriate care. If so, it is important to determine the environment in which the injury occurred because it may help identify the type of organism responsible for the infection. Significant medical conditions should be noted, as should all medications being taken—especially antibiotics. Open wounds over the metacarpophalangeal (MP) or proximal interphalangeal (PIP) joints of the dominant hand in a young male must be considered a bite wound until proved otherwise.

Erythema, heat, and swelling are nonspecific signs of inflammation that are often present in an established infection. Important clues about the location of the infection can be obtained by determining the site of maximum tenderness in relation to the compartments of the hand. Radiographs should be examined for foreign bodies, osteomyelitis, and fractures. Air density in the soft tissues may indicate gas gangrene, a rapidly progressive and destructive infection caused by clostridial or other anaerobic gas-producing microorganisms.

Drainage from wounds should be evaluated with a Gram stain and culture before antibiotics are prescribed. Initial cultures always should test for both aerobic and anaerobic microorganisms. Special culture media may be required when certain pathogens such as fungi, atypical mycobacteria, and viruses are suspected.[16]

Although the concept of quantitative bacteriology dates back to World War I, a definitive technique for wound assessment was developed only in recent years.[31] It has been determined that approximately 10^5 bacteria per gram of tissue are required to sustain a clinical infection. However, tissue is rendered more susceptible to bacterial invasion by crushing, shredding, chemical injury, and the presence of penetrating foreign bodies.[26] Patients with more severe infections should be evaluated with a complete blood count and a blood glucose test to screen for diabetes.[34]

CLASSIFICATION

There are four possible types of infection in the hand, depending on the kind of tissue involved: (1) superficial spreading (cellulitis and lymphangitis), (2) subcutaneous abscess, (3) synovial sheath, and (4) fascial space. Patients usually have one type of infection or another, but in rare cases, some combination may exist.[4,19,20] It is vitally important to distinguish an acute spreading infection involving the skin, subcutaneous tissue, or lymphatics from a localized abscess or closed-space infection because the respective approaches to the treatment of these two entities are in direct opposition.[23,32]

PRINCIPLES OF MANAGEMENT

Prophylaxis is the most important factor in the management of hand infections. Few significant infections develop after a severe open injury because prompt and appropriate wound care is usually administered. Most cases involve an apparently trivial injury that was either neglected or treated inadequately.

Primary care of open wounds of the hand begins with gentle irrigation to remove debris and foreign bodies, débridement of devitalized tissue, and the application of a dressing to protect against secondary contamination.[23] After infection has established itself in a hand wound, the anatomic boundaries of the infected area should then be defined because the type of infection present determines treatment. Treatment may include supportive measures, antimicrobial therapy, wound care, surgical drainage, and/or physical therapy to regain motion and prevent contractures.[25,28,44]

When the infection is accompanied by acute inflammation, it is helpful to immobilize the affected areas in a protected position to prevent the infection from spreading through the tissue planes, decrease pain and edema, and prevent joint contractures. A local finger splint that supports the interphalangeal (IP) joints in extension can be used when the infection is localized to a single digit. If the infection involves the palm, MP joint region, or larger areas of the hand, a whole-hand splint is worn to protect against flexion contractures of the MP joint and contractures of the thumb-index web space. Moist heat can increase local circulation and antibiotic delivery and is especially useful in the treatment of superficial spreading infections.

After the acute inflammation has subsided, the patient should begin active and passive range-of-motion (ROM) exercises to tolerance. Early ROM along with elevation and compression wraps can help control edema, which is critical to controlling pain and preventing fibrosis and contracture. Retrograde massage is to be avoided in the presence of an active infection because it may cause the infection to spread proximally.

The use of antibiotics depends on the clinical situation. Minor infections often resolve with supportive measures alone. Oral antibiotics are effective in the management of superficial infections, and intravenous antibiotics play a critical role in the treatment of severe infections. The choice of drug is based on the culture results, but initial therapy is directed against the most likely pathogens. A first-generation cephalosporin is generally prescribed because it is effective against most staphylococci and streptococci. Patients who are immunocompromised or have devitalized wounds are more prone to severe infections and should receive broader antibiotic coverage, preferably by the intravenous route. The detailed aspects of antimicrobial therapy are beyond the scope of this discussion, and the interested reader is referred to specialized texts on the subject.[12,29,34,35]

Tetanus prophylaxis is essential in all wounds with soil, animal, oral, or fecal contamination. The patient with a tetanus-prone wound who has never been immunized should be administered 0.5 ml of absorbed tetanus toxoid along with 250 to 500 units of tetanus immune globulin intramuscularly at different injection sites with different syringes. Penicillin also may be considered.[22]

Fascial space, tendon sheath, and joint space infections require emergent surgical drainage. These potentially devastating conditions are usually best treated in the operating room under general anesthesia and tourniquet control. Incisions are made to provide adequate drainage, with care taken to avoid extending the infection to adjacent uninfected spaces. Standard sterile technique and precautions are required to prevent secondary contamination by more virulent microorganisms.[19]

Unlike closed-space infections, superficial spreading infections, cellulitis, and lymphangitis are not treated surgically unless a necrotic abscess or necrotic tissue develops. Instead, they are managed with an initial period of rest, immobilization, and elevation. Moist warm heat can be applied to the area to increase the local blood supply and antibiotic delivery.

TYPES OF INFECTIONS
Superficial spreading infections

Cellulitis. Cellulitis is a superficial infection of the skin and subcutaneous layer and is characterized by the absence of pus or localized abscess (Fig. 22-1). An area of the dorsum of the finger or hand is usually involved, and the organism responsible is usually streptococcal. Typically, there is a history of a scratch, minor cut, or puncture. The affected area is warm, erythematous, and tender. Treatment involves supportive measures, including elevation, splinting, warm compresses, and administration of antibiotics with activity against *Streptococcus.* If the patient has systemic symptoms or a compromised immune system, hospitalization and intravenous antibiotics may be appropriate. After the acute inflammation is controlled, ROM exercises should be initiated to further assist in edema control and prevent joint stiffness.

Lymphangitis. Lymphangitis is much less common than cellulitis but is one of the most serious and rapidly

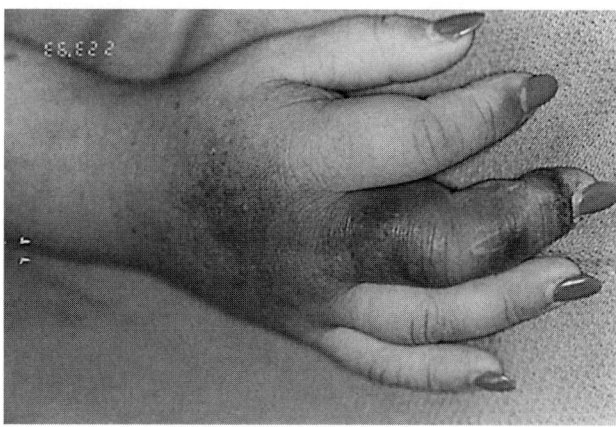

Fig. 22-1. Cellulitis. Swelling and redness are present over the dorsum of the middle finger. Note the extension over the back of the hand.

progressing types of hand infection. Lymphangitis often develops from a trivial injury that has been neglected. It also can result from direct inoculation of an extremely virulent organism—usually *Streptococcus.* The organism spreads quickly through the lymphatics and may produce a generalized infection within a few hours.[32] Red streaking develops from the site of inoculation up the hand and forearm, along the pathways of the lymphatic channels. If untreated, an abscess may form about the elbow or in the axilla near the lymph nodes. Prompt recognition and hospitalization are essential. Treatment includes parenteral antibiotics with activity against *Streptococcus,* immobilization, elevation, and warm moist compresses. Unlike closed-space infections, surgical drainage is reserved for cases in which there is definite evidence of localized pus and abscess formation or tissue necrosis.[23]

Subcutaneous abscesses

Paronychias. Bacterial infection of the nail fold and/or nail plate is one of the most common infections in the hand. It begins as a cellulitis of the skin surrounding the nail plate (the eponychium and paronychium) and progresses to pus formation. Acute pyogenic paronychias usually are caused by *S. aureus.* In late cases, the abscess may extend to all three borders of the nail fold (run-around abscess) or spread beneath the nail plate (Fig. 22-2).[22] The treatment of early paronychias consists of warm soaks and antibiotics. However, surgical drainage is necessary after an abscess has formed. If pus has accumulated beneath the nail, partial or complete nail plate removal may be necessary to achieve adequate drainage.

Chronic paronychias differ from the acute forms in that the offending organisms usually include *Candida albicans* along with the pyogenic bacteria (Fig. 22-3). Individuals with occupational exposure to moisture appear to be more

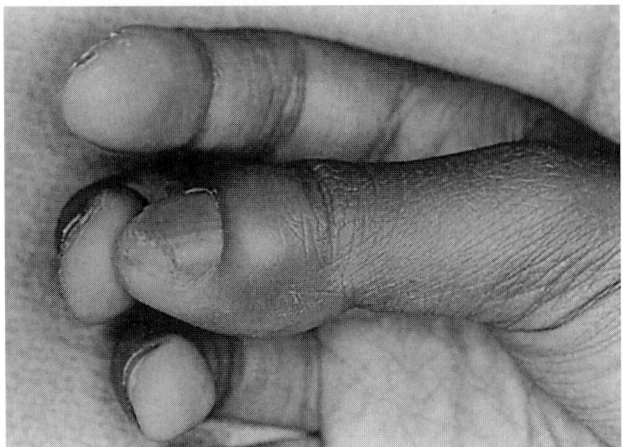

Fig. 22-2. This acute paronychia involving the proximal nail fold will require incision and drainage.

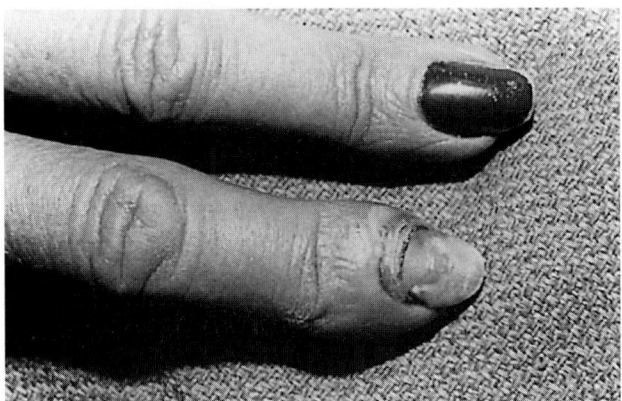

Fig. 22-3. Chronic paronychia caused by a combination of bacterial and fungal microorganisms.

prone to the chronic variety.[7] The treatment of this condition, which has been less successful than that for acute paronychias, involves partial or complete nail plate removal. Often, long periods of topical antimicrobial agents are needed. Keyser and Eaton[21] have recommended eponychial marsupialization, which requires removing an elliptical segment of skin in the proximal nail fold and permitting adequate drainage from the infected proximal nailbed.

Felons. The distal pulp of the finger has specialized fibrous septa that extend from the skin to the bone, forming many tiny separate compartments. Because of the fixed septa, infection or swelling of the pulp produces a marked increase in pressure with severe throbbing and pain. A felon is a deep infection of the pad of the finger that involves these compartments. There is usually a history of a puncture wound or other open injury. Pus is formed in a closed space under pressure, causing intense pain, throbbing, marked tenderness, redness, and tense swelling over the fingertip pad. Treatment consists of surgical drainage. The incision

may be made directly over the point of the abscess or through its midlateral aspect. After drainage, the wound may be kept open with a loose pack that can be removed for finger soaks.[7,26,35]

Subepidermal abscesses. Subcutaneous abscesses are localized collections of pus at the subcuticular level. They can occur in the palm or on the volar pads of the fingers between the flexor creases (Fig. 22-4). Like felons, they are caused by *S. aureus.* The abscess will usually point toward the skin, and it resolves rapidly with simple incision and drainage. If left untreated, it may track deep and invade the flexor sheath or deep compartment of the palm.[34]

Flexor sheath infections

Infections within the flexor sheath, or purulent flexor tenosynovitis, are among the most destructive and devastating of all infections in the hand. They usually develop after a puncture wound over the flexor crease at the level of the IP or MP joint, where the skin is separated from the flexor sheath by only a thin layer of subcutaneous tissue (Fig. 22-5, *A*). This condition also can result from direct extension of a pulp-space infection. Hematogenous spread has occurred in rare cases. *Staphylococcus* or *Streptococcus* is usually responsible, but other organisms such as mycobacteria and *Neisseria gonorrhoeae* also can be causative agents.

The flexor tendon sheath is a closed space rich in synovial fluid and provides an excellent environment for bacterial growth. After inoculation, the infection spreads rapidly within the confines of the sheath. Even if this type of infection is identified and treated early, it may produce permanent adhesions and scarring and severely limit flexor tendon gliding and motion.[2] Sufficient pressure may build to produce tendon necrosis, destruction of the flexor sheath, and extension of pus into the subcutaneous space.

Flexor tenosynovitis can be recognized by the four cardinal signs of Kanavel[20]: (1) flexed posture of the digit, (2) uniform swelling of the digit, (3) tenderness over the length of the involved tendon sheath, and (4) severe pain on attempted hyperextension of the digit (Fig. 22-6).

Infection of the flexor sheath represents a true hand surgery emergency. Prompt recognition is crucial to avoiding rapid progression of the infection and destruction of the flexor tendon and sheath. For the most part, treatment involves emergent surgical decompression and drainage with irrigation catheters within the flexor sheath (Fig. 22-5, *B*). Patients are hospitalized, and parenteral antibiotics are administered.

In rare cases when the symptoms and infection are recognized early (i.e., within 24 hours), a brief trial of parenteral antibiotics, immobilization, and elevation may be attempted, and resolution might be achieved without surgery. However, if the signs of infection do not resolve rapidly, surgical treatment is required.[22,34]

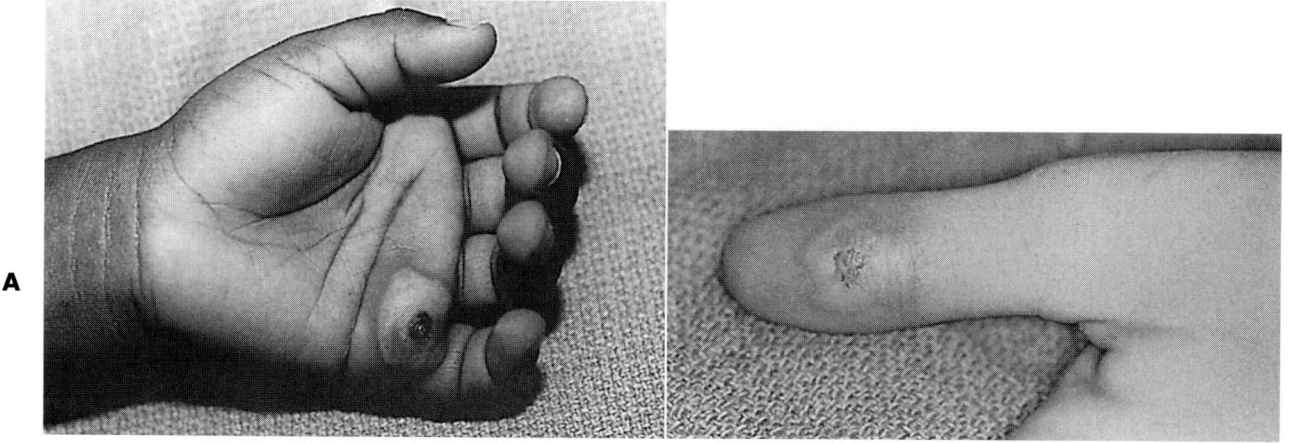

Fig. 22-4. Subepidermal abscess of the distal palm (**A**) and volar pad of the thumb (**B**).

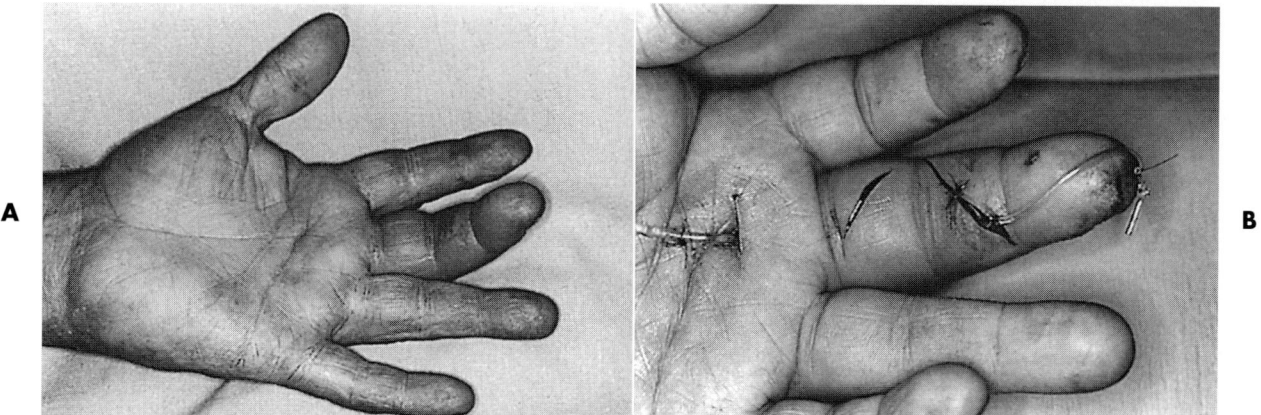

Fig. 22-5. Flexor sheath infection. **A,** The hand is shown 24 hours after a puncture wound over the proximal interphalangeal crease in the middle finger. **B,** Treatment involved open irrigation and drainage of the flexor sheath in the finger and palm.

Fascial-space infections

As mentioned earlier, there are five fascial spaces in which pus can accumulate: (1) the dorsal subcutaneous, (2) dorsal subaponeurotic, (3) hypothenar, (4) thenar, and (5) midpalmar. Accurate diagnosis and treatment relies on knowing the boundaries of these spaces and the most common routes of extension of each. Fascial space infections must be differentiated from the two other serious purulent hand infections—those of the flexor sheath and lymphangitis.

Treatment consists of surgical drainage, which is best done in the operating room under general anesthesia and tourniquet control. Incisions are made to provide adequate drainage, with care taken to avoid extending the infection to adjacent uninfected spaces. Standard sterile technique and precautions are used to prevent secondary contamination by more virulent microorganisms.[5,10,19]

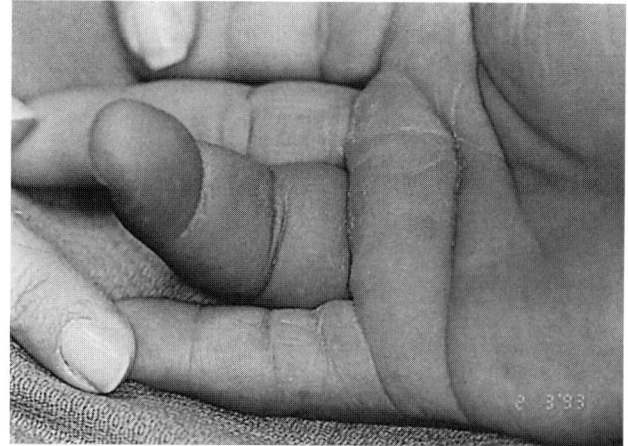

Fig. 22-6. The cardinal signs of Kanavel—flexed posture of the digit, uniform swelling, tenderness over the flexor sheath, and pain on hyperextension—indicate the presence of a purulent flexor sheath infection.

COMMON SOURCES OF INFECTION
Human bites

Depending on the status of an individual's oral hygiene, human saliva may contain as many as 42 species of bacteria and up to 10^8 organisms per milliliter.[9,38,40] As such, the human mouth has been compared with a cesspool.[38] The bacteria commonly isolated from human bite wounds include streptococci, staphylococci and other micrococci, spirochetes, *Clostridium, Bacteroides, Fusobacterium, Neisseria,* and other gram-negative species. More rarely, this route has transmitted *Actinomyces, Treponema pallidum,* hepatitis B virus, and *M. tuberculosis.*[8,9,26,30] Hand wounds contaminated by human saliva are caused by biting, fist-to-mouth contact, nail biting, and accidental penetration by a toothpick or dental instrument.[38] Wounds that are caused by fist-to-mouth contact have the highest incidence of complications, and they usually occur over the dorsal aspect of the third, fourth, or fifth metacarpal joint. This area is especially susceptible to infection because the thin pliant skin over the knuckle provides only a thin barrier to the ligaments, synovial space, and articular cartilage over the metacarpal head.[30]

The injury usually occurs during an evening brawl when the patient is inebriated, and he or she is too embarrassed to seek treatment until several days later (Fig. 22-7, *A* and *B*). This delay calls for an aggressive approach to treatment to prevent a progressive and severe infection. The wound must be vigorously cleansed and debrided (Fig. 22-7, *C*) and the patient administered broad-spectrum antibiotics intravenously. Wound care, whirlpool therapy, and ROM exercises must be initiated early to prevent severe tissue fibrosis and contractures. The wound is left open to heal by secondary intention.

Animal bites

Dogs are responsible for 90% of animal bite wounds, with cats being a distant second (5%).[41] The incidence of infection associated with the latter, however, is nearly three times as great. This kind of injury may result in a rapidly progressing cellulitis or lymphangitis, especially if treatment is not obtained.[27] *Pasteurella* species, especially *P. canis* in dog bites and *P. multocida* subspecies in cat bites, are isolated from the wounds most often.[27,43] The laboratory should be notified in advance of the suspicion of *Pasteurella* species to optimize identification (Fig. 22-8). Treatment involves cleansing the wound and débridement of any devitalized or necrotic tissue. The wound is left open, and the patient given either combination therapy with penicillin and a first-generation cephalosporin or clindamycin and a fluoroquinolone for *P. multocida* infection.[25,27,41,43]

Intravenous drug abuse

Intravenous drug abusers commonly develop abscesses over the dorsum of the hand or forearm at the sites of

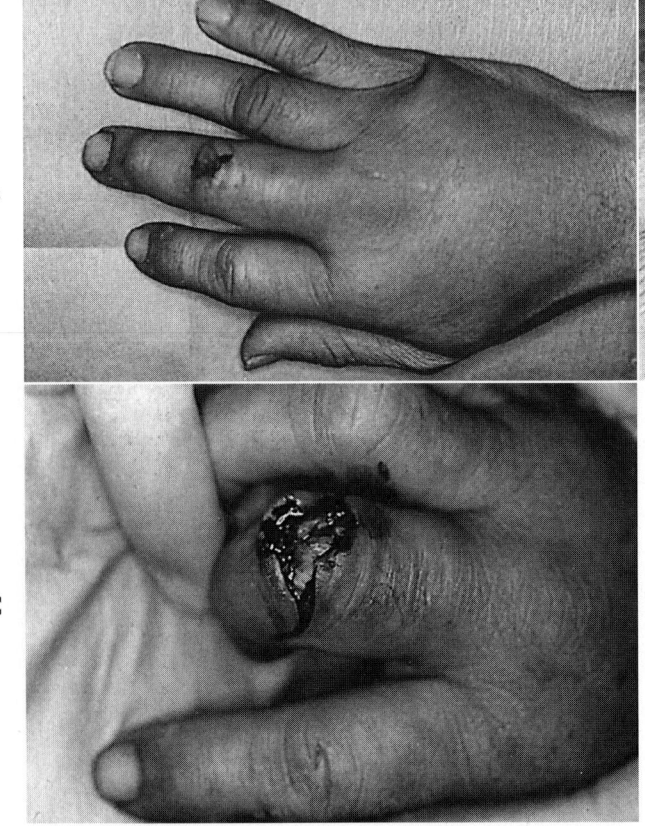
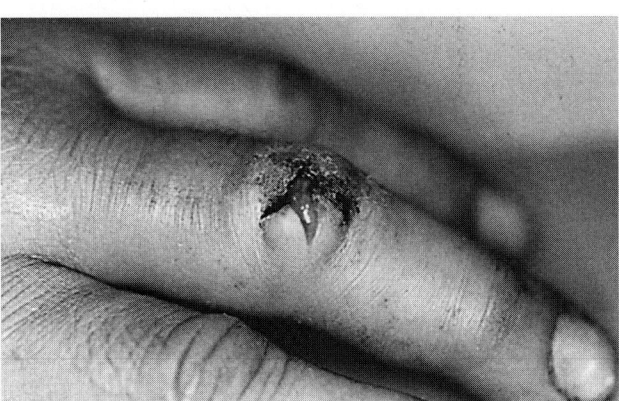

Fig. 22-7. A, Appearance of a human bite wound in a bar patron 2 days after a brawl. **B,** There is pus and necrosis of the extensor tendon and surrounding tissues. **C,** Treatment involved surgical irrigation and débridement. Note the extensive involvement of the articular cartilage of the proximal interphalangeal joint.

attempted venous access (Fig. 22-9). These infections are caused by the introduction of various pathogens and local chemical necrosis from the extravasation of injected materials. Management of the intravenous drug abuser is complicated because he or she is extremely unreliable and usually seeks treatment only when the infection has reached an advanced stage. Treatment is also more difficult because this individual is often debilitated and has an altered immune response secondary to malnutrition, chronic infection with human immunodeficiency virus[14,33] or some other pathogen, or both.

Subcutaneous abscesses are incised, drained, and allowed to close secondarily. Infections of the flexor sheath, joint space, and fascial space should be identified and surgically decompressed through appropriate incisions. Broad-spectrum antibiotics should be instituted immediately and the antimicrobial therapy modified when the culture results are obtained. Because of their poor compliance, these patients should be hospitalized until their acute infection is under control.

Certain drug abusers—desperate individuals and those in whom no injectable veins remain—may use their radial or ulnar artery as a dangerous alternative site for drug injection. In these patients, the major problem is chemical vasculitis rather than infection. Distal necrosis of the digit or hand with dry gangrene and ischemic pain are present.[39] Supportive measures are used to treat this problem and consist of antibiotics and wound care. Necrosis in the region supplied by the artery and amputation usually follow.

Mycobacteria

Mycobacterial infections in the hand may be caused by any one of several species *(M. tuberculosis, M. marinum, M. avium, M. intracellulare)* and most often present as indolent processes that affect the skin, flexor tendon sheaths, carpal canal, or extensor tendons and synovium on the dorsum of the wrist. Infections caused by *M. tuberculosis* have a clinical presentation similar to that of rheumatoid arthritis (Fig. 22-10). There is often a delay between the onset of symptoms and diagnosis, and many patients will have no history of pulmonary involvement.[1,6]

Of the atypical mycobacteria, *M. marinum* is most often responsible for hand infections.[15,17] This organism is a common contaminant of warm water environments, and exposure typically occurs when the patient suffers a skin abrasion or puncture wound while at the beach, lake, river, or pool, or when working with a fish tank. The infection presents as either a chronic skin ulceration or a localized tenosynovitis along the digital flexor sheath, carpal tunnel, or extensor tendons over the dorsum of the wrist (Fig. 22-11).[24,37] *M. marinum* must be cultured on special media at 30° to 32° C, so the laboratory must be apprised of its possible presence. Deep infections are treated by surgical synovectomy and prolonged antituberculous medication.

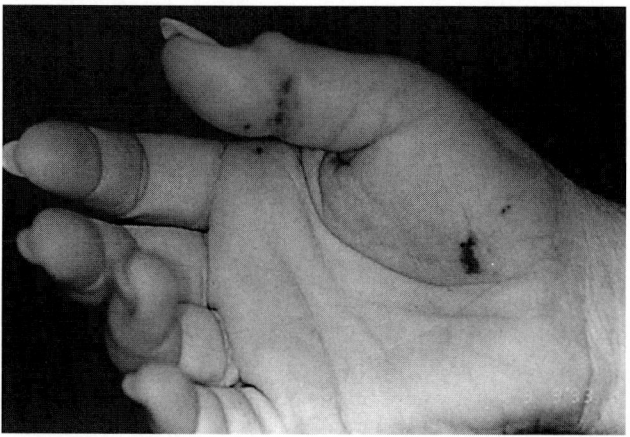

Fig. 22-8. Multiple puncture wounds from cat bites, with secondary cellulitis. *Pasteurella multocida* was cultured from the wound drainage.

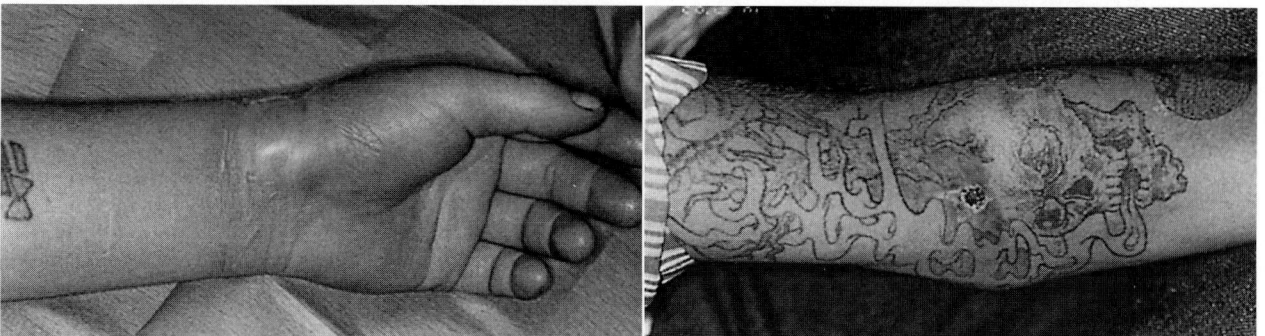

A

B

Fig. 22-9. Infection secondary to intravenous drug abuse. **A,** Subcutaneous abscess over the volar radial wrist in a young female drug addict. Note the scars indicating sites of past infection and surgical débridement. **B,** Appearance of a subcutaneous abscess in the antecubital fossa after surgical drainage. The infection had developed after intravenous injection of cocaine. Multiple tattoos may mask needle marks, or "tracks."

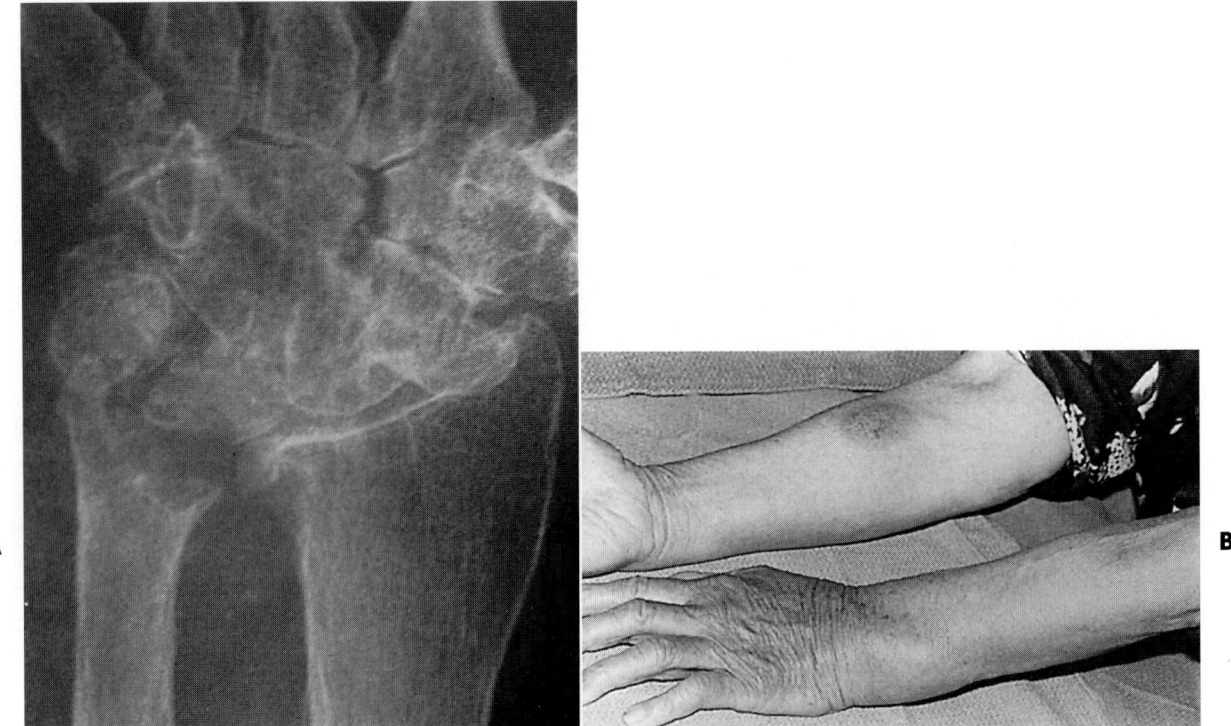

Fig. 22-10. This woman from Southeast Asia presented with isolated wrist pain that was thought to be secondary to inflammatory arthritis. **A,** Radiographs demonstrated bony destruction. **B,** The soft tissue over the wrsit was swollen, and the purified protein derivative (PPD) skin test on the opposite forearm was positive. Surgical specimens revealed acid-fast bacilli, and cultures were positive for *Mycobacterium tuberculosis.*

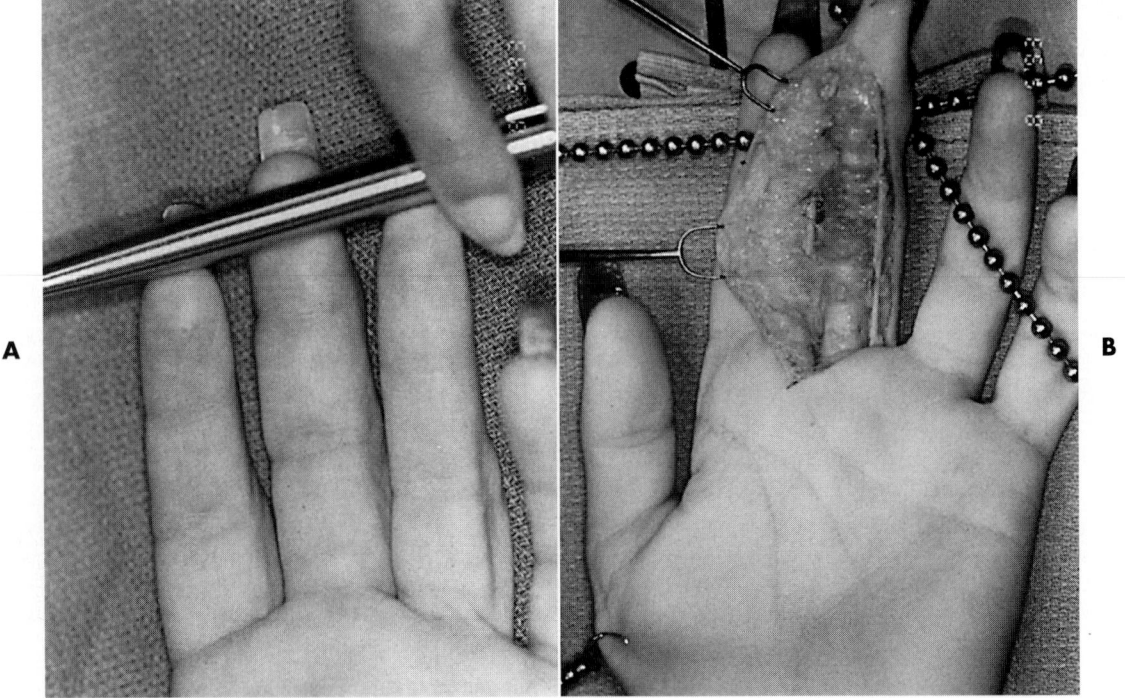

Fig. 22-11. A, Chronic *Mycobacterium marinum* infection involving the flexor sheath of the middle finger. **B,** Surgical exposure of the flexor sheath demonstrated extensive tenosynovitis.

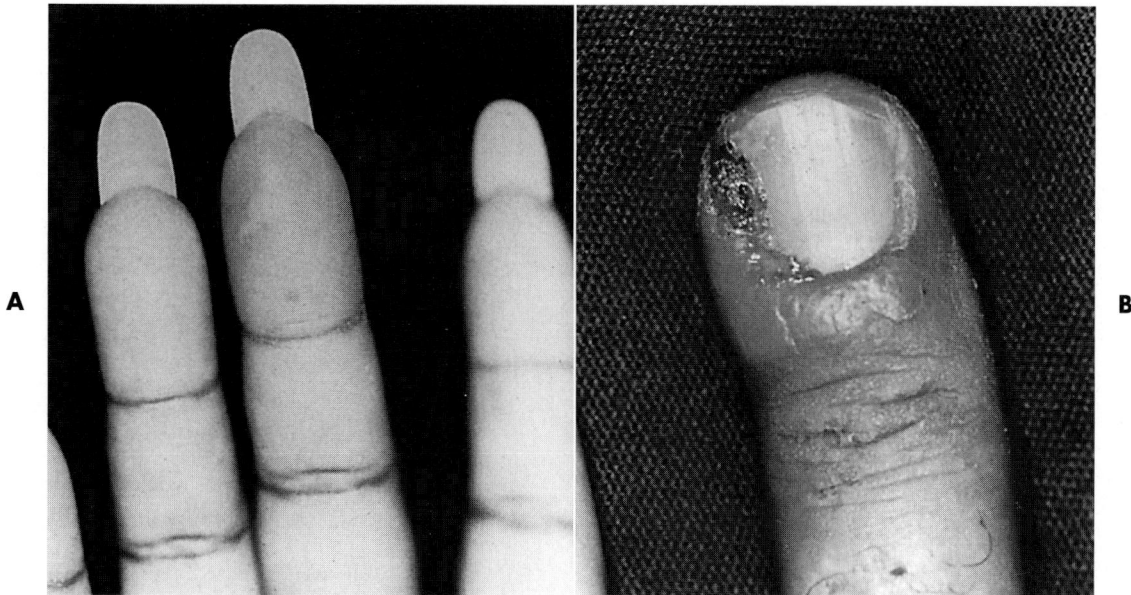

Fig. 22-12. **A,** Herpesvirus lesions in the distal pad of the middle finger in a respiratory therapist. **B,** Herpesvirus vesicles around the nailfold with a secondary bacterial infection that developed after incision and drainage.

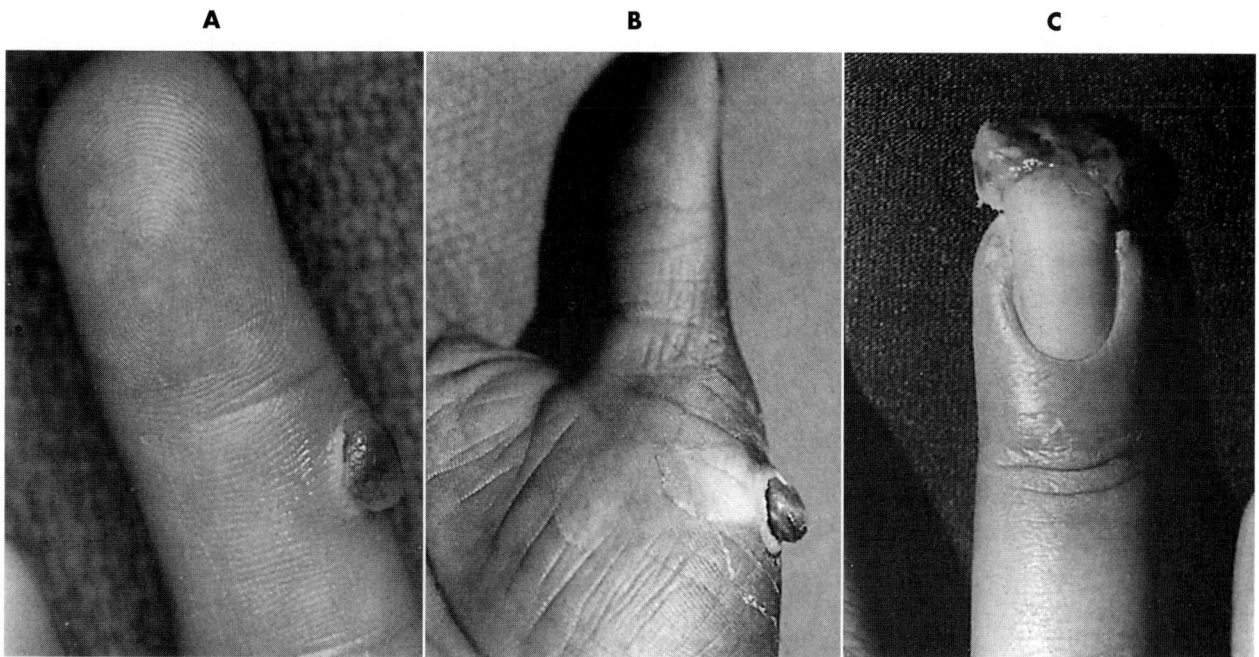

Fig. 22-13. Pyogenic granuloma. **A** and **B,** Typical appearance of the lesion. **C,** This large lesion of the distal tip of the ring finger developed after the patient sustained a puncture wound.

Viruses

Herpetic whitlow is a superficial infection that appears as one or more vesicles on or near the finger pad, and it is often seen in medical and dental personnel (Fig. 22-12, *A*). There may or may not be a history of herpes simplex infection elsewhere in the body. The diagnosis can be made on the basis of the clinical appearance and confirmed using the fluorescent antibody test. If recognized and left to run its 2- to 4-week course, this type of infection is self-limited. Incision and drainage should be avoided because it prolongs recovery and may lead to bacterial superinfection (Fig. 22-12, *B*).[7,11,18,36]

Pyogenic granuloma

A pyogenic granuloma is a growth of granulation tissue above the skin caused by a chronic low-grade infection or foreign body. Continuously moist local environments and bandages favor their development. These infections are common and appear as red friable growths that bleed readily with little provocation (Fig. 22-13). Simple curettage and cauterization with silver nitrate may be performed in the office and is usually curative. Operative excision may be necessary for larger lesions.[22,25]

SUMMARY

The first consideration of hand infections is prophylaxis. One must provide appropriate care for all open hand wounds, whether trivial or extensive. The established hand infection severity and progression is determined by host factors and the characteristics of the organism. Infections of the hand can be classified based on the type of tissue involved. Common pathogens and sources of transmission must be recognized. Infections involving the hand, if neglected, may become one of the most disabling of all conditions affecting the upper extremity. Treatment involves a combination of immobilization, antibiotics, moist heat delivery, and surgical decompression and debridement.

REFERENCES

1. Benkeddache YL, Gottesman H: Skeletal tuberculosis of the wrist and hand: a study of 27 cases, *J Hand Surg* 7:593, 1982.
2. Boles SD, Schmidt CC: Pyogenic flexor tenosynovitis, *Hand Clin* 14:567, 1998.
3. Boyes JH: *Bunnell's surgery of the hand,* ed 5, Philadelphia, 1970, JB Lippincott.
4. Bunnell S: *Surgery of the hand,* Philadelphia, 1944, JB Lippincott.
5. Burkhalter WE: Deep space infections, *Hand Clin* 5:553, 1989.
6. Bush DC, Schneider LH: Tuberculosis of the hand and wrist, *J Hand Surg* 9A:391, 1984.
7. Canales FL, Newmeyer WL, Kilgore ES: The treatment of felons and paronychia, *J Hand Surg* 5:515, 1989.
8. Coleman DA: Human bite wounds, *Hand Clin* 5:561, 1989.
9. Faciszewski T, Coleman DA: Human bite wounds, *Hand Clin* 5:561, 1989.
10. Flynn JE: Clinical and anatomical investigations of deep fascial space infections of the hand, *Am J Surg* 55:467, 1942.
11. Gill JJ, Arlette J, Buchan K: Herpes simplex virus infection of the hand, *Am J Med* 84:89, 1988.
12. Glass KD: Factors related to the resolution of treated hand infections, *J Hand Surg* 7:388, 1982.
13. Glickel SZ: Hand infections in patients with acquired immunodeficiency syndrome, *J Hand Surg* 13A:770, 1988.
14. Gonzalez MH, et al: Upper extremity infections in patients with the human immunodeficiency virus, *J Hand Surg* 23A:348, 1988.
15. Gunther SS, Levy CS: Mycobacterial infections, *Hand Clin* 5:591, 1989.
16. Hausman MR, Lisser SP: Hand infections, *Orthop Clin* 23:171, 1992.
17. Hurst LC, et al: *Mycobacterium marinum* infections of the hand, *J Hand Surg* 12A:428, 1987.
18. Hurst LC et al: Herpetic whitlow with bacterial abscess, *J Hand Surg* 16A:311, 1991.
19. Kanavel AB: An anatomical, experimental, and clinical study of acute phlegmons of the hand, *Surg Gynecol Obstet* 1:221, 1905.
20. Kanavel AB: *Infections of the hand—a guide to the surgical treatment of acute and chronic suppurative process in the fingers, hand, and forearm,* Philadelphia, 1912, Lea & Febiger.
21. Keyser J, Eaton RG: Surgical cure of chronic paronychia by eponychial marsupialization, *Plast Reconstr Surg* 58:66, 1976.
22. Kilgore ES: Hand infections, *J Hand Surg* 8A:723, 1983.
23. Koch SL: Acute rapidly spreading infections following trivial injuries of the hand, *Surg Gynecol Obstet* 69:277, 1934.
24. Leddy JP: Infections of the upper extremity, *J Hand Surg* 11A:294, 1986.
25. Linscheid RL, Dobyns JH: Common and uncommon infections of the hand, *Orthop Clin* 6:1063, 1975.
26. Linscheid RL, Dobyns JH: Bone and soft tissue infections of the hand and wrist. In Evarts CM, editor: *Surgery of the musculoskeletal system,* ed 2, New York, 1990, Churchill Livingstone.
27. Lucas GL, Bartlett DH: Pasteurella multocida infection in the hand, *Plast Reconstr Surg* 67:49, 1981.
28. Mancini LH, Fort LK: Rehabilitation of the infected hand, *Hand Clin* 5:635, 1989.
29. Mann RJ: *Infections of the hand,* Philadelphia, 1988, Lea & Febiger.
30. Mann RJ, Hoffeld TA, Farmer CB: Human bites of the hand: twenty years' experience, *J Hand Surg* 2:97, 1977.
31. Marshall KA, et al: Quantitative microbiology: its application to hand injuries, *Am J Surg* 131:730, 1976.
32. Mason ML: Infections of the hand, *Surg Clin North Am* 455, 1942.
33. McAuliffe JA, Seltzer DG, Hornicek FJ: Upper-extremity infections in patients seropositive for human immunodeficiency virus, *J Hand Surg* 22A:1084,1997.
34. McGrath MH: Infections of the hand. In McCarthy JG, editor: *Plastic surgery,* Philadelphia, 1990, WB Saunders.
35. Milford L: Infections of the hand. In Crenshaw AH, editor: *Campbell's operative orthopedics,* ed 7, St Louis, 1987, Mosby.
36. Newmeyer WL: *Primary care of hand injuries,* Philadelphia, 1979, Lea & Febiger.
37. Phillips, SA, et al: *Mycobacterium marinum* infections of the finger, *J Hand Surg* 20B:801, 1995.
38. Rayan GM, Flournoy DJ: Hand infections, *Contemp Orthop* 20:41, 1990.
39. Reyes FA: Infections secondary to intravenous drug abuse, *Hand Clin* 5:629, 1989.
40. Shields C, et al: Hand infections secondary to human bites, *J Trauma* 15:235, 1975.
41. Snyder CC: Animal bite wounds, *Hand Clin* 5:571, 1989.
42. Spinner M: *Kaplan's functional and surgical anatomy of the hand,* ed 3, Philadelphia, 1984, JB Lippincott.
43. Talan DA: Emergency medicine animal bite infection study group, *N Engl J Med* 340:85, 1999.
44. Tsai E, Failla JM: Hand infections in the trauma patient, *Hand Clin* 15:373,1999

Part V

FRACTURES AND JOINT INJURIES TO THE HAND

Chapter 23

FRACTURES: GENERAL PRINCIPLES OF SURGICAL MANAGEMENT

Paul N. Krop

"It is extremely important that the surgeon caring for fractures should understand the principles and something of the practical working of massage and mobilization. . . . The objectives in administering relaxed or passive movement may be summarized as follows:

1. Joints are kept supple.
2. The formation of pathological bands and adhesions is prevented.
3. Repair of all normal structures, even of bone, is hastened.
4. The elasticity of the muscles is maintained.
5. The circulation of the venous blood and of the lymph is assisted materially, and hence the removal of waste products by extravasation and of edema is hastened.
6. The restoration of any disorganization of the motor system is probably assisted very materially—the main fact is effecting repair of injured structures.
7. The joint sense is reeducated, or its loss is prevented, as the case may be, and thus the main link in the reflex of coordinated movement is restored or maintained.
8. The way is paved for instituting active movement."

Charles Locke Scudder
The Treatment of Fractures, 1939

The care of fractures of the hand and of the upper extremity has long been a challenge to physicians and therapists. These practitioners have understood the need for stable fixation, be it by external casts or by more invasive techniques, including external fixators, percutaneous pins, and open re-

duction with more rigid fracture fixation.* Because of the close relationship between fractures in the hand and upper extremity and crucial overlying soft tissue structures, it is paramount that we have a thorough knowledge of the surrounding soft tissue envelope.[18,105,110] Because fractures often involve injuries to these structures from both within and without, surgeons must understand how to repair them if traumatized, and therapists must be aware of techniques to restore gliding of these tissues. The goal is early restoration of joint movement[84] and, ultimately, complete rehabilitation of the injured upper extremity, including reincorporation of the part into the total activities of the patient.

Accordingly, both surgeon and therapist need to take a thorough history of the patient, including an assessment of the general health history, occupation, and avocations. The history of previous injuries or symptoms in the injured extremity also will be important in knowing how to rehabilitate the fracture in question.

CLASSIFICATION OF FRACTURES
Location

Fractures can be classified according to several criteria (Table 23-1). They may be defined according to location in the bone. When this involves a long bone such as a

*References 4, 17, 19, 21, 24, 32, 38, 54, 87, 90, 94, 109.

Table 23-1. Examples of ways in which fractures are classified

Criteria	Examples/comments
Location in the bone	Diaphyseal, metaphyseal, articular (articular fractures may be further classified)
Angle of fracture through the bone	Transverse, oblique or spiral, stellate, longitudinal
Number of fragments	Simple, comminuted (comminuted fragments may be further classified by geometric appearance)
Skin closed or open	Closed, open (open fractures are classified further by severity of soft tissue injury)

metacarpal or phalanx, they can be described as being diaphyseal (in the midportion of the shaft of bone), metaphyseal (in the area of bony flare close to the articular surface), or articular when they involve the end of the bone and enter the joint (Fig. 23-1, *A*). If articular, they may be designated as condylar (Fig. 23-1, *B*), T-condylar (Fig. 23-1, *C*) or Y-condylar (Fig. 23-1, *D*). They may be fractures of the rim of the joint, which often denote an avulsion of a portion of capsule, collateral ligament, or tendon (Fig. 23-1, *E*). Because the gliding surface of articular cartilage is crucial for joint performance, accurate reduction of articular fractures is paramount.[61,68] Joint surface displacement in a vertical direction away from (or into) the joint has been shown to contribute to the development of posttraumatic arthritis[22] (Fig. 23-1, *F*). A "step-off" of up to 2 mm is considered by some authors[68] the maximum allowable displacement to allow good joint function and low chance of posttraumatic arthritis. By most standards today, less than 2 mm of displacement is recommended and no incongruity is desirable.[80]

Angle of fracture

Next, fractures should be described according to the angle of the fracture line through bone, such as transverse, oblique, or spiral (Fig. 23-1, *G*); stellate (or starlike), with fracture lines radiating out from some central point; or longitudinal (Fig. 23-1, *H*).

Simple or comminuted

Furthermore, fractures should be classified according to whether they are simple, producing two major fracture fragments, or comminuted, producing multiple fragments. Fragments may be further characterized according to geometric appearance. The typical butterfly fragment is one in which a pie-shaped fragment appears to be taken out of both major fragments at the site of a major transverse or oblique fracture line (see Fig. 23-1, *G*).

Closed or open

Finally, fractures are characterized by whether they are closed or open. Open fractures in which the soft tissue envelope has been violated have been subclassified by Gustilo et al.[52] according to the severity of the soft tissue injury.

- A type I open fracture is one in which there is a puncture wound without significant gross contamination, less than 1 cm in size, and with the fracture being noncomminuted.
- Type II open fractures have a laceration greater than 1 cm in size with minimal to moderate soft tissue crush, and the fracture is still characterized as a simple one.
- Type III open fractures are divided into three subsets. Type IIIA has extensive soft tissue laceration or crush, but there is still adequate soft tissue coverage of bone. Type IIIB has extensive soft tissue loss that likely will leave bone uncovered unless covered by later skin grafting or flaps. Type IIIC injuries have associated arterial injury requiring repair or reconstruction. Type III fractures often (but not necessarily) involve significant comminution of bone.

Successful management of open fractures requires great attention to detail. The fracture wound must be cultured and prophylactic antibiotics begun.[51,102] Antibiotics are chosen according to the patient's history, the location of the fracture within the body, and the milieu in which the fracture occurred. The tetanus toxoid status of the patient must be ascertained and the appropriate tetanus booster or tetanus immunization given as needed. A thorough debridement of the wound to remove devitalized tissues and gross debris should be performed.[102] Pulsatile lavage systems have helped improve the cleansing of the wound and often will be used by the operating room team.

The objective of the hand surgeon in caring for the open fracture is to provide the greatest opportunity for the soft tissues to reestablish their protective envelope over bone. A thorough assessment of the status of all the soft tissues, including skin, muscle and tendon, and neurovascular structures, also is performed at this stage, and vital structures are repaired. If possible, loose soft tissue skin coverage may be accomplished on an initial debridement and repair of the type IIIA wound. However, in a type III wound in which gross contamination has been present and doubts remain as to the ability to fully cleanse the wound or to assess vascularity, the wound should be left open.[102] Later debridement and closure, skin graft, or flap coverage can be carried out after soft tissues appear to be healthy. Fracture fixation in type III wounds often necessitates the use of external fixators to avoid the placement of large metallic devices in the contaminated wound or to maintain length when bone loss is significant.[9,89] The placement of external fixation pins remote to the site of

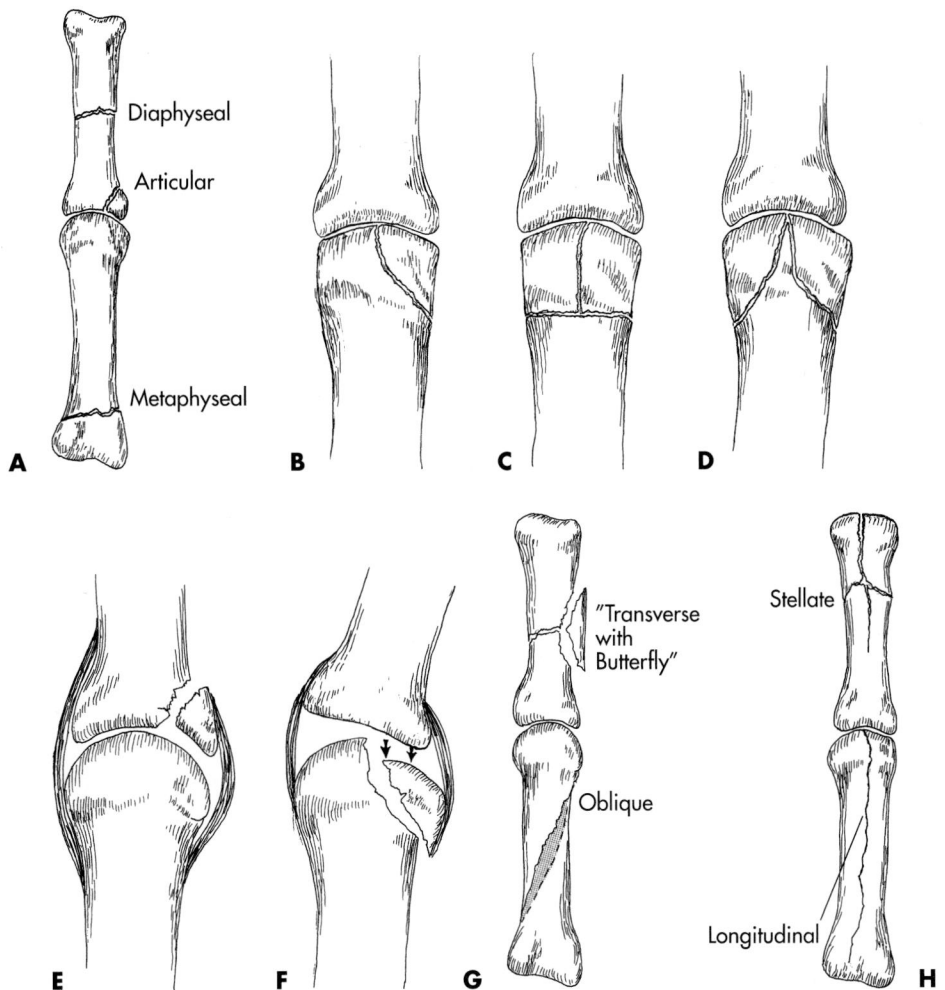

Fig. 23-1. Fracture types. Fractures may be classified according to their location in the bone: diaphyseal, metaphyseal, and articular (**A**); condylar (**B**); T-condylar (**C**); Y-condylar (**D**); articular avulsion (**E**); and articular depression (**F**). Fractures also may be described according to the angle of the fracture line through the bone: transverse with "butterfly" and oblique (**G**) and stellate or longitudinal (**H**).

injury avoids this dilemma and often can provide stable fixation to allow early motion. Plate or intermedullary fixation may be chosen, depending on the fracture site, and may be used initially if it is thought that the wound can be converted from "dirty" to "clean" and soft tissue coverage is adequate.[102]

It is obvious that as fractures increase in their severity, the complications increase. Not only does the likelihood of infection increase, but the possibility of avascular necrosis or loss of blood supply to fragments in a comminuted wound increases, and the chance of delayed union and thus implant fixation failure increases. The soft tissue envelope certainly must be considered as a casualty of such complicated fractures, as adhesions binding soft tissue planes to fracture sites will be common. Thus not only the reestablishment of bony stability but also the repair of essential soft tissue

gliding structures and their early mobilization through proper therapy will be crucial for success.[18]

FACTORS AFFECTING UNION RATES

Union may be delayed for a variety of causes. As already suggested, fractures that are comminuted or open have a higher rate of delayed union or nonunion, a result of damage to the blood supply of bone caused by higher levels of energy imparted in open or comminuted fractures. Of course, further loss of blood supply through surgical approaches that can further injure blood supply may, indeed, delay union despite the expected benefit of this approach. Steroids have been shown to decrease bone mass and delay healing of various wounds. The protein wasting that occurs during corticosteroid use may be partially reversed by physical training,[37] and thus a good argument can be made for a general fitness program for patients who are receiving steroids and are concomitantly healing from such an injury. Smokers have a decreased rate of healing in certain fractures, including those of the spine,[16] and this difference is significant. It is surmised that the absorption of carbon monoxide from smoke produces a lowering of oxygen tensions and decreased oxygen delivery to the sites of healing and thus promotes the production of fibrous or cartilaginous tissue at the healing site rather than bone. Vasospasm also occurs as a result of the nicotine, which may, in addition, decrease oxygen delivery to the periphery. Nutritional factors, including abuse of substances such as alcohol, also contribute to delayed union. Diabetes and other diseases that affect the turnover of basement membrane or affect blood supply may decrease the healing of bony injuries.

Factors that may speed healing therefore include controlling the aforementioned diseases or habituations and maximizing nutritional support for the patient. This is especially true in patients in whom multiple fractures have produced a serious negative nitrogen balance that may take weeks to reverse. These patients may require intravenous hyperalimentation, nutritional support, and other measures.

Stable compression loading of fractures, such as can be accomplished with internal fixation devices, can improve fracture healing and functional recovery. Such stability can allow early guarded loading of the fracture site and early range of motion of adjacent joints. The application of electrical stimulation to facilitate fracture healing has also been researched extensively, and pulsed electromagnetic fields have been shown to successfully treat delayed unions or nonunions.[14,34] However, there have not yet been large prospective double-blind studies to prove conclusively that electrical stimulation increases the rate of healing in uncomplicated fractures. Accordingly, electrical fields have been applied to fracture care generally only for delayed unions or nonunions.

SOFT TISSUE ENVELOPE

Even in closed injuries, the soft tissue envelope can be significantly traumatized by a blunt external blow or from within by fracture edges. This can include lacerations of the floor of flexor sheaths or damage to flexor[113] and extensor tendons themselves,[86] stripping of the periosteal blood supply to bone, damage to neurovascular structures,[113] and injury to ligaments that may produce significant joint instability.[81] Injury to all of these must be evaluated by the hand surgeon carefully at the time of fracture to assess the need to repair these structures as well as care for the fracture itself. Examination of the hand by the therapist as a part of the initial therapy evaluation must include a look at the function of these structures so that proper attention can be paid to reestablishing the gliding function of tendons and nerves. Immobilization of muscle-tendon units during fracture healing (even without laceration) leads to considerable dysfunction requiring rehabilitation.[12,65]

Finally, vigilant observation by the surgeon and therapist is needed to look for signs of compartment syndrome developing after any bony injury.[20] Compartment syndrome is a clinical state in which the pressure within an enclosed muscular (or bony-and-muscular) compartment rises above the level at which the arterial perfusion pressure of the compartment can maintain positive blood flow through the compartment.[2] As a result, viability of any tissues within the compartment may be lost and necrosis begins. Such a syndrome may be present acutely after fracture, vigorous exercise,[10] or burns,[95] or it may occur chronically, producing borderline ischemia to muscle and nerve in the compartment, which may not be detected until later. The surgeon and therapist should be aware of the signs of compartment syndrome, including the classic pain, pallor, paresthesias, and pulselessness. Pulselessness generally occurs only very late in the syndrome, so reliance on the other factors is paramount.[42] Inordinate pain, especially that worsened by passive stretch of muscle within the compartment, is probably the most useful clinical finding.[76] If a compartment syndrome is suspected, intracompartmental pressure monitoring should be performed, and if intracompartmental pressure is elevated dangerously, fasciotomy should be conducted.[53,77,79,93,112] If a wound dressing appears to be constrictive or if a cast is in place and is contributing to compression of compartments, the external device should be loosened or removed while fracture support is maintained, and the part should be elevated to the level of the heart. Overzealous elevation actually can decrease tissue perfusion and worsen some compartment syndromes.[75] The examination of the hand or forearm to evaluate for compartment syndrome should especially involve palpation of the various muscle compartments for teseness and tenderness and the passive pain stretch tests. Forearm muscular compartments can be tested by passively stretching flexors or extensors. This should include passive extension or flexion of the wrist and the digits, including metacarpophalangeal (MP) and interphalangeal (IP) joints. Testing for intrinsic muscle compartment compression syndromes should involve putting the digits through abduction and adduction while the MP joints are maintained in extension and the proximal interphalangeal (PIP) joint is maintained in flexion. The adductors of the thumb can be tested by passive palmar and radial abduction of the thumb, and the remainder of the thenar muscles can be tested by radial abduction and retroposition dorsal to the plane of the palm. The hypothenar muscle can be tested by adducting the little digit and extending it, thus stretching the intrinsic flexor and providing abduction of this digit.[36,54]

Except for measurement of intracompartmental pressure, the finding of pain on passive stretch is far more important than other classic signs of compartment syndrome because these classic signs may not occur until long after muscle necrosis and even late fibrosis has occurred.[106] *Immediate attention* to a possible compartment syndrome is necessary to avert the disastrous effects of Volkmann's ischemic contracture.[28]

Gunshot wounds produce composite tissue damage and are a significant challenge to treat. Bony loss is common and begs immediate stabilization, either through provisional K-wire fixation or definitive external fixator placement. Soft tissue control and reconstruction usually requires multiple debridements and may be followed by bone grafting, if needed. Early plate and screw fixation may be used with or without bone grafting if a low-velocity missile wound exists and may actually improve functional outcome by allowing early rehabilitation.[45]

Soft tissue complications may take other forms less severe than muscular compartment necrosis, including joint stiffness and carpal tunnel syndrome as seen in Colles' fracture.[24,71,73,104] Carpal tunnel pressures may be significantly altered by wrist position extremes in the treatment of Colles' fracture.[40]

Timing of fracture reduction

Displaced fractures, recognized early, are usually reduced and started on therapy. But what if discovered late? Delays in treatment often prompted by labyrinthine referral routes caused by insurance roadblocks have changed the presentation. Definitive delayed open reduction and internal fixation of impending malunions (e.g., 1 month after fracture) often results in greater function than when waiting until well after fracture healing to perform the malunion correction.[70] Late open reduction of displaced articular fractures often results in improved function and diminished pain if done before posttraumatic arthritis has begun.[63]

ARTICULAR INJURY

Fractures that affect joints may injure them in several ways. The ligamentous support of the joint itself may be injured by avulsion of ligament attachment points from bone with or without bony fragments.

Direct articular injury may include direct blunt contusions to cartilage surfaces or lacerations to them by penetrating injuries. The latter are usually treated by debridement, as much as is possible, at an open operative procedure to repair the overlying laceration and assess damage. When bone and cartilage have been avulsed from an articular surface as a composite, they may be secured in place by open reduction and may revascularize as part of the healing process. Such articular fragments may be held in place with small metal pins, which are countersunk, or by polydioxanone pins, which are resorbable and which may be cut off flush at the fracture surface or countersunk.[29,88]

Indeed, polydioxanone has been found equal to metal pins in the fixation of hand fractures with respect to bending and compression loads, although not in torsion.[29a] Joint injuries may require special studies, including computed tomography (CT) or arthrography,[6] to further define them.

Unlike fractures in the metaphysis or diaphysis, articular fractures may not be left significantly displaced, and more than 1 to 2 mm of displacement often spells doom for an articular fracture if one expects a near-normal recovery.[68] A step-off greater than this usually requires operative reduction. Other factors the surgeon considers are the age of the patient, the location within the particular joint, and the resultant angular deformity that may be left in the joint.[13,14,33,101] An unreduced articular step-off may further overload a particular condyle by compressive weight bearing and hasten the demise of the condyle (see Fig. 23-1, *F*).

Just as important as accurate, stable reduction in an articular injury is early motion. Mooney and Ferguson[83] and later Salter et al.[96,98] demonstrated the biologically beneficial effects of continuous passive motion on the healing of full-thickness defects in articular cartilage. Immediate continuous motion after the production of joint surface injuries was shown to significantly improve joint resurfacing and range of motion when compared with immobilization or intermittent caged activity of experimental animals. These studies further confirm the impression of others (e.g., Scudder, quoted in the introduction of this chapter) that early movement will produce a superior result when fracture stability can be provided.

CHOICES FOR FRACTURE FIXATION
Closed reduction versus open reduction and internal fixation

What are the factors that affect the choice of fracture support? Do we use closed reduction and cast (splint), percutaneous pins, external fixators, or open reduction and internal fixation? Fractures that are thought to be stable are considered good choices for treatment with closed methods.[91] Stable fractures are those in which muscular forces are not likely to displace the fragments or in which the fracture lines are not articular and not likely to be displaced with motion. Fracture of the fifth metacarpal neck (the "boxer's" fracture), in which significant angular deformity is still associated with an excellent clinical result, is a good example of a fracture that is almost always treated with closed methods. Relatively short-term cast or splint immobilization in this fracture is the rule, with rapid recovery of function and good overall results.[60] Distal phalangeal fractures often require only conservative management, unless significant articular avulsions destabilize the joint.[111,115]

The fracture that is already displaced and has an unstable pattern, such as the oblique second or fifth metacarpal shaft fracture (in which shortening or rotary deformity is likely), is much more likely to require some form of internal fixation.[50,56,58] Fear of neurovascular compromise or laceration with ongoing fracture instability is another factor that may direct the surgeon toward an operative approach to prevent further injury. Long bone fractures, such as both bones of the forearm, commonly

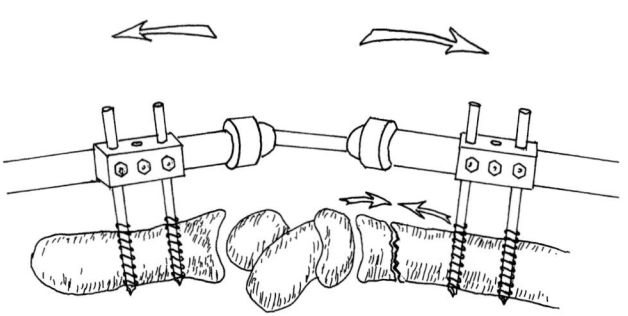

Fig. 23-2. External fixator.

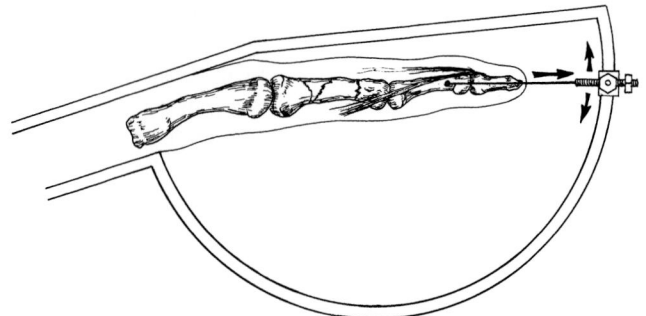

Fig. 23-3. Options for internal fixation.

fit this category and require operative intervention to allow early mobilization, prevent further deformity, and prevent nerve or vessel injury.

External fixation. After it is decided to fix a fracture because it is unstable, requires early mobilization for good results, or is already displaced, how does one choose from the various options for fracture fixation? What makes an external fixator versus a plate-and-screw combination the treatment of choice for a given fracture?

External fixators probably began as skeletal pins incorporated into plaster.[23] They are devices in which traction is applied to a fracture that is under a compressive load to prevent it from shortening or to hold a reduction carried out by either open or closed means. The principle of the external fixator is to provide longitudinal traction to prevent fracture shortening or angulation, while allowing muscle and tendon units to resume function across the fracture site[1,9,27,64,103] (Fig. 23-2).

Some fractures (e.g., comminuted articular fractures) may require a combination of external fixation and supplemental internal fixation for maximum fracture reduction and stability. Fractures in which significant comminution has occurred (and thus in which the placement of internally fixing plate, screws, or pins may be difficult) often are best treated by placing an external fixator across the fracture to bring it out to length and to neutralize the compressive forces of muscle-tendon units. Through pulling on ligamentous attachment points (ligamentotaxis), bony fragments may be brought out to length and held in position while healing occurs. If significant impaction of the fractures has occurred with bony defects remaining after the fracture has been reduced, bone grafting may be needed to fill the void. The use of an external fixator in this situation also may prevent the trauma of a surgical exposure that may further compromise blood supply to the fractured parts.

Examples of external fixators used in the hand and forearm include the Synthes, Agee, Orthofix, and Hoffman designs, which are useful in both the forearm and hand. These devices allow the treatment of a broad range of

fracture types and bone sizes, from forearm bones to phalanges in the hand. Some allow variable compression or distraction to be carefully adjusted during treatment before removing the device, and some allow mobilization of joints while still maintaining traction across the fracture sites.

A series of ingenious manufactured or made-on-site splints have been detailed in recent literature. Most allow early motion under intradigital traction and have been especially useful for comminuted fractures around the PIP joint or middle phalanx. Although they require some time to construct in the operative room, they are generally inexpensive and made from readily available materials.[3,26,39,44,78,85]

There have been a variety of approaches to the care of the pins at the site of percutaneous pin fixation or external fixator pin entry. Most current recommendations include daily cleansing with peroxide to remove crusts and application of topical antibiotic ointment. Other authors have recommended initial application of antibiotic ointment and simple coverage with an adherent dressing over the pin sites to allow a protective crust to form that will inhibit the ingress of bacteria. Perhaps most likely to cause drainage and pin-tract infection is the motion of soft tissues about the pin site as the part is put through its range-of-motion exercises. Indeed, the complications of the use of percutaneous pins or external fixators are mostly those of transfixation of soft tissues between skin and bone, which prevent gliding and produce fibrosis.

Perhaps the greatest indication for external fixation is an open fracture in which there is significant soft tissue injury, or the case with tissue loss in which the placement of relatively large internal devices, such as plates and screws, would be considered an additional infection risk. The placement of an external fixator across a fracture site in this situation allows stabilization of the fracture and further treatment of the skin and soft tissue loss by appropriate debridement and possible later grafting or skin flaps. Unstable fractures of the phalanges that are too comminuted to internally fix may benefit from simple[31,41,82] or dynamic traction that also allows early motion[92,99] (Fig. 23-3).

Internal fixation. The indications for internal fixation include the following:

1. Displaced fractures irreducible by closed manipulation
2. Articular fractures that are displaced more than a minimal amount
3. Fractures in which early motion is essential (including articular fractures or fractures in which the soft tissue envelope has been injured and requires early mobilization for soft tissue gliding)
4. Fractures with an unusually high incidence of nonunion or malunion without open reduction/internal fixation, including some scaphoid fractures and fractures of both bones of the forearm in adults
5. Open or closed fractures that are unstable and likely to displace

Options available to the surgeon for internal fixation devices (Fig 23-4), with their advantages and disadvantages, are listed in Table 23-2 and are detailed by a number of authors.* Some fractures defy adequate fixation by the aforementioned methods and may require a silicone implant for load sharing,[107] although such applications are not common.

With this information in mind, the therapist and surgeon can collaborate on a therapeutic approach after surgical fixation, with its inherent strengths and weaknesses, to maximize early motion and rehabilitative efforts. The hand therapist is a frequent observer of the external fixator or the percutaneously placed pin that has been left protruding and can help alert the surgeon early when problems arise. Such observations include pin-tract redness, drainage, or loosening of the pin. These findings may necessitate cultures, appropriate antibiotics, and possibly exploration and drainage of the pin site. Early pin removal may be necessary to prevent or treat osteomyelitis. The importance of close cooperation of members of the hand care team in this situation cannot be overemphasized.

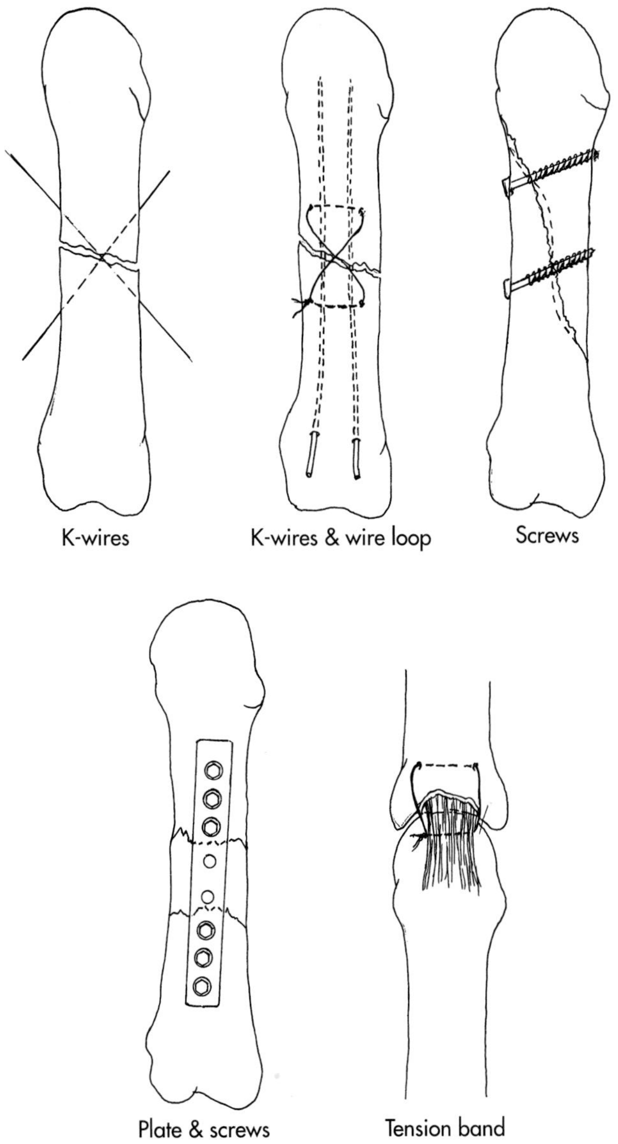

Fracture healing—clinical signs

The process of fracture healing and repair goes through a series of phases that can be clinically judged by both physical exam and x-ray. These phases include (1) development of hematoma and traumatic inflammation, (2) organization, (3) union by callus, and (4) remodeling of callus and bony union.[15] An assessment of fracture healing can help the physician and therapist decide when to increase activity levels. The initial two fracture phases produce significant swelling, pain, and local tenderness. In this period, extravasation of blood and serum from the fracture as well as the overlying injured soft tissues occurs. Generally, by the seventh to tenth day after injury, this has reached its peak and

*References 5, 8, 11, 30, 35, 62, 66, 74, 108.

K-wires   **K-wires & wire loop**   **Screws**

Plate & screws   **Tension band**

Fig. 23-4. Options for internal fixation.

has begun to subside as the fracture hematoma organizes and vascular and fibrous ingrowth into the hematoma begins. Callus formation has thus begun and forms a "rubbery" mass at the fracture interface. Provided that fracture fixation or immobilization has been achieved by this point, the pain should diminish significantly.

From this point forward, associated swelling, pain, and tenderness generally diminish rapidly as the callus matures. It is the resolution of much of the edema and tenderness that signals that one can begin to add significant forces across the fracture and be confident that displacement of the fracture will be unlikely. Generally, by the fourth to sixth week in most fractures in adults (and the third to fourth week in most fractures in children in the hand and forearm), forces of active and active-assisted range of motion can be increased.

Table 23-2. Fracture fixation options

Device	Advantages	Disadvantages
K-wires (percutaneous or buried)	Minimal exposure, minimal penetration of bone	Relatively weak fixation[7,48]
Circlage wires	Minimal exposure	Requires long spiral fracture[49]
K-wires and wire loop combination	Greater strength than K-wire alone; greater compression of fracture	Greater exposure of the fracture site required[43,46,72]
Tension band wires	Excellent for small avulsion fracture	None[60]
Screws	Provide rigid compression loading of fracture sites	Greater exposure required for drilling[25]
Plate-and-screw combinations	Greater rigidity of fixation	Wider exposure with greater tissue dissection and potential compromise of blood supply[30]
Polydioxanone	Resorbable; especially good in articular application	Less rigid fixation[88]

However, this always depends on the full assessment of the fracture and considerations of the initial stability, type of reduction used, general health and reliability of the patient, and x-ray appearance. A simple, cursory examination of the part and the acknowledgment that tenderness has resolved will never signal the time to throw caution to the wind and begin vigorous unprotected activities.

Pediatric fractures

Fractures in children can be described in a manner similar to those in adults in terms of location within the shaft of the bone and whether a fragment of bone has been avulsed from a corner of a joint, or whether the fracture involves the articular surface at all. However, when fractures cross ossification centers and the combination of epiphysis and physis, they become more critical (Fig. 23-5). Accurate reduction of such fractures is important, although the remodeling capabilities in children far exceed those in adults. Fractures that do cross the epiphyseal lines have been classified by Salter and Harris[97] (Fig. 23-6). Epiphyseal injuries occur 34% more commonly in the hand than elsewhere in the skeleton, according to Hastings and Simmons.[57] Understanding the anatomy of the metaphysis-physis-epiphysis relationships is important in understanding the classification of Salter and Harris. Injuries that damage the epiphysis, such as the Salter III, IV, and V, are more likely to result in growth abnormalities or growth cessation. Lack of accurate reduction of these latter injuries may leave an articular incongruity in addition to the angular deformity that may result if Salter I and II injuries are not reduced. Accordingly, some Salter III, IV, and V fractures will require open reduction and internal fixation for accurate reconstitution of the joint surface. Similarly, some Salter I and II fractures will require open reduction if they cannot be reduced by closed methods. Those that do require operative intervention are more likely to be referred to the hand therapist for early protected motion and may be more of a rehabilitation challenge.[47,69,114]

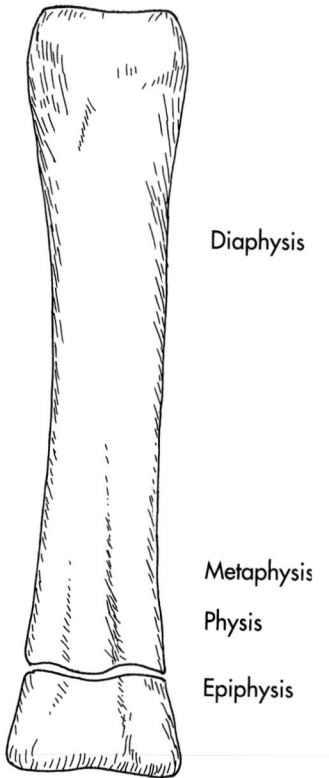

Fig. 23-5. Long bone in children.

Be especially aware of the displaced Salter I fracture at the proximal end of proximal or middle phalanges. These are often difficult to see as they usually occur in the very young.[55] Imaging these in children younger than 5 years of age may require sedation when performing a CT scan.

Late soft tissue issues

Some fractures in the hand and wrist develop contractures despite the best of fracture fixation and rehabilitation. These are usually preordained to be difficult because of soft tissue injury or their location near joints. Schneider[100] believes that

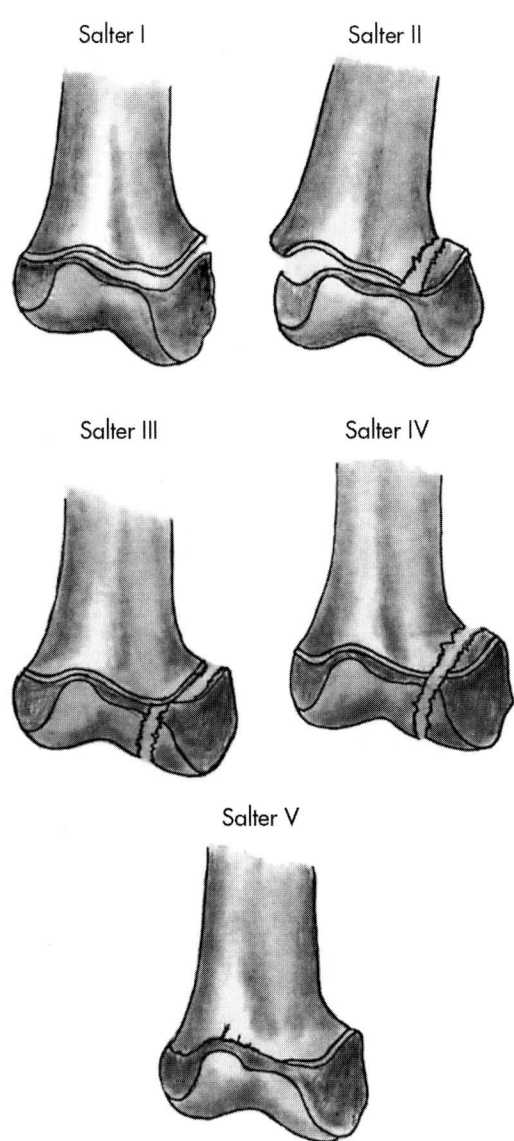

Salter I   Salter II

Salter III   Salter IV

Salter V

Fig. 23-6. Salter-Harris classification of physeal fractures.

when blood supply and sensation remain good, and in a well motivated patient, that an aggressive soft tissue release or resection may be in order. This often includes dorsal and palmar capsulectomies and tenolysis under sedation with local block. Of course, this is followed by a well-designed hand therapy program.[100]

SUMMARY

Fracture care, from initial assessment through completion of hand therapy, is a challenge that requires an understanding of the anatomy and physiologic process of fracture repair. It also demands a thorough knowledge of the nonoperative and operative treatment options available to the treating physician and hand therapist. A good dialog and comfortable working relationship between these two hand care profes-

sionals will help optimize the outcome in difficult fractures of the hand and upper extremity.

"There is no class of injuries which a practitioner approaches with more doubt and misgiving than fractures, or one which demands a greater amount of ready knowledge, self-reliance, and consummate skill. . . . I certainly know none which requires a more thorough knowledge of topographical anatomy, a nicer sense of discrimination, a calmer judgment, a more enlarged experience . . . in a word, none which requires a higher combination of surgical tact and power."

Samuel D. Gross
A System of Surgery, volume II, 1859

REFERENCES

1. Agee J: Unstable fracture dislocation of the proximal interphalangeal joint: treatment with the force couple splint, *Clin Orthop* 214:101, 1987.
2. Ashton H: The effect of increased tissue pressure on blood flow, *Clin Orthop* 113:15, 1975.
3. Bain GI, et al: Dynamic external fixation for injuries of the proximal interphalangeal joint, *J Bone Joint Surg* 80B:1014, 1998.
4. Barton NJ: Fractures of the hand, *J Bone Joint Surg* 66B:159, 1984.
5. Beach DM, et al: The stability of internal fixation in the proximal phalanx, *J Hand Surg* 11A:672, 1986.
6. Bell MJ, et al: Fracture of the ulnar sesamoid of the metacarpophalangeal joint of the thumb: an arthrographic study, *J Hand Surg* 10B:379, 1985.
7. Belsky MR, Eaton RG, Lane LB: Closed reduction and internal fixation of proximal phalangeal fractures, *J Hand Surg* 9A:725, 1984.
8. Belsole R: Physiological fixation of displaced and unstable fractures of the hand, *Orthop Clin North Am* 11:393, 1980.
9. Bilos ZJ, Eskestrand T: External fixator in use in comminuted gunshot fractures of the proximal phalanx, *J Hand Surg* 4:357, 1979.
10. Bird CB, McCoy JW Jr: Weight-lifting as a cause of compartment syndrome in the forearm: a case report, *J Bone Joint Surg* 65A:406, 1983.
11. Block DM, et al: Comparison of internal fixation techniques in metacarpal fractures, *J Hand Surg* 10A:466, 1985.
12. Booth FW: Physiologies and biochemical effects of immobilization of muscle, *Clin Orthop* 219:15, 1987.
13. Bora WF, Didizian NH: The treatment of injuries to the carpometacarpal joint of the little finger, *J Bone Joint Surg* 56A:1459, 1974.
14. Bora WF, Osterman AC, Brighton CT: The electrical treatment of scaphoid nonunion, *Clin Orthop* 161:33, 1986.
15. Brand RA: Fracture healing. In Evarts CM, editor: *Surgery of the musculoskeletal system*, vol 1, New York, 1983, Churchill Livingstone.
16. Brown CW: The rate of pseudarthrosis (surgical nonunion) in patients who are smokers and patients who are nonsmokers: a comparison study, *Spine* 11:942, 1986.
17. Brown PW: The management of phalangeal and metacarpal fractures, *Surg Clin North Am* 53:1393, 1973.
18. Burkhalter W: Mutilating injuries of the hand, *Hand Clin* 2:45, 1986.
19. Burton RI, Eaton RG: Common hand injuries in the athlete, *Orthop Clin North Am* 4:809, 1973.
20. Burton RI, Miller RJ: Compartment syndromes. In Evarts CM, editor: *Surgery of the musculoskeletal system*, vol 1, New York, 1983, Churchill Livingstone.
21. Butler B Jr: Complications of treatment of injuries to the hand. In Epps CH, editor: *Complications in orthopaedic surgery*, Philadelphia, 1978, JB Lippincott.

22. Clendenin MB, Smith RJ: Fifth metacarpal hamate arthrodesis for post-traumatic osteoarthritis, *J Hand Surg* 9:374, 1984.

23. Cole JM, Obletz BE: Comminuted fractures of the distal end of the radius treated by skeletal transfixion in plaster cast: an end result study of 33 cases, *J Bone Joint Surg* 48A:931, 1966.

24. Colles A: On the fracture of the carpal extremity of the radius, *Edinburgh Med Surg J* 10:182, 1814.

25. Crawford GP: Screw fixation for certain fractures of the phalanges and metacarpals, *J Bone Joint Surg* 58A:487, 1976.

26. de Soras X, et al: Pins and rubbers traction system, *J Hand Surg* 22B:730, 1997.

27. Dickson RA: Rigid fixation of unstable metacarpal fractures using transverse K-wires bonded with acrylic resin, *Hand* 7:284, 1975.

28. Eaton RG, Green WT: Volkman's ischemia, a volar compartment syndrome of the forearm, *Clin Orthop* 113:58, 1975.

29. Eitoussi F, Ip WY, Chow SP: External fixation for comminuted phalangeal fractures: a biomechanical cadaver study, *J Hand Surg* 21:760, 1996.

29a. Eitoussi F, et al: Biomechanical properties of absorbable implants in finger fractures, *J Hand Surg* 23B:79, 1996.

30. Fernandez DL: Correction of post-traumatic wrist deformity in adults by osteotomy, bone grafting, and internal fixation, *J Bone Joint Surg* 64A:1164, 1982.

31. Fitzgerald JAW, Kohn MA: The conservative management of fractures of the shafts of the phalanges of the finger by combined traction-splintage, *J Hand Surg* 9B:303, 1984.

32. Flatt AE: *Fractures the care of minor hand injuries,* ed 3, St Louis, 1972, Mosby.

33. Foster RJ, Hastings H II: Treatment of Bennett, Rolando, and vertical intraarticular trapezial fractures, *Clin Orthop* 214:121, 1987.

34. Frykman GK, et al: Treatment of nonunited scaphoid fractures by pulsed electromagnetic field and cast, *J Hand Surg* 11A:344, 1986.

35. Fyfe IS, Mason S: The mechanical stability of internal fixation of fractured phalanges, *Hand* 11:50, 1979.

36. Garfin SR: Anatomy of the extremity compartments. In Mubarak SJ, Haigers AR, editors: *Compartment syndromes and Volkmann's contractures: monographs in clinical orthopaedics,* vol 3, Philadelphia, 1981, WB Saunders.

37. Garrel DR et al: Effects of moderate physical training on prednisone induced protein wasting: a study of whole body and bone protein metabolism, *Metabolism* 37:257, 1988.

38. Gaul JS Jr: Management of acute hand injuries, *Ann Emerg Med* 9:139, 1980.

39. Gaul JS Jr, Rosenberg SN: Fracture-dislocation of the middle phalanx at the proximal interphalangeal joint: repair with a simple intradigital traction-fixation device, *Am J Orthop* 27:682, 1998.

40. Gelberman RH, Szabo RM, Masterson WW: Carpal tunnel pressures and wrist position in patients with Colles' fractures, *J Trauma* 24:747, 1984.

41. Gelberman RH, Vance RM, Zahaib GS: Fractures of the base of the thumb: treatment with oblique traction, *J Bone Joint Surg* 61A:260, 1979.

42. Gelberman RH, et al: Compartment syndromes of the forearm: diagnosis and treatment, *Clin Orthop* 161:252, 1981.

43. Gingrass R, Fehring B, Matloub H: Intraosseous wiring of complex hand fractures, *Plast Reconstr Surg* 66:383, 1980.

44. Godwin Y, Arnstein PM: A cheap, disposable external fixator for comminuted phalangeal fractures, *J Hand Surg* 23B:84, 1998.

45. Gonzalez MH, Hall M, Hall RF Jr: Low-velocity gunshot wounds of the proximal phalanx: treatment by early stable fixation, *J Hand Surg* 23:150, 1998.

46. Gordon L, Montanto EH: Skeletal stabilization for digital replantation surgery, use of intraosseous wiring, *Clin Orthop* 214:72, 1987.

47. Grad JB: Children's skeletal injuries, *Orthop Clin North Am* 17:437, 1986.

48. Green DP, Anderson JR: Closed reduction and percutaneous pin fixation of fractured phalanges, *J Bone Joint Surg* 55A:1651, 1973.

49. Gropper PT, Bower V: Cerclage wiring of metacarpal fractures, *Clin Orthop* 188:203, 1984.

50. Grundberg AB: Intramedullary fixation for fractures of the hand, *J Hand Surg* 6:568, 1981.

51. Gustilo R, Anderson J: Prevention of infection in the treatment of one thousand and twenty-five open fractures of the long bones, *J Bone Joint Surg* 58A:543, 1976.

52. Gustilo R, et al: Analysis of 511 open fractures, *Clin Orthop* 66:148, 1969.

53. Halpern AA, Nagel DA: Compartment syndromes of the forearm: early recognition using tissue pressure measurements, *J Hand Surg* 4:258, 1979.

54. Halpern AA, et al: Compartment syndrome of the interosseous muscles, *Clin Orthop* 140:23, 1979.

55. Hashizume H, et al: Dorsally displaced epiphyseal fracture of the phalangeal base, *J Hand Surg* 21B:136, 1996.

56. Hastings H: Unstable metacarpal and phalangeal fracture treatment with screws and plates, *Clin Orthop* 214:37, 1987.

57. Hastings H II, Simmons BP: Hand fractures in children: a statistical analysis, *Clin Orthop* 188:120, 1984.

58. Heim U, Pfeiffer KM, in collaboration with Meuli HC: *Small fragment set manual: technologies recommended by the ASIF Group,* ed 2, New York, 1982, Springer-Verlag.

59. Hubbard LF: Fractures of the hand and wrist. In Evarts CM, editor: *Surgery of the musculoskeletal system,* vol 1, New York, 1983, Churchill Livingstone.

60. Hunter JM, Cowen NJ: Fifth metacarpal fractures in a compensation clinic population, *J Bone Joint Surg* 52A:1159, 1970.

61. Isani A: Small joint injuries requiring surgical treatment, *Orthop Clin North Am* 17:407, 1986.

62. Iselin F, Thevenin R: Fixation of fractures of the digits with intramedullary flexible screws, *J Bone Joint Surg* 65A:1096, 1974.

63. Jebson PJ, Blair WF: Correction of malunited Bennett's fracture by intra-articular osteotomy: a report of two cases, *J Hand Surg* 22:441, 1997.

64. Johnson V: External fixation for dislocated Colles' fracture, *Acta Orthop Scand* 54:878, 1983.

65. Jokl P, Konstadt S: The effects of limb immobilization on muscle function and protein composition, *Clin Orthop* 174:222, 1983.

66. Jupiter JB, Koniuch MP, Smith RJ: The management of delayed union and non-union of the metacarpals and phalanges, *J Hand Surg* 10A:457, 1985.

67. Jupiter JB, Sheppard JE: Tension wire fixation of avulsion fractures in the hand, *Clin Orthop* 214:113, 1987.

68. Knirk JL, Jupiter JB: Intraarticular fractures of the distal end of the radius in young adults, *J Bone Joint Surg* 68A:647, 1986.

69. Lee BS, Esterhai JL Jr, Das M: Fracture of the distal radial epiphysis characteristics and surgical treatment of premature, post-traumatic epiphyseal closure, *Clin Orthop* 185:90, 1984.

70. Lester B, Mellik A: Impending malunions of the hand. Treatment of subacute, malaligned fractures, *Clin Orthop* 327:55, 1996.

71. Lindscheid RL, Dobyns JH: Athletic injuries of the wrist, *Clin Orthop* 198:141, 1985.

72. Lister G: Intraosseous wiring of the digital skeleton, *J Hand Surg* 3:427, 1978.

73. Lucas GL, Sachtjen KM: An analysis of hand function in patients with Colles' fractures treated by Rush rod fixation, *Clin Orthop* 155:172, 1981.

74. Massengill JB, et al: A phalangeal fracture model: quantitative analysis of rigidity and failure, *J Hand Surg* 8:383, 1983.

75. Matsen FA, Krugmire RB Jr, King RV: Increased tissue pressure and its effects on muscle oxygenation in the level and elevated human limbs, Nicholas Andry Award, *Clin Orthop* 144:311, 1979.

76. Matsen FA, Rorabeck CH: Compartment syndromes, *AAOS Instruc Course Lect* 38:463, 1989.

77. Matsen FA III, Winquist RA, Krugmire RB Jr: Diagnosis and management of compartmental syndromes, *J Bone Joint Surg* 62A:286, 1980.

78. McCulley SJ, Hasting C: External fixator for the hand: a quick, cheap and effective method, *J R Coll Surg Edinb* 44:99, 1999.

79. McDermott AGP, Marble AE, Yabsley RH: Monitoring acute compartment pressure with the STIC catheter, *Clin Orthop* 190:192, 1984.

80. McElfresh EC, Dobyns JH: Intra-articular metacarpal head fractures, *J Hand Surg* 8:383, 1983.

81. Melone CP Jr: Joint injuries of the fingers and thumb, *Emerg Med Clin North Am* 3:319, 1985.

82. Moberg E: The use of traction treatment for fractures of phalanges and metacarpals, *Acta Chir Scand* 99:341, 1949-1950.

83. Mooney V, Ferguson AB: The influence of immobilization and motion on the formation of fibrocartilage in the repair granuloma after joint resection from the rabbit, *J Bone Joint Surg* 48A:1145, 1966.

84. Mooney V, Stills M: Continuous passive motion with joint fractures and infections, *Orthop Clin North Am* 18:1, 1987.

85. Mullett JH, et al: Use of the "S" Quattro dynamic external fixator in the treatment of difficult hand fractures, *J Hand Surg* 24B:350, 1999.

86. Murahami Y, Todani K: Traumatic entrapment of the extensor pollicis longus tendon in Smith's fracture of the radius: case report, *J Hand Surg* 6A:238, 1981.

87. O'Brien ET: Fractures of the hand and wrist region. In Rockwood CA, Wilkins KE, King RE, editors: *Fractures in children,* Philadelphia, 1984, JB Lippincott.

88. Papagelopoulos PJ, Giannarakos DG, Lyritis GP: Suitability of biodegradable polydioxanone materials for the internal fixation of fractures, *Orthop Rev* 585, 1993.

89. Peimer CA, Smith RJ, Leffert RD: Distraction fixation in the primary treatment of metacarpal bone loss, *J Hand Surg* 6:111, 1981.

90. Posner MA: Injuries to the hand and wrist in athletes, *Orthop Clin North Am* 8:593, 1977.

91. Pritsch M, Engel J, Farin I: Manipulation and external fixation of metacarpal fractures, *J Bone Joint Surg* 63A:1289, 1981.

92. Quigley TB, Urist MR: Interphalangeal joints: method of digital skeletal traction which permits active motion, *Am J Surg* 73:175, 1947.

93. Rowland SA: Fasciotomy: the treatment of compartment syndrome. In Green DP, editor: *Operative hand surgery,* New York, 1993, Churchill Livingstone.

94. Ruby LK: Common hand injuries in the athlete, *Orthop Clin North Am* 11:819, 1980.

95. Salisbury RD, McKeel DW, Mason AD: Ischemic necrosis of the intrinsic muscles of the hand after thermal injuries, *J Bone Joint Surg* 56A:1701, 1974.

96. Salter RB, Bell RS, Keeley FW: The protective effect of continuous passive motion on living articular cartilage in acute septic arthritis: an experimental investigation in the rabbit, *Clin Orthop* 159:223, 1981.

97. Salter RB, Harris WR: Injuries involving the epiphyseal plate, *J Bone Joint Surg* 45A:587, 1963.

98. Salter RB, et al: The biologic effects of continuous passive motion on the healing of full thickness defects in articular cartilage: an experimental investigation in the rabbit, *J Bone Joint Surg* 62:12, 1980.

99. Schenck R: Dynamic traction and early passive movement for fractures of the proximal interphalangeal joint, *J Hand Surg* 11A:850, 1986.

100. Schneider LM: Tenolysis and capsulectomy after hand fractures, *Clin Orthop* 327:72, 1998.

101. Seno N, et al: Fractures of the base of the middle phalanx of the finger: classification, management, and long-term results, *J Bone Joint Surg* 79:758, 1997.

102. Shaw WW, et al: Symposium: management of type III extremity fractures, *Contemp Orthop* 25:2, 1992.

103. Stark RH: Treatment of difficult PIP joint fractures with a mini-external fixation device, *Orthop Rev* 22:609, 1993.

104. Stewart HD, Innes AR, Burke RD: The hand complications of Colles' fractures, *J Hand Surg* 10B:103, 1985.

105. Strickland JW, et al: Fractures influencing digital performance after phalangeal fracture. In Strickland JW, Steicken JB, editors: *Difficult problems in hand surgery,* St Louis, 1982, Mosby.

106. Sunderaraj GD, Mani K: Pattern of contracture and recovery following ischemia of the upper limb, *J Hand Surg* 10B:155, 1985.

107. Swanson AB, Jaeger SH, LaRochelle D: Comminuted fracture of the radial head. The role of silicone implant replacement arthroplasty, *J Bone Joint Surg* 63A:1039, 1981.

108. Vanik RK, et al: The comparative strengths of internal fixation techniques, *J Hand Surg* 9A:216, 1984.

109. Watson FM Jr: Fractures in the hand, metacarpals and phalanges, *Emerg Med Clin North Am* 3:293, 1985.

110. Weeks PM, Wray RC: *Management of acute hand injuries: a biological approach,* ed 2, St Louis, 1978, Mosby.

111. Weiner RL, Fakharzadeh FF, Rosenstein RG: Open treatment of fingertip amputations, *Contemp Orthop* 24:549, 1992.

112. Whitesides TE Jr, et al: Tissue pressure measurements as a determinant for the need of fasciotomy, *Clin Orthop* 113:43, 1975.

113. Wong FY, Pho RW: Median nerve compression, with tendon ruptures after Colles' fracture, *J Hand Surg* 9B:139, 1984.

114. Wood VE: Fractures in the hand in children, *Orthop Clin North Am* 7:527, 1976.

115. Zacher JB: Management of injuries of the distal phalanx, *Surg Clin North Am* 64:747, 1984.

Chapter 24

MANAGEMENT OF NONARTICULAR FRACTURES OF THE HAND

Beth A. Purdy
Robert Lee Wilson

PATIENT EVALUATION

Fractures of the hand skeleton are more common than any other area of the body. The hand is made vulnerable as the primary instrument of human vocation, avocation, and expression. Therefore the treatment of hand injuries must take into account the person to whom the injury has occurred.

Hand dominance, age, occupation, and avocations all may direct treatment choices and outcome. The initial history should note the specific mechanism of injury, the time elapsed and treatment applied, and whether the injury was work-related. Associated illness, such as diabetes, immunocompromise, or peripheral vascular disease should also be noted. Allergies or medication intolerances are identified, as is tetanus immunization status.

Examination of a patient with a hand injury includes, at minimum, the entire limb. In penetrating injuries such as gunshot wounds or stabbings, or in cases of altered mental status, a complete physical examination is required.

Specific examination of the hand begins with inspection, noting the precise location of swelling, ecchymosis, abrasions, or lacerations, as well as obvious deformity. Gentle palpation should localize the point of maximal tenderness. A common temptation in cases of dramatic wounds or deformity is to focus the examination exclusively on the obvious, ignoring more subtle findings elsewhere in the hand or limb.

Rotational deformity is best evaluated with finger flexion (Fig. 24-1), but in cases where the injury prevents it, careful inspection of the plane of the nails, with close comparison with the other hand, offers a less exact assessment. Circulation is documented with capillary refill, warmth, and Allen's test at the wrist or digits when appropriate. Sensory evaluation includes, at minimum, light touch sensitivity, but may also document static or dynamic two-point discrimination, or monofilament threshold testing.

Ligament stability should be tested gently, but approached cautiously before radiographic evaluation to avoid inadvertent fracture displacement and unnecessary discomfort. Finally, tendon function is systematically evaluated.

Radiographic evaluation must include at least three views of the hand or digit. When evaluating a finger fracture, the lateral view offers the greatest information on joint alignment, and care must be taken to obtain a "perfect" lateral, even if it requires multiple attempts. Lateral views of the hand should always fan the fingers for maximal efficiency. Even when only spot views of a single digit are obtained, a single posteroanterior (PA) view of the hand should also be included to screen for other abnormalities such as previous trauma or degenerative arthritis.

PRINCIPLES OF TREATMENT

Total active range of motion (AROM) is the gold standard by which all hand injuries are measured, and stiffness in the

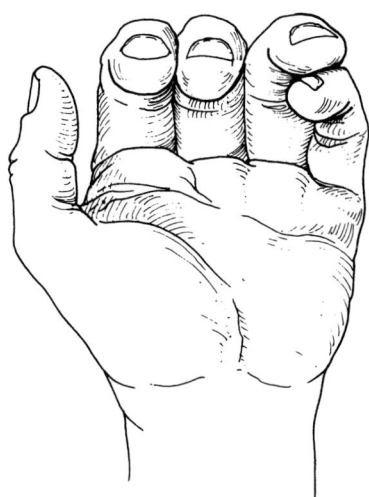

Fig. 24-1. Diagram of a malrotated ring finger.

hand is the adversary to be avoided. Treatment choices therefore are guided by the pursuit of motion. Fracture stability is first evaluated, and then associated soft tissue injury. The method that successfully stabilizes the fracture and most gently treats the soft tissue, allowing *early mobilization*, is the treatment of choice. The timing of treatment is crucial, yet often is compromised by delays in referrals to a hand surgeon by primary "gatekeepers" in the managed health care context. An interesting study by Davis and Stothard[9] defending early referral of all finger fractures to a hand surgeon found that almost 30% of fractures not treated by a hand surgeon had gross errors in treatment. These included failure to recognize open fractures or appropriately treat them with antibiotics, and inappropriate splinting. Impending malunions of hand fractures are also becoming more frequent with delays in definitive treatment, severely limiting clinical choices. These often require aggressive surgical treatment with correction of malalignment and early mobilization for return of function.[20]

Complications of open treatment

Early mobilization of unstable fractures demands rigid fixation. However, much has been written about the hazards associated with the use of plates and screws in the treatment of hand fractures. For instance, Stern et al.[31] reported on the use of 2.7- and 2.0-mm screws and plates in the treatment of metacarpal and phalangeal fractures, with complications seen in 67% of proximal phalanx platings and 34% of metacarpal platings. A relationship was seen between complications and the degree of soft tissue injury. No infections were noted. Complications included malunion, ruptured flexor tendons, and nonunion, which all were related to the technical application of the hardware. Stiffness was also a common complication, although formal mobilization was not begun in some cases until 21 days after surgery. A subsequent review by Page and Stern[27] again noted that complications of

---

proximal phalanx fixation were in excess of those of metacarpals. Many complications continued to be related to technique. One of the greatest disadvantages of plate fixation was its bulk, which interferes with the extensor apparatus. Their conclusion, after noting improvements in profile and configuration of modern plates, was that the primary determinant of outcome was not the plates themselves, but the circumstances in which they were used.

Hastings[18] also noted a high rate of complications with the use of plates and screws and categorized them according to errors in management (Box 24-1).

Chen et al.[7] outlined the many advantages of rigid internal fixation in the context of acute complex hand injury. The indications included unstable fractures, segmental defects, and extreme comminution. They believed that primary internal fixation, even in the face of extreme soft tissue injury, laid the foundation for tendon and neurovascular recovery. The resultant stable construct can minimize joint stiffness and tendon adhesions, and achieve rapid recovery with appropriate postoperative mobilization.

Open fractures in the hand

The close juxtaposition of the bony skeleton of the hand to the skin, combined with the propensity of the hand for injuries at work and play, makes open fracture common. Gustilo and Anderson's[17] classification of open fractures has been the prognostic gold standard for many years, but its application to hand injuries has required some imagination. McLain et al.[21] applied it to open hand fractures with minor modifications and, surprisingly, their conclusions did not demonstrate delay in treatment as a predictor for deep infection. They did note that *Staphylococcus aureus* was the most common infecting organism, but greater than one third were polymicrobial. Further classifications have been proposed, focusing on the specific soft tissue injury or contamination (Box 24-2 and Table 24-1).

Classification and prediction of outcome as presented by Chow et al.[8] was based on a prospective study of 245 open digital fractures. Associated flexor tendon injuries had the gravest prognosis. In this series, the incidence of infection and nonunion was not related to the character of the fracture or the severity of the soft tissue injury. Swanson et al.[32] also remarked that the rate of infection appeared unrelated to high-energy injuries; concomitant tendon, nerve, or vascular injury; and large wound size. In a review of 75 open hand

<table>
<tr><td colspan="2">

Box 24-2   Swanson classification of open hand fractures[32]

</td></tr>
<tr><td>

Type I

Clean wound without significant contamination or delay in treatment

and

No significant systemic illness

</td><td>

Type II

Contamination with gross dirt, debris, human or animal bites, warm lake/river injury, barnyard injury;

Delay in treatment greater than 24 hours;

or

Significant systemic illness (e.g., diabetes, rheumatoid arthritis, alcoholic hepatitis)

</td></tr>
</table>

Table 24-1. Chow classification of open digital fractures[8]

Type	Soft tissue injury	Expected outcome (%)		
		Good	Fair	Poor
I	Nil	41.7	32.5	25.8
	Digital nerve	38.5	38.5	23.1
II	Extensor tendon	18.8	31.2	50.0
	Extensive skin loss	15.0	40.0	45.0
III	Flexor tendon	0.0	0.0	100.0
	Two or more components	4.5	22.7	72.7

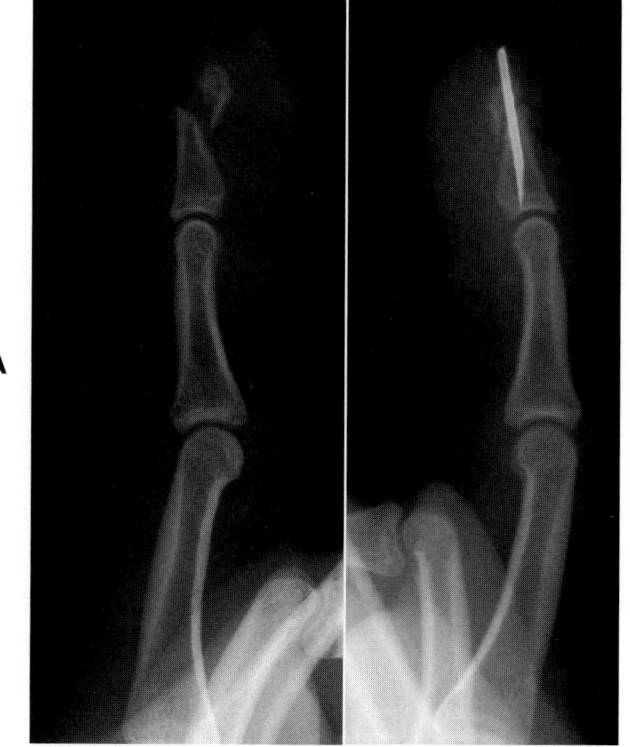

A   **B**

Fig. 24-2. A, Crush injury with obvious bony and soft tissue injury sustained when finger was caught between a forklift and a wall. **B,** Following irrigation and debridement, nailbed repair and grafting, and stabilization with a longitudinal 18-gauge needle.

fractures, Duncan et al.[12] found that the result attained at 6-month and 7-year follow-up did correlate with the level of associated soft tissue injury. Phalangeal fractures, especially proximal phalanx, fared much worse than metacarpal fractures. Results were further worsened when associated with tendon injury.

DISTAL PHALANX FRACTURES

Distal phalanx fractures are most commonly associated with crush injuries and often result in lacerations of the nailbed (Fig. 24-2). Kaplan's[19] classification has survived in its simplicity since 1940, describing longitudinal, tuft, and transverse fractures (Fig. 24-3). Tuft and longitudinal fractures generally have inherent stability and require immobilization for comfort only. Associated nailbed injuries at most may require nail plate removal and repair, and at least may require nail trephination to relieve the painful pressure of a subungual hematoma.

Even most transverse fractures have some stability afforded by the support of the fibrous septa connecting the skin to the bone. Occasionally, instability requires longitudinal pinning with either a K-wire or a needle (Fig. 24-4).

Open injuries necessitate careful debridement, tetanus prophylaxis, and appropriate antibiotic coverage. These injuries often result in severe hypersensitivity; therefore early attention must be paid to an aggressive desensitization program.

Distal phalanx injuries in children are complicated by the proximal physis. In toddlers, an axial load, such that would result in a mallet injury in an adult, can dorsally dislocate the

epiphysis. This epiphysis does not begin ossification until 22 to 36 months of age, making radiographic diagnosis difficult. Clinical suspicion is raised by the presence of a dorsal mass. If left untreated, it results in loss of longitudinal and circumferential growth, as well as nail abnormalities from associated injury to the germinal matrix.[34]

In children with Salter I or II injuries to the distal phalanx, the associated open soft tissue injury is often overlooked. The nail and underlying bed and sterile matrix can herniate dorsal to the nail fold. Persistence of this untreated can result in osteomyelitis and permanent nail growth deformities. Irrigation and debridement, followed by reduction and repair of the nailbed, is necessary. Supplementation

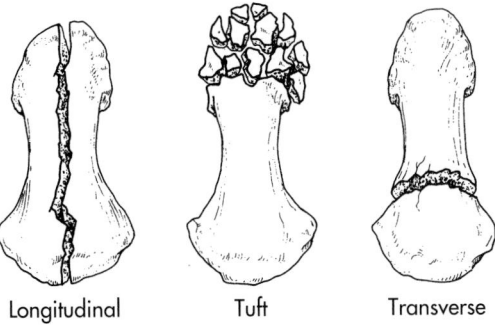

Fig. 24-3. Kaplan's classification of fractures of the distal phalanx based on location and fracture pattern.

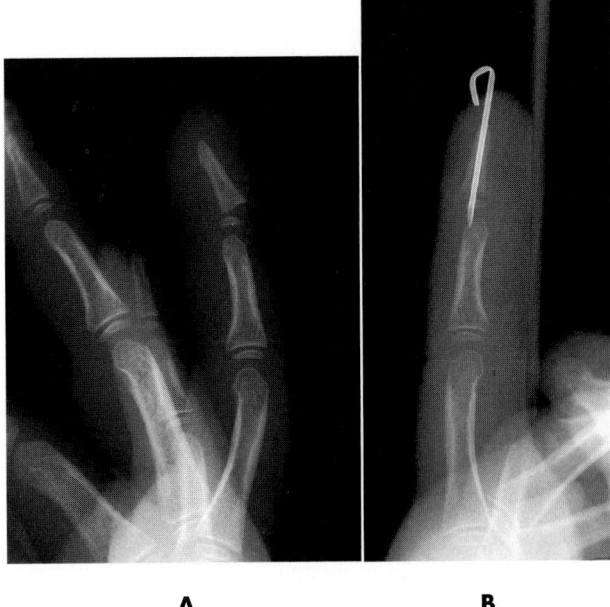

Fig. 24-5. A, Missed open physeal injury, seen 10 days after the incident. **B,** After irrigation and debridement of open fracture, nailbed repair, and pinning with an 18-gauge needle.

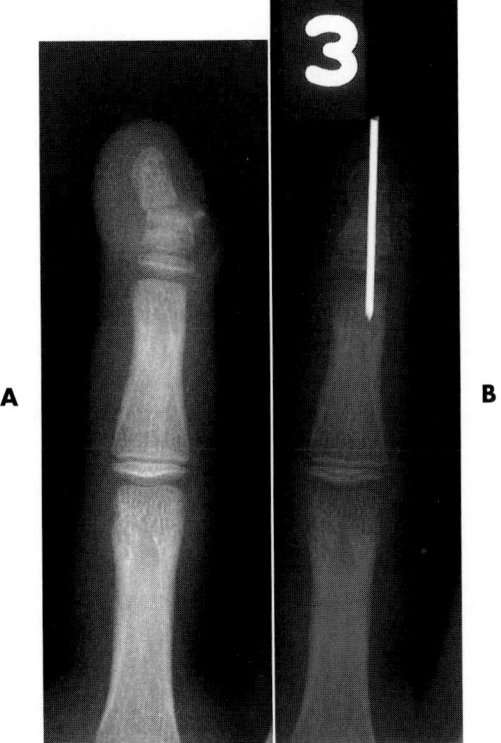

Fig. 24-4. A, This 12-year-old boy sustained a crush injury to his right middle finger, resulting in an open fracture of the distal phalanx and a nailbed injury. **B,** After irrigation, debridement, nailbed repair, and pinning.

with a longitudinal wire for stability is sometimes needed (Fig. 24-5).

Therapy concerns after distal phalanx fractures

The most common problems that occur after distal phalanx fractures, particularly following a crush injury, are pain and hypersensitivity. Limited motion at the distal interphalangeal (DIP) joint, most noticeably flexion, may also develop. A desensitization program should be initiated, with the patient beginning with rubbing the pulp and tapping the tip of the injured digit. This is initiated as soon as the skin healing is stable enough to tolerate it. Splinting of distal

phalanx fractures is rarely required for greater than 3 weeks, and in the case of isolated tuft fractures, often may be less. The patient will next progress to resistive pinch and grasping activities. A variety of modalities can be used including fluidotherapy, vibration, transcutaneous electrical nerve stimulation, and fabric manipulation. When the fracture has healed and the distal phalanx can be remobilized, exercises should be directed at the DIP joint. If both passive and active motion at the distal joint are decreased, a dynamic flexion splint may be helpful. Another technique is to tape the DIP joint in the flexed position for short periods, particularly when the patient is at rest. A rubber glove can be used to stretch both interphalangeal (IP) joints into flexion and should be used for only brief periods of time (3 to 5 minutes). When attempting to regain flexion, care must be taken that the activities are not so vigorous that an extensor lag occurs.

MIDDLE AND PROXIMAL PHALANX FRACTURES
Etiology

Middle and proximal phalanx fractures have been shown to be most common in 10- to 29-year-olds, with sport injuries as the leading cause. Accidental falls are the most common etiology in the elderly population. People ages 40 to 69 years are most frequently injured by machinery.[11]

Biomechanics

Middle phalanx fracture angulation is influenced by position relative to the broad flexor digitorum superficialis insertion along the proximal one third of the middle phalanx.

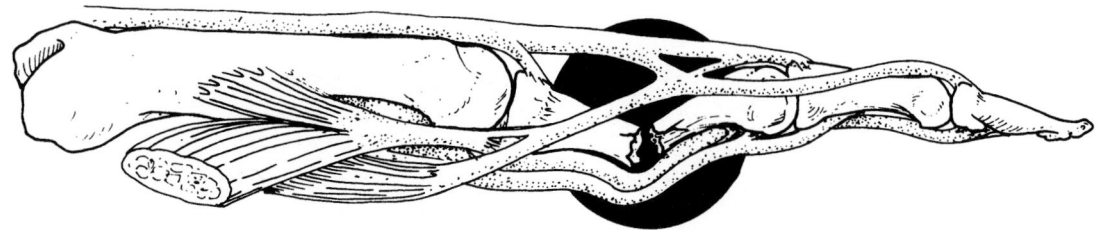

Fig. 24-6. Diagram showing the deforming forces of the intrinsic muscles that result in an apex volar angulation of proximal phalanx fractures.

Fractures distal to that insertion will tend to deform apex volar, and those proximal will rotate apex dorsal, relative to which fragment is controlled by the superficialis.

Proximal phalanx fractures are more indirectly influenced by the interossei, whose vectors flex the proximal fragment and extend the distal one, resulting in apex volar angulation (Fig. 24-6). This will result in decreased extension of the proximal interphalangeal (PIP) joint from laxity of the extensor, and secondary flexion contractures. Vahey, Wegner, and Hastings[33] demonstrated a linear relationship between proximal phalanx shortening by angulation and resultant extensor tendon redundancy with every 1 mm of discrepancy leading to 12 degrees of PIP extensor lag. This was without consideration for the almost certainly associated extensor adhesion, which would further exacerbate the lag (Table 24-2).

The intimate proximity of the proximal and middle phalanges to the flexor sheath and extensor apparatus is functional genius under healthy conditions, but adhesions relative to the hemorrhage of fracture, abrasions of the tendons, and malaligned fragments can present a sometimes insurmountable therapeutic challenge in maintaining mobility. Agee[1] succinctly outlined an optimal repair as one that results in restoration of anatomy with a method permitting active IP motion with tendon gliding during healing.

Phalangeal neck fractures

Fractures of the middle or proximal phalanx neck are seen most frequently in children. Newington et al.[25] reviewed five cases of proximal phalanx neck fractures with 180-degree rotational deformity. These occurred when the finger was caught in a door or drawer and then sharply withdrawn. All cases required open reduction, with the phalangeal head found herniated through a rent in the dorsal capsule, and the volar plate invaginated into the PIP joint. Full recovery was seen in all cases. Newington's group strongly recommend against the application of a distracting force when attempting to reduce those fractures that are rotated less than 180 degrees. The dorsal origin of the collateral ligament will spin the rotating fragment volarly, completing the 180-degree turn.

In contrast, Mintzer et al.[23] offered a case report of a missed middle phalangeal neck fracture in a 7-year-old boy

Table 24-2. Proximal phalanx angulation and proximal interphalangeal (PIP) lag

Average apex palmar angulation	PIP lag
16 degrees	10 degrees
27 degrees	24 degrees
46 degrees	66 degrees

erroneously treated with a splint. The fragment was 100% dorsally displaced at presentation 10 weeks after injury. Complete remodeling was seen within 15 months after injury, with normal motion and no rotational deformity.

Neck fractures of the proximal or middle phalanges generally are treated with percutaneous pin fixation after closed reduction with maximal IP joint flexion (Fig. 24-7). In adults, unstable periarticular phalangeal neck fractures also may be treated successfully with a minicondylar plate, as outlined by Ouellette and Freeland.[26] Placement of the plate laterally minimized interference with the extensor mechanism. Hardware prominence is the most common complication. With anatomic restoration achieving stability and early motion, good and excellent recoveries can be expected.

Phalangeal shaft fractures

Stable fractures of the proximal or middle phalangeal shafts can be treated with functional splinting and close clinical and radiographic follow-up. Unstable fractures require more aggressive treatment, and therein lies tremendous debate regarding the treatment options available. As previously emphasized, techniques resulting in stable fixation with minimal resultant tendon adhesions are ideal; open techniques using plates or screws are demanding, but when used appropriately fulfill that criteria, and early mobilization and tendon gliding is achieved. Pun et al.[29] prospectively followed proximal and middle phalanx fractures, openly treated. Nine complications in 52 fractures were directly related to technique or implant, such as penetration of the articular surface by a condylar blade plate. The dismayed appraisal by Pun's group was that the technique showed no benefit over K-wire fixation.

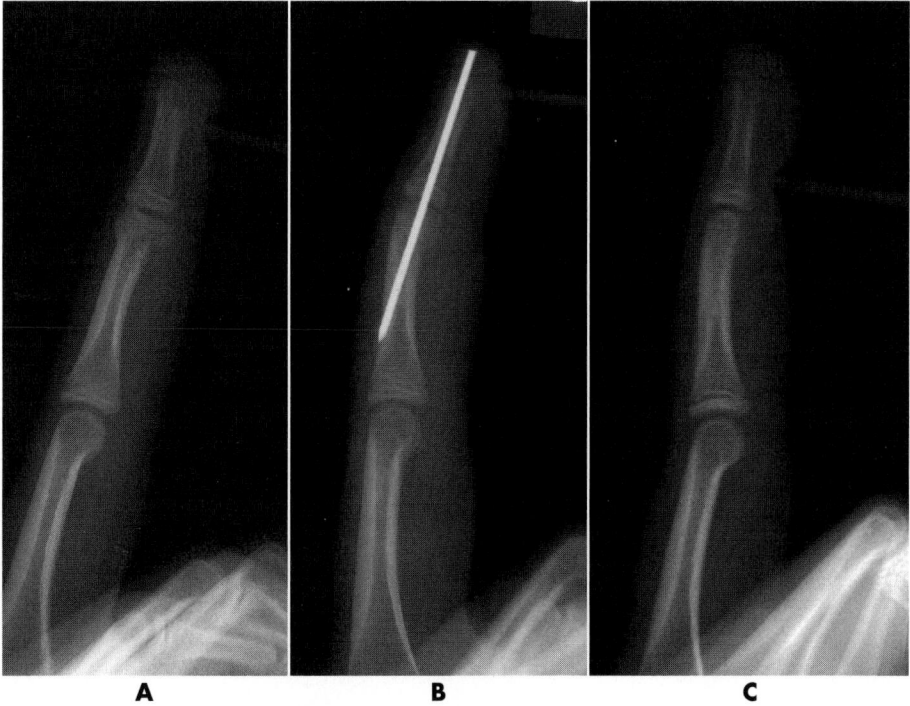

Fig. 24-7. A, Rotated phalangeal neck fracture in a 12-year-old girl. **B,** After closed reduction and percutaneous pinning. **C,** Fracture healing 6 weeks postoperatively.

A technique of intramedullary nailing has been presented by Gonzalez et al.[14,16] for the treatment of transverse or oblique fractures without bicortical comminution and excluding long oblique or spiral fractures. Small 0.8-mm-diameter rods were introduced through drill holes, packing the intramedullary space snugly. Immediate postoperative PIP motion was begun in a "clam-digger" splint. Total AROM averaged 238 degrees.

Complications of pin fixation were highlighted by Botte et al.[6] in a review of pins placed around the hand and wrist. They reported a 69% complication rate in the phalanges, including infection, loosening, loss of fixation, nonunion, and impaled flexor tendon. Superficial or pin tract infections accounted for the greatest percentage of complications (Fig. 24-8).

External fixation is another possible treatment of complex phalangeal extraarticular fractures. Their use is considered in the context of severe comminution, bony defects, or complex soft tissue wounds requiring access for care (e.g., gunshot wounds). External fixators offer stable but not rigid fixation and, with care in pin placement, result in minimal soft tissue trauma. Their bulk often interferes with surrounding digits, pin tract infection is of concern, and fracture reduction is less precise than with open techniques.[24] Availability of appropriately sized fixators for

use in the hand is improving. Shehadi[30] reviewed 26 cases of metacarpal and phalangeal fractures treated with an external fixator composed of K-wires and plastic tubing filled with methylmethacrylate. The pins were placed midlaterally. He reported no rotational deformities, loss of reduction, or pin tract infections.

Finally, open reduction and internal fixation with screws and/or plates offers stability in construct with the resultant opportunity for early mobilization. Obvious disadvantages, as previously stated, include a high level of required technical skill and soft tissue disruption necessary for exposure. Multiple studies exist recounting the pitfalls and perils of plate and screw fixation, especially in the phalanges.[12,18,27,31] We believe that most of the complications outlined (malunion, nonunion, loss of fixation, flexor tendon rupture from screw penetration, and postoperative stiffness) represent surgical inattention to detail and lack of appropriate mobilization postoperatively.

Bosscha and Snellen[5] treated 47 metacarpal and phalangeal fractures with AO minifragment screws and plates, treating the phalangeal fractures postoperatively with a soft bandage, and formally mobilizing at 3 weeks. Of both the metacarpal and phalangeal fractures, 92% had excellent recovery of total active flexion. The current availability of appropriately sized implants, reduction tools, and clear

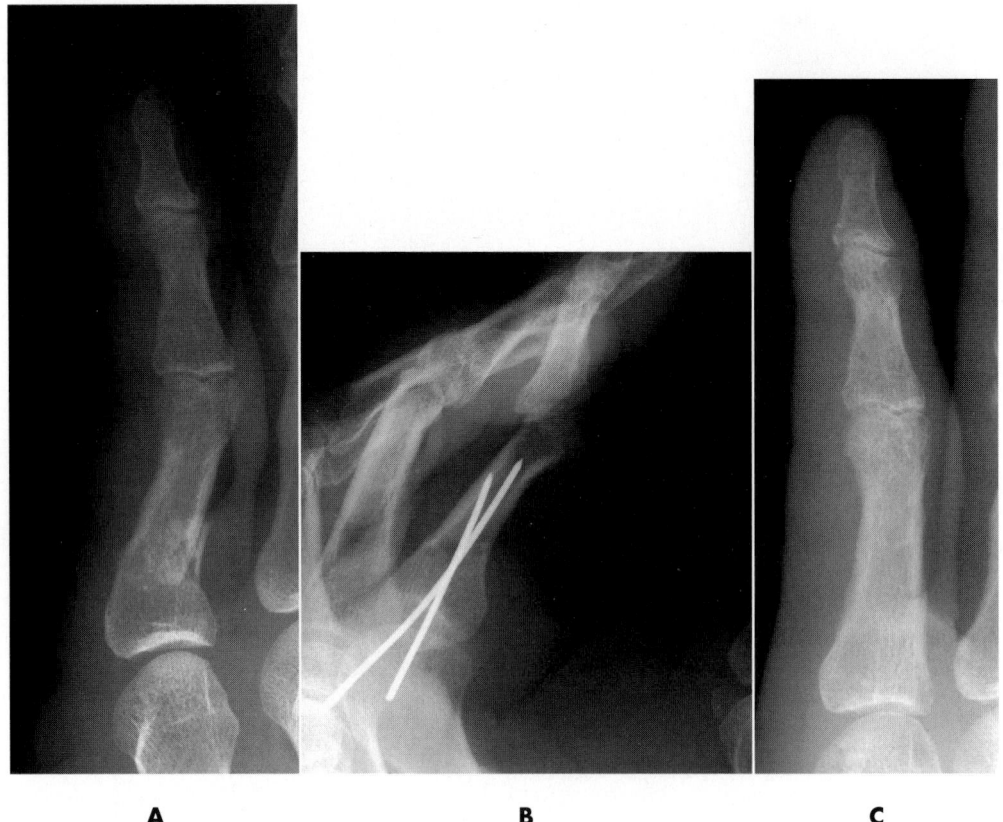

A   **B**   **C**

Fig. 24-8. A, This 51-year-old plumber caught his right index finger between a wrench and an adjacent pipe. **B,** After closed reduction and pinning. **C,** Five months after injury with return of nearly full range of motion.

intraoperative fluoroscopy has greatly expanded the application. For example, the Synthes Hand Modular set (Synthes USA Corporation, Paoli, Pennsylvania) offers four separate trays with differing sizes of screws and plates (Figs. 24-9 and 24-10).

Therapy considerations after proximal and middle phalangeal fractures

When planning a treatment program, the therapist must have a clear understanding of the fracture's pattern, location, deforming forces, soft tissue involvement, and any associated injuries. If the fracture has been treated surgically, the therapist needs to understand the technique of immobilization of the fracture fragments and whether a stable construct has been achieved.

When a proximal phalanx fracture has been rendered absolutely stable, the patient can be promptly remobilized. At 24 to 72 hours after surgery, the patient should be referred to therapy, the bulky surgical dressing removed, and the wounds evaluated. Prime considerations include regaining PIP joint mobility, controlling edema, and avoiding flexion contractures. AROM and PROM exercises are initiated (the latter by the therapist), and these should emphasize tendon gliding over the area of the fracture and PIP joint extension.

The patient should be placed in a hand-based resting splint with the metacarpophalangeal (MP) joints flexed and the IP joints extended (e.g., in the safe or clam-digger position). This splint should remain in place between exercise periods and at night. On occasion, a splint holding the digit in extension at the IP joints may be satisfactory. Dynamic splinting and taping the digits in flexion may be necessary to improve joint motion. When the wounds are healed and the sutures are removed, scar remobilization techniques are initiated and Coban can be used to diminish edema. Splinting to protect the fracture usually can be discontinued 4 to 6 weeks after surgery, except when the patient is participating in contact sports. Protection can be achieved with buddy taping and light resistive exercises should be initiated. At 6 to 8 weeks, heavy resistance and strengthening exercises are started.

If absolute fracture stability cannot be achieved through internal fixation (because of comminution, bone loss, and the like), early active and passive motion may not be allowed. However, if the surgeon believes that sufficient stability has been achieved to allow a gentle remobilization program, this may be initiated at 3 to 10 days. As previously mentioned, edema control is a prime consideration and the patient will require protective splinting and directed exercises. For prox-

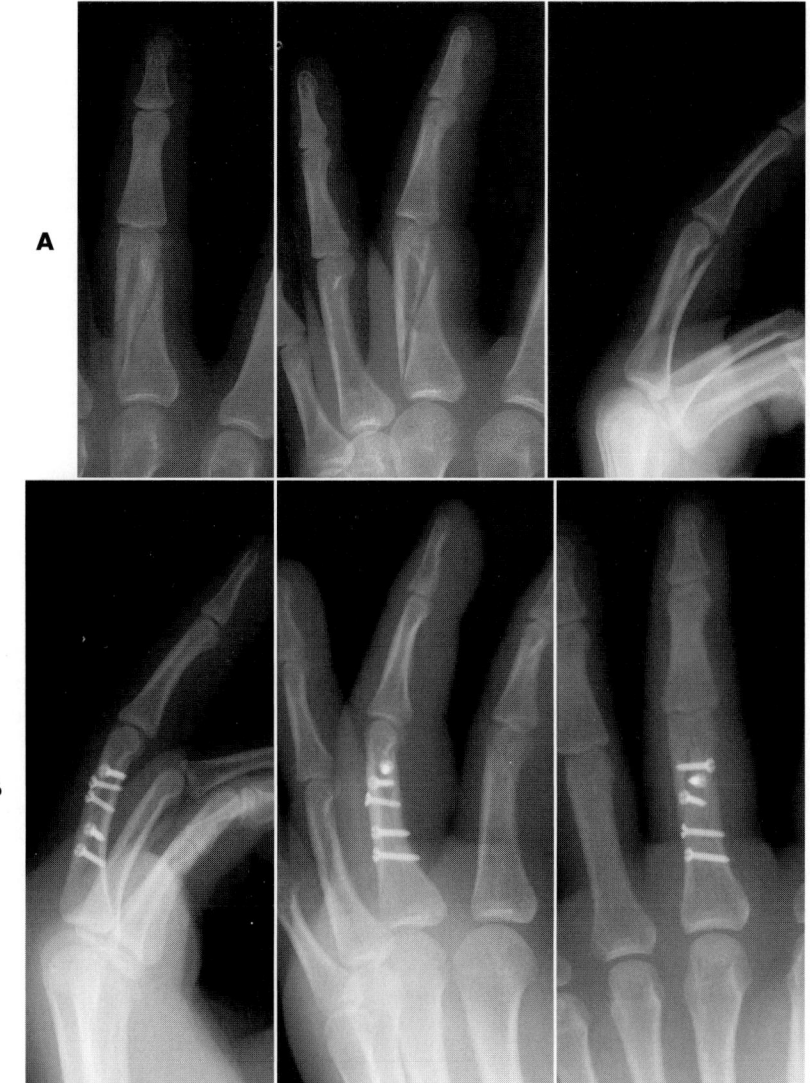

Fig. 24-9. A, Comminuted spiral fracture of the proximal phalanx in a 29-year-old laborer. **B,** After open reduction and screw fixation obtaining stable anatomic fixation. Mobilization was begun on postoperative day 2 with nearly full recovery of motion.

imal phalanx fractures involving the base or midportion, a hand-based splint as previously mentioned is used. For more distal fractures at the head and neck, a digital splint to maintain IP joint extension is provided. With all proximal phalanx fractures, active, active assistive, and passive motion at the IP joints is the main focus. With fractures involving the more proximal portion of the proximal phalanx, the therapist or the patient can provide supplemental support to the fracture with manual pressure. When treating more distal fractures (proximal phalanx head or neck), prompt active motion at the MP joint is initiated. By 3 weeks, AROM is carried out at all joints with protective splinting between exercises and at night. When the surgeon believes the fracture is sufficiently healed clinically, the therapist may include a PROM program and dynamic splinting, if needed.

The most serious complication that can happen after a proximal phalanx fracture is the occurrence of a fixed PIP joint flexion contracture. Contractures at this joint occur because of the relatively weak extension force in comparison with the strong flexion force and is compounded by the normal resting flexion posture of the PIP joint.[35] To prevent this, the PIP joint should be splinted in full extension. A dynamic PIP joint extension splint should be initiated at the first sign of a flexion deformity as long as the fracture is sufficiently healed. The second complication is limited active PIP joint extension when the patient has full passive extension of this joint secondary to adherence of the extensor mechanism at the fracture site. The best therapy procedure for this complication is extensor mechanism blocking exercises using a splint that will prevent MP joint hyperex-

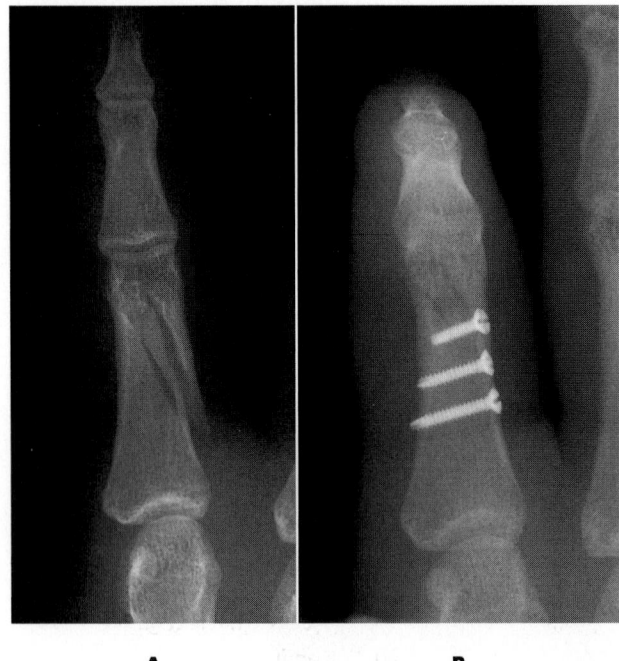

Fig. 24-10. A, Spiral fracture of the proximal phalanx in a 19-year-old landscaper. **B,** After open reduction and screw fixation through a lateral approach. Full motion was achieved postoperatively with an aggressive mobilization program.

tension. This will allow concentration of the extension force at the PIP joint. Extrinsic and intrinsic extensor muscle stimulation occasionally will prove helpful. Limited flexion at both the MP and PIP joints may occur as a result of secondary capsuloligamentous tightness. To overcome such problems, a dynamic flexion assist splint, the application of a continuous passive motion machine, or taping the fingers into the flexed position may prove helpful.

When flexor tendon adherence occurs at the fracture site, limiting active flexion of the digit, muscle stimulation of the flexors may be necessary. Tendon gliding exercises are also appropriate.

Middle phalanx fractures, although uncommon, can result in limited motion at both the PIP and DIP joints. The primary objective after middle phalanx fractures is to realize full motion at the two more proximal joints (MP and PIP). The goal is to achieve a "superficialis hand" with full flexion of the MP and PIP joints. If lengthy rest splinting extends to the proximal phalanx, the PIP joint will become stiff. A middle phalanx fracture may require a longer period to consolidate, but when stabilized with a pin, early active and gentle passive motion can be carried out at the PIP joint.

A PIP flexion contracture is not uncommon after a fracture involving the middle phalanx base. To prevent this, the splint should rest the PIP joint in full extension. When a PIP joint flexion contracture occurs, a dynamic extension splint should be used. Limited motion at the DIP joint is common, particularly with fractures in the distal half of the middle phalanx. The DIP joint must be splinted in full extension and remobilized with blocking exercises. If the program is too vigorous, a flexion deformity or an extension lag at the DIP joint will occur and the joint motion must be monitored constantly. To treat an extension contracture at the DIP joint, a dynamic flexion splint may be used or the IP joints of the finger may be taped into flexion. This technique should be applied for 20 to 30 minutes four times a day, and at night if tolerated. If the flexor digitorum profundus tendon becomes adherent over the middle phalanx, limited active DIP flexion can occur. Profundus tendon blocking exercises and electrical stimulation to the profundus tendon can be used.

METACARPAL FRACTURES
Etiology

The highest incidence of metacarpal fractures is found in 10- to 29-year-old males. In a 1994 review by deJonge et al.,[10] of almost 4000 metacarpal fractures, motor vehicle and bicycle accidents were found to be the major determinants in all age groups. In our experience, clenched fist injuries seem to hold predominance.

Anatomic considerations

Injuries to the metacarpals may compromise basic structural support of the hand, and treatment must include attention to the natural arches of the hand (Fig. 24-11). Slight rotational deformities at the metacarpal level will be exaggerated with full flexion of the phalanges. The intricate extensor mechanism, with its limited excursion, is very sensitive to shortening of greater than 3 mm, and can result in an extensor lag. In contrast, extensor adhesion at the metacarpal level will lead to significant loss of finger flexion or extrinsic tightness.

Metacarpal base fractures

Extraarticular fractures of the metacarpal base are often stable. Their healing is hastened by their metaphyseal location, and in the stable setting may be treated with splinting for 3 to 4 weeks. In cases of displacement, angulation, and/or shortening, closed reduction and pinning or open reduction may be required (Fig. 24-12).

Metacarpal shaft fractures

Metacarpal fractures, as with fractures of all long bones, are subject to displacement, angulation, rotation, and shortening. Shortening in the central middle and ring finger metacarpals is limited by the distal support of the transverse intermetacarpal ligaments. Angulation is almost always apex dorsal, from the vector applied by the interossei and the long flexors. With the apex dorsal angulation, significant displacement is frequent. Comminution, when present, is often volar, contributing to the angulation and instability. Short oblique

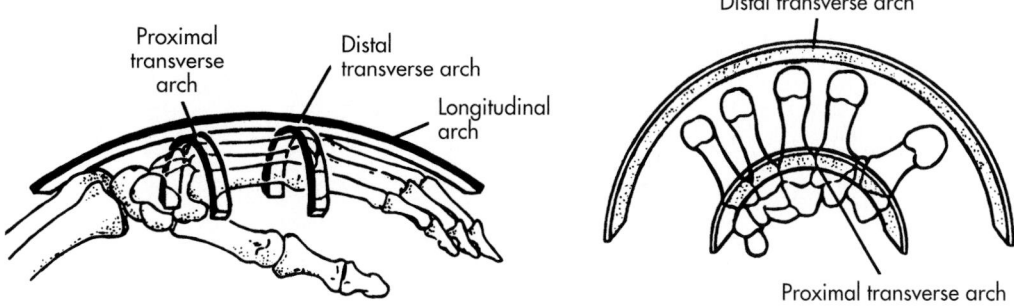

Fig. 24-11. A diagram of the longitudinal, proximal transverse, and distal transverse arches of the hand. The longitudinal arch extends through the metacarpal and phalanges of the middle finger. The proximal transverse arch is located at the base of the metacarpals, and the distal transverse arch is located through the metacarpal heads. (Courtesy the American Society of Surgery of the Hand.)

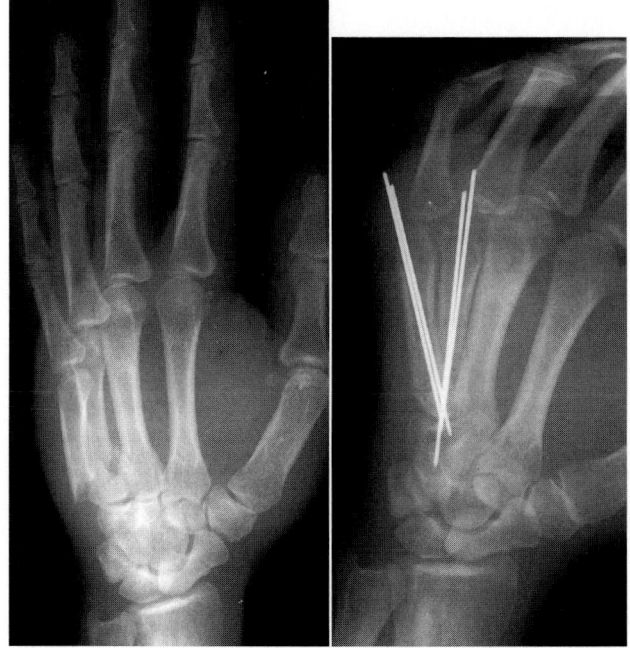

A

B

Fig. 24-12. **A,** This 45-year-old male hit a door in anger, suffering extraarticular fractures of the fourth and fifth metacarpals. The injury was 3 weeks old at presentation. **B,** After open reduction and pinning.

or spiral fractures from a torquing injury need very minimal shortening to result in significant rotational deformity.

Stable fractures of the metacarpal diaphysis are usually treated with immobilization for 3 to 5 weeks, holding the injured finger and an adjacent one, leaving the IP joints free and the MP joints flexed to 70 degrees. This is followed by a period of intermittent protective splinting in coordination with mobilization. Close radiographic and clinical follow-up is necessary to monitor for changes in reduction or the development of a rotatory deformity.

McMahon et al.[22] compared treatment with a standard plaster splint with application of a compressive glove and early mobilization for stable metacarpal fractures. The rationale behind the use of the glove was that it offered controlled compression of the soft tissues, which would in turn stabilize the fractures. Additional benefit would be control of swelling and the ability to mobilize the hand freely. Indeed, they found significant decrease in swelling and stiffness, each as independent variables.

Indications for internal fixation have been clearly outlined by Ashkenaze and Ruby.[4] These include inability to achieve or maintain an adequate reduction, any rotational malalignment, marked comminution, or excessive angulation. Relative indications were fractures seen on a delayed basis or marked associated soft tissue trauma. Hastings[18] added multiple fractures as a clear indication, and clarified unstable fractures as displaced transverse, short oblique, or short spiral fractures, as well as those with a segmental defect.

Methods of fixation range from K-wire fixation to screws and plates. Transverse or short oblique fractures are amenable to plate fixation, using a lag screw across the fracture if possible (Fig. 24-13). At least four cortices should be engaged on each side of the fracture. Plates should be applied dorsally to provide the greatest rigidity to a dorsal apex load, as shown by Prevel et al.[28] Gonzalez et al.[15] reviewed the technique of intramedullary nailing of 98 metacarpal fractures, filling the medullary canal with 0.8-mm blunted nails. Postoperatively, a clam-digger splint was applied with immediate IP motion. They concluded that nailing afforded excellent results when proper selection of fractures and good surgical technique were applied.

Long oblique or spiral fractures are nicely treated with screw fixation, when the length of the fracture is at least twice the width of the diaphysis (Fig. 24-14).

Metacarpal neck fractures

Metacarpal neck fractures are most common on the ulnar side of the hand, and most frequently occur from clenched fist trauma. A high suspicion must be maintained for associated human bite wounds, which certainly will result in

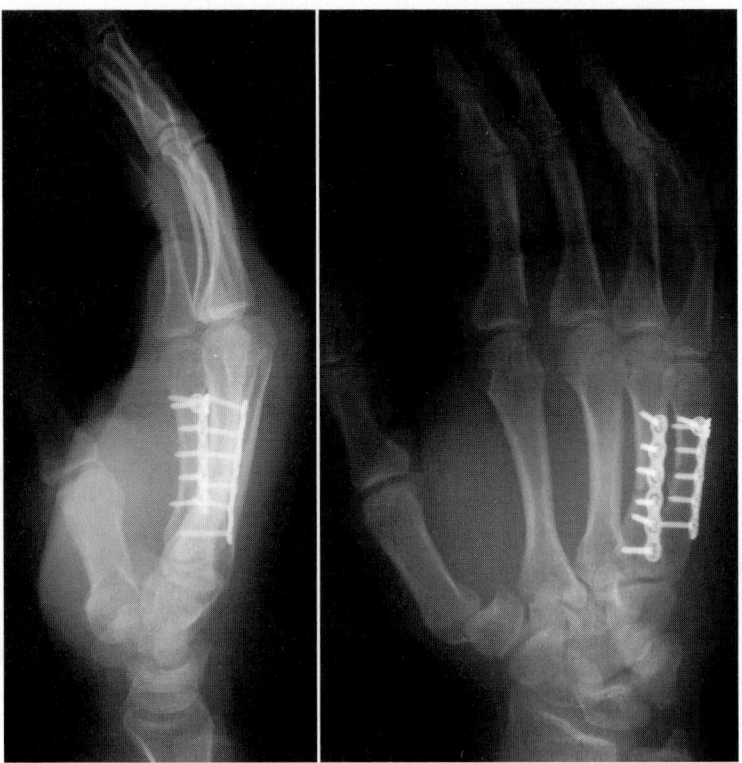

Fig. 24-13. A crush injury of the right hand in a 45-year-old resulted in open fractures of the fourth and fifth metacarpal shafts. Immediate open treatment followed by aggressive mobilization resulted in full return of motion and fracture healing.

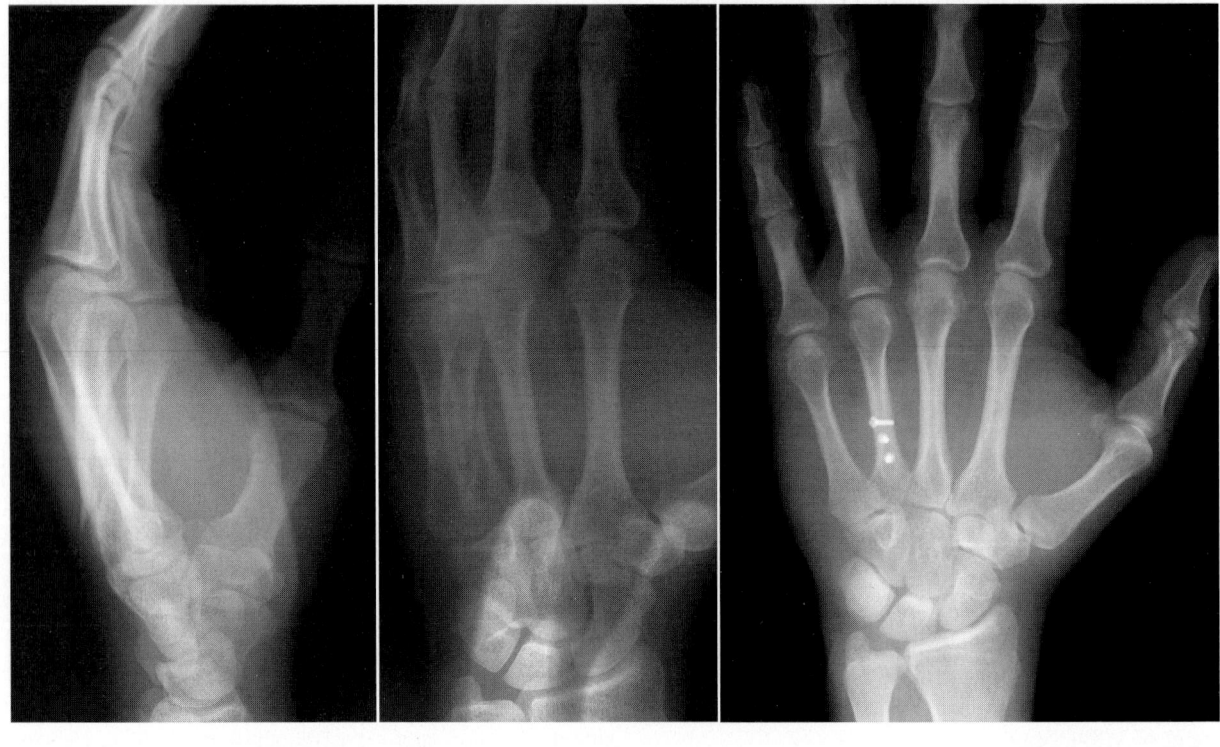

A   B

Fig. 24-14. A, Short spiral fracture of the ring metacarpal sustained in a brawl. **B,** Anatomic stable screw fixation.

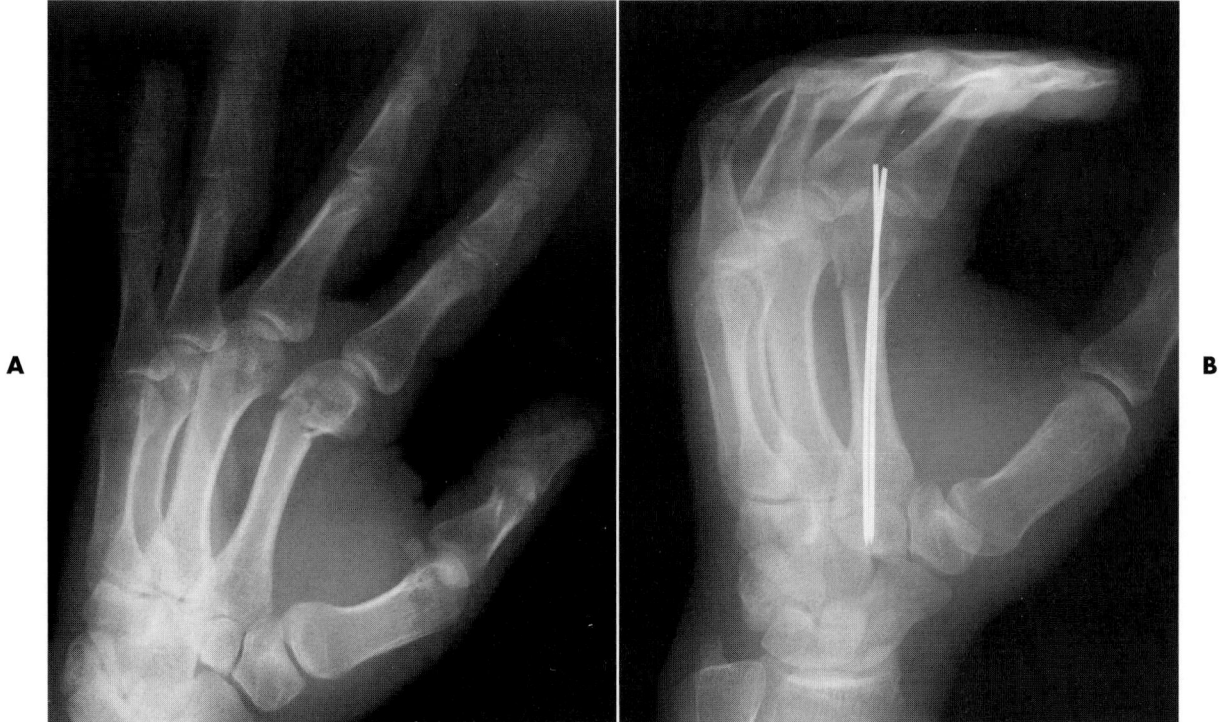

Fig. 24-15. A, Index metacarpal neck fracture in a 25-year-old male, sustained in a motor vehicle accident. **B,** Following closed reduction and pinning.

local sepsis. These require incision, arthrotomy, irrigation, and possible extensor tendon repair. Antibiotic coverage appropriate for both skin and oral flora is also necessary. Any laceration over the metacarpal head in association with a metacarpal neck fracture should be presumed to be a human bite wound with deep inoculation into the MP joint until proven otherwise.

The mobility of the fourth and fifth carpometacarpal joints has classically allowed for greater acceptance of persistent angulation on the ulnar side of the hand. Index and middle finger metacarpal neck fractures with angulation greater than 10 to 15 degrees are very poorly tolerated and often require operative treatment (Fig. 24-15).

Tremendous variability in treatment recommendations for fifth metacarpal neck fractures exist in the literature. Anatomic purists focus on the alteration in mechanical advantage by the relative shortening and resultant vector changes and muscle length, and recommend tolerance of less than 30 degrees of angulation.[2] Many other studies present a more pragmatic view, seeking to find if any treatment beyond temporary activity modification is necessary. Ford et al.[13] prospectively studied 62 fractures with angulation up to 70 degrees, treating them with early active motion only. Ford's group reported that the acute discomfort resolved in a few days, with some pain after vigorous activity persisting to some degree during the early months following injury. The lump on the dorsum of the hand was unchanged at a year

after injury. No patient was bothered by palmar prominence or weakness, either subjectively or by clinical measure. Arafa et al.[3] also reported an excellent return to even manual labor within 4 weeks, using a similar treatment plan.

In the selection of the appropriate treatment, the personality of both the patient and the fracture must be appraised. In the setting of multiple previous clenched fist injuries and a declared propensity to continue in that vein, conservative treatment would seem ideal. This may be less appropriate in a highly skilled musician whose hand may adapt less readily to its required task. Whatever treatment is chosen, whether early active motion only, reduction/immobilization, or internal fixation, mobilization of the IP joints must begin immediately. This leaves the only remaining hurdle following fracture healing to be the mobilization of the MP joint.

Therapy concerns after metacarpal fractures. Before a therapy program can be established for metacarpal fractures, the stability of the fracture fragments must be known. Fractures that are unstable after closed reduction or a comminuted fracture that is only partially stabilized with percutaneous or internal fixation will not permit an active motion program within the first few weeks. Fractures with stable or semirigid fixation will allow protected early AROM and a gentle passive motion program by the therapist. Fractures in this class include those that have been stabilized with percutaneous Kirschner wires and those that have been internally fixed with a plate and screws, a tension band, or a lag screw. A stable fracture construct achieved through compression of the fracture fragments will allow both early AROM and PROM. The therapist needs to understand the location and type of fracture and the degree of the soft tissue injury. Complex wounds that include extensor tendon disruptions and ligament injuries to the small joints will require special considerations. Postinjury edema associated with metacarpal fractures can pose a major difficulty.

Metacarpal fractures that are rigidly stabilized can be remobilized at 24 to 72 hours after surgery. Initial considerations include edema control as well as AROM and PROM exercises. The exercise program should include isolated extensor digitorum exercises as well as independent MP joint flexion and composite flexion of the fingers. Between exercise periods and at night, the hand should be splinted in the safe or intrinsic plus position. This splint should include the fingers and the wrist. After the postoperative pain is controlled, flexion taping and a dynamic flexion splint may be used for limitations in MP flexion. Scar remodeling techniques are begun at 2 weeks. By 4 weeks, the protective splint is discontinued and gentle resistant exercises are started. Buddy taping is used as needed. At 6 weeks, the patient is started on a more vigorous exercise program and this includes the use of weights and the work simulator. When dorsal scarring poses a problem, a silicone elastomer pressure splint may be applied and scar mobilization techniques can be used. If the fracture is not rigidly fixed, sufficient stability may be present to allow an early active and active assistive ROM program. The patient or the therapist may provide additional support to the area of the fracture. When incomplete stability is achieved, PROM exercises are not initiated until 3 to 4 weeks after injury and these are initially directed toward the MP joint. Dynamic flexion splinting and active exercises can be initiated at 4 weeks.

When the fracture remains unstable, the doctor treating the patient should be consulted about the time table for remobilization. In general, AROM should be initiated by 3 to 4 weeks.

The most common complication following a metacarpal fracture is disproportionate dorsal edema. This can be managed by retrograde massage, compressive splinting, a compression glove (e.g., Isotoner), and occasionally, Coban wrapping. Tendon adherence to a metacarpal fracture is an unusual complication. However, if the patient has a combined injury that includes trauma to the extensor tendons, skin, and soft tissue, as well as fractures, all of these tissues may adhere to one another. For patients with these complex injuries, consideration should be given to an early passive motion and remobilization program. (See Chapter 31.) If extensor tendon adherence does occur, the program should include isolated extensor digitorum communis exercises, for example, MP extension while holding the PIP joints taped in a flexed position, scar massage, electrical stimulation directed toward the extensor tendons, and periodic extension splinting with outriggers. This splint will assist MP extension, while providing resistance to MP flexion—the motion that will provide a force directed at the extensor tendon at the point of adherence.

MP joint extension contractures can occur if the proximal joints are not splinted in flexion during the immediate postinjury period. Dynamic flexion splints are indicated. Intrinsic tightness can develop and the patient should be carefully evaluated for this complication. When present, intrinsic stretching exercises and dynamic IP joint flexion with the proximal phalanx stabilized may improve this condition.

THERAPY CONSIDERATION AFTER THUMB FRACTURES

Loss of motion following fractures to the thumb is often greater than in the fingers. Fortunately, the thumb is better able to compensate for any residual deformity than stiffness in the fingers. One often overlooked complication following a thumb metacarpal fracture is adduction of the first metacarpal. Postfracture or postoperative splinting must not allow a contracture of the thumb web space.

Remobilization and therapy after fractures to the thumb is similar in principle to that for the fingers. Mild angulation of the thumb metacarpal fracture is acceptable because of compensatory motion at the trapeziometacarpal joint. Loss of motion at the MP joint of the thumb results in substantially less decrease in function than a similar loss of motion at a finger MP joint.

Metacarpal fractures that are rigidly stabilized are treated with a prompt remobilization program. Fractures that have less than rigid fixation or ones treated by cast immobilization alone should begin a remobilization program at 3 to 4 weeks depending on the clinical signs of fracture healing. The patient is placed in a thumb spica splint and started with active and active assistive ROM exercises and a gentle passive motion program by the therapist. As noted previously, any splinting program should prevent a first web contracture. With increasing comfort on the patient's part, the splint may be discontinued and a strengthening program initiated.

Phalangeal fractures at the thumb are managed in a similar manner to those of the fingers.

SUMMARY

Treatment of nonarticular fractures of the hand is a challenge balancing stability and mobility. Treatment is guided by the personality of the fracture, the biomechanics involved, and the person to whom the injury occurred. Communication among the surgeon, therapist, and patient is essential for an excellent result, with that result easily impacted by any of the participants. The simplest technique achieving the most stable constrict allowing the earliest mobilization is the treatment of choice and must be individualized for each unique injury.

REFERENCES

1. Agee J: Treatment principles for proximal and middle phalangeal fractures, *Orthop Clinic North Am* 23:35, 1992.
2. Ali A, Hamman J, Mass DP: The biomechanical effects of angulated boxer's fractures, *J Hand Surg* 24A:835, 1999.
3. Arafa M, et al: Immediate mobilization of fractures of the neck of the fifth metacarpal, *Injury* 17:277, 1986.
4. Ashkenaze DM, Ruby LK: Metacarpal fractures and dislocations, *Orthop Clinic North Am* 23:19, 1992.
5. Bosscha K, Snellen JP: Internal fixation of metacarpal and phalangeal fractures with AO minifragment screws and plates: a prospective study, *Injury* 24:166, 1993.
6. Botte MJ, et al: Complications of smooth pin fixation of fractures and dislocations in the hand and wrist, *Clin Orthop* 276:194, 1992.
7. Chen SHT, et al: Miniature plates and screws in acute complex hand injury, *J Trauma* 37:237, 1994.
8. Chow SP, et al: A prospective study of 245 open digital fractures of the hand, *J Hand Surg* 16B:137, 1991.
9. Davis TRC, Stothard J: Why all finger fractures should be referred to a hand surgery service: a prospective study of primary management, *J Hand Surg* 15B:299, 1990.
10. deJonge JJ, et al: Fractures of the metacarpals: a retrospective analysis of incidence and aetiology and a review of the English-language literature, *Injury* 25:365, 1994.
11. deJonge JJ, et al: Phalangeal fractures of the hand: an analysis of gender and age-related incidence and aetiology, *J Hand Surg* 19B:168, 1994.
12. Duncan RW, et al: Open hand fractures: an analysis of the recovery of active motion and of complications, *J Hand Surg* 18A:387, 1993.
13. Ford DJ, Ali MS, Steel WM: Fractures of the fifth metacarpal neck: is reduction or immobilization necessary? *J Hand Surg* 14B:165, 1989.
14. Gonzalez MH, Hall RF: Intramedullary fixation of metacarpal and proximal phalangeal fractures of the hand, *Clin Orthop* 327:47, 1996.
15. Gonzalez MH, Igram CM, Hall RF: Flexible intramedullary nailing for metacarpal fractures, *J Hand Surg* 20A:382, 1995.
16. Gonzalez MH, Igram CM, Hall RF: Intramedullary nailing of proximal phalangeal fractures, *J Hand Surg* 20A:808, 1995.
17. Gustilo RB, Anderson JT: Prevention of infection in the treatment of one thousand and twenty-five open fractures of long bones, *J Bone Joint Surg* 58A:453, 1976.
18. Hastings H: Unstable metacarpal and phalangeal fracture treatment with screws and plates, *Clin Orthop* 214:37, 1987.
19. Kaplan L: The treatment of fractures and dislocations of the hand and fingers: technic of unpadded casts for carpal, metacarpal, and phalangeal fractures, *Surg Clin North Am* 20:1695, 1940.
20. Lester B, Mallik A: Impending malunions of the hand, *Clin Orthop* 327:55, 1996.
21. McLain RF, Steyers C, Stoddard M: Infections in open fractures of the hand, *J Hand Surg* 16A:108, 1991.
22. McMahon PJ, Woods DA, Burge PD: Initial treatment of closed metacarpal fractures, *J Hand Surg* 19B:597, 1994.
23. Mintzer CM, Waters PM, Brown DJ: Remodelling of a displaced phalangeal neck fracture, *J Hand Surg* 19B:594, 1994.
24. Nagy L: Static external fixation of finger fractures, *Hand Clin* 9:651, 1993.
25. Newington DP, Craigen MA, Bennet GC: Children's proximal phalangeal neck fractures with 180 degrees rotational deformity, *J Hand Surg* 20B:353, 1995.
26. Ouellette EA, Freeland AE: Use of the minicondylar plate in metacarpal and phalangeal fractures, *Clin Orthop* 327:38, 1996.
27. Page SM, Stern PJ: Complications and range of motion following plate fixation of metacarpal and phalangeal fractures, *J Hand Surg* 23A:827, 1998.
28. Prevel CD, et al: Mini and micro plating of phalangeal and metacarpal fractures: a biomechanical study, *J Hand Surg* 20A:44, 1995.
29. Pun WK, et al: Unstable phalangeal fractures: treatment by AO screw and plate fixation, *J Hand Surg* 16A:113, 1991.
30. Shehadi SI: External fixation of metacarpal and phalangeal fractures, *J Hand Surg* 16A:544, 1991.
31. Stern PJ, Wieser MJ, Reilly, DG: Complications of plate fixation in the hand skeleton, *Clin Orthop* 214: 59, 1987.
32. Swanson TV, Szabo RM, Anderson DD: Open hand fractures: prognosis and classification, *J Hand Surg* 16A:101, 1991.
33. Vahey JW, Wegner DA, Hastings H: Effect of proximal phalangeal fracture deformity on extensor tendon function, *J Hand Surg* 23A:673, 1998.
34. Waters PM, Benson LS: Dislocation of the distal phalanx epiphysis in toddlers, *J Hand Surg* 18A:581, 1993.
35. Wilson RL, Reynolds CC: Joint stiffness in the hand. In McFarlane RM, editor: *Unsatisfactory results in hand surgery,* Edinburgh; New York, 1987, Churchill-Livingstone.

Chapter 25

MANAGEMENT OF JOINT INJURIES AND INTRAARTICULAR FRACTURES

Peter J. Campbell
Robert Lee Wilson

The small joints of the hand are characterized by their wide range of motion and inherent stability. The diverse positions that the hand and individual fingers can obtain exposes them to varying degrees of trauma.[15] Unfortunately, many of these injuries are considered trivial and go unrecognized or untreated until the sequelae of stiffness or instability seriously restricts hand function (Fig. 25-1). The goal of both the physician and therapist is early recognition of the injured structures, whether bony or ligamentous, and initiation of appropriate treatment that will offer protection and allow early range of motion (ROM) of the involved joints.

PROXIMAL INTERPHALANGEAL JOINT

The proximal interphalangeal (PIP) joint functions essentially as a hinge joint, allowing an arc of motion in excess of 100 degrees. Minor incongruencies exist between the articular surfaces of the proximal and middle phalanges, resulting in a slight amount of translational and rotational motion.[6] Condylar asymmetry produces approximately 9 degrees of supination during flexion. Stability of the PIP joint is achieved both by articular congruency and the surrounding retaining ligaments[6,63] (Fig. 25-2). Most important are the radial and ulnar collateral ligaments with their attachment to the volar plate (VP). The proper collateral ligaments (PCL) have an eccentric origin on the lateral aspect of the proximal phalanx. These fibers then course volarly and distally to insert on the lateral tubercles of the middle phalanx. A smaller, thinner, accessory collateral ligament (ACL) courses from the PCL, attaching

to the VP. The VP is a thick, fibrocartilaginous structure on the palmar aspect of the PIP joint. The area where all three of these structures converge at the middle phalanx is important anatomically to joint stability. This has been termed by Bowers as the *critical corner*.[6] As the PIP joint flexes, tension increases on the PCLs as they stretch over the wider portion of the proximal phalanx. The ACLs fold into synovial recesses, and the VP migrates proximally to allow maximal joint flexion. Conversely, with the joint in full extension, the ACL becomes taut and the strong lateral attachments of the VP prevent hyperextension of the PIP joint.

Several tendons cross the PIP joint and offer added dynamic stability (Fig. 25-3). The central extensor tendon (CET) attaches to the dorsal tubercle of the middle phalanx. The lateral bands, which receive contribution from the intrinsic musculature, pass volar to the metacarpophalangeal (MP) joint axis, converging to form the terminal extensor tendon, which is dorsal to the PIP joint axis. The transverse retinacular ligament (TRL) courses from the volar border of the lateral band to the lateral aspect of the flexor sheath enshrouding the PIP joint and collateral ligaments. The TRL effectively functions to prevent dorsal displacement of the lateral bands.

The oblique retinacular ligament (ORL) of Landsmeer courses parallel but distal to the lateral bands. This ligament takes origin from the flexor sheath adjacent to the proximal phalanx coursing distally, volar to the PIP joint axis, and inserting dorsally at the terminal extensor tendon. As the PIP joint is extended, the ORL tightens, aiding in concomitant

396

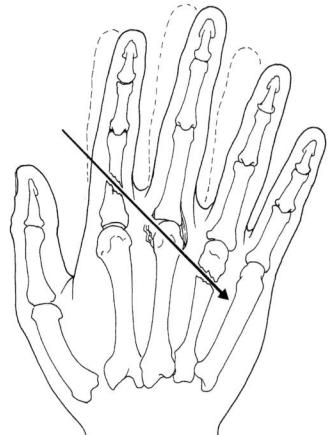

Fig. 25-1. Although digital fractures usually can be demonstrated on radiographs, an intervening injury to a joint's soft tissue supports can be anticipated only by determining the direction or line of force creating the fractures. Careful examination of the joint should specify the extent of damage and allow appropriate simultaneous treatment with management of the fractures.

PIP and distal interphalangeal (DIP) joint extension. The oblique retinacular ligament also helps prevent PIP joint hyperextension.

Evaluation

A complete examination includes a thorough history regarding the mechanism of injury, presence of any initial deformity, primary treatment received, and time elapsed since the traumatic episode. Physical examination begins with inspection, looking specifically for the amount and location of swelling, ecchymosis, or gross deformity. Palpation is carried out in a systematic, organized fashion to localize specific areas of tenderness about the PIP joint. The use of a rubber eraser on a pencil tip is often helpful (Fig. 25-4).

Radiographic examination is obtained before assessing joint stability or functional ROM. If no serious fracture is noted, functional ROM is tested.[15] The patient is asked to actively flex and extend the finger while the examiner notes any instability. Radial and ulnar stress is then applied and compared to the contralateral uninjured joint. Any questionable instability should be confirmed with stress radiographs. A digital block using a local anesthetic can be used to aid in examination of the acutely injured joint (Fig. 25-4, *B*).

Collateral ligament injuries

Angular force applied to the extended PIP joint can injure the collateral ligaments. This more commonly occurs on the radial aspect of the digit. After functional ROM and stress testing are carried out, the degree of injury can be graded (Table 25-1).

Grade I injuries represent a sprain with damage to individual fibers; however, the ligament itself remains intact. The joint remains stable through a full, active range of

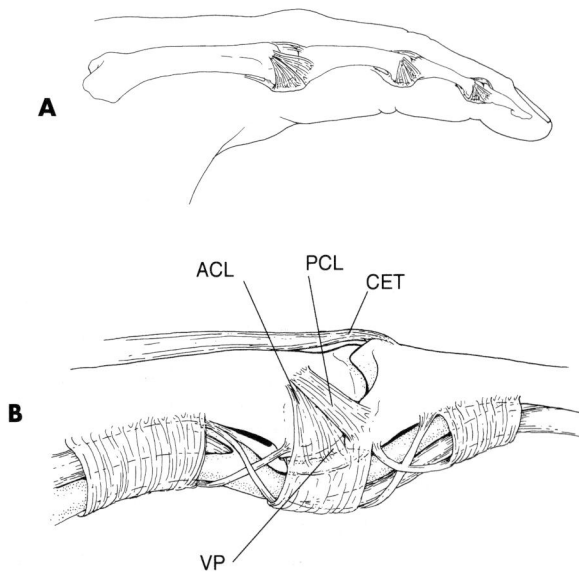

Fig. 25-2. A, Lateral view of metacarpophalangeal (MP), proximal interphalangeal (PIP), and distal interphalangeal (DIP) joints demonstrating the capsuloligamentous structures. **B,** PIP joint. The major retaining ligaments of the PIP joint include the proper and accessory collateral ligaments *(PCL* and *ACL),* the volar plate *(VP),* and the dorsal capsule with its central extensor tendon *(CET).* The VP acts as a gliding surface for the flexor tendon.

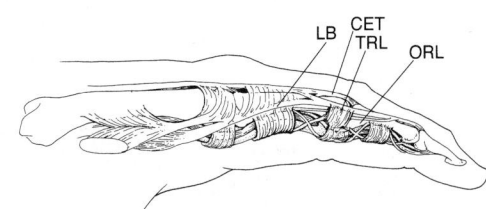

Fig. 25-3. Many structures give supplemental stability to the proximal interphalangeal joint. These include the central extensor tendon *(CET),* the lateral bands *(LB),* the transverse retinacular ligament *(TRL),* and Landsmeer's oblique retinacular ligament *(ORL).*

motion (AROM), and passive stress testing shows no instability.[63] Treatment for this stage includes immobilization in full extension or slight flexion until the acute discomfort subsides, usually within the first week. The joint is then protected by buddy taping to the adjacent finger to allow early ROM, preventing further ligament damage and providing pain relief (Fig. 25-5).

Grade II injuries represent a complete disruption of the collateral ligament. The joint will be stable through AROM but will show instability on passive stress testing. Radiographically, this is represented by greater than 20 degrees of lateral angulation when compared with the contralateral, uninjured digit.[25] These injuries require splint protection for 2 to 4 weeks. Early ROM may be initiated, but angular stress on the digit must be avoided.

Grade III injuries involve complete disruption of the collateral ligament and associated injury to either the volar or dorsal capsular structures. The patient generally describes the joint as having dislocated, pointing in either a lateral, dorsal, or volar direction. Nonoperative treatment can be considered if a congruous reduction can be obtained and the joint remains reduced through an AROM program. However, many authors recommend early operative intervention.[7,25]

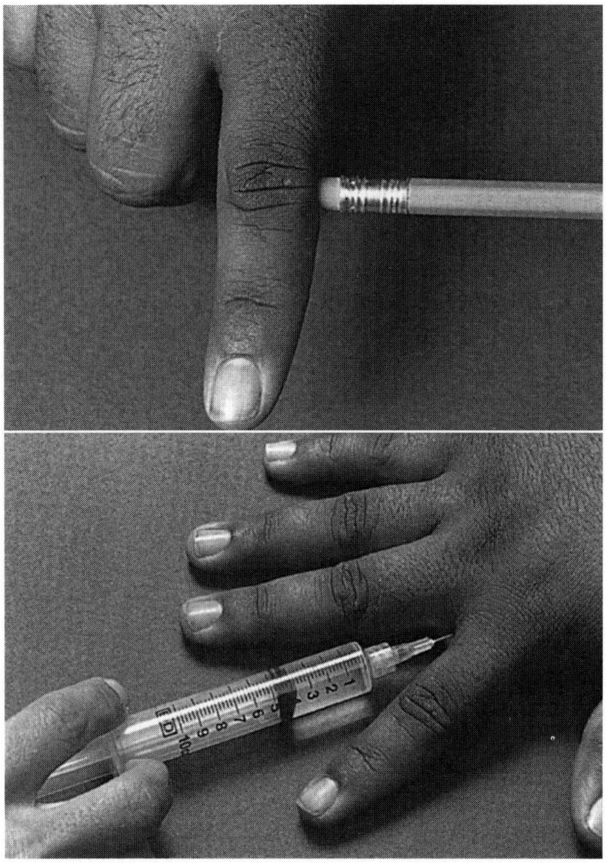

Fig. 25-4. Examination of the injured proximal interphalangeal joint. Specific area(s) of tenderness about each major retaining ligament should be localized (**A**). A metacarpal block may be helpful before functional range-of-motion testing in the acutely injured joint that is painful (**B**).

The most common sequelae following collateral ligament injuries are pain and loss of motion. Full, functional flexion can generally be obtained, but a flexion contracture limiting full extension is not uncommon.[62]

Therapy considerations. The principal goals of therapy are to prevent further injury to the ligament and to prevent joint stiffness by initiating an early joint remobilization program. Edema can be a primary impediment to remobilization. Initially, digital edema may be controlled with a RICE program—*r*est, *i*ce, *c*ompressive wraps, and *e*levation, along with retrograde massage (Fig. 25-6). The patient must be instructed on a home exercise program and counseled on what activities to avoid. Even mild grade I ligament injuries may remain symptomatic for up to 6 months; this is much better accepted by the patient who is informed early of what to expect. ROM exercises should be performed for periods of 3 to 5 minutes and repeated on an hourly schedule during the course of the day. The frequency of an exercise program needs to be based on the amount of pain and swelling that occurs. Iontophoresis or cortisone injection should be considered if ROM reaches a plateau with persistent swelling and incomplete motion (Fig. 25-7, page 401). Static splinting at night is effective for maintaining the achieved joint extension. Often, a flexion contracture develops, and a dynamic splinting program is necessary. This should not be initiated until sufficient healing has occurred (6 to 8 weeks for grade III injuries). Various prefabricated splints are available. If the joint remains relatively supple, recommended splints include the LMB spring wire, reverse knuckle bender or a Capener splint (Fig. 25-8, *A*, page 401). For the less compliant joint, a Joint Jack, Dynasplint, or custom low-profile dynamic extension splint would be more appropriate (Fig. 25-8, *B*, page 401). Prefabricated splints are convenient but must fit well to be effective. The goal of the dynamic splinting program is to apply a low load over a long duration. Pain tolerance and compliance need to be considered for each patient and the program tailored on an individual basis.

Dorsal dislocations

Hyperextension force applied to an extended finger is the most common joint injury of the hand. An Eaton type I injury

Table 25-1. Ligament injuries involving the proximal interphalangeal joint

	Grade I	Grade II	Grade III
Pathology	Sprains/diffuse fiber disruption	Complete disruption of one CL	Complete disruption of one CL as well as volar and/or dorsal structures
Functional ROM testing	Active → stable	Active → stable	Active → unstable
	Passive → less than 20 degrees of angulation	Passive → more than 20 degrees of angulation	Passive → unstable
Treatment	Immobilize, slight flexion 3-10 days, and buddy taping	Immobilize 3-4 weeks, may begin early protected motion	Closed treatment if stable after reduction versus early open treatment

CL, Collateral ligament; *ROM,* range of motion.

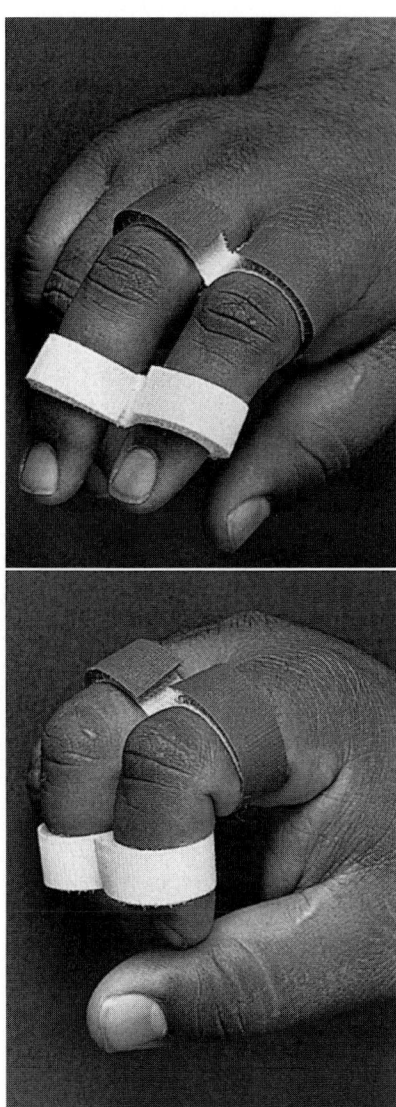

Fig. 25-5. Velcro straps can be fabricated in the clinic and used instead of taping.

represents injury to the central attachment of the VP on the middle phalanx.[16] The lateral attachments, or critical corner, remains intact. A type II injury occurs as the force continues, causing avulsion of the VP distally and a tear between the accessory and proper collateral ligament. A type III injury represents instability both volarly and laterally and presents as a dorsal dislocation. The VP usually fails at its insertion on the middle phalanx, and radiographically a small avulsion chip fracture may be noted in this location (Fig. 25-9, *A*). Occasionally, a dorsal dislocation will be irreducible by closed means, and this may represent soft tissue interposed within the joint.[3,29]

If the joint can be reduced and remain stable, treatment consists of extension block splinting[35] such as a *figure-of-eight splint* (Fig. 25-10). This should place the joint in

approximately 20 degrees of flexion to prevent recurrent dorsal dislocation. Active flexion is initiated immediately, and range is increased as pain and swelling allow. The extension block is removed at approximately 3 weeks, and extension exercises are initiated.

If the PIP joint does not remain reduced following closed reduction, a dorsal extension block splint is placed in the amount of flexion required to maintain reduction.[35] If greater than 25 degrees of flexion is required to maintain reduction, operative intervention is indicated.[7,25] Surgical options available to maintain reduction and allow early ROM include dynamic skeletal traction,[38,49,56] extension block pinning,[58] open reduction and internal fixation of large bony avulsion fragments,[55] force couple splint,[2] or VP arthroplasty[16] (Fig. 25-11, page 403).

Early complications following dorsal dislocations are recurrent dislocation or subluxation. Late sequelae include a residual flexion contracture. This may be confused with a boutonnière deformity. However, the extensor tendon has not been injured, and this can be differentiated clinically because the DIP joint remains flexible. The flexion contracture following this type of capsular injury has been described as a pseudoboutonnière deformity.[34]

Volar dislocations

Volar dislocation of the PIP joint is a rare injury and usually involves disruption of the central slip with a tear between the central tendon and either lateral band. The collateral ligament often disrupts from the origin on the proximal phalanx. If the middle phalanx proceeds to rotate on the contralateral intact collateral ligament, a volar rotatory subluxation occurs. These are commonly irreducible injuries because the proximal phalanx buttonholes through the rent between the central slip and lateral band.[44] Attempted reduction using standard distraction on the dislocated finger only "tightens the noose," preventing reduction. Gentle closed reduction should be attempted by passively extending the wrist to relax the extrinsic extensor tendons and passively flexing the MP joint to relax the intrinsic component of the lateral bands.[57] The joint may then be reduced by "pushing" the middle phalanx into reduction as opposed to pulling on the fingertip.[41] These injuries often require surgery to obtain reduction,[29] and repeated attempted closed reduction should be discouraged.

Treatment of volar dislocations following reduction depends on the integrity of the central slip tendon (Fig. 25-9, *C*). If the central slip remains intact, a short period of immobilization is instituted, followed by a controlled early motion program. However, if the central slip is found to be avulsed, treatment consists of 6 weeks of full-time PIP joint extension splinting or open tendon repair. The DIP joint is not immobilized and AROM or passive range of motion (PROM) is encouraged to prevent contracture of the oblique retinacular ligaments. Unfortunately, the central slip avulsion often goes unrecognized and results in a progressive boutonnière deformity.

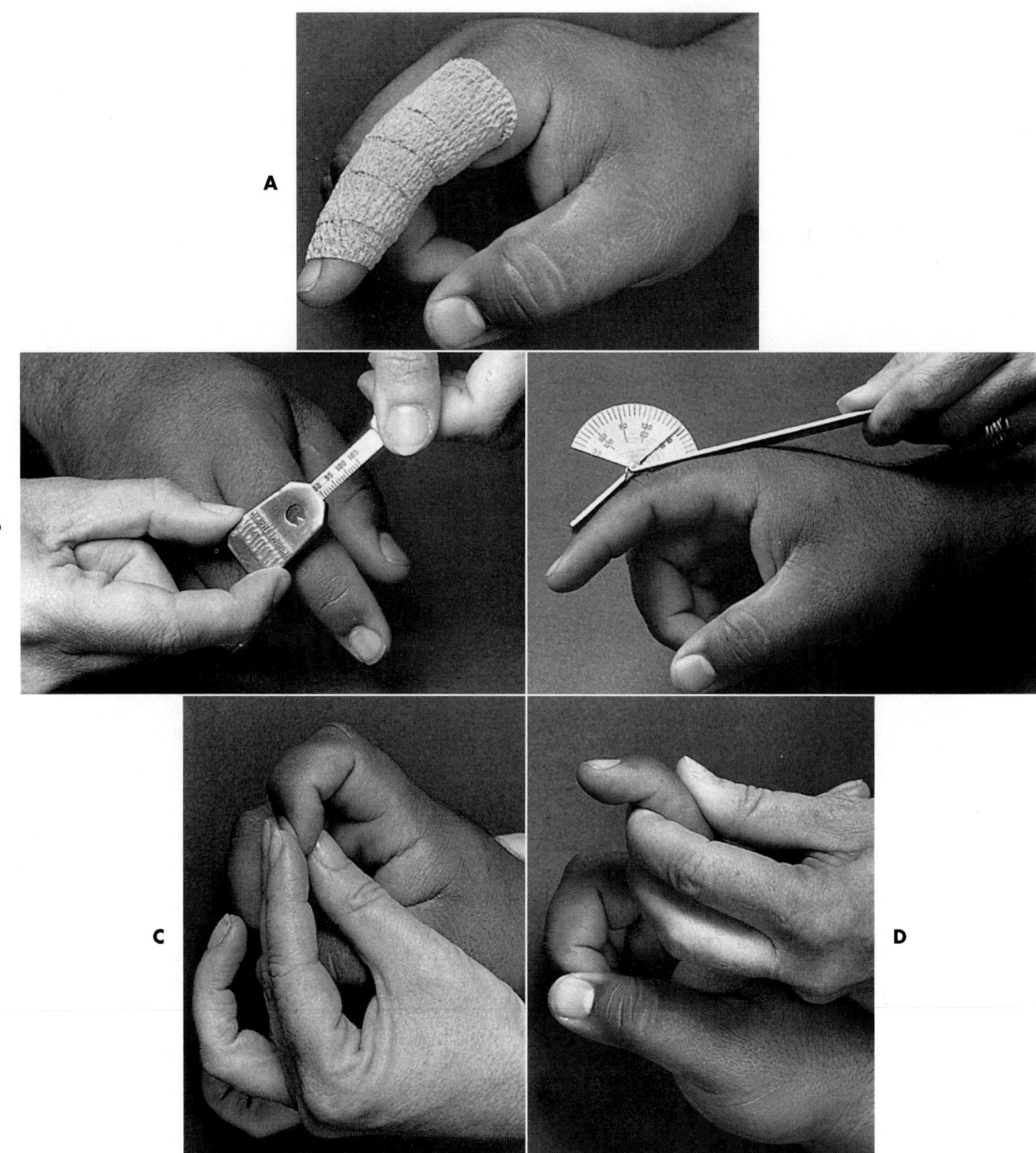

Fig. 25-6. A, Coban wrap is an effective means of edema control in the injured joint. **B,** Weekly evaluations that include circumference and joint motion measurements are important to determine the direction of treatment. **C,** Intrinsic stretching is carried out through simultaneous interphalangeal joint flexion and metacarpophalangeal joint extension. **D,** Retinacular ligament stretching involves obtaining maximal distal joint flexion with proximal interphalangeal joint extension.

Intraarticular fractures

Fractures of the PIP joint can involve the head of the proximal phalanx and/or the base of the middle phalanx (Box 25-1). The goals of treatment of intraarticular fractures of the PIP joint are to obtain anatomic alignment and to achieve a stable construct to allow early ROM, if possible. Avulsion fragments associated with dislocations have been

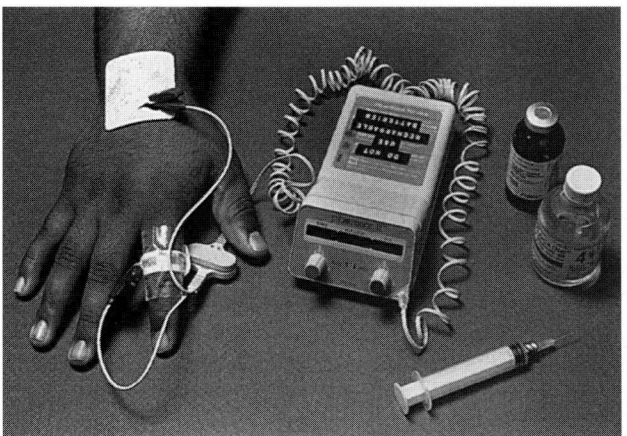

Fig. 25-7. Dexamethasone in combination with lidocaine is administered with direct current iontophoresis.

discussed previously and are treated in association with efforts to maintain joint stability. Intraarticular fractures of the proximal phalanx are generally of three types.[32] Type I fractures are unicondylar, nondisplaced, and stable. Type II fractures are oblique and tend to displace and shorten, allowing angulation of the PIP joint. Type III injuries are bicondylar fractures and are inherently unstable.

Treatment of nondisplaced fractures requires splint immobilization for the first 2 to 3 weeks. This is followed by a protected, AROM program. PROM is generally not initiated until 6 weeks after injury. An experienced hand therapist may initiate earlier gentle PROM as pain permits. The PIP joint should be maintained in extension between exercise sessions during the first few weeks. Dynamic or static extension splinting may be required should a flexion deformity develop.

Any displacement of the articular surface greater than 1 mm requires reduction.[52] Surgical options include closed reduction with percutaneous pin fixation, dynamic external fixation,[3] or open reduction and internal fixation. Minifragment screws are now available that allow stable, internal fixation on even very small fracture fragments. Screw fixation is superior to percutaneous pinning because it allows for early active and active assisted ROM without impeding the surrounding capsule and tendons.

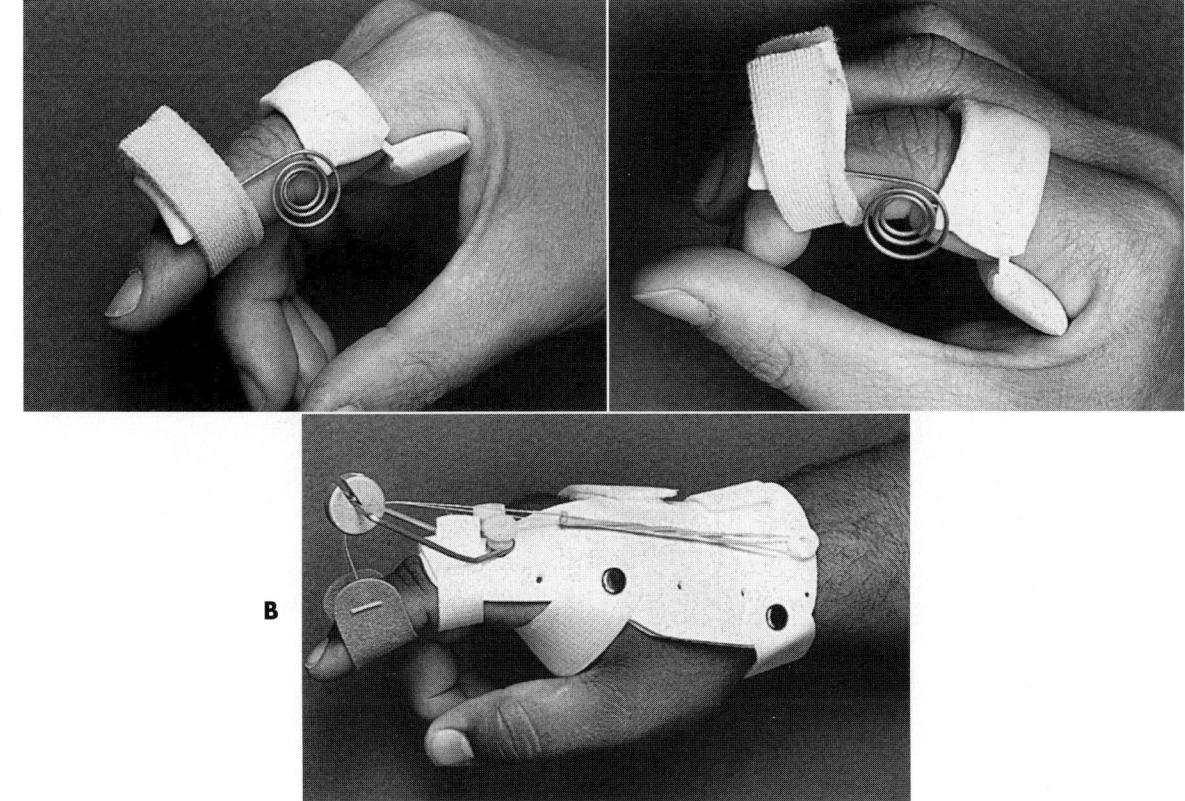

Fig. 25-8. A, A Capener splint allows motion but at the same time allows for a dynamic extension force. **B,** A low-profile splint contoured directly to the patient's hand allows for a custom fit.

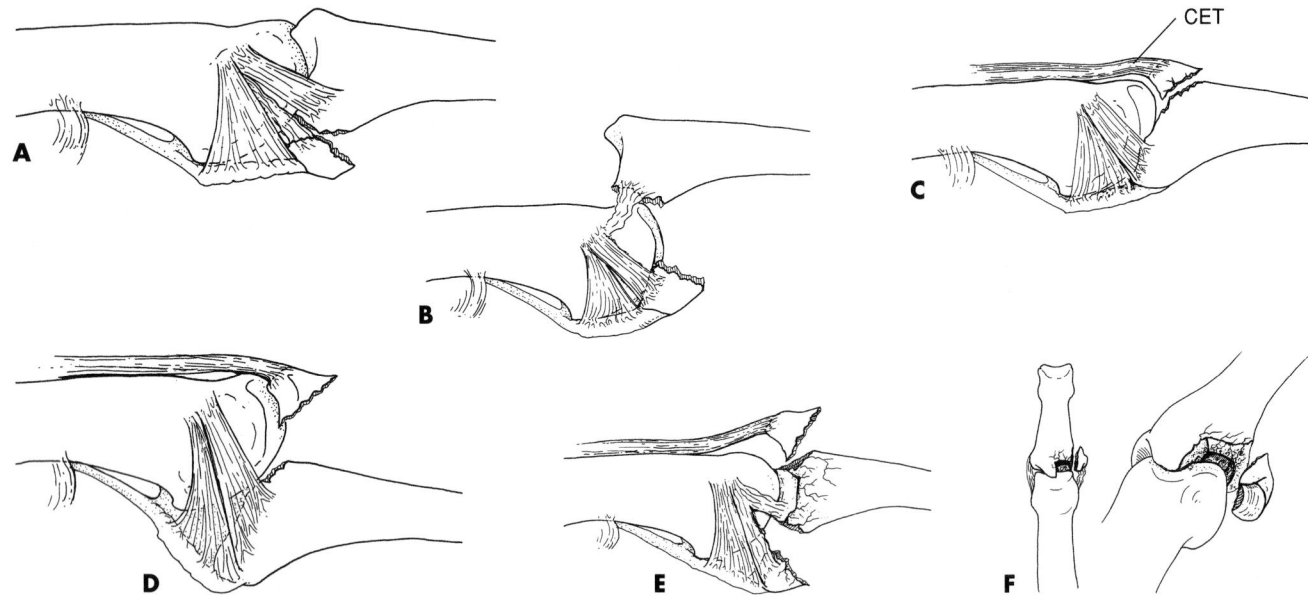

Fig. 25-9. A, Avulsion fracture of the volar base of the middle phalanx. The volar plate remains attached to the fracture fragment. **B,** Intraarticular volar fracture with dorsal dislocation. With 40% articular involvement, the middle phalanx displaces dorsally, decreasing tension in the collateral ligament fibers that remain attached to the shaft at the middle phalanx. **C,** Avulsion fracture of the dorsal lip. The central extensor tendon *(CET)* remains attached to the fracture fragment. **D,** Intraarticular dorsal fracture with volar dislocation. The dorsal support is lost, and the middle phalanx displaces volarly. **E,** Pilon fracture. An axial loading force causes depression of the central articular surface, while the remainder of the articular surface shatters and displaces. **F,** A lateral compression fracture, caused by axial and angulatory forces, produces depression of the lateral articular surface by the proximal phalanx condyle.

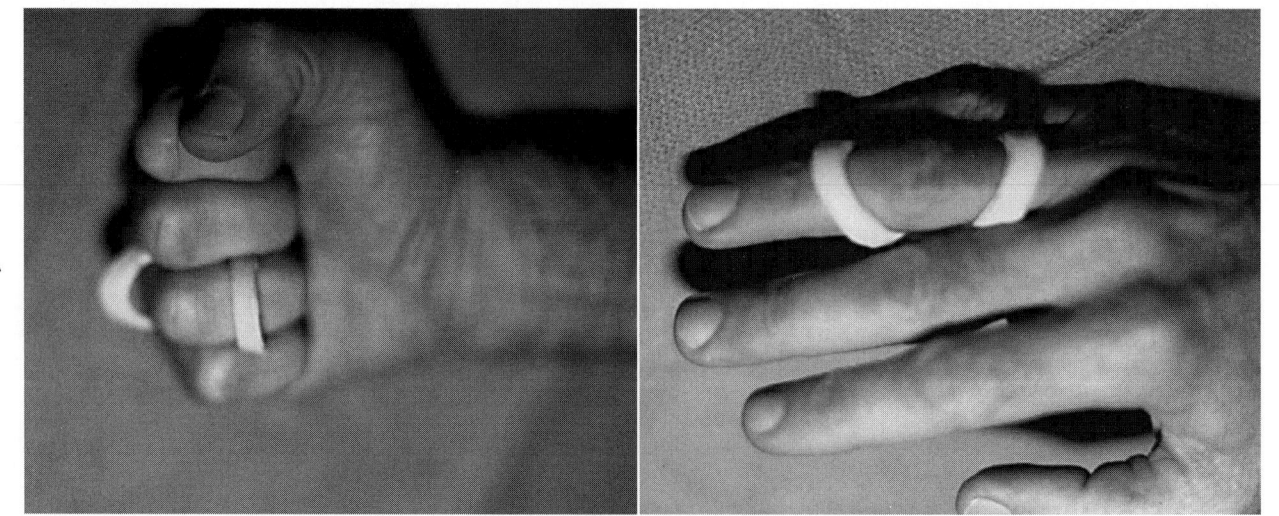

Fig. 25-10. A, Figure-of-eight splint, **B,** Figure-of-eight splint prevents hypertension while allowing full flexion.

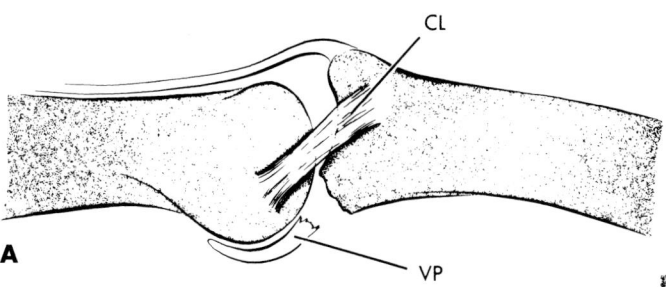

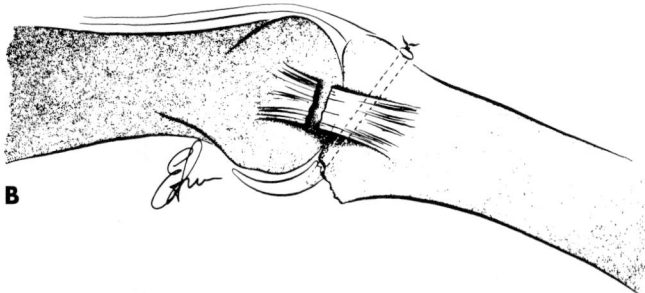

Fig. 25-11. Volar plate arthroplasty. **A,** Any dorsal capsule adhesions or collateral ligament *(CL),* contractures must be released. **B,** Small fracture fragments are removed and volar plate *(VP)* is advanced into defect with wire suture.

Box 25-1   Fractures of the middle phalanx base

Avulsion fractures of the volar base
Volar fractures with dorsal subluxation-dislocation
Avulsion fractures of the dorsal lip
Dorsal fractures with volar subluxation-dislocation
Lateral compression fractures
Pilon fractures

Compression fractures can occur on the articular surface of the middle phalanx, resulting in either a central pilon depression (Fig. 25-9, *E*) or a lateral compression (Fig. 25-9, *F*). Treatment of this injury often requires bone grafting to supplement the metaphyseal void that results following reduction of the articular surface. The construct is generally tenuous, and remobilization cannot be initiated until fracture healing has occurred. In contrast, dynamic skeletal traction offers the ability to maintain reduction and allow early ROM.[38,49,55] This requires a compliant patient and close radiographic follow-up to ensure maintenance of reduction.

Therapy considerations. The focus of rehabilitation following intraarticular fractures is to maintain fracture reduction and begin ROM as soon as possible.[61] This requires direct communication between the surgeon and therapist on a patient-by-patient basis.

Fractures with tenuous fixation require splint protection and later treatment of the expected contracture that develops. Stable internal fixation (assessed intraoperatively) should be followed with immediate AROM and PROM exercises. The joint should be splinted in full extension between exercise sessions. Emphasis initially must be on active extension exercises. Blocking the MP joint in slight flexion enhances the extensor tendon function to the PIP joint (Fig. 25-12).

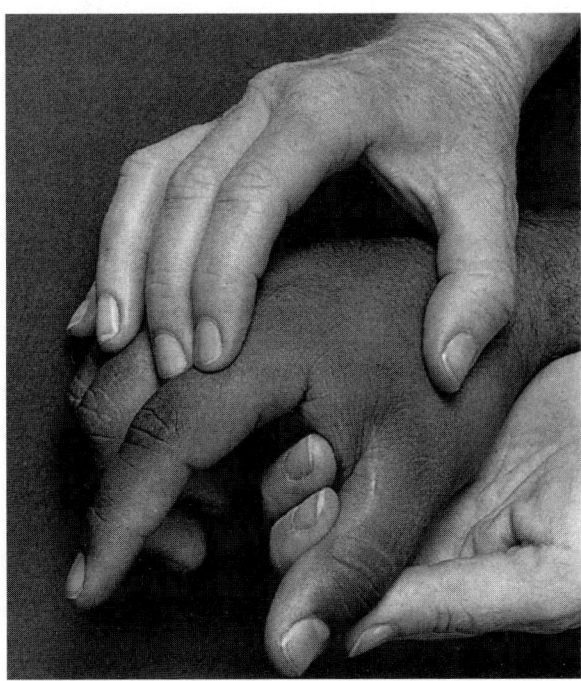

Fig. 25-12. Maximum extension of the proximal interphalangeal joint may be obtained by blocking the metacarpophalangeal joint in flexion.

Abduction and adduction exercises should be applied for the intrinsic muscles. Fixed PIP joint contractures must be treated promptly with dynamic splinting (see Fig. 25-8).

THUMB INTERPHALANGEAL AND FINGER DISTAL INTERPHALANGEAL JOINTS

The anatomy of the interphalangeal (IP) joint of the thumb and DIP joints of the fingers are similar to that of the PIP joint, that being a bicondylar, ginglymus joint with stout capsular ligaments. Dynamic stability also is offered by

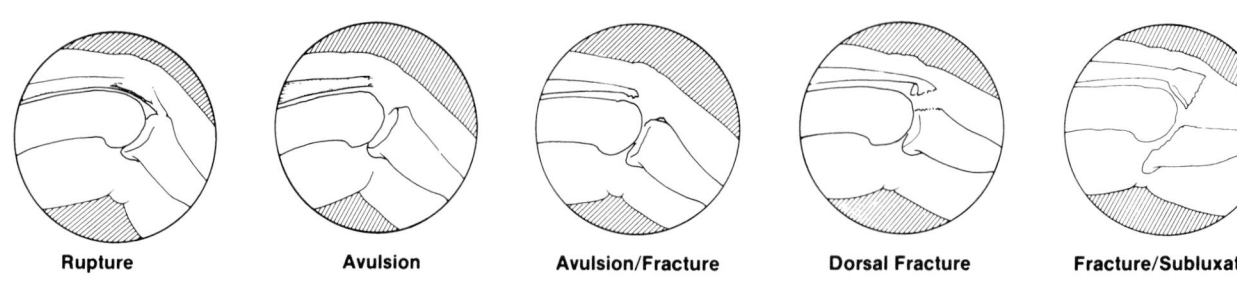

Rupture   Avulsion   Avulsion/Fracture   Dorsal Fracture   Fracture/Subluxation

Fig. 25-13. Mallet deformity can be produced from extensor tendon rupture, avulsion of terminal extensor tendon, or avulsion of bone with extensor tendon. Dorsal fracture of distal phalanx and fracture-subluxation, although not tendon injuries, can present as mallet deformities. (From Management of acute extensor injuries. In Hunter JM, Schneider LH, Mackin EJ, editors: *Tendon surgery in the hand,* St Louis, 1987, Mosby.)

attachments of the terminal flexor and extensor tendons to the distal phalanx. Injury to these distal joints can involve the osseous structures, capsuloligamentous structures, tendons, and the nail bed. A distal phalanx fracture or fracture dislocation associated with a large subungual hematoma represents an open fracture and must be recognized. This is a common injury in skeletally immature patients and represents an open fracture through the distal phalanx physis known as a *Seymour fracture*.[48] As with examination of the PIP joint, a digital block may be necessary to assess ROM and joint stability. Radiographs should include posteroanterior (PA), lateral, and oblique views, with stress views as indicated.

Avulsion of the terminal extensor tendon from its insertion on the dorsal aspect of the distal phalanx presents as an extensor lag to the distal joint, called a *mallet injury*.[60] This injury occurs when a sudden flexion force is applied to an extended DIP joint. The distal phalanx assumes a flexed position, and the patient is unable to actively extend the joint. Passive extension remains intact. Hyperextension commonly is noted at the PIP joint because of the tendon imbalance. This is known as a *swan-neck deformity*. These injuries may be purely tendinous or associated with an avulsion fracture fragment (Fig. 25-13). Radiographs should be obtained to rule out a bony injury or volar subluxation of the DIP joint. Indications for open reduction and internal fixation include the presence of a large fracture fragment, fragment displacement of more than 2 mm, an extensor lag over 35 degrees, or volar subluxation of the DIP joint.[33,59] Postoperative management of this fracture is similar to treatment for an acute closed tendon injury. This requires the distal joint to be splinted in full extension continuously for 4 to 6 weeks. Patient education cannot be overemphasized. Hyperextension of the DIP joint is to be avoided because this position decreases the microcirculation to the injured tendon.[46] It is imperative that the PIP joint be free and ROM encouraged. A prefabricated (Fig. 25-14) or custom-made mallet splint with an open pulp space allows for use of the finger with tactile feedback during the splinting program. The patient is weaned from the splint over the following 2 to 4 weeks as remobilization is initiated. This requires close observation

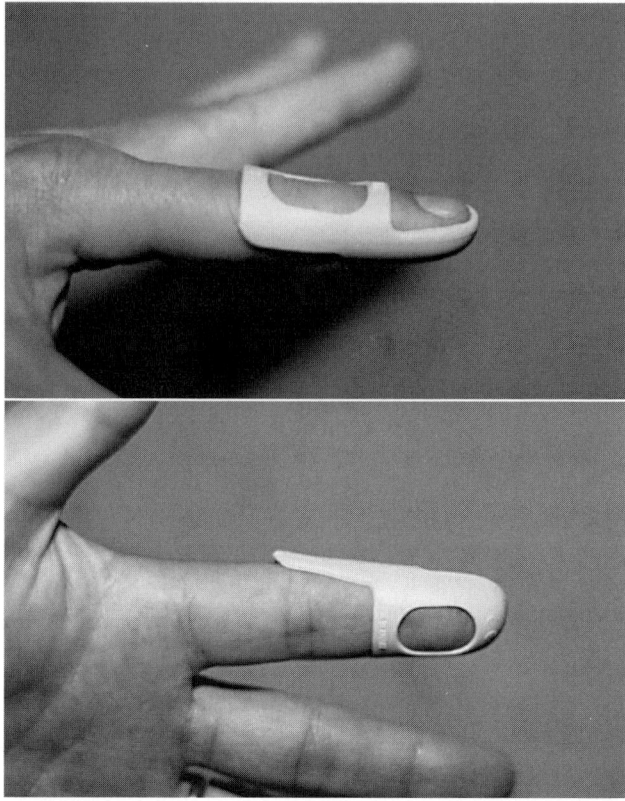

Fig. 25-14. Mallet splint. (Link America Inc., Hanover, New Jersey.)

for any extensor lag.[54] For several months, splinting may be required at night and during any athletic activities.

A hyperextension force to the flexed DIP joint may produce an avulsion of the flexor digitorum profundus or flexor pollicis longus tendon at its insertion to the distal phalanx.[64] This most commonly occurs in the ring finger and is known as a *rugger jersey injury*. The patient will be unable to actively flex the involved DIP joint. Tenderness along the flexor sheath to the level of the palm is common. Radiographs should be obtained to evaluate for evidence of a bony avulsion fragment. Three types of avulsion injuries have been described.[30] In type I, the tendon retracts into the palm beneath the A_1 pulley. A substantial amount of blood supply to the tendon is lost with rupture of the vincular system. This injury requires prompt operative intervention within the first 7 to 10 days before the musculotendinous unit becomes contracted. Type II injury is the most common type, with the tendon retracting to the level of the PIP joint. Further retraction is limited by the intact vinculum at this location. A type III injury represents an avulsion with a large, bony fragment. Generally, the fragment catches on the A_4 pulley, and radiographs show the fragment to be just proximal to the DIP joint. This requires open reduction and internal fixation of the bony fragment. Rehabilitation is similar to zone I flexor tendon repairs and requires significant patient compliance and close observation by the therapist.

Dislocations of the distal IP joints and thumb IP joint are rare injuries. Dorsal dislocations that can be reduced are splinted in neutral or slight flexion for 1 to 2 weeks. This is followed by an active and active-assisted flexion program. PROM can be initiated at 4 to 6 weeks. Radial or ulnar stress should be avoided if there is a concomitant collateral ligament injury. A splint is worn on the distal joint for protection for 4 to 6 weeks.

Volar dislocations represent avulsion of the terminal extensor tendon and are treated as a mallet injury. Open dislocations and irreducible dislocations require open reduction.

METACARPOPHALANGEAL JOINTS 2 TO 5

The MP joints are injured less frequently than the PIP joint. This is partly because of the increased mobility of the MP joint, which helps dissipate disruptive forces. The metacarpal head is narrow on the dorsal aspect and widens volarly. The PCLs have an eccentric dorsal origin and tighten during joint flexion, which allows stability during pinch and grasp. When the joint is placed in full extension, these ligaments are lax, allowing approximately 30 degrees of lateral motion. The VP is continuous with the deep transverse metacarpal ligament and, as opposed to the PIP joint, has a weak proximal attachment.

Collateral ligament injuries

Collateral ligament injuries occur after a forceful radial or ulnar stress to the joint. This most commonly occurs to the radial collateral ligament. Clinically, point tenderness occurs over the injured ligament or instability to ulnar stress occurs with the joint in flexion. Radiographs may show an avulsion fracture from the metacarpal origin. An arthrogram can be performed in equivocal cases and will show extravasation of dye at the site of the ligament tear.[24]

Treatment of acute injuries requires immobilization of the MP joints in 50 degrees of flexion for 3 weeks. This is followed by a protected ROM program using buddy taping for an additional 3 to 6 weeks. The tendency is to want to immobilize the joint in full flexion to prevent an extension

contracture. However, this position would place the injured ligament under maximal tension and would interfere with the healing process. Surgical intervention is required for avulsion fragments that are greater than 2 mm displaced or when gross instability is present with rotatory and palmar subluxation of the joint. Remobilization techniques should emphasize extremes of motion and avoidance of any angular stress to the damaged ligament until point tenderness has resolved. Should an extension contracture occur, a gentle dynamic flexion program can be initiated.

Metacarpophalangeal joint dislocations

Dorsal MP joint dislocation commonly occurs after a hyperextension force to the digit. The VP fails proximally, allowing the finger to dislocate dorsally. These dislocations commonly are associated with metacarpal head fractures and must not be overlooked. Dislocations are categorized as either simple or complex. Simple dislocations present with the proximal phalanx rotated dorsally in 60 to 90 degrees of hyperextension. It is termed a *simple* dislocation because it usually can be reduced by closed manipulation. Rehabilitation following reduction encourages early mobilization with a dorsal extension block splint. Some patients have persistent pain on the volar aspect of the joint at the level of the A_1 pulley. Extension stretching, deep heat modalities, and phonophoresis may be required.

More commonly, a complex, or irreducible, dislocation occurs. This is caused by failure of the VP proximally, which becomes interposed dorsal to the metacarpal head, preventing reduction. Clinically, the proximal phalanx is less hyperextended than in a simple dislocation. A dimpling of the skin may be noticed on the palm at the volar aspect of the MP joint.[14] Radiographs may show a widened joint space with interposition of the sesamoid. This requires surgical reduction, which can be approached either volarly or dorsally.[5] The dorsal approach offers less risk of iatrogenic neurovascular injury. Reduction is achieved as the VP is retracted from the joint. This often requires incision through the VP longitudinally to allow reduction. Postoperatively, the joint is immobilized in greater than 50 degrees of flexion, and a prompt remobilization program is initiated with an extension block splint.

Volar MP joint dislocations are rare. These generally can be reduced by closed manipulation. Failure to obtain closed reduction is usually due to a proximal avulsion of the dorsal capsule or distal avulsion of the VP, either of which become interposed within the joint, blocking reduction. Rehabilitation requires prompt remobilization.

Metacarpophalangeal joint fractures

MP joint fractures occur from an axially directed force and may be associated with a joint dislocation. Radiographs are required for evaluation of the fracture pattern. A Brewerton view obtained with MP joints in a flexed position with the dorsum of the proximal phalanx on the x-ray plate is helpful in delineating collateral ligament avulsion fractures.[62] Treatment depends on fracture displacement. Any articular incongruity must be corrected. Internal fixation is obtained with K-wires, minifragment screws, or interfragmentary screws, such as the Herbert or mini-Acutrack screw.[21] The goal of internal fixation is to obtain rigid stable fixation without impeding tendon or ligament motion to allow for early ROM. Severely comminuted metacarpal or proximal phalanx articular fractures are very difficult to treat with open reduction and internal fixation. Alternatives include skeletal traction or primary silicone MP joint arthroplasty.[31] Arthroplasty should not be considered in the index finger because it is destined to fail as a result of the high sheer stresses that occur during lateral pinch.

CARPOMETACARPAL JOINTS 2 TO 5

Injuries to the carpometacarpal (CMC) joints often go unrecognized. These injuries can vary from a ligamentous sprain to a complex fracture-dislocation involving multiple joints. Trauma to these joints generally results from an axial load such as striking an object with a closed fist or a combination of axial loading and a lever type force in either flexion or extension.[62] The radial CMC joints of the index and middle finger articulate with the trapezoid and capitate and have very little mobility. The fourth and fifth metacarpals articulate with the hamate and have 15 to 30 degrees of flexion, respectively. These joints have strong dorsal, palmar, and intermetacarpal ligamentous support. This is further reinforced by the attachment of the wrist flexor and extensor tendons to the second, third, and fifth metacarpals.

Sprains of the individual CMC joints are diagnosed by point tenderness in this location with or without comparative laxity on performing stress maneuvers compared with the opposite hand. Diagnosis can be confirmed by injecting a local anesthetic into the involved joint, resulting in temporary pain relief. Dorsal extension block splinting of the MP joints with the wrist in neutral or slight extension is usually successful in eliminating these symptoms. Failure to recognize these injuries can lead to progressive pain and weakness.

Dorsal dislocation or fracture-dislocations of the fifth CMC joint are most common. An intraarticular fracture leaving a small radial intraarticular component reduced in the hamate fossa is analogous to a Bennett's fracture of the thumb.[40] Displacement of the metacarpal shaft occurs in a dorsal ulnar direction because of the unopposed pull of the extensor carpi ulnaris. A radiograph should include a 30-degree pronated view that profiles the fifth CMC joint. Computed tomography or linear tomography is helpful in equivocal cases. Volar dislocations are less common and usually are caused by a crushing type of injury. The deep motor branch of the ulnar nerve courses just volar to the fifth CMC joint and can be injured in these rare dislocations. Treatment of the acute injury consists of attempted closed reduction using longitudinal traction and direct pressure over the dislocated metacarpal. If a palpable reduction is achieved, postreduction radiographs are obtained. A stable reduction can be treated with 4 weeks of cast immobilization with the wrist in slight extension. Unstable dislocations or fracture-dislocations require percutaneous K-wire fixation to maintain reduction. Postreduction radiographs in multiple planes need to be critically assessed to ensure articular congruency. Inadequate reduction may be due to interposed capsule or small fracture fragments, and open reduction would be required. Multiple CMC dislocations[20] represent more extensive soft tissue injury. These dislocations are most commonly dorsal, and treatment is the same as an isolated fifth CMC dislocation with pin fixation of each injured joint. The deep palmar arch is situated volar to the third CMC joint and may be injured with palmar dislocation of this ray.

Therapy consideration

K-wires are maintained for 6 weeks, and the hand is protected with a dorsal extension block splint with the MP joints in flexion and the wrist in slight extension. Early PROM and AROM exercises to the IP joints should be instituted to prevent stiffness. Intrinsic stretching also should be included. Following pin removal, the patient begins a remobilization program, including PROM and AROM of the MP and CMC joints. Progressive grip strengthening and resistive exercises are added as the ROM improves.

Chronic or unrecognized injuries to the CMC joint often lead to pain with weakness of grip, carpal bossing, ganglion formation, and CMC arthrosis. Late options for treatment include joint debridement, excision of osteophytes, arthrodesis,[11] or interposition arthroplasty.[18]

THUMB METACARPOPHALANGEAL JOINT

The thumb MP joint functions principally as a hinge, or ginglymus joint. The arc of motion in the sagittal plane is variable, ranging from 6 to 86 degrees. More spherical metacarpal heads have greater degrees of flexion. This ROM is usually symmetric bilaterally.[50] The radial condyle of the metacarpal head is slightly wider than the ulnar condyle, which allows for a slight pronation with flexion. Like the finger MP joints, the PCL are tightest in full flexion and are relatively lax in full extension. Lateral movement of the MP joint is variable and ranges from 0 to 20 degrees with the joint in full extension.[4,23,27]

Palmarly, the VP provides strong support and is attached firmly at the base of the proximal phalanx. Dynamic stability is offered by insertion of the thenar musculature through the sesamoid bones in the distal portion of the VP. The adductor pollicis inserts into the ulnar sesamoid and adductor aponeurosis. The abductor pollicis brevis (APB) and flexor pollicis brevis (FPB) insert into the radial sesamoid and abductor aponeurosis. Further support is offered dorsally by the extensor pollicis longus and extensor pollicis brevis

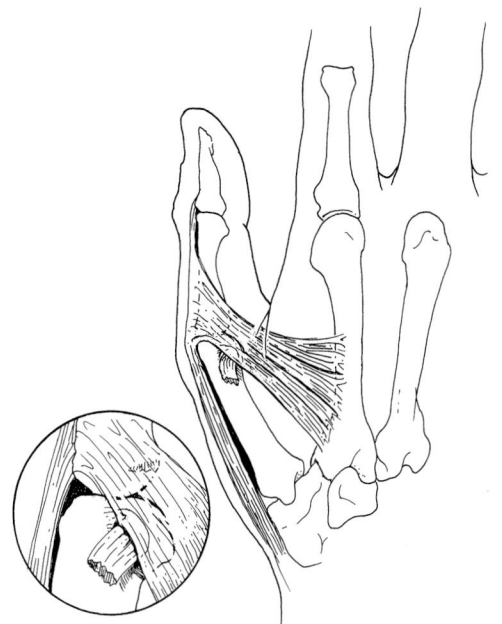

Fig. 25-15. Diagram and enlargement of the Stener lesion. A hyperabduction force results in complete rupture of the ulnar collateral ligament at its distal insertion, with displacement proximally. The adductor aponeurosis blocks the ligament from returning to its insertion site, thus preventing adequate healing.

(EPB) tendons, and volarly by the flexor pollicis longus tendon.

Ulnar collateral ligament injuries

Ulnar collateral ligament injuries occur 10 times more frequently than injuries to the radial collateral ligament.[39,45] The mechanism of injury is generally forced radial deviation and hyperextension. This is a common injury when falling to an outstretched hand while holding a ski pole, and has been referred to as *skier's thumb*. The more common acronym, *gamekeeper's thumb*,[10] is derived from the injury to the thumb of British gamekeepers incurred by repetitive trauma while killing rabbits. This recurrent stress to the ulnar collateral ligament of the gamekeeper often resulted in chronic instability because of attenuation of the ulnar collateral ligament. In an acute injury, the ulnar collateral ligament is usually detached from its distal insertion on the proximal phalanx. Injuries to the VP, ACL, and dorsal capsule also may occur. If the ulnar collateral ligament is completely disrupted and a significant radial deviation force is applied to the MP joint of the thumb, the ligament displaces superficial to the adductor aponeurosis. The interposition of the adductor aponeurosis will not allow normal healing of the ligament to its insertion. The displaced ligament often can be palpated clinically and is called a *Stener's lesion* (Fig. 25-15).[1,53] The goal during examination of the patient is to distinguish between a partial and complete ligament tear. Point tenderness is present along the ulnar and

volar aspect of the MP joint. If examined early, before significant swelling has occurred, the Stener's lesion may be palpable proximal to the MP joint. Gentle radial stress should be applied to the MP joint both in extension and 30 degrees of flexion, with comparison to the contralateral thumb. A local anesthetic can be used if pain limits accurate testing. Often, a partial ligament tear will cause more discomfort than a complete tear on stress testing. PA, lateral, and oblique radiographs should be obtained to evaluate for the presence of an avulsion fracture. Stress radiographs are helpful in equivocal cases (Fig. 25-16). A complete ligament tear is characterized by instability or laxity exceeding 35 degrees (or 15 degrees greater than the contralateral thumb). The presence of a nondisplaced small avulsion fragment should not discourage gentle stress testing. Failure to recognize the ligament tear may lead to long-term instability. Arthrograms, ultrasound,[22] and magnetic resonance imaging[19,22] have been used in diagnosis. These tests are expensive but may be indicated to confirm evidence of a serious ligament injury in the equivocal case.

Partial ligament injuries, or nondisplaced and stable avulsion fractures are treated in a hand-based thumb spica cast with the IP joint free for 2 to 4 weeks. The IP joint is exercised while in the thumb spica cast.[43] At 2 to 4 weeks, if the patient is pain free, a removable splint can be fabricated. The MP joint is then mobilized with active and active-assisted ROM over 3 to 4 weeks. Key pinch exercises can be initiated early; however, tip pinch should be avoided for approximately 8 weeks. Strengthening should be encouraged. Obtaining terminal ROM is not as important as obtaining a stable, pain-free joint.

Complete ligament disruptions with instability or displaced intraarticular fracture fragments are treated surgically with open reduction and internal fixation of the fracture fragment, or direct repair of the ulnar collateral ligament to its insertion on the proximal phalanx can be done.[13,26] Arthroscopic reduction of the Stener's lesion has also been reported.[47] Often, a pin is placed across the MP joint in slight overcorrection to prevent any stress on the repair site. The patient is treated postoperatively in a thumb spica cast. The pin is removed at 4 weeks and a protected ROM program initiated.

Therapy considerations. Remobilization of the IP joint of the thumb begins immediately postoperatively, while in a thumb spica cast. This helps prevent tendon adhesions from occurring at the extensor hood. Following cast removal, the IP and trapeziometacarpal (TMC) joints are vigorously exercised with AROM. The MP joint is started on a gentle, passive motion program and progressed to active assisted ROM over a 2- to 4-week period. Lateral, or key pinch strengthening, is started initially; however, tip pinch should be avoided for approximately 8 weeks. A thumb spica splint should be used when not exercising to prevent an adduction contracture of the first web space and to prevent an abduction

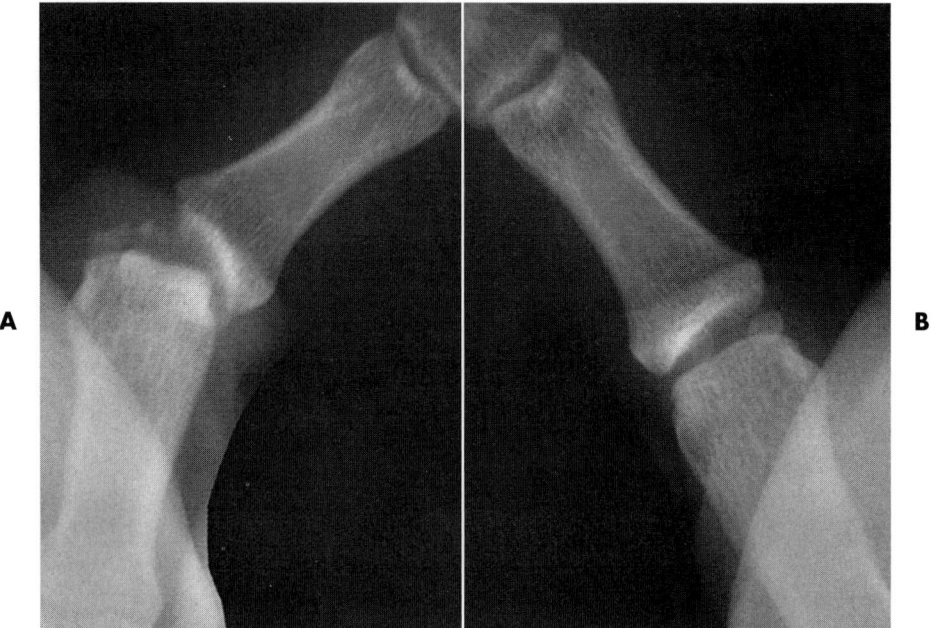

Fig. 25-16. Comparative stress radiography of a 32-year-old skier who sustained injury to the left thumb metacarpophalangeal (MP) joint (**A**) during a fall. Note the amount of displacement and an associated chip fracture. The right thumb MP joint (**B**) is normal.

force on the MP joint. The patient is progressively weaned from the splint over a 2- to 6-week period. Mild discomfort at the ulnar aspect of the MP joint may be present for 3 to 4 months after surgical repair.

Radial collateral ligament injuries

Injury to the radial collateral ligament at the MP joint of the thumb is less common than injury to the ulnar collateral ligament. The mechanism of injury is usually forced adduction or rotation of the thumb metacarpal. As opposed to the ulnar collateral ligament, the radial collateral ligament generally ruptures in the midsubstance of the ligament. The abductor aponeurosis is broad and prevents displacement of the torn ligament; therefore no Stener's lesion is present on the radial aspect of the thumb. Examination will show point tenderness over the dorsal radial joint line. Occasionally, the thumb is hyperpronated. Patients may complain of pain with pressure applied to the thumb in the adducted position, such as opening a jar.[36] Because the torn ligament is not displaced, many treat a partial or complete ligament injury with immobilization for 4 weeks, followed by a ROM program. Instability greater than 30 degrees or volar subluxation of the MP joint are indications for operative repair of the ligament. Rehabilitation is similar to that of the ulnar collateral ligament injury except the thumb is protected from adduction stress and initiation of tip pinch strengthening can begin earlier.

Dislocations

Sudden forceful hyperextension of the thumb MP joint may result in rupture of the proximal VP. As with MP joint dislocations in the fingers, dislocation can be characterized as simple (reducible) or complex (irreducible). Complex dislocations are those in which the metacarpal head tears through the palmar plate proximal to the sesamoids and becomes entrapped between the intrinsic muscles. Radiographs should be obtained before joint manipulation or reduction is attempted. A postreduction radiograph should be obtained after successful reduction. Increased space between the metacarpal head and proximal phalanx or displacement of the sesamoid bones is suggestive of interposed VP. Complex dislocations require open reduction. ROM and stability should be tested following closed reduction. A successful reduction should be immobilized 3 weeks in a short opponens splint with the MP joint in 20 to 30 degrees of flexion. Splint protection and rapid remobilization are then required. Emphasis should be placed on strengthening and functional activities rather than trying to achieve maximal flexion.

Dorsal capsular injuries

Injuries to the dorsal MP joint capsule and EPB tendon are rare injuries that result from isolated hyperflexion. Pain is recognized over the dorsal capsule[28] and is reproduced by forceful, passive flexion. This generally can be treated

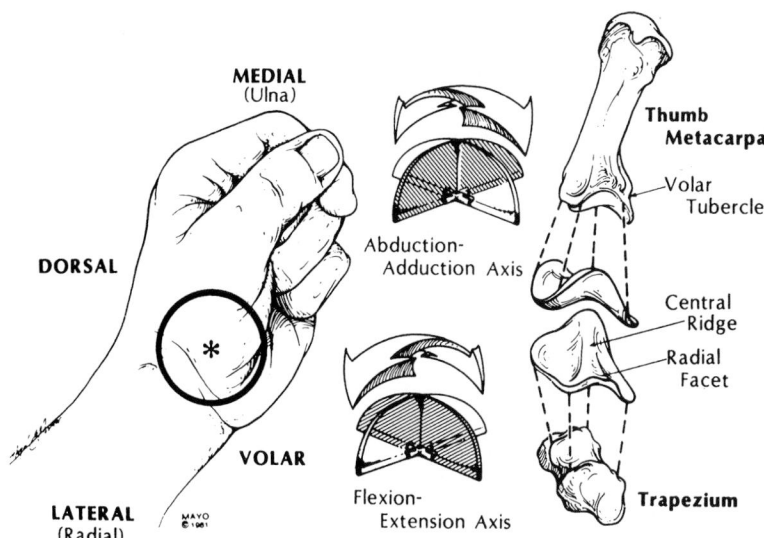

Fig. 25-17. The articular surfaces of the trapezium and metacarpal base are saddle-shaped. This unique configuration allows for motion in the abduction-adduction plane as well as the flexion-extension plane. (From Cooney WP, et al: *J Bone Joint Surg* 63A:1371, 1981.)

successfully by short-term splint immobilization, antiinflammatories, and local therapy modalities. Surgical exploration with imbrication of the capsule is indicated for patients with recalcitrant pain.[28] Rarely, the MP joint may dislocate volarly with interposition of the dorsal capsule or extensor tendons, requiring open reduction.[37]

TRAPEZIOMETACARPAL JOINT

The TMC joint provides the thumb its greatest mobility and function. The articular surfaces are composed of a saddle-shaped joint forming interlocking reciprocal biconcave articular surfaces. This unique articulation allows for motion in the flexion/extension plane as well as abduction, adduction, and pronosupination[12] (Fig. 25-17). Joint stability is offered by four capsular ligaments. The most important ligament is the anterior oblique or volar oblique ligament, which extends from the trapezial tubercle to the volar beak of the first metacarpal.[15] This ligament offers stability for lateral or key pinch, becoming taut in flexion, adduction, and supination.[42] Other important ligaments are the dorsoradial, the posterior oblique, and the intermetacarpal ligament.[4] A slip of the abductor pollicis longus (APL) is the sole tendon that inserts to the base of the first metacarpal.

Trapeziometacarpal joint dislocations

A pure dorsal dislocation of the TMC joint is a rare injury. The mechanism of injury is a longitudinal force applied to the partially flexed metacarpal shaft.[15] The dorsoradial and anterior oblique ligaments are torn or avulsed with a small, bony fragment.

Diagnosis of the ligament injury can be suspected by localized tenderness and can be confirmed with radiographs, including stress views. Partial ligament injuries are treated

with cast immobilization for 4 weeks, followed by a gentle, progressive AROM program. Complete ligament tears with instability or noted dislocations require operative intervention and ligamentous repair. Results of closed reduction and percutaneous pinning have been unsatisfactory, with a high incidence of recurrent instability.[51]

Trapeziometacarpal joint fractures

The most common intraarticular fracture pattern is an avulsion fracture from the volar aspect of the first metacarpal base, called a *Bennett's fracture*[8] (Fig. 25-18, *A*). The strong, anterior oblique ligament remains intact and attached to the bony fragment. The metacarpal shaft is displaced dorsally and radially by the unopposed force of the APL tendon, extrinsic thumb extensors, and adductor pollicis.[17]

The goal of treatment is to obtain anatomic joint congruity.[8] Closed reduction may be successful with longitudinal traction and pronation of the thumb. This is secured with K-wire fixation under fluoroscopic guidance.[56] Fracture fragments that involve more than 30% of the articular surface or fractures that cannot be reduced by closed means require open reduction and internal fixation.[56] Minifragment screw fixation of large fragments allows stable reduction and early, AROM exercises postoperatively. Splint protection will be required until fracture healing.

Comminuted intraarticular T- or Y-shaped fractures of the first metacarpal base are called *Rolando's fractures* (Fig. 25-18, *B*). The mechanism of injury is more of a direct axial load with less metacarpal flexion. This fracture often requires open reduction and internal fixation with the use of multiple K-wires, minifragment plate, or tension band wiring. Severely comminuted fractures that are not amenable to internal fixation may be treated with longitudinal skeletal traction[17] or external fixation.[9]

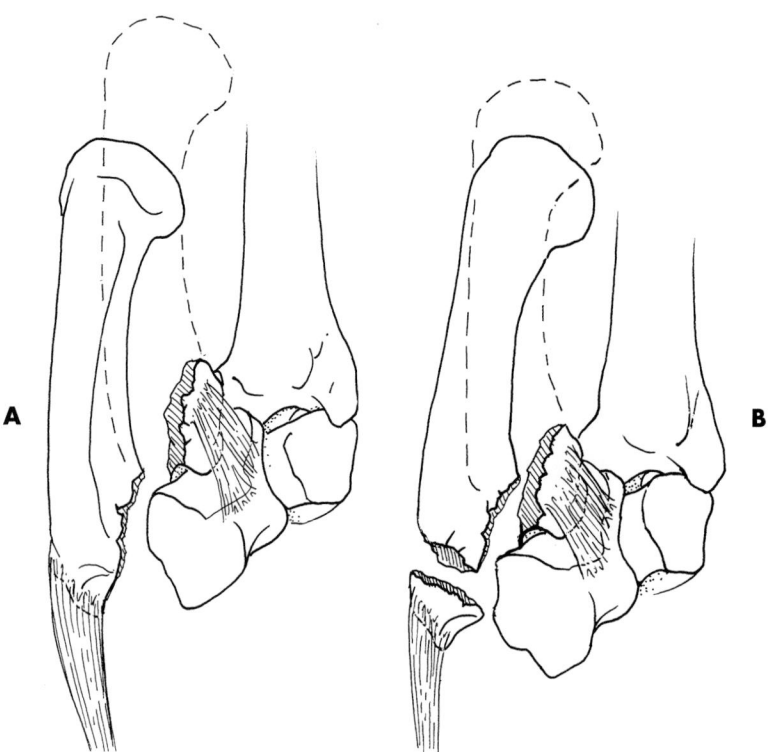

Fig. 25-18. A, Bennett's fracture. The fracture occurs through the beak of the metacarpal, with the intact anterior oblique ligament stabilizing the small fragment. The metacarpal shaft is displaced proximally secondary to the strong muscle and tendon attachments. **B,** Rolando's fracture. This is a T- or Y-shaped intraarticular fracture, frequently with even more comminution than demonstrated here.

SUMMARY

A thorough understanding of the possible injuries that occur to the small joints in the hand allows the individual treating the patient to appropriately assess the patient's condition and establish a satisfactory management program. Direct communication between the surgeon and the therapist is vital. The immobilization period required to allow sufficient healing and the remobilization program differ at each joint, for each patient, and for each injury. Patient education, early mobilization, and prolonged protection are essential components in the management of small joint injuries.

ACKNOWLEDGMENT

We wish to thank Sue Brown for her help in the preparation of this manuscript.

REFERENCES

1. Abrahamsson SO: Diagnosis of displaced ulnar collateral ligament of the metacarpophalangeal joint of the thumb, *J Hand Surg* 15A:457, 1990.
2. Agee JM: Unstable fracture dislocations of the proximal interphalangeal joint of the fingers: a preliminary report of a new treatment technique, *J Hand Surg* 3A:386, 1978.
3. Bain GI: Dynamic external fixation for injuries of the proximal interphalangeal joint, *J Bone Joint Surg* 80B:1014, 1998.
4. Barmakian JT: Anatomy of the joints of the thumb, *Hand Clin* 8:683, 1992.
5. Bohart PG: Complex dislocations of the metacarpophalangeal joint, *Hand Clin* 4:491, 1988.
6. Bowers WH: The anatomy of the interphalangeal joints. In Bowers WH, editor: *The interphalangeal joints,* Edinburgh, 1987, Churchill Livingstone.
7. Bowers WH: Injuries and complications of injuries to the capsular structure of the interphalangeal joints. In Bowers WH, editor: *The interphalangeal joints,* Edinburgh, 1987, Churchill Livingstone.
8. Breen T: Intra-articular fractures of the basilar joint of the thumb, *Hand Clin* 4:491, 1988.
9. Buchler E: Comminuted fractures of the basilar joint of the thumb: combined treatment by external fixation, limited internal fixation, and bone grafting, *J Hand Surg* 6:556, 1991.
10. Campbell CS: Gamekeeper's thumb, *J Bone Joint Surg* 37A:148, 1955.
11. Clendenin MD, Smith RJ: Fifth metacarpal hamate arthrodesis for post-traumatic osteoarthritis, *J Hand Surg* 9A:374, 1984.
12. Cooney WP, et al: The kinesiology of the thumb trapezio-metacarpal joint, *J Bone Joint Surg* 63A:1371, 1981.
13. Downey DJ: Acute gamekeeper's thumb: quantitative outcome of surgical repair, *Am J Sports Med* 23:222, 1995.
14. Dutton RO: Complex dorsal dislocation of the thumb MP joint, *Clin Orthop April:*160, 1982.
15. Eaton RG: *Joint injuries of the hand,* Springfield, Ill, 1971, Charles C. Thomas.
16. Eaton RG: Volar plate arthroplasty for the proximal interphalangeal joint: a review of ten years' experience, *J Hand Surg* 5A:260, 1980.

17. Foster RJ: Treatment of Bennett, Rolando and vertical intra-articular trapezial fractures, *Clin Orthop* 214:121, 1987.
18. Gainor BJ: Tendon arthroplasty of the fifth carpometacarpal joint for treatment of post traumatic arthritis, *J Hand Surg* 16A:520, 1991.
19. Harper MT: Gamekeepers thumb: diagnosis of UCL injury using MRI, MR arthrography and stress radiography, *J Magn Reson Imaging* 6:322, 1996.
20. Hartwig RH: Multiple carpometacarpal dislocations, *J Bone Joint Surg* 61A:906, 1979.
21. Hastings H: Treatment of closed articular fractures of the metacarpophalangeal joint and proximal interphalangeal joints, *Hand Clin* 4:503, 1988.
22. Hergan K: Pitfalls in sonography of the gamekeepers thumb, *Eur Radiol* 7:65, 1997.
23. Imaeda T: Functional anatomy and biomechanics of the thumb, *Hand Clin* 8:9, 1992.
24. Ishizuki M: Injury to collateral ligament of metacarpophalangeal joint of a finger, *J Hand Surg* 13A:456, 1988.
25. Kiefhaber TR: Lateral stability of the proximal interphalangeal joint, *J Hand Surg* 11A:661, 1986.
26. Kozin S: Treatment of thumb ulnar collateral ligament ruptures with the mitek bone anchor, *Ann Plastic Surg* 35:1, 1995.
27. Kraemer BA: Anatomy affecting the metacarpal and phalangeal bones. In Gilula LA, editor: *The traumatized hand and wrist,* Philadelphia, 1992, WB Saunders.
28. Krause J: Isolated injuries to the dorsoradial capsule of the thumb metacarpophalangeal joint, *J Hand Surg* 21A:428, 1996.
29. Kung G: Irreducible dislocation of the proximal interphalangeal joint of the finger, *J Hand Surg* 23B:252, 1998.
30. Leddy J: Avulsion of the profundus tendon insertion in athletes, *J Hand Surg* 2:66, 1977.
31. Light TR: Management of intra-articular fractures of the MP joint, *Hand Clin* May:303, 1994.
32. London PS: Sprains and fractures involving the interphalangeal joints, *Hand* 3:155, 1971.
33. Lubahn JD: Mallet finger fractures: a comparison of open and closed technique, *J Hand Surg* 14A:394, 1989.
34. McCue FC, et al: A pseudoboutonnière deformity, *Hand* 7:166, 1975.
35. McElfresh EC: Management of fracture-dislocation of the proximal interphalangeal joints by extension-block splinting, *J Bone Joint Surg* 54A:1705, 1972.
36. Miller RJ: Dislocations and fracture dislocations of the metacarpophalangeal joint of the thumb, *Hand Clin* 4:45, 1988.
37. Miyamoto M: Volar dislocation of the metacarpophalangeal joint of the thumb: a case report, *J Hand Surg* 11B:51, 1986.
38. Morgan JP: Dynamic digital traction for unstable comminuted intra-articular fracture/dislocation the proximal interphalangeal joint, *J Hand Surg* 20A:565, 1995.
39. Moutet F: Les entarses de la metacarpo-phalangienne due pouce a une experience de plus de 1000 cas, *Ann Chir Main Memb Super* 8:99, 1989.
40. Neichajev I: Dislocation intra-articular fracture of the base of the fifth metacarpal: a clinical study of 23 patients, *Plast Reconstr Surg* 75:406, 1985.
41. Oni O: Irreducible buttonhole dislocation of the proximal interphalangeal joint of the finger, *J Hand Surg* 10B:100, 1985.
42. Pellegrini VD Jr: Fractures at the base of the thumb, *Hand Clin* 4:87, 1988.
43. Pichora DR: Gamekeeper's thumb: a prospective study of functional bracing, *J Hand Surg* 14A:567, 1989.
44. Posner MA: Irreducible volar dislocation of the proximal interphalangeal joint of the finger caused by interposition of an intact central slip, *J Bone Joint Surg* 60A:133, 1978.
45. Posner MA: Metacarpophalangeal joint injuries of the thumb, *Hand Clin* 8:713, 1992.
46. Rayan GM: Skin necrosis complicating mallet finger splinting and vascularity of the distal interphalangeal joint overlying skin, *J Hand Surg* 12A:548, 1987.
47. Ryu J: Arthroscopic treatment of acute complete thumb metacarpophalangeal ulnar collateral ligament tears, *J Hand Surg* 20A:1037, 1995.
48. Seymour N: Juxta-epiphyseal fracture of the terminal phalanx of the finger, *J Bone Joint Surg* 48B:347, 1966.
49. Schenck RR: Dynamic traction and early passive movement for fracture of the proximal interphalangeal joint, *J Hand Surg* 11A:850, 1986.
50. Shaw SJ: The range of motion of the metacarpophalangeal joint of the thumb and its relationship to injury, *J Hand Surg* 17B:164, 1992.
51. Simonian P: Traumatic dislocation of the thumb carpometacarpal joint: early ligamentous reconstruction vs. closed reduction and pinning, *J Hand Surg* 21A:802, 1996.
52. Stark HH: Troublesome fractures and dislocations of the hand. In *AAOS instructional course lectures,* vol 19, St Louis, 1970, Mosby.
53. Stener B: Displacement of the ruptured ulnar collateral ligament of the metacarpophalangeal joint of the thumb, *J Bone Joint Surg* 44B:869, 1962.
54. Stern PJ: Complications and prognosis of treatment of mallet finger, *J Hand Surg* 13A:329, 1988.
55. Stern PJ: Pilon fractures of the proximal interphalangeal joint, *J Hand Surg* 16A:844, 1991.
56. Stern PJ: Fractures of the metacarpals and phalanges. In Green DP, editor: *Operative hand surg,* ed 3, vol 1, New York, 1993, Churchill Livingstone.
57. Thompson JS, Eaton RG: Volar dislocation of the proximal interphalangeal joint, *J Bone Joint Surg* 2:232, 1977.
58. Viegas S: Extension block pinning for proximal interphalangeal joint fracture/dislocations: preliminary report of a new technique, *J Hand Surg* 17A:896, 1992.
59. Wehbe MD: Mallet fractures, *J Bone Joint Surg* 66A:658, 1984.
60. Wilson RL: Mallet finger. In Hunter JM, Schneider LH, Mackin EJ, editors: *Tendon surgery in the hand,* St Louis, 1987, Mosby.
61. Wilson RL, Carter M: Joint injuries in the hand: preservation of proximal interphalangeal joint function. In Hunter J, et al: *Rehabilitation of the hand,* St Louis, 1978, Mosby.
62. Wilson RL, Liechty BW: Complications following small joint injuries, *Hand Clin* 2:329, 1986.
63. Wilson RL, McGinty LD: Common hand and wrist injuries in basketball players, *Clin Sports Med* 12:265, 1993.
64. Wilson RL, et al: Flexor profundus injuries treated with staged profundus grafting, *J Hand Surg* 5:74, 1980.

Part VI

TENDON INJURIES

Chapter 26

PRIMARY CARE OF FLEXOR TENDON INJURIES

Randall W. Culp
John S. Taras

Restoring digital function after flexor tendon injury continues to be one of the great challenges in hand surgery.* In recent years, important advancements in our understanding of tendon anatomy,[22,23] biomechanics,[51,52,137] nutrition,† adhesion formation,[43,56,64,65,120] and tendon repair techniques have led to enhanced results after flexor tendon repair. Despite the many gains, problems of stiffness, scarring, and functional impairment persist in frustrating the most experienced hand surgeon.

ANATOMY

Appreciation of the anatomy of the flexor tendons[51] as well as the flexor retinacular sheath[22-25,50,83] is critical for the surgeon dealing with flexor tendon injuries. The flexor digitorum profundus (FDP) arises from the proximal volar and medial surfaces of the ulna, the interosseous membrane, and occasionally the proximal radius. Along with the flexor pollicis longus (FPL), the FDP forms the deep muscle layer in the flexor compartment of the proximal forearm. In the midforearm, the muscle belly separates into a radial and ulnar bundle. In the distal third of the forearm, the radial bundle forms the index finger profundus tendon, and the ulnar bundle forms the profundus tendon to the ulnar three digits. The profundus tendons pass through the carpal canal, occupying the floor of the tunnel.

After traversing the carpal canal, the profundus tendons diverge to the digits. The lumbrical muscles originate at this level. The profundus tendons enter the flexor sheath deep to the superficialis tendons at the level of the metacarpopha-

langeal (MP) joint. At the midproximal phalanx level, the profundus tendon becomes more palmar as it passes through the bifurcating superficialis tendon. It continues distally to insert into the palmar base of the distal phalanx.

Innervation of the FDP occurs through the anterior interosseous branch of the median nerve for the index and occasionally the long finger. The ulnar nerve innervates the FDP to the ring and small fingers. The flexor digitorum superficialis (FDS) originates from two separate heads. The humeroulnar head arises from the medial humeral epicondyle and the coronary process of the ulna. The radial head arises from the proximal shaft at the radius. In the proximal forearm, it occupies the intermediate layer of the flexor compartment superficial to the flexor profundus. In the middle third of the forearm, four separate muscles are identified. Four distinct tendons are seen in the distal third of the forearm. The superficialis to the small finger is variable and may be absent in 21% of patients.[4] At the carpal tunnel level, the long and ring finger superficialis tendons lie superficial and central to those of the index and small, which lie deeper and more peripheral.

At the level of the MP joint, the superficialis tendon enters the flexor sheath palmar to the profundus tendon. At the proximal third of the proximal phalanx, the superficialis bifurcates around the profundus tendon. The two slips reunite deep to the profundus tendon at Camper's chiasm, with 50% of fibers decussating and 50% remaining ipsilateral. The superficialis tendon then inserts through the radial and ulnar slips into the proximal metaphysis of the middle phalanx.

Innervation of the superficialis muscle is provided solely by the median nerve. The FPL originates from the proximal

---

*References 12, 13, 59-63, 106, 133, 152-154.
†References 36, 39, 44, 84, 85, 138.

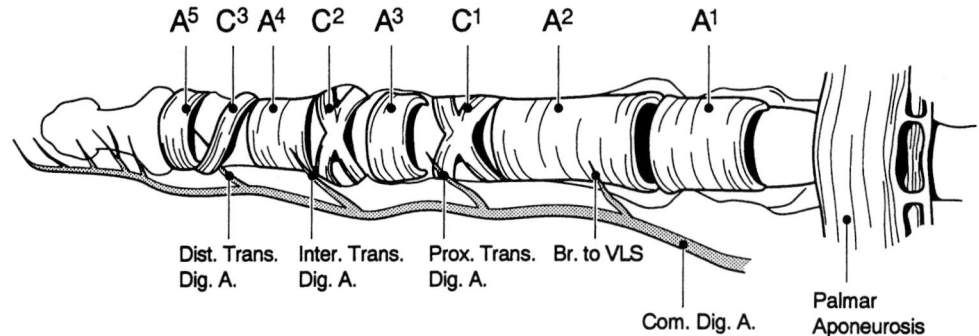

Fig. 26-1. Flexor digital retinacular sheath and flexor tendon vascular supply.

radius and interosseous membrane. In the proximal third of the forearm, it lies radially in the deep layer of the flexor compartment. At the carpal tunnel level, it lies on the radial floor. After traversing the carpal tunnel, it enters the palm by emerging between the adductor pollicis and the flexor pollicis brevis (FPB). It enters the flexor sheath of the thumb as the sole tendon and inserts at the proximal palmar base of the distal phalanx. The FPL is innervated by the anterior interosseous branch of the median nerve.

The digital flexor sheath is a synovial-lined fibroosseous tunnel. This system functions to hold the flexor tendons in close opposition to the phalanges, ensuring efficient mechanical function in producing digital flexion. The flexor sheath is composed of synovial and retinacular tissue components, each with separate and distinct functions.[24] The synovial component of the sheath consists of a visceral, or epitenon, layer that envelops the flexor tendon and a parietal, or outer, layer that lines the walls of the flexor sheath. These two layers are contiguous at the ends of the sheath, creating a double-walled, hollow tube that surrounds the flexor tendons. In the index, long, and ring fingers, the membranous sheath begins at the MP joint and ends at the distal phalanx. The synovial sheath at the thumb and small fingers continues proximally into the carpal tunnel as the radial and ulnar bursae, respectively.[22,25] The function of the synovial sheath is to provide a low-friction gliding system and provide nutrition to the tendon.

The retinacular portion of the sheath is characterized by fibrous bands that overlay the synovial sheath in segmental fashion[22,23,50,83] (Fig. 26-1). Thickened transverse bands are termed *annular* pulleys, and thin flexible areas of crisscrossing fibers are termed *cruciate* pulleys. Stronger, broader annular pulleys provide mechanical stability to the system, ensuring optimal joint flexion for a given amount of tendon excursion. The more flexible cruciate pulleys permit flexibility to the system. The following pulleys have been identified: the palmar aponeurosis pulley, five annular pulleys, and three cruciate pulleys. The palmar aponeurosis pulley is formed from the transverse fibers of the palmar aponeurosis.[23,83] It is located at the beginning of the

membranous sheath and is anchored on each side of the sheath by vertical septa that attach to the deep transverse metacarpal ligament. The first annular pulley (A_1) arises from the volar plate of the MP joint. The second annular pulley (A_2) arises from the volar aspect of the proximal half of the proximal phalanx. The first cruciate pulley (C_1) extends from the A_2 to the third annular pulley (A_3), which arises from the volar plate of the proximal interphalangeal (PIP) joint. The fourth annular pulley (A_4) arises from the middle phalanx and is connected proximally to the A_3 pulley by the second cruciate pulley (C_2). The fifth annular pulley (A_5) arises from the volar plate of the distal interphalangeal (DIP) joint. It is connected proximally to the A_4 pulley by the third cruciate pulley (C_3). Not all of the elements of the flexor sheath can be identified as described, particularly A_3 and A_5, which can be indistinct or absent.

The pulley system of the thumb is distinct from that of the digits[25] (Fig. 26-2). One oblique and two annular pulleys have been identified. The first annular pulley of the thumb (A_1) arises from the palmar plate of the MP joint, and the second annular pulley (A_2) arises from the palmar plate of the interphalangeal (IP) joint. The oblique pulley originates and inserts on the proximal phalanx in close association with the insertion of the adductor pollicis tendon.

Anatomic and clinical studies have demonstrated that the A_2 and A_4 pulleys are the most important components of the flexor sheath, their presence ensuring biomechanical efficiency of the system.[24,51,52] A_3 and the palmar aponeurotic pulleys become important only when A_2 and A_4 have been damaged.[23,24,52,83] The loss of all or portions of the pulley system may lead to flexor bowstringing. This leads to an increased mechanical moment arm, which can create late flexion contractures. In addition, increased flexor tendon excursions are required to produce full digital flexion. In the thumb, the oblique pulley is the most important. Its loss results in decreased IP joint motion. Incompetence of both the A_1 and oblique pulleys of the thumb leads to a 30% loss of IP joint motion.[25]

Flexor tendon excursions in the zone of the retinacular sheath in cadaveric specimens have been calculated.[104]

Chapter 26 Primary care of flexor tendon injuries **417**

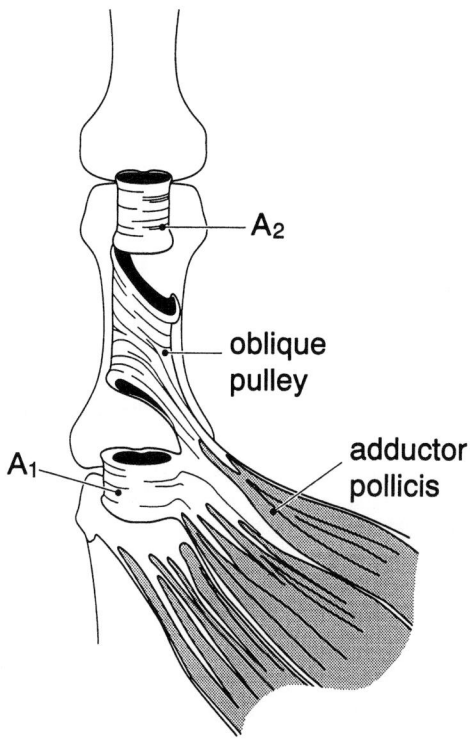

Fig. 26-2. Flexor retinacular sheath of the thumb.

Passive MP joint motion produces no relative motion of the tendons to the sheath. DIP joint motion produces excursion of the FDP on the FDS of 1 mm for 10 degrees of flexion. PIP joint motion produces excursion of the FDS and the FDP together of 1.3 mm for 10 degrees of flexion relative to the retinacular sheath. Recently, postrepair clinical motion studies have demonstrated that in marked tendons this calculated excursion decreases.[140] DIP joint motion of 10 degrees produces excursion of the FDP of only 0.3 mm, and PIP motion of 10 degrees produces excursion of the FDP and superficialis of 1.2 mm. This may explain why DIP motion is often suboptimal after flexor tendon repair.

NUTRITION

Flexor tendon nutrition appears to occur through both direct vascular supply* (see Fig. 26-1) and synovial diffusion.[30,78,82-87,94,101] Proximal to the digital sheath, a longitudinal blood supply originates from within the proximal muscle tissue and is carried distally through the peritenon. Within the sheath, transverse branches of the digital arteries passing through the vincular system add segmental blood supply.[111] These branches include a proximal vessel to the vinculum longus superficialis, a proximal digital transverse artery, an IP transverse digital artery, and a distal transverse digital artery. As the transverse branches pass to the midline, they merge to carry palmarly into the

---

*References 2, 8, 28, 48, 77, 98-100, 111, 113, 117, 147, 180.

tendons via the vincula. The vinculum profundus brevis is a short triangular pedicle supplying the profundus tendon near its insertion. A similar short vinculum supplies the superficialis tendon at the neck of the proximal phalanx, but here the vessels continue to form the vinculum longus to the profundus tendon. The superficialis receives additional blood supply from the vinculum longus superficialis at the base of the proximal phalanx. Both tendons receive additional blood supply from their distal osseous attachments. Throughout the sheath, vessels enter the tendon from the dorsal surface, with the palmar third remaining relatively avascular.[77] This anatomic fact has led to the surgical technique of palmar placement of sutures within the tendon to preserve blood supply. Finally, an avascular watershed zone of the FDP has been identified between the longitudinal and vincular vessels at the midproximal phalanx level.[48,77]

In addition to nourishment of the flexor tendons by vascular perfusion, experiments have demonstrated the importance of diffusional nutrition by the synovial fluid.[30,78,82-87,94] Radioisotope tracer studies suggest a greater role of diffusion than perfusion.[84,86] In addition, strong evidence has demonstrated that the superficial layers of isolated segments of tendon can heal in an isolated synovial environment without direct vascularity.[25,46,85] This finding has led some authors to recommend sheath repair to restore synovial fluid.[71-73] The relative significance of these dual nutritional pathways in the normal and repaired flexor tendon has yet to be completely clarified. Recent studies suggest that synovial diffusion associated with neovascularization of the healing site in the absence of ingrowth of peripheral vessels may play a role in the nourishment of the healing tendon.[36]

FLEXOR TENDON HEALING

The subject of flexor tendon healing has traditionally been associated with controversy. Two theories have been proposed to help explain observed experimental phenomena. The first, the extrinsic healing theory, suggests that tendon healing occurs through cells extrinsic to the tendon through a fibroblastic response from surrounding tissue.[90,114,115,121-123] This theory presupposes the necessity of surrounding peritendinous adhesions to allow complete healing of the tendon; thus immobilization after flexor tendon repair was encouraged. Experimental clinical evidence of adhesions at the repair site has supported this concept. The sequence of healing by extrinsic mechanism begins with the ingrowth of capillaries and fibroblasts from 0 to 4 days, formation of collagen fibers from 4 to 21 days, and scar remodeling after 21 days.

The second theory, intrinsic healing, suggests that healing is possible in the absence of cells and tissue extrinsic to the tendon.* More recent experimental and clinical evidence to

---

*References 2, 29, 32, 33, 38-40, 70, 75, 78, 87, 91, 95, 142.

support this concept includes rounded ends of unrepaired tendons, tendon healing in the absence of adhesions, and in vitro healing of tendons in isolated, cell-free environments. Controlled mobilization of repaired tendons to allow healing but to prevent peritendinous adhesions was the stated advantage of this healing theory. The sequence of intrinsic healing begins with the inflammatory phase, from 0 to 3 days, with proliferation and thickening of epitenon cell layers. At 5 to 7 days, collagen formation and early vascular ingrowth ensue. A fibrous callus is noted at 10 days, and proliferation ingrowth of endotenon tenocytes occurs at 2 to 3 weeks.

Although the relative roles of each type of tendon healing remain to be elucidated, in the clinical situation, tendons probably heal by a combination of extrinsic and intrinsic cellular activity.[32,56,153] The more intrinsic healing that occurs, the less peritendinous adhesions theoretically would be formed. This concept forms the basis of controlled mobilization programs after tendon repair.

ZONES OF INJURY

One must consider the level of injury when performing flexor tendon repair. Five anatomic zones of injury have been identified based on Verdan's original description of the flexor tendon system[63,165-168] (Fig. 26-3). The level of injury should be recorded in relation to the position of tendon laceration in the sheath, with the finger in the extended position.

Zone 1 extends from the insertion of the FDS at the middle phalanx to that of the FDP at the distal phalanx. Injuries in this level may involve lacerations or avulsions of the FDP. Zone II involves that region in which both the FDS and FDP travel within the flexor sheath from the A$_1$ pulley to the insertion of the FDS. This zone has previously been termed "no man's land" by Bunnell because of the worse prognosis associated with treatment of flexor tendon injuries at this level.[12] A more descriptive term may be "some man's land" because the more experienced hand surgeon can obtain satisfactory results with appropriate care. Zone III comprises the area between the distal border of the carpal tunnel and the A$_1$ pulley of the flexor sheath. Besides the common digital nerves, vessels, and both flexor tendons, the lumbrical muscles reside in this zone. Zone IV consists of that segment of flexor tendons covered by the transverse carpal ligament within the carpal tunnel. Concomitant injuries to the median and ulnar nerves may be associated with flexor tendon injuries in this zone. Zone V extends from the flexor musculotendinous junction in the forearm to the proximal border of the transverse carpal ligament. Associated neurovascular injuries may compromise results in this region as well.

The flexor tendon system in the thumb is predicated on only one flexor tendon. Zone I is at the insertion area of the FPL. Zone II coincides with the flexor retinaculum of the thumb, from the neck of the metacarpal to the neck of the

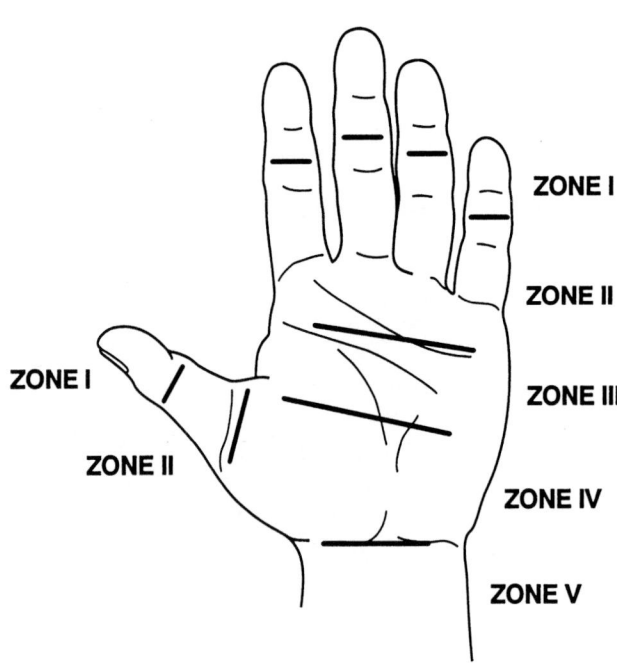

Fig. 26-3. Zone classification of flexor tendon injuries.

proximal phalanx. Zone III is the area of the thenar muscles. Zone IV represents the area of the carpal canal. Finally, zone V is the anatomic area from the musculotendinous junction of the FPL to the transverse carpal ligament.

DIAGNOSIS

A knowledge of flexor tendon anatomy is necessary to accurately diagnose acute injury. In the cooperative patient, diagnosis is usually not difficult. Because of the common muscle origin of the flexor profundi, FDS function can be assessed only by restraining the profundi by completely extending the other digits. Independently functioning superficialis is demonstrated by full flexion of the PIP joint of the affected finger. This test often is not applicable to the index finger because of the independent muscle belly of the FDP. The FDS to the index finger can be demonstrated through pulp-to-pulp pinch with the thumb and index finger.

Demonstration of PIP joint flexion of the index finger with the DIP joint fully extended or hyperextended documents superficialis function to the index finger. As noted earlier, the FDS of the small finger is variable and can be absent in 21% of patients.[4] The FDP function is demonstrated by active flexion of the DIP. Active flexion of the IP joint of the thumb indicates an intact FPL. If when performing these tests the patient demonstrates motion but experiences pain, the surgeon must entertain the possibility of partial flexor-tendon injury.

In the uncooperative or unconscious patient or a child, additional diagnostic signs may be helpful. In the normal

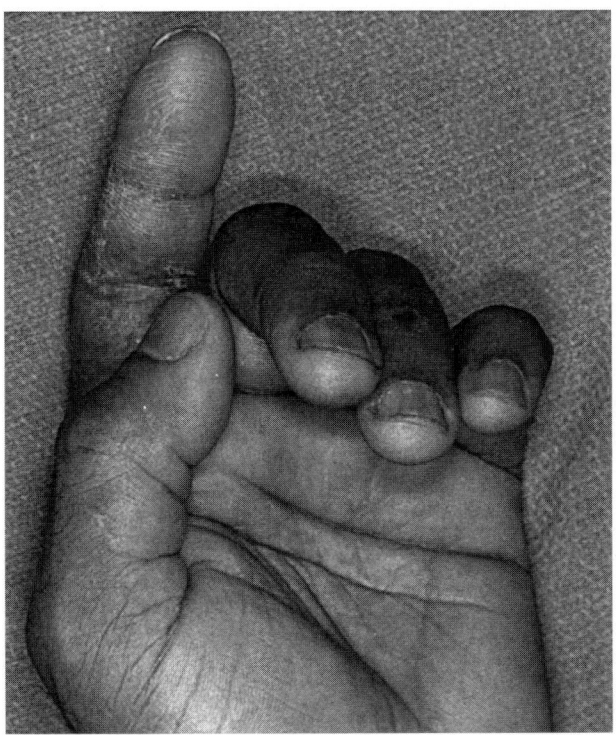

Fig. 26-4. Laceration of the index finger. Posture of the index finger in extension suggests complete laceration of the flexor digitorum profundus and superficialis.

hand, a cascade of flexion of the digits is noted, increasing as one proceeds from the index to the small fingers. Abnormal posture or change in the normal cascade can indicate flexor tendon injury (Fig. 26-4). In addition, squeezing the forearm musculature to demonstrate flexion of the digits may be helpful. Finally, assessing tenodesis of flexor tendons with the wrist in extension will demonstrate loss of finger flexion if flexor tendons are severed.

The examiner is responsible for determining that the flexor tendons are intact before dismissing the patient. If the examiner is uncertain, exploration of the wound under operating room conditions may be required. The actual level of tendon laceration depends on the position of the fingers when the injury occurred. If the injury occurred with the finger in extension, the skin wound and both tendons will be lacerated at the same level. In fingers injured in flexion, the tendon injury will be distal to the skin wound. In addition, the FDP will be lacerated at a level different from that of the superficialis tendon because of their different excursions.

INDICATIONS AND CONTRAINDICATIONS

Although there has been some controversy in the past over the efficacy of primary repair of flexor tendons, particularly in zone II,[7,12,13,92] immediate or delayed primary repair is currently advocated for flexor tendon injuries with

only few exceptions.* The advantages of primary repair over secondary grafting include less extensive surgery, decreased periods of disability, and restoration of normal tendon length.[167]

Specific contraindications to immediate or delayed primary repair include severe contamination where infection is a possibility.† In addition, loss of palmar skin overlying the flexor system generally precludes tendon repair,[59,61] although there have been some recent reports of concomitant tendon repair and soft tissue coverage procedures.[35] Another contraindication to primary repair is extensive damage to the flexor retinacular, where pulley reconstruction and one- or two-stage tendon reconstruction probably will be required.[134] Concurrent fracture or neurovascular injury, however, does not necessarily contraindicate tendon repair. If fracture stabilization can be obtained, flexor tendon repair generally should ensue.

Researchers have effectively demonstrated that repair of both the FDP and the FDS rather than the FDP alone, even in zone II injury, will provide the most optimal result.[31,34,63,66,168] Advantages of repairing and maintaining the FDS include maintenance of vincular blood supply to the FDP, retaining of a smooth gliding surface for the FDP, independent motion of the digit with stronger flexion power, and decreased possibility of hyperextension deformities of the PIP joint.

Schneider et al.[136] have demonstrated that tendon repair as long as 3 weeks after injury exhibited outcomes similar to those tendons repaired more acutely. Although not statistically significant, repairs performed within the first 10 days tended to be superior. Recently, animal studies also have supported improved tendon excursion with early repairs.[45] These studies demonstrate that, although tendon repair is not emergent, repair within the first few days after injury appears warranted.

OPERATIVE TECHNIQUE
General considerations

Flexor tendon repair must be performed only by trained surgeons who know the anatomy of the flexor tendon system and the potential pitfalls of surgical repair. Repair is performed under regional or general anesthesia in a bloodless field. The use of 2- to 4-power loupe magnification will decrease inadvertent nerve or vessel injury. Lateral or palmar zigzag (Bruner) incisions are performed, depending on the surgeon's preference. The Bruner incision, our preferred approach, offers excellent exposure but can cause scarring over the palmar surface of the digit.[9,10] The midlateral incision is technically more demanding and may interfere with transverse digital branches supplying the vincula but

*References 34, 59-63, 66, 74, 79, 102, 108, 116, 133, 135, 141, 152, 154, 155, 164.
†References 59, 61, 135, 152, 154, 155.

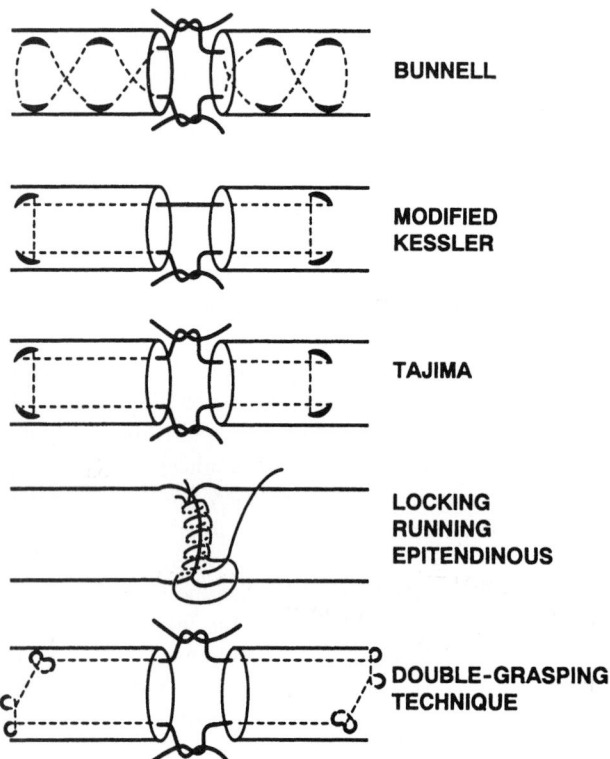

BUNNELL

MODIFIED
KESSLER

TAJIMA

LOCKING
RUNNING
EPITENDINOUS

DOUBLE-GRASPING
TECHNIQUE

Fig. 26-5. Suture techniques used in flexor tendon repairs.

has the advantage of decreased scarring over the flexor surface, which can lead to improved rehabilitation.[66] Delicate instrumentation is required; pinching or crushing of the flexor tendon or sheath will inevitably lead to suboptimal results.[12,13] We generally prefer to handle the tendon at its cut end only, avoiding grasping of the epitenon, which can create later epitendinous adhesions. Minimal debridement of tendon ends is not usually required but may be performed if necessary using a knife or nerve-cutting instrument. Many suture techniques have been described.[53-55,88,131,161,170] Traditionally, many surgeons prefer a modified Kessler grasping-type core stitch, based on the excellent studies by Urbaniak and others.[57,162,178] A 3-0 or 4-0 braided synthetic material placed in the volar third of the tendon is preferred by most surgeons. The Tajima modification of the modified Kessler grasping stitch is also popular; suture knots are tied within the repair site, with a separate stitch for each cut tendon end. Alternatively, a double-grasping modification of the Tajima suture can be used. Locking loops have been shown to possibly increase strength of repair.[47] Most authors currently recommend at least a four-strand core repair, crossing the repair site with an epitendinous suture augmentation. A variety of core suture designs have been described, ranging from four to eight strands crossing the repair site (Fig. 26-5). Adding a horizontal mattress suture to the traditional suture is one convenient method to that end. Multiple strand sutures swedged to a single needle, used in

the traditional Tajima position, has been described. This provides the immediate four-strand suture strength and the added advantage of ease of placement. A 3-0 or 4-0 Ethibond suture is used. A running locking epitendinous suture of 6-0 nonabsorbable monofilament material is used at the repair site. Recent studies have demonstrated that the epitendinous suture significantly increases the strength of the repair.[69,89,129,169,170] The superficialis tendon is repaired using either a Tajima-type stitch or a simpler mattress suture, depending on the size of the tendon and the location of the laceration. Several techniques are available to atraumatically retrieve retracted tendon ends. With the wrist and MP joints placed in maximal flexion, flexor muscle bellies may be milked manually to deliver the tendon ends.

If this fails, alternatives are available. If a tendon end is visible in the flexor sheath, one may use a skin hook. The hooked end is slid along the surface of the sheath until it has passed the tendons, and the hook is then turned toward the tendons, engaging the most superficial one. As the instrument is pulled distally, the tendons may follow. The tendons then can be held in position by a Keith or 25-gauge hypodermic needle placed through the skin and A_2 pulley area for later repair.

Another commonly used technique uses a catheter (pediatric feeding tube, red rubber tube, or Hunter rod), which is passed distal to proximal alongside the flexor tendons, which are left in situ. The catheter is sutured to both tendons 2 cm proximal to the A_1 pulley through a second palmar incision. The catheter is advanced distally to deliver tendon ends into the repair site. A 25-gauge hypodermic needle is passed transversely through the skin and A_2 pulley to maintain tendon position. Core sutures are then placed. The catheter tendon suture is then cut in the palm and withdrawn.[149]

A final technique often used again uses a catheter that is passed from distal to proximal through the flexor sheath. A Tajima stitch is placed into the tendon end, and the other end of the suture is placed into the end of the catheter. The catheter and suture, followed by the tendons, are pulled distally through the flexor sheath. Further retraction of tendons is prevented again by transfixing them to the skin and A_2 pulley with a 25-gauge hypodermic needle.

For all of these techniques, the anatomic relationship of the profundus to the superficialis tendons must be maintained.[72] One anatomic point that may aid the surgeon in maintaining this orientation and preventing tendon twisting is the fact that the vincula insert on the dorsal surface of the tendons.

Every attempt is made to preserve all pulleys of the flexor retinacular sheath. Small surgical windows into the sheath often are required to identify tendon ends. Whether the sheath should be subsequently repaired is controversial.* Theoretic support for repair includes tendon gliding and

*References 2, 43, 71, 73, 117-120, 127.

nutrition. To date, no clinical studies have documented superiority of repair versus resection of the sheath.[2,73] In addition, one prospective study comparing the two techniques demonstrated no superiority of sheath repair.[127] Currently, we favor sheath repair using 6-0 or 7-0 monofilament suture if there has been minimal loss of sheath substance and the repair can be performed easily without constriction of the sheath or the tendon repair.

TREATMENT OF ACUTE FLEXOR TENDON INJURIES
Zone I

In zone I, distal to the FDS insertion, only the FDP tendon is injured. The patient maintains PIP joint flexion but loses DIP flexion. Although adequate finger function can be maintained without repair in some circumstances, early direct repair is desirable. This is particularly true as one proceeds from the radial (precision grip) to the ulnar (power grip) side of the hand. In addition, the superficialis of the small finger is absent in a significant percentage of individuals, necessitating repair of the lacerated FDP tendon in that digit. With early repair, digital function can be near normal.

If more than 4 weeks have elapsed, direct repair usually cannot be performed because of contracture of the FDP muscle belly. Another pitfall in this zone that must be avoided is injury to the normally functioning FDS caused by excessive surgical manipulation. Finally, the surgeon must not advance the profundus tendon more than 1 cm at this level of injury to afford repair.[80] This leads, particularly in the ulnar three digits, to unacceptable flexion contractures of the affected digit as well as incomplete flexion of the neighboring digits; this has been termed *quadrigia syndrome.*[166]

There are three patterns of lacerations in zone I. The first is where the short vincula of the FDP remain intact. Although this pattern is rare, the FDP remains just proximal to its insertion. Direct repairs can be performed late with this pattern of injury. The second pattern presents with the long vincula of the FDP intact. The severed end of the tendon lies at the FDS decussation. The prognosis for early repair is good. Finally, the FDP can retract into the palm, with both vincula being ruptured. Loss of vincular blood supply has occurred. This repair requires more extensive surgical dissection and early repair. When this pattern of injury is diagnosed late, alternative treatments such as observation, tendon graft, DIP tenodesis, and arthrodesis must be entertained.

Surgical technique in zone I injuries. A volar zigzag incision from the PIP joint crease to distal to the DIP joint is performed. Every effort is made to preserve the A_4 pulley. If only a short distal stump of FDP remains, opening the tendon sheath at the C_3, A_5 pulley level may be required. If the proximal FDP stump has retracted to the level of the PIP joint, a window at the C_2 pulley may be fashioned to retrieve

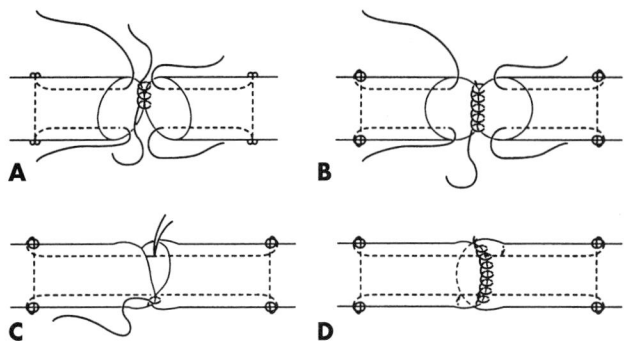

Fig. 26-6. A sequence of flexor tendon repair. **A,** Core suture has been placed in each tendon end. A running, locking epitendinous suture is begun on the back wall. **B,** The back wall epitendinous suture is completed. **C,** Core suture is tightened with knots in the repair site, avoiding gapping or buckling. **D,** Completion of epitendinous suture.

it. If the proximal profundus has retracted to the level of the palm, the zigzag incision may be extended proximally, or a separate transverse incision in the palm proximal to the A_1 pulley may be required. Retracted proximal FDP tendon ends are retrieved atraumatically as described previously. If the injury is recent, the FDP may be passed through the FDS decussation. In older lacerations, one slip of the superficialis may be sacrificed to facilitate passage of the FDP through a tight flexor sheath. Under no circumstances should a normal FDS be completely excised to repair the FDP.

Every effort is made to repair to the distal tendon stump to avoid overadvancement. Tajima or double-grasping 3-0 or 4-0 sutures are placed in each tendon end. We often begin the repair by performing the "back wall" epitendon stitch, first using 6-0 nylon in running, locking fashion. The Tajima core stitch is then tied, followed by completion of the remainder of the palmar epitendinous suture (Fig. 26-6). This avoids the necessity to "flip" the repair to complete the epitendinous suture. As previously discussed, the FDP is not advanced more than 1 cm to permit repair. If the repair catches at the end of the A_4 pulley, a small portion of the sheath may be resected.

If the distal stump is extremely short or nonexistent, the tendon will have to be repaired to the distal phalanx (Fig. 26-7). One develops a periosteal flap at the base of the distal phalanx, carefully avoiding the palmar plate of the DIP joint. The cortex is prepared with a curette to provide a bleeding bone surface that will encourage tendon-to-bone healing. A synthetic monofilament suture, such as 3-0 Prolene, is inserted into the tendon in "unlocked" fashion to facilitate later removal. Keith needles are drilled obliquely in the radial and ulnar aspects of the bone surface, exiting through the nail plate distal to the germinal matrix. Suture ends are placed in the Keith needles. The Keith needles are withdrawn, and the sutures are tied over the nail with a button. The pull-out suture and button are removed 4 to 6 weeks after initial repair. Alternatively, a bone anchor can be

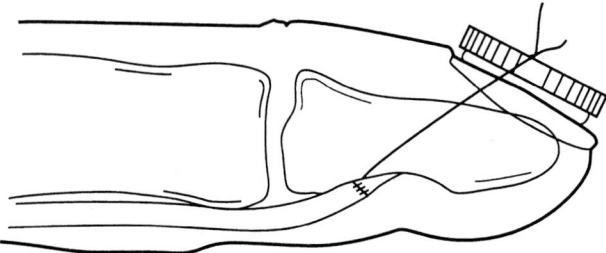

Fig. 26-7. Reinsertion technique for flexor digitorum profundus laceration at distal phalanx in zone I injury.

deployed at the distal phalanx level. The length of the bone anchor must avoid the nailbed.

Zone II

Classically termed "no man's land," injuries at zone II are associated with the greatest technical difficulties in obtaining maximal function. Atraumatic technique is nowhere more important than in zone II, where both flexor tendons are confined in the flexor retinacular sheath. Early repair of both the FDP and FDS is indicated when wound conditions permit.

Surgical technique in zone II injuries. The area is exposed with a volar zigzag or midlateral incision incorporating the laceration (Fig. 26-8). One identifies the flexor sheath, carefully protecting the neurovascular bundles. If nerve injury is identified, the nerve is prepared for repair after repair of the flexor tendons. Every effort must be made to maintain the annular pulleys, especially some portion of the A_2 and A_4 pulleys. If possible, repair should be made through windows in the cruciate-synovial areas through small lateral or transverse incisions. The distal profundus and superficialis tendons usually can be identified and delivered into the wound by acutely flexing the digit. The proximal tendons are atraumatically identified and delivered into the wound by one of the methods previously described. When retrieving the proximal tendons, one should maintain the superficialis and profundus tendons together so as not to interrupt their vascular connections. In zone II, the surgeon must understand the spiral nature of the FDS as it bifurcates around the profundus to reinsert on the middle phalanx at Camper's chiasm. If the superficialis is lacerated after its bifurcation, proximal and distal ends can rotate 180 degrees in different directions. If this anatomic orientation is not corrected, excursion of the profundus tendon can be suboptimal.

After the tendons are delivered into the wound, a Keith or 25-gauge hypodermic needle is placed across the skin and annular pulley to maintain position. A 3-0 or 4-0 core suture is placed in a fashion to produce at least a four-strand core repair. Although traditionally the suture has been placed volarly in the tendon to avoid the blood supply, recent studies show some biomechanical benefit to dorsal placement.[148,150] Before tying the core suture, we again perform the

epitendinous locking 6-0 nylon "back wall" suture. This is followed by tying of the core suture, then the completion of the remainder of the epitendinous suture in its volar portion. The alternative is to tie the core suture in its entirety and then complete the epitendinous locking 6-0 nylon suture by flipping the tendon. If the superficialis is lacerated distal to its bifurcation, mattress or figure-of-eight sutures usually suffice. If the superficialis is lacerated proximal to the bifurcation, a standard Tajima suture is used. The flexor retinaculum is repaired with 6-0 or 7-0 Prolene if possible. If this cannot be achieved and a bulky repair is snagging on a pulley, a portion of the pulley should be either excised or laterally released to allow unimpaired motion after surgery. Finally, at the proximal level of the flexor sheath, one may consider converting a zone II to a zone III injury by excising the A_1 pulley. This is particularly appropriate if a bulky repair is performed at the A_1 pulley level. If pulleys require reconstruction, we currently favor staged tendon reconstruction at this level.

Zone III

Injuries at zone III carry a good prognosis because zone III is located out of the fibroosseous sheath and therefore is less prone to adhesion formation. Injuries to the common digital nerves may accompany the tendon injury. Both superficialis and profundus tendons should be repaired. Delayed primary repair can be performed up to 3 weeks or more after injury because the proximal end of the profundus tendon is held by the lumbrical origin.

Surgical technique in zone III injuries. The zigzag approach to the palm is used. Excision of local palmar fascia may be necessary for exposure. Careful protection of associated neurovascular structures is essential. Repair of both tendons with 3-0 or 4-0 core suture and a 6-0 locking running epitendinous nylon suture is standard.

Zone IV

Flexor tendon injuries in zone IV (within the carpal tunnel) are less common because of the anatomic protection of the medial and lateral bony pillars as well as the stout transverse carpal ligament. Injuries to the median and ulnar nerves, ulnar artery, and superficial palmar arch are often associated because of their proximity to the flexor tendons. If possible, repair of all tendons should be undertaken. If swelling precludes repair of all tendons, the superficialis to the small finger can be excised. If anatomic confines preclude even further repair, all the superficialis tendons can be excised as necessary. Delayed primary repair should be performed within 3 weeks because myostatic contraction prevents repair after this.

Surgical technique in zone IV injuries. The area is approached through a volar zigzag incision incorporating a carpal tunnel–type incision. One may consider a Z-plasty lengthening of the transverse carpal ligament for later repair, although some authors have not found bowstringing to be a

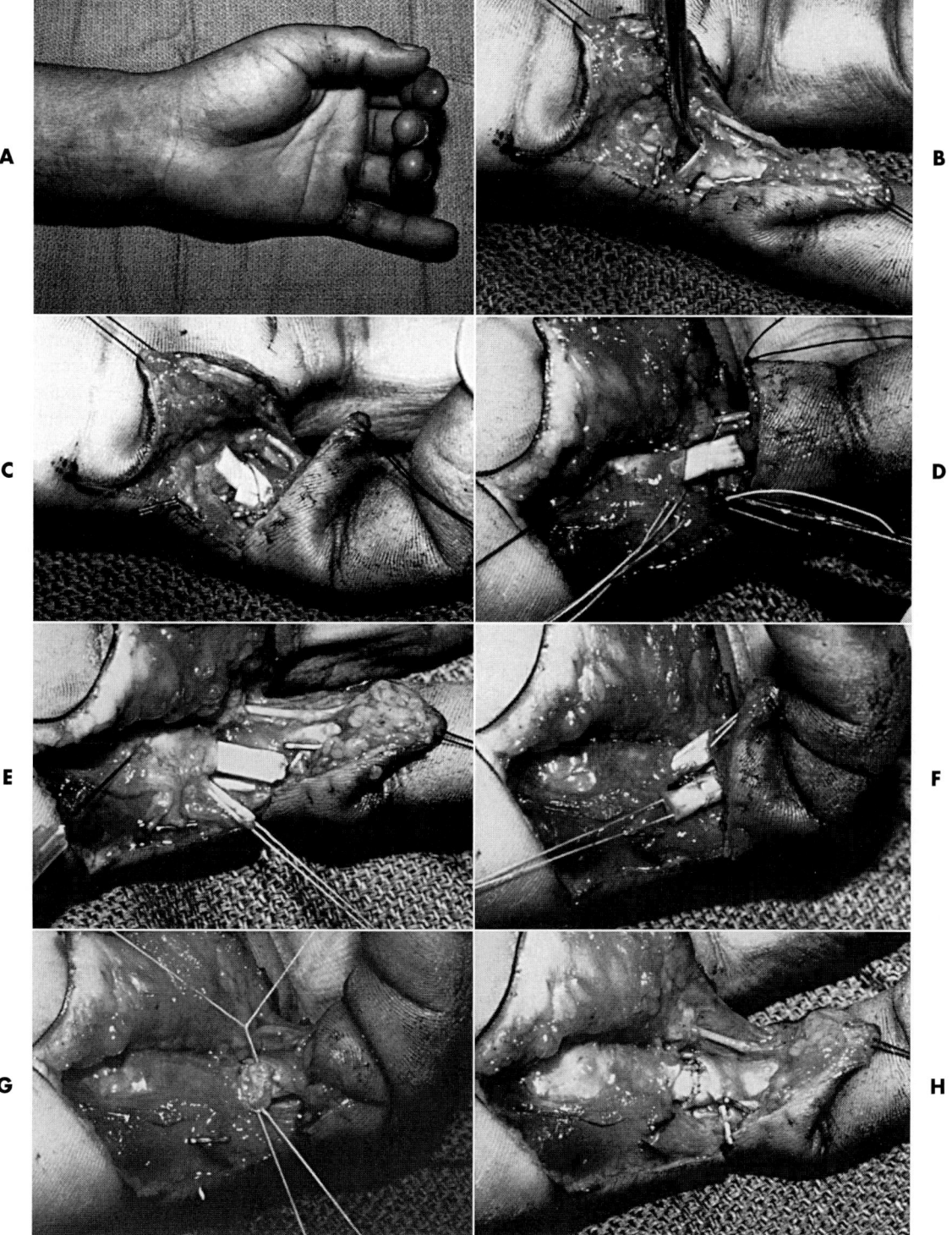

Fig. 26-8. A, Laceration of the flexor digitorum profundus and superficialis, ulnar digital nerve of the small finger in zone II. **B,** Ulnar digital nerve is identified with microclips; flexor retinacular sheath is preserved. **C,** Distal tendon ends are easily identified by flexing the digit. **D,** Proximal tendon ends are atraumatically retrieved. Temporary fixation of the proximal tendon ends with a hypodermic needle facilitates placement of the core suture and repair. **E,** Suture in flexor digitorum superficialis slip. Spiral relationship of superficialis to profundus must be maintained at this level. **F,** Core sutures in place proximally and distally. **G,** Back wall epitendinous suture placed; core sutures tightened. **H,** Repair complete.

problem if appropriate postoperative splinting with the wrist in neutral position is performed.[66] If the motor branch of the ulnar nerve is lacerated, one should consider repairing it first because it is the deepest structure requiring repair in the wound. All flexor tendons are repaired with a 3-0 or 4-0 core suture. Frequently, swollen or hemorrhagic synovium must be resected to allow repair. Closing the transverse carpal ligament without a Z-plasty lengthening is not wise because it may constrict the median nerve. After surgery, a controlled mobilization program with the wrist near neutral position and the MP joints flexed to 70 degrees is maintained to prevent bowstringing and avoid placing stress on nerve repairs.

Zone V

Deep forearm lacerations proximal to the transverse carpal ligament typically involve multiple structures, including tendons, median and ulnar nerves, and the radial and ulnar arteries. Primary repair of all structures is recommended. Return of satisfactory motion is the rule in this zone, but it may take several months.

Surgical technique in zone V. A zigzag or curvilinear approach is used. Depending on the level of laceration, a carpal tunnel release may be performed. A Tajima or double-grasping–type suture is often used after using 3-0 Ethibond suture because of the caliber of tendon at this level. Double-stranded sutures are especially helpful at this level in the case of multiple tendon lacerations because a four-strand core repair can be accomplished quickly. A surgical caveat in this zone if multiple tendons and nerves are lacerated is to identify and tag structures as one progresses from superficial to deep. This avoids the mistake of mismatching proximal and distal tendon ends because the proximal tendon ends can lose their normal anatomic alignment as the dissection is performed. Circumferential epitendon suture can be performed if time permits, although it is not necessary if multiple tendons require repair during a long procedure.

Flexor pollicis longus

The anatomic differences between the FPL and the digital tendons and sheath have been described. The FPL spans only two digital joints and travels alone in its flexor sheath. These factors may explain improved results in FPL repair.[109,110,163] The FPL has only one vincula and no associated lumbrical muscles; therefore lacerations in zones I and II of the FPL are more likely to retract proximally to the palm or wrist level. Direct repair of the FPL is recommended at all levels as wound conditions permit if no more than 3 or 4 weeks have elapsed since the injury.

Surgical technique for flexor pollicis longus. Lacerations in zones I and II of the FPL again are approached in a volar zigzag incision. The flexor sheath is identified, and windows are made for identification of the tendon ends as required. The A_1 or oblique pulley must be maintained to prevent late bowstringing.

If the tendon is lacerated at its insertion, a pull-out suture to the distal phalanx, as previously described, is used. More proximally in the thumb, if the proximal tendon end is easily identified, it is usually still being held by an intact vinculum. If the proximal tendon is not identified in the thumb, it is retracted into the palm or wrist. We prefer not to explore the carpal tunnel or thenar eminence to retrieve the proximal end for risk of damaging sensory or motor branches of the thumb; rather, a separate transverse or curvilinear incision in the distal forearm is used to identify the proximal tendon. Passing a tube or catheter from the distal incision to the proximal one, using one of the techniques described earlier, can atraumatically retrieve the tendon. Standard end-to-end repair is accomplished with an additional epitendon suture.

Partial flexor tendon lacerations

The treatment of partial flexor tendon lacerations is highly controversial.* Early experimental studies demonstrated that if more than 50% of a tendon is divided, rupture is likely under applied stress.[105] Other reported complications of untreated partial flexor tendon lacerations include triggering, rupture, and entrapment.[58,132] On the other hand, several researchers have noted that placement of core sutures into a largely intact tendon will weaken the tendon, increasing the likelihood of tendon rupture.[175,179] More recently, researchers have demonstrated that early protected mobilization after partial tendon lacerations demonstrated improved tensile strengths. In addition, they recommended repair of partial flexor tendon lacerations when more than 60% of the width of the tendon is divided.[6,19,20]

Surgical technique for partial flexor tendon lacerations. A volar zigzag approach is again used. The flexor tendon sheath is identified, and the partial laceration is evaluated. It has been our practice, based on the available data, to repair partial lacerations greater than 50% with a modified Kessler core suture followed by an epitendinous 6-0 suture. Lacerations of 25% to 50% are repaired with a 6-0 running epitendinous suture. Partial lacerations of less than 25% are treated by minimal handling of the tendon and beveling of sharp edges to prevent catching. A dynamic controlled mobilization program is used postoperatively.

Closed rupture of the flexor digitorum profundus tendon

Rupture of the FDP is caused by forced extension at the DIP joint while the profundus muscle is maximally contracting. The injury commonly occurs in football or rugby players as they grab an opponent's jersey. The patient describes pain and swelling over the area of distal avulsion. Because the superficialis still provides function to the PIP joint, the injury is often missed and the opportunity for early repair lost. Radiographs should always be obtained because,

---

*References 11, 49, 58, 103, 105, 132, 171, 175, 177, 179.

occasionally, a fragment of distal bone is also avulsed, which can localize the profundus tendon end.

Although any digit, including the thumb, has been reported to be involved, this injury most often involves the ring finger. Several theories have been advanced to explain the propensity for the ring finger to be involved. These include a lack of independent extension of the ring finger because of its junctura tendinae and another demonstrating that the ring finger has the weakest profundus insertion.[81]

Avulsion of the profundus tendon has been classified by Leddy into three main types.[66,67] In type I, the tendon retracts into the palm, where a substantial blood supply is lost because of vincular rupture. Tendon repair must be early, within 7 to 10 days, before it becomes contracted. In type II avulsions, the tendon retracts to the PIP joint. The vincula are intact, and some synovial nutrition remains intact. Although early repair is recommended, repair up to 3 months after surgery can result in satisfactory results. Type III injuries involve a large bone fragment. The A_4 pulley prevents retraction of the tendon. Early reinsertion or, with large fragments, open reduction and internal fixation will provide satisfactory results. Finally, type IIIA injuries describe a simultaneous avulsion of the profundus tendon and a fracture fragment distally.[14,66,146] This injury requires open reduction and internal fixation of the bony fragment and reinsertion of the avulsed tendon.

If a case of flexor profundus avulsion is missed and left untreated beyond the period of repair, options for treatment include observation, tendon grafting, a DIP joint tenodesis, or arthrodesis.[66]

Surgical technique for closed rupture of flexor profundus tendon. A palmar zigzag or midlateral incision is used, exposing the flexor sheath just proximal to the PIP joint to the insertion of the profundus tendon. For a type I injury, a transverse window is made just distal to the A_2 pulley. If the tendon is not seen, it has retracted into the palm. Therefore an additional incision is required in the palm proximal to the A_1 pulley. The proximal tendon is atraumatically passed through the sheath and the superficialis decussation by one of the methods described previously. It is then reinserted into the distal phalanx through a periosteal flap with 3-0 nonlocking Prolene suture tied over a button on the nail plate distal to the germinal matrix. Again, a bone anchor can also be used. For type II injuries, the tendon end is noted at the incision just distal to the A_2 pulley, held by its vincula. No palmar incision is required. The tendon is reinserted distally as described. For type III or type IIIA incisions, the bony fragment is noted just distal to the A_4 pulley. The transverse sheath incision distal to the A_2 pulley is not required. Open reduction and internal fixation of the bony fragment usually provides satisfactory results. In the case of a IIIA injury, after open reduction and internal fixation of the bone fragment, the distal tendon is reinserted as described previously.

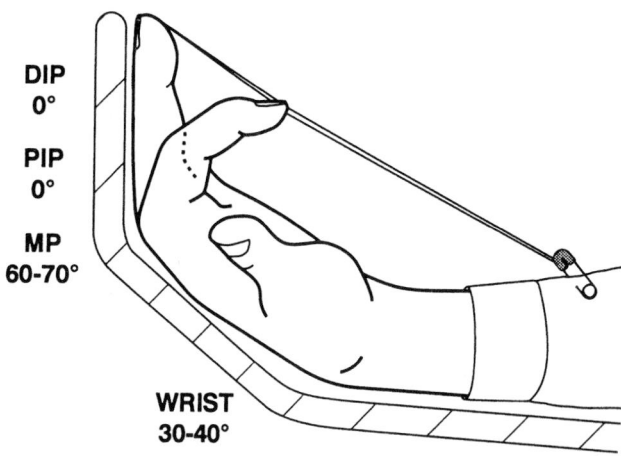

Fig. 26-9. Position of dorsal hood splint for dynamic early protected motion. *DIP,* Distal interphalangeal; *MP,* metacarpophalangeal; *PIP,* proximal interphalangeal.

REHABILITATION

Traditionally, immobilization of 3 to 4 weeks with the wrist in 30 to 40 degrees of flexion, the MP joint at 70 degrees of flexion, and IP joints in extension was used with flexor tendon injuries. This method may be useful for a noncompliant patient or a child and does decrease the likelihood of gap formation. However, the technique is associated with a slower return of strength and adhesion formation.[157] This has led to the use of early mobilization programs that attempt to allow tendon healing but decreased surrounding adhesion formation.[74,157] Researchers have demonstrated that repair tendons stressed through an early mobilization program heal faster, gain tensile strength faster, and have less adhesions and better excursion than unstressed repairs.[37,38,46,174] Some type of early mobilization program is currently the accepted postoperative treatment after flexor tendon repair.

Several general techniques for early controlled mobilization have been developed. They all share the use of a dorsal splint that maintains the wrist palmarly flexed at approximately 30 degrees, MP joints flexed at 70 degrees, and IP joints in extension (Fig. 26-9). If nerve repairs have been performed, the IP joints may be flexed 10 degrees, depending on the tension of nerve repair. Kleinert and others have popularized the dynamic splint.[62,74] Kleinert uses a rubber band attached to the fingernail to provide dynamic passive flexion against which the patient actively extends (see Fig. 26-9). The original splint, which has been occasionally associated with flexion contractures, has been modified more recently.* The Duran technique[15,26] consists of passive flexion and extension exercises of each IP joint, with the addition of gentle active motion at 4 to 5 weeks. This protocol is based on the observation that 3 to 5 mm of tendon excursion is necessary to prevent adhesion

*References 18, 27, 96, 97, 143, 144, 155, 172.

formation. Chow and others have described superior results from using a combination of both of the previously described techniques.[16,17,128] Finally, the use of a continuous passive motion device after flexor tenorrhaphy has been described.[11,46]

Our primary flexor tendon rehabilitation program is divided into four phases. The rate at which individuals progress through the phases is determined by observable and palpable scarring as well as by how well the tendon is gliding when it is tested at 4 weeks.

The early phase of treatment extends 4 to 6 weeks from the time of repair. Within the first few days of repair, the postoperative dressing is debulked, with care being taken to maintain the flexed posture of the wrist and MP joints. If the dorsal plaster splint continues to fit well, it can be used to support the hand. If the plaster splint is unsuitable, a splint of thermoplastic material is fabricated. Elastic thread traction is applied to sutures placed through the nail at surgery or to a hook bonded to the nail plate. The elastic traction thread is secured 3 inches proximal to the wrist. Occasionally, a palmar pulley is used. Tension is adjusted to allow full active finger extension within the splint and to pull the finger into the palm with extensor muscle relaxation. The patient is instructed to perform hourly exercises of 10 repetitions of full extension of the digit while awake, and passive DIP joint, PIP joint, and MP joint flexion four times each day with 10 repetitions each. Elastic thread traction can be maintained throughout the entire early phase or removed at night with the IP joint splinted in extension. Removal of the splint and active flexion are prohibited. Scar massage is initiated when the sutures are removed. If IP joint flexion contractures are found to develop during treatment, the MP flexion within the splint can be increased to facilitate active IP joint extension, and elastic thread traction should be suspended during the night. In addition, static extension splinting can be used for persistent IP joint flexion contractures.

The dorsal splint is removed, and the patient is placed in a wristlet at 4 to 6 weeks after repair. Passive extension exercises are continued against elastic thread traction that allows full extension of the digits with the wrist in neutral. Place-and-hold exercises are initiated. Tendon gliding exercises of hook fist, straight fist, and full fist are started at 6 to 8 weeks. These exercises are designed to produce maximal glide of the profundus and superficialis tendons with respect to each other and through their total excursion. A dynamic IP joint extension splint can be used at this point to address IP joint flexion contractures. Blocking exercises and strengthening are initiated at 8 weeks.

COMPLICATIONS

Despite the use of early controlled mobilization, adhesion formation remains the most common complication after flexor tendon surgery. Surgical tenolysis is the treatment of choice if an appropriate period of therapy has failed (3 to 6 months).[154,173,176] Tendon rupture after primary repair is uncommon. Although rupture can occur late, it is usually noted around the seventh to tenth postoperative day. Early reexploration and repair is the treatment of choice.[1,66,112] If the FDP is advanced and repaired greater than 1 cm, quadrigia syndrome can develop.[80,166] This is based on the limited proximal excursion of the remaining FDP tendons, which have a common muscle belly. A flexion contracture of the affected digit is noted, and the patient often complains of a weak grasp because of lack of full motion of surrounding digits.

FUTURE

Early active mobilization or controlled active motion is now established as a reliable method for the postoperative management of flexor tendon repairs.[5,139,168] Several factors must be considered when it is used in clinical practice. The tensile strength of the suture material must be adequate, and the design of the suture must enable it to withstand active mobilization without rupture or gapping. Several recent studies have addressed these issues.* It is clear from those studies that the strength of a tendon repair is roughly proportional to the number of strands that cross the repair site.[159] Multiple core suture designs have been described. It is believed that at least a four-strand core repair, plus an epitendinous suture, is required for early active motion postoperatively. This knowledge must be tempered by the fact that the work of flexion is also proportional to the amount of suture material present at the repair site.[3] In addition, several new techniques have been developed for the epitendinous stitch, which has assumed an increasingly important role both in ultimate strength and prevention of gap formation after flexor tendon repair.[69,89,129,169,170]

Another fruitful area of future research is the biochemical modification of adhesion formation after flexor tendon repair.[56,64,65,107,158] Recently, experimental studies have implied decreased adhesion formation with the use of nonsteroidal antiinflammatory medications.[64,65,158]

REFERENCES

1. Allen BN, et al: Ruptured flexor tenorrhaphies in zone II: repair and rehabilitation, *J Hand Surg* 12:18, 1987.
2. Amadio PC, et al: The effect of vincular injury on the results of flexor tendon surgery in zone 2, *J Hand Surg* 10A:626, 1985.
3. Aoki M, et al: Work of flexion after tendon repair, *J Hand Surg* 20B:310, 1995.
4. Austin GJ, Leslie BM, Ruby LK: Variations of the flexor digitorum superficialis of the small finger, *J Hand Surg* 14A:262, 1989.
5. Balctir A, et al: Flexor tendon repair in zone II followed by early active mobilization, *J Hand Surg* 21B:624, 1996.
6. Bishop AT, Cooney WP, Wood MB: Treatment of partial flexor tendon lacerations: the effect of tenorrhaphy and early protected mobilization, *J Trauma* 26:301, 1986.

*References 21, 41, 42, 68, 93, 124-126, 130, 131, 145, 160.

7. Boyes JH, Wilson JN, Smith JW: Flexor-tendon ruptures in the forearm and hand, *J Bone Joint Surg* 42A:637, 1960.
8. Brockis JG: The blood supply of the flexor and extensor tendons of the fingers in man, *J Bone Joint Surg* 35B:131, 1953.
9. Bruner JM: The zig-zag palmar-digital incision for flexor-tendon surgery, *Plast Reconstr Surg* 40:571, 1967.
10. Bruner JM: Surgical exposure of the flexor pollicis longus tendon, *Hand* 7:241, 1975.
11. Bunker TD, Potter B, Barton NJ: Continuous passive motion following flexor tendon repair, *J Hand Surg* 14B:406, 1989.
12. Bunnell S: Repair of tendons in the fingers and description of two new instruments, *Surg Gynecol Obstet* 26:103, 1918.
13. Bunnell S: Repair of tendons in the fingers, *Surg Gynecol Obstet* 35:88, 1922.
14. Buscemi MA, Page BJ: Flexor digitorum profundus avulsions with associated distal phalanx fractures: a report of four cases and review of the literature, *Am J Sports Med* 15:366, 1987.
15. Cannon NM, Strickland JW: Therapy following flexor tendon surgery, *Hand Clin* 1:147, 1985.
16. Chow JA, et al: Controlled motion rehabilitation after flexor tendon repair and grafting, *J Bone Joint Surg* 70B:591, 1988.
17. Chow JA, et al: A splint for controlled active motion after flexor tendon repair, *J Hand Surg* 15A:645, 1990.
18. Cooney WP, Lin GT, An KN: Improved tendon excursion following flexor tendon repair, *J Hand Ther* April-June:102, 1989.
19. Cooney WP, et al: Management of acute flexor tendon injury in the hand, *AAOS Instr Course Lect* 34:373, 1985.
20. Cooney WP, et al: Partial flexor tendon lacerations. In Hunter JM, Schneider LH, Mackin EJ, editors: *Tendon surgery in the hand,* St Louis, 1987, Mosby.
21. Cullen KW, et al: Flexor tendon repair in zone 2 followed by controlled active mobilization, *J Hand Surg* 14B:392, 1989.
22. Doyle JR: Anatomy of the flexor tendon sheath and pulley system, *J Hand Surg* 13A:473, 1988.
23. Doyle JR: Anatomy and function of the palmar aponeurosis pulley, *J Hand Surg* 15A:78, 1990.
24. Doyle RF, Blythe W: The finger flexor tendon sheath and pulleys: anatomy and reconstruction. In American Academy of Orthopaedic Surgeons: *Symposium on tendon surgery in the hand,* St Louis, 1975, Mosby.
25. Doyle RF, Blythe W: Anatomy of the flexor tendon sheath and pulleys of the thumb, *J Hand Surg* 2:149, 1977.
26. Duran RJ, Houser RG: Controlled passive motion following flexor tendon repair in zones 2 and 3. In American Academy of Orthopaedic Surgeons: *Symposium on flexor tendon surgery in the hand,* St Louis, 1975, Mosby.
27. Edinburg M, Widgerow AD, Biddulph SL: Early postoperative mobilization of flexor tendon injuries using a modification of the Kleinert technique, *J Hand Surg* 12A:34, 1987.
28. Edwards DA: The blood supply and lymphatic drainage of tendons, *J Anat* 80:147, 1946.
29. Eiken O, Hagberg L, Lundborg G: Evolving biologic concepts as applied to tendon surgery, *Clin Plast Surg* 8:1, 1981.
30. Eiken O, Lundborg G, Rank F: The role of the digital synovial sheath in tendon grafting, *Scand J Plast Reconstr Surg* 9:182, 1975.
31. Ejeskar A: Finger flexion force and hand grip strength after tendon repair, *J Hand Surg* 7:61, 1982.
32. Flynn JE, Graham JH: Healing following tendon suture and tendon transplants, *Surg Gynecol Obstet* 360:467, 1962.
33. Furlow LT: The role of tendon tissues in tendon healing, *Plast Reconstr Surg* 57:39, 1976.
34. Gault DT: A review of repaired flexor tendons, *J Hand Surg* 12B:321, 1987.
35. Gault DT, Quaba AA: The role of cross-finger flaps in the primary management of untidy flexor tendon injuries, *J Hand Surg* 13B:62, 1988.
36. Gelberman RH, Khabie V, Cahill CJ: The revascularization of healing flexor tendons in the digital sheath, *J Bone Joint Surg* 73A:868, 1991.
37. Gelberman RH, et al: The influence of protected passive mobilization on the healing of flexor tendons: a biochemical and microangiographic study, *Hand* 13:120, 1981.
38. Gelberman RH, et al: Effects of early intermittent passive mobilization on healing canine flexor tendons, *J Hand Surg* 7:170, 1982.
39. Gelberman RH, et al: Flexor tendon healing and restoration of the gliding surface: an intrastructural study in dogs, *J Bone Joint Surg* 65A:70, 1983.
40. Gelberman RH, et al: The early stages of flexor tendon healing: a morphologic study of the first fourteen days, *J Hand Surg* 10A:776, 1985.
41. Gelberman RH, et al: The excursion and deformation of repaired flexor tendons treated with protected early motion, *J Hand Surg* 11A:106, 1986.
42. Gelberman RH, et al: Flexor tendon repair, *J Orthop Res* 4:119, 1986.
43. Gelberman RH, et al: Influences of flexor sheath continuity and early motion on tendon healing in dogs, *J Hand Surg* 15A:69, 1990.
44. Gelberman RH, et al: Fibroblast chemotaxis after tendon repair, *J Hand Surg* 16A:686, 1991.
45. Gelberman RH, et al: Healing of digital flexor tendons: importance of the interval from injury to repair, *J Bone Joint Surg* 73A:66, 1991.
46. Gelberman RH, et al: Influences of the protected passive mobilization interval on flexor tendon healing, *Clin Orthop* 264:189, 1991.
47. Hatanaka H, Manske PR: Effect of the cross-sectioned area of locking loops in flexor tendon repair, *J Hand Surg* 24A:751, 1999.
48. Hergenroeder PT, Gelberman RH, Akeson WA: The vascularity of the flexor pollicis longus tendon, *Clin Orthop* 162:298, 1982.
49. Hitchcock TF, et al: New technique for producing uniform partial lacerations of tendons, *J Orthop Res* 7:451, 1989.
50. Hunter JM, et al: The pulley system, *J Hand Surg* 5:283, 1980.
51. Idler RS: Anatomy and biomechanics of the digital flexor tendons, *Hand Clin* 1:3, 1985.
52. Idler RS, Strickland JW: The effects of pulley resection on the biomechanics of the proximal interphalangeal joint, *Univ Pa Orthop J* 2:20, 1986.
53. Ikuta Y, Tsuge K: Postoperative results of looped nylon suture used in injuries of the digital flexor tendons, *J Hand Surg* 10B:67, 1985.
54. Kessler I: The "grasping" technique for tendon repair, *Hand* 5:253, 1973.
55. Kessler I, Nissim F: Primary repair without immobilization of flexor tendon division within the digital sheath, *Acta Orthop Scand* 40:587, 1969.
56. Ketchum LD: Effects of triamcinolone on tendon healing and function, *Plast Reconstr Surg* 47:471, 1971.
57. Ketchum LD: Suture materials and suture techniques used in tendon repair, *Hand Clin* 1:43, 1985.
58. Kleinert HE: Should an incomplete severed tendon be sutured? *Plast Reconstr Surg* 57:235, 1976.
59. Kleinert HE, Cash SL: Management of acute flexor tendon injuries in the hand, *AAOS Instr Course Lect* 34:361, 1985.
60. Kleinert HE, Kutz JE, Cohen MJ: Primary repair of zone 2 flexor tendon lacerations. In American Academy of Orthopaedic Surgeons: *Symposium on tendon surgery in the hand,* St Louis, 1975, Mosby.
61. Kleinert HE, Schepels S, Gill T: Flexor tendon injuries, *Surg Clin North Am* 61:267, 1981.
62. Kleinert HE, et al: Primary repair of flexor tendons in "no man's land," *J Bone Joint Surg* 49A:577, 1967.

63. Kleinert HE, et al: Primary repair of flexor tendons, *Orthop Clin North Am* 4:865, 1973.

64. Kulick MI, Smith S, Hadler K: Oral ibuprofen: evaluation of its effect on peritendinous adhesions and the breaking strength of a tenorrhaphy, *J Hand Surg* 11A:110, 1986.

65. Kulick MI, et al: Injectable ibuprofen: preliminary evaluation of its ability to decrease peritendinous adhesions, *Ann Plast Surg* 13:459, 1984.

66. Leddy JP: Flexor tendons: acute injuries. In Green DP, editor: *Green's operative hand surgery,* New York, 1993, Churchill Livingstone.

67. Leddy JP, Packer JW: Avulsion of the profundus insertion in athletes, *J Hand Surg* 2:66, 1977.

68. Lee H: Double loop locking suture: a technique of tendon repair for early active mobilization, *J Hand Surg* 15A:945, 1990.

69. Lin GT, et al: Biomechanical studies of running suture for flexor tendon repair in dogs, *J Hand Surg* 13A:553, 1988.

70. Lindsay WK, Thomson HG, Walker FG: Digital flexor tendons: an experimental study, *Br J Plast Surg* 13:1, 1960.

71. Lister GD: Incision and closure of the flexor tendon sheath during primary tendon repair, *Hand* 15:123, 1979.

72. Lister GD: Pitfalls and complications of flexor tendon surgery, *Hand Clin* 1:133, 1985.

73. Lister GD, Tonkin M: The results of primary flexor tendon repair with closure of the tendon sheath, *J Hand Surg* 11A:767, 1986.

74. Lister GD, et al: Primary flexor tendon repair followed by immediate controlled mobilization, *J Hand Surg* 2:441, 1977.

75. Lundborg G: Experimental flexor tendon healing without adhesion formation, *Hand* 8:235, 1976.

76. Lundborg G, Holm S, Myrhage R: The role of the synovial fluid and tendon sheath for flexor tendon nutrition, *Scand J Plast Reconstr Surg* 14:99, 1980.

77. Lundborg G, Myrhage R, Rydevik B: The vascularization of human flexor tendons within the digital synovial sheath region: structural and functional aspects, *J Hand Surg* 2:417, 1977.

78. Lundborg G, Rank F: Experimental intrinsic healing of flexor tendons based upon synovial fluid nutrition, *J Hand Surg* 3:21, 1978.

79. Madsen E: Delayed primary suture of flexor tendons cut in the digital sheath, *J Bone Joint Surg* 52B:264, 1970.

80. Malerich MM, et al: Permissible limits of flexor digitorum profundus tendon advancement: an anatomic study, *J Hand Surg* 12A:30, 1987.

81. Manske PR, Lesker PA: Avulsion of the ring finger flexor digitorum profundus tendon: an experimental study, *Hand* 10:52, 1978.

82. Manske PR, Lesker PA: Nutrient pathways of flexor tendon in primates, *J Hand Surg* 7:436, 1982.

83. Manske PR, Lesker PA: Palmar aponeurosis pulley, *J Hand Surg* 8:259, 1983.

84. Manske PR, Lesker PA: Biochemical evidence of flexor tendon participation in the repair process: an in vitro study, *J Hand Surg* 9B:117, 1984.

85. Manske PR, Lesker PA: Histologic evidence of intrinsic flexor tendon repair in various experimental animals: an in vitro study, *Clin Orthop* 182:297, 1984.

86. Manske PR, Lesker PA: Diffusion as a nutrient pathway to the flexor tendon. In Hunter JM, Schneider LH, Mackin EJ, editors: *Tendon surgery in the hand,* St Louis, 1987, Mosby.

87. Manske PR, et al: Intrinsic flexor-tendon repair, *J Bone Joint Surg* 66A:385, 1984.

88. Mashadi ZB, Amis AA: The effect of locking loops on the strength of tendon repair, *J Hand Surg* 16B:35, 1991.

89. Mashadi ZB, Amis AA: Strength of the suture in the epitenon and within the tendon fibres: development of stronger peripheral suture technique, *J Hand Surg* 17B:172, 1992.

90. Mason ML, Allen HS: The rate of healing of tendons: experimental study of tensile strength, *Ann Surg* 113:424, 1941.

91. Mass DP, Tuel RJ: Intrinsic healing of the laceration site in human superficialis flexor tendons in vitro, *J Hand Surg* 16A:24, 1991.

92. Matev I, et al: Delayed primary suture of flexor tendons cut in the digital theca, *Hand* 12:158, 1980.

93. Mathews JP: Early mobilisation after flexor tendon repair, *J Hand Surg* 14B:363, 1989.

94. Matthews P: The pathology of flexor tendon repair, *Hand* II:233, 1979.

95. Matthews P, Richards H: Factors in the adherence of flexor tendon after repair: an experimental study in the rabbit, *J Bone Joint Surg* 58B:230, 1976.

96. May EJ, Silfverskiöld KL, Sollerman CJ: Controlled mobilization after flexor tendon repair in zone II: a prospective comparison of three methods, *J Hand Surg* 17A:942, 1992.

97. May EJ, Silfverskiöld KL, Sollerman CJ: The correlation between controlled range of motion with dynamic traction and results after flexor tendon repair in zone II, *J Hand Surg* 17A:1133, 1992.

98. Mayer L: The physiological method of tendon transplantation. I. Historical: anatomy and physiology of tendons, *Surg Gynecol Obstet* 22:182, 1916.

99. Mayer L: The physiological method of tendon transplantation. II. Operative technique, *Surg Gynecol Obstet* 22:298, 1916.

100. Mayer L: The physiological method of tendon transplantation. III. Experimental and clinical experiences, *Surg Gynecol Obstet* 22:472, 1916.

101. McDowell CL, Snyder DM: Tendon healing: an experimental model in the dog, *J Hand Surg* 2:122, 1977.

102. McFarlane RM, Lamon R, Jarvis G: Flexor tendon injuries within the finger, *J Trauma* 8:987, 1988.

103. McGeorge DD, Stilwell JH: Partial flexor tendon injuries: to repair or not, *J Hand Surg* 17B:176, 1992.

104. McGrouther DA, Ahmed MR: Flexor tendon excursions in "no-man's land," *Hand* 13:129, 1981.

105. McMaster PE: Tendon and muscle ruptures: clinical and experimental studies on the causes and locations of subcutaneous rupture, *J Bone Joint Surg* 15:705, 1933.

106. Meals RA: Current concepts review of flexor tendon injuries, *J Bone Joint Surg* 67A:817, 1985.

107. Meyers SA, et al: Effect of hyaluronic acid/chondroitin sulfate on healing of full-thickness tendon lacerations in rabbits, *J Orthop Res* 7:683, 1989.

108. Nielsen AB, Jensen PO: Primary flexor tendon repair in "no man's land," *J Hand Surg* 9B:279, 1984.

109. Noonan KJ, Blair WF: Long-term follow-up of primary flexor pollicis longus tenorrhaphies, *J Hand Surg* 16A:653, 1991.

110. Nunley JA, et al: Direct end-to-end repair of flexor pollicis longus tendon lacerations, *J Hand Surg* 17A:118, 1992.

111. Ochiai N, et al: Vascular anatomy of flexor tendons: I. Vincular system and blood supply of the profundus tendon in the digital sheath, *J Hand Surg* 4:321, 1979.

112. Parkes A: The "lumbrical plus" finger, *J Bone Joint Surg* 53B:236, 1971.

113. Peacock EE: A study of the circulation in normal tendons and healing grafts, *Ann Surg* 149:415, 1959.

114. Peacock EE: Fundamental aspects of the wound healing relating to the restoration of gliding function after tendon repair, *Surg Gynecol Obstet* 2:119, 1964.

115. Peacock EE: Biological principles in the healing of long tendons, *Surg Clin North Am* 45:461, 1965.

116. Peacock EE, Madden JW, Trier WC: Postoperative recovery of flexor tendon function, *Am J Surg* 122:686, 1971.

117. Penington DG: The influence of attendance sheath integrity vincula blood supply on adhesion formation following tendon repairing in hands, *Br J Plast Surg* 32:302, 1939.

118. Peterson WW, Manske PR, Lesker PA: The effect of flexor sheath integrity on nutrient uptake by primate flexor tendons, *J Hand Surg* 11A:413, 1986.

119. Peterson WW, et al: Effect of flexor sheath integrity on tendon gliding: a biomechanical and histologic study, *J Orthop Res* 4:458, 1986.

120. Peterson WW, et al: Effect of various methods of restoring flexor sheath integrity on the formation of adhesions after tendon injury, *J Hand Surg* 15A:48, 1990.
121. Potenza AD: Tendon healing within the flexor digital sheath in the dog, *J Bone Joint Surg* 44A:49, 1962.
122. Potenza AD: The healing of autogenous tendon grafts within the flexor digital sheath in dogs, *J Bone Joint Surg* 46A:1462, 1964.
123. Potenza AD: Flexor tendon injuries, *Orthop Clin North Am* 1:355, 1970.
124. Pruitt DL, Manske PR, Fink B: Cyclic stress analysis of flexor tendon repair, *J Hand Surg* 16A:701, 1991.
125. Riaz M, et al: Long term outcome of early active mobilization following flexor tendon repair in zone II, *J Hand Surg* 24B:157, 1999.
126. Robertson GA, Al-Qattan MM: A biomechanical analysis of a new interlock suture technique for flexor tendon repair, *J Hand Surg* 17B:92, 1992.
127. Saldana MJ, et al: Flexor tendon repair and rehabilitation in zone II open sheath technique versus closed sheath technique, *J Hand Surg* 12A:1110, 1987.
128. Saldana MJ, et al: Further experience in rehabilitation of zone II flexor tendon repair with dynamic traction splinting, *Plast Reconstr Surg* 87:543, 1991.
129. Sanders WE: Advantages of "epitenon first" suture placement technique in flexor tendon repair, *Clin Orthop* 280:198, 1992.
130. Savage R: The influence of wrist position on the minimum force required for active movement of the interphalangeal joints, *J Hand Surg* 13B:262, 1988.
131. Savage R, Risitano G: Flexor tendon repair using a "six strand" method of repair and early active mobilization, *J Hand Surg* 14B:396, 1989.
132. Schlenker JD, Lister GD, Kleinert HE: Three complications of untreated partial laceration of flexor tendon: entrapment, rupture, and triggering, *J Hand Surg* 6:392, 1981.
133. Schneider LH, Bush DC: Primary care of flexor tendon injuries, *Hand Clin* 5:1853, 1993.
134. Schneider LH, Hunter JM: Flexor tendons: late reconstruction. In Green DP, editor: *Green's operative hand surgery,* New York, 1983, Churchill Livingstone.
135. Schneider LH, McEntee PE: Flexor tendon injuries: treatment of the acute problem, *Hand Clin* 2:119, 1986.
136. Schneider LH, et al: Delayed flexor tendon repair in no-man's land, *J Hand Surg* 2:452, 1977.
137. Schuind F, et al: Flexor tendon forces: in vivo measurements, *J Hand Surg* 17A:291, 1992.
138. Seradge H: Elongation of the repair configuration following tendon repair, *J Hand Surg* 8:182, 1983.
139. Silfverskiöld KL, May EJ: Flexor tendon repair in zone II with a new suture technique and an early mobilization program combining passive and active flexion, *J Hand Surg* 19A:53, 1994.
140. Silfverskiöld KL, May EJ, Tornvall AH: Flexor digitorum profundus tendon excursions during controlled motion after flexor tendon repair in zone II: a prospective clinical study, *J Hand Surg* 17A:122, 1992.
141. Singer M, Maloon S: Flexor tendon injuries: the results of primary repair, *J Hand Surg* 13B:269, 1988.
142. Skoog T, Persson B: An experimental study of the early healing of tendons, *Plast Reconstr Surg* 13:384, 1954.
143. Slattery PG: The modified Kleinert splint in zone II flexor tendon injuries, *J Hand Surg* 13B:273, 1988.
144. Slattery PG, McGrouther DA: A modified Kleinert controlled mobilization splint following flexor tendon repair, *J Hand Surg* 9B:217, 1984.
145. Small JO, Brennen MD, Colville J: Early active mobilization following flexor tendon repair in zone 2, *J Hand Surg* 14B:383, 1989.
146. Smith JH: Avulsion of a profundus tendon with simultaneous intraarticular fracture of the distal phalanx, *J Hand Surg* 6:600, 1981.
147. Smith JW: Blood supply of tendons, *Am J Surg* 109:272, 1965.
148. Soejima O, et al: Comparative mechanical analysis of dorsal versus palmar placement of core suture for flexor tendon repair, *J Hand Surg* 20A:801, 1995.
149. Sourmelis SG, McGrouther DA: Retrieval of the retracted flexor tendon, *J Hand Surg* 12B:109, 1987.
150. Stein T, et al: A randomized biomechanical study of zone II human flexor tendon repairs analyzed in an in vitro model, *J Hand Surg* 23A:1046, 1998.
151. Steinberg DR: Acute flexor tendon injuries, *Orthop Clin North Am* 23:125, 1992.
152. Strickland JW: Management of acute flexor tendon injuries, *Orthop Clin North Am* 14:827, 1983.
153. Strickland JW: Flexor tendon injuries. Part 1: anatomy, physiology, biomechanics, healing, and adhesion formation around a repaired tendon, *Orthop Rev* 15:21, 1986.
154. Strickland JW: Flexor tendon injuries. Part 2: flexor tendon repair, *Orthop Rev* 15:49, 1986.
155. Strickland JW: Biologic rationale, clinical application, and results of early motion following flexor tendon repair, *J Hand Ther* April-June: 71, 1989.
156. Strickland JW: Flexor tendon surgery. Part 2: free tendon graft and tenolysis, *J Hand Surg* 14B:368, 1989.
157. Strickland JW, Glogovac SV: Digital function following flexor tendon repair in zone II: a comparison of immobilization and controlled passive motion techniques, *J Hand Surg* 5:537, 1980.
158. Szabo RM, Younger E: Effects of indomethacin on adhesion formation after repair of zone II tendon lacerations in the rabbit, *J Hand Surg* 15A:480, 1990.
159. Thurman RT, et al: Two-, four-, and six-strand zone II flexor tendon repairs: an in situ biomechanical comparison using a cadaver model, *J Hand Surg* 23A:261, 1998.
160. Trail IA, Powell ES, Noble J: The mechanical strength of various suture techniques, *J Hand Surg* 17B:89, 1992.
161. Tsuge K, Ikuta Y, Matsuishi Y: Intra-tendinous tendon suture in the hand: a new technique, *Hand* 7:250, 1975.
162. Urbaniak JR, Cahill JD, Mortenson RA: Tendon suturing methods: analysis of tensile strengths. In American Academy of Orthopaedic Surgeons: *Symposium on tendon surgery in the hand,* St Louis, 1975, Mosby.
163. Urbaniak JR, Goldner JL: Laceration of the flexor pollicis longus tendon: delayed repair by advancement, free graft or direct suture, *J Bone Joint Surg* 55A:1123, 1973.
164. Vahvanen V, Gripenberg L, Nuutinen P: Flexor tendon injury of the hand in children, *Scand J Plast Reconstr Surg* 15:43, 1981.
165. Verdan C: Primary repair of flexor tendons, *J Bone Joint Surg* 42A:647, 1960.
166. Verdan C: Practical considerations for primary and secondary repair in flexor tendon injuries, *Surg Clin North Am* 44:951, 1964.
167. Verdan C: Primary and secondary repair of flexor and extensor tendon injuries. In Flynn JE, editor: *Hand surgery,* Baltimore, 1966, Williams & Wilkins.
168. Verdan C: Half a century of flexor-tendon surgery: current status and changing philosophies, *J Bone Joint Surg* 54A:472, 1972.
169. Wade PJF, Muir IFK, Hutcheon LL: Primary flexor tendon repair: the mechanical limitations of the modified Kessler technique, *J Hand Surg* 11B:71, 1986.
170. Wade PJF, Wetherell RG, Amis AA: Flexor tendon repair: significant gain in strength from the Halsted peripheral suture technique, *J Hand Surg* 14B:232, 1989.
171. Weeks PM: Invited comment on "three complications of untreated partial lacerations of flexor tendon: entrapment; rupture, and triggering," *J Hand Surg* 64:396, 1981.
172. Werntz JR, et al: A new dynamic splint for postoperative treatment of flexor tendon injury, *J Hand Surg* 14A:559, 1989.
173. Whitaker JH, Strickland JW, Ellis RK: The role of flexor tenolysis in the palm and digits, *J Hand Surg* 2:462, 1977.

174. Woo SL-Y, et al: The importance of controlled passive mobilization on flexor tendon healing, *Acta Orthop Scand* 52:615, 1981.

175. Wray RC, Holtmann B, Weeks PM: Clinical treatment of partial tendon lacerations without suturing and with early motion, *Plast Reconstr Surg* 59:231, 1977.

176. Wray RC, Moucharafieh B, Weeks PM: Experimental study of the optimal time for tenolysis, *Plast Reconstr Surg* 61:184, 1978.

177. Wray RC, Ollinger H, Weeks PM: Effects of mobilization on tensile strength of partial tendon lacerations, *Surg Forum* 26:557, 1975.

178. Wray RC, Weeks PM: Experimental comparison of techniques of tendon repair, *J Hand Surg* 5:144, 1980.

179. Wray RC, Weeks PM: Treatment of partial tendon lacerations, *Hand* 12:163, 1980.

180. Young L, Weeks PM: Profundus tendon blood supply within the digital sheath, *Surg Forum Plast Surg* 21:504, 1971.

Chapter 27

POSTOPERATIVE MANAGEMENT OF FLEXOR TENDON INJURIES

Karen M. Stewart Pettengill
Gwendolyn van Strien

Postoperative management of the repaired flexor tendon requires substantial preparation by the hand therapist. The well-prepared therapist understands the anatomy, physiology, biomechanics, and normal and pathologic healing not only of the flexor tendons but also of all adjacent structures. A tendon injury does not occur in isolation; it is always accompanied by injury to skin or other soft tissue structures and often to bone or nerve. In addition to understanding these structures and how they heal, the therapist evaluates tendon function through palpation, observation, and measurement. When the patient is referred for therapy, the surgeon communicates to the therapist the particulars of injury and of surgical and medical management; the therapist then questions both surgeon and patient to obtain any additional information. On the basis of all these factors, the therapist, in consultation with the referring surgeon, selects the appropriate therapeutic approach and modifies treatment when needed.

This chapter presents fundamental tendon management concepts and then reviews flexor tendon anatomy, biomechanics, and mechanisms of nutrition and healing. Following that is an examination of the three approaches to tendon management, with protocols that exemplify each.

FUNDAMENTAL CONCEPTS
Goal: a strong repair that glides freely

Normal tendon function requires free gliding of the tendon without hindrance from surrounding tissues. Each tendon glides through a given amplitude of excursion to flex the digit completely and with adequate power. Because so many structures lie in such a constricted space within the hand, scar adhesions between adjacent structures can occur very easily after injury or surgery. Tendon adhesions can limit excursion to such an extent that tendon function is seriously compromised; intertendinous adhesions can further decrease function.

As it glides, a tendon encounters a certain normal amount of resistance or drag from surrounding tissues. For the first weeks after a repair, that drag is increased considerably by normal posttraumatic or postoperative edema, lacerated tissues, and the extra bulk of sutures and newly forming scar. Given the low strength of a newly repaired tendon, extra care must be taken to allow for this increased drag during all exercise.

In addition to unobstructed gliding, the tendon repair requires enough strength to withstand the normal forces acting on the tendon during daily activity. If subjected to excessive stress during early phases of healing, the repair may rupture or the tendon ends may pull apart without complete rupture. The gap may be filled with scar, but not only will it be weaker than a healthy repair, but it also will elongate the tendon, in effect putting the tendon on slack. An elongated tendon requires even greater excursion to function as it should. Gap formation also has been shown to provoke increased adhesion formation in immobilized tendon repairs, although the functional significance of such gaps appears to be less in the repair that has been mobilized early.[44,94] Therefore our goal is for the tendon to heal without rupture or gap formation, with sufficient strength and excursion for daily activities.

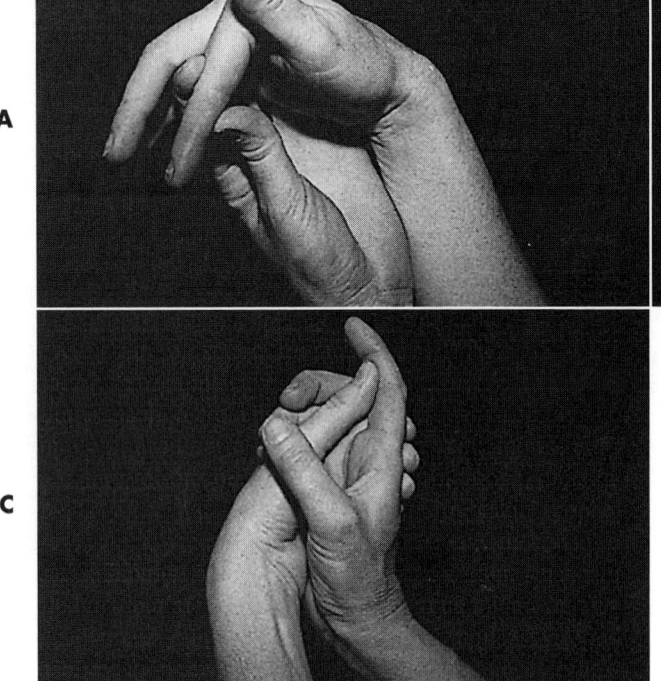

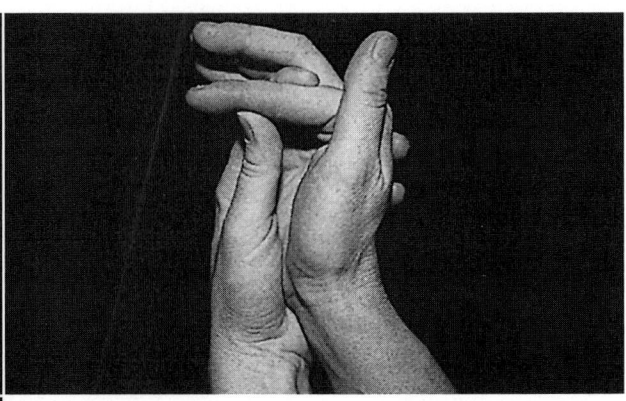

Fig. 27-1. A, The proximal interphalangeal joint (PIP) joint can be extended completely when the wrist and metacarpophalangeal joint (MP) joints are flexed. This means that there are no periarticular or articular restrictions to PIP extension. **B,** The PIP still can be extended completely when the wrist is extended, but we see the distal interphalangeal joint begin to flex, reflecting some tightening of the flexor digitorum profundus tendon. **C,** When the MP and wrist are extended simultaneously, the PIP cannot be extended, indicating probable flexor tendon adhesions in the palm or at the level of the MP joint or the proximal phalanx. (From Stewart KM: Tendon injuries. In Stanley BG, Tribuzi SM, editors: *Concepts in hand rehabilitation,* Philadelphia, 1992, FA Davis.)

Evaluating tendon function

To plan effective therapy, the therapist evaluates tendon function in several ways. The most obvious is measurement of active and passive range of motion (AROM and PROM, respectively). If passive flexion greatly exceeds active flexion, the tendon is not functioning adequately. The repair may have ruptured or elongated, or it may be adherent. This alone is not enough information, however. The therapist now palpates along the course of the tendon to detect impediments to smooth gliding. Such impediments may be very subtle; patience and experience are needed to accurately assess glide, but this is one of the therapist's most valuable skills.

An adherent tendon usually will exhibit some excursion, however limited, but the entire excursion may be taken up by flexion of a single joint. For example, an adherent flexor digitorum profundus (FDP) tendon may produce active flexion of the distal interphalangeal (DIP) joint when the proximal interphalangeal (PIP) joint and metacarpophalangeal (MP) joint are held passively in extension, but when the proximal joints are left free, the limited excursion may not be sufficient to produce flexion at all joints.

An adherent tendon also limits passive composite extension because it is in effect tethered to tissues at one level or more and cannot passively glide to allow full extension. Fig. 27-1 illustrates this phenomenon. The therapist evaluating limitations in motion also differentiates between those caused by impaired tendon function and those caused by articular or periarticular involvement.

Three approaches to tendon management. Each postoperative tendon management protocol falls within one of the following three categories.

Immobilization. These protocols call for complete immobilization of the tendon repair, generally for 3 to 4 weeks, before beginning active and passive mobilization.

Early passive mobilization. These protocols involve passively mobilizing the repair early (usually within the first week, often within 24 hours), either manually (by therapist and/or patient) or by dynamic flexion traction. Passive flexion pushes the tendon proximally, and limited active or passive extension pulls the tendon distally.

Early active mobilization. These protocols mobilize the repair (within a few days of repair) through active contraction of the involved flexor, with caution and within carefully prescribed limits.

ANATOMY

Flexor tendon anatomy has been described in Chapters 3 and 26. Following is a brief discussion of anatomic features pertinent to postoperative management.

The flexor tendons commonly are described according to the zones defined by the International Federation of Societies for Surgery of the Hand (IFSSH) Committee on Tendon Injuries (Fig. 27-2), which apply to the two finger flexors (FDP and flexor digitorum superficialis [FDS]), and the single extrinsic thumb flexor (flexor pollicis longus [FPL]). The distinguishing anatomic characteristic of *zone 5* is the musculotendinous junction in the distal third of the forearm.

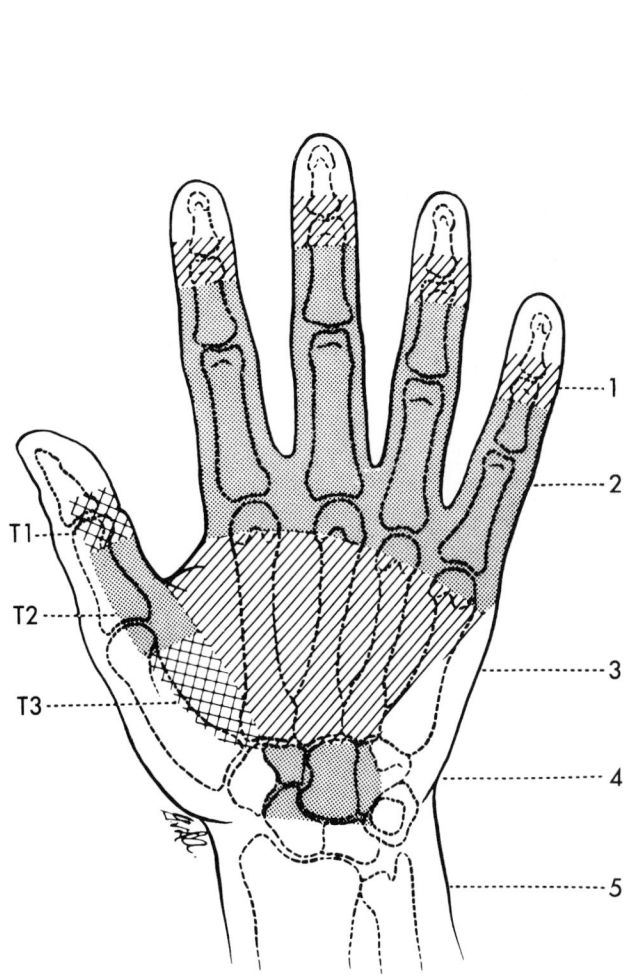

Fig. 27-2. Flexor tendon zones of the hand. (From Kleinert HE, Schepel S, Gill T: *Surg Clin North Am* 61:267, 1981.)

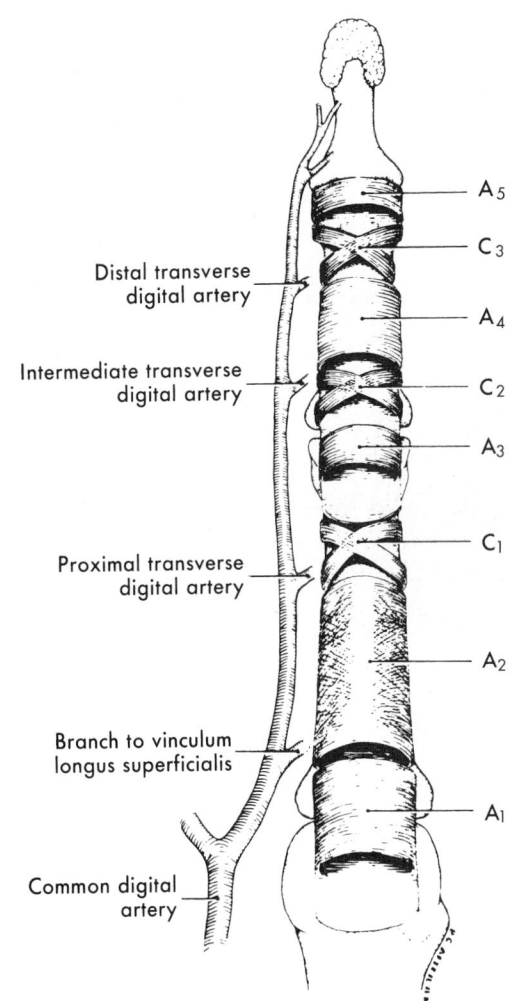

Fig. 27-3. The fibroosseous tunnel or pulley system, with five annular pulleys (A_1 to A_5) and three cruciform pulleys (C_1 to C_3). Note the width of the A_2 and A_4 pulleys. (From Schneider LH: *Flexor tendon injuries,* Boston, 1985, Little, Brown.)

In *zone 4,* the tendons pass through the carpal tunnel. Here the tendons are surrounded by synovial sheaths that provide lubrication, nutrition, and protection from the overlying flexor retinaculum, which holds the tendons within the carpal canal.

Zone 3 (and *zone T3* of FPL) lies distal to the carpal tunnel. While in zone 3 the synovial sheaths of FPL and of FDP and FDS to the fifth digit continue (known respectively as the *radial* and *ulnar bursae*), and the flexors to the second, third, and fourth digits here emerge from the synovial sheath as they pass from beneath the flexor retinaculum. At this level, the lumbricals take their origin from the FDP tendons of the second through fourth digits.

Zone 2 (and T2) is bounded proximally by the beginning of the separate digital synovial sheaths (and continuations of the radial and ulnar bursae) and distally by the FDS insertion. Overlying the synovial sheath is the fibroosseous tunnel, with thickened portions called *pulleys:* annular

pulleys A_1 through A_3 and cruciate pulleys C_1 and C_2 (Fig. 27-3). In the thumb (T2) are the A_1 and oblique pulleys. The pulleys function as restraints or guides to the tendons, rather like the loops on a fishing rod. Without the restraint of the pulleys, the tendon would pull away from bone with each muscle contraction, and "bowstringing" (Fig. 27-4) would result. Investigators have measured the effect of pulley resection on the flexor function and excursion. The data revealed that the A_2 and A_4 pulleys are most important for achieving normal tendon function, although partial resection may not significantly effect function.[71,75] As the tendons enter zone 2, FDS overlies FDP. FDS splits to allow FDP to pass through, and the two slips of FDS merge deep to FDP and split again before inserting in the middle of the proximal phalanx (this elaborate decussation is known as *Camper's chiasma*). Also within zone 2 are the vinculum longus and vinculum brevis to the FDS and vinculum longus to FDP; the vincula are folds of me-

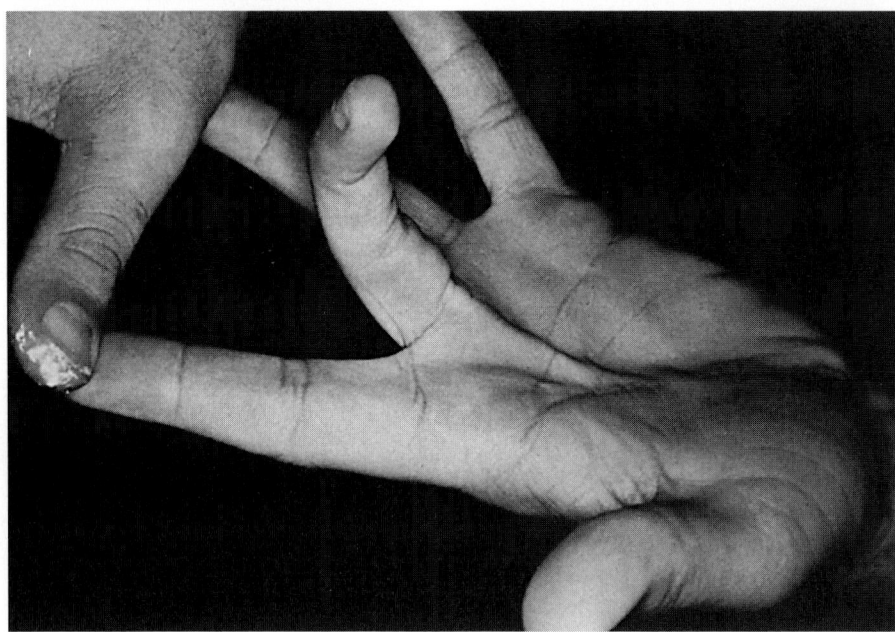

Fig. 27-4. Bowstringing of the flexor tendons is illustrated in this patient with absent pulleys because of a childhood injury.

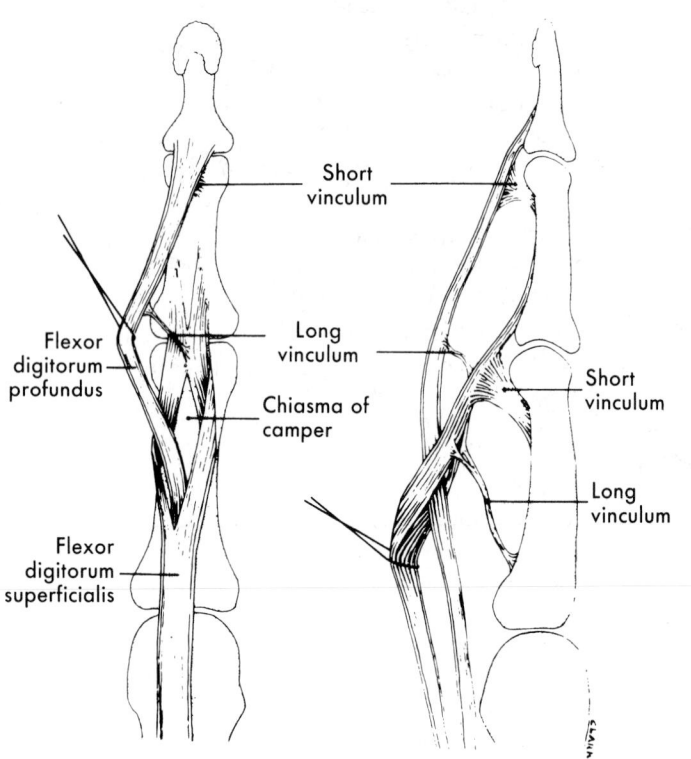

Fig. 27-5. The flexor digitorum superficialis lies volar to the flexor digitorum profundus as the tendons enter the sheath. At the level of the proximal phalanx, the superficialis tendon splits and the two slips pass around dorsal to the profundus tendon, merging and splitting again before inserting on the middle phalanx (Camper's chiasm). Both tendons have a short and long vinculum. The vinculum longus profundus is a continuation of the vinculum brevis superficialis. (From Schneider LH: *Flexor tendon injuries,* Boston, 1985, Little, Brown.)

sotenon carrying blood supply to the flexor tendons (described in more detail in later text) (Fig. 27-5).

Zone 1 extends from the insertion of FDS to the insertion of FDP at the base of the distal phalanx and includes the A_4, C_3, and A_5 pulleys. The synovial sheath ends in this zone. In the thumb, zone T1 includes the insertion of FPL and the A_2 pulley.

NUTRITION

There are three main sources of blood supply to a flexor tendon. The two less important sources are the proximal vessels entering at the musculotendinous junction and the distal bony insertion of the tendon. The third and most important source of blood supply comes from vessels in the surrounding tissues.

Two different areas are described for the third source of blood supply. In the forearm and proximal palm, where the tendon is not surrounded by a retinaculum, an abundance of vessels enter the tendon at random from the surrounding tissues. Within the pulley system, the small vessels originating from the surrounding tissues enter the tendon through mesotenon extensions called *vincula*. The vincular anatomy and the points of entry into the flexor tendons can vary from digit to digit.

Two types of vincula are described for each tendon: the vinculum longus and vinculum brevis (see Fig. 27-5). Both superficialis and profundus tendons have a vinculum brevis. The vinculum longus for the profundus tendon is a continuation of the vinculum brevis superficialis. The small vessels entering the vincula originate from four transverse communicating arteries, which branch from the two digital arteries. The vincular vessels communicate with the intratendinous vessels (one arteriole and one or two venules) that lie longitudinally within the tendon and originate in the palm. These longitudinally oriented vessels are located in the dorsal half of each tendon, leaving the volar side of the tendon relatively avascular. Areas of relative avascularity between the segmental vincular blood supply have been described as "watershed," or critical tendon zones.[4]

In zone 2, where the tendons are surrounded by the pulley system and there are areas of relative avascularity, tendon nutrition comes from two sources—the blood supply and synovial diffusion.

Investigators have shown that under certain conditions synovial fluid can provide the essential nutrition for tendon viability and the elements necessary for healing after tendon injury,[1,57] even if detached from all blood supply. These studies demonstrated the role of synovial diffusion as an important pathway for tendon nutrition.

Synovial fluid is apparently "forced" into the tendon under influence of high pressure against the pulleys during active flexion of the finger.[4,112] The pumping mechanism, under influence of pressure of the tendon against the firm resistance of the pulleys, has been compared with the mechanism of synovial diffusion in articular cartilage.

A delicate balance between the two nutritional pathways (blood supply and synovial diffusion) is found within the tendon sheath. Nutrition to the aforementioned watershed areas is supplied mostly by diffusion from the synovium. When injury occurs in these relatively avascular areas, the balance is disturbed and excessive adhesion formation often is seen. The adhesions bring the additional blood supply to the tendon necessary for the healing process, yet they limit free tendon glide. Injury to the vincular system also affects the nutritional balance, compromises tendon healing, and causes adhesion formation.

BASIC CONCEPTS OF TENDON HEALING

Histologically, tendon consists of connective tissue, and its function is to link muscle to bone. It is made up of collagen bundles, with only a small amount of proteoglycans and elastic fibers. The collagen bundles are longitudinally oriented parallel bundles surrounded by epitenon.

After a tendon is lacerated and repaired, the entire wound actually involves more than just the tendon. All surrounding tissues, such as skin, subcutaneous tissues, and underlying tissues, also are involved in the wound healing process. The following describes wound healing in the immobilized tendon. In the first few days after repair, the wound is filled with a cicatrix, consisting of ground substance and many types of cells. Scar formed in the first 3 weeks will "glue" all involved tissue layers together, and independent function is lost. Peacock[72] described this as the one-wound concept.

Three phases are described for wound healing: the exudative or inflammatory phase, the fibroplasia phase, and the collagen remodeling or maturation phase.

The exudative phase starts immediately after injury. Tensile strength of the immobilized tendon repair diminishes in the first 3 to 5 days because of softening of the tendon ends.[44,64] Immediately after injury, an inflammatory reaction changes the permeability of the vascular system. As a result, there is an influx of leukocytes and macrophages, among other inflammatory elements, in the wound area. Macrophages stimulate growth and migration of fibroblasts.

During the second phase, fibroblasts migrate to the wound area and start production of tropocollagen approximately 5 days after injury. Tropocollagen is a triple-helix molecule with little tensile strength. After the weak hydrogen bonds of the tropocollagen molecule are replaced by stronger cross-links between the three strands of the helix, collagen fibers are formed, and tensile strength starts to develop. The collagen molecules form a randomly oriented network, creating a bond between all tissues in the wound. From day 5 to day 21, tensile strength increases as the collagen matures and the intramolecular cross-linking continues.

Intermolecular cross-linking between collagen fibrils can start during the second phase of wound healing, but it usually starts approximately 21 days after injury. This coincides with the beginning of the third phase of wound healing (the remodeling phase), which starts 3 weeks after injury and continues until 6 months or a year after injury. In the remodeling phase, the tissues are differentiated, and dense, unyielding scar can be changed into more favorable scar. Scar remodeling is characterized by a balance between collagen production and collagen lysis. The randomly oriented collagen between tendon ends, under the influence of stress, is slowly replaced by newly formed collagen oriented along the long axis of the tendon, thus providing increased tensile strength. The randomly oriented fibers of the scar between tendon and surrounding tissues, however, must become loose and filmy to regain gliding function.

When an adhesion-bound tendon gains motion, it is usually not because adhesions are broken, but rather because they are lengthened or changed under influence of stress. Brand[13] stated that if living tissue is subjected to slight tension for a relatively long period of time, "the living cells will sense the strain and the collagen fibers will be actively and progressively absorbed and laid down again with modified bonding patterns." This model may be the explanation for clinical observations that repaired tendons, under the influence of gentle stress, regain motion and restoration of gliding surfaces during the collagen remodeling process.

Many researchers have attempted to improve the quality of tendon healing by influencing quantity and type of adhesion formation. To limit fixed adhesions, weak healing is needed between tendon and surrounding tissues. In contrast, strong healing is needed between the tendon ends to transmit muscle power. This type of differential wound healing seems necessary to recover a free-gliding and functioning tendon after flexor tendon repair.

Extrinsic versus intrinsic healing

Three possible mechanisms of tendon healing are discussed in the literature: the intrinsic mechanism, the extrinsic mechanism, and a combination of the two.

Extrinsic healing depends on formation of adhesions between tendon and surrounding tissue. These adhesions provide the blood supply and the cells (in particular, fibroblasts) needed for tendon healing. Unfortunately, they also prevent the tendon from gliding. The research supporting this mechanism of healing suggests that the tendon has no active role in the healing process, whereas adhesion formation is vital to tendon healing.[77,78]

Intrinsic healing occurs between the tendon ends only, without formation of limiting adhesions. This type of healing relies on the synovial fluid for nutrition and does not result in restricted motion of the tendon. The cells needed for tendon healing are supplied by the epitenon and endotenon itself.[1,37,57,60]

A third group of investigators believe the tendon probably heals through a combination of both intrinsic and extrinsic processes.[59,87,89] Although experimental research demonstrates that tendon healing is possible by either intrinsic or extrinsic means, in actual practice adhesions are seen to varying degrees and the healing response is probably a balance between intrinsic and extrinsic healing mechanisms.

Effects of motion on tendon healing

Beneficial effects of early mobilization and stress applied to tendon anastomoses have been demonstrated in several laboratory experiments. Although concluding that the risks outweighed the potential benefits, in 1941 Mason and Allen[64] noted that motion created a stronger repair in the wrist flexor tendons of some of their canine subjects. Tensile strength increased after the seventh day, especially when mobilization was protected.

Gelberman et al.[32-36] performed a series of experimental studies of early passive mobilization of tendons in dogs. The authors reported that compared with tendons subjected to immobilization or delayed mobilization, the tensile strength and excursion of mobilized tendons were superior, probably as a result of improved intrinsic healing, and consequently restored gliding surfaces. The studies by Gelberman et al.[32-36] support the hypothesis that motion has a beneficial effect on tendon nutrition, tenocyte metabolism, or both.

In 1987, Hitchcock et al.[44] studied healing of chicken flexor profundus tendons, comparing immobilized tendons and those allowed immediate controlled mobilization. They found that the immobilized tendons healed as described by previous investigators,[64] with a decrease in strength as tendon ends softened during the exudative phase as early as 5 days after repair. In contrast, the mobilized tendons did not go through a definable exudative phase, but rather gained strength, appearing to heal through intrinsic mechanisms, with a notable lack of adhesion formation. On the basis of their study, the authors recommended that repairs be mobilized as early as possible, within 1 or 2 days of repair. A study by Feehan and Beauchene,[31] also in a chicken model, found that early passive mobilization does not decrease strength and may enhance healing efficiency of repaired tendons.

POSTOPERATIVE MANAGEMENT PROTOCOLS
Factors affecting healing and rehabilitation

Many variables may affect the outcome of a tendon repair. Among these are individual patient characteristics, factors related to injury or surgery, and factors related to therapy.

Patient-related factors

Age. The only documented age-related factor is the number of vincula, which decreases as the patient grows older.[3] As a result, larger areas within the tendon will lack blood supply, with a consequent decrease in healing potential. In addition, in theory, cell aging could lead to decreased healing capacity of tenocytes.[4]

General health and healing potential. In general, patients in good health heal well. Certain lifestyles or dietary habits adversely affect healing. For example, a cigarette smoker may experience delayed healing caused by the vasoconstrictive effect of tobacco. Patients with a large intake of coffee can expect similar effects.[109]

Rate and quality of scar formation. In practice, clinicians often observe that of two patients with virtually identical injury, surgery, and therapy one may form scar rapidly and heavily and have great difficulty mobilizing the tendon as a result, while the other may form scar slowly and then form very light scar. The latter patient runs a greater risk of tendon rupture.

Patient motivation. The patient's motivation and ability to follow the postoperative program are critical factors in determining the end result of a primary flexor tendon repair. One cannot expect careful and conscientious performance of the therapy program by a patient who does not understand his or her central role in rehabilitation. Each patient's goal is different and often is dictated by his or her occupation. The therapist must identify the patient's goals and make them a part of the overall therapy goals.

Patient education can decrease the danger of rupture, prevent overzealous patients from exercising too much or too forcefully, and perhaps help less-motivated patients understand the importance of adhering to the home program.

Socioeconomic factors. A patient's family life, his or her economic status, and other socioeconomic factors can help or hinder in rehabilitation. The patient may have no health insurance and no income or may be supporting a family but is unable to work. The patient's family may be unsupportive of his or her rehabilitation efforts or may simply be unable to help the patient. The patient may live alone and be unable to handle all of his or her daily responsibilities while performing a complex home program. If these factors are not taken into account in planning treatment, therapy may fail.

Injury- and surgery-related factors

Level of injury. The effect of injury varies from one level of injury to another.

In zone 1, the tendon does not have a great excursion (only 5 to 7 mm), so loss of even a small amount of excursion can be functionally limiting. These injuries also are prone to adhesion of the repair to the A_4 or A_5 pulley and attenuation of the repair.

Zone 2 is still known as "no man's land," so called because for so long results of tendon repair at this level were virtually doomed to failure. Although surgical and therapeutic intervention has evolved to a point at which we now often can achieve excellent results, the risks are many and must be carefully considered. With so many structures packed into the confines of the fibroosseous tunnel, adhesions are highly likely between FDP and FDS; between tendon and sheath; and between tendon and bony, vascular, and other soft tissue structures. If tendons have retracted (in a delayed repair or if the finger was in flexion during injury so that muscle contraction pulled the proximal tendon stump into the palm), the tendon must be retrieved, inevitably contributing intraoperative trauma. In cases of delayed repair, the tendon may have shortened since injury and thus may be repaired under some tension. In addition, damage to the pulleys may compromise tendon function, and injury to the vincula may compromise nutrition. Finally, loss of even a few millimeters of tendon excursion can mean a considerable functional deficit. It is no wonder that so much time and effort have been expended in designing postoperative protocols to control adhesion formation, facilitate adequate nutrition and healing, and attain maximum excursion in the zone 2 injury.

Zone 3 lacerations are susceptible to adhesions to adjacent tendons, lumbricals, and interossei, and to overlying fascia and skin. Zone 4 injuries are at risk for adhesion to synovial sheaths, to each other, and to the other structures lying within the constricted carpal tunnel space. As with zone 2 injuries, intertendinous adhesions will limit differential glide and thus can severely limit hand function. Tendon injuries in zone 5 commonly become markedly adherent to overlying skin and fascia, but these adhesions generally are not problematic because adhesions form between the tendon and paratenon. Because the paratenon is a loose connective tissue, adhesions are not as restrictive as those that form between tendon and the firm, well-anchored flexor retinaculum or fibroosseous tunnel.

Unfortunately, adhesion formation in this zone is often very heavy, possibly in part because the limited vascularity stimulates formation of adhesions to supply nutrition to the healing tendon. Wherever tendons lie in close proximity (as within the fibroosseous tunnel of zone 2 and in the carpal tunnel in zone 4), they will tend to form intertendinous adhesions, which limit independent digit function as well as overall digit flexion and strength.

Type of injury. The nature of the injury is another important determinant of final outcome. In an untidy laceration or crush, subsequent infection may prolong the inflammatory process and delay healing. Crushing or blunt injuries usually cause more associated injuries to surrounding tissues and lead to more scar formation. Crush injuries also commonly involve vascular injury, and this can impair healing, especially with injury to the vincula. When adjacent injured tissues must be protected (as with fractures or injuries to neurovascular bundles), treatment is modified, and this may compromise the ultimate result.

An isolated FDP injury heals with fewer adhesions, partly because only a single repair, rather than two contiguous repairs, is prone to intertendinous adhesion. If FDS is injured, the likelihood of vincular damage is greater and vascularity is impaired, thus again increasing the risk of adhesion formation (see Fig. 27-5).

The prognosis also may be better for a partial laceration than for a complete laceration because vascularity generally will be better preserved. There is controversy in the literature about whether to repair the partial laceration.[11,68,69] Triggering or entrapment may occur when the irregular surface of an untreated partially lacerated tendon catches on the sheath, and theoretically the unrepaired partially lacerated tendon may rupture.

If the finger was flexing powerfully when injured, the contracting muscle will pull the proximal portion proximally like a rubber band cut under tension. The vincula may be ruptured or stretched, impairing vascularity. The surgeon must retrieve the proximal tendon stump before repair. The very retrieval may be traumatic to the tendon and surrounding sheath.

Position of the finger when injured also will affect outcome in that a given point on the tendon glides proximally during flexion and distally during extension. For example, suppose a test tube breaks in a patient's hand, lacerating the FDP and FDS of one finger. The finger is flexed when injured. If the digit is extended, the cut distal portion of each tendon could be pulled distally by as much as 3 or 4 cm, depending on the excursion of the tendon in that patient and the actual level of injury.

Sheath integrity. The sheath and pulleys often are involved in a zone 1 or 2 injury. There is some disagreement about repair of this system.

Injury to the pulley system decreases the mechanical advantage of the tendon, as has been demonstrated.[71,75] Pulley injury also affects tendon nutrition because of the role the pulleys play in synovial diffusion. As discussed previously, the pulleys create a firm opposing surface for the avascular volar side of the tendon during flexion. If this "pumping mechanism" between the tendon and pulley indeed resembles the diffusion in articular cartilage, then pulley repair is imperative for optimal tendon healing conditions.

With the exception of the pulleys, synovial sheath repair may not improve the healing of repaired flexor tendons. Several studies have shown no advantage to sheath repair.[38,73,74,76] Apparently a single cell layer much like the sheath regenerates in the first postoperative days.[74,89] Many surgeons will attempt to repair the sheath, however, to prevent the possibility of triggering of the tendon-repair site on the open sheath.

Surgical technique. Meticulous surgical technique can minimize the amount of additional tissue trauma and hematoma, thereby reducing the number of adhesions. Excessive postoperative hematoma causes increased inflammatory and cellular responses. An increase in the amount of hematoma therefore may increase the number of adhesions surrounding the repaired tendon.

Tissues must be handled delicately. Potenza[79] has demonstrated that even the marks of the forceps on the epitenon can trigger adhesion formation. The effect of different surgical variables on adhesion formation in repaired tendons also has been investigated.[65] The authors demonstrated an increase in adhesion formation when suture material was added to a gliding tendon. Injury to the sheath and splinting were other variables investigated and found to increase adhesion formation. Sutures may "strangulate" the intratendinous vessels and provoke adhesion formation. In fact, sutures often are placed in the relatively avascular volar aspect of the tendon to avoid damage to the dorsally placed intratendinous vessels.

Suture strength is a crucial variable. It was only when both strong and atraumatic sutures were developed that early mobilization could be contemplated. The suture must be strong enough to prevent gapping while allowing gentle stress to the repair. Today's development of early active mobilization techniques depends even more heavily on adequate suture strength. Although a discussion of specific sutures is beyond the scope of this chapter, several recently developed sutures clearly are strong enough to withstand early active mobilization if performed with carefully controlled force. The literature indicates that given a grasping suture, technically well placed, strength is directly proportional to the number of strands crossing the repair.[104,105,117] Several studies also have indicated that a well-designed

circumferential suture will add strength to any repair.* Suture knot placement also may add strength.[7,80] Another consideration is the work of flexion, or resistance to gliding caused by placement, bulk, or other design aspects of the core or circumferential suture.[6,8,9,52]

Timing of repair. The longer a tendon repair is delayed, the more difficult the rehabilitation may be.[40] By 2 weeks after injury, the cut tendon ends will have scarred down to surrounding tissues and must be dissected free before repair. In addition, the entire musculotendinous unit shortens and pulls the tendon proximally; this may place tension on the repair and increase the risk of gapping or rupture; shortening also increases the risk of later flexion contractures.

Therapy-related factors

Timing. As noted, an immobilized tendon repair loses strength initially, whereas early mobilization strengthens the repair. Therefore, if early mobilization is to be used, therapy should begin as soon as possible. If mobilization begins at 1 week after repair, the repair will already have weakened enough to be greatly at risk for rupture or deformation. Adhesions also will have begun to form, adding to the stress placed on the weakened repair. A 1995 study by Tottenham et al.[107] found better results in patients whose repaired zone 2 tendons were mobilized passively within 1 week than in those mobilized between 1 and 3 weeks after repair. However, in a severely edematous digit, starting early mobilization on the day of surgery would be dangerous. Inflammation and edema will subside after a day or so of rest and elevation in the compressive postoperative dressing, and this will reduce the work of flexion.[43]

Another aspect of timing is progression according to tendon healing status. Although not always described as such, every protocol can be divided into three phases or stages. The early stage is a protective period that includes the inflammatory and fibroplasia phases and sometimes the beginning of the remodeling phase of wound healing, when the repair is at its weakest. This lasts for 3 to 4 weeks. Next is the intermediate stage, when stress to the tendon is increased, either by mobilizing for the first time, or by decreasing protection during mobilization. The late stage generally begins at 6 to 8 weeks and continues to the end of therapy. Stress to the tendon is increased, and muscle strengthening and job simulation are added gradually.

Technique. As the following discussion makes clear, the postoperative rehabilitation technique must be selected with care to match the needs of the patient. Not every tendon injury can be treated with the identical protocol, and often the best approach is a combination of techniques from various protocols.

Expertise. The therapist's expertise must be taken into account in selecting a therapy protocol. No therapist should undertake a treatment program without sufficient preparation, experience, and any supervision needed. This may seem

---

*References 52, 55, 62, 63, 81, 90, 111.

evident, but despite the multitude of available options for tendon management, many therapists attempt to use protocols that they simply do not understand. Nowhere is it more vital to have a full understanding of rationale for treatment than in tendon management.

The uninformed reader may be misled easily by results of various studies presented in the literature. In addition to evaluating research design, instrumentation, and other components of any study, keep the following factors in mind as you read with a critical eye.

Obviously, an in vitro study would have more potential limitations in clinical application than would an in vivo study. The same is true of cadaver versus living tissue studies. Similarly, a study with human subjects is more clinically meaningful than one with an animal model, even if the animal is anatomically comparable. Terms such as *active mobilization* should be defined (do the authors mean active extension or active flexion?).

Two papers cannot be compared unless the results are reported according to the same criteria. The following are a few of the commonly used systems for evaluating flexor tendon results

In the Strickland system,[106] intended for use in zones 1 and 2, assessment is based on total active motion (TAM) of the IP joints only (sum of DIP and PIP flexion minus sum of DIP and PIP extension deficit) divided by 175 degrees (considered "normal" IP TAM) and multiplied by 100 to give a percentage of normal motion. MP joints are excluded from measurement because full MP motion can be recovered even when tendon gliding is poor. Ratings follow:

Excellent	85% to 100%	150+ degrees
Good	70% to 84%	125 to 149 degrees
Fair	50% to 69%	90 to 124 degrees
Poor	<50%	<90 degrees

In the Modified Strickland system,[103] the same TAM calculation is made, but the ratings are not as strict:

Excellent	75% to 100%	132+ degrees
Good	50% to 74%	88 to 131 degrees
Fair	25% to 49%	44 to 87 degrees
Poor	<25%	<44 degrees

In the American Society for Surgery of the Hand (ASSH) system,[5] TAM (including MP joints) is divided by 260 degrees and expressed as a percentage, or TAM is compared with the contralateral finger for a percentage of that patient's norm. The ASSH rating of results is the strictest of all TAM systems.

Excellent	100%
Good	75% to 99%
Fair	50% to 74%
Poor	<50%

The Buck-Gramcko system[15] assigns point values to total flexion in both degrees and centimeters from the palm, and

to extension deficit (in degrees). Classification is again excellent (14 or 15 points), good (11 to13 points), fair (7 to 10 points), or poor (0 to 6 points).

In any study, the rupture rate should be no more than 10% to be acceptable, and then only in a high-risk experimental program or high-risk population. The percentage of ruptures should be considered in light of the number of tendons and number of fingers in the study, and the study should indicate whether the rupture rate is figured on the basis of number of fingers or number of tendons.

Following are the rationale, indications, and representative protocols for each of the three basic approaches to flexor tendon management: immobilization, early passive mobilization, and early active mobilization. The discussion of immobilization is the most concrete and detailed, including concepts and techniques that may be used in other approaches.

Immobilization

Rationale and indications. No matter how sophisticated our therapeutic and surgical care becomes, there probably will always be a need for immobilization of flexor tendon repairs in some circumstances. Early mobilization protocols are appropriate for alert, motivated patients who understand the exercise program and precautions. For this reason, immobilization is still the treatment of choice for patients younger than 10 years of age, those with cognitive deficits, and those who for any other reason are clearly unable or unwilling to participate in a complex rehabilitation program. These patients will benefit far more from protection of the repair until adequate healing and adhesion formation have taken place. Some tendons also must be immobilized to protect other injured structures. It may be difficult to mobilize these repairs later on because of heavy adhesion formation. On the other hand, adhesions may lend additional support to the immobilized repair, which is theoretically weaker than a repair treated with early immobilization. Therefore, if the patient is overzealous or ignores precautions when first allowed to move the tendon, there is a built-in margin of safety.

In some cases the patient is not referred to therapy for a postoperative splint but simply remains in the postoperative cast until sent to therapy at 3 to 4 weeks after surgery. Therefore all therapists must be prepared to treat the immobilized tendon with skill and care.

Protocol. The following protocol is based on that developed by Cifaldi Collins and Schwarze[20] and is designed to provide guidelines for sufficiently aggressive therapy after mobilization. This protocol includes several techniques and concepts applicable to all flexor tendon management, regardless of the approach used.

Early stage (from 0 to 3 or 4 weeks)

Splint. The dorsal forearm-based postoperative splint or cast holds the wrist in 10 to 30 degrees of flexion, the MP joints in 40 to 60 degrees of flexion, and the interphalangeal (IP) joints in full extension.

There are three ways of making a fist:

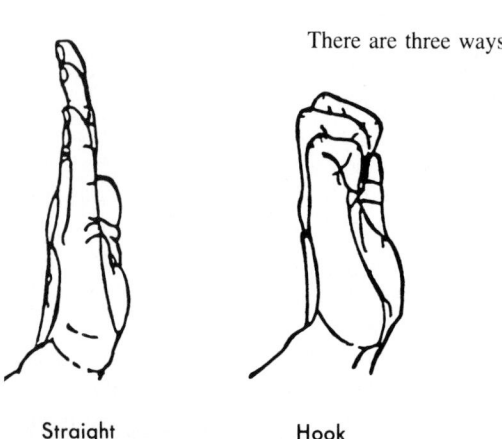
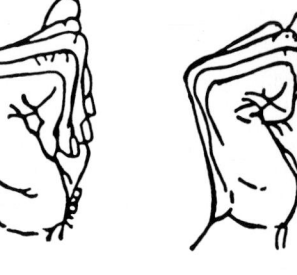

Straight   Hook   Straight   Fist

Fig. 27-6. The three different positions of tendon gliding exercises: hook fist, straight fist, and full fist.

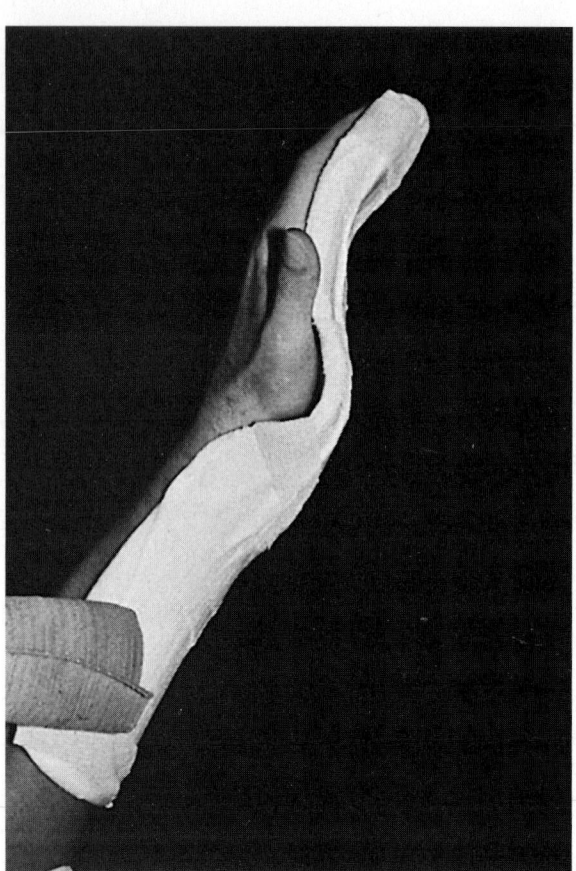

Fig. 27-7. A forearm-based splint or plaster "stretcher" maintains maximum comfortable extension at night. It will be serially remolded or remade to accommodate gains in extension.

Exercise. At home patients perform range-of-motion (ROM) exercise to uninvolved joints (elbow, shoulder) to prevent stiffness. The splint is worn 24 hours a day except for therapy visits one to two times a week, when the splint may be removed for gentle protected PROM by the therapist. For protected PROM, the therapist holds adjacent joints in flexion while extending and flexing each joint. Thus, for

example, for PIP extension, the wrist and MP and DIP joints are kept flexed to give some slack to the flexor tendons. If the adjacent MP and DIP joints were allowed to remain extended during PIP extension, the slack would be taken up and PIP extension might stretch or rupture a repair at proximal phalanx level. The concept of protected passive motion is applied in all flexor tendon management protocols. Often, after prolonged protection in MP flexion, patients develop intrinsic tightness. Therefore, in addition to protected isolated ROM of all joints, we perform protected intrinsic stretch exercises (wrist flexed maximally while MP joints are held in neutral and IP joints are gently flexed passively).

During the therapy session, the therapist may remove the splint to clean the patient's skin and, after the sutures are removed and the incision is well healed, perform massage to the scar. As the scar heals, massage may help control both skin and tendon adhesions. Elastomer or other pressure dressings are helpful for flattening unusually bulky scars but generally should be used only at night to avoid restricting mobility during the day. In some patients, such pressure can be applied during the early stage without removing the splint.

Intermediate stage (starting at 3 to 4 weeks)

Splint. At 3 to 4 weeks, the splint is modified to bring the wrist to neutral (0 degrees). The patient is taught to remove the splint hourly for exercise.

Exercise. With the wrist at 10 degrees of extension, the patient performs 10 repetitions of passive digit flexion and extension, followed by 10 repetitions of active differential tendon gliding exercises (Fig. 27-6). These exercises elicit maximum total and differential flexor tendon glide at wrist/palm level.[113] The straight fist, with MP and PIP joints flexed but DIP joints extended, elicits maximum FDS glide in relation to surrounding structures. The full fist, with MP, PIP, and DIP joints flexed, does the same for the FDP tendon. In the hook fist, with MP joints extended while IP joints are flexed, maximum differential gliding between the two tendons is achieved. For the Cifaldi Collins and Schwarze[20]

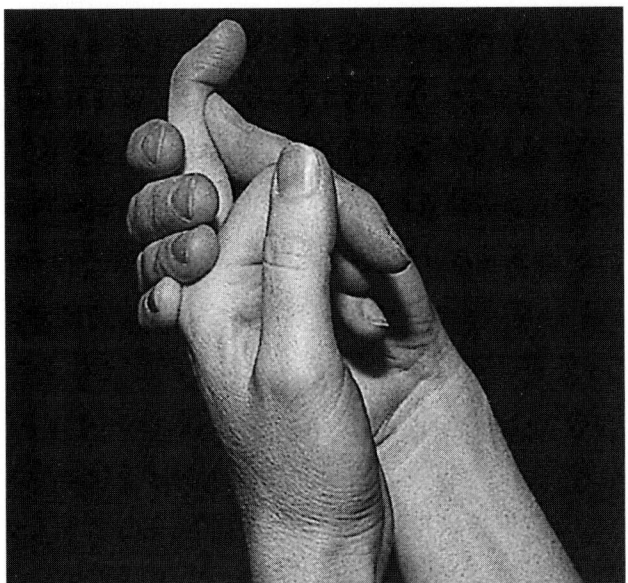

Fig. 27-8. Blocking exercise for flexor digitorum profundus gliding. The proximal interphalangeal joint (PIP) is gently maintained in passive PIP extension to prevent flexor digitorum superficialis glide. Blocking exercises are performed carefully, avoiding forceful distal interphalangeal joint flexion that may apply excessive stress to newly healed tendons. (From Stewart KM: *Hand Clin* 7:447, 1991.)

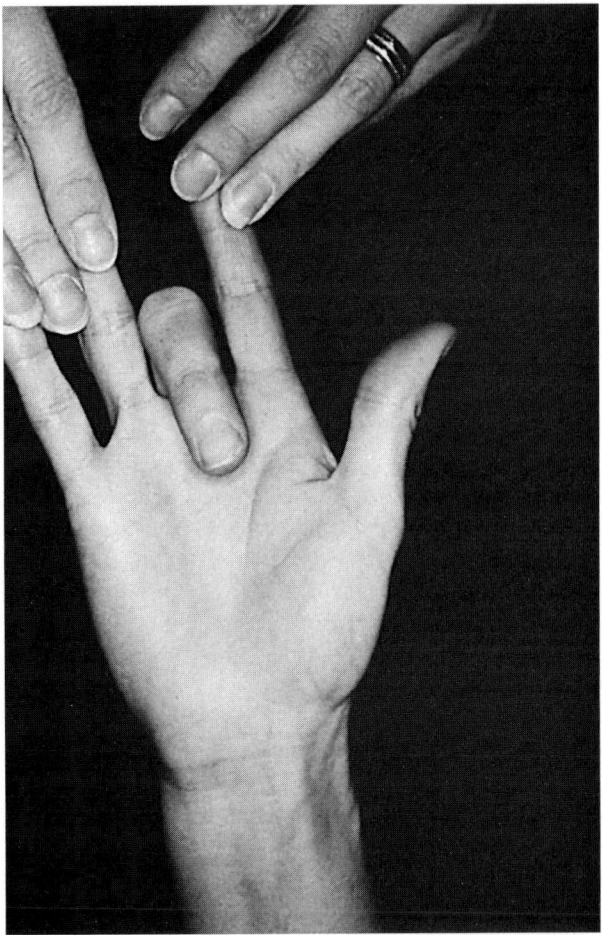

Fig. 27-9. Active isolated superficialis exercise: flexing one finger at a time at the proximal interphalangeal joint while holding the other fingers in extension with the uninvolved hand.

protocol, the exercises incorporate tenodesis: The wrist extends when the digits flex and flexes when the digits extend, increasing the excursion attained.

After 3 or 4 days of these exercises, tendon function is evaluated. The therapist measures active and passive flexion, totaling the degrees of flexion achieved at MP and IP joints for total active and passive flexion. If there is a discrepancy of more than 50 degrees between total active and total passive flexion, poor gliding and heavy adhesion formation are assumed and the patient is moved on to the next phase of therapy. If the discrepancy is less than 50 degrees, the patient continues with the current phase of therapy until 6 weeks after repair.

Late stage (starting at 4 to 6 weeks)

Splint. The dorsal blocking splint is discontinued. If flexor muscle–tendon unit shortening is a problem, a forearm-based palmar nighttime splint may be worn, holding wrist and fingers in maximum comfortable extension (Fig. 27-7). The splint, made of plaster or thermoplastic material, is serially remade or adjusted to accommodate for any improvements in extension. Within 1 week, if improvement is not noted, dynamic or static progressive extension splints may be introduced, using very gentle tension initially. Later, with a resistant PIP flexion contracture (not uncommon in zone 2 injuries), serial cylinder casting may be needed.

Exercise. The patient begins gentle blocking exercises for isolated FDP and FDS glide. For isolated FDP gliding, the MP and PIP joints are held in extension, thus preventing FDS glide, while the FDP functions alone to flex the DIP joint (Fig. 27-8). For isolated FDS glide, the adjacent fingers are held in full extension, thus holding FDP tendons (which have a common muscle belly) at their full length and making it virtually impossible for them to assist as the FDS flexes the PIP joint (Fig. 27-9). The index finger often has a separate FDP muscle belly, allowing FDP glide even when the adjacent middle finger is held in extension, but the patient often can be taught to use only the FDS tendon, with extension of the middle finger as a cue.

Blocking exercises can be dangerous for a newly healed tendon if not performed correctly. This is true particularly in the case of isolated DIP flexion. If the patient does not concentrate on flexing only the DIP, but instead "fights" the fingers holding the PIP in extension, this active exercise becomes a strongly resisted exercise. When the finger is edematous and the FDP tendon is gliding poorly, the patient may have difficulty resisting the temptation to exercise too vigorously. Patient education includes the danger of rupture with overzealous blocking exercise; some patients may not be appropriate candidates for blocking until 2 or 3 weeks later, when the tendon repair is stronger.

Blocking exercises are performed four to six times a day, with 10 repetitions, in addition to the passive exercise and active differential flexor tendon gliding introduced in the previous stage. After 1 week, if active flexion has not improved, the program is upgraded to include towel walking (flexing fingers individually in turn to gather a towel on a flat surface), light pick-ups, and gentle putty squeezing (no more than 10 repetitions with the lightest putty).

In another week, sustained grip activities may be added, followed by light-resistance grip exercisers, putty scraping, and use of heavier putty. The patient also may be instructed to begin lifting heavier objects at home (e.g., a quart of milk). The decision as to when to step up the amount of resistance and functional use is not easy. There are no rules! This is where the therapist's skill comes into play, including the understanding of tendon healing and the ability to evaluate tendon function precisely. Greater resistance to flexion will elicit a stronger muscle contraction and therefore assist in stretching tendon adhesions and improving glide, but excessive resistance may rupture a tendon even as late as 3 months after injury. In general, the more adherent the tendon, the safer it is to apply resistance to glide. The tendon that is gliding well does not need that additional resistance. Smoothly gliding tendons should not receive even light resistance until 7 or 8 weeks, and most tendons are not ready for heavy resistance (e.g., lifting more than 10 pounds, using heavy putty) and manual labor job simulation until 10 to 12 weeks.

One of the most common mistakes made by patients is overdoing resistive exercise or a favorite activity, however light the resistance to flexion involved. This can provoke inflammation and lead to increased fibrosis and stiffness. Patients may develop trigger fingers (stenosing tenosynovitis) through excessive repetitive gripping or squeezing (as with putty exercise). The therapist must not only warn patients of this danger but also routinely palpate for triggering at the A_1 pulley.

Treating adhesion problems. Restrictive adhesions are the most common complication after immobilization of the repaired flexor tendon. Several techniques for mobilizing the adherent tendon are all aimed at gradually lengthening adhesions to allow greater glide. The object is not to break adhesions, because this internal trauma may lead to greater fibrosis and new adhesions. To select the best method of treatment, the therapist first identifies the location and extent of adhesions, as described earlier (see Fundamental Concepts: Evaluating Tendon Function). A forearm-based dynamic extension splint might be used, for example, in the presence of extensive FDP and FDS adhesions of three fingers in zones 2 through 4: The wrist and MP and IP joints all could be placed at maximum extension to stretch adhesions, and the splint also could be used for exercise, resisting differential tendon gliding. Such a splint would be unnecessarily complex for a single FDP tendon repair adherent only in the distal portion of zone 2. In this case a PIP flexion contracture could be addressed with a finger-based dynamic splint or cylinder cast, and limitations in flexion could be addressed with frequent blocking, putty scraping, or sustained grip activities such as dowel sanding, use of a rake or other garden implement, or bicycling. Some patients find it helpful to carry with them at all times a lipstick, a pill bottle, or other small cylinder that they can barely grip. Frequently throughout the day, they grip the cylinder 10 times for 10 to 30 seconds.

Precise identification of adhesions assists in planning precise intervention: If a single FDS tendon is adherent, exercise could focus on gliding of that single tendon, with or without resistance (Fig. 27-9). If all FDS tendons are adherent, DIP extension splints may be worn during active and resistive exercises to aid in eliciting FDS glide.

Neuromuscular electrical stimulation may be used to provoke a stronger muscle contraction; this would be appropriate within 1 week of initiating resisted exercise. Ultrasound may provide deep heat combined with stretch or active tendon gliding to stretch adhesions. Interested readers are referred to Chapters 107 and 109. Superficial and deep scar respond well to soft tissue mobilization techniques such as cross-frictional massage. The patient also may actively contract the affected muscle while massaging over the adherent tendon; the tendon will pull proximally while the patient gently pushes the skin distally, stretching local adhesions.

Early passive mobilization

Rationale and indications. If applied with care, early passive mobilization (starting within a few days of repair) has been shown to produce superior results, apparently because early mobilization inhibits restrictive adhesion formation, promotes intrinsic healing and synovial diffusion, and produces a stronger repair, preventing the decrease in tensile strength of repairs noted in immobilized tendons by Mason and Allen and by Urbaniak.* In a study using metal markers in repaired flexor tendons, Silfverskiöld et al.[93] demonstrated that measurable passive excursion occurs with passive IP joint flexion. Related studies by May et al.[67] and Silfverskiöld et al.[92] found a statistically significant correlation between early passive IP joint flexion and later active flexion measured in long-term follow-up.

Protocols. There are two basic types of early passive mobilization protocols. One approach is based on the work of Kleinert,[49,50] and the other on that of Duran and Houser.[25,26] Hand specialists have worked many variations

---

*References 32, 37, 39, 44, 51, 64, 108.

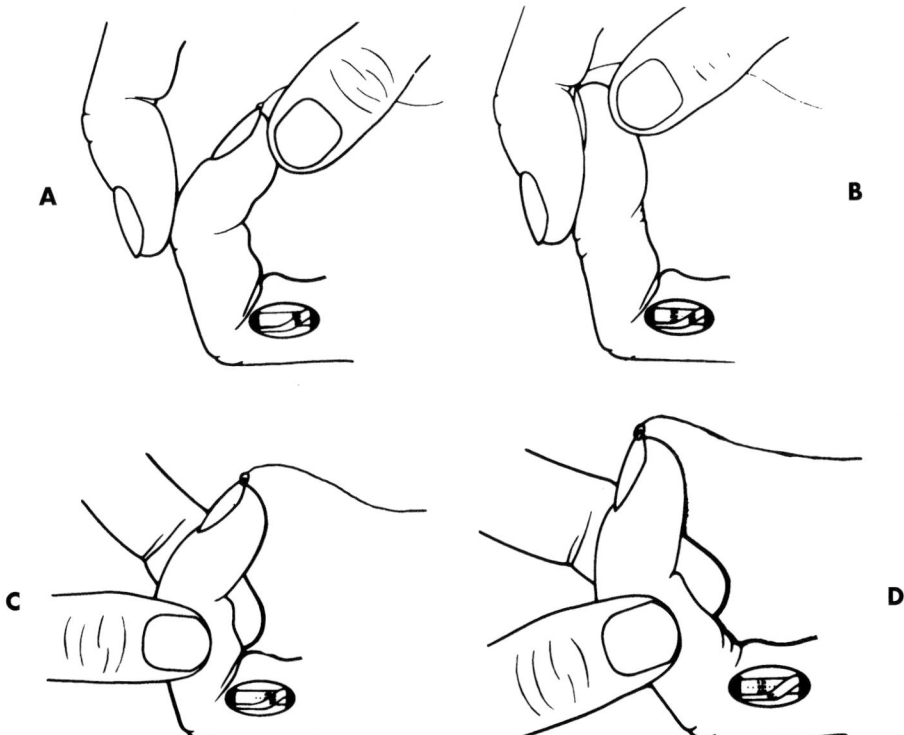

Fig. 27-10. Duran and Houser's exercises for passive flexor tendon gliding. With the metacarpophalangeal joint (MP) and proximal interphalangeal joint (PIP) flexed **(A),** the distal interphalangeal joint (DIP) is passively extended **(B),** thus moving the flexor digitorum profundus repair distally, away from a flexor digitorum superficialis repair. Then with DIP and MP flexed **(C),** the PIP is extended **(D);** both repairs glide distally away from the site of repair and any surrounding tissues to which they might otherwise form adhesions. (From Duran RJ, et al: Management of flexor tendon lacerations in zone 2 using controlled passive motion postoperatively. In Hunter JM, et al, editors: *Rehabilitation of the hand,* ed 3, St Louis, 1990, Mosby.)

on these two approaches, and in fact, few therapists adhere closely to one protocol or the other.[24,29,66,102]

In both approaches, a forearm-based dorsal blocking splint, applied at surgery, blocks the MP joints and wrist in flexion to place the flexor tendons on slack, and the IP joints are left free or allowed to extend to neutral within the splint. The plaster splint may be replaced with a thermoplastic splint within 1 or 2 weeks. The splint allows passive flexion of the fingers but does not allow extension beyond the limits of the splint. Dynamic traction maintains the fingers in flexion to further relax the tendon and prevent inadvertent active flexion. The dynamic traction may be provided by rubber bands, elastic threads, springs, or other devices; the traction is applied to the fingernail either by placing a suture through the nail in surgery or by gluing to the fingernail a dress hook, Velcro, a piece of soft leather or moleskin, or the rubber band itself.

Duran and Houser

Early stage (from 0 to 4.5 weeks)

SPLINT. The wrist is held in 20 degrees of flexion and the MP joints in a relaxed position of flexion.

EXERCISE. Duran and Houser[25] determined through clinical and experimental observation that 3 to 5 mm of glide was sufficient to prevent formation of firm tendon adhesions; the exercises (6 to 8 repetitions twice a day) are designed to achieve this. With MP and PIP joints flexed, the DIP joint is passively extended, thus moving the FDP repair distally, away from an FDS repair. Then with DIP and MP joints flexed, the PIP is extended; both repairs glide distally away from the site of repair and any surrounding tissues to which they might otherwise form adhesions (Fig. 27-10).

Intermediate stage (from 4.5 weeks to 7.5 or 8 weeks)

SPLINT. After 4.5 weeks, the splint is replaced with a wrist band to which rubber band traction is attached (Fig. 27-11).

EXERCISE. Active extension exercises begin within the limitations imposed by the wrist band. Active flexion (blocking, FDS gliding, and fisting) is initiated on removal of the wrist band at 5.5 weeks.

Late stage (starting at 7.5 to 8 weeks). Resisted flexion waits until 7.5 to 8 weeks. The program is upgraded following the principles outlined under the earlier section on Immobilization.

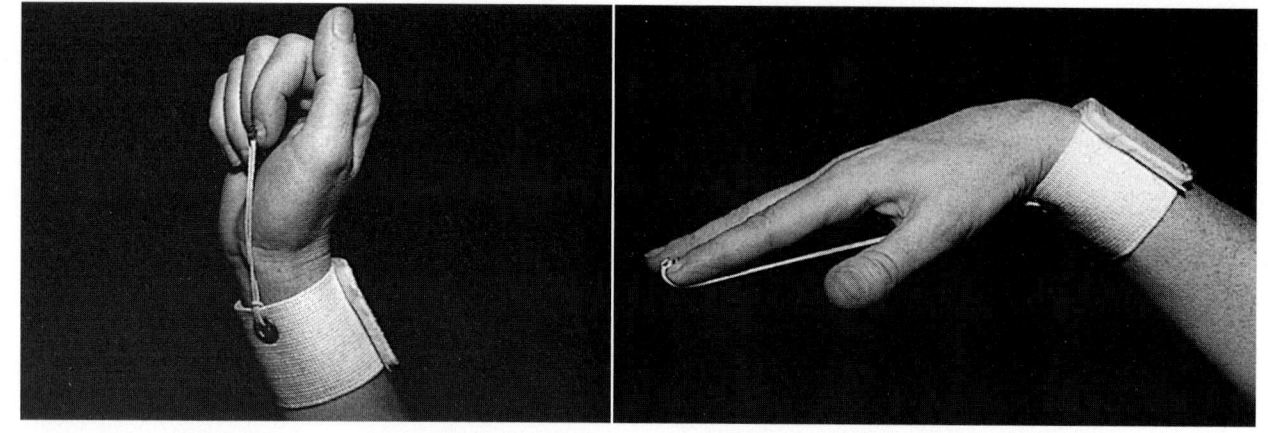

Fig. 27-11. Elastic traction from the wrist band prevents simultaneous wrist and finger extension. **A,** When the wrist is extended, the fingers are passively flexed by the elastic traction. **B,** When the fingers extend, the wrist is passively flexed. (From Stewart KM: Tendon injuries. In Stanley BG, Tribuzi SM, editors: *Concepts in hand rehabilitation,* Philadelphia, 1992, FA Davis.)

Modified Duran. The Duran protocol is not commonly used in its standard form by hand therapists, but many have adopted the use of the wrist band as a way of protecting the tendon after discontinuing the dorsal blocking splint. Some therapists (including us) now use what is often called a *modified Duran approach.* This is to apply a dorsal protective splint (we prefer 40 to 50 degrees at the MP joints and from 20 degrees of extension to 20 degrees of flexion at the wrist, depending on the quality of the repair and other factors), with the IP joints allowed to extend to neutral in the splint) but to omit the rubber band traction and strap the IP joints in extension between exercises or at night (Fig. 27-12). Patients perform passive individual and composite flexion and extension, active composite extension exercises (manually blocking the MP in greater flexion for more complete active IP extension), and the passive flexion and extension exercises advocated by Duran and Houser. In therapy only, the splint is removed for careful protected tenodesis exercises (passive or assisted simultaneous wrist flexion and finger extension, alternating with simultaneous wrist extension and finger flexion). Obviously, performance of tenodesis exercises depends on the zone of injury and relative safety of this maneuver for the patient.

Kleinert. Duran and Houser use dynamic traction to rest the digit in flexion, but Kleinert uses the rubber band to resist full active extension, based on findings of electromyographic silence in the flexors during resisted digit extension.[49,56] Others have questioned this finding in more recent research, as later noted.

The original protocol will not be described in detail because it is no longer used much in the original form. More recent adaptations are summarized later under Achieving Maximum Passive Tendon Excursion.

Splint. In the original Kleinert protocol, the dorsal blocking splint blocked the wrist in 45 degrees of flexion and the MP joints in 10 to 20 degrees (since modified to 40

degrees). Rubber band traction was directed to the fingernail from the wrist or just proximal to the wrist.

Exercise. Every hour, the patient actively extends the fingers to the limits of the splint 10 times, allowing the rubber bands to flex the fingers.

At 3 to 6 weeks (depending on the quality of tendon glide) gentle active flexion may begin (intermediate stage), although resisted exercise waits until 6 to 8 weeks (late stage).

Variations on early passive mobilization

Prevention of PIP flexion contractures. When the fingers are maintained in PIP flexion with dynamic traction, PIP flexion contractures often result. One solution is to remove the traction at night and strap the fingers in IP extension.[66,85,101] Therapists employ variations on night and intermittent day splinting to correct incipient PIP flexion contractures in both Kleinert and modified Duran protocols, particularly if a delicate digital nerve repair or other injury has mandated splinting the PIP in slight flexion.[85,100] A static PIP extension splint may be inserted between the dorsal blocking splint and the dorsum of the finger to address this problem when it first develops. However, prevention is the best treatment.

Another reason for PIP flexion contractures may be the difficulty of extending the injured finger fully against excessive resistance. Recent studies[21,110] indicate no advantage to increasing the strength of dynamic flexion traction; in fact, these electromyogram (EMG) studies disagree with that of Lister et al.,[56] finding that flexor contraction is inconsistently inhibited no matter how great the resistance to extension (thus throwing some doubt on any use of resisted extension in early passive mobilization programs). Studies have shown that rubber bands offer increasing resistance because finger extension stretches the elastic further.[16,19,115] Burge and Brown[16] found that this increase could be moderated by use of a palmar pulley or by positioning the MP in no more than 20 degrees of flexion. Patients may be

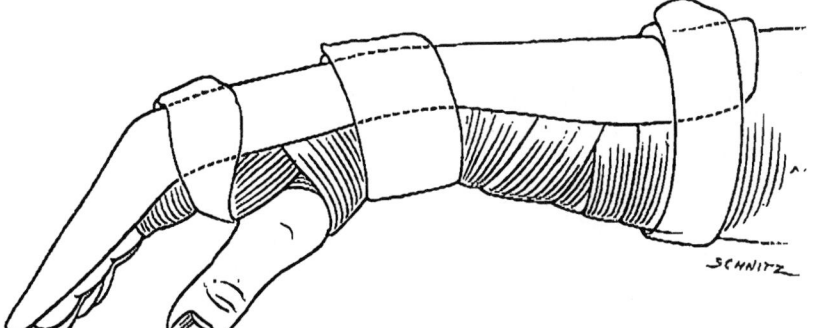

Fig. 27-12. Dorsal blocking splint used for modified Duran protocol. Wrist and metacarpophalangeal joints are flexed, and fingers are strapped in interphalangeal joint extension when not exercising. (From Cannon N: *Indiana Hand Center Newslett* 1:13, 1993.)

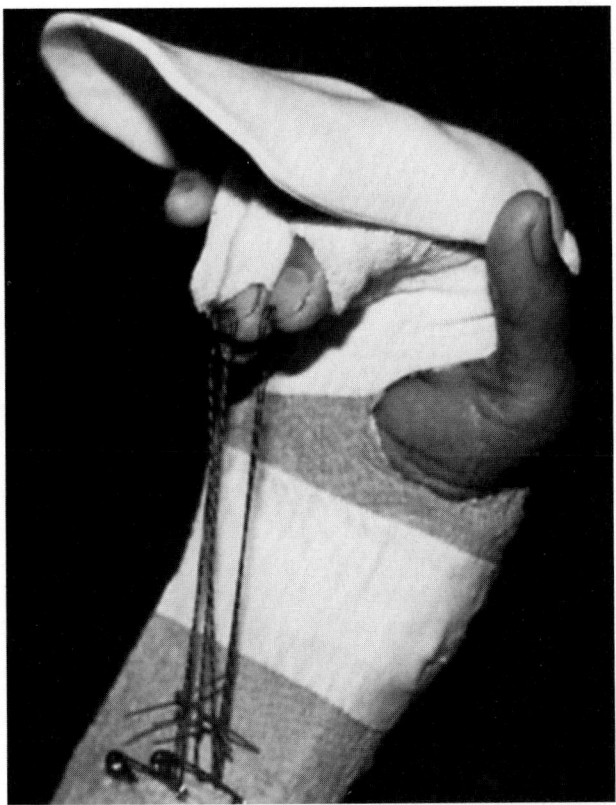

Fig. 27-13. In the Kleinert splint as originally designed, the metacarpophalangeal joint and proximal interphalangeal joint are held in flexion by rubber band traction, but the distal interphalangeal joint rests in almost complete extension.

instructed to manually release some rubber band tension during exercise to ease extension.

Another proposed solution is to change the means of dynamic traction within the splint design. In the Washington regimen,[18,19,24] two rubber bands are used, one of which is cut in half so that it forms a single strand. Before performing active extension exercises, the patient detaches proximally the intact rubber band so that only the single strand elastic resists extension, making full extension easier to achieve. The finger rests in complete flexion to the distal palmar

crease (DPC) when not exercising. A splint design proposed by Werntz et al.[115] incorporates a coiled lever to offer a more constant resistance and make full extension easier to achieve. However, this splint is not commonly used, given the less expensive alternatives available.

Achieving maximum passive tendon excursion. Mc-Grouther and Ahmed[70] found that complete excursion of the FDP tendon and differential excursion between FDP and FDS could be accomplished only through flexion of the DIP; later this principle also was found to be true for the FPL.[14] In other words, to achieve glide of a repair, it is necessary to flex the joints distal to the repair. The cadaver study of FDP excursion in zone 2 by Horibe et al.[45] confirmed the importance of distal joint flexion but also found that PIP flexion appears to produce the greatest excursion relative to the tendon sheath. Silfverskiöld et al., in their series of in vivo studies, initially found results agreeing with Horibe's.[93] Later studies[95] used a larger number of cases and found a significant correlation between controlled passive DIP, ROM, and FDP excursion. All of these studies taken together suggest that early passive mobilization programs should incorporate the greatest possible degree of flexion in the IP joints.

In the standard dynamic flexion splint as first designed by Kleinert, the rubber band traction is directed from the wrist or distal forearm to the fingernail. This flexes the MP joint and, to a lesser extent the PIP joint, but leaves the DIP in virtual extension (Fig. 27-13). Slattery and McGrouther[96] proposed adding a palmar pulley to redirect dynamic traction and thus fully flex the DIP joint (Fig. 27-14). This has become standard practice with zone 2 FDP injuries. Brown and McGrouther[14] later suggested that similarly, in FPL lacerations, the thumb MP joint should be immobilized and efforts directed toward mobilizing the IP joint.

Comparative studies. May et al.[66] have put forward an early passive mobilization protocol that they call the "four-finger" method. They support this with a prospective study comparing three methods of postoperative flexor tendon management. For all three methods, the wrist was flexed 30 to 45 degrees and the MP joints 50 to 70 degrees. For the first two groups, the splint extended to the fingertips and allowed

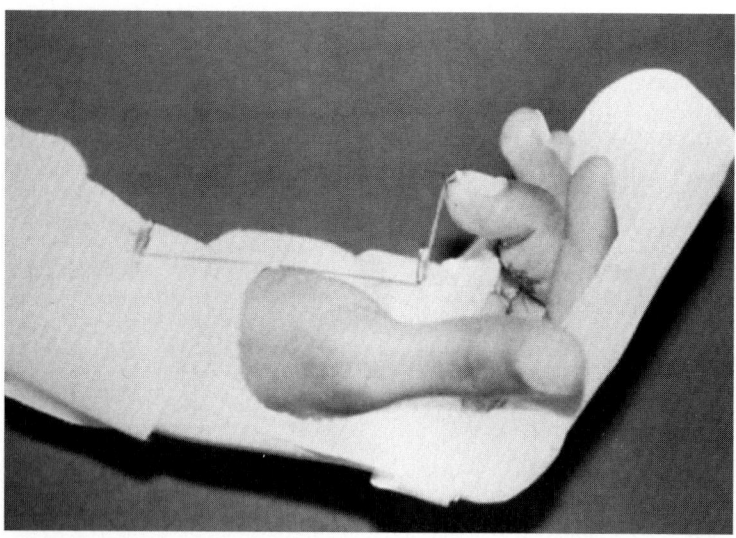

Fig. 27-14. A simple palmar pulley can be provided by a safety pin attached to a palmar strap at distal palmar crease level. The line passes through the "eye" of the safety pin to direct the pull precisely.

full IP extension. Rubber band traction passed through a palmar pulley, and patients performed hourly active IP extension exercises. In the second group, patients added manual passive flexion and extension to each repetition of the exercises. In the third group, there were several different elements. The dorsal splint extended only to the PIP joints to ensure that PIP extension was not limited. All four fingers were included in traction, even if not injured. A thicker rubber band was used to ensure maximum passive flexion, and as in the second group, manual pressure to all four fingers was used to attain the final degrees of passive flexion during exercise. Patients were instructed to use the uninvolved hand to decrease resistance from the rubber bands by pulling them distally during the active extension part of the exercises. The exercises were otherwise the same as in the other two groups. At night, the rubber bands were detached, and a volar component was added holding the IP joints in extension.

For all three groups, the splint was discontinued at 4 weeks, and active flexion and extension were initiated (intermediate stage). Resistance to flexion was added at 6 weeks (late stage) and progressed to blocking and heavier resistance at 8 weeks. Dynamic extension for any flexion contractures was initiated at 6 weeks. Most patients returned to work at 10 to 12 weeks.

May et al.[66] found that the third group (the four-finger group) had significantly better results, which the authors attributed to inclusion of all four fingers in traction and strapping in extension at night. Although all of the components of this program (including all four fingers in traction, strapping in IP extension at night, releasing rubber band tension during exercise, applying a manual "push" into full flexion, splint extending only to the PIP joint, and using a palmar bar) have been tried by various therapists, May's study supports this combination of interventions nicely and offers a sound rationale for each.

Cooney et al.[22,46] conducted a cadaver study comparing the total FDP, total FDS, and differential FDP/FDS excursion obtained at three levels (zones 2, 3, and 5) using three different methods. The first was original Kleinert traction directed from the distal forearm. The second was a splint with a palmar pulley. Third was a new splint using synergistic wrist motion to produce a dynamic tenodesis effect: wrist flexion producing finger extension and wrist extension producing finger flexion. The study found that although all three splints produced adequate total excursion (judged according to Duran and Houser's recommended 3 to 5 mm), the Brooke Army splint produced more than did the Kleinert, and the synergistic wrist motion splint produced the greatest excursion of all. Surprisingly, in view of the previously cited tendon excursion studies,[45,70,93] the traditional Kleinert splint produced more differential gliding than did the Brooke Army; the synergistic wrist motion splint again outperformed both of the other splints. To date, no clinical trials have been published on this particular splint design. Nonetheless, we can draw two important inferences from this study: (1) More research is needed to resolve the conflicts in the literature regarding tendon excursion, and (2) we need to define the optimal total and differential excursion of the healing tendon. Without this information we cannot choose the most effective protocol. In the meantime, many therapists now incorporate guarded wrist tenodesis exercise (under therapist supervision) in the first stage of therapy.

Continuous passive motion. A multicenter study has examined the effect of increasing the duration and number of repetitions of daily passive motion exercise through the use of continuous passive motion (CPM) after repairs in zone 2.[41] The authors propose that the superior results in the CPM group may be attributable to the far greater duration and number of repetitions of passive mobilization. Using CPM for management of flexor tendons is cumbersome in most settings, and we do not know of any hand therapists currently

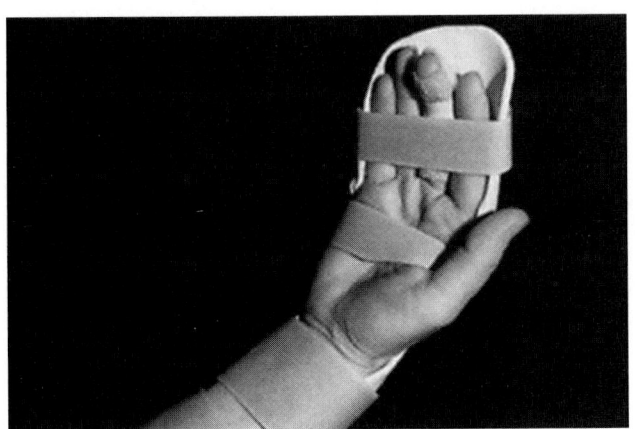

Fig. 27-15. A static dorsal distal interphalangeal joint flexion splint is worn on the involved finger. (From Stewart KM: *Hand Clin* 7:447, 1991.)

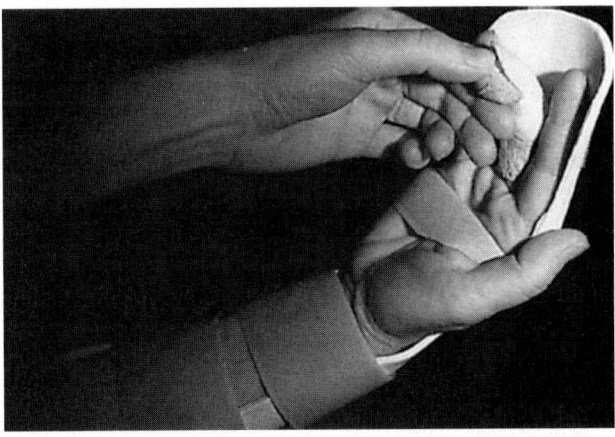

Fig. 27-16. The distal interphalangeal joint can be further flexed passively to 75 degrees to provide 4 mm passive excursion of flexor digitorum profundus. (From Stewart KM: *Hand Clin* 7:447, 1991.)

using this approach. However, the authors of the CPM study suggest that similar results could be obtained with "traditional" techniques using increased duration or repetitions of exercise.

Early passive mobilization in zone 1. The early passive mobilization protocols were developed primarily for zone 2 flexor tendon injuries to decrease the unacceptable rate of adhesion formation, secondary joint stiffness, and other complications so common after repairs at this level. The same programs have produced improved results in other zones as well, apparently because even where adhesions are a less significant problem, controlled stress improves healing and scar remodeling. There is little in the literature regarding specific variations in approach depending on the level of injury, but hand specialists can readily identify functional and anatomic differences that dictate changes in treatment.

Evans[29] has developed such a protocol for zone 1 flexor tendon injuries. Pointing out a number of functional and anatomic features of the FDP and problems specific to healing at this level, distal to the insertion of the FDS, the author proposes certain measures to control gap formation, elongation of the repair, and adhesion formation at specific sites.

Early stage (from 0 to 3 weeks)

SPLINT. The dorsal blocking splint holds the wrist at 30 to 40 degrees of flexion and blocks the MP joints at 30 degrees, with full extension permitted at the IP joints. A separate finger-based dorsal static splint holds the DIP of the affected finger in 45 degrees of flexion (Fig. 27-15). This splint is taped onto the finger proximal to the DIP crease, allowing further manual passive flexion of the joint (Fig. 27-16).

The DIP flexion splint allows passive excursion of the zone 1 repair within a range calculated to produce 4 mm of excursion without stressing the repair excessively. At the same time, the tendon repair at rest is positioned proximal to the site of injury to reduce chances of adhesion to injured tissues. The DIP splint also counteracts the effect of the

oblique retinacular ligament, which tightens with PIP extension and pulls the DIP into extension.

The 30-degree MP flexion position is designed to decrease the viscoelastic effect of the lumbrical on the profundus tendon. With greater MP flexion, the lumbricals shorten and FDP can glide distally, thus impeding efforts to position the repair site proximal to its normal resting position. At the same time, this MP position allows modified passive hook-fist exercise, which has been shown to produce (at least with active motion) the greatest differential tendon glide.[113]

EXERCISE. Passive exercises include DIP flexion to 75 degrees (see Fig. 27-16), composite flexion, and modified hook fist (MP joints can be extended only to 30 degrees within the splint, but DIP and PIP joints can be fully flexed). In addition, the patient uses the other hand to block the MP in full flexion while actively extending the PIP completely. Finally, with the distal strap holding the adjacent fingers in extension, the patient uses the other hand to place the PIP of the affected finger in flexion and then actively maintains the position with a gentle contraction, including place-hold FDS gliding to prevent adhesions between FDS and FDP, particularly at the chiasma of Camper (Fig. 27-17). The therapist also takes the splint off to perform limited passive wrist extension with passive finger flexion and passive hook-fisting with the wrist hyperflexed passively. These exercises are designed to increase the passive tendon excursion as well as maintain wrist and MP joint mobility and prevent intrinsic tightness (through the hook-fist position).

Intermediate and late stages (starting at 3 weeks). After 3 weeks, gentle active exercise begins with place-hold fisting, and the DIP flexion splint is discarded. The program is progressed to include tenodesis wrist exercises, hook fists, and gentle DIP flexion blocking for FDP glide by 4 weeks, before instituting activities and other exercises, following a schedule similar to that of other early passive mobilization protocols. Splinting and other techniques to regain DIP extension are not instituted until 4.5 weeks. From this point

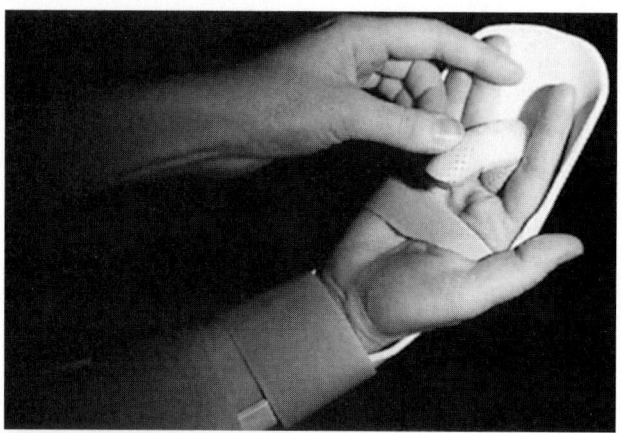

Fig. 27-17. Place-hold gliding of the uninjured flexor digitorum superficialis tendon. (From Stewart KM: *Hand Clin* 7:447, 1991.)

forward, the program progresses in the same manner as other early mobilization protocols. Some of the techniques described by Evans[29] have been used by other therapists, but the rationale has not hitherto been described so completely as it relates to the level of injury. The published results are promising, and our experience with the protocol has been gratifying.

Other adaptations. Many authors speak of varying programs according to the needs of the patient, and this we all know to be at the heart of our specialty.[28,85,101] Some patients appear to scar more heavily than others; tendon glide is extremely limited even after close adherence to a program that has worked well for other patients. These patients may start active or resistive exercise earlier, and their programs may be more vigorously pursued, under the close supervision of an attentive hand therapist. Other patients demonstrate virtually full active motion as early as 3 weeks. These patients already have achieved their ROM and appear to have no adhesions limiting tendon glide. They also may have formed very tenuous scar between the coapted tendon ends and run a high risk of rupture; therefore such patients are protected with further splinting, and when active motion is initiated, it is done so cautiously and the program is modified in response to both visually observed and palpated tendon glide, again under the careful supervision of a hand therapist. The inexperienced therapist initially should follow a highly structured protocol such as the May or modified Duran protocol, using guidelines such as those given by Cifaldi Collins and Schwarze[20] to judge when a tendon is ready for the next phase of therapy. Over time, however, it is incumbent on all therapists to learn the rationale for such guidelines and to develop the skill of making such judgments without relying on protocol structure.

Comparing protocols and current trends. As previously noted, all early passive mobilization protocols use a dorsal blocking splint for at least 3 weeks, and all involve some form of passive flexion and active extension. Except

for the Duran, all use frequent exercise (every 1 to 2 hours). Over the years, there has been a tendency to use less and less wrist flexion; severe wrist flexion angles are uncomfortable and lead to difficulty regaining wrist extension. In the zone 4 or 5 injury, excessive flexion can lead to serious flexion contractures. The experienced hand therapist, who can evaluate soft tissue condition and understands the stresses placed on the tendon, may remove the dorsal blocking splint in therapy during the first few weeks to perform passive tenodesis exercises, with the dual goal of improving tendon glide and preventing secondary wrist stiffness. When zone 2 repair status does not pose an unacceptable risk, gentle MP extension by the therapist, combined with IP and wrist flexion, can prevent intrinsic tightness from developing.

Among the splints with dynamic flexion traction, there is a general trend toward incorporation of a palmar pulley to increase DIP and composite flexion in zone 2. There are two large differences, however, between protocols using dynamic traction, exemplified by the opposite approach of the May protocol, and that used by Thomes (personal communication, 1993). Both of these protocols, as discussed, involve a palmar pulley. May believes that better ultimate tendon glide is achieved through strapping in IP extension at night and inclusion of all four fingers in dynamic traction, even for a single finger flexor tendon injury. In contrast, Thomes advocates resting the tendon at its shortest length, in full flexion, and leaving the uninvolved fingers out of dynamic traction. The argument for strapping in extension is to prevent flexion contractures, which significantly limit ultimate TAM and thus limit the functional result. Thomes believes this danger is adequately countered by emphasizing active and passive IP extension exercise. Others avoid strapping in extension for fear that a patient may inadvertently flex the digits against the palmar strap and rupture or elongate the repair.

There are two completely opposite arguments for including all fingers in dynamic traction. One is that such protection will prevent inadvertent flexion of the adjacent finger by keeping it in a flexed position; because FDP tendons share a common muscle belly and FDS tendons may tend to act together in spite of having more distinct bellies, active flexion of an uninvolved finger may provoke a muscle contraction in the involved finger. This probably does occur, but is such a contraction harmful or helpful? If the patient is not actually attempting to make fists and use the hand for normal activities, such limited stress actually may increase the strength of the repair and improve excursion rather than cause deleterious repair deformation or rupture. Many therapists have observed that their best results are in those patients who "cheat" just a little on their programs with light and intermittent flexion. May[66] believes that when all fingers are included in traction, passive flexion is easier to attain; she also believes that with this technique, patients are more prone to involuntarily flex actively. Thomes (personal communication, 1993) and Evans (personal communication, 1993) believe that leaving the adjacent uninvolved fingers free is more likely to produce involuntary flexion and also allows patients to "cheat" in a beneficial manner.

Obviously, the choice between one protocol and another is a matter of assessment of the patient (i.e., compliance, ability to attend therapy regularly), the surgery (strength of suture, factors impairing healing or gliding), and the therapist (experience and skill). It is far better to take a conservative approach as an inexperienced therapist; the more experienced therapist tends to become more aggressive as he or she learns how to assess progress and consider all circumstances.

Early active mobilization

Rationale. Early mobilization protocols are applied to recently injured, edematous tendons with added bulk at the suture sites. The tendons are mobilized within surrounding sheath or other structures that are also edematous and that often do not provide a smooth gliding surface. In early passive mobilization programs, the tendon is pushed proximally; as has been pointed out, this is akin to pushing a piece of cooked linguine down a tube. The tendon is likely to fold or bunch up rather than glide. Early active mobilization involves active contraction of the injured flexor muscle, pulling the tendon proximally, and logically this should produce better glide. Certainly, the results of such programs so far have been very encouraging, supporting the observation made earlier that some of the best early passive mobilization results come when patients "cheat" and add a little active motion. Previously cited studies[22,45,46,92] found that passive IP flexion does provide passive FDP glide. However, one study found that while passive PIP flexion "mobilized the tendon with an efficiency of 90%" compared with active motion, the efficiency of DIP flexion was only 36%.[93] This could mean a poorer prognosis for zone 2 FDP injuries over the middle phalanx when managed with passive mobilization.

Kubota et al.,[51] investigating the breaking strength and increase in cellular activity produced by early mobilization and tension to tendon repairs, found that early mobilization without tension on the repair was not as effective as a combination of the two (such as would occur in active mobilization). We can conclude that active mobilization would produce a stronger repair with better excursion, especially at the level of the middle phalanx. Furthermore, if the tendon attains better excursion, this will increase the "milking" effect and thus enhance the nutrition through synovial diffusion.

Repair techniques have improved vastly in recent years: We now have stronger, less bulky sutures that glide much more easily. Clearly, whenever feasible, early active mobilization is preferable to early passive mobilization. The literature is growing rapidly and contains a diversity of postoperative approaches.* It can be difficult to sort out the relative value of one approach over another or to select the appropriate patient for early active mobilization. This should not stop the experienced therapist or surgeon from exploring this promising avenue, as long as we remember one caveat: Just as a piece of cooked linguine will bunch up if pushed through a tube, it will also tear if pulled too hard! Early active mobilization is only appropriate if both therapist and surgeon possess skill and experience in tendon management, if they communicate closely with each other, if the suture used was of adequate strength, and if the patient is highly reliable and understands the program thoroughly.

Protocols. Most early active mobilization protocols were developed for zone 2 injuries. Almost all protocols use a dorsal blocking splint like those used for early passive mobilization protocols. The Coventry protocol[48] uses a wrist splint only, but as published, it is not described in enough detail for the purposes of this chapter. Exercises and exercise frequency vary, but all protocols protect the tendon by limiting active flexion for the first 3 to 6 weeks. Following is a discussion of the distinctions between a few selected protocols. Some of these protocols undoubtedly have been updated since publication. Wherever possible, changes in protocols have been incorporated in the following material.

Active mobilization

Allen/Loma Linda. Although references have been made to early active mobilization for years, one of the first well-documented early active mobilization protocols using current surgical technique (an atraumatic, grasping suture with minimal bulk) was published in 1987 by Allen et al.[2] and has been used by their group for several years. That protocol involves splinting the wrist at 30 degrees and MP joints at 60 to 70 degrees with rubber band flexion traction. For the first 3 weeks (early stage), hourly gentle active flexion and extension exercises (10 repetitions) are performed in the splint with rubber band traction attached. At 3 weeks, the splint is replaced with a wrist cuff as used in the Duran protocol, and wrist AROM is initiated (intermediate stage). The program progresses to dowel gripping and unresisted weight well exercise at 5 weeks, with progressive resistive exercise as needed (late stage). However, if tendon gliding is poor (TAM less than 20 degrees at the DIP joint or less than 30 degrees at the PIP joint), this stage begins at 3 weeks. Patients begin light activities at 6 weeks.

Belfast and Sheffield. A group of related early active mobilization programs have been published by authors from the United Kingdom. Two similar original protocols[23,97] were modified subsequently by other authors.[10,27,42,118] Following is one of the more detailed of the recently published versions by Gratton.[42]

---

*References 2, 10, 12, 17, 23, 30, 42, 48, 53, 54, 58, 61, 83, 97, 98, 102, 104, 105, 118.

EARLY STAGE (FROM 0 TO 4 OR 6 WEEKS)

SPLINT. The postoperative cast maintains the wrist at 20-degree flexion and MP joints at 80 to 90 degrees of flexion, allowing full IP extension. The cast extends 2 cm beyond the fingertips to inhibit use of the hand. A radial plaster "wing" wraps around the wrist just proximal to the thumb to prevent the cast from migrating distally. On initiation of therapy, the postoperative dressing is debulked to allow exercise.

EXERCISE. For zone 3 injuries, therapy is initiated 24 hours after repair, but zone 2 repairs are allowed to rest until 48 hours after surgery to allow postoperative inflammation to subside. Exercises, performed every 4 hours within the splint, include all digits and consist of two repetitions each of full passive flexion, active flexion, and active extension. The first week's goal is full passive flexion, full active extension, and active flexion to 30 degrees at the PIP joint and 5 to 10 degrees at the DIP joint. Active flexion is expected to gradually increase over the following weeks, reaching 80 to 90 degrees at the PIP joint and 50 to 60 degrees at the DIP joint by the fourth week. In the presence of joint stiffness, passive exercises are increased to every 2 hours. A pen could be placed behind the proximal phalanx to block the MP in flexion for greater IP active extension if flexion contractures develop.

INTERMEDIATE STAGE (STARTING AT 4 TO 6 WEEKS)

SPLINT. The splint is discontinued at 4 weeks if tendon glide is poor (not achieving expected goals given above), at 5 weeks for most patients, or at 6 weeks for patients with unusually good tendon gliding (full fist developing within the first 2 weeks). Three weeks after splinting is discontinued, any residual flexion contractures are treated with finger-based dynamic extension splints.

EXERCISE. The only exercise specified for this period is protected passive IP extension (with the MP held in flexion) in the presence of flexion contractures. Presumably, patients continue active flexion and extension exercises, and the program progresses from this point as it would for any tendon protocol, adding light resistance first as warranted by difficulty attaining tendon glide, and then stepping up resistance (late stage) for strengthening. Small et al.[8] do speak of using blocking exercises to increase tendon glide at 6 weeks, and Cullen et al.[23] initiate progressive resistive

exercise and heavier hand use at 8 weeks, with full function expected by 12 weeks.

Active-hold/place-hold mobilization

Strickland/Cannon. Various authors[30,86,88,108] have attempted to quantify the force or muscle tension of the flexors during such motions as passive and active flexion and flexion against varying amounts of resistance. Each author has used a different method and arrived at different numbers. For their early mobilization protocol, Strickland[104,105] and Cannon[17] have assumed forces similar to those measured by Urbaniak et al.[108]: for FDP, 500 g for passive motion (Urbaniak, 200 to 300 g) and 1500 g for "light grip" (Urbaniak, 1500 g for flexion against moderate resistance). For FDS, the values would be 15% to 30% of the values for FDP. Their protocol assumes that some margin must be allowed for postoperative edema and other factors, and they rely on tensile strength of 2150 to 4300 g during the first 3 weeks with the Tajima repair plus a horizontal mattress (or an equivalent four-strand suture[105]) and a running lock epitendinous suture. They further decrease the load on the tendons by holding the wrist in extension and keeping the MP joints flexed for active flexion exercise. This is based on work by Savage,[86] which found that the force required for active digit flexion decreased when the wrist was held at 45 degrees of extension and the MP joints at 90 degrees of flexion.

This protocol is, properly speaking, an "active-hold" or "place-hold active mobilization" protocol. The digits are passively placed in flexion, and the patient then maintains the flexion with a gentle muscle contraction. Patients learn to use only minimal force by practicing with the uninjured hand and also use biofeedback to monitor the strength of contraction (less than 10 mV on a Cyborg model biofeedback unit).

EARLY STAGE (FROM 0 TO 4 WEEKS)

SPLINTS. Two different splints are used. A dorsal blocking splint is worn most of the time, with the wrist at 20 degrees of flexion and MP joints at 50 degrees (see Fig. 27-12). The exercise splint has a hinged wrist, allowing full wrist flexion, but wrist extension is limited to 30 degrees. Full digit flexion and full IP extension are allowed, but MP extension is limited to 60 degrees. The splint used for distal FPL repairs (zone T1) is similar but allows IP extension to only 25 degrees (as in the Evans zone 1 protocol) to

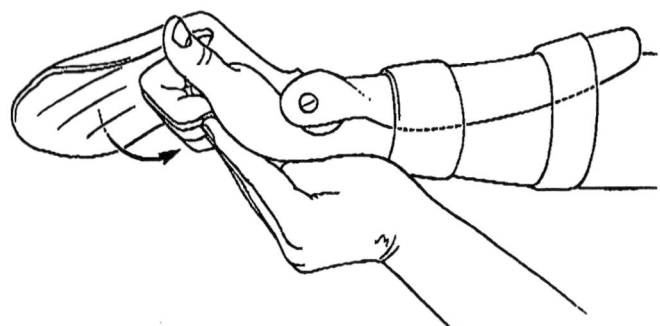

Fig. 27-18. The patient extends the wrist actively with simultaneous passive digit flexion. (From Cannon N: *Indiana Hand Center Newslett* 1:13, 1993.)

prevent repair deformation and problems with glide deep to the A$_2$ pulley.

EXERCISE. Every hour, patients perform the Strickland version of modified Duran exercises (15 repetitions of PROM to the PIP and DIP joints and the entire digit) in the dorsal blocking splint, followed by 25 repetitions of place-hold digit flexion in the tenodesis splint. The patient extends the wrist actively with simultaneous passive digit flexion (Fig. 27-18) and actively maintains digit flexion for 5 seconds (Fig. 27-19). The patient then relaxes and allows the

wrist to flex and digits to extend within the limits of the splint (Fig. 27-20).

INTERMEDIATE STAGE (FROM 4 WEEKS TO 7 OR 8 WEEKS)

SPLINT. Tenodesis splint is discontinued. Patient still wears dorsal blocking splint except for tenodesis exercises.

EXERCISE. The tenodesis exercises (Fig. 27-21) continue every 2 hours with 25 repetitions followed by 25 repetitions of active flexion and extension exercise for wrist and digits, avoiding simultaneous wrist and digit extension. FDS gliding also may be added. At 5 to 6 weeks, blocking and

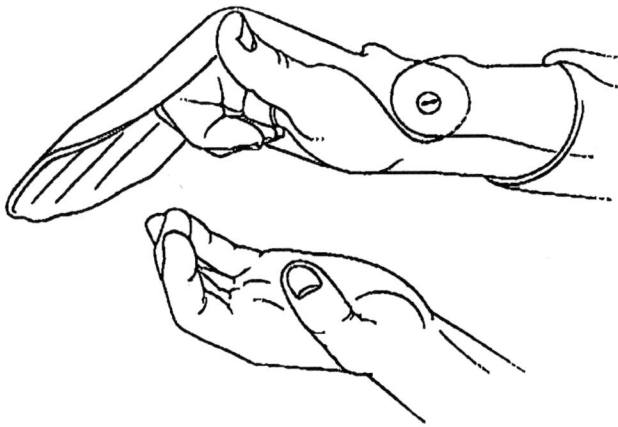

Fig. 27-19. The patient maintains digit flexion with a gentle active muscle contraction. (From Cannon N: *Indiana Hand Center Newslett* 1:13, 1993.)

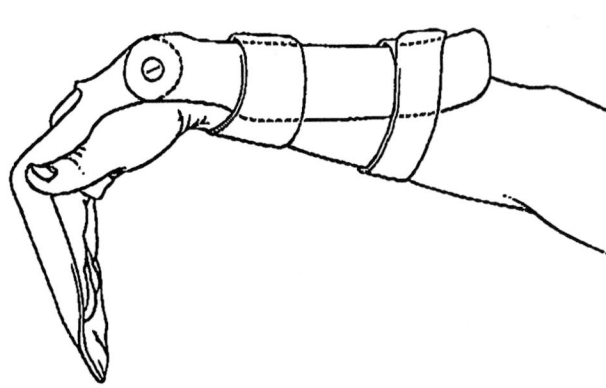

Fig. 27-20. The wrist is allowed to relax into flexion with simultaneous digit extension (limited to 60 degrees at the metacarpophalangeal joints). (From Cannon N: *Indiana Hand Center Newslett* 1:13, 1993.)

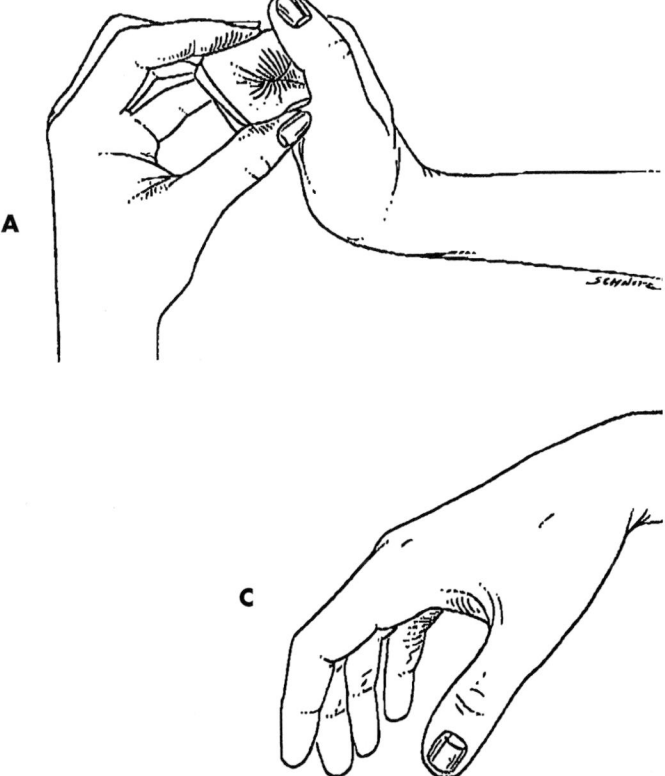

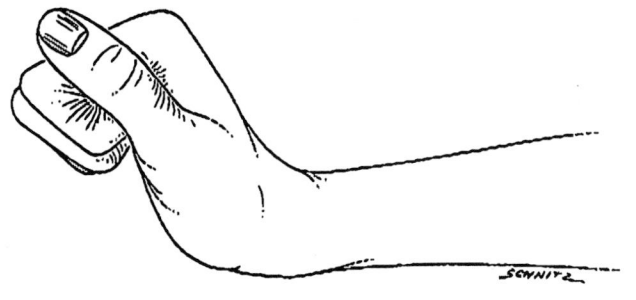

Fig. 27-21. The exercise splint is discontinued at 4 weeks, but the patient continues tenodesis exercises. **A,** The wrist is extended, with passive digit flexion, maintained actively **(B).** **C,** The patient then allows the wrist to relax into flexion with simultaneous digit extension. (From Cannon N: *Indiana Hand Center Newslett* 1:13, 1993.)

hook fists may be added if needed to improve tendon gliding.

LATE STAGE (STARTING AT 7 TO 8 WEEKS)

SPLINT. The splint is discontinued.

EXERCISE. Progressive resistive exercise is initiated. The patient gradually resumes activities of daily living, with no restrictions by 14 weeks. FPL is moved more aggressively than digit flexors (putty exercises are initiated by 7 weeks), and flexors to the small finger are moved the least aggressively, in the light of the authors' clinical observation that repairs of these tendons are the most prone to deformation and rupture.

Silfverskiöld and May.[91] These authors have added an active-hold component to their previously published early passive mobilization protocol (see the four-finger protocol of May et al.[66] discussed previously in Comparative Studies) in patients whose zone 2 FDP tendons were repaired with a modified Kessler core suture and a new epitenon suture (the "cross-stitch.") The wrist is splinted in neutral instead of 30 to 45 degrees of flexion, but the splint is otherwise identical to the early passive mobilization protocol (MP joints in 50 to 70 degrees flexion and splint extending only to the PIP joints). Exercises are similar to those outlined for the four-finger program, but after using the uninvolved hand to push the fingers of the involved hand into full flexion, the patient uses an active muscle contraction to maintain flexion of the involved fingers for 2 to 3 seconds. The program is progressed in the same manner as the four-finger protocol. In a prospective clinical study of 47 patients with 56 injured fingers, the authors demonstrated promising results.

Evans and Thompson.[30] Evans and Thompson have examined the biomechanical aspects of early active-hold mobilization using the concept of "minimal active muscle-tendon tension" (MAMTT), "the minimal tension required to overcome the viscoelastic resistance of the antagonistic muscle-tendon unit. They calculated the drag encountered by each flexor tendon, the force necessary to overcome that drag, and the force normally exerted by the finger in flexion in various positions. Two central findings were that flexion forces increase dramatically at the end of the flexion range (in a full fist) and when digit flexion is combined with wrist flexion. The authors then surveyed currently used tendon repair sutures and designated guidelines for early place-hold mobilization of the tendon with any suture used in combination with an epitenon running suture. They presented a retrospective review of 165 tendons (both flexor and extensor tendons) treated with their guidelines.

Note that this is not a protocol, but a set of guidelines to be used by a therapist in planning treatment. The therapist must know the strength of the suture, recognize any unusual factors such as severe edema, and decide whether this approach is appropriate. He or she must consider the anticipated potential drop in tensile strength of the repair between day 5 and day 15 and adapt the program accordingly.

The MAMTT exercises are performed only under a therapist's supervision, while the patient follows an early passive mobilization program at home (which protocol is not specified by the authors; a dorsal blocking splint and rubber band traction into flexion are used). For MAMTT exercise, the splint is removed. The wrist is passively placed in 20-degree extension and the finger passively flexed to 83 degrees at the MP joint, 75 degrees at the PIP joint, and 40 degrees at the DIP joint. The patient is then asked to maintain the position with as gentle a muscle contraction as possible. The force of the muscle contraction is measured with a small (less than 150 g) Haldex pinch gauge. A loop of string passes perpendicularly around the gauge arm of the pinch meter and around the finger tip. The patient flexes the finger with a force of 50 g or less.

Unlike the Strickland/Cannon protocol, the Evans and Thompson guidelines suggest that few patients can perform this program at home. However, Evans (personal communication, 1993) states that she has patients perform active-hold exercises with the uninvolved fingers at home, thus probably eliciting some active muscle-tendon tension in the involved fingers.

Timing initiation of early active mobilization. Based on studies indicating that early motion increases repair strength,[33,44,51] most published protocols start motion at 24 to 48 hours after surgery. Halikis et al.[43] have recently published a study comparing work of flexion (i.e., resistance to flexion imposed by surrounding edematous tissues) in immobilized repairs to those mobilized immediately, those mobilized at 3 days, and those mobilized at 5 days. They found that the work of flexion increased significantly in tendons mobilized immediately, whereas work of flexion increased the least for tendons initiating active mobilization at 3 days. This calls into question the assumption that immediate mobilization is crucial to a good result.

Our preferred approach

We prefer to start therapy with postoperative splint application as soon as possible after surgery. We splint the wrist in neutral and the MP joints at 40 degrees and strap IP joints in extension between exercises. If we are using active mobilization, we will delay initiation until 2 to 4 days after surgery to allow inflammation to subside somewhat and reduce the work of flexion. We always precede active flexion with edema control measures and passive flexion to reduce tissue resistance, and we always integrate a modified Duran approach with active mobilization. For example, patients may begin with a modified Duran program at home and active flexion only in therapy, with active flexion added to the home program only when we are sure the patient is able to follow instructions safely. We are much more cautious using early active mobilization with little finger injuries because in our experience they are more likely to rupture.

We start in therapy with assisted or place-hold flexion, using synergistic wrist motion/tenodesis. If the patient does not understand the concept of tenodesis or appears to be flexing with excessive force, the following technique may be helpful. The patient sits with elbow on the table, wrist relaxed forward into flexion. The patient is instructed to extend the wrist while keeping the fingers relaxed. If he or she is able to do this, the fingers will automatically assume a midflexion position. If instead the patient extends his or her fingers along with the wrist, the patient is asked to extend the wrist while touching the fingers to the thumb or grasping a light object such as a pencil held by the therapist. Often, a functional grasp is much easier for an apprehensive patient to comprehend than a structured exercise. At home, active or place-hold flexion exercises may be performed either with the splint on (the wrist is at neutral in the splint) or with the splint removed or replaced with a simple dorsal wrist splint limiting wrist extension to 20 degrees. Generally, the patient performs 10 repetitions of modified Duran exercises hourly, and four to six times a day performs 10 repetitions of passive flexion followed by 3 to 5 repetitions of active flexion. The number of repetitions and frequency of exercise must be tailored to the patient.

Patients are gradually weaned out of the splint, beginning at 3 to 5 weeks, depending on the quality of motion and the patient's reliability. They begin using their injured hands at 4 to 6 weeks for very light functional prehension (e.g., assisting the uninjured hand to carry light objects, turning the pages of a book, playing cards, eating light finger foods such as popcorn). This should be relatively easy because these patients have achieved good excursion through early active mobilization. When possible, functional motions are used in place of exercise: "piano playing" on the tabletop, towel walking, paper crumpling, handling dice, grasping handfuls of packing "popcorn" or large beans, handling light objects of varying size and shape. As needed, tendon gliding exercises and blocking can be added. Any PIP flexion contractures or flexor tightness should be addressed early, by changing nighttime splinting (at 3 to 5 weeks) to serial static extension or by using a PIP cylinder cast.

There are many ways to mobilize tendons actively in the first few weeks. Many hand therapists use a combination of the published protocols. Therapists should read the literature and make decisions based on a detailed understanding not only of the protocols but also of their rationales, indications, and relative effectiveness. Of particular importance is that some studies were performed with a patient population that was hospitalized initially and could be seen by the therapist several times a day in the first few days.

A special case: multiple tendon and nerve lacerations in zone 5

Laceration of multiple flexor tendons in zone 5 presents a special problem in management. As noted earlier, in zone 5 (from proximal edge of carpal tunnel to the musculotendinous junction) the flexor tendons lie in close proximity both to each other and to major nerves (median and ulnar) and arteries (radial and ulnar). This type of injury has been labeled "spaghetti wrist," "suicide wrist," and "full house syndrome" by various authors.* As with all flexor tendon injuries besides those in zone 2, there is little in the literature to indicate the best postoperative management. However, to design the appropriate program, we can draw on experience, a good understanding of how the involved structures heal, and both specific and related literature.

The psychosocial ramifications of such injuries are significant, but luckily not insurmountable. A certain percentage of these injuries result from suicide attempts, so one might expect a poor prognosis because of psychologic and emotional issues. However, some authors have found favorable results and improved psychologic status after such injuries. Many sustain these injuries on broken glass, often when an angry young man punches his fist through a glass window. Again, the immaturity and poor impulse control of the patient would seem to predict compromised results, but youth is to the patient's advantage, with some authors noting better results in younger patients.

These patients, correctly handled, generally attain satisfactory or full-digit flexion because the extrasynovial tendons can produce full flexion with excursion limited by relatively heavy adhesions to the overlying skin and surrounding tissues. Independent FDS glide is difficult to achieve but has not been found to impair function. In fact, recent research indicates that in the normal hand, FDS may not glide as independently as one might assume. Wrist and digit extension are commonly limited to some extent by flexor adhesions. There may be limitations in isolated wrist extension as well as in composite wrist and digit extension. In most cases, either passive extension can be regained over time through diligent treatment, or the patient finds that the lack of extension is not a functional impairment.

A greater problem is reinnervation. Both sensory and intrinsic muscle reinnervation are needed for a full functional recovery. One small study suggests that injuries to the ulnar nerve may have a poorer prognosis than injuries to the median nerve.[116] In any case, in addition to impaired flexor tendon function, these patients lack part or all of their intrinsic muscle function (depending on which nerve is injured) as well as median and/or ulnar nerve sensibility. Unless and until reinnervation occurs, patients may injure their insensate fingers when attempting to use their hands normally and may have difficulty with prehension and strong grip because of lack of normal sensory feedback. They will lack full grip strength and pinch strength in the absence of intrinsic muscle power and will miss the control and balance afforded by the intrinsics for fine dexterity. If not carefully managed, over time, they may develop deformities (e.g., "claw hand" or "ape hand," PIP flexion contractures, thumb adduction contracture) that are both unattractive and an impediment to function.

*References 47, 82, 99, 114, 116, 118.

The literature includes both early passive mobilization* and early active mobilization[118] approaches. As always, the approach should be selected according to the individual patient characteristics, with preference given to early mobilization of some sort. All of the published protocols keep the wrist in some flexion, but as with injuries at other levels, the recent trend is toward less wrist flexion. Too much wrist flexion can make it difficult to regain extension with an injury so close to the wrist and to the flexor retinaculum, a prime source for flexor adhesions.

Our preference is to protect the patient with the wrist as close to a neutral position as possible and MP joints flexed about 40 degrees. Holding the MP joints in flexion might encourage some intrinsic tightness, which is a bonus when a long wait for return of nerve function is expected. Nerves repaired under tension must be very carefully protected with more wrist flexion.

Early management is similar to that for injuries in other zones, with the following special considerations. As soon as possible after active mobilization is initiated, the program should include differential tendon gliding. Because passive extension is so often a problem, these patients may need nighttime serial static extension splinting (see Fig. 27-7) as early as 4 weeks after repair and dynamic extension splinting during the day beginning within the following week. The flexor tightness often limits the "clawing" produced by intrinsic palsies, but if not, an "anticlaw" splint of some sort (preventing MP hyperextension but allowing full wrist and finger flexion) may be needed to prevent development of a full-fledged claw deformity. The therapist also may opt to forgo intrinsic stretch exercises in the protective stage so that some intrinsic tightness will be allowed to develop, as noted previously.

SUMMARY

This chapter reviews the fundamentals of tendon management and explores a range of management approaches. No single source can prepare the clinician to treat the repaired flexor tendon. Readers are urged to read both the original references cited in the discussion of each protocol and the research that validates each approach.

As we study suture strength and gliding properties, measure muscle-tendon force, gather data, and choose the protocol based on scientific principles, we must not lose sight of the most important variable of all: the patient. After all, our job is patient care. Without a motivated patient who is able to participate fully in his or her rehabilitation, all our efforts will be in vain. So understanding is really the key to effective postoperative management of the flexor tendon— understanding the scientific basis for our intervention and understanding the patient.

*References 47, 82, 84, 99, 114, 116.

REFERENCES

1. Abrahamsson SO, Lundborg G, Lohmander LS: Tendon healing in vivo: an experimental model, *Scand J Plast Reconstr Surg Hand Surg* 23:199, 1989.
2. Allen BN, et al: Ruptured flexor tendon tenorrhaphies in zone II: repair and rehabilitation, *J Hand Surg* 12A:18, 1987.
3. Amadio PC, Hunter JM: Prognostic factors in flexor tendon surgery in zone 2. In Hunter JM, Schneider LH, Mackin EM, editors: *Tendon surgery in the hand,* St Louis, 1987, Mosby.
4. Amadio P, Jaeger S, Hunter J: Nutritional aspects of tendon healing. In Hunter J, et al, editors: *Rehabilitation of the hand,* ed 3, St Louis, 1990, Mosby.
5. American Society for Surgery of the Hand (ASSH): *Clinical Assessment Committee Report,* 1976, American Society for Surgery of the Hand.
6. Aoki M, et al: Canine cadaveric study of flexor tendon repair using tendon splint: tensile strength and the work of flexion, *Nippon Seikeigeka Gakkai Zasshi* 69:332, 1995.
7. Aoki M, et al: Effect of suture knots on tensile strength of repaired canine flexor tendons, *J Hand Surg* 20B:72, 1995.
8. Aoki M, et al: Work of flexion after flexor tendon repair according to the placement of sutures, *Clin Orthop* Nov:205, 1995.
9. Aoki M, et al: Work of flexion after tendon repair with various suture methods. A human cadaveric study, *J Hand Surg* 20B:310, 1995.
10. Bainbridge LC, et al: A comparison of post-operative mobilization of flexor tendon repairs with "passive flexion-active extension" and "controlled active motion" techniques, *J Hand Surg* 19B:517, 1994.
11. Bishop AT, Cooney WP, Wood MB: Treatment of partial flexor tendon lacerations: the effect of tenorrhaphy and early protected mobilization, *J Trauma* 26:301, 1986.
12. Boulas HJ, Strickland JW: Strength and functional recovery following repair of flexor digitorum superficialis in zone 2, *J Hand Surg* 18B:22, 1993.
13. Brand PW: *Clinical mechanics of the hand,* St Louis, 1985, Mosby.
14. Brown CP, McGrouther DA: The excursion of the tendon of flexor pollicis longus and its relation to dynamic splintage, *J Hand Surg* 9A:787, 1984.
15. Buck-Gramcko D, Dietrich FE, Gogge S: Evaluation criteria in follow-up studies of flexor tendon therapy, *Handchirurgie* 8:65, 1976.
16. Burge PD, Brown M: Elastic band mobilisation after flexor tendon repair; splint design and risk of flexion contracture, *J Hand Surg* 15B:443, 1990.
17. Cannon N: Post flexor tendon repair motion protocol, *Indiana Hand Center Newslett* 1:13, 1993.
18. Chow J, et al: A combined regimen of controlled motion following flexor tendon repair in "no man's land," *Plast Reconstr Surg* 79:447, 1987.
19. Chow J, et al: A splint for controlled active motion after flexor tendon repair: design, mechanical testing and preliminary clinical results, *J Hand Surg* 15A:645, 1990.
20. Cifaldi Collins D, Schwarze L: Early progressive resistance following immobilization of flexor tendon repairs, *J Hand Ther* 4:111, 1991.
21. Citron ND, Forster A: Dynamic splinting following flexor tendon repair, *J Hand Surg* 12B:96, 1987.
22. Cooney WP, Lin GT, An K-N: Improved tendon excursion following flexor tendon repair, *J Hand Ther* 2:102, 1989.
23. Cullen KW, et al: Flexor tendon repair in zone 2 followed by controlled active mobilisation, *J Hand Surg* 14B:392, 1989.
24. Dovelle S, Heeter P: The Washington regimen: rehabilitation of the hand following flexor tendon injuries, *Phys Ther* 69:1034, 1989.
25. Duran R, Houser R: Controlled passive motion following flexor tendon repair in zones 2 and 3, *AAOS symposium on tendon surgery in the hand,* St Louis, 1975, Mosby.

26. Duran R, et al: Management of flexor tendon lacerations in zone 2 using controlled passive motion postoperatively. In Hunter J, et al, editors: *Rehabilitation of the hand,* ed 3, St Louis, 1990, Mosby.

27. Elliot D, et al: The rupture rate of acute flexor tendon repairs mobilized by the controlled active motion regimen, *J Hand Surg* 19B:607, 1994.

28. Evans R: Management of the healing tendon: what must we question? *J Hand Ther* 2:61, 1989.

29. Evans R: A study of the zone I flexor tendon injury and implications for treatment, *J Hand Ther* 3:133, 1990.

30. Evans RB, Thompson DE: The application of force to the healing tendon, *J Hand Ther* 6:266, 1993.

31. Feehan LM, Beauchene JG: Early tensile properties of healing chicken flexor tendons: early controlled passive motion versus postoperative immobilization, *J Hand Surg* 15A:63, 1990.

32. Gelberman RH, Manske PR: Factors influencing flexor tendon adhesions, *Hand Clin* 1:35, 1985.

33. Gelberman RH, Woo SL-Y: The physiological basis for application of controlled stress in the rehabilitation of flexor tendon injuries, *J Hand Ther* 2:66, 1989.

34. Gelberman RH, et al: The influence of protected passive mobilization on the healing of flexor tendons: a biochemical and microangiographic study, *Hand* 13:120, 1981.

35. Gelberman RH, et al: Effects of early intermittent passive mobilization on healing canine flexor tendons, *J Hand Surg* 7A:170, 1982.

36. Gelberman RH, et al: The early stages of flexor tendon healing: a morphologic study of the first fourteen days, *J Hand Surg* 10A:776, 1985.

37. Gelberman RH, et al: Flexor tendon repair, *J Orthop Res* 4:119, 1986.

38. Gelberman RH, et al: Influences of flexor sheath continuity and early motion on tendon healing in dogs., *J Hand Surg* 15A:69, 1990.

39. Gelberman RH, et al: Fibroblast chemotaxis after tendon repair, *J Hand Surg* 16A:686, 1991.

40. Gelberman RH, et al: Healing of digital flexor tendons: importance of the interval from injury to repair: a biomechanical, biochemical, and morphological study in dogs, *J Bone Joint Surg* 73A:66, 1991.

41. Gelberman RH, et al: Influences of the protected passive mobilization interval on flexor tendon healing: a prospective randomized clinical study, *Clin Orthop* Mar:189, 1991.

42. Gratton P: Early active mobilization after flexor tendon repairs, *J Hand Ther* 6:285, 1993.

43. Halikis MN, et al: Effect of immobilization, immediate mobilization, and delayed mobilization on the resistance to digital flexion using a tendon injury model, *J Hand Surg* 22A:464, 1997.

44. Hitchcock TF, et al: The effect of immediate constrained digital motion on the strength of flexor tendon repairs in chickens, *J Hand Surg* 12A:590, 1987.

45. Horibe S, et al: Excursion of the flexor digitorum profundus tendon: a kinematic study of the human and canine digits, *J Orthopaed Res* 8:167, 1990.

46. Horii E, et al: Comparative flexor tendon excursion after passive mobilization: an in vitro study, *J Hand Surg* 17A:559, 1992.

47. Hudson DA, de Jager LT: The spaghetti wrist. Simultaneous laceration of the median and ulnar nerves with flexor tendons at the wrist, *J Hand Surg* 18B:171, 1993.

48. Kitsis CK, et al: Controlled active motion following primary flexor tendon repair: a prospective study over 9 years, *J Hand Surg* 23B:344, 1998.

49. Kleinert HE, Kutz JE, Cohen MJ: Primary repair of zone 2 flexor tendon lacerations. In *AAOS symposium on tendon surgery in the hand,* St Louis, 1975, Mosby.

50. Kleinert HE, et al: Primary repair of lacerated flexor tendons in no-man's-land, *J Bone Joint Surg* 49A:577, 1967.

51. Kubota H, et al: Effect of motion and tension on injured flexor tendons in chickens, *J Hand Surg* 21A:456, 1996.

52. Kubota H, et al: Mechanical properties of various circumferential tendon suture techniques, *J Hand Surg* 21B:474, 1996.

53. Lee H: Double loop locking suture: a technique of tendon repair for early active mobilization. Part I, *J Hand Surg* 15A:945, 1990.

54. Lee H: Double loop locking suture: a technique of tendon repair for early active mobilization. Part II, *J Hand Surg* 15A:953, 1990.

55. Lin GT, et al: Biomechanical studies of running suture for flexor tendon repair in dogs, *J Hand Surg* 13A:553, 1988.

56. Lister GD, et al: Primary flexor tendon repair followed by immediate controlled mobilization, *J Hand Surg* 2A:441, 1977.

57. Lundborg G, Rank F, Heinau B: Intrinsic tendon healing: a new experimental model, *Scand J Plast Reconstr Surg* 19:113, 1985.

58. MacMillan M, Sheppard JE, Dell PC: An experimental flexor tendon repair in zone II that allows immediate postoperative mobilization, *J Hand Surg* 12A:582, 1987.

59. Manske PR: Flexor tendon healing, *J Hand Surg* 13B:237, 1988.

60. Manske PR, et al: Intrinsic restoration of the flexor tendon surface in the nonhuman primate, *J Hand Surg* 10A:632, 1985.

61. Marin Braun F, et al: Reparation du flechisseur profond et du long flechisseur du pouce par la "fixation en rappel." Resultats d'une serie de soixante-dix-sept cas, *Annales de chirurgie de la Main et du Membre Superieur* 10:13, 1991.

62. Mashadi ZB, Amis AA: The effect of locking loops on the strength of tendon repair, *J Hand Surg* 16B:35, 1991.

63. Mashadi ZB, Amis AA: Strength of the suture in the epitenon and within the tendon fibres: development of stronger peripheral suture technique, *J Hand Surg* 17B:172, 1992.

64. Mason J, Allen H: The rate of healing of tendons: an experimental study of tensile strength, *Ann Surg* 113:424, 1941.

65. Matthews P, Richards H: Factors in the adherence of flexor tendons after repair. An experimental study in the rabbit, *J Bone Joint Surg* 58B:230, 1976.

66. May EJ, Silfverskiold KL, Sollerman CJ: Controlled mobilization after flexor tendon repair in zone II: a prospective comparison of three methods, *J Hand Surg* 17A:942, 1992.

67. May EJ, Silfverskiold KL, Sollerman CJ: The correlation between controlled range of motion with dynamic traction and results after flexor tendon repair in zone II, *J Hand Surg* 17A:1133, 1992.

68. McCarthy DM, et al: Effect of partial laceration on the structural properties of the canine FDP tendon: an in vitro study, *J Hand Surg* 20A:795, 1995.

69. McGeorge DD, Stilwell JH: Partial flexor tendon injuries: to repair or not, *J Hand Surg* 17B:176, 1992.

70. McGrouther DA, Ahmed M: Flexor tendon excursions in "no man's land," *Hand* 13:129, 1981.

71. Mitsionis G, et al: Feasibility of partial A2 and A4 pulley excision: effect on finger flexor tendon biomechanics, *J Hand Surg* 24A:310, 1999.

72. Peacock EE: Biological principles in the healing of long tendons, *Surg Clin North Am* 45:2, 1965.

73. Peterson WW, Manske PR, Lesker PA: The effect of flexor sheath integrity on nutrient uptake by chicken flexor tendons, *Clin Orthop* Dec:259, 1985.

74. Peterson WW, Manske PR, Lesker PA: The effect of flexor sheath integrity on nutrient uptake by primate flexor tendons, *J Hand Surg* 11A:413, 1986.

75. Peterson WW, et al: Effect of pulley excision on flexor tendon biomechanics, *J Orthop Res* 4:96, 1986.

76. Peterson WW, et al: Effect of flexor sheath integrity on tendon gliding: a biomechanical and histologic study, *J Orthop Res* 4:458, 1986.

77. Potenza AD: Tendon healing within the flexor digital sheath in the dog: an experimental study, *J Bone Joint Surg* 44A:49, 1962.

78. Potenza AD: Critical evaluation of flexor tendon healing and adhesion formation within artificial digital sheaths. An experimental study, *J Bone Joint Surg* 45A:1217, 1963.

79. Potenza AD: Prevention of adhesions to healing digital flexor tendons, *JAMA* 187:99, 1964.

80. Pruitt DL, Aoki M, Manske PR: Effect of suture knot location on tensile strength after flexor tendon repair, *J Hand Surg* 21A:969, 1996.

81. Pruitt DL, Manske PR, Fink B: Cyclic stress analysis of flexor tendon repair, *J Hand Surg* 16A:701, 1991.

82. Puckett CL, Meyer VH: Results of treatment of extensive volar wrist lacerations: the spaghetti wrist, *Plast Reconstr Surg* 75:714, 1985.

83. Riaz M, et al: Long term outcome of early active mobilization following flexor tendon repair in zone 2, *J Hand Surg* 24B:157, 1999.

84. Rogers GD, et al: Simultaneous laceration of the median and ulnar nerves with flexor tendons at the wrist, *J Hand Surg* 15A:990, 1990.

85. Rosenblum N, Robinson S: Advances in flexor and extensor tendon management, *Clin Phys Ther* 17:17, 1986.

86. Savage R: The influence of wrist position on the minimum force required for active movement of the interphalangeal joints, *J Hand Surg* 13B:262, 1988.

87. Schepel S J: Intrinsic healing of flexor tendons in primates. In Hunter JM, Schneider LH, Mackin EJ, editors: *Tendon surgery in the hand,* St Louis, 1987, Mosby.

88. Schuind F, et al: Flexor tendon forces: in vivo measurements, *J Hand Surg* 17A:291, 1992.

89. Seyfer AE, Bolger WE: Effects of unrestricted motion on healing: a study of posttraumatic adhesions in primate tendons, *Plast Reconstr Surg* 83:122, 1989.

90. Silfverskiöld KL, Andersson CH: Two new methods of tendon repair: an in vitro evaluation of tensile strength and gap formation, *J Hand Surg* 18A:58, 1993.

91. Silfverskiöld KL, May EJ: Flexor tendon repair in zone II with a new suture technique and an early mobilization program combining passive and active flexion, *J Hand Surg* 19A:53, 1994.

92. Silfverskiöld KL, May EJ, Oden A: Factors affecting results after flexor tendon repair in zone II: a multivariate prospective analysis, *J Hand Surg* 18A:654, 1993.

93. Silfverskiöld KL, May EJ, Tornvall AH: Flexor digitorum profundus tendon excursions during controlled motion after flexor tendon repair in zone II: a prospective clinical study, *J Hand Surg* 17A:122, 1992.

94. Silfverskiöld KL, May EJ, Tornvall AH: Gap formation during controlled motion after flexor tendon repair in zone II: a prospective clinical study, *J Hand Surg* 17A:539, 1992.

95. Silfverskiöld KL, May EJ, Tornvall AH: Tendon excursions after flexor tendon repair in zone. II: results with a new controlled-motion program, *J Hand Surg* 18A:403, 1993.

96. Slattery P, McGrouther D: A modified Kleinert controlled mobilization splint following flexor tendon repair, *J Hand Surg* 9B:34, 1984.

97. Small JO, Brennen MD, Colville J: Early active mobilisation following flexor tendon repair in zone 2, *J Hand Surg* 14B:383, 1989.

98. Steelman P: Treatment of flexor tendon injuries: therapist's commentary, *J Hand Ther* 12:149, 1999.

99. Stefanich RJ, et al: Flexor tendon lacerations in zone V, *J Hand Surg* 17A:284, 1992.

100. Stegink Janson C, Minerbo G: A comparison between early dynamically controlled mobilization and immobilization after flexor tendon repair in zone 2 of the hand, *J Hand Ther* 3:20, 1990.

101. Stewart KM: Tendon injuries. In Stanley BG, Tribuzi SM, editors: *Concepts in hand rehabilitation,* Philadelphia, 1992, FA Davis.

102. Stewart Pettengill K: Postoperative therapy concepts in management of tendon injuries: early mobilization. In Hunter JM, Schneider LH, Mackin EJ, editors: *Tendon and nerve surgery in the hand: a third decade,* St Louis, 1997, Mosby.

103. Strickland JW: Flexor tendon injuries. Part 5. Flexor tenolysis, rehabilitation and results, *Orthop Rev* 16:137, 1987.

104. Strickland JW: Flexor tendon injuries: I. Foundations of treatment, *J Am Acad Orthopaedic Surg* 3:44, 1995.

105. Strickland JW: Flexor tendon injuries: II. Operative technique, *J Am Acad Orthopaedic Surg* 3:55, 1995.

106. Strickland JW, Glogovac SV: Digital function following flexor tendon repair in zone 2: a comparison study of immobilization and controlled passive motion, *J Hand Surg* 5A:537, 1980.

107. Tottenham VM, Wilton-Bennett K, Jeffrey J: Effects of delayed therapeutic intervention following zone II flexor tendon repair, *J Hand Ther* 8:23, 1995.

108. Urbaniak JR, Cahill JD, Mortenson RA: Tendon suturing methods: analysis of tensile strengths, *AAOS symposium on tendon surgery in the hand,* St Louis, 1975, Mosby.

109. van Adrichem LNA, et al: The acute effect of cigarette smoking on the microcirculation of a replanted digit, *J Hand Surg* 17A:230, 1992.

110. van Alphen JC, Oepkes CT, Bos KE: Activity of the extrinsic finger flexors during mobilization in the Kleinert splint, *J Hand Surg* 21A:77, 1996.

111. Wade PJ, Wetherell RG, Amis AA: Flexor tendon repair: significant gain in strength from the Halsted peripheral suture technique, *J Hand Surg* 14B:232, 1989.

112. Weber ER: Nutritional pathways for flexor tendons in the digital theca. In Hunter JM, Schneider LH, Mackin EJ, editors: *Tendon surgery in the hand,* St Louis, 1987, Mosby.

113. Wehbe MA, Hunter JM: Flexor tendon gliding in the hand. II: differential gliding, *J Hand Surg* 10A:575, 1985.

114. Weinzweig N, et al: "Spaghetti wrist": management and results [published erratum appears in *Plast Reconstr Surg* Aug, 1998 following table of contents], *Plast Reconstr Surg* 102:96, 1998.

115. Werntz J, et al: A new dynamic splint for postoperative treatment of flexor tendon injury, *J Hand Surg* 14:559, 1989.

116. Widgerow AD: Full-house/spaghetti wrist injuries: analysis of results, *S Afr J Surg* 28:6, 1990.

117. Winters SC, et al: The effects of multiple-strand suture methods on the strength and excursion of repaired intrasynovial flexor tendons: a biomechanical study in dogs, *J Hand Surg* 23A:97, 1998.

118. Yii NW, Urban M, Elliot D: A prospective study of flexor tendon repair in zone 5, *J Hand Surg* 23B:642, 1998.

Chapter 28

TENOLYSIS: DYNAMIC APPROACH TO SURGERY AND THERAPY

Lawrence H. Schneider
Sheri B. Feldscher

The surgical release of nongliding adhesions that form along the surface of a tendon after injury or repair is a useful procedure in the salvage of tendon function.* Tendon adhesions occur whenever the surface of a tendon is damaged either through the injury itself, be it laceration or crush, or by surgical manipulation.[22,41] At any point on the surface of a tendon where violation occurs, an adhesion will form in the healing period.[25,32] Whenever these adhesions cannot be mobilized by therapy techniques, tenolysis should be considered. This procedure is as demanding as tendon repair itself and cannot be undertaken lightly. It represents another surgical onslaught in an area of previous trauma and surgery. If the procedure is unsuccessful, the patient's hand may show no improvement or may even be worse. The risk of further decreasing the circulatory supply and innervation to an already deprived finger is a real one. Rupture of the lysed tendon, a disastrous complication, is another hazard of tenolysis.

PREOPERATIVE EVALUATION FOR TENOLYSIS

Patient selection is a vital aspect in successful tenolysis. The patient should have been in an adequate therapy program combining active motion techniques with gentle passive motion exercises for approximately 3 months after tendon repair or injury, and progress should be at a standstill. This time interval allows for wound healing and maturation while the patient is trying to elongate the adhesions that have formed.[55] The patient's level of cooperation in a postoper-

ative program also can be evaluated during this interval. A patient unable to wholly commit himself or herself to the program should be rejected for lysis.

At 3 months[55] if the range of movement attained is regarded by patient and surgeon as inadequate, discussion is entered into regarding the risks and rewards of lysis in view of the functional demands and needs of the patient. A realistic picture must be drawn. A cold, insensate finger will not be improved even if a full range of motion (ROM) could be regained. The decision to perform tenolysis is often subjective. For example, 50% of a normal ROM may be reasonable to accept, especially in an aged person, a person with functional demand, or one who has concurrent joint surface injury or degenerative arthritis. The presence of adequate skin cover is another prerequisite for this surgery. Ideally, the patient who would be best suited would be one whose repaired tendon had a localized adhesion that limited gliding. On release, a full ROM is regained. However, this is the uncommon situation. More commonly, the adhesions involve a long segment of the involved tendon and require extensive exposure for release. Joint contracture, which can occur secondary to the tendon fixation, also may require simultaneous correction and thus further complicates the surgery and the patient's recovery.[49]

SURGICAL TECHNIQUE

After the patient meets the criteria established, lysis is performed under local anesthesia to allow full evaluation during the procedure itself.[18] It is through this technique that one can determine whether release of the offending tendon

*References 8, 17, 20, 36, 37, 42, 44, 50, 54.

457

system adhesions is adequate to restore motion or the patient also requires surgical release of the joints. At times it is necessary to turn the hand over and release the opposing tendon system also. This situation is not uncommon in crushing injuries, especially if there are associated phalangeal fractures. All patients for flexor lysis have been prepared for the possibility of staged tendon reconstruction if a reasonable flexor mechanism cannot be salvaged.[16,39]

The local anesthesia used is 1% or 2% lidocaine, infiltrated locally in the skin or as a digital block at the metacarpal level. Nerve blocks at the wrist also can be used, but with resultant paralysis of the intrinsic muscles, some benefits of this technique are sacrificed.

The administration of intravenous medication relieves anxiety and alleviates tourniquet pain. Many anesthetic agents that can be administered intravenously have been useful in achieving sedation and comfort while allowing active participation in the operative procedure. This medi-

cation is given as needed for the patient's comfort and as allowed by the patient's condition. Monitoring of the vital signs by experienced anesthesia personnel in an operating room environment is necessary. Careful titration of the medication is also necessary because overuse depresses the patient's function and his or her ability to cooperate. With proper dosage, the tourniquet can be tolerated for as long as 1 hour. The dissection proceeds rapidly, and the patient's ROM is repeatedly reevaluated until tourniquet paralysis intervenes at 20 to 25 minutes. If further dissection is needed, it is continued as necessary and evaluation is carried out after the tourniquet is released and hemostasis is obtained. If additional surgery is deemed necessary, reinflation can be carried out and dissection continued until completed. The surgeon can directly determine whether the tendon motor actually is effective and flexor pulleys are adequate. It can be determined whether the lysed tendon appears healthy or whether a tendon graft, usually conducted in two stages, is

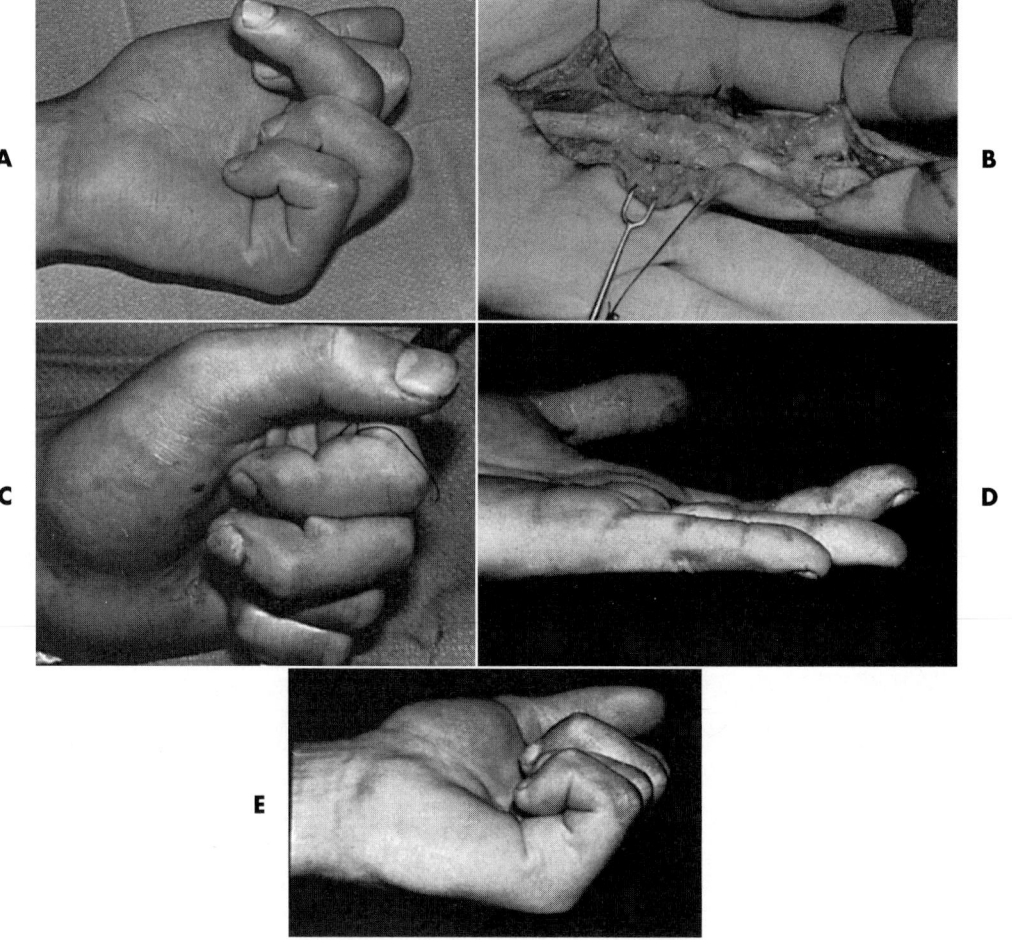

Fig. 28-1. Flexor lysis. A 17-year-old boy severed both flexor tendons in his left long finger. After primary repair of his flexor digitorum profundus, he had minimal pull-through of his flexor system at 4 months after repair. **A,** Attempted flexion of the left long finger. **B,** During tenolysis, massive adhesions were found at the repair site. **C,** After lysis under local-sedation technique, he obtained excellent active flexion with hand lying on a table. **D** and **E,** Through an active therapy program, he maintained the gains accomplished through surgery. Photographs of extension and flexion taken at 3 months after surgery.

advisable. When lysis has successfully restored active range of motion (AROM) that is deemed acceptable, the wounds are closed and a dressing is applied. An early postoperative motion program is planned.

Foucher et al.[9] have published their postoperative technique after tenolysis in which they briefly immobilize the operated fingers in flexion. On the second postoperative day, under local anesthesia, they bring the fingers passively into extension. Hand therapy is then instituted. They showed good gains in ROM in difficult cases. We have no experience in this technique, and the reader is referred to their article.[9]

More recently, Goloborod'ko[15] has published his protocol for the postoperative management of the tenolysis patient. Similar to the technique of Foucher et al.,[9] the operated digit is maintained in a flexed position during which time some soft adhesions do form between the lysed tendon and surrounding tissues. On the first postoperative day, the digit is passively extended under local anesthesia, disrupting the soft adhesions. The patient is then asked to actively flex the digit into the palm. The digit is maintained in this flexed

position with bandages. These manipulations are continued once daily for 5 to 6 postoperative days, following which, tendon gliding exercises[51,53] are begun. Flexion bandaging continues nightly for the next 10 to 12 days. Each morning, the digit is passively and fully extended. Dynamic extension splinting is used to manage flexion contractures. Goloborod'ko's work shows promising results. However, caution is advised because of an increased likelihood of tendon rupture.

Summary of current surgical technique

Flexor lysis[37-39]

1. Make a zig-zag incision; if necessary, be prepared to expose the entire course of the tendon.
2. Preserve pulleys as possible.
3. Release joints if significant contractures exist.
4. Look carefully at the site of the tendon repair or injury. The surgeon should be wary of a gapped tendon that has filled in with scar tissue. Although one may succeed in carving a tendonlike structure out of this scar tissue, when

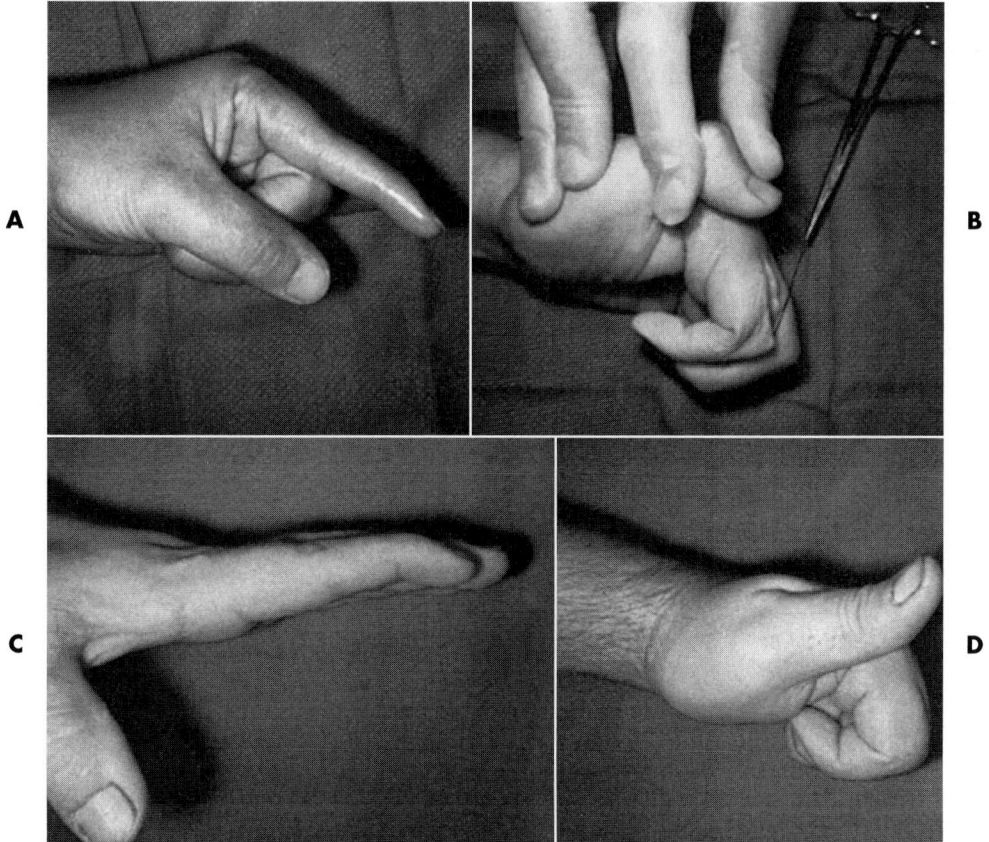

Fig. 28-2. Extensor lysis. A 42-year-old man severed his extensor mechanism over the proximal interphalangeal joint of his left index finger. After repair, extension contracture persisted despite active exercise program. **A,** Fixed extension posture of the finger before lysis. **B,** On an operating table, after lysis of tendon adhesions and release of dorsal capsule of the proximal interphalangeal joint, he could flex actively to 90 degrees. **C** and **D,** Range of motion was retained with therapy as shown at 3 months after tenolysis.

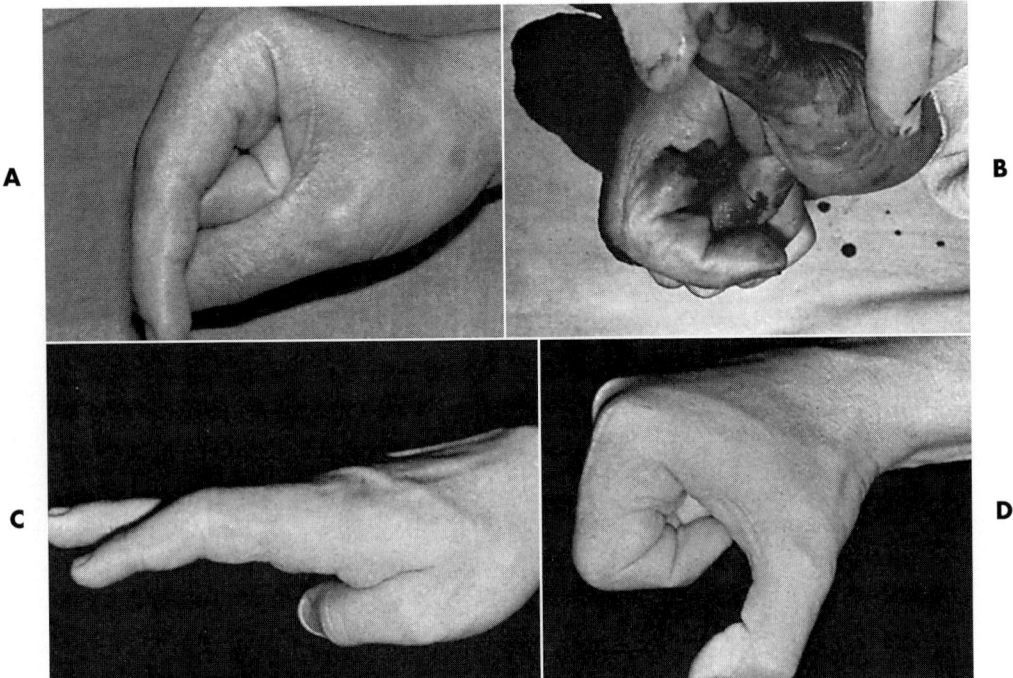

Fig. 28-3. Combined extensor and flexor lysis. A 35-year-old man sustained a crush injury to his right index finger. His extensor system primarily was involved. His finger became contracted in extension, and he had only 20 degrees of flexion from a straight position at the proximal interphalangeal joint (PIP). **A,** Maximum active flexion at the PIP joint. **B,** Lysis of extensor tendon system with release of PIP joint dorsal capsule returned passive flexion, but active flexion was not regained until volar exposure revealed adhesions of the flexor tendons. With release of these adhesions, he regained active flexion as shown here. **C,** Active extension was maintained at 4 months. **D,** Active flexion also was possible at 4 months.

a large gap is present, the tendon will be too long and lose mechanical efficiency and have an increased chance of rupturing (see item number 5).

5. Preoperatively prepare the patient for possibility of staged tendon reconstruction to be done at the same sitting when tenolysis is recognized as unlikely to succeed.[16,36,39]

Flexor lysis (Fig. 28-1) after failed direct repair has been more successful than after failed tendon graft, a finding that further stresses the advantages of direct repair, done early, in flexor injuries when wound conditions allow.[8,41]

Extensor lysis

1. Make a curvilinear incision over adherent area (Fig. 28-2).
2. Perform tenolysis, attempting to preserve continuity of the tendon.
3. Joint releases, particularly dorsal capsulotomies, are often needed.
4. Try to preserve some segment of the dorsal retinaculum at wrist.

When both flexor and extensor tendons are involved in adhesions, the prognosis is notably poorer, but finger salvage can occasionally be achieved (Fig. 28-3).

POSTOPERATIVE MANAGEMENT

The procedures surrounding the tenolysis operation are as vital as the lysis itself. Complications are not uncommon, but they can be minimized when a knowledgeable postoperative hand therapy program is implemented. Referral information should include (1) the integrity of the lysed tendon; (2) intraoperative AROM, if available; (3) intraoperative passive range of motion (PROM); (4) additional procedures performed (e.g., capsulectomy); (5) vascularity of the digit; and (6) the surgeon's prognosis for motion. This information then dictates the postoperative treatment program. For example, tendons of good integrity can undergo more vigorous postoperative therapy programs, whereas tendons of poor quality have an increased likelihood of rupture and require a protected ROM program designed to maximize tendon excursion while minimizing the stress applied to the lysed site.[36-39]

Postoperative week 1

Tenolysis demands immediate AROM.[49] It is initiated in the operating room and recovery area on the day of surgery. When possible, the patient is also seen in therapy on the day

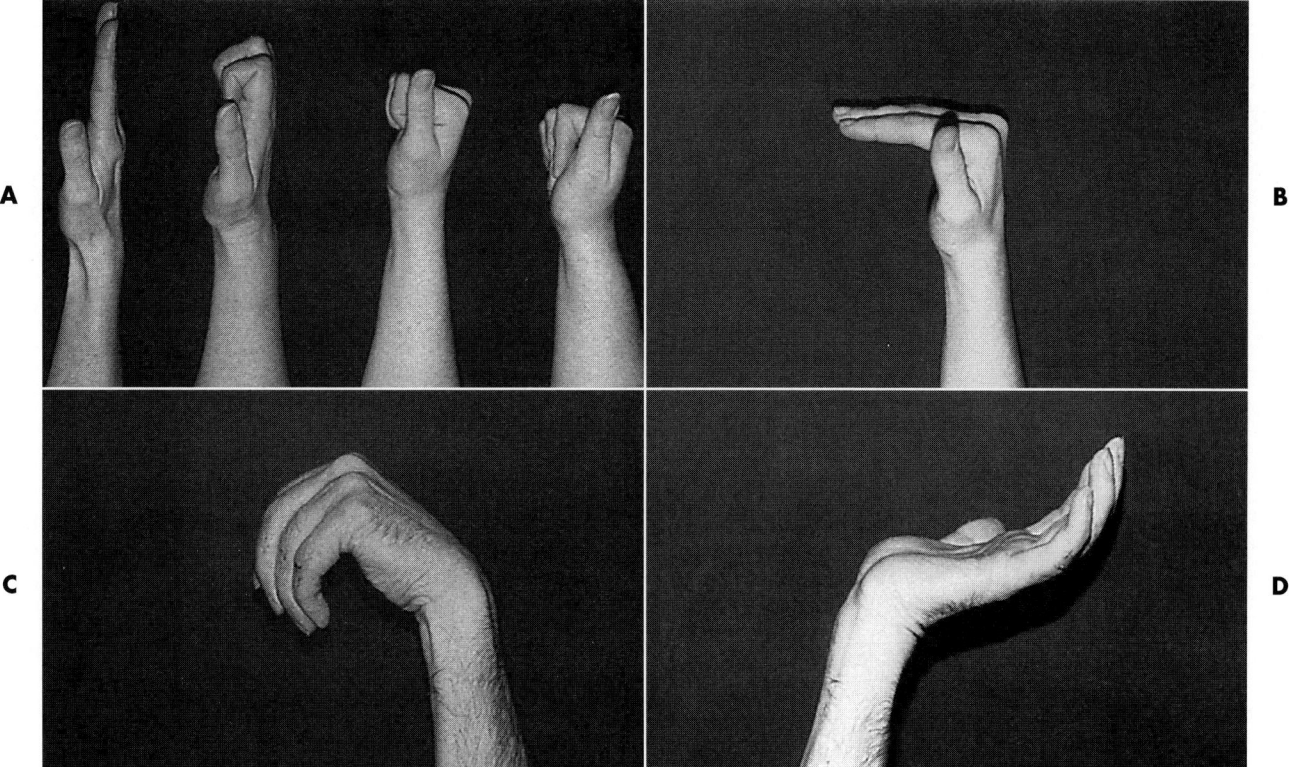

Fig. 28-4. A, Tendon gliding exercises allow for the flexor tendons to glide to their maximum potential. **B,** "Tabletop" position can be included to maximize metacarpophalangeal joint motion. **C** and **D,** Incorporation of wrist range of motion further increases tendon excursion.

of surgery. A more detailed therapy program is initiated on the first postoperative day. Ideally, the patient is seen in therapy daily for the first 5 postoperative days.

The first 5 days are crucial in the postoperative management. Inflammation occurs during the process of tissue healing and may result in associated edema and discomfort. Intraoperative ROM should be achieved in therapy as soon as possible in an effort to prevent the recurrence of binding adhesions.

Evaluation. Universal wound precautions must be implemented at all times. Evaluation and treatment are performed with the involved hand on a sterile drape. The therapist wears sterile gloves. Initial evaluation includes assessment of the wound, edema, AROM, PROM, and level of discomfort.

The bulky dressing applied at surgery is removed; the adherent dressing covering the incision is left undisturbed to protect the wound. The status of the wound is noted. At the end of the treatment session, a dry sterile gauze pad is reapplied to the incision. This is held in place by a tube bandage if a digit is involved and a gauze wrap if the incision extends into the palm or forearm. The newly applied dressing should not be removed until the next treatment session with the therapist. Postoperative dressings should be protective but nonrestrictive. Full AROM must be possible within the confines of the dressing.

Circumferential measurements for edema are recorded with a tape measure over the dressing. Measurements of AROM and PROM also are taken. The distance from the fingertips to the distal palmar crease is recorded during active flexion.

The patient's subjective reports of discomfort may be assessed with one of the many available pain assessments. Such assessments provide valuable information regarding the patient's level of pain tolerance and his or her ability to participate fully in the program.

Treatment. Initial treatment includes AROM, PROM, edema control, splinting if necessary, and home program instruction.

Active range of motion. Preoperatively, patients should have been instructed in the postoperative therapy regimen. They are warned that the postoperative therapy program will begin immediately after surgery and that it will be vigorous. Despite such warning, patients often are reluctant to exercise the recently operated finger because of discomfort. The therapist must be supportive, understanding, and encouraging. Both the patient and therapist must work together, giving forth their best effort to achieve a maximal result. The patient must understand that if he or she exercises consistently and frequently, each exercise session will get easier as ROM improves and stiffness begins to decrease.

Gentle active exercises begun during the first postoperative visit include tendon gliding exercises (TGEs)[51-53] and "place-hold" exercises. Occasionally, digital blocking ex-

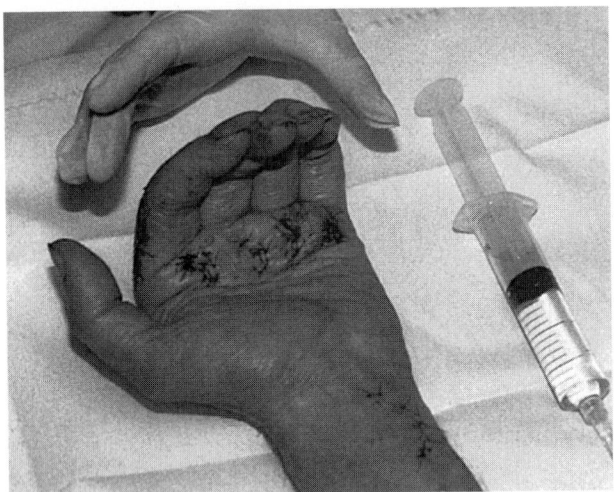

Fig. 28-5. This "place-hold" exercise is performed by the patient placing his fingers into slight flexion, using the uninvolved hand. The patient maintains the fist, using his own muscle power.

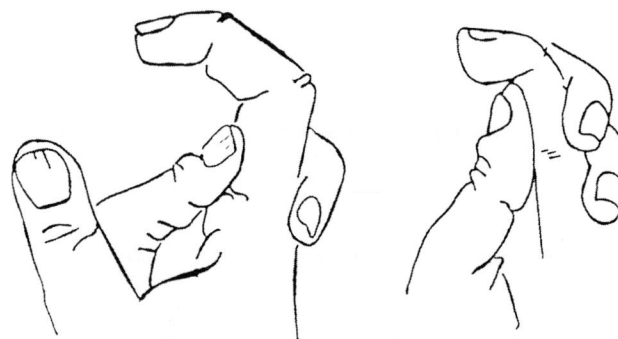

Fig. 28-6. Blocking exercises increase active range of motion by better directing the available tendon excursion to the target joint.

ercises and individual flexor digitorum superficialis (FDS) glides may be added, but they are usually reserved until the second postoperative week.

1. TGEs (Fig. 28-4, *A*) include full extension, a hook-fist, a full-fist, and a straight-tip–fist position.[53] In addition, a tabletop position (Fig. 28-4, *B*) can be included to maximize metacarpophalangeal (MP) joint motion. TGEs provide maximal differential gliding of the flexor digitorum profundus (FDP) and FDS tendons to minimize adhesions between the tendons and between the FDP and bone. Initially, these exercises are performed with the wrist in a neutral position; all TGEs begin from a position of neutral wrist and finger extension. Composite wrist and digit flexion (Fig. 28-4, *C*) are followed by simultaneous wrist and digit extension (Fig. 28-4, *D*), which may be added later to increase tendon excursion.

2. Place-hold exercises (Fig. 28-5) are performed by having the patient place his or her fingers into three positions: slight flexion, moderate flexion, and maximal flexion using the uninvolved hand. At each position, the patient releases the "helping" hand and maintains the fist, using his or her own muscle power.

   Cannon[2] and Strickland[42,43,46] have described their "frayed exercise program" for use with patients having poor tendon integrity intraoperatively who require protection against rupture. This protected ROM program involves place-hold exercises performed in full flexion, followed by active extension to 0 degrees to passively maximize excursion of the long flexors. Place-hold exercises are the only active flexion exercises performed. These exercises apply less tensile loading on the operated tendon than other active exercises, yet they provide the same tendon excursion that

is produced when the patient actively flexes the digit to end range. The benefits of this program include decreased pain, decreased rupture rate, and ease in maintaining excursion of the lysed tendon. This program also may be used with patients experiencing crepitus or synovitis postoperatively when rupture is a concern. As the tendon heals and gains in strength, gentle active exercises may be added progressively to the program when indicated by the surgeon.

3. Two different blocking exercises (Fig. 28-6) are performed on each digit in turn: (1) active flexion of the proximal interphalangeal (PIP) joint while holding (blocking) the MP joint in extension, and (2) active distal interphalangeal (DIP) joint flexion while holding (blocking) the MP and PIP joints in extension. Blocking exercises increase AROM by allowing the available tendon excursion to be better directed to the target joint.

4. Active PIP joint extension is performed while holding (blocking) the MP joint in a hyperflexed position with the uninvolved hand. The hyperflexed MP joint facilitates PIP joint extension. This exercise is performed to encourage PIP joint extension in instances when the PIP joint has a flexion contracture or is at risk to develop one.

5. Isolated FDS glides (Fig. 28-7) are performed with the patient's hand supinated on a flat surface. The therapist manually holds all the digits in extension except the digit being flexed. The patient is instructed to actively flex the PIP joint into the palm. This exercise requires isolated function of the FDS and enhances differential tendon gliding between the FDS and FDP tendons.

Passive range of motion. Gentle passive exercises are incorporated into the exercise program when joint stiffness

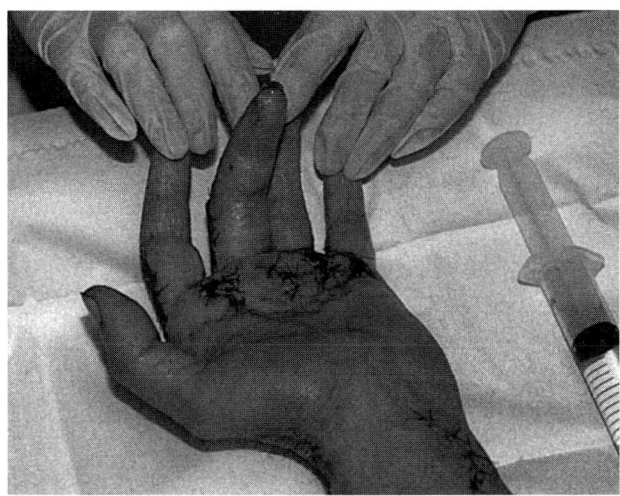

Fig. 28-7. Flexor digitorum superficialis (FDS) glides allow for isolated function of the FDS tendon and promote differential gliding between the FDS and flexor digitorum profundus tendons.

is present. Caution must be used when performing these exercises. Overly vigorous ROM can result in increased pain and inflammation that will only impede recovery.[23,40,45]

Edema control. Edema, a normal reaction to trauma, must be controlled early because persistent edema may result in significant tissue scarring and fibrosis.[45] Uncontrolled edema will lead to restrictions in ROM and tendon excursion.

Edema control includes elevation of the hand above the level of the heart to minimize limb dependency.[40] If elevation does not control edema sufficiently, other measures may be considered. Cold packs may be applied to the involved extremity three to four times per day for approximately 15 to 20 minutes with the hand in elevation. When one is applying cold packs, the wound must be kept dry and sterile and vascular status must be monitored.

Coban is applied without tension in a figure-of-eight, distal-to-proximal fashion to digits with good vascularity. Coban may be worn full-time (if needed), except during wound care. If ROM is impeded by Coban, it should be removed during exercise.

Isotoner gloves may be worn by patients (with good digital vascularity) who have excessive edema present throughout the hand.

An exercise that is very effective in controlling edema and in promoting active tendon excursion is overhead pumping. This exercise entails the patient elevating the involved extremity overhead and making a firm fist 10 times per hour.

Splinting. Splinting may be required to achieve or maintain the ROM gained in surgery, to rest violated tissues between periods of exercise to allow healing to occur, or to protect weakened tendons or repaired pulleys.

Patients who have had flexion contractures released at the time of tenolysis require static extension splinting of the

involved joint(s) (Fig. 28-8). Extension splints initially may be worn full-time, except during exercise and wound care. As extension improves, the daily wearing schedule may be gradually reduced, but nighttime extension splinting may be necessary for up to 6 months.[40] Splints designed to increase or maintain PROM must be monitored carefully. Too much stress applied too early can increase pain and inflammation.

Pulleys are rarely reconstructed at the time of tenolysis. When they are, they require protective splinting. Before any active motion is initiated, a pulley ring, constructed of felt and Velcro, is applied over the reconstructed pulley. After edema subsides, a thermoplastic ring is fabricated. Some patients elect to wear a metal ring instead of the thermoplastic ring for greater durability and improved aesthetics. Direct pressure applied over the reconstructed pulley by the patient's uninvolved hand during exercises also may be used to protect the pulley. The pulley ring is worn full-time for 6 months after repair.

When dynamic or serial static extension splinting is required, two pulley rings are fabricated to maintain adequate protection of the repaired pulley. One pulley ring is fabricated with the splint in place to counteract the passive extension forces of the extension outrigger; the second is fabricated without the splint in place and is worn during exercises.[40]

Home program instruction. The patient is instructed in a home program consisting of 5 to 10 repetitions of each active exercise performed hourly. Exercises are upgraded according to patient tolerance and progress. Patients who are unable to tolerate the exercise program because of persistent discomfort require a modified program consisting of a decreased number of repetitions and frequency of exercises (i.e., 3 repetitions performed every other hour). This allows continued tendon gliding through the lysed area without further increasing discomfort. Patients are instructed to actively hold the end position of each exercise for 5 seconds to increase total end-range time and to extend and flex the digits fully and strongly to maximize tendon excursion.[51] Gentle passive exercises at each joint of the involved digits are performed for 5 to 10 repetitions, four times per day. Edema control is included in every home program.

Postoperative weeks 2 to 3

As the proliferative phase of wound healing begins, fibroblasts enter the wound along fibrin strands and begin to synthesize scar tissue. The wound begins to rapidly gain strength as scar tissue forms. Edema and discomfort are now decreasing, and intraoperative AROM should have been achieved. Gains in AROM may become more difficult to achieve or maintain as restrictive adhesions begin to reform.

Evaluation. Evaluation includes assessment of the wound and/or scar, edema, AROM, PROM, discomfort, activity of daily living (ADL) performance, and sensibility (if necessary). After the wound is well healed, the scar is assessed for thickness and mobility. Thickened, immobile scars will restrict tendon gliding and require immediate intervention. Edema may be assessed using either circumferential or volumetric measures after the wound is well healed. AROM, PROM, and discomfort are assessed as previously described. ADL performance may be assessed via observation and patient interview. Sensibility may be assessed using Semmes-Weinstein monofilaments.

Treatment. Treatment goals now include maintenance of AROM as collagen bonds begin to form, edema control, scar management, functional use of the involved hand, and independence with ADLs.

AROM exercises are continued with upgrades as tolerated. PROM exercises are continued, if necessary, for persistent joint stiffness. After the sutures are removed, fluid-flushing massage, performed in a distal-to-proximal direction, may be added to the program to further decrease edema. Splinting techniques are continued as previously described, with modifications as needed to account for increasing AROM and decreasing edema. Scar management,[56] if necessary, is initiated when the sutures are removed. An elastomere mold is fabricated or silicone gel sheet, worn nightly to help soften thickened, immobile scars.

The home program now includes deep friction massage performed four to five times per day along the scar line. Deep friction massage is performed to help soften the scar and maintain tissue mobility as collagen bonds form and gain in strength. Fluid-flushing massage may be performed for 5 to 10 minutes four times per day, if needed to decrease edema. Light ADLs may be initiated to encourage functional use of the involved hand.[40]

Postoperative weeks 4 to 6

The proliferative phase of wound healing is now ending, and scar remodeling is in process. During scar remodeling, the pattern of the collagen fibers becomes more organized and forms parallel to the wound surface. This further enhances tensile strength.

The wound should now be well healed, scars are beginning to soften, edema and discomfort are decreased or absent, AROM is equivalent to or greater than that achieved during surgery, and strength is improving.

Evaluation. Evaluation includes assessment of the scar, edema, AROM, PROM, and grip and pinch strength.

Treatment. Treatment goals are to maintain AROM as collagen bonds continue to form and gain in strength, to

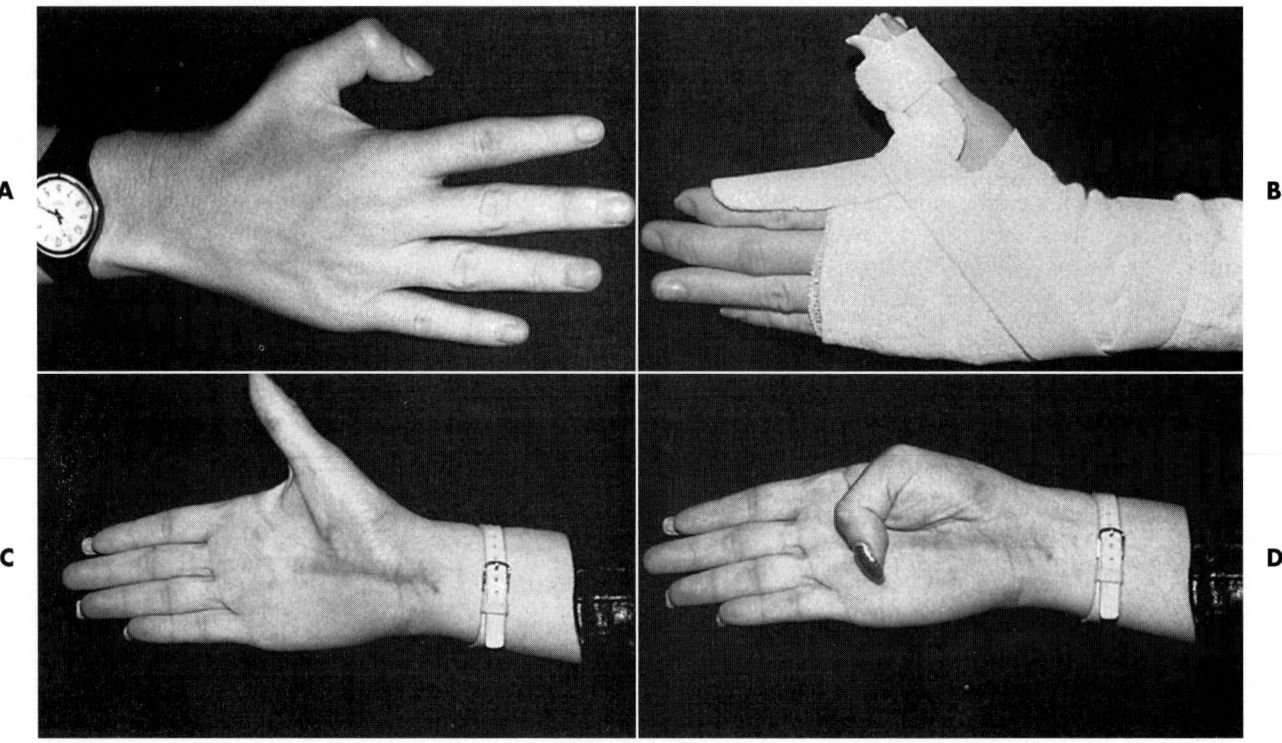

Fig. 28-8. This 30-year-old right-hand dominant bartender slipped and fell at work. This resulted in lacerations of her right flexor pollicis longus tendon in zone III; median nerve, proximally from the palm to digit I; radial and digital nerves to digit I; and radial digital nerve to digit II. **A,** At 3 months status after primary repair, thumb active range of motion (AROM) was metacarpophalangeal 20/65; and interphalangeal 30/55. **B,** A web stretcher was fabricated after lysis and worn nightly to maintain the gains achieved in range of motion. **C** and **D,** The patient was discharged at 8 weeks after surgery with AROM within normal limits.

continue scar management, and to increase grip and pinch strength.

AROM, PROM, and splinting are continued, with upgrades as tolerated. If edema persists, additional techniques such as string wrapping may be used. Scar management techniques are continued to remodel the collagen fibers. If the surgeon reports that tendon integrity is good, sustained gripping exercises may be initiated earlier, at 3 to 4 weeks after surgery, and later progressed to increase resistance.[40] Some examples of these activities are dowel squeezes, foam squeezes, and isometric exercises. If tendon integrity is poor, sustained gripping exercises are added to the program only when indicated by the surgeon.

The home program now includes sustained gripping exercises in addition to active exercises, deep friction massage, and light ADLs. Passive exercises and edema control techniques are continued if needed. The home program should be reevaluated regularly, and exercises that are no longer needed should be eliminated from the program.

At 6 weeks, graded grip strengthening exercises and progressive resistive exercises are initiated during treatment and at home. Whole-body conditioning now must be considered as return to work is approaching. Aerobic exercise such as walking and bicycle riding are recommended to increase whole body strength and endurance.

Postoperative weeks 7 to 8

The focus of treatment now begins to shift toward preparation for return to work via job simulation, work hardening, and on-site job visits.

Evaluation. Evaluation includes assessment of ROM and strength. In addition, the patient's abilities in comparison with job demands are functionally assessed. Such evaluation may include assessment of lifting, carrying, pushing/pulling, and reaching. In addition, prehension skills, material/tool handling, and endurance may be assessed.

Treatment. The treatment goals include maintaining ROM and maximizing strength while initiating light job simulation. The goal is to return the patient to work at approximately 8 to 12 weeks after tenolysis, depending on job requirements.

Heavy resistive exercises may be initiated at 8 weeks.

ANCILLARY MODALITIES

Additional modalities may be indicated as treatment adjuncts to enhance patient performance.

Transcutaneous electrical nerve stimulation

Transcutaneous electrical nerve stimulation (TENS) (Fig. 28-9, A) may be applied to the involved extremity immediately after tenolysis to manage postoperative discomfort.[4] Presterilized, disposable electrodes are placed along the peripheral nerve distribution supplying the affected area. The patient is instructed in the operation of the unit at home. After pain relief has been achieved, the daily wearing time is gradually reduced and the patient is weaned from the unit.

Marcaine catheter

Another method to reduce postoperative discomfort is an indwelling polyethylene catheter (Fig. 28-9, B) that provides a local anesthetic.[17] The catheter is inserted at the time of the surgical procedure, proximal to the incision, over the sensory nerve branches.[36-38] The patient slowly instills small amounts (1 to 2 ml)[37,40] of local anesthetic (Bupivacaine 0.25% or 0.5%)[17] into the area every 4 hours.[37,40] At each

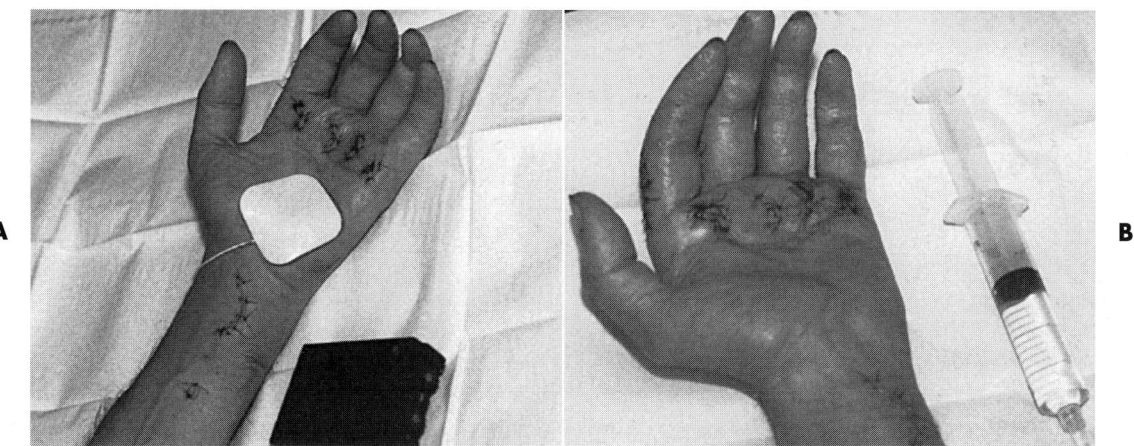

Fig. 28-9. Transcutaneous electrical nerve stimulation (**A**) or Marcaine catheter (**B**) may be used to manage the postoperative discomfort that in some cases prevents the patient from exercising.

dressing change, an antibiotic ointment is applied to the catheter entrance site. The catheter is left in place for approximately 5 to 7 days, during which time the patient is on a regimen of oral antibiotics.[40] Although this technique is effective in reducing postoperative discomfort, we have found that it is being used with less frequency in recent years.

Continuous passive motion

McCarthy et al.[26] studied continuous passive motion (CPM) as a treatment adjunct to tenolysis. They found that CPM was associated with an increase in tendon rupture and in the terminal force necessary to flex the phalanx actively. Histologically, it appeared that the passive motion elicited a hypergranular response that weakened the tendons and decreased the motion. In their study, CPM was continued for 5 consecutive days without removal for AROM.

Tenolysis protocol demands immediate AROM to maximize tendon excursion and enhance tensile strength and nutrition of the muscle-tendon unit.[2,14,24,51] CPM is recommended for use following tenolysis as a treatment adjunct, not as a replacement for AROM. Cannon[2] has identified indications for initiating CPM following tenolysis. These include patients whose PROM is not fully supple preoperatively; patients in whom pain and/or edema persist longer than expected with the initial injury; patients with excessive scarring following the initial injury; patients requiring extensive tenolysis from the digital level proximally to the muscle belly in the forearm; and patients who are apprehensive and fearful of moving the digit. In addition, we have found it to be beneficial with patients who have had joint contractures released at the time of lysis. Nothing is more important than active motion postoperatively, and it is the primary activity in the program for the posttenolysis patient.

The CPM device is applied shortly after the surgery and worn throughout the first 3 postoperative weeks, whenever the patient is not actively exercising the involved digits. Studies have shown the clinical benefits of CPM include increased AROM and PROM,[2,10-12] decreased pain,[5,21,35] decreased edema,[21] and the prevention of joint stiffness.[35]

Neuromuscular electrical stimulation

Neuromuscular electrical stimulation (NMES) may be implemented after tenolysis to increase tendon excursion, muscle strength, and AROM via the facilitation of muscle contractions.[2,3,47] It may be initiated by the end of the first postoperative week if the patient is not independently demonstrating strong active muscle contractions, if PROM exceeds AROM, and if the surgeon reports that tendon integrity is good.

Verification of tendon integrity is essential if NMES is being considered. NMES at high intensities is equivalent to the performance of resistive exercises. A weakened tendon may be unable to tolerate such strong muscle contractions

before 6 to 8 weeks and may rupture if such tension is applied too soon. Caution also must be used with NMES to avoid overexercise, which could result in an inflammatory response and further impede recovery. NMES is continued until the goal of full AROM is achieved or when progress reaches a plateau.

Electromyographic biofeedback

Electromyographic (EMG) biofeedback[1,30] may be used after tenolysis to restore functional coordinated movement, motivate the patient, redirect attention away from postoperative discomfort, and/or facilitate muscular relaxation. Biofeedback also may be used in conjunction with electrical stimulation to further enhance muscular activity.

Ultrasound

Ultrasound may be initiated at approximately 4 to 5 weeks after tenolysis to increase collagen tissue extensibility and blood flow, decrease pain, improve joint mobility, and enhance tendon gliding.[27,28,48] When used in conjunction with hot packs, ultrasound may provide greater elevation of tissue temperature.[29]

The use of ultrasound on healing tendons remains controversial. Studies on tendon healing suggest that the time at which ultrasound is initiated in the course of tendon healing is critical.[2,13,19,27,34] Gan et al.[13] recently compared the effects of early and late ultrasound treatments. They found ultrasound to be beneficial early in the healing process of flexor tendons. Other recent findings indicate that ultrasound may increase rate of repair, collagen synthesis, and breaking strength of healing tendons.[19,33] Many of the available studies on ultrasound have been conducted in various animal models using a variety of parameters, making it difficult to draw conclusions and make applications to the clinical setting.

Dosage parameters for ultrasound use vary throughout the literature. A frequency of 3.0 MHz is recommended for treatment of the hand[7] and in treating tissues 1 to 2 cm from the skin surface.[27,28] A frequency of 1.0 MHz is used to affect deeper structures.[27,28,31] The strength of an ultrasound beam is determined by its intensity. The weakest beam or lowest possible intensity that produces the desired effect should be used when treating patients. To enhance tissue healing, ultrasound should be used in the range of 0.1 to 0.5 W/cm^2.[31] An intensity of 0.5 W/cm^2 may be used with acute and subacute injuries.[27] A continuous or pulsed-wave mode is selected, depending on the stage after injury and the desired therapeutic effect. Continuous-wave ultrasound is appropriate for use once the surgeon has determined it safe to perform a strong active contraction of the lysed tendon.[28] Continuous-wave ultrasound may be contraindicated if circulation is compromised, sensibility is altered, or edema is uncontrolled and a thermal effect is not desirable. Recent findings in the literature indicate that low-intensity pulsed ultrasound may be most appropriate to resolve acute and subacute inflammation; promote healing of open wounds; promote tissue healing; and enhance repair in tendon, nerve, and bone.[6,7,31] More research is needed to determine optimal dosage parameters to achieve maximal benefits of ultrasound following tenolysis.

In summary, tenolysis is a very demanding procedure both surgically and therapeutically. In some cases, it is the final option for our patients. For this procedure to be successful, the patient, surgeon, and therapist all must work cooperatively and diligently to achieve a freely gliding tendon.

REFERENCES

1. Blackmore SM, Williams DA: The use of biofeedback in hand rehabilitation. In Hunter JM, Mackin EJ, Callahan AD, editors: *Rehabilitation of the hand: surgery and therapy,* ed 4, St Louis, 1995, Mosby.
2. Cannon NM: Enhancing flexor tendon glide through tenolysis and hand therapy, *J Hand Ther* 2:122, 1989.
3. Cannon NM, Strickland JW: Therapy following flexor tendon surgery, *Hand Clin* 1:147, 1985.
4. Cannon NM, et al: Control of immediate postoperative pain following tenolysis and capsulectomies of the hand with TENS, *J Hand Surg* 8:626, 1983.
5. Chow J, Schenck RR: Early continuous passive movement in hand surgery, *Curr Surg* 46:97, 1989.
6. Enwemeka CS, Rodriguez O, Mendosa S: The biomechanical effects of low-intensity ultrasound on healing tendons, *Ultrasound Med Biol* 16:801, 1990.
7. Fedorczyk JM: Heat and cold in hand rehabilitation. In Michlovitz SL, editor: *Thermal agents in rehabilitation,* ed 3, Philadelphia, 1996, FA Davis.
8. Fetrow KO: Tenolysis in the hand and wrist, *J Bone Joint Surg* 49A:667, 1967.
9. Foucher G, et al: A postoperative regime after flexor tenolysis, *J Hand Surg* 18B:35, 1993.
10. Frank C, et al: Physiology and therapeutic value of passive joint motion, *Clin Orthop* 185:113, 1984.
11. Frykman GK, Unsell RS, Yahiku H: *Continuous passive motion machine after metacarpophalangeal implant resection arthroplasties,* scientific sessions, Seattle, 1989, American Society for Surgery of the Hand.
12. Frykman GK, et al: *CPM improves ROM after PIP and MP capsulectomies: a controlled prospective study* (abstract), scientific sessions, Seattle, 1989, American Society for Surgery of the Hand.
13. Gan BS, et al: The effects of ultrasound treatment on flexor tendon healing in the chicken limb, *J Hand Surg* 20B:809, 1995.
14. Gelberman RH, et al: The influence of protected passive mobilization on the healing of flexor tendons: a biochemical and microangiographic study, *Hand* 13:120, 1981.
15. Goloborod'ko SA: Postoperative management of flexor tenolysis, *J Hand Ther* 12:4, 1999.
16. Hunter JM, Salisbury RE: Flexor tendon reconstruction in severely damaged hands, *J Bone Joint Surg* 53A:829, 1971.
17. Hunter JM, Seinsheimer F III, Mackin EJ: Tenolysis: pain control and rehabilitation. In Strickland JW, Steichen JB, editors: *Difficult problems in hand surgery,* St Louis, 1982, Mosby.
18. Hunter JM, et al: A dynamic approach to problems of hand function, *Clin Orthop* 104:112, 1974.
19. Jackson BA, Schwane JA, Starcher BC: Effect of ultrasound therapy on the repair of Achilles tendon injuries in rats, *Med Sci Sports Exer* 23:171, 1991.
20. Jupiter JB, Pess GM, Bour CJ: Results of flexor tendon tenolysis after replantation in the hand, *J Hand Surg* 14:35, 1989.
21. LaStayo PC: Continuous passive motion for the upper extremity. In Hunter JM, Mackin EJ, Callahan AD, editors: *Rehabilitation of the hand: surgery and therapy,* ed 4, St Louis, 1995, Mosby.
22. Lindsay WK, Thomson HG: Digital flexor tendons: an experimental study, *Br J Plast Surg* 12:289, 1960.
23. Mackin EJ: Benefits of early tendon gliding after tenolysis. In Hunter JM, Schneider LH, Mackin EJ, editors: *Tendon surgery in the hand,* St Louis, 1987, Mosby.
24. Mason ML, Allen HS: The rate of healing of tendons, *Ann Surg* 113:424, 1941.
25. Matthews P, Richards H: Factors in the adherence of flexor tendons after repair, *J Bone Joint Surg* 58B:230, 1976.
26. McCarthy JA, et al: Continuous passive motion as an adjunct therapy for tenolysis, *J Hand Surg* 11B:88, 1986.
27. McDiarmid T, Ziskin MC, Michlovitz SL: Therapeutic ultrasound. In Michlovitz SL, editor: *Thermal agents in rehabilitation,* ed 3, Phila, 1996, FA Davis.
28. Michlovitz SL: Use of ultrasound in upper extremity rehabilitation. In Hunter JM, Mackin EJ, Callahan AD, editors: *Rehabilitation of the hand: surgery and therapy,* ed 4, St Louis, 1995, Mosby.
29. Miller LE, et al: Sequential use of hot packs and ultrasound, *Phys Ther* 59:559, 1979.
30. Nelson RM, Currier DP: *Clinical electrotherapy,* ed 2, Norwalk, Conn, 1991, Appleton & Lange.
31. Nussbaum E: The influence of ultrasound on healing tissues, *J Hand Ther* 11:140, 1998.
32. Potenza AD: Critical evaluation of flexor tendon healing and adhesion formation within artificial digital sheaths, *J Bone Joint Surg* 45A:1217, 1963.
33. Ramirez A, et al: The effect of ultrasound on collagen synthesis and fibroblast proliferation in vitro, *Med Sci Sports Exerc* 29:326, 1997.
34. Roberts M, Rutherford JH, Harris D: The effect of ultrasound on flexor tendon repairs in the rabbit, *Hand* 14:17, 1982.
35. Salter RB: The biologic concept of CPM of synovial joints, *Clin Orthop* 242:12, 1989.
36. Schneider LH: *Flexor tendon injuries,* Boston, 1985, Little, Brown.
37. Schneider LH: Flexor tenolysis. In Hunter JM, Schneider LH, Mackin EJ, editors: *Tendon surgery in the hand,* St Louis, 1987, Mosby.
38. Schneider LH, Hunter JM: Flexor tenolysis. In *AAOS symposium on tendon surgery in the hand,* St Louis, 1975, Mosby.
39. Schneider LH, Hunter JM: Flexor tendons: late reconstruction. In Green DB, editor: *Operative hand surgery,* New York, 1988, Churchill Livingstone.
40. Schneider LH, Mackin EJ: Tenolysis: dynamic approach to surgery and therapy. In Hunter JM, et al, editors: *Rehabilitation of the hand,* ed 3, St Louis, 1990, Mosby.
41. Schneider LH, et al: Delayed primary flexor tendon repair in no man's land, *J Hand Surg* 2:452, 1977.
42. Strickland JW: Flexor tenolysis, *Hand Clin* 1:121, 1985.
43. Strickland JW: Flexor tendon injuries. Part 5: flexor tenolysis, rehabilitation and results, *Orthop Rev* 16:137, 1987.
44. Strickland JW: Flexor tenolysis: a personal experience. In Hunter JM, Schneider LH, Mackin EJ, editors: *Tendon surgery in the hand,* St Louis, 1987, Mosby.
45. Strickland JW: Biologic rationale, clinical application, and results of early motion following flexor tendon repair, *J Hand Ther* 2:2, 1989.

46. Strickland JW: Flexor tendon surgery. Part 2: free tendon grafts and tenolysis, *J Hand Surg* 14:368, 1989.

47. Takai S, et al: The effects of frequency and duration of controlled passive mobilization on tendon healing, *J Orthop* 9:705, 1991.

48. Taylor Mullins PA: Use of therapeutic modalities in upper extremity rehabilitation. In Hunter JM, Mackin EJ, Callahan AD, editors: *Rehabilitation of the hand: surgery and therapy,* ed 4, St Louis, 1995, Mosby.

49. Verdan CE: Tenolysis. In Verdan CE, editor: *Tendon surgery of the hand,* Edinburgh, 1979, Churchill Livingstone.

50. Verdan CE, Crawford GP, Martini-Benkeddache Y: The valuable role of tenolysis in the digits. In Cramer LM, Chase RA, editors: *Symposium on the hand,* vol 3, St Louis, 1971, Mosby.

51. Wehbe MA: Tendon gliding exercises, *Am J Occup Ther* 41:164, 1987.

52. Wehbe MA, Hunter JM: Flexor tendon gliding in the hand. Part I: in vivo excursions, *J Hand Surg* 10A:570, 1985.

53. Wehbe MA, Hunter JM: Tendon gliding, *Orthop Rev* 14:49, 1985.

54. Whitaker JH, Strickland JW, Ellis RK: The role of flexor tenolysis in the palm and digits, *J Hand Surg* 2:462, 1977.

55. Wray RC, Moucharafieh B, Weeks PM: Experimental study of the optimal time for tenolysis, *Plast Reconstr Surg* 61:184, 1978.

56. Wray RC, et al: Effects of stress on the mechanical properties of tendon adhesions, *Surg Forum* 25:520, 1974.

Chapter 29

STAGED FLEXOR TENDON RECONSTRUCTION

James M. Hunter
Evelyn J. Mackin

Part I: staged flexor tendon reconstruction

James M. Hunter*

INDICATIONS/CONTRAINDICATIONS

Transformation of the scarred, postinjury flexor tendon complex to a gliding, pliable, functional system can be accomplished by the two-stage tendon graft method using the Hunter tendon implant (Wright Medical Technology, Inc., 5677 Airline Road, Arlington, Tennessee 38002, 901-867-9971) at stage I. This method permits the "linchpin" factors to take place by permitting new anatomic reconstruction of pulleys and fibrous sheathing around the tendon implant. The results are improved gliding biomechanics and a fluid flow through a synovial nutrition system that can maintain gliding of active and passive implants and ultimately nourish the stage II tendon graft free of restricting adhesions. This concept permits the surgeon and therapist to achieve maximum functional gains in rehabilitation of the hand because stage II surgery can be delayed for extended periods of time.[2,3]

Staged tendon reconstruction

A tendon implant is indicated in the following situations: (1) as a temporary segmental spacer in certain damaging injuries where primary tendon repair is not likely to give a good result; (2) in scarred tendon beds where a one-stage tendon graft can be predicted to fail; and (3) in salvage situations where, despite predicted degrees of stiffness, scarred tendon bed, and reduced nutrition, useful function

can be returned. This procedure has been used successfully in extensor tendon reconstruction, reconstruction of the severely mutilated hand, and construction of tendon systems in congenital anomalies with deficient tendon systems. Any tendon transfer (i.e., opponens transferre) that would have to transverse a suboptimal bed should be considered for this procedure. This procedure also may be indicated for grafting of a profundus tendon through an intact superficialis when the profundus tendon bed is scarred. In a Boyes grade V or VI salvage finger,[3] particularly when the adjacent finger has been amputated, the passive or active tendon may be used to create a *superficialis finger*. In this procedure, arthrodesis is performed on the distal joint, and the distal juncture of the implant is to the middle phalanx.

In acute trauma, the tendon implant also may be used if the wounds have been adequately debrided and rendered surgically clean. When the injury requires simultaneous fracture fixation and flexor and extensor tendon repair, the use of a tendon implant in the flexor system should be considered.

A timely indication for the two-stage procedure has been in replantation surgery. In multiple digital amputations, the use of the implant in the flexor system at the time of replantation may significantly simplify the postoperative rehabilitation. A full-length tendon implant, or even a short spacer, can maintain the fibroosseous canal and regenerate a flexor sheath in damaged areas after the fracture or fusion has healed and the neurovascular status is stabilized. The passive flexion and active extension have helped rehabilitate both the flexor and extensor systems simultaneously and have significantly improved the function of replanted digits. If the replantation is proximal to zone II or at wrist level, it is reasonable to repair the flexor tendons proximally and place extensor implants dorsally, because the wrist is usually flexed to protect the neurovascular repairs. Again, the postoperative rehabilitation is simplified.

*Part I reproduced from Hunter JM: Staged flexor tendon reconstruction. In Strickland JW, editor: *Master techniques in orthopaedic surgery, the hand,* Philadelphia, 1998, Lippincott-Raven.

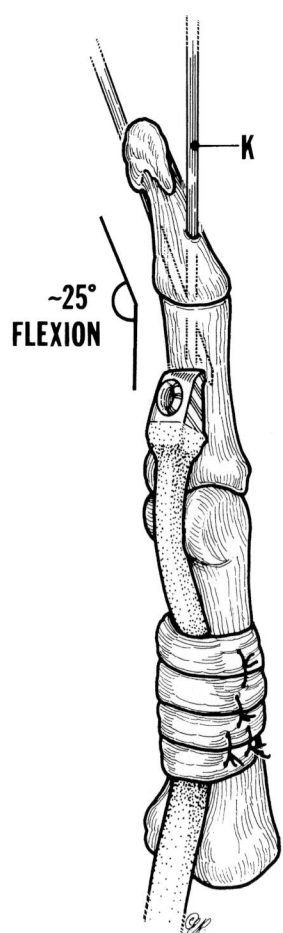

~25°
FLEXION

K

Fig. 29-1. Superficialis finger. The active tendon is fixed distally to the base of the middle phalanx. The A₂ pulley has been reconstructed, and the distal interphalangeal joint has been fused in 25 degrees of flexion. *K,* K-wire. (From Hunter JM: Staged flexor tendon reconstruction. In Strickland JW, editor: *Master techniques in orthopaedic surgery, the hand,* Philadelphia, 1998, Lippincott-Raven.)

Acute infection is an absolute contraindication to this procedure. Appropriate surgical and antimicrobial treatment and subsequent wound healing will allow the procedure to be carried out later without complication. Finally, the digit that has borderline nutrition, bilateral digital nerve injuries, and joint stiffness may be better treated by amputation rather than reconstruction.

Active tendon implants

An active tendon or passive tendon implant may be indicated in the following situations: (1) as a temporary segmental spacer in selected primary injuries where conditions are unfavorable or impossible for tendon repair; (2) in scarred tendon beds where a one-stage tendon graft would most likely fail; and (3) in salvage situations where useful functions can be returned despite predicted stiffness, scarred tendon beds, and reduced nutrition. If an injury requires simultaneous fracture fixation and flexor and extensor

tendon repair, the implant should be considered for the flexor system. The only absolute contraindication to this procedure is acute infection.

The following are indications for an active tendon rather than a passive tendon: (1) a patient with the proper motivation for compliance with the rehabilitation protocol, (2) an extensor system that functions well enough to balance the predictive flexion of the finger, and (3) patient understanding that a superficialis finger reconstruction with distal interphalangeal (DIP) joint arthrodesis may be needed if the DIP joint extensor tendon function is not adequate or if more than two pulleys will require reconstruction. The active tendon, when used in the hand injury requiring multiple reconstructive procedures, can be an important choice for patient morale.

Superficialis finger reconstruction

The superficialis finger concept is based on the principle of a one-tendon/two-joint finger. The distal fixation of the implant is on the proximal aspect of the middle phalanx, and the proximal implant juncture is in the forearm, as previously described. In addition, tenodesis or fusion of the DIP joint is done, and pulley reconstruction then can be performed at the proximal phalanx (Fig. 29-1). Indications for the superficialis finger include the following: (1) reconstruction of more than two pulleys is needed; (2) extensor tendon control of the DIP joint is poor; (3) arthritis of the DIP joint is present; (4) there are multiple finger injuries in one hand and partial or complete amputations of adjacent fingers; and (5) vascular deficiencies of the finger are present.

PREOPERATIVE PLANNING
Examination: passive tendon

The preoperative assessment includes a careful analysis of dismembered parts of the hand and deficient sensibility patterns because these will significantly affect final results. Sensibility loss should be studied carefully before flexor tendon reconstruction, and the nutritional status should be reviewed by the Allen test. The need for skin grafts, which will affect contractures of the fingers, also should be examined carefully at this time. It is important to record ranges of joint motion and the ability to extend digits actively within those ranges and to look at how far the finger pulp comes from the distal palmar crease.

Pencil sketches showing range of motion (ROM) and lack thereof are helpful. The sketches also should include the site of injury and other abnormalities, such as needed skin grafting. Additional sites of injury beyond the finger (i.e., palm and forearm) should be recorded, because these will affect the position of the tendon implant.

Types of Hunter tendon implants

Passive gliding implant system. Two basic types of Hunter tendon implants have evolved from the experience gained in experimental and clinical trials during the past 25

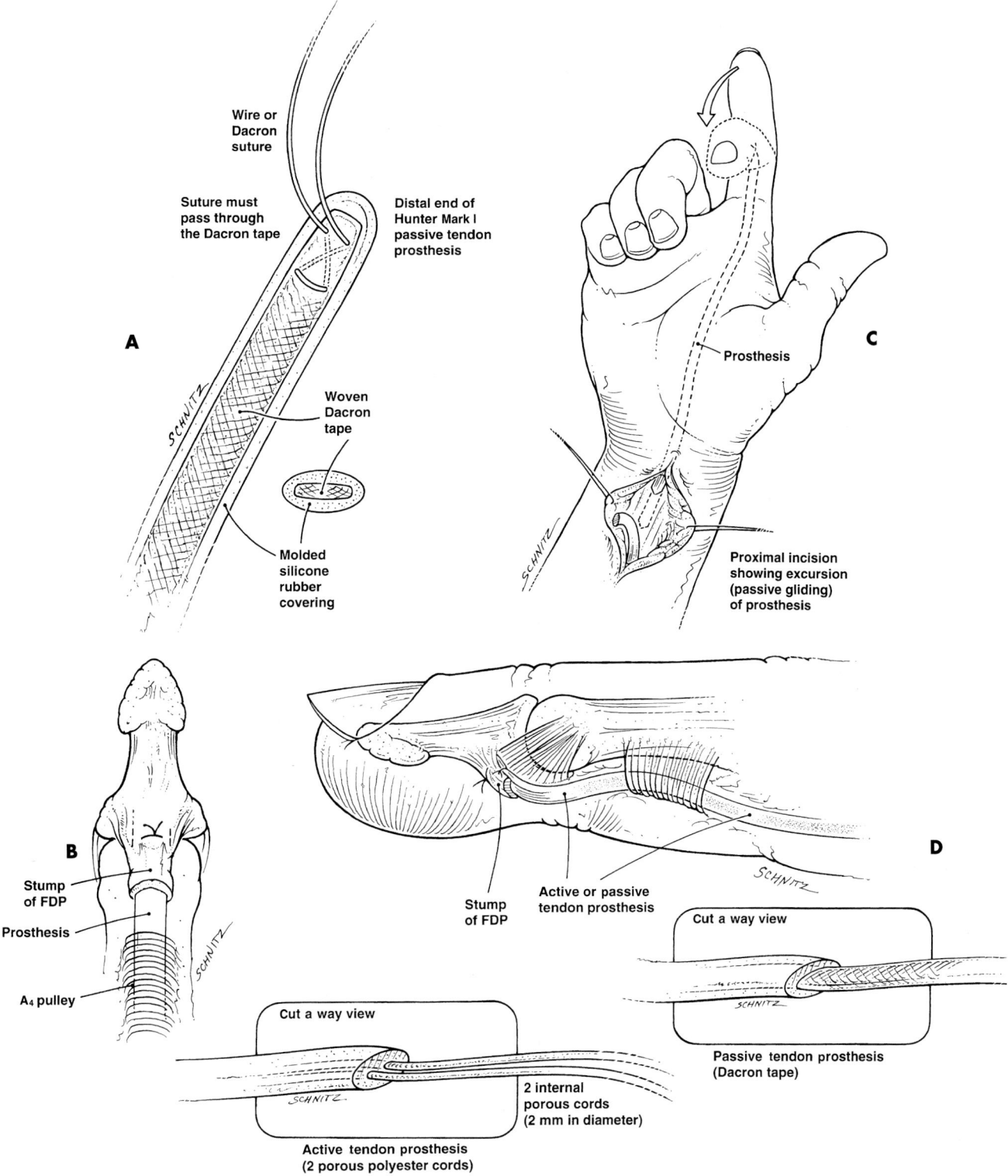

Fig. 29-2. Passive gliding system using the Hunter tendon prosthesis. Stage I: placement of tendon prosthesis after excision of scar and formation of pulleys. **A,** Figure-of-eight suture in distal end of prosthesis. **B,** Distal end of prosthesis sutured to stump of profundus tendon and adjacent fibrous tissue on distal phalanx. **C** and **D,** Prosthesis in place showing free gliding and excursion of its proximal end during passive finger flexion. *FDP,* Flexor digitorum profundus. (From Hunter JM: Staged flexor tendon reconstruction. In Strickland JW, editor: *Master techniques in orthopaedic surgery, the hand,* Philadelphia, 1998, Lippincott-Raven.)

years: passive implants (Mark I) and active implants (Mark II and III). All the implants have a core of woven Dacron that is pressure molded into a radiopaque medical-grade silicone rubber. The surface finish is smooth, and the cross-sectional design is ovoid to aid optimal tendon sheath development. The term *passive gliding implant system*[3] implies that the distal end of the implant is fixed securely to bone or tendon while the proximal end glides freely in the proximal palm or forearm (Figs. 29-2 and 29-3). Movement of the implant is produced by active extension and passive flexion of the digit. A new biologic sheath begins to form around the implant during the period of gliding that follows: stage I surgery. The new sheath progresses through a 4-month phase of biologic maturity and develops a fluid system that supports gliding and nutrition gliding for the tendon graft after stage II. Usually, 3 to 4 months after stage I surgery, the sheath is mature and the implant can be electively replaced by a tendon graft (Figs. 29-4 and 29-5 and Plate 31). The passive implant incorporates design characteristics of firmness and flexibility to permit secure distal fixation and to minimize the buckling effect during the passive push phase of gliding.

Silicone rods are not reinforced and therefore tend to coil and buckle during flexion. Distal fixation is a problem with a simple silicone rod; eventual loosening of the rod results in synovitis and proximal migration. All Hunter implants, active and passive, have been designed with a woven Dacron core to eliminate these problems so that results can be predictable.

The two passive tendon implants available differ only in their distal juncture. One implant has a stainless steel distal metal end plate that is attached to the distal phalanx by a screw. It provides excellent fixation to bone, eliminating loosening and proximal migration of an implant, the number one cause of sheath synovitis. It also provides the added benefit of shortening the second-stage procedure. The screw hole in the distal phalanx acts as a guide hole that is further enlarged in an oblique fashion for the acceptance of the tendon graft. The Woodruff and the 2-mm AO bone screws are available in various sizes. The length of the screw is determined from the preoperative roentgenogram. A pilot hole is drilled at a 15- to 20-degree angle to the DIP joint with a 1.5 drill. The bone cutter should not be used because self-cutting of the bone is needed. The length of the screw should be sufficient to engage the dorsal cortex of the phalanx, but not pass beyond it, because to do so could result in pain dorsally. The tip of the screw should be proximal to the germinal matrix of the nail so as not to cause a nail deformity. This implant is available in 6-, 5-, 4-, and 3-mm diameters. The lengths are either 23 or 25 cm. These implants can be trimmed proximally to the appropriate length.

The passive tendon implant without a screw-fixation terminal device is held in place with a 4-0 nonabsorbable suture that is woven through the distal end of the implant; this distal end is secured under the profundus stump (see Fig. 29-2). Care must be taken to place the suture through the central Dacron core. The distal juncture is also reinforced with two lateral sutures of Dacron. This implant is available in the following sizes: 3 mm × 23 cm, 4 mm × 23 cm, 5 mm × 25 cm, and 6 mm × 25 cm. This implant can also be shortened and should be trimmed at the distal end.

The passive tendon implant is indicated for the young patient with an open epiphyseal plate. A 3-mm tendon implant is often used. The digital end is sutured to the stump of the profundus. Once again, the sutures must be placed in the Dacron core because if the sutures are just in silicone rubber, the distal end will loosen during passive mobilization after the stage I surgery.

Active tendon implant types. Four types of active tendon, one fixed and three adjustable lengths, are available (Fig. 29-6). The fixed-length implant consists of a metal plate distally, a porous-cord silicone flexible shaft, and a preformed porous-cord silicone loop proximally. It is available in 16-, 18-, 20-, and 22-cm lengths and 4-mm overall diameter. The adjustable-length implant is useful when extremely short or long tendon defects are encountered. It allows for length adjustment by pulling the silicone away from the two porous woven polyester cords, allowing for shortening of the implant (Figs. 29-7 to 29-9). Care must be taken not to damage the fine polyester weave while peeling away the silicone. Three designs are available (Table 29-1).

SURGICAL TECHNIQUE
Reconstruction of scarred flexor tendon bed using the basic Dacron reinforced implant

The damaged flexor tendons and their scarred sheath are exposed. In the finger, this is done through a midlateral incision or the zigzag incision of Bruner. In the palm, exposure is accomplished through transverse incision or through a proximal continuation of Bruner zigzag incision. In the forearm, an ulnarly curved volar incision is made to expose the proximal portions of the flexor tendons and their musculotendinous junctions (see Fig. 29-2). A stump of the profundus tendon, 1 cm long, is left attached to the distal phalanx. Scarred tendons, sheath, and retinaculum then are excised. Contracted or scarred lumbricals always should be excised to prevent the paradoxical motion of the lumbrical that is seen after some tendon grafts. This motion causes the finger to extend rather than flex as the patient attempts to flex the finger completely.

Undamaged portions of the flexor fibroosseous retinaculum that are not contracted are retained. Any portion of the retinaculum that can be dilated instrumentally with a hemostat is also preserved; the remainder is excised. The retinacular pulley system (see Figs. 29-1 and 29-2) should be preserved or reconstructed proximal to the axis of motion of each joint; otherwise, normal gliding of the tendon will not

Text continued on page 476

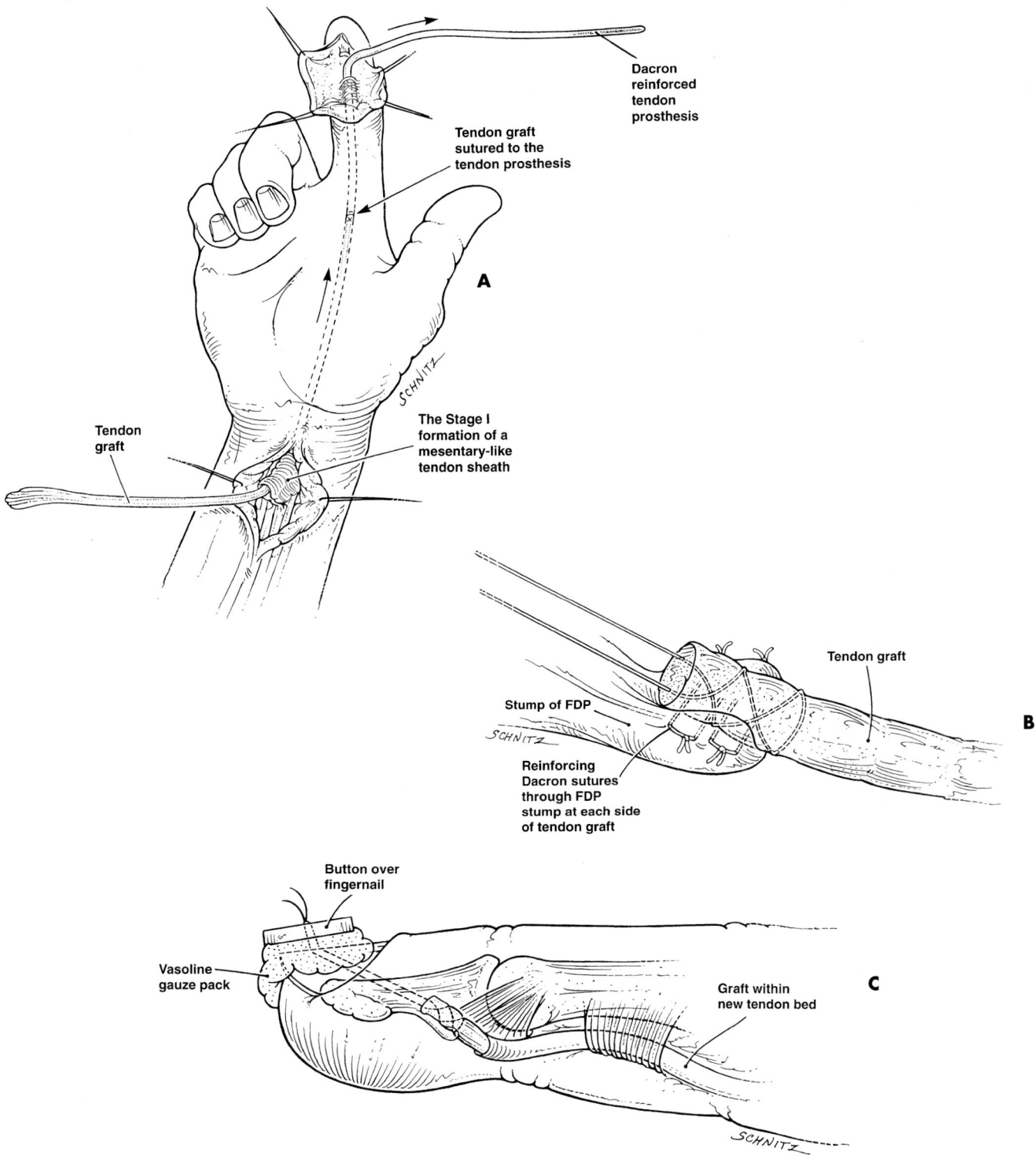

Fig. 29-3. Stage II: removal of prosthesis and insertion of tendon graft. **A,** Graft has been sutured to the proximal end of the prosthesis and then pulled distally through the new tendon bed (note mesentery-like attachment of new sheath visible in the forearm). **B,** Distal anastomosis. Bunnell pull-out suture in distal end of tendon graft. **C,** Distal anastomosis. Complete Bunnell suture with button over fingernail (reinforcing sutures are usually placed through the stump of the profundus tendon). *FDP,* Flexor digitorum profundus. (From Hunter JM: Staged flexor tendon reconstruction. In Strickland JW, editor: *Master techniques in orthopaedic surgery, the hand,* Philadelphia, 1998, Lippincott-Raven.)

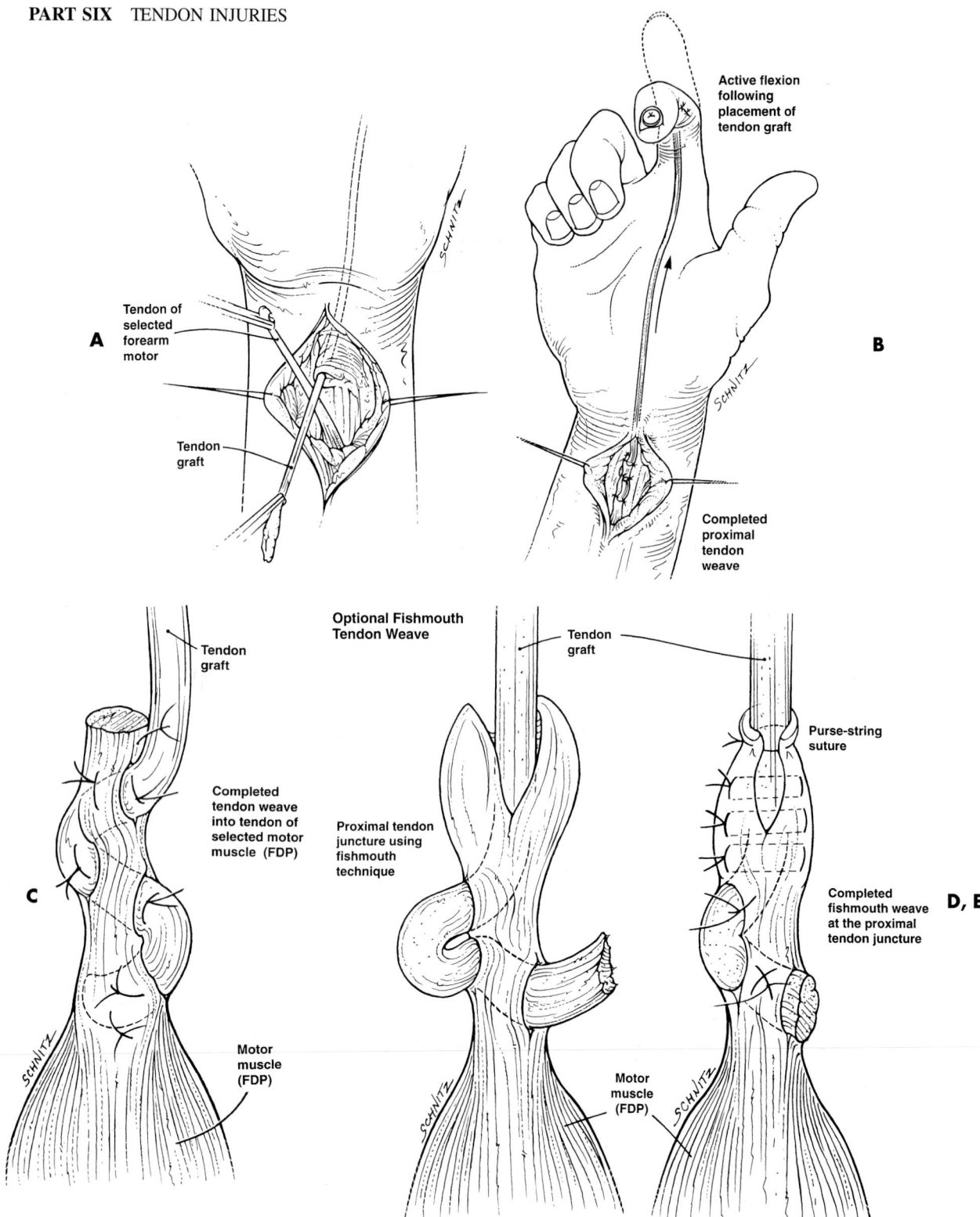

Fig. 29-4. Passive gliding system using the Hunter tendon implant. Stage II: removal of prosthesis and insertion of tendon graft. **A,** Proximal anastomosis measuring excursion of tendon graft and selecting motor (if the procedure is performed under local anesthesia, the true amplitude of active muscle contraction can be measured). **B,** Proximal anastomosis. Graft is threaded through tendon motor muscle two or three times for added strength. **C,** Proximal anastomosis. Stump is fish-mouthed after the method of Pulvertaft; the tension is adjusted, and one suture is inserted as shown (further adjustment of the tension can be accomplished simply by removing and shortening or lengthening as necessary). **D,** Proximal anastomosis. After appropriate tension has been selected, the anastomosis is completed. **E,** Proximal anastomosis. Technique when graft is anastomosed to common profundus tendon. *FDP,* Flexor digitorum profundus. (From Hunter JM: Staged flexor tendon reconstruction. In Strickland JW, editor: *Master techniques in orthopaedic surgery, the hand,* Philadelphia, 1998, Lippincott-Raven.)

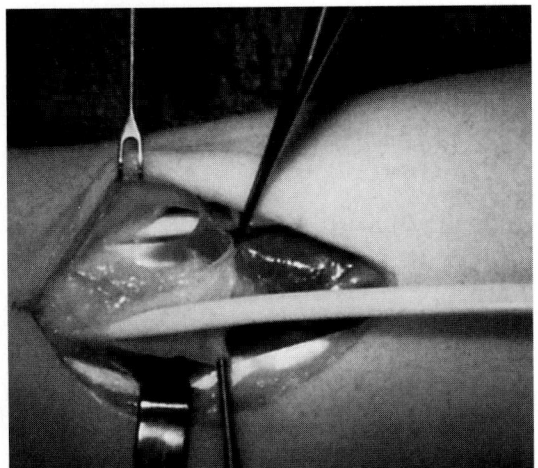

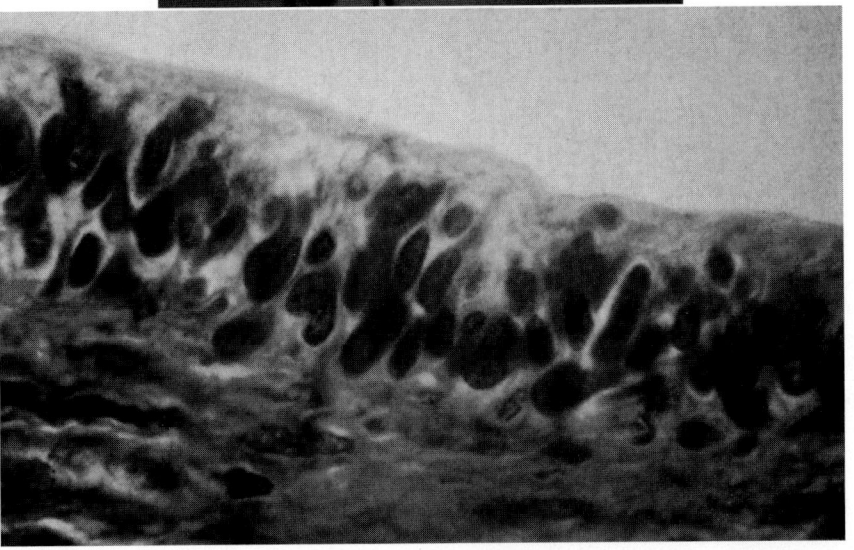

Fig. 29-5. Stage II: **A,** New sheath around Hunter passive tendon at 4 months in forearm. **B,** Pseudosheath at 4 months in forearm; high-power histology. Ready for tendon graft. (From Hunter JM: Staged flexor tendon reconstruction. In Strickland JW, editor: *Master techniques in orthopaedic surgery, the hand,* Philadelphia, 1998, Lippincott-Raven.)

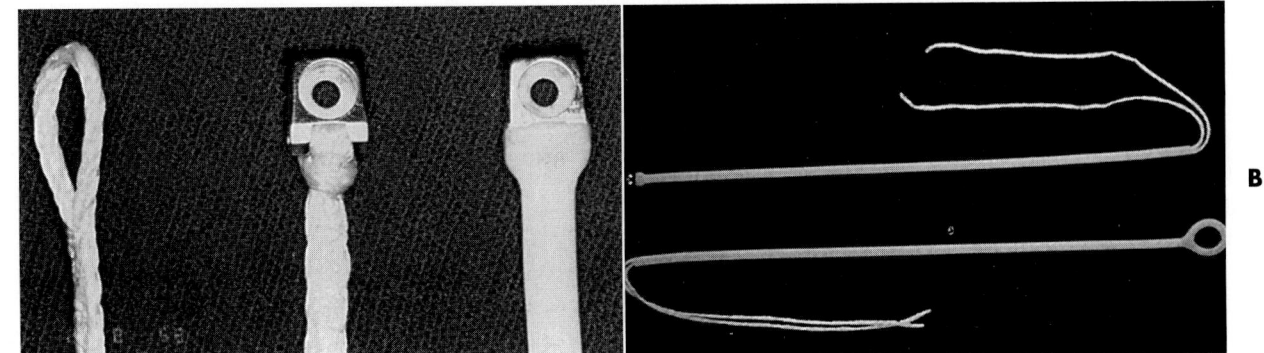

Fig. 29-6. A, Types of active tendon implants. **B,** Fixed-length implant with plate distally and loop proximally; adjustable-length implant with plate distally and porous cords proximally; adjustable-length implant with porous cords distally and loop proximally. (From Hunter JM: Staged flexor tendon reconstruction. In Strickland JW, editor: *Master techniques in orthopaedic surgery, the hand,* Philadelphia, 1998, Lippincott-Raven.)

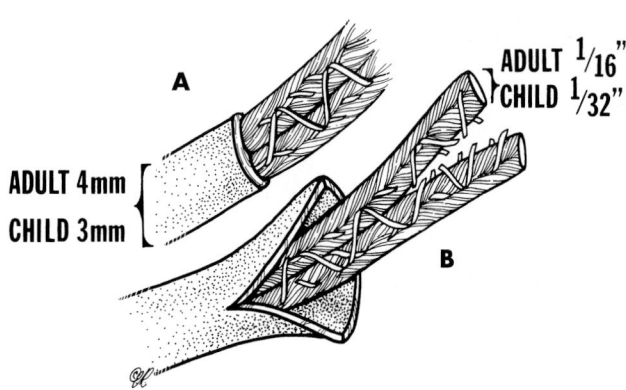

Fig. 29-7. Shortening of the implant. A, The silicone is divided sharply and then peeled back to reveal the polyester cords. B, The cords then are separated by dividing those stitches that keep the cords held together. The total width is 4 mm for the adult implant and 3 mm for the child implant. Each porous cord is ¹⁄₁₆ inch for the adult implant and ¹⁄₃₂ inch for the child implant. (From Hunter JM: Staged flexor tendon reconstruction. In Strickland JW, editor: *Master techniques in orthopaedic surgery, the hand,* Philadelphia, 1998, Lippincott-Raven.)

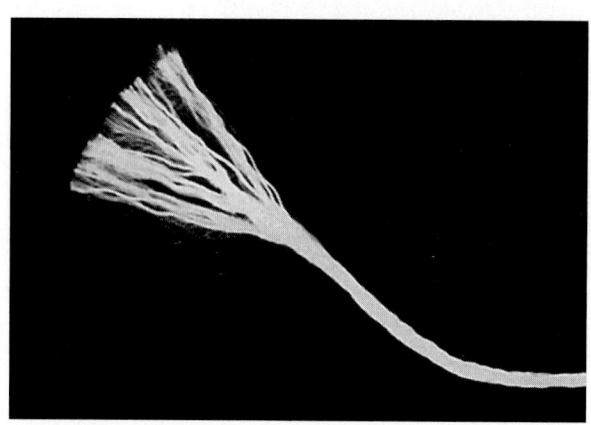

Fig. 29-8. A magnified view shows the helical configuration of the polyester weave. (From Hunter JM: Staged flexor tendon reconstruction. In Strickland JW, editor: *Master techniques in orthopaedic surgery, the hand,* Philadelphia, 1998, Lippincott-Raven.)

be restored. Four pulleys are preferred: one proximal to each of the three finger joints and one at the base of the proximal phalanx.

The distal end of the prosthesis is sutured beneath the stump of the profundus tendon after resecting all but the most distally attached fibers of the tendon (see Fig. 29-2). A figure-of-eight suture of no. 32 and 34 monofilament stainless steel wire (3-0 Ethibond) on an atraumatic taper-cut needle is used. In addition, medial and lateral sutures of no. 35 multifilament wire are passed through the tendon, prosthesis, and fibroperiosteum for further fixation. Any excess of profundus tendon is resected. Traction then is

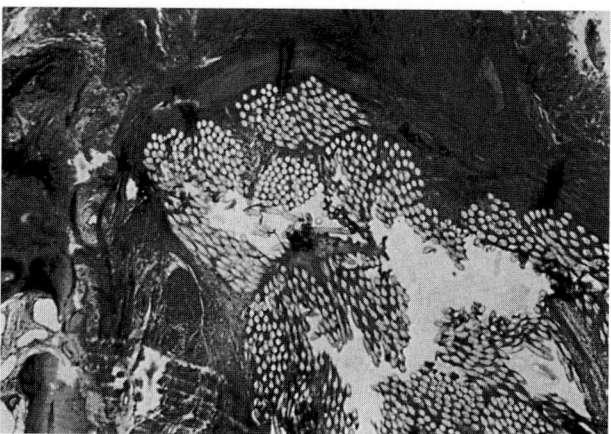

Fig. 29-9. Histologic cross section of porous polyester tendon. Collagenous ingrowth is seen between the fibers. (From Hunter JM: Staged flexor tendon reconstruction. In Strickland JW, editor: *Master techniques in orthopaedic surgery, the hand,* Philadelphia, 1998, Lippincott-Raven.)

Table 29-1. Types of adjustable-length active tendon implants

Distal fixation	Proximal fixation
Metal plate	Two free porous cords
Two free porous cords	Porous-cord silicone loop
Two free porous cords	Two free porous cords

Note: All have 27-cm shafts.

applied on the proximal end of the prosthesis in the forearm to ensure that the attachment of the prosthesis is distal to the DIP joint and its volar plate and that there is no binding of the tendon during flexion and extension. The prosthesis is also observed during passive flexion and extension of the finger (see Fig. 29-2) to ensure that it glides freely with no binding or buckling distal to some part of the pulley system that may be too tight. If any portion of the system is tight, it must be removed and replaced with a new pulley constructed from a free tendon graft.

The proximal end of the prosthesis also should be observed during passive flexion and extension to ensure that it glides properly (see Fig. 29-2). The proximal end of the prosthesis should be in the forearm so that the newly formed sheath extends to the region of the musculotendinous junction of the motor muscle (see Figs. 29-2 and 29-3). The proximal end may be placed superficial or deep to the antebrachial fascia or deep in one of the intermuscular planes. The track for the prosthesis can be fashioned by separating connective tissues and tendon mesenteries with the moistened gloved finger. The track must permit free passive gliding of the prosthesis during passive flexion and extension of the finger. If such a track cannot be established by spreading and adjusting the tissues, the prosthesis should be shortened so that, when the finger is fully extended, the proximal end of the prosthesis lies proximal to the flexion crease at the wrist. When multiple prostheses are threaded through the carpal canal, the superficialis tendons are generally removed from the canal.

Finally, before the wound is closed, traction should be applied to the prosthesis again and the amount of active finger motion determined and recorded (see Fig. 29-3). Importantly, if this maneuver does not produce full flexion, it may be necessary to modify the pulley system.

A small amount of barium sulfate is incorporated in Dacron-reinforced active and passive implants so that their function can be checked roentgenographically at 6 weeks and again just before insertion of the tendon graft. Antero-posterior and lateral roentgenograms of the hand and distal half of the forearm are made with the fingers and wrist in full extension and full flexion. These roentgenograms will demonstrate how much the proximal end of the prosthesis moves with respect to the distal end of the radius. If there is full ROM of the wrist and all finger joints, an excision of 5 to 6 cm is not unusual (see Figs. 29-3 and 29-4).

Stage II tendon grafting following active or passive implants

The interval between stages I and II should be 2 to 6 months, or long enough to permit maturation of the tendon bed to the point where it can nourish and lubricate the gliding tendon graft and until maximum softening of the tissues and mobilization of the stiff joints has been achieved. Each case must be individualized, and the decision to do the second-stage procedure must be made by the surgeon on the basis of the findings in the hand.

Before stage II surgery, the limits of extension and flexion of the finger must be accurately measured and recorded to establish the base for postoperative care. A short midlateral or Bruner zigzag incision then is made to locate the distal end of the prosthesis, where it is attached to the distal phalanx. This attachment is left intact, and a second ulnarly curved volar incision is made in the forearm through the original stage I incision to expose the proximal end of the prosthesis and the musculotendinous junction of the superficialis or profundus tendon, which is used as a motor for the tendon graft. With the prosthesis still in place, excursion of the proximal end of the prosthesis as the finger is moved from full extension to full flexion also should be measured as an additional check on the amount of excursion that the motor muscle must have to provide full finger motion.

The palmaris longus tendon works for short tendon grafting: thumb, fifth finger, and sublimus fingers. Longer grafts may be required for longer fingers. A long tendon graft is obtained from one leg (preferably, the plantaris) but if this is missing, a long-toe extensor tendon may be used. If a toe extensor must be used, the graft is obtained using a modified Brand tendon stripper and two or more incisions so that the portion of the tendon proximal to the retinaculum is obtained. Any attached fat or muscle is removed, and one end

of the graft is sutured to the proximal end of the passive implant with a catgut or polyester suture (see Fig. 29-3, *A*). Leaving the distal end of the prosthesis attached to the distal phalanx, the remainder of the prosthesis with the attached tendon graft is pulled distally, thereby treading the graft through the new sheath. The prosthesis then is removed and discarded. Free motion of the graft in the sheath can be confirmed by grasping each end of the graft with a hemostat and pulling it proximally and distally.

The tendon graft is secured to the distal phalanx using a Bunnell-type wire suture, with the button on the fingernail, and medial and lateral reinforcing sutures through the profundus tendon stump (see Fig. 29-3). Traction is applied to the proximal end of the graft, and the predicted range of active flexion, measured as the distance of the finger pulp from the distal palmar crease, is determined. After this maneuver, attachment of the graft to the distal phalanx is inspected to check the security of the fixation.

Scar tissue from previous surgery, antebrachial fascia, and muscle fascia are excised to minimize motion-restricting adhesions. When the firm fascia is carefully dissected away from the newly formed tendon sheath, the sheath is found to be soft, with loose mesentery-like attachments to the surrounding tissues. The sheath should be resected far enough distally that there will be no scar in the region of the tendon suture of the anastomosis; this is not always possible, however. In this event, the sheath is either dissected away completely so that there is no contact between the anastomosis and the sheath, or the sheath may be left open so that one side of the anastomosis glides on the sheath (see Fig. 29-4).

For the index finger, when either the superficialis or the profundus muscle is available as a motor, the graft is anastomosed to the proximal segment of the motor tendon according to the method of Pulvertaft (see Fig. 29-4). However, for the long, ring, and little fingers, the graft is woven through the oblique stab incisions in the common profundus tendon, securing the different tendons together as one tendon unit (see Fig. 29-4).

It is essential to adjust the length of the graft accurately. The excursion of the prosthesis during flexion and extension has already been determined. The excursion of the tendon graft should be checked by pulling on the graft, starting with the finger in full extension (see Fig. 29-4). Having determined the excursion necessary to produce a full range of flexion, the excursions of the available motors then are determined, and the one with the requisite excursion is selected.

The tension of the graft is adjusted so that, with the wrist in neutral, the involved finger rests in slightly more flexion than that of the adjacent fingers (see Fig. 29-22). When the anastomosis has been completed, the tension is checked with the wrist in both flexion and extension to assess the tenodesis effect and to ensure that the tension of the graft is correct. If the patient is under local anesthesia, after the distal anastomosis is completed and the distal wound is closed, the

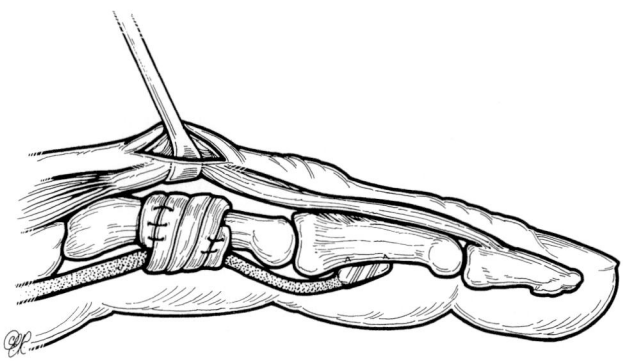

Fig. 29-10. Pulley reconstruction in a superficialis finger. A retractor is placed into a split that is made centrally in the extensor hood. This is accomplished via a dorsal skin incision to retract the extensor hood to allow for passage of the free tendon graft. Four loops are used to reconstruct the A₂ pulley. (From Hunter JM: Staged flexor tendon reconstruction. In Strickland JW, editor: *Master techniques in orthopaedic surgery, the hand,* Philadelphia, 1998, Lippincott-Raven.)

graft is sutured tentatively to the motor tendon and, after the tourniquet has been deflated for 10 to 15 minutes, the patient is asked to flex and extend the finger. If the predicted amount of active flexion is not achieved, the tension of the graft is readjusted or a motor with more excursion is selected. When the best possible function has been achieved, the anastomosis is completed, and the wound is closed and dressed.

Stage I: the active tendon implant

This technique is divided into two stages, although stage II may be delayed for months or years. Stage I is similar to stage II using the passive tendon implant, and the same indications are used. The major differences are the exact type of implant and the placement of the proximal junction to an active motor tendon for early function.

Implant positioning. The distal component is passed from the palm through the finger pulleys using a no-touch technique, which can be facilitated by moistening the device with Ringer's solution. The implants with porous cords distally or proximally are easily passed, whereas those with a distal metal plate are more difficult. Wet umbilical tape or heavy nonabsorbable, nonmetallic suture is threaded through the screw hole. Both ends of the tape or suture are used to guide the distal component through the A₁ and A₂ pulleys. In most cases, the A₄ retinaculum needs to be cut along the periosteal rim on the middle phalanx to allow the implant to pass. The A₄ pulley should be repaired with multiple sutures using small drill holes if necessary.

Pulley reconstruction. As with the passive tendon technique, stage I is the time for pulley reconstruction, if it is necessary. The flexor retinaculum must be reconstructed and of adequate strength to support the strong vector forces of the active flexor tendon implant. A free tendon graft is wrapped around the bone (Fig. 29-10). The tendon is passed under the extensor tendon hood for A₂ and A₄ pulley

reconstruction. At least two wraps are recommended for adequate strength to allow early active motion. If possible, four wraps are preferred for A₂ reconstruction. A separate small dorsal skin and extensor tendon incision will allow a retractor to be placed to lift the extensor tendons to facilitate passing the free graft under the extensor tendon hood. After the graft has been wrapped, it is held with sutures connecting each wrap. The tendon graft pulley placed in the dorsal synovial bed under the extensor tendon will remain soft and flat during function.

Proximal implant placement. Next, the implant is passed proximally from palm to forearm through the carpal canal. If necessary, a tendon passer can be used (see Fig. 29-19). The diameter of the passer should be slightly larger than that of the implant. Again, the implant with porous cords is easily passed proximally, whereas the implant with a silicone loop may be more difficult proximally. A wet umbilical tape can be looped through the implant loop and brought into the forearm on a tendon passer. It is imperative to protect the silicone coating on the loop during this process.

Distal fixation: metal plate (active or passive implants). The distal component must be fixed to allow strong, durable, immediate juncture. With the joint identified, the base of the distal phalanx is stripped of volar periosteum, and the following steps are performed (Fig. 29-11). The point where the screw should enter the bone is measured. The ideal position of the component is with its proximal edge 3 mm distal to the joint. This position is marked. The plate then is centered over the marked bone (Fig. 29-11, *A*). The dorsum of the patient's finger is placed on a firm part of the operative table, and a bone impacter is positioned against the plate and "struck firmly," which drives the four sharp spikes into the bone so that the plate is secure and evenly aligned on the bone. A 1.5-mm drill bit is passed through both cortices of bone at an angle 15 degrees dorsal to the joint line (Fig. 29-11, *B*), and a lateral radiograph is taken. The drill should have missed the joint and base of the nail and should be in the central portion of the cortical bone.

A 2-mm AO screw is recommended (Fig. 29-11, *C*). Holding the joint securely, the proper 1.5-mm-diameter hole is drilled, and the proper screw length is chosen. The distal end is secured by carefully turning the screw through both cortices of bone to thumb tightness. The screw should appear dorsally with less than 1 mm protruding. The screw fit should be firm all the way, and final fixation should be secure. If the final screw turns are loose, the system may not endure cyclic force. If the screw fixation is not firm, it should be either reinserted more distally in bone or fixed with twisted wires (see following discussion). Importantly, the four metal spikes on the metal end of the implant do the hard work, and the screw merely holds the plate securely in place. The profundus tendon stump should be drawn over the distal component and sutured laterally to provide a soft tissue buffer to prevent irritation of the overlying skin (Fig. 29-11, *D*). In the superficialis finger procedure, a strip of superficialis tendon may be drawn over the distal component and

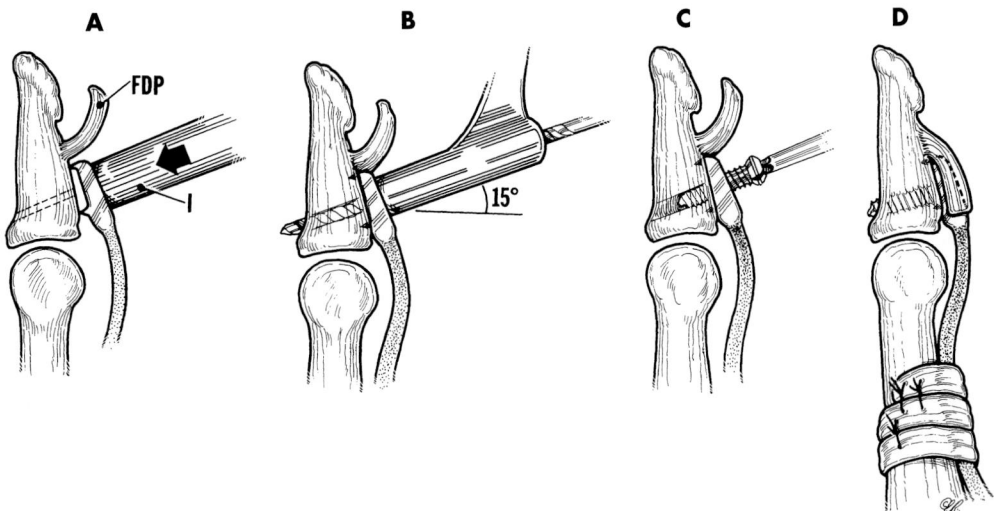

Fig. 29-11. Distal implant fixation, screw technique. **A,** The plate is centered over the marked bone and a bone impactor is used to strike the plate firmly to secure it to the distal phalanx. **B,** A 1.5-mm drill bit is passed through both cortices of bone at an angle 15 degrees dorsal to the joint line. The drill should miss the joint and base of the nail and be in the central portion of the cortical bone. **C,** A 2-mm screw is used to securely fix the plate. **D,** The profundus tendon stump then is drawn over the distal component and sutured laterally to provide a soft tissue buffer to prevent irritation of the overlying skin. Reconstruction of the A$_4$ pulley is also shown. *FDP,* Flexor digitorum profundus stump; *I,* bone impactor. (From Hunter JM: Staged flexor tendon reconstruction. In Strickland JW, editor: *Master techniques in orthopaedic surgery, the hand,* Philadelphia, 1998, Lippincott-Raven.)

sutured laterally at the middle phalanx level. The tourniquet is released, the wounds are irrigated, and the distal incision is closed.

The distal component is also designed to allow fixation by two twisted wires through the bone as well as the screw. If the bone has been fractured or shows osteoporosis, wiring is preferred. Also, if the bone is deformed during preparation for screw insertion, the wire fixation by two drill holes is preferred (Fig. 29-12). The distal metal component with spikes must be held securely to bone to prevent movement and wire fracture. Fixation must be strong enough to prevent the tendency of the plate to lift off the distal phalanx (Fig. 29-13).

The active tendon may be fixed to the distal phalanx for a one-tendon, three-joint finger or to the middle phalanx for a one-tendon, two-joint finger (the superficialis finger).

Distal fixation: two porous cords (active tendon only). In this technique, the porous cords are passed through drill holes in the bone, which may be facilitated with a Swanson tendon passer. The polyester cords then are tied with a square knot that is reinforced with 3-0 Ethibond Dacron sutures. It is extremely important that a taper-cut needle be used for the reinforcing stitch because a cutting needle will damage the polyester fibers. Fixation with helical porous cords is uniquely useful for salvage when a proximal interphalangeal (PIP) joint arthroplasty with intramedullary stems is necessary in superficialis finger reconstruction (Fig. 29-14). It is also useful for the small finger and in young people where the metal plate may be too large.

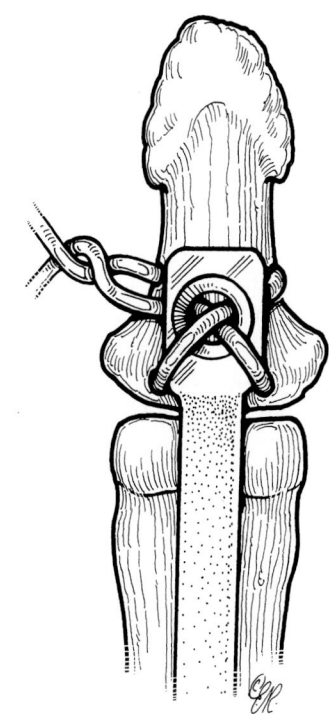

Fig. 29-12. Distal implant fixation, wire technique. The wire is passed in a figure-of-eight through drill holes to secure the plate. The wire should pass over the proximal portion of the plate to prevent this from lifting up during active finger flexion. (From Hunter JM: Staged flexor tendon reconstruction. In Strickland JW, editor: *Master techniques in orthopaedic surgery, the hand,* Philadelphia, 1998, Lippincott-Raven.)

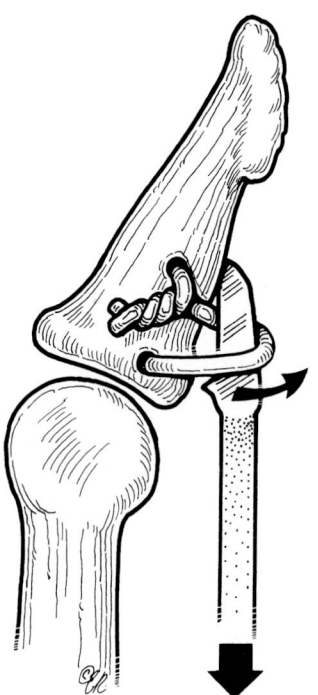

Fig. 29-13. Potential problem with distal fixation. As the distal interphalangeal joint is actively flexed, the force of the tendon tends to pull up the proximal aspects of the plate. It is extremely important to hold down the proximal portion of the plate with the wire. (From Hunter JM: Staged flexor tendon reconstruction. In Strickland JW, editor: *Master techniques in orthopaedic surgery, the hand,* Philadelphia, 1998, Lippincott-Raven.)

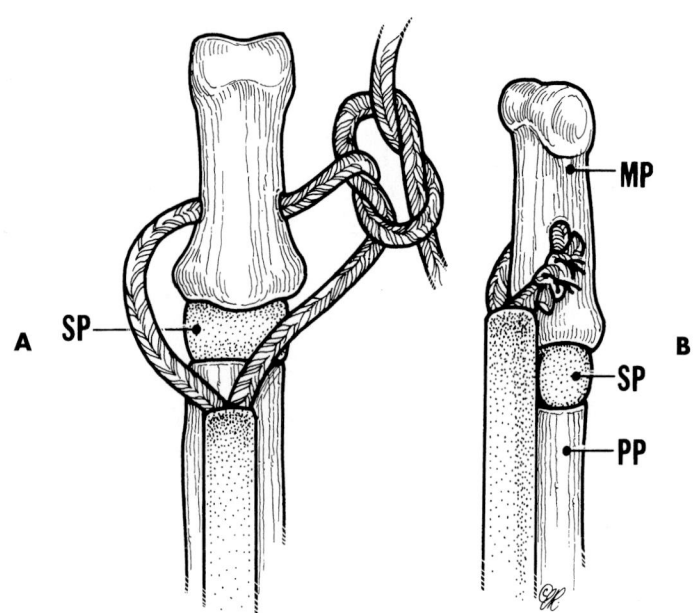

Fig. 29-14. Distal implant fixation: porous-cord technique with Swanson proximal interphalangeal (PIP) implant. **A,** The porous cords are passed through the previously drilled hole in the middle phalanx and tied with a square knot. **B,** The square knot is reinforced with 3-0 nonabsorbable sutures. The stump of the superficialis tendon then can be sutured down over the implant (not shown). *MP,* Middle phalanx; *PP,* proximal phalanx; *SP,* Swanson PIP implant. (From Hunter JM: Staged flexor tendon reconstruction. In Strickland JW, editor: *Master techniques in orthopaedic surgery, the hand,* Philadelphia, 1998, Lippincott-Raven.)

Proximal fixation: loop method (active tendon only).
The length of the motor tendon must be sufficient to pass through the proximal loop and return proximally for at least two 90-degree passes through the tendon. Desired excursion of the motor tendon is 4 cm for the flexor digitorum profundus and 3 cm for the flexor digitorum superficialis. If the patient can be aroused from anesthesia, an accurate assessment of the muscle amplitude is possible. Otherwise, the traditional technique of passively flexing and extending the wrist to obtain a cascade of the fingers is effective. The operated finger should be slightly more flexed than the adjacent fingers.

The selected motor tendon is passed through the implant loop and then through a small longitudinal split in the tendon (Fig. 29-15). One suture is placed through the tendon for temporary fixation. The tension then is tested by moistening the implant surface with saline, followed by wrist flexion and extension. The finger should lie in extension during wrist flexion and show a position of slight flexion over balance with the adjacent fingers on wrist extension. If this is acceptable, a second suture is placed and the tendon is turned 90 degrees through one or two additional longitudinal splits in the tendon. Tendon balance is retested to ensure that there has been no loss of tendon tension.

Proximal fixation: two porous cords (active tendon only). The helical porous cords are woven into the lateral borders of the tendon with a free needle or a sharp tendon presser and fixed with 3-0 Ethibond sutures at points of exit (Fig. 29-16). Tendon balance is tested, as previously described, after the first two sutures and is readjusted if necessary. After three or four passes, the cords can be tied securely with a square knot and reinforced with 3-0 Ethibond sutures. The free ends are cut with 200° F electric cautery. Only taper-cut needles should be used during all reinforcement procedures because cutting needles will seriously damage the delicate polyester weave. The final balance of the fingers is again checked. When satisfactory tendon tension has been achieved, the proximal juncture is tucked beneath the muscle folds and the muscle is gently closed over the juncture with 5-0 sutures.

Stage II: active tendon replacement

A short Bruner zigzag incision is made to locate the distal end of the device where it is attached to the phalanx. This

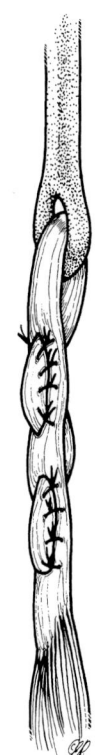

Fig. 29-15. Proximal implant fixation, loop technique. The tendon is passed through the porous-cord silicone loop and then sutured to itself. Several weaves are made for firm fixation. Tension is checked after the first weave. (From Hunter JM: Staged flexor tendon reconstruction. In Strickland JW, editor: *Master techniques in orthopaedic surgery, the hand,* Philadelphia, 1998, Lippincott-Raven.)

attachment is left intact, and a second ulnarly curved incision is made through the previous stage I incision in the distal volar forearm to expose the proximal end of the device.

Either the palmaris longus, plantaris, or long-toe extensor tendon is obtained for use as the graft. The proximal end of the implant is removed from the motor tendon by cutting the polyester-reinforced silicone loop. If the proximal weave technique has been used, the cords are cut through at the sheath juncture. When the implant and tendon have been sufficiently separated, the proximal end of the implant is trimmed to a straight edge. One end of the tendon graft is sutured to the proximal end of the implant. The distal end of the implant is left attached to the distal phalanx, and the rest of the implant with the attached tendon graft is pulled distally. The distal end of the implant is now removed, and the graft is freed for distal juncture to bone. This procedure is completed by following established techniques for tendon grafting. One important exception is that the connective tissue around the proximal juncture should be carefully preserved and closed around the new tendon graft juncture with fine sutures. When the proximal tendon anastomosis is completed, great care is taken to preserve the sheath and

peritenon (see Fig. 29-21). First, the peritenon is gently pushed proximally until the musculotendinous junction is exposed; then, after completion of the anastomosis, the peritenon is pulled distally and sutured to the proximal end of the newly formed sheath or to the surrounding tissues as far distally as possible. The wound is irrigated with sterile saline solution and then closed, and the final dressing is applied, with a plaster splint to maintain the wrist and metacarpophalangeal (MP) joints in moderate flexion and the interphalangeal (IP) joints in slight flexion.

POSTOPERATIVE MANAGEMENT
Stage I

Following skin closure, a standard postoperative hand dressing is applied, with the wrist and MP joints in moderate flexion (40 to 50 degrees) and the IP joints in slight flexion (20 to 30 degrees). In this position, the new sheath will be formed proximally and free excursion of the prosthesis distally will be possible when passive motion is begun at 3 weeks. Where there are joint contractures before insertion of the prosthesis, intermittent dynamic splinting may be required to prevent recurrence of the contracture. This periodic elastic traction on the fingers, while the wrist and MP joints are maintained in position by splinting, may be started during the first postoperative week. Gentle passive motion of all joints is started gradually during the second to fourth weeks and PIP contracture control is now introduced. Regular passive stretching, under the supervision of the hand therapist, is begun in the fifth week and the patient is taught at this time to flex the finger whenever possible, using an adjacent finger hooked over the damaged one. Usually, by the sixth week, range of passive motion is improved.

Stage II

Therapy begins the first postoperative day and is the same as for a one-stage tendon graft. Usually by 8 weeks, patients are permitted full activities with restrictions on full-power grip until 12 weeks after surgery.

The immature mesothelial sheath is formed around the tendon implant by 72 hours and becomes a functioning organ by 4 weeks; 4 to 5 months usually are required for hand reconditioning. As time passes, with the tendon implant actively gliding in the digit, the motor unit becomes stronger, ROM is maximized, and soft tissue becomes more pliable. The digit is better prepared for stage II.

The interval between stage I and stage II can be quite variable. The active tendon implant should be retained for at least 4 months to allow for maturing of the proximal juncture and biologic softening of connective tissues. If the proximal juncture fails, stage II surgery still can be delayed if there is full passive gliding on radiographic examination and there are no signs of synovitis. Patients who have returned to work and a normal lifestyle can benefit beyond 1 year before stage II tendon grafting. Indeed, stage II may be delayed indefinitely.

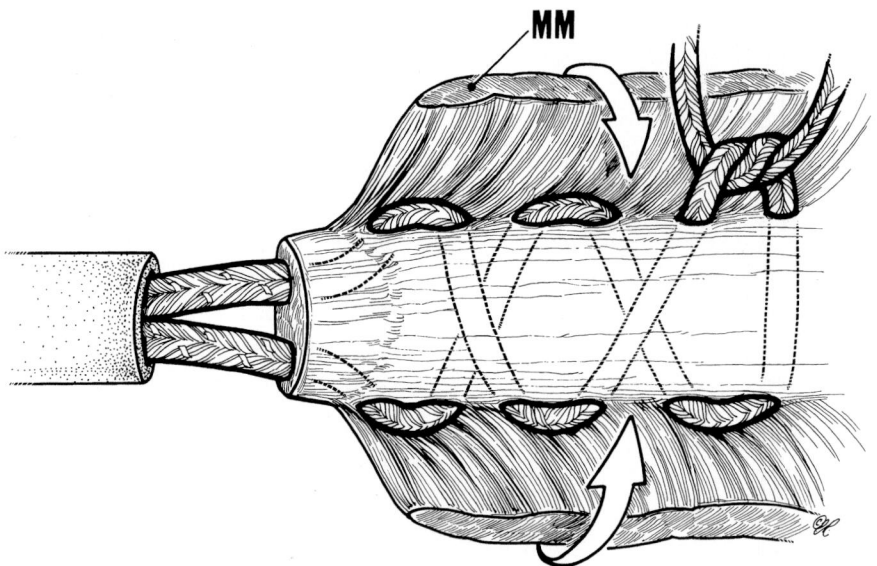

Fig. 29-16. Proximal implant fixation, porous-cord technique. The cords are woven through the proximal tendon in a criss-cross fashion after the muscle has been stripped off into the musculotendinous junction. The cords then are tied with a square knot that is then reinforced. The muscle is then repaired over the cords with fine absorbable sutures. *MM,* Muscle. (From Hunter JM: Staged flexor tendon reconstruction. In Strickland JW, editor: *Master techniques in orthopaedic surgery, the hand,* Philadelphia, 1998, Lippincott-Raven.)

Postoperatively, the patient's hand is kept in a protective dorsal splint with the wrist in 30 degrees of flexion, the MP joints at 70 degrees, and the IP joints in full extension. Early mobilization with elastic-band traction begins the first postoperative day. Postoperative therapy is similar to that after stage I. In patients who develop rapid function, the splint will be maintained for approximately 12 weeks to guard the distal and proximal junctures as adhesions are reduced by gliding function.

Stage II tendon grafting. Early protected active flexion of the grafted finger is encouraged while a padded dorsal splint prevents sudden forceful extension. The wrist is splinted in 30 degrees and the MP joints in 40 degrees. Each patient is instructed at the first postoperative dressing, usually after 5 to 7 days, to splint the MP joints while the PIP and DIP joints are actively flexed and extended. Intermittent splinting is continued during the fourth week while the suture and button are still in place. At the fifth or sixth week, the button wire is removed, and light, active supervised stretching exercises are encouraged. Some vigorous patients with full excursion of the graft may require splinting during the sixth to eighth weeks to protect the proximal anastomosis from excessive stress. If stubborn contractures were present before tendon grafting, a supervised program of passive stretching and splinting of the stiff joints may be required after the fifth week. Patients should achieve a full range of active motion during the sixth to twelfth weeks. Intensive training in active exercises during this period, personally supervised by the operating surgeon, are essential. *The goal after stage II is to match the ROM gained after stage I with active flexion by way of the tendon graft in the new gliding bed and the base of the active tendon juncture bed* (see Figs. 29-27 and 29-28).

COMPLICATIONS
Stage I

Loosening of the distal attachment is the number one cause of problems such as sheath synovitis and implant migration. Careful fixation of the metal end plate at stage I eliminates this complication. The silicone rod used in the first reconstructions in 1960 often showed loosening because reinforced rubber does not hold sutures well. In the United States, all passive and active implant designs were reinforced for secure suturing or had metal end plates after 1966.

Synovitis of the new flexor tendon sheath may occur around a gliding implant or a tendon graft. In either instance, a smear or culture is required to rule out infection if the swelling does not resolve with rest. Swelling of the sheath is an early sign of a mechanical change in implant gliding function. This is the time to review radiographs, in flexion and extension, and to look for separation of the distal juncture of the implant, buckling of a tight pulley, or actual migration of the implant. Implant migration to a forearm compartment is usually silent and may be identified only before stage II tendon grafting by a forearm roentgenogram.

Early management with antibiotic therapy or rest for swelling of the flexor sheath could eliminate infectious tenosynovitis. Implant synovitis can be controlled by rest because it is usually a mechanical problem in an early phase. If neglected, however, it will erupt with inflammation and sheath pressure through a previous wound site (the so-called blister that is similar to a pyrogenic granuloma). Once opened to the outside, it represents a true infection; treatment is implant removal with scalene and triple antibiotic wound irrigation, followed by replacement of a new implant or tendon graft. Silicone tendon implants are similar to silicone joint implants: Delayed removal of a mechanically unstable implant progresses to chronic changes and deterioration of adjacent bone and soft tissue. After removal of the implant, a return visit 3 to 6 months later for reevaluation for reconstruction is recommended.

Pulley rupture. Pulley rupture occurs at stage I with an active tendon and represents a sagging-out of the old original pulley or a weak grafted pulley. Pulley replacement is now indicated at stage II tendon grafting.

Stage II tendon graft complications

Several complications may be noted after stage II. Pulley failure and adhesions may be brought on by faulty tendon graft gliding. This complication occurs more commonly with the passive gliding implant. The pulley strength does not really come under evaluation until the sixth or eighth week in therapy, and rupture occurs during training, despite finger and external pulley support. Pulley reconstruction around the biologic sheath will be required later. Pulley failure may herald adhesions at the proximal juncture, restricting gliding during the eighth to twelfth weeks of postoperative recovery. Eventual tenolysis will be necessary around the proximal tendon juncture. Tendon graft rupture is rare and, when it occurs, it is late. The distal juncture and proximal juncture separation that follows violent activity (i.e., a fight or fall) is the most likely cause of tendon graft rupture. Rupture in midgraft is very rare: Three occurred in a series of more than 700 staged cases. The distal and proximal tendon rupture treatment is immediate repair; functional salvage is expected. The rare midgraft rupture will require replacement with either a new tendon graft or an active tendon implant.

ILLUSTRATIVE CASES FOR TECHNIQUE

Two case studies, both males in their early 20s, are reviewed to emphasize two specific indications for staged flexor tendon reconstruction: In case study 2, the flexor tendon injury was followed by a failed primary repair. In case study 1, the flexor tendon injury was compounded by three failed surgeries.

Case study 1: stage I. Active tendon reconstruction following failed reconstruction

The patient, a 21-year-old male tree surgeon and guitar player, sustained a zone II injury with a tree saw, compound fractures of the proximal phalanx, and destruction of the flexor tendon system of the right index finger. His surgeries consisted of (1) primary repair of double tendon laceration, digital nerve repair, and reduction of proximal phalanx fracture; (2) fractures healed from his second operation (flexor tenolysis for

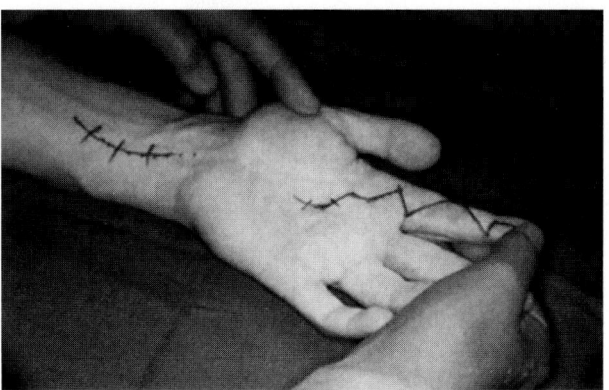

Fig. 29-17. Case study 1. Incision for stage I reconstruction: nutrition, sensation, and passive range of motion are satisfactory at the time of surgery. (From Hunter JM: Staged flexor tendon reconstruction. In Strickland JW, editor: *Master techniques in orthopaedic surgery, the hand,* Philadelphia, 1998, Lippincott-Raven.)

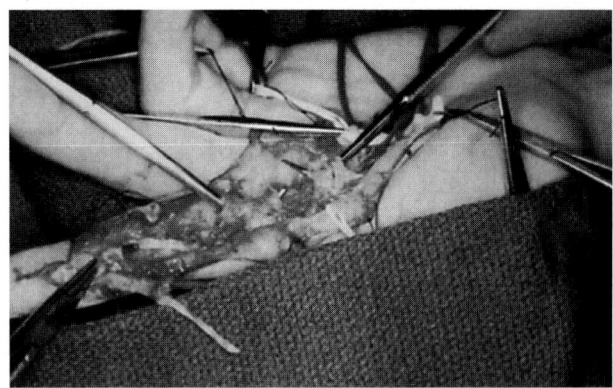

Fig. 29-18. Case study 1. Exploration of flexor tendon bed of right index finger. The tendon bridge graft is removed at the distal part of the wound. Three key pulleys are preserved, with metal instruments identifying the pulleys. *Note:* The A_2 pulley eventually failed by rupture, requiring late reconstruction after stage II grafting. (From Hunter JM: Staged flexor tendon reconstruction. In Strickland JW, editor: *Master techniques in orthopaedic surgery, the hand,* Philadelphia, 1998, Lippincott-Raven.)

failed primary repairs); and (3) a second flexor tenolysis and bridge grafting of damaged tendons using available superficialis tendon, with two suture lines adjacent to the site of injury. The patient had achieved no useful function in his right index finger. He was self-referred after being told by his surgeon that nothing further could be accomplished.

Before making an incision for stage I reconstruction, nutrition, sensation, and passive range of motion (PROM) were assessed and found to be satisfactory (Fig. 29-17 and Plate 32). The flexor tendon bed of the right index finger was explored and the tendon bridge graft was removed at the distal part of the wound (Fig. 29-18 and Plate 33). Three key pulleys were preserved, with metal instruments identifying the pulleys. The A_2 pulley eventually failed by rupture, requiring late reconstruction after stage II grafting.

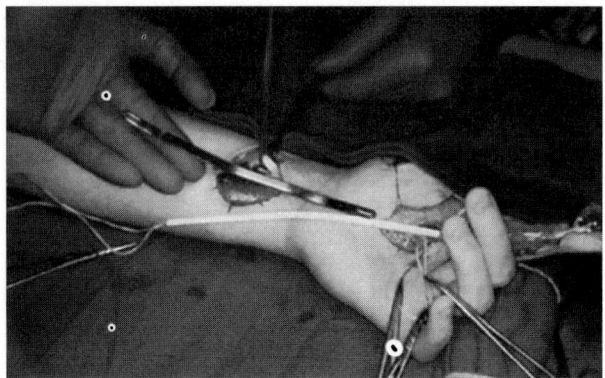

Fig. 29-19. Case study 1. Flexor tendon bed has been prepared by removing all scar tissue and preserving the pulleys. Digital nerves are identified by yellow vessel loops. Long active tendon implants are being sized on the hand (note metal plate distal and two porous cords proximal). An Ober tendon passer is shown and is used to guide the proximal end of the tendon implants to the palm and into the forearm. The loop retractor holds the profundus tendon to the index in the forearm (this is the future motor tendon). (From Hunter JM: Staged flexor tendon reconstruction. In Strickland JW, editor: *Master techniques in orthopaedic surgery, the hand,* Philadelphia, 1998, Lippincott-Raven.)

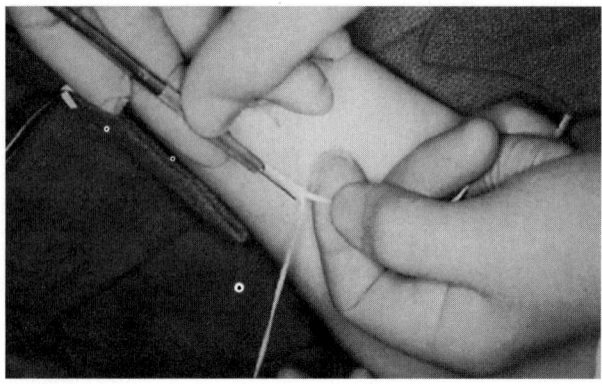

Fig. 29-20. Case study 1. Preparing the length of the active tendon: silicone rubber is trimmed away and two Dacron cords are separated. (From Hunter JM: Staged flexor tendon reconstruction. In Strickland JW, editor: *Master techniques in orthopaedic surgery, the hand,* Philadelphia, 1998, Lippincott-Raven.)

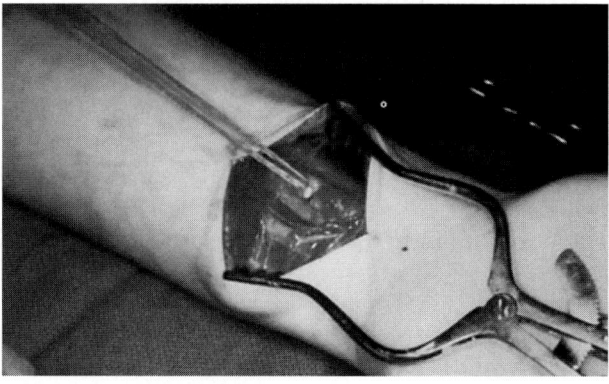

Fig. 29-21. Case study 1. Proximal junction completed between tendon implant and flexor to determine the profundus tendon of the index finger in the forearm: two Dacron cords are divided using hot cautery, with the distal end completed first by fixing the metal plate of the distal phalanx with a screw. Finally, the muscle of the flexor profundus of the index finger will gently cover the juncture. (From Hunter JM: Staged flexor tendon reconstruction. In Strickland JW, editor: *Master techniques in orthopaedic surgery, the hand,* Philadelphia, 1998, Lippincott-Raven.)

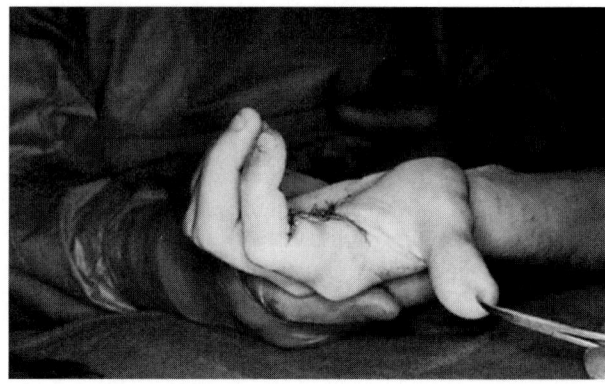

Fig. 29-22. Case study 1. Stage I: complete tendon balance is noted with wrist in the neutral position. (From Hunter JM: Staged flexor tendon reconstruction. In Strickland JW, editor: *Master techniques in orthopaedic surgery, the hand,* Philadelphia, 1998, Lippincott-Raven.)

The flexor tendon bed was prepared by removing all scar tissue and preserving the pulleys (Fig. 29-19 and Plate 34). First, the digital nerves were identified by yellow vessel loops and the long active tendon implants sized on the hand (note the metal plate distal and two porous cords proximal). An Ober tendon passer then was used to guide the proximal end of the tendon implants to the palm and into the forearm while the loop retractor held the profundus tendon to the index in the forearm (the future motor tendon). Next, the length of active tendon was prepared. The silicone rubber was trimmed away and two Dacron cords separated (Fig. 29-20 and Plate 35).

The proximal junction then was completed between tendon implant and flexor to determine the profundus tendon of the index finger in the forearm. Two Dacron cords were divided using hot cautery, with the distal end completed first by fixing the metal plate of the distal phalanx with a screw. Finally, the muscle of the flexor profundus of the index finger gently covered the juncture (Fig. 29-21 and Plate 36). Finished stage I demonstrates complete tendon balance with wrist in the neutral position (Fig. 29-22 and Plate 37).

Four months postoperatively, a radiograph of the finger in extension shows the proximal end of the tendon implant just proximal to the wrist (silicone rubber on surface of implant

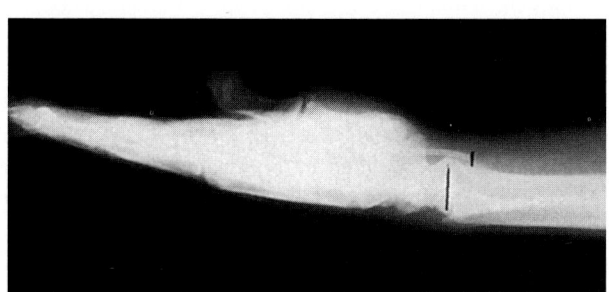

Fig. 29-23. Case study 1. Stage 1: postoperative at 4 months, monitored radiographically. The finger is in extension. Note the proximal end of the tendon implant just proximal to the wrist (silicone rubber on surface of implant contains 0.025% barium for radiographic identification). (From Hunter JM: Staged flexor tendon reconstruction. In Strickland JW, editor: *Master techniques in orthopaedic surgery, the hand,* Philadelphia, 1998, Lippincott-Raven.)

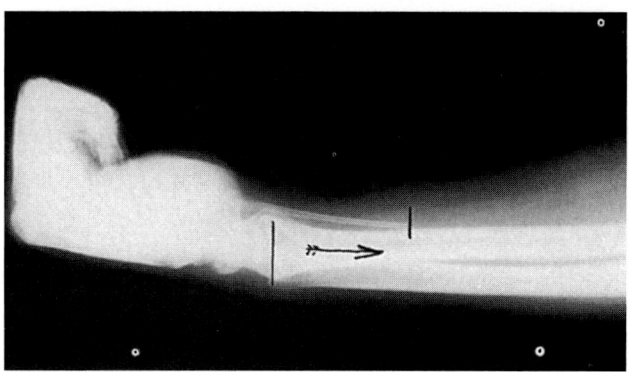

Fig. 29-24. Case study 1. Stage I: postoperative at 4 months. The right index finger is in active flexion. Active tendon function is easily documented radiographically. The excursion of the muscle tendon juncture is measured from a fixed point at the wrist. The patient is now ready for stage II or return to light-duty work. (From Hunter JM: Staged flexor tendon reconstruction. In Strickland JW, editor: *Master techniques in orthopaedic surgery, the hand,* Philadelphia, 1998, Lippincott-Raven.)

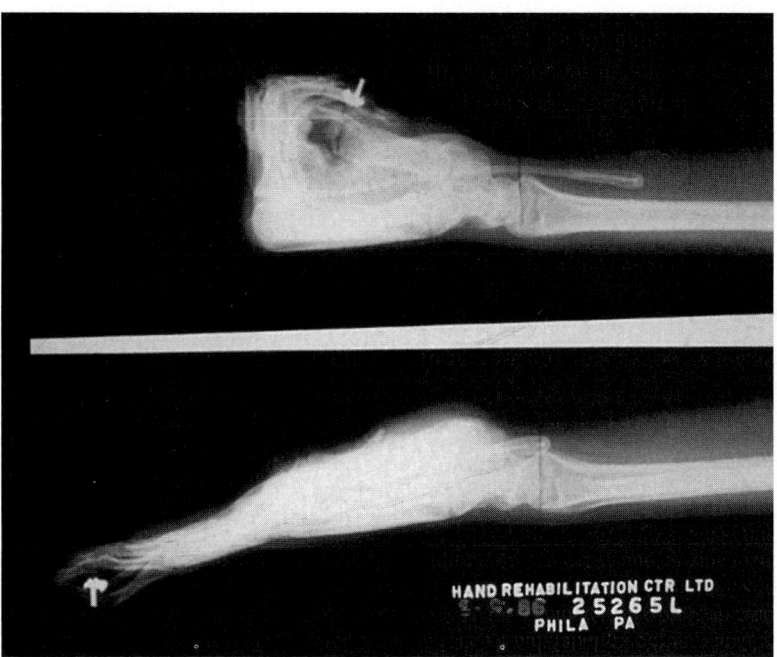

Fig. 29-25. Case study 2. Radiograph shows function before stage II. (From Hunter JM: Staged flexor tendon reconstruction. In Strickland JW, editor: *Master techniques in orthopaedic surgery, the hand,* Philadelphia, 1998, Lippincott-Raven.)

contains 0.025% barium for radiographic identification (Fig. 29-23). The right index finger is in active flexion, and active tendon function is easily documented on radiograph (Fig. 29-24). The excursion of the muscle tendon juncture is measured from a fixed point at the wrist. The patient is now ready for stage II or return to light-duty work and the delayed stage II programs.

Case study 2: stage II. Flexor tendon reconstruction following a failed primary repair

The patient, a 22-year-old right-handed male college student, presented for a stage I flexor tendon reconstruction of the right index finger following a failed primary repair. He hoped to miss as little time from college as possible. The patient worked between stages I and II.

Radiographs show function before stage II (Fig. 29-25). The active tendon implant used was a fixed-length type with a metal plate and screw in the distal phalanx and loop-to-loop juncture to profundus tendon in the index finger in the proximal forearm. The excursion of the tendon implant could be seen in the forearm, and the function of the finger is ¼

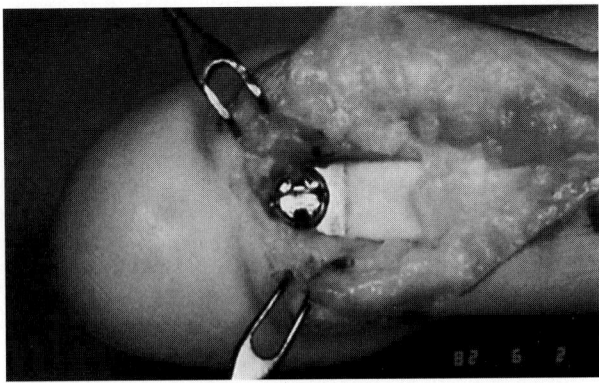

Fig. 29-26. Case study 2. Active tendon: fixed-length type with metal plate and screw in distal phalanx and loop-to-loop juncture to profundus tendon in index finger in the proximal forearm. The excursion of the tendon implant is seen in the forearm and the function of the finger is ¼ inch of the distal palmar crease. At the time of stage II, the distal end is opened, showing metal screw and plate. This will be replaced by tendon grafting. (From Hunter JM: Staged flexor tendon reconstruction. In Strickland JW, editor: *Master techniques in orthopaedic surgery, the hand,* Philadelphia, 1998, Lippincott-Raven.)

inch of the distal palmar crease. At the time of stage II reconstruction, the distal end of the finger was opened, showing the metal screw and plate (Fig. 29-26 and Plate 38). This will be replaced by tendon grafting.

The biologic bed is shown at stage II with the biologic profundus tendon at the right and the artificial tendon loop at the left in the forearm (Fig. 29-27, *A,* and Plate 40, *A*). Note the soft connective tissues as they move from flexion to midextension to full extension. This connective tissue interface, at stage II, should be disturbed as little as possible because it permits 4 cm of active tendon excursion (Fig. 29-28 and Plate 39).

All soft tissue was preserved and the graft was ready to glide within the tendon sheath, to the left, into the finger (see Fig. 29-28 and Plate 39). Note the stage II tendon graft at the left and the junctures to the profundus tendon of the index finger at the right. This shows the preservation of the connective tissue structure that existed around the proximal juncture of the tendon implant. This reconnected tissue is held in the retractor at the top and will be gently closed with a 5-0 suture. Using this method, the stage II proximal tendon graft juncture will have little, if any, restrictive adhesions (see Figs. 29-4 and 29-5 and Plate 31).

Nine months after stage II tendon grafting, full extension and full flexion are demonstrated (Fig. 29-29 and Plate 41). The patient performed light-duty work between stages I and II, and returned to light-duty work 12 weeks after stage II flexor tendon reconstructive surgery.

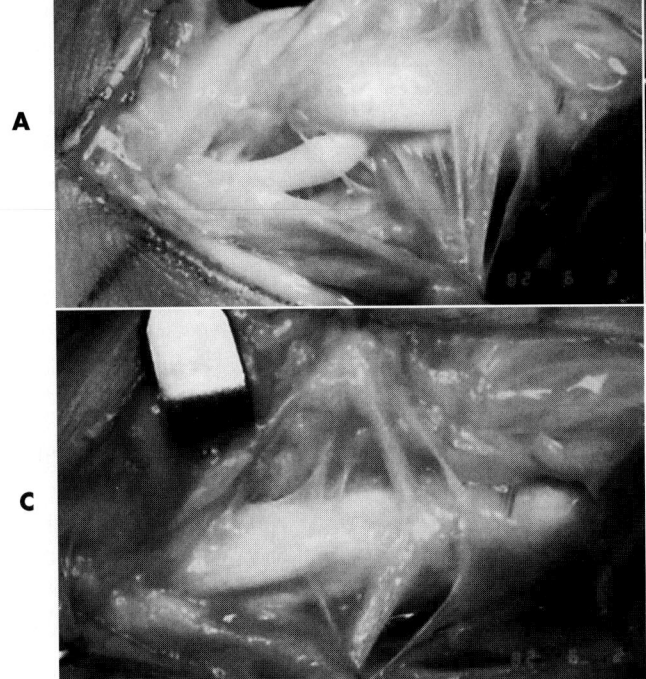

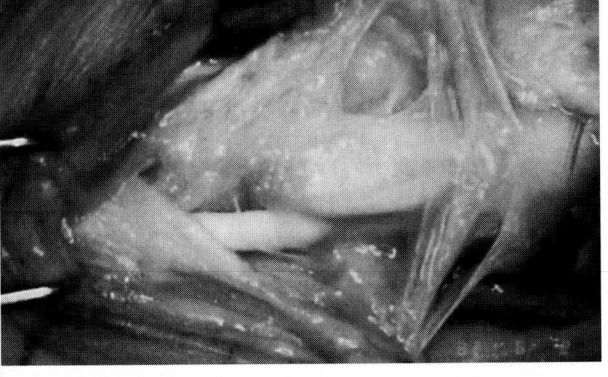

Fig. 29-27. Case study 2. The biologic bed is shown at stage II with the biologic profundus tendon at the right and the artificial tendon loop at the left in the forearm. Note the soft connective tissues as they move from flexion **(A)** to midextension **(B)** to full extension **(C).** This connective tissue interface, at stage II, should be disturbed as little as possible; it permits 4 cm of active tendon excursion. (From Hunter JM: Staged flexor tendon reconstruction. In Strickland JW, editor: *Master techniques in orthopaedic surgery, the hand,* Philadelphia, 1998, Lippincott-Raven.)

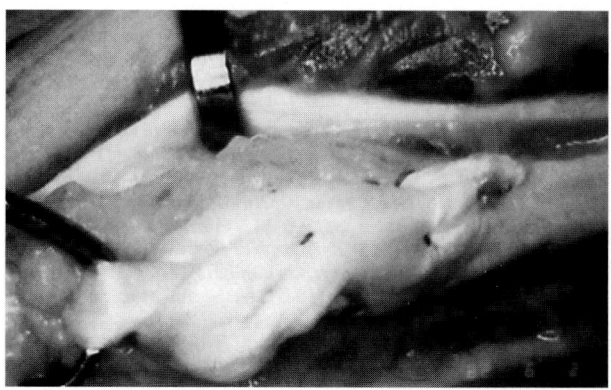

Fig. 29-28. Case study 2. Stage II tendon graft at the left and the junctures to the profundus tendon of the index finger at the right. This important illustration shows the preservation of the connective tissue structure that existed around the proximal juncture of the tendon implant. All soft tissue is preserved; the graft is ready to glide within the tendon sheath, to the left, into the finger. This reconnected tissue is held in the retractor at the top and will be gently closed with a 5-0 suture. Using this method, the stage II proximal tendon graft juncture will have little, if any, restrictive adhesions. (From Hunter JM: Staged flexor tendon reconstruction. In Strickland JW, editor: *Master techniques in orthopaedic surgery, the hand,* Philadelphia, 1998, Lippincott-Raven.)

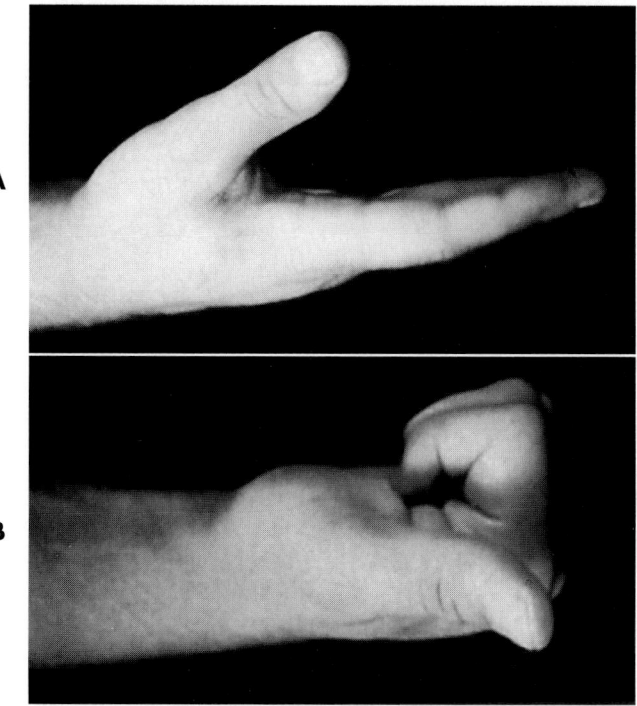

A

B

Fig. 29-29. A and **B,** Case study 2. Follow-up of the patient 9 months after stage II tendon grafting: full flexion. The patient has been at light-duty work between stages I and II, and returned to light-duty work 12 weeks after stage II flexor tendon reconstructive surgery. (From Hunter JM: Staged flexor tendon reconstruction. In Strickland JW, editor: *Master techniques in orthopaedic surgery, the hand,* Philadelphia, 1998, Lippincott-Raven.)

Part II: staged tendon reconstruction: postoperative therapy

Evelyn J. Mackin

PASSIVE TENDON IMPLANT[3]
Stage I

During the first 3 weeks after operation, the patient's hand is kept in a protective dorsal blocking splint. The postoperative dressing is an important detail because it must permit hand therapy in the immediate postoperative period. We prefer dressings of minimal bulk because they permit complete passive digital flexion. The dorsal forearm-based splint is applied to extend 2 cm beyond the fingertips with the wrist flexed to 30 degrees, the metacarpophalangeal (MP) joints flexed to 60 to 70 degrees, and the interphalangeal (IP) joints in full extension. It is essential that the splint allow full active extension of the IP joints. The splint is worn 24 hours a day. Light protected exercise is initiated in the first week and consists of gentle passive flexion and light finger trapping. Ten repetitions of each exercise are performed four times a day (Fig. 29-30, *A-C*).

During these early weeks, the patient is seen in therapy two or three times a week, when the splint may be removed for gentle passive range of motion (PROM) by the therapist. The therapist measures the passive flexion and active and passive extension of the involved digits.

If a proximal interphalangeal (PIP) or distal interphalangeal (DIP) joint flexion contracture existed before stage I, it is likely to recur postoperatively. If a contracture does begin to recur, it should be treated immediately by application of a static IP joint extension splint within the dorsal splint to subject the contracted joints to gentle passive extension. Splinting to correct flexion contractures and to prevent further contractures must be integrated into the therapy program during the entire reconstruction. Nighttime splinting for persistent flexion contractures may need to continue for 6 months after stage II.

One also must pay attention to early signs of synovitis caused by an overzealous patient or aggressive therapist. Patient education often can prevent an overzealous patient from exercising too much or too frequently. It can also help the less motivated patient to understand the importance of adhering to the home program. Discomfort in the involved digit, swelling along the volar aspect of the finger, decreased range of motion (ROM), and swelling at the incision site in the forearm should be reported to the surgeon. If synovitis develops, resolution usually can be achieved by temporarily discontinuing the exercise program and by immobilization in a resting splint. If synovitis is not remedied by rest, the stage II procedure should be performed earlier. The therapist should know that aggressive and forceful manipulation of the tissues can cause synovitis and that continued mobili-

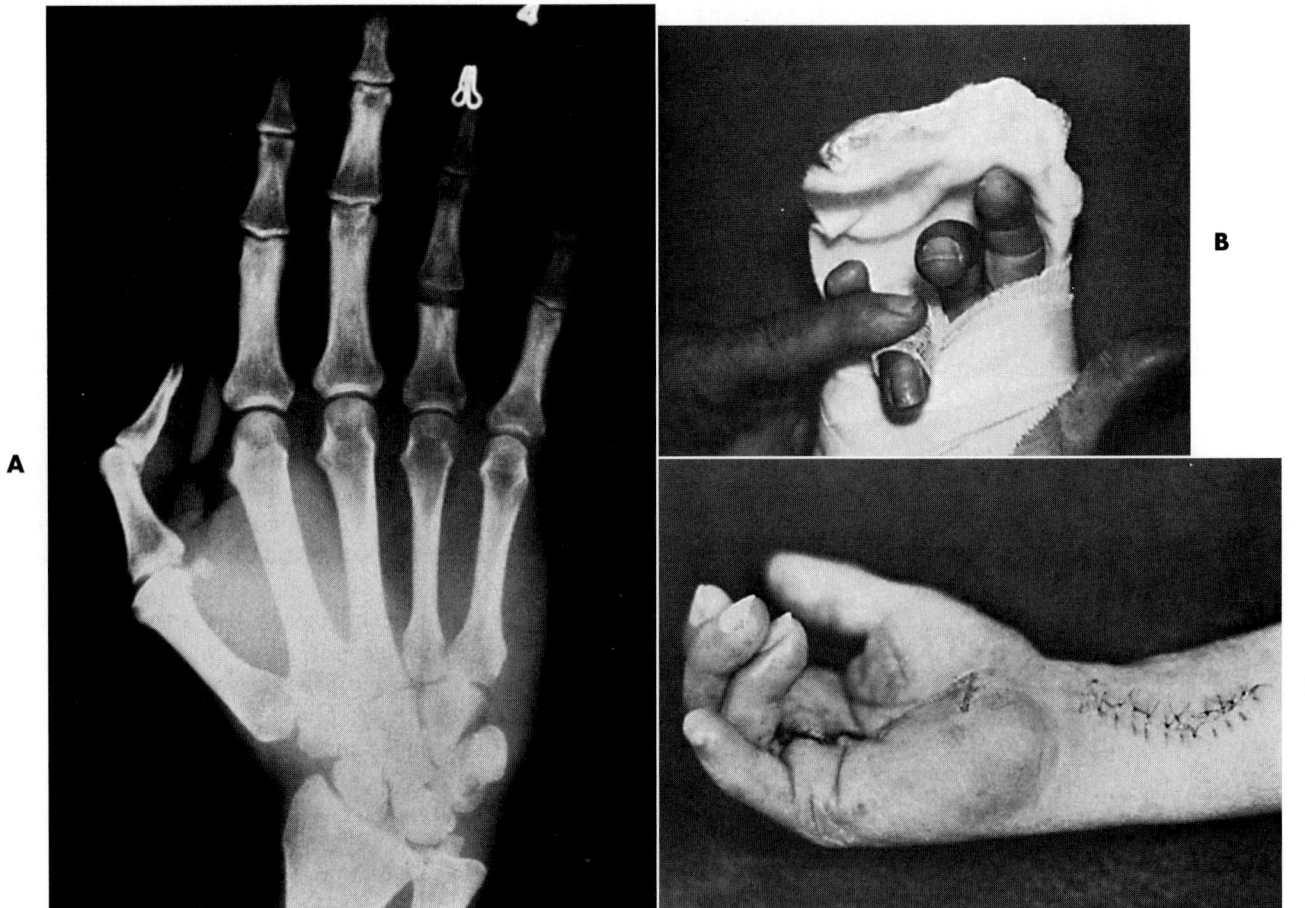

Fig. 29-30. A, Microsurgical replantation of the ring finger, with insertion of a Swanson silastic implant in the proximal interphalangeal (PIP) joint. The patient, a 49-year-old right-handed welder, sustained a band saw amputation of the left ring finger at the PIP joint, with partial amputation of the small finger at the distal interphalangeal (DIP) joint. The patient had a myocardial infarction 3 days after discharge from the hospital; there was no previous cardiac history or any indication of cardiac distress while in the hospital. As a result, therapy was not initiated until 7 weeks after replantation. By then the wound had healed; however, the delay in beginning therapy resulted in an adhered flexor tendon system in the ring finger, limiting active flexion. Thus the patient became a candidate for staged tendon reconstruction. **B,** Gentle passive motion was initiated the first week after stage I surgery. **C,** Finger trapping. Strapping the involved finger to the adjacent normal finger incorporates the involved finger into useful function. *Continued*

zation in the face of synovitis results in a thickened sheath. The result will be a recurrence of contractures and a loss of motion.

The protective postoperative splint is removed after 3 weeks, and programmed activity continues with the PROM exercise and a finger-trapping program. A Velcro trapper is added to the finger-trapper exercise (Fig. 29-30, *D* and *E*). By strapping the involved finger to the adjacent normal finger, one incorporates the former into useful function. After the incisions have healed, lanolin massage alleviates dryness and softens the tissues. At 6 weeks, with the use of the trapper, some patients may be able to return to work, depending on their job requirements.

The goals of hand therapy during the period between stages I and II are to obtain good mobility of the joints,

passive flexion of the digit to the distal palmar crease (or motion equal to that obtained at stage I surgery), correction of flexion contractures, and a viable gliding system. The hand should be in its best possible condition before stage II surgery (Fig. 29-30, *F*).

Stage II

Early passive mobilization protocol. After surgery, the patient's hand is again kept in a protective dorsal forearm-based splint with the wrist in 30 degrees of flexion, the MP joints flexed to 70 degrees, and the IP joints in full extension. The therapist must be certain that the patient can fully extend the IP joints within the splint. The dressings are essentially the same as those used after stage I surgery. If the dressings do not permit full passive digital flexion, some of

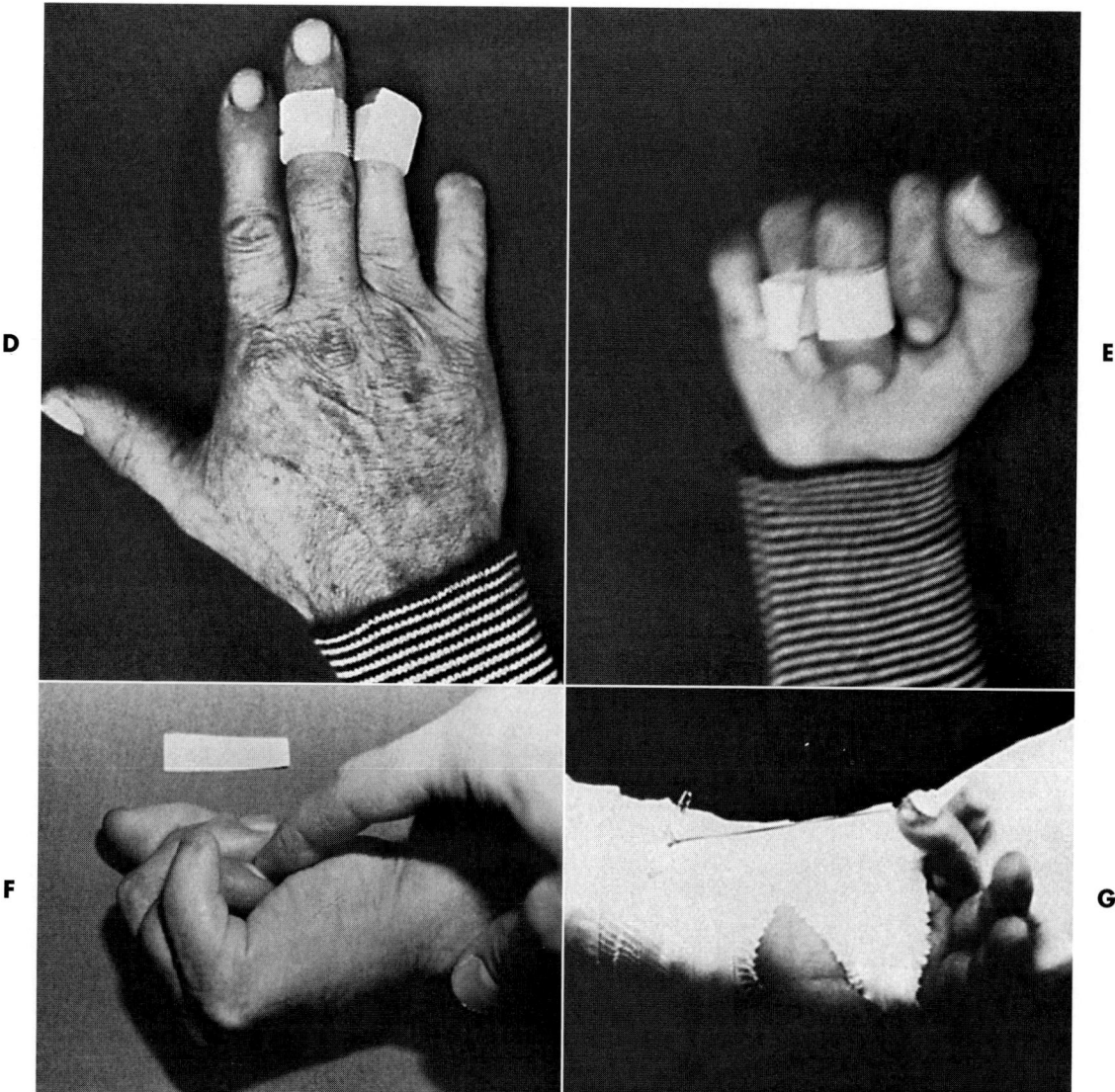

Fig. 29-30, cont'd. D, Extension. **E,** Flexion. **F,** Condition of the patient's finger improved: finger was supple with good skin condition; active potential of 1.5 cm was achieved (1.5 cm at stage I surgery), Tinel's sign was present at the finger tip, and radiograph revealed good excursion of the tendon implant. **G,** Dynamic splinting was initiated the first day after stage II surgery. Active extension and passive flexion were performed with elastic band attached to the fingernail.

Continued

the dressing may have to be removed, but when that is done, the splint may not fit as securely. If that is the case, additional adhesive tape or Coban tape should be applied across the forearm, wrist, and palm to ensure that the patient's hand will not slip proximally within the splint and thereby put tension on the newly sutured junctures. Often, a thermoplastic splint is made for the patient if the plaster cast does not fit securely or does not allow full active extension of the IP joints.

Early passive mobilization has improved tendon gliding in primary tendon repair. We have applied the concept of early passive mobilization to patients undergoing staged tendon grafting by using dynamic flexion traction to provide passive flexion and allow active extension within the dorsal

splint. One advantage of dynamic flexion traction using an elastic band is that it facilitates tendon and joint movement without requiring active pull on the flexor tendon. Another advantage is that the digit's resting position in passive flexion protects the grafted tendon from sudden active flexion (e.g., if the patient jerks his or her fingers during sleep or if the patient falls).

We prefer to wait until the patient attends therapy on the first postoperative day before fitting him or her with an elastic band so that the quality, positioning, and tension of the hand can be accurately established. The elastic band should be attached approximately 3 inches proximal to the wrist crease on the volar aspect of the forearm dressing, with

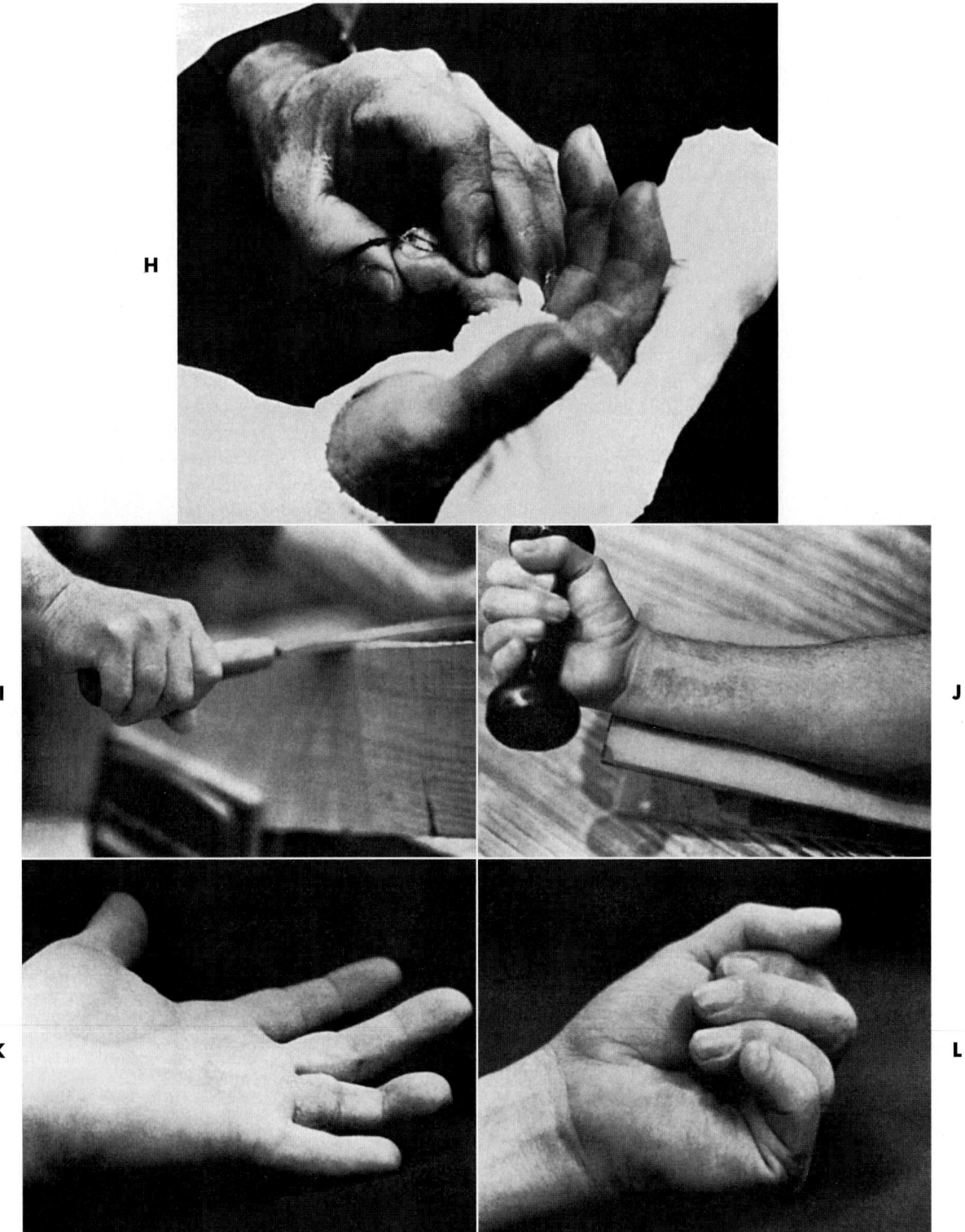

Fig. 29-30, cont'd. H, Gentle passive extension of the DIP joint. Metacarpophalangeal and PIP joint flexion decreases tension at the tendon juncture. **I,** Tendon and joint reconstruction enables the patient to use his ring finger as a stabilizer when using a tool in a sustained-grip activity. **J,** Grip strengthening at 3 months. **K,** Extension and **(L)** flexion at 12 weeks after surgery. Considering the severe nature of this patient's amputation injury, the subsequent tissue ischemia, the unique problems of establishing adequate circulation to the replanted part, the development of a new functionally adapted fibrous capsule for the Swanson silastic implant and tendon gliding after the two-stage tendon reconstruction using a Hunter passive tendon implant, and the myocardial infarction, this patient has come a long way.

the involved digit in its normal alignment. The distal attachment of the elastic band is to a monofilament suture placed through the fingernail at surgery. The tension of the hand is important. It should be adjusted so that it pulls the finger into flexion at rest and yet permits the antagonist muscles to actively fully extend the finger within the limits of the dorsal splint; this prevents the development of flexion contractures. The patient is instructed to actively extend the finger and then reciprocally relax it as the elastic band brings it back into flexion. This exercise is repeated 10 times every waking hour (Fig. 29-30, *G*). We have found that standard rubber bands are not always suitable for this purpose. Often, the tension of a standard rubber band will hold the fingers in the appropriate flexion at rest but will not allow the patient to actively extend his or her finger fully against the tension of the band. Patients may be instructed to manually release some rubber band tension during the exercise to ease tension. Failure to completely extend the PIP and DIP joints will result in flexion contractures. Elastic thread is a much better alternative for dynamic traction. A single strand can be used and will more easily allow full active IP joint extension. As the digit becomes stronger in active extension, a double strand can be used to increase the tension.

Gentle passive flexion of each IP joint also is performed. Ten repetitions are performed several times a day. Manual passive flexion of the DIP joint must be performed carefully. Previous operations and excessive passive "cranking" may cause attenuation of the extensor tendon; thus, as we strive to achieve passive DIP joint flexion, we also emphasize active DIP joint extension.

Particular attention should be paid to controlling contractures of the DIP and PIP joints. Salvage fingers may have poor extensor tendon function because of tendon attenuation or adhesions from previous surgeries. Consequently, these fingers are especially prone to recurrent contractures. Early treatment of incipient flexion contractures is of primary importance. If the dorsal splint does not allow full extension of the PIP joint, the patient can manually hold down the proximal phalanx of the involved finger to a greater degree, thereby facilitating active extension of the IP joints. An alternative is for the therapist to place a felt block behind the proximal phalanx during exercise to flex the MP joint so that when the patient actively extends the involved digit, full extension of the IP joints is facilitated.

When the surgeon and the therapist are alerted to the development of PIP or DIP flexion contractures, passive extension of the IP joints may be initiated as early as the first postoperative week. For protected PROM, tension is taken off the tendon juncture by flexion of the adjacent joint. The MP and PIP joints are held down in flexion while the PIP joint is gently extended with the uninvolved hand. If there is evidence of contracture formation at the DIP joint, the therapist may support the MP and PIP joints in flexion and gently extend the DIP joint (Fig. 29-30, *H*). These passive extension exercises should be included in the patient's home program. Care is taken to avoid simultaneous extension of the PIP and DIP joints. Ten repetitions of each exercise are repeated four times daily.

Persistent flexion contractures may require a proximal joint wedge (Fig. 29-30, *G* and *H*) or a PIP joint passive extension splint. A proximal joint wedge placed behind the proximal phalanx or an Alumafoam splint that positions the MP joint in greater flexion and gently pulls the contracted IP joint into extension with a Velcro strap is custom fitted within the postoperative dorsal splint. The wedge or splint should be worn intermittently during the day. The exact schedule depends on the feel of the contracture (i.e., whether it will quickly or slowly respond to stretching). In our experience, this technique of passive stretching minimizes problems with flexion contractures and enhances overall tendon function.

The patient is seen weekly by the surgeon during the first 3 to 4 postoperative weeks. Gentle, active tendon pull-through is checked at those visits. Full excursion of the tendon graft within the first 3 to 4 postoperative weeks indicates minimal adhesion formation. In such cases, the tendon junctures are at greater risk of rupturing if stressed by active motion. Those patients who move exceptionally well (to 70% of the final goal) during the first 3 weeks are protected in the dorsal splint. The 3 to 4 weeks in the dorsal splint may be extended to 6 weeks to minimize the chance of rupture.

When the dorsal splint is removed, usually at 4 weeks, the patient's hand is maintained in a wristlet with elastic band traction attached to the fingernail suture. The wristlet permits full active extension of the IP and MP joints with the wrist in neutral position. The elastic band pulls the fingers back into flexion at rest. The hourly active extension exercises against the rubber band are continued with the wrist held in neutral. Active wrist dorsiflexion is performed with the fingers resting in flexion to avoid tension on the tendon junctures. Contracture control is continued. Passive flexion and extension exercises are continued as during the earlier weeks, four times a day with 10 repetitions of each exercise. Soft tissue massage continues.

At surgery, the proximal end of the tendon graft is attached to the motor tendon. Distally, the tendon is attached to bone. The button and wire holding the tendon in place are not removed for a minimum of 6 weeks, at which time physiologic union has taken place. If the patient is doing well, with good tendon glide, the button is not removed for 12 weeks. The better the patient is doing, the longer the button is kept in place.

At 6 weeks, the wristlet is removed and the patient begins light activity. The initiation of active flexion exercise depends on how well the tendon is gliding. When adhesions seem to be restricting motion, we begin active flexion earlier (e.g., at 4 weeks), but we have held the patient back when active flexion is excellent. Finger blocking and active differential tendon gliding exercises may be initiated at this time.

Tendon gliding exercises. With the wrist at 10 degrees of extension, the patient performs 10 repetitions of passive digit flexion and extension, followed by 10 repetitions of active differential tendon gliding exercises. These exercises elicit maximum total and differential flexor tendon glide at wrist/palm level. The straight fist, with MP and PIP joints flexed but DIP joints extended, elicits maximum flexor digitorum superficialis (FDS) glide in relation to surrounding structures. The full fist, with MP, PIP, and DIP joints flexed, does the same for the flexor digitorum profundus (FDP) tendon. In the hook fist, with MP joints extended and IP joints flexed, maximum differential gliding between the two tendons is achieved.

Contracture control at 6 weeks can become more aggressive. Dynamic splinting may be needed for some patients. When the contracture is caused by tendon tightness, a plaster stretcher is the choice of treatment (see Chapter 113).

At 8 weeks, the patient may begin light, supervised grip strengthening activities, such as sanding and filing in woodworking (Fig. 29-30, *I*). Progressive weight-resistance exercises and heavy-resistance exercises are not permitted until 3 months after surgery (Fig. 29-30, *J-L*), when the emphasis is on return to work.

Early active motion protocol

If the tendon bed was judged to be in excellent condition and the graft junctures were strong during surgery, an active flexion protocol may be initiated without the use of an elastic band in the first postoperative week, with passive hold exercises in the dorsal splint. The splinting guidelines for this method of early motion are essentially the same as those for early motion using elastic band traction. The protective dorsal splint holds the wrist in 30 degrees of flexion, the MP joints in 70 degrees of flexion, and IP joints in full extension.

To perform the passive hold exercise, the patient must relax the forearm muscles of the involved extremity. The patient gently presses the fingers into flexion with the uninvolved hand and then tries to actively, lightly hold the fingers in flexion. The rationale for the passive hold is that it takes less force to maintain an already flexed finger in flexion than to actively pull the finger into flexion from an extended position, and the benefits of tendon excursion are the same as those derived from active flexion. We ask the patient to perform this exercise in full flexion and at two ranges of partial flexion (i.e., slight flexion, midflexion, and full flexion). Three repetitions at each range are performed three to four times a day. In addition, gentle passive flexion of the IP joints is performed several times a day within the dorsal splint. If the patient begins to glide the tendon very early and excellent tendon pull-through is demonstrated, we slow him or her at 2 weeks by applying elastic band traction. The patient still can perform the passive hold exercise, but the elastic band traction program adds protection.

The program from week 6 to week 12 is essentially the same as that described for the early passive mobilization program, including wristlet and graded strengthening. One continues to devote attention to the prevention of flexion contractures.

MOLESKIN SLING

When a nylon suture cannot be attached to the tip of the fingernail at surgery (e.g., because the fingernail is absent),

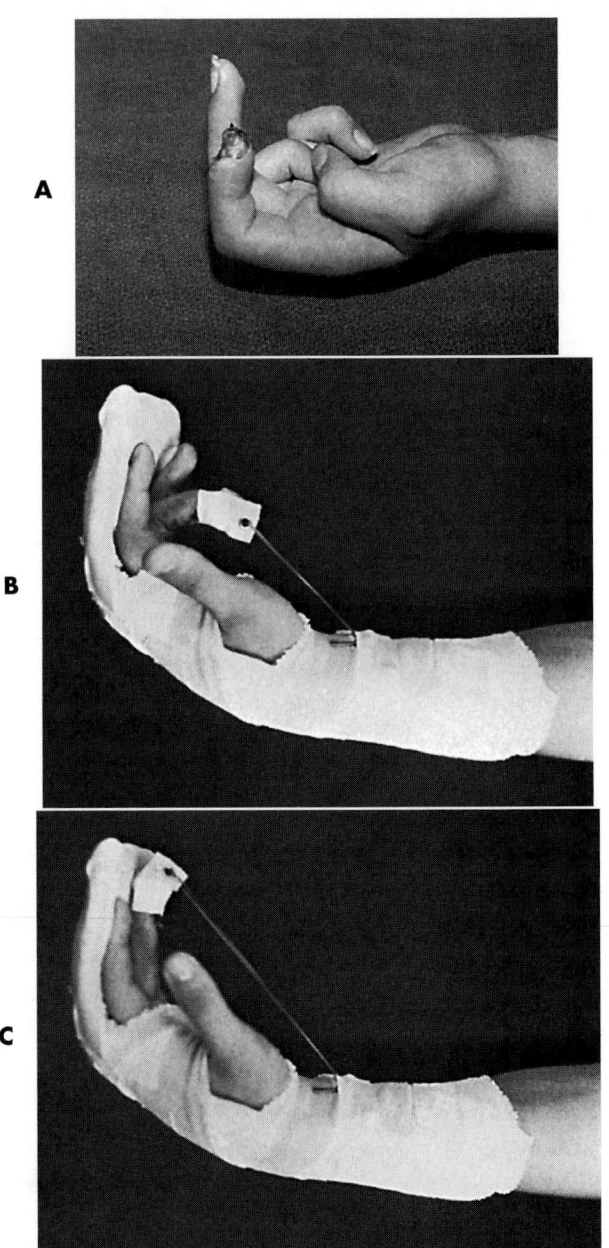

Fig. 29-31. Moleskin sling may be used to provide elastic band traction. **A,** This patient with loss of the nail plate requires moleskin to attach the elastic band. **B** and **C,** Another patient demonstrates passive flexion and extension using the moleskin sling.

a sling of moleskin can be used to provide an attachment point for elastic band traction around the button and wire. Tincture of benzoin is applied to the finger to help the moleskin adhere. The sling is applied laterally on the finger from the midphalanx to the fingertip. A segment of moleskin approximately 3 inches long and ½ inch wide is folded in half, and an eyelet is punched through at the folded end. An S-hook, made from a paper clip, is hooked through the eyelet opening, and an elastic band is attached to it and to a safety pin on the volar surface of either the forearm dressing or a wrist cuff (Fig. 29-31, *A, B,* and *C*).

ACTIVE TENDON IMPLANT[3]
Stage I

A careful and structured postoperative program is required to facilitate orderly pseudosheath development around the tendon implant and to prepare the patient's hand for return to work (Fig. 29-32, *A*). Therapy is initiated on the first postoperative day and is similar to that for a stage II tendon graft with early active mobilization, although slightly more rigorous. It begins with the passive hold exercise described previously (Fig. 29-32, *B, C,* and *D*). Hand dressings must permit full passive flexion of the digit into the palm. At 2 weeks, when the patient demonstrates good tendon gliding, elastic band traction is added. The passive hold exercise is continued, but as stated previously, the elastic band adds protection.

If pulleys were reconstructed at stage I surgery, the postoperative program must take them into account. Pulley reconstruction at stage I using a passive tendon implant attached only distally does not require protection because the patient will be performing only passive motion. Reconstructed pulleys in the presence of an active tendon implant must be protected with a pulley ring so that the active motion of the implant does not stretch the pulley repair (Fig. 29-32, *E* and *F*). Protection during the first postoperative days may be provided by either a Velcro and felt pulley ring or support with pressure from a finger of the opposite hand (Fig. 29-33). When postoperative edema decreases, the soft pulley ring can be replaced with a thermoplastic pulley ring and, eventually, a metal ring in some cases (Fig. 29-34, *A-F*). Pulley reconstruction is as sensitive as tendon repair and should be protected for 6 months.

If the patient does not have full active IP joint extension, a contracture-control program must be initiated during the first postoperative week. A felt wedge is fitted behind the proximal phalanx within the dorsal splint. The pulley ring provides a counterforce over the reconstructed pulley, preventing its attenuation as the contracted joint is gently pulled into extension (Fig. 29-32, *G* and *H*).

Light grip strengthening is begun with foam squeeze after the third postoperative week, and light putty squeezing is permitted after 4 weeks; 10 repetitions are performed several times a day (Fig. 29-32, *I*). The passive hold exercise is continued. Overzealous use of the digit soon after surgery is to be avoided because this may result in a synovitis. This complication generally responds to rest and splinting.

At 6 weeks, the protective dorsal splint may be removed and a wristlet and elastic band traction applied; these permit wrist extension to neutral and full extension of the MP and IP joints. An active patient may need a dorsal splint for an additional 2 weeks. By 8 weeks, patients usually are permitted full activities, with restrictions on full-power grip until 12 weeks. During weeks 8 to 12, the goal is improvement of strength and endurance through the beginning of putty exercise and light, sustained grip activities (woodworking), progressing to the weight-well and resistance exercise. A return-to-work program is initiated.

The immature mesothelial sheath is formed around the tendon implant by 4 weeks and becomes mature by 4 months. A minimum of 4 to 6 months is required between stages I and II to facilitate hand reconditioning. If tendon and joint function are satisfactory, stage II often is delayed for up to 2 years or longer. As time passes with the tendon implant in the digit, the motor unit becomes stronger, ROM is maximized, and soft tissue becomes more pliable, thus making the digit better prepared for stage II.

Stage II

Stage II surgery consists of removal of the active tendon implant, insertion of a tendon graft through the pseudosheath, and initiation of postoperative therapy to facilitate gliding of the graft to achieve maximum digital motion. After surgery, the patient's hand is kept in a protective dorsal forearm-based splint with the wrist in 30 degrees of flexion, the MP joints flexed to 70 degrees, and the IP joints in full extension. Early mobilization with elastic band traction begins the first postoperative day. The patient actively extends the finger and then reciprocally relaxes it, permitting the elastic band to flex the digit. Ten repetitions of this exercise are performed every hour. Gentle passive motion is performed; 10 repetitions are performed several times a day, with care given to avoiding extensor tendon attenuation by overstretching. Attention continues to be devoted to controlling the development of contractures. Postoperative therapy is similar to that after stage I. However, because very early pain-free gliding generally occurs, protective splinting may be extended beyond the usual 6-week period if necessary to protect against excessive force on the tendon junctures (Fig. 29-34, *G*). Initiation of the wristlet at 6 weeks after surgery may be delayed until 8 weeks, and active exercise at 8 weeks may be delayed until 10 weeks. Timetables always should be adjusted according to the patient's progress (Fig. 29-34, *A-G*).

THE SUPERFICIALIS FINGER[1,2]

The superficialis finger technique, originally described by Osborne,[5] was used as a means of salvage for the finger

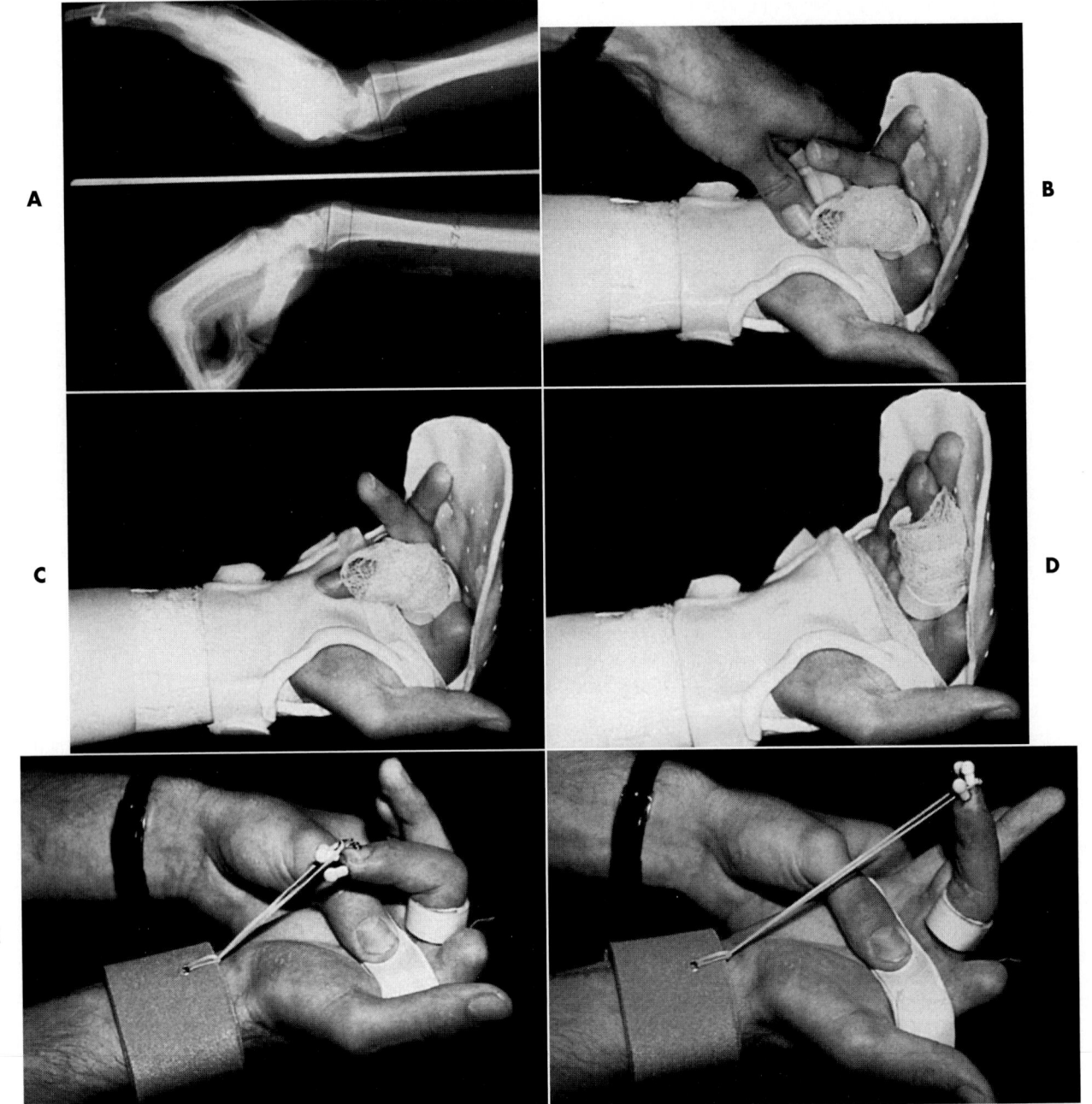

Fig. 29-32. A, Superficialis finger. The patient, a 23-year-old right-dominant surveyor, incurred a severe injury to his right hand with a log splitter. **B** through **F,** The index finger was shattered and unsalvageable. The long finger was amputated and replanted. Vascularity was reestablished to the long finger, but the tendons were badly damaged and not repaired primarily. Subsequently, the patient underwent a tendon graft procedure 8 months after injury. A swan-neck deformity developed, and the patient underwent a secondary revision 8 months later. Approximately 2 years after injury, the patient was seen at the Philadelphia Hand Center. He had good neurovascular function in the finger but lacked active flexion. He had maintained good passive range of motion, which made the finger salvageable for flexor reconstruction. It was thought that the patient could benefit from tendon reconstruction using the active tendon implant and superficialis finger reconstruction. The flexor tendon graft was excised. A volar plate advancement tenodesis was performed to prevent hyperextension of the proximal interphalangeal (PIP) joint. The distal interphalangeal joint was arthrodesed. The active tendon implant was inserted, and the A_2 and A_4 pulleys were reconstructed. A dorsal protective splint was applied at surgery. Therapy was begun with passive hold exercise. Elastic band traction was added in therapy on the first postoperative day. Wristlet and elastic band traction were applied 6 weeks after surgery. Reconstructed A_1 and A_2 pulleys are protected with pulley rings. Direct digital pressure from the uninvolved hand adds support to the reconstructed A_4 pulley during the early training program.

Continued

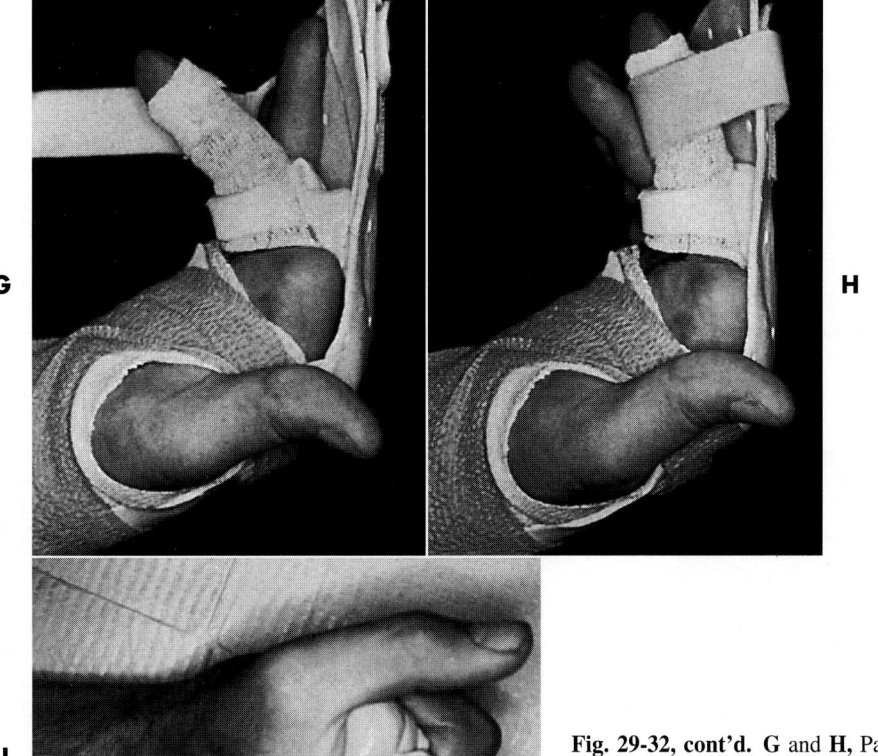

Fig. 29-32, cont'd. G and H, Passive extension of PIP joint. A felt wedge places the proximal phalanx in more flexion. With the felt wedge in place, the Velcro strap gently pulls the PIP joint into 220 degrees of extension. Volar plate reconstruction prohibits further PIP extension at this time in the therapy program. I, Resistive exercises were initiated 12 weeks after surgery.

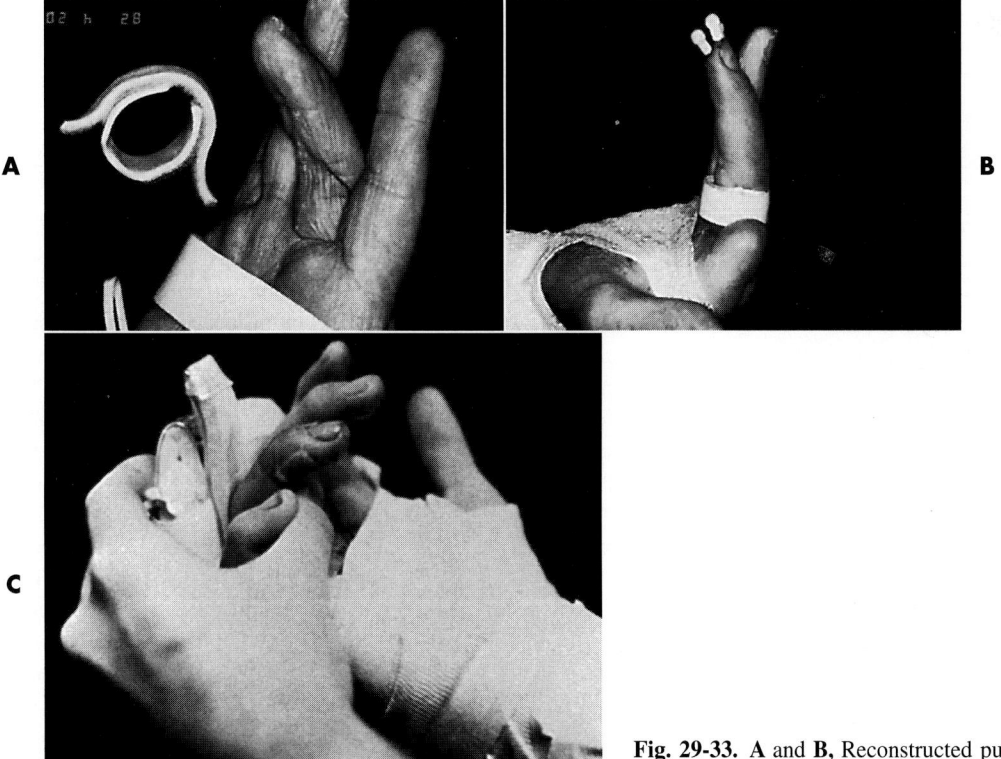

Fig. 29-33. A and B, Reconstructed pulley supported with a Velcro and felt pulley ring during active flexion. C, Pulley supported with pressure from a finger from the opposite hand.

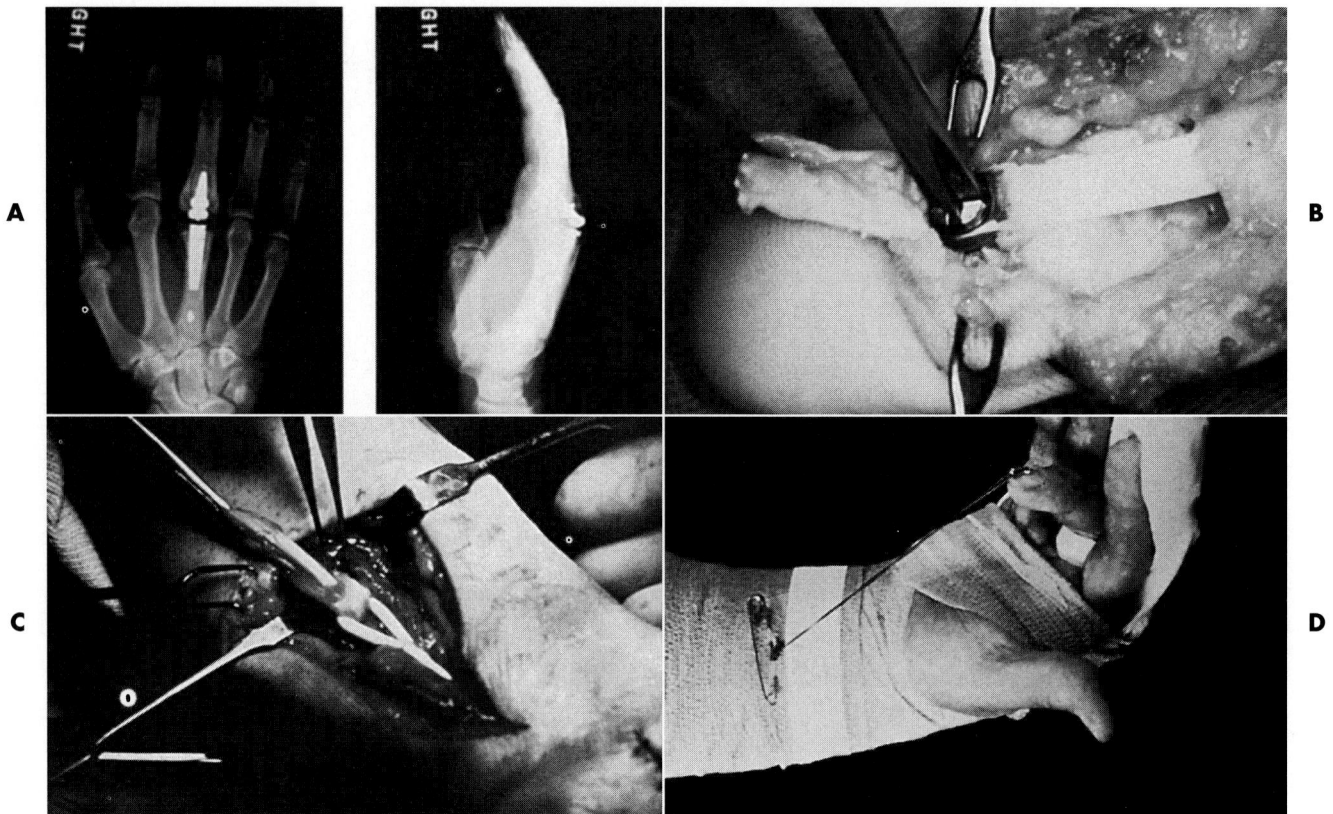

Fig. 29-34. A, Metallic implant arthroplasty for degenerative arthritis performed on a 54-year-old right-dominant man. Approximately 4 years after surgery he lost motion, and pain developed in the digit. Evaluation at the Philadelphia Rehabilitation Center disclosed that the implant had fractured and perforated the proximal phalanx volarly, with rupture of the flexor digitorum profundus and flexor digitorum superficialis tendons of the long finger. Stage I surgery involved insertion of a Swanson joint implant and a Hunter active tendon implant. **B,** Stainless steel distal metal end plate is attached to the distal phalanx by screw fixation. The profundus stump is drawn over the distal component and sutured laterally to provide a soft tissue buffer, preventing irritation of the overlying skin. **C,** Preformed silicone-coated Dacron loop for motor tendon unit juncture. **D,** Postoperative dorsal protective splint and elastic band traction. Velcro and felt pulley ring protects the reconstructed pulley. Active extension/passive flexion.   *Continued*

affected by severe adhesions or failed tendon graft procedures.

Emphasis on restoring motion to the PIP joint with sacrifice of motion at the DIP joint is based on the concept that the PIP joint has the largest arc of motion and makes the greatest contribution of functional ROM of the fingers. The principles of superficialis staged tendon reconstruction and secondary tendon grafting are strictly followed and well described in the literature.[1,2,4] Therapy postoperatively is simplified because of decreased excursion required for PIP flexion as well as the decreased potential for adhesions (see Fig. 29-32, *A-I*).

SUMMARY

With a Hunter passive or active tendon, before stage I surgery, all patients should undergo hand therapy to mobilize stiff joints, minimize joint contractures, and maximally improve the condition of the soft tissue. Extensor imbalance should be noted. The timing of stage I surgery should be based on the judgment of the surgeon and hand therapist, the success of preoperative splinting, and patient motivation.

The two-stage tendon graft procedure using the Hunter passive tendon implant has proved to be a consistently reliable method of salvaging scarred tendon systems. The pseudosheath that forms after the first surgical stage nourishes the subsequently placed tendon graft. This fluid nutrition system and early protected gliding of the graft notably reduce the likelihood of postoperative adhesions, which, along with the release of contractures, reconstruction of the pulleys, and supervised therapy, maximize postoperative digital motion (Fig. 29-34, *A-G*).

The Hunter active tendon can be used in all two-stage reconstructions. The technique may have its greatest value in workers who are permitted to return to their occupations for

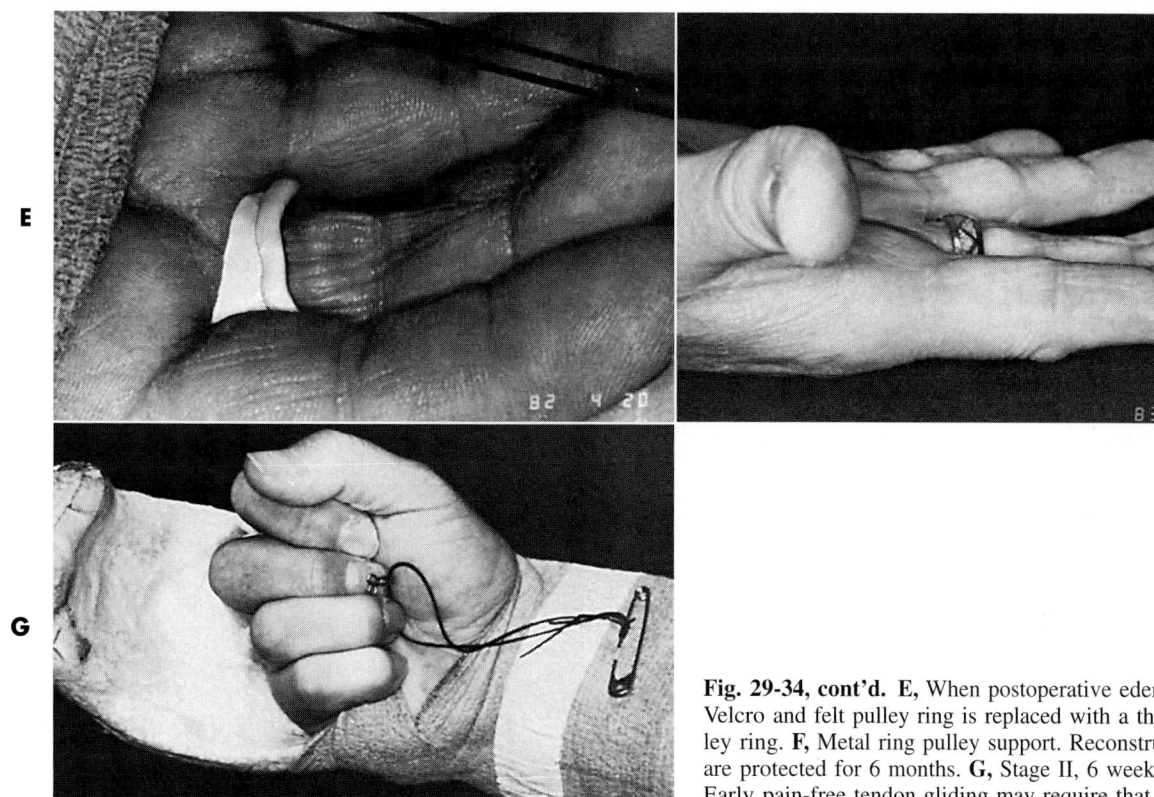

Fig. 29-34, cont'd. E, When postoperative edema decreases, Velcro and felt pulley ring is replaced with a thermoplastic pulley ring. **F,** Metal ring pulley support. Reconstructed pulleys are protected for 6 months. **G,** Stage II, 6 weeks after surgery. Early pain-free tendon gliding may require that protective splinting be extended beyond the 6-week period.

extended periods while a new sheath is forming throughout the finger, palm, and forearm. The active tendon implant adds the interface between the muscle tendon in the forearm so that the proximal juncture matures while the new sheath is forming. By the time stage II surgery is to be performed, which could be a year or two after stage I, the finger is in much better condition and the patient's morale and motivation should have substantially improved. The active tendon implant program shows sufficient clinical predictability to be considered a viable alternative when dealing with the problems that follow flexor tendon injury or disease.

REFERENCES

1. Hunter JM: Reconstruction of flexor tendon function and strength: the Hunter active tendon sublimus finger method. In Hunter JM, Schneider LH, Mackin EJ, editors: *Tendon and nerve surgery in the hand: a third decade,* St Louis, 1997, Mosby.
2. Hunter JM, Salisbury RE: Flexor tendon reconstruction in severely damaged hands, *J Bone Joint Surg* 53A:829, 1971.
3. Hunter JM, et al: Staged tendon reconstruction using passive and active tendon implants. In Hunter JM, Mackin EJ, Callahan AC, editors: *Rehabilitation of the hand: surgery and therapy,* ed 4, St Louis, 1995, Mosby.
4. Kobus JK, Kirkpatrick WH: The superficialis finger: an alternative in flexor tendon surgery. In Hunter JM, Mackin EJ, Callahan AC, editors: *Rehabilitation of the hand: surgery and therapy,* ed 4, St Louis, 1995, Mosby.
5. Osborne G: The sublimis tendon replacement technique in tendon injuries, *J Bone Joint Surg* 42B:647, 1960.
6. Wehbe MA, Hunter JM: Flexor tendon gliding in the hand: part II differential gliding, *J Hand Surg* 10A:575, 1985.

BIBLIOGRAPHY

Hunter JM, Auliano PI: Salvage of scarred tendon system using passive and active Hunter tendon implants. In Jupiter JB, editor: *Flynn's hand surgery,* 4 ed, Philadelphia, 1991, Lippincott Williams & Wilkins.
Hunter JM, Maser SA: Active tendon implants. In Balderston RA, Kirkpatrick WH, editors: *Operative techniques in orthopaedics,* vol 3(4), Philadelphia, 1993, WB Saunders.
Hunter TJM: Artificial tendons: early development and application, *Am J Surg* 109:325, 1965. (Republished in Hunter JM, Schneider LH, Mackin EJ: *Tendon surgery of the hand,* part 2, St Louis, 1987, Mosby.)

Chapter 30

THE EXTENSOR TENDONS:
ANATOMY AND MANAGEMENT

Erik A. Rosenthal

Normal hand function mirrors the integrity of the extensor tendons. Their contribution to the balance, power, dexterity, and range of hand activities is fundamental; any restraint on them will be reflected in a proportional loss of function. The effect of an injury on the extensor tendons is often regarded less seriously than a flexor tendon injury. The treatment and rehabilitation of the injury often are believed to be less intricate, less time-consuming, and associated with a relatively favorable prognosis compared with flexor tendon injuries. However, experience demonstrates that injuries to the extensor tendons can be equally complex, time-consuming, frustrating, and disappointing.

The extensor muscles to the digits are weaker, and their capacity for work and their amplitude of glide are less than their flexor antagonists, yet they require a latitude of motion that is not necessary for flexor function. The extensor tendons distal to the extensor retinaculum are relatively thin, broad structures that present a disproportionately large surface vulnerable to injury and susceptible to the formation of restraining scar. The complex interrelationships within the intricately designed extensor tendons of the digits increase their susceptibility to functional disarray after injury. Any violation of the extensor tendons or their investments introduces the potential for a functional deficiency.

DORSAL FASCIA

An appreciation of the fascial anatomy of the forearm and hand is helpful for the design of surgical procedures and for modification of a rehabilitation program after an injury.

The fascia of the forearm is divided into superficial (pars superficialis) and deep (pars profunda) layers.[27] The extensor retinaculum at the wrist level consists of supratendinous and infratendinous layers that originate from the pars profunda of the forearm fascia. The supratendinous portion consists of multidirectional woven fibers that wrap around the wrist. The proximal fibers of the supratendinous retinaculum on the radial side merge with the forearm fascia over the palmaris longus; the central fibers insert onto the radius; and the distal fibers attach to the thenar fascia. The supratendinous retinaculum on the ulnar side wraps around the distal ulna but does not attach to it. The proximal ulnar fibers of the supratendinous retinaculum pass over the flexor carpi ulnaris (FCU) and merge with the forearm fascia, the central fibers attach on the triquetrum and pisiform, and the distal fibers attach to the hypothenar fascia. Six vertical septa attach the supratendinous retinaculum to the distal radius and partition the first five dorsal compartments. These define fibroosseous tunnels that position and maintain the extensor tendons and their synovial sheaths relative to the axis of wrist motion in the proximal pole of the capitate. The sixth septum separates the extensor digiti quinti (EDQ) from the extensor carpi ulnaris (ECU) and is attached proximally to the ulnar border of the distal radius but not to the ulna.[27,165] This radial attachment blends with the origin of the dorsal distal radioulnar ligament and the origin of the ulnocarpal complex,[123,165] forming a ligament confluence that is analogous to the assemblage nucleus described for the palmar ligaments adjacent to the finger metacarpophalangeal (MP) joints.[165,182]

The brachioradialis tendon forms the floor of the first compartment; the periosteum of the radius forms the floor of the second and third. The infratendinous retinaculum forms the floor of the fourth and fifth compartments. The ECU, in the sixth compartment, is in a separate tunnel formed from the infratendinous retinaculum, separated from the supratendinous retinaculum by loose areolar tissue. This

Plate 31. Stage II: **A,** New sheath around Hunter passive tendon at 4 months in forearm. **B,** Pseudosheath at 4 months in forearm; high-power histology. Ready for tendon graft. (From Strickland JW, editor: Master techniques in orthopaedic surgery. In: *The hand,* Philadelphia, 1998, Lippincott-Raven.)

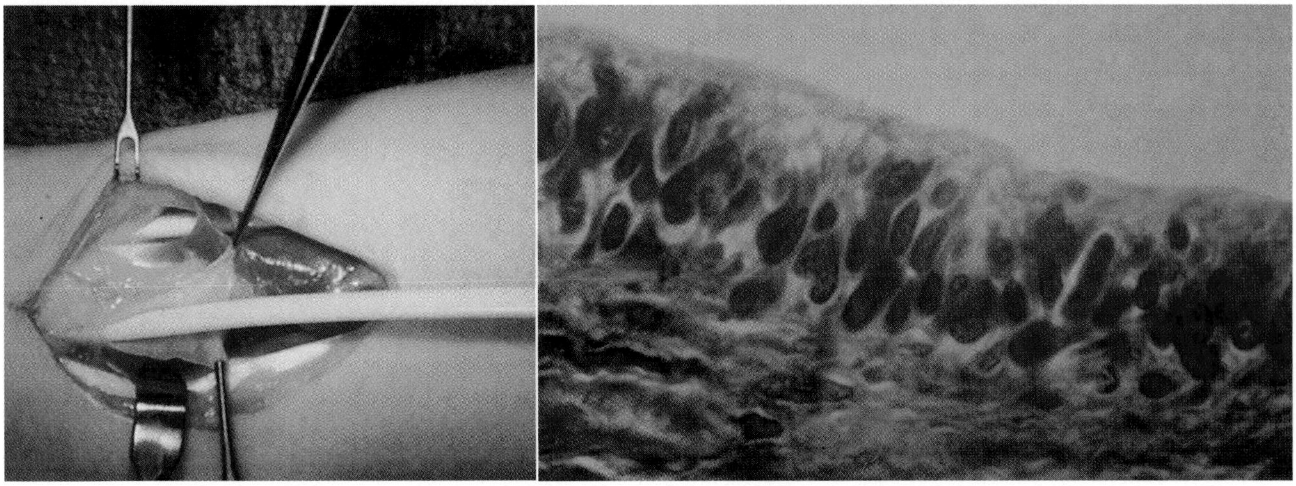

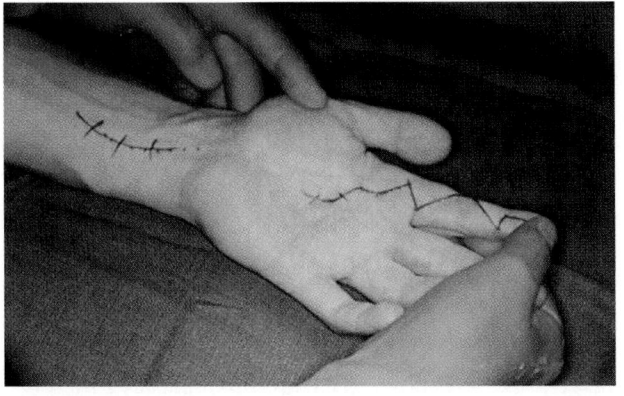

Plate 32. Case study 1. Incision for stage I reconstruction: nutrition, sensation, and passive range of motion are satisfactory at the time of surgery. (From Strickland JW, editor: Master techniques in orthopaedic surgery. In: *The hand,* Philadelphia, 1998, Lippincott-Raven.)

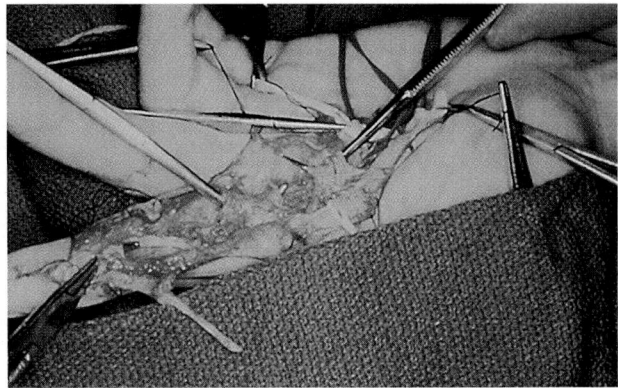

Plate 33. Case study 1. Exploration of flexor tendon bed of right index finger. The tendon bridge graft is removed at the distal part of the wound. Three key pulleys are preserved, with metal instruments identifying the pulleys. *Note:* The A_2 pulley eventually failed by rupture, requiring late reconstruction after stage II grafting. (From Strickland JW, editor: Master techniques in orthopaedic surgery. In: *The hand,* Philadelphia, 1998, Lippincott-Raven.)

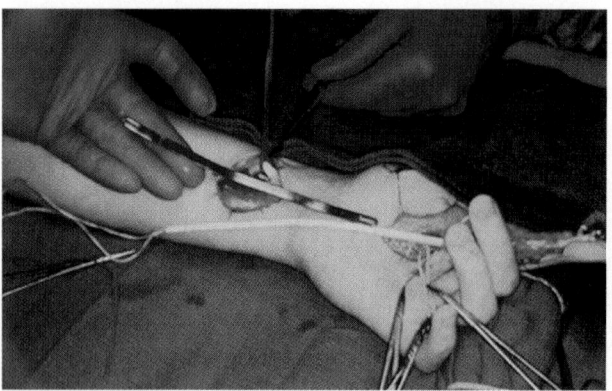

Plate 34. Case study 1. Flexor tendon bed has been prepared by removing all scar tissue and preserving the pulleys. **A,** Digital nerves are identified by yellow vessel loops. **B,** Long active tendon implants are being sized on the hand (note metal plate distal and two porous cords proximal). **C,** An Ober tendon passer is shown and is used to guide the proximal end of the tendon implants to the palm and into the forearm. **D,** The loop retractor holds the profundus tendon to the index in the forearm (this is the future motor tendon). (From Strickland JW, editor: Master techniques in orthopaedic surgery. In: *The hand,* Philadelphia, 1998, Lippincott-Raven.)

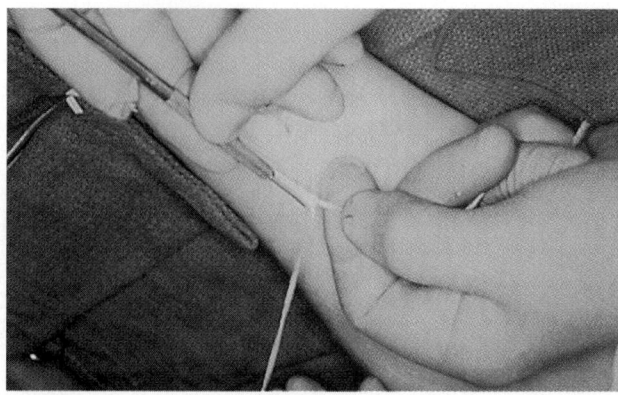

Plate 35. Case study 1. Preparing the length of the active tendon: silicone rubber is trimmed away and two Dacron cords are separated. (From Strickland JW, editor: Master techniques in orthopaedic surgery. In: *The hand,* Philadelphia, 1998, Lippincott-Raven.)

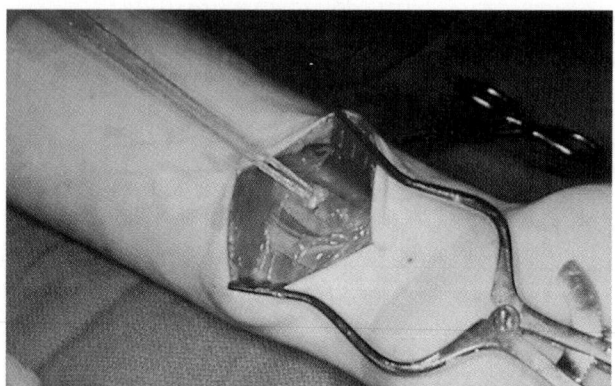

Plate 36. Case study 1. Proximal junction completed between tendon implant and flexor to determine the profundus tendon of the index finger in the forearm: two Dacron cords are divided using hot cautery, with the distal end completed first by fixing the metal plate of the distal phalanx with a screw. Finally, the muscle of the flexor profundus of the index finger will gently cover the juncture. (From Strickland JW, editor: Master techniques in orthopaedic surgery. In: *The hand,* Philadelphia, 1998, Lippincott-Raven.)

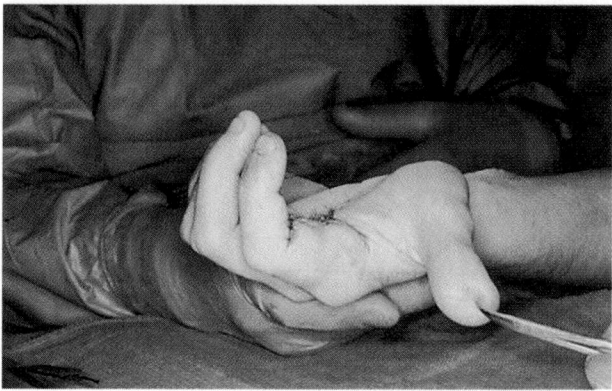

Plate 37. Case study 1. Stage I: complete tendon balance is noted with wrist in the neutral position. (From Strickland JW, editor: Master techniques in orthopaedic surgery. In: *The hand,* Philadelphia, 1998, Lippincott-Raven.)

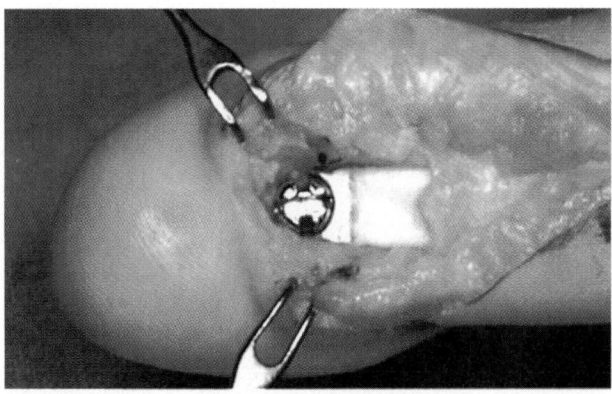

Plate 38. Case study 2. Active tendon: fixed-length type with metal plate and screw in distal phalanx and loop-to-loop juncture to profundus tendon in index finger in the proximal forearm. The excursion of the tendon implant is seen in the forearm and the function of the finger is ¼ inch of the distal palmar crease. At the time of stage II, the distal end is opened, showing metal screw and plate. This will be replaced by tendon grafting. (From Strickland JW, editor: Master techniques in orthopaedic surgery. In: *The hand,* Philadelphia, 1998, Lippincott-Raven.)

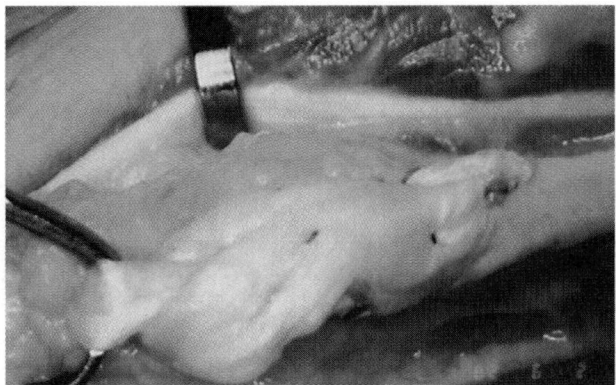

Plate 39. Case study 2. Stage II tendon graft at the left and the junctures to the profundus tendon of the index finger at the right. This important illustration shows the preservation of the connective tissue structure that existed around the proximal juncture of the tendon implant. All soft tissue is preserved; the graft is ready to glide within the tendon sheath, to the left, into the finger. This reconnected tissue is held in the retractor at the top and will be gently closed with a 5-0 suture. Using this method, the stage II proximal tendon graft juncture will have little, if any, restrictive adhesions. (From Strickland JW, editor: Master techniques in orthopaedic surgery. In: *The hand,* Philadelphia, 1998, Lippincott-Raven.)

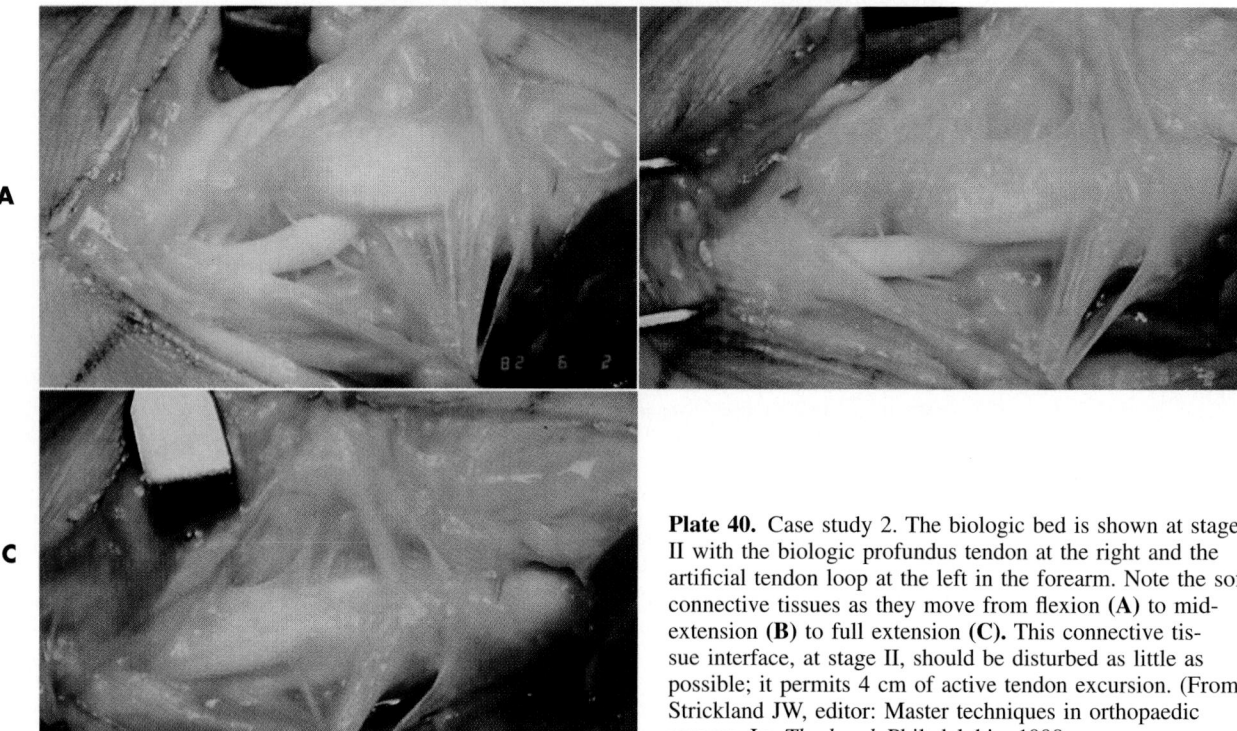

Plate 40. Case study 2. The biologic bed is shown at stage II with the biologic profundus tendon at the right and the artificial tendon loop at the left in the forearm. Note the soft connective tissues as they move from flexion **(A)** to mid-extension **(B)** to full extension **(C).** This connective tissue interface, at stage II, should be disturbed as little as possible; it permits 4 cm of active tendon excursion. (From Strickland JW, editor: Master techniques in orthopaedic surgery. In: *The hand,* Philadelphia, 1998, Lippincott-Raven.)

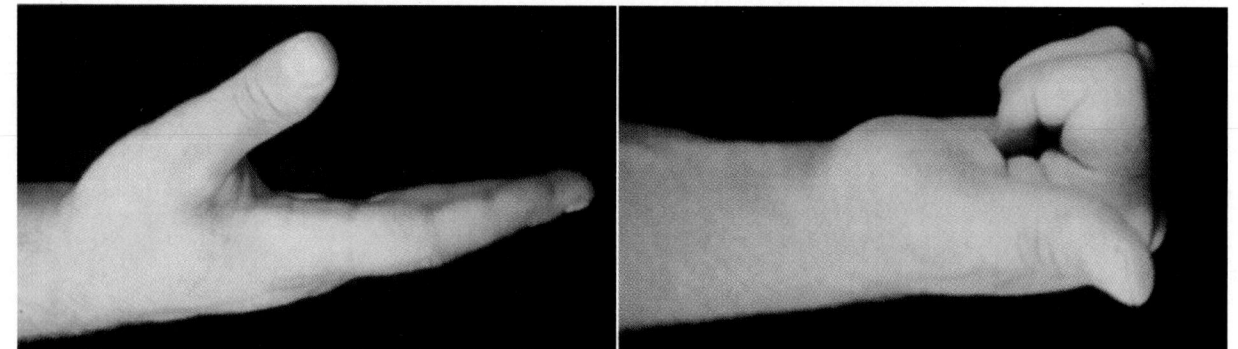

Plate 41. A and **B,** Case study 2. Follow-up of the patient 9 months after stage II tendon grafting: full flexion. The patient has been at light-duty work between stages I and II, and returned to light-duty work 12 weeks after stage II flexor tendon reconstructive surgery. (From Strickland JW, editor: Master techniques in orthopaedic surgery. In: *The hand,* Philadelphia, 1998, Lippincott-Raven.)

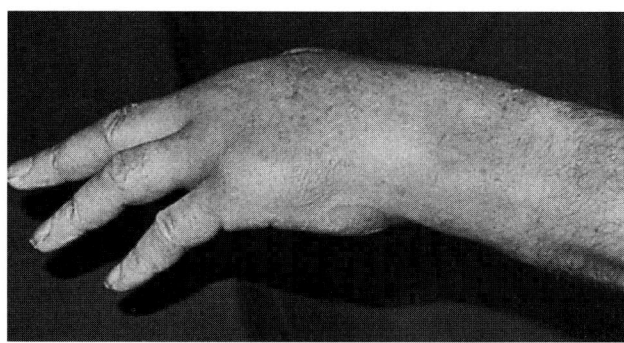

Fig. 30-1. Distension of dorsal skin and fascia reverses transverse metacarpal arch and tethers digits in extension.

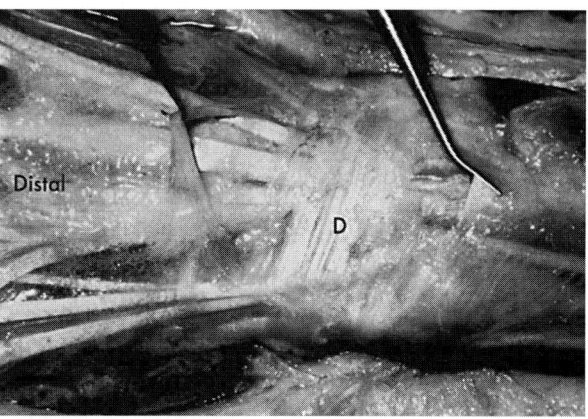

Fig. 30-2. Anatomy of deep dorsal fascia. Probe elevates deep fascia proximally while hook holds deep fascia distal to fibers of extensor retinaculum. Areolar peritendinous fascia, the paratenon, envelops extensor tendons distal to the extensor retinaculum. Fascia contributes to efficiency of tendon excursion and intrinsic tendon circulation. *D,* Extensor retinaculum.

lack of attachment to the supratendinous retinaculum permits unrestricted ulnar rotation during pronation and supination. The fixed tunnel, or *subsheath*,[123] exists only distal to the ulnar head[27,73] and attaches to the triangular fibrocartilage complex (TFCC),[166] triquetrum, pisiform, and fifth meta-carpal. This tunnel maintains the straight course of the ECU between the ulnar styloid and the fifth metacarpal during forearm pronation and supination. The ECU slips dorsal to the ulnar styloid and outside its groove during supination. The ECU is dynamically stabilized proximal to the fixed sheath by a fascial sling, the linea jugata, that tightens during supination and opposes further tendon displacement.[165]

The pliable skin over the dorsum of the hand lacks the fascial septa that stabilize the palmar skin. The skin redundancy associated with digital extension is consumed during grip. This tightening of the dorsal skin compresses the underlying dorsal veins and lymphatics, providing an efficient venous and lymphatic pump.

The superficial dorsal fascia of the hand is composed of a variable fatty layer and a deeper membranous layer that contains the dorsal veins, superficial lymphatics, and sensory branches of the radial and ulnar nerves. The superficial fascia is loosely attached to the deep fascia, with the interface representing a potential space. Dorsal subcutaneous bleeding and lymphedema tether the fingers in extension and the thumb in extension/supination. The pump mechanism is hampered, swelling increases, and grip becomes restrained further. Dorsal cicatrix also restrains normal grip mechanics. The penalty for uncontrolled dorsal swelling is secondary joint stiffness with tightness of the MP joints and dorsal fascia of the thumb web (Fig. 30-1).

The extensor retinaculum continues distally as the deep fascia over the dorsum of the hand (Fig. 30-2). This deep fascia is composed of two layers, a dorsal supratendinous layer and a deep infratendinous layer. They define a closed fascial space bordered by the synovial sheaths of the extensor tendons proximally, the index and fifth metacarpals, and the metacarpal heads distally. The flattened finger

extensor tendons course between these two layers of the deep fascia, invested in a vascularized film of peritendinous fascia, the *paratenon*. The infratendinous layer of the deep fascia rests on the interosseous fascia (Fig. 30-3).

The peritendinous fascia is represented in the embryonic hand and is believed to give rise to the extensor tendons. Anatomic variations in the extensor tendons may reflect developmental variations in the precursor of adult paratenon.[26,60,67,120] This transparent vascular membrane permits gliding of the extensor tendons within the small tolerances of the two layers of the deep fascia. The response to certain traumatic conditions demonstrates a prodigious capacity for generating scar tissue and adhesions (see subsequent discussion of Secrétan's disease).

The extensor tendons receive their blood supply through vascular mesenteries—mesotendons—that are analogous to the vincula of the flexor tendons.[184] Branches of the radial and ulnar arteries, perforating dorsal branches of the anterior interosseous artery, and vessels originating in the deep palmar arch are carried to the tendons in these flexible folds of delicate fascia. The mesotendons are longer and are adapted to a longer tendon excursion where the extensor tendons are synovial beneath the extensor retinaculum but are significantly shorter within the deep fascial pocket over the metacarpals.[183] The intratendinous vascular architecture of the extensor tendons is similar throughout.[168] Synovial diffusion, which provides 70% of the nutrition, is the major nutritional pathway for the extensor tendons beneath the extensor retinaculum. Vascular perfusion through the meso-tendons provides significantly less (30%). No significant contribution is made by the longitudinal intratendinous vasculature.[99] The contribution of the deep fascia to the intrinsic nutrition of the extensor tendons may parallel the role of the fibroosseous sheath in synovial diffusion of the flexor tendons.[99,184]

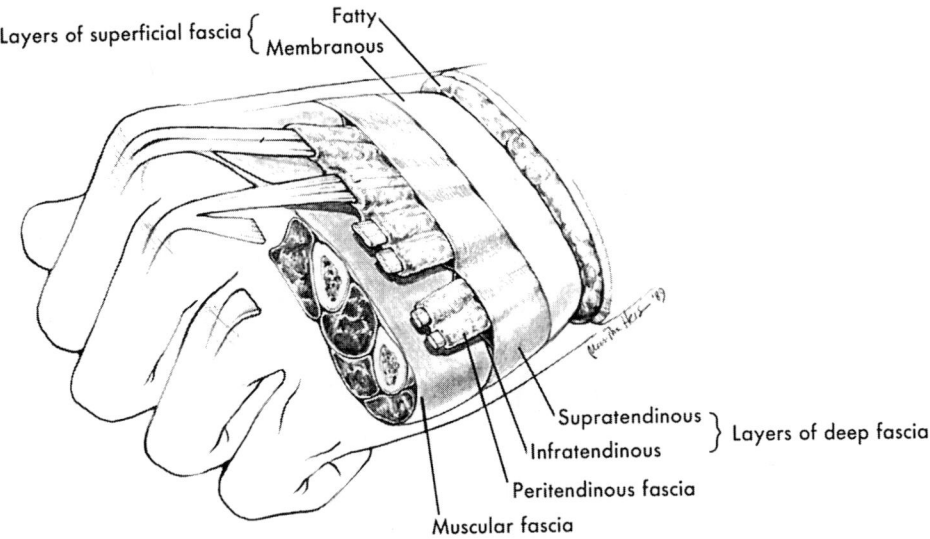

Layers of superficial fascia { Fatty
Membranous

Supratendinous } Layers of deep fascia
Infratendinous
Peritendinous fascia
Muscular fascia

Fig. 30-3. Dorsal fascia of hand. (Redrawn from Anson BJ, et al: *Surg Gynecol Obstet* 81:327, 1945.)

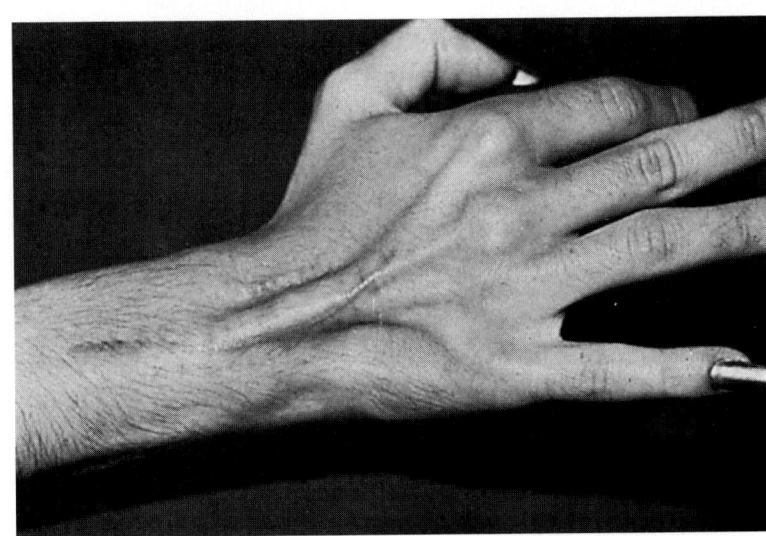

Fig. 30-4. Dorsal bowing and reduced effective extensor excursion as a result of removal of dorsal retaining layers. A portion of the extensor retinaculum must be retained to preserve function and avoid disfigurement.

The dorsal fascia contributes another function to the extensor tendons. The supratendinous layer constitutes a dorsal pulley that promotes efficient distal transfer of the inherent strength and amplitude of the extensor muscles. Selective removal of portions of the dorsal fascia is compatible with retained function. A portion of the extensor retinaculum should be retained at the level of the radiocarpal and ulnocarpal joints. The tendon excursion required to achieve a given degree of wrist extension is doubled by resecting the extensor retinaculum.[123] Excessive removal results in unsightly bowing and altered extensor kinetics. Patients may compensate for bowstringing and decreased extensor power by not endeavoring to extend the fingers when the wrist is extended (Fig. 30-4).

Extensor tenosynovectomy of the first dorsal compartment for stenosing tenosynovitis should preserve the volar attachment of the extensor retinaculum to the distal radius and limit fascial release distal to the radial styloid. Disruption of the volar attachment of the first compartment permits palmar displacement of the first compartment tendons during wrist flexion. An extended release distal to the radial styloid can introduce tendon bowing that changes normal thumb mechanics. First metacarpal abduction by the abductor pollicis longus (APL) is then weakened. Extensor pollicis brevis (EPB) bowing increases its moment arm for first metacarpal extension but may also lessen thumb MP joint extension (Fig. 30-5).

The dressing applied after an operative procedure should contribute to the control of hand edema and discourage hematoma formation. Sterile Dacron batting (Mountain Mist, Stearns & Foster, Cincinnati, Ohio), immersed in saline solution and applied wet about the wound, provides

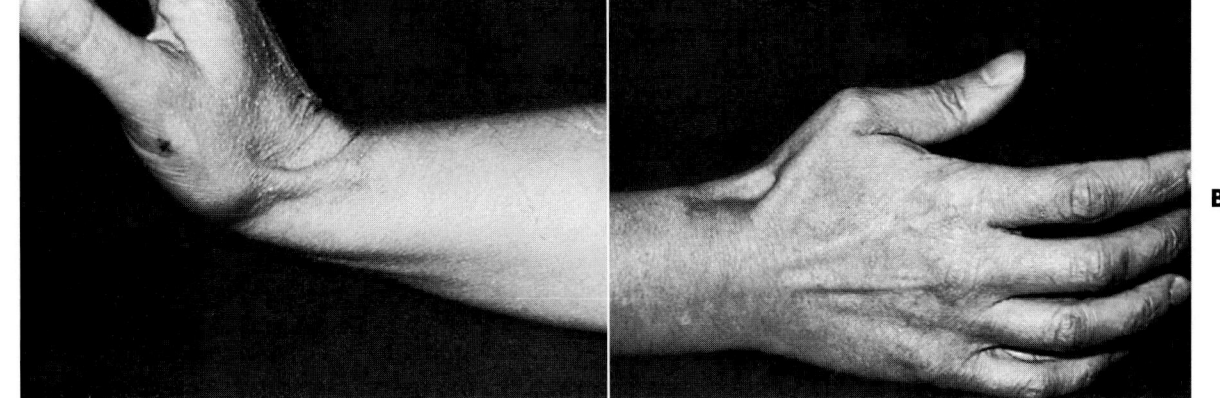

Fig. 30-5. Thumb imbalance reflecting removal of extensor retinaculum and deep fascia, retaining abductor pollicis longus and extensor pollicis brevis. **A,** Displacement of tendons and bowing with wrist extension/flexion. **B,** Exaggerated extension of first metacarpal with extension lag at metacarpophalangeal joint resulting from alteration of moment arms and decreased effective excursions of these tendons. Deep fascia distal to the radius should be retained when the extensor retinaculum is released over the first dorsal compartment.

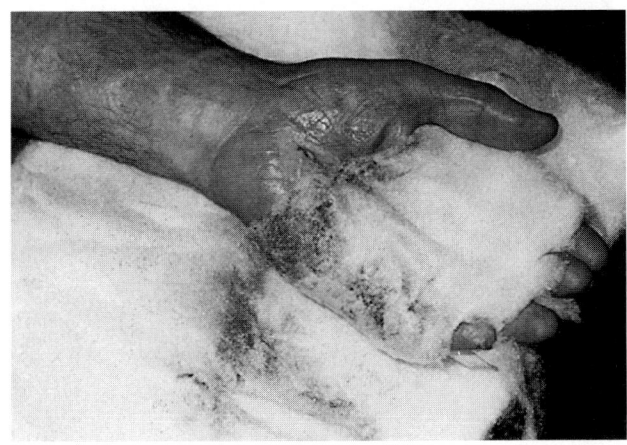

Fig. 30-6. Wet polyester batting makes comfortable, gently compressive dressing and disperses blood away from wound.

comfortable, gently compressive immobilization of the hand and promotes diffusion of expressed blood away from the wound (Fig. 30-6).

WRIST EXTENSOR TENDONS

The wrist extensor tendons are the key to balanced hand function and the success of rehabilitation after injury. Positional grip depends on the selective stabilizing forces of the three wrist extensor tendons. The digital extensor tendons, in the absence of the wrist extensor tendons, can secondarily induce wrist extension. However, this substitution lacks normal power and is devoid of flexibility in spatial positioning of the hand. Wrist extension is then the obligate follower of finger extension, an unnatural functional sequence.

The stations of the extensor carpi radialis longus (ECRL), extensor carpi radialis brevis (ECRB), and ECU are fixed relative to the axis of wrist motion in the second, third, and sixth dorsal compartments, respectively, at the level of the distal radius and ulna (Fig. 30-7). The three wrist extensor muscles have different masses, cross-sectional areas, fiber lengths, and moment arms.[5,14,24,75] These differences are manifested in varying performances and contributions to wrist motion.*

The ECRB, with the longest extension moment arm and the largest cross-sectional area, is the strongest and most efficient wrist extensor. The ECRL extends proximal to the elbow and has the longest muscle fibers and the largest mass, and thus it has the greatest capacity for sustained work. It extends and radially deviates the wrist and opposes the FCU. The ECU has the longest moment arm for ulnar deviation but is most effective as an ulnar deviator with the forearm positioned in pronation. The radial wrist extensors have an amplitude of 37 mm during wrist flexion/extension; the ECU has 18 mm.[12] These three muscles with different anatomic endowments are cerebrally integrated to balance wrist extension, flexion, and ulnar and radial deviation.

---

*Mass or volume of muscle fibers is proportional to work capacity. Cross-sectional area of all fibers is proportional to maximum tension. Average fiber length is proportional to potential excursion. Moment arm is the perpendicular distance from the axis of motion.[10]

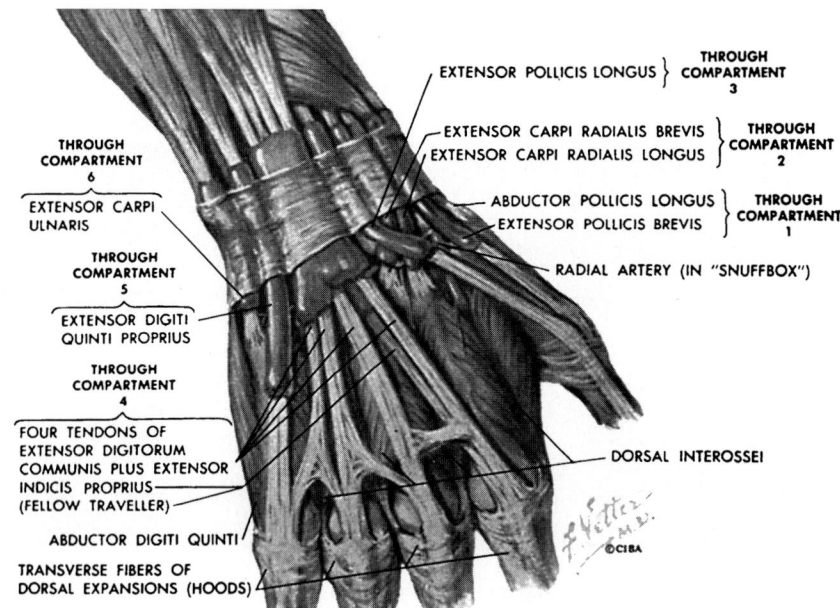

Fig. 30-7. Extensor tendon anatomy. (From Lampe EW: *Surgical anatomy of the hand,* Summit, NJ, 1969, CIBA Pharmaceutical.)

The ECU is unique among the wrist extensor tendons. It exhibits some degree of contraction during all phases of wrist motion. Its variable potential for wrist extension depends on the position of forearm rotation. During pronation, the normal tendon rests on the medial (ulnar) side of the ulnar head and stabilizes the wrist: It is a strong ulnar deviator and balances the tension of all tendons radial to the axis of wrist motion (in the proximal end of the capitate) but is a relatively weak wrist extensor. When the forearm is supinated, its moment arm for wrist extension lengthens and the ECU becomes a more efficient wrist extensor.[181]

The tendon of the ECU inserts distally on the base of the fifth metacarpal. It is firmly stabilized distal to the ulnar head, from the base of the ulnar styloid to the triquetrum, by its own fibroosseous sheath, a strong collar of synovial-lined deep fascia that is separate from the overlying supratendinous layer of the extensor retinaculum.[87,155] The ECU fibroosseous sheath, or subsheath, has a broad, strong connection with the underlying TFCC. Release of the TFCC increases excursion and bowstringing of the ECU during wrist extension[166] (Fig. 30-8).

Proximally, the ECU tendon is stabilized dynamically by a longitudinal thickened band of the forearm fascia, the *linea jugata,* that originates from the ulnar styloid and courses obliquely proximally and medially. The tendon assumes an ulnar-directed obtuse angle during supination. The apex of the angle is at the transition point between the proximal dynamic stabilizer, the linea jugata, and the distal fixed stabilizer, the *subsheath.* This angle becomes increasingly acute as forearm supination and ulnar wrist deviation increases. Contraction of the ECU, forearm supination, and ulnar wrist deviation increase ulnar-directed stresses on the

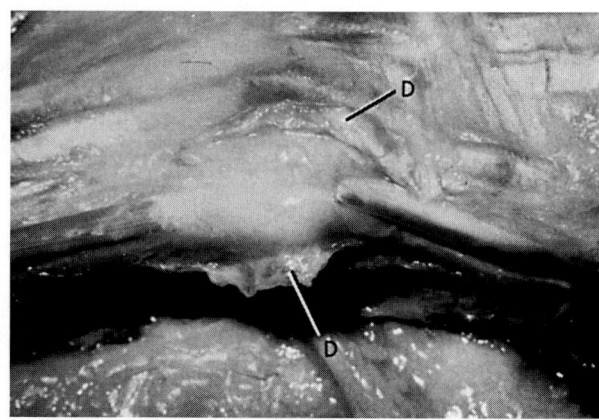

Fig. 30-8. Sixth dorsal compartment. Supratendinous extensor retinaculum is seen reflected. Extensor carpi ulnaris tendon fixed distal to ulna by synovial-lined tunnel of fascia derived from infratendinous retinaculum. Angulation of tendon increases displacement forces during supination. Insertion of tendon on fifth metacarpal to right. *D,* Extensor retinaculum.

ECU that are opposed by the subsheath, the extensor retinaculum, and the linea jugata.[18,165]

Attrition of the ECU from stress-induced tenosynovitis with partial tendon rupture is a source of chronic ulnar wrist pain.[23] The deep fascial tunnel of the ECU can rupture, permitting subluxation of the tendon during forearm rotation.[30,127] This painful condition reflects a specific anatomic deficiency. Reconstruction with a radially based flap from the extensor retinaculum is feasible in patients when symptoms persist despite conservative treatment.[18]

Rupture of the ECU tendon over the distal ulna has been reported from forced supination. Erosion of the floor of the

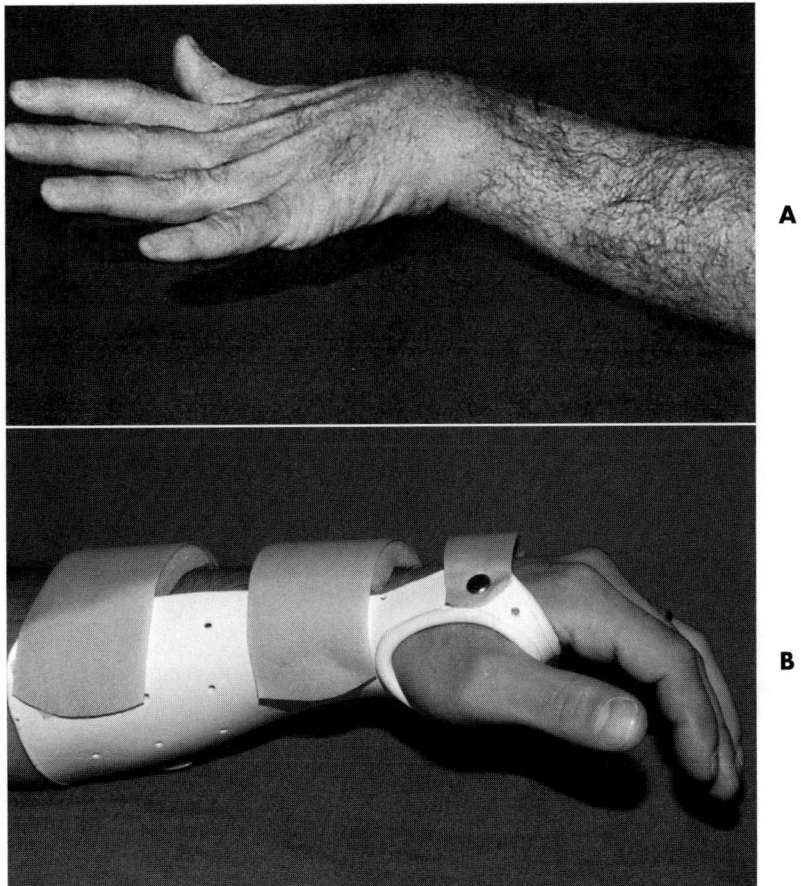

Fig. 30-9. Loss of wrist extensor function after trauma. There was no direct insult to wrist extensors. **A,** Substitution pattern using digital extensors to extend wrist. **B,** Early splinting and reeducation of wrist extensors are necessary.

sixth extensor compartment from an ulnar osteophyte is a variable finding but may contribute to attrition of the tendon. The ruptured tendon can be reconstituted with an intercalary free tendon graft.[112]

The ECU contributes a rare anomalous tendon slip to the EDQ extensor hood. This connection between two tendons with differential excursions can impede simultaneous flexion of the small finger and wrist and produce painful dysfunction. Resection of the anomalous tendon is then indicated.[6]

Wrist extensor function may deteriorate after an injury to the hand or wrist without direct trauma to the wrist extensor tendons. A wrist drop occurs, and a pattern substituting the digital extensors is adopted to implement extension of the wrist. This centrally mediated inhibition of the wrist extensor tendons should be detected early and supportive wrist splinting initiated. The wrist is supported in slight extension, permitting digital flexion and extension while the wrist extensors are being retrained. Extending the wrist against resistance while the digits are fully flexed is helpful in this pursuit. The natural synergy between the wrist extensors and digital flexors facilitates recovery (Fig. 30-9).

Laceration of the ECU introduces a significant imbalance in some patients. The inability to balance the tension of the radial wrist extensors produces persistent radial deviation of the wrist. Extension in ulnar deviation is precluded, grip is weak, and most functions are performed awkwardly (Fig. 30-10, *A*). Laceration of the radial wrist extensors also interferes with balanced spatial positioning of the hand and dexterity of grip (Fig. 30-10, *B*). All three wrist extensor tendons contribute significantly to normal function, and each should be repaired after injury.

FINGER EXTENSOR TENDONS
Proximal to MP joints (zones VIII, VII, and VI)

The extensor tendons of the MP joints of the fingers are the extensor digitorum communis (EDC), the extensor indicis proprius (EIP), and the EDQ. The tendons of the EDC and EIP pass beneath the extensor retinaculum within synovial sheaths in the fourth dorsal compartment, then diverge as they course distally, where they blend with the sagittal bands over the MP joints of the fingers. They flatten distally between the layers of the deep fascia. The EDC

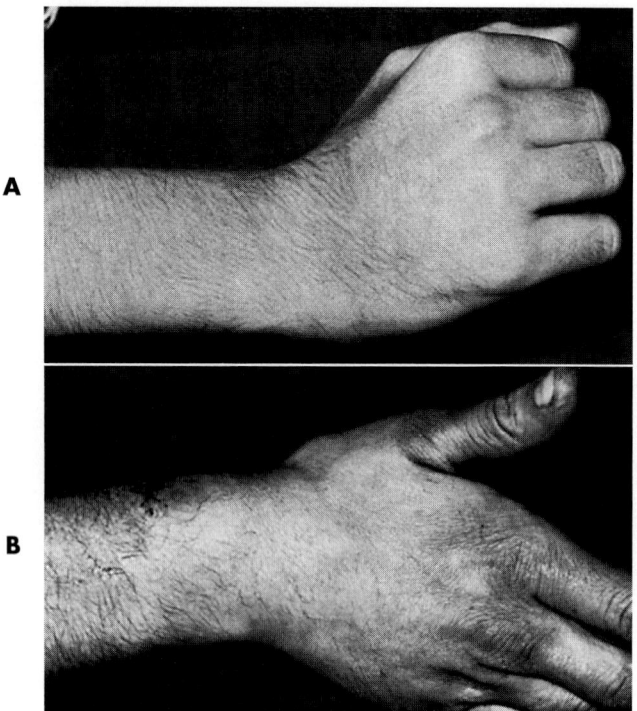

Fig. 30-10. **A,** Interruption of extensor carpi ulnaris (ECU) introduces imbalance of wrist extensors. Therapy after repair requires awareness of multiple facets of normal ECU function. **B,** Laceration of radial wrist extensor tendons. Inability to deviate wrist radially introduces major deficiency in spatial positioning of hand and grip strength.

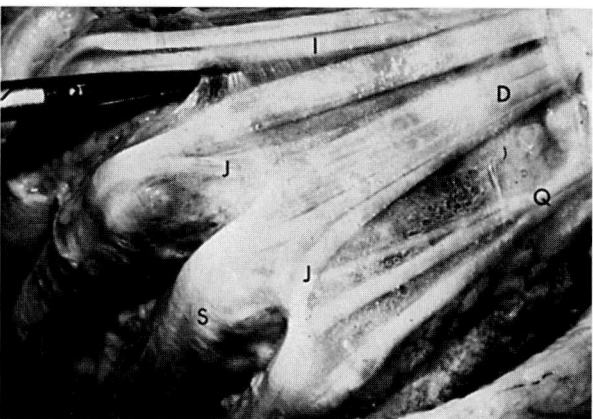

Fig. 30-11. Extensor tendon anatomy. Deep fascia has been removed. Instrument lifts vestige of junctura tendinum to index extensor tendons. *D,* Extensor digitorum communis; *I,* extensor indicis proprius; *J,* junctura tendinum; *Q,* extensor digiti quinti; *S,* sagittal bands over ring metacarpophalangeal joint. Juncturae tendinum dynamically stabilize extensor tendons during grip.

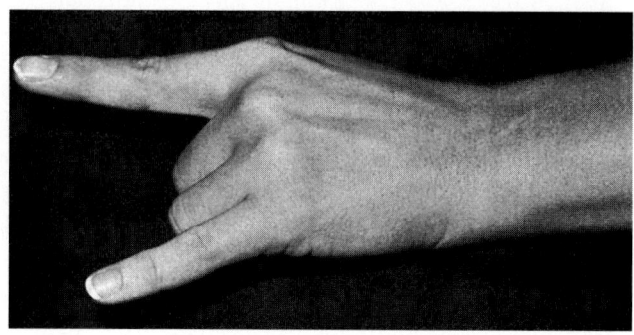

Fig. 30-12. Extensor indicis proprius and extensor digiti quinti have independence of function from separate muscles. No distal tethering exists with flexion of other fingers. Extensor digitorum communis to index finger may have separate muscle belly with individual nerve supply.

contributes substantial tendons to the index, long, and ring fingers, giving a variable slip to the small finger. Extension of the MP joints of the long, ring, and small fingers depends on the position of the adjacent fingers; independent extension is lacking[103,172] (Fig. 30-11). Extensor autonomy is less in the long finger and least in the ring finger. Loss of extensor autonomy has been attributed to fibrous connecting bands within the muscle belly of the EDC in the forearm[72] as well as to the integrity of the juncturae tendinum.[172] A separate muscle belly of the EDC to the index finger with individual nerve supply from the posterior interosseous nerve can preserve independent index finger extension after the EIP has been transferred.[111]

The excursion of the extrinsic finger extensor tendons approximates 50 mm: 31 mm with wrist flexion/extension, 16 mm with MP joint motion, 3 to 4 mm with proximal interphalangeal (PIP) joint motion, and 3 to 4 mm with distal interphalangeal (DIP) joint motion.*

The EIP and EDQ have independent muscles that allow independent function. Extension of the index and small fingers is readily performed, irrespective of flexed positions

*DIP joint motion only imparts motion to the extensor tendon over the proximal phalanx when the PIP joint is restrained. Normally, terminal tendon excursion is dissipated at the level of the PIP joint by the migration of the lateral bands and does not affect the extensor tendon more proximally.

of the other fingers (Fig. 30-12). The EIP may contribute a rare, anomalous tendon to the thumb: the extensor pollicis and indicis communis tendon.[26] An anomalous muscle originating from the dorsal compartment of the forearm and inserting into the extensor hood of the long finger, the *extensor medii proprius,*[171] is analogous to the EIP.[178] When the EIP splits and inserts into both index and long fingers, the anomaly is termed the *extensor indicis et medii communis.*[171]

Juncturae tendinum. The juncturae tendinum are broad intertendinous connections that diverge from the EDC tendon to the ring finger. These bands connect with the EDC tendons to the long, small, and variably, index fingers. The EDQ commonly receives a significant contribution, but the EIP does not.[171,173] The connection with the EDC tendon to the index finger extensor tendons is frequently only a vestige (see Fig. 30-11). These bands assist extension of adjacent connected fingers by transferring forces during extension, enabling the extensor tendons to function as a

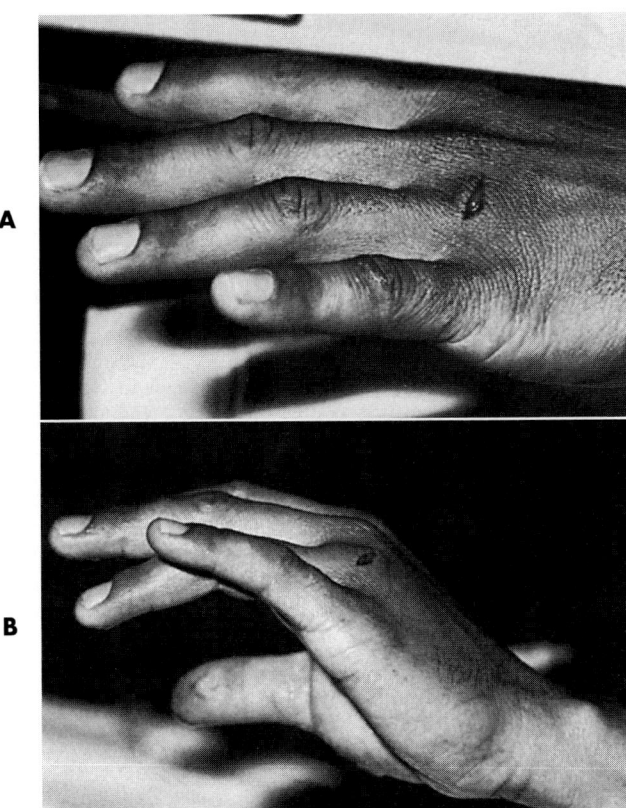

Fig. 30-13. Laceration of extensor tendon to ring finger. **A,** No apparent deficit with wrist in neutral. Metacarpophalangeal joint extension accomplished through fascial connection. **B,** Deficit is apparent when function is tested with combined wrist and finger extension.

unit.[103,171] Laceration of an extensor tendon proximally may be obscured by the contribution of these bands. Demonstration of a full range of potential motion with direct visualization of the injured tendon is required before the possibility of a lacerated tendon can be dismissed (Fig. 30-13). A junctura between the index EDC and extensor pollicis longus (EPL) is an anatomic variant. Thumb interphalangeal (IP) joint flexion restrains index finger extension when this variant exists.[161]

The extensor tendons to the fingers diverge distal to the extensor retinaculum. During finger flexion these tendons glide distally and separate. The juncturae tendinum assume a more transverse orientation and develop increased tension as they displace distally. They dynamically stabilize the fingers by transmitting forces to the radial sagittal bands of the index and long fingers and to the ulnar sagittal bands of the ring and small fingers. Active grip thus contributes to the stability of the transverse metacarpal arch and to the centralization of the extensor tendons over the dorsum of the MP joints.[1]

The role of the juncturae and the normal displacements of the finger extensor tendons are applied during reconstruction for extensor tendon ruptures. Distal ends of ruptured tendons

are sutured to intact adjacent tendons. Tension at the tendon junction is adjusted with the fingers held in slightly less than full flexion. This ensures that the sutured tendons are sufficiently oblique for transmission of active extension forces and that tendon separation will not be restricted during finger flexion (Fig. 30-14).

Extensor digiti quinti. The extensor tendons to the small finger have significant anatomic features.[141] The EDQ gains attachment to the abductor tubercle of the base of the proximal phalanx through insertion of its ulnar tendon into the abductor digiti quinti (ADQ) tendon (Fig. 30-15). Some patients with ulnar palsy who are incapable of MP joint hyperextension and do not develop a claw deformity acquire an abduction deformity of the small finger (Wartenberg's sign) from paralysis of the third palmar interosseous muscle. Their abducted small finger is associated with an oblique junctura from the ring finger, a weak biomechanical link. The EDQ is relatively unopposed and abducts the small finger. Patients who do not acquire this deformity have a transverse orientation of the junctura, a biomechanically forceful link that opposes the deformity.[9]

An oblique junctura from the ring finger will permit continued extension of the small finger after interruption of the EDQ more proximally. The patient often is unaware of any deficit until the decreased strength and lost autonomy are demonstrated. This situation is seen commonly in patients with rheumatoid arthritis (Fig. 30-16).

Tendon ruptures. The wrist and finger extensor tendons are exposed to entrapment by fractures of the distal radius[66,97,113] and dislocations of the distal ulna.[122] Attrition with delayed rupture has been reported from multiple conditions, including anomalous extensor brevis manus muscle,[64,134] Madelung's deformity,[57] tophaceous pyrophosphate deposition,[69] rheumatoid tenosynovitis, nonrheumatoid dorsal subluxation of the distal ulna,[57] granulomatous tenosynovitis, extraskeletal osteochondroma,[105] Kienbock disease,[105] nonunion scaphoid fracture,[57] instability of the distal ulna after excessive surgical resection,[114] fixation screws,[105] and nonunion fracture of Lister's tubercle.

Secrétan's disease. Hard, brawny edema involving the dorsum of the hand has stimulated controversy since it was described in 1901.[146] The condition follows trauma to the dorsum of the hand, often pursues a protracted course, and has been associated with an unfavorable surgical prognosis.[138] It has been considered synonymous with factitious, or self-induced, edema.[129,152] Monetary gain and compensation award have been considered significant causative factors. The anatomy of the dorsum of the hand and the clinical observations at surgery support the contention that there is a specific pathologic entity involving peritendinous fibrosis about the extensor tendons and juncturae tendinum, within the confines of the layers of the deep fascia after trauma, which is different from factitious dorsal edema.[130,132] The form and distribution of the fibrosis

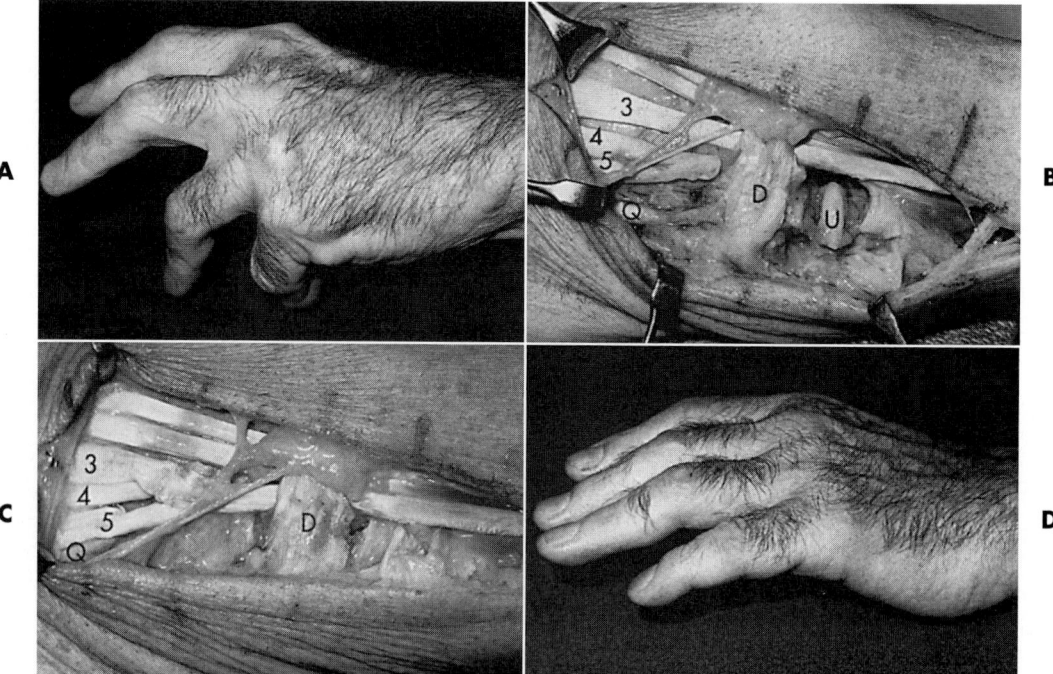

Fig. 30-14. Ruptured extensor tendons to ring and small fingers in 65-year-old man with caput ulnae syndrome caused by rheumatoid arthritis. **A,** Active extension deficit. **B,** Distal ends of ruptured extensor digiti quinti (EDQ) and extensor digitorum communis (EDC) to ring and small fingers lie distal to retained strip of extensor retinaculum. Deformed ulnar head has eroded joint capsule. **C,** Adjacent suture of EDC from ring and small fingers into EDC to long finger, and EDQ into EDC to small finger. Tendon junction is flat, and sutures are tied beneath tendon. **D,** Active extension 6 months after reconstruction. Finger flexion was retained. *D,* Extensor retinaculum; *Q,* EDQ; *U,* ulnar head; *3,* EDC to long finger; *4,* EDC to ring finger; *5,* EDC to small finger.

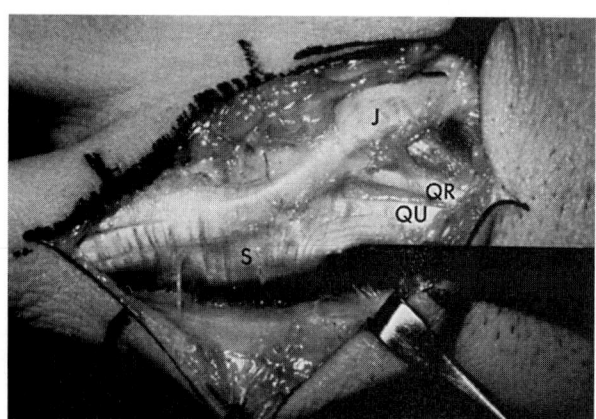

Fig. 30-15. Extensor tendon insertion at metacarpophalangeal joint of small finger. Extensor digiti quinti (EDQ) gains attachment to lateral tubercle of proximal phalanx through insertion of its ulnar tendon into abductor digiti quinti tendon. *J,* Junctura tendinum; *QR,* radial tendon EDQ; *QU,* ulnar tendon EDQ; *S,* sagittal bands.

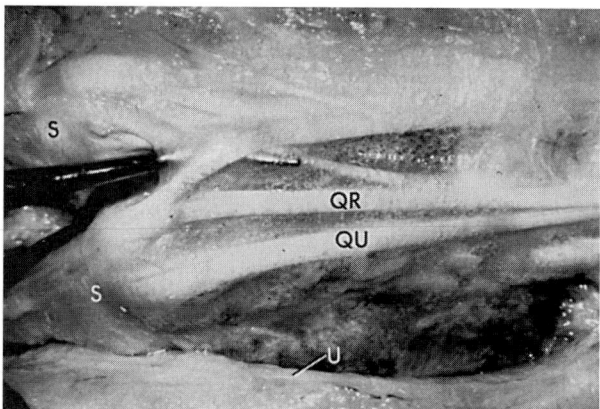

Fig. 30-16. Extrinsic extensor tendons to the small finger. Deep fascia has been removed. Instrument lifts oblique junctura to small finger. This oblique connection may mask rupture of the extensor digiti quinti (EDQ) proximally. *QR,* Radial tendon EDQ; *QU,* ulnar tendon EDQ; *S,* sagittal bands; *U,* dorsal sensory branch of ulnar nerve.

conform to the fascial anatomy already described.[68] The inelastic peritendinous scar restricts excursion of the finger extensor tendons and their juncturae, blocking longitudinal and transverse tendon glide. Surgical, psychologic, and rehabilitative treatment are necessarily integrated. This condition presents a diverse spectrum of clinical challenges with a cautious prognosis.

MP joints and distal (zones V, IV, III, II, and I)

The form and complexity of the extensor tendons change at the level of the sagittal bands that shroud the MP joints of the fingers. Distally, they consist of a continuous sheet of precisely oriented fibers that transmit tension. This fiber array wraps the finger skeleton in the form of a bisected cone that is composed of a tendon system, which transmits tension and imparts motion, and a retinacular system, which stabilizes the tendon system. An alteration in the alignment or length of the proximal or middle phalanges of the fingers changes the normal adjustment of forces within the tendon systems and permits the retinacular system to foreshorten.[86] The imbalance within the tendon system establishes deformities; the tightening of the retinacular system fixes these deformities and resists correction.

The broad, fibrous dorsal hood of the finger MP joints consists of fibers from the juncturae tendinum, sagittal bands, and extensor tendon. The extensor tendon is nested between two layers of the sagittal bands: a thin superficial layer and a thick, deep layer. These two layers blend laterally to form a single, substantial layer.[63,65] This blend of fibers is strong except in the long finger, where the superficial sagittal layer and the deep extensor attachments are relatively weak.[76] Ulnar displacement forces are greatest with the MP joints in full extension, decrease during the first 60 degrees of flexion, then progressively increase with greater flexion. Relatively little force is needed to maintain a normally located extensor tendon. Significantly higher restraining forces are required to prevent added displacement of a tendon that is displaced ulnarward; an ulnar-displaced tendon tends to displace further with increased MP joint flexion.[76] Sagittal band rupture can occur during full extension or with grip, is more likely with ulnar wrist deviation, and usually involves the radial sagittal fibers. In the long finger, the extensor tendon can separate from the underlying sagittal band and displace without sagittal band rupture.

The extensor tendons have a variable insertion on the base of the proximal phalanx that is not significant for extension of the fingers.[71,86,169] This insertion, if present, centralizes the extensor tendon but contributes little to the normal kinematics of finger extension. There is a linear relationship between excursion of the extensor tendons over the dorsum of the hand and the angle of motion of the MP joints.[5,32] Extension of the MP joint is achieved through the sagittal bands, vertically oriented fibers that shroud the capsule and

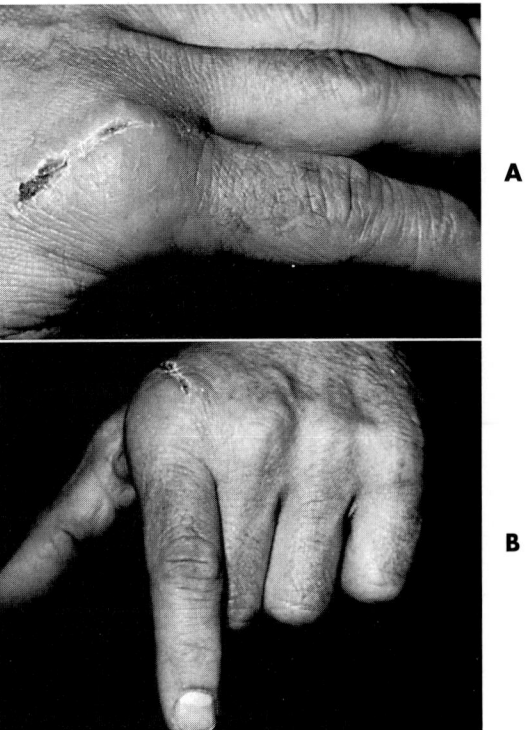

Fig. 30-17. Laceration of radial sagittal bands of index finger without repair. Deformity has developed. **A,** Ulnar displacement with palmar subluxation of extensor digitorum communis results in palmar subluxation with incomplete extension of metacarpophalangeal joint. **B,** Deformity includes ulnar angulation and supination of injured finger.

collateral ligaments, connecting the extensor tendons with the volar plate and proximal phalanx on both sides of the joint.[56] These broad bands constitute functional slings that pass between the joint capsule and the intrinsic muscles (see Fig. 30-16). They cover the axis of joint motion during extension and pass distal to the axis of motion during flexion. They stabilize the extensor tendons over the dorsum of the MP joints during flexion, complementing the juncturae tendinum.[182]

Laceration or closed rupture of the sagittal bands disrupts the stability of the extensor tendons over the MP joints. The extensor tendon displaces ulnarward during flexion. Active extension then produces ulnar angulation of the MP joint with supination of the finger. A painful snap may accompany extension as the extensor tendon relocates dorsally. Tightness develops that maintains the ulnar deviation deformity, prevents dorsal relocation of the extensor tendon, and precludes full active extension of the MP joint (Fig. 30-17).

Distal to the sagittal bands, the lumbrical and interosseous muscles contribute proximal vertical and distal oblique fibers to the extensor tendon over the proximal phalanx (Fig. 30-18). The vertical fibers transmit flexor forces to the proximal phalanx, which flex the MP joint. The oblique

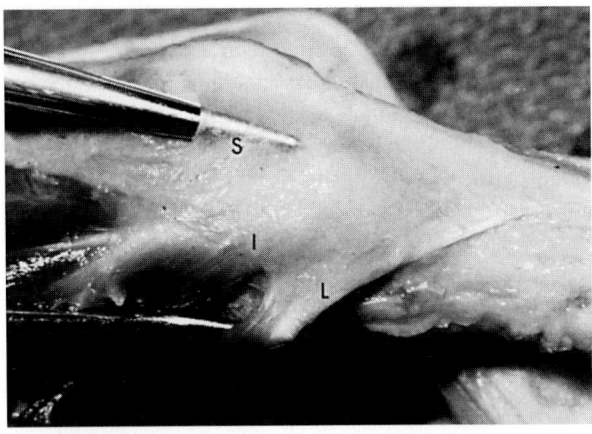

Fig. 30-18. Extrinsic and intrinsic tendons merge about the radial side of the index finger metacarpophalangeal (MP) joint. Sagittal bands effect MP joint extension. Interosseous and lumbrical muscles transmit tension through dorsal apparatus and lateral bands for MP joint flexion and interphalangeal joint extension. *I,* Interosseous tendon; *L,* lumbrical tendon; *S,* sagittal bands.

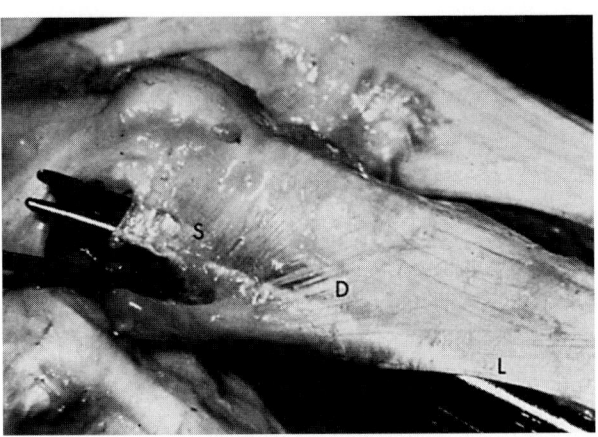

Fig. 30-19. Dorsal apparatus of the finger. Hook retracts interosseous muscle. Sagittal bands separate intrinsic muscles from metacarpophalangeal joint capsule. Sagittal bands and oblique fibers of intrinsic tendon transmit extension forces. Vertical fibers of intrinsic tendons transmit flexion forces. Delicate fibers are vulnerable to interference by scar. *D,* Vertical fibers of intrinsic tendon; *L,* oblique fibers of intrinsic tendon; *S,* sagittal bands.

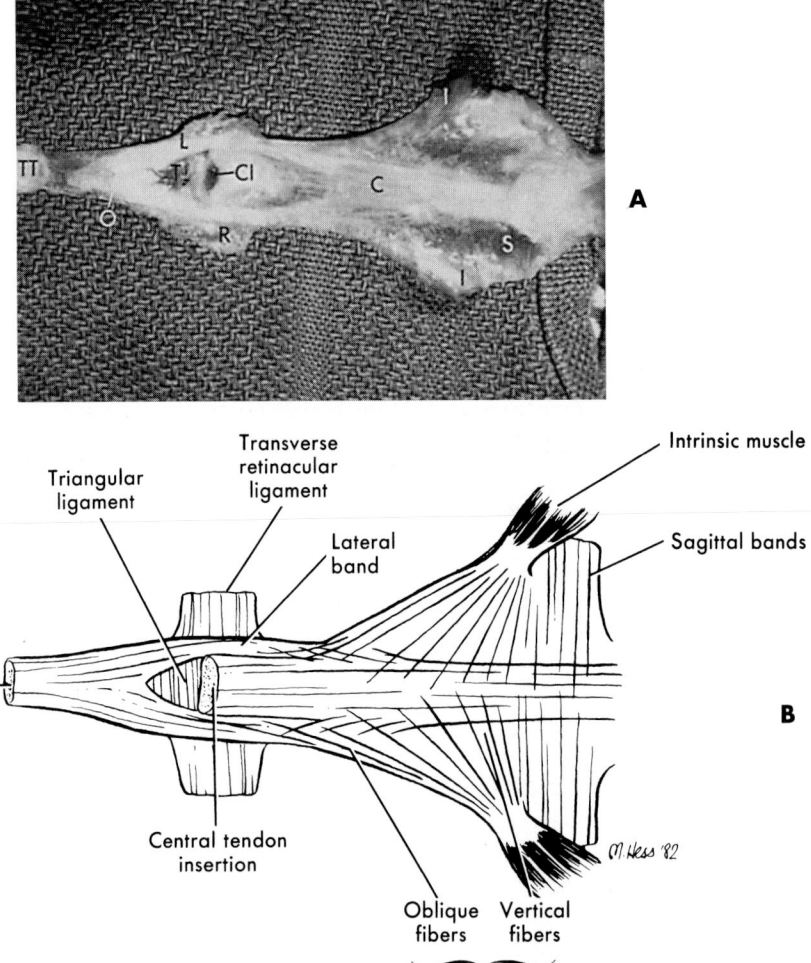

Fig. 30-20. Extensor tendons in fingers are represented by continuous sheet of specialized fibers that are stabilized by retinacular ligaments. **A,** Deep side of extensor tendon complex. Terminal tendon is at left. **B,** Schematic drawing of **A.** *C,* Central tendon; *CI,* central tendon insertion; *I,* intrinsic tendon; *L,* lateral band; *O,* oblique retinacular ligament; *R,* transverse retinacular ligament; *S,* sagittal bands; *T,* triangular ligament, *TT,* terminal tendon.

Triangular ligament

Transverse retinacular ligament

Intrinsic muscle

Lateral band

Sagittal bands

Terminal tendon

Central tendon insertion

Oblique fibers

Vertical fibers

Intrinsic tendon

M. Hess '82

fibers transmit extension forces to the PIP and DIP joints. This combined sheet of extrinsic and intrinsic motored fibers over the proximal phalanx is appropriately termed the *dorsal apparatus* because it contributes to both flexion and extension[151] (Fig. 30-19). The extrinsic extensor tendons are primarily extensors of the MP joints. They are capable of secondarily extending the IP joints only if hyperextension of the MP joint is prevented. The intrinsic tendons flex the MP joints and extend the IP joints.[93,95]

The extensor mechanism about the proximal phalanx is a complex assembly of multidirectional fibers that present a variable spatial orientation during PIP joint flexion. The fiber connections between the central tendon and lateral bands criss-cross in separate layers. The fibers from the central tendon pass superficial to those from the intrinsic lateral bands. Descent of the lateral bands during flexion is accompanied by an increase in the longitudinal angle between these crossing fibers, analogous to the expansion of a taut mesh.[145] These geometric changes are caused by changes in the orientation of the fibers rather than by changes in the length of individual fibers.[44] The delicacy of this fiber interplay accentuates the vulnerability of the extensor tendons in the fingers to the restraints of scar. The extrinsic extensor tendon continues as the central tendon to insert on the dorsal base of the middle phalanx with medial fibers from the intrinsic tendons.

The conjoined lateral bands represent the continuation of the oblique fibers of the intrinsic tendons, supplemented by lateral fibers from the central extensor tendon (Fig. 30-20). The lateral bands continue distally, converging over the middle phalanx as a single terminal tendon that inserts on the dorsal base of the distal phalanx (Fig. 30-21).

The lateral bands normally lie dorsal to the axis of motion of the PIP joints during extension and descend to cover the axis of joint motion during flexion. This shift of the lateral bands permits synchronized motion of both PIP and DIP joints by compensating for the difference in the radii—or moment arms—of both joints. The smaller DIP joint would extend disproportionately relative to the PIP joint without the compensation provided by the shifting of the lateral bands.[151,182]

Retinacular ligaments. The retinacular ligaments consist of fibers that encircle the finger obliquely about the PIP joint. They originate proximally from the flexor fibroosseous sheath and palmar plate and course dorsally and distally about the joint. Their function is analogous to that of the sagittal bands about the MP joints. Fibers palmar to the lateral bands—the transverse retinacular ligaments—contribute to axial stability of the PIP joint, restrain dorsal displacement of the lateral bands, and assist descent of the lateral bands during flexion. Dorsally, these fibers connect the lateral bands: Proximal fibers cover the insertions of the central tendon and medial fibers of the intrinsic tendons; more distal fibers connect the converging

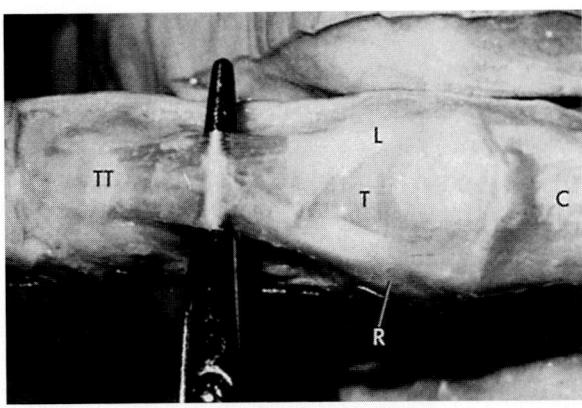

Fig. 30-21. Extensor tendon anatomy about proximal interphalangeal (PIP) and middle phalanx. Central tendon (continuation of extrinsic extensor tendon) courses deep to proximal, transversely oriented retinacular fibers to insert on the dorsal base of the middle phalanx. More distal retinacular fibers (the triangular ligament) normally restrain descent of the lateral bands during PIP joint flexion. Scarring of these fibers can impair PIP joint flexion. Instrument lifts the merged conjoined lateral bands that insert as the terminal extensor tendon to the left. Dissection of the extensor tendon over the middle phalanx invites scarring that may restrict distal interphalangeal joint motion. *C,* Central tendon; *L,* conjoined lateral band; *R,* transverse retinacular ligament; *T,* triangular ligament; *TT,* terminal tendon.

conjoined lateral bands. These distal fibers constitute the triangular ligament. Preservation of these dorsal retinacular ligaments after rupture or surgical division of the central tendon retains active extension of the PIP joint without development of a boutonnière deformity. Interruption of the transverse retinacular ligaments fosters dorsal displacement of the lateral bands with development of a swan-neck deformity.

The oblique retinacular ligaments originate from the flexor fibroosseous sheath at the proximal phalanx, pass palmar to the axis of the PIP joint deep to the transverse retinacular ligament, and insert on the dorsal base of the distal phalanx adjacent to the terminal extensor tendon.[52] Distal fibers interdigitate with the terminal tendon before inserting, an important anatomic feature that influences the clinical presentation of the mallet tendon lesion[156,182] (Fig. 30-22).

The oblique retinacular ligaments probably contribute little to DIP joint extension in the normal finger.[55,147] The position of its proximal fibers depends on the position of the PIP joint. They are below the joint axis only when the PIP joint is flexed. Passive extension of the PIP joint does not normally increase tension through the oblique retinacular ligaments.[31] They may stabilize the loaded finger tip when fully flexed under certain circumstances, such as the intrinsic-plus position with the DIP joint flexed during chuck pinch or when fingering the E string of a violin.[7] They can

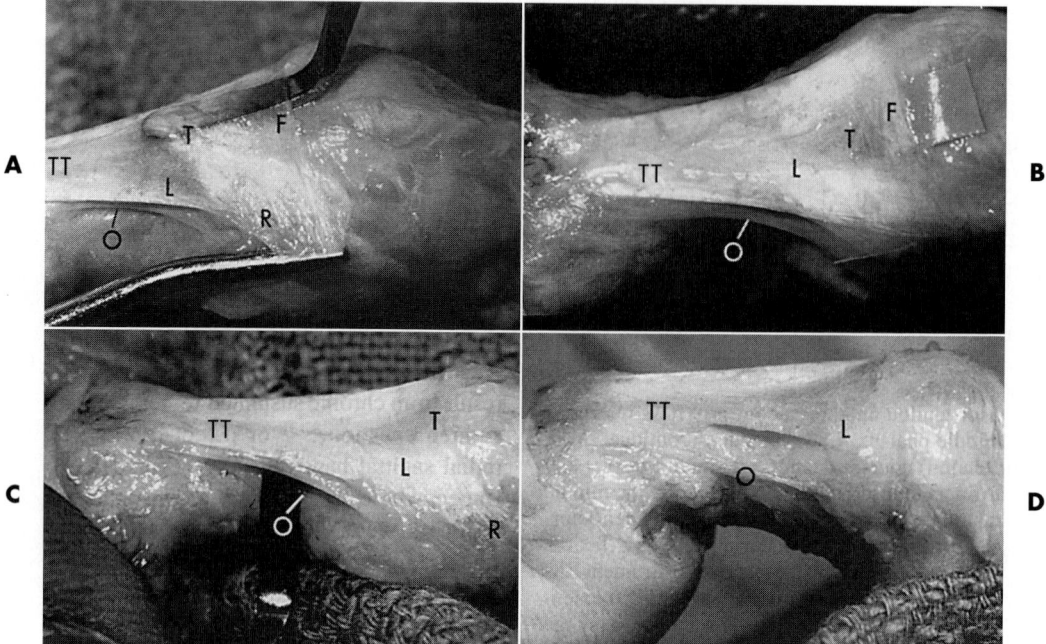

Fig. 30-22. Anatomy of the retinacular ligaments in the fingers. **A,** Vertical fibers about the proximal interphalangeal joint. These continuous fibers influence the descent and ascent of the lateral bands during flexion and extension. **B,** Fibers bridging the lateral bands dorsally restrain palmar migration during flexion. The rubber sheet is beneath the dorsal retinacular fibers and superficial to the central tendon insertion. **C** and **D,** Oblique retinacular ligament. Fibers are oriented in the axis of the finger. Proximal fibers pass beneath the transverse retinacular ligament palmar to the axis of the joint. Distal fibers mix with the lateral bands and terminal tendon. *F,* Dorsal fibers; *L,* lateral band; *O,* oblique retinacular ligament; *R,* transverse retinacular ligament; *T,* triangular ligament; *TT,* terminal tendon. (Adapted from Rosenthal EA: Extensor surface injuries. In Bowers WH, editor: *The interphalangeal joints,* London, 1987, Churchill Livingstone.)

contribute significantly to deformity in the imbalanced finger or when they have been altered by scar.

The terminal tendon alone is capable of completely extending the distal phalanx. The dorsal rectangular segment of the collateral ligaments of the DIP joints can support the distal phalanx in 45 degrees of flexion. In the absence of the terminal tendon, the fully flexed distal finger joint will passively return to midflexion because of the collateral ligaments assisted by the dorsal capsule and oblique retinacular ligaments. Only the terminal tendon can complete extension of this joint.[148]

EXTENSOR TENDON INJURIES ABOUT THE MP JOINTS (ZONE V)

Closed soft tissue injuries about the MP joints of the fingers jeopardize the extensor tendons, sagittal bands, dorsal joint capsule, collateral ligaments, and adjacent intrinsic tendons. Closed fractures of the metacarpal and sprain fractures of the MP joints develop swelling and pain, which must be differentiated from soft tissue injuries by careful clinical and radiographic examination. Radiographs for evaluation of swelling and tenderness after injury of the finger MP joints should include posteroanterior (PA), lateral,

and Brewerton views* to eliminate the possibility of occult marginal fractures.

Differential diagnosis

Subluxation of the extensor tendon. Subluxation of the extensor tendon at this level was described in 1868.[90] It may result from chronic sustained forces,[13,58,121] tendon attrition, sudden exertion,[8,139] or direct trauma.[163] Rupture of the radial sagittal bands usually occurs,[179] except in the long finger, where the extrinsic extensor tendon may dislodge from its weak attachment to the underlying sagittal fibers.[63,76] A partial arcuate tear in the ulnar sagittal bands with chronic pain and swelling over the MP joint without displacement of the extensor tendon also has been described.[82] Radial displacement of the extensor tendon is rare.[135] A chronically painful traumatic rupture of the dorsal capsule without rupture of the overlying sagittal bands can occur; repair of the capsule is then indicated.

*An anteroposterior tangential view of the metacarpal heads, useful for visualizing the fossae of origin of the collateral ligaments. The dorsum of the extended fingers rests on the cassette, with the MP joints in 65 degrees of flexion. The x-ray beam is perpendicular to the cassette and directed 15 degrees from the ulnar side.

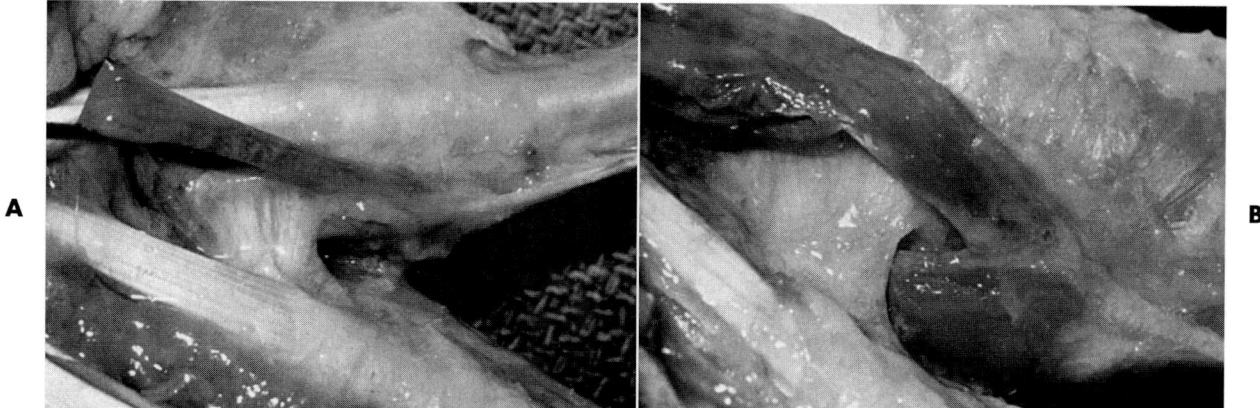

Fig. 30-23. Lumbrical and interosseous muscles merge distal to deep transverse metacarpal ligament: the anatomic basis of saddle syndrome. **A,** Hook lifts third lumbrical palmarward from ligament connecting palmar plates of long and ring finger metacarpophalangeal joints. **B,** Lumbrical merges with second palmar interosseous muscle distally. Adhesions between the ligament and intrinsic tendons may produce painful intrinsic dysfunction.

Displacement of the tendon in the acute injury is commonly obscured by swelling. Extensor tendon subluxation with ulnar finger angulation of the index, long, or ring finger may not appear immediately and will not develop with a partial rupture of the radial sagittal bands. Ulnar angulation of the small finger is opposed by the junctura tendinum. Tenderness, swelling, and ecchymosis are suggestive of sagittal fiber rupture in the acute case.

Conservative nonoperative treatment, including cast immobilization of the wrist with MP joints in the neutral position for 4 weeks, has been successful for treatment of the acute injury.[135] However, surgery is appropriate when complete rupture of the sagittal bands is apparent—the extensor tendon has subluxated and the finger is angulated— and in the chronic recurrent case. Precise reconstitution of the normal anatomic relationships restores a balance that may be only wishful with closed methods.

Surgical repair of a sagittal band defect with extensor subluxation was first described by Haberern.[50] Repair of the radial[77] or ulnar[82] sagittal bands and a variety of surgical tenodeses that maintain the centralized extensor tendon have been described for operative correction of imbalance and dysfunction that persist despite adequate nonoperative treatment.[21,29,35,79,101,104,179]

Saddle syndrome. The interosseous and lumbrical tendons converge distal to the deep transverse metacarpal ligament radial to the MP joint of the long, ring, and small fingers (Fig. 30-23). Consolidation of these tendons by restraining adhesions about the deep transverse metacarpal ligament after closed injuries has been descriptively termed the *saddle syndrome*.[22] This uncommon chronic condition is characterized by persistent pain with grip. Direct and compression tenderness between the adjacent metacarpal

necks, painful active intrinsic function (MP joint flexion with IP extension) against resistance, and pain with eliciting the intrinsic tightness test (passive flexion of the IP joints while the MP joints are supported in extension) support this diagnosis. Intrinsic restraint can be lateralized by deviating the finger away from the side being tested (see Fig. 30-57). Intrinsic tenolysis, including resection of the distal margin of the deep transverse metacarpal ligament through a palmar incision, is indicated when symptoms persist.[22,175]

Collateral ligament rupture. Early diagnosis is apparent when the fully flexed MP joint is unstable to lateral deviation. Normally, this joint is most stable in full flexion. Partial ruptures are painful when tested but retain stability. Radiographs are essential. Closed treatment is indicated initially for soft tissue injuries; significant joint fractures are replaced and internally stabilized. Closed sprains that continue to be painful after immobilization and supportive nonoperative treatment may require surgery.

Chronic tendon adhesions. Inelastic adhesions between the extensor hood, intrinsic tendons, and underlying capsule may be the source of persistent painful swelling with loss of motion. Thickening of the dorsal joint capsule may develop beneath the scarred extensor hood. Chronic thickening of the extensor hood from repeated trauma, reported in students of karate, has been termed *hypertrophic infiltrative tendinitis* (HIT syndrome).[46] Painful active motion, an extrinsic tenodesis (the extensor-plus phenomenon [see Fig. 30-56]), and positive intrinsic tightness test all are possible findings when adhesions consolidate the extrinsic and intrinsic tendons about the finger MP joints.[136] Tenolysis that selectively defines the extrinsic and intrinsic tendon systems, in combination with a dorsal capsulectomy when necessary, liberates the tethered tendons (Fig. 30-24).

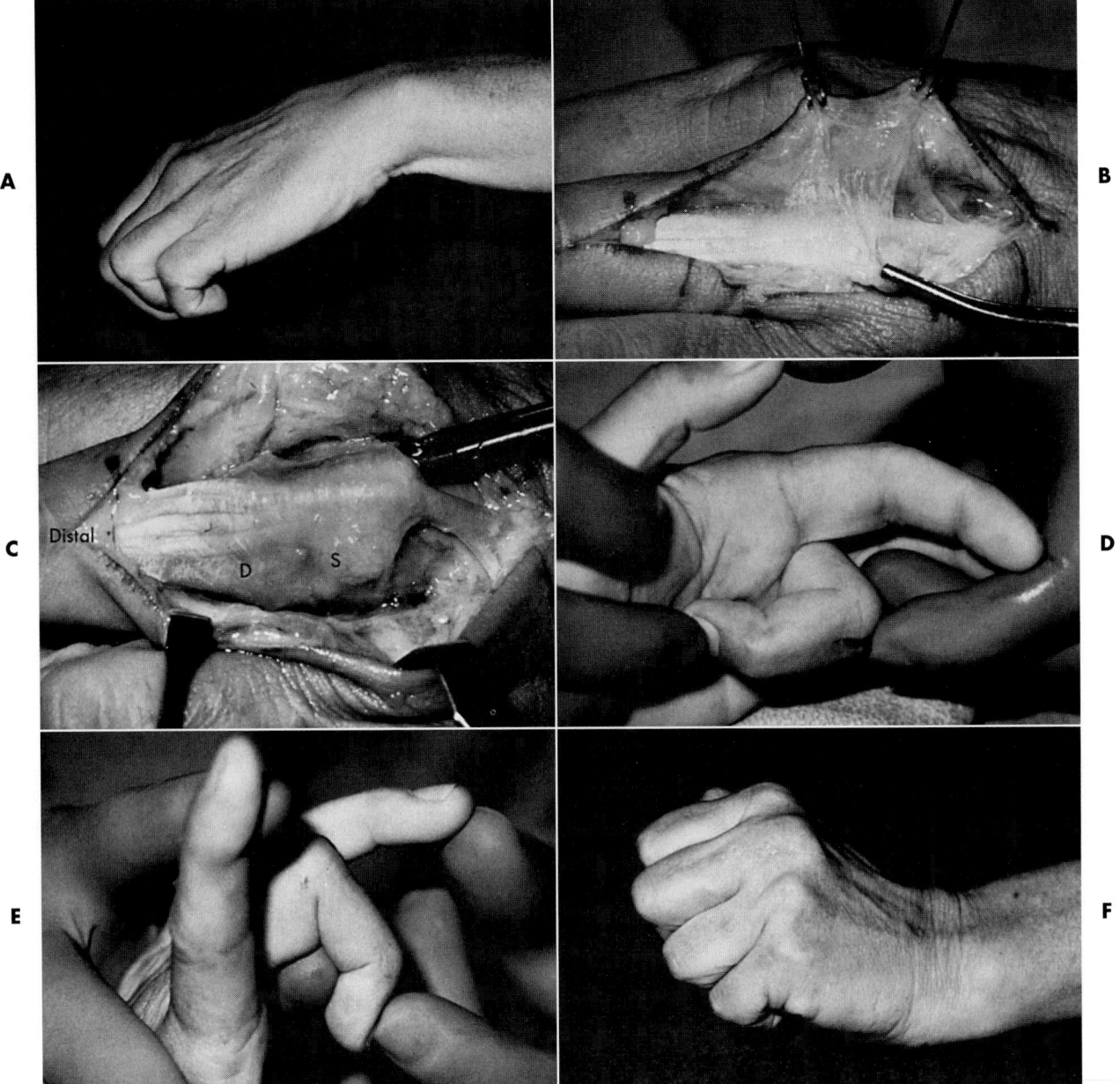

Fig. 30-24. Extrinsic and intrinsic dysfunction from scarring caused by focal crush injury about long finger metacarpophalangeal (MP) joint in a 54-year-old woman. **A,** Limited, painful grip 6 months after injury. Extrinsic tenodesis and positive intrinsic tightness test were elicited. **B,** Dorsal exposure over MP joint. Adhesions between skin flap and extensor hood are evident. **C,** Anatomic structures clearly defined after tenolysis. Instrument is beneath radial sagittal bands and dorsal apparatus. **D,** Extrinsic tenodesis has been eliminated. **E,** Intrinsic tightness test is negative. **F,** Voluntary grip after wound healing and rehabilitation. *D,* Dorsal apparatus; *S,* ulnar sagittal bands.

EXTENSOR TENDON INJURIES ABOUT THE PIP JOINTS (ZONE III)

Interruption of the extensor tendons at the PIP joint may result from lacerations, closed trauma, burns, rheumatoid synovitis, or tightly applied casts and splints. The deformities that develop reflect a distortion of forces that are normally balanced by tendon and retinacular systems. Early deformities are reversed more easily than lasting ones that have developed ligament and tendon tightness. Persistent deformities acquire a resistance to correction that adversely influences the prognosis for treatment.

Functional anatomy

The central tendon is the primary extensor of the PIP joint. The intrinsic tendons contribute medial slips that insert on the dorsal lip of the middle phalanx adjacent to the central tendon and receive lateral slips from the extrinsic tendon to form the conjoined lateral bands. The lateral bands normally descend during flexion and cover the axis of joint motion, where they are incapable of initiating extension. In this position, they do not transmit much tension and initially do not generate a significant deforming flexor moment to the PIP joint.[44] The central tendon alone is capable of initiating extension of the flexed joint. Tension through the lateral bands increases progressively as they migrate dorsally during extension; their contribution to PIP joint extension increases with dorsal displacement. Dorsally stationed lateral bands can maintain extension of the PIP joint. Normally, the lateral bands are relaxed when the PIP joint is fully flexed, tethered by the central tendon and incapable of extending the DIP joint. In moderate (30- to 40-degree) PIP joint flexion, there is weak but evident transfer of tension through the lateral bands to the DIP joint. This can be demonstrated clinically by holding the MP joint in neutral and the PIP joint in moderate flexion: a weak active extension of the DIP joint is evident.

The transverse retinacular ligaments and their dorsal fibers connect the lateral bands and have functional similarities to the sagittal bands about the MP joint; they contribute to extension of the PIP joint. Translation of the lateral bands is controlled by the fibers of the retinacular ligaments. Descent is limited by the dorsal fibers of the retinacular ligament (the triangular ligament); dorsal displacement is restrained by the transverse retinacular ligament. The palmar plate and the flexor superficialis tendon resist hyperextension.

Pathologic anatomy

Disruption of the central tendon interferes with normal active extension of the PIP joint. Initiation of extension of the flexed joint is lost. The final 15 to 20 degrees of active extension also is lost. This can be demonstrated by actively extending the fingers while the wrist and MP joints are supported in flexion: It infers disruption of the central tendon

with potential for development of a boutonnière deformity.[20] The positioned PIP joint can be maintained in extension by the lateral bands while they remain dorsal.

Release of the central tendon allows the finger extensor mechanism to slide proximally. This increases forces transmitted to the middle phalanx through the transverse retinacular ligaments and to the distal phalanx through the lateral slips, conjoined lateral bands, and terminal tendon. Active extension of the DIP joint then can be demonstrated while the MP joint is held in neutral with the PIP joint in full flexion.[36] Hyperextension of the PIP joint is resisted by the transverse retinacular ligaments that restrain dorsal displacement of the lateral bands during extension and by the flexor superficialis tendon and palmar plate. These observations form the anatomic rationale for surgical tenotomy of the central tendon in selected patients with a mallet finger deformity.[107]

The dorsal fibers of the retinacular ligament (triangular ligament) significantly influence the sequence of events after rupture of the central tendon. Partial tears of the triangular ligament retain sufficient control of the lateral bands to ensure dorsal positioning during extension with a favorable prognosis for return of extensor function after closed treatment. However, partial tears extend if unprotected motion continues after an injury.[110] Complete tear of the triangular ligament, combined with interruption of the central tendon, eliminates control of both joint extension and the lateral bands. This situation initiates an imbalance that results in a fixed deformity unless diligent treatment intercedes. Passive extension of the PIP joint implies that the lateral bands have relocated dorsally, the retinacular ligaments have not tightened, and closed treatment can proceed.

The finger is vulnerable to combined tissue injuries that involve the extensor tendons, collateral ligaments, and palmar plate when the flexed PIP joint is subjected to torsional stress.[48] Axial instability with extensor tendon rupture after a closed injury is an indication for primary surgery. Loss of active and passive extension of the PIP joint occurs when a lateral band becomes trapped beneath the condylar flare of the proximal phalanx. This is another indication for primary operative intervention (Fig. 30-25).

Examination of the injured PIP joint

The finger deformity and distribution of swelling are important indicators that infer the location and nature of the injury. Palpation with the fingertip or a pencil eraser can precisely locate tenderness. Radiographs should include PA, true lateral, and both oblique views of the injured finger.

Active extension of the PIP joint should be evaluated against gravity and against resistance with the MP joint in neutral.[133] Only the central tendon can initiate extension of the fully flexed PIP joint. The lateral bands alone can maintain extension of the passively extended joint if they rest dorsal to the axis of joint motion, but they cannot initiate

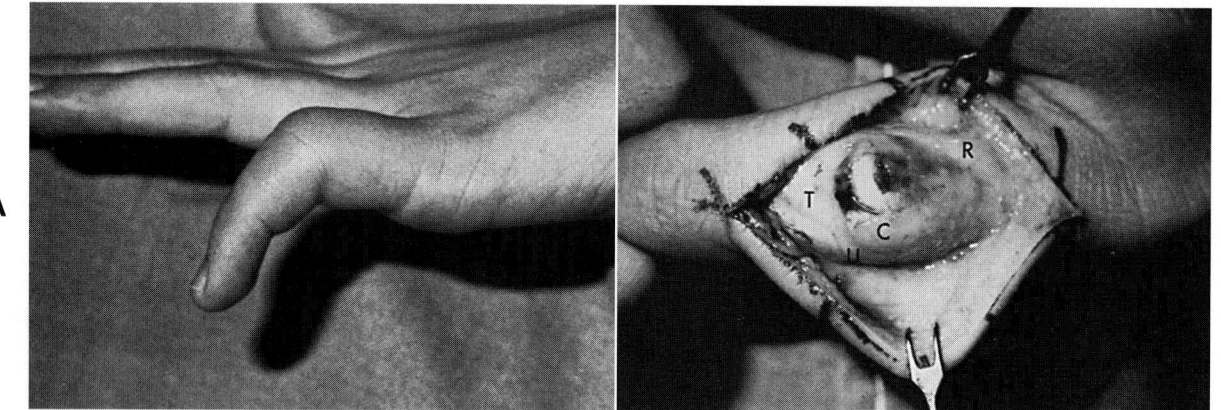

Fig. 30-25. Closed rupture of extensor tendon about the proximal interphalangeal (PIP) joint. Active and passive extension were limited. There was no resistance to flexion of distal joint. **A,** Clinical posture of injured finger. **B,** Operative findings: central tendon ruptured with herniation of head of proximal phalanx; triangular ligament was preserved. Radial lateral band is trapped beneath condyle of proximal phalanx. Inability to passively extend PIP joint is indication for primary operative repair in extensor tendon injuries at this level. *C,* Central tendon; *R,* radial lateral band; *T,* triangular ligament; *U,* ulnar lateral band.

extension of the completely flexed joint. A single lateral band can maintain extension even when the other lateral band and the triangular ligament are torn. Inability to initiate active extension of the fully flexed PIP joint is consistent with interruption of the central tendon.

Integrity of the central tendon also can be tested by a tenodesis mechanism. The wrist and MP joint are held in flexion, and active PIP joint extension is tested. A 15- to 20-degree extension lag at the PIP joint suggests injury to the central tendon with the potential for development of a boutonnière deformity.[20]

Assess DIP joint extension while the PIP joint is moderately flexed (30 to 40 degrees) and fully flexed.[36] The lateral bands normally do not transmit tension to the DIP joint when they have descended to the axis of joint motion during full PIP joint flexion; transmitted tension increases progressively as the PIP joint is extended. The lateral bands cannot extend the DIP joint while the PIP joint is fully flexed and only weakly extend the DIP joint when the PIP joint is partially flexed, unless the central tendon is interrupted. Relatively strong DIP joint extension, compared with adjacent normal fingers, with the PIP joint fully flexed or partially flexed is consistent with interruption of the central tendon and retention of at least one lateral band. DIP joint extension cannot be executed when both lateral bands have been interrupted.

The lateral bands are normally weak extensors of the DIP joint when the PIP joint is in full extension. Increased tension, compared with adjacent normal fingers, with passive flexion of the DIP joint while the PIP joint is fully extended implies interruption of the central tendon with proximal slide of the extensor tendons.

The therapist should assess axial stability for both sides of the joint as well as hyperextension stability. Axial instability is consistent with collateral ligament rupture. Oblique hyperextension can rupture the proximal attachments of the palmar plate with localized tenderness but with normal initial x-ray films. Early motion with protective splinting is required to prevent the development of a pseudoboutonnière deformity.[89,102] Axial instability combined with extensor tendon rupture defines a combined tissue injury and is an indication for primary operative repair.[48]

Boutonnière deformity

The boutonnière deformity develops after an injury to the extensor mechanism and specifically denotes flexion of the PIP joint with hyperextension of the DIP joint. The head of the proximal phalanx herniates through a defect in the extensor mechanism after rupture of the central tendon and dorsal fibers of the retinacular ligament (triangular ligament).[23] An analogous deformity occurs in the thumb with MP flexion and IP extension. The mechanisms of closed injury include involuntary forceful flexion of an actively extended digit, blunt trauma to the dorsum of the joint, and dislocation of the joint with tearing of the extensor tendons and stabilizing ligaments.

Interruption of the central tendon and triangular ligament permits proximal displacement of the extensor mechanism and palmar shift of the lateral bands. The unopposed flexor digitorum superficialis (FDS) flexes the PIP joint. The extrinsic extensor tendon, released from the middle phalanx, transfers forces through the sagittal bands that enhance extension of the MP joint. Both extrinsic and intrinsic

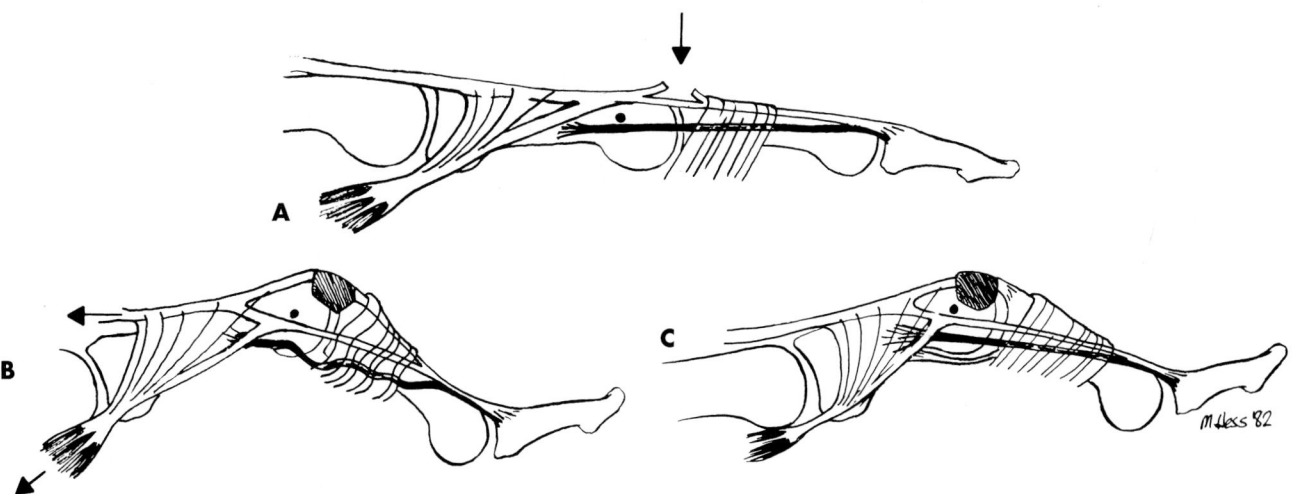

Fig. 30-26. Development of boutonnière deformity. **A,** Injury involves insertion of central extensor tendon at base of middle phalanx with interruption of dorsal fibers of transverse retinacular ligament. **B,** Middle phalanx is pulled into flexion by flexor digitorum superficialis. Lateral bands displace palmarly over axis of joint and become flexors of this joint. At this stage, palmar plate ligaments and oblique and transverse retinacular ligaments are loose. The deformity can be reversed with relative ease. **C,** Established deformity with shortening of extensor tendons and tightening of palmar plate ligaments and oblique and transverse retinacular ligaments. Retinacular tightness test is positive. Passive correction of deformity is resisted. Reversal of deformity at this stage is slow and represents a significant commitment by surgeon and therapist.

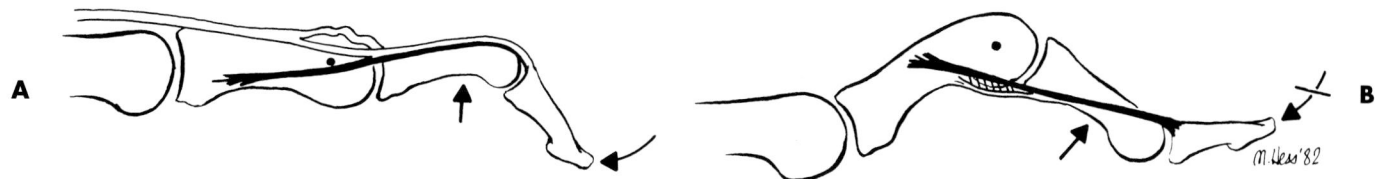

Fig. 30-27. Testing for tightness of oblique retinacular ligament. **A,** Passive extension of middle phalanx with passive flexion of distal phalanx is performed without resistance in normal finger: a negative test. **B,** Contracture of oblique retinacular ligament, with resistant flexion of proximal interphalangeal (PIP) joint and hyperextension of distal interphalangeal joint. Distal joint cannot be passively flexed when extension of PIP joint is passively increased: a positive test.

muscles transmit exaggerated forces through the conjoined lateral bands that extend the DIP joint. The transverse retinacular ligaments, oblique retinacular ligaments, and check ligaments of the palmar plate are loose early in the evolution of the deformity (Fig. 30-26, *A* and *B*). The test for retinacular tightness is negative, and the deformity is reversible passively (Fig. 30-27, *A*). The lateral bands return to their normal dorsal station and can maintain extension. Prognosis after splinting is most favorable during this early phase.

The lateral bands descend progressively, and the PIP joint cannot be maintained in full extension. An active extension lag develops that is passively correctable while the transverse and oblique retinacular ligaments and palmar plate remain supple and have not foreshortened (Fig. 30-26, *B*).

The palmarly displaced lateral bands become fixed to the underlying collateral ligaments and joint capsule while the retinacular ligaments and palmar plate tighten and oppose

passive correction (Fig. 30-26, *C*). The DIP joint loses active flexion, develops hyperextension, and progressively loses passive flexion. The retinacular tightness test is then positive (Fig. 30-27, *B*). The deformity is fixed and cannot be reversed without sustained effort. Treatment of the fixed deformity is complicated, and the prognosis is altered (Fig. 30-28).

Nonoperative treatment

Closed extensor tendon injuries about the PIP joint must be accurately appraised and closely monitored (Table 30-1). Prescribed treatment is designed for a specific injury. A palmar injury with potential for a pseudoboutonnière deformity is approached differently from a dorsal injury with potential for a classic boutonnière deformity. Swelling and dorsal tenderness should be considered an indication of an injury to the extensor tendons even when examination suggests intact structures. Partial ligament and tendon tears

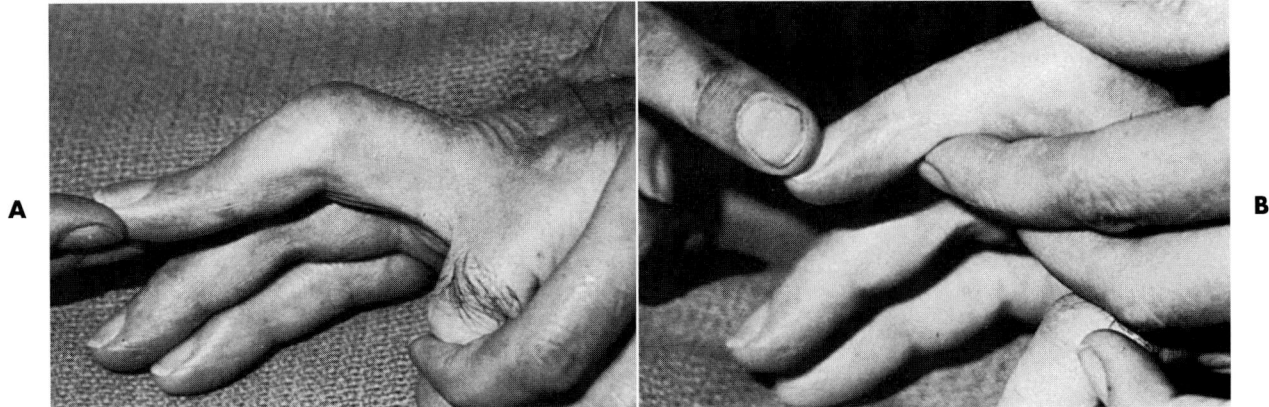

Fig. 30-28. Established boutonnière deformity. **A,** Fixed flexion deformity of proximal interphalangeal (PIP) joint with hyperextension of distal interphalangeal (DIP) joint. **B,** Resistant passive flexion of DIP joint with attempted extension of PIP joint from tightness of retinacular ligaments augmented by tightness of extensor tendons through displaced lateral bands.

Table 30-1. Treatment of closed injuries of the extensor tendons of the proximal interphalangeal (PIP) joint

Clinical findings	• Suggestive examination • Active extension • Passive extension • No fracture	• Active extension loss • Passive extension • No fracture	• Active extension loss • Passive extension loss • ± Axial instability • ± Fracture
Treatment	Splint PIP joint Reassess in 1 week	Splint PIP joint for 6 wk Possible K-wire	Primary repair Open reduction fracture Possible second-stage tendon reconstruction

From Rosenthal EA: Extensor surface injuries at the proximal interphalangeal joint. In Bowers WH, editor: *The hand and upper limb, vol 1—the interphalangeal joints,* London, 1987, Churchill Livingstone.

may extend unless the injured digit is protected.[110] The PIP joint is splinted in extension, and the digit is reassessed in 1 week. DIP joint motion is permitted during this period. A repeat normal functional examination of the finger implies that complete tendon rupture has not occurred. However, splinting is continued for an additional 2 weeks if swelling, tenderness, or ecchymosis is noted during reexamination. Splinting is discontinued after 3 weeks if the patient continues to demonstrate intact extensor tendons and no deformity has developed.

Splint or digital cast for a closed extensor tendon injury about the PIP joint treated without operative intervention immobilizes the PIP joint in neutral. The MP joint and DIP joint are left free. Active distal joint flexion synergistically relaxes the intrinsic and extrinsic extensor tendon muscles. A 3- to 4-mm glide is imparted to the central tendon through the lateral bands while the PIP joint is restrained.[61] The oblique retinacular ligament also is exercised through continued distal joint motion.

A splinting program recommended for treatment of the established boutonnière deformity should be tailored to fit the tissue requirements of the patient. The physician and therapist should be familiar with the anatomy of the extensor tendons and the pathomechanics of the deformity being

treated. Initial splinting supports the PIP joint in neutral while permitting active flexion of the DIP joint. This is continued without interruption for 6 weeks. Carefully monitored flexion of the PIP joint is then initiated. The PIP joint is supported in extension for an additional 2 to 4 weeks, when active motion is not being pursued. The requirements for continued support of the PIP joint reflect postural stability of the finger. Splinting is reinstituted if an extensor lag or boutonnière deformity recurs. Splinting is recommended only at night, when PIP joint extension can be sustained, and if there has been no deterioration during subsequent visits.

The time required for rehabilitation of the boutonnière deformity by splinting can be prolonged. Resistant cases can require attention and supervision for 6 to 9 months after injury. Tissue maturation with realization of the full potential function of the finger may not be achieved for a full year (Fig. 30-29).

Operative treatment

Primary operative repair is indicated for the acute closed injury with loss of passive extension of the PIP joint and in combined tissue injuries when central tendon rupture is associated with joint instability. Severe soft tissue injuries associated with fractures may require staged reconstruction.

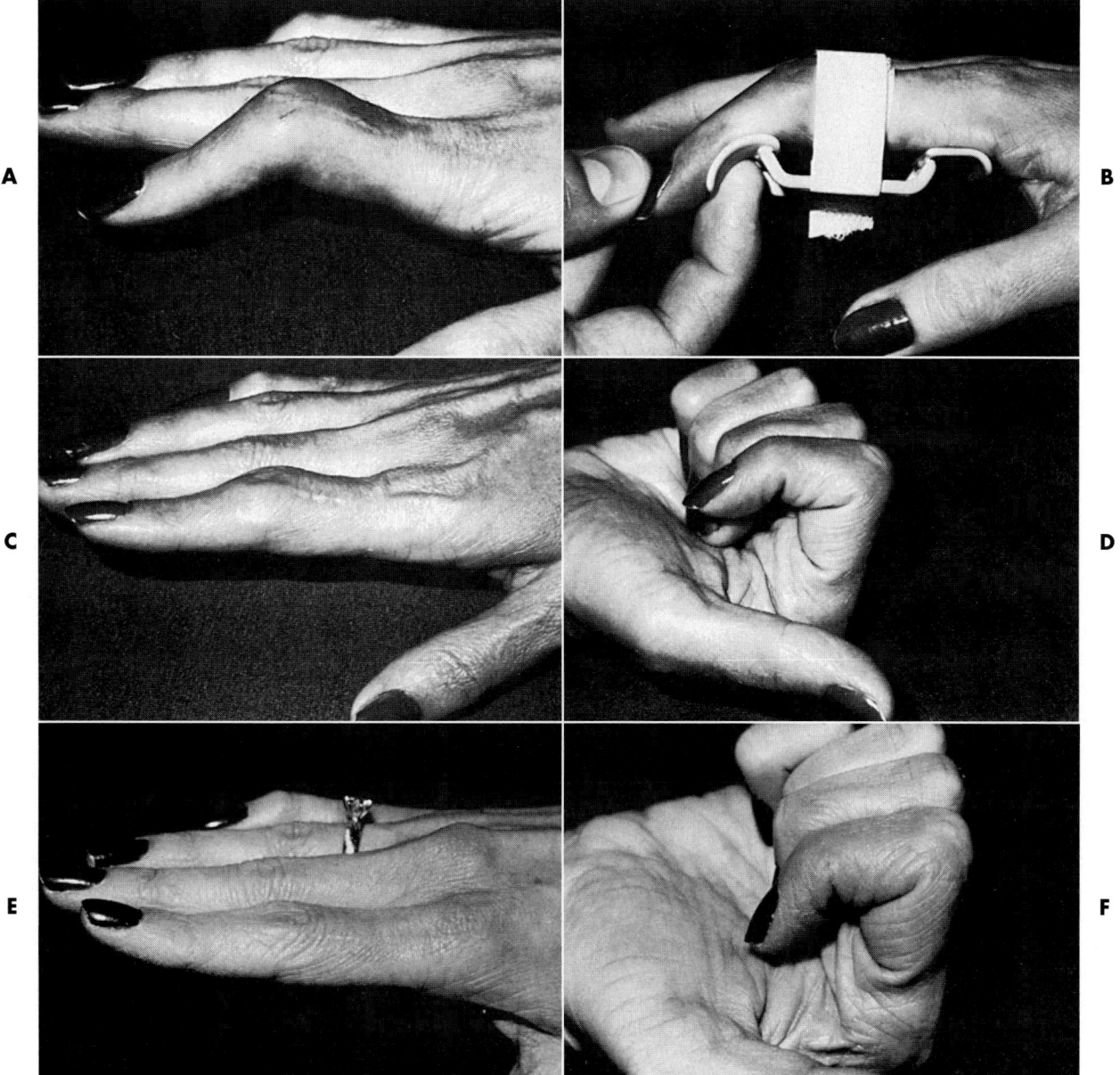

Fig. 30-29. Conservative treatment of boutonnière deformity. Laceration of extensor tendons with delayed primary treatment and wound infection. **A,** Fixed deformity with resistant flexion of proximal interphalangeal joint and extension of distal interphalangeal joint. **B,** Supervised serial static splinting designed to reestablish extension of proximal and flexion of distal joint deformities. (Splint marketed as New Extension Finger Splint in six sizes by Christensen Orthopedic Supply Company [COSCO], Hermosa Beach, California.) **C,** Five months after program was instituted, active extension with normal power was present. Tissue softening is progressing. Dorsal bump presents cosmetic disfigurement. **D,** Active flexion after 5 months. **E,** Complete extension with mature soft tissues and reduced disfigurement after 3 years. **F,** Active flexion after 3 years.

The fracture is repaired primarily, then tendon restoration is performed as a separate procedure after the fracture has healed.

Electing surgery for the chronic boutonnière deformity is an individualized decision. A mild (less than 30 degrees) flexion deformity of the PIP joint has variable individual effect and may not significantly interfere with grasp or finger function. The cosmetic deformity is often disliked by patients but may not be sufficient to motivate a request for reconstruction. A comfortable, useful range of active flexion of both IP joints provides excellent function despite the persistence of a slight flexion deformity of the PIP joint.

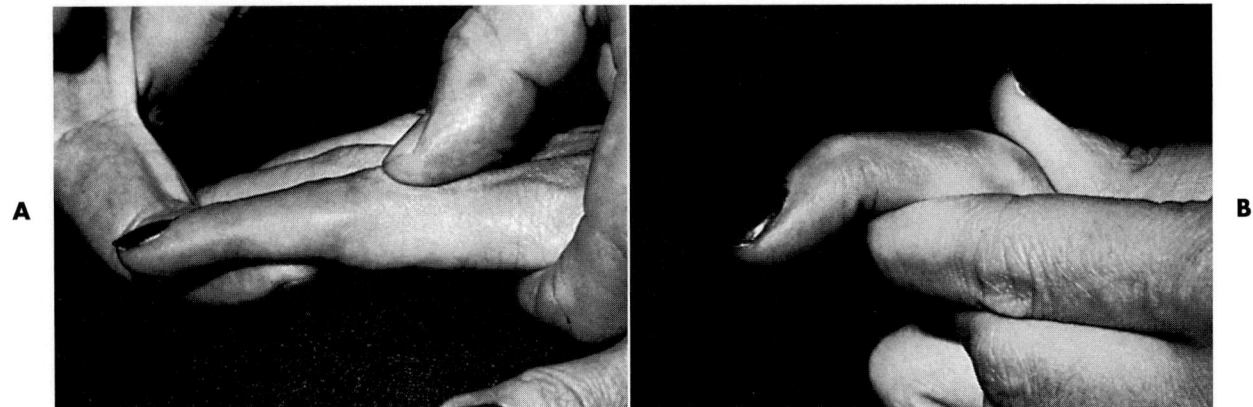

Fig. 30-30. Passive correction of boutonnière deformity before surgery improves prognosis. **A,** Reversal of flexion deformity of proximal interphalangeal (PIP) joint. **B,** Active flexion of distal interphalangeal joint with complete passive extension of PIP joint confirms sufficient lengthening of extensor tendons and retinacular ligaments for appropriate consideration of surgery.

More severe deformities do create functional impairments. A large portion of the handicap with an established boutonnière deformity reflects loss of distal joint flexion. Candidates for surgery should be selected carefully after evaluating their symptoms, deformity, anticipated improvement from treatment, and compliance. Selection as a candidate for surgery implies a willingness to participate in a closely supervised, often prolonged, rehabilitation program after surgery.

PIP joint flexion deformity should be reversed and active DIP joint flexion should be restored before surgery (Fig. 30-30). The results from surgery are better when joint deformities are corrected preoperatively.[67] Mature, hard, resistant scar occasionally demonstrates a surprising plasticity when subjected to tension for long periods of time. Extensor tendon reconstructions alone will not improve the passive correction that preoperative treatment has gained (Fig. 30-31). Fingers that cannot be corrected by means of splinting and supervised therapy require extensive surgical releases that introduce new imbalances capable of promoting additional future deformity (Fig. 30-32).

The method for operative repair will be determined by the condition of the central tendon and lateral bands. Elliott's anatomic reconstruction requires an adequate central tendon and both lateral bands.[33,34] Littler and Eaton[96] restored PIP joint extension by reefing both lateral bands over the dorsum of the PIP joint and central tendon remnant. The lumbrical tendon and oblique retinacular ligament were preserved to maintain DIP joint extension. Matev's method has application when the central tendon is deficient and permits rebalancing of both PIP and DIP joints[100] (Fig. 30-33). Other innovative techniques have been promulgated to replace variable deficiencies of the skin/subcutaneous envelope, central tendon, and lateral bands when correcting the boutonnière deformity. Intact lateral bands may be mobilized then approximated centrally over the dorsum of the PIP joint without interrupting the terminal tendon when there has been loss of substance of the central tendon.[2,59] Mobilized lateral bands can be reinforced by folding both transverse retinacular ligaments dorsally.[140] A lost central tendon also can be replaced by reinserting a single lateral band,[94] by a distally reversed segmental tendon graft from proximal extensor tendon,[153] by transfer of a lateral band from an adjacent finger,[154] by free tendon graft bridging the central tendon insertion with proximal extrinsic extensor tendon[118] or the intrinsic tendons,[16] by interposition of the tendon of FDS that is passed dorsally through the normal insertion of the central tendon,[157] by an intercalary palmaris longus free tendon graft that includes the deep forearm fascia,[42] and by an arterialized tendocutaneous flap containing a lateral band.[70] The works by Burton[19] and Rosenthal[137] are recommended for expanded discussions of operative management of deformities from extensor tendon injuries about the PIP joint.

EXTENSOR TENDON INJURIES AT THE DIP JOINT (ZONE I)

Mallet finger is synonymous with interruption of the extensor tendon mechanism at the level of the DIP joint. The term is not descriptive but has gained universal acceptance for the deformity that results (Fig. 30-34).

The terminal extensor tendon represents the distal extension of the merged lateral bands that insert on the dorsal base of the distal phalanx. The more central fibers of the tendon are bordered by the distal extensions of the oblique retinacular ligaments that insert on the lateral base of the distal phalanx adjacent to the terminal tendon.[182] The interweaving of adjacent tendon and ligament fibers before insertion contributes to the success with treatment of central fiber injuries at this level.

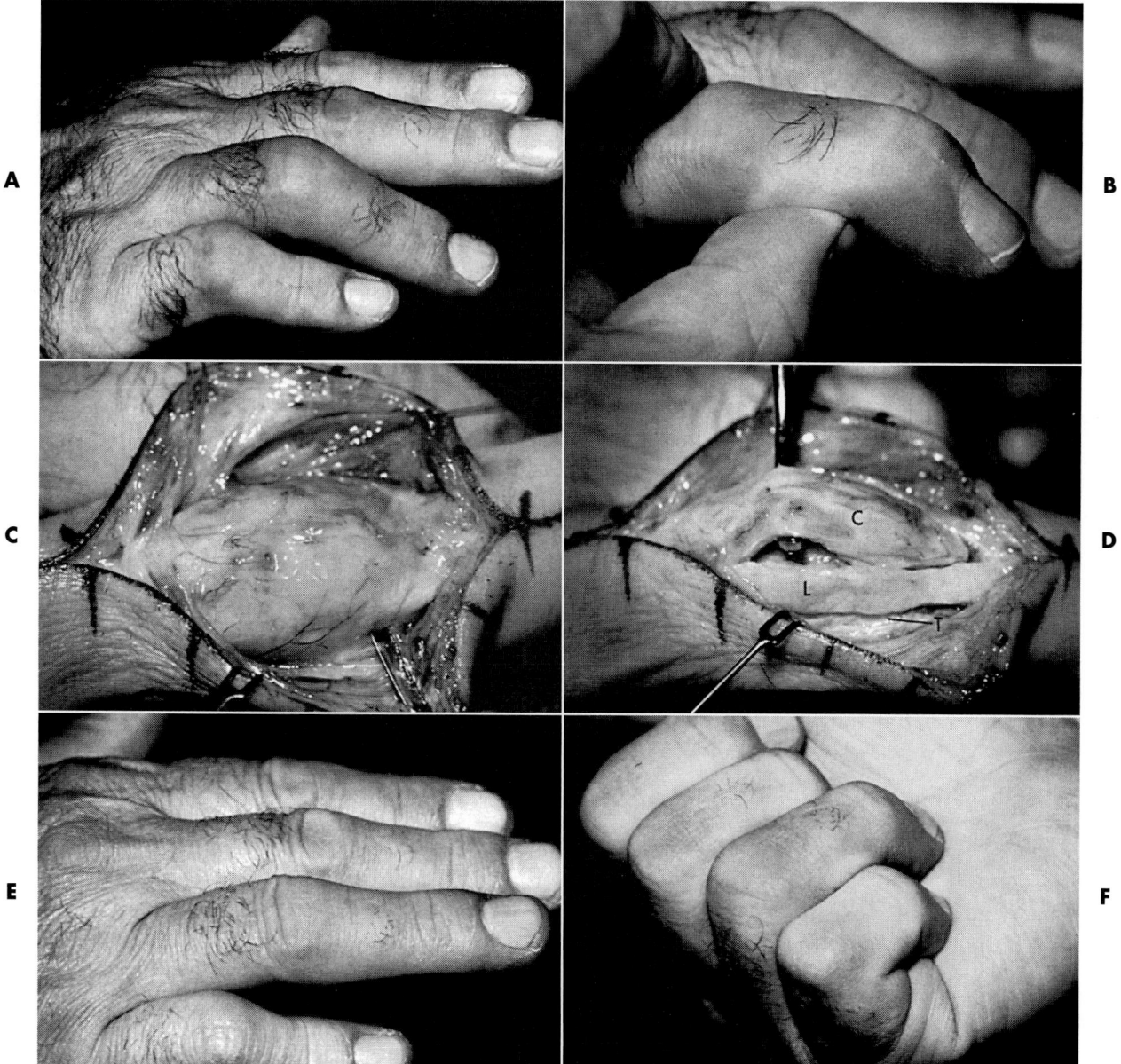

Fig. 30-31. Chronic boutonnière deformity with functional impairment. Closed ring finger injury in 67-year-old man initially treated with 2 weeks of splinting. Regression followed removal of splint. **A,** Posture when first evaluated. Passive correction of proximal interphalangeal (PIP) joint was achieved with splinting. **B,** Active distal interphalangeal joint flexion with PIP joint in neutral confirms reversal of tendon and ligament tightness. **C,** Normal tendon anatomy about PIP joint transformed by scar; subluxated ulnar lateral band is adherent to capsule. **D,** Elevator lifts central tendon created from scarred tissue. Lateral bands were surgically defined. Thick transverse retinacular ligaments were incised. Proximal and distal joint extensor tendons were functionally rebalanced. **E,** Active extension 7 months after surgery lacks 20 degrees. **F,** Active flexion at 7 months. *C,* Central tendon; *L,* lateral band; *T,* transverse retinacular ligament.

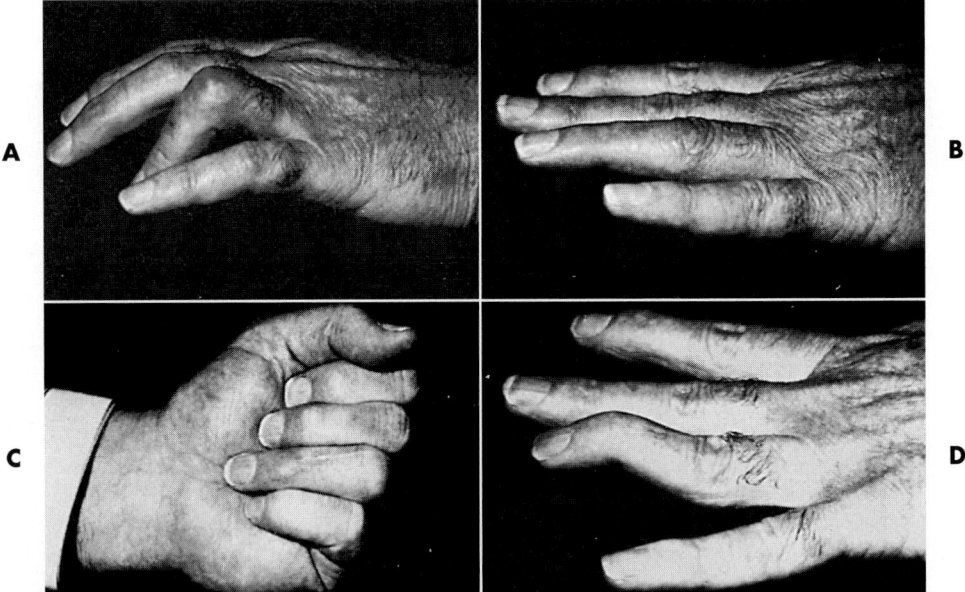

Fig. 30-32. Man, 45 years old, with closed injury of extensor tendons at proximal interphalangeal (PIP) joint. Unsuccessful surgery 3 months after injury for uncorrected boutonnière deformity. Surgery included suture of lateral bands dorsally with terminal tendon tenotomy. **A,** Fixed deformity when first seen 4 months after surgery. **B,** Clinical extension 6 months after anatomic reconstruction of central tendon, palmar plate release, and resection of accessory collateral ligaments of PIP joint. The extensor tendon over the middle phalanx was not disturbed. **C,** Active flexion 6 months after surgery. **D,** Posture 9 years after reconstruction. Swan-neck deformity has developed from hyperextension instability of the PIP joint. The distal interphalangeal joint actively flexed. Mature scar retains some plasticity when subjected to chronic tensions. Extensive surgical releases introduce a potential for imbalances beyond those in original deformity.

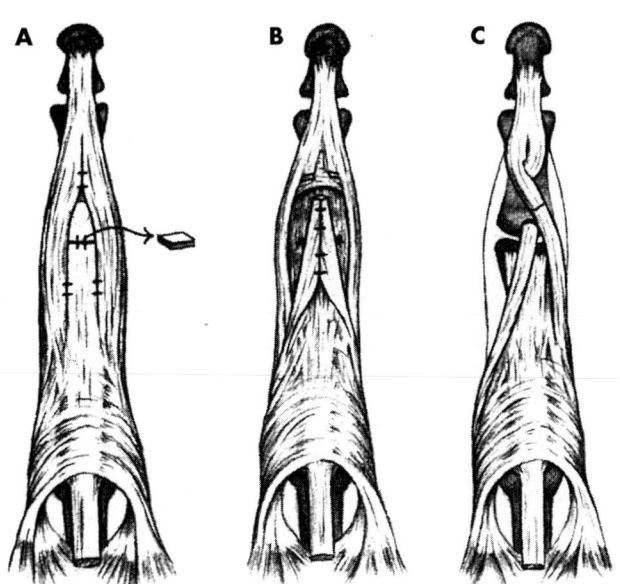

Fig. 30-33. Operative methods for reconstruction of the chronic boutonnière deformity. **A,** Anatomic reconstruction described by Elliott.[34] **B,** Replacement of the central tendon with lateral bands that are folded dorsally and inserted on the base of the middle phalanx, described by Littler.[96] **C,** Matev[100] method for reconstructing central tendon and adjusting terminal tendon using both lateral bands. (From Rosenthal EA: Extensor surface injuries at the proximal interphalangeal joint. In Bowers WH, editor: *The hand and upper limb,* vol 1, *The interphalangeal joints,* London, 1987, Churchill Livingstone.)

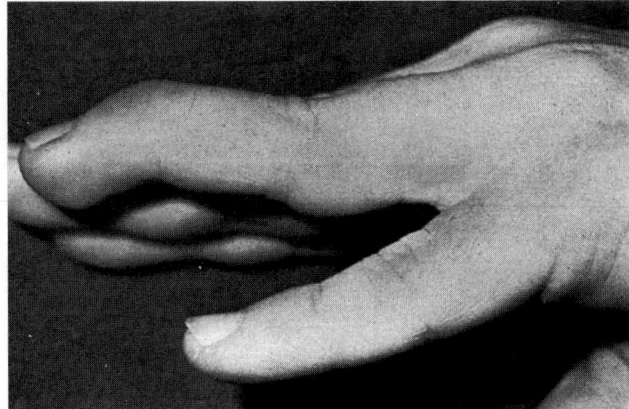

Fig. 30-34. Mallet finger with hyperextension deformity of proximal interphalangeal joint. Interruption of terminal tendon concentrates extension forces at middle phalanx. Swan-neck deformity with mallet tendon lesion has wide range of severity.

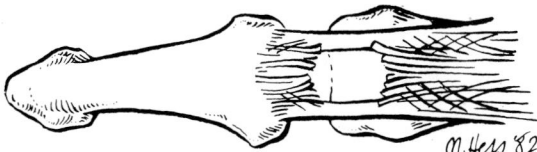

Fig. 30-35. Mallet tendon lesion. Shredding or tearing of terminal tendon occurs proximal to its insertion, over trochlea of the middle phalanx. Central fibers that insert on dorsal beak of the distal phalanx have the greatest moment arm for distal joint extension, are subject to greater tension during passive distal joint flexion, and rupture first. More lateral fibers that insert closer to the axis of joint motion are less efficient extensors, are subject to less stress, and may be preserved. Interweaving between lateral extensor tendon fibers and oblique retinacular ligament may maintain some continuity of the extensor tendon with the distal phalanx.

Patterns of injury

The patterns of closed injuries depend on the position of the DIP joint at the time of injury and the direction of the injuring force. The treatment depends on the type of injury.

Passive flexion of the distal phalanx is resisted by tension through the terminal tendon through the initial 45 degrees of DIP joint flexion. The oblique retinacular and collateral ligaments are normally relaxed through this range. Direct trauma to the partially flexed distal phalanx ruptures (frays) the central fibers of the terminal tendon over the trochlea of the middle phalanx.[156] These central fibers that insert on the dorsal beak of the distal phalanx have the largest moment arm for distal joint extension and are the most efficient terminal tendon fibers for active extension. Lateral border terminal tendon fibers that insert on the distal phalanx closer to the axis of joint motion are less efficient distal joint extensors, are subject to less stress during passive joint flexion, and may be preserved. The oblique retinacular ligaments are not under tension and remain intact. The interwoven border fibers of tendon and ligament retain some anatomic continuity with the base of the distal phalanx (Fig. 30-35). The partial active distal joint extension that these patients retain is from preserved lateral terminal tendon fibers. Recoil of passively flexed distal joint is by the collateral ligaments of the joint and retinacular ligaments.[148] The extension lag is passively correctable. This is a pure tendon lesion.

Both the terminal tendon and the oblique retinacular ligaments are under tension when the DIP joint is flexed beyond 45 degrees. Passive flexion of the distal phalanx while tension is transmitted through the terminal tendon produces a dorsal avulsion fracture with total interruption in the functional continuity of the extensor tendon[160] (Fig. 30-36).

A longitudinal impaction force that hyperextends the DIP joint creates a large articular fracture of the base of the distal phalanx[88] (Fig. 30-37, A). This is a significant joint injury. The effect on extensor tendon function is often small, without a mallet deformity. The large dorsal fragment retains collateral ligament attachments to the middle phalanx. Dorsal fractures of more than one third of the base of the

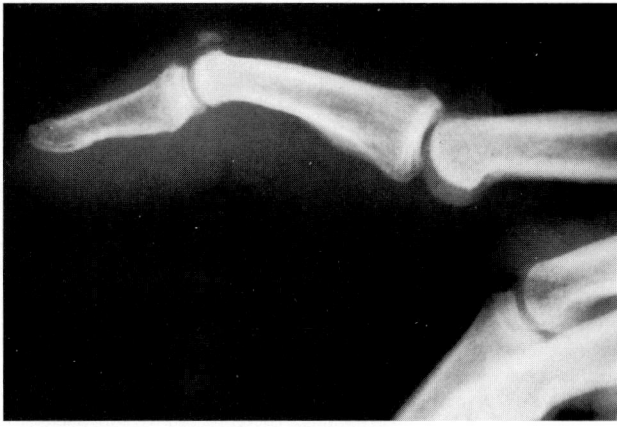

Fig. 30-36. Total interruption of terminal extensor tendon insertion with adjacent retinacular ligaments may be associated with a small dorsal avulsion fracture. This produces a mallet deformity. Residual extension of distal interphalangeal joint results from retained lateral tendon fibers.

distal phalanx may be unstable.[159,177] The degree of instability relates to disruption of collateral ligament attachments to the distal fracture fragment. A stable distal fragment flexes; the unstable distal fragment is pulled proximally by the flexor profundus and subluxates palmarward (Fig. 30-37, B). Patients are inclined to dismiss the injury as trivial and may not seek early treatment.

Development of deformity

Interruption of the terminal tendon insertion permits retraction of the extensor tendons proximally. This transfers tension to the central tendon and conjoined lateral bands. The central tendon (via its bony insertion) and the lateral bands (via the transverse retinacular ligaments) concentrate extension forces on the middle phalanx. The palmar plate resists hyperextension of the PIP joint. The retinacular ligaments are initially lax. Hyperextension of the PIP joint develops if the palmar plate is lax. The flexor digitorum profundus (FDP) flexes the DIP joint, and a mild swan-neck deformity develops. The severity of the deformity is inversely proportional to the stability of the palmar plate at the PIP joint (Fig. 30-38). The swan-neck deformity from a mallet tendon lesion usually is not severe enough to impart difficulties with finger flexion unless hyperextension of the PIP joint is advanced.

Treatment

Closed injuries. The mallet tendon lesion without fracture should be treated with uninterrupted immobilization of the DIP joint in slight hyperextension for 6 weeks.[29,160] The PIP joint is not immobilized. The classical treatment proposed by Smillie,[150] which immobilized the PIP joint in flexion and the DIP joint in hyperextension, is no longer advocated. Hyperextension may produce dorsal skin blanching with cutaneous and terminal tendon ischemia. The safe

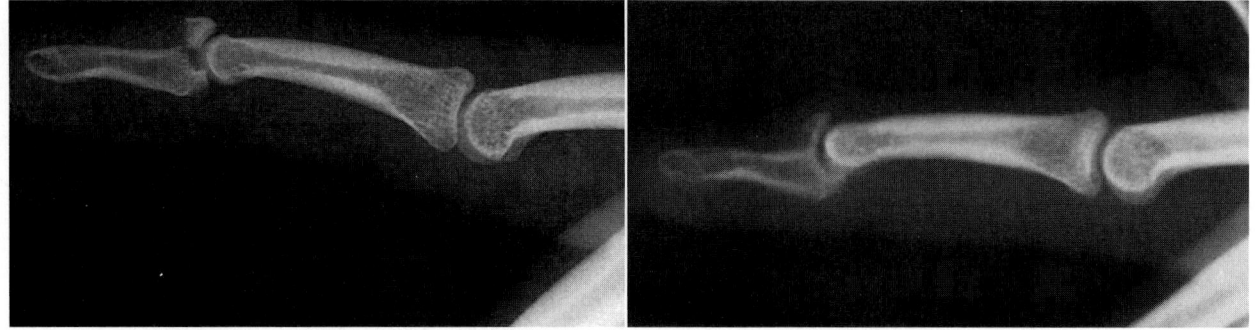

Fig. 30-37. Impaction hyperextension injury produces major articular fracture with potential instability of distal interphalangeal joint, usually without mallet deformity. **A,** Radiograph at time of injury. Patient was treated with digital casting for 3 weeks followed by 3 weeks of splinting. **B,** Three months after injury. Early remodeling with persistent palmar subluxation is evident; traumatic arthritis is established. Major articular distal joint injuries are unstable. Despite significant potential for remodeling, operative reduction with internal stabilization is meritorious.

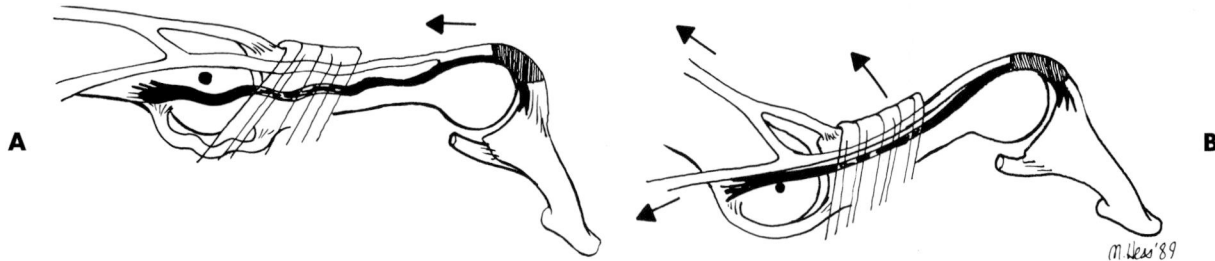

Fig. 30-38. Development of mallet deformity. **A,** Interruption of extensor tendon over distal interphalangeal joint permits unopposed flexion of joint by flexor digitorum profundus (FDP) tendon. Loss of distal restraint permits proximal slide of extensor tendons. Oblique retinacular ligaments and lateral bands become slack. Palmar plate at the proximal interphalangeal (PIP) joint resists hyperextension. **B,** Concentration of extension forces from extrinsic and intrinsic muscles transmitted through central tendon, lateral bands, and transverse retinacular ligaments produces hyperextension at PIP joint. Hyperextension increases as palmar plate yields. Transposed dorsal lateral bands and tight oblique retinacular ligaments resist flexion until forced palmarly over condylar flares of proximal phalanx from extreme flexion of distal joint by FDP.

position for splinting is individualized; dorsal skin should not blanch in the splinted position.[128] Reliable patients can be treated with splinting; others may require K-wire pinning. Some patients require adjustment of the attitude of the splinted joint as the swelling of injury subsides and further extension is tolerated.

Carefully supervised treatment is successful in restoring DIP joint extension and reducing extension lag when treatment is initiated early (within 2 weeks of injury) or is delayed (beyond 4 weeks of injury).[43] A favorable prognosis is more predictable with earlier treatment than with delayed treatment even though successful delayed treatment has been reported. K-wire pinning under metacarpal neck block anesthesia with mini C-arm control is the most secure and predictable treatment for mallet tendon injuries. The risk of pin tract infection increases the longer the pin is retained and the more actively the patient uses the digit during the treatment period. Cutting the distal end of the pin beneath the skin is a worthwhile precaution that lessens the risk of

infection and permits more normal function. However, this precaution requires a secondary operative procedure to remove the pin.

Numerous designs for mallet splints have been promoted. Variations in digital contour, distal joint extensibility, and swelling after injury justify use of splints that are individually crafted for each injured finger. A carefully molded digital QuickCast (Sammons Preston, Inc., Bolingbrook, Illinois) that immobilizes only the DIP joint is a stable immobilizing method that avoids risk of positional lapses during splint changes. These casts reduce swelling, but are even more effective when applied over Coban (3M Health Care, St. Paul, Minnesota). The cast needs to be replaced periodically to ensure skin hygiene throughout immobilization. Dorsal splinting of the DIP joint with a foam-padded aluminum splint does not encroach on the tactile palmar surface of the finger and avoids localized pressure over the site of tendon injury (Fig. 30-39). A better splint can be made by thinning the foam of commercially available material.

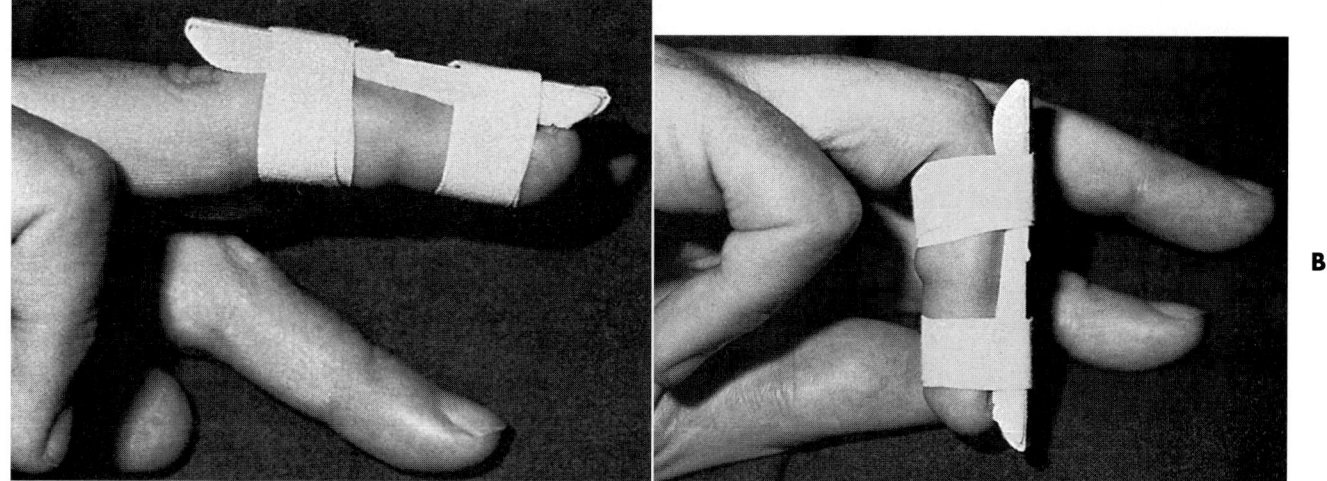

Fig. 30-39. Dorsal splint for mallet finger. **A,** Splint maintains distal joint in slight hyperextension. Hyperextension is an individual determination. **B,** Proximal interphalangeal (PIP) joint motion is encouraged throughout the 6 weeks of uninterrupted splinting that is recommended for initial treatment of mallet finger. PIP joint flexion has little effect on the distal tendon injury with the distal interphalangeal joint in hyperextension in the normal finger.

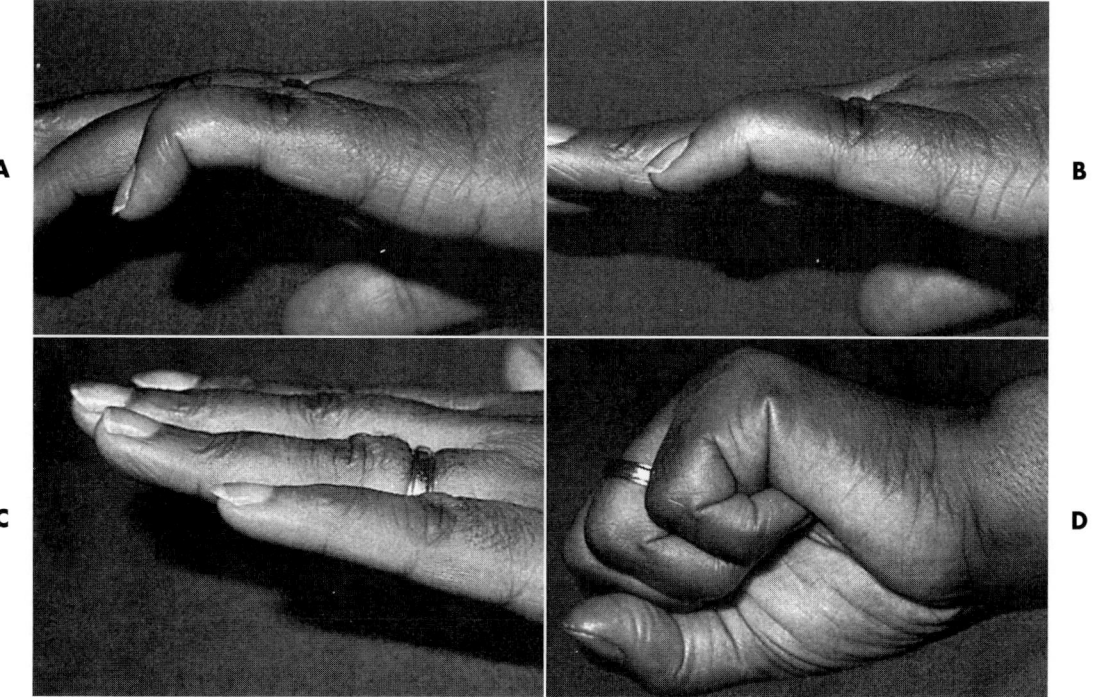

Fig. 30-40. Chronic mallet deformity from blunt injury in 54-year-old woman. **A,** Resting attitude of 70 degrees. **B,** Active extension to 55 degrees, suggesting potential benefit from splinting. **C,** Active extension after 7 weeks of uninterrupted splinting and additional 4 weeks of night splinting. **D,** Active flexion.

Cloth adhesive tape between the foam and skin reduces maceration. The splint may be changed periodically by the insightful patient; other patients require more frequent visits to the physician or therapist. The traditional Stack splint has been windowed to permit evaporation of moisture and pulp contact during splinting.[158] Perforated thermoplastic splints

with Velcro straps also are available.[78] Active motion of the PIP joint is continued throughout the period of splinting; this flexion reduces tension at the site of injury. Distal joint motion is begun after 6 weeks of continuous splinting. Night splinting of the distal joint is continued for an additional 4 weeks after distal joint motion is begun (Fig. 30-40).

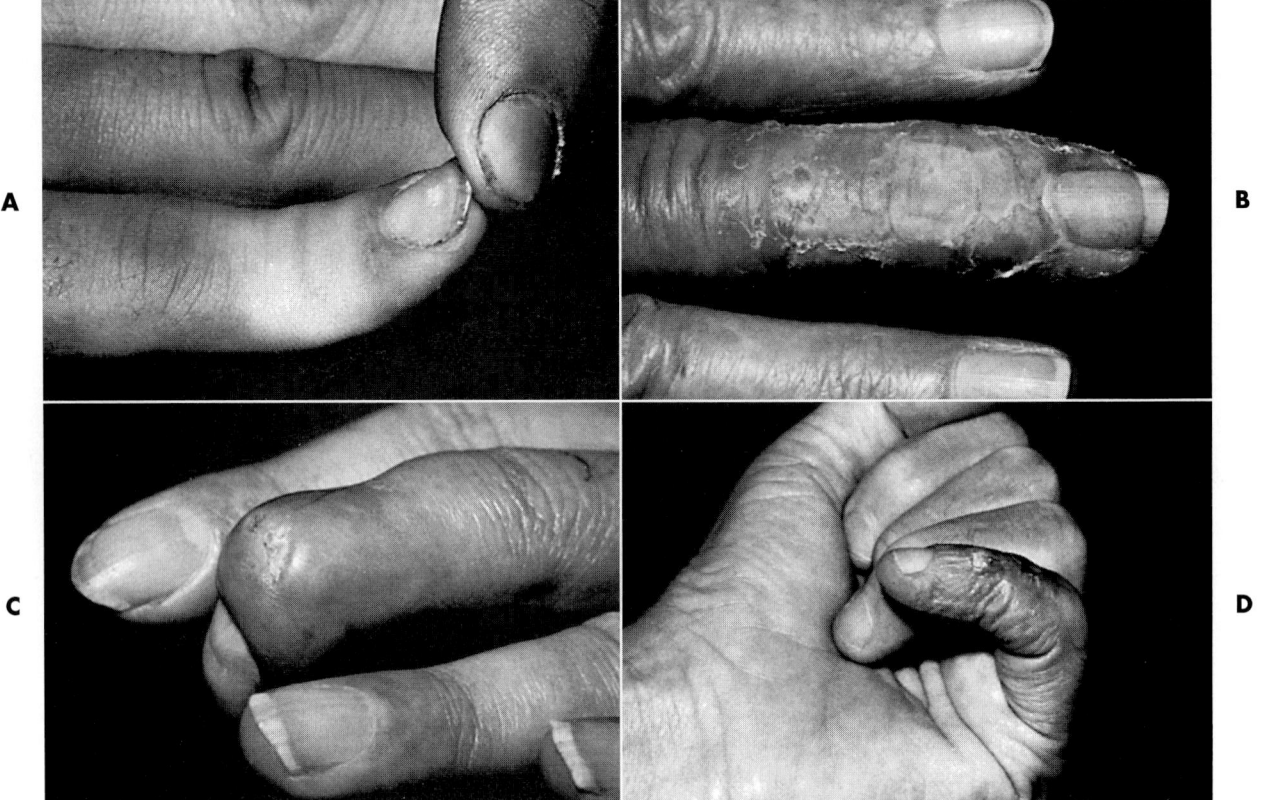

Fig. 30-41. Complications of treatment for mallet finger deformity. **A,** Dorsal skin blanching signifies ischemia of subcutaneous tissues and terminal tendon. **B,** Maceration of dorsal skin beneath splint from neglect. Secondary infection can develop. **C,** Chronic pyarthrosis with necrosis of terminal tendon after surgery. Middle phalanx projects through scar. **D,** Tenodesis of extensor tendons with osteomyelitis of middle phalanx after surgery. Distal joint is subluxated.

Full-time splinting should be reinstituted if clinical regression occurs after active distal joint motion is begun.

Loss of active extension—an *extension lag*—and decreased distal joint flexion from terminal tendon scarring are both complications from closed treatment of the mallet tendon lesion.[142] Dorsal skin maceration or necrosis is a complication of improper splinting. A 45% incidence of complications associated with closed treatment of mallet finger injuries has been reported.[162]

The clinical result may not be realized for at least 6 months after injury.[17] An early extension lag can decrease as the healing tendon scar contracts.[158] Pulvertaft[126] observed that 60% of patients obtained satisfactory results with splintage and 20% more will improve sufficiently over time to be acceptable.

Treatment of the distal tendon avulsion fracture is the same as that described for a pure tendon lesion. Positioning the distal joint in slight extension returns the distal phalanx to the small proximal fragment. Success can be monitored by comparing lateral radiographs taken before and after splinting. Calcification of the bridging callus may form a dorsal beak that nonetheless represents functional continuity of the extensor tendon and usually is not symptomatic.

Nonoperative treatment of larger articular fractures of the distal phalanx has been recommended because of the significant capacity of the distal phalanx to remodel its articular surface and the incidence of complications after surgery.[143,177] The most common impairment after open reduction of a major articular fracture of the distal phalanx is decreased flexion of the DIP joint from a scar tenodesis over the middle phalanx.[53] Additional complications from surgery for this injury are wound infection, thinning of the dorsal skin, joint injury, nail bed injury, pulp fibrosis, pain, and dysesthesias.[124] A 53% incidence of complications after operative treatment of mallet fingers has been reported[162] (Fig. 30-41).

Despite the capacity for these injured joints to remodel with nonoperative treatment,[176] an accurate approximation of the fracture fragments has merit.[119,159] Reapproximation of the distal phalanx to the retracted proximal fragment can be performed through a transverse incision localized over the fracture site without disturbing the terminal tendon proximal to the joint. The dorsal capsule proximally should not be disturbed. An oblique 0.028 K-wire compresses the fracture site and prevents proximal retraction of the terminal tendon.[92] The palmar surface of the dorsal fragment can be notched to accommodate the wire, which stabilizes the distal joint. This delicate procedure is demanding technically and represents a challenge in precision. The wires are removed after 6 weeks, and active motion is begun. Night splinting is continued for

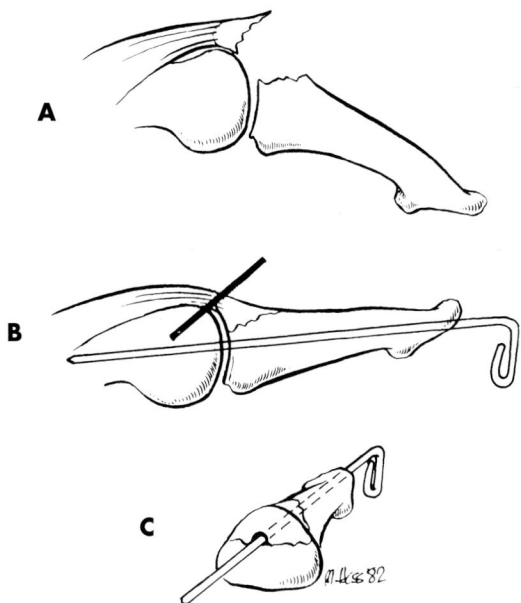

Fig. 30-42. Operative method for major articular fracture of distal interphalangeal joint. **A,** Injury represents significant interruption of articular surface with potential instability. Effect on extensor tendons may be small. **B,** Accurate reduction of fracture fragments. Longitudinal wire stabilizes distal joint in neutral or slight extension. Oblique buttress wire compresses fracture site and prevents retraction of proximal fragment by extensor tendon. **C,** Palmar surface of proximal fragment may be notched to accommodate K-wire.

2 to 4 weeks until absence of an extension lag is ensured (Fig. 30-42).

Chronic mallet finger deformity may implicate only the DIP joint or may present with an imbalance collapse of the entire finger—a swan-neck deformity. Favorable results have been reported after secondary suture repair and also with plication of the terminal tendon scar, a *tenodermodesis*.[62,81] The terminal tendon has a small excursion, and the tenodesis that is created may restrict distal joint motion. This procedure is contraindicated in the presence of a fixed flexion contracture, joint instability, or osteoarthritis. If the distal joint is unsightly or intrusive, arthrodesis of the DIP joint in neutral position is a reliable procedure that provides a painless, stable, cosmetically improved finger.

The chronic mallet finger with a swan-neck deformity presents a more complex problem. Surgery to rebalance the finger should not be considered unless both joints are healthy and the joint deformities are passively correctable. The finger can be rebalanced by tenotomy of the central tendon insertion at the PIP joint.[11,55] The lateral slips to the intrinsic tendons and at least one of the transverse retinacular ligaments must be preserved. The lateral slips maintain terminal tendon continuity with the extrinsic extensor tendon. The transverse retinacular ligaments resist PIP joint hyperextension from dorsal displacement of the lateral bands. Both transverse retinacular ligaments can be preserved by releasing the central tendon through a longitudinal incision in the extensor tendon proximal to the dorsal fibers of the retinacular ligament. An extensor tenolysis over the middle phalanx is needed if distal joint position is not improved after the tenotomy. The extension lag noted at the PIP joint after this procedure can be reduced with appropriate splinting. Ultimate improvement may not be realized for a full year[49] (Fig. 30-43).

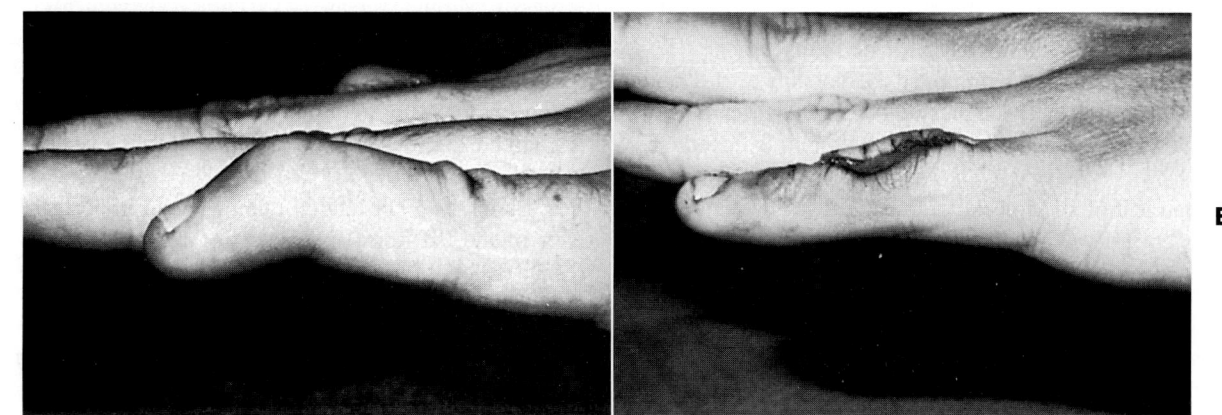

Fig. 30-43. Tenotomy of central tendon insertion on middle phalanx for treatment of selected patients with passively correctable mallet deformity. Tenotomy permits readjustment of tensions through extensor tendons, reversing extensor deficiency at the distal interphalangeal joint and reducing hyperextension forces at the proximal interphalangeal joint. **A,** Preoperative view of patient with history of three ruptures of the terminal tendon while playing football and two previous surgical attempts at anatomic reconstruction. **B,** Active extension after tenotomy of central tendon with tenolysis over middle phalanx. Both transverse retinacular ligaments were preserved.

Swan-neck deformity in a mallet finger with significant hyperextension of the PIP joint may be rebalanced with reconstruction of an oblique retinacular ligament using a free tendon graft.[80,167] The tendon graft passes from the dorsum of the distal phalanx around the digit palmar to the flexor sheath and is attached proximal to the PIP joint. This reverses both distal joint flexion and proximal joint hyperextension.

Open injuries. Lacerations of the terminal tendon should be approximated. Intramedullary K-wire pinning of the DIP joint in slight hyperextension will coapt the tendon ends in tidy wounds without the need for tendon sutures.[84] Divided tendons that require suture repair are approximated with fine 5-0 or 6-0 braided, white nonabsorbable sutures. Interrupted figure-of-eight or horizontal mattress sutures are selected, depending on the consistency of the tendon ends. A relatively avascular critical zone exists in the terminal tendon 11 to 16 mm proximal to the osseotendinous junction, where the tendon is compressed over the head of the middle phalanx during flexion. This may influence healing after repair in this area.[174] The DIP joint is pinned because the repair initially depends on the integrity of the sutures. Motion is begun after 6 weeks. The distal joint is supported by splinting between active motion sessions for an additional 2 weeks. Development of an extensor lag indicates the need for further supportive splinting. There is no compelling rationale for an early motion protocol after repair of zone I or II extensor tendon injuries at this time.

SWAN-NECK DEFORMITY

The collapse deformity of the fingers that is metaphorically called the *swan-neck deformity* is a postural deformity with numerous causes. The deformity results from an imbalance of forces within the finger that creates an instability, with collapse between the proximal, middle, and distal phalanges. Hyperextension of the PIP joint with flexion of the DIP joint, the swan-neck deformity, is the postural deformity that results.

The swan-neck deformity that follows the mallet finger tendon injury is one example of such an imbalance. However, the pathomechanics of swan-neck deformity from other causes result in similar distortions of the finger extensor tendons and retinacular and capsular ligaments. The initiating factor may be increased forces through the extensor or intrinsic tendons, PIP joint instability, loss of the FDS tendon, or release of distal extensor attachment.

The basic mechanism in the swan-neck deformity was discussed relative to the mallet finger. The severity of this deformity increases and is more difficult to reverse with other etiologies: the transverse retinacular ligaments stretch, triangular ligament fibers shorten, and the lateral bands displace dorsally where they are tethered. The hyperextended PIP joint then resists flexion. A self-sustaining deformity is established as the oblique retinacular ligaments displace dorsally and shorten. Contracted oblique ligaments and lateral bands cannot traverse the condyles of the

proximal phalanx during flexion. PIP joint flexion, which normally anticipates flexion of the distal joint, is then preceded by distal joint flexion: Synchronized IP joint flexion is halted. Distal joint flexion proceeds without flexion of the PIP joint until sufficient force develops in the FDP tendon to overcome resistance by the structures dorsal to the PIP joint. An abrupt flexion then occurs as the lateral bands snap over the condyles of the PIP joint. These are the pathomechanics of an established swan-neck deformity. Joint deterioration from rheumatoid synovitis or injury hinders treatment further.

The numerous causes of swan-neck deformity may be grouped anatomically by the pathway through which the deformity is initiated:

- Extrinsic tendon tightness
- Intrinsic tendon tightness
- Articular
- Distal tendon release

Normal variants

People with normally hypermobile IP joints can produce swan-neck deformities of all fingers voluntarily by contracting their finger intrinsic muscles. Aside from the curiosity they may attract, these hands represent normal variants and do not need treatment.

Extrinsic tendon tightness

Tightness through the central tendon hyperextends the middle phalanx. Cerebral palsy with spasticity of the EDC is a dynamic cause in this category.

Flexion deformity of the wrist and subluxation of the finger MP joint both tighten the extrinsic extensor tendon by lengthening the dorsal skeleton. MP joint subluxation can result from rheumatoid synovitis, intrinsic contracture, or excessive surgical release of the collateral ligaments. In each instance, PIP joint hyperextension (resistance to passive flexion) increases with MP joint flexion. This is an important distinction from intrinsic tightness.

Extensor tendon scarring over the dorsum of the hand that produces an extensor plus tenodesis increases tension through the central tendon while the MP joint is flexed (see Fig. 30-57).

Treatment of swan-neck deformity caused by conditions in this category is incomplete unless the proximal abnormality is corrected. Hyperextension of the PIP joint is a distal deformity that stems from a more proximal imbalance.

Intrinsic tendon tightness

Increased tension through the intrinsic tendons can produce palmar subluxation of the MP joint and hyperextension of the PIP joint in the fingers. Deformity is resisted by the glenoidal segments of the collateral ligaments at the MP joint and the palmar plate and FDS at the PIP joint. Spasticity in cerebral palsy, rheumatoid arthritis, ischemic intrinsic muscle contracture, and posttraumatic intrinsic tightness all produce deformity by increasing tightness through the intrinsic tendons. Tendon transfers for weakness or claw deformity in the ulnar palsied hand can initiate swan-neck deformity by this same pathway. Less severe tightness exhibits a positive distal intrinsic tightness test (see Fig. 30-58). Advanced tightness affects the MP joint in addition to the PIP joint.

Treatment of conditions in this category is directed toward release of the intrinsic tightness and rebalancing of the deformities. The procedures selected depend on the stage of the condition and the joints that are deformed. For example, flexor tenosynovectomy combined with distal intrinsic resections may suffice in rheumatoid disease with stable MP joints. Otherwise, proximal intrinsic tenotomy with MP joint arthroplasty also may be necessary to rebalance the fingers.

Articular

Rupture of the palmar plate of the PIP joint permits hyperextension, which may progress without early protective splinting. The treatment is reattachment of the palmar plate that has avulsed distally. This is feasible in longstanding ruptures and has been successfully performed as long as 10 years after injury.

Synovitis of the MP or PIP joints can destabilize fingers. Rheumatoid and psoriatic arthritis are the most commonly seen forms. Lupus arthritis results in joint deformity by a different mechanism but does not develop synovitis with cartilage erosion. Periarticular inflammation stimulates adhesions to the tendons, sagittal bands, and retinacular ligaments. This category of swan-neck deformities is difficult to treat because deteriorated joints are involved with adherent, displaced extensor tendons.

Distal tendon release

Release of the terminal extensor tendon concentrates extensor tension on the middle phalanx through the central tendon after a mallet tendon lesion. Hyperextension deformity with fracture of the middle phalanx has the same result; the distal extensor tendon is functionally lengthened. Prognosis for distal joint motion after fracture repositioning is guarded in cases that develop a tenodesis over the fracture site.

Loss of the FDS tendon eliminates an important stabilizer of the PIP joint. The severity of the deformity that results depends on the inherent stability of the palmar plate. This tendon should be divided as far proximally as possible when used for tendon transfer to preserve maximum tendon attachments within the flexor fibroosseous sheath proximal to the PIP joint.

THUMB EXTENSOR TENDONS

The EPL is the most mobile of the digital extensor tendons. Its 58-mm longitudinal excursion exceeds that of

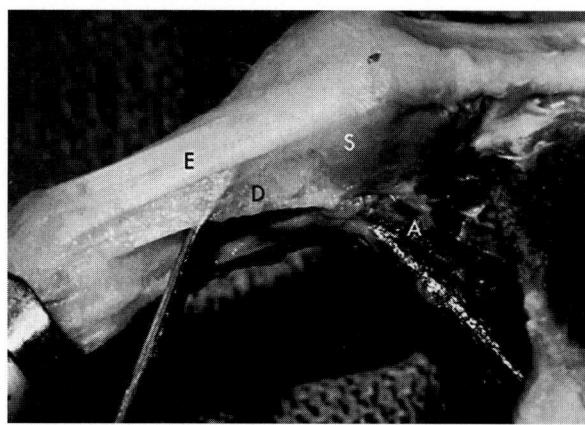

Fig. 30-44. Extensor apparatus of thumb. Adductor pollicis contributes to expansion of dorsal apparatus and assists extension of interphalangeal joint. Vertical fibers about metacarpophalangeal joint resemble the transverse retinacular ligaments of the fingers. *A,* Adductor pollicis muscle; *D,* dorsal apparatus; *E,* extensor pollicis longus over proximal phalanx; *S,* fibers representing homologue of transverse retinacular ligament.

the other digital extensor tendons.[5] (The EPL has a total excursion of 58 mm: 35 mm with wrist motion, 15 mm with MP motion, and 8 mm with flexion/extension of the IP joint.) A 13-mm medial/lateral translation of the tendon distal to the radius occurs with flexion/extension of the first metacarpal. The EPL supinates and adducts the thumb, extends the thumb MP joint with the EPB, extends the thumb IP joint with the dorsal hood fibers from the thumb intrinsic muscles, and is the only tendon capable of hyperextending the IP joint. Hyperextension of the IP joint normally precedes extension of the MP joint when the EPL is activated.[67]

The APL and EPB tendons are secured over the lateral border of the distal radius within the first dorsal fibroosseous compartment. Distal to the extensor retinaculum they pass beneath the superficial layer of the deep fascia. Fasciotomy distal to the extensor retinaculum during surgery for stenosing tenosynovitis of the extensor tendons (de Quervain's disease) may alter the balance of forces about the thumb.[180] Radial bowing of the APL and EPB tendons produces an exaggerated extension of the first metacarpal with an extension lag of the MP joint (see Fig. 30-5).

Extensor tendon anatomy about the MP joint resembles that of the finger PIP joint. Transverse fibers, similar to the transverse retinacular ligaments, shroud the capsule and attach to the flexor fibroosseous sheath.[106] The adductor pollicis on the ulnar side and the abductor pollicis brevis on the radial side contribute dorsal expansions that stabilize the extensor tendons and transfer extension forces to the IP joint (Fig. 30-44). The intrinsic muscles of the thumb thus are able to extend the IP joint to neutral but are not capable of hyperextension.

The EPB usually inserts on the dorsal base of the proximal phalanx but commonly has a second insertion into

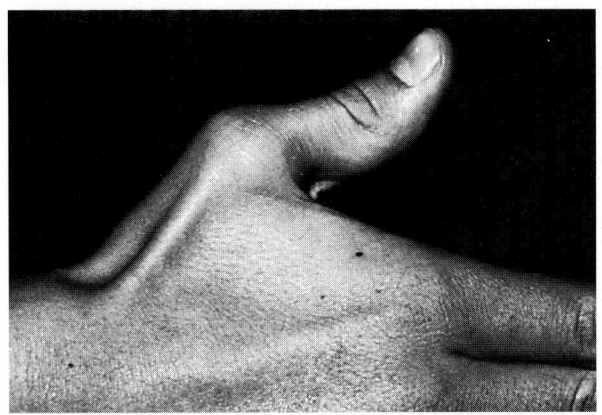

Fig. 30-45. Rupture of extensor pollicis brevis and dorsal fibers of extensor apparatus produce loss of metacarpophalangeal (MP) joint extension. Displacement of extensor pollicis longus (EPL) may accentuate flexion of MP joint and contributes to hyperextension of interphalangeal joint. EPL tendon is identified clearly.

the EPL.[73] It extends the first metacarpal and the MP joint. Interruption of the EPB introduces extension weakness at the base of the proximal phalanx. As the MP joint flexes, increased tension develops through the EPL, which hyperextends the IP joint (Fig. 30-45).

The EPL can extend the MP joint through the fibers of the dorsal apparatus. Diastasis or rupture of these fibers permits palmar displacement of the tendon. The tendon flexes the MP joint when displaced below the axis of joint motion, which exaggerates extension forces at the IP joint. This extrinsic-minus deformity, common with rheumatoid arthritis, is analogous to the boutonnière deformity of the finger.

Closed injuries

Rupture EPL. The EPL is subject to continued stress during performance of normal activities. Tenosynovitis has been attributed to overuse in the classic drummer's palsy.

Fig. 30-46. Rupture of extensor pollicis longus at level of Lister's tubercle. Tendon is not clinically apparent. Loss of metacarpophalangeal joint extension is most significant functional loss. Demonstrated extension of interphalangeal joint is by intrinsic muscles through their contribution to dorsal apparatus.

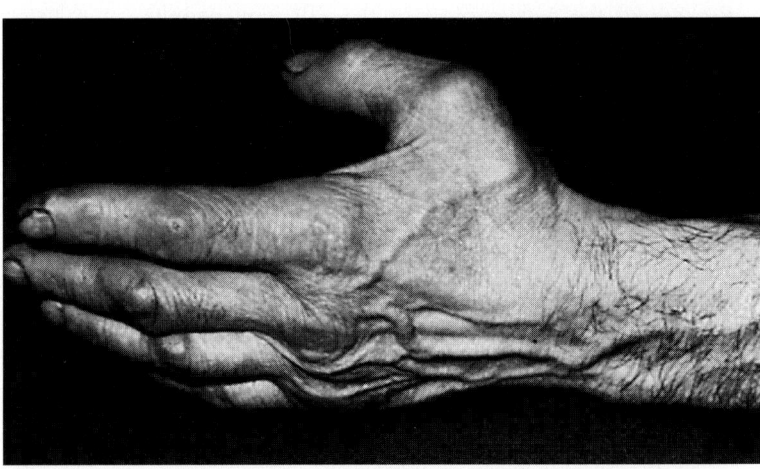

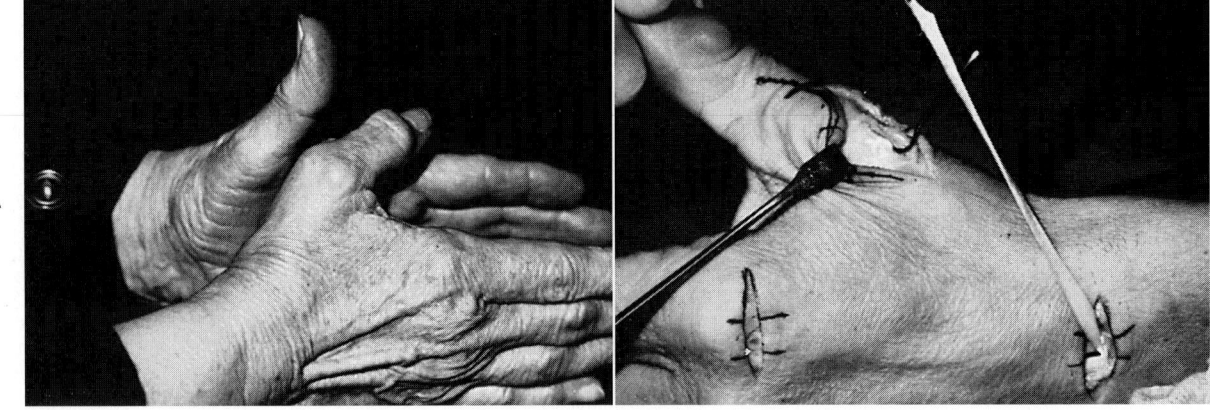

Fig. 30-47. Ruptured extensor pollicis longus (EPL). **A,** Loss of metacarpophalangeal extension and interphalangeal joint hyperextension. **B,** Reconstruction with extensor indicis proprius (EIP) transfer. EIP has excursion comparable with EPL. Course of the tendon transfer simulates vector of ruptured tendon.

Musicians with impairment of this tendon experience difficulty with dexterous maneuvers. Thumb-under transpositions on the piano keyboard or manipulations of a string-board are severely hindered with a painful affliction involving the EPL.[25]

The tendon usually ruptures at the level of the distal radius beneath the extensor retinaculum. Rheumatoid synovitis and fractures of the distal radius, often undisplaced, are common predisposing conditions; surgery of the distal radius,[149] uremia, diabetes, and local steroid injections are less commonly implicated.[51] The cause of the rupture is believed to be ischemia of a segment of the tendon that normally has poor vascularity. Microangiographic studies suggest that pressure from the effusion that accompanies synovitis or a fracture impedes the intrinsic nutrition in this tendon segment.[37] Oral anabolic steroids have been associated with tendon fiber dissociation with calcification and rupture.[83]

The most disabling impairment after rupture of the EPL is extension lost at the MP joint (Fig. 30-46). The origin of the EPL is long, and the muscle retains some contractility after tendon rupture. The myostatic tightness that develops with attritional rupture can be overcome by strong thenar and thumb flexor antagonists after reconstruction. Successful rehabilitation with an intercalated free tendon graft that bridges the ruptured tendon ends depends on the potential function of the retracted muscle.[54] EIP tendon transfer—rerouted superficial to the deep fascia distal to the extensor retinaculum and sutured to the EPL at the MP joint of the thumb—is technically easier, requires only one tendon repair, and simulates the normal vector of the EPL.[144] The EIP and EPL have comparable mean fiber length and tension fraction.[14,24] The index finger usually retains independent extension from the EDC after transfer (Fig. 30-47).

Rupture insertion EPL. Closed rupture of the EPL mimics the mallet tendon injury of the finger. Loss of full active extension of the IP joint with localized dorsal swelling occurs. Incomplete extension after flexion is from intact lateral tendon fibers. Treatment is by uninterrupted dorsal splinting with the IP joint in hyperextension for 6 weeks. Subsequent night splinting for an additional 2 to 4 weeks is usually recommended. The position of splinting should not create skin blanching.[28,109,125]

FRACTURES AND EXTENSOR TENDON DEFORMITY
Metacarpals

Fractures initiate deformity through the extensor tendons by mechanically fixing the tendon, disrupting normal tendon mechanics and promoting adhesions. Skeletal architecture and the disposition of the extensor tendons about the skeleton influence fracture displacement and predetermine the deformity that results. The metacarpals and the phalanges arch dorsally. Transverse fractures of the metacarpals flex because of the interosseous muscles. Spiral fractures flex and rotate, and the distal fragment displaces palmarward. The flexed metacarpal head positions the MP joint in hyperextension. The dorsal fracture apex mechanically alters zone VI tendons. The lengthened dorsal skeleton increases tension transmitted distally by the extrinsic extensor tendons. MP joint hyperextension is accentuated by increased tension through the extensor tendon. The PIP joint then reciprocally flexes; this is an extension lag. If the dorsal capsule and MP joint collateral ligaments shorten, a dorsal MP joint contracture ensues. The deformity is an extensor-plus claw deformity (Fig. 30-48).

Proximal phalanx

The extrinsic extensor tendon and the distal fibers of the digital extensor mechanism are situated dorsally about the proximal phalanx. Transverse fractures of the proximal phalanx develop hyperextension at the fracture site. Segmental fractures permit linear shortening caused by loss of bone support. In spiral fractures, the distal fragment rotates, migrates proximally, and tilts dorsally, a combination of

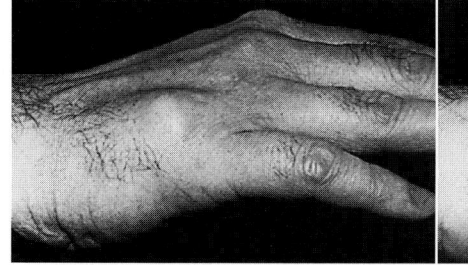 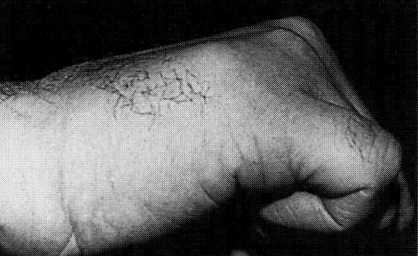 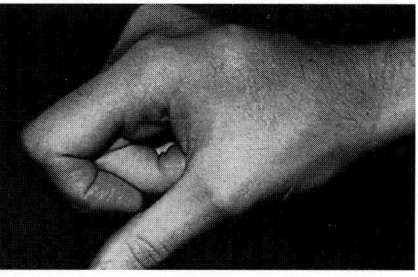

A   **B**   **C**

Fig. 30-48. Deformity and extensor tendon dysfunction from malunion of metacarpal fracture. **A** and **B,** Malunion fracture of fifth metacarpal. **A,** Dorsal bump is apex of fracture. The distal fragment is flexed and the metacarpophalangeal (MP) joint is hyperextended. Active MP joint extension. **B,** Finger flexion is restricted as a result of extensor tendon tightness and dorsal capsular contracture of MP joint. **C,** Malunion fracture index metacarpal. Dorsally angulated index metacarpal fracture mechanically impedes extensor tendon glide and restricts MP joint flexion. There is little dorsal tightness of the MP joint.

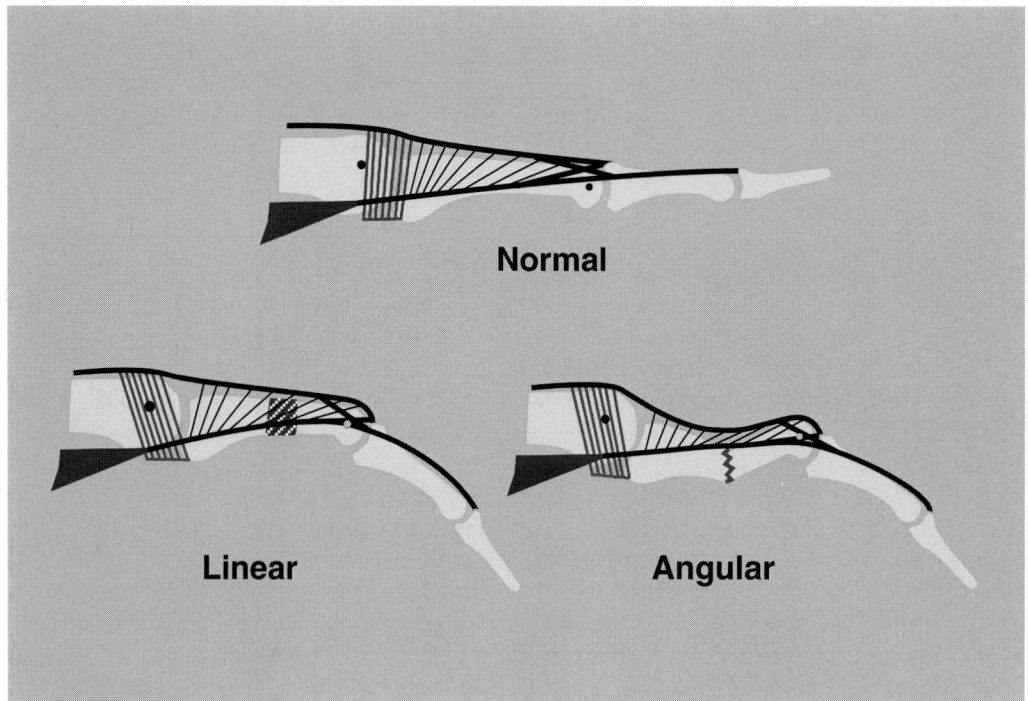

Fig. 30-49. Tension in the digital extensor mechanism and balance between the extrinsic and intrinsic tendon fibers are maintained normally by the integrity of the proximal phalanx. Segmental bone loss produces linear shortening. Unstable fractures of the proximal metaphysis and shaft permit dorsal angulation that results in angular shortening. Both conditions functionally lengthen the digital extensor mechanism with extension lag at the interphalangeal joints. The ability to compensate for shortening—the *extensor reserve*—is limited. The intrinsic tendons have small excursions and the extrinsic tendon is restrained by the sagittal bands that attach to the palmar plate and proximal phalanx.

angular and linear shortening. Each condition relaxes the extensor mechanism, functionally lengthens the tendons and weakens IP extension. An extension lag of the PIP joint results. The MP joint then hyperextends by the sagittal bands as the extensor mechanism shifts proximally in a compensatory effort to achieve PIP extension through the central tendon. The ability of the extensor mechanism to compensate for proximal phalangeal shortening—the *extensor tendon reserve*—is limited by the volar attachments of the sagittal bands. Extensor tendon reserve has been 2 to 6 mm in cadaver studies[170] (Fig. 30-49). Fractures of the proximal phalanx and associated adhesions may also impede flexor tendons within the fibroosseous sheath. Realignment of the proximal phalanx restores balance to the extensor mechanism and reverses MP joint hyperextension. It is difficult to balance a finger through the tendons without restoring skeletal length and alignment first. Preservation of proximal phalangeal length and alignment remains a primary objective after injury (Fig. 30-50).

Middle phalanx

The middle phalanx hyperextends after transverse fractures because of the dorsally situated extensor tendons and

oblique retinacular ligaments. Proximal fragment flexion is accentuated by the insertion of the FDS tendon. Spiral fractures permit skeletal shortening that relaxes the extensor tendon distally. The resulting deformity is an extension lag of the DIP joint with increased PIP joint extension. Flexion of the proximal fragment increases the extension moment by the central tendon and accentuates PIP joint extension. The deformity is resisted by the palmar-stabilizing ligaments of the PIP joint. PIP joint hyperextension results in a swan-neck deformity.

EXTENSOR TENDON SEPARATION: CONFRONTING THE TENDON GAP

Disruption of a tendon is normally followed by a phased healing sequence. Blood vessels and fibroblasts capable of collagen production migrate into the wound. Protein aggregates and collagen fibers unite the tendon ends by approximately day 4. Tendon remodeling then progresses under the influence of biophysical and biochemical factors. The ideal flexor tendon repair reestablishes continuity of collagen fibers and establishes a smooth gliding surface. The requirements for a functioning extensor tendon repair are less stringent. Bridging collagen alone is necessary for function.[98]

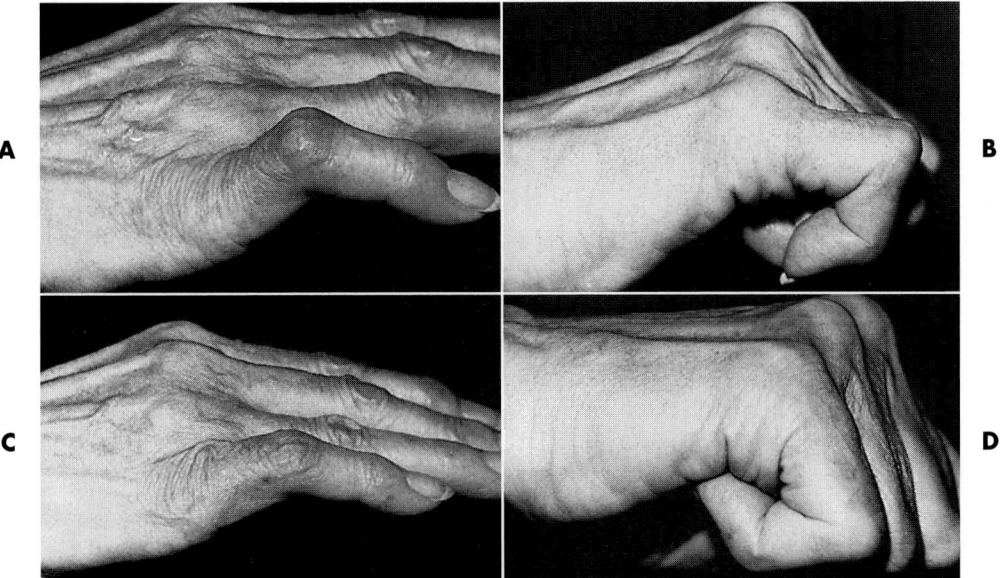

Fig. 30-50. Deformity and extensor tendon dysfunction from malunion fracture of the proximal phalanx. Hyperextension of the proximal phalanx fracture functionally lengthens extensor tendons, creating extension lag of the proximal interphalangeal joint with reciprocal hyperextension of metacarpophalangeal (MP) joint in 72-year-old woman. **A,** Active extension 6 months after injury. **B,** Active flexion. Longstanding hyperextension has created a dorsal MP joint contracture that blocks flexion. **C,** Active extension 6 months after correctional osteotomy of the proximal phalanx demonstrates improved extensor tendon balance. **D,** Active flexion.

Investigators have pondered the balance between immobilization and controlled motion after extensor tendon repair. Mobilization of repairs after 1 day of splinting stretched the repair sites and produced an extension lag. Immobilization for 3 weeks produced stiffness and decreased flexion. Ten days was once considered optimal immobilization.[164] Long-term results of extensor tendon lacerations treated with repair and conventional splinting for 3 to 4 weeks have been disappointing. Good to excellent results (total active motion, 230 degrees) were achieved in 64% of patients without associated injuries, but in only 45% with associated injuries. Distal zones I to IV had significantly poorer results than proximal zones V to VIII. The percentage of fingers that lost flexion exceeded the percentage that lost extension.[115] Modification of the biophysical environment of the healing tendon through controlled tension has improved the quality of tendon healing and clinical results. Experience with early protected motion after flexor tendon repairs was applied to extensor tendon injuries with improved results.* Methods that were effective in proximal extensor zones V to VIII have been refined and successfully adapted for more distal zones III and IV.[61] The biomechanical[108] and electro-physiologic[3,116] rationale for the success of these early motion protocols has facilitated the implementation of these methods in the clinical arena. At this time there is still no justification for an early motion protocol in zone 1 or 2 extensor tendon repairs or after repair of a wrist extensor tendon.

The tensile strength of tendon has been compared with that of steel. The strength at the musculotendinous junction approximates 10% of the strength of tendons. Tensile strength of a healed tendon approximates that of the musculotendinous junction.[74] The junction of the repaired tendon remains the weakest link in the muscle-tendon unit. Separated tendons resist passive approximation after the healing process has begun; distal joint repositioning is not a predictable means of reapproximating them (Fig. 30-51). A larger gap heals slower than a smaller one and is weaker when healed. Treatment strives to minimize the effect of the tendon gap.

Muscle lacerations

Muscle belly lacerations without repair result in a gap that disrupts the parallel arrangement of endomysial tubes, prevents muscle regeneration, and heals by scar formation. Excessive gapping increases resting muscle length and

*References 4, 15, 38-40, 85, 91, 131.

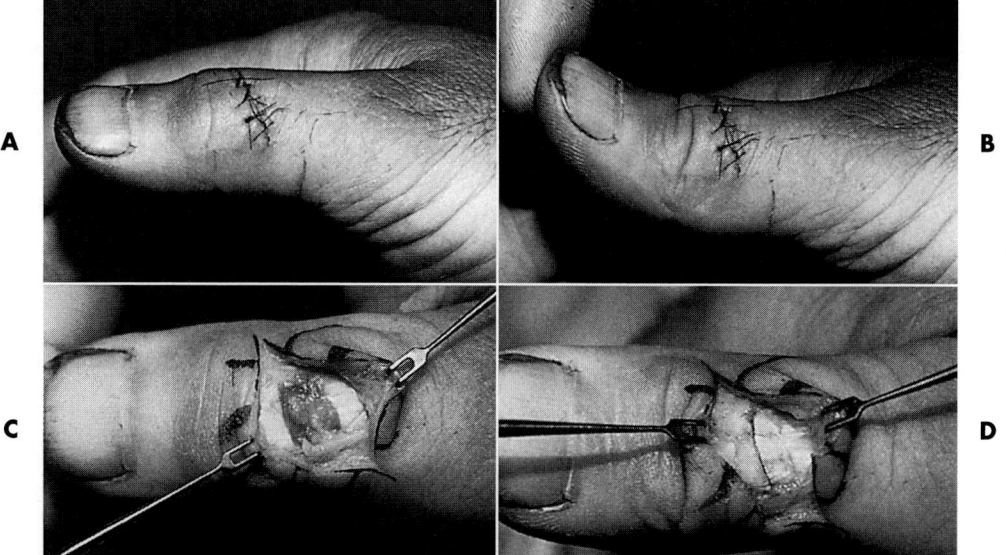

Fig. 30-51. Laceration of the extensor pollicis longus (EPL) tendon in thumb zone II, 10 days after primary wound repair without tendon repair. **A,** Active extension of the interphalangeal (IP) joint lacks hyperextension capability because of loss of EPL. **B,** Joint mobility demonstrates the passive potential. **C,** Tendon gap is bridged by early elements of tendon healing. The tendon ends will not accurately approximate by passive positioning of the IP joint distally. **D,** The tendon gap has been evacuated and the tendon ends accurately approximated. Tendon strength is improved and adhesions are diminished by minimizing the tendon gap.

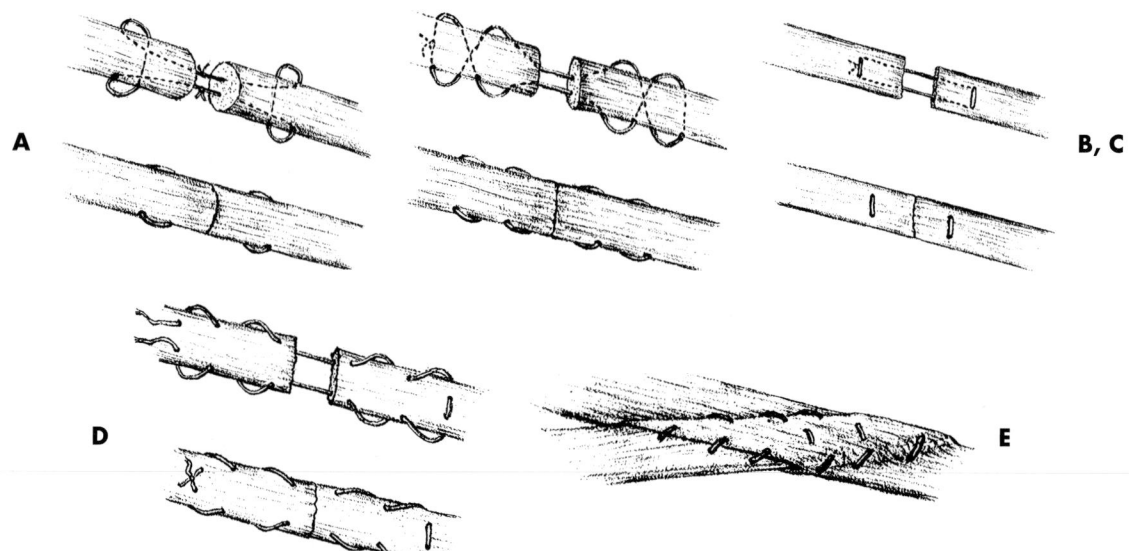

Fig. 30-52. Suture techniques for extensor tendon repair. Braided, white, synthetic nonabsorbable 3-0 or 4-0 sutures such as Mersilene* or Ethibond* are used, depending on the caliber of the tendon. The junction suture is 6-0. **A,** Peripheral grasping suture is applicable for round or oval tendons. Placement of sutures with respect to intratendinous vasculature is less critical with extensor tendons. **B,** The classic Bunnell weave suture, also useful for cylindrical or oval tendons, is technically easy to insert. Kleinert's modification uses a single paired loop on each side of the tendon junction. **C,** The horizontal mattress suture is weaker than weave sutures, but has application for broad, flat tendons with longitudinal fibers. This suture does not crimp the tendon but can foreshorten the tendon if it is tied too tightly. **D,** The modified baseball stitch combines a central horizontal mattress with a continuous peripheral grasping technique that approximates broad, flat tendons without creating a constriction deformity. **E,** Adjacent tendons are joined by passing the proximal end of a disrupted tendon through a cleft in an intact tendon. Multiple sutures are tied deep to the tendon. The result is a flat junction that is not clinically conspicuous. (Mersilene and Ethibond, Ethicon, Inc., Somerville, New Jersey.)

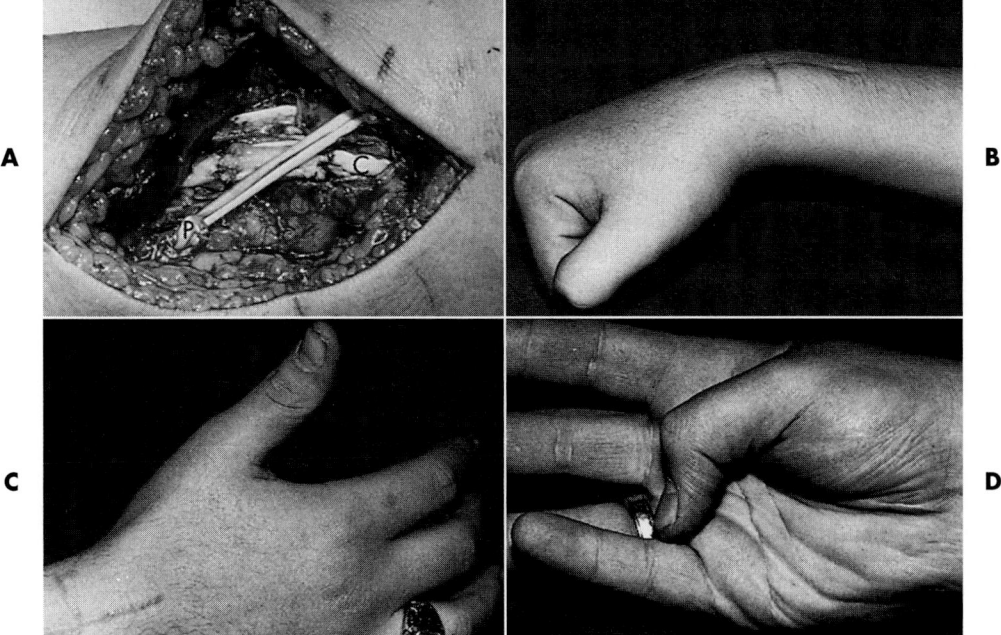

Fig. 30-53. Free tendon grafts used to bridge tendon gaps caused by myostatic tightness in lacerated extensor carpi radialis longus (ECRL) and extensor pollicis longus (EPL) tendons in zone VI in 15-year-old boy 4 weeks after injury. Extensor carpi radialis brevis was not injured. **A,** Tendon grafts bridge gaps in lacerated tendons and avoid tendon repair with excessive tension. **B,** Wrist flexion 7 months after repair. **C,** Active EPL function. **D,** There is no restriction of thumb flexion by the EPL. *C,* ECRL; *P,* EPL.

decreases effective contraction. Completely lacerated muscles in animals recover 50% of their ability to produce tension and 80% of their normal excursion.[47] Through-and-through, free tendon grafts are effective approximators of lacerated muscle bellies: 41% of treated patients regained grade 5 muscle strength after repair.[10]

Extensor tendon repairs

Accurate repair aspires to minimize the tendon gap. There have been significant problems with strength and quality of extensor tendon repairs. Sutured extensor tendons are roughly 50% as strong as flexor tendons, largely because of reduced tendon dimension and lack of collagen cross-linking. All tested repair techniques in zone VI cadaver tendons produced tendon shortening with restrained MP joint motion caused by the repair. The Kleinert modification of the Bunnell method and the Kessler techniques were the strongest.[117]

Selection of suture caliber and method is determined clinically by the cross-sectional configuration and stiffness of the tendon. Braided, white nonabsorbable sutures are preferred. Pigmented, monofilament nonabsorbable sutures are unattractive when visible beneath thin skin, and their hard knots can create erosive lesions.[79] Knots are tied deep to the extensor tendons when there is a paucity of subcutaneous fat or the skin is thin. A Kessler peripheral grasping or Bunnell weave suture is used for round or oval tendons, such as the EPL, EIP, or EDQ. A horizontal mattress suture is weaker and gaps when tested[117] but is nevertheless preferred for small, flat tendons, such as the juncturae tendinum or the lateral bands about the PIP joint. The baseball stitch[74] has been modified to pass through the tendon ends and is preferred for broad, thin tendons, such as the EDC in zone VI (Fig. 30-52). The extensor hoods over the MP joints are substantial structures composed of longitudinal tendon and transverse sagittal band fibers that hold simple or figure-of-eight sutures well. The central tendon and terminal tendon insertions are structurally stiffer than other fibers in the finger extensor apparatus[45] and can be sutured securely. Large gaps may be unavoidable without introducing intolerable tension and must then be bridged. Interposition free tendon grafts, described for the EPL,[54] have broader application (Fig. 30-53).

The functional pseudotendon

Dehiscence of a tendon repair or failure to repair a tendon creates a large void between the tendon ends. The gap fills with scar that bears little physical resemblance to a normal tendon. This pseudotendon lacks the glide flexibility of a normal tendon but has sufficient structural integrity to function adequately after it has been surgically liberated (Fig. 30-54).

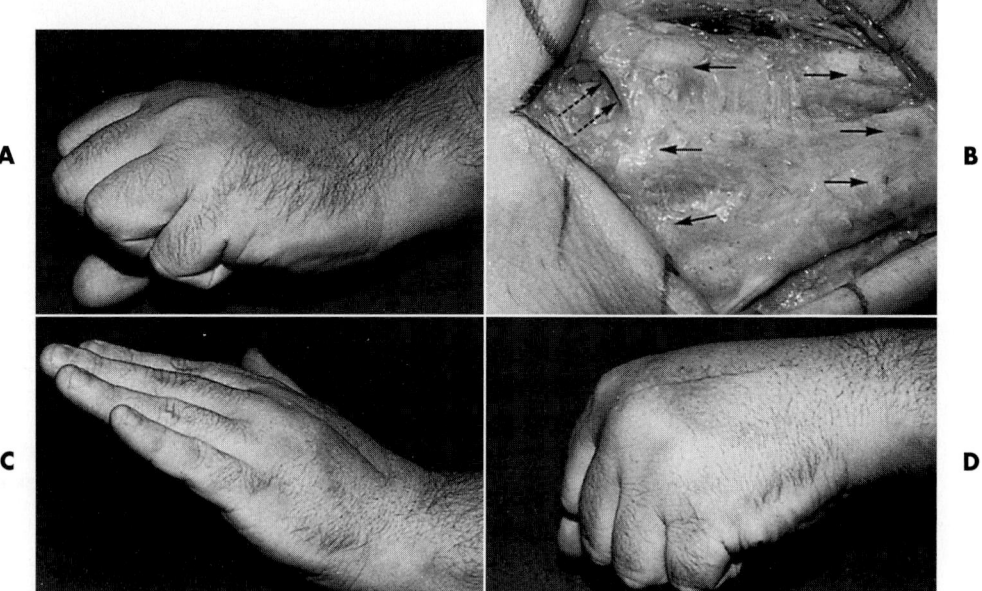

Fig. 30-54. The functional pseudotendon. Restricted grip in 33-year-old man seen 10 months after primary repair of extensor tendons to index, long, and ring fingers in zone VI. **A,** Grip lacks combined metacarpophalangeal and proximal interphalangeal joint flexion, an extensor-plus tenodesis. **B,** Extensor tenolysis has defined a functional sheet of scar—the pseudotendon—that bridges the dehisced ends of the repaired extensor tendons. Black monofilament sutures are visible in the proximally retracted tendons to the right. Tendon individuality had been lost, but potential for unified finger function was retained. **C,** Active extension 9 weeks after tenolysis. **D,** Active flexion. *Solid arrows,* Ends of dehisced tendon repairs; *dotted arrows,* margins of functional pseudotendon after tenolysis.

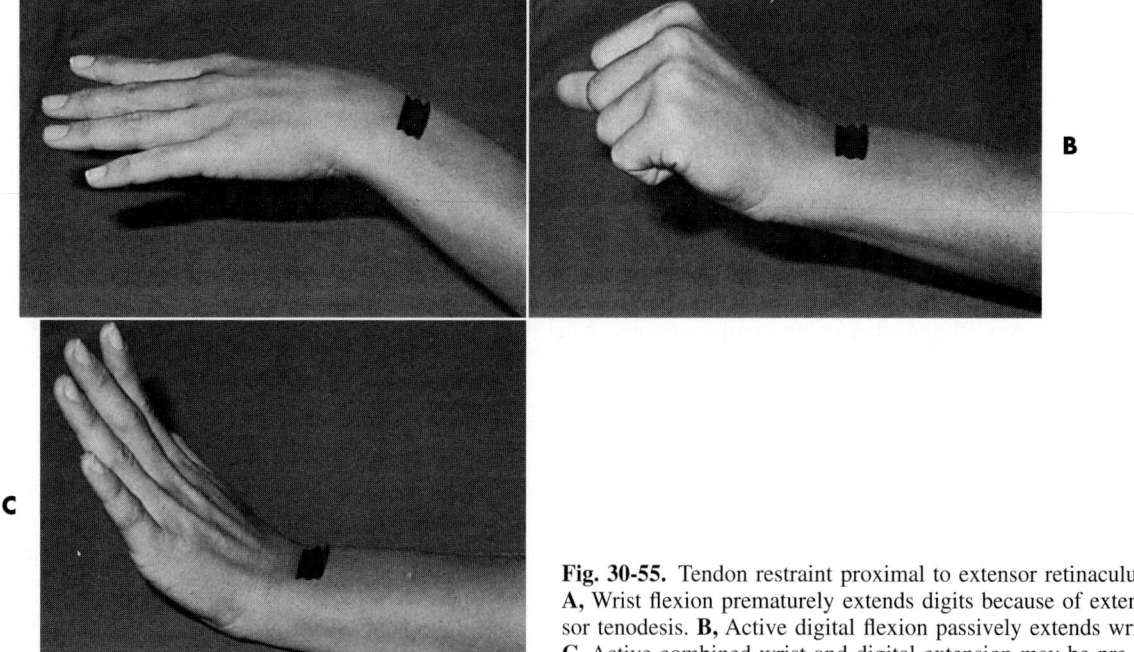

Fig. 30-55. Tendon restraint proximal to extensor retinaculum. **A,** Wrist flexion prematurely extends digits because of extensor tenodesis. **B,** Active digital flexion passively extends wrist. **C,** Active combined wrist and digital extension may be preserved if glide is not obstructed proximally.

PATTERNS OF RESTRAINT FROM SCARRED EXTENSOR TENDONS

Injured extensor tendons are prone to restraint from scar formation and can be difficult to rehabilitate. Their disproportionately large surface area and comparatively less excursion, strength, and capacity for sustained tension compared with flexor tendons introduce special challenges after injury and reparative surgery.

Sites of blockage from tendon adhesions can be localized by comparing active and passive ranges of motion. Skin adherence, localized induration, and dimpling reliably indicate the location of restraining scar. The following discussions relate to the extensor tendons and retinacular systems. These principles cannot be applied unless the joints are passively mobile.

Proximal to extensor retinaculum

Scar adhesions of the finger extensor tendons proximal to the extensor retinaculum restrain combined wrist and finger flexion. A reciprocal wrist extension/finger flexion grip pattern may develop; active finger flexion passively extends the wrist while active wrist extension permits the fingers to flex further by reducing the distance between the blockage and the extensor tendon insertions. Passive wrist flexion initiates a tenodesis that passively extends the fingers. Only wrist flexion is impaired when the wrist extensor tendons alone are involved (Fig. 30-55).

Distal to extensor retinaculum

Neither active nor passive wrist motion is impaired. The pattern of scar restraint at this level depends on whether the scar glides, as with a bulky tendon repair, or is anchored to the deep fascia. Gliding scar limits motion because of its inability to pass beneath the deep fascia or extensor retinaculum. Combined wrist and finger extension is restricted. Wrist extension may be enhanced by flexing the fingers first. This pulls the impeding scar distally, further from the distal edge of the abutting ligament, and permits additional wrist extension before the scar is again blocked by the extensor retinaculum proximally (Fig. 30-56).

Anchored scar fixing the digital extensor tendons to the deep fascia produces an extensor-plus phenomenon. This tenodesis passively extends the IP joints of the finger as the MP joint is flexed. As the IP joints flex, the tenodesis is transferred proximally and the MP joints passively extend. Active and passive reciprocity exists between the MP and IP joints. Combined MP and IP joint flexion is prevented (Fig. 30-57).

Intrinsic tightness versus tendon scarring

Tightness of the intrinsic muscles and adhesions adjacent to the extensor hood about the MP joint that involve the intrinsic tendons both can interfere with finger flexion. Active and passive flexion may be painful with either condition. Scar involving the extensor hood can produce a clinical picture that is indistinguishable from an intrinsic contracture by clinical testing. Intrinsic tightness is tested by passively extending the finger MP joint while flexing the IP joints—the intrinsic tightness test described by Finochietto.[41] The radial and ulnar intrinsic muscles of each finger may be evaluated separately by deviating the finger away from the side being tested. Intrinsic restraint suggested by testing may be the

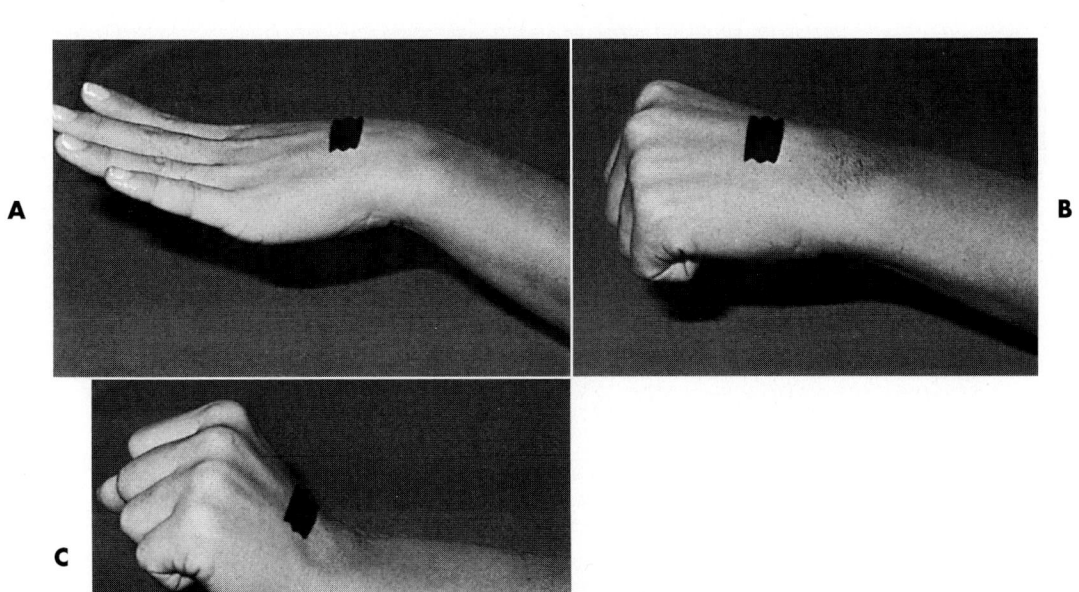

A

B

C

Fig. 30-56. Gliding scar distal to extensor retinaculum. **A,** Bulky scar abuts extensor retinaculum, preventing simultaneous wrist and finger extension. **B,** Finger flexion before wrist extension increases potential for wrist extension. **C,** Wrist and finger flexion may not be impaired.

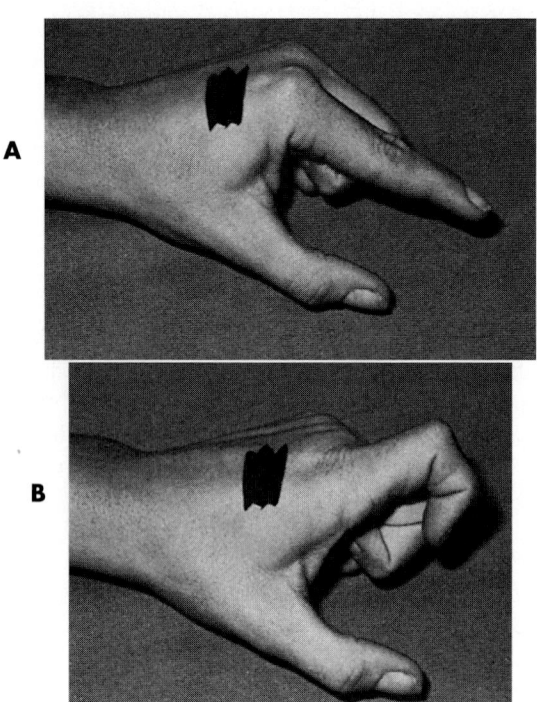

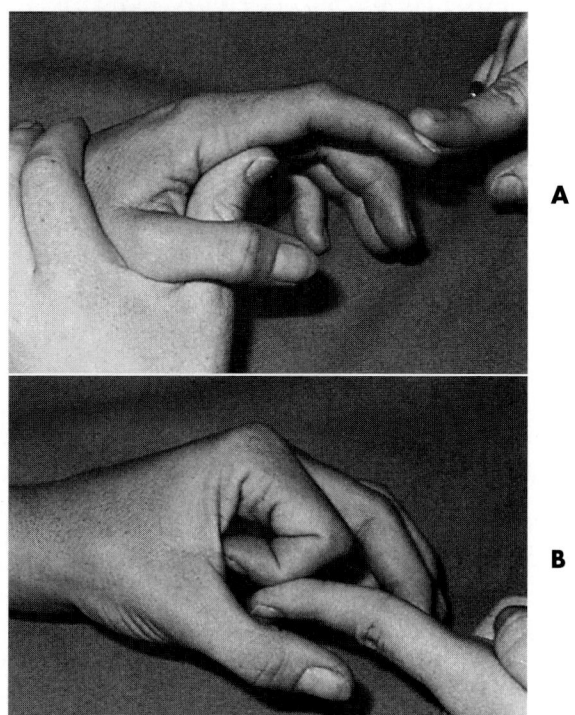

Fig. 30-57. Extensor-plus finger tenodesis caused by restrained extensor tendons proximal to metacarpophalangeal (MP) joints. **A,** Active and passive flexion of MP joint produces passive tenodesis with extension of interphalangeal (IP) joints. **B,** Active or passive IP joint flexion passively extends MP joints.

Fig. 30-58. Intrinsic-plus test (Finochietto[41]). **A,** Passive flexion of interphalangeal (IP) joints while metacarpophalangeal (MP) joint is supported in neutral tests for tightness through the distal intrinsic tendons. The radial and ulnar intrinsics can be individually tested by deviating finger away from side being tested. **B,** MP joint flexion relaxes intrinsic muscles, lessens tension through extensor tendons, and decreases resistance to passive IP joint flexion.

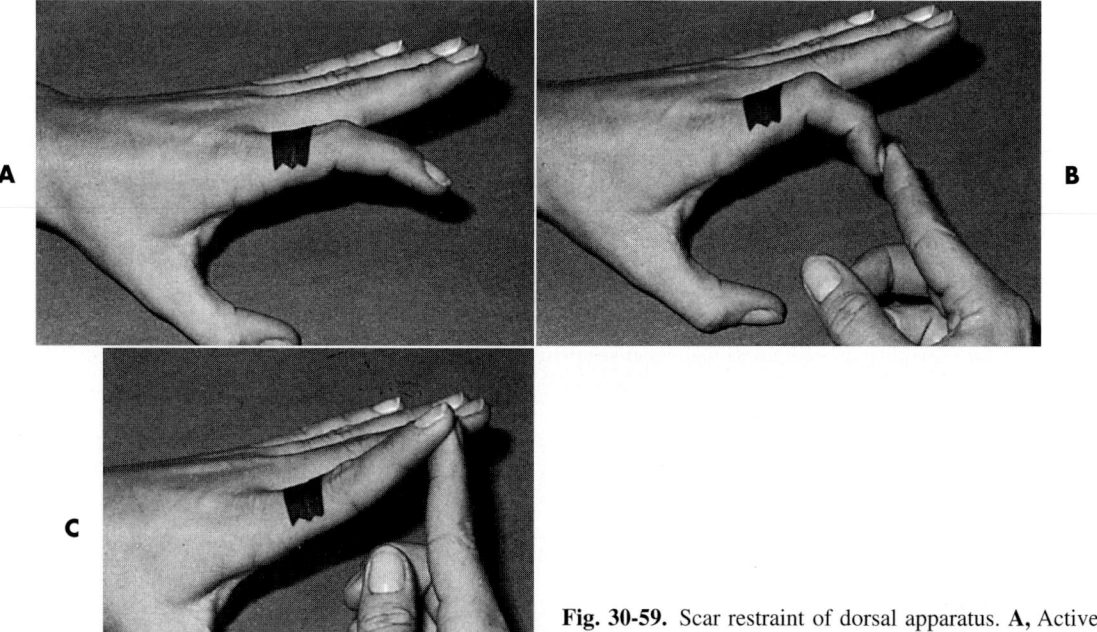

Fig. 30-59. Scar restraint of dorsal apparatus. **A,** Active extension beyond resting position is prevented. **B,** Active and passive flexion is resisted, often feeling "springy." **C,** Passive extension is present if interphalangeal joints are healthy.

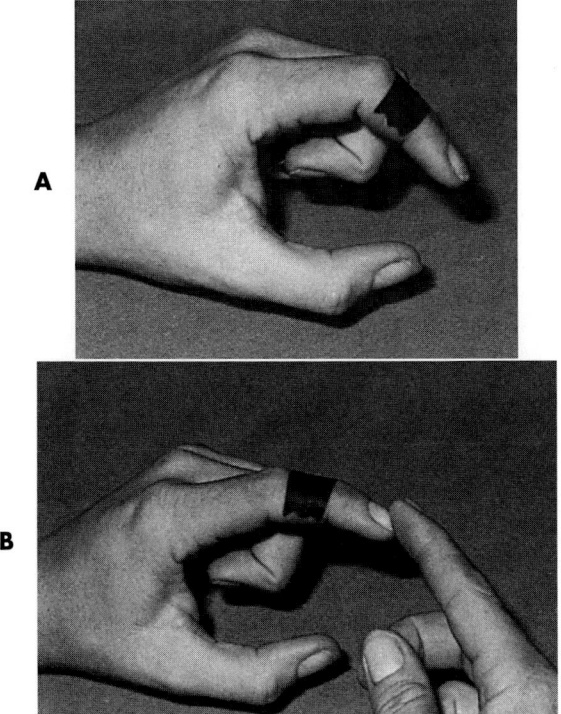

Fig. 30-60. Extensor tendon restraint over middle phalanx. **A,** Active distal joint flexion is lacking. Extension lag may be present. **B,** Passive distal joint flexion is "springy" or blocked. Associated resistance of proximal interphalangeal joint flexion infers restraint of lateral bands and triangular ligament.

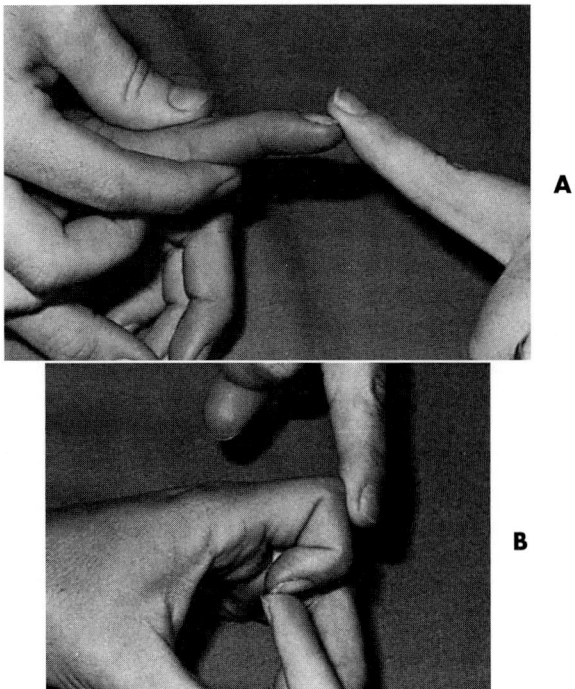

Fig. 30-61. Retinacular tightness test or intrinsic-plus phenomenon. **A,** Oblique retinacular ligament tightness is tested by passively flexing distal joint while proximal interphalangeal (PIP) joint is supported in neutral. Resistance is relative and should be compared with normal fingers. Relative resistance indicates a positive test. **B,** Combined flexion of both interphalangeal joints is present normally and with mild ligament tightness. Test depends on the position of the PIP joint.

result of muscle contracture or adhesions of the intrinsic tendons distally. Careful clinical examination often can differentiate scarring about the intervolar plate ligaments, the *saddle syndrome,* from scarring about the extensor hood at the MP joint. The location of swelling and tenderness is helpful in differentiating these conditions. The discernment may not be absolute before surgery; it is then made at the time of tenolysis (Fig. 30-58).

Proximal phalanx

Scarring of the extensor tendons over the proximal phalanx can restrict the extrinsic central tendon, intrinsic expansions, or the entire dorsal apparatus. The resting position of the PIP joint reflects the position of the extensor tendons when motion is finally arrested. Active extension of the PIP joint beyond the resting position is lacking. Frequently, an extension lag is present, and passive correction to neutral is possible. Active and passive flexion of the PIP joint is blocked; there is often an elastic or springy quality of restrained joint motion during testing (Fig. 30-59).

Flexion of the PIP joint also can be blocked by scarring of the triangular ligament. This restrains the lateral bands dorsally and can consolidate the lateral bands with the central tendon insertion. Proximal IP joint flexion is blocked in both instances: in the first, palmar descent by the lateral

bands is prevented; in the second, a tenodesis with the central tendon exists. Flexion of the DIP joint is usually restricted when flexion of the PIP joint is blocked by these conditions.

Middle phalanx

Scarring of the extensor tendon over the middle phalanx restrains flexion of the DIP joint. Active and passive flexion restraint that is unrelated to the position of the PIP joint implies scarring of the extensor tendon. The retinacular ligaments usually are involved also (Fig. 30-60). These ligaments have little influence on the normal finger but play a significant role in the scarred or imbalanced finger by limiting distal joint motion and fostering deformity. A tight oblique retinacular ligament produces a positive retinacular tightness test, also called an *intrinsic intrinsic-plus phenomenon.*[7] Normally, there is some passive flexion of the DIP joint while the PIP joint is supported in extension. Shortening or scarring of the oblique retinacular ligament restrains distal joint flexion. This restraint depends on the position of the PIP joint—increased PIP joint flexion diminishes DIP joint flexion—which differentiates this from fixation of the extensor tendon. Capsular contracture of the DIP joint can also restrict distal joint motion that is independent of PIP joint position. An integrated assessment of the history, clinical findings, and x-ray films assists in compiling a definitive appraisal (Fig. 30-61).

REFERENCES

1. Agee J, Guidera M: The functional significance of the juncturae tendinum in dynamic stabilization of the metacarpophalangeal joints of the fingers, ASSH Proceedings, *J Hand Surg* 5:288, 1980.
2. Aiche A, Barsky AJ, Weine DL: Prevention of boutonnière deformity, *Plast Reconstr Surg* 46:164, 1970.
3. Allieu Y, Asencio G, Rouzand J-C: Protected passive mobilization after suturing of the extensor tendons of the hand. In Tubiana R, editor: *The hand,* vol 3, Philadelphia, 1988, WB Saunders.
4. Allieu Y, et al: Suture des tendons extensuers de la main avec mobilisation assisteé a propos de 120 cas, *Rev Chir Orthop* 70:69, 1984.
5. An K-N, et al: Tendon excursion and moment arm of index finger muscles, *J Biomech* 16:419, 1983.
6. Barfred T, Adamsen S: Duplication of the extensor carpi ulnaris tendon, *J Hand Surg* 11A:423, 1986.
7. Bendz P: The functional significance of the oblique retinacular ligament of Landsmeer: a review and new proposals, *J Hand Surg* 10B:25, 1985.
8. Bin Iftikhar T, et al: Spontaneous rupture of the extensor mechanism causing ulnar dislocation of the long extensor tendon of the long finger, *J Bone Joint Surg* 66A:1108, 1984.
9. Blacker GJ, Lister GD, Kleinert HE: The abducted little finger in low ulnar palsy, *J Hand Surg* 1:190, 1976.
10. Botte MJ, et al: Repair of severe muscle belly lacerations using a tendon graft, *J Hand Surg* 12A:406, 1987.
11. Bowers HW, Hurst LC: Chronic mallet finger: the use of Fowler's central slip release, *J Hand Surg* 3:373, 1978.
12. Boyes JH: *Bunnell's surgery of the hand,* ed 5, Philadelphia, 1970, JB Lippincott.
13. Bracey DJ, Jeffreys TE: Habitual extensor tendon dislocation, *Hand* 11:284, 1979.
14. Brand PW, Beach RB, Thompson DE: Relative tension and potential excursion of muscles in the forearm and hand, *J Hand Surg* 6:206, 1981.
15. Browne EZ, Ribik CA: Early dynamic splinting for extensor tendon injuries, *J Hand Surg* 14A:72, 1989.
16. Bunnell S: *Surgery of the hand,* ed 3, Philadelphia, 1956, JB Lippincott.
17. Burke F: Mallet finger, *J Hand Surg* 13B:115, 1988 (editorial).
18. Burkhart SS, Wood MB, Linscheid RL: Post traumatic recurrent subluxation of the extensor carpi ulnaris tendon, *J Hand Surg* 7:1, 1982.
19. Burton RI: Extensor tendons: late reconstruction. In Green DP, editor: *Operative hand surgery,* ed 2, New York, 1988, Churchill Livingstone.
20. Carducci AT: Potential boutonnière deformity: its recognition and treatment, *Orthop Rev* 10:121, 1981.
21. Carroll C, Moore JR, Weiland AJ: Posttraumatic ulnar subluxation of the extensor tendons: a reconstructive technique, *J Hand Surg* 12A:227, 1987.
22. Chicarilli ZN, et al: Saddle deformity: posttraumatic interosseous-lumbrical adhesions—review of eighty-seven cases, *J Hand Surg* 11A:210, 1986.
23. Chun S, Palmar AK: Chronic ulnar wrist pain secondary to partial rupture of the extensor carpi ulnaris tendon, *J Hand Surg* 12A:1032, 1987.
24. Cooney WP: Tendon transfer for median nerve palsy, *Hand Clin* 4:155, 1988.
25. Crabb DJ: Hand injuries in professional musicians: a report of six cases, *Hand* 12:200, 1980.
26. Culver JE Jr: Extensor pollicis and indicis communis tendon: a rare anatomic variation revisited, *J Hand Surg* 5A:548, 1980.
27. De Leeuw B: The stratigraphy of the dorsal wrist region as basis for an investigation of the position of the extensor carpi ulnaris in pronation and supination of the forearm, thesis, Leiden, 1962, Luctor et Embergo.
28. Din KM, Meggitt BF: Mallet thumb, *J Bone Joint Surg* 65B:606, 1983.
29. Doyle JR: Extensor tendons: acute injuries. In Green DP, editor: *Operative hand surgery,* ed 2, New York, 1988, Churchill Livingstone.
30. Eckhardt WA, Palmer AK: Recurrent dislocation of the extensor carpi ulnaris tendon, *J Hand Surg* 6:629, 1981.
31. El-Gammal TA, et al: Anatomy of the oblique retinacular ligament of the index finger, *J Hand Surg* 18A:717, 1993.
32. Elliot D, McGrouther DA: The excursions of the long extensor tendons of the hand, *J Hand Surg* 11B:77, 1986.
33. Elliott RA: Injuries to the extensor mechanism of the hand, *Orthop Clin North Am* 1:335, 1970.
34. Elliott RA: Boutonnière deformity. In Cramer LM, Chase RA, editors: *Symposium of the hand,* St Louis, 1971, Mosby.
35. Elson RA: Dislocation of the extensor tendons of the hand: report of a case, *J Bone Joint Surg* 49B:324, 1967.
36. Elson RA: Rupture of the central slip of the extensor hood of the finger: a test for early diagnosis, *J Bone Joint Surg* 68B:229, 1986.
37. Engkvist O, Lundborg G: Rupture of the extensor pollicis longus tendon after fractures of the lower end of the radius: a clinical and microangiographic study, *Hand* 11:76, 1979.
38. Evans RB: Therapeutic management of extensor tendon injuries, *Hand Clin* 2:157, 1986.
39. Evans RB, Burkhalter WE: Early passive motion in complex extensor tendon injury. Second International Meeting of American Society of Hand Therapists, Boston, 1983.
40. Evans RB, Burkhalter WE: A study of the dynamic anatomy of extensor tendons and implications for treatment, *J Hand Surg* 11A:774, 1986.
41. Finochietto R: Retracción de Volkmann de los músculos intrínsecos de las manos, *Bol Trab Soc Cir Buenos Aires* 4:31, 1920.
42. Flatt AE: *Care of the arthritic hand,* ed 4, St Louis, 1983, Mosby.
43. Garberman S, Diao E, Peimer CA: Mallet finger: results of early versus delayed closed treatment, *J Hand Surg* 19A:851, 1994.
44. Garcia-Elias M, et al: Extensor mechanism of the fingers. I. A quantitative geometric study, *J Hand Surg* 16A:1130, 1991.
45. Garcia-Elias M, et al: Extensor mechanism of the fingers. II. Tensile properties of components, *J Hand Surg* 16A:1136, 1991.
46. Gardner RC: Hypertrophic infiltrative tendinitis (HIT syndrome) of the long extensor: the abused karate hand, *JAMA* 211:1009, 1970.
47. Garrett WE, et al: Recovery of skeletal muscle after laceration and repair, *J Hand Surg* 9A:683, 1984.
48. Garroway RY, et al: Complex dislocations of the proximal interphalangeal joint, *Orthop Rev* 13:21, 1984.
49. Grundberg AB, Reagan DS: Central slip tenotomy for chronic mallet finger deformity, *J Hand Surg* 12A:545, 1987.
50. Haberern JP: Ueber sehnenluxationen, *Deutsche Zeitschrift Chir* 62:191, 1902.
51. Haher JN, et al: Bilateral rupture of extensor pollicis longus, *Orthopedics* 10:1577, 1987.
52. Haines RW: The extensor apparatus of the finger, *J Anat* 85:251, 1951.
53. Hamas RS, Horrell ED, Pierret GP: Treatment of mallet finger due to intra-articular fracture of the distal phalanx, *J Hand Surg* 3A:361, 1978.
54. Hamlin C, Littler JW: Restoration of the extensor pollicis longus tendon by an intercalated graft, *J Bone Joint Surg* 59A:412, 1977.
55. Harris C: The Fowler operation for mallet finger deformity, *J Bone Joint Surg* 48A:63, 1966.

56. Harris C: The functional anatomy of the extensor mechanism of the finger, *J Bone Joint Surg* 54A:713, 1972.
57. Harvey FJ, Harrey PM: Three rare causes of extensor tendon rupture, *J Hand Surg* 14:957, 1989.
58. Harvey FJ, Hume KF: Spontaneous recurrent ulnar dislocation of the long extensor tendons of the fingers, *J Hand Surg* 5A:492, 1980.
59. Hellman K: Die wiederherstellung der strecksehnen im berich der ingermittelgelenke, *Langenbeck's Archiv Klin Chir* 309:36, 1964.
60. Hollinshead WH: *Anatomy for surgeons: the back and limbs,* ed 2, vol 3, New York, 1969, Harper & Row.
61. Hung LK, et al: Early controlled active mobilization with dynamic splintage for treatment of extensor tendon injuries, *J Hand Surg* 5A:251, 1990.
62. Iselin F, Levame J, Godoy J: A simplified technique for treating mallet fingers: tenodermodesis, *J Hand Surg* 2A:118, 1977.
63. Ishizuki M: Traumatic and spontaneous dislocation of extensor tendon of the long finger, *J Hand Surg* 15A:967, 1990.
64. Ishizuki M, Furuya K, Kumakura T: Extensor digitorum brevis manus associated with attrition rupture of a common extensor tendon, *J Hand Surg* 11A:582, 1986.
65. Ishizuki M, et al: The anatomy of the extensor apparatus of the hand and traumatic ulnar dislocation of the extensor tendons of the fingers, *J Jpn Soc Surg Hand* (in Japanese) 2:97, 1985.
66. Itoh Y, et al: Extensor tendon involvement in Smith's and Galeazzi's fractures, *J Hand Surg* 12A:535, 1987.
67. Jackson WT, et al: Anatomical variations in the first extensor compartment of the wrist: a clinical and anatomical study, *J Bone Joint Surg* 68A:923, 1986.
68. Johansson SH: *Peritendinous fibrosis of the dorsum of the hand,* Fifth World Congress of Plastic and Reconstructive Surgery, London, 1971, Butterworth.
69. Jones A, et al: Tophaceous pyrophosphate deposition with extensor tendon rupture, *Br J Rheum* 31:421, 1992.
70. Joshi BB: A salvage procedure in the treatment of the boutonnière deformity caused by contact burn and friction injury, *Hand* 14:33, 1982.
71. Kaplan EB: Functional significance of the insertion of the extensor digitorum communis in man, *Anat Rec* 92:293, 1945.
72. Kaplan EB: Anatomy, injuries and treatment of extensor apparatus of the hand and digits, *Clin Orthop* 13:24, 1959.
73. Kaplan EB: *Functional and surgical anatomy of the hand,* ed 2, Philadelphia, 1965, JB Lippincott.
74. Ketchum LD, Martin N, Kappel D: Factors affecting tendon gap and tendon strength at the site of tendon repair, *Plast Reconstr Surg* 59:708, 1977.
75. Ketchum LD, et al: The determination of moments for extension of the wrist generated by muscles of the forearm, *J Hand Surg* 3:205, 1978.
76. Kettelkamp DB, Flatt AE, Moulds R: Traumatic dislocation of the long-finger extensor tendon: a clinical, anatomical and biochemical study, *J Bone Joint Surg* 53A:229, 1971.
77. Kilgore ES, et al: Correction of ulnar subluxation of the extensor communis, *Hand* 7:272, 1975.
78. Kinninmonth AW, Holburn F: A comparative controlled trial of a new perforated splint and a traditional splint in the treatment of mallet finger, *J Hand Surg* 11B:261, 1986.
79. Kinninmonth WG: A complication of the buried suture, *J Hand Surg* 15:959, 1990.
80. Kleinman WB, Petersen DP: Oblique retinacular ligament reconstruction for chronic mallet finger deformity, *J Hand Surg* 9A:399, 1984.
81. Kon M, Bloem JJ: Treatment of mallet fingers by tenodermodesis, *Hand* 14:174, 1982.
82. Koniuch MP, et al: Closed crush injury of the metacarpophalangeal joint, *J Hand Surg* 12A:750, 1987.
83. Kramhøft M, Solgaard DP: Spontaneous rupture of the extensor pollicis longus tendon after anabolic steroids, *J Hand Surg* 11B:87, 1986.
84. Kus H: Nahtolose Rekonstruktion des streckshene bei hammerfinger (sutureless reconstruction of the extensor tendon in mallet finger), *Handchir Mikrochir Plast Chir* 16:231, 1984.
85. Labourea JP, Renevey A: Utilisation d'un appareil personnel de contention et de rééducation segmentaire élastique de la main type "crabes," *Ann Chir* 25:165, 1980.
86. Landsmeer JMF: The anatomy of the dorsal aponeurosis of the human finger and its functional significance, *Anat Rec* 104:31, 1949.
87. Landsmeer JMF: *Atlas of anatomy of the hand,* New York, 1976, Churchill Livingstone.
88. Lange RH, Engber WD: Hyperextension mallet finger, *Orthopedics* 6:1426, 1983.
89. Lee BS: Pseudo-boutonnière deformity, its pathogenesis and treatment, *Orthop Rev* 11:81, 1982.
90. Legouest L: Société impériale de chirugie, *Gazette de hôpitaux* 138, 1868.
91. Lemke T, Crayen P, Maroske D: Funktionelle behandlung der strecksehnenverletzung an der hand, *Chirurg* 55:264, 1984.
92. Light TR: Buttress pinning techniques, *Orthop Rev* 10:49, 1981.
93. Linscheid RL, An K-N, Gross RM: Quantitative analysis of the intrinsic muscles of the hand, *Clin Anat* 4:265, 1991.
94. Littler JW: Principles of reconstructive surgery of the hand. In Converse JM, editor: *Reconstructive plastic surgery,* Philadelphia, 1964, WB Saunders.
95. Littler JW: The finger extensor mechanism, *Surg Clin North Am* 47:415, 1967.
96. Littler JW, Eaton RG: Redistribution of forces in the correction of the boutonnière deformity, *J Bone Joint Surg* 49A:1267, 1967.
97. Mackay I, Simpson RG: Closed rupture of extensor digitorum communis tendon following fracture of the radius, *Hand* 12:214, 1980.
98. Manske PR: Flexor tendon healing, *J Hand Surg* 13B:237, 1988.
99. Manske PR, Ogata K, Lesker PA: Nutrient pathways to extensor tendons of primates, *J Hand Surg* 10B:8, 1985.
100. Matev I: Transposition of the lateral slips of the aponeurosis in treatment of longstanding "boutonnière deformity" of the fingers, *Br J Plast Surg* 17:281, 1964.
101. McCoy FJ, Winski AJ: Lumbrical loop operation for luxation of the extensor tendons of the hand, *Plast Reconstr Surg* 44:142, 1969.
102. McCue FC, et al: A pseudo-boutonnière deformity, *Hand* 7:166, 1975.
103. Mestagh H, et al: Organization of the extensor complex of the digits, *Anat Clin* 7:49, 1985.
104. Michon J, Vichard P: Luxation latérales des tendons extenseurs en regard de l'articulation métacarpo-phalangiénne, *Rev Med de Nancy* 86:595, 1961.
105. Miki T, et al: Rupture of the extensor tendons of the fingers: report of three unusual cases, *J Bone Joint Surg* 68A:610, 1986.
106. Milford LW: *Retaining ligaments of the digits of the hand,* Philadelphia, 1968, WB Saunders.
107. Milford LW: *The hand,* St Louis, 1971, Mosby.
108. Minamikawa Y, et al: Wrist position and extensor tendon amplitude following repair, *J Hand Surg* 17A:268, 1992.
109. Miura T, Nakamura R, Shuhei R: Conservative treatment for a ruptured extensor tendon on the dorsum of the proximal phalanges of the thumb (mallet thumb), *J Hand Surg* 11A:229, 1986.
110. Montant R, Baumann A: Rupture luxation of the extensor apparatus of the finger of the first interphalangeal articulation, *Rev d'Orthop* 25:5, 1938.
111. Moore JR, Weiland AJ, Valdata L: Independent index extension after extensor indicis proprius transfer, *J Hand Surg* 12A:232, 1987.
112. Moran S, Ruby LK: Nonrheumatoid closed rupture of extensor carpi ulnaris tendon, *J Hand Surg* 17A:281, 1992.
113. Murakami Y, Todani K: Traumatic entrapment of the extensor pollicis longus tendon in Smith's fracture of the radius: case report, *J Hand Surg* 6A:238, 1981.

114. Newmeyer WL, Green DP: Rupture of digital extensor tendons following distal ulnar resection, *J Bone Joint Surg* 64A:178, 1982.

115. Newport ML, Blair WF, Steyers CM Jr: Long-term results of extensor tendon repair, *J Hand Surg* 15A:961, 1990.

116. Newport ML, Shukla A: Electrophysiologic basis of dynamic extensor splinting, *J Hand Surg* 17A:272, 1992.

117. Newport ML, Williams CD: Biomechanical characteristics of extensor tendon suture techniques, *J Hand Surg* 17A:1117, 1992.

118. Nichols HM: Repair of extensor tendon insertions in the fingers, *J Bone Joint Surg* 33A:836, 1951.

119. Niechajev IA: Conservative and operative treatment of mallet finger, *Plast Reconstr Surg* 76:580, 1985.

120. Ogura T, Inoue H, Tanabe G: Anatomic and clinical studies of the extensor digitorum brevis manus, *J Hand Surg* 12A:100, 1987.

121. Ovesen OC, Jensen EK, Bertheussen KJ: Dislocation of extensor tendons of the hand caused by focal myoclonic epilepsy, *J Hand Surg* 12B:131, 1987.

122. Paley D, McMurty RY, Murray JF: Dorsal dislocation of the ulnar styloid and extensor carpi ulnaris tendon into the distal radioulnar joint: the empty sulcus sign, *J Hand Surg* 12A:1029, 1987.

123. Palmer AK, et al: The extensor retinaculum of the wrist: an anatomical and biomechanical study, *J Hand Surg* 10B:11, 1985.

124. Patel MR, Desai SS, Bassini-Lipson L: Conservative management of chronic mallet finger, *J Hand Surg* 11A:570, 1986.

125. Primiano GA: Conservative treatment of two cases of mallet thumb, *J Hand Surg* 11A:233, 1986.

126. Pulvertaft RG: Mallet finger: discussion. In Stack HG, Bolton H, editors: *The proceedings of the second hand club,* London, 1975, British Society for Surgery of the Hand.

127. Rayan GM: Recurrent dislocation of the extensor carpi ulnaris in athletes, *Am J Sports Med* 11:183, 1983.

128. Rayan GM, Mullins PT: Skin necrosis complicating mallet finger splinting and vascularity of the distal interphalangeal joint overlying skin, *J Hand Surg* 12A:549, 1987.

129. Reading G: Secrétan's syndrome: hard edema of the dorsum of the hand, *Plast Reconstr Surg* 65:182, 1980.

130. Redfern AB, Curtis RM, Shaw Wilgis EF: Experience with peritendinous fibrosis of the dorsum of the hand, *J Hand Surg* 7:380, 1982.

131. Regnard PJ, et al: Extensor tendon injuries: presentation of a series of ninety-nine cases, *Ann Chir Main* 4:55, 1985.

132. Riordan DC: Peritendinous fibrosis of the extensor tendons, *J Bone Joint Surg* 47A:632, 1965.

133. Riordan DC: In Dobyns JH, Chase RA, Amadio PC, editors: *Year book of hand surgery,* St Louis, 1988, Mosby.

134. Riordan DC, Stokes HM: Synovitis of the extensor of the finger associated with extensor digitorum brevis manus muscle: a case report, *Clin Orthop* 95:278, 1973.

135. Ritts GD, Wood MB, Engber WD: Nonoperative treatment of traumatic dislocations of the extensor digitorum tendons in patients without rheumatoid disorder, *J Hand Surg* 10A:714, 1985.

136. Rosenthal EA: Tenolysis, AAOS Sound Slide Program no 719, 1978, American Academy of Orthopaedic Surgeons.

137. Rosenthal EA: Extensor surface injuries at the proximal interphalangeal joint. In Bowers WH, editor: *The hand and upper limb,* vol 1, *The interphalangeal joints,* London, 1987, Churchill Livingstone.

138. Saferin WH: Secrétan's disease, *Plast Reconstr Surg* 58:703, 1976.

139. Saldana MJ, McGuire RA: Chronic painful subluxation of the metacarpal phalangeal joint extensor tendons, *J Hand Surg* 11A:420, 1986.

140. Salvi V: Technique for the buttonhole deformity, *Hand* 1:96, 1969.

141. Schenck RR: Variations of extensor tendons of the fingers, *J Bone Joint Surg* 46A:103, 1964.

142. Schneider LH: Complications in tendon injury and surgery, *Hand Clin* 2:361, 1986.

143. Schneider LH: Commentary, *J Hand Surg* 18A:608, 1993.

144. Schneider LH, Rosenstein RG: Restoration of extensor pollicis longus function by tendon transfer, *Plast Reconstr Surg* 71:533, 1983.

145. Schultz RJ, Furlong J II, Storace A: Detailed anatomy of the extensor mechanism of the proximal aspect of the finger, *J Hand Surg* 6:493, 1981.

146. Secretan H: Œdéma dur et hyperplasie traumatique du métacarpe dorsal, *Rev Med Suisse Romande* 21:409, 1901.

147. Shrewsbury MM: A systematic study of the oblique retinacular ligament of the human finger: its structure and function, *J Hand Surg* 2:194, 1977.

148. Shrewsbury MM, Johnson RK: Ligaments of the distal interphalangeal joint and the mallet position, *J Hand Surg* 5:214, 1980.

149. Siegel D, Gebhardt M, Jupiter JB: Spontaneous rupture of the extensor pollicis longus tendon, *J Hand Surg* 12A:1106, 1987.

150. Smillie IS: Mallet finger, *Br J Surg* 24:439, 1937.

151. Smith RJ: Balance and kinetics of the fingers under normal and pathological conditions, *Clin Orthop* 92:104, 1974.

152. Smith RJ: Factitious lymphedema of the hand, *J Bone Joint Surg* 57A:89, 1975.

153. Snow JW: Use of a retrograde tendon flap in repairing a severed extensor tendon in the PIP joint area, *Plast Reconstr Surg* 51:555, 1973.

154. Snow JW: A method for the reconstruction of the central slip of the extensor tendon of a finger, *Plast Reconstr Surg* 57:455, 1976.

155. Spinner M, Kaplan EB: Extensor carpi ulnaris: its relationship to the stability of the distal radioulnar joint, *Clin Orthop* 68:124, 1970.

156. Stack HG: Mallet finger, *Hand* 1:83, 1969.

157. Stack HG: Buttonhole deformity, *Hand* 3:152, 1971.

158. Stack HG: A modified splint for mallet finger, *J Hand Surg* 11B:263, 1986.

159. Stark HH: Troublesome fractures and dislocations of the hand, *Instruct Course Lect* 19:130, 1970.

160. Stark HH, Bayer JH, Wilson JN: Mallet finger, *J Bone Joint Surg* 44A:1061, 1962.

161. Steichen JB, Petersen DP: Junctura tendinum between extensor digitorum communis and extensor pollicis longus, *J Hand Surg* 9:674, 1984.

162. Stern PJ, Kastrup JJ: Complications and prognosis of treatment of mallet finger, *J Hand Surg* 13A:329, 1988.

163. Straus FH: Luxation of extensor tendons in the hand, *Ann Surg* III:135, 1940.

164. Stuart D: Duration of splinting after repair of extensor tendons in the hand: a clinical study, *J Bone Joint Surg* 47A:72, 1965.

165. Taleisnik J, et al: The extensor retinaculum of the wrist, *J Hand Surg* 9A:495, 1984.

166. Tang JB, Ryu J, Kish V: The triangular fibrocartilage complex: an important component of the pulley for the ulnar wrist extensor, *J Hand Surg* 23A:986, 1998.

167. Thompson JS, Littler JW, Upton J: The spiral oblique retinacular ligament (SORL), *J Hand Surg* 3:482, 1978.

168. Tubiana R: *The hand,* vol 1, Philadelphia, 1981, WB Saunders.

169. Tubiana R, Valentin P: The anatomy of the extensor apparatus of the fingers, *Surg Clin North Am* 44:897, 1964.

170. Vahey JW, Wegner DA, Hastings H: Effect of proximal phalangeal fracture deformity on extensor tendon function, *J Hand Surg* 23A:673, 1998.

171. Von Schroeder HP, Botte MJ: The extensor medii proprius and anomalous extensor tendons to the long finger, *J Hand Surg* 16A:1141, 1991.

172. Von Schroeder HP, Botte MJ: The functional significance of the long extensors and juncturae tendinum in finger extension, *J Hand Surg* 18A:641, 1993.

173. Von Schroeder HP, Botte MJ, Gellman H: Anatomy of the juncturae tendinum of the hand, *J Hand Surg* 15A:595, 1990.

174. Warren RA, Kay NRM, Norris SH: The microvascular anatomy of the distal digital extensor tendon, *J Hand Surg* 13B:161, 1988.

175. Watson HK, Ritland GD, Ghung EK: Post traumatic interosseous lumbrical adhesions, a cause of pain and disability in the hand, *J Bone Joint Surg* 56A:79, 1974.

176. Weinberg H, Stein HC, Wexler M: A new method of treatment for mallet finger, *Plast Reconstr Surg* 58:347, 1976.

177. Wehbé MA: Junctura anatomy, *J Hand Surg* 17A:1124, 1992.

178. Wehbé MA, Schneider LH: Mallet fractures, *J Bone Joint Surg* 66A:658, 1984.

179. Wheeldon FT: Recurrent dislocation of extensor tendons in the hand, *J Bone Joint Surg* 36B:612, 1954.

180. White GM, Weiland AJ: Symptomatic palmar tendon subluxation after surgical release for de Quervain's disease: a case report, *J Hand Surg* 9A:704, 1984.

181. Youm Y, Thambyrajah K, Flatt AE: Tendon excursion of wrist movers, *J Hand Surg* 9A:202, 1984.

182. Zancolli EA: *Structural and dynamic basis of hand surgery,* ed 2, Philadelphia, 1979, JB Lippincott.

183. Zbrodowski A: Vascularization and anatomical model of the meso-tendons of the extensor digitorum and extensor indicis muscles, *J Anat* 130:697, 1980.

184. Zbrodowski A, Gajisin S, Grodecki J: Vascularization of the tendons of the extensor pollicis longus, extensor carpi radialis longus and extensor carpi radialis brevis muscles, *J Anat* 135:235, 1982.

Chapter 31

CLINICAL MANAGEMENT OF EXTENSOR TENDON INJURIES

Roslyn B. Evans

Problems that accompany the complex extensor tendon injury or mismanagement of the simple extensor injury are well known to the hand specialist. Most functional problems to tendon systems are associated with the tendon's response to injury and repair, and despite decades of research on the subject, the problem of restrictive scar formation remains one of the most unpredictable factors contributing to postoperative morbidity.[110] Over the past two decades, the techniques of early controlled motions initially applied to flexor tendon management have been slowly incorporated into standard postoperative care for the extensor system. We have learned, with clinical studies and experience, that (1) extensor tendons in all zones (except zone I) tolerate controlled *active* motion, (2) gapping and rupture are rarely an issue in carefully applied postoperative regimens that control forces and excursion, (3) we probably can allow more digital joint motion with injury in zones V through VII than had previously been thought possible, (4) wrist position is critical to decreasing resistive forces from the flexor system and is a factor in true tendon excursion gained with digital motion, (5) we have probably been moving these tendons *actively* all along within the confines of their dynamic splints, and (6) early referral to therapy with attention to splint geometry and applied stress is a critical variable to outcomes.

The new studies on postoperative management technique* are basically just a verification of earlier studies† that demonstrate that these tendons tolerate and do better with early motion. The only difference in protocols is simply some variation in splint design and in attempts to incorporate an active component into postoperative regimens.* The principals of treatment are the same as with the last writing of this chapter: Initiate therapy by postoperative day 3, rest the tendon short (the repair site proximal to its normal resting position), and control excursion with a splint design that allows at least 5 mm (or more) of motion at the repair site.

A current literature search on tendon healing from the last 5 years of the twentieth century into the new millennium yields a number of articles on tissue engineering,† the effects of mechanical stress on tendon healing,‡ and some experimental work on the effects of electrical modalities and ultrasound (US)[163,165] that will be of interest to the serious student of tendon management.

The concept of tissue engineering is based on the manipulation of cellular and biochemical mediators that will positively affect protein synthesis and improve tissue remodeling. Woo et al.[219] have predicted that the combination of cell therapy with growth factor application via gene transfer will offer new opportunities to improve tendon and ligament healing. Even though these new biologic therapies show much promise for facilitating bone and fibrous tissue healing in the future, Buckwalter and Grodzinsky[27] remind us that none has been proven to offer the beneficial effects comparable to those produced by the loading of healing tissues. These same investigators point out that one of the most important concepts in orthopedics in this century is the understanding that loading accelerates healing of bone, fibrous tissue, and skeletal muscle,[27] and thus we can surmise that early controlled motion to the healing tendon remains our best current treatment for tendon repair.

*References 36, 96, 132, 191, 194, 195.
†References 3, 24, 33, 49-52, 55, 92, 109, 153, 171, 207.

*References 51, 54, 91, 111, 183, 191.
†References 11, 31, 32, 48, 83, 100, 102, 105, 127, 219.
‡References 10, 26, 27, 95, 101, 104, 114, 161, 186.

Most basic scientific and clinical research on tendon has been focused on the synovial flexor tendon, which has posed the most problems with restoration of functional gliding after repair. Clinicians have perhaps been too liberal in their application of some of these basic science studies to clinical application in the extensor system. Nonetheless, despite the histologic, metabolic, and nutritional differences between the two tendon systems[1] and within the different levels of the extensor system,[65] the fact is that all tendon is a type of dense connective tissue that functions to transmit muscle force to the skeleton, and to perform its work requirement, all tendon must glide relative to its surrounding tissues.

After injury to tendon at any level in either flexor or extensor system, the wound response and subsequent problems of maintaining tendon excursion are the same.[5] A blood clot forms, a nonspecific inflammatory response occurs, the clot becomes populated with fibroblasts and advancing capillary buds, and collagen and ground substance are produced that will heal the deficit but that also may limit the tendon's normal gliding ability.[5,103] Loss of fiber gliding of tendon and neighboring connective tissues with resulting functional deficits of strength, mobility, and coordination impede the tendon's ability to transmit muscle force to bone with mechanical efficiency.[93] Rehabilitation of a healing tendon is simply reestablishing its ability to glide and transmit force without creating gapping or rupture at the repair site.

The purpose of this chapter is to define the problems that follow injury to the different extensor tendon levels and to offer solutions to these problems based on current experimental and clinical research in the areas of tendon repair techniques, tendon healing, true tendon excursions, and the application of force to the healing extensor tendon. Anatomy and surgical management of the extensor tendon are elegantly described in Chapter 30.

The first section, General Considerations, is dedicated to a current literature review of basic science and clinical studies that support early motion for the healing tendon. Although this material may seem complex to the student or inexperienced therapist, it is essential information for any therapist or physician who assumes the responsibility of caring for an injured tendon. Treatment by protocol is appropriate only if there are no variables. Unfortunately, in the real clinical situation we are required to treat tendons with associated injury to bone, joint, nerve, and vessel in patients with associated metabolic, immunosuppressive, or personality problems, often referred by the nonspecialized surgeon, whose surgical technique and timing further complicate the case. This requires the therapist to be able to adjust treatment parameters based on a solid knowledge of wound healing, tendon repair tensile strength, and the effects of immobilization and early motion on the biochemistry and biomechanics of the healing tendon.

The questions once posed to me as a young therapist by Dr. Paul Brand—when, how often, how far, and how much

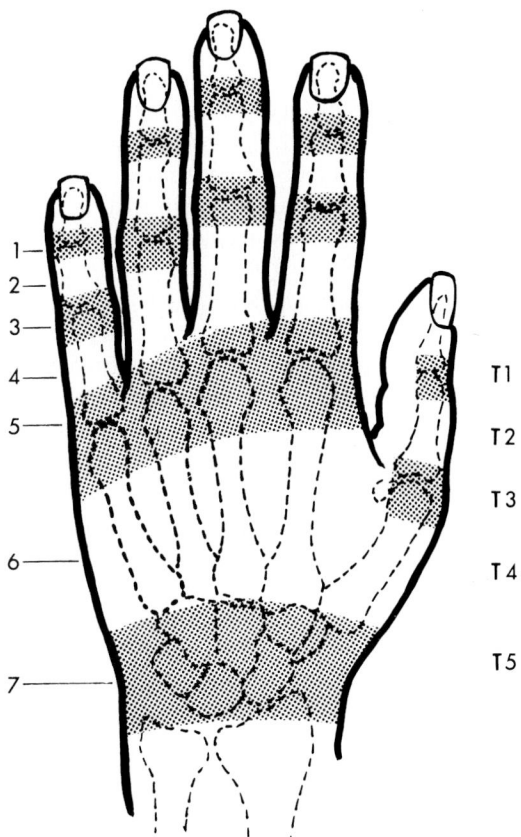

Fig. 31-1. Extensor tendon zones as defined by the Committee on Tendon Injuries for the International Federation of the Society for Surgery of the Hand. (From Kleinert HE, Schepel S, Gill T: *Surg Clin North Am* 61:267, 1981.)

when applying stress to healing connective tissue—are addressed in this chapter. These questions should be a part of the hand clinician's clinical decision-making process with each tendon case if quality of care is to be delivered.

The second section, Clinical Management of Extensor Tendon Injuries, is dedicated to management by level of injury. Within this section, general guidelines for treatment by immobilization, early passive motion, and early active motion are defined in terms of splinting and stress application.

GENERAL CONSIDERATIONS

Characteristics of the extensor tendon vary at each level, dictating variations in treatment. The committee on tendon injuries for the International Federation of the Society for Surgery of the Hand defines extensor tendon injury by delineating seven zones for the extrinsic finger extensors and five zones for the thumb extensors[113] (Fig. 31-1).

Schedules for immobilization, the application of controlled stress, and progressive resistive exercises depend on the tensile strength of the repair technique and the stage of wound healing as they relate to the physiologic and biomechanical differences of the tendon in its different zones or anatomic levels. Guidelines for treatment based on the biochemical and biomechanical requirements of this system must be altered to accommodate the circumstances of the individual patient and injury. The surgeon should apprise the therapist of the quality of the repair, the type of repair, alterations in tendon length, the integrity of the tissue, the status of surrounding tissues, and any additional pathologic conditions that might alter the amount of controlled stress that the healing tendon can accommodate. The patient should be evaluated in terms of anticipated compliance. This information will influence any variation from suggested timing of immobilization and mobilization schedules. Therapeutic management should be considered in terms of the biochemical and biomechanical events of wound healing and the effects that our management techniques have on these events. Management of the inflammatory state; timing of stress application; the judicious application of controlled stress; and the effects of active versus passive motion, splint geometry, the position of exercise, external load application with stress application, and the duration of exercise all influence either positively or negatively the healing and remodeling of this fibrous connective tissue.

Controlling inflammation

The importance of early repair,[75] nontraumatic surgery, prevention of infection, and edema control as a means of minimizing the inflammatory response after injury is well documented in the literature (see Chapters 12 and 22). The fibroblastic response and ultimately the amount of collagen that is produced at the wound site will be proportional to the local inflammatory response.[211] Complex dorsal injuries will be accompanied by significant edema and may require bulky, compressive dressings between therapy sessions for the first 5 to 7 days, but injuries with less tissue response can be lightly dressed and placed in early motion splints by 24 hours after surgery. The digits should be individually wrapped with a single layer of Coban to control digital edema for as long as any extra volume of fluid is present about the proximal interphalangeal (PIP) joint, a time that may exceed 8 to 12 weeks after repair for the digital injury. Twenty-four-hour elevation, motion for the uninvolved joints, and controlled motion for the involved joints will help control edema but require precise participation by the patient. Patient education, complete with explanations of anatomy, wound healing, and precautions, is a critical component of rehabilitation. Most people want to get well and will comply if they understand the importance of their actions. This requires time, patience, knowledge, and firm control on the part of the health care provider.

Management of the open or cleanly incised and sutured wound is defined in detail in Chapter 19. Careful cleansing, protection of the wound microenvironment, and proper dressing will speed epithelialization and enhance macrophage activity so that time in the inflammatory stage is

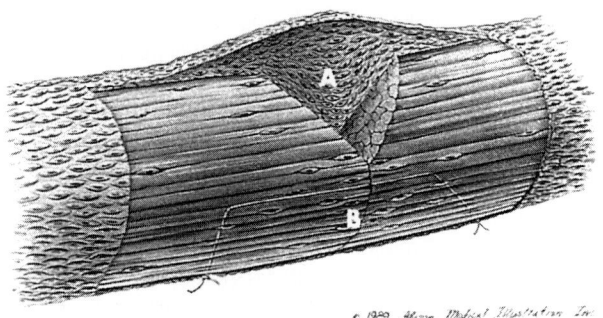

Fig. 31-2. Schematic drawing of a tendon repair. Area *A* represents the epitenon, where increased extrinsic healing is associated with gap formation. Area *B* represents the endotenon, where increased intrinsic tendon healing is associated with precise coadaptation at the repair site. (Redrawn from Gelberman RH, et al: *J Hand Surg* 10A:776, 1985.)

minimized. Exposed wounds tend to be more inflamed and necrotic than occluded wounds.[211] In the later stages, the dermis of exposed wounds is more fibroblastic, fibrotic, and scarred.[123,211]

The position of immobilization

The tendon repair site should be positioned by splinting proximal to its normal resting position during the first 3 weeks of healing to minimize stress at the repair site and thus decrease the chances for gap formation. Gap formation has been associated with increased adhesion formation and poorer clinical results[45,72,122,159,177] (Fig. 31-2). It has recently been demonstrated (in an experimental flexor tendon study) that gapping of more than 3 mm at a repair site does not increase the prevalence of adhesions or impair range of motion (ROM), but it does prevent the accrual of strength and stiffness that normally occurs with time.[77] Any gapping at the repair site could result in elongation of the tendon callus, which is particularly critical in zones I to IV, where the tendon moment arms and excursions are small.[22] Extensor lag in any zone at 3 or 4 weeks is much more difficult to overcome than extensor tightness and can be prevented by precise positions of immobilization.[57,196]

The effects of immobilization

Biomechanical and biochemical changes in immobilized connective tissue (tendon, ligament, and cartilage) have been studied primarily in the animal model in various joints.[71,139,156,214-216,218] We must interpret the information gained from these experimental studies with caution as we attempt to alter clinical treatment based on basic science studies in the nonhuman model and more often than not on synovial flexor tendon.

The negative effects of total immobilization during the inflammatory and fibroblastic stages of healing on tendon biochemistry are a loss of glycosaminoglycan concentration, loss of water, decreased fibronectin (FN) concentration, and decreased endoteneon healing.* Biomechanically, the immobilized tendon loses tensile strength in the first 2 weeks after repair,[63,84,136,204] and it loses gliding function by the first 10 days after repair.[70,71,169,217,218]

The effects of controlled stress

Many elegant studies have demonstrated the positive influence of stress on healing tendon, with documented improvement of tensile strength, improved gliding properties, increased repair-site DNA, and accelerated changes in peritendinous vessel density and configuration.† Motion may enhance the diffusion of synovial fluid within the tendon in synovial regions.[139,208] Stress-induced electrical potentials may increase the connective tissue healing potential.[9,15,195] Studies have demonstrated that early passive motion in a clinically relevant tendon-repair model increases FN concentration[6] and fibroblast chemotaxis[73] at the tendon repair site. These basic science studies are strengthened by clinical studies that demonstrate the benefit of controlled motion over immobilization for both the repaired flexor and extensor tendon.‡

The effect of timing

Time from injury to repair of intrasynovial flexor tendons, considered as an isolated variable, has been demonstrated to have a significant effect on the function of tendon in dogs. Tendons repaired immediately were significantly improved over tendons repaired at 7 or 21 days with respect to angular rotation and linear excursion, but there were no significant differences in total concentration of collagen at the sites of repair or in the levels of reducible Schiff-base cross-links in tendons from the three groups.[75]

Gelberman et al.[66,71] demonstrated in the canine model that immobilized tendons become bound by adhesions by the tenth day after repair but that tendons that are immediately mobilized have early restoration of gliding surface without adhesion ingrowth.

Preliminary experimental studies indicate that timing in relation to stress during the early inflammatory stage of wound healing is critical. An experimental study on chicken flexor tendons has demonstrated that tendons treated with controlled passive motion have significantly improved tensile strength by 5 days after repair compared with digits treated with immobilization.[84] The magnitude of difference in strength between the two groups increased with time. The authors of that study concluded that immediate constrained digital motion after repair allows progressive tendon healing without the intervening phase of tendon softening or weakening described in the classic study by Mason and Allen in 1941.[136]

*References 6, 7, 27, 63, 66, 74, 84, 114, 215, 216, 218.
†References 15, 63, 65, 67-71, 73, 74, 84, 95, 101, 104, 114, 178, 186, 205, 212, 216, 217.
‡References 4, 24, 33, 36, 37, 44, 49-55, 59, 91, 92, 96, 111, 112, 119, 132, 138, 153, 171, 183, 184, 188, 190, 191, 194, 195, 207.

In another study of early tensile properties of healing chicken flexor tendons, early controlled passive motion was found to improve healing efficiency.[64] Results of this study indicated that controlled-passive-motion tendons had significantly greater values for rupture load, stress, and energy absorbed when compared with immobilized tendons.

FN, which appears to be an important component of the early tendon repair process, has been localized in a clinically relevant tendon repair model. Fibroblast chemotaxis and adherence to the substrate in the days after injury and repair appear to be directly related to FN concentration.[74] Early passive motion has been correlated with an increased FN concentration in the tendon repair model of the previous study.[6] FN concentration in mobilized tendon was found to be twice that of immobilized tendon by 7 days after surgery. Iwuagwu and McGrouther[101] recently determined that load applied the first five days postoperative resulted in better orientation and fewer fibroblasts in repaired tendons.

We have no studies on the effect of immediate motion on the healing of the in vivo human tendon, and one must recognize that most of the experimental tendon work is performed on the synovial flexor tendon in animal models. However, these basic science studies offer some documentation that increased cellular activity and strengthening will occur with very early motion during the immediate postrepair period and emphasize the critical relationship between the application of force and timing. "Early motion" at 7 to 10 days after surgery may indeed not be early motion at all. By the end of the first week, the window of time may have been lost for the biochemical advantages of immediate motion, and by the tenth day after surgery, the immobilized tendon may be surrounded by dense adhesions.

The duration of exercise

The duration of the daily controlled-passive-motion interval has been determined to be a significant variable in a clinical study of repaired flexor tendons. A prospective multicenter clinical study of 51 patients with flexor tendon repair has determined that greater durations of daily controlled passive motion after flexor tendon repair resulted in increased active interphalangeal (IP) joint motion at a mean time of 6 months after surgery.[76] Two groups of patients treated with continuous passive motion (CPM) and traditional early passive motion were compared in terms of IP motion. The authors concluded that the duration of the daily controlled motion interval is a significant variable in postrepair flexor tendon excursion.[76]

In a related study, designed to determine the effects of frequency and duration of controlled passive motion on the healing flexor tendon after primary repair, adult mongrel dogs were studied as two groups based on the frequency of passive motion.[192] Results indicated that gliding function in both groups was similar, but tensile properties, as represented by linear slope, ultimate load, and energy absorption, were significantly improved in the higher-frequency group.

The authors concluded that the frequency of controlled passive motion in postoperative tendon management protocols is a significant factor in accelerating the healing response after tendon repair, and higher-frequency controlled passive motion has a beneficial effect.[192]

These studies offer some proof that "more is better" in the early healing phase. However, in my clinical experience, the very aggressive patient who exercises excessively may develop inflammation and synovitis within the synovial areas of both flexor[56] and extensor systems if tendon gliding is limited by adhesions that would increase friction or if the tendon is still swollen from increased metabolic activity associated with healing. Patient compliance is a significant and often difficult-to-control variable with these postoperative regimens. Dobbe et al.[42] have developed a device to record duration of exercise that is attached to the postoperative splints. This concept may prove to have clinical relevance by improving patient compliance.

Extensor tendon excursion

Tendon excursion in the early healing phases of tendon rehabilitation should be limited to a range that is great enough to provide the stress necessary to stimulate biochemical changes at the repair site and to provide some proximal migration of the repair site to control the collagen bonds as they are formed in the peritendinous region, yet small enough that it does not create gapping or rupture at the repair site. Researchers have raised the question of actual tendon excursion with passive motion.[88,89,134,138,143] Some tendon researchers now believe that a component of controlled active motion may be necessary to create some proximal migration of a tendon repair site and that passive motion may only cause the repair site to fold or buckle instead of gliding proximally. This is the rationale for controlled early active motion as opposed to controlled passive motion in postoperative management of the repaired tendon. References to tendon excursion in the next section with cadaveric measurement, measurement by radians, and intraoperative measurement all refer to the relationship of passive joint motion to tendon excursion.

The tendon migration necessary to maintain functional glide and stimulate cellular activity may be in the range of 3 to 5 mm. Duran and Houser[44] recommended this passive excursion range for the flexor tendons in the digital sheath and thought that 3 to 5 mm is sufficient to prevent dense adhesions. Gelberman et al.,[72] in an earlier study, suggested that 3 to 4 mm of passive excursion is necessary to stimulate the intrinsic repair process without creating significant repair-site deformation with flexor tendons. More recent studies have indicated that 1.7 mm of tendon excursion is sufficient to prevent adhesion formation in canine tendon and that additional excursion provides little added benefit.[179] Early active and passive motion allowing an estimated 5 mm of excursion has proven to be successful with extensor tendon repairs in zones V, VI, VII, T-IV, and T-V.[49,50,55,58]

Table 31-1. Excursions for digital extensor tendons as reported by Bunnell

	Total	Wrist	MP	PIP	DIP
Extensor digitorum communis					
Index	54 mm	38 mm	15 mm	2 mm	0
Long	55 mm	41 mm	16 mm	3 mm	0
Ring	55 mm	39 mm	11 mm	3 mm	0
Small	35 mm	20 mm	12 mm	2 mm	0
	Total	Wrist	CMC	MP	IP
Extensor pollicis longus					
Thumb	58 mm	33 mm	7 mm	6 mm	8 mm

From Boyes JH: *Bunnell's surgery of the hand,* Philadelphia, 1970, JB Lippincott.
CMC, Carpometacarpal; *DIP,* distal interphalangeal; *MP,* metacarpophalangeal; *PIP,* proximal interphalangeal.

and approximately 4 mm of active excursion with extensor repair in the digital zones III and IV.[51,57]

To safely apply stress to a healing tendon, the therapist must understand tendon excursion as it relates to joint motion and understand tendon tensile strengths as they relate to suture techniques and healing schedules. This requires either a general working knowledge of tendon excursions as cited in the literature or the ability to calculate individual tendon excursions with Brand's technique of using the radian concept and corresponding joint moment arms.[20]

Literature review of extensor tendon excursions

Reported extensor tendon excursions are variable but within a consistent range.* Differences may exist between the individual extensor digitorum communis (EDC) tendons, as well as from person to person. Variables also are found in the method of study, as well as the size of the hand or joint being examined.[20,22] Cadaveric studies are limited by the absence of normal biochemistry and muscle tone.

Bunnell's cadaver studies of excursions[19] provide detailed information and closely correlate with those described by Brand.[20] Bunnell assigned values for individual finger tendons at each metacarpophalangeal (MP), PIP, and distal interphalangeal (DIP) joint, with the wrist in a neutral position[19] (Table 31-1). The excursions become smaller as the joint size (and thus the tendon moment arm) decreases.

Excursions for the digital extensor in zones III and IV are small but may be slightly more than those reported by Bunnell, who calculated the EDC excursion to be 2 mm for the index finger, 3 mm for the long finger, 3 mm for the ring finger, and 2 mm for the small finger.[19] In other cadaveric studies, Tubiana[199] cites 8 mm, Valentine[202] cites 7 to 8 mm, Zancolli[220] cites 6 mm, and DeVoll and Saldana[40] cite up to 5 mm of tendon excursion at this level.

*References 19, 20, 107, 187, 199, 202.

An et al.[8] calculated tendon excursion and the moment arm of cadaver index finger joints during rotation and found that excursion and joint displacement were not always linear. Excursion of the extensor digitorum at the PIP level with a mean motion of 89.5 degrees was 5.58 mm. Micks and Reswick[141] determined that the extensor moment arm at the PIP joint is not constant and increases with the position of flexion.

Elliot and McGrouther[46] investigated the mathematic relationship between extensor tendon excursion and joint motion in seven cadaver hands and found this relationship to be linear for all joints in all five rays of the hand. They found that excursion of the middle slip over the proximal phalanx is in effect the excursion of the extensor digitorum that accompanies PIP joint movement. They calculate excursion per 10 degrees for each joint with all other joints immobile and all surrounding structures released. The mean motion per 10 degrees was 0.8 mm for the index, long, and ring PIP joints and 0.6 mm for the small PIP joint. This would translate to 2.4 mm of excursion for the index, long, and ring fingers; 1.8 mm of excursion for the small finger; and 1.8 mm of excursion for the small finger per 30 degrees of PIP motion. Their findings are contrary to those of An et al.[8,141]

Calculating excursions with radians and moment arms

Brand[20] describes a constant relationship between joint motion and tendon excursion at both the MP and PIP joints. A fairly constant extensor tendon moment arm (the perpendicular distance from the joint axis to the extensor tendon) exists at both joint levels. Although not precisely constant, the extensor tendon moment arm does not change dramatically with joint motion.[20] Brand calculated the mean moment arm for the index MP joint to be 10 mm in cadaver studies and for the middle finger PIP joint to be 7.5 mm.[20] The moment arm will vary as joint size varies, but these figures give us a working base to calculate approximate extensor tendon excursion.

Tendon excursion can be calculated geometrically with radians.[20] A radian is the angle that is created when the radius laid along the circumference of a circle is joined by a line at each end to the center of the circle (Fig. 31-3). This angle always equals 57.29 degrees (one radian). This segment of the circumference of the circle is always equal to the radius of the circle when the working angle is 57.29 degrees.

To calculate extensor tendon excursion at the MP joint level, consider the head of the metacarpal in terms of a circle (Fig. 31-4, *A*). The moment arm of the extensor tendon (or the perpendicular distance between the MP joint axis, or center of the circle, and the extensor tendon) will be equal to the excursion of the extensor tendon if the MP joint is moved through one radian, or 57.29 degrees. Using Brand's figure of 10 mm for an average extensor tendon moment arm in the index finger,[20] MP joint motion of 57.29 degrees would yield 10 mm of extensor tendon excursion (see Fig. 31-4, *A*). To obtain the 5 mm of excursion suggested by Duran and

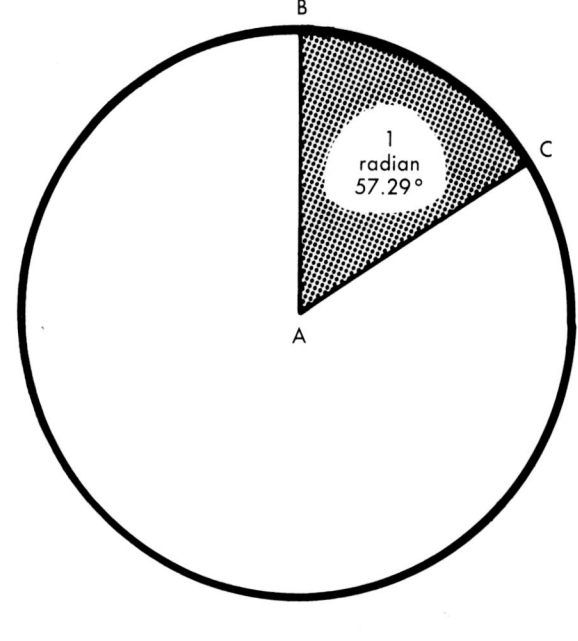

A = Axis

AB = Radius

AB = BC

BAC = 57.29°

Fig. 31-3. A radian is the angle that is created when the radius laid along the circumference of a circle is joined by a line at each end to the center or axis of the circle. Angle *BAC* equals 1 radian, or 57.29 degrees.[20,21]

Houser[44] and Gelberman et al.[72] to minimize extrinsic adhesions, the joint would need to be moved through 0.5 radian, or 28.64 degrees of rotation[55] (Fig. 31-4, *B*).

Because joint size varies, the therapist must consider that it is the constant relationship of tendon excursion to angular rotation and the length of the moment arm that is important. A smaller joint with a smaller moment arm will produce less tendon excursion with the same joint motion. For example, if the MP joint of the small finger has a moment arm of 7.5 mm, angular change of 0.5 radian, or 28.64 degrees, will produce 3.75 mm of glide. To obtain the necessary excursion to maintain tendon glide in the smaller ulnar joints or in smaller hands, one must move these joints through more than 0.5 radian of rotation.[55]

Calculation by simple equation of safe parameters for controlled motion

Evans and Burkhalter[55] proposed a simple equation for determining excursion of the extrinsic finger extensors in zones V, VI, and VII in the initial biomechanical study supporting early passive motion in these zones: Joint motion divided by tendon excursion for that particular joint is equal

INDEX
E D C Excursion calculated at M P level by radians

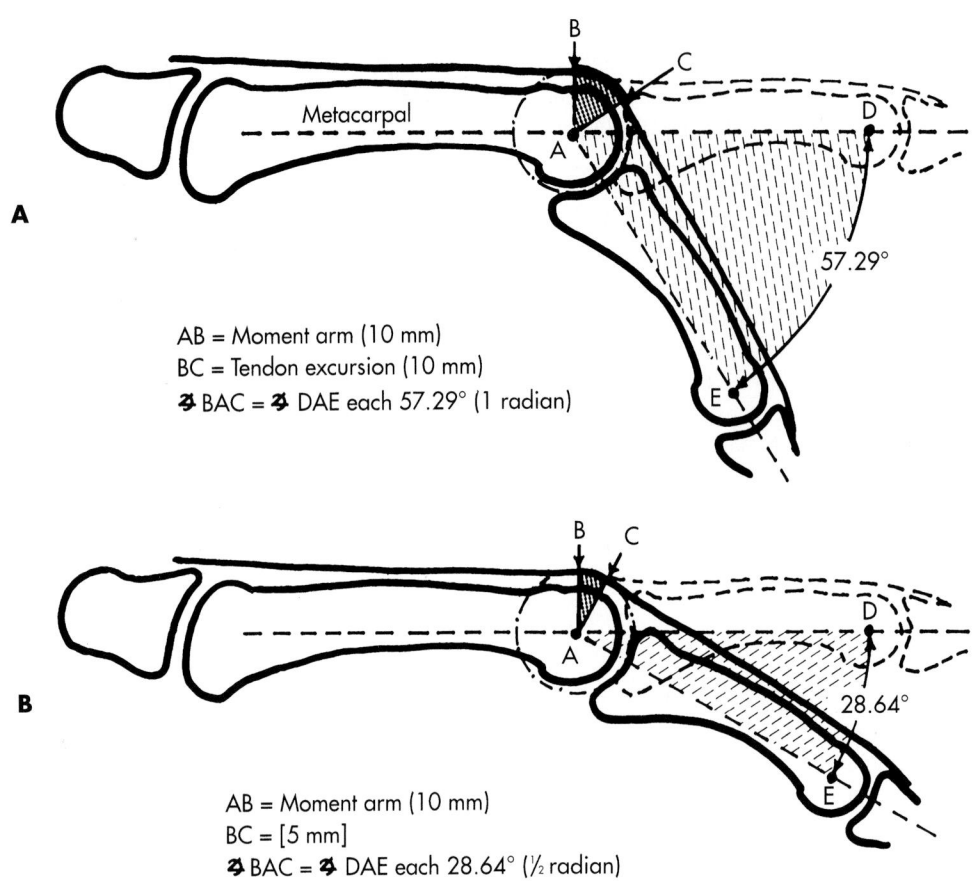

AB = Moment arm (10 mm)
BC = Tendon excursion (10 mm)
∢ BAC = ∢ DAE each 57.29° (1 radian)

AB = Moment arm (10 mm)
BC = [5 mm]
∢ BAC = ∢ DAE each 28.64° (½ radian)

Fig. 31-4. A, If the head of the metacarpal is considered in terms of a circle, the moment arm of the extensor tendon is equal to the radius of that circle. If metacarpophalangeal joint motion equals 57.29 degrees, or 1 radian, extensor tendon excursion is equal to the moment arm, or *AB = BC.* If the moment arm equals 10 mm, angular change of 57.29 degrees effects 10 mm of extensor tendon excursion.[55] **B,** Angular change of 0.5 radian, 28.3 degrees, effects the 5 mm of extensor tendon excursion recommended for the early passive motion program.[55] (**A,** From Evans RB, Burkhalter WE: *J Hand Surg* 11:774, 1986.)

to the number of degrees of motion required to effect 1 mm of tendon glide.

Joint motion (degrees)/Tendon excursion (mm) = degrees/mm

Application of this equation is contingent on total joint motion and total tendon excursion for each individual finger at the MP level and the amount of excursion considered safe and effective for providing controlled stress to the healing tendon.

The suggested equation is applied with these average values for MP joint motion: 85 degrees, index; 88 degrees, long; 90 degrees, ring; and 92 degrees, small finger.[55] Excursions used were those described by Bunnell,[19] because he measured each finger separately (see Table 31-1). Controlled stress allowing 5 mm of passive glide, as

suggested by Duran and Houser[44] and substantiated by intraoperative measurements in the pilot study,[55] was determined to be a safe and effective excursion (Table 31-2).

Extensor tendon excursions were investigated in eight fresh cadaveric limbs.[143] The authors found that if the wrist is extended more than 21 degrees, the extensor tendon glides with little or no tension in zones V and VI throughout a full simulated grip to full passive extension. On the basis of this cadaveric study, the authors recommend that up to 6.4 mm of tendon can be safely debrided in these zones and that full grip can be permitted postoperatively if the wrist is splinted in more than 45 degrees of extension. Their study emphasizes the importance of wrist position to tendon excursion, but their conclusions based on cadaveric study should be applied to the clinical situation with caution.

Table 31-2. Calculation for extensor digitorum communis excursion at the metacarpophalangeal level

---

Index $\dfrac{85 \text{ degrees}}{15 \text{ mm}}$ = 5.66 degrees per mm × 5 mm = 28.3 degrees

Long $\dfrac{88 \text{ degrees}}{16 \text{ mm}}$ = 5.5 degrees per mm × 5 mm = 27.5 degrees

Ring $\dfrac{90 \text{ degrees}}{11 \text{ mm}}$ = 8.18 degrees per mm × 5 mm = 40.9 degrees

Small $\dfrac{92 \text{ degrees}}{12 \text{ mm}}$ = 7.66 degrees per mm × 5 mm = 38.33 degrees

---

From Evans RB, Burkhalter WE: *J Hand Surg* 11A:774, 1986.

Intraoperative measurement

Evans and Burkhalter[55] measured extensor tendon excursion intraoperatively and found by gross measurement that 30 degrees of MP motion effected 5 mm of extensor glide in zones V, VI, and VII, supporting our calculations by radians with the predescribed equation. This more limited amount of motion has worked well in my 20 years of clinical experience with early motion of extensor tendons, but others[24,143] believe that full digital flexion should be considered safe within the confines of splints that hold the wrist in extension and fingers controlled in dynamic extension traction.

Cadaveric studies and mathematic equations do not consider biology. We have no study to date that describes extensor tendon excursion after repair in vivo to give us accurate measurements for passive or active motion, but intraoperative measurement may be more accurate than cadaveric study.

Excursion of the central slip measured in radians

The same calculation techniques can be applied to the PIP joint and central slip excursion and are used to establish safe parameters for immediate early active motion for central slip repairs (discussed later).[57] Biomechanically, the excursion of the extensor tendon at the level of the PIP joint is proportional to angular changes of the joint.[20] The mean moment arm for the extensor tendon of the long-finger PIP joint has been determined to be 7.5 mm.[20] Therefore PIP joint motion of 57.29 degrees, one radian, would effect 7.5 mm of excursion in the freely gliding tendon. One half (0.5) radian, or 28.65 degrees, would effect 3.75 mm of excursion[57] (Fig. 31-5).

There is some disagreement in the literature regarding the extensor moment arm at the PIP joint. Micks and Reswick[141] determined that the extensor moment arm at the PIP joint is not constant and increases with flexion. Brand[20] found the moment arm of the extensor to be fairly constant at this level, unchanging with motion. An et al.[8] found that excursion and joint displacement were not always linear at the PIP joint, but Elliot and McGrouther[46] found that relationship to be linear.

The protocol for early motion for the extensor zones III, IV, V, VI, and VII[51,55,57,58] requires only 30 to 40 degrees of joint motion at the respective MP or PIP joints; therefore the changes in the extensor moment arms are small and unlikely to be significant enough to alter the calculation of excursion.

Excursion of the extensor pollicis longus

Excursions for the extensor pollicis longus (EPL) tendon vary in the literature from 25 to 60 mm.[19,107,187] The simple angular arrangement of the flexion/extension axis at the MP level of the fingers does not exist for the EPL in zones T-IV and T-V. Calculating excursion mathematically is complicated by the oblique course that the tendon takes at Lister's tubercle, by the moments of adduction and external rotation at the carpometacarpal (CMC) level, and by the fact that alterations in thumb position alter the moment arms at each joint.[20,106] Evans and Burkhalter[55] measured EPL excursion intraoperatively to determine the amount of joint motion necessary to create 5 mm of glide for the early motion pilot study and found that with the wrist neutral and the thumb MP joint extended, 60 degrees of IP joint motion effected 5 mm of tendon excursion at Lister's tubercle.

True tendon excursion

The question of actual tendon excursion with passive motion has been raised.[88,134,138] Experimentally (intact fresh frozen cadaver specimens), passive motion in flexor tendons has been demonstrated to be almost half that of theoretically predicted values under conditions of low tendon tension[89]; investigators have shown that actual tendon excursion will be equal to the predicted tendon excursions of earlier studies[44,201] only when more than 300 g of tension is applied to the repair site.[89] Similar studies correlating in vivo tendon tension and tendon excursion for the extensor system have not been performed, but cadaver studies suggest that the tendons may buckle only in zones V, VI, and VII with digital joint motion from flexion to extension.[143]

The concept of using immediate active motion after tendon repair is simply an attempt to ensure that the repair site does glide proximally. Some clinicians now think that an as yet undefined degree of active tension at a repair site may be necessary to create a proximal migration of the healing tendon and that passive motion may only cause the tendon to buckle, fold, or roll up at the repair site.[134,143] The use of immediate active motion as a means of restricting limiting adhesions and improving tendon gliding is neither new[81,82,115,120] nor widely accepted in clinical practice, but it is now the subject of renewed interest in tendon management programs.* Stronger suture techniques that are designed for active motion have been developed for flexor

---

*References 37, 49, 51, 52, 54, 57, 59, 91, 92, 111, 119, 183, 184, 189-191, 194.

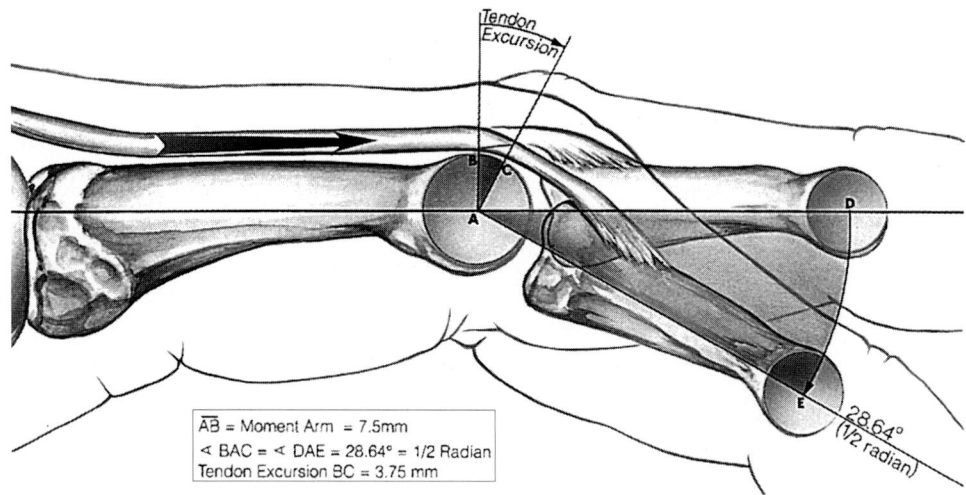

Fig. 31-5. Excursion of the central slip (zone III) as calculated by radians. *AB* = the moment arm of the central slip. Angle *BAC* = 0.5 radian, or 28.64 degrees. If the proximal interphalangeal joint is moved through 0.5 radian, the central slip excursion will equal one half the moment arm, or 3.75 mm. The average moment arm of the middle finger central slip is 7.5 mm as measured by Brand and Hollister.[20] (From Evans RB, Thompson DE: *J Hand Ther* Oct-Dec:193, 1992.)

tendon repairs* and for extensor system repairs.[90,131] Favorable clinical results with active motion programs have been reported for both the flexor system† and the extensor system.[51,52,54,91,111,183,191]

Tendons rehabilitated in dynamic extension splints intended for passive motion programs in reality probably move actively throughout the early healing phases, so the discussion of "active versus passive" tendon excursion is most likely a moot point for extensors in zones V, VI, and VII when rehabilitated in such splints. Newport and Shukla[150] performed electromyographic (EMG) studies on a group of normal volunteers to determine the level of activity present in the EDC within the confines of a dynamic extension splint. Their study validates what most therapists observe clinically—that most patients move their repaired and splinted extensor tendons actively within the dynamic extension splint and within the exercise regimen that is intended to provide active flexion and passive extension. They found that if the MP joints were splinted in 0 degrees of extension, the EDC tendons were active within the dynamic extension splint; however, if the MP joints were splinted in modest flexion (20 degrees), the extensor tendons were quiescent during the active flexion exercise.[150] The authors of that study use this information to recommend that the MP joints be splinted in 20 degrees of flexion to prevent active motion of the repaired tendon. I would use their information to support dynamic splinting of the MP joints at 0 degrees of extension to facilitate some physiologic active

motion at the repair site. I believe that the MP joints should be splinted at 0 degrees, not only to prevent extensor lag but also to create some active tension and true proximal migration of the repair site.

The application of force

Force application is the sum of muscle contraction and viscoelastic drag of the tissues. Viscoelastic drag is the sum of the antagonistic muscle tension, resistance from the periarticular support systems, edema, and adhesions.[22] Resistance from Coban wraps or bandaging also must be considered as an increased force application in early active motion programs. A safety margin must be established in which the force application (or the stress applied to the tendon) is less than the tensile strength of the tendon with all early motion programs.

Force application at the repair site

Internal tendon forces as they relate to various joint angles and applied external loads are defined for the flexor and extensor tendons in two scientific articles on early active motion for both tendon systems.[57,58] The results of these biomechanical analyses are presented in a series of mathematic models that negate resistance from the antagonistic muscle-tendon group and any other drag and apply a known external force. The force analysis of the EDC with the wrist in an extended position and no external load is calculated so that conservative estimates of tendon forces can be made (Fig. 31-6). With the digital joints in a neutral position, tensions on the EDC are zero, but as the digits are extended, the forces rise to 1200 g. These forces would drop

*References 25, 118, 140, 175, 180, 190.
†References 14, 37, 53, 59, 74, 119, 181, 184, 190.

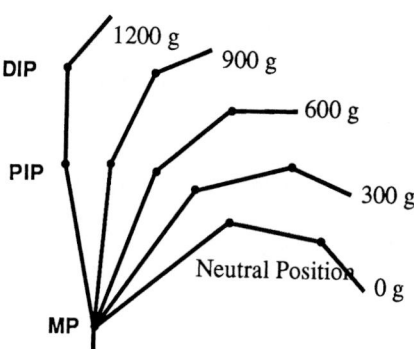

Fig. 31-6. This schematic demonstrates the force analysis of the extensor digitorum communis (EDC) in various joint angles with the wrist extended. Note that with the metacarpophalangeal *(MP)*, proximal interphalangeal *(PIP)*, and distal interphalangeal *(DIP)* joints in a neutral position, no force (0 g) is transmitted to the EDC, but that as extension angles for these joints increase, the forces are elevated to as much as 1200 g. With the wrist flexed, these forces are greatly diminished. (From Evans RB, Thompson DE: *J Hand Ther* 6:270, 1993.)

dramatically if the wrist were placed in 20 degrees of flexion (the position recommended for early active controlled motion) because resistance from the flexor tendons would be reduced by wrist position.[57,58,174] The force applied to the extensor tendon at both MP and PIP joint levels with active extension of 30 degrees of flexion to 0 degrees of extension (at either joint) has been calculated mathematically to be approximately 300 g if the wrist is positioned at 20 degrees of flexion.[57,58]

Tensile strength of extensor tendon repairs

The tensile strength of freshly sutured tendon depends on the strength of the suture material, the suture method, the balance between the strands and knot, the number of strands, the size of the tendon, and the addition of a circumferential suture to a core suture.* Several studies[90,149,151,221] have investigated the mechanical strengths of tendon repair techniques and suture materials for the extensor system. Newport and Williams[151] reported on the biomechanical characteristics of extensor tendon suture at 2-mm gapping and at failure. The mattress suture gapped 2 mm at 488 g and failed at 840 g; figure-of-eight gapped at 587 g and failed at 696 g; Kessler gapped at 1353 g and failed at 1830 g; and Bunnell gapped at 1425 g and failed at 1985 g.[151]

Most studies on repair tensile strengths report the strength in newtons (N), but as therapists, we usually calculate the forces of dynamic splints, torque ROM, and the force of

motion in grams. Evans and Thompson[58] reviewed a large number of studies on the strengths of the various repairs and translated newtons into grams to assist therapists as they assess the strength of the particular repair they are treating (1 kg = 9.8 N, or 1 g = 0.01 N; conversion of newtons to grams: N divided by 9.8 × 1000 = g). Comparisons of these studies are difficult because of the many variables (subject, material, technique of repair, and method of testing) studied.

The load at which a tendon gaps is the number that we must recognize, particularly with the controlled active motion programs. Gap formation has been associated with increased adhesion formation and poorer clinical results.* Although most surgeons believe that gapping above 1 to 3 mm is incompatible with a good result,[45,122,159,177] investigators have demonstrated in an in vivo study that gaps of up to 10 mm in a repaired flexor digitorum profundus (FDP) are compatible with a good functional ROM when passive motion programs are used.[181] Gelberman et al.[77] have recently demonstrated that a gap at a repair site of more than 3 mm does not increase the prevalence of adhesions or impair ROM but does prevent the accrual of strength and stiffness that normally occurs with time.

Adjusting the equation

The equations for force application and tensile strength just described must be adjusted to consider the increased resistance from postsurgical edema, stiff joints, and bandaging and to allow for a possible drop in tensile strength in the repaired tendon. The estimated tensile strength of the repair may decrease as much as 25% to 50% by postoperative days 5 to 15[1] in the unstressed tendon[36,201]; however, tendon subjected to immediate or very early controlled motion may not experience this drop in tensile strength.[6,63,74,84,114] The estimated force application to the repair site with the early active motion protocols may need to be doubled to account for the resistance from drag.[21]

The effect of complex injury

There is a relationship between the amount of tissue damage and biologic response that is a basic phenomenon of wound healing.[211] Increased inflammation associated with severe injury increases the work requirement of the macrophage, and the number of macrophage cells necessary to meet the metabolic demands of the injury determines the number of fibroblasts that are signaled into the wound for repair. Collagen deposition can be expected to be proportional to the number of fibroblasts, or collagen-producing factories, present in the wound bed.[211]

Rothkopf et al.[169] studied mechanical trauma and immobilization in the canine flexor tendon model to study adhesion formation associated with complex injury. These researchers defined *complex tendon injury* as one associated

*References 78, 121, 130, 197, 201, 206, 219.

*References 45, 71, 72, 122, 159, 177.

with crush injury, concomitant nerve injury, or tendon injury treated with immobilization. Their experimental model demonstrated significant decreases in tendon excursions and an increase in work requirement to effect tendon excursion in the complex injury. This experimental model in the animal flexor tendon may have implication for the human flexor or extensor tendon.

We all have observed clinically that the more complex injury can be expected to cause more complications associated with increased fibroblastic response and that immobilization of the complex injury will add to those complications. Many authors have endorsed the use of early motion with the complex injury,[26,29,55,57,210] but there are few clinical reports in the literature on early motion for the complex tendon injury, and most clinical results refer to clean lacerations. This area deserves more study.

CLINICAL MANAGEMENT OF EXTENSOR TENDON INJURIES
Zones I and II

A lesion of the terminal extensor tendon results in a flexion deformity of the DIP joint, commonly referred to as the *mallet* or *baseball* finger. Treatment and prognosis of the mallet finger depend on associated tissue injury and age of the lesion before treatment.[98,210] These injuries may be open or closed, with or without associated fracture or fracture dislocation. In many cases, conservative treatment with splint immobilization is sufficient to restore tendon continuity.[98,210] However, open injury, associated fracture, or chronic deformity may require direct repair or K-wire fixation[43,210] (see also Chapter 30).

Most authors recommend approximately 6 to 8 weeks of continuous extension splinting for the DIP joint only with both conservative and operative treatment.[43,210] Dagum and Mahoney[38] have recommended that the wrist be splinted with a simple wrist control splint in addition to the distal joint splint to prevent gapping in zone I; however, in my clinical experience this does not seem to be necessary. Katzman et al.,[108] in a cadaveric study of gap formation in mallet fingers, determined that joint motion proximal to the DIP joint and retraction of the intrinsics did not cause a tendon gap in a finger with mallet lesion, supporting the concept that one joint splinting is sufficient for these injuries. Honner[87] recommends some limited active flexion at 4 weeks, with continuous splinting between exercise periods for an additional 4 weeks. The DIP joint can be immobilized with commercially available Stack splints, aluminum-padded splints, or molded thermoplastic splints (Fig. 31-7). Splint application is most often volar to the level of the PIP joint. A wide plastic tape placed across the dorsal aspect of the DIP joint will act as a counterpressure and will hold the DIP joint in complete extension. I prefer to use Transpore tape by 3M with a small square of moleskin lining the portion of the tape that is directly over the DIP joint. Dorsal immobilization permits more freedom of the PIP joint and

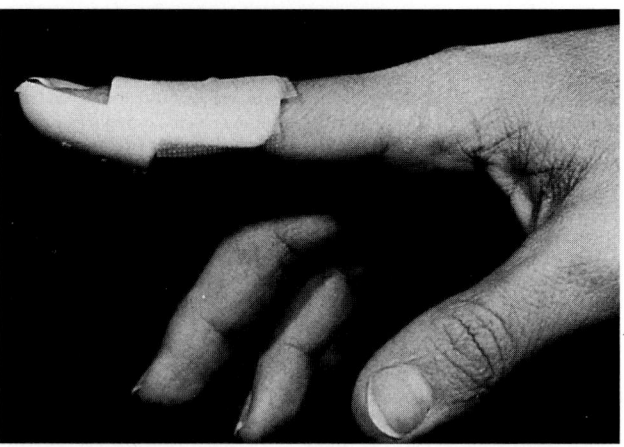

Fig. 31-7. A stack splint for zone I extensor tendon injury immobilizes the distal joint in slight hyperextension. (From Evans RB: *Hand Clin* 2:157, 1986.)

allows the fingertip its sensory function; however, in my hands, dorsal splinting (Fig. 31-8) has not been as effective as volar splinting.

Splint position and skin integrity should be monitored carefully. The distal joint should be immobilized at 0 degrees of extension or slight hyperextension.[43,162] Extreme hyperextension jeopardizes circulation to the dorsal skin by stretching the volar vasculature, which provides nutrition to the area distal to the termination of the dorsal vessels, and may create skin necrosis.[129] Rayan and Mullins,[162] in a study of skin necrosis complications associated with mallet finger splinting, suggested a position of hyperextension less than the angle that causes skin blanching, a precursor of skin necrosis. They determined the average total passive hyperextension of the distal joint to be 28.3 degrees and found that circulation to the dorsal skin was compromised when the distal joint was splinted at more than 50% of its total hyperextension. Splint immobilization that allows even slight flexion will result in extensor lag because the tendon callus will heal in an elongated position.[99]

Skin maceration is a problem with these injuries. It is difficult for patients to keep the affected hand dry for 6 to 8 weeks, and most patients find it irksome to be so limited by a one-joint injury. They must be instructed in proper splint application, skin care, technique for maintaining the DIP joint in extension during cleansing (I usually teach them to use the ipsilateral thumb to hold the DIP joint in hyperextension while cleansing with the contralateral hand), splinting, and splint adjustment to make sure that the distal joint always rests in complete extension. The splints can be lined with moleskin to absorb perspiration, and patients should be instructed to change the lining if it becomes damp. The DIP joint must be held in hyperextension while the patient changes the splint lining. I provide two distal joint splints; one can be worn while showering. The splint must be adjusted as edema decreases to provide a precise fit.

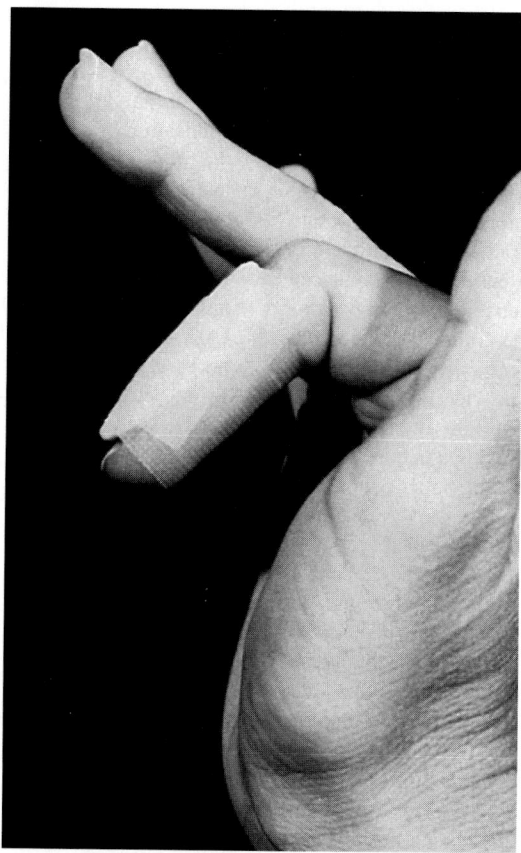

Fig. 31-8. Dorsal immobilization of the distal joint permits more freedom of the proximal interphalangeal joint and allows the fingertip its sensory function. (From Evans RB: *Hand Clin* 2:157, 1986.)

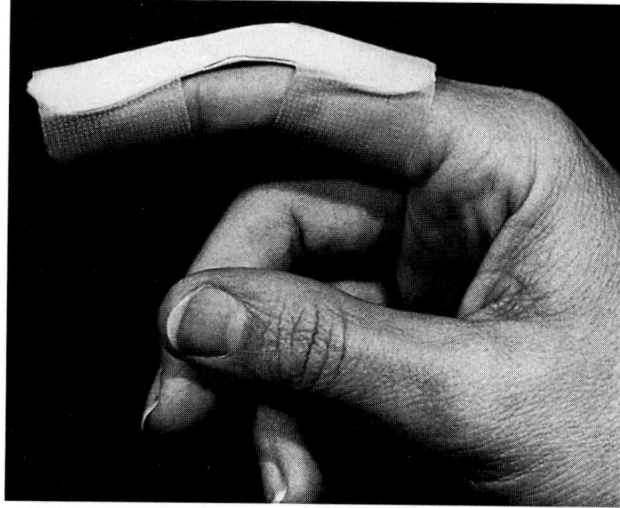

Fig. 31-9. The proximal interphalangeal joint should be splinted in slight flexion in the mallet finger that develops a swan-neck posture to advance the lateral bands. (From Evans RB: *Hand Clin* 2:157, 1986.)

During the immobilization phase, the patient should be seen weekly for wound care when necessary, for adjustment of the fit of the splint, and for maintenance of motion in the unaffected joints. The distal joint must be held in extension continuously during splint adjustments to prevent attenuation of the healing tendon.

If the PIP joint develops a posture of slight hyperextension, the PIP joint should be splinted at 30 to 45 degrees of flexion while the DIP joint is held at complete extension (Fig. 31-9). This position will advance the lateral bands and may assist in closer approximation of the torn extensor tendon at the DIP joint.[167] Doyle[43] describes a treatment for the mallet finger with plaster casting of the PIP joint at 60 degrees and the DIP joint in slight hyperextension. He points out that in most cases, PIP immobilization is not necessary for these injuries but that casting both the PIP and DIP joints is a workable solution for patients who are unreliable or who are unable to understand or perform the correct application of a splint.[43] Bunnell explained the rationale for the 60-degree flexion angle of the PIP. In this position, the lateral bands are advanced a distance of 3 mm.[19] This much flexion could result in flexor contracture of the PIP joint, and clinically 30 to 45 degrees of PIP flexion has worked well for me. Flexion

contracture of the PIP joint has not been a problem with PIP flexion splinting at these angles in my practice. Splinting the PIP joint may not be necessary beyond the first few weeks, after which the long splint can be exchanged for a shorter one-joint splint for the DIP.

After 6 weeks of uninterrupted splinting in extension, very gentle active flexion exercises are initiated. The opposing FDP is a powerful musculotendinous unit and will easily overpower the more fragile terminal extensor tendon. Brand and Hollister[20] calculated the work capacity of the extensors to be less than one third of that of the flexors; therefore flexion increments should be obtained gradually with the initial emphasis on active extension. Because the moment arm of the extensor tendon at this level is small, so also is extensor tendon excursion.[19,20,107,187]

Instructions to the patient should be very specific. During the first week of mobilization, no more than 20 to 25 degrees of active flexion of the distal joint should be allowed. Exercise duration is empirically prescribed at 10 to 20 repetitions every couple of hours. During the second week, if no lag has developed, distal joint flexion to 35 degrees may be allowed. The overly ambitious patient will benefit from a template exercise splint with specific angles of motion preset to prevent overstretching of the terminal tendon (Fig. 31-10). If the distal joint is tight in extension, the oblique retinacular ligaments may need to be stretched by manual immobilization of the PIP joint at 0 degrees of extension while the DIP joint is actively or passively flexed.[43]

If an extensor lag develops, resplinting is indicated and exercises are delayed for a few weeks.[43,210] Splinting between exercise sessions is recommended during the first 2 weeks of mobilization (a total of 8 to 10 weeks after injury), and night splinting should be continued for an additional 4 weeks after intermittent daytime splinting is discontinued.

Early active or passive motion is not accepted practice for the tendon at this level, where excursions are small and where the tendon tissue becomes stiffer and more cartilaginous.[20,65] However, because of inconsistent clinical results with these injuries and problems of loss of both flexion and extension, earlier motion techniques are now being investigated. Nakamura and Nanjyo[146] published their experience with surgical intervention with a wire implant and K-wire pinning for 3 weeks in 15 patients with fresh mallet fingers (average time from injury to surgery, 19.4 days) without associated fractures. The K-wire is removed at 3 weeks, and distal joint motion in gradually increased increments is allowed. The wire in the tendon stumps is removed at 5 weeks. Nakamura and Nanjyo[146] report improved ROM and fewer complications with this technique, which also reduces immobilization time.

Prehension and coordination activities should supplement ROM exercise. Desensitization of a painful fingertip may be necessary with crush injuries or nailbed injuries before the patient will incorporate the digit into prehension activities (see Chapter 35). Exercise may gradually proceed to resistive grasp and pinch activities. Flexion angles should be increased only if complete extension is maintained, and full flexion should not be attempted before 3 months.

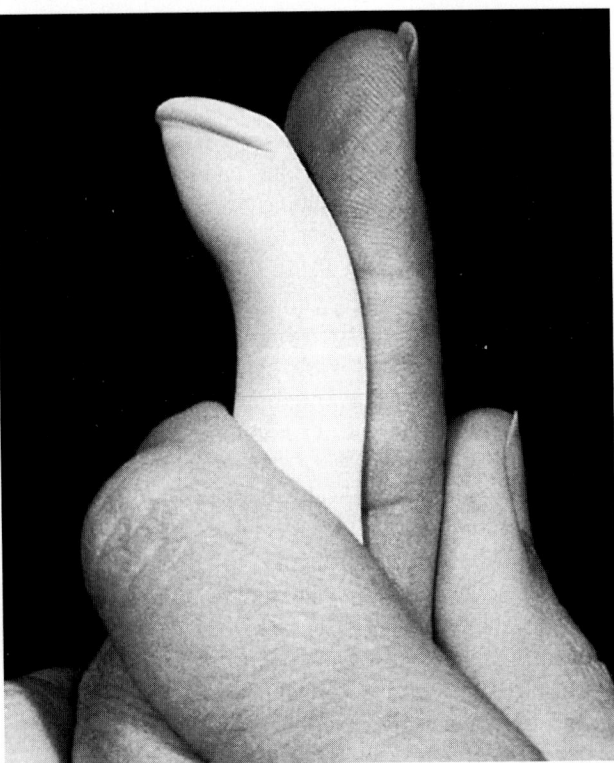

Fig. 31-10. A template exercise splint will set limits for graded flexion and prevent overstretching of the terminal extensor tendon in the overly ambitious patient. (From Evans RB: *Hand Clin* 2:157, 1986.)

Therapy for the zone I and II extensor tendon injury is primarily educational. If the patient understands the nature of the injury and the rationale for treatment, he or she should be able to perform most of the therapy independently.

Zones III and IV

Extensor injuries in zones III and IV may result in a boutonnière deformity (see Chapter 30). The natural progression of the zone III extensor injury is well defined in the literature.* Untreated, the lacerated middle band will retract, allowing the lateral bands to carry the full force of the extrinsic extensor tendon. The lateral bands migrate palmarward, act as flexors of the PIP joint, and with an increase in effort to extend the PIP joint, actually hyperextend the DIP joint. With time, the tendon and the retinacular tissues tighten and accommodate to the change in joint posture, tightening to a point where they resist even passive correction of the deformity. The relationship of the zone III tendon over the PIP joint and the zone IV tendon over the proximal phalanx to the lateral bands does differ, creating different tensions in these two zones as the distal joint is flexed[57,93,220]; however, for all practical purposes, I treat both zones with the same splinting and motion techniques and hereafter refer to this injury as zone III or central slip.

Traditional management of the zone III tendon injury

The literature contains conflicting opinions concerning direct repair and immobilization with K-wire versus conservative management of the open zone III injury. However, most authors recommend conservative treatment of the acute closed injury at this level with uninterrupted immobilization of the PIP joint at 0 degrees for 6 weeks.[43,176,210] Open and repaired injuries are mobilized as early as 3 to 4 weeks by some authors, with protective splinting between exercise sessions and graded increments in ROM allowed between 3 and 6 weeks[49,97,185]; however, most authors recommend continuous splinting for 6 weeks before motion is initiated.[43,64] Traditional management of this injury often calls for immobilization of the more proximal joints in extension as well as the PIP joint; however, I have never immobilized more than the digit (PIP and DIP joints) unless the zone IV injury is very proximal, approaching zone V, and have not found this to be a problem clinically. With either operative or nonoperative treatment, it is critical that the splint position of the PIP joint be at absolute 0 degrees; otherwise, there will be some tension at the repair site, possibly creating some gapping, which may result in tendon healing in an elongated position.[51,57]

The PIP joint can be immobilized with a volar static thermoplastic splint with a counterpressure directly over the PIP joint applied with Transpore tape (Fig. 31-11) or with a circumferential finger cast (Fig. 31-12, *A*). The finger cast is always the treatment of choice with the closed injury,

*References 19, 43, 64, 116, 124, 168, 200, 210, 220.

especially if the PIP joint is tight in flexion or if the digit is swollen. The circumferential pressure will decrease edema, and the pressures that the cast imposes will serve to elongate the tight volar structures.[62] The finger cast is preferable when noncompliance is suspected.

Finger casting is an art and requires some practice before this treatment is imposed on a patient (see Chapter 114). Casting material can be applied directly to the skin with the closed injury and encouraged to remain there with an application of benzoin to the skin before casting. With the open wound, a sterile contact layer and tube gauze dressing are applied first. If the wound area or skin is fragile, a small square of closed-cell adhesive foam can be applied directly over the PIP joint to disperse pressure before the fast-setting plaster is applied. Circulation should be monitored during cast application and for at least 20 minutes before the patient leaves the clinic. Casted digits that are cool, slightly

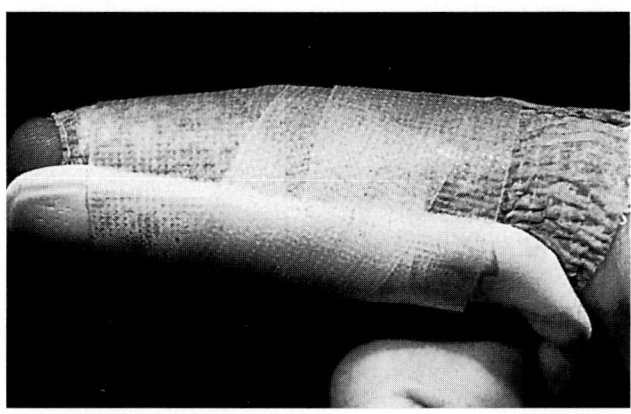

Fig. 31-11. The involved digit is splinted in a volar static thermoplastic splint, immobilizing the proximal and distal interphalangeal joints at absolute 0 degrees. Dorsal pressure is applied over both joints with 1-inch Transpore tape (Velcro straps will not maintain as much pressure).

discolored, or throbbing should be recast before the patient leaves the clinic. The patient should be instructed that if the finger swells or becomes painful at home, the cast should be removed by soaking the casted digit in warm water until the material softens and can be slipped off the digit. A digital static extension splint supplied by the therapist as a backup should then be applied until the next therapy appointment. Finger casts must be removed and replaced during the first 7 to 10 days for wound care and as edema decreases to ensure a proper fit.

If the lateral bands require no surgical repair, the distal joint is left free to prevent distal joint tightness, loss of extensibility of the oblique retinacular ligaments, and lateral band adherence.[220] Distal joint motion should be encouraged. If the lateral bands are repaired, the DIP joint also can be immobilized for 4 to 6 weeks[43]; however, this can result in significant loss of distal joint motion, and I would start lateral band gliding exercises by the third week.

Active distal joint flexion, combined with static splinting of the PIP joint in extension and the DIP joint in flexion, or intermittent traction into flexion provides improved extensibility to the oblique retinacular ligaments for the digit with limited distal joint flexion (Fig. 31-12, *B*).

Mobilization schedules for treatment by immobilization vary from 3 to 6 weeks for the open and repaired injury to 5 to 6 weeks for the closed boutonnière. Proponents of this approach recommend progressive gentle flexion exercises between weeks 3 and 6 with protective extension splinting between exercise sessions.[43,210] PIP joint flexion exercises for both the open and repaired central slip or the closed boutonnière should be initiated with caution because the immobilized extensor tendon will have little tensile strength and most likely will be adherent over the proximal phalanx, limiting gliding and elevating tension at the level of repair. The first week of mobilization (regardless of whether motion

A 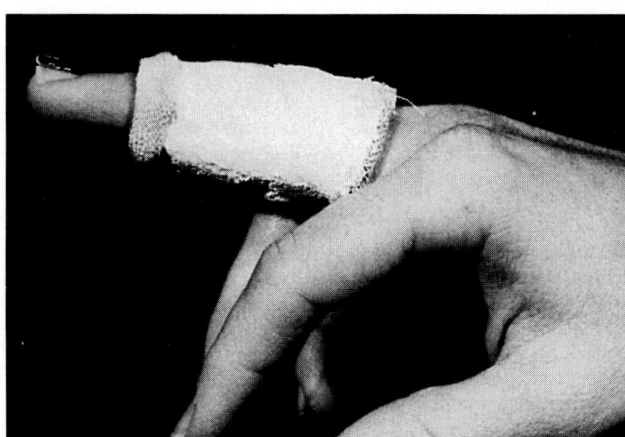 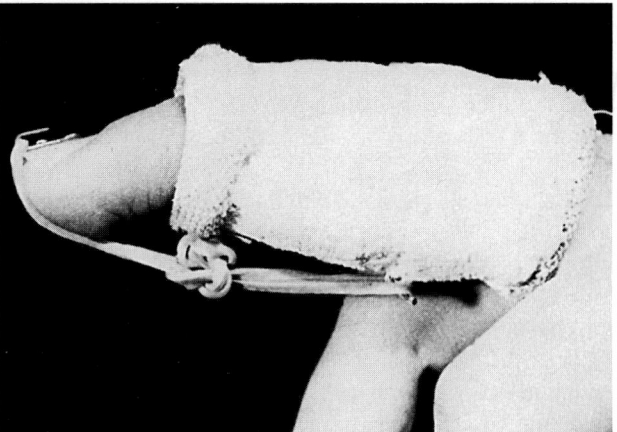 **B**

Fig. 31-12. A, A cylinder plaster cast immobilizes the proximal interphalangeal joint at 0 degrees of extension. The circumferential pressure of the cast is effective in reducing digital edema. **B,** Gentle intermittent traction can be incorporated into the digital cast to stretch the distal joint periarticular structures if the oblique retinacular ligaments are tight. (From Evans RB: *Hand Clin* 2:157, 1986.)

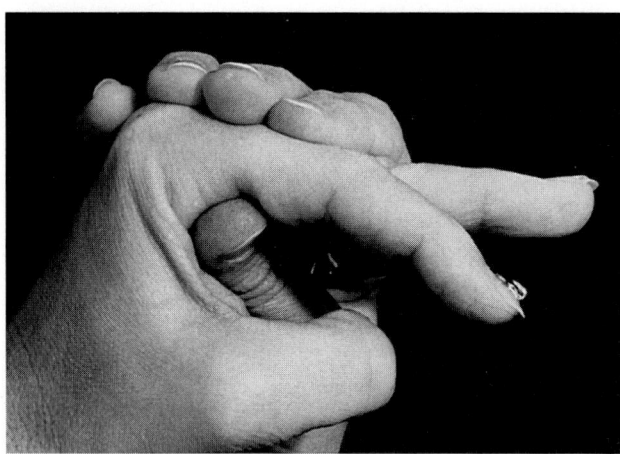

Fig. 31-13. The proximal phalanx of the affected digit is held manually in flexion as the patient relaxes the proximal interphalangeal (PIP) joint into mild flexion and then actively lifts the joint to full extension. With the metacarpophalangeal (MP) joint flexed, PIP joint extension is primarily affected through the interossei,[125,126] possibly with some contribution from the lumbrical,[202] but with little contribution from the extensor digitorum communis.[182] Tension on the central tendon is decreased with MP flexion because of sagittal band distal migration.[220] PIP exercise should also be performed with the MP held at 0 degrees of extension to direct increased forces to the central slip.

is started at week 3, 4, 5, or 6) should emphasize active PIP joint extension with an exercise position of the MP joint at 0 degrees of extension and PIP flexion to no more than 30 degrees. If no lag develops, motion can progress to 40 to 50 degrees by the second week of motion, thereafter adding 20 to 30 degrees per week. Forceful flexion exercises are not appropriate, and development of lag should be addressed with increased extension splinting and decreased increments of flexion (Fig. 31-13).

If there is no extensor lag, flexor forces can be directed to the stiff PIP joint by (1) applying a forearm-based dynamic splint that blocks the MP joint in extension and applies a light traction (less than 250 g) to the midphalanx level, (2) applying a hand-based exercise splint that blocks the MP joint in extension and encourages PIP joint flexion in the hook fist position, or (3) splinting the distal joint, manually supporting the proximal phalanx, and actively flexing the PIP joint (Fig. 31-14).

Digital swelling can be controlled with Coban wraps. Scars can be softened with massage and silicone gel sheeting (SGS) or elastomer molds applied with pressure. Exercises should emphasize blocking of individual joints and grasping activity. Osteoarthritic fingers with inflammation and incomplete hook fist position should not engage in repetitive grasping activity that requires acute composite flexion because this may encourage triggering in the flexor system.[56]

The chronic or fixed boutonnière deformity will require splinting and exercise to regain passive motion for both IP joints before surgery.[176] Treatment for the chronic boutonnière is well described by a number of authors.[43,97,167,176]

Immediate active short arc motion for the repaired central slip

The acutely repaired central slip injury treated traditionally with 4 to 6 weeks of immobilization is often compromised by problems of extensor tendon lag, insufficient extensor tendon excursion, joint stiffness, and loss of flexion. Newport et al.,[148] in a report of long-term results of extensor tendon repair, found that extensor tendon injuries within the digit treated with immobilization had high percentages of fair and poor results as compared with those of more proximal injuries; they also found that injuries in zones III and IV had higher percentages of resultant extensor lag (35%) and loss of flexion (71%). They note that there is little margin for adhesion formation or shortening of the extensor tendon on the dorsum of the digit if a reasonable result is to be obtained.[148] Verdan[204] observed that extensor injury over the proximal phalanx produced the worst results; Lovett and McCalla[128] found the highest percentages of extensor lag in zones III and IV.

The following factors may negatively influence the final outcome of the acutely repaired and immobilized central slip injury: (1) the broad tendon-bone interface in zone IV, (2) resting of the tendon at less than absolute 0 degrees of extension during immobilization, and (3) the effects of stress deprivation on the connective tissue (tendon, cartilage, ligament) of the PIP joint.[51,57]

The broad tendon-bone interface in zone IV. Brand et al.[22] have noted that there is no other area in the human body with a ratio of tendon to bone as unfavorable as over the proximal phalanx. This adverse ratio has been credited as the primary cause of surgical failures after attempts to free the dorsal expansion.[22] The broad tendon-bone interface, along with the intimacy of the periosteum and the extensor tendon and the complex gliding requirements of the extensor system in zones III and IV, results in functional problems associated with adhesions.[168]

Zone III injuries tend to be complex, which compounds the problems of scar formation. In a clinical series of open and repaired central slip injuries of 64 digits that I treated from 1985 to 1992, 79.6% were associated with injury to adjacent soft tissue, the PIP joint, or the distal joint.[51] Other clinicians have reported similar findings.[148,168,210] We all have observed clinically, and investigators have demonstrated experimentally[169] that the complex injury treated with immobilization can be expected to produce problems associated with increased fibroblastic response.

Considering these factors, we may hypothesize that a major problem in mobilization of the zone III extensor tendon injury is tendon-to-bone adherence in zone IV. The immobilized repair in zone III devoid of the benefits of greater intrinsic healing and strengthening associated with early motion may attenuate or gap when motion is initiated at 4 to 6 weeks because its proximal segment in zone IV is nongliding (Fig. 31-15). This increased resistance or drag from adhesion in zone IV elevates the extensor tension in

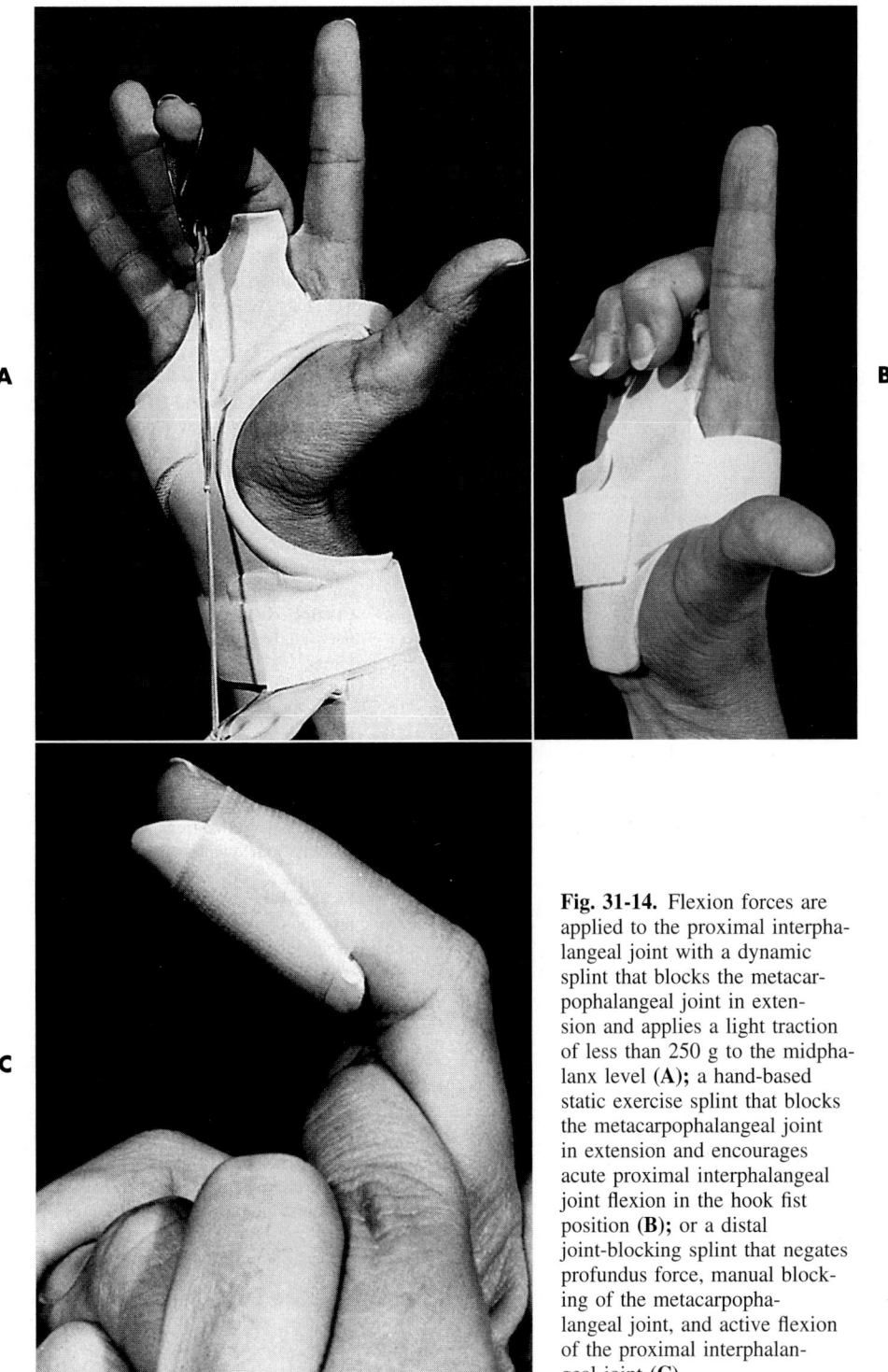

Fig. 31-14. Flexion forces are applied to the proximal interphalangeal joint with a dynamic splint that blocks the metacarpophalangeal joint in extension and applies a light traction of less than 250 g to the midphalanx level (**A**); a hand-based static exercise splint that blocks the metacarpophalangeal joint in extension and encourages acute proximal interphalangeal joint flexion in the hook fist position (**B**); or a distal joint-blocking splint that negates profundus force, manual blocking of the metacarpophalangeal joint, and active flexion of the proximal interphalangeal joint (**C**).

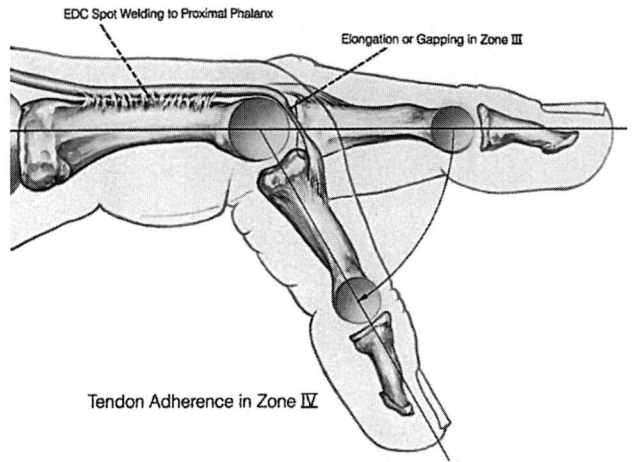

EDC Spot Welding to Proximal Phalanx

Elongation or Gapping in Zone III

Tendon Adherence in Zone IV

Fig. 31-15. Schematic drawing illustrating the problem of tendon-to-bone adhesions after injury to the dorsal digital extensor mechanism. The broad tendon-bone interface in zone IV and the intimacy of periosteum and extensor tendon yield functional gliding problems in the zone III injury. The zone III portion of the tendon (the repaired central slip) may gap or attenuate in late mobilization programs because its more proximal segment is adherent and nongliding. The increased resistance in zone IV increases force application in zone III and may exceed the tensile strength of the repair. *EDC,* Extensor digitorum communis. (From Evans RB, Thompson DE: *J Hand Ther* 5:190, 1992.)

zone III, which may exceed the tensile strength of the repair. This can be observed clinically in the immobilized central slip that begins to lose motion in extension as flexion is gained with late mobilization programs.

Resting the tendon at functional length during immobilization. The anatomy of the PIP joint favors flexion.[18] The normal resting position of the PIP joint is between 30 and 40 degrees of flexion.[22] In this position, the central slip, with a larger moment arm, and the lateral bands, with a smaller moment arm, are at equal tension.[22] An edematous PIP joint will posture in 30 to 40 degrees because in this position the joint will more comfortably accommodate the increased volume from edema. A schematic drawing on the effects of edema on the dorsal PIP joint and overlying skin can help us visualize the effect of effusion or edema under the central slip[20] (Fig. 31-16). The increase in volume could increase the moment arm of the central slip and thus tension on the repair.[20,22]

A common problem with these injuries is incorrect splinting that allows some flexion of the PIP joint during the healing phase, resulting in extensor lag. Alumafoam splints with adhesive tape proximal and distal to the PIP joint encourage swelling and allow the joint to rest in flexion; finger casts that are not checked frequently allow the PIP to rest in flexion as edema decreases. In my experience, unmonitored splinting is more often than not ineffective.

The splint position necessary to prevent gap formation and attenuation of the repair is absolute 0 degrees of extension. This position brings the repair site proximal to its

normal resting position and reduces repair-site tension (see Fig. 31-11).

Connective tissue stress deprivation. Total immobilization of 4 to 6 weeks can impose injury on uninjured cartilage and ligament. Although biochemical and biomechanical changes in immobilized connective tissue have been studied primarily in the animal model in various joints,[213,214] results of these studies have influenced our thinking on the subject of stress application to healing connective tissue in the human. The information gained from these experimental studies must be interpreted with caution as we attempt to alter clinical treatment based on basic science studies in the nonhuman model.

The biochemical and biomechanical effects of stress deprivation versus controlled motion for tendon are briefly reviewed in the first segment of this chapter. Similar changes take place in immobilized ligament and cartilage.[213] Stress deprivation for ligament results in alterations in collagen cross-linking synthesis and degradation, as well as in loss of water and proteoglycan content.[3,7,9,12] Nonligamentous injuries treated with immobilization can produce ligament-length problems, and there is evidence that ligament structures can shorten, limiting joint motion.[9,209] Investigators have demonstrated that ligaments under no tension are associated with the contractile protein actin and will actually shorten.[18,39] Authors have postulated that immobilization may decrease the normal stress-generated electrical potentials in the dense connective tissue of ligament and that this could be interpreted by the fibroblast as a signal to degrade the older collagen molecules and synthesize newer, shorter collagen molecules, which will shorten the ligament structure.[9]

The relationship between motion and cartilage metabolism cannot be ignored. Joint motion is important to maintaining articular cartilage homeostasis. The substances required by the chondrocytes for normal metabolism are derived from synovial fluid.[28,145] The transport of these nutrients through cartilage occurs by diffusion, convection, or both, and the combination of motion and joint loading is essential to nutrient transport by convection.[28,80,133,145] Joint immobilization then would decrease nutrient transport to cartilage. Prolonged immobilization will result in decreased mechanical properties, disorganized ultrastructure, and biochemical alterations similar to those noted in ligament.[3,7] Experimentally, CPM has been found to produce a tissue that histochemically and morphologically resembles hyaline cartilage in healing rabbit cartilage.[172,173] Therefore immobilization at the PIP joint level, where cartilage is the thinnest of any joint in the body, should be avoided if possible.

Anatomic considerations for the short arc motion program. The exercise position for the short arc motion (SAM) program is 30 degrees of wrist flexion, 0 degrees of MP joint extension, and PIP joint motion from 0 degrees of extension to 30 degrees of flexion and active return to 0 degrees of extension. Only the digital joints (PIP and DIP) of the affected digits are splinted between the active component exercise, allowing complete motion of the wrist and MP joints. The distal joint is flexed to 25 to 30 degrees while the PIP joint is held at 0 degrees if the lateral bands are repaired and to full flexion while the PIP is at 0 degrees if the lateral bands are not repaired.

The elastic components of the surrounding soft tissue, as well as the active muscle forces, must be considered when calculating active force and resistance to a repaired tendon in the healing phase. Tubiana[198] makes the point that the coordination of motions in the hand depends on active and passive factors of the more proximal joints. The passive factors include the restraining action of the ligaments and muscular viscoelasticity, and the active factors include the dynamic balance between antagonistic muscles.[198] Therefore we must consider the effect of joint positional changes and contributions from the surrounding soft tissues when reducing or increasing the work requirement of the EDC.

Anatomic influences for the zone III extensor tendon have been analyzed in detail in the support paper for SAM[57] and are only briefly reviewed here.

The action of the middle or central extensor tendon, which inserts on the base of the middle phalanx, functions in some regard to extend all three phalanges. It extends the middle phalanx on which it inserts except when the MP joint is in hyperextension, it contributes to extension of the proximal phalanx when the PIP joint is flexed, and it contributes to distal joint extension through the coordinating action of the oblique retinacular ligaments.[198,203]

Wrist position influences tension in the extrinsic tendons because of the viscoelasticity of the antagonist muscle-tendon unit.[20,35,174,198] Passive tension is minimal when the muscle is short and increases as the muscle lengthens.[174] The movements of wrist flexion and finger extension are synergistic; finger extension is effectively increased as the wrist flexes.[203,220] The position of wrist flexion reduces the passive tension of the digital extrinsic flexors.[21] Although this position may increase passive tension in the extensor system as the muscle-tendon unit lengthens, the actual force required of the extensor communis to extend the digital joints is reduced by the reduction of viscoelastic flexor forces.[174] The action of the interossei muscles with the wrist flexed may further reduce work requirement of the digital extensor mechanism in active extension of the IP joints. Close and Kidd[34] have concluded that the interossei do contract with IP joint extension even when no resistance is applied if (1) all fingers are extended simultaneously or (2) the finger is extended with the wrist flexed.

Active wrist extension is synergistic with finger flexion. With the digital splint taped in place between exercise sessions, unrestricted motion can take place in the wrist and MP joint. As the wrist extends, the MP joint will flex because of the viscoelastic pull of the flexors. The sagittal bands glide distally with MP flexion, actually reducing tension on the central slip.[220] Tubiana[198] states that the movement of

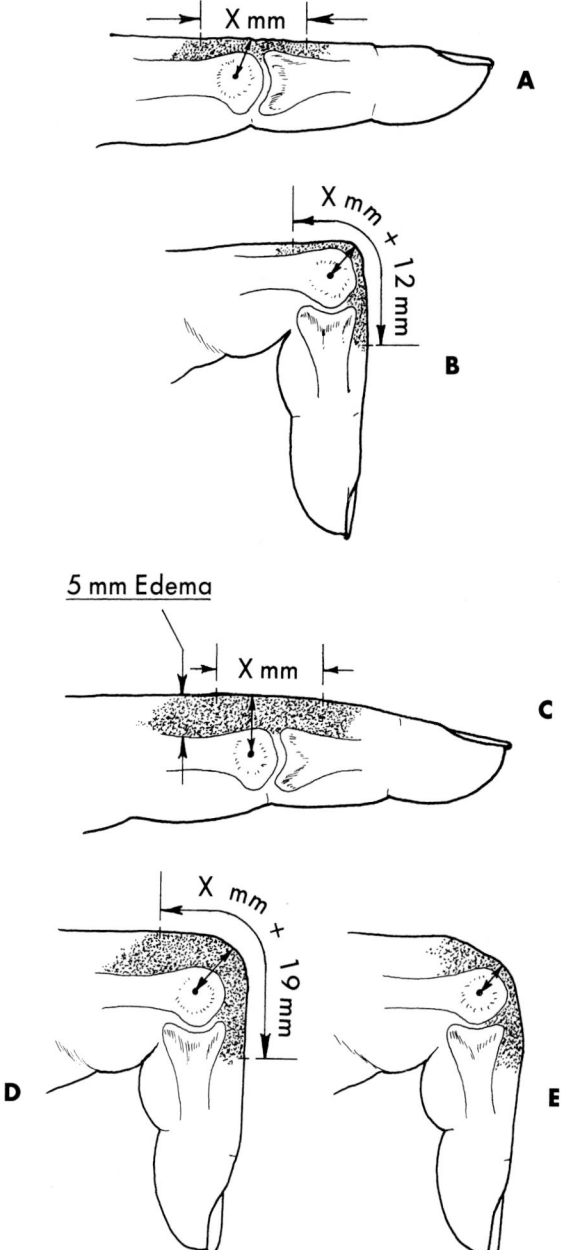

Fig. 31-16. Schematic drawing by Brand illustrating the effects of a 5-mm increase in the diameter of a finger from edema and its effect on the dorsal skin. **A** and **B,** Dorsal skin requires 12 mm of lengthening for 90 degrees of flexion. **C** and **D,** With 5 mm thickness of edema, skin requires 19 mm of lengthening for 90 degrees of flexion. **E,** With continuing torque, slowly applied, the edema fluid moves around, permitting the skin to cross closer to the joint axis requiring less stretch. This illustration will help the reader visualize the effects of protein and cellular edema that may collect under the central slip, which would increase the moment arm of the tendon and possibly contribute to attenuation of the repair or a resting posture of slight flexion. (From Brand PW: *Clinical mechanics of the hand,* St Louis, 1985, Mosby.)

the phalanges can be independent of wrist position through the action of the interossei.

Based on these anatomic considerations, the recommended position for the wrist with the SAM protocol is 30 degrees of flexion during PIP exercise. This position reduces flexor resistance, facilitates interossei function to extend the PIP, and thus reduces the work requirement of the EDC with active extension of the PIP joint.

MP joint positional changes from complete extension to complete flexion glide the sagittal bands and interosseous hood proximal and distal by 16 mm[203] to 20 mm.[220] As the sagittal bands glide distally with MP joint flexion, the EDC is able to transmit virtually no force distal to the MP joint because of its insertion on the dorsal hood/sagittal band complex.[182] Tension on the central tendon is decreased with MP flexion because of sagittal band distal migration.[220] This same observation has been noted by others in a study of central slip tension measured intraoperatively.[170] With the MP joint flexed, PIP extension is affected primarily through the interossei,[125,126] possibly with some contribution from the lumbrical,[202] but with little contribution from the EDC.[182]

The sagittal bands glide proximally with MP joint extension.[220] The attachment of the dorsal hood with the MP joint extended is slack and allows distal transmission of power to the central slip region.[182] Long[125,126] has determined by EMG that the lumbrical is electrically active with the MP joint extended, thus contributing to IP joint extension. Indirectly, the lumbrical contributes to IP joint extension by reducing the viscoelastic resistance of the FDP. Lumbrical contraction pulls the profundus distal, reducing the work requirement of the antagonistic extensor. Thus the lumbricals neutralize the viscoelastic tension of the profundi during digital extension.[125,126,182]

Although Long[125,126] has determined by EMG that the interossei are silent with the MP extended, Valentine[202] has determined by anatomic dissection that if the MP joint is extended, contraction force of the interossei is transmitted directly to the lateral bands, which in turn extend the IP joints. As mentioned, Close and Kidd[34] have demonstrated that the interossei will contract if all the MP joints are extended simultaneously or if the wrist is in flexion.

Thus the position of MP extension facilitates transmission of EDC force distal to the central slip region with proximal migration of the sagittal bands[182,220] while minimizing the work requirement of the EDC through the contribution of the lumbricals and interossei.[125,126,202]

Distal joint motion is an important aspect of this protocol to maintain excursion of the lateral bands and of the oblique retinacular ligaments. The DIP joint is unrestrained during the active PIP exercise of 30 degrees. With simultaneous flexion of the PIP and DIP joints, gliding of the terminal tendon is not transferred to the extensor communis but is taken up by the volar slide of the lateral bands.[203] The terminal tendon slackens through the action of the lateral

band migration when the PIP joint is flexed, facilitating DIP flexion. Zancolli[220] observed in two cadaveric dissections that when the FDP acts, both IP joints flex (linked flexion); the middle phalanx flexes before the distal phalanx; and during the course of flexion, the angle of flexion of the middle joint is greater than the distal joint.

Distal joint extension is facilitated by combined action of the EDC, action of the lateral bands, and tenodesis of the oblique retinacular ligament.[124,203] Active PIP joint extension, which is initiated by the long extensor, creates tension in the oblique retinacular ligament, which assists DIP joint extension. DIP joint extension then is completed as the lateral bands rise dorsally and finally reach the same tension as the central tendon.[124]

Therefore the moderate PIP joint flexion of 30 degrees with the DIP joint unrestrained in the SAM protocol may create no more than an estimated 1 to 2 mm of excursion of both lateral bands and terminal tendon, based on lateral band excursion cited by Zancolli[220] and Littler and Thompson.[124]

If the lateral bands are repaired, DIP joint flexion to 30 degrees with the PIP joint held at 0 degrees of extension will facilitate a minimal excursion for these structures. If the lateral bands are not repaired, the DIP joint may be flexed fully with the PIP joint held at 0 degrees of extension. Flexion of the DIP joint with the PIP restrained imparts 3 to 4 mm of distal migration to the EDC in zone IV through the action of the lateral bands in their attachment to the EDC proximal to zone III. This exercise position then actually reduces tension at a zone III repair site while creating distal migration of the zone IV tendon.

Clinical application of immediate active short arc motion for the repaired central slip. Based on the assessment of problems associated with the immobilized zone III and IV repaired extensor tendon, I developed an early motion protocol in 1988 that uses immediate active short arc motion for the repaired central slip. The protocol is as follows.

Except during exercise, the involved digit is immobilized in a volar static thermoplastic splint that immobilizes only the PIP and DIP joints (see Fig. 31-11). The splint is taped directly over the PIP and DIP joints with a 1-inch Transpore (3M) plastic tape to ensure that both of these joints rest at absolute 0 degrees extension.

Two exercise template splints are used by the patient during exercise sessions to control stress application and excursion for the repaired central slip. Template splint 1 (Fig. 31-17, A) for PIP joint motion is a volar static splint fabricated with a 30-degree flexion angle for the PIP joint and a 20- to 25-degree angle for the DIP joint. The template splint 2 (Fig. 31-18, A) for DIP joint flexion is a volar static splint for the proximal and middle phalanx with the PIP joint at 0 degrees and the DIP joint free.

The patient is instructed to remove the immobilization splint every waking hour for an empirical 20 repetitions of PIP and DIP joint exercise. The wrist is positioned at 30

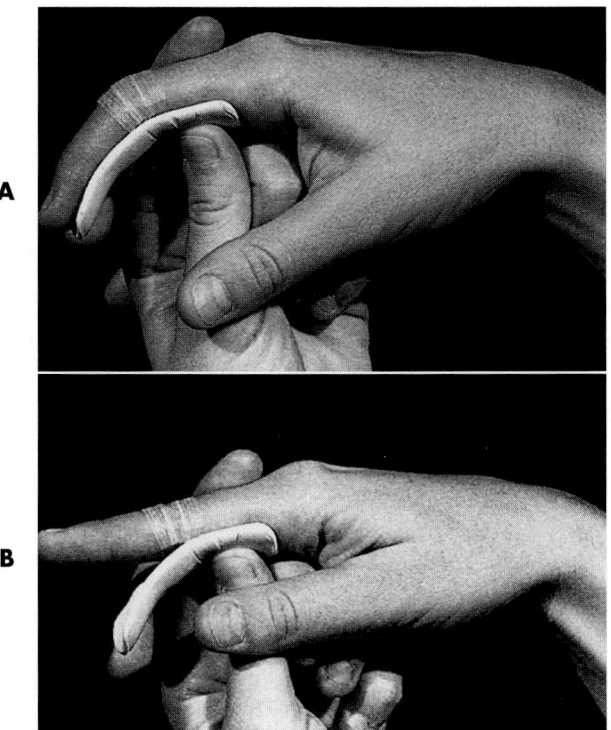

Fig. 31-17. A and **B,** Template splint 1 allows 30 degrees at the proximal interphalangeal (PIP) joint and 20 to 25 degrees at the distal interphalangeal joint, preventing the patient from stretching the repair site by allowing only the precalculated excursion of the central slip. The wrist is positioned in 30 degrees of flexion, the digit is supported at the proximal phalanx by the contralateral hand, and the PIP joint is actively flexed and extended in a controlled range of motion. (From Evans RB: *J Hand Surg* 19A:992, 1994.)

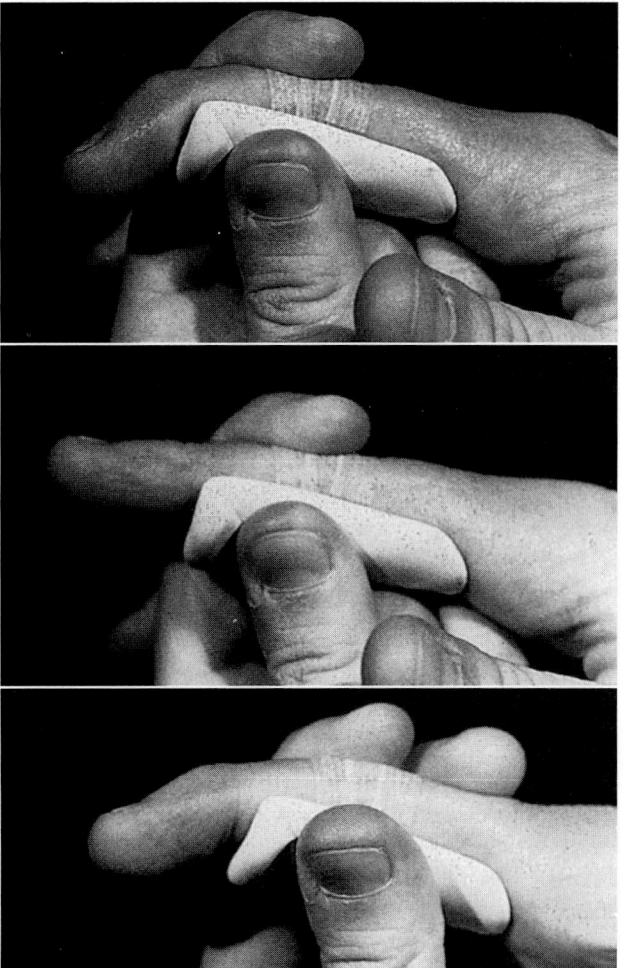

Fig. 31-18. A through **C,** Template splint 2 immobilizes only the proximal interphalangeal joint, allowing isolated distal joint motion to create gliding of the lateral bands. If the lateral bands are not repaired, the distal joint is fully flexed and extended (**A, B**). If the lateral bands are repaired, the distal interphalangeal joint is flexed only to 30 to 35 degrees (**C**). (From Evans RB: *J Hand Surg* 19A:993, 1994.)

degrees of flexion, and the MP joint is positioned at 0 degrees of extension to very slight flexion. The patient is instructed to manually support the MP joint in template splint 1, which allows the PIP joint to flex to 30 degrees and the unrestrained DIP joint to flex to 20 to 25 degrees. The patient will actively flex and extend the PIP joint through this 30-degree range with 20 repetitions (see Fig. 31-17, *A* and *B*). The patient is instructed that each repetition should be performed slowly and sustained briefly in a fully extended position. Template splint 2 is then applied with manual pressure to stabilize the PIP joint at 0 degrees (see Fig. 31-18, *A*). If the lateral bands are not repaired, the distal joint is flexed fully and extended to 0 degrees (see Fig. 31-18, *A* and *B*); if the lateral bands are repaired, the distal joint is flexed only to 30 to 35 degrees (visually monitored by the patient) with active extension emphasized (see Fig. 31-18, *C*).

The patient is instructed in a technique of controlled active motion that applies very low internal tendon tension with the active extension exercise. For the program to be effective, the patient must understand that the exercise must be performed in the prescribed position (wrist, 30 degrees flexion; MP joint, 0 degrees to slight flexion; with PIP and DIP joints moving within the guidelines of the template

splints), that the repetitions are to be performed slowly and frequently, and that the position of the immobilization splint must be absolutely precise with the PIP and DIP joints resting at 0 degrees.

The application of force in this position with only the weight of the finger as resistance and no allowance for drag from tight joint structures or edema is approximately 300 g.[57,58] When the PIP joint is moved actively through the 30-degree range (approximately one half radian, 28.65 degrees), extensor tendon excursion in zones III and IV is approximately 3.75 mm[57] (see Fig. 31-5).

At 2 weeks after surgery, the template splint 1 is altered to allow 40 degrees at the PIP joint if no extensor lag has developed. The PIP joint angle can be changed to 50 degrees by the third postoperative week and up to 70 to 80 degrees by the end of the fourth week if the PIP joint is actively extending to 0 degrees. If an extensor lag develops, flexion increments should be more modest and active extension exercise and extension splinting should be emphasized. In my clinical experience, by 4 weeks after surgery, the average PIP joint moves actively approximately 60 to 70 degrees, and by the sixth week, from 3 degrees of extension to 88 degrees of flexion. The stiff PIP joint at 4 weeks can be splinted intermittently into flexion, but static extension splinting for the digit should continue until week 5 or 6. By the fifth week, composite flexion exercises and gentle strengthening are appropriate; PIP joints treated with the SAM protocol often are ready for discharge by week 6, and the patient is allowed to strengthen with a home program.

The wrist joint, MP joint, and uninvolved digits are free to move through a range of motion with a natural tenodesis effect taking place (wrist extension and finger flexion, and wrist flexion and finger extension), with only the affected PIP and DIP joints of the injured digits immobilized (Fig. 31-19, *A* and *B*). General practices for wound care and edema control with Coban wraps, ice, and elevation should be followed. Controlled mobilization with active exercise and gentle distraction techniques to avoid cartilage-cartilage abutment, and dynamic flexion traction with less than 250 g of tension, will help elongate periarticular structures, promote tendon glide, and ultimately reestablish PIP joint motion at the fourth and fifth postoperative weeks. Flexion must not be regained at the expense of losing extension; therefore increases in stress application and flexion angles should not be attempted unless extension is complete.

Comparison study of immobilization and short arc motion

The results of open and repaired central slip injuries (64 digits, 55 patients) I treated from 1985 to 1992 with two entirely different protocols were analyzed.[51] Group I was treated with 3 to 6 weeks of immobilization (defined in the section on traditional management of zone III and IV injuries), and group II was treated with SAM (as described in the immediately preceding paragraphs), initiated between days 2 and 11. The two groups were further subdivided into simple injury (only tendon) or complex injury (associated injury to bone, cartilage, or DIP joint). The results of this preliminary study are summarized in Table 31-3 and continue to be supported by my clinical experience with these injuries treated since that time. The conclusion from the clinical study[51] is that open and repaired central slip injuries treated with SAM yield statistically superior results when compared with those treated by 3 to 6 weeks of immobilization in regard to extensor lag, total active motion (TAM) (Strickland-Glogovac formula,[188] which calculates only the PIP and DIP joint motion), and treatment time ($p < .01$; t-test). The greater extensor lag in the immobilization group may be due to improper splinting during the immobilization phase

and attenuation of the repair during mobilization because of extensor tendon adherence in zone IV.

Zones V and VI

Extensor tendons in zones V and VI can be managed postoperatively by immobilization,[43,160] controlled passive motion,[4,24,33,55] or the controlled active tension technique.[58] Considering the previously described benefits of controlled motion for the healing tendon, I could not recommend total immobilization for tendon at any level except zone I and II and T-I, T-II extensor. However, total immobilization may be necessary with the very young or noncompliant patient and may be acceptable treatment for the simple injury for a period of 3 weeks. The abundant and mobile soft tissue that characterizes the dorsum of the hand facilitates the reestablishment of tendon glide in this area and creates a forgiving environment for simple tendon injury treated with total immobilization. Total immobilization should not be consid-

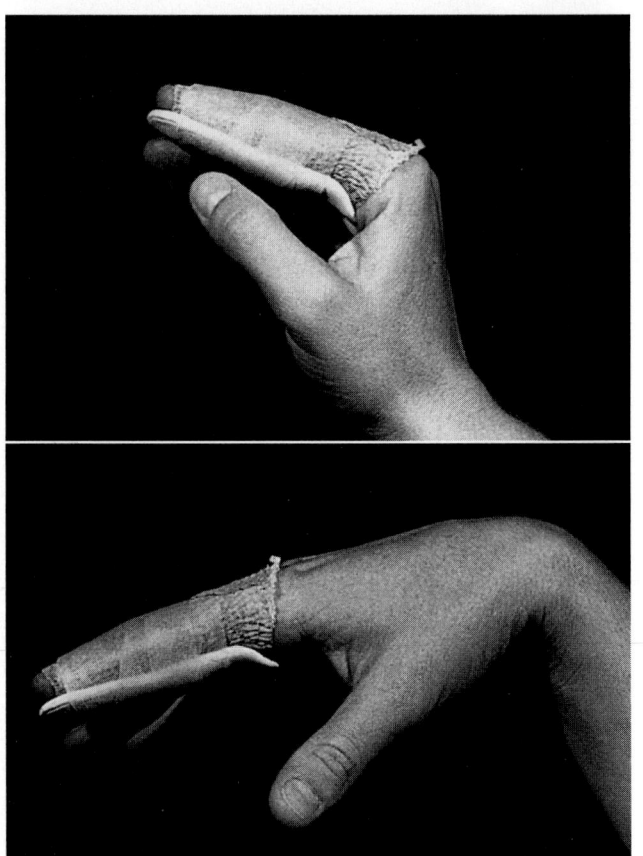

A

B

Fig. 31-19. **A** and **B,** The wrist and metacarpophalangeal joints, as well as the uninvolved joints, are free to move through all available ranges of motion. The natural tenodesis action of wrist extension and finger flexion, as well as wrist flexion and finger extension, will create proximal and distal migration of the sagittal bands but place minimal stress on the repair site, which is protected by the position of proximal interphalangeal joint extension. (From Evans RB: *J Hand Surg* 19A:993, 1994.)

ered with extensor tendon injury associated with crush injury where the paratenon would be extensively involved, with injury to the periosteum or adjacent soft tissues, or in hands with osteoarthritic or rheumatoid joints.[55]

Atraumatic surgical technique, preservation of the paratenon,[154] and proper postoperative immobilization minimize problems in the rehabilitation phase. Edema control is important to decrease complications of adhesion formation and shortening of periarticular structures that may result from the accumulation of protein and fluid in the extravas-

cular space.[85] The extensor tendons have 11 to 16 mm of excursion in zones V and VI,[19] requiring protection of both wrist and digital joints within the immobilizing or controlled-motion splints to prevent excessive tension at the repair.

Treatment by immobilization

The therapist's concerns during the first 3 postoperative weeks for extensor tendon repairs treated by immobilization are for wound care, edema control, and proper postoperative

Table 31-3. Final results and statistical analysis for SAM and treatment by immobilization for the repaired central slip

Results	Group I (immobilization)	Group II (SAM)	Statistical significance of *t* test	Statistical significance of chi square
Number of digits	38	26		
Mean age	39.9	42.2	>.5, NS	
% Male sex	86.8%	80.8%		>.5 NS
% Complex injury	76.3%	76.9%		>.5 NS
Mean day motion initiated	32.9	4.59	<.001, significant	
Mean day injury to discharge	76.07	51.38	<.001, significant	
PIP extension lag on first motion day	13°	3°	<.01, significant	
PIP extension lag on discharge day	8.13°	2.96°	<.01, significant	
PIP motion at 6 weeks	44°	88°	<.001, significant	
PIP motion at discharge	72°	88°	<.01, significant	
Total active motion (PIP and DIP) at discharge	110.7°	131.5°	<.01, significant	
DIP motion at discharge	37.63°	45°	<.01, significant	

From Evans RB: *J Hand Surg* 19A:994, 1994. *DIP,* Distal interphalangeal; *NS,* not significant; *PIP,* proximal interphalangeal.

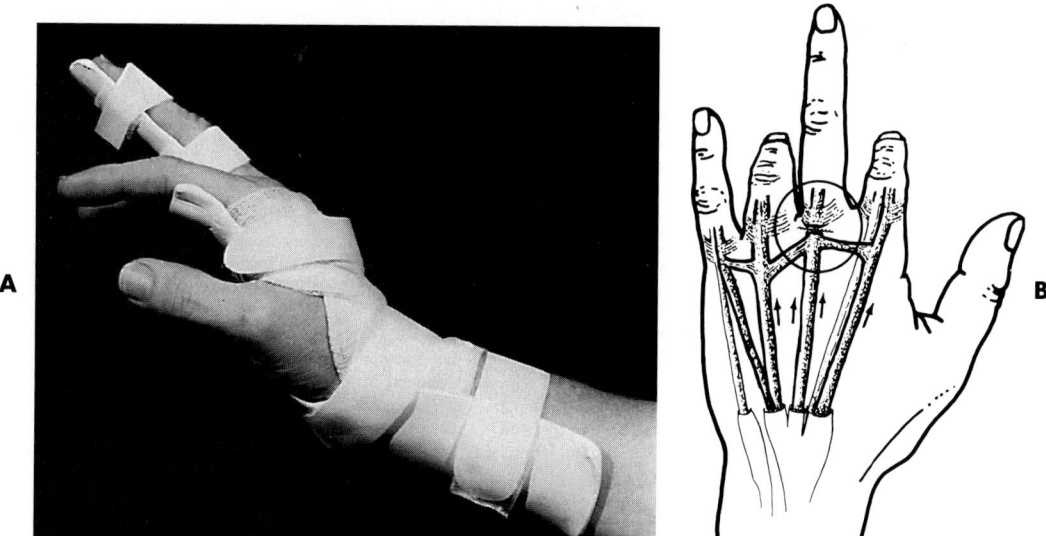

Fig. 31-20. A, Repair to the extensor digitorum communis distal to the juncturae in the long finger can be adequately protected with splinting that rests the long metacarpophalangeal joint at 0 degrees and adjacent metacarpophalangeal joints at 30 degrees of flexion. This position relieves tension at the repair site while maintaining some extensibility of the collateral ligaments of the uninvolved fingers. **B,** Tension can be reduced on the anastomosis of the extensor digitorum communis when the repair site is distal to the juncturae tendinum if the adjacent fingers are held in mild flexion. This position advances the proximal end of the severed tendon by a force of the intertendinous connection. (From Beasley RW: *Hand injuries,* Philadelphia, 1981, WB Saunders.)

immobilization to protect the repaired structures from rupture or elongation. The position of immobilization should be 40 to 45 degrees of wrist extension, 0 to 20 degrees of MP joint flexion, and 0 degrees of IP joint flexion. Many authors[43,86,160,163] recommend splinting the MP joints in mild flexion to retain the integrity of the collateral ligaments. However, in my clinical experience, splinting the MP joints in mild flexion with the immobilization technique will result in MP extensor lag. The early motion programs that splint the MP joints at 0 degrees between exercise sessions yet allow some MP joint motion solve the problem of collateral ligament tightness versus extensor lag.[55]

Simple laceration to the extensor indicis proprius (EIP) and extensor digiti minimi (EDM) requires immobilization of only the repaired tendons.[60,203] However, with the EDC, one must consider the juncturae tendinum, which, while functioning to dynamically stabilize the MP joints, also limits independent function of these tendons[2,60] (see Chapter 30). If the repair site is proximal to the interconnecting tendon, all fingers should be splinted in extension. If it is distal to the interconnection, the adjacent fingers can be immobilized in 30 degrees of flexion (Fig. 31-20, A). The latter position permits advancement of the proximal end of the severed tendon by a force of the intertendinous connection, thus actually reducing tension on the anastomosis[13] (Fig. 31-20, B).

The therapist should assess the digital joints in the immobilized hand for stiffness during dressing changes and splint rechecks during the first 3 postoperative weeks. The therapist should manually place the wrist in full extension while supporting all digital joints at 0 degrees. The therapist then can carefully assess the feel of each MP joint by gently moving the index and long fingers from slight hyperextension to 30 degrees of flexion, and the ring and small fingers from hyperextension to 38 to 40 degrees of flexion (Fig. 31-21). This protected motion will create approximately 3 to 5 mm of tendon excursion and will not jeopardize the repair.[55] These excursions are calculated mathematically by radians and are explained in Table 31-2. If the MP joints seem excessively stiff and do not easily tolerate this much motion, the surgeon and therapist should consider passive motion during supervised therapy sessions or dynamic splinting instead of static splinting to allow some controlled passive motion by the patient.[49,55]

The PIP joints can be assessed with the wrist and MP joints held in extension. There is little excursion created in zones V and VI with IP joint motion.[19,20] An extensor tendon amplitude study on eight cadaver hands demonstrated that if the wrist is held in more than 21 degrees of extension, the extensor tendon glides with little or no tension in zones V and VI throughout full simulated grip to full passive extension.[143] The authors of that study suggest that full passive flexion is safe with these injuries if the wrist is extended. However, I do not think that this much excursion

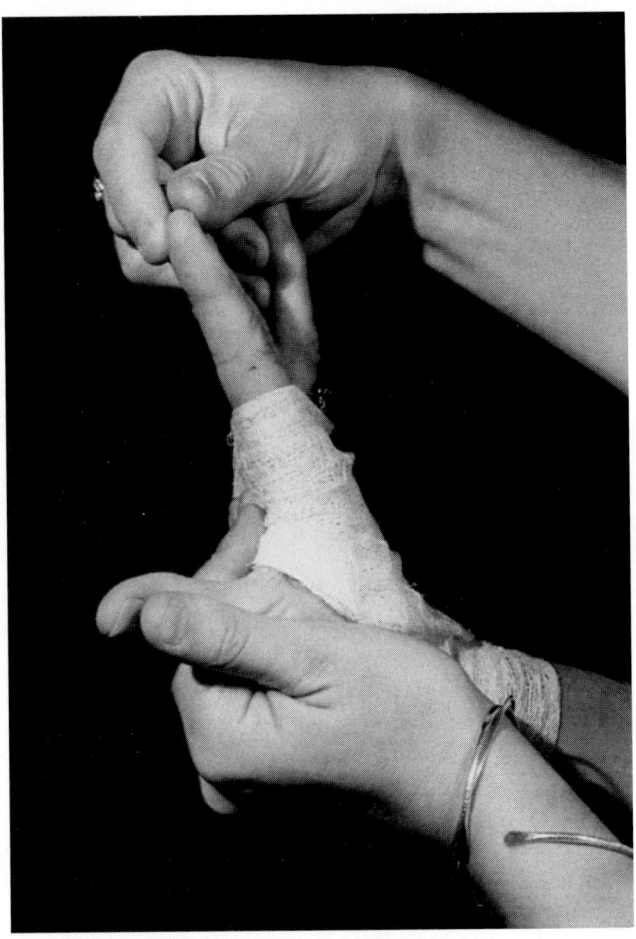

Fig. 31-21. The hand treated with immobilization techniques should be assessed during the first and second postoperative weeks to determine whether excessive stiffness is developing at the metacarpophalangeal or proximal interphalangeal joint levels. The wrist and digits are held passively in maximum extension as the therapist passively moves the metacarpophalangeal joints from hyperextension to 30 degrees of flexion for the index and long fingers, and 40 degrees for the ring and small fingers. Unyielding periarticular structures may require a change in splint position or in treatment approach to early passive motion.

is necessary, and I will outline another approach to maintaining tendon excursion in the section on early passive motion. Each IP joint can be passively and individually moved through a complete ROM while the wrist and MP joints are held in extension.[55] A solution to the problem of stiff IP joints associated with arthritis or swelling from the more proximal injury, when treatment by immobilization is chosen, is to cut away the immobilizing splint under each PIP joint to allow active and passive motion at this level (Fig. 31-22, A). These joints should rest in extension between exercise sessions to prevent problems of extensor lag and PIP flexion contracture, a sequela of resting the swollen PIP joint in flexion. A removable volar component can be applied

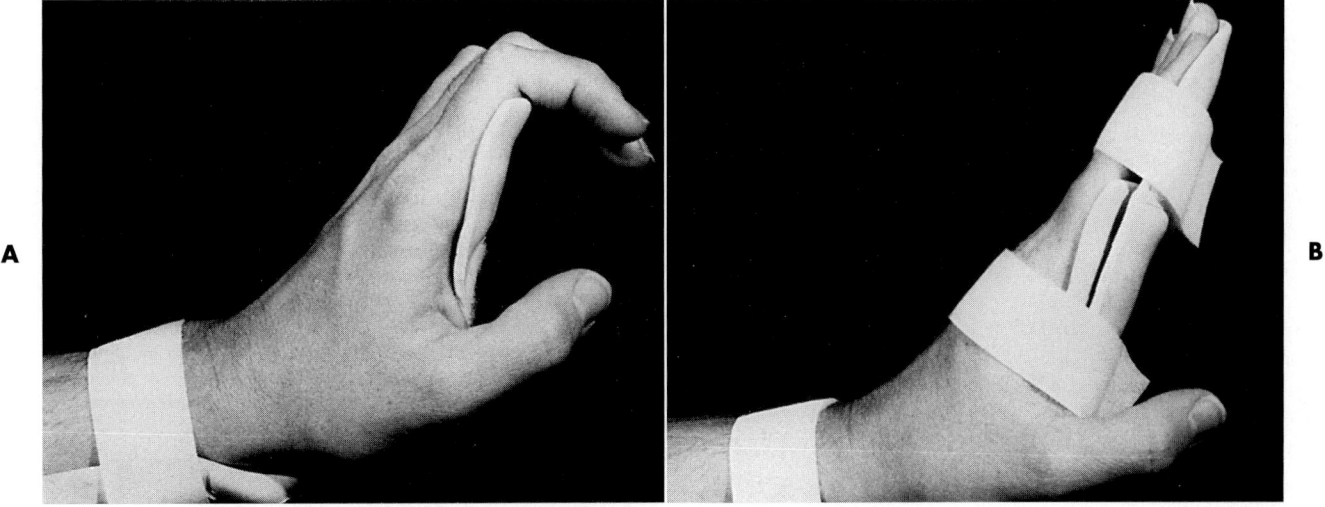

Fig. 31-22. A, A static extension splint that immobilizes the wrist and metacarpophalangeal joints in extension allows motion of the proximal and distal interphalangeal joints without jeopardizing repairs in zones V, VI, and VII. **B,** A removable extension component is applied between exercise sessions to prevent volar plate tightness and extension lag, problems that are associated with swollen proximal interphalangeal joints that rest in flexion.

to the splint to rest the IP joints in extension between exercises (Fig. 31-22, *B*).

Guarded active motion should be initiated by the third postoperative week. The immobilized tendon at 3 weeks should be considered to have little tensile strength from endotenon healing,[63,84,114,136,201] but some strength from peritendinous adhesions associated with immobilization.[71,157] The patient should be instructed to protect the repair by proper joint positioning during exercise and splint protection between exercise sessions.

As with any hand injury, one begins treatment by cleansing and softening the skin and instructing the patient in self-care. The hand may be washed or debrided in a small portable whirlpool in which the wrist and fingers can be supported in extension. The patient is instructed in retrograde massage techniques to reduce edema and to soften the scar. SGS or Otoform can be used to soften the scar (see Chapter 19). Micropore paper tape worn continuously on dry skin in a longitudinal fashion from approximately 2 weeks until 2 months postoperative will reduce hypertrophic scarring by minimizing wound tension. This technique has been found to be as effective as the use of silicone gel sheeting and is much less expensive.[147,164]

Gentle active and active assistance exercise during the third to fourth week should emphasize extension at the MP joint with the wrist in a neutral to slightly flexed position to decrease elastic resistance from the antagonistic flexor system,[58] and MP joint flexion from 40 to 60 degrees should be performed with the wrist held in an extended position to maintain MP collateral ligament extensibility without overstressing the anastomosis. This synergistic play of simulta-

neous wrist flexion and MP joint extension, and wrist extension with MP joint flexion, will allow for active tendon excursion and ligament excursion without placing excessive force on the repair site. The IP joints may be exercised through a complete range with the wrist and MP joints extended. The repairs can be protected between exercise sessions with a dynamic extension splint that supports the wrist at approximately 20 degrees of extension and the fingers dynamically at 0 degrees (Fig. 31-23).

Duration of exercise is for the most part an empirical decision. As discussed in the first section of this chapter, we have one clinical study on management of flexor tendon injuries that demonstrates improved motion with increased duration of motion[76] but no study on the extensor tendon. I usually instruct the patient to perform each exercise with 10 to 20 repetitions every waking hour. Patients are warned not to overexercise because this may cause inflammation of the tissues.

By the fourth week, composite flexion can be attempted with the wrist extended. Individual finger extension exercise and the "claw," or intrinsic-minus, position will direct controlled stress to the extrinsic extensors[60,203] (Fig. 31-24, *A*). Dynamic flexion splinting for application of stress to the stiff MP or PIP joints should be initiated as early as the third week if joint motion is less than 30 to 40 degrees with a "hard end-feel," and by the fourth week with motion limited in the range of 50 to 60 degrees. Force can be directed to the stiff MP joint during active exercise by negating long flexor forces with volar digital extension splints taped directly over the PIP joint during intrinsic-plus exercise (Fig. 31-24, *B*). Stiff IP joints should be splinted with a separate splint that

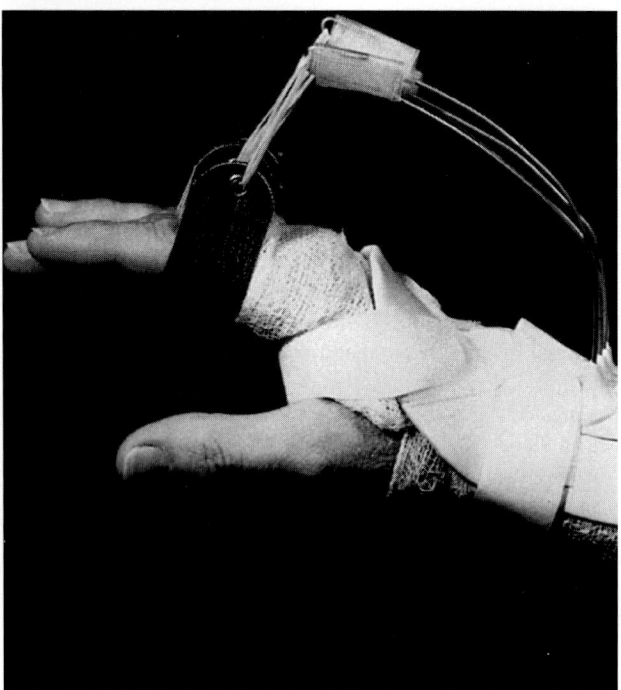

Fig. 31-23. A dorsal dynamic extension splint that rests the metacarpophalangeal joints at 0 degrees and allows controlled flexion will prevent excessive stress at the repair site while encouraging joint motion and increased tendon excursion.

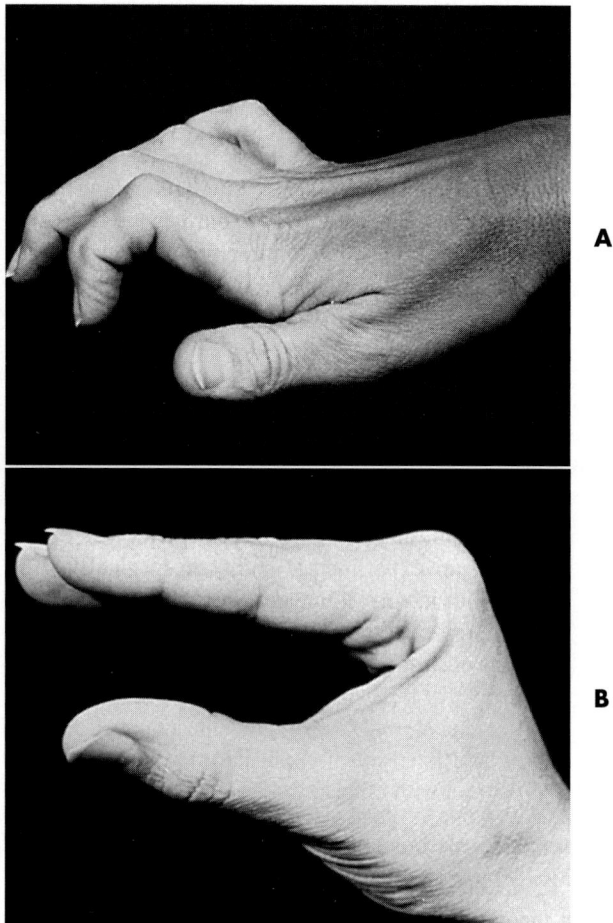

Fig. 31-24. A, The intrinsic-minus or "claw position" will isolate the extrinsic extensors during exercise. **B,** The intrinsic-plus position will direct force to the metacarpophalangeal collateral ligaments without placing excessive stress on repairs in zones V, VI, or VII if the wrist is extended during exercise.

blocks the MP joints in extension between the third and fourth weeks to direct forces to the periarticular structures, but by the fourth to fifth week combinations of both MP and PIP joint traction (MP flexion cuffs and nail traction) can be used to direct forces along the length of the extensor tendons.

Composite finger flexion can be facilitated with the use of graded dowels between 4 and 5 weeks. By the sixth week, postoperative composite finger and wrist flexion exercises will be tolerated by the repaired tendon and mild strengthening can be added to the exercise regimen. A 1-pound weight for wrist flexion/extension exercise and for pronation/supination can be used for several weeks to increase the tensile strength of the tendons and also to strengthen the extensor carpi radialis brevis (ECRB) and flexor carpi ulnaris (FCU). These muscles, weakened by immobilization and disuse, will make the patient who returns to sports activities or manual labor without strengthening prone to develop lateral or medial epicondylitis. Forearm strengthening should be performed with fewer repetitions (10 repetitions, three times per day, with gradual increments over a 2- to 3-week period, to 20 repetitions four times per day). The BTE work simulator or other computerized exercise equipment can be used for mild strengthening but should be supplemented with a home program. In today's medical-economic climate, it is often not possible to follow a repaired tendon for 6 weeks, and treatment by immobilization that usually produces more complications of tendon adherence and joint stiffness should be considered only when

the health care provider believes no other option is available. The patient should be advised that strong resistive exercise should be delayed until the tenth to twelfth week, when the tendon has regained near-normal tensile strength.

The modalities of heat, cold, high-voltage galvanic stimulation, or whirlpool can be used as hand volume and joint stiffness dictate. Functional electrical stimulation on a light setting can be used by the fourth week as a type of biofeedback and applied with more force directed to the extensor muscle by the fifth week, and even to the flexor system by the fourth to fifth week when composite flexion becomes a goal. At present, the use of US with the healing tendon is still questionable,[152] although basic science studies indicate that US may have a role on a limited basis at low intensity during the earliest stages of wound healing.[47,94] The use of US during the early stages of wound healing has been shown to increase ROM, decrease scar formation, and have no adverse effect of decreased strength in an experimental study of surgically repaired flexor tendons in zone II in the white leghorn chicken animal model.[94] However, the effect of US on the healing human tendon has not yet been established, although clinical studies are currently under way. US should not be used for tendon management until clinical guidelines in regard to timing, duration, and intensity of application have been established and supported with clinical studies.

Treatment with early passive motion

I established a controlled early passive motion program for the healing extensor tendon in zones V, VI, and VII in 1979 to reduce the postoperative problems associated with the complex injury. Precise guidelines for correlating tendon excursion with joint motion were defined in a study of the biomechanics and excursions of the extensor system[55] and are outlined in the first segment of this chapter. The rationale for applying controlled stress to the healing extensor tendon is the same as that for the flexor tendon: to promote intrinsic healing and to encourage longitudinal reorientation of adhesions associated with extrinsic healing.[66,68,76,103,137,157]

Although the simple dorsal injury often is discounted at this level, significant problems of adherent tendon and extensor lag can result from immobilization, improper splint position, and inattention during the first 3 weeks of healing. Rosenthal[167] discusses the inflammatory response of the extensor paratenon (characterizing the extensor tendons in the extrasynovial zones V and VI) when disturbed, especially in the complex extensor tendon injury, and notes that the paratenon has a prodigious capacity for generating scar tissue and adhesions. Peacock,[156] in a study of the effects of enveloping tendon transfers with paratenon, observed that transplanted paratenon abounds in collagen-synthesizing cells. The observed physiologic response of disturbed paratenon is an increased production of adhesions in surrounding tissues.[156,157,199] This increase may explain proliferative adhesion formation in the extrasynovial extensor tendon injury in zones V and VI, particularly with crushing injury in which the enveloping paratenon is widely disturbed.

Although in my earlier reports I suggested using early passive motion in these zones only for extensor injuries associated with periosteal injury, crush, or associated soft tissue injury,[49,55] I now recommend early motion for simple injury as well. Clinically, we observe that even the simple injury treated with immobilization can become problematic, and the biochemical and biomechanical benefits of early motion cannot be disputed.

Clinical application. Controlled stress is applied to the extrinsic tendons 24 hours to 3 days after surgery by allowing the repaired tendons to glide 5 mm within a forearm-based dynamic extension splint. Stress is relieved at the repair site for the finger extensors by positioning the wrist at approximately 40 to 45 degrees of extension. Splinting the wrist in a neutral position, as suggested by Minamikawa et al.,[143] will rest the repair site distal to its normal resting

position and will result in extensor lag. The MP and IP joints rest at 0 degrees in dynamic extension slings (Fig. 31-25, *A*). I prefer to use a moving high-profile outrigger made of spring steel (as opposed to a static outrigger, which provides motion only through rubber band or monofilament), which is bent at a right angle at the point of attachment and applied to the splint with Polyform proximal to the dorsal retinaculum. The counterforce from the resistance of the weight of the fingers is then proximal to the wound, and the moving outriggers offer less resistance to active flexion than would a static outrigger (Fig. 31-25, *B*). The use of a high-profile outrigger, as opposed to a low-profile outrigger, is supported by the work of Boozer et al.[17] An interlocking palmar blocking splint will permit only the predetermined angular changes at the MP joint level (see Table 31-2).

The patient is instructed to actively flex the digits at the MP joint until the fingers touch the volar splint and then to relax the digits, allowing the extensor outrigger to passively return the finger joints to 0 degrees (see Fig. 31-25, *A* and *B*). The patient is instructed to repeat this exercise at least 20 times each waking hour. If the patient has difficulty flexing the fingers at the MP joint level or if the proximal IP joints do not rest at 0 degrees within the extension slings, a volar digital extension splint should be fitted to each problematic digit and slipped inside each finger cuff to ensure that motion takes place at the MP joint. A low-profile outrigger with stop beads to control excursion can be used, but for the reasons stated previously, I prefer to use a high-profile, moving outrigger (Fig. 31-25, *C* and *D*).

The patient is seen in therapy for wound care, splint adjustments, controlled passive motion for the IP joints, and wrist tenodesis exercises. With the wrist and MP joints fully extended, minimal excursion takes place at the IP joint levels, and each digital joint can be moved passively through a complete ROM without creating excessive stress or gapping to repairs at any level from zone V and proximal. Isolated exercise for the digital joints is especially important with the edematous or arthritic hand. Cooney et al.[35,89] have emphasized the importance of wrist tenodesis exercises with flexor tendon protocols to increase passive excursion of the repair site. I have applied their concept of tenodesis to the extensors with these parameters: The joints are moved passively in supervised therapy sessions with simultaneous maximum wrist extension and MP joint flexion to 40 degrees, followed by simultaneous wrist flexion to 20 degrees with all digital joints held at 0 degrees. This concept of wrist tenodesis can be supported by the previously mentioned cadaver study on extensor tendons,[143] in which investigators demonstrated that if the wrist is extended more than 21 degrees, the extensors glide with little or no tension in zones V and VI throughout full simulated grip to full passive extension.

One must take care to ensure that the ulnar MP joints do not rest in hyperextension, compromising the transverse metacarpal arch or creating problems for MP joint collateral

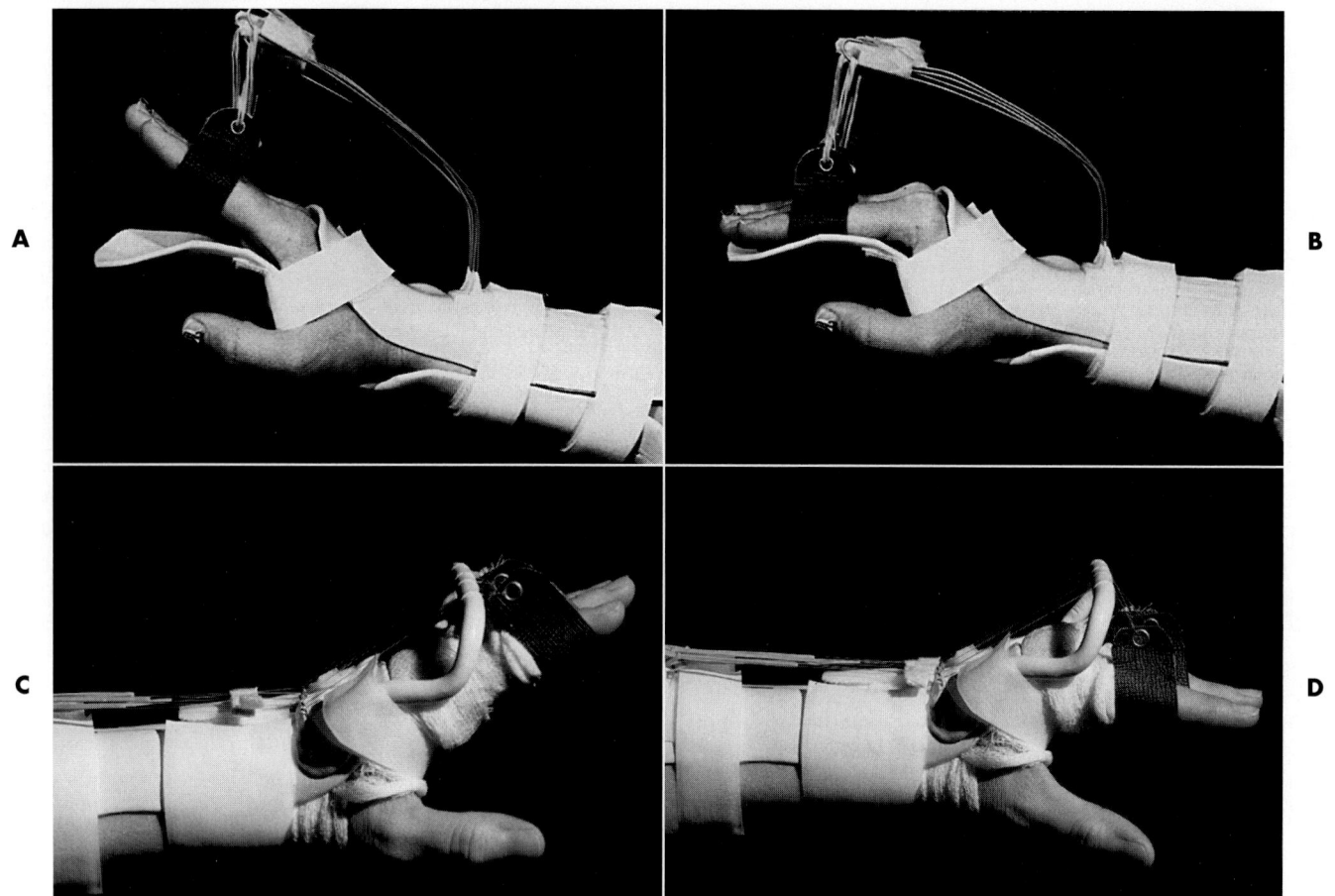

Fig. 31-25. A, A dorsal forearm-based dynamic extension splint immobilizes the wrist at 45 degrees of extension and rests all finger joints at 0 degrees to position the repair site proximal to its normal resting position to prevent gapping and extensor lag. A volar block permits only the predetermined metacarpophalangeal joint flexion, allowing slightly more flexion for the ulnar digits to achieve the necessary tendon excursion. **B,** The patient actively flexes the digits to the volar block an empirical 20 repetitions each waking hour to create approximately 5 mm of passive excursion for the extensor tendons. Dynamic traction returns the digits to 0 degrees, but most patients inadvertently actively extend within the slings as well. **C,** Low-profile dynamic splint that rests the digital joints at 0 degrees. **D,** The desired motion at the MP joint is controlled by a stop bead that limits rubber band and monofilament line excursion. (**A,** From Evans RB, Burkhalter WE: *J Hand Surg* 11A:774, 1986.)

ligament extensibility. The patient may be instructed to remove the dorsal outrigger component and to secure the volar component by repositioning the Velcro straps to simplify dressing activities. The digits must rest at the 0-degree position at all other times, however, to prevent gapping or elongated tendon callous healing and extensor lag. I occasionally fit the patient with a second volar static extension splint with the MP joints positioned at 0 degrees for sleeping. The patient follows the active flexion, passive extension exercise regimen at home within the confines of the dynamic extension splint and volar block.

This regimen is followed for 21 days, at which time the volar block is removed and increased digital joint motion and tendon excursion are permitted within the dynamic extension splint. Splint protection is necessary for another 2 to 3 weeks, with the dynamic extension component only in the daytime

and the static volar component at night. The protocols for exercise, modalities, and dynamic flexion splinting as outlined in the section on management by immobilization can be followed at the 3-week period for tendons treated with early passive motion. In my clinical experience, these patients will have composite finger flexion by the fourth to fifth weeks and composite finger and wrist flexion by the sixth week with no lag.

Treatment by immediate active tension. The application of force with minimal active tension as a means of managing the repaired extensor tendon postoperatively is divided into two exercise components[54,58]: (1) Slow, repetitious passive motion should be performed until passive torque[23] at the end arc of extension is less than 200 to 300 g of force, before the active component of exercise is employed. Slow passive force reduces resistance and helps

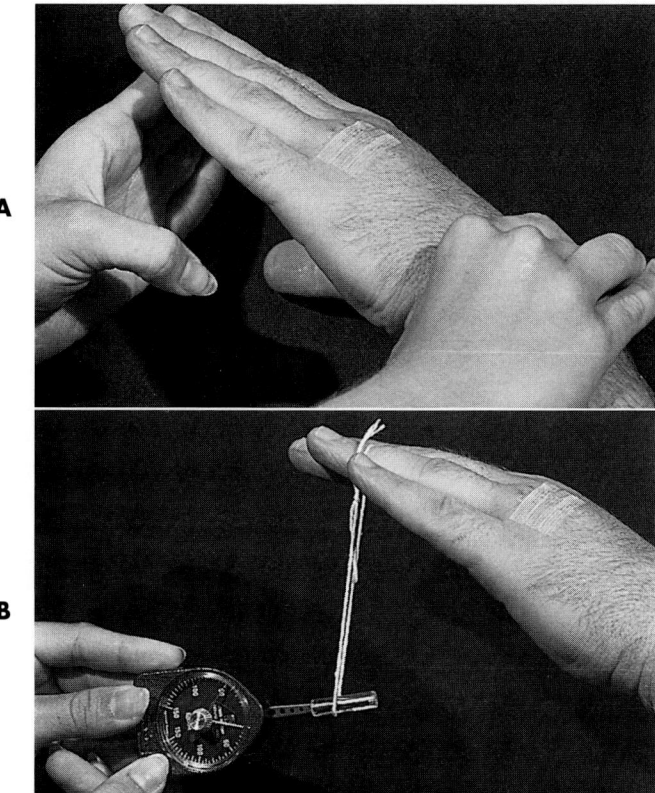

Fig. 31-26. A, Passive extension for repairs in extensor zones V, VI, and VII with the wrist slightly extended to reduce the drag from edema, tight joints, and the antagonistic flexors. **B,** The active hold component (MAMTT) is carefully controlled. External load is measured with a small calibrated Haldex pinch meter in the active hold position with the wrist flexed to 20 degrees and the digital joints extended. The patient is allowed to apply active force in the range of 25 to 50 g in the prescribed joint position under therapist supervision. (From Evans RB, Thompson DE: *J Hand Ther* 6:276, 1993.)

displace the high-molecular-weight fluids of edema[21] (Fig. 31-26). (2) The "active hold" component is then performed with the hand passively placed by the therapist in a position of 20 degrees of wrist flexion with all digital joints at 0 degrees, and the patient is asked to gently maintain this position to create some minimal active tension in the extensor system. The MP joint is moved actively, from 30 degrees of flexion to 0 degrees of extension, while the wrist is held in 20 degrees of flexion, with all repairs at the MP level and proximal. A calibrated small Haldex pinch meter (less than 150 g) can be used to demonstrate to the patient how gentle the forces of extension must be and can also provide the therapist with a repeatable and reliable technique for applying force to a tendon repair site. A string applied to the gauge arm of the pinch meter at a 90-degree angle and then around the digit at a 90-degree angle can be used to

measure external load application[58] (Fig. 31-26, *B*). The external force should be applied in the range of 0 to 25 g with joint angles as previously described. Force applied to repair sites in zones V, VI, and VII with these joint angles and with no external load except the weight of the finger has been calculated mathematically to be in the range of 300 g when drag is excluded.[58] The active component of treatment should be performed in the hands of the therapist after passive exercise in extension to reduce resistance of the antagonistic flexors. The active component is usually performed in my hands 20 or so times during a therapy session, three times per week for the first 3 weeks.

Active motion is supplemented in therapy with wrist tenodesis exercises as described earlier. I have not allowed the patients to come out of their protective splints at home for either the active component or wrist tenodesis exercise. The active component of this regimen is supplemented by the patient with the same dynamic splint (see Fig. 31-25, *A* and *B,* or *C* and *D*) and passive protocol described in the previous section on passive motion. The frequency of therapy visits depends on the status of the MP and PIP joints. Digital joints that are swollen or that have limited motion may require that the patient be treated daily during the first few weeks; otherwise, the patients will be seen two or three times a week. Digits held in extension slings are moving actively to some degree, inadvertently or otherwise,[58,150] so we can assume that the tendon does experience some proximal migration within the dynamic extension splint. Treatment between 3 and 12 weeks with a gradual increase in excursion and resistance is the same as that outlined in the section on treatment by immobilization for zones V and VI.

Timing is a critical component of active motion programs. The preferred protocol is to initiate some active tension by 24 hours after surgery. Although tension at the repair site may be elevated from edema and hematoma,[117] at this early stage suture is strong,[201] and no collagen bonds have formed that would limit tendon glide.[75] Presumably, it is safer to move a tendon at 24 hours after surgery than it is at day 5 or 10, when adhesions have formed and drag is increased. Experimentally, investigators have demonstrated that very early stress at a repair site may prevent the anticipated drop in tensile strength.[6,63,74,84,114]

Clinical results. I have compared the results of tendons treated with controlled active motion with tendons referred to me late that were treated with immobilization, and also to tendons treated from 1979 to 1990 with the passive motion technique (Tables 31-4 and 31-5). Tendons treated with wrist tenodesis and active motion demonstrated modest improvement (average, 9 degrees of TAM) over those treated with passive motion in a series that included both simple and complex injury but demonstrated significant improvement over treatment by immobilization (average improvement in TAM, 56 degrees[58]). The similarity in the results of active and passive techniques again is probably because tendons treated with the "passive" technique do, in fact, move

Table 31-4. Clinical results, primary repair of the extensor system

Zone	No. of Patients	No. of Tendons	Immediate minimal active muscle tendon tension			Days from surgery to discharge	ROM Strickland-Glogovac	TAM* ROM	Extensor lag
			Mean age	% Male	% Complex				
III, IV	28	32	42	80%	77%	51	135 degrees		3 degrees
V, VI	14	24	40	56%	41%	50		249 degrees	0 degrees
Immobilization†									
III, IV	30	38	40	87%	76%	77	111 degrees		8 degrees
V, VI	8	15	50	86%	60%	80		193 degrees	31 degrees
VII	1	4	38	100%	100%	50		210 degrees	20 degrees
T-III, T-IV, T-V	6	6	38	100%	50%	53		120 degrees	5 degrees

From Evans RB, Thompson DE: *J Hand Ther* 6:278, 1993.
*TAM = MP + PIP + DIP − extensor lag.
†1990, 1991, 1992, 1993.
No tendon seen early in this time tx only c̄ Passive Motion.

Table 31-5. Clinical results of extensor tendons as reported in two earlier clinical studies

Zone	Early passive motion* (pilot study, 1986)			
	No. of Patients	No. of Tendons	% Complex	TAM
IV, V, VI	36	66	100%	210 degrees
Multicenter Study 1989 (Early passive motion)†				
V, VI	32	50	0%	240 degrees
V, VI	16	35	100%	237 degrees
VII	8	17		242 degrees
T-IV, T-V	8	8	56%	116 degrees
(Immobilization 1989)				
V, VI	6	9	100%	185 degrees, 30 degrees extensor lag
VII	3	12	100%	188 degrees

From Evans RB, Thompson DE: *J Hand Ther* 6:281, 1993.
*Evans RB, Burkhalter WE: *J Hand Surg* 11A:774, 1986.
†Evans RB: *Phys Ther,* 6B:1041, 1989.

Table 31-6. Excursions for the wrist extensors as reported by Bunnell

	Flexion	Extension	Radial deviation	Ulnar deviation
ECRL	16 mm	21 mm	8 mm	16 mm
ECRB	16 mm	21 mm	4 mm	12 mm
ECU	14 mm	4 mm	3 mm	22 mm

From Boyes JH: *Bunnell's surgery of the hand,* Philadelphia, 1970, JB Lippincott.
ECRL, Extensor carpi radialis longus; *ECRB,* extensor carpi radialis brevis; *ECU,* extensor carpi ulnaris.

The moment arms and consequently tendon excursions are greatest for the digital extensor tendons at the wrist level[20] (Table 31-6). EDC excursions, as measured by Bunnell, at the wrist level vary as much as 20 mm from the small finger to the radial three fingers (see Table 31-1). The wrist extensors also vary significantly from tendon to tendon and with lateral motion as opposed to flexion and extension[19] (Table 31-6). Note the large excursions with the ECU in ulnar deviation as opposed to radial deviation and extension.

The relationship between tendon excursion and joint motion has been shown to be approximately linear for the long extensors at the wrist and at the finger joints.[20,46] Elliot and McGrouther[46] have provided a set of values for the long extensors that provide a basis for calculation of tendon excursions that are helpful as we establish controlled motion and splinting protocols. The excursions of the EIP and the EDC to the index finger were found to be indistinguishable during movement of the wrist and MP joints, as were the EDM and EDC for the small finger.[46] At the wrist joint, the slips of the EDC to the middle and long fingers are bound closely together, moving in unison[46] and obligating us to splint both of these fingers even when only one tendon is repaired.

actively at times. In a continuous series from 1993 to present, no extensor tendon treated with the active hold technique has ruptured.

Zone VII

The extensor tendons are synovial at the wrist, where they pass through six fibroosseous canals as they gain entrance to the hand.[43,166,167] The synovial sheaths and dorsal retinaculum act as pulleys, maintaining the relationship of tendon to bone while allowing for changes in direction. The synovial sheaths also may be important to tendon nutrition at this level.[16,135,222]

The extrinsic digital tendons at this level can be treated with any of the three techniques described for zones V and VI. Problems of adhesion formation in this synovial level are much the same as for zone II flexor tendons; therefore treatment by early passive motion or controlled active motion is especially important in this region. The wrist should be splinted in at least 40 to 45 degrees of extension and the digits held in dynamic traction at 0 degrees to allow the tendons to rest proximal to their normal resting position between exercise sessions to prevent extensor lag (see Fig. 31-25, *A* and *B*). Wrist tenodesis exercises should allow the wrist to come to only approximately 10 degrees of extension for the repaired EDC and to no more than 20 degrees of extension for the repaired wrist tendons to prevent excessive stress at the repair site(s) during the first 3 weeks of healing. Multiple repairs of the EDC require differential tendon gliding exercises from the earliest treatments. One can accomplish this by moving one digit at a time into flexion at the MP joint level while all other digits are held in extension, but it may be important to move the long and ring fingers together because of their interconnection at the wrist.[46] The MP joints can be moved from 30 to 40 degrees during the first 3 weeks, progressing to 40 to 60 degrees by week 4, and 70 to 80 degrees by week 5 while the wrist is extended. Very moderate wrist flexion with approximately 50% composite finger flexion is added to the excursion exercises by the fourth week, progressing to attempts at simultaneous composite finger flexion and complete wrist flexion by 6 weeks after surgery. Again, time schedules for duration of splinting, exercise, and the application of force for excursion and strengthening are as outlined in detail in the section on zones V and VI. The extensor tendon at this level is fairly large; therefore it will have more tensile strength after repair than would a smaller tendon at a more distal level. The work requirement of the wrist tendons also is greater than that of digital tendons at a more distal level; therefore return to normal loading for the wrist tendons should be delayed a few weeks beyond the schedules outlined for digital extensor tendons.

If treatment by immobilization is chosen, both the wrist and MP joints must be splinted in extension for repair of the digital tendons (Fig. 31-27). To prevent PIP joint tightness, extensor lag, or excessive force with active extension, a removable component such as described in Fig. 31-22 can be used. Active extension with the wrist held in extension elevates force at the repair site dramatically,[58] and forces in this position may exceed the tensile strength of the repair. Extension of the PIP joints with the wrist and MP joints held in extension should be passive; active extension will be safe if the hand is removed from the splint and the wrist is held in a neutral position to slightly flexed position.[58]

Treatment by immobilization will undoubtedly lead to tendon adherence to the synovial sheaths. Problems of limited tendon excursion and increased friction from adhesions that limit excursion may cause inflammatory problems

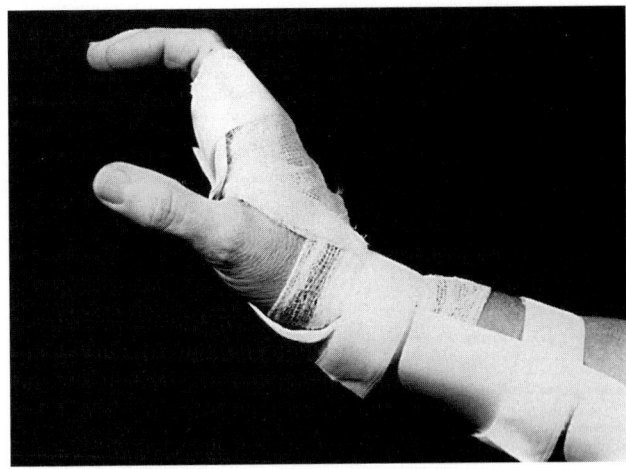

Fig. 31-27. Repair of the digital extensors in zone VII treated by immobilization requires immobilization of the wrist and metacarpophalangeal joints.

with hand-intensive activities and often lead to long rehabilitation programs, the need for combined wrist and digital flexor splinting, and tenolysis.

Adhesions proximal to the dorsal carpal ligament restrict combined wrist and digital flexion because the tendons will not glide distally under the dorsal pulley. Wrist flexion creates an exaggerated tenodesis effect of the digital extensors, depriving the patient of power grip. Scar distal to the retinaculum permits composite wrist and digital flexion but prevents composite wrist and digital extension because the tendons cannot glide proximally under the dorsal pulley. These problems can be minimized by proper postoperative splinting and early motion programs that use dynamic splints and controlled wrist tenodesis exercises. Micropore paper tape prevents tension to the incision line and is extremely effective in preventing hypertrophic scar if worn continuously from week 2 until week 8.[147,164] SGS, applied very early, as soon as the skin wound is epithelialized, appears to discourage scar formation and to reduce the density of subcutaneous adhesion. This physiologic mechanism is as yet unexplained (see Chapter 19), but I have had excellent clinical results with this material, especially when applied during early wound healing. Dense scar also can be treated with elastomer molds applied with pressure or with mechanical stress applied to the tendons in all arcs of motion by the sixth week with either exercise or splinting.

Treatment with early passive motion or controlled active motion is as described for the zone V and VI repair, with splinting and the active hold component. With repairs to the digital tendons, the therapist may position the wrist at approximately 20 degrees of flexion and digits at 0 degrees of extension while the patient gently maintains this position. However, if a wrist extensor tendon is involved, the wrist should not be moved beyond approximately 10 to 20 degrees of extension, and then the therapist should realize that forces at the repair site are increased with this change in wrist

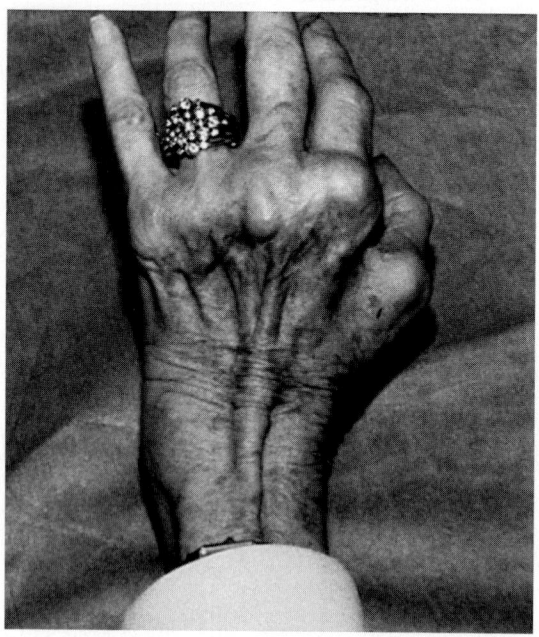

Fig. 31-28. Disruption of the dorsal carpal ligament increases the moment arm of the extensor tendons, resulting in lost mechanical efficiency and an extensor lag at the metacarpophalangeal joint.

position because of increased resistance of the antagonistic flexors.[58]

Disruption or extensive excision of the dorsal carpal ligament increases the moment arm of the extensor tendons and decreases mechanical efficiency.[16,20,193,198] Bowstringing of the extensor tendons at the wrist level translates to an extensor lag at the MP joint (Fig. 31-28). Boland[16] correlated loss of the extensor retinaculum with extensor lag of only 2 to 4 degrees at the wrist level, but as much as 70 degrees at the MP joint level, depending on the width of the retinacular fascia lost. With decreased mechanical efficiency, the workload of the extensor tendons is increased, especially during activities requiring sustained wrist and finger extension. Therefore the therapist should be aware that (1) with an absent or diminished dorsal retinaculum, it may not be possible to correct lag at the MP joint with therapy, and (2) altered biomechanics resulting from adhesions or lost pulley may result in cumulative trauma problems. Treatment should be adjusted appropriately.

The work capacity and load requirements for the wrist extensors are great, requiring protective splinting for as long as 8 weeks.[20] Tendon excursion of the three wrist extensors as it relates to flexion/extension and radioulnar deviation will determine the parameters for controlled motion programs (see Table 31-6). The wrist tenodesis exercises have been previously described for the first 3 weeks of healing. By the third to fourth week, repaired wrist tendons, which may be expected to have approximately 25% to 30% of their tensile strength,[136,201] may be moved actively from 0 degrees to full extension with gravity eliminated. Larger tendons with more

surface area for suturing will have more tensile strength than repairs at the more distal levels. The EDC tendons may be used to assist the wrist tendons during the first week of active exercise to bear some of the external load and possibly decrease stress at the wrist tendon anastomosis.

Increments in wrist flexion should be added slowly from week 5 to week 8. The same caution should be used with lateral motions. For example, the ECU has 22 mm of excursion in ulnar deviation, 3 mm in radial deviation, 4 mm in extension, and 14 mm in flexion.[19] To effect maximum excursion of the ECU, the wrist should be exercised into ulnar and radial deviation, with the forearm both supinated and pronated.[19,86,198] The patient may develop a tendency to lift the wrist with the EDC tendons, much like the pattern that we see after wrist fractures. Stress during exercise in the later stages of rehabilitation must be directed to the wrist tendons by excluding finger extension during exercise or functional electrical stimulation.

The thumb

The thumb extensor tendons are divided into five zones[113] (see Fig. 31-1). Injuries in T-I and T-II are treated similarly to injuries of zones I and II of the finger.[41,43,210] Reports in the literature on the mallet thumb indicate that the injury is rare and that opinions differ concerning surgical repair versus conservative treatment with splinting.[41,43,144,155,158] Zone T-I injuries require that the IP joint be splinted for 8 weeks continuously at 0 degrees or slight hyperextension with conservative management, and 5 to 6 weeks with operative repair. Both approaches require an additional 2 to 4 weeks of splint immobilization between exercise sessions. Increments in flexion as mobilization is initiated should be no more than 20 degrees per week and delayed if extensor lag develops. IP joint extension splinting should be continued between exercise periods and at night for an additional 2 to 3 weeks. Pinching and gripping activity with mild resistance can be initiated between the sixth and eighth weeks, depending on the duration of immobilization.

Zone T-II injuries are immobilized with a hand-based static splint that immobilizes the MP and IP joints at 0 degrees and radially extends the thumb. Active motion can be initiated in the short arc (25 to 30 degrees) by the third week, progressing slowly with more joint motion for the next 3 weeks. The problems of tendon-to-bone adherence will be similar to the digit over the proximal phalanx. Splint protection between exercise sessions is needed for a total of 6 weeks.

Injuries in zones T-III and T-IV should be splinted with the thumb MP joint at 0 degrees and slight abduction and the wrist at 30 degrees of extension. Care must be taken that the MP joint does not rest in hyperextension or that the immobilizing splint does not migrate distally, hyperextending this joint. Regaining flexion at the MP joint level is difficult in either case and may extend required rehabilitation. If the MP joint is tight in hyperextension, dynamic

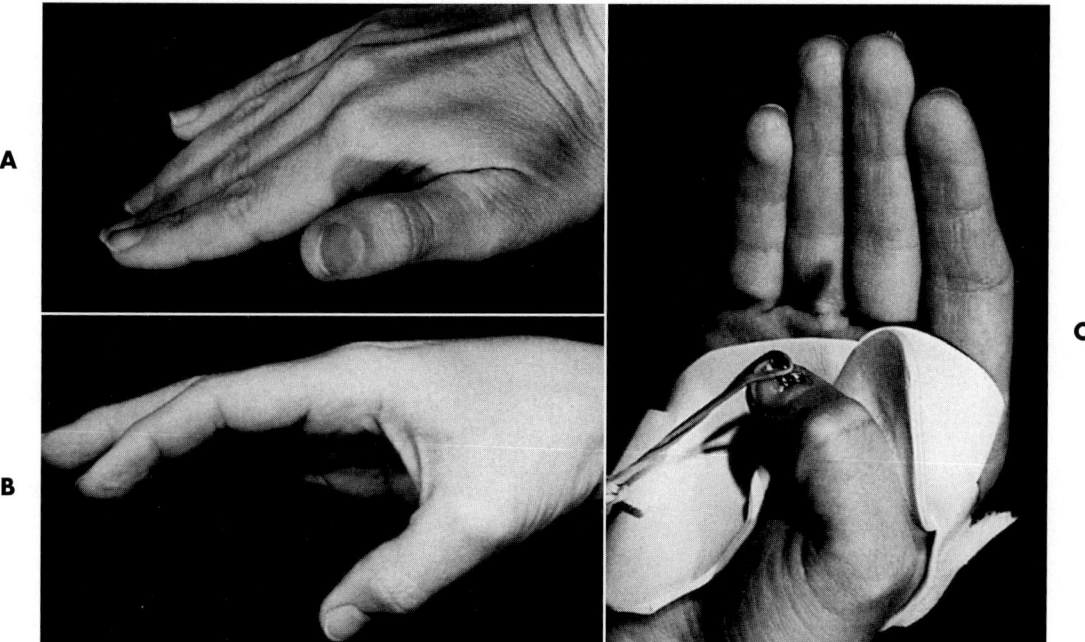

Fig. 31-29. A, The thumb should be exercised from complete retropulsion with the wrist extended to, **B,** simultaneous abduction and flexion with the wrist flexed to obtain complete excursion of the extensor pollicis longus tendon by the sixth week. **C,** Combinations of abduction and flexion splinting may be necessary for the thumb splinted incorrectly with adduction of the carpometacarpal joint and hyperextension of the metacarpophalangeal joint during the immobilization phase.

splinting for the MP joint with a gentle traction and joint mobilization techniques that use simultaneous axial distraction and flexion will help elongate the periarticular structures so that flexion can be regained.

Zone T-V injuries create difficult rehabilitation problems. Dense adhesions frequently limit excursion of the EPL at the retinacular level.[55] Improper immobilization in which the MP joint is hyperextended or in which insufficient web space is maintained will create extension contracture of the MP joint, first-web contracture, and problems in regaining ligamentous extensibility and tendon glide.[55,210] Dynamic flexion splinting of the MP joint with the wrist and first metacarpal extended is appropriate treatment for MP joint extension contracture between weeks 3 and 4 if the rubber band traction is less than 250 g and the anastomosis is protected from excessive stress by proper positioning of the proximal joints. Combinations of abduction and flexion splinting and exercise are appropriate between weeks 4 and 5 for excursion problems at this level (Fig. 31-29).

Early motion. Repair of the EPL in zone T-V always should be considered complex because the tendon at this level is synovial. The anticipated problems of maintaining excursion should be addressed with some type of controlled early motion—passive, controlled active motion, or combinations of both.

Excursions for the EPL vary in the literature from 25 to 60 mm and are subject to many variables.[19,20,187] Excursion of this tendon cannot be calculated by the radian technique because the ratio of tendon excursion to joint motion is not linear. The simple angular arrangement of the flexion/extension axis at the MP joint level of the fingers does not exist for the EPL in zones T-IV and T-V. Calculating excursion is complicated by the oblique course that the tendon takes at Lister's tubercle, by the moments of abduction and external rotation, and by the fact that alterations in thumb position alter moment arms at each joint.[20,106] Therefore Evans and Burkhalter[55] measured the EPL intraoperatively and determined that, with the wrist in a neutral position and the thumb MP joint extended to 0 degrees, 60 degrees of IP joint motion effected 5 mm of tendon excursion at the level of Lister's tubercle. Extending the wrist beyond approximately 30 degrees most likely would change the excursion with IP motion.

The early passive motion technique requires dynamic splinting that immobilizes the wrist in extension, the MP joint at 0 degrees, and the IP joint at 0 degrees in dynamic traction. The volar component of the splint is cut away at the IP joint, allowing the prescribed 60 degrees of IP motion to take place (Fig. 31-30). I have altered my original approach to these injuries by adding other motions while the patient is in my hands. Passive motion by the patient is supplemented in therapy with controlled passive motion to the MP joint of approximately 30 degrees while the wrist is held in maximum extension and the IP joint is held at 0 degrees; by abduction and adduction motions for the CMC joint in a 50% to 60% range; and by wrist tenodesis exercise in which the

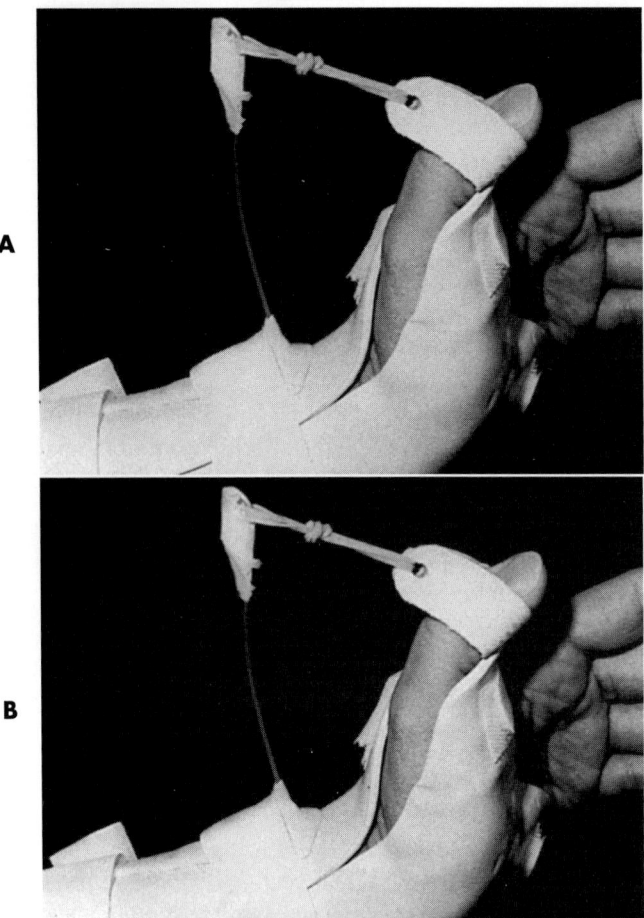

A

B

Fig. 31-30. A, The repaired extensor pollicis longus in zones IV and V is splinted with the wrist extended, carpometacarpal joint in neutral, metacarpophalangeal joint at 0 degrees, and interphalangeal joint resting at 0 degrees of extension in the dynamic traction. **B,** The patient actively flexes the distal joint through its available range (not to exceed 60 degrees) intermittently every hour to effect the 5 mm of glide at the level of Lister's tubercle (From Evans RB, Burkhalter WE: *J Hand Surg* 11A:774, 1986).

wrist is moved to a 0-degree position while the thumb kinetic chain is held in maximum extension, the thumb is relaxed, and the wrist is moved to full extension. To ensure that the tendon repair site is truly migrating proximally, I also add a component of "active hold." After the passive exercise, which will help minimize drag by reducing the resistance of edema and joint stiffness, the wrist is placed in 20 degrees of flexion while the CMC, MP, and IP joints are held in extension and the patient is asked to gently maintain this position. The wrist position of minimal flexion reduces the elastic drag of the antagonistic flexor pollicis longus (FPL) and thus reduces the internal force applied to the repair with the active hold portion of the exercise.[58] The patient may come out of the protective splint during exercise and for showering during the third to fourth weeks, but splint protection should be maintained otherwise. Each joint

should be moved actively into graded increments of flexion while all other joints in the thumb and the wrist are held in extension during the third and fourth weeks. By the fifth week, composite thumb flexion and opposition exercises may be initiated. Modalities and schedules for adding resistance for the tendon at this level are the same as for the digit. Continuous repetitive motions or overuse of therapy putty may inflame the tendons in the first dorsal compartment, creating a de Quervain's tendonitis in the overambitious patient trying to regain flexion.

Considerations for the rheumatoid tendon

Tendon rehabilitation in the rheumatoid hand is complicated by altered biomechanics created by lost pulleys, subluxed tendons, imbalances between the intrinsic and extrinsic tendon systems,[30,61] the effects of immobilization on the diseased joints, and the integrity of the tendon before rupture or laceration.[61,142]

The type of repair—end-to-end anastomosis, suture of the distal stump to an adjacent tendon, or tendon transfer—will affect the immobilization and early motion schedules. The therapist should estimate the tensile strength of the repair based on the type of suture used,[58] adjust this number to accommodate a decrease in strength that may be associated with each postoperative day, and adjust again for delayed healing that could be associated with poor tissue or steroid use. I have used the SAM program successfully for extensor reconstruction in the rheumatoid hand in zone III and have used early motion with the stronger repairs in zones V, VI, VII, and T-V (e.g., a modified Kessler or Bunnell with an epitenon stitch, or a Pulvertaft weave with tendon transfer). The application of force with passive motion or active motion should be calculated as outlined earlier in this chapter and then applied only if there is a safety margin between the tensile strength of the repair and the application of force with controlled motion. Early motion to the distal joints will be especially important in these hands to prevent a loss of joint motion. These patients often have more problems with postsurgical bleeding or hematoma because of their medications, so again early motion is important to control adhesions as they form. Extensor lag with all zones will be more of an issue in the rheumatoid hand, so it is especially important to allow these tendons to heal with no tension in the position of immobilization. Splint protection probably should exceed that cited earlier for normal tendons by a few weeks.

Repairs in zones V, VI, and VII associated with intrinsic tightness should be splinted with the MP joints at 0 degrees and the fingers free at the PIP joints and distal during the immobilization stage. This position protects the repairs but puts the digits in a position for intrinsic stretch. If the dynamic extension splint for early passive motion is used and there are swan-neck deformities, the digits should be splinted within their slings with a dorsal static two-joint splint that positions the PIP joints in 30 degrees of flexion

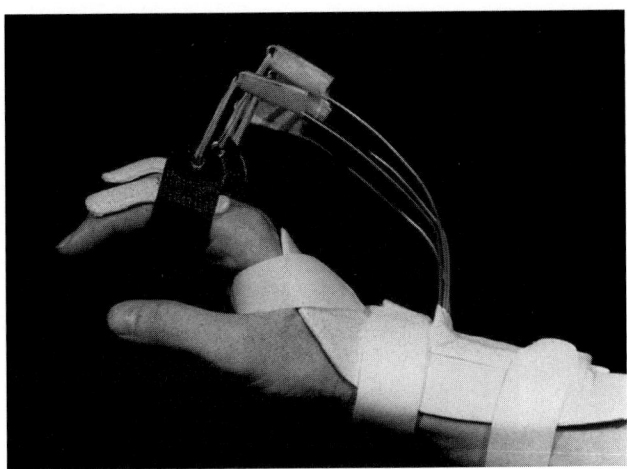

Fig. 31-31. Swan-neck deformities should be counterbalanced with digital splinting to help transmit extensor forces to the zone V and VI levels when active extension exercise is initiated.

(Fig. 31-31). This splint arrangement allows proximal joint flexion, inhibits the swan deformity, and helps transmit the forces of passive motion to the more proximal zones. This same digital splint arrangement should be continued in the active stages of rehabilitation. The goal with extensor repair in the more proximal zones associated with swan-neck deformity is to facilitate MP extension, PIP joint flexion, and intrinsic stretch.

SUMMARY

Extensor tendon management after surgery has changed dramatically over the past decade from prolonged periods of immobilization to shorter periods of immobilization, controlled passive motion programs, and minimal active muscle-tendon tension programs. Investigators have demonstrated clinically that extensor tendon in all zones except I, II, T-I, and T-II benefit from immediate short arc motion at the joint associated with the repair and some controlled motion at the wrist level. The concepts of immediate motion are supported biochemically in experimental studies, biomechanically through excursion studies, through mathematic analysis of excursion and force application, and through analysis of tendon repair tensile strengths. Meticulous care in the control of edema, postoperative splinting, and controlled motion programs will greatly improve the results of both the simple and complex extensor tendon injury not only in terms of function achieved but in terms of time and expense.

REFERENCES

1. Abrahamsson SO: Matrix metabolism and healing in the flexor tendon: experimental studies on rabbit tendon, *Scand J Plast Reconstr Surg Hand Surg Suppl* 23:1, 1991.
2. Agee J, Guidera M: The functional significance of the juncturae tendineae in dynamic stabilization of the metacarpophalangeal joints of the fingers. ASSH proceedings, *J Hand Surg* 5:288, 1980.
3. Akeson WH, et al: Collagen cross-linking, alterations in joint contractures: changes in the reducible cross-links in periarticular connective tissue collagen after nine weeks of immobilization, *Connect Tissue Res* 5:15, 1977.
4. Allieu Y, Ascenio G, Rouzaud JC: Protected passive mobilization after suturing the extensor tendons of the hand: a survey of 120 cases. In Hunter JM, Schneider LH, Mackin EJ, editors: *Tendon surgery in the hand,* St Louis, 1987, Mosby.
5. Amadio PC: Tendon and ligament. In Cohen IK, Diegelmann RF, Lindblad WJ, editors: *Wound healing: biochemical and clinical aspects,* Philadelphia, 1992, WB Saunders.
6. Amiel D, et al: Fibronectin in healing flexor tendons subjected to immobilization or early controlled passive motion, *Matrix* 2:184, 1991.
7. Amiel D, et al: The effect of immobilization on collagen turnover in connective tissue: a biochemical-biomechanical correlation, *Acta Orthop Scand* 53:325, 1982.
8. An KN, et al: Tendon excursion and moment arm of index finger muscles, *J Biomech* 16:419, 1983.
9. Andriacchi T, et al: Ligament: injury and repair. In Woo SL-Y, Buckwalter JA, editors: *Injury and repair of the musculoskeletal soft tissues,* Park Ridge, Ill, 1988, American Academy of Orthopaedic Surgeons.
10. Aoki M, Ogiwara N, Nabeta Y: Early active motion and weightbearing after cross-stitch Achilles tendon repair, *Am J Sports Med* 26:794, 1998.
11. Aspenberg P, Forslund C: Enhanced tendon healing with GDF 5 and 6, *Acta Orthop Scand* 70:51, 1999.
12. Bassett AL: Effect of force on skeletal tissues. In Downey JA, Darling RC, editors: *Physiological basis of rehabilitation medicine,* Philadelphia, 1971, WB Saunders.
13. Beasley RW: *Hand injuries,* Philadelphia, 1981, WB Saunders.
14. Becker H: Primary repair of flexor tendons in the hand without immobilization: preliminary report, *Hand* 10:37, 1978.
15. Becker H, Diegelman RF: The influence of tension on intrinsic tendon fibroplasia, *Orthop Rev* 13:65, 1984.
16. Boland D: Anatomical and biomechanical observations of the extensor retinaculum. Scientific poster session, 41st annual meeting of the American Society of Hand Surgeons, New Orleans, Feb 1986.
17. Boozer JA, Sanson MS, Soutas-Little RW: Comparison of the biomechanical motions and forces of high versus low-profile dynamic splinting, *J Hand Ther* 7:171, 1994.
18. Bowers WH: The anatomy of the interphalangeal joints. In Bowers WH, editor: *The interphalangeal joints,* New York, 1987, Churchill Livingstone.
19. Boyes WH: *Bunnell's surgery of the hand,* Philadelphia, 1970, JB Lippincott.
20. Brand PW, Hollister A: *Clinical mechanics of the hand,* ed 2, St Louis, 1993, Mosby.
21. Brand PW, Thompson DE: Mechanical resistance. In Brand PW, Hollister A, editors: *Clinical mechanics of the hand,* ed 2, St Louis, 1993, Mosby.
22. Brand PW, Thompson DE, Micks JE: The biomechanics of the interphalangeal joints. In Bowers WH, editor: *The interphalangeal joints,* New York, 1987, Churchill Livingstone.
23. Breger-Lee D, Bell-Krotoski J, Brandsma JW: Torque range of motion in the hand clinic, *J Hand Ther* 3:14, 1990.
24. Browne EZ, Ribik CA: Early dynamic splinting for extensor tendon injuries, *J Hand Surg* 14A:72, 1989.
25. Brunelli G, Vigasio A, Brunelli F: Slip-knot flexor tendon suture in zone II allowing immediate mobilization, *Hand* 15:352, 1983.
26. Buckwalter JA: Effects of early motion on healing of musculoskeletal tissues, *Hand Clin* 12:13, 1996.
27. Buckwalter JA, Grodzinsky AJ: Loading of healing bone, fibrous tissue and muscle: implications for orthopaedic practice, *J Am Acad Orthop Surg* 7:291, 1999.

28. Buckwalter J, et al: Articular cartilage, injury and repair. In Woo SL-Y, Buckwalter JA, editors: *Injury and repair of the musculoskeletal soft tissues,* Park Ridge, Ill, 1988, American Academy of Orthopaedic Surgeons.

29. Burkhalter WE: Wound classification and management. In Hunter JM, et al, editors: *Rehabilitation of the hand,* ed 3, St Louis, 1990, Mosby.

30. Burkhalter WE: Altered dorsal mechanics in the rheumatoid hand, *J Hand Ther* 2:114, 1989.

31. Chang J, et al: Molecular studies in flexor tendon wound healing: the role of basic fibroblast growth factor gene expression, *J Hand Surg* 23A:1052, 1998.

32. Chang J, et al: Studies in flexor tendon wound healing: neutralizing antibody to TGF-beta 1 increases postoperative range of motion, *Plast Reconstr Surg* 105:148, 2000.

33. Chow JA, et al: Postoperative management of repair of extensor tendons of the hand…dynamic splinting versus static splinting, *Orthop Trans* 11:258, 1987.

34. Close JR, Kidd CC: The functions of muscles of the thumb, the index, and the long finger, *J Bone Joint Surg* 51A:1601, 1969.

35. Cooney WP, Lin GT, An KN: Improved tendon excursion following flexor tendon repair, *J Hand Ther* 2:102, 1989.

36. Crosby CA, Wehbe MA: Early protected motion after extensor tendon repair, *J Hand Surg* 24A:1061, 1999.

37. Cullen KW, et al: Flexor tendon repair in zone II followed by controlled active mobilization, *J Hand Surg* 14B:392, 1989.

38. Dagum AB, Mahoney JL: Effect of wrist position on extensor mechanism after disruption separation, *J Hand Surg* 19A:584, 1994.

39. Dahners LE: Ligament contraction. A correlation with cellularity and actin staining, *Trans Orthop Res Soc* 11:56, 1986.

40. DeVoll JR, Saldana MJ: Excursion of finger extensor elements in zone III. Presented at the annual meeting of the American Association for Hand Surgery, Toronto, 1988.

41. Din KM, Maggitt BF: Mallet thumb, *J Bone Joint Surg* 66B:606, 1983.

42. Dobbe JG, et al: A portable device for finger tendon rehabilitation that provides an isotonic training force and records exercise behavior after finger tendon surgery, *Med Biol Eng Comput* 37:396, 1999.

43. Doyle JR: Extensor tendons…acute injuries. In Green DP, editor: *Operative hand surgery,* ed 4, New York, 1999, Churchill Livingstone.

44. Duran RJ, Houser RG: Controlled passive motion following flexor tendon repair in zones II and III. In *The American Academy of Orthopaedic Surgeons: symposium on tendon surgery in the hand,* St Louis, 1975, Mosby.

45. Ejeskar A, Irstam L: Elongation in profundus tendon repair. A radiological and clinical study, *Scand J Plast Surg* 15:61, 1981.

46. Elliot D, McGrouther DA: The excursions of the long extensor tendons of the hand, *J Hand Surg [Br]* 11:77, 1986.

47. Enwemeka CS, Rodriguez O, Mendoza S: The biomechanical effects of low intensity ultrasound on healing, *Ultrasound Med Biol* 16:807, 1990.

48. Evans CH: Cytokines and the role they play in the healing of ligaments and tendons, *Sports Med* 28:71, 1999.

49. Evans RB: Therapeutic management of extensor tendon injuries, *Hand Clin* 2:157, 1986.

50. Evans RB: Clinical application of controlled stress to the healing extensor tendon: a review of 112 cases, *Phys Ther* 68:1041, 1989.

51. Evans RB: Early active short arc motion for the repaired central slip, *J Hand Surg* 19A:991, 1994.

52. Evans RB: Immediate active short arc motion following extensor tendon repair, *Hand Clin* 11:483, 1995.

53. Evans RB: Rehabilitation techniques for applying immediate active tension to zone I and zone II flexor tendon repairs, *Tech Hand Upper Extremity Surg* 1:286, 1997.

54. Evans RB: Rehabilitation techniques for applying immediate active tension to the repaired extensor system, *Tech Hand Upper Extremity Surg* 3:139, 1999.

55. Evans RB, Burkhalter WE: A study of the dynamic anatomy of extensor tendons and implications for treatment, *J Hand Surg* 11A:774, 1986.

56. Evans RB, Hunter JM, Burkhalter WE: Conservative management of the trigger finger: a new approach, *J Hand Ther* 1:59, 1988.

57. Evans RB, Thompson DE: An analysis of factors that support early active short arc motion of the repaired central slip, *J Hand Ther* 5:187, 1992.

58. Evans RB, Thompson DE: The application of stress to the healing tendon, *J Hand Ther* 6:262, 1993.

59. Evans RB, Thompson DE: Immediate active short arc motion following tendon repair. In Hunter JM, Schneider LH, Mackin EJ, editors: *Tendon and nerve surgery in the hand: a third decade,* St Louis, 1997, Mosby.

60. Fahrer M: Interdependent and independent actions of the fingers. In Tubiana R, editor: *The hand,* vol 1, Philadelphia, 1981, WB Saunders.

61. Flatt AE: *Care of the arthritic hand,* ed 4, St Louis, 1983, Mosby.

62. Flowers K, La Stayo P: Effect of total end range time on improving passive range of motion, *J Hand Ther* 7:150, 1994.

63. Freehan LM, Beauchene JG: Early tensile properties of healing chicken flexor tendons: early controlled passive motion versus postoperative immobilization, *J Hand Surg* 15A:63, 1990.

64. Froelich JA, Akelman E, Herndon JH: Extensor tendon injuries at the proximal interphalangeal joint. In Burton RI, editor: *Hand clinics,* Philadelphia, 1988, WB Saunders.

65. Garcia-Elias M, et al: Extensor mechanism of the fingers. II. Tensile properties of components, *J Hand Surg* 16A:1136, 1991.

66. Gelberman RH, Manske PR: Effects of early motion on the tendon healing process: experimental studies. In Hunter JM, et al, editors: *Tendon surgery in the hand,* St Louis, 1987, Mosby.

67. Gelberman RH, et al: The effects of mobilization on the vascularization of healing flexor tendons in dogs, *Clin Orthop* 153:283, 1980.

68. Gelberman RH, et al: The influence of protected passive mobilization on the healing of flexor tendons: a biomechanical and microangiographic study, *Hand* 13:120, 1981.

69. Gelberman RH, et al: Effects of intermittent passive mobilization on healing canine flexor tendons, *J Hand Surg* 7:170, 1982.

70. Gelberman RH, et al: Flexor tendon healing and restoration of the gliding surface: an ultrastructural study in dogs, *J Bone Joint Surg* 65A:70, 1983.

71. Gelberman RH, et al: The early stages of flexor tendon healing: a morphologic study of the first fourteen days, *J Hand Surg* 10A:776, 1985.

72. Gelberman RH, et al: The excursion and deformation of repaired flexor tendons treated with protected early motion, *J Hand Surg* 11A:106, 1986.

73. Gelberman RH, et al: Influences of flexor sheath continuity and early motion on tendon healing in dogs, *J Hand Surg* 15A:69, 1990.

74. Gelberman RH, et al: Fibroblast chemotaxis after repair, *J Hand Surg* 16A:686, 1991.

75. Gelberman RH, et al: Healing of digital flexor tendons: importance of time between injury and operative repair: a biomechanical, biochemical, and morphological study in dogs, *J Bone Joint Surg Am* 73:66, 1991.

76. Gelberman RH, et al: Influences of the protected passive mobilization interval on flexor tendon healing: a prospective randomized clinical study, *Clin Orthop* 264:189, 1991.

77. Gelberman RH, et al: The effect of gap formation at the repair site on the strength and excursion of intrasynovial flexor tendons. An experimental study on the early stages of tendon-healing in dogs, *J Bone Joint Surg* 81A:975, 1999.

78. Haddad RJ, et al: Comparative mechanical analysis of a looped suture tendon repair, *J Hand Surg* 13A:709, 1988.

79. Hagberg L, Selvik G: Tendon excursion and dehiscence during early controlled mobilization after flexor tendon repair in zone II: an x-ray stereophotogrammetric analysis, *J Hand Surg* 16A:669, 1992.

80. Hall B, Newman S: *Cartilage, molecular aspects,* Boca Raton, Fla, 1991, CRC Press.
81. Harmer TW: Tendon suture, *Boston Med Surg J* 177:808, 1917.
82. Harmer TW: Certain aspects of hand surgery, *N Engl J Med* 214:613, 1936.
83. Harwood FL, et al: Regulation of alpha(v)beta3 and alpha5beta1 integrin receptors by basic fibroblast growth factor and platelet-derived growth factor BB in intrasynovial flexor tendon cells, *Wound Repair Regen* 7:381, 1999.
84. Hitchcock TF, et al: The effect of immediate constrained digital motion on the strength of flexor tendon repairs in chickens, *J Hand Surg* 12A:590, 1987.
85. Hobby J: Postoperative edema. In Tubiana R, editor: *The hand,* Philadelphia, 1985, WB Saunders.
86. Holdeman V: Rehabilitation of extensor tendon injuries. In Hunter JM, et al, editors: *Rehabilitation of the hand,* St Louis, 1987, Mosby.
87. Honner R: Acute and chronic flexor and extensor mechanism injuries at the distal joint. In Bowers WH, editor: *The interphalangeal joints,* New York, 1987, Churchill Livingstone.
88. Horibe S, et al: Excursion of the human flexor digitorum profundus tendon: a kinematic study of the human and canine digits, *J Orthop Res* 8:167, 1990.
89. Horii E, et al: Comparative flexor tendon excursions after passive mobilization: an in vitro study, *J Hand Surg* 17A:559, 1992.
90. Howard RF, Ondrovic L, Greenwald DP: Biomechanical analysis of four-strand extensor tendon repair techniques, *J Hand Surg* 22A:838, 1997.
91. Howell JW, et al: Immediate controlled active motion following zone 4-7 extensor tendon repair. American Society of Hand Therapists Annual Meeting, Orlando, Fla, September 1999.
92. Hung LK, et al: Early controlled active mobilization with dynamic splintage for extensor tendon injuries, *J Hand Surg* 15A:251, 1990.
93. Hurlbut PT, Adams BD: Analysis of finger extensor mechanical strains, *J Hand Surg* 20A:832, 1995.
94. Huys S, et al: The effects of ultrasound on flexor tendon healing in the chicken limb, *J Hand Surg* 20B:809, 1995.
95. Ikegami H: Experimental study on the effects of tension-reduced early mobilization on extensor tendon healing, *Nippon Seikeigeka Gakkai Zasshi* 69:493, 1995.
96. Ip WY, Chow SP: Results of dynamic splintage following extensor tendon repair, *J Hand Surg* 22B:283, 1997.
97. Iselin F: Boutonniere deformity treatment. In Hunter JM, Schneider LH, Mackin EJ, editors: *Tendon and nerve surgery: a third decade,* St Louis, 1997, Mosby.
98. Iselin F: Reconstruction techniques for treating mallet finger. In Hunter JM, Schneider LH, Mackin EJ, editors: *Tendon surgery in the hand,* St Louis, 1987, Mosby.
99. Iselin F, Lerame J, Godoy J: A simplified technique for treating mallet fingers: tenodermodesis, *J Hand Surg* 2:118, 1977.
100. Ishii Y, et al: Effects of hyperbaric oxygen on procollagen messenger RNA levels and collagen synthesis in the healing of rat tendon laceration, *Tissue Eng* 5:279, 1999.
101. Iwuagwu FC, McGrouther DA: Early cellular response in tendon injury: the effect of loading, *Plast Reconstr Surg* 102:2064, 1998.
102. Jann HW, Stein LE, Slater DA: In vitro effects of epidermal growth factor or insulin-like growth factor on tenoblast migration on absorbable suture material, *Vet Surg* 28:26, 1999.
103. Joyce ME, Lou J, Manske PR: Tendon healing: molecular and cellular regulation. In Hunter JM, Schneider LH, Mackin EJ, editors: *Tendon and nerve surgery in the hand: a third decade,* St Louis, 1997, Mosby.
104. Jrvinen TA, et al: Mechanical loading regulates tenascin-C expression in the osteotendinous junction, *J Cell Sci* 112:315, 1999.
105. Kang HJ, Kang ES: Ideal concentration of growth factors in rabbit's flexor tendon culture, *Yonsei Med J* 40:26, 1999.
106. Kapandji IA: Biomechanics of the thumb. In Tubiana R, editor: *The hand,* Philadelphia, 1985, WB Saunders.
107. Kaplan EB: *Functional and surgical anatomy of the hand,* ed 2, Philadelphia, 1965, JB Lippincott.
108. Katzman BM, et al: Immobilization of the mallet finger: effects of the extensor tendon, *J Hand Surg* 24B:1:80, 1999.
109. Kerr CD, Burczak JR: Dynamic traction after extensor tendon repair in zones 6, 7, 8: a retrospective study, *J Hand Surg* 14B:21, 1989.
110. Khan U, et al: Differences in proliferative rate and collagen lattice contraction between endotenon and synovial fibroblasts, *J Hand Surg* 23A:266, 1998.
111. Khandwala AR, et al: A comparison of dynamic extension splinting and controlled active mobilization of complete divisions of extensor tendons in zones 5 and 6, *J Hand Surg* 25B:140, 2000.
112. Kleinert HE, Kutz JE, Cohen MJ: Primary repair of zone II flexor tendon lacerations. In *AAOS symposium on tendon surgery in the hand,* St Louis, 1975, Mosby.
113. Kleinert HE, Verdan C: Report of the committee on tendon injuries, *J Hand Surg* 8:795, 1983.
114. Kubota H, et al: Effect of motion and tension on injured tendons in chickens, *J Hand Surg* 21A:456, 1996.
115. Lahey F: A tendon suture which permits immediate motion, *Boston Med Surg J* 188:851, 1923.
116. Landsmeer JMF: The anatomy of the dorsal aponeurosis of the human figure and its functional significance, *Anat Rec* 104:31, 1949.
117. Lane JM, Black J, Bora FW: Gliding function following flexor tendon injury: a biomechanical study of rat tendon function, *J Bone Joint Surg* 58A:985, 1976.
118. Lee H: Double loop locking suture: a technique of tendon repair for early active mobilization. Part I, *J Hand Surg* 15A:945, 1990.
119. Lee H: Double loop locking suture: a technique of tendon repair for early active mobilization. Part II, *J Hand Surg* 15A:953, 1990.
120. Lexer E: Verwethung der freien sehnentransplantation, *Arch Klin Chir* 98:818, 1912.
121. Lin GT, et al: Biomechanical studies of running suture for flexor tendon repair in dogs, *J Hand Surg* 13A:553, 1988.
122. Lindsay WK, Thompson HG, Walker FG: Digital flexor tendons: an experimental study. Part II. The significance of a gap occurring at the line of suture, *Br J Plast Surg* 13:1, 1960.
123. Linsky CB, Rovee DT, Dow T: Effect of dressing on wound inflammation and scar tissue. In Dineen P, Hildick-Smith G, editors: *The surgical wound,* Philadelphia, 1981, Lea & Febiger.
124. Littler JW, Thompson JS: Surgical and functional anatomy. In Bowers WH, editor: *The interphalangeal joints,* New York, 1987, Churchill Livingstone.
125. Long CH: Intrinsic-extrinsic muscle control of the finger electromyographic studies, *J Bone Joint Surg* 52A:853, 1970.
126. Long CH: Electromyographic studies of hand function. In Tubiana R, editor: *The hand,* vol 1, Philadelphia, 1981, WB Saunders.
127. Lou J, et al: In vivo gene transfer and overexpression of focal adhesion kinase (pp125 FAK) mediated by recombinant adenovirus-induced tendon adhesion formation and epitenon cell change, *J Orthop Res* 15:911, 1997.
128. Lovett WL, McCalla MA: Management and rehabilitation of extensor tendon injuries, *Orthop Clin North Am* 44:811, 1983.
129. Macht SD, Watson HK: The Moberg volar advancement flap for digital reconstruction, *J Hand Surg* 5:372, 1980.
130. MacMillan M, Sheppard JE, Dell PC: An experimental flexor tendon repair in zone II that allows immediate postoperative mobilization, *J Hand Surg* 12A:582, 1986.
131. Madden KN, et al: Resorbable and non-resorbable augmentation devices for tenorrhaphy of xenografts in extensor tendon deficits: 12 week study, *Biomaterials* 18:225, 1997.
132. Maddy LS, Meyerdierdierks EM: Dynamic extension assist splinting of acute central slip lacerations, *J Hand Ther* 10:206, 1997.
133. Mak AF: The apparent viscoelastic behavior of articular cartilage, the contributions from the intrinsic matrix viscoelasticity and interstitial fluid flows, *J Biomech Eng* 108:123, 1986.

134. Manske PR: Flexor tendon healing, *J Hand Surg* 13B:237, 1988.

135. Manske PR, Lesker PA: Nutrient pathways to extensor tendons within the extensor retinacular compartments, *Clin Orthop* 181:234, 1983.

136. Mason ML, Allen HS: The rate of healing tendons: an experimental study of tensile strength, *Ann Surg* 113:424, 1941.

137. Matsui T, Hunter JM: Injury to the vascular system and its effect on tendon injury in no man's land. In Hunter JM, Schneider LH, Mackin EJ, editors: *Tendon and nerve surgery in the hand: a third decade,* St Louis, 1997, Mosby.

138. Matthews JP: Early mobilization after flexor tendon repair, *J Hand Surg* 14B:363, 1989.

139. McDowell CL, Snyder DM: Tendon healing: an experimental model in the dog, *J Hand Surg* 2:122, 1977.

140. Messina A: The double armed suture: tendon repair with immediate mobilization of the fingers, *J Hand Surg* 17A:137, 1992.

141. Micks J, Reswick J: Confirmation of differential loading of lateral and central fibers of the extensor tendon, *J Hand Surg* 6:462, 1981.

142. Millender LH, Nalebuff EA, Feldon PG: Rheumatoid arthritis. In Green DP, editor: *Operative hand surgery,* ed 2, New York, 1988, Churchill Livingstone.

143. Minamikawa Y, et al: Wrist position and extensor tendon amplitude following repair, *J Hand Surg* 17A:268, 1992.

144. Miura T, Ryogo N, Shuhei T: Conservative treatment for a ruptured extensor tendon on the dorsum of the proximal phalanges of the thumb (mallet thumb), *J Hand Surg* 11A:229, 1986.

145. Mow V, Rosenwasser M: Articular cartilage: biomechanics. In Woo SL-Y, Buckwalter JA, editors: *Injury and repair of the musculoskeletal soft tissues,* Park Ridge, Ill, 1988, American Academy of Orthopaedic Surgeons.

146. Nakamura K, Nanjyo B: Reassessment of surgery for mallet finger, *Plast Reconstr Surg* 93:141, 1994.

147. Niessen FB, et al: The use of silicone occlusive sheeting (Sil-K) and silicone occlusive gel (Epiderm) in the prevention of hypertrophic scar formation, *Plast Reconstr Surg* 102:1962, 1998.

148. Newport ML, Blair WF, Steyers CM: Long-term results of extensor tendon repair, *J Hand Surg* 15A:961, 1990.

149. Newport ML, Pollack GR, Williams CD: Biomechanical characteristics of suture techniques in extensor zone IV, *J Hand Surg* 20A:650, 1995.

150. Newport ML, Shukla A: Electrophysiologic basis of dynamic extensor splinting, *J Hand Surg* 17A:272, 1992.

151. Newport ML, Williams D: Biomechanical characteristics of extensor tendon suture techniques, *J Hand Surg* 17A:1117, 1992.

152. Nussbaum E: The influence of ultrasound on healing tissues, *J Hand Ther* 11:140, 1998.

153. O'Dwyer FG, Quinton DN: Early mobilization of acute central slip injuries, *J Hand Surg* 15B:404, 1990.

154. Pan Z, Wang C, Zhou W: The effect of repair of paratenon in tendon healing, *Cjung Kuo Hsiu Fu Chung Chien Ko Tsa Chih* 11:279, 1997.

155. Patel MR, Desai SS, Bassini-Lipson L: Conservative management of the mallet finger, *J Hand Surg* 11A:570, 1986.

156. Peacock EE: Collagen metabolism during healing of long tendons. In Hunter JM, et al, editors: *Tendon surgery in the hand,* St Louis, 1987, Mosby.

157. Potenza AD: Concepts of tendon healing and repair. In *American Academy of Orthopaedic Surgeons symposium on tendon surgery in the hand,* ed 2, St Louis, 1975, Mosby.

158. Primano GA: Conservative treatment of two cases of mallet thumb, *J Hand Surg* 11A:233, 1986.

159. Pruitt DL, Manske PR, Fink B: Cyclic stress analysis of flexor tendon repair, *J Hand Surg* 16A:701, 1991.

160. Purcell T, et al: Static splinting of extensor tendon repair, *J Hand Surg* 25B:180, 2000.

161. Rantanen J, Hurme T, Kalimo H: Calf muscle atrophy and Achilles tendon healing following experimental tendon division and surgery in rats: comparison of postoperative immobilization of the muscle tendon complex in relaxed and tension positions, *Scand J Med Sci Sports* 9:57, 1999.

162. Rayan GM, Mullins PT: Skin necrosis complicating mallet finger splinting and vascularity of the distal interphalangeal joint overlying skin, *J Hand Surg* 12A:548, 1987.

163. Reddy GK, et al: Biochemistry and biomechanics of healing tendon: part II. Effects of combined laser therapy and electrical stimulation, *Med Sci Sports Exerc* 30:794, 1998.

164. Reiffel RS: Prevention of hypertrophic scars by long-term paper tape application, *Plast Reconstr Surg* 96:1715, 1995.

165. Robotti E, et al: The effect of pulsed electronic fields on flexor tendon healing in chickens, *J Hand Surg* 24B:56, 1999.

166. Rosenthal EA. Dynamics of the extensor system. In Hunter JM, Schneider LH, Mackin EJ, editors: *Tendon and nerve surgery in the hand: a third decade,* St Louis, 1997, Mosby.

167. Rosenthal EA: The anatomy and management of extensor tendons. In Hunter JM, et al, editors: *Rehabilitation of the hand,* ed 4, St Louis, 1997, Mosby.

168. Rosenthal EA: Extensor surface injuries at the proximal interphalangeal joint. In Bowers WH, editor: *The interphalangeal joints,* New York, 1987, Churchill Livingstone.

169. Rothkopf DM, et al: An experimental model for the study of canine flexor tendon adhesions, *J Hand Surg* 16A:694, 1991.

170. Rouzaud JC, et al: Mesure de la tension differentielle du systeme extenseur au niveau de la PIP. Paris, France, Second International Congress, International Federation of Societies of Hand Therapists, May 19, 1992.

171. Saldana MJ, et al: Results of acute zone III extensor tendon injuries treated with dynamic extension splinting, *J Hand Surg* 16A:1145, 1999.

172. Salter RB, et al: Continuous passive motion and the repair of full-thickness articular cartilage defects: a one-year followup, *Trans Orthop Res Soc* 7:167, 1982.

173. Salter RB, et al: The biological effect of continuous passive motion on healing of full-thickness defects in articular cartilage: an experimental study in the rabbit, *J Bone Joint Surg* 61A:1232, 1980.

174. Savage R: The influence of wrist position on the minimum force required for active movement of the interphalangeal joints, *J Hand Surg* 13B:262, 1988.

175. Savage R, Ristano G: Flexor tendon repair using a "six strand" method of repair and early active mobilization, *J Hand Surg* 14B:396, 1989.

176. Schneider LH, Smith KL: Boutonnière deformity. In Hunter JM, Schneider LH, Mackin EJ, editors: *Tendon surgery in the hand,* St Louis, 1987, Mosby.

177. Seradge H: Elongation of the repair configuration following flexor tendon repair, *J Hand Surg* 8:182, 1983.

178. Seyfer AE, Bolger WE: Effects of unrestricted motion on healing: a study of post traumatic adhesions in primate tendons, *Plast Reconstr Surg* 83:122, 1989.

179. Silva MJ, et al: Effects of increased in vivo excursion on digital range of motion and tendon strength following flexor tendon repair, *J Orthop Res* 17:777, 1999.

180. Silverskiold KL, Anderson CH: Two new methods of tendon repair: an in vitro evaluation of tensile strengths and gap formation, *J Hand Surg* 18A:58, 1993.

181. Silverskiold KL, May EJ, Tornvall AH: Gap formation during controlled motion after flexor tendon repair in zone II: a prospective clinical study, *J Hand Surg* 17A:539, 1992.

182. Simmons BP, De La Caffiniere JY: Physiology of flexion of the fingers. In Tubiana R, editor: *The hand,* vol 1, Philadelphia, 1981, WB Saunders.

183. Slater RR Jr, Bynom DK: Simplified functional splinting after extensor tenorrhaphy, *J Hand Surg* 22A:445, 1997.

184. Small JO, Brennen MD, Colville J: Early active mobilization following flexor tendon repair in zone II, *J Hand Surg* 14B:383, 1989.

185. Spinner M, Choi BY: Anterior dislocation of the proximal interphalangeal joint, a cause for rupture of the central slip of the extensor mechanism, *J Bone Joint Surg* 52A:1329, 1970.

186. Stehnno-Bittel L, et al: Biochemistry and biomechanics of healing tendon: part I. Effects of rigid plaster casts and functional casts, *Med Sci Sports Exerc* 30:788, 1998.

187. Steindler A: *Kinesiology of the human body under normal and pathological conditions,* Springfield, Ill, 1964, Charles C Thomas.

188. Strickland JW, Glogovac SV: Digital function following flexor tendon repair in zone II: a comparison of immobilization and controlled passive motion techniques, *J Hand Surg* 5:537, 1980.

189. Strickland JW: Flexor tendon injuries. I. Foundations of treatment, *J Am Acad Orthop Surg* 3:44, 1995.

190. Strickland JW: Flexor tendon injuries. II. Operative treatment, *J Am Acad Orthop Surg* 3:55, 1995.

191. Sylaidis P, Youatt M, Logan A: Early active mobilization for extensor tendon injuries, *J Hand Surg* 22B:594, 1997.

192. Takai S, et al: The effects of frequency and duration of controlled passive mobilization on tendon healing, *J Orthop Res* 9:705, 1991.

193. Taleisnik J, et al: The extensor retinaculum of the wrist, *J Hand Surg* 9A:495, 1984.

194. Thomas D, Moutet F, Guinard D: Postoperative management of extensor tendon repairs in zones V, VI and VII, *J Hand Ther* 9:309, 1996.

195. Thomes LJ, Thomes LJ: Early mobilization method for surgically repaired zone III extensor tendons, *J Hand Ther* 8:195, 1995.

196. Thorngate S, Ferguson DJ: Effect of tension on healing of aponeurotic wounds, *Surgery* 44:619, 1958.

197. Trail IA, Powell ES, Noble J: The mechanical strength of various suture techniques, *J Hand Surg* 17B:89, 1992.

198. Tubiana R: Architecture and functions of the hand. In Tubiana R, editor: *The hand,* vol 1, Philadelphia, 1981, WB Saunders.

199. Tubiana R: Tendon lesions: anatomical, pathological and biological considerations. In Tubiana R, editor: *The hand,* vol 3, Philadelphia, 1988, WB Saunders.

200. Tubiana R: Anatomy of the extensor tendon system. In Hunter JM, Schneider LH, Mackin EJ, editors: *Tendon and nerve surgery in the hand: a third decade,* St Louis, 1997, Mosby.

201. Urbaniak JR, Cahill JP, Mortenson RA: Tendon suturing methods: analysis of tensile strength. In *American Academy of Orthopaedic Surgeons symposium on tendon surgery in the hand,* St Louis, 1975, Mosby.

202. Valentine P: The interossei and the lumbricals. In Tubiana R, editor: *The hand,* vol 1, Philadelphia, 1981, WB Saunders.

203. Valentine P: Physiology of extension of the fingers. In Tubiana R, editor: *The hand,* vol 1, Philadelphia, 1981, WB Saunders.

204. Verdan CE: Primary and secondary repair of flexor and extensor tendon injuries. In Flynn JE, editor: *Hand surgery,* Baltimore, 1966, Williams & Wilkins.

205. Viidik A: Tensile strength properties of Achilles tendon systems in trained and untrained rabbits, *Acta Orthop Scand* 40:261, 1969.

206. Wade PJF, Wetherell RG, Amis AA: Flexor tendon repair, significant gain in strength from the Halstead peripheral suture technique, *J Hand Surg* 14B:232, 1989.

207. Walsh MT, et al: Early controlled motion with dynamic splinting versus static splinting for zones III and IV extensor tendon lacerations: a preliminary report, *J Hand Ther* 7:232, 1994.

208. Weber ER: Nutritional pathways for flexor tendons in the digital theca. In Hunter JM, Schneider LH, Mackin EJ, editors: *Tendon surgery in the hand,* St Louis, 1987, Mosby.

209. Wilson CJ, Dahners LE: An examination of the mechanism of ligament contracture, *Clin Orthop* 227:286, 1988.

210. Wilson RL, Fleming F: Treatment of acute extensor tendon injuries. In Hunter JM, Schneider LH, Mackin EJ, editors: *Tendon and nerve surgery in the hand. A third decade,* St Louis, 1997, Mosby.

211. Wiseman DM, et al: Wound dressings: design and use. In Cohen IK, Diegelman RF, Lindblad WJ, editors: *Wound healing. Biochemical and clinical aspects,* Philadelphia, 1992, WB Saunders.

212. Woo SL-Y: Mechanical properties of tendons and ligaments. I. Quasi-static and nonlinear viscoelastic properties, *Biorheology* 19: 385, 1982.

213. Woo SL-Y, Buckwalter JA, editors: *Injury and repair of the musculoskeletal soft tissues,* Park Ridge, Ill, 1988, American Academy of Orthopaedic Surgeons.

214. Woo SL-Y, Mow VC, Lai WM: Biomechanical properties of articular cartilage. In Skalak R, Chein S, editors: *Handbook of bioengineering,* New York, 1987, McGraw-Hill.

215. Woo SL-Y, et al: The biomechanical and biochemical properties of swine tendons: long term effects of exercise on the digital extensors, *Connect Tissue Res* 7:177, 1980.

216. Woo SL-Y, et al: The effects of exercise on the biomechanical and biochemical properties of swine digital flexor tendons, *J Biomech Eng* 103:51, 1981.

217. Woo SL-Y, et al: The importance of controlled passive mobilization on flexor tendon healing: a biomechanical study, *Acta Orthop Scand* 52:615, 1981.

218. Woo SL-Y, et al: Mechanical properties of tendons and ligaments. II. The relationships of immobilization and exercise on tissue remodeling, *Biorheology* 19:397, 1982.

219. Woo SL, et al: Tissue engineering of ligament and tendon healing, *Clin Orthop* 367(suppl):S312, 1999.

220. Zancolli EA: *Structural and dynamic bases of hand surgery,* ed 2, Philadelphia, 1979, JB Lippincott.

221. Zatitisc N, Mazzer N, Barbieri CH: Mechanical strengths of tendon sutures: an in vitro comparative study of six techniques, *J Hand Surg* 23B:228, 1998.

222. Zbrodowski A, Gajisin S, Grodecki J: Vascularization and anatomical model of the mesotenons of the extensor digitorum and extensor indicis muscles, *J Anat* 130:697, 1980.

Part VII

ACUTE NERVE INJURIES

Chapter 32

NERVE RESPONSE TO INJURY AND REPAIR

Kevin L. Smith

CLASSIFICATION OF NERVE INJURY

There are many diverse causes of peripheral nerve dysfunction, and most treatments are outside the scope of the hand surgeon and therapist. Although some of the sequelae of nerve dysfunction can be treated surgically (e.g., tendon transfer or decompression), essentially only traumatic peripheral nerve injuries—transection, crush, compression, and stretch—can be repaired or reconstructed surgically. Because each particular type of nerve injury carries with it a different prognosis; it is important to fully appreciate the effects of each kind of nerve injury and the extent to which they effect the nerve cell, axon, and target organ. With this knowledge, the surgeon and therapist can offer the patient reasonable advice regarding prognosis and the expected results of surgical reconstruction.[118]

Two complementary schemes of classification of peripheral nerve injury are in common use today, and the result of retrospective analysis of the vast experience of Seddon[146] and Sunderland.[163] These classification schemes are based on the degree of disruption of the internal structures of the peripheral nerve—this being closely correlated with prognosis for recovery. The three-part classification scheme devised by Seddon is the less complicated of the two. The mildest form of nerve injury, a localized conduction block, is categorized as a *neuropraxic* injury. Axonal continuity is maintained in this level of injury, and nerve conduction is preserved proximal and distal to the lesion. Recovery is rapid and complete within weeks.[29,72,152,157]

Axonotmesis is the next category of nerve injury. These injuries are more severe, and damage is sufficient to disrupt the continuity of axons within the peripheral nerve. Axonal disruption leads to wallerian degeneration of the distal axon, and the time required to recover depends on the distance

from the injury to the end-organ. Prognosis for functional recovery remains good because the continuity of the supportive connective tissue, satellite cells, and basement membrane remains.[29,72,152,157]

The most severe type of injury in the Seddon classification is the neurotmetic injury. There is complete anatomic disruption of the peripheral nerve, and no recovery can be expected without microcoaptation of the severed nerve ends. Distal degeneration occurs in all of the peripheral nerve axons, and some degree of proximal degeneration occurs.[152]

The classification scheme developed by Sunderland is similar to that of Seddon, but emphasis is placed on the integrity of the fascicular structure of the nerve and the categories are expanded to five[163,165,171] (Fig. 32-1). Sunderland's *first-degree* injury is identical to the *neuropraxic* injury of Seddon. In first-degree injuries, there is a localized conduction block but no disruption of antegrade or retrograde axoplasmic transport. Axonal viability is maintained, and the distal nerve remains capable of stimulation. Clinically, there is a decrease or absence of motor or sensory function that can last from minutes to months.[29,146,163] Second-degree injury is the equivalent of the axonotmetic injury. The axon is severed or severely damaged, and distal (wallerian) degeneration occurs. Because the supporting connective tissue structures remain intact, axonal regeneration is end-organ specific and clinical return of function requires only the time needed for axonal growth.

The third category of Seddon, neuropraxia, correlates with the third-, fourth-, and fifth-degree injuries of the Sunderland classification. In the third-degree injury, nerve fibers are severed along with their endoneurial covering, but the perineurium remains intact. Regeneration occurs, but the reinnervation of target organs is haphazard because

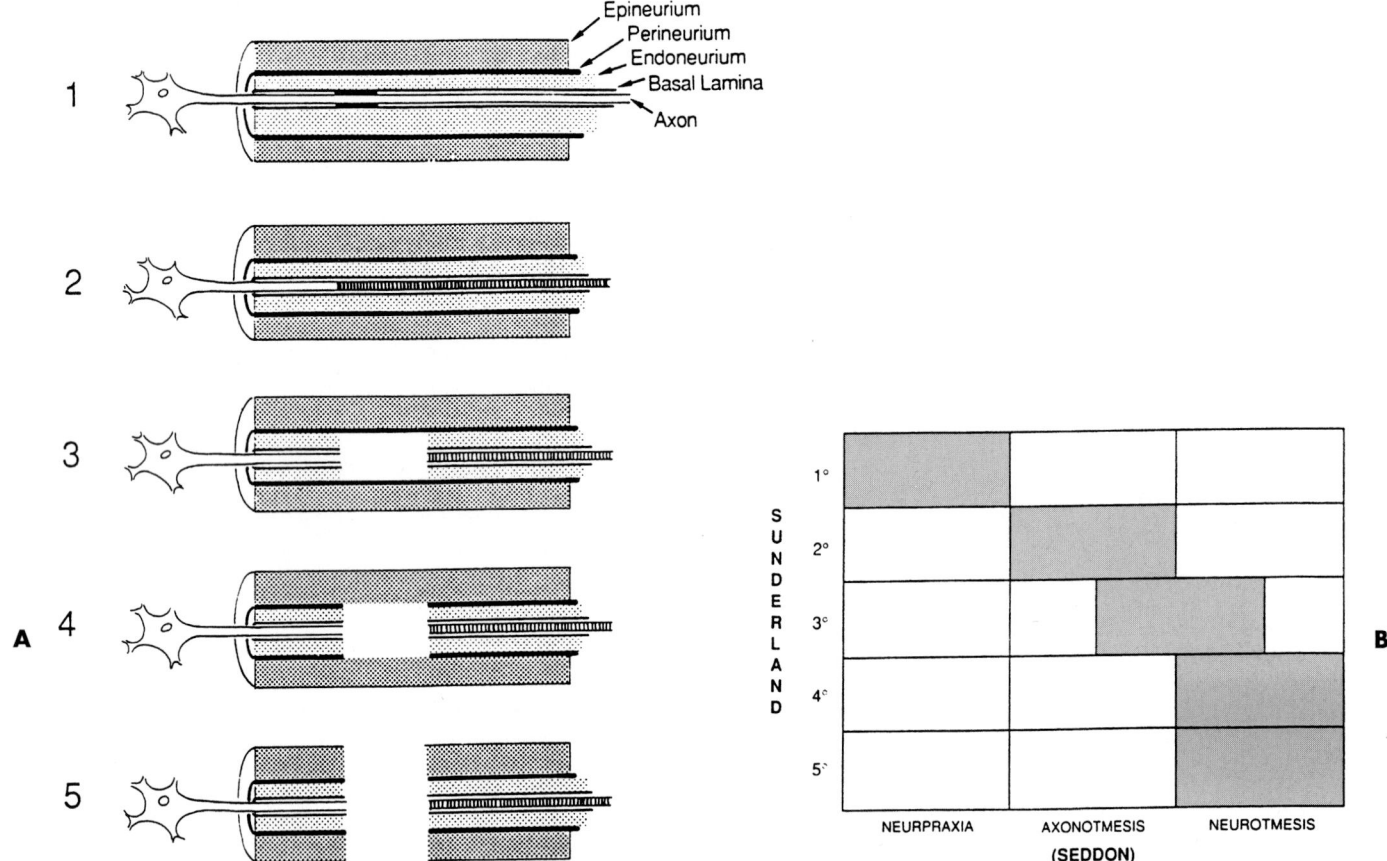

Fig. 32-1. A, Sunderland's classification of nerve injury. *1,* First-degree injury—local conduction blockage with minimal structural disruption. Prognosis: complete recovery within days/months. *2,* Second-degree injury—complete axonal disruption with wallerian degeneration. Basal lamina remains intact. Prognosis: complete recovery in months. *3,* Third-degree injury—axonal and endoneurial disruption with interruption of the basal lamina. Prognosis: intrafascicular axonal admixture with regeneration yields mild/moderate functional reduction. *4,* Fourth-degree injury—axonal, endoneurial, and perineurial disruption. Prognosis: moderate to severe functional loss caused by interfascicular axonal admixture. Microsurgical manipulation can improve prognosis. *5,* Fifth-degree injury—complete structural disruption. Prognosis: no return without microsurgical manipulation. **B,** Comparison of Sunderland's and Seddon's classifications. First-degree injuries correspond to neuropraxic injuries. Second-degree injuries are axonotmetic. Third-degree injuries may be either axonotmetic or neurotmetic, and fourth- and fifth-degree injuries are neurotmetic. (**A** modified from Horn KL, Crumley RL: *Otolaryngol Clin North Am* 17:321, 1984. **B** from Terzis JK, Smith KL: *The peripheral nerve: structure, function and reconstruction,* New York, 1990, Raven Press.)

of *intrafascicular* mixing of the growing axons. The fourth-degree classification includes those nerves in which a more severe injury disrupts the perineurium. Extensive damage to the endoneurial architecture worsens the prognosis for target-specific regeneration because there is extensive *interfascicular* mixing of growing axons. Externally, the epineurium remains intact and the continuity of the nerve trunk is maintained. There is far more extensive intraneural scarring than with lower levels of injury. The fifth-degree injury is the most extensive and refers to complete disruption of the nerve trunk, with little hope of spontaneous recovery of function.[157,163]

It is unfortunate that traumatic nerve injuries infrequently present with clearly defined degrees of injury. Except in severe transection injuries (fourth- and fifth-degree lesions, where all components are, by definition, damaged), nerve injuries have components of first-, second-, and third-degree injuries. For this reason, clinical presentation of nerve injury confronts the surgeon and therapist with a confusing array of findings. Depending on the nerve involved, complex injuries can be clinically confusing, with rapid return of function of a few fibers lending false hope for a favorable outcome.[163,169]

END-ORGAN DENERVATION CHANGES

As long as a nerve cell body remains alive, it has an unlimited potential for regeneration. This is not the case for the sensory or motor end-organ. Peripheral nerve end-organs *require* innervation to stay viable. The loss of the trophic stimulus of the nerve axon dooms the end-organ to atrophy and eventual death. However, this deterioration does differ in time for each kind of end-organ, and the understanding of the pathophysiology of end-organ degeneration will help determine the time constraints for surgical reconstruction.

Sensory end-organs

The response of the sensory end-organ to denervation varies along the continuum from atrophy to frank degeneration and disappearance. This response not only is time dependent but also depends on the life cycle of the receptor in question. Muscle spindles, which undergo no further division after differentiation, respond to denervation by atrophy. Other cell types that are characterized by a short life cycle and high turnover—such as the taste bud—respond to denervation by degeneration and complete disappearance within 1 to 2 weeks.[182] The integrity of sensory receptors apparently depends on an intact nerve fiber, although there need not necessarily be efferent impulses. Spinal ganglia, severed of their connections with the spinal cord, are able to maintain sensory structures as long as the axon is intact.[140] The three most common sensory end-organs—the Meissner corpuscle, the Merkel cell-neurite complex, and the Pacinian corpuscle—have similar responses to denervation. As a result of wallerian degeneration, the axon terminal progressively degenerates over time and is absent by 9 months. The lamellar components of the Meissner corpuscles and the Pacinian corpuscles become atrophic but never completely disappear, as do the supporting structures of the Merkel cell-neurite complex.[15,36,48,83,131] The Merkel cells seem to reduce in number, become atrophic, and possibly even become differentiated into transitional cells or keratinocytes after denervation.[47] If the sensory receptor does proceed to complete degeneration after long-term denervation, it is lost to the receptor pool because the adult mammal appears to have lost the ability to form new sensory receptors de novo.[35,128] The muscle spindle, innervated with both motor and sensory fibers, responds in a similar fashion. When the gamma innervation is severed, the polar regions become atrophic, while the central sensory component (nuclear bag or chain regions) remains intact. When the dorsal roots, which supply the sensory portions, are injured, the central regions decrease in size, lose their equatorial collections of nuclei, and are eventually replaced by striated muscle.[182]

Motor end-organs

After the denervation of skeletal muscle, many changes are apparent. Clinically, the muscle ceases to function and there is gross muscle atrophy. Muscle atrophy after nerve injury results in a decrease of total muscle weight, a loss of total protein, and an overall reduction in muscle cross-sectional area.[34] There is not a decrease in the number of individual muscle fibers, even though there is a relative increase in the amount of connective tissue stroma.[163] Rates of atrophy can vary widely, with reports of as much as a 40% decrease in muscle mass within 1 to 3 weeks of denervation.[140] This does not represent an irreversible degradation, however, and anecdotal reports have documented successful restoration of function after 22 years of denervation.[40] Realistically, however, functional reinnervation is unlikely after 2 years of denervation. Denervated muscles can be made to function by external electrical stimulation, and this can prevent some of the changes caused by denervation.[92-94,137,193] However, the role functional electrical stimulation plays in the reconstruction and rehabilitation of the peripheral nerve injury remains to be seen.

MECHANISMS OF NERVE INJURY

Whenever a patient has sustained a peripheral nerve injury, the treating physician and therapist must fully understand the nature of the injury and the mechanism by which the nerve was injured. Each different type of injury carries with it a different prognosis, and at the time of acute injury, the clinical findings of numbness, paralysis, paresthesia, or pain shed little light on the pathophysiology and ultimate prognosis. By knowing the mechanism of the injury and the pathologic changes produced by that injury, the clinician may better predict the outcome and be better able to plan the care and ultimate reconstruction of the patient's nerve injury.

Nerve injuries can result from many different mechanisms. They can result from compression by internal forces (e.g., tumors, fracture, callus) or by external forces (tourniquet or "crutch palsy"), or from ischemia, traction, x-radiation, inadvertent injection injury, or electrical injury. Although each mechanism represents a different type of injury, all of the injuries result from either mechanical deformation, ischemia-induced metabolic failure, or both.

The first category of injuries result from mechanical deformation. These lesions encompass the entire spectrum of nerve injury from first-degree neuropraxic injuries to fifth-degree injuries. In general, the effects of mechanical deformation depend on the rate of application of the deforming forces, the area of the nerve over which they are applied, and the magnitude of the forces. The regional anatomy of the nerve and its adjacent structures, as well as the nerve's proximity to underlying bone and unyielding fascial bands, must be considered. Internal nerve anatomy also is important. Peripheral nerves organized as a single fascicle are much more vulnerable to injury than nerves consisting of many fascicles surrounded by a larger amount of protective connective tissue.

The mechanisms of injury creating mechanical deformation include acute and chronic compression, crush, and stretch. All of these lesions involve some degree of vascular injury. Occlusion of the supporting vasculature accompanies any deformation and may remain after the release of the deforming force.[142] Recovery may depend on the degree of resultant ischemia that persists.

When a peripheral nerve is subjected to a severe, abruptly applied deforming force, three grades of injury may result. There may be a rapidly reversible physiologic block, a local demyelinating block, or wallerian degeneration.[57] Although it is not completely understood which mechanism— mechanical deformation or ischemia—causes the injury, each factor has some role, and they are probably additive.[8]

Acute compression

Acute compression injuries are especially amenable to experimental examination and can be reproducibly created by the use of a pneumatic tourniquet.[141] At low pressures (up to 30 mm Hg), impaired venular flow is observed[142] and endoneurial fluid pressures are seen to be up to three times normal.[101] Physiologically, decreased nerve conduction velocities are noted.[67] At pressures of 60 mm Hg, nerve-fiber viability is endangered by the creation of a local metabolic block, secondary to ischemia. In addition, at this level of compression, mechanical deformation within the nerve fiber is seen. At higher levels of compression (90 mm Hg and higher), there is even greater mechanical deformation of the axon and the supporting structures (Schwann cells), as well as collapse of the intraneural microcirculation, which is likely to persist upon the release of the deforming force.[101,144]

Application of a tourniquet at pressures above systolic but at levels insufficient to cause cellular damage results in progressive centripetal sensory loss and paralysis within 30 to 40 minutes.[87] In these first-degree neuropraxic injuries, the earliest pathophysiologic change is the inability of the nerve to transmit repeated impulses. Although the exact defect is unknown, ischemia from compression surely creates anoxic block of ionic and axonal transport. In addition, compression at high levels causes narrowing of the involved axons, increased endoneurial fluid pressure, and subsequent intraneural edema.[75,153] The classic examples of acute neuropraxic compression neuropathy include the transient conduction block, typified by paresthesias, that results from local pressure on a peripheral nerve. This causes the familiar sensation that one's leg or arm "goes to sleep." The conduction block rapidly recovers when the pressure is relieved or posture altered. When a motor nerve is involved, the sensation is one of "pseudocramps."[124]

With extended tourniquet application at suprasystolic pressures, motor deficits and mild sensory losses occur. There is a higher degree of impairment in faster-conducting larger axons (primarily motor, proprioceptive, and light-touch fibers), whereas the smaller and nonmyelinated axons (pain, temperature, and autonomic function) are spared.[159] Higher levels of compression yield a longer-lasting conduction block caused by focal demyelination without disruption

of axonal continuity. This local conduction block is caused by mechanical deformation (nodal intussusception).[57,123] Higher levels of pressure on a nerve create further mechanical deformation, which results in the shearing of the mesaxonal Schwann cell from the adaxonal portion of the cell. This damages the myelin, which then degenerates and leaves an area of exposed axon. Conduction is not restored until remyelination is complete,[57,123,183] and function returns in most cases by 3 to 6 weeks.[183] Because axonal continuity is maintained, there is little, if any, target-organ degeneration. Because of the differential susceptibility of axons, complete paralysis (large fibers) can occur without loss of cutaneous sensibility (smaller myelinated and unmyelinated fibers).[51]

Long periods of compression or high levels of pressure over a relatively small area of a peripheral nerve can produce a crushing injury that may be second, third, or even fourth degree. These are *lesions-in-continuity,* and the prognosis for recovery depends on the magnitude of the intraneural disruption. When the crush injury is axonotmetic, the axonal basement membrane remains intact, and regeneration progresses with an exact target-organ match and good recovery. Although recovery can be delayed, most patients have achieved 50% return by 4 months.[141] When the crush injury is neurotmetic (third or fourth degree), function is mildly or moderately reduced by the failure of some axons to achieve a proper end-organ match. Axonal admixture as well as increased amounts of intraneural scar prevents complete return of function and budding axons can become lost in the interposed scar and develop a neuroma-in-continuity.

Chronic compression

Injury created by low-grade chronic compression differs from the acute compression injury in all aspects of etiology, histology, and clinical presentation. The susceptibility of peripheral nerves to chronic compression is a function of internal anatomy. Proximal nerves, which contain many fascicles and an abundant amount of supportive connective tissue, are much less vulnerable to compression than distal nerves. Within each nerve, peripheral fascicles are more affected than central fascicles, and within each fascicle, peripheral axons are more likely to be injured than the central ones.[164] There is also a greater susceptibility to compression if the patient is afflicted with malnutrition, alcoholism, diabetes, or renal failure.

Histologic assessment of chronic nerve compression shows myelin-sheath asymmetry, epineurial fibrosis, perineurial thickening, and in severe stages, endoneurial fibrosis. Larger fibers appear to "drop out." There is some wallerian degeneration, and simultaneous regeneration of axons is seen.[164] In contradistinction to the acute compressive neuropathy that creates nodal intussusception, the terminal loops of the inner lamellae of the thinned myelin near the entrapment become detached from the axon at the node and retract. An abundance of myelin appears at the opposite end of the internode, which produces bulbous paranodal swelling. The detachment and subsequent myelin retraction leave multiple consecutive internodes demyelinated. This partially accounts for the reduced conduction velocity seen in nerves injured by chronic compression. The conduction block seen in acute compression injuries is rarely seen in these chronic lesions.[18]

Chronic compression also affects the vascular supply of the involved segment. In pressures as low as 30 mm Hg, impaired venular flow is observed, ultimately leading to congestion and anoxia. This induced ischemia leads to further vascular dilation, nerve swelling, and more compression, beginning a vicious cycle.[165] The rapid reversibility of some chronic compression injuries supports the vascular etiology.[49] Axoplasmic flow is decreased in chronic compressive injuries, and even when the force is insufficient to create a demyelinating lesion, there is a profound effect on the function of the nerve. Distal to the compressive force, the nerve becomes more sensitive to low levels of pressure. Multiple subclinical levels of compression along any given nerve can lead to symptoms of compressive neuropathy. This *double crush syndrome* implies that serial constraints of axoplasmic flow are additive in nature.[147,186] Histologic changes are observed in nerves subject to chronic compression. Epineurial fibrosis and perineurial thickening are noted, and there is a decrease in the number of large axons in the periphery of the affected fascicles. There is proteinaceous intraneural edema from the loss of the blood-nerve barrier within which fibroblasts proliferate and ultimately render the nerve segment permanently scarred and potentially anoxic.[60] *Late* chronic compression injuries are more likely to require extensive external neurolysis (and sometimes even internal neurolysis) than early lesions because of the extensive nature of the *intraneural* scar.

Patients with chronic compression injuries often report the sensation of pain, but this can arise along any area of the affected nerve's course and is often a misleading diagnostic sign. A more useful diagnostic sign that correlates with the site of compression is the Tinel's sign.[102]

At surgical exploration, the affected nerve often is seen to be swollen, edematous, and hyperemic proximal to the area of compression. The nerve underlying the compression is often pale and narrow.[115] At the time of surgical decompression, almost all patients obtain relief of their pain, although improvement in conduction delay takes weeks or months to return.[60]

Stretch injury

Peripheral nerves must incorporate within their structure the ability to accommodate changes in joint position. To do this, nerves have the inherent ability to stretch, recoil, and glide within their beds on their loose mesoneurial attachments.[66,108,109,194] Under conditions of minimal tension, the nerve fibers assume an undulating course within the fascicle. As longitudinal tension is applied to the nerve, the nerve slides within the bed and begins to take up the load and become stressed. The epineurium—an elastic structure—begins to elongate by "stretch," and the fascicles within completely straighten out. Upon release of the longitudinal tension, the nerve recoils and resumes its natural resting length.[66,114,164,178] As long as the nerve remains free to glide within its bed, significant stretch can be tolerated without injury. Normal excursions of nerves vary greatly, from a maximum of 15.3 mm (average for the brachial plexus) to a minimum of 1.15 mm (average for a digital nerve).[108,109,194] When a nerve is injured (through compression, scar, entrapment, or adhesions) and is subsequently anchored by scar to its bed, it can be subjected to "overstretch" traction injury during normal physiologic demands. There are also certain traumatic states that can exceed the normal nerve excursion or limits of elasticity and therein create injury.[194] A nerve achieves its strength through the perineurium. This layer has three orientations of collagen fibers in its outer sheath: circumferential, longitudinal, and oblique.[174,178] As longitudinal tension is applied, the perineurium lengthens, but at the expense of the cross-sectional area. This creates an increase in the intrafascicular pressure along the entire length of the nerve.[168,194] As long as the perineurium remains intact, the nerve maintains its elastic characteristics, but intraneural damage occurs far below the point of mechanical failure.[168] The elastic limit, or allowable stretch limit, is about 20%. At that level, there can be one or many areas of intraneural tearing, with axonal and fascicular disruption and areas of hemorrhage. Fibroblastic proliferation follows, which ultimately leads to intraneural scarring.[37,66,122]

Although the true incidence of nerve stretch injuries is unknown, these injuries are commonly associated with traumatic events, such as fractures, dislocations, obstetric trauma, and occasionally inadvertent retraction during surgery. Of nerve injuries associated with fractures, 95% occur in the upper extremities, and of the five most commonly injured nerves, 58% are radial, 18% ulnar, 16% peroneal, 6% median, and 2% sciatic.[59] In a prospective study of 648 nerve traction lesions in which the nerve was seen to be in continuity at the time of surgery, Omer[127] reported that 70% achieved spontaneous recovery. In low-velocity gunshot wounds, 69% recovered between 3 and 8 months. Patients with high-velocity gunshot wounds also recovered 69% of the time, but these lesions took up to 9 months to recover. Nerve injuries associated with fractures and dislocations recovered spontaneously between 1 and 4 months in 83% of the patients, and in patients with nerve traction (stretch) injuries, 86% recovered in 3 to 6 months.[127]

Not all traction injuries are traumatic. Some are the result of attempts to overcome an excessive nerve gap during reconstruction. This may be by stretch on the nerve stumps to achieve coaptation or by positioning the joints in flexion and creating the traction by the progressive postoperative extension of the joints. The progressive extension may lead to an ischemic injury or even exceed the elastic limits of the nerve.[69] It has been shown that some length can be gained with slow stretch over time.[168] This finding has been exploited using tissue expansion techniques that allow progressive nerve lengthening before nerve reconstruction to overcome nerve gaps. When caring for a patient with a major traction injury, we must be aware of the fact that the injury can affect the entire length of the nerve. The most clinically significant injury may be remote from the actual site of extremity injury, and this may test even the most astute diagnostician.

Ischemic injury

The peripheral nerve requires a continuous and adequate supply of oxygen for aerobic metabolism to drive the normal functions of axoplasmic transport; maintain cell integrity; and remain primed for the generation, maintenance, and restoration of the membrane potentials necessary for conduction of impulses. To accomplish this goal, the nerve has an elaborate dynamic plexus of blood vessels composed of two integrated but functionally independent systems.[99] The peripheral nerve can survive relatively long anoxic periods with a rapid recovery of function,[33,97,98] but longer periods of acute ischemia or chronic hypoxia may produce irreversible injury. Muscle weakness, pain, paresthesias, hypersensitivity, and sensory deficits all are symptoms of ischemic nerve lesions.[76,163,184] Ischemic injury may result from three different pathologic processes. There may be large vessel occlusion, arteriolar angiopathy, or nutrient capillary disease. Large vessel occlusion caused by conditions such as trauma or embolism is amenable to medical management or direct surgical reconstruction. Arteriolar and capillary disease is indirectly approached by attempts at improving the nerve environment (e.g., flap reconstruction of the nerve bed) or by release of the offending perineurial and intraneural scar (or both).[42,143] Some of the pathologic states that affect the arteriolar (50 to 400 µm in diameter) vessels are necrotizing angiopathic disorders such as polyarteritis nodosa, rheumatoid arthritis, Churg-Strauss syndrome, Wegener's granulomatosis, and thromboangiitis obliterans (Buerger's disease). All of these disease states affect the epineurial arterioles and result in patchy occlusion and ischemic nerve damage.[3,41,42,139]

The length of time the ischemic insult persists is the most important determinant of anoxic damage. Within the first 10 minutes of nerve ischemia, there is a rapid decrease in the membrane resting potential and electrical resistance. By 15 minutes, the action potential decreases and there is a further decrease in the resting potential, which blocks conduction.[105] There is a complete loss in conductivity by 30 to 40 minutes.[57] Reoxygenation brings recovery within 1 to 2 minutes, and recovery is usually complete by 10 minutes. This implies that the pathologic insult of ischemia is a metabolic phenomenon and not a morphologic one. In chronically ischemic nerves, there is segmen-

tal demyelination[41,44,81] and irreversible axonal infarction may occur.[68,82] If regeneration occurs, there is a favorable prognosis because the intraneural destruction leaves the axonal basement membrane intact. This ensures directed axonal regrowth and proper nerve–end-organ connectivity.[195]

The question of tolerance to ischemia becomes very important when the issue of replantation or free tissue transfer is raised. A normal nerve apparently can tolerate up to 8 hours of warm ischemia (room temperature) and suffer little morphologic damage. Nutrient blood flow is rapidly restored upon revascularization. After 8 hours, there is a breakdown of the blood-nerve barrier, and the resultant influx of proteinaceous fluid negatively affects nerve regeneration by ultimately stimulating fibroblastic proliferation and subsequent intraneural scar.[98] For more proximal amputations in which there is a significant amount of muscle involved, the tolerance to ischemia of the nerve is not of clinical importance because the target organs suffer irreversible damage before the nerves. However, injured nerve fibers are more susceptible to induced ischemia than are normal nerves. This may be because there is a reduction in axoplasmic flow in the injured nerve (especially if severed).[58]

Electrical injury

An electrical injury to the upper extremity can run the gamut from minor to life-threatening and is associated with a significant percentage of resultant amputations (32.5%).[38] The severity of these injuries depends on the current pathway and the relevant features of voltage level, tissue resistance, and current duration. The neurologic defects following electrical injury are usually immediate in onset and, for reasons incompletely understood, more commonly involve motor nerves. Most injured nerves show some recovery over time, but complete resolution of significant injuries is rare.[136] The major pathologic change in the electrically injured nerve is one of coagulation necrosis resulting from the generation of heat energy. The electrical current follows the path of least resistance, and resistance to flow increases in various tissues in the following order: nerve, blood vessel, muscle, skin, tendon, fat, and bone.[134,151] The electrical injury therefore preferentially follows the neurovascular bundles and creates deep tissue destruction along these pathways. Flash thermal burns at the entrance and exit sites accompany these injuries. In 22% of reported cases of electrical burns, direct nerve destruction was the initial result of the injury.[38] In nondestructive lesions, electrical injuries are found to cause an increase in threshold stimulus and a loss of amplitude of the response to supramaximal stimulation. Although some of these changes were reversible, the electrical injury left a persistent increase in latency and decreased conduction velocity.[185] Severe injuries can lead to patchy necrosis of the entire nerve as well as central necrosis.

Hemorrhage and subarachnoid bleeding also are common.[38,85,132,151,155] If the nerve is not destroyed, total demyelination in a multifocal distribution is seen, and blood vessels in the vasa nervorum sustain significant damage, thus creating a late ischemic injury.

Complicating electrical injury are violent tetanic contractures that can result in hemorrhage, muscle rupture, and broken bones. Late changes principally result from chronic ischemic changes associated with vascular damage and progressive perineurial fibrosis. Unlike the previously mentioned vascular pathology, this chronic ischemic injury may respond to neurolysis and revascularization of the nerve (e.g., muscle flap, omental transfer).[134,155]

Radiation injury

As radiation treatment becomes more precise and refined, its use as a treatment modality in the therapy for cancer is increasing. With it come increasing survival rates for patients with cancer and also greater opportunity to observe the late effects of radiation injury on surrounding soft tissues and nerves. In the past, orthovoltage radiation (less than 1 million volts) was the standard, and this technique had very shallow tissue penetration. There were marked skin changes that limited the total dose of radiation before significant nerve damage could result. Today, megavoltage radiation (1 million to 35 million volts) has allowed increased penetrance to deeper tissue planes with minimal apparent skin damage, and the result is a much higher dose of radiation to the adjacent structures within the field.[160]

Radiation injury to the peripheral nerve is poorly understood. Injury results from direct cell injury and indirectly from damage caused to the supportive vascular and connective tissues. These injuries are synergistic.[100] Fortunately for neural tissue, there is relative stability in cellular population (i.e., there is little mitotic activity, and therefore little biologically significant damage occurs at the genetic encoding level) until attempts at neural regeneration.[121,150] Cellular damage is more pronounced if the radiation follows a nerve injury that stimulates the cellular supportive proliferation.[95]

Radiation injury is permanent and does not seem to abate with time. Histologically, there is axonal dropout and patchy loss of myelin within the radiated segment. Attempts at Schwann cell proliferation yield a decreased total number of cells that produce abnormally thin myelin sheaths. An increased nerve cross-sectional area implies that there is persistent intraneural edema associated with abnormal endoneurial vessel permeability. Late examination reveals marked intraneural and perineurial fibrosis with apparent fibrous replacement of fascicles and a marked amount of thick pale scar.[28,95,100,160] Because of the common use of radiation in the treatment of cancers of the breast, brachial plexus radiation injury has been the most extensively studied type of radiation injury. The incidence of brachial plexopathy varies greatly, depending on the mode of delivery and the total dosage. In one series, using 4 MV radiation, 15% of patients developed neu-

rologic symptoms after 5775 rads; after 6300 rads, the percentage increased to 73%.[160] After radiation given by a 15-MV betatron, 22% of patients receiving between 400 and 5000 rads developed an actinic plexopathy, increasing to 47% after 550 to 6600 rads.[52] The latent period between radiation and the onset of symptoms of plexopathy has ranged from as short as 5 months to as long as 20 years, with a mean latency of 4.25 years.[28,173]

Pain is by far the most common presentation of brachial plexopathy, with as many as 80% of patients reporting some amount. Fifty percent of patients describe their pain as severe. Sixty-six percent of patients presented with muscle weakness and atrophy, and this sign was often associated with marked upper extremity lymphedema. Most of the patients with sensory and motor deficits presented with median and ulnar involvement.[28,173]

The typical patient who presents to the hand surgeon with upper extremity pain and who has had radiation for the treatment of a carcinoma presents a diagnostic dilemma. The problem is in distinguishing an actinic plexopathy from local recurrence or metastatic involvement of the nerves by tumor. Both present with like signs and symptoms and have the same mean onset. Both progress steadily over years, but progression of the plexopathy without the development of other metastatic sites is the best presumptive evidence for a radiation-induced lesion. In all surgical cases, absence of metastatic disease must be confirmed by liberal biopsy.[80,86,173,176] The strongest indication for surgical intervention in radiation-induced nerve injury is intractable pain, but surgery should not be approached in a cavalier fashion. Downgrading of function is a likely outcome because the compromised nerves will not tolerate much surgical manipulation. The goals of surgical intervention should be to gently excise the strangulating fibrotic scar and to improve the vascularity of the involved nerves by transposition to an improved bed or by flap reconstruction.

Injection injuries

The peripheral nerve is vulnerable to direct injection in many circumstances, and this can result in permanent damage to the nerve. It is common to inject various substances in the immediate vicinity of nerves when administering local anesthetic agents for regional anesthesia or injecting steroid preparations for the local treatment of inflammatory conditions. In addition, the intramuscular injection of materials such as antibiotics can result in inadvertent injection into an underlying peripheral nerve. Most of these injuries could be avoided by knowledge of the surface and underlying anatomy.[89] When a nerve injection injury occurs, the patient can experience severe pain at the site of injection that radiates to the distribution of the nerve. This is often associated with a neurologic deficit—sensory, motor, or both.[53,55,74,103] Injection injury was thought to be caused by mechanical needle injury, allergic neuritis, ischemia, and the development of circumferential scar, as well as the intraneural deposition of neurotoxic substances. Several studies have shown that only the intraneural injection of neurotoxic substances causes significant nerve-fiber injury. Only with diazepam, chlordiazepoxide, chlorpromazine, and benzylpenicillin was extrafascicular injection associated with nerve injury. The most severe injuries were related to the intrafascicular injection of meperidine, diazepam, chlorpromazine, hydrocortisone, triamcinolone hexacetonide, procaine, and tetracaine. Less severe, but still significant, injuries were produced by gentamicin, cephalothin, methylprednisolone, triamcinolone acetonide, lidocaine (worse if with epinephrine), and bupivacaine hydrochloride with epinephrine.[54,56,74,103,148] Several of these drugs contain similar buffers, and these may be the offending agents.[24,27] Acutely, axonal dropout and wallerian degeneration are seen. Alterations of the blood-nerve barrier change the normal endoneurial environment and may lead to late changes caused by the attendant swelling, ischemia, and intraneural scar. By 8 weeks after injury, there is severe intraneural fibrosis associated with minimal external scar.[54,55]

When a peripheral nerve injection injury occurs, observation is indicated for the first 3 months, with electrophysiologic studies obtained about 6 weeks after the injury.[74] Early surgical exploration with irrigation of the offending agent or external neurolysis is not recommended. Because the damage is intraneural, extraneural manipulations do not address the pathology. If there is no clinical recovery by 4 months, exploration is indicated. An internal neurolysis procedure should be done to decompress the scarred fascicles, and several months should be allowed to elapse to see what functional recovery follows. If little improvement is gained, one should perform resection of the neuroma-incontinuity followed by reconstruction.[26,31,74.]

Laceration injury

Nerve laceration is likely to be one of the most common injuries the peripheral nerve surgeon treats. Lacerations are either complete or partial, and all are fifth-degree neurotmetic lesions. A sharp instrument causes most such injuries, but some are associated with sharp bone fragments in a closed fracture. All are associated with a clearly defined neural motor or sensory deficit that will not improve without surgical intervention. Approximately 20% of all nerve lacerations that appear to be complete are in fact only partial lacerations, with contusion and stretch being responsible for the neuropraxic or axonotmetic deficit of the remaining intact fascicles.[31]

Nerve lacerations are essentially low-velocity crush injuries isolated to very small areas of the involved nerve. Even under ideal conditions, a divided nerve will have some component of crush injury in the proximal and distal stumps, which must be treated by careful debridement at the time of surgical reconstruction.[77]

PERIPHERAL NERVE REGENERATION

Any injury to a peripheral nerve results in a predictable sequence of events affecting the distal and the proximal nerve stumps. Distally, wallerian degeneration is noted by the disruption of the axon and the preparation by the remaining Schwann cell sheath to accept growing axons. Proximally, the axon undergoes limited degeneration up to the last preserved internode. If the injury is severe, neuron death can occur and the entire axon degenerates. If not severe, the cell body exhibits central chromatolysis, which represents the shift of the cell metabolism from maintenance to a regenerative mode designed to generate structural proteins.[149] These new structural proteins are transported to the end of the injured nerve axon and assembled there to bulge into a growth cone by the end of 24 hours. Anterograde growth then begins at the level of the last preserved internode by the advancement of the tip of the growth cone. There is also sprouting of collaterals from the growth cone and from the nodes of Ranvier up to several segments proximal to the axon tip.[26,50,62] After the first 24 hours, some of the sprouting axons have reached the area of injury and have begun to penetrate the developing scar at the site of injury. Accompanying the axonal sprouts are Schwann cells derived from the replication of the terminal satellite cells.[157] Axonal growth appears to be a result of random filopodial protrusion. When a suitably adhesive substrate is contacted by the filopodium, adherence occurs, and then, through some transmembrane event, contact guidance propels the axon in that direction.[86,190,191] Many axonal sprouts can grow down the nerve fiber in this fashion, but when one reaches a target organ, the others degenerate and the contacting axon matures.[20] The axonal growth might not be entirely directed by mechanical or random means. The type of guidance may be neurotropic (guiding) or neurotrophic (nutrient) factors.[63] Investigators have demonstrated that the growth cone has a high level of endocytotic activity and that there is a rapid internalization of exogenous materials that are then rapidly transported back to the cell body.[19] Perhaps the budding axons follow a gradient of nutrient or tropic chemicals to the target organ.[6,125] Of course, impenetrable scar at the level of injury or along the distal nerve fiber will prevent any axon from reaching its target.

Changes in the distal axon

After a nerve injury that results in wallerian degeneration (second degree and above), the Schwann cells provide phagic degradation of the myelin and axonal debris, and they proliferate within the remaining basal lamina and become longitudinally arranged bands ready to accept the advancing regenerating axons.[149,177] While the axons are growing down the distal axon, an additional layer of endoneurial collagen is deposited. This ultimately narrows the regenerating axon.[174] In addition, there are quantitatively more Schwann cells per unit length of regenerated axons, resulting in an overall decreased internodal distance.[30,177]

Without the regenerating axon, the distal nerve fiber is not stimulated to maintain its anatomic, metabolic, and functional integrity, and eventually there is irreversible shrinkage of the endoneurial tube. By 2 years, the nerve fiber has shrunk to only 1% of its normal size. The blood supply also contracts and, even after optimal regeneration, never exceeds 80% of its original cross-sectional area.[39,167] The rate of nerve regeneration is inversely proportional to the distance from the cell body and can be followed by measuring the speed of the advancing Tinel's sign. Reported rates of regeneration are 8.5 mm per day in the upper arm, 6 mm per day in the proximal forearm, 1 to 2 mm per day at the wrist, and 1 to 1.5 mm per day in the hand.[163,180]

After the regenerating axon reaches its target organ and begins to mature, the single axon is then enfolded by the Schwann cells, which were aligned and served to guide the regenerating fiber.[1] The axon is enfolded from proximal to distal, and the myelination is predetermined by the parent axon and not by the end-organ.[21]

The degree of injury greatly affects the prognosis for recovery. In second-degree injuries, the single axon is guided by its basal lamina. The endoneurial tube leads the regenerating axon directly to its proper target organ, and there is no chance of misrouting. End-organ specificity is maintained.[71] When an injury disrupts the basal lamina (third degree and higher), end-organ–specific regeneration is no longer possible, neighboring axons intermingle, and misrouting can occur. Only as a random event will there be exact end-organ–specific regeneration. In third-degree injuries, fascicular integrity remains and prognosis depends on the level of the lesion and the proximity of the nerve to its target organs. The more proximal the injury, the greater the fascicular heterogeneity and the greater the likelihood of axonal admixture. If the lesion is distal (near the end-organ), there is axonal homogeneity and the prognosis for a reasonable functional return is good.[31] When a fourth-degree lesion occurs, the fascicular separation allows greater stump retraction, but the intact epineurium limits the extent of the interposed scar. Budding axons sprout and become entangled in the scar tissue, few axons find their way through this mass, and if they do, distal connectivity is haphazard.[21,39,117,118] Clinically, these are seen as neuroma-in-continuity lesions and are masses of misdirected axons within scar bound by the intact epineurium.[77] Fifth-degree lesions are those in which there is a complete separation of the entire nerve trunk. There is an attempt at regeneration, but because of the loss of continuity of the epineurium, there is no possibility of connectivity with the distal stump, and the budding axons grow into scar and Schwann cell masses at the severed end of the nerve, forming an *amputation neuroma*.[157,192] Without surgical intervention (coapting the stumps of the severed

nerve), there is no hope of spontaneous regeneration of the fifth-degree lesion.

Factors that influence regeneration

Peripheral nerve reconstruction is built on a foundation of principles that, when followed, facilitate the natural regenerative process of the nerve. Regeneration of the peripheral nerve after injury is influenced by mechanical forces, delay to repair, the patient's age, and the level of the injury. Mechanical interference to nerve regeneration is in the form of scar tissue and inappropriate topographic orientation. The nerve axon has the greatest likelihood of accurate regeneration when minimum scar is interposed between the severed nerve ends and if there is accurate alignment of the fascicles. This increases the probability that the regenerating axons will enter their native nerve fibers and achieve appropriate connectivity.[149] Delay before reconstruction is another important factor. The capacity for a nerve cell body to regenerate is essentially unlimited as long as cell death does not occur. It is the passage of time, however, that eliminates the possibility for regeneration by time-related changes in the distal nerve segment (scar and progressive decrease in diameter) and in the target organs (atrophy and degeneration).[163] There is little question that there is a consistently better functional return in the young after nerve injury.[5]

Rates of nerve regeneration are age related. They decline with increasing age and may be related to the decreasing rates of slow axonal transport with age.[7] In addition, trophic mechanisms seem to function over greater distances in the young, and this may facilitate more accurate end-organ connectivity.[149] The differences in the quality of return of sensibility between the young and old may be attributable to the diminution in receptor populations that occurs naturally in the old (at least for populations of Meissner corpuscles).[138] Last, the consistently better functional outcomes in the young may result from greater central plasticity. This is the cortical ability to relearn or reorganize spatially disrupted input and thereby overcome the inexact peripheral connectivity.[43]

The injury level (proximal versus distal) is one of the greatest factors in determining the prognosis for successful outcome of regeneration. Proximal injuries generally carry a worse prognosis than distal injuries. In a proximal injury, regenerative demand on the cell body is greater because the axon must regenerate for a greater distance. Also, in proximal injuries there is a greater likelihood of neuronal death.[17,18] Second, if the injury is proximal, there is a greater distance to the target organ, and in the time the axon takes to regenerate over the great distance to the end-organ, considerable atrophy or degeneration may have occurred.[17,31,64] Intraneural topography also plays an important role. The more proximal the nerve, the greater the fascicular heterogeneity. In higher-level injuries, there is more axonal mixing during regeneration; this makes appropriate target-organ connectivity difficult if not impossible.[163] The cause of the nerve injury is important, and the associated structures—skin, bone, joint, and vascular system—must be stabilized before any definitive reconstruction. Devitalized tissues must be debrided, bones must be stabilized, and blood vessels (when injured) must be repaired. Severe injuries may result in multilevel nerve lesions from traction, compression, or ischemia. As an injury increases in severity, there is more scarring around the nerve and its bed, thereby decreasing the quality of regeneration. In addition, a patient in an unstable condition may require delay in the repair. Nerve repair or reconstruction should not be performed in the absence of good skin cover, skeletal stability (ideally with supple joints), and without correction of vascular insufficiency. Infection should be aggressively treated, and adjunctive procedures such as flap coverage should be performed if they will facilitate earlier nerve reconstruction.

Reinnervation

Reinnervation of a target organ involves much more than just axonal regeneration and connectivity. After an axon reaches the target organ, neuromuscular junctions and the axon terminus of sensory receptors must be reestablished, and this does not occur if there is an axon–target organ mismatch. Because of the randomness of regeneration for all of the higher-level injuries, there are five potential outcomes of regeneration. An axon may achieve exact reinnervation by establishing continuity with its native target organ. If the end-organ is not irreversibly damaged, return of function can be essentially normal. If the end-organ has degenerated, there will be no useful return of function. The wrong receptor may be reinnervated within the proper territory, resulting in improper input, or the axon may achieve connectivity with the appropriate receptor in the wrong territory and create false localization. Finally, the axon may be frustrated and not achieve end-organ connectivity, thereby rendering the results of regeneration fruitless.

When a regenerating motor axon reaches a denervated muscle, reinnervation generally occurs at old motor end-plates.[16,133,140] The axon then sprouts and reinnervates contiguous muscle fibers, creating histochemically uniform *giant* motor units.[116] Recovery of motor function does not immediately occur upon reestablishment of the neuromuscular junctions. There is an 18-day delay before nerve stimulation will produce contraction, and another 5 days before functional reflex activity can occur.[65] Recovery of *functional* activity best correlates with the return of the *gamma efferent control* of the intrafusal fibers.[179] Without adequate gamma return, the muscle function is downgraded clinically by imprecision of motion despite good return.[73]

The recovery of sensibility occurs in a repeatable orderly sequence that correlates with the morphology of the reinnervated receptor populations. The perception of pain and temperature precede the return of touch, and the touch submodalities recover in the following sequence: 30-Hz

frequencies, moving touch, constant touch, and finally 256-Hz stimuli.[35]

PERIPHERAL NERVE RECONSTRUCTION

Over the past two decades, the therapeutic approach toward the patient with nerve injury has significantly changed, facilitated by new technologies of intraoperative electrodiagnosis, by better instruments and magnification, and by better understanding of peripheral nerve structure and function. *Atraumatic* nerve handling and suture techniques have improved the potential for nerve reconstruction. Awareness of fascicular anatomy has made the results of nerve repair more precise, and the appreciation of the untoward effects of tension at the repair site has made nerve interposition grafting commonplace. After reconstruction, knowledge of the patterns of sensory recovery has led to elaborate schemes of sensory reeducation that enable more functional use.

Timing

There are no absolute rules regarding the timing of nerve repair, and the decisions should be made after careful consideration of the nature of the injury, the condition of the patient, and the status of the associated injuries. Nerve injuries can be divided into two broad categories. First are those injuries in which there is a suspected transection. These must be handled with primary reconstruction if all conditions permit. Second are those injuries in which the nerve is expected to be in-continuity or in which there are multilevel lesions or marked contusion. These injuries require secondary reconstruction. By definition, primary repair is that which is done within 48 hours of injury. Early secondary repairs are those performed within the first 6 weeks, and late secondary repairs are performed after 3 months.[31,77,78,113] If the limits of the nerve injury can be delineated, there is a definite advantage to performing repair or reconstruction primarily. If the repair is performed within 4 days, electrical stimulation can be used to identify distal fascicles and nerve stump retraction is limited. If the repair is delayed beyond 4 days, wallerian degeneration has progressed and electrical stimulation is not possible. If the wound is contaminated or if there is a soft tissue deficit or fracture, nerve repair must be delayed until a clean stable wound can be obtained. With adequate debridement, soft tissue reconstruction, and fracture stabilization, the nerve repair can be done simultaneously. If a primary nerve repair fails because it is done under poor conditions, the patient is likely to obtain a worse result than if repair had been delayed until a secondary repair could be done under good conditions.

There are times when the surgeon should delay repair or reconstruction after an injury. These are when there is an expected first-, second-, or third-degree injury. No surgical reconstruction is better than an intact fascicle, and time should be allowed to elapse for the resolution of low-grade lesions. It is appropriate to allow 8 to 16 weeks for the resolution of nontransecting blunt or stretch injuries. The greatest advantage of primary nerve reconstruction is the saving of time.[113] The great disadvantage is the inability to detect the precise extent of the nerve injury, especially if there is an undetected traction or multilevel injury. If repair is done under the latter circumstances (undetected injury), some function can return with time, but the surgeon is then faced with the decision to reoperate in hopes of achieving greater return or to wait for improvement that is not likely to come. A great advantage of all secondary repairs is that the surgeon and the operating team can perform the surgery electively, without fatigue, and under proper operating room conditions, making it perhaps easier to achieve a more meticulous microcoaptation.

Nerve repair technique

Exploration after an injury always should be done under tourniquet control if possible. This allows for more accurate dissection and identification of the lesion. Nerve microcoaptation does not require a bloodless field as long as the structures are properly positioned and tagged. In fact, it is sometimes preferable to deflate the tourniquet before the microsurgical repair to obtain homeostasis because this can be difficult to accomplish after a nerve repair without jeopardizing the coaptation.

Nerve lesions should be approached with wide exposure, proximal and distal. The nerve is dissected from the uninjured to the injured areas of the nerve, with attempt made to preserve all vascular attachments. For lacerations, high magnification is used to determine the fascicular pattern of the nerve; this allows the orientation of both the proximal and distal ends of the nerve to be appreciated. High magnification also should be used to perform the fascicular dissection for lesions that are in-continuity. As the lesion is reached, fascicles that do not contribute to the neuroma can be carefully freed from the offending scar and involved fascicles. Electrical stimulation or intraoperative electrodiagnosis can be used to determine which of the fascicles retain sufficient conduction and can be spared. The fascicles that contribute to the neuroma then can be resected and repaired or reconstructed with interposition grafts.

End-to-end coaptation

The most commonly used technique for peripheral nerve microcoaptation is the *epineurial repair* technique (Fig. 32-2).[171] This technique is applied to the completely transected nerve, and its advantages are simplicity, rapid execution time, and minimal requirement for magnification. The cut nerve end is debrided carefully and serially sectioned until the axoplasmic outflow mushrooms under positive intrafascicular pressure and the fascicular pattern is identified and is relatively free of scar.[13] The same is done for the distal stump, and then, with the nerves lying without tension next to one another, the magnification is increased to 25 power and 10-0 nylon sutures are placed in the

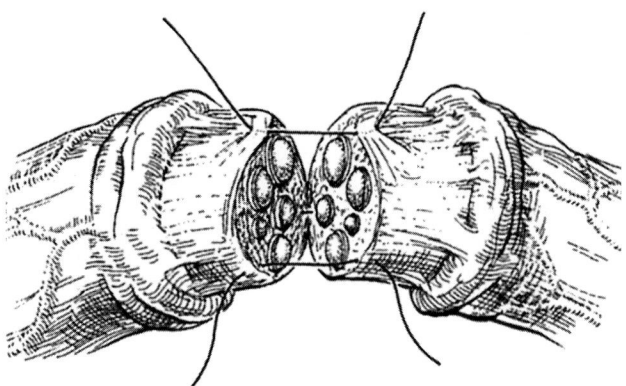

Fig. 32-2. Epineurial repair. Diagrammatic representation of the microcoaptation. The outer epineurium is resected proximally and distally. After careful alignment of the nerve stumps, sutures are placed in the inner epineurium. Two or three tension-relieving sutures can be used if necessary, using 8-0 nylon, and the coaptation is completed using 10-0 nylon. (From Terzis JK, Smith KL: *The peripheral nerve: structure, function and reconstruction,* New York, 1990, Raven Press.)

epineurium, as one carefully realigns the fascicular bundles to achieve exact coaptation. A minimum number of sutures are used to complete the repair. Usually, 8 or 10 sutures are necessary for a large nerve and as few as 2 sutures for a small one. If the nerve gap is so large that the first 10-0 suture cannot hold the nerve ends in apposition, one or two guide sutures of 8-0 can be used.

The leading causes of failure of the epineurial repair are gapping, overriding, buckling, and straddling of the fascicle ends. Even slight tension can create a significant intraneural gap, which is quickly filled with scar tissue, making regeneration difficult at best.[9,45,162]

The second common technique of peripheral nerve reconstruction is the *perineurial repair* (Fig. 32-3). A great deal of discussion focuses on whether an *epineurial repair* or a *perineurial repair* (fascicular repair) is the preferred method of peripheral nerve reconstruction, but numerous articles report no difference in the regeneration and functional recovery associated with either technique.[22,23,79,130] When significant debridement is required before microcoaptation, fascicular matching is improved with this technique; it is also used extensively when interposition grafts are indicated.

Under high magnification, the nerve ends are prepared and the epineurium is dissected away. Fascicles are separated, and coaptation is performed between matching fascicles, with sutures placed into the inner epineurium. Sutures are carefully placed so as not to enter the endoneurium. The great advantage of the perineurial technique is the accurate coaptation of similar-size fascicles. The greatest disadvantage is the stimulation of greater amounts of intraneural scar by increased dissection and foreign material (suture).[84,130,166,187]

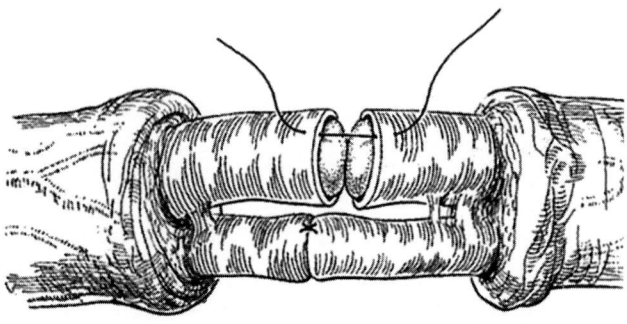

Fig. 32-3. Perineurial (fascicular) repair. Diagrammatic representation of the microcoaptation. The outer and inner epineurium is dissected from the proximal and distal stumps. Fascicles and fascicular groups are aligned, and the coaptations are performed with the minimum number of 10-0 nylon sutures necessary (as few as two). Note the care taken to place the sutures within the inner epineurium or perineurium and not to violate the endoneurium. (From Terzis JK, Smith KL: *The peripheral nerve: structure, function and reconstruction,* New York, 1990, Raven Press.)

Tension and nerve grafting

After any nerve injury in which there is a gap between the nerve endings, either after trauma or as required by debridement, the surgeon faces a dilemma. Should the nerve gap be bridged by extensive mobilization and stretch (with the nerve repair under tension); should the defect be bridged with a nerve graft, forcing the axons to cross two coaptations[170]; or should the limb be postured in flexion to bring the nerve ends together and then slowly returned to full extension in hopes of stretching the nerves out to length?

Tension at the site of coaptation invites the proliferation of scar tissue at the repair. As the scar matures, it tends to constrict the regenerating axons within.[31] If the joints are flexed, mobilization can create a second traction lesion in the already injured nerve. If the regenerating axons manage to cross the suture line and grow down the nerve fiber, they are unlikely to achieve functional reinnervation in a great number of cases. Studies have shown that repeated stretching of a sutured nerve fails to elongate, and instead, repetitive traction injuries result.[69,70]

Comparing the results of nerve grafting with those of coaptation under tension, Millesi determined that there was little interposed scar at the coaptation if the nerve was repaired without tension, with or without a graft. Electrophysiologic studies supported the use of grafts in lieu of coaptation under tension and showed excellent recovery even in the face of two suture lines.[112,115,120]

Nerve grafting is approached surgically like any nerve exploration. The nerve ends are exposed and prepared, and a suitable donor nerve (commonly the sural nerve) is harvested and cut to length. Depending on the caliber of the injured nerve, the number of interposition grafts is chosen to match the cross-sectional area. Fascicular matching is conducted, and the perineurial repairs are done.

Alternatives to nerve grafting

Autogenous nerve grafting is no longer the only approach available to reconstruct the nerve gap. The nerve gap can be mechanically shortened by nerve-lengthening techniques (tissue expansion or nerve distraction)[104] or bridged by tubes of biologic or nonbiologic materials. To avoid donor site morbidity from autogenous nerve harvest, interest has been rekindled in various tubulization techniques and in homografting (transplant). Like an autogenous nerve graft, the nonneural tube offers a conduit for the budding axons, and growing nerves can be directed across a nerve gap to achieve connectivity with the distal nerve stump. Examples of conduits currently in use are constructed from polyglycolic acid, autogenous vein, and amnion.[25,161] Results of reconstruction with conduits of short nerve gaps (less than 3 cm) in digital nerves show functional results equal to tensionless coaptations, thereby making this technique quite advantageous in view of the elimination of donor site morbidity.[189] However, the maximum gap that can presently be bridged with a conduit seems to be 3 cm and reconstruction with conduits requires 2 to 3 weeks of splinting in the postoperative period. Promising results have also been obtained with tissue-expansion techniques. Slow expansion of wallerian-degenerated nerve results in accelerated Schwann cell proliferation and increased vascularity that seems to facilitate nerve regeneration.[126] Permanent elongation of 30% could be achieved with expansion techniques yielding results of repair equal to tensionless primary nerve coaptation. However, the proximal segment tolerated expansion better than the distal segment.[154]

With successful repair, the progressing Tinel's sign can follow regeneration as the budding axons travel along the nerve. It is important to follow the punctum maximum because this delineates the most distal extent of the majority of axons. If the Tinel's sign fails to progress and remains at the site of coaptation, this is an indication for reexploration and repair. If Tinel's sign stalls distally to the repair, one must assume there is a second lesion previously unknown.

After the nerve repair, it is important that the nerve coaptation be protected for 7 to 10 days by immobilization. Then, during the period of nerve regeneration, therapy should concentrate on keeping the affected areas supple, mobile, and ready to accept the growing axons. As soon as sensory reinnervation is seen, sensory reeducation programs should begin.

SUMMARY

Over the last decades, peripheral nerve reconstructive surgery has evolved from rather crude reapproximation of severed nerve ends performed without much regard for tension or topographic orientation, to technically precise methods of surgery for which better understanding of the intraneural anatomy has allowed better fascicular alignment and has led to improved results. These still fall below the ideal of axon-to-axon realignment, however. Perhaps in the future, new understanding of tropic and trophic manipulations will allow us to achieve even better results and achieve exact target-organ reinnervation, and techniques of tensionless suture, less coaptation, and scar manipulation will serve to eliminate fibrotic interference with regeneration.

Today, we can appreciate that the nerve cell has an essentially unlimited regenerative capability. It is the job of the surgeon to perform as precise a repair after a nerve injury as possible, and it is the job of the therapist to assist the patient in the maintenance of the end-organs by protective splinting, range-of-motion therapy, massage, and modalities as indicated, to achieve the best possible functional results after nerve injuries and repair.

REFERENCES

1. Aguayo AJ, Bray GM: Cell interactions studied in the peripheral nerves of experimental animals. In Dyck PJ, et al, editors: *Peripheral neuropathy,* Philadelphia, 1989, WB Saunders.
2. Barchi RL: Excitation and conduction in nerve. In Sumner AJ, editor: *The physiology of peripheral nerve disease,* Philadelphia, 1980, WB Saunders.
3. Barker NW: Lesions of peripheral nerves in thrombangiitis obliterans, *Arch Intern Med* 62:271, 1938.
4. Barr ML, Hamilton JD: A quantitative study of certain morphological changes in spinal motor neurons during axon reaction, *Comp Neurol* 89:93, 1948.
5. Birch R, Achan P: Peripheral nerve repairs and their results in children, *Hand Clin* 16:579, 2000.
6. Bisby M: Changes in composition of labelled protein transported by motor axons during their regeneration, *J Neurobiol* 11:435, 1980.
7. Black MM, Lasek RJ: Slowing of the rate of axonal regeneration during growth and maturation, *Exp Neurol* 63:108, 1979.
8. Bora FW, Osterman AL: Compression neuropathy, *Clin Orthop* 163:20, 1982.
9. Bora FW, Pleasure DE, Didizian NA: A study of nerve regeneration and neuroma formation after nerve suture by various techniques, *J Hand Surg* 1:138, 1976.
10. Bostock H, Sears TA: Continuous conduction in demyelinated mammalian nerve fibers, *Nature* 263:786, 1976.
11. Bostock H, Sears TA: The internodal axon membrane: electrical excitability and continuous conduction in segmental demyelination, *J Physiol (Lond)* 280:273, 1978.
12. Bradley WG: *Disorders of peripheral nerves,* Oxford, 1974, Blackwell Scientific.
13. Braum RM: Epineurial nerve suture, *Clin Orthop* 163:50, 1982.
14. Bristow WR: Injuries of peripheral nerves in two world wars, *Br J Surg* 34:333, 1947.
15. Brown A, Iggo A: The structure and function of cutaneous "touch corpuscles" after nerve crush, *J Physiol* 165:28, 1963.
16. Brown MC, Holland RL, Hopkins WG: Motor nerve sprouting, *Annu Rev Neurosci* 4:17, 1981.
17. Brown PW: Factors influencing the success of the surgical repair of peripheral nerves, *Surg Clin North Am* 52:1137, 1972.
18. Brown WF, et al: The location of conduction abnormalities in human entrapment neuropathies, *Can J Neurol Sci* 3:111, 1976.
19. Bunge MB: Initial endocytosis of peroxidase or ferritin by growth cones of cultured nerve cells, *J Neurocytol* 6:407, 1977.
20. Bunge RP, Bunge MB: Tissue culture observations relating to peripheral nerve development, regeneration, and disease. In Dyck PJ, et al, editors: *Peripheral neuropathy,* Philadelphia, 1984, WB Saunders.
21. Cabaud HE, Rodkey WG, Nemeth TJ: Progressive ultrastructural changes after peripheral nerve transection and repair, *J Hand Surg* 7:353, 1982.
22. Cabaud HE, Rodkey WG, McCarroll HR: Peripheral nerve injuries: studies in higher nonhuman primates, *J Hand Surg* 5:201, 1980.
23. Cabaud HE, et al: Epineurial and perineurial fascicular nerve repairs: a critical comparison, *J Hand Surg* 1:131, 1976.
24. Chino N, Award EA, Kopttke FJ: Pathology of propylene glycol administered by perineural and intramuscular injection in rats, *Arch Phys Med Rehabil* 55:33, 1974.
25. Chiu David: Autogenous venous nerve conduits: a review, *Hand Clinics* 15:667, 1999.
26. Clark WK: Surgery for injection injuries of peripheral nerves, *Surg Clin North Am* 52:1325, 1972.
27. Clark WK: Discussion of Mackinnon SE et al: Peripheral nerve injection injury with steroid agents, *Plast Reconstr Surg* 69:490, 1982.
28. Clodius L, Uhlschmidt G, Hess K: Irradiation plexitis of the brachial plexus. In Terzis JK, editor: *Microreconstruction of nerve injuries,* Philadelphia, 1987, WB Saunders.
29. Coctaldo JE, Ochoa JL: Mechanical injury of peripheral nerves, fine structure and dysfunction, *Clin Plast Surg* 11:9, 1984.
30. Cragg BG, Thomas PK: The conduction velocity of regenerated peripheral nerve fibers, *J Physiol (Lond)* 171:164, 1964.
31. Daniel RK, Terzis JK: Principles, practices, and techniques of peripheral nerve surgery. In Daniel RK, Terzis JK, editors: *Reconstructive microsurgery,* Boston, 1977, Little, Brown.
32. Daniel RK, Terzis JK: *Reconstructive microsurgery,* Boston, 1977, Little, Brown.
33. Daube JR, Dyck PJ: Neuropathy due to peripheral vascular diseases. In Dyck PJ, et al, editors: *Peripheral neuropathy,* vol 2, Philadelphia, 1984, WB Saunders.
34. Davis HL, Kiernan JA: Effect of nerve abstract on atrophy of denervated or immobilized muscles, *Exp Neurol* 72:582, 1981.
35. Dellon AL: *Evaluation of sensibility and reeducation of sensation in the hand,* Baltimore, 1981, Williams & Wilkins.
36. Dellon AL, Witebsky FG, Terrill RE: The denervated Meissner corpuscle: a sequential histologic study after nerve division in the Rhesus monkey, *Plast Reconstr Surg* 46:182, 1975.
37. Denny-Brown D, Hoherty MM: Effects of transient stretching of peripheral nerve, *Arch Neurol Psychiatr* 54:116, 1945.
38. Di Vencenti FC, Moncrief JA, Pruitt BA: Electrical injuries: a review of 65 cases, *J Trauma* 9:497, 1977.
39. Ducker TB, Kempe LG, Hayes GJ: The metabolic background for peripheral nerve surgery, *J Neurosurg* 30:270, 1969.
40. Duel AB: Clinical experiences in the surgical treatment of facial palsy by autoplastic nerve grafts, *Arch Otolaryngol* 16:767, 1932.
41. Dyck PJ, Conn DL, Okazaki H: Necrotizing angiopathic neuropathy: three-dimensional morphology of fiber degeneration related to sites of occluded vessels, *Mayo Clin Proc* 47:461, 1972.
42. Dyck PJ, et al: Pathologic alterations of the peripheral nervous system of humans. In Dyck PV, et al, editors: *Peripheral neuropathy,* Philadelphia, 1984, WB Saunders.
43. Dykes RW: Central consequences of peripheral nerve injuries, *Ann Plast Surg* 13:412, 1984.
44. Eames RA, Lange LS: Clinical and pathological study of ischemic neuropathy, *J Neurol Neurosurg Psychiatry* 30:215, 1967.
45. Edsage S: Peripheral nerve suture: a technique for improved intraneural topography, *Acta Chir Scand Suppl* 331:1, 1964.
46. Engh CA, Schofield BH: A review of the central response to peripheral nerve injury and its significance in nerve regeneration, *J Neurosurg* 37:198, 1972.

47. English KB: Cell types in cutaneous type I mechanoreceptors (Haarscheiben) and their alterations with injury, *Am J Anat* 141:105, 1974.

48. English KB: The ultrastructure of cutaneous type I mechanoreceptors (Haarscheiben) in cats following denervation, *J Comp Neurol* 172:137, 1977.

49. Eversman WW, Ritsick JA: Intraoperative changes in motor nerve conduction latency in carpal tunnel syndrome, *J Hand Surg* 3:77, 1978.

50. Foreman DS, Berenberg RA: Regeneration of motor axons in the rat sciatic nerve studied by labelling with axonally transported radioactive proteins, *Brain Res* 156:213, 1978.

51. Fowler TJ, Danta G, Gilliatt RW: Recovery of nerve conduction after a pneumatic tourniquet, observations on the hind limb of the baboon, *J Neurol Neurosurg Psychiatry* 35:638, 1972.

52. Frischbier HJ, Lohbeck HD: Strahlenchaden nach elektronentherapie beim mammacarcinom, *Strahlentherapie* 139:684, 1970. Cited in reference 26.

53. Gentili F, Hudson AR, Hunter D: Clinical and experimental aspects of injection injuries of peripheral nerves, *Can J Neurol Sci* 7:143, 1980.

54. Gentili F, et al: Peripheral nerve injection injury: an experimental study, *Neurosurgery* 4:244, 1979.

55. Gentili F, et al: Early changes following injection injury of peripheral nerves, *Can J Surg* 23:177, 1980.

56. Gentili F, et al: Nerve injection injury with local anesthetic agents: a light and electron microscopic, fluorescent microscopic, and horseradish peroxidase study, *Neurosurgery* 6:263, 1980.

57. Gilliatt RW: Acute compression block. In Sumner AJ, editor: *The physiology of peripheral nerve disease,* Philadelphia, 1980, WB Saunders.

58. Gilliatt RW, Wilson TG: Schemic sensory loss in patients with peripheral nerve lesions, *J Neurol Neurosurg Psychiatry* 17:104, 1954.

59. Goodall RJ: Nerve injuries in fresh fractures, *Texas State J Med* 52:93, 1956.

60. Goodman HV, Gilliatt RW: The effect of treatment on median nerve conduction in patients with the carpal tunnel syndrome, *Ann Phys Med* 6:137, 1961.

61. Grafstein B: The nerve cell body's response to axotomy, *Exp Neurol* 48:32, 1975.

62. Grafstein B, McQuarrie IG: Role of the nerve cell body in axonal regeneration. In Cotman CW, editor: *Neuronal plasticity,* New York, 1978, Raven Press.

63. Gunderson RW, Barrett JN: Characterization of the turning response of dorsal root neurites toward nerve growth factor, *J Cell Biol* 87:546, 1980.

64. Gutman E, Gutman L: Factors affecting the recovery of sensory function after nerve lesions, *J Neurol Neurosurg Psychiatry* 5:117, 1942.

65. Gutman E, Young JZ: The reinnervation of muscle after various periods of atrophy, *J Anat (Lond)* 18:15, 1944.

66. Haftek J: Stretch injury of peripheral nerve, acute effects of stretching on rabbit peripheral nerve, *J Bone Joint Surg* 52B:354, 1970.

67. Hargens AR, et al: Peripheral nerve conduction block by high muscle compartment pressure, *J Bone Joint Surg* 61A:192, 1979.

68. Hess K, et al: Acute ischemic neuropathy in the rabbit, *J Neurol Sci* 44:19, 1979.

69. Highet WB, Holmes W: Traction injuries to the lateral popliteal nerve and traction injuries to peripheral nerves after suture, *Br J Surg* 30:212, 1943.

70. Highet WB, Saunders FK: The effect of stretching nerves after suture, *Br J Surg* 30:355, 1943.

71. Horch K: Guidance of regrowing sensory axons after cutaneous nerve lesions in the rat, *J Neurophysiol* 42:1437, 1979.

72. Horn KL, Crumley RL: The physiology of nerve injury and repair, *Otolaryngol Clin North Am* 17:321, 1984.

73. Hubbard JH: The quality of nerve regeneration. Factors independent of the most skillful repair, *Surg Clin North Am* 52:1099, 1972.

74. Hudson AR: Nerve injection injuries. In Terzis JK, editor: *Microreconstruction of nerve injuries,* Philadelphia, 1987, WB Saunders.

75. Jewett DL: Functional blockade of impulse tissues by acute nerve compression. In Jewett DL, McCarroll HR, editors: *Nerve repair and regeneration,* St Louis, 1980, Mosby.

76. Karnash LJ: Sciatic causalgia due to nerve trunk ischemia, *J Nerv Ment Dis* 84:283, 1936.

77. Kline DG: Timing for exploration of nerve lesions and evaluation of the neuroma-in-continuity, *Clin Orthop* 163:42, 1982.

78. Kline DG, Hackett ER: Reappraisal of timing for exploration of civilian peripheral nerve injuries, *Surgery* 78:54, 1975.

79. Kline DG, Hudson AR, Bratton BR: Experimental study of fascicular nerve repair with and without epineurial closure, *J Neurosurg* 54:513, 1981.

80. Kori SH, Foley KM, Posner JB: Brachial plexus lesions in patients with cancer; clinical findings in 100 cases, *Neurology* 29:583, 1979.

81. Korthals JK, et al: Peripheral demyelination after transient ischemia, *Neurology* (NY) 34:168, 1984.

82. Korthals JK, Korthals MA, Wisniewski HM: Peripheral nerve ischemia. Part 2: accumulation of organelles, *Ann Neurol* 4:487, 1978.

83. Kurosumi K, Kurosumi U, Inoue K: Morphological and morphometric studies with the electron microscope on the Merkel cells and associated nerve terminals in normal and denervated skin, *Arch Histol* 42:243, 1979.

84. Kutz JE, Shealy G, Lubbers L: Interfascicular nerve repair, *Orthop Clin North Am* 12:277, 1981.

85. Langworthy OR: Histological changes in nerve cells following injury, *Bull Johns Hopkins Hosp* 47:11, 1930.

86. Letourneau PC: Cell-to-substratum adhesion and guidance of axonal elongation, *Dev Biol* 44:92, 1975.

87. Lewis T, Pickering GW, Rothschild P: Centripetal paralysis arising out of arrested blood flow to the limb, including notes on a form of tingling, *Heart* 16:1, 1931.

88. Lieberman AR: The axon reaction: a review of the principle features of perikaryal response to axonal injury, *Int Rev Neurobiol* 14:49, 1971.

89. Lindner DW, Gurjian ES: Injuries of nerves. Clinical aspects. In Vinken PJ, Bruyn GW, editors: *Handbook of clinical neurology: diseases of nerves,* New York, 1970, Elsevier.

90. Lindsay WK, Walker FG, Farmer AW: Traumatic peripheral nerve injuries in children. Results of repair, *Plast Reconstr Surg* 30:462, 1962.

91. Lipsztein R, Dalton JF, Bloomer WD: Sequelae of breast irradiation, *JAMA* 253:3582, 1985.

92. Lomo T, Rosenthal J: Control of ACh sensitivity by muscle activity in the rat, *J Physiol* 221:493, 1972.

93. Lomo T, Westgaard RH: Control of ACh sensitivity in rat muscle fibers, *Cold Spring Harb Symp Quant Biol* 40:263, 1975.

94. Lomo T, Westgaard RH: Further studies on the control of ACh sensitivity by muscle activity in the rat, *J Physiol* 225:603, 1975.

95. Love S: An experimental study of peripheral nerve regeneration after x-irradiation, *Brain* 106:39, 1983.

96. Lubinska L: Early course of wallerian degeneration in myelinated nerve fibers of the rat phrenic nerve, *Brain Res* 130:47, 1979.

97. Lundborg G: Structure and function of the intraneural microvessels as related to trauma, edema formation and nerve function, *J Bone Joint Surg* 57:725, 1975.

98. Lundborg G: Intraneural microvascular pathophysiology as related to ischemia and nerve injury. In Daniel RK, Terzis JK, editors: *Reconstructive microsurgery,* Boston, 1977, Little, Brown.

99. Lundborg G: The intrinsic vascularization of human peripheral nerves: structure and functional aspects, *J Hand Surg* 4:34, 1979.

100. Lundborg G, Schildt B: Microvascular permeability in irradiated rabbits, *Acta Radiol (suppl)* (Stockh) 10:311, 1971.

101. Lundborg G, et al: Median nerve compression in the carpal tunnel—functional response to experimentally induced controlled pressure, *J Hand Surg* 7:252, 1982.
102. Mackinnon SE, Dellon AL: Experimental study of chronic nerve compression, *Hand Clin* 2:639, 1986.
103. Mackinnon SE, et al: Peripheral nerve injection injury with steroid agents, *Plast Reconstr Surg* 69:482, 1962.
104. Margiotta MS, et al: A nerve distraction model in the rat, *Ann Plast Surg* 40:486, 1998.
105. Maruhashi J, Wright EB: Effect of oxygen lack in the single isolated mammalian (rat) nerve fiber, *J Neurophysiol* 30:434, 1967.
106. McDonald WI: Physiological consequence of demyelination. In Sumner AJ, editor: *The physiology of peripheral nerve disease,* Philadelphia, 1980, WB Saunders.
107. McEwan LE: Median and ulnar nerve injuries, *Aust NZ J Surg* 32:89, 1962.
108. McLellan DL: Longitudinal sliding of the median nerve during hand movements, *Lancet* 1:663, 1975.
109. McLellan DL, Swash M: Longitudinal sliding of the median nerve during movements of the upper limb, *J Neurol Neurosurg Psychiatry* 39:566, 1976.
110. Miller RG: Acute vs. chronic compression neuropathy, *Muscle Nerve* 7:420, 1984.
111. Millesi H: Treatment of nerve lesions by fascicular free nerve grafts. In Michon J, Moberg E, editors: *Traumatic nerve lesions,* Edinburgh, 1975, Churchill Livingstone.
112. Millesi H: Interfascicular nerve grafting, *Orthop Clin North Am* 12:287, 1981.
113. Millesi H: Reappraisal of nerve repair, *Surg Clin North Am* 61:321, 1981.
114. Millesi H: The nerve gap: theory and clinical practice, *Hand Clin* 2:651, 1986.
115. Millesi H: Nerve grafting. In Terzis JK, editor: *Microreconstruction of nerve injuries,* Philadelphia, 1987, WB Saunders.
116. Mira JC: Quantitative studies of the regeneration of rat myelinated fibres: variations in the number and size of regenerating nerve fibres after repeated localized freezings, *J Anat (Lond)* 129:77, 1979.
117. Mira JC: Degeneration and regeneration of peripheral nerves: ultrastructural and electrophysiological observation, quantitative aspects and muscle changes during reinnervation, *Intern J Microsurg* 3:102, 1981.
118. Mira JC: Effects of repeated denervation of muscle reinnervation. In Terzis JK, editor: *Microreconstruction of nerve injuries,* Philadelphia, 1987, WB Saunders.
119. Mohammad J, et al: Modulation of peripheral nerve regeneration: a tissue-engineering approach. The role of amnion tube conduit across a 1-centimeter nerve gap, *Plast Reconstr Surg* 105:660, 2000.
120. Moneim MS: Interfascicular nerve grafting, *Clin Orthop* 163:65, 1982.
121. Muruyama Y, Myirea MM, Logothetis J: Neuropathy following irradiation. An unusual late complication of radiotherapy, *AJR Am J Roentgenol* 101:216, 1967.
122. Nobel W: Peroneal palsy due to hematoma in the common peroneal nerve sheath after distal torsional fractures and inversion ankle sprains, *J Bone Joint Surg* 48A:1484, 1966.
123. Ochoa J, Fowler TJ, Gilliatt RW: Anatomical changes in the peripheral nerves compressed by a pneumatic tourniquet, *J Anat* 113:433, 1972.
124. Ochoa JL, Torebjork HE: Paresthesia from ectopic impulse generation in human sensory nerves, *Brain,* 103:835, 1980.
125. Ochs S: Fast axoplasmic transport in the fibers of chromatolysed neurons, *J Physiol (Lond)* 255:249, 1976.
126. Ohkaya S, Hirata H, Uchida A: Repair of nerve gap with the elongation of wallerian degenerated nerve by tissue expansion, *Microsurgery* 20:126, 2000.
127. Omer GE: Injuries to nerves of the upper extremity, *J Bone Joint Surg* 54A:1615, 1974.
128. Omer GE: Nerve response to injury and repair. In Hunter JM, et al, editors: *Rehabilitation of the hand,* St Louis, 1984, Mosby.
129. Onne L: Recovery of sensibility and sudomotor activity in the hand after nerve suture, *Acta Chir Scand Suppl* 300:1, 1962.
130. Orgel MG: Epineurial versus perineurial repair of peripheral nerves. In Terzis JF, editor: *Microreconstruction of nerve injuries,* Philadelphia, 1987, WB Saunders.
131. Palmer P: Ultrastructural alterations of Merkel cells following denervation, *Anat Rec* 151:396, 1965.
132. Panse F: Electrical lesions of the nervous system. In Vinken PJ, Bruyn GW, editors: *Handbook of clinical neurology,* vol 7, New York, 1970, Elsevier.
133. Pockett S, Slack JR: Source of stimulus for nerve terminal sprouting in partially denervated muscle, *Neuroscience* 7:3173, 1982.
134. Ponten B, Erickson U, Johansson S: New observations on tissue changes along the pathway of the current in an electrical injury, *Scand J Plast Reconstr Surg* 4:75, 1970.
135. Powell HC, Myers RR: Pathology of the peripheral myelinated axon. In Adachi M, Hirano A, Aronson SM, editors: *The pathology of the myelinated axon,* New York, 1985, Igaku-Shoin.
136. Pruitt BA: Other complications of burn injury. In Artz CP, Moncrief JA, Pruitt BA, editors: *Burns: a team approach,* Philadelphia, 1979, WB Saunders.
137. Purvis D, Sakmann B: The effect of contractile activity on fibrillation and extrajunctional acetylcholine sensitivity in rat muscle maintained in organ culture, *J Physiol* 224:237, 1974.
138. Ridley A: Silver staining of the innervation of Meissner corpuscles in peripheral neuropathy, *Brain* 91:539, 1968.
139. Roberts JT: The effect of occlusive arterial diseases of the extremities on the blood supply of nerves. Experimental and clinical studies on the role of the vasa nervorum, *Am Heart J* 35:369, 1948.
140. Rosenthal J: Trophic interactions of neurons. In Bookhart JM, Mountcastle VB, editors: *Handbook of physiology,* Bethesda, Md, 1977, American Physiological Society.
141. Rudge P: Tourniquet paralysis with prolonged conduction block: an electrophysiological study, *J Bone Joint Surg* 56B:716, 1974.
142. Rydevik B, Lundborg G, Bagge U: Effects of graded compression on intraneural blood flow; an in vivo study on rabbit tibial nerve, *J Hand Surg* 6:3, 1981.
143. Rydevik B, Lundborg G, Nordborg C: Intraneural tissue reactions induced by internal neurolysis, *Scand J Plast Reconstr Surg* 10:3, 1976.
144. Schnapp B, Mugnaini E: Membrane architecture of myelinated fibers seen by freeze-fracture. In Waxman SG, editor: *Physiology and pathology of axons,* New York, 1974, Raven Press.
145. Schut L: Nerve injuries in children, *Surg Clin North Am* 52:1307, 1972.
146. Seddon HJ: Three types of nerve injury, *Brain* 66:237, 1943.
147. Seiler WA, et al: Double crush syndrome: experimental model in the rat, *Surg Forum* 34:596, 1983.
148. Selander D, et al: Local anesthetics: importance of mode of application, concentration, and adrenaline for the appearance of nerve lesions, *Acta Anaesthesiol Scand* 23:127, 1979.
149. Selzer ME: Regeneration of the peripheral nerve. In Sumner AJ, editor: *The physiology of peripheral nerve disease,* Philadelphia, 1980, WB Saunders.
150. Shack RB, Lynch JB: Radiation dermatitis, *Clin Plast Surg* 14:391, 1987.
151. Silversides J: The neurologic sequelae of electrical injury, *J Can Med Assoc* 91:195, 1964.
152. Simpson JA: Nerve injuries, general aspects. In Vinken PJ, Bruyn GW, editors: *Handbook of clinical neurology, diseases of nerves,* New York, 1970, Elsevier.
153. Sjostrand J, McLean WG, Frizell M: The application of axonal transport studies to peripheral nerve problems. In Omer G, Spinner M, editors: *Management of peripheral nerve problems,* Philadelphia, 1980, WB Saunders.

154. Skoulis TG, et al: Nerve expansion. The optimal answer for the short nerve gap. Behavioral analysis, *Clin Orthop* 314:84, 1995.

155. Solem L, Fischer RP, Strate RG: The natural history of electrical injury, *J Trauma* 17:487, 1977.

156. Souttar HS: Nerve injuries in children, *Br Med J* 2:349, 1945.

157. Spencer PS: Morphology of the injured nerve. In Daniel RK, Terzis JK, editors: *Reconstructive microsurgery,* Boston, 1977, Little, Brown.

158. Spencer PS, Thomas PK: Ultrastructural studies of the dying-back process. II. The sequestration and removal by Schwann cells and oligodendrocytes of organelles from normal and diseased axons, *J Neurocytol* 3:763, 1974.

159. Stain RE, Olson WH: Selective damage of larger diameter peripheral nerve fibers by compression, *Exp Neurol* 47:68, 1975.

160. Stoll BA, Andrews JT: Radiation-induced neuropathy, *Br Med J* 1:834, 1966.

161. Strauch B: Use of nerve conduits in peripheral nerve repair, *Hand Clin* 16:123, 2000.

162. Sunderland S: Factors influencing the course of regeneration and the quality of the recovery after nerve suture, *Brain* 75:19, 1952.

163. Sunderland S: *Nerves and nerve injuries,* Edinburgh, 1968, E & S Livingstone.

164. Sunderland S: *Nerves and nerve injuries,* Edinburgh, 1973, E & S Livingstone.

165. Sunderland S: Nerve lesion in the carpal tunnel syndrome, *J Neurol Neurosurg Psychiatry* 39:615, 1976.

166. Sunderland S: The pros and cons of funicular nerve repair, *J Hand Surg* 4:201, 1979.

167. Sunderland S, Bradley KC: Denervation atrophy of the distal stump of a severed nerve, *J Comp Neurol* 93:401, 1950.

168. Sunderland S, Bradley KC: Stress-strain phenomena in human peripheral nerve trunks, *Brain* 84:102, 1961.

169. Terzis JK: *Microreconstruction of nerve injuries,* Philadelphia, 1987, WB Saunders.

170. Terzis JK, Faibisoff B, Williams HB: The nerve gap: suture under tension versus graft, *Plast Reconstr Surg* 56:166, 1975.

171. Terzis JK, Smith KL: *The peripheral nerve: structure, function and reconstruction,* New York, 1990, Raven Press.

172. Terzis JK, Strauch B: Microsurgery of the peripheral nerve, *Clin Orthop* 133:39, 1987.

173. Thomas JE, Colby MY: Radiation-induced or metastatic brachial plexopathy, *JAMA* 222:1392, 1972.

174. Thomas PK: The connective tissue of peripheral nerve: an electron microscopic study, *J Anat* 97:35, 1963.

175. Thomas PK: The deposition of collagen in relation to Schwann cell basement membrane during peripheral nerve regeneration, *J Cell Biol* 23:375, 1964.

176. Thomas PK, Holdorff B: Neuropathy due to physical agents. In Dyck PJ, et al, editors: *Peripheral neuropathy,* vol 2, Philadelphia, 1984, WB Saunders.

177. Thomas PK, Landon DN, King RHM: Normal structure of the peripheral nerve. In Adams JH, Corcellis J, Duchen LW, editors: *Greenfield's neuropathology,* New York, 1984, John Wiley & Sons.

178. Thomas PK, Olson Y: Microscopic anatomy and function of the connective tissue components of peripheral nerve. In Dyck PJ, et al, editors: *Peripheral neuropathy,* Philadelphia, 1984, WB Saunders.

179. Thulin CA: Electrophysiological studies of peripheral nerve regeneration with special reference to small diameter (gamma) fibers, *Exp Neurol* 2:598, 1960.

180. Tinel J: The sign of "tingling" in lesions of the peripheral nerves, *J Presse Med* 23:388, 1915. (Translated in *Arch Neurol* 24:574, 1971.)

181. Torvik A, Skjorten F: Electron microscopic observations on nerve cell regeneration and degeneration after axon lesions. I. Changes in the nerve cell cytoplasm, *Acta Neuropathol (Berl)* 17:248, 1971.

182. Tower SS: Atrophy and degeneration in the muscle spindle, *Brain* 55:77, 1932.

183. Trojaborg W: Rate of recovery in motor and sensory fibers of the radial nerve: clinical and electrophysiological aspects, *J Neurol Neurosurg Psychiatry* 33:625, 1970.

184. Truge K: Management of established Volkmann's contracture. In Green DP, editor: *Operative hand surgery,* New York, 1982, Churchill Livingstone.

185. Ugland OM: Electrical injuries to peripheral nerves in animals: a preliminary report, *Acta Chir Scand* 131:432, 1966.

186. Upton ARM, McComas AJ: The double crush syndrome in nerve entrapment syndromes, *Lancet* 2:359, 1973.

187. Urbaniak JR: Fascicular nerve suture, *Clin Orthop* 163:57, 1982.

188. Watson WE: An autoradiographic study of the incorporation of nucleic acid precursors by neurons and glia during nerve degeneration, *J Physiol* 180:741, 1965.

189. Weber R, et al: A randomized prospective study of polyglycolic acid conduits for digital nerve reconstruction in humans, *Plast Reconstr Surg* 106:1036, 2000.

190. Weiss P: Nerve patterns. The mechanics of nerve growth, *Growth* 5(suppl):163, 1941.

191. Weiss P: The technology of nerve regeneration: a review. Sutureless tubulation and related methods of nerve repair, *J Neurosurg* 1:400, 1944.

192. Westgaard RH: Influence of activity on the passive electrical properties of soleus muscle fibers in the rat, *J Physiol* 225:683, 1975.

193. Wilgis EF, Murphy R: The significance of longitudinal excursion in peripheral nerves, *Hand Clin* 2:761, 1986.

194. Woltman HW, Wilder RM: Diabetes mellitus: pathologic changes in the spinal cord and peripheral nerves, *Arch Intern Med* 44:576, 1927.

195. Yates SK, Hurst LM, Brown WF: The pathogenesis of pneumatic tourniquet paralysis in man, *J Neurol Psychiatr* 44:759, 1981.

Chapter 33

THERAPIST'S MANAGEMENT OF PERIPHERAL-NERVE INJURIES

Terri M. Skirven
Anne D. Callahan

Rehabilitation of the individual with a peripheral-nerve lesion requires the full repertoire of the therapist's skills and judgment. A nerve injury often results in long-term and severe functional limitations. Motor power, sensibility, and sympathetic function all may be disrupted, and unless managed properly, fixed postural deformities may result. This chapter (1) discusses nerve anatomy, nerve response to injury, and classification of nerve injuries; (2) facilitates an understanding of the treatment goals and priorities during the acute, recovery, and chronic phases following nerve injury; and (3) discusses treatment techniques that are unique to nerve injuries, including motor retraining, splinting, sensory reeducation, and desensitization.

ANATOMY REVIEW

A peripheral nerve consists of a bundle or bundles of nerve fibers or axons whose cell bodies are in the spinal cord or ganglia just outside the spinal cord. The cell bodies of motor nerve fibers are in the anterior column of the spinal cord; sensory nerve fibers originate in the dorsal root ganglia; sympathetic fibers are axons of cell bodies in the sympathetic ganglia of the autonomic nervous system[25] (Fig. 33-1).

Some fibers are myelinated, others are thinly myelinated or unmyelinated. Each fiber is enclosed completely by a protective sheath or tube of connective tissue called *endoneurium* or *the endoneurial tube.* In addition to enclosing each fiber, the endoneurium also serves as packing tissue between individual fibers. It is elastic and resists stretch, thus acting to protect the individual fibers from

stretch. After nerve injury, as the wallerian degeneration occurs, the axons waste away distal to the level of injury and for a short distance proximal to it. The endoneurial tubes remain to serve as guiding tubes for regenerating axons to their terminal endpoints.[25]

Nerve fibers occur in groups or bundles of varying size called *funiculi* (singular: funiculus). Each funiculus is ensheathed by *perineurium,* which is a denser and stronger connective tissue than endoneurium. This perineurium provides a protective cushion against external compression of the funiculus that it surrounds. Each funiculus usually contains a mixture of motor, sensory, and sympathetic fibers, but it also may contain only one or two types of fibers.[25]

The funiculi are packed loosely in connective tissue called *epineurium,* which also forms the outermost layer of the nerve (Fig. 33-2). The elasticity of the epineurium protects the fibers against stretch. The amount of epineural tissue increases at joints to provide more of a cushion against compressive forces at joints.[25]

NERVE RESPONSE TO INJURY

Nerve response to injury proceeds in two phases.[3] The first phase involves the disintegration of the axon and the breakdown of its myelin sheath, a process that is referred to as *wallerian degeneration.* This degeneration occurs distal to the level of injury.

What remains distally are the empty Schwann sheaths and endoneurial tubes that subsequently undergo some degree of shrinkage and collapse with a decrease in the fascicular cross-sectional area. Degeneration also occurs at the motor

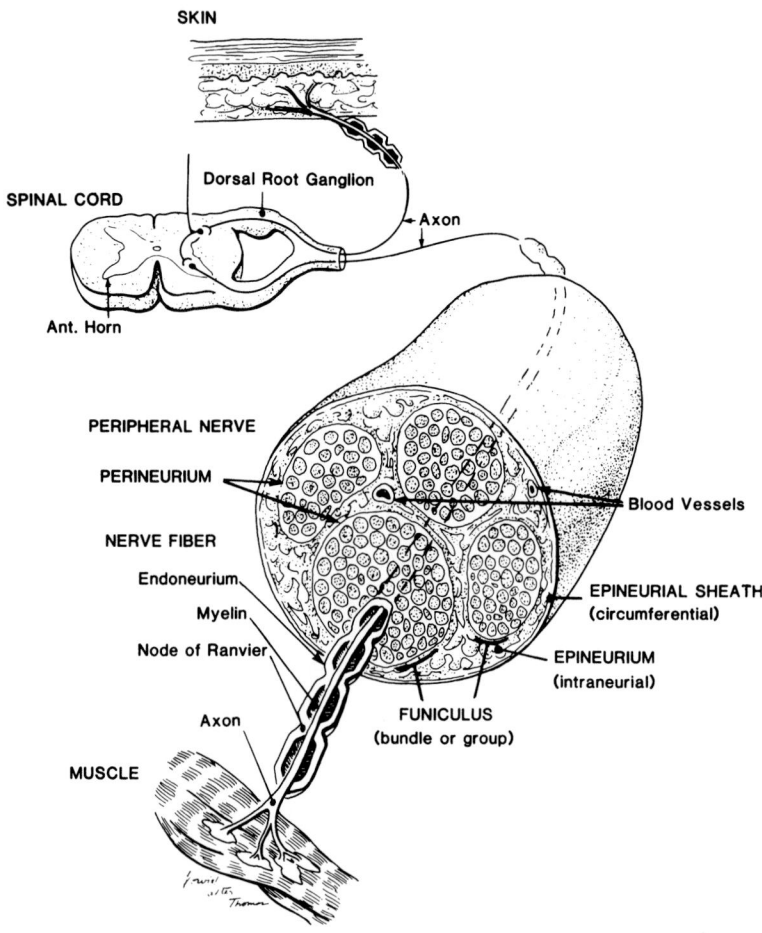

Fig. 33-1. Schematic anatomy of a peripheral nerve. (From Omer GE: Acute management of peripheral nerve injuries. In Mackin EJ, editor: *Hand clinics: hand rehabilitation,* Philadelphia, 1986, WB Saunders.)

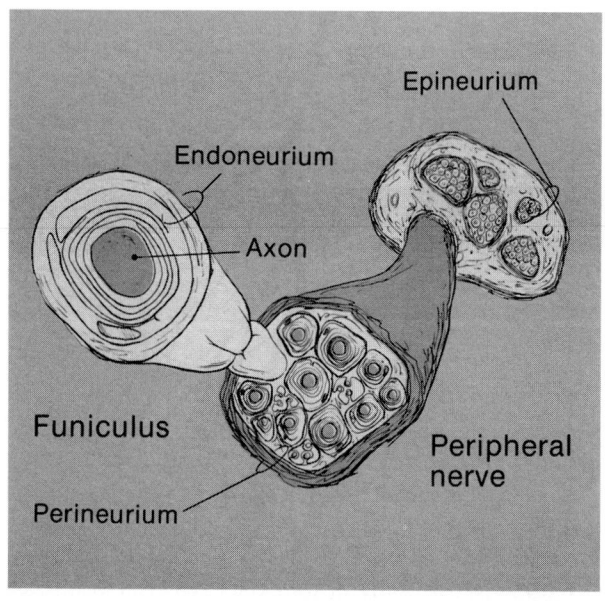

Fig. 33-2. The funiculi are loosely packed in connective tissue called epineurium, which also forms the outermost layer of the nerve.

and sensory end receptors. The second phase of the nerve's response to injury involves neuronal regeneration with sprouting of the axon. For nerve regeneration to be successful, the axon must cross the injury site and enter the same endoneurial tube. The rate of regeneration is 1 to 3 mm/day after an initial latency of 3 to 4 weeks with additional delays at the injury site and at the end organ.[17]

The process of nerve regeneration is complicated by many factors. These factors may include shrinkage of the endoneurial tubes, preventing reentry of the sprouting axons; scarring at the injury site, short-circuiting the progress of the sprouting axons; mismatching of the motor, sensory, and sympathetic fibers; and degeneration of the motor or sensory end receptors. Consequently, even under the most favorable of conditions, severance of a peripheral nerve usually results in some degree of residual deficit.

CLASSIFICATION OF NERVE INJURIES

Nerve injuries are classified according to the extent of injury to the axon and the connective tissue sheath. Sunderland[25] has classified five degrees of nerve injury (Fig. 33-3) and noted the implications for recovery of each. Any

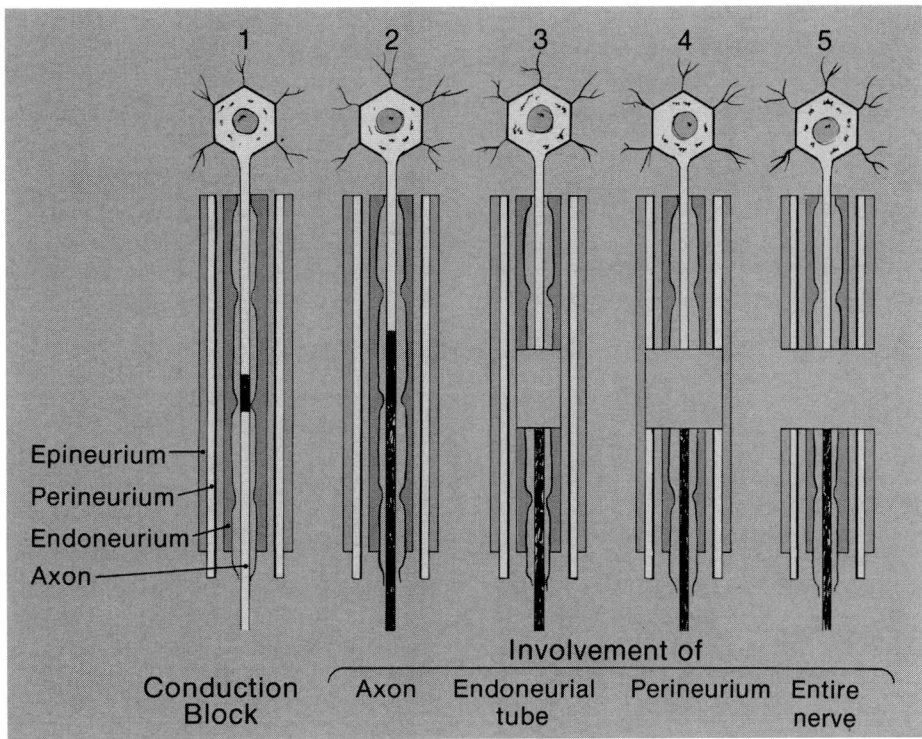

Fig. 33-3. Sunderland's five degrees of nerve injury.

agent of injury can account for degrees 1 through 4 of injury; only mechanical means can cause a fifth-degree injury.

First degree

With first-degree injury, axonal conduction is interrupted but all structures remain intact. There is temporary loss of nerve function in the following order, which proceeds from largest to smallest fiber-diameter involvement: motor, proprioception and vibration, touch, pain, and sudomotor function. Recovery is spontaneous and complete.[25] This degree of injury corresponds to Seddon's "neuropraxia."[20]

Second degree

In second-degree injury, injury to the nerve results in interruption of axons, but not of endoneurium, perineurium, or epineurium. Although wallerian degeneration of the axons occurs, recovery is spontaneous and good because the endoneurial tubes are intact, allowing the regenerating axons to resume their former pathway to their terminal endings.[25]

Third degree

With third-degree injury, the axons and their endoneurial tubes are no longer in continuity. Thus the interiors of the funiculi are involved. Recovery is spontaneous but less complete than in first- or second-degree injuries, because even though the regenerating axons remain with their original funiculus, scarring may prevent them from bridging the area of damage and reentering their original endoneurial tubes. Thus a regenerating axon might fail to

enter a tube at all. It might enter a functionally different tube (e.g., a sensory axon might enter a tube that terminates in a sweat gland). It might enter a functionally similar tube but one that terminates at a different point than the axon previously innervated. All of these possibilities result in faulty reinnervation, residual motor and sensory deficits, and possibly, the need for sensory reeducation. Sunderland[25] states that this degree of injury often occurs in entrapment lesions.

Fourth degree

The extent of fourth-degree injury is such that even the strong perineurium is no longer in continuity. The amount of scarring and internal disorganization is much greater than in previous levels because more tissue has been injured and the integrity of the fiber bundles is lost. Some spontaneous, but hardly useful, recovery may occur. Surgical excision and repair of the involved segment is required to allow functional healing to occur, but residual deficits will occur as a result of scarring and faulty regeneration and reinnervation.[25]

Fifth degree

The entire nerve trunk including the epineurium and all internal structures is transected in fifth-degree injury. Surgical repair is required, but under the most favorable conditions, residual motor and sensory deficits will persist as a result of scarring and faulty regeneration and reinnervation.[25] This degree of injury compares with Seddon's

Table 33-1. Comparison of Seddon and Sunderland classifications of nerve injuries: clinical findings

	Pathology	Motor	Sensory	Treatment	Recovery	Therapy implications
Neurapraxia (Seddon) First degree (Sunderland)	Anatomic and axonal continuity	Complete paralysis	Minimal loss	Observation	Complete	Short-term, focused
Second degree (Sunderland) Axonotmesis (Seddon)	Transection axon but endoneurium intact	Complete paralysis	Complete loss	Observation	Usually complete	Moderate intervention
Third degree (Sunderland)	Transection axon—loss of endoneurial tube continuity but perineurium intact (traction lesion)	Complete paralysis	Complete loss	Surgical intervention may be required	Incomplete	Moderate
Fourth degree (Sunderland)	Continuity of nerve trunk via epineurium but severe disorganization (neuroma in continuity)	Complete paralysis	Complete loss	Surgical intervention	Incomplete	Long-term comprehensive
Neurotmesis (Seddon)	Loss of nerve trunk continuity, complete disorganization	Complete paralysis	Complete loss	Surgical intervention mandatory	Never complete	Long-term comprehensive
Fifth degree (Sunderland)	Loss of nerve trunk continuity, complete disorganization	Complete paralysis	Complete loss	Surgical intervention mandatory	Never complete	Long-term comprehensive

"neurotomesis."[20] Seddon also has described a system of classification that Bowers et al.[4] has compared with Sunderland's classification (Table 33-1).

FACTORS AFFECTING PROGNOSIS FOR RECOVERY

In addition to the amount of scar and internal disorganization that occurs after nerve injury, several additional factors affect the prognosis for recovery, some of which are discussed in the following sections.

Nature of the injury

A clean, simple laceration results in less damage than a dirty laceration. A crush or stretch injury can result in irreparable damage along a considerable length of the nerve. Avulsion lesions are potentially the most damaging, especially if nerve roots are avulsed.

The higher the level of injury to the axon, the more difficult it becomes for the cell body to participate in axonal regeneration. In addition, there is more mixing of motor, sensory, and sympathetic fibers within funiculi high in the nerve; therefore the opportunity for mismatching of endoneurial tubes and regenerating axons is greater. The higher the lesion, the longer the distal muscle fibers and sensory end organs will remain denervated and undergo processes of atrophy and fibrosis.[24]

Age

Children have far better functional recovery after suture than adults, although the exact reasons for this are unknown.

Mixed versus unmixed nerves

In third-degree or worse injuries, in which the endoneurial tubes are no longer intact, the prognosis for functional recovery is better if the fibers within a given funiculus are unmixed. This would allow regenerating axons to enter functionally similar tubes, even if not to their original termination point. In cases of mixed fibers within a funiculus, the amount of nonfunctional regeneration is far greater.

Motor versus sensory recovery

According to Omer,[17] denervated muscles can remain viable for up to 3 years. However, in that time, atrophy and fibrosis could prevent functional reinnervation from taking place. Sensory end organs appear to degenerate more quickly than motor end organs. A delay of greater than 6 months between injury and suture will adversely affect the potential for recovery.[17]

It is realistic to conclude that, except for minor injuries, the preinjury state cannot be restored completely in adults. The goal of therapy is to maximize motor and sensibility recovery and to assist in compensation for residual deficits.

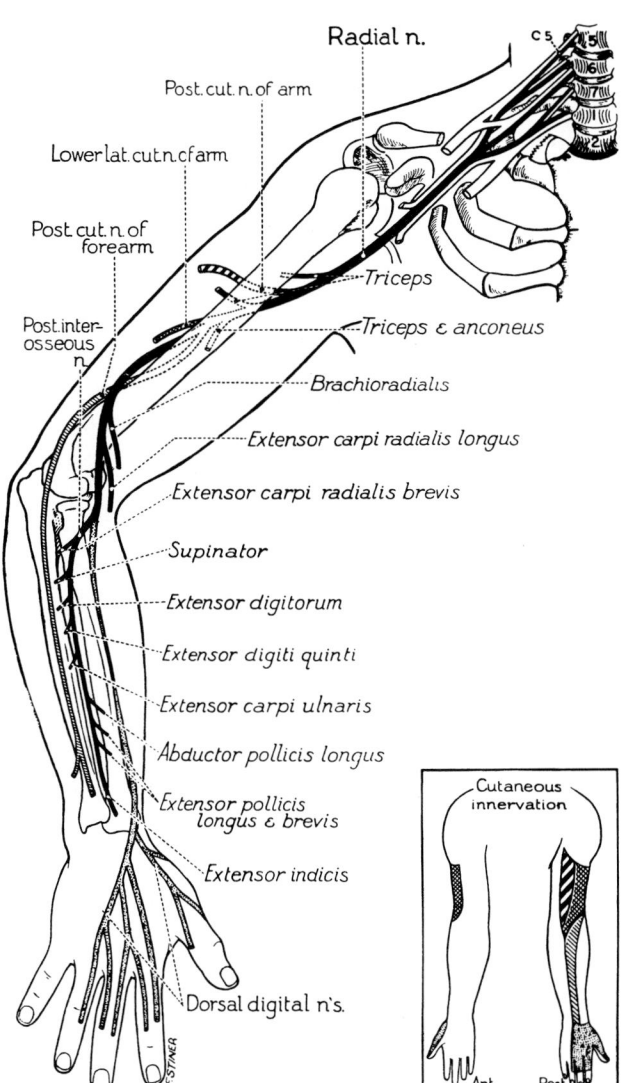

Radial n.

Post. cut. n. of arm

Lower lat. cut. n. of arm

Post. cut. n. of forearm

Post. inter-osseous n.

Triceps

Triceps & anconeus

Brachioradialis

Extensor carpi radialis longus

Extensor carpi radialis brevis

Supinator

Extensor digitorum

Extensor digiti quinti

Extensor carpi ulnaris

Abductor pollicis longus

Extensor pollicis longus & brevis

Extensor indicis

Dorsal digital n's.

Cutaneous innervation

Ant. Post.

Fig. 33-4. The course and distribution of the radial nerve. (From Haymaker W, Woodhall B: *Peripheral nerve injuries: principles of diagnosis,* Philadelphia, 1953, WB Saunders.)

SPECIFIC NERVE LESIONS
Radial nerve

Radial-nerve injuries may be associated with fractures of the humeral shaft, fracture and dislocation of the elbow, fractures of the upper third of the radius, and compression of the nerve at the level between the radial head and the supinator muscle. The latter type of compression is referred to as *radial tunnel syndrome.*

Motor, sensory, and functional loss associated with radial-nerve lesions depends on the exact site of injury (Fig. 33-4). With forearm-level lesions, the following muscles are involved:

- Extensor carpi ulnaris
- Extensor digitorum communis
- Extensor digiti minimi
- Abductor pollicis longus

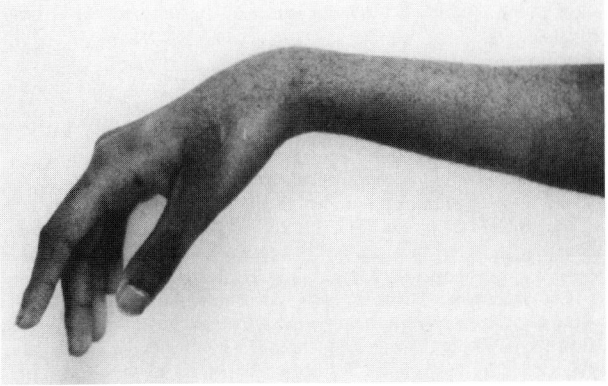

Fig. 33-5. Wrist drop deformity resulting from radical-nerve injury. (From Stanley BG, Tribuzi SM, editors: *Concepts in hand rehabilitation,* Philadelphia, 1992, FA Davis.)

- Extensor pollicis longus
- Extensor pollicis brevis
- Extensor indicis proprius

The functional deficit includes loss of metacarpophalangeal (MP) joint extension of all digits, of thumb radial abduction and extension, and of ulnar wrist extension. The sensory loss involves the dorsal aspect of the thumb and the dorsum of the second, third, and half of the fourth ray to the level of the proximal interphalangeal (PIP) joint. If the posterior interosseous nerve branch is solely involved with forearm-level lesions, no cutaneous sensory deficit will occur.

With lesions at the elbow level, the motor loss involves all of the aforementioned muscles with the addition of the following:

- Supinator
- Extensor carpi radialis longus
- Extensor carpi radialis brevis

The functional loss includes loss of ulnar and radial wrist extension and weakened supination, as well as loss of MP joint extension, thumb extension, and radial abduction. The sensory loss is the same.

With lesions just proximal to the elbow, the motor loss will include the brachioradialis as well as all of the aforementioned muscles, and the additional functional deficit is weakened elbow flexion. Lesions in the upper arm involve all of the aforementioned, with the addition of the triceps. Functionally, elbow extension is lost. The classic deformity associated with radial-nerve lesions is the wrist drop deformity (Fig. 33-5). Hand grip is compromised significantly as a result of the loss of wrist extensors, which position and help stabilize the wrist during grasp.

Median nerve

Median-nerve injuries can be associated with humeral fractures, elbow dislocations, distal radius fractures, and

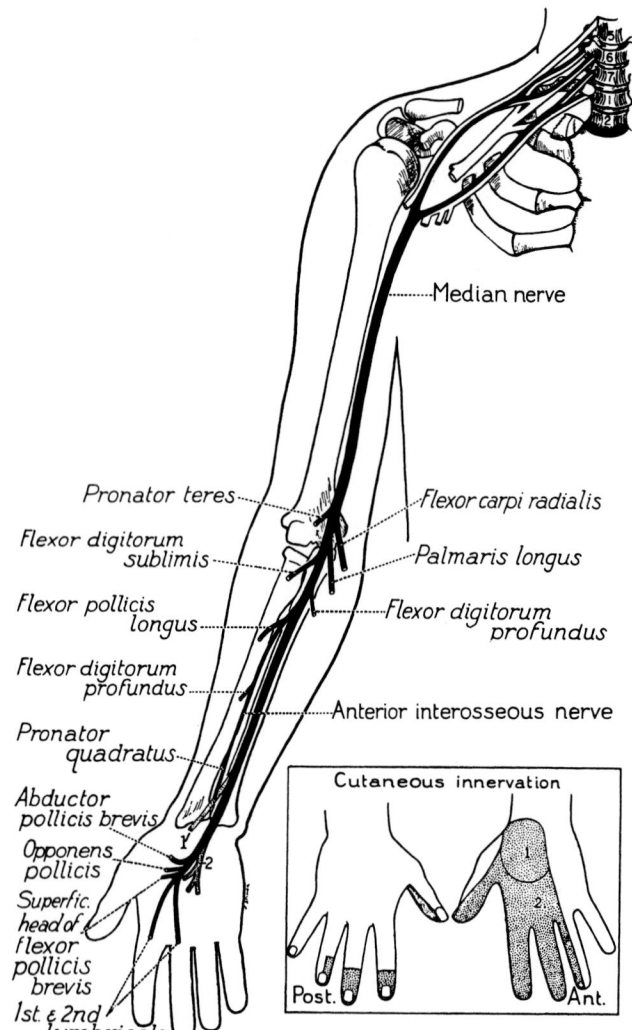

Fig. 33-6. The course and distribution of the median nerve. (From Haymaker W, Woodhall B: *Peripheral nerve injuries: principles of diagnosis,* Philadelphia, 1953, WB Saunders.)

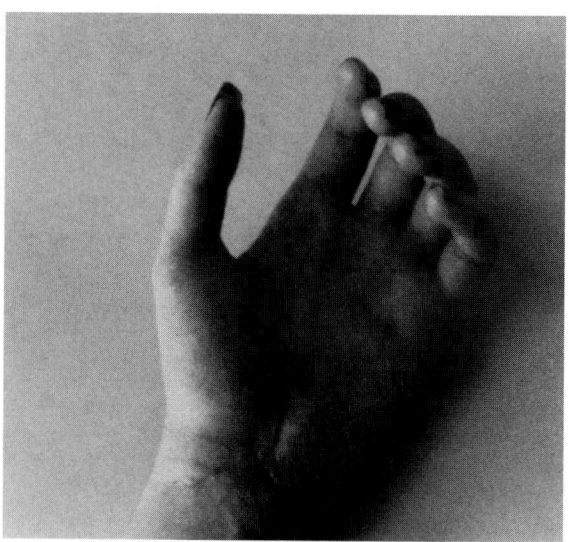

Fig. 33-7. Median-nerve palsy with flattened thenar eminence. (From Stanley BG, Tribuzi SM, editors: *Concepts in hand rehabilitation,* Philadelphia, 1992, FA Davis.)

dislocations of the lunate into the carpal canal, as well as knife and glass lacerations of the volar wrist. Compression of the median nerve can occur at the carpal canal (carpal tunnel syndrome), between the two heads of the pronator teres in the forearm (pronator syndrome), and compression of the anterior interosseous nerve in the forearm.

Deficits associated with median-nerve lesions depend on the site of the injury (Fig. 33-6). With a low or wrist-level lesion, the following muscles are involved:

- Opponens pollicis
- Abductor pollicis brevis (APB)
- Flexor pollicis brevis (FPB; superficial head)
- First and second lumbricales

Functionally, thumb opposition is lost, compromising activities requiring fine prehension. Sensory loss involves the volar surface of the thumb, index, long, and radial half of the ring fingers, and the dorsal surface of the distal phalanges of the thumb, index, long, and radial half of the ring fingers with some variations.

With a high-level lesion at the elbow or above, in addition to the aforementioned, the following muscles also are involved:

- Pronator teres
- Flexor carpi radialis
- Flexor digitorum superficialis
- Palmaris longus
- Flexor pollicis longus (FPL)
- Flexor digitorum profundus (FDP) to the index and long fingers
- Pronator quadratus

Functionally, pronation and wrist flexion is weakened, and thumb and index interphalangeal (IP) joint flexion is lost in addition to the loss of thumb opposition. The sensory loss is the same with a high-level lesion.

The median nerve gives off the anterior interosseous branch in the forearm approximately 8 cm distal to the elbow. Involvement of this branch affects the FPL and the FDP to the index finger and occasionally the long finger, and the pronator quadratus. There is no cutaneous sensory loss at this level.

The characteristic deformity associated with median-nerve injuries is sometimes called the *ape* or *simian hand* (Fig. 33-7). The thenar eminence is flattened, with the thumb lying to the side of the palm with loss of the ability to oppose and palmarly abduct the thumb. Secondarily, the web space may contract with loss of the span of the thumb. Fingertip

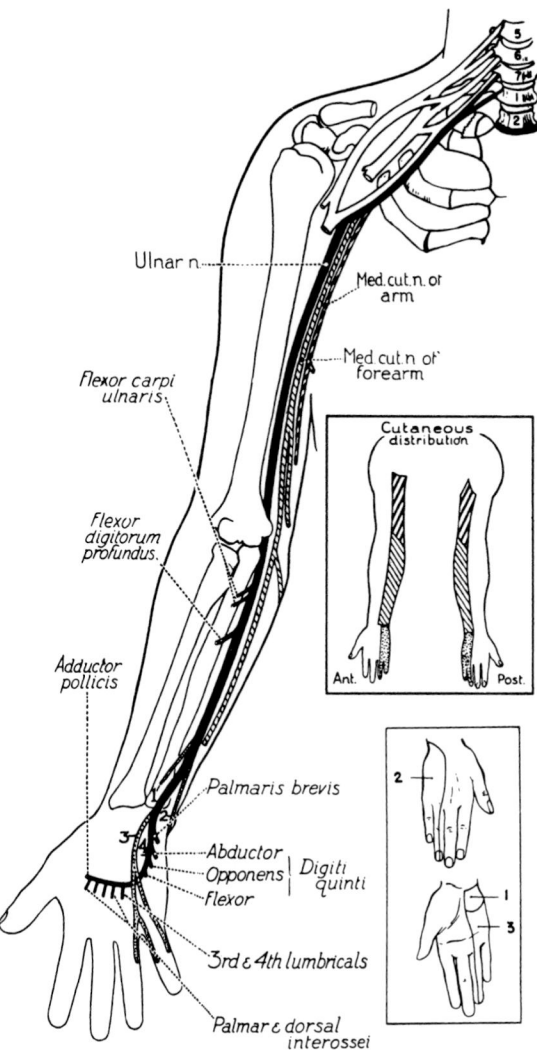

Fig. 33-8. The course and distribution of the ulnar nerve. (From Haymaker W, Woodhall B: *Peripheral nerve injuries: principles of diagnosis,* Philadelphia, 1953, WB Saunders.)

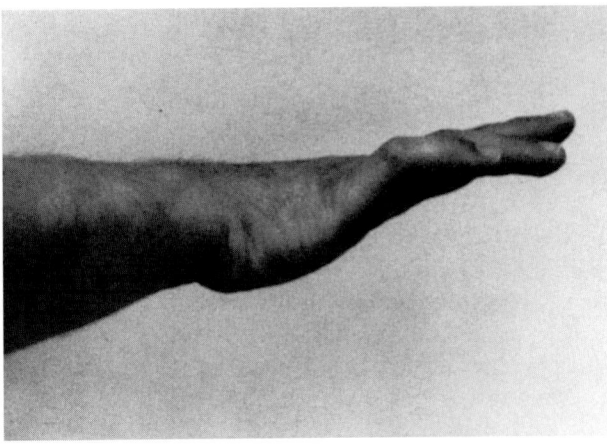

Fig. 33-9. Claw deformity associated with ulnar-nerve injury. (From Stanley BG, Tribuzi SM, editors: *Concepts in hand rehabilitation,* Philadelphia, 1992, FA Davis.)

- Opponens digiti minimi
- Lumbricales to the fourth and fifth digits
- Dorsal interossei
- Palmar interossei
- FPB (deep head)
- Adductor pollicis

With ulnar-nerve deficits, functional grip and pinch are affected. With attempts at lateral pinch, the thumb substitutes for the loss of the adductor with the FPL, resulting in flexion of the IP joint during attempts at pinch. This posture is called *Froment's sign.* Finger abduction and adduction are lost and the ability to actively flex the MP joints of the ring and small fingers with simultaneous active IP extension is not possible. Because of the loss of the intrinsics, there is a decrease in power grip and a loss of fine prehension. This sensory loss involves the superficial terminal branch of the ulnar nerve, which supplies sensation to the volar surface of the ulnar aspect of the palm distally, and the volar surface of the small and ulnar half of the ring fingers.

With a high-level lesion—that is, one at or above the elbow—the following muscles also are involved:

- Flexor carpi ulnaris
- FDP to the ring and small fingers

Functionally, the clinical picture is the same with hand grip further weakened by the loss of the profundus to the ring and small fingers. Sensory loss involves both the palmar and dorsal cutaneous branches of the ulnar nerve in addition to the superficial terminal branch. These branches innervate the dorsal surface of the small and ulnar half of the ring fingers, and the proximal palm on the ulnar side.

The characteristic deformity associated with ulnar-nerve lesions is the claw deformity (Fig. 33-9). The ring and small fingers rest in a posture of MP joint hyperextension and IP joint flexion. This posture results from the loss of the

prehension is lost because of the loss of the thenar intrinsics, as well as the loss of sensibility of the volar radial side of the hand.

Ulnar nerve

Ulnar-nerve injuries can be associated with fractures of the medial epicondyle of the humerus and the olecranon of the ulna. Glass and knife lacerations of the wrist can involve the ulnar nerve as well. Common sites of compression are within Guyon's canal at the wrist level and within the cubital tunnel proximally.

Deficits associated with an ulnar-nerve lesion depend on the site of injury (Fig. 33-8). With a low or wrist-level lesion, the following muscles are involved:

- Abductor digiti minimi
- Flexor digiti minimi

balancing influence of the intrinsic muscles on the extrinsic flexors and extensors. In addition, there is atrophy of the interossei with hollowing between the metacarpals and flattening of the hypothenar area.

EVALUATION

Nerve injuries can result in deficits in muscle strength, in protective and discriminative sensibility, and in sympathetic function. Postural disturbances of the hand result from muscle imbalance, and this along with muscle weakness can lead to a loss of joint mobility and the formation of joint and soft tissue contractures. These sequelae have a serious impact on hand function and self-care, work, and leisure activities. Therefore the essential elements of the therapist's evaluation include a thorough history, manual muscle testing, range-of-motion (ROM) evaluation, sensibility examination, evaluation of sympathetic function, and an analysis of the impact of the injury on the patient's functional status. A careful evaluation serves to set a baseline from which to gauge the process of reinnervation, as well as to judge the effectiveness of therapy. Ongoing reevaluation allows monitoring of the patient's status to ensure that loss of joint mobility does not develop as a result of muscle weakness and to monitor for signs of damage to insensate skin.

The following sections cover important details in the evaluation of the nerve-injured hand.

History

The history should include the following:

- Patient name
- Sex
- Date of evaluation
- Age (The prognosis is better in the child than in the adult.)
- Dominance (The degree of sensibility and coordination deficit in a median-nerve lesion may require a change of dominance.)
- Occupation (Occupation may be a contributing factor to a compression lesion or a cumulative trauma disorder. A median-nerve lesion will impair performance in a job that requires manual dexterity. An ulnar-nerve lesion will impair the manual laborer's ability to perform grasp activities, especially if strength is required. Protective sensibility might be adequate for some occupations, whereas others require fine discriminative sensibility.)
- Avocational interests (The same considerations are true as for occupation.)
- Nature of injury (Suggests the extent of damage and the relative amount of scarring that might interfere with axonal regeneration.)

- Level of injury (Prognosis is better for lower-level lesions.)
- Date of injury/repair (Whether the injury is recent or old and how long it has been since repair helps in assessing whether current deficits are "reasonable" at this time or suggest that regeneration is no longer occurring.)
- Patient's description of problems, including problems in activities of daily living (ADLs) (The examiner should not bias the response by asking leading questions. Ask the patient to be more specific about terms such as "numbness" and "it feels dead." Problems in ADLs might suggest the need for an assistive splint or adaptive equipment.)

Sympathetic function

The sympathetic fibers are concerned with vasomotor, sudomotor (sweat), pilomotor ("gooseflesh" response), and trophic (nourishment) functions in the upper extremity. The area of autonomic sympathetic supply closely corresponds to, but is smaller than, the area of cutaneous supply of a nerve. This is because the autonomic fibers travel closely with the cutaneous fibers on their way to the periphery. The return of sympathetic function does not necessarily imply return of cutaneous sensibility. However, the absence of sympathetic function immediately after nerve injury or in long-term cases of injury does tend to imply absence of significant sensibility.[18,19,23,26]

Certain changes in sympathetic function are seen immediately or very early after nerve injury; others occur 3 to 6 weeks after injury or even later as continued effects of impaired vasomotor and trophic function.

Examination of sympathetic function is accomplished by observation and palpation with comparison to ipsilateral and contralateral skin (see Chapter 14).

Motor function

When evaluating motor function after nerve injury, one must consider the expected pattern of motor return as regeneration progresses. The principles of muscle testing must be adhered to, and the examiner must be observant for trick motions during manual muscle testing.

Expected pattern of motor return. Following nerve repair, there is a latent period of 3 to 4 weeks, after which axonal regeneration occurs at the rate of approximately 1 mm/day.[17] Muscle reinnervation occurs in the order in which the muscles were originally innervated. An early sign of motor reinnervation is sensitivity of a previously insensitive muscle to pressure.[24] As reinnervation continues, the muscle undergoes several stages of recovery:

- Observable and palpable contracture without production of motion

- Ability to "hold" a test position without being able to produce that position
- Ability to move the joint through the test motion
- Ability to move the joint through the test motion and hold the position against resistance[15]

Manual muscle testing. For accuracy in muscle testing, certain principles should be followed:

- Stabilize the joint proximal to the joint being tested.
- Be aware of limitations in passive range of motion (PROM), muscle shortening, or contractures that could interfere with motion of the part being tested.
- Place the joint in the test position and ask the patient to "hold." Observe for compensatory motions distally or proximally that indicate substitution attempts. If the position is held accurately, apply resistance gradually until the muscle can no longer hold or full resistance is achieved.
- Apply resistance near the distal end of the bone on which the muscle inserts.
- Follow a standard grading scale to record results (e.g., "0 through 5" or "absent through normal").

Trick motions in manual muscle testing.[15,24] Anomalous nerve supply can account for unexpected performance of a test motion by a prime mover (e.g., the ulnar nerve might provide full innervation of opponens pollicis, thus allowing it to function in the presence of an injured median nerve). Apparent performance of a test motion by other than the prime mover can occur in several ways.

Rebound. If the antagonistic muscle strongly contracts then relaxes, joint motion in the opposite direction will occur. This is termed *rebound.* For example, if the extensor pollicis longus muscle contracts strongly then relaxes, slight flexion of the thumb IP joint will occur, simulating contraction of the FPL.[25]

Supplementary action. Some muscles, by virtue of their line of pull, can produce a joint motion in the absence of the prime mover, but it will not be a perfect reproduction. For example, in the absence of wrist flexors, abductor pollicis longus can flex the wrist. This is called *supplementary action.*[15]

Antagonist. Strong contraction of an antagonistic muscle can result in apparent contraction of an agonistic muscle by passive pull on the tendon of that agonistic muscle. This occurs when the agonist muscle is a two-joint muscle. For example, when the wrist is strongly dorsiflexed against resistance, the fingers assume a flexed position because their tendons have been stretched over the volar aspect of the dorsiflexed wrist and do not have sufficient length to allow the finger joints to remain in extension.[15]

Common tendons. Tendinous slips of an intact muscle into the tendinous insertion of a denervated muscle can reproduce the motion of the denervated muscle. When the intact muscle contracts, it pulls on the insertion of the denervated muscle. For example, APB muscle sends a slip into the tendon of the extensor pollicis longus and can produce thumb IP extension in the presence of a denervated extensor pollicis longus muscle.

Testing for median-nerve function.[15,24] Signs of low median-nerve involvement include atrophy of the thenar eminence and a resting posture of the thumb pulp in the plane of the palm of the hand. If the long flexors are involved, a "benediction" posture of the index and long fingers can be observed, and there will be wasting of the medial epicondyle muscle mass (secondary also to involvement of pronator teres and flexor carpi radialis).

The following tips are helpful during muscle testing:

- *Pronation:* The pronator teres can be palpated; the pronator quadratus cannot. Brachioradialis can pronate the forearm sufficiently from a position of supination to allow gravity to complete the motion. Failure to stabilize the arm can result in substitution by internal rotation.
- *Wrist flexion:* This can occur by a combination of flexor carpi ulnaris and abductor pollicis longus, although this will tend to occur with ulnar deviation of the wrist.
- *Finger flexion:* FDP can have anomalous innervation.
- *Thumb-tip flexion:* Function of the FPL should be tested with the thumb in palmar adduction and the wrist in neutral. This is to eliminate possible trick flexion achieved by the abductor pollicis longus, which by abducting the thumb while the wrist is hyperextended can exert a passive tendon pull on the FPL tendon.
- *Palmar abduction of thumb:* APB function should be tested with the thumb in a vertical plane perpendicular to the index finger to eliminate substitution by the abductor pollicis longus. Some palmar abduction with thumb pronation can sometimes be performed by the ulnar head of the FPB by virtue of its attachment into the metacarpal. A strong short FPB will enhance this substitute motion.
- *Thumb opposition:* Haymaker and Woodhall[15] note that in normal opposition of the thumb to the fifth finger, both fingertips are extended as they meet pulp-to-pulp and the fingers form a vertical arch. In the absence of opponens pollicis, pseudoopposition can occur by a combination of FPB (deep head), which acts to flex the thumb carpometacarpal and MP joints, and adductor pollicis, which acts to slide the thumb across the palm. The result is that the flexed thumb advances to the lateral aspect of the fifth finger and rotation does not take place.
- *MP flexion of the index and long fingers:* The intrinsic muscles can compensate for the paralyzed muscles. Anomalous or double innervation of the lumbrical to the long finger is common.[24]

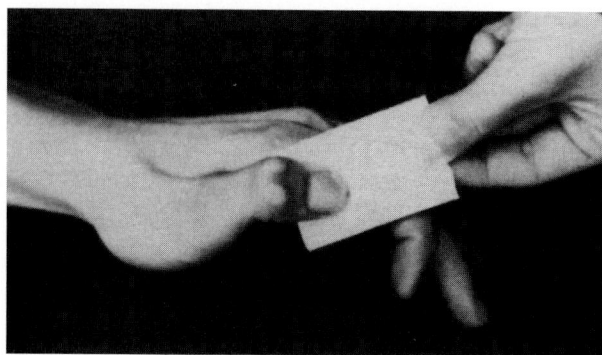

Fig. 33-10. Froment's sign.

- *IP extension of the index and long fingers:* The movement usually will be weak but present because of intact interossei.

Testing for ulnar-nerve function.[15,24] Signs to look for in a low ulnar-nerve lesion are atrophy of the intrinsics, which in advanced cases, can be seen as "hollows" between the metacarpals; atrophy of the hypothenar eminence; clawing of the ring and small fingers, with less clawing in the index and long fingers because of their intact lumbricals; and a posture of abduction of the small finger resulting from unopposed action of the extensor digiti quinti tendon in the absence of adduction of the small finger. In high ulnar-nerve lesions, the clawing in the digits will be lessened because of the paralysis of the FDP, but as that muscle undergoes reinnervation the clawing will increase. In a high lesion, there also will be wasting on the medial aspect of the upper forearm.

The following guidelines are helpful during muscle testing:

- *Thumb adduction:* This motion should be tested by requiring that the thumb remain in contact with the palm to eliminate substitution by the medial fibers of the APB, which can adduct the thumb across the palm but only with some simultaneous abduction away from the palm.[24]

  From a position of abduction, the thumb can be adducted against the radial aspect of the palm by the extensor pollicis longus and be swept across the palm by the FPL. The signs of this are visible contraction of the extensor pollicis longus tendon and flexion of the terminal joint of the thumb.[25] These signs are accentuated when adduction is attempted against resistance (Froment's sign) (Fig. 33-10). The extensor pollicis longus tendon by itself can also hold the thumb in adduction against resistance.[24]
- *Finger abduction:* The tendons of the extensor digitorum can abduct the fingers if simultaneous MP extension also is allowed. Even if it is not allowed, the index

and small fingers can still be extended by their respective extensor digitorum tendons. Therefore the best test is to require radial and ulnar abduction of the middle finger without the finger lifting from the test surface.[25]

- *Finger adduction:* The finger flexors can adduct the fingers if simultaneous MP flexion is permitted. Therefore the motion should be tested on a flat surface, which prevents finger flexion. Even in this case, adduction of the index finger might still occur by action of the extensor indicis proprius. Adduction of the fifth finger cannot be supplemented by substitute motions.
- *MP flexion:* The first and second lumbricals compensate for the index and long fingers. The third lumbrical might be innervated by the median nerve, thus permitting flexion of the ring MP joint. The flexor digitorum sublimis tendon in the ring and small fingers might flex the MP joints, but only with simultaneous PIP joint flexion.[25]
- *IP joint extension:* In the index and long fingers, this motion will be present but weak. In the ring and small fingers, it can occur only by extensor digitorum communis action when the MP joints are prevented from hyperextending.

Testing for radial-nerve function. According to Sunderland,[24] every radial-nerve motion can be observed in complete lesions of the nerve except that of the abductor pollicis longus. However, the patient will be unable to simultaneously extend the wrist and fingers or to radially abduct the extended thumb. The examiner should look for a "drop wrist" when the elbow is flexed and pronated and should look for wasting of the dorsal arm (triceps), at the lateral supracondylar muscle mass (brachioradialis, extensor carpi radialis longus and brevis), and on the dorsum of the forearm (finger and thumb extensors and the ulnar wrist extensor).[24]

- *Elbow extension:* This can occur with the assistance of gravity.
- *Supination:* This can occur by action of the biceps.
- *Wrist extension:* This can occur with finger flexion because of the passive pull on the extensor digitorum tendons. This tendon pull acts to lift the wrist. However, the wrist will not be able to be lifted if the fingers are simultaneously held in extension.
- *Finger extension:* Tension on the tendons of extensor digitorum will produce passive finger extension at the MP joints, which occurs with wrist flexion.
- *Thumb extension:* A slip of the APB into the extensor pollicis longus tendon can result in extension of the terminal joint. Palmar abduction may accompany this motion.

Sensibility function

When evaluating sensibility after nerve injury, the examiner must consider the expected pattern of return.

Following an initial latent period of 3 to 4 weeks, axonal regeneration progresses at a rate of approximately 1 mm/day.[24] Sensibility recovery occurs in the following sequence: deep pressure and pinprick (protective sensation), moving touch, static light touch, and discriminative (functional) touch.[7,22,24] At first, a stimulus will be poorly localized and may radiate proximally or distally. Accurate localization is among the last sensibility functions to recover.[21]

Many tests are in clinical use today. Tests are chosen based on whether they can provide information on the following questions, which relate to the sequence of recovery: Is regeneration occurring? What is the area of sensibility dysfunction? Is protective sensation present? Is light touch present? Is discriminative sensibility present?

Whichever tests are selected for use, the examiner should use the same methods of administration at each test session to help make serial tests as reliable as possible. Testing should also be done in a quiet room, free of visual and auditory distractions. Tests typically included in the sensibility battery for peripheral-nerve injuries include Tinel's sign; sharp/dull discrimination; Semmes-Weinstein light-touch deep-pressure testing; two-point discrimination, both static and moving; and Moberg Pick-up Test (see Chapter 14).

Pain

Finally, pain is addressed as part of the therapist's assessment. Severe, burning pain in the distribution of the injured nerve, referred to as *causalgia,* may be associated with a nerve injury. Neuromas may also be a source of extreme pain when touched and may develop at the site of the injury. Clinical features of the patient's pain are documented, such as the time of onset following the injury, the quality of pain and its distribution, and precipitating factors.

THERAPEUTIC MANAGEMENT

The remainder of this chapter focuses on the rehabilitation of nerve injuries during the acute, recovery, and chronic phases. The *acute* phase refers to the early postinjury and postsurgery time when the focus is on healing and prevention. The *recovery* phase refers to the period of reinnervation when retraining and reeducation are stressed. The *chronic* phase refers to that time when the potential for reinnervation has peaked and the patient is left with significant residual deficits. The emphasis during this phase is on compensatory function.

Acute phase

The objectives of the therapist's management during the acute phase are primarily protection and prevention: protection of the traumatized or surgically repaired nerve and prevention of joint contracture and further injury secondary to decreased sensibility. Table 33-2 highlights information

Table 33-2. Referral information and treatment implications

Required information	Treatment implications
Nerve involvement	
A. Specific nerve injured	A. Indicates sensory and motor impairment; provides focus for evaluation
B. Classification and level of injury	B. Indicates prognosis and facilitates goal setting
C. Mechanism of injury; clean versus crush	C. Indicates degree of tissue reaction and scar to anticipate more damage with crush injuries than with clean lacerations
D. Other structures involved	D. Treatment protocols must be integrated to allow appropriate management for all injured structures
Surgical management	
A. Date of repair	A. Nerve repairs protected from stress for 3-5 wk
B. Position of joints to allow relaxation of the nerve juncture	B. Tension at the nerve juncture can compromise results; relaxation of the nerve juncture achieved by flexing the joints across which the nerve passes
C. Type of repair	C. Early repair is superior to late repair; with nerve grafts, axons must regenerate across junctures

important for the therapist to obtain at the time of referral and the therapy implications. The types of diagnoses seen during this phase may include an acute nerve compression, postsurgical decompression and release, and postsurgical repair of a lacerated nerve.

Period of immobilization. The purpose of postoperative immobilization or splinting is to (1) minimize tension at the repair site, (2) protect the nerve from disruption, and (3) in the case of nerve compression or following decompression, immobilize or splint to minimize and facilitate the resolution of the inflammatory reaction.

Splinting following nerve repair may be done by the attending physician or the therapist with either a plaster cast or a removable plastic splint. The choice usually is made by the physician, who considers the reliability of the patient and his or her lifestyle. Positioning, whether with casting or splinting, is done with joints flexed or extended to avoid tension at the repair site. For example, with a median-nerve repair, the wrist may need to be flexed. The specific position of the splint and duration of use is determined by the surgeon and communicated to the therapist. In general, immobilization is maintained for 3 to 4 weeks after nerve repair, at which time tensile strength of the nerve is great enough to withstand stress. An important consideration when splinting the hand with compromised sensation is the potential for skin breakdown. Splints must be fabricated carefully to avoid pressure areas, and the patient must be instructed to monitor the skin for any signs of breakdown, such as redness or blistering. Splinting following a nerve compression or contusion is done to rest the involved area to facilitate the resolution of the inflammation reaction. If applied acutely, the splint is worn continuously for 1 to 2 weeks and then intermittently thereafter. The splint is positioned to allow a minimum of pressure on the nerve at the site of compression. For example, with carpal tunnel syndrome, the wrist is positioned in neutral to slight extension, which minimizes pressure on the median nerve.[2]

During the period of immobilization, the therapist must monitor the status of the unimmobilized joints and instruct the patient in ROM exercises to ensure maintenance of joint mobility.

Postimmobilization. The priorities of the therapy program after immobilization are to recover ROM lost during the period of immobilization, to enhance function, and to educate the patient in a program of protection and prevention.

Increase of range of motion. ROM exercises are directed at recovering the motion lost during the phase of immobilization. For example, with a low median- or ulnar-nerve repair, the wrist is positioned in flexion during the phase of immobilization and the patient may have restricted wrist extension when permitted to begin exercises. Exercises are directed at gradually recovering wrist extension, generally starting with active range of motion (AROM).

Passive and active-assisted ROM exercises are introduced depending on the patient's progress as well as on specific precautions relevant to the individual case. For example, if the patient is recovering ROM at a satisfactory rate with the active program, PROM exercises may not be necessary. However, if progress is slow (i.e., less than a 5-degree gain per week), PROM exercises may begin. In any case, aggressive stretching exercises are avoided to protect the repaired nerve from a potentially harmful maximum stretch. Occasionally, specific ROM limits will be imposed by the surgeon to protect a nerve repaired under tension or when a nerve gap has had to be overcome with more extensive joint positioning. In these cases, the therapy approach may be to increase incrementally the amount of ROM allowed by a specific number of degrees on a week-to-week basis; for example, following median-nerve repair under tension, wrist extension may be permitted at a rate of 10 degrees per week. Splints may be serially adjusted to ensure that ROM limits are not exceeded.

Enhancement of function. Splinting is also used at this stage, with the aim to enhance function. When the nerve injury results in muscle paresis or paralysis and muscle imbalance disrupts the normal resting posture of the hand, soft tissue and joint contractures may result, as well as overstretching of the weakened muscle by the pull of its

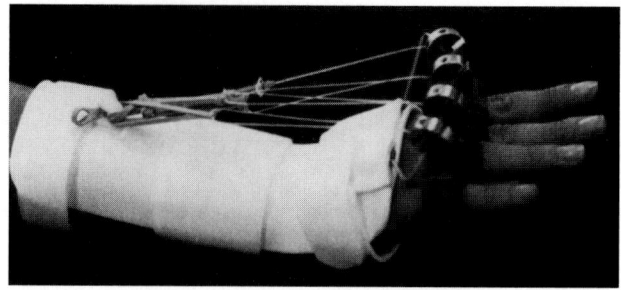

Fig. 33-11. Phoenix outrigger. (From Stanley BG, Tribuzi SM, editors: *Concepts in hand rehabilitation,* Philadelphia, 1992, FA Davis.)

antagonist. Splinting is used to restore the normal resting posture and to prevent secondary joint contractures. By restoring a more normal posture, the splint also may enhance function. With each nerve injury, specific requirements must be fulfilled. The exact style of splint, the material from which it is made, and the method of construction is, to some extent, secondary as long as the splint resolves the problem and is acceptable to the patient.

Radial-nerve splints. The critical problem with radial-nerve palsy is the loss of wrist extension. The wrist rests in a flexed posture, which puts the wrist extensors at risk for overstretching. In addition, the MP joints rest in a more extended position when the wrist is flexed, resulting from the tension placed on the extensor digitorum communis across the flexed wrist. This extended MP joint position, if unrelieved, may result in shortening of the collateral ligaments and hence extension contractures of the MP joints.

The splint applied must support the wrist in extension. A simple wrist cock-up splint or a Futuro splint may be used. There is also a loss of MP joint extension because of the involvement of the extrinsic finger extensors. The wrist splint can be made to include the MP joints, supporting them in neutral or slight flexion. However, supporting the MP joints limits full flexion and may result in a loss of MP joint flexion if not monitored closely. Many patients prefer a wrist splint without MP joint support and report satisfactory function.

A dynamic splint with an outrigger to assist finger and thumb extension can also be used to allow a full arc of finger motion. The splint can be made dorsally with the wrist supported in a slight degree of extension. The commercially available low-profile Phoenix outrigger can be used to provide the extension assist (Fig. 33-11). Colditz[12] has developed a splint for radial-nerve palsy that reestablishes the normal tenodesis pattern of the hand. The splint includes a dorsal trough with a low-profile outrigger that extends across the wrist to the level of the proximal phalanges. Finger loops are worn around each proximal phalanx, and nylon cord is directed from these loops through channels on the outrigger and pulled to a proximal attachment point on

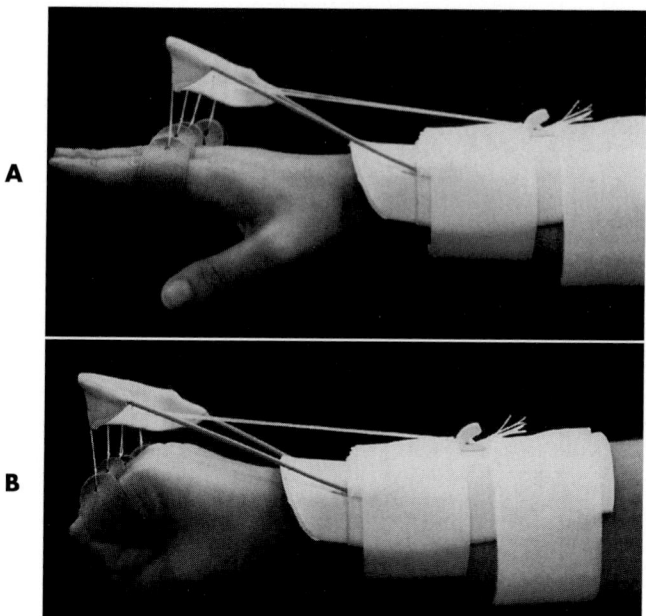

Fig. 33-12. A, Splint for radial-nerve palsy designed by Colditz, which reestablishes the tenodesis pattern of the hand. **B,** With digital flexion, the wrist is brought into extension. (From Stanley BG, Tribuzi SM, editors: *Concepts in hand rehabilitation,* Philadelphia, 1992, FA Davis.)

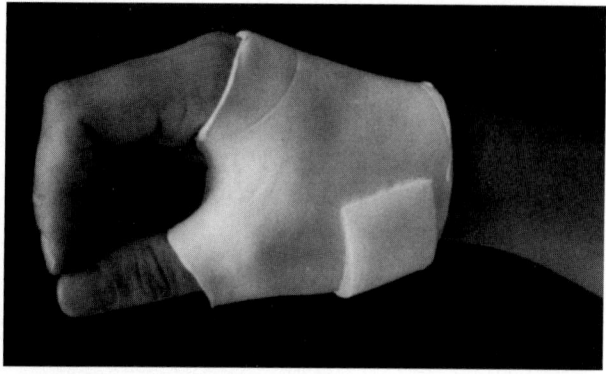

Fig. 33-13. Opponens splint for the median-nerve palsy. (From Stanley BG, Tribuzi SM, editors: *Concepts in hand rehabilitation,* Philadelphia, 1992, FA Davis.)

the dorsal base of the splint (Fig. 33-12). When the digits are flexed, tension on the cord brings the wrist into extension, and when the wrist is flexed, the digits are pulled into extension (see Fig. 33-12).

For the splinting program to be successful, the specific splint chosen, whether static or dynamic, must be one that is functional for the patient but also cosmetically acceptable. Some patients reject a dynamic splint as being too bulky or attention getting and will not wear it, preferring a static splint. When the dominant extremity is involved, the functional requirement usually takes precedence and a dynamic splint often is the best choice. When the nondominant extremity is involved, the functional requirement may be less, and the patient's concern for cosmesis may lead to the choice of a static splint. At night, a simple wrist splint is sufficient to position the wrist and allow the fingers to fall into a normal resting posture.

Median-nerve splints. Median-nerve injury results in loss of the ability to position the thumb in opposition to the fingers and to palmarly abduct the thumb. Splinting is needed to facilitate thumb and finger prehension and to maintain the thumb web space. A hand-based splint that positions the thumb in palmar abduction and opposition to the index and long fingers can be used (Fig. 33-13).

However, some patients find that they do just as well without a splint and can use compensatory motions to substitute for the absent thenar intrinsics. If the opponens splint is not used, the web space must be maintained either

with a web spacer splint (Fig. 33-14) worn at night or with conscientious web stretching, or both. If a web space contracture does develop, serial web space splinting would be indicated to restore the web space.

Ulnar-nerve splints. The loss of the interossei and the fourth and fifth lumbricales with ulnar-nerve injury results in a claw deformity. The resting position is one of MP joint hyperextension with PIP and distal interphalangeal (DIP) joint flexion owing to the unopposed action of the extrinsic flexors and extensors. The posture is more pronounced with the ring and small fingers because the index and long finger lumbricales are median innervated. The deformity initially may be passively correctable, but left untreated, fixed flexion contractures may result at the PIP and DIP joint levels. Functionally, the patient will have difficulty with grasp because he or she will be unable to extend the fingers in approaching objects to be grasped. Splinting is needed to provide a counterbalance for the extrinsic muscles that will help prevent the development of flexion contractures and allow extension at the IP joints to facilitate grasp.

A dorsal hand-based splint that blocks MP joint hyperextension can be fabricated. With the MP joint blocked, the extensor digitorum can exert its pull distally and extension is then possible at the IP joints. The splint is fabricated to allow full digital flexion (Fig. 33-15). Another option is a figure-of-eight design fabricated from a ½- to ¾-inch-wide piece of double thermoplastic material approximately 12 inches long (Fig. 33-16). A simple alternative is to limit MP joint hyperextension using finger cuffs over the proximal phalanges with elastics volarly and proximally attached to a wrist strap or band (Fig. 33-17). When the patient extends, the cuff limits MP joint hyperextension, and then IP joint extension is possible. If PIP flexion contractures have already developed, dynamic, serial static, or three-point extension splinting is needed to correct the deformity and restore passive PIP joint extension.

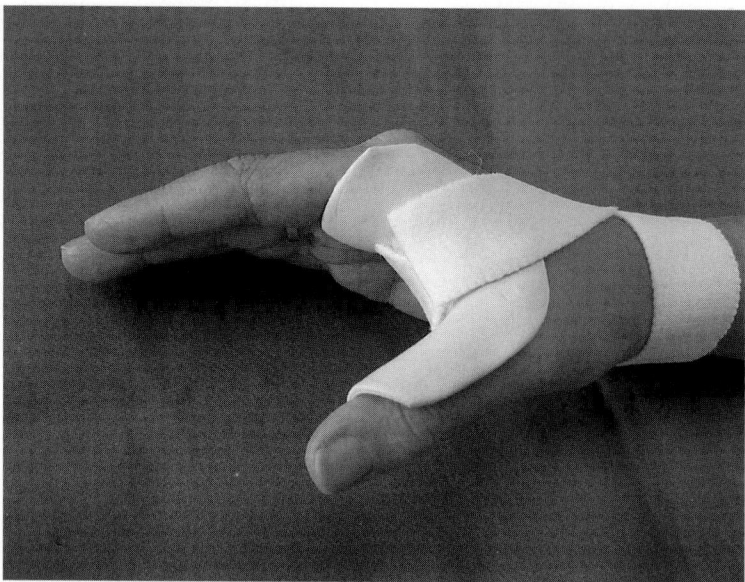

Fig. 33-14. Thumb web spacer splint to be worn at night.

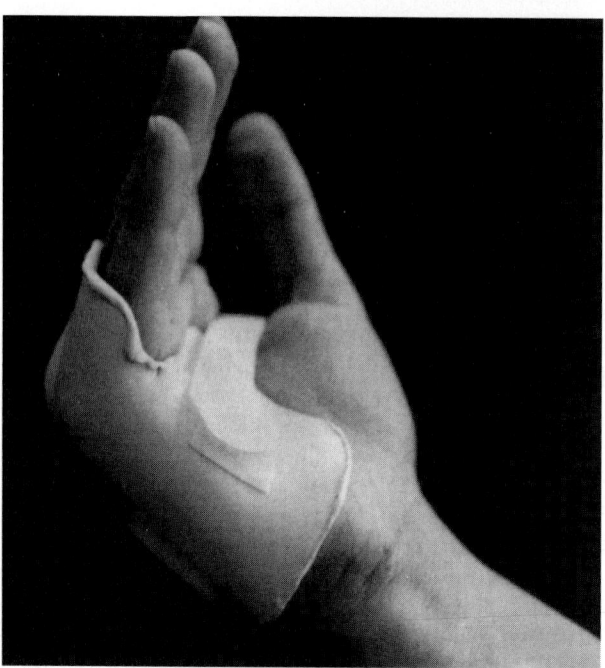

Fig. 33-15. Splint used to counteract the claw deformity of ulnar-nerve palsy. (From Stanley BG, Tribuzi SM, editors: *Concepts in hand rehabilitation,* Philadelphia, 1992, FA Davis.)

Patient education. A fully informed and involved patient is one of the most important ingredients for a successful rehabilitation program. The therapist's early sessions with the patient should be focused on education. A simplified explanation of nerve function and the consequences of injury, as well as what outcomes can be expected, needs to be covered. Patients must be aware of the slow rate of nerve regeneration and the guarded prognosis with complete and

high lesions to adjust their expectations accordingly. Communication between the therapist and surgeon is essential to ensure that the same information is being conveyed.

A clear, simple, and realistic home program also must be a part of this early education process. What the patient does outside of the therapy clinic is just as important as the supervised therapy sessions. Patients must know what deformities they are at risk for and what measures they need to take for preventing these. The therapist must work with the patient in developing a schedule of exercise and splint use that is reasonable within the context of the patient's lifestyle but that achieves the goals of therapy.

The patient also must know the risks related to the loss of sensation. For example, because of the loss of sensation, the patient is susceptible to thermal injuries and those from sharp or abrasive objects. Because of the loss of feeling, the patient may grip objects with more force and may sustain the grip longer, resulting in skin breakdown and blister formation. Once injury has occurred, healing may take longer than usual because of the decreased nutrition and vascularity of denervated skin.[24]

The patient must be instructed to avoid handling very hot, cold, sharp, or abrasive objects. When tools or other objects are being used, sustained grasp must be avoided, tools should be changed frequently, tool handles should be built up to distribute pressure, and protective work gloves must be worn. Regular skin inspection is stressed, with prompt treatment of any wounds or blisters that may result from daily activities or from improperly fitting or applied splints. Brand[5,6] recommends daily soaks and oil massage to compensate for the dryness of the skin and reduced compliancy under pressure that occurs because of the loss of sweating function of the skin that normally maintains moistness and protects the skin from cracking.

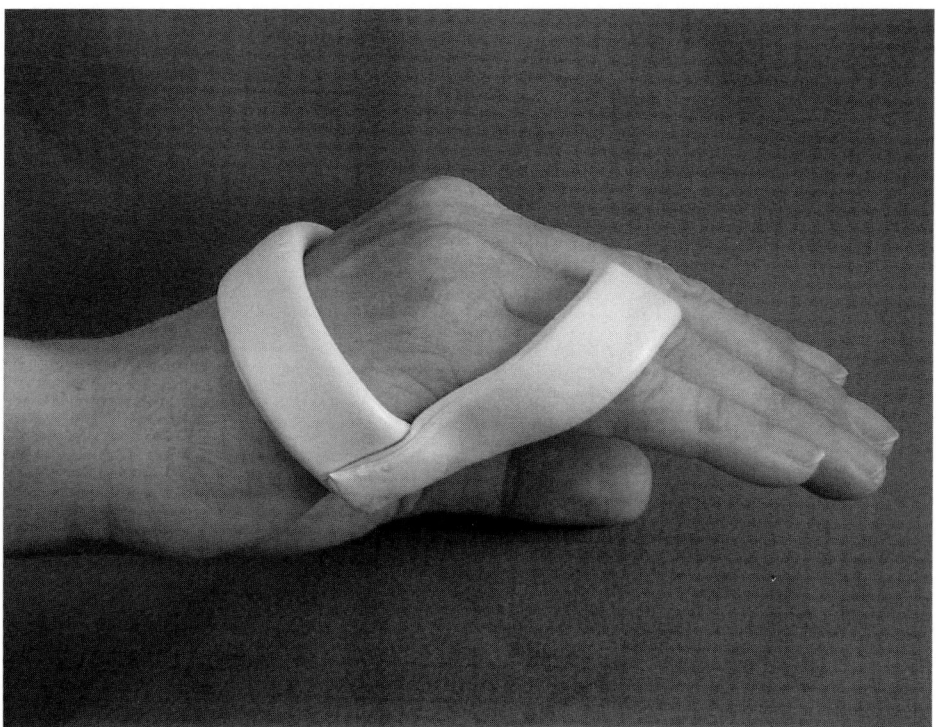

Fig. 33-16. This splint is a figure-of-eight design fabricated from ½- to ¾-inch-wide piece of double thermoplastic material approximately 12 inches long.

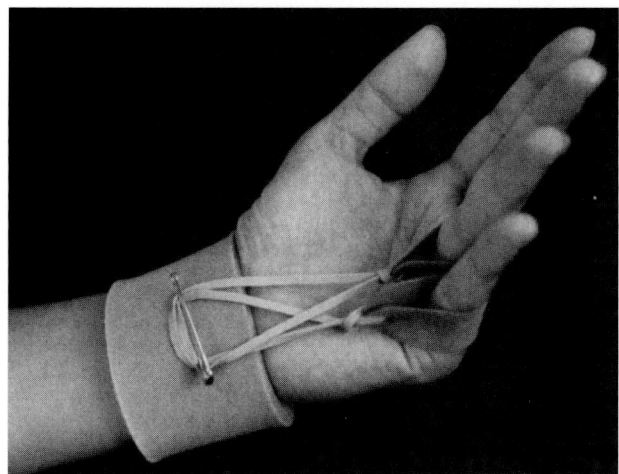

Fig. 33-17. Alternative method for splinting an ulnar-nerve palsy to counteract clawing. (From Stanley BG, Tribuzi SM, editors: *Concepts in hand rehabilitation,* Philadelphia, 1992, FA Davis.)

Recovery phase

Once clinical signs of reinnervation become apparent, the therapy program and treatment goals must be reestablished. With the return of sensory and motor function, retraining and reeducation become important. As muscles are reinnervated, therapy is designed to enhance the recovery of strength and control. As skin receptors are reinnervated, techniques of desensitization and reeducation are applied to normalize and maximize the recovery of functional sensibility.

Motor retraining. Motor retraining begins at the earliest evidence of muscle reinnervation. Before this time, passive exercises are important to maintain joint ROM and muscle-tendon length. Some clinicians also advocate the use of electrical stimulation to forestall the deterioration of denervated muscle. The rationale is that the recovery of muscle strength following reinnervation will be more complete if the physiologic muscle integrity is maintained with electrical stimulation. However, research support for this theory is limited, and the use of electrical stimulation for denervated muscle is not a universally agreed-upon practice. However, once reinnervation begins, electrical stimulation may be used to give the patient the proprioceptive feedback of the recovering muscle. Active and active-assisted exercises are provided for the function the muscle is primarily responsible for. Position-and-hold exercises are helpful at this stage. For example, the involved joint or joints are placed in the desired position, and the patient is asked to hold the position through contraction of the target muscle. During this exercise, electrical stimulation of the muscle can enhance the patient's efforts. Biofeedback can also help by increasing the patient's awareness of minute contractions through visual and auditory feedback. Initially, the therapy sessions must be kept short to avoid fatigue. As the patient demonstrates increasing control, isotonic exercises are introduced. Functional activities are incorporated into the program to provide practice in coordinating movement patterns and to further increase strength and endurance. Progressive resistive exercise is also used to increase

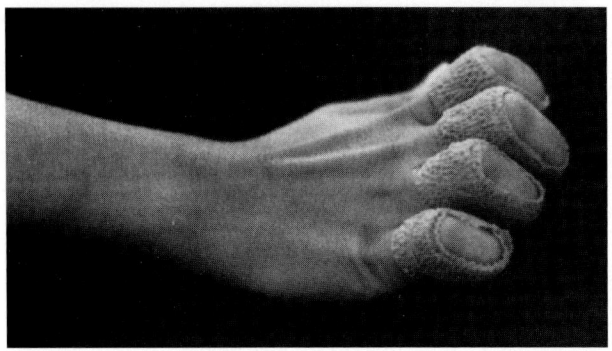

Fig. 33-18. Exercise for the extensor digitorum communis. (From Stanley BG, Tribuzi SM, editors: *Concepts in hand rehabilitation,* Philadelphia, 1992, FA Davis.)

strength and endurance and to increase strength when the target muscle reaches the fair grade.

Key exercises for the radial-nerve lesions involve wrist, finger, and thumb extension. Wrist extensor muscle activity is easily monitored using biofeedback, a useful technique during the early stages of motor return. During the retraining of the finger extensors, intrinsic substitution should be eliminated by preventing IP extension while attempting MP joint extension. Coban wrap can be used to position the IP joints in flexion when isolating extensor digitorum communis activity (Fig. 33-18). Key exercises for median-nerve lesions involve the thenar intrinsic muscles. The thumb is positioned in opposition, and the patient is asked to hold it this way. Positioning and holding in palmar abduction is also practiced. A circular object such as a jar lid can be placed perpendicularly in the palm and the patient can attempt to trace the perimeter of the jar lid with the thumb, a motion that requires the action of the opponens and the APB (Fig. 33-19). Finger abduction and adduction exercises are key with ulnar-nerve lesions. The patient's hand is placed palm down on a flat surface that can be dusted with powder to eliminate friction, and abduction and adduction of the digits is attempted. Lateral pinching exercises are also important and involve activity of the first dorsal interosseous muscle and the adductor pollicis.

Desensitization. Regeneration of a sensory nerve is often associated with dysesthesia. A light touch of the involved area may range from being mildly irritating to extremely painful in the case of neuroma formation. Desensitization has been described by several authors[1,10,14] as being helpful in reducing this hypersensitivity. *Desensitization* refers to the process of lessening reactivity to an external stimulus through the use of a graded series of modalities and procedures. Treatment begins with exposure to a stimulus that is slightly irritating but tolerable, and as tolerance increases, more noxious stimuli are introduced. Barber[1] has developed a structured approach to the evaluation and treatment of hypersensitivity. Three sensory modalities are used in Barber's approach: textures, contact

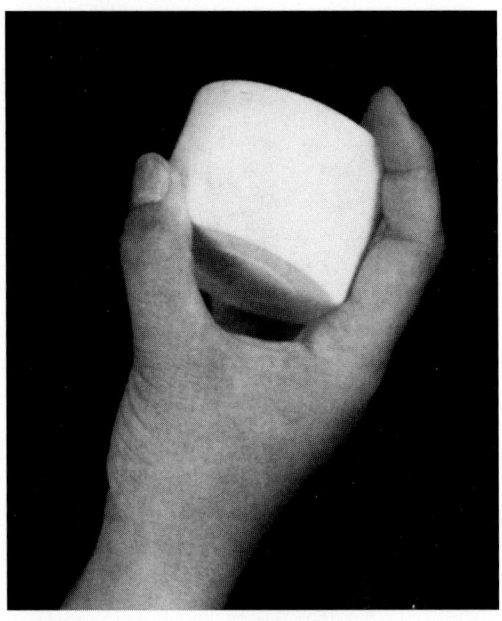

Fig. 33-19. Exercise used to assist the rotatory action of the opponens pollicis. (From Stanley BG, Tribuzi SM, editors: *Concepts in hand rehabilitation,* Philadelphia, 1992, FA Davis.)

particles, and vibration. In the testing phase, the patient is instructed to rank a series of each of these modalities ranging from the least to the most irritating.

For example, 10 different types of textures fixed to dowels are organized by the patient from the least to the most irritating (Fig. 33-20). Particulate materials, from cotton to sharp-edged cubes, are arranged in 3-pound coffee cans. Vibratory stimulus is applied with a commercially available vibrator and is ranked according to the cycles per second (cps), the duration of application, and whether the stimulus is intermittent or sustained. After arranging the hierarchy, the patient selects a tolerable but mildly irritating stimulus from each of the three modalities and uses this to desensitize the involved area. The textures are rubbed, tapped, or rolled over the area; the hand is immersed in the particulate materials; and the vibratory stimulus is applied in either a continuous or intermittent fashion. Treatment is performed daily, three or four times a day, for 10 minutes a session. When the stimulus becomes tolerable, the next in the series is used. Maximum progress occurs when the most irritating of the series is tolerated. Barber[1] reviewed a series of 124 patients who participated in the desensitization program at the Downey Hand Center between March 1980 and March 1982. The length of treatment averaged 7 weeks and was initiated an average of 8 to 13 weeks after injury. Barber found that all 124 patients improved to the extent that they were discharged from treatment and were able to return to work. They all showed improvement in some aspect of the hand sensitivity test.

Sensory reeducation. The prognosis for recovery of discriminative sensibility following nerve injury is generally

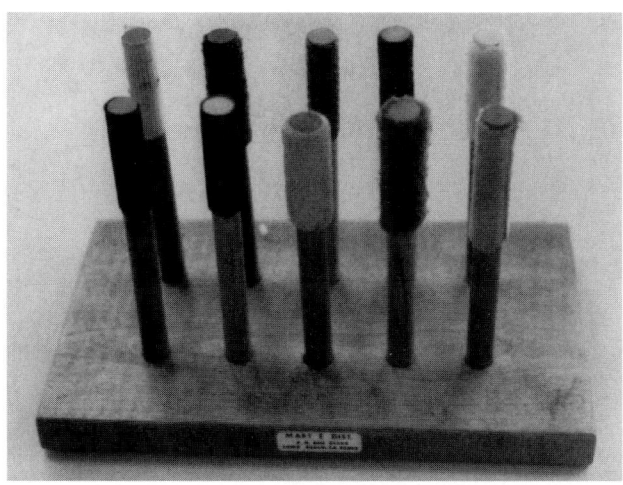

Fig. 33-20. Graded textures fixed to dowels used in a desensitization program. (From Stanley BG, Tribuzi SM, editors: *Concepts in hand rehabilitation,* Philadelphia, 1992, FA Davis.)

considered poor. This poor prognosis is because, during nerve regeneration, the axon may be blocked by scar at the suture line, a neuroma may form, or the axon may enter a different endoneurial tube or may reinnervate a different end organ. Consequently, when the affected area is stimulated, the patient will be unable to interpret the stimulus correctly because the nerve impulses received by the brain will be altered compared with the preinjury pattern; that is, the stimulus may be applied at one place on the hand and be perceived at another place. Cortical reorganization is needed to improve tactile discriminative ability, and sensory reeducation has been proposed by many investigators as an effective approach to the problem.[13,27] As defined by Dellon,[13] sensory reeducation is one of several methods that help the patient with a sensory deficit learn to reinterpret the altered pattern of neural impulses elicited by stimulation of the involved area of skin.

Dellon[13] identified a pattern of sensory recovery following nerve injury. Pain is the first to recover, followed by perception of vibration of 30 cps, the perception of moving touch, constant touch, and vibration of 256 cps. The return proceeds from proximal to distal. When the perception of 30 cps and moving touch have returned to a particular area, the first phase of Dellon's sensory reeducation program can begin. The goal of the first phase is to reeducate the localization of the stimulus- and submodality-specific perceptions (e.g., moving versus constant touch). The eraser end of a pencil is used to stimulate the specific area or zone. A moving-touch stimulus is used initially and a visual and tactile matching process is used. Stimulation of the affected area of the hand is performed with the patient's vision occluded, and patients are asked to localize where they were touched. If the response was incorrect, the stimulation is repeated with the patient's eyes open, and patients concentrate on matching the tactile impression with the visual

image. Finally, the stimulation is repeated with the patient's eyes closed, and patients concentrate on matching what they are feeling with what they have just seen.

When the patient can perceive constant touch, this same approach is used to reeducate localization of this touch submodality. Once moving and constant touch are perceived at the fingertips with good localization, the second phase of Dellon's program begins. The goal of this phase is the recovery of tactile recognition. Familiar household objects that vary in size, shape, and texture are used. A similar visual-tactile matching process is used during this phase. As recognition improves, the patient is challenged to discriminate more subtle differences.

Callahan[11] divides her sensory reeducation into two types: protective and discriminative. The goal of protective sensory reeducation is to educate the patient in techniques of compensation for the loss of protective sensory input, as discussed under patient education, and begins during the acute phase of management. Discriminative sensory reeducation is similar to Dellon's[13] approach, with training tasks involving localization and graded discrimination of textures, shapes, and objects.

Training methods. Training must be done in a quiet room to maximize attention and concentration of the patient. The training task consists of identification of the nature or location of a stimulus or performance of a task with vision occluded. In all cases, the training methods are essentially the same:

- First, the task is attempted with the eyes closed.
- Second, the patient opens his or her eyes and checks to see if the task was performed correctly.
- If it was, he or she closes his or her eyes and attempts to carry out another task.
- If incorrect, the patient repeats the same task with eyes open so that he or she might integrate vision with tactile experience and commit both to memory.
- Finally, the patient closes his or her eyes again and attempts the same task for reinforcement of what was just learned while his or her eyes were open.[9]

Training tasks.[9] Training tasks chosen will depend on the therapist's evaluation of present discrimination skills. Emphasis is placed on training of the fingertips because these are the sensory surfaces most involved in discriminative function. A consideration in choosing a task is whether it requires significant motor function. As much as possible, activities should be designed so that they can be carried out independently by the patient. The variety of tasks is limited only by the therapist's ingenuity and imagination. Examples are presented here:

- *Localization of a stimulus:* At first, the stimulus is blunt and delivered with firm pressure. Grading is achieved by using a stimulus delivered with increasingly lighter pressure.

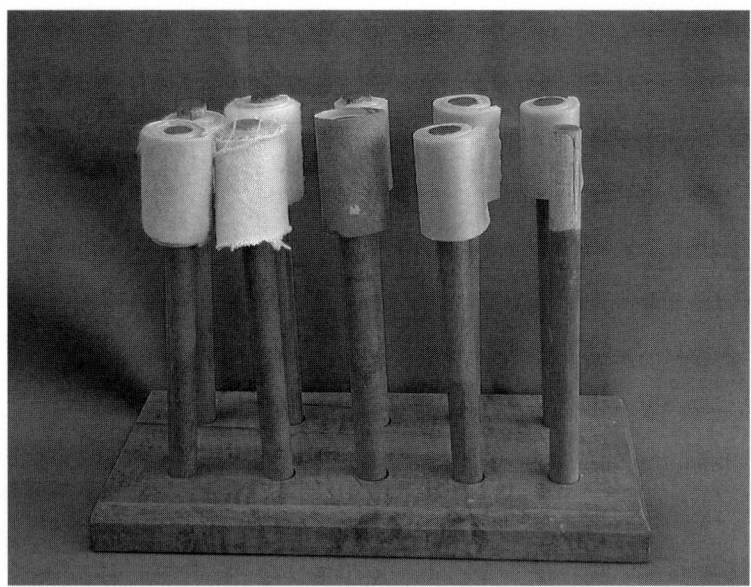

Fig. 33-21. Identical and different grades of sandpaper are attached to opposite ends of several wood dowels.

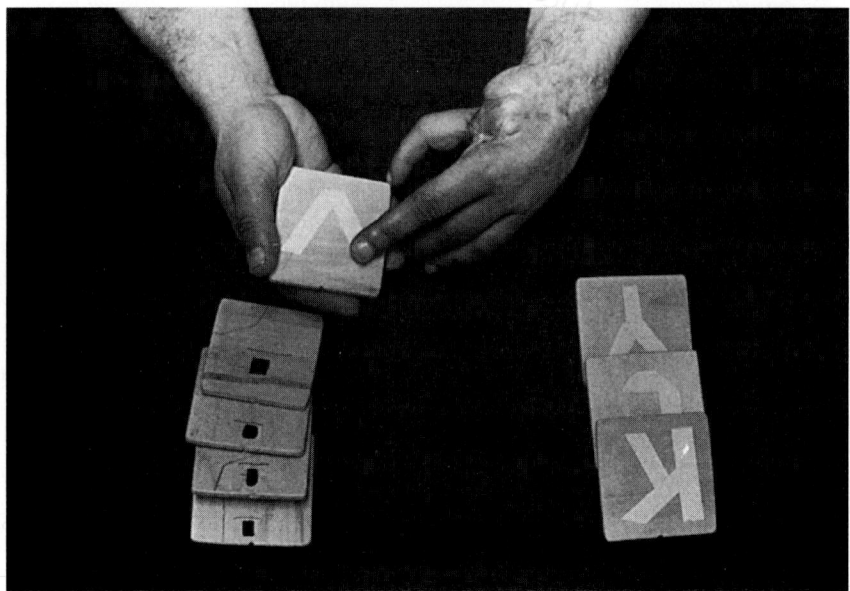

Fig. 33-22. Identification of Velcro letters superimposed on small wooden blocks. Grading is achieved by setting a time limit and by requiring identification of three-dimensional letters.

- *Identification of sandpaper on dowels:* Identical and different grades of sandpaper are attached to opposite ends of several wood dowels. The patient is required to state whether two ends of a dowel successively applied to a small area of skin are of the same grade or different. The activity is made more difficult by using similar grades of sandpaper and by using a light pressure when applying the stimulus to the skin (Fig. 33-21).
- *Identification of textures:* At first, the patient is required simply to match a sample texture with one of a small

group of different textures. Grading is achieved by requiring a match from a larger group of textures and by requiring description or identification of the texture.
- *Identification of Velcro letters superimposed on small wooden blocks:* Grading is achieved by setting a time limit and by requiring identification of three-dimensional letters (Fig. 33-22).
- *Braille designs and finger mazes:* The patient is required to use an involved fingertip to trace over and identify features on a braille design (e.g., a house) or to

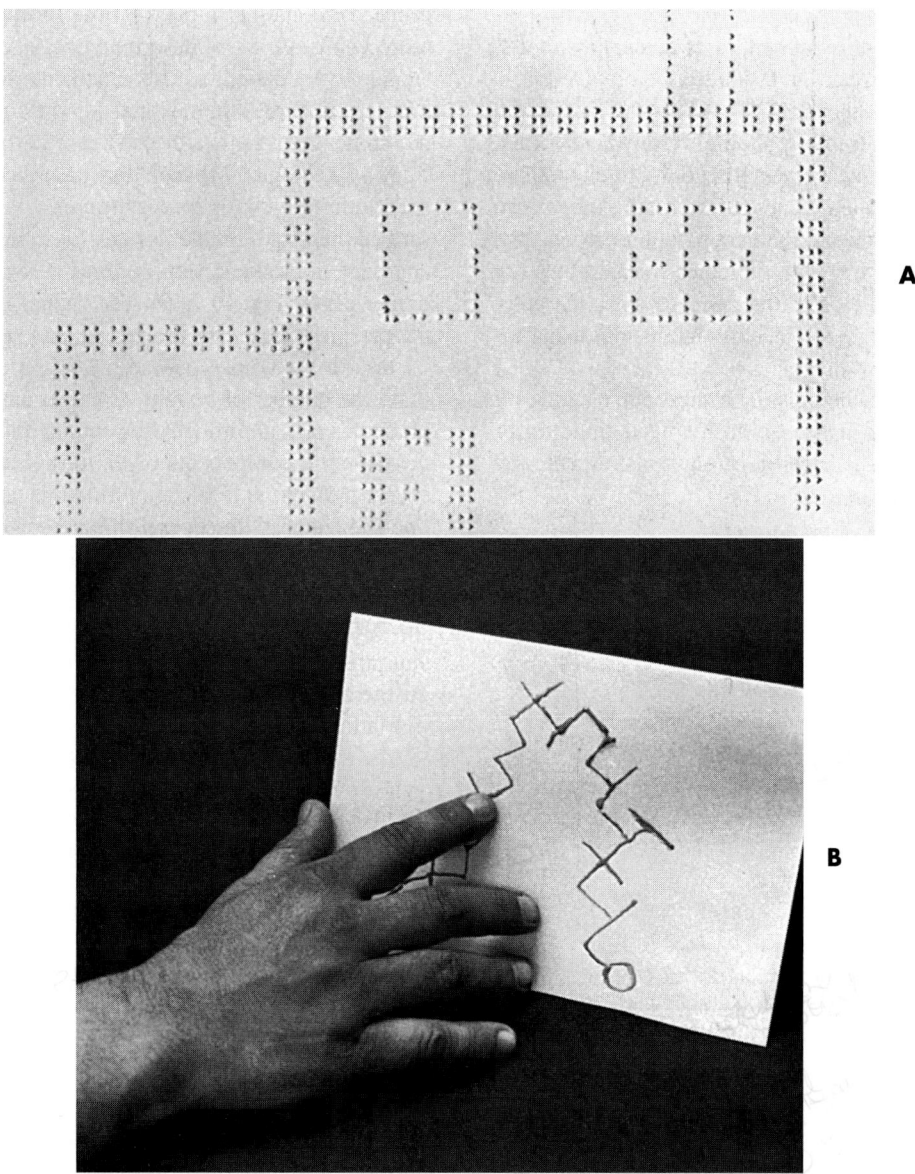

Fig. 33-23. Braille designs and finger mazes. Patient is required to use an involved fingertip to trace over and identify features on a Braille design or to trace over a finger maze made from raised epoxy glue on cardboard to reach a particular "destination" in the maze.

trace over a finger maze made from raised epoxy glue on cardboard to reach a particular "destination" in the maze (Fig. 33-23). Grading is achieved by using closer spacing in the braille designs or by making the finger mazes more intricate.

- *Picking up objects from a background medium:* At first, large objects must be retrieved from a background medium such as sand. Grading is achieved by setting a time limit and by using smaller objects in a coarser background medium, such as Styrofoam chips.
- *Identification of everyday objects:* At first, large dissimilar objects are used. Grading is achieved by

setting a time limit and by using smaller, more similar objects.
- *ADL tasks and work-simulated tasks:* The patient is required to perform selected tasks with vision occluded. Grading is achieved by setting a time limit and by making the tasks more intricate.

Chronic phase

When the patient's progress has peaked and there are significant and functionally limiting residual deficits, the focus of the therapy program turns toward compensation. A complete inventory of the patient's functional abilities and limitations is taken.

Adaptive techniques and assistive equipment are suggested, when appropriate, to allow independent function in self-care, work, and leisure activities. For example, the patient with a median-nerve injury may require a buttonhook to fasten buttons. Splinting alternatives are explored that improve function and are practical and cosmetic for long-term use. Splints previously provided during the acute and recovery phases are reevaluated and refabricated or modified as needed. The goals of splinting at this stage are essentially the same as for earlier phases but have a greater emphasis on the splint's ability to improve function and its practicality for long-term use.

Surgical alternatives are considered at this stage, including nerve exploration and grafting, joint fusions, and tendon transfers. If there has been minimal or no nerve regeneration and satisfactory compensatory function has not developed, tendon transfers may be appropriate.

Tendon transfers. Tendon transfer is a technique that involves the application of motor power of one muscle to another weaker or paralyzed muscle by transfer of its tendinous insertion. This procedure does not add to, but rather redistributes, power in an attempt to improve function. The therapist can play an important role both before and after surgery. Preoperatively, full PROM must be obtained because incomplete PROM may compromise the results of the transfer. Maintaining optimal soft tissue status is also important. Tissues and scars must be supple and mobilized. The donor muscle is strengthened preoperatively, and isolated control is emphasized. This muscle will be performing a new function that can only approximate the lost motion; it must be in optimal condition to maximize results. Finally, a realistic attitude on the patient's part must be fostered. The tendon transfer is a palliative procedure. Return to normal, full ROM is not expected.

Postoperatively, tendon transfers are immobilized for 3 to 5 weeks. During this protected phase, the therapist may be asked to fabricate a splint that places the hand and wrist in a position that minimizes tension on the transfer. In addition, attention is paid to the uninvolved joints to ensure maintenance of ROM, and edema control techniques are used as needed.

Mobilization of the transfer begins after 3 to 5 weeks of splinting or casting. Active movement of the transfer before this time could result in elongation or rupture at the site of the tendon juncture because the strength and maturation of the healing tissue is insufficient to allow active movement. The patient attempts the desired motion through contraction on the donor muscle.

When first attempting to use the muscle in its new role, the patient should focus on the motion that the donor muscle did before the transfer. For example, with a pronator teres to radial wrist extensor tendon transfer, the patient should attempt wrist extension while thinking about and initiating pronation. Biofeedback and electrical stimulation of the

donor muscle can be used to increase the patient's awareness and isolated control. Overstretching of the transfer can occur at this stage if exercise is done too vigorously in the direction opposite to that of the transfer. For example, after tendon transfer to restore wrist and finger extension is performed, flexion exercises are performed cautiously, avoiding simultaneous wrist and finger flexion and postponing passive flexion exercises until later stages of therapy. Protective splinting is continued during this stage to prevent overloading of the tendon junctures that can occur with inadvertent and unsupervised activity of the hand. Splinting also supports the desired position of the hand during this early phase when the tendon transfer may not be fully functioning or strong. The splint is removed only for exercise and hygiene. In addition, massage is begun to mobilize the scars and soft tissue to reduce edema. Adhesions can occur anywhere along the route of the transfer but are most often at the incision and must be treated early with massage to avoid binding of the transfer and compromise of the functional result. The patient is instructed to carry out a home program using all of the aforementioned techniques.

After 6 to 8 weeks, when the tendon juncture sites are strong enough to withstand stress, passive exercises and functional activities can be added to the program and the splint can be decreased to night use only. Strengthening with putty and other forms of resistive exercise can begin after 8 to 12 weeks. The specific exercises and activities are individualized according to the transfer.

A basic familiarity with the most common tendon transfers for the wrist and hand is essential. This includes knowledge of the purpose of the transfer, the donor muscle used, and the early precautions to be observed (Table 33-3).

CLINICAL DECISION MAKING: CASE STUDY

B.W. is a 25-year-old right hand–dominant man who sustained a glass laceration of the ulnar, volar aspect of the right wrist, resulting in a complete laceration of the palmar branch, the superficial terminal branch, and the deep terminal motor branch of the ulnar nerve at the level of the pisiform, with loss of a 1-cm segment from the superficial terminal branch. Injury occurred when the patient slipped and fell onto a trash bag filled with wine bottles.

B.W. underwent a primary microsurgical repair of the ulnar nerve with anastomosis of all three divisions. Application of a bulky dressing with a dorsal plaster splint was applied with the wrist flexed at 50 degrees to prevent tension at the repair site of the nerve.

Therapeutic management, acute phase

Evaluation. B.W. was referred for hand therapy and splinting 5 weeks after repair when his cast was removed. Before this time, the cast had been repositioned once in a lesser degree of flexion. Referral was for splinting, exercise, and patient education. The initial evaluation included

Table 33-3. Common tendon transfers

Level	Function	Transfer	Early precautions
Radial nerve	Wrist extension	Pronator teres to extensor carpi radialis longus and brevis	Avoid simultaneous wrist and digital flexion to prevent overstretch of the transfer
	Finger extension	Flexor carpi ulnaris or flexor carpi radialis to extensor digitorum communis	
	Thumb extension	Palmaris longus or flexor digitorum superficialis to extensor pollicis longus	
Median nerve	Opposition	Flexor digitorum superficialis, palmaris longus, or extensor digiti minimi	Avoid simultaneous wrist, thumb, and finger extension
	Thumb IP flexion (high lesions)	Brachioradialis to flexor pollicis longus	
	DIP flexion of index (high lesions)	Flexor digitorum profundus of the long, ring, and small fingers to the flexor digitorum profundus of the index finger	
Ulnar nerve	Correct claw (control MP joint hyperextension)	Flexor digitorum superficialis, extensor indicis proprius, extensor digiti minimi to intrinsics	Avoid full MP joint extension; avoid simultaneous finger, thumb, and wrist extension
	Thumb adduction	Flexor digitorum superficialis or extensor carpi radialis longus to adductor pollicis	
	Index abduction	Abductor pollicis longus, extensor carpi radialis longus, or extensor indicis proprius to first dorsal interossei	
	DIP flexion of the long, ring, and small fingers (high lesions)	Side-to-side tenodesis of flexor digitorum profundus of index	

DIP, Distal interphalangeal; *IP,* interphalangeal; *MP,* metacarpophalangeal.

medical, social, and vocational history; AROM and PROM evaluations; manual muscle test; sensibility examination; and a functional evaluation of ADLs.

Problems identified included the following:

1. Paralysis of the ulnar nerve–innervated intrinsics resulting in loss of active IP joint extension of the ring and the small fingers; loss of thumb adduction, and loss of abduction and adduction of the digits; and resting of the ring and small fingers in a claw posture
2. Secondary limitations of the wrist in extension because of prolonged positioning in flexion during cast immobilization, with a tight and adherent volar scar
3. Loss of protective sensibility of the ulnar side of the palm and ulnar volar half of the ring finger and volar surface of the small finger; loss of sympathetic function over the same area
4. ADL difficulties secondary to the impairment of the dominant function of the right hand

Establishing treatment priorities. The initial program focuses on recovery of ROM lost during cast immobilization, prevention of a fixed claw deformity, a protective

sensory reeducation program, and regular monitoring for the return of ulnar-nerve function.

1. *Recovery of ROM:* Active, active-assisted, and passive ROM exercises were provided to recover wrist extension. A volar splint was used initially to support the wrist in maximum extension and was adjusted to increase the position of the wrist toward greater extension as the patient improved.
2. *Prevention of deformity:* Splinting and patient education were used to prevent the development of a fixed claw deformity. A small, hand-based splint was provided, with a dorsal block limiting hyperextension of the MP joints of the fourth and fifth fingers but allowing full flexion. Initially, that was worn in conjunction with the wrist splint. IP joint extension was possible with this splint through the action of the extensor digitorum communis. B.W. was thoroughly instructed in the potential for the deformity and the necessity for using the splint continuously, and for daily monitoring to ensure that PIP joint flexion contractures were not developing.
3. *Protective sensory reeducation:* B.W. was instructed to avoid very hot or cold, abrasive or sharp objects; to

avoid sustained grasp; to change his grip frequently when working with tools; and to build up handles of tools. Recovery of sensation was monitored regularly, and discriminative sensory reeducation was begun when the perception of moving and constant touch was present. Localization exercises were performed with a visual tactile matching process. B.W. performed these exercises at home four times a day for 5 to 10 minutes each session.

4. *Monitoring for return of ulnar-nerve function:* Periodic sensory and motor tests were performed to allow appropriate upgrading of the program and introduction of more challenging intervention strategies.

Therapeutic management: recovery phase

Reevaluation. Repeated measurements of ROM reflected recovery of full wrist ROM after 4 weeks of therapy. At 5 months, manual muscle testing revealed trace to poor strength of the adductor digiti minimi. Protective sensibility had returned to the ulnar aspect of the palm and ring and small digits with localization increasing in accuracy.

Reestablishing treatment priorities. The focus of therapy during this phase was on motor retraining and further sensory reeducation.

1. *Motor retraining:* As strength increased from poor to fair, active and active-assisted exercises for the interossei, hypothenars, fourth and fifth lumbricales, and thumb adductor were provided, with progression to light resistance when a fair-plus grade of strength was achieved. General putty gripping and pinching exercises, as well as resistance for abduction and adduction of the fingers, was provided. During the earlier phases of reinnervation, biofeedback and electrical stimulation were used to increase B.W.'s awareness of muscle contraction and to augment his efforts.

2. *Sensory reeducation:* Discriminative sensory reeducation exercises included texture, shape, and size discrimination exercises using the ulnar palm and ring and small fingers. In addition, discrimination of objects embedded in rice was done, using the ring and small fingers to search for the objects, and the thumb and ring and small fingers were used to pick the object out of the rice.

Follow-up status

At 1 year after nerve repair, B.W. demonstrated full ROM of the wrist and hand. Manual muscle testing reflected activity of all ulnar innervated intrinsics in the good range of strength.

Grip and pinch strength were still 20% less than on the uninvolved side. Sensibility examination reflected recovery of localization and of protective and light touch sensibility, but two-point discrimination was 12 mm at the tip of the small finger and on the ulnar half of the tip of the ring finger. B.W. has resumed his previous work and leisure activities.

SUMMARY

The management of the patient with a peripheral-nerve injury challenges the full range of the therapist's knowledge and skills. A thorough understanding of nerve anatomy, nerve response to injury, classification of nerve injuries, and specific nerve lesions is necessary to establish a frame of reference.

A careful assessment is essential to the treatment planning process and includes manual muscle testing, ROM evaluation, sensibility examination, evaluation of sympathetic function, and an analysis of the impact of the injury on the patient's functional status. Goals are set and treatment is provided according to the phases of nerve recovery.

During the acute phase, the objectives of the therapist's management include protection of the traumatized or surgically repaired nerve to allow healing, prevention of joint contracture, and avoidance of further injury secondary to decreased sensibility. These objectives are accomplished through the use of protective and functional splints, ROM exercises, and patient education in safety precautions for decreased sensation. During the recovery phase, retraining and reeducation become important. As muscles are reinnervated, exercise, biofeedback, and electrical stimulation are used to enhance the recovery of strength and control. As skin receptors are reinnervated, desensitization is used to reduce hypersensitivity and sensory reeducation is needed to improve tactile discrimination. In the chronic stage, when progress has peaked and functional deficits remain, the focus of therapy is on compensation for loss of function. Techniques include the use of assistive devices, adaptive methods, and functional splints. Finally, tendon transfers may be performed to redistribute remaining power, with hand therapy being important both before and after surgery. Full passive motion, supple and nonadherent tissues, and isolated control and strength of the donor muscle are preoperative goals. Postoperatively, emphasis is on initial protection of the transfer through splints and reeducation of the tendon transfer to perform its new functions.

REFERENCES

1. Barber LM: Desensitization of the traumatized hand. In Hunter JM, et al, editors: *Rehabilitation of the hand,* St Louis, 1990, Mosby.
2. Baxter-Petralia P: Therapist's management of carpal tunnel syndrome. In Hunter JM, et al, editors: *Rehabilitation of the hand,* St Louis, 1990, Mosby.
3. Beasley R: *Hand injuries,* Philadelphia, 1981, WB Saunders.
4. Bowers WH, et al: Nerve suture and grafting, *Hand Clin* 5:447, 1989.
5. Brand PW: Rehabilitation of the hand with motor and sensory impairment, *Orthop Clin North Am* 4:1135, 1973.
6. Brand PW: Clinical mechanics of the hand, St Louis, 1985, Mosby.
7. Bunnell S: *Surgery of the hand,* ed 5, Philadelphia, 1970, JB Lippincott.

8. Callahan AD: Sensibility testing: clinical methods. In Hunter JM, et al, editors: *Rehabilitation of the hand,* ed 2, St Louis, 1984, Mosby.

9. Callahan AD: Methods of compensation and reeducation for sensory dysfunction. In Hunter JM, et al, editors: *Rehabilitation of the hand,* ed 2, St Louis, 1984, Mosby.

10. Callahan AD: Nerve injuries in the upper extremity. In Malick MH, Kasch MC, editors: *Manual on management of specific hand problems,* Pittsburgh, 1984, AREN Publications.

11. Callahan AD: Methods of compensation and re-education for sensory dysfunction. In Hunter JM, et al, editors: *Rehabilitation of the hand,* St Louis, 1990, Mosby.

12. Colditz JC: A dynamic radial palsy splint, *J Hand Ther* 1:3, 1988.

13. Dellon AL: *Evaluation of sensibility and re-education of sensation,* Baltimore, 1981, Williams & Wilkins.

14. Hardy MA, Moran CA, Merritt WH: Desensitization of the traumatized hand, *VA Med* 109:134, 1983.

15. Haymaker W, Woodhall B: *Peripheral nerve injuries: principles of diagnosis,* ed 2, Philadelphia, 1967, WB Saunders.

16. Moberg E: Functional sensory testing. Presented at the Symposium: Management of the Insensitive Hand, US Public Health Service Hospital, Carville, Va, March 29-31, 1983.

17. Omer G: Nerve response to injury and repair. In Hunter JM, et al, editors: *Rehabilitation of the hand,* St Louis, 1990, Mosby.

18. Onne L: Recovery of sensibility and sudomotor activity in the hand after nerve suture, *Acta Chir Scand* 300(suppl):1, 1962.

19. Perry JF, et al: Protective sensation in the hand and its correlation to the Ninhydrin Sweat Test following nerve laceration, *Am J Phys Med* 53:113, 1974.

20. Seddon HJ: Three types of nerve injury, *Brain* 66:238, 1943.

21. Seddon HJ, editor: *Peripheral nerve injuries,* London, 1954, Her Majesty's Printing Office.

22. Seddon HJ: *Surgical disorders of the peripheral nerves,* ed 2, New York, 1975, Churchill Livingstone.

23. Stromberg WB, et al: Injury of the median and ulnar nerves: one hundred and fifty cases with an evaluation of Moberg's Ninhydrin Test, *J Bone Joint Surg* 43A:717, 1961.

24. Sunderland S: *Nerves and nerve injuries,* London, 1968, E & S Livingstone.

25. Sunderland S: The nerve lesion in the carpal tunnel syndrome, *J Neurol Neurosurg Psychiatr* 39:615, 1976.

26. vonPrince K, Butler B: Measuring sensory function of the hand in peripheral nerve injuries, *Am J Occup Ther* 21:385, 1967.

27. Wynn Parry CB: *Rehabilitation of the hand,* London, 1973, Butterworth.

BIBLIOGRAPHY

Basmajian JV: *Biofeedback: principles and practice for clinicians,* Baltimore, 1979, Williams & Wilkins.

Cannon NM, et al: *Manual of hand splinting,* New York, 1985, Churchill Livingstone.

Fess EE: Rehabilitation of the patient with peripheral nerve injury. In Mackin EJ, editor: *Hand clinics: hand rehabilitation,* Philadelphia, 1986, WB Saunders.

Haymaker W, Woodhall B: *Peripheral nerve injuries,* Philadelphia, 1953, WB Saunders.

Omer GE: Acute management of peripheral nerve injuries. In Mackin EJ, editor: *Hand clinics: hand rehabilitation,* Philadelphia, 1986, WB Saunders.

Peacock EE: *Wound repair,* Philadelphia, 1984, WB Saunders.

Toth S: Therapist's management of tendon transfers. In Mackin EJ, editor: *Hand clinics: hand rehabilitation,* Philadelphia, 1986, WB Saunders.

Tubiana R: *Examination of the hand and upper limb,* Philadelphia, 1984, WB Saunders.

Chapter 34

SPLINTING THE HAND WITH A PERIPHERAL-NERVE INJURY

Judy C. Colditz

Splinting the hand with a peripheral-nerve injury is both easy and difficult. The ease of splinting results from the readily recognizable and often identical deformities. Therefore, unlike many other hand injuries, the deformities resulting from isolated peripheral nerve paralysis are usually effectively splinted using standard splinting designs. The difficulty, however, in splinting peripheral nerve paralysis arises from the impossibility of building a static external device that substitutes for the intricately balanced muscles the splint attempts to replace.

PRINCIPLES OF SPLINTS

The purposes common to all splints used for peripheral nerve injuries are as follows:

1. To keep denervated muscles from remaining in an overstretched position
2. To prevent joint contractures
3. To prevent the development of strong substitution patterns
4. To maximize functional use of the hand

Overstretching of muscles

In all cases of isolated upper extremity peripheral nerve injury, the denervated muscle group will have normal unopposed antagonist muscles still present. These normal muscles will continuously overpower the denervated muscles and maintain them on constant stretch. A muscle undergoing reinnervation must first overcome this stretched position and achieve a normal resting length before it is able to contract enough to bring about joint motion. Short periods during which the unopposed muscles overpower the denervated muscles will not cause harm, but a denervated muscle

constantly held in a stretched position decreases the potential for early return of normal muscle activity. A denervated muscle protected by appropriate splinting allows the earliest perception of returning motion. Properly executed splints will enhance returning muscle function instead of allowing substitution patterns.

Joint contractures

Joints held continually in one position cannot experience the habitual movement of the capsular structures. Even without accompanying trauma, prolonged immobility will result in restriction of joint motion.[1-3,14,15,22,26] To maintain motion, the joint must be frequently taken through its full range. It is not adequate to immobilize joints at one extreme at night and the other extreme during the day. Although positional splinting at night can be useful, it is the full active motion of joints during the day that maintains joint lubrication and accompanying soft tissue glide.

Substitution patterns

In an isolated peripheral nerve injury, there is no opposing force to the intact active muscle group and muscle imbalance is created. Without an external splinting constraint, the patient constantly reinforces the strength of the normal muscles and overpowers the denervated muscles. An excellent example is low median palsy, in which the intact flexor pollicis longus (FPL) and extensor pollicis longus (EPL) carry the thumb back and forth across the palm in an adducted position (Fig. 34-1). With the opponens pollicis (OP) and abductor pollicis brevis (APB) absent, the extrinsic muscle pattern becomes dominant in the motor cortex. As the OP and APB are reinnervated, they have difficulty participating in thumb motion because the stronger extrinsic muscles con-

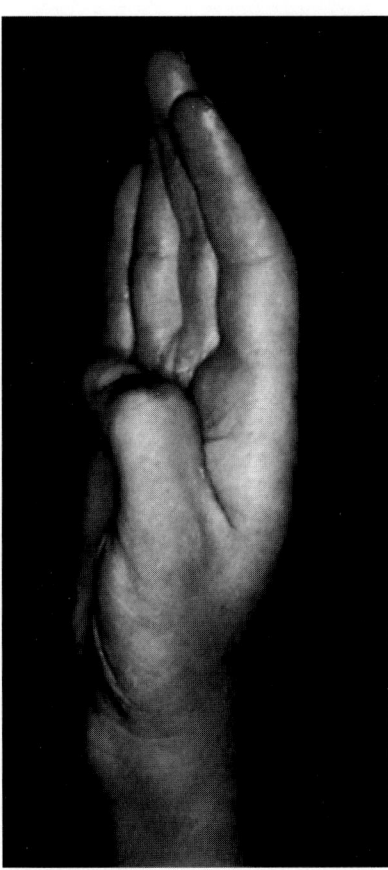

Fig. 34-1. In low median palsy, the thumb is carried back and forth across the palm in an adducted position by extrinsic muscles because of the absence of the opponens pollicis and the abductor pollicis brevis.

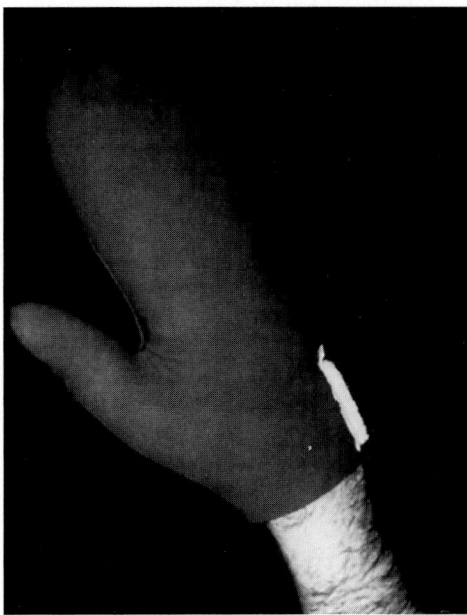

Fig. 34-2. In the nerve-injured hand, a neoprene mitten aids in cold tolerance.

tinue to dominate. If substitution patterns are prevented, the patient is able to isolate and strengthen returning musculature earlier.

Functional use of the hand

A peripheral-nerve lesion with significant sensory loss prevents functional use of the hand even when a splint substitutes for absent muscles. The combination of sensory loss and motor imbalance in median and ulnar nerve lesions makes it impossible to use the hand normally. A splint can assist in maximizing function only when the sensibility returns to a functional level.

Cold intolerance is common with peripheral-nerve injuries, particularly during reinnervation. Protective neoprene mittens, gloves, or finger sleeves are helpful for patients in colder climates or for those who work in cold environments (Fig. 34-2).

SPLINT REQUIREMENTS
Design

Splints should be kept as simple as possible. Bulky splints, if worn by the patient, will impede function of the

hand rather than reinforce it. Early after the nerve injury, it is acceptable to cover a denervated sensory area with the splint. In cases of partial nerve laceration or returning sensibility, the tactile surfaces should be left free if possible.

Splints for peripheral-nerve injuries should not totally immobilize any joint. For example, splinting of the wrist in radial palsy with a static wrist immobilization splint prevents the returning wrist extensor muscles from gaining strength or excursion while in the splint.

Splint timing

Many peripheral-nerve injuries are associated with accompanying trauma to skin, tendon, bone, or vascular structures. Tension on the healing tissues must be avoided immediately after injury to allow adequate healing. Thereafter, glide of tendons and joint movement take precedence over splinting for the peripheral-nerve deformity. The peripheral-nerve splint will often restrict full tendon excursion. For example, in a laceration at the wrist involving the median and ulnar nerves and wrist and finger flexor tendons, the wrist must be held in some flexion immediately postoperatively to prevent tension at the repair sites. Only as wrist motion is gained and excursion of the flexor tendons is achieved will the claw deformity of the fingers be evident. The initial adherence of the flexor tendons at the wrist will create tenodesis of the finger flexors, providing a built-in splint. Only when the deformity becomes clinically evident should one splint for it. In longstanding denervation in which joint contractures have already developed, one must first splint to regain joint motion before splinting the dynamic deformity.

SPECIFIC NERVE LESIONS

It is easiest to understand the deformity of a pure lesion of the three primary upper extremity peripheral nerves: ulnar, median, and radial. Combined nerve injuries, especially when associated with other injuries, require more skill to determine treatment priorities, although the splinting principles are the same.

Ulnar nerve

Low lesion. Laceration of the ulnar nerve at the wrist (low ulnar palsy) results in denervation of the majority of the intrinsic muscles of the hand (Fig. 34-3). The ulnar nerve innervates all of the hypothenar muscles: abductor digiti minimi, flexor digiti minimi, and the opponens digiti minimi. The ulnar border of the transverse metacarpal arch is lost. Absence of the dorsal and volar interossei muscles creates the inability to abduct and adduct the fingers, causing loss of the fine manipulative power of the hand. In addition to the loss of the interossei, the ring and little fingers also lose function of the lumbricales, removing any intrinsic muscle balancing force in these two digits. The extrinsic muscles dominate.

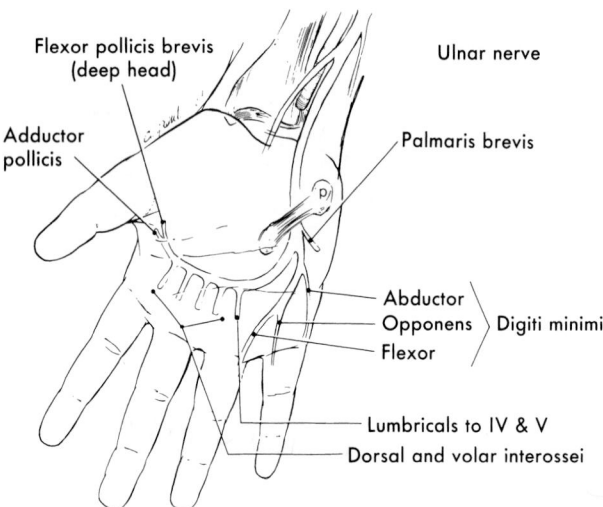

Fig. 34-3. The path of the ulnar nerve in the hand and the muscles involved in low ulnar palsy.

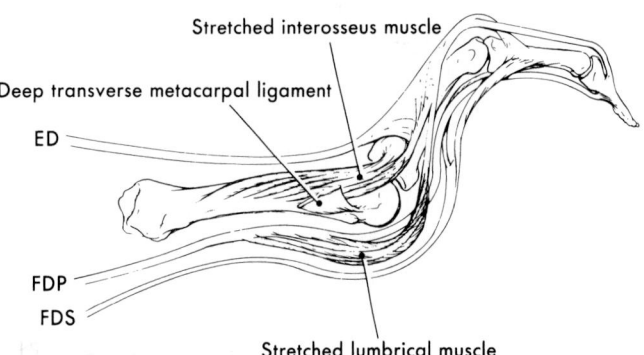

Fig. 34-4. In ulnar palsy, the loss of intrinsic muscle control in the ring and little fingers allows the metacarpophalangeal joints to hyperextend. The denervated muscles are stretched in this claw position. *ED,* Extensor digitorum communis; *FDP,* flexor digitorum profundi; *FDS,* flexor digitorum superficialis.

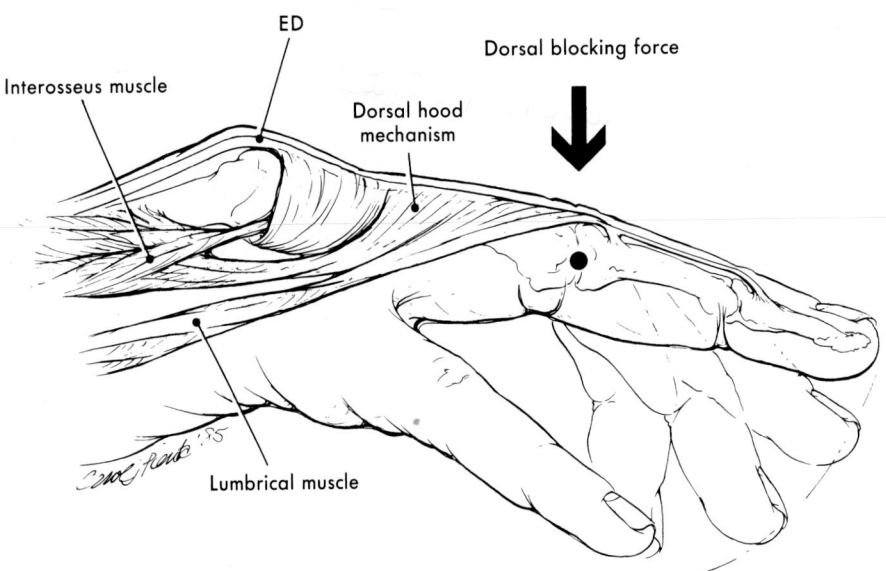

Fig. 34-5. A blocking force over the dorsum of the proximal phalanx prevents metacarpophalangeal hyperextension and allows the extrinsic extensor to transmit power to the interphalangeal joints when the intrinsic muscles are absent. *ED,* Extensor digitorum communis.

The resulting deformity is clawing of the ring and little fingers. The intrinsic muscles normally flex the metacarpophalangeal (MP) joint and extend the interphalangeal (IP) joints. When they are absent, there are no prime flexors of the MP joint. Because there is no intrinsic muscle control in these digits, the tension of the long flexors is opposed only by the extrinsic extensors, which primarily extend the MP joints (Fig. 34-4). In this claw position, both the lumbricales and the interossei are held in a stretched position. The patient can flex the MP joints actively, but only after the IP joints are fully flexed. The greatest functional loss is the inability to open the hand in a large span to grasp objects and the inability to handle small objects with precision.

The loss of the powerful adductor pollicis and the deep head of the flexor pollicis brevis removes one of the key supports of the thumb MP joint during pinching. The thumb may demonstrate Froment's sign: extension or hyperextension of the MP joint with hyperflexion of the IP joint.[16] Splinting cannot easily assist this deformity because stabilizing the thumb is difficult without restricting other essential mobility.

The goal in splinting ulnar palsy is to prevent overstretching of the denervated intrinsic muscles of the ring and little fingers. The ring and little finger MP joints must be prevented from fully extending (Fig. 34-5). Any splint that blocks the MP joints in slight flexion prevents the claw deformity by forcing the extrinsic extensors to transmit force into the dorsal hood mechanism of the finger. This extends the IP joints in the absence of active intrinsic muscle pull (Fig. 34-6). The dorsal block should be molded carefully to distribute pressure over the dorsum of each proximal phalanx and should end exactly at the axis of the proximal interphalangeal (PIP) joint.

A bulky splint that blocks the MP joints will impede function of the hand. In isolated low ulnar palsy, two thirds of the palmar surface of the hand has intact median nerve sensibility. Ulnar palsy splints should cover a minimal surface of the palm. Total finger flexion must also remain unimpeded. Early after injury, the MP joint block can be incorporated into the immobilization splint that prevents tension on the nerve and tendon repairs at the wrist. When wrist movement is allowed, a small molded thermoplas-

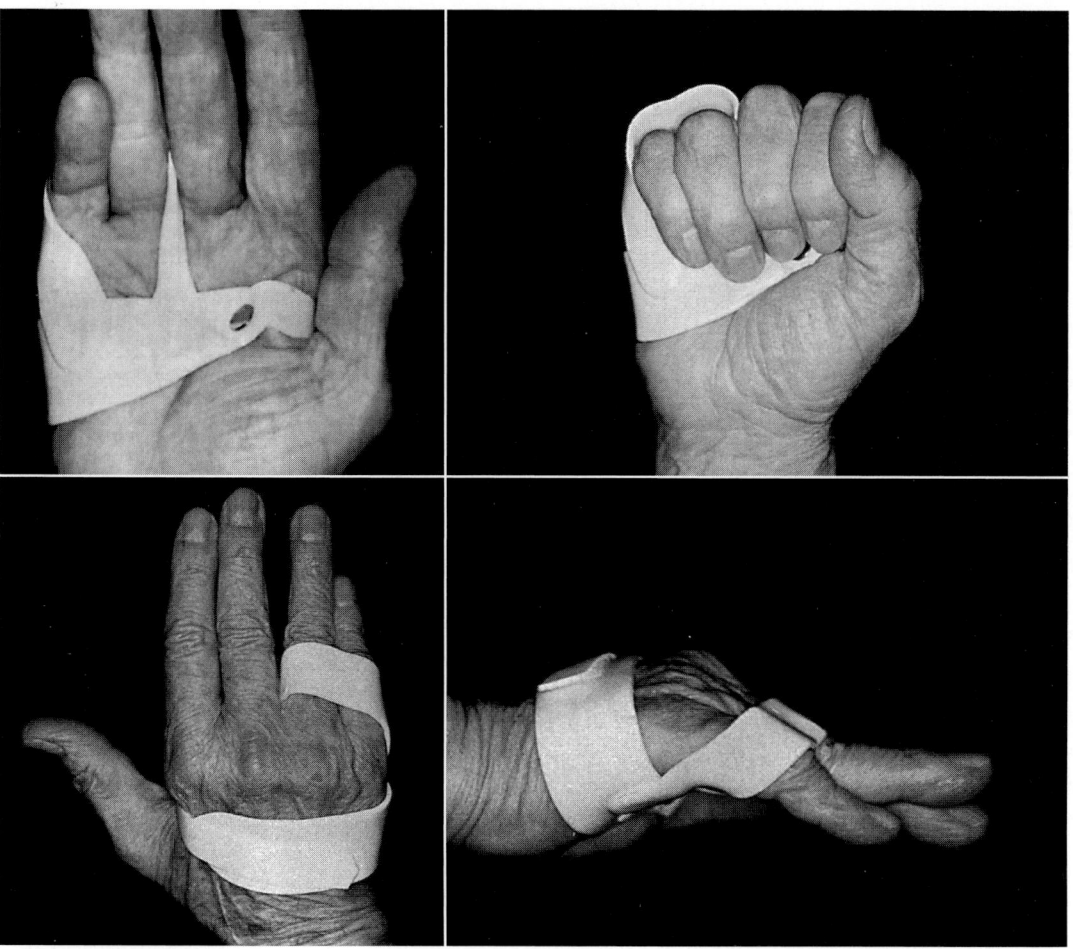

Fig. 34-6. This ulnar palsy splint blocks hyperextension of the metacarpophalangeal joints but allows full flexion of all finger joints.

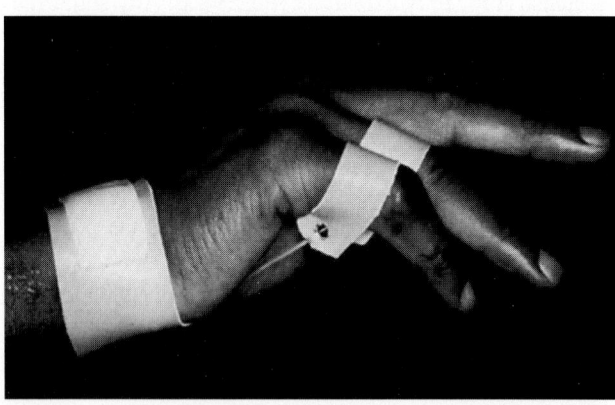

Fig. 34-7. An ulnar palsy splint may be made of leather wrist and finger cuffs with a static line to block metacarpophalangeal hyperextension.

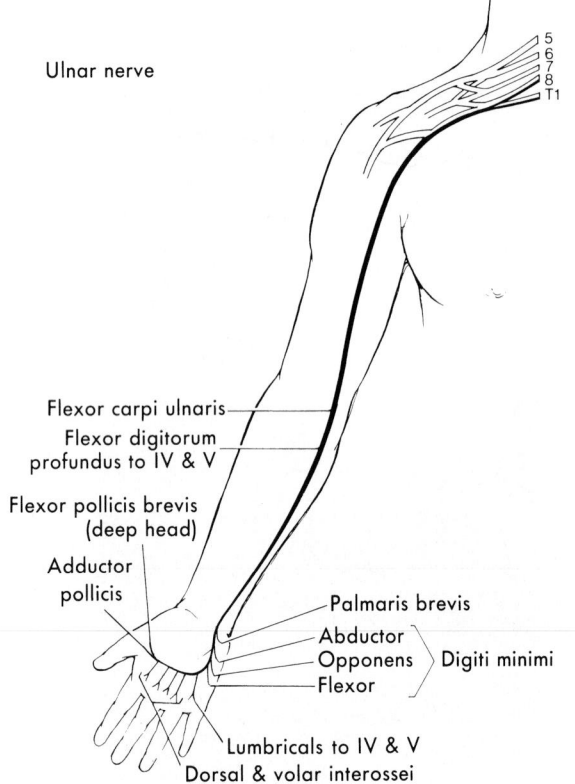

Fig. 34-8. The path of the ulnar nerve and the muscles involved in high ulnar palsy.

tic splint (see Fig. 34-6) or leather splint can be applied (Fig. 34-7).

Some authors advocate a spring wire splint with a coil at the axis of the MP joint that allows full MP extension and follows the joint through the full MP flexion.[7,8] This splint

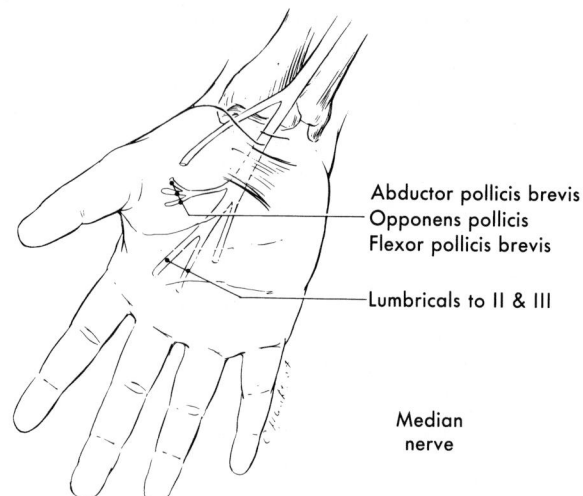

Fig. 34-9. Low median palsy involves the intrinsic muscles of the thumb and index and long fingers.

construction is challenging because the tension of the spring must be exact. It must be strong enough to block MP extension when the patient attempts finger extension while also following the arc of the proximal phalanx when the MP joint flexes. Therapists who apply a dynamic force for MP flexion (e.g., the Bunnell knuckle-bender splint[5]) are missing the concept of blocking MP hyperextension. In such a splint, the patient hyperextends actively against the force of the rubber bands, which gives resistance and proprioceptive input to the extrinsic extensors, strengthening them. Unless one is able to construct a coil splint with precise tension, it is recommended that static splinting that prevents the MP joint from hyperextending be applied.

Ulnar palsy splints will not create flexion contractures of the MP joint. Every time the splint is removed for skin care, the extrinsic extensor will still hyperextend the MP joint.

High lesion. High ulnar palsy lesions are commonly a result of trauma at or above the elbow. In addition to the muscles previously mentioned in low ulnar palsy, the flexor digitorum profundi (FDP) of the ring and little fingers and the flexor carpi ulnaris are absent in a high lesion (Fig. 34-8). With absence of the FDP and all intrinsic muscles to the ring and little fingers, clawing in the high ulnar nerve lesion is rarely present. As reinnervation of the FDP occurs, clawing becomes evident and splinting becomes mandatory rather than optional. The same MP hyperextension restriction splint is used for both the high and low ulnar palsy lesions (see Fig 34-5). In a high lesion, the patient must maintain full passive IP flexion of the ring and little fingers when the FDP is absent.

Median nerve

Low lesion. A laceration of the median nerve at the wrist produces low median palsy, a devastating injury. The median nerve innervates the majority of the thenar muscles and

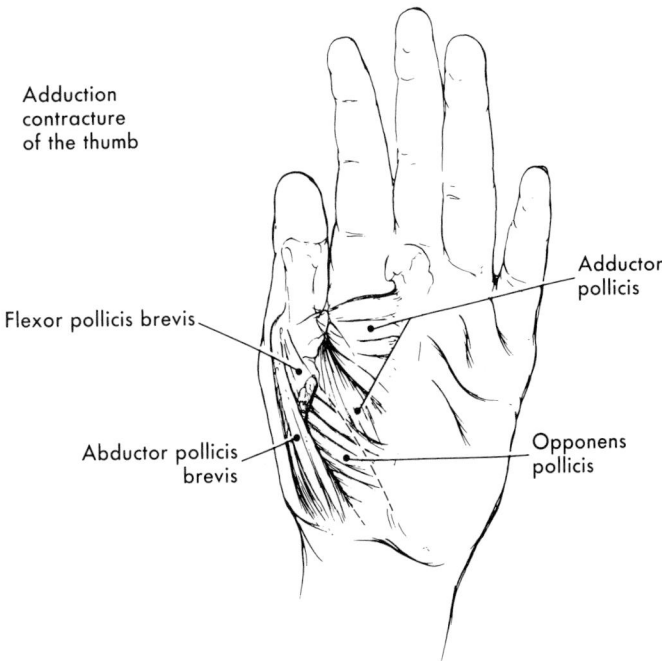

Fig. 34-10. An adduction contracture of the thumb in median palsy is caused by an unopposed adductor pollicis muscle.

provides sensibility to the radial three and one half digits. Motor loss is present in only the radial portion of the hand (Fig. 34-9). Loss of the OP and APB renders it impossible to pull the thumb away from the palm. The thumb is carried across the palm in an adducted position (see Fig. 34-1). If the adduction deformity is not obvious, the nerve injury may be partial or one may be observing the not uncommon cross-innervation from the ulnar nerve. In low median palsy, the lumbrical muscles of the index and long fingers are also absent. Because the ulnarly innervated palmar and dorsal interossei are still present, clawing is nearly always absent in these two digits; only in combined median and ulnar palsy is clawing of the index and long fingers present (along with the ring and little fingers).

Adduction contractures of the thumb are the most common deformity following a low lesion of the median nerve. To provide a balance to the unopposed adductor pollicis, some means of holding the first metacarpal abducted from the second metacarpal is necessary (Fig. 34-10). Thumb abduction splinting prevents the OP and APB from resting in a stretched position and reinforces early return of their action. Abduction splinting also maintains the soft tissue length of the first web space. Much of the functional abduction of the thumb requires the elongation of the soft tissue of the entire first web.

It is difficult to maintain the full length of the first web space while still allowing MP flexion of the index finger. A night splint that holds the index finger extended and the thumb abducted is helpful in maintaining the motion necessary for functional abduction of the thumb (Fig. 34-11).

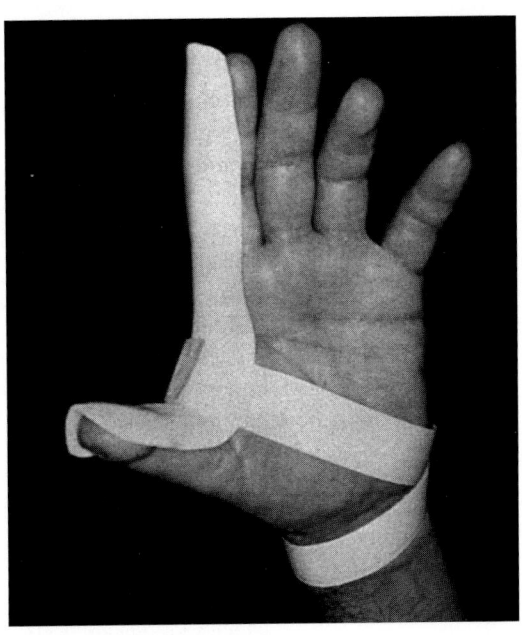

Fig. 34-11. Night splint for full abduction of the thumb web.

A small daytime splint made of neoprene, leather, or thermoplastic material is used during the day to hold the thumb in a stable opposed, but less than fully abducted, position (Fig. 34-12). If a daytime splint prevents full flexion of the MP joint of the index finger, it can lead to an unnecessary extension contracture of this joint.

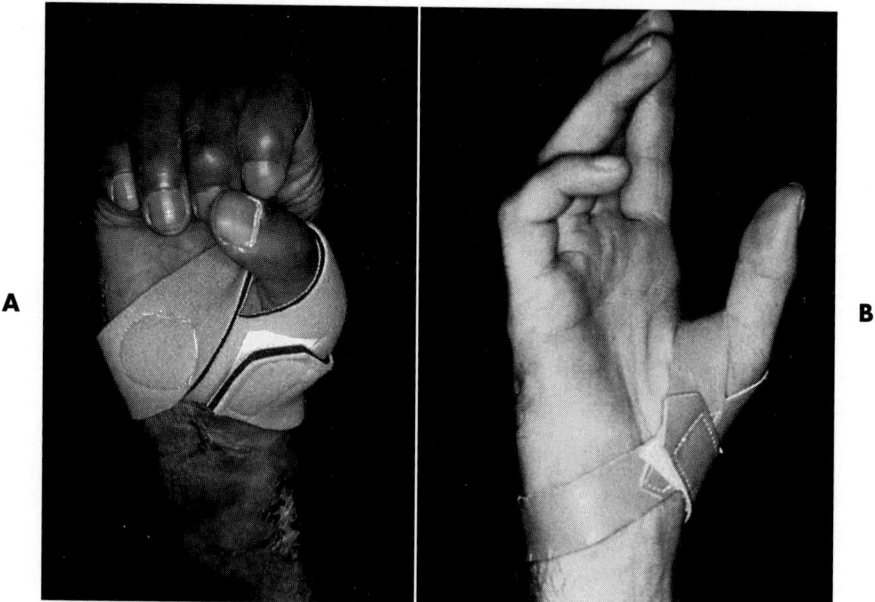

Fig. 34-12. Neoprene **(A)** or leather **(B)** splint for maintaining functional abduction of the thumb while awaiting median nerve return.

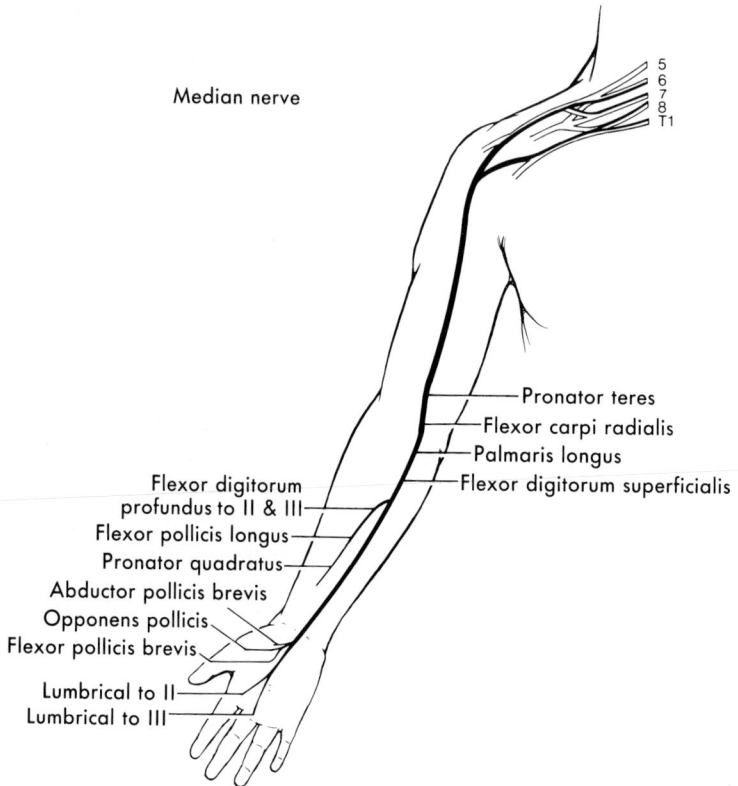

Fig. 34-13. High median palsy robs the radial aspect of the hand of the majority of flexor muscle function.

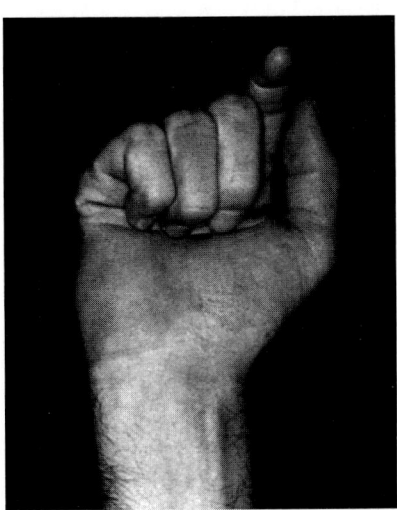

Fig. 34-14. In high median palsy, the long finger is carried into flexion because of the common flexor profundus muscle belly.

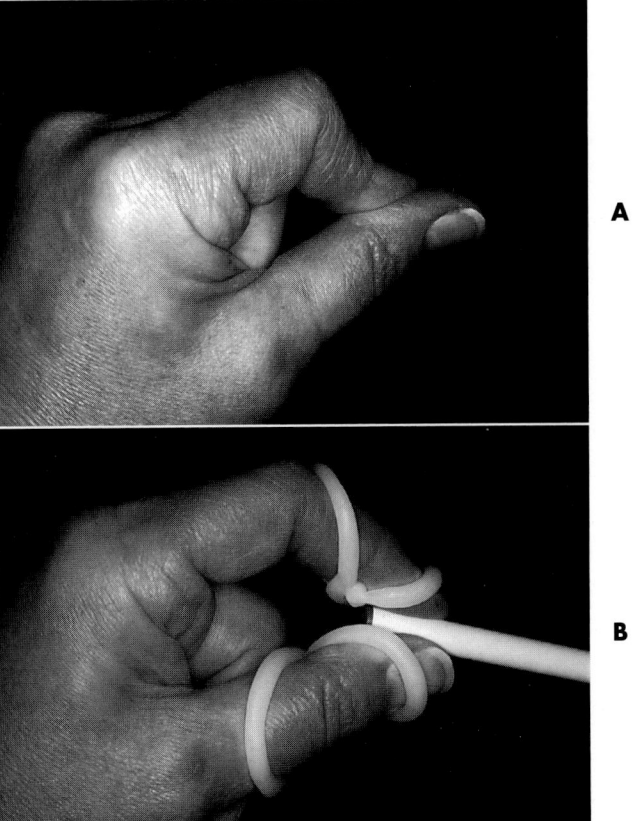

Fig. 34-15. A, Fingertip pinch is impossible in anterior nerve palsy. **B,** Small splints that prevent joint extension re-create fingertip pinch.

The thumb, index, and long fingers are the prime digits for manipulating objects. In median palsy, loss of sensibility in these digits makes it extremely difficult for the patient to use the hand for normal activity. Because reinnervation proceeds proximally to distally, it is common that the motor return precedes full sensory return. At times the splint may be discontinued before sensory return reaches maximum. For this reason, early after a median nerve repair at the wrist, one need not hesitate to cover the palm to position the thumb. As the nerve regenerates, a small leather or neoprene splint (see Fig. 34-12) positions the thumb in slight abduction and opposition so that the strong extrinsic flexor and extensor does not overpower the returning thenar intrinsic muscles.

In many adults, especially those with a high nerve lesion, OP function often does not return even though sensibility may recover to a protective level. In these patients a tendon transfer to restore thumb opposition increases functional thumb use.

High lesion at the elbow. High median nerve injuries result from injury to the nerve at or near the elbow. In these lesions, loss of the FDP of the index and long fingers and the flexor digitorum superficialis to all fingers robs the hand of all except minimal gross grasp function (Fig. 34-13). It is often difficult to maintain passive flexion of the index finger. Buddy taping it to the long finger does not provide adequate passive motion. Even though the long finger appears to flex actively, it is actually being carried along into flexion as part of the common muscle belly of the profundi of the long, ring, and little fingers (the ring and little FDP are innervated by the ulnar nerve) (Fig. 34-14).

Active pronation is also lost with denervation of the pronator teres and pronator quadratus, but slight abduction of the arm allows gravity to assist with pronation.

In the adult patient with a high median or ulnar nerve lesion, normal motor and sensory return is rare. Splinting high-level deformities to maintain passive range of motion is appropriate in preparation for tendon transfers. Although no splint need be cumbersome if correctly designed, some authors suggest very early tendon transfers as an internal splint to prevent the need for cumbersome external devices.[4,6,18,20]

High lesion: anterior interosseous nerve. The median nerve bifurcates distal to the elbow, just after it passes between the two heads of the pronator (see Fig. 34-13). One branch continues with sensory and motor fibers to the hand. The other purely motor branch, the anterior interosseous nerve, terminates in the forearm as it innervates the FDP of the index and long fingers, the FPL, and the pronator quadratus.

Absence of anterior interosseous nerve function prevents the patient from successfully transmitting force to the tips of the index and long fingers, as well as the thumb. This can

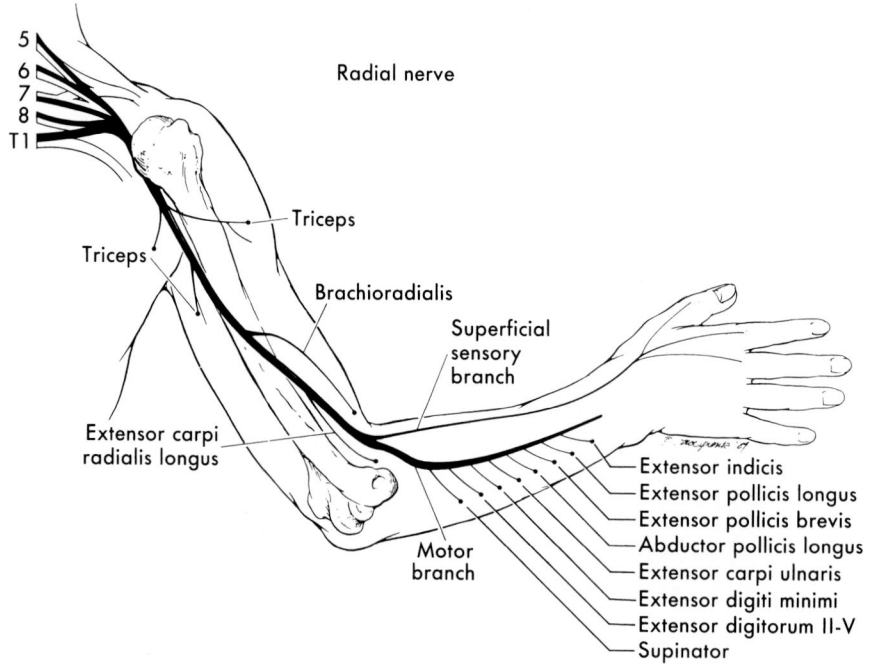

Fig. 34-16. The path of the radial nerve and the muscles it innervates. (Modified from Colditz J: *J Hand Ther* 1:19, 1987.)

most easily be demonstrated by asking the patient to pinch the thumb tip against the index tip. The index distal interphalangeal (DIP) joint and the thumb IP joint fall into extension or hyperextension (Fig. 34-15, *A*). In isolated anterior interosseous nerve palsy, all intrinsic muscles are normal and sensibility throughout the hand is intact. Thus the primary functional loss is the inability of the thumb tip to transmit force because the remainder of the thumb is functioning normally.

While awaiting return of anterior interosseous nerve function, splinting the thumb IP joint (and perhaps also the index DIP joint) allows the patient to continue writing, dressing, and performing other pinching activities. The splint blocks joint extension but can allow further flexion. Either a temporary custom molded thermoplastic splint (Fig. 34-15, *B*) or a more streamlined and durable sterling silver Siris splint (Silver Ring Splint Company, P.O. Box 2856, Charlottesville, Virginia) may be used as a functional splint until definitive nerve return occurs or tendon transfer is completed.

Radial nerve

High lesion. Unlike the median and ulnar nerve, the radial nerve is more commonly injured at the higher level where it spirals around the humerus (Fig. 34-16). Injury at the spiral groove of the humerus is most commonly associated with humeral fractures and direct compression. Sensory loss with radial nerve palsy is of little functional concern because it lies over the dorsoradial aspect of the hand. In isolated radial palsy, the entire palmar surface of the

hand retains normal sensibility. Injury at or below the spiral groove spares the innervation of the triceps, leaving elbow function intact. There is absence of all wrist and finger extensors as well as the supinator, but all flexor and intrinsic muscles in the hand retain full function.

Unlike patients with median or ulnar nerve palsy, in whom sensory and intrinsic muscle loss impedes hand function, the patient with radial palsy has the potential for relatively normal use of the hand. For this to be possible, a splint must be appropriately designed to harnesses wrist motion while allowing finger flexion. Although some authors advocate early tendon transfers to eliminate the need for external splinting, this is not the standard management of radial palsy.[6,20,21,23,25] Radial nerve palsy often recovers spontaneously; therefore effective splinting may be needed for months during regeneration.

The primary functional loss in radial palsy is inability to stabilize the wrist in extension so that the finger flexors can be used normally. The loss of the wrist and finger extensors destroys the essential reciprocal tenodesis action vital to the normal grasp-and-release pattern of the hand (Fig. 34-17). The ideal splint re-creates this natural harmony of tenodesis action: finger extension with wrist flexion and wrist extension with finger flexion. Many authors suggest the use of a static wrist support splint.[11-13,19] Wrist immobilization splints do not address the problem of absent finger and thumb extension. Any grasp or release activity must be assisted by the uninvolved hand. Wrist immobilization splints also commonly cover the valuable palmar sensibility.

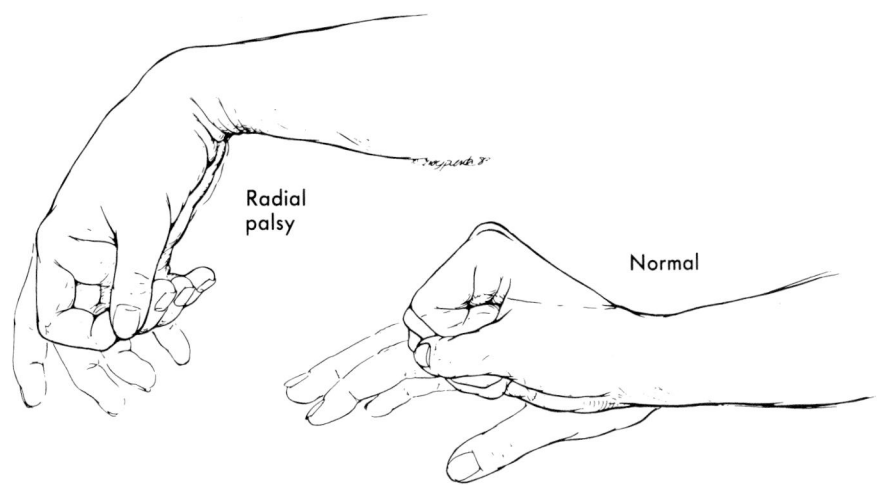

Fig. 34-17. Radial palsy robs the hand of the normal reciprocal tenodesis action. (From Colditz J: *J Hand Ther* 1:19, 1987.)

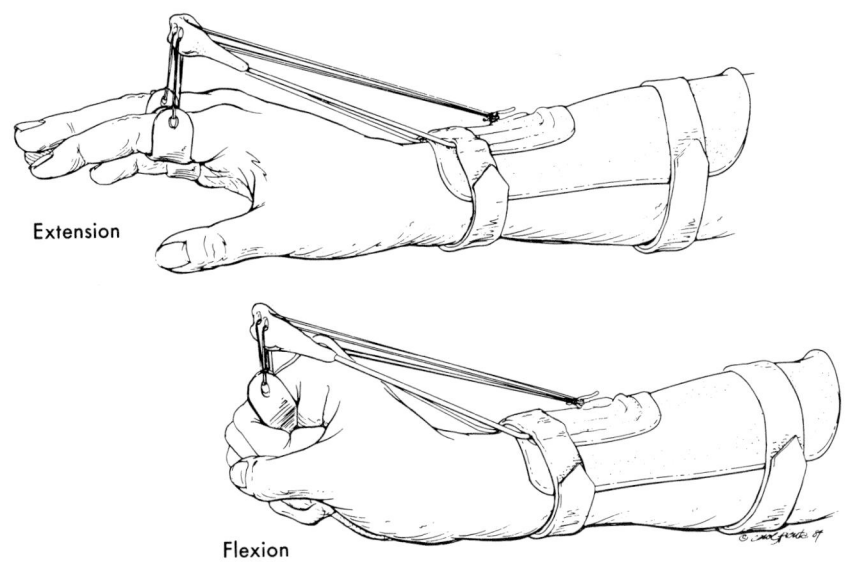

Fig. 34-18. Radial palsy splint that re-creates normal tenodesis action by the use of a static line. (From Colditz J: *J Hand Ther* 1:19, 1987.)

A splint first described by Crochetiere et al.[10] and a modified design described by Hollis[17] and Colditz[9] provide a static nylon cord rather than dynamic rubber bands to suspend the proximal phalangeal area (Fig. 34-18). This splint allows full finger flexion. Because the wrist never drops below neutral, the powerful flexors have the ability to bring the wrist into slight extension. During relaxation, gravity drops the wrist and the blocking force of the loops under the proximal phalanges achieves extension of the MP joints. Full finger extension is accomplished by the intrinsic muscles acting in concert with the blocking action of the splint. Because the splint receives a facsimile of the normal tenodesis motion, training is rarely required for the patient to adapt to the splint.

The EPL, extensor pollicis brevis, and abductor pollicis longus are extrinsic muscles that lie on the dorsoradial surface of the forearm. They are taken off maximum stretch when the splint harnesses the wrist. In this splint the thumb is not included in the outrigger system because of the awkwardness of an outrigger projecting radially. Occasionally, the absence of the extrinsic extensor and abductor muscles of the thumb allows it to rest under the index finger, impeding finger flexion. In such circumstances, a small splint is used to immobilize the thumb MP joint in extension but allow unrestricted thumb carpometacarpal (CMC) and IP joint motion. The intrinsic muscles of the thumb can extend the IP joint in the absence of the extrinsic extensors.

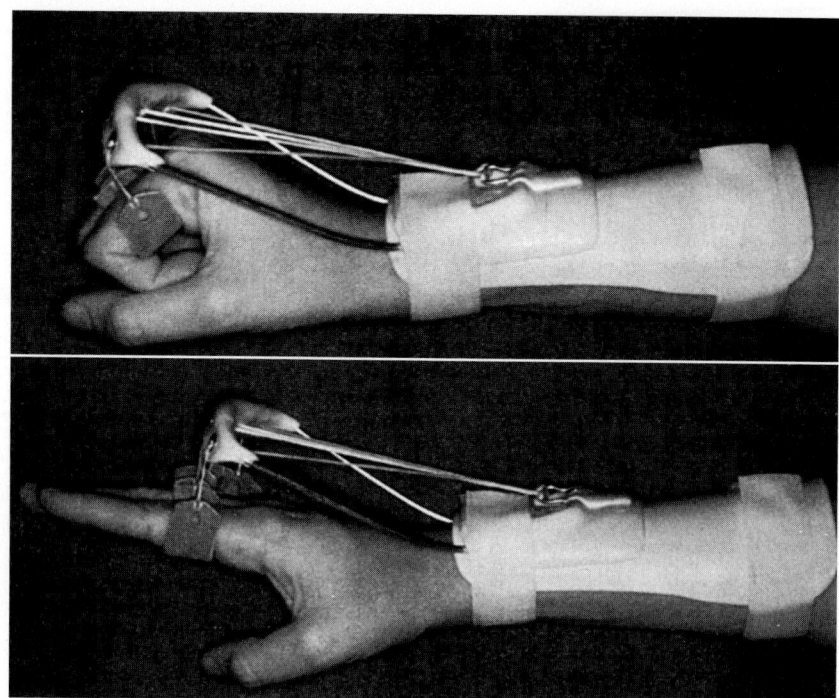

Fig. 34-19. Radial palsy splint allows full flexion and extension of the fingers.

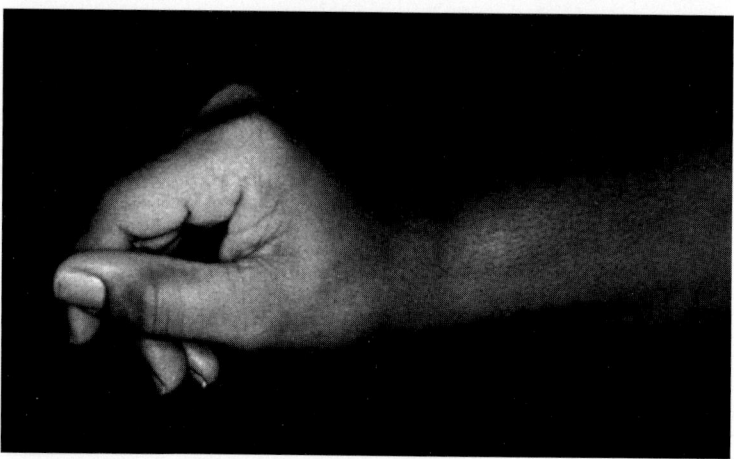

Fig. 34-20. Posture of the hand with posterior interosseous palsy shows radial wrist extension.

The advantages of this splint design are numerous. The suspension design allows partial wrist motion and full finger motion (Fig. 34-19). It maintains the normal hand arches as the thumb and ring and little CMC joints are unimpeded. This free motion is impossible in static splints or when rigid bars hold the metacarpal or proximal phalangeal area. Most strikingly, this splint has an absence of splinting material on the palmar surface, allowing normal grasp. The greatest advantage of this splint is its comparatively low profile, which allows it to be used effectively by the patient in the daily routine.

As function begins to return, the splint facilitates strengthening of the wrist extensors instead of impeding

them. One should be cautioned against designs for dynamic wrist and finger extension because the powerful unopposed flexors often overcome the force of the dynamic splint during finger flexion.

Low lesion: posterior interosseous nerve. After the radial nerve crosses the elbow and plunges below the supinator, it divides, forming the posterior interosseous branch (deep motor) and the superficial sensory branch (see Fig. 34-16). Posterior interosseous palsy is the isolated involvement of the deep motor branch of the radial nerve. In posterior interosseous palsy, radial wrist extension is nearly always spared and brachioradialis function will always be present. Clinical presentation will be strong radial deviation

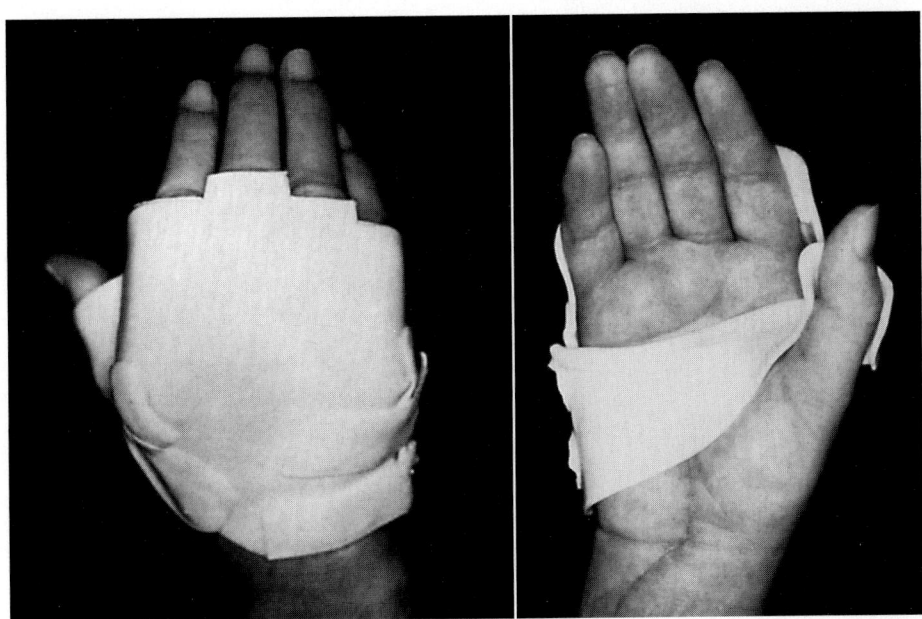

Fig. 34-21. A median/ulnar palsy splint must have a firm palmar bar to provide a point of counterforce to effectively prevent metacarpophalangeal joint hyperextension and position the thumb in abduction.

of the wrist during attempted wrist extension (Fig. 34-20). Attempted finger extension will demonstrate a pattern of MP flexion and IP extension in view of the absent extensor digitorum communis, extensor digiti minimi, and extensor indicis proprius muscles and the intact interosseous and lumbrical muscles.

Although the clinical picture differs from that of the high radial nerve lesion, the same mechanics for splinting apply to the low lesion. The splint design described earlier allows the radial wrist extensors to function normally to stabilize the wrist during finger flexion. Finger extension is achieved by the patient dropping the wrist into flexion, as the statically suspended proximal phalanges area supports the MP joints in extension. No joint has been unnecessarily immobilized, and the normal tenodesis pattern of the hand is maintained.

In the unusual circumstance of a partial lesion of the posterior interosseous nerve, normal finger extension can be harnessed to lift a weak finger. A custom thermoplastic splint molded under the weak finger or fingers and over the adjacent normal fingers at the proximal phalanx may be of functional value to the patient and hasten the return of the isolated weak muscle.

MIXED NERVE LESIONS

Mixed nerve lesions provide the ultimate splinting challenge. Because multiple nerve involvement nearly always accompanies trauma to many other structures, a balance between increasing glide of soft tissues and constraint splint-ing for the denervated muscles is required. Monitoring the kinesiologic balance of motion is the guidepost for splinting.

The most common mixed lesion is concurrent injury to the median and ulnar nerves, because they both lie on the palmar surface of the wrist. Division of these nerves robs the hand of all intrinsic muscles, and clawing of all four digits is present. A splint must block MP hyperextension. Likewise, there are no intrinsic muscles stabilizing the thumb, and the thumb should be held in an abducted position (Fig. 34-21).

When only the radial nerve is functioning, one may harness wrist extension power into finger flexion by fitting the Rehabilitation Institute of Chicago tenodesis splint.[24] This splint can occasionally be applicable to the mixed nerve palsy patient to provide both a minimal grasp function and to maintain some range of finger flexion (Fig. 34-22).

In combined lesions in which muscle loss requires periodic static splinting, it is essential that the patient frequently remove the splint and carry out passive ranging of the joints. In isolated nerve injuries, one muscle group is denervated with the antagonist still working. In combined lesions, the imbalance may not be so simple. As the nerve return changes the muscle balance, splinting needs change.

The possible combinations of mixed nerve lesions are endless. A complete manual muscle test and a clear clinical picture of the balance of motion are the only guides to determining the splinting regimen.

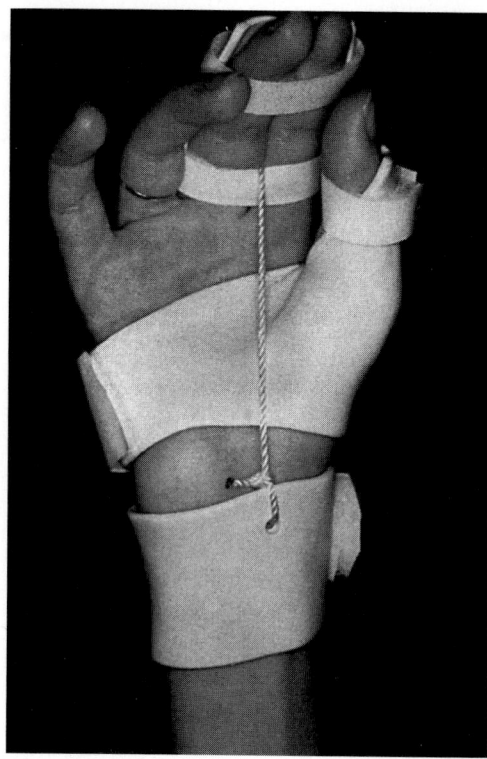

Fig. 34-22. The Rehabilitation Institute of Chicago tenodesis splint harnesses the power of wrist extension into functional pinch.

CONCLUSION

Splinting deformities that result from isolated nerve injuries in the upper extremity requires knowledge of normal and pathologic kinesiology. One must understand the correct design and mechanics of splints. A thorough knowledge of the anatomy and the expected course of reinnervation, as well as manual muscle testing skill, are necessary to evaluate the nerve-injured hand. The external constraints of splinting should maximize the balance of motion while awaiting return. Changes in splinting must occur in response to muscle and sensory return to assist in maximizing function.

REFERENCES

1. Akeson WH, Amiel D, Woo SLY: Immobility effects on synovial joints: the pathomechanics of joint contracture, *Biorheology* 17:95, 1980.
2. Akeson WH, et al: Effects of immobilization on joints, *Clin Orthop Rel Res* 219:28, 1987.
3. Amiel D, et al: The effect of immobilization on collagen turnover in connective tissue: a biochemical-biomechanical correlation, *Acta Orthop Scand* 53:325, 1982.
4. Brand PW: Tendon transfers in the forearm. In Flynn JE, editor: *Hand surgery,* ed 3, 1982, Baltimore, Williams & Wilkins.
5. Bunnell S: Splints for the hand. In Edwards JW, editor: *Orthopaedic appliance atlas,* vol 1, Ann Arbor, Mich, 1952, AAOS.
6. Burkhalter WE: Early tendon transfer in upper extremity peripheral-nerve injury, *Clin Orthop Rel Res* 104:68, 1974.
7. Cannon NM, et al: *Manual of hand splinting,* New York, 1985, Churchill Livingstone.
8. Capener N: Lively splints, *Physiotherapy* 53:371, 1967.
9. Colditz JC: Splinting for radial nerve palsy, *J Hand Ther* 1:18, 1987.
10. Crochetiere W, Granger CV, Ireland J: The "Granger" orthosis for radial nerve palsy, *Orthop Pros* 29:27, 1975.
11. Ellis M: Orthoses for the hand. In Lamb DW, Kuczynski K, editors: *The practice of hand surgery,* Oxford, 1981, Blackwell Scientific.
12. Falkenstein N, Weiss-Lessard S: *Hand rehabilitation: a quick reference guide and review,* St Louis, 1999, Mosby.
13. Fess EE, Philips CA: *Hand splinting, principles and methods,* ed 2, St Louis, 1987, Mosby.
14. Finsterbush A, Freidman B: Reversibility of joint changes produced by immobilization in rabbits, *Clin Orthop Rel Res* 111:290, 1975.
15. Frank C, et al: Physiology and therapeutic value of passive joint motion, *Clin Orthop Rel Res* 185:113, 1984.
16. Froment J: La prehension dans les paralysies, du nerf cubital et la signe du ponce, *Presse Med* 409, 1915.
17. Hollis I: Innovative splinting ideas. In Hunter JM, et al, editors: *Rehabilitation of the hand,* St Louis, 1978, Mosby.
18. Imbriglia JE, Hagnerg WC, Baratz ME: Median nerve reconstruction. In Peimer CA, editor: *Surgery of the hand and upper extremity,* New York, 1996, McGraw-Hill.
19. McKee P, Morgan L: *Orthotics in rehabilitation,* Philadelphia, 1998, FA Davis.
20. Omer GE Jr: Tendon transfers for reconstruction of the forearm and hand following peripheral nerve injuries. In Omer GE Jr, Spinner M, editors: *Management of peripheral nerve problems,* Philadelphia, 1980, WB Saunders.
21. Omer GE Jr: Early tendon transfers as internal splints after nerve injury. In Hunter JM, Schneider LH, Mackin EJ, editors: *Tendon surgery in the hand,* St Louis, 1987, Mosby.
22. Peacock EEJ: Some biochemical and biophysical aspects of joint stiffness: role of collagen synthesis as opposed to altered molecular bonding, *Ann Surg* 164:1, 1966.
23. Reid RL: Radial nerve palsy, *Hand Clin* 4:179, 1988.
24. Sabine C, Sammons F, Michela B: Report of development of the RIC plastic tenodysis splint, *Arch Phys Med Rehabil* 40:513, 1959.
25. Wheeler DR: Reconstruction for radial nerve palsy. In Peimer CA, editor: *Surgery of the hand and upper extremity,* New York, 1996, McGraw-Hill.
26. Woo SL-Y, et al: Connective tissue response to immobility: correlative study of biomechanical measurements of normal and immobilized rabbit knees, *Arthritis Rheum* 18:257, 1975.

Chapter 35

SENSORY REEDUCATION

Elaine Ewing Fess

Sensory reeducation is an important aspect of returning patients who have sustained peripheral nerve injuries to productive lives. After peripheral nerves have been repaired and nerve regeneration has progressed to the point that patients are able to perceive some touch or pressure stimuli, they often experience difficulty in using their hands because they have problems identifying objects they grasp. Their sense of touch, although marginally present, is distorted, and visual cues are needed to compensate for their impaired touch. Commonly voiced complaints are, "I can feel coins in my pocket but I can't tell one coin from another" or "When I'm working on my car and I need a tool, I have to look to be sure I am picking up the right one. I can't just reach over and pick up the tool I need by touching it."

The ability to identify objects following peripheral nerve repair is predictably problematic because of the number of axons involved and the specific distances and courses these regenerating axons must traverse to reach their termination points. Despite excellent surgical skill and ever-evolving more refined nerve repair techniques, even in the best of circumstances, routes taken by regenerating axons are often different from their original preinjury pathways, producing disappointing and sketchy functional sensibility capacities because of inconsistent and often more sparse axonal termination sites. To use a computer analogy, the patient has a newly rewired, lower-grade keyboard—the reinnervated hand. The patient's brain, the computer hard drive, is not recognizing transmissions from the new keyboard. Upper extremity rehabilitation specialists play an essential role in assisting postperipheral nerve repair patients to learn to use their recently distorted and still changing "touch communication systems" by helping them recognize the new message patterns their brains are receiving from their recovering hands.

According to Webster's Third International Dictionary, *reeducation* means, "to train . . . in an effort to replace or restore lost competence."[19] Wynn Parry,[22] a pioneer in sensory reeducation concepts, describes reeducation as "teaching the patient to lay down new response patterns in the brain to these abnormal stimuli so that he can relate his abnormal sensation to the nature of the surface of the object tested, which will have pre-injury patterns of response stored in the brain." Responsible for popularizing the concept of sensory reeducation in the United States and further expanding the knowledge base upon which its underlying principles are founded, Dellon[5] defines sensory reeducation as "a method or combination of techniques that help the patient with a sensory impairment learn to re-interpret the altered profile of neural impulses reaching his conscious level after his injured hand has been stimulated." In other words, the patient is learning the new touch code that the hand is sending to the brain.

Contemporary sensory reeducation theory and techniques have evolved over time, combining elements from various disciplines. Although intuitively interdependent, three central components contribute to present sensory reeducation's conceptual foundation. Following peripheral nerve repair, functional sensibility of the hand improves (1) over time, (2) with use, and (3) with training.

Surgeons and therapists have long recognized that their patients are better able to tactilely perceive and identify objects with the passage of time. In 1957, Nicholson and Seddon[14] helped focus this impression when they reported that the percentage of their ulnar-nerve repair patients attaining a +3 sensory score progressively increased from 5% of the patients at 1 year, to 15% at 3 years, and to 21% at 5 years after repair. Identifying the importance of occupation and early use, Davis,[4a] in 1949, reported that peripheral-nerve repair patients who early in their postoperative rehabilitation programs exercised and used their hands more frequently exhibited better sensory recovery of their involved hands than those who did not. He also correlated functional recovery success with job satisfaction. Bowden,[2] in discussing recovery after nerve injuries noted, in 1954, that "there is an indication that constant usage may lead to greater manual dexterity." In 1970, Honner et al.[9] found that better results were achieved with skilled workers as compared with semiskilled or manual workers. Supporting the concept that sensibility can be improved with training, independent studies have documented that blind subjects who read braille had better two-point discrimination than their control group counterparts.[1,8] Dellon[5] notes that "constant activity is the sensory reeducation that provides a physiologic face-lift to the . . . wrinkled hand."

Since Wynn Parry's introduction of the first formal sensory reeducation program in 1966,[21] acceptance of the important role sensory reeducation programs provide in rehabilitating patients who have sustained peripheral nerve injuries has grown to the point that these programs are routine in most hand and upper extremity rehabilitation centers. Research studies continue to document and increase knowledge regarding the effectiveness and application of sensory reeducation endeavors.

In a controlled study of patients recovering from median-nerve repair at the wrist level, Imai et al.[10,11] reported a statistically significant better result ($p < .003$) in patients who received sensory reeducation than in those who did not. They also found that despite these improvements, normal sensibility thresholds were not achieved. The same authors, in a later similar study, found that paresthesias were diminished and that object recognition was statistically better in patients who received sensory reeducation training. Based on these two studies, the investigators concluded that a program of sensory reeducation in adults who have had median-nerve repair at the wrist minimizes discomfort and improves sensibility.[10,11]

With refinement of microneurovascular techniques, transfer of innervated soft tissue has expanded appreciation for and use of sensory reeducation techniques. Regarding sensory potential for donor sites, Brown et al.[3] reported that "sensory reeducation protocol demonstrated that even these normal values may be improved." Shieh et al.[17] compared two randomly selected groups of patients with replanted or revascularized digits in which one group participated in a sensory reeducation and the second group, the control received no sensory reeducation. With an average duration of 18.8 weeks of sensory reeducation, at 1-year follow-up, the sensory reeducation group exhibited significantly better sensibility as measured by two-point discrimination and Semmes-Weinstein monofilaments.[17] In a study of patients who had toe-to-thumb transfers, Leung[12] found that in less than 1 year, patients who participated in sensory reeducation programs attained better results than those in a control group who had dropped their reeducation programs. Furthermore, for the patients who continued with their sensory reeducation, two-point discrimination on their transplanted toes—

now thumbs—was better than that which the toes had had before undergoing surgical transplantation.[12] Gickman and Mackinnon[7] identified factors that influence digital sensibility following replantation. These factors include age, level and mechanism of injury, digital blood flow, cold intolerance, and postoperative sensory reeducation.[7]

Importance of age is further documented in a study by Paletta and Senay[15] in which four pediatric subjects had radical excision of lipofibromatotous hamartomas of the median and ulnar nerves. The 20-year follow-up found moving two-point discrimination was normal in the two patients who had resection distal to the wrist and abnormal in the older patient and the patient whose resection was at wrist level. Presence of compensatory sensibility despite the fact that electromyographic studies demonstrated no sensory regeneration speaks strongly to the extraordinary reeducation capabilities in children younger than 2 years of age.[15] In another study, Tajima and Imai[18] compared a pediatric group of median-nerve repairs with an adult group with similar repairs and concluded that "the capacity for peripheral neural regeneration and cerebral plasticity in children is such that excellent recovery of functional sensation in the hand can occur without the need for sensory reeducation."

When sensory reeducation should begin and how long it lasts are intriguing questions. Wei and Ma[20] report statistically significant ($p < .0001$) improvement in 22 toe transfers in which sensory reeducation programs were begun an average of 38 months (range, 13 to 98 months) after transfer. After an average of 3.3 months of sensory reeducation, each of the transfers was reported to have 7-mm static and 6-mm moving two-point discrimination.[20] In 1998, when investigating long-term effects of sensory reeducation intervention, Shieh et al.[16] found that patients with replanted or revascularized digits who had participated in sensory reeducation programs for 1.5 years postoperatively were evaluated 1 year after they discontinued their reeducation programs. A second similar group of patients who never had sensory reeducation were also evaluated at the same time format. "After cessation of sensory reeducation, the degree of moving two-point discrimination became significantly worse in the formal sensory-reeducated group ($p < .05$) and significantly improved in the group without sensory reeducation initially ($p < 5$), whereas it showed a nonsignificant change of Semmes-Weinstein threshold both in the group with formal sensory reeducation and without sensory reeducation. Sensory retraining did influence the progressive change of moving two-point discrimination, but not in a parallel way with the Semmes-Weinstein threshold test."[16]

SENSORY REEDUCATION PROGRAMS

Currently, four basic sensory reeducation programs may be found in the literature. These include strategies described by Wynn Parry,[21,22] Dellon,[5,6] Callahan,[4] and Nakada and Uchida.[13] Each approach has individually distinct treatment facets and methods of evaluation, and all four have common elements upon which they agree. Although these sensory reeducation programs are reviewed briefly, in-depth descriptions and analyses are beyond the scope of this chapter. Readers are directed to the cited references for more detailed information about these innovative methods. To better underscore the historical fundamental differences and similarities between the four programs, their original formats are described. With the passage of time, program distinctions become less defined as each system continues to evolve to meet the ever-changing opportunities afforded by new information and better insights.

The focus of Wynn Parry's sensory reeducation program is directed toward reorganization of central connections through graded stimuli, including shapes, weights, textures, and games, and localizations. Progress is assessed through two-point discrimination, time for object recognition, time for texture recognition, and time for correct localization. Dellon's sensory reeducation strategy is divided into early and late phases. During the early phase, focus is directed at reeducating submodality-specific perceptions and incorrect localization. The late phase guides recovery of tactile gnosis or recognition. Progress is assessed with 30-cps tuning fork, moving touch, constant touch, and 256-cps tuning fork. Callahan's program introduces the important concept of compensation for lack of protective sensation through eight guidelines for teaching patients to prevent damage to their hands from use. She also describes a discriminative reeducation process using localization tasks and graded discrimination tasks. Nakada and Uchida introduce two more important variables—proximal vibration sense and muscle tension sense—with five interventional stages, including feature detection and recognition of objects, correction of prehension patterns, control of grasping force, maintenance of grip force during proximal joint movement, and manipulation of objects. Nakada and Uchida incorporate the Semmes-Weinstein monofilaments, 256-cps and 30-cps vibration, temperature, and pain testing in her program.

Wynn Parry, Dellon, and Callahan all recognize and describe patients who may best benefit from their respective programs. Wynn Parry[21] writes that patients who are "cooperative, well motivated, and need their sensation for everyday activities . . . [and] have appreciation of sensation in fingers" do well with sensory reeducation endeavors. He also notes that children almost always have good results.[21] Dellon[5] states that sensory reeducation may be initiated "when 30-cps vibration and moving touch have returned to an area." Callahan's defines two groups of patients for her program: (1) those with severely diminished or lacking protective sensation and (2) those who perceive touch and temperature but lack discriminative sensation. Return of touch perception to the fingertips at the level of the 4.31 Semmes-Weinstein monofilament or better is a requisite for the second group. She observes, as have others, that

well-motivated intelligent patients who are able to concentrate achieve better results with sensory reeducation methods.[4] In contrast, Nakada and Uchida do not define entry-level criteria for their system. Instead, they convincingly present a case study of a blind woman with no measurable protective sensation, a seeming worst-case scenario that has surprising results.

Similarities of the four sensory reeducation programs include incorporation of localization tasks, graded stimulus tasks, and recognition tasks. Three of the four systems define minimum entry-level or prerequisite criteria and all describe methods of assessment, although Nakada and Uchida's assessment techniques are not specific to her program. Interestingly, these four important programs span 30 years of development from Wynn Parry's introduction of the first formal sensory reeducation program in 1966 to Nakada and Uchida's equally innovative contribution in 1997. Each system in turn introduces unique and valuable concepts that directly affect and improve patient care. These programs also facilitate greater understanding of the multifaceted peripheral nervous system and its equally complex and integrated relationship within the central nervous system.

SENSORY EDUCATION EQUIPMENT

Unlike many aspects of therapy that have gone high-tech, sensory reeducation equipment, for the most part, maintains a humble profile in therapy departments. Some prepackaged touch or weight reeducation products are available commercially, but patients seem to enjoy the "home-made" concoctions their therapists devise for them more. Sensory reeducation practice (not assessment) is one of the few remaining areas in therapy that does not require strict standardization of protocols, procedures, and equipment for successful treatment.* Emphasis is placed on common everyday items, and in the current climate of managed care, home programs are essential foundations for sensory reeducation programs. Although reeducation equipment is available in therapy departments, it is often used to show patients how to set up their own programs at home, rather than for specific clinic-based therapy sessions. Because of the frequency of sessions required (i.e., multiple times a day) and its extended duration over time, sensory reeducation intervention is not economically amenable to contemporary therapy clinics. Instead, patients are taught the fundamentals of sensory reeducation and shown examples of equipment that they may assemble at home. Emphasis on home programs has an added benefit in that when patients are involved in creating and setting up their own home programs they have more acceptance of the programs and their participation is better. Home programs can also be fun

---

*Note: Assessment tools used to evaluate peripheral nerve injury patients must meet very specific measurement criteria including NIST standards. See Chapter 16.

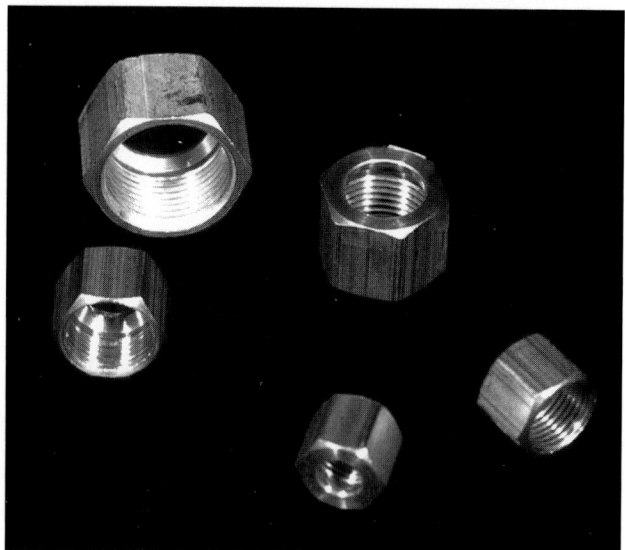

Fig. 35-1. Similar objects with differing sizes may be rank ordered by size from largest to smallest or they may be matched according to size. Metal objects also introduce fine temperature gradations because they are perceived to be "cooler" than like objects of other materials such as wood or rubber.

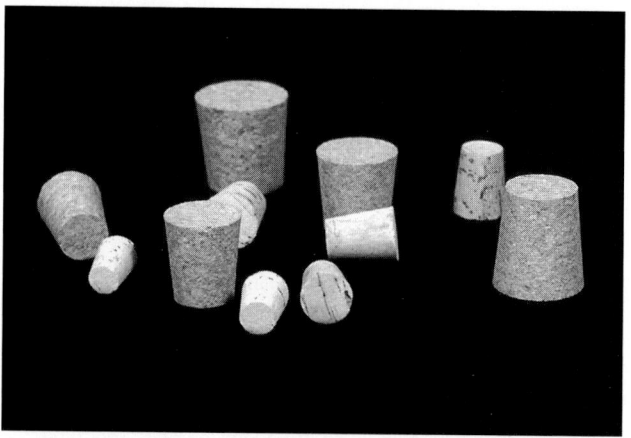

Fig. 35-2. Because of their lightweight corks of different sizes, these objects rank toward the more difficult end of sensory reeducation options. Patients need relatively good sensibility acuity before they are able to master this type of object.

learning experiences for staff. Patients often devise novel and very appropriate new sensory reeducation tools that may be shared with other sensory reeducation patients. *Fair warning:* Patients have been known to come up with some not-so-good creations as well.

Sensory reeducation equipment generally falls into one of three general categories: localization tools, graded stimulus tools, or recognition tools. Objects used in sensory reeducation are limited only by therapists' imaginations and understanding of the basic concepts involved in sensory reeducation. Common items become treatment inspirations when viewed through the eyes of knowledgeable and experienced therapists. Hardware stores, toy stores, and fabric stores yield intriguing bits and pieces of materials and paraphernalia. When properly organized, these odd assemblages of seemingly unrelated scraps become innovative, effective treatment tools. Objects that provide shape, size (Figs. 35-1 and 35-2), texture (Fig. 35-3), weight (see Fig. 35-2), temperature, and/or figure/ground stimuli (Fig. 35-4) are included in sensory reeducation training. In addition, the environments in which these objects are placed may be changed, allowing a continuum of tasks ranking from easy to very difficult mediums in which patients are asked to find "hidden" objects using their affected hands (see Fig. 35-4).

For patients who have moderate to severe limitations of finger or thumb range of motion, it is important to incorporate objects of appropriate size into their sensory reeducation programs. Gluing graded textures or smaller objects to dowels or wooden tongue depressors allows patients with limited digital motion to carry out their sensory

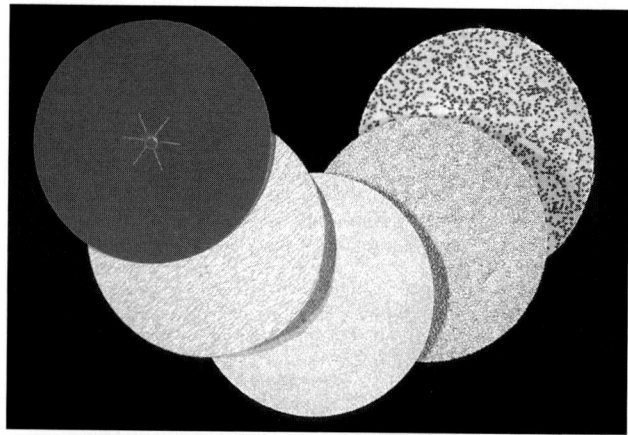

Fig. 35-3. Sand papers are manufactured in different grades of textures which makes them easily adapted to create sensory reeducation graded stimulus tasks. *A precaution:* The grit from some sand papers is easily dislodged making them inappropriate choices for patients with open wounds.

reeducation programs within the functional limitations imposed by restricted motion. Desensitization tasks may also be necessary for patients who have tactile defensive responses in addition to impaired sensibility capacity.

Generally speaking, sensory reeducation programs advance from gross tasks to more refined tasks as patients become more sophisticated in their abilities to perceive a variety of tactile stimuli. Each patient has individual requirements for which his or her specific sensory reeducation programs must be adapted. As noted earlier, patients who are motivated and actively have buy-in into their

Chapter 35   Sensory reeducation   **639**

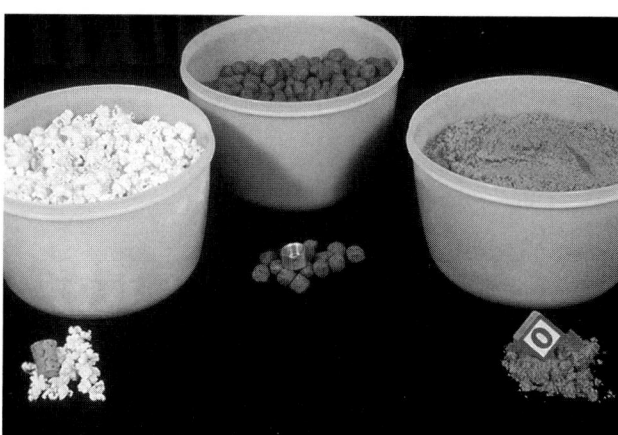

Fig. 35-4. Objects may be hidden in contact particle or milieu bowls for patients to find using their affected hands. Small corks in a popcorn bowl are very difficult for patients to find. Note the child's block on the far right. Raised letters on blocks may be used in recognition tasks.

programs achieve better results with sensory reeducation techniques. Although some patients require very little formal direction, intuitively understanding that use is the key to improved sensory awareness of their affected hands, most candidates for sensory reeducation programs benefit from formal instruction and periodic routine follow-up visits to the therapy clinic.

FUTURE CONSIDERATIONS

Advancement of one's sensory reeducation knowledge base depends on additional prospective, randomized trial research studies using assessment instruments that have proven statistical reliability and validity. The 1998 study by Shieh et al.[16] cited earlier in this chapter is an excellent example of research that opens the future to many more exciting and challenging questions. Were their results due to the fact that one of the two assessment instruments used in their study lacks force control, or more intriguing, is there an inherent difference in the phenomenon the two instruments measure? Nakada and Uchida's blind patient case study speaks loudly to the fact that we do not yet have all the answers when it comes to understanding sensibility and the neurophysiologic basis of sensory reeducation programs. We now have a more stable base from which we may say that sensory reeducation programs are effective, but this is not enough. The next questions are why and how are they

effective. In looking forward, we must also look back and acknowledge the many contributions of those individuals whose investigations have brought us to our present understanding of sensibility.

REFERENCES

1. Almquist E: The effect of training on sensory function. In Mickon J, Moberg E, editors: *Traumatic nerve lesions of the upper extremity,* Edinburgh, 1975, Churchill Livingstone.
2. Bowden REM: Factors influencing function recovery. In Seddon H, editor: *Peripheral nerve injuries,* London, 1954, Her Majesty's Stationery Office.
3. Brown C, et al: The sensory potential of free flap donor sites, *Ann Plast Surg* 23:135, 1989.
4. Callahan A: Methods of compensation and reeducation for sensory dysfunction. In Hunter J, Mackin E, Callahan A, editors: *Rehabilitation of the hand: surgery and therapy,* vol 1, St Louis, 1995, Mosby.
4a. Davis DR: Some factors affecting the results of treatment of peripheral nerve injuries, *Lancet* 1:877, 1949.
5. Dellon A: *Evaluation of sensibility and re-education in the hand,* Baltimore, 1981, Williams & Wilkins.
6. Dellon L: *Somatosensory testing and rehabilitation,* Bethesda, Md, 1997, American Occupational Therapy Association.
7. Glickman LT, Mackinnon SE: Sensory recovery following digital replantation, *Microsurgery* 11:236, 1990.
8. Heinrichs R, Moorhouse J: Touch perception in blind diabetic subjects in relation to the reading of braille type, *N Engl J Med* 280:72, 1969.
9. Honner R, Fragiadakis E, Lamb D: An investigation of the factors affecting the results of digital nerve division, *Hand* 2:21, 1970.
10. Imai H, Tajima T, Natsuma Y: Interpretation of cutaneous pressure threshold (Semmes-Weinstein monofilament measurement) following median nerve repair and sensory reeducation in the adult, *Microsurgery* 10:142, 1989.
11. Imai H, Tajima T, Natsumi Y: Successful reeducation of functional sensibility after median nerve repair at the wrist (see comments), *J Hand Surg* 16A:60, 1991.
12. Leung PC: Sensory recovery in transplanted toes, *Microsurgery* 10:242, 1989.
13. Nakada M, Uchida H: Case study of a five-stage sensory reeducation program, *J Hand Ther* 10:232, 1997.
14. Nicholson O, Seddon H: Nerve repairs in civil practice: results of therapy of median and ulnar nerve lesions, *Br Med J* 2:1065, 1957.
15. Paletta FX, Senay LC Jr: Lipofibromatous hamartoma of median nerve and ulnar nerve: surgical treatment, *Plast Reconstr Surg* 68:915, 1981.
16. Shieh SJ, Chiu HY, Hsu HY: Long-term effects of sensory reeducation following digital replantation and revascularization, *Microsurgery* 18:334, 1998.
17. Shieh SJ, et al: Evaluation of the effectiveness of sensory reeducation following digital replantation and revascularization, *Microsurgery* 16:578, 1995.
18. Tajima T, Imai H: Results of median nerve repair in children, *Microsurgery* 10;145, 1989.
19. *Webster's third new international dictionary of the English language unabridged,* Springfield, Mass, 1981, Merrian-Webster.
20. Wei FC, Ma HS: Delayed sensory reeducation after toe-to-hand transfer, *Microsurgery* 16:583, 1995.
21. Wynn Parry C: Rehabilitation of the hand, London, 1966, Butterworth & Company.
22. Wynn Parry C: Rehabilitation of the hand, ed 3, London, 1973, Butterworth & Company.

Part VIII

COMPRESSION NEUROPATHIES

Chapter 36

CARPAL TUNNEL SYNDROME

Edward P. Hayes
Karen Carney
Jennifer Wolf
Jennifer Moriatis Smith
Edward Akelman

Compression of the median nerve at the wrist, or carpal tunnel syndrome (CTS), is the most common upper extremity compressive neuropathy. Recent data have indicated that CTS may affect approximately 0.1% of the population of the United States per year.[124] The Bureau of Labor Statistics has estimated that in 1997, there were 29,200 cases of CTS that required time off from work.*

This clinical entity was first described by Paget in 1854,[98] as a sequela of trauma to the wrist. Later autopsy studies by Marie and Foix in 1913[83] demonstrated median-nerve neuromas at the transverse carpal ligament. These authors postulated that such neuromata could be relieved by transection of the transverse carpal ligament. Several surgeons contributed case reports detailing the use of carpal tunnel release in small numbers of patients in the early twentieth century. In 1965, George Phalen reviewed a large number of patients with CTS in the literature. Phalen presented his initial experience with 654 hands, including the diagnostic workup and the surgical results. He noted that "the median nerve is easily compressed by any condition that increases the volume of the structures within the carpal tunnel."[101]

ANATOMY

The carpal tunnel is an inelastic structure located at the wrist. Its floor is composed of the concave arch of the carpal bones. The hook of the hamate, triquetrum, and pisiform constitute the ulnar border, whereas the radial aspect includes the trapezium, scaphoid, and the fascia over the

flexor carpi radialis (FCR).[107] The roof of the carpal tunnel is made up of the deep forearm fascia, the transverse carpal ligament, and the distal aponeurosis of the thenar and hypothenar muscles. The transverse carpal ligament extends from the scaphoid tuberosity and trapezium to attach to the pisiform and the hook of the hamate.[27,124] The contents of the carpal tunnel consist of the median nerve and nine flexor tendons. The flexor pollicis longus (FPL), four flexor digitorum profundus (FDP), and four flexor digitorum superficialis (FDS) tendons pass through the carpal tunnel, with the nerve lying superficially and anteroradially in the tunnel (Fig. 36-1).

At the distal edge of the carpal tunnel, the median nerve most commonly divides into six branches: two common digital nerves, three proper digital nerves, and the recurrent motor branch, which innervates the thenar musculature. The nerve gives off the palmar cutaneous branch proximally and radially, approximately 5 cm proximal to the wrist crease. This branch travels with the main nerve for 1.4 to 2.6 cm and then penetrates the antebrachial fascia between the palmaris longus and FCR. It emerges subcutaneously, usually proximal to the wrist crease, to innervate the palm.[32,123]

Multiple variations of median nerve anatomy have been described. These include various high divisions of the median nerve, persistence of the median artery, anomalous muscle attachments, and cross-connections with the ulnar nerve, and all are rare.[73] More commonly seen are variations in the branching and courses of the recurrent motor branch (Fig. 36-2) and the palmar cutaneous branch.[12,32,108,123] An awareness of these variations is essential when performing surgical release of the carpal tunnel.

*American Academy of Orthopaedic Surgery Bulletin, April 2000, p. 5.

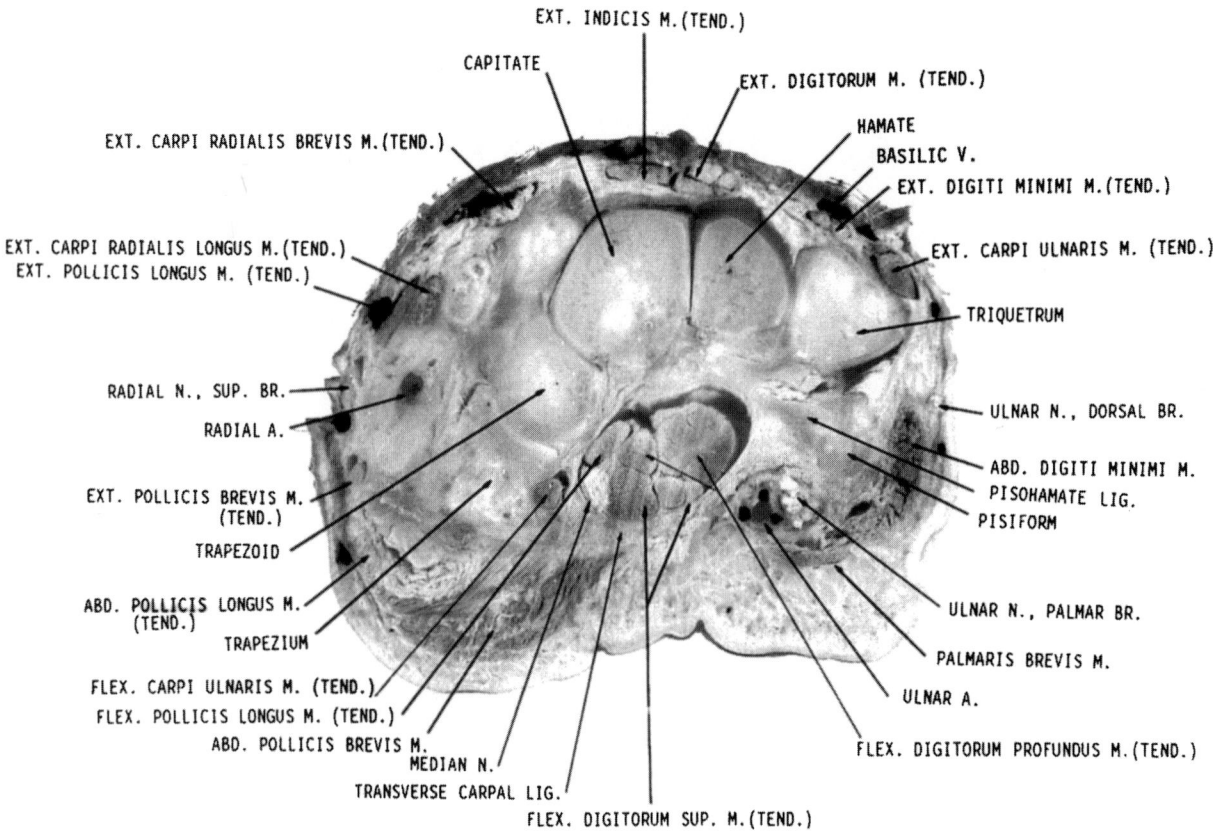

Fig. 36-1. Cross section of the wrist at the carpal tunnel.

PATHOGENESIS
Factors influencing pressure in the carpal canal

The causes of CTS may be divided into three general areas: the anatomy of the carpal tunnel proper, both systemic and local, pathophysiologic disorders, and CTS related to functional use. In general, any disorder that decreases the cross-sectional area of the carpal tunnel or that produces increased carpal tunnel canal volume content may cause CTS. Systemic conditions that primarily affect the blood vessels or cells of the nerve, such as diabetes or the overuse of alcohol; systemic inflammatory conditions such as rheumatoid arthritis; or conditions that affect blood pressure or edema in the carpal tunnel may cause CTS. Although controversial, repetitive motions involving the wrist in flexion, extension, and ulnar deviation, as well as digital flexion and extension, may cause CTS.

Recent scientific discussion has included the role of the lumbricals as space-occupying structures within the carpal tunnel when the fingers are flexed, leading to compression of the median nerve. If this is indeed the case in some patients,

standard wrist immobilizing splints may not be adequate for these patients because they allow full digital flexion.

The lumbrical muscles originate distal to the carpal tunnel with the fingers held in extension, but they lie within the carpal canal when the fingers are actively flexed by the proximal retraction of the FDP tendon.[28,115] This may contribute to compression of the median nerve in the canal, especially if there is hypertrophy of the lumbricals, as in the hands of manual laborers. Cobb et al.[28] measured lumbrical incursion in four finger positions: full extension, 50% finger flexion, 75% finger flexion, and 100% finger flexion. The lumbrical muscles were distal to the proximal aspect of the hook of the hamate (the most constrictive area of the carpal tunnel) only when the digits were in full extension or 50% finger flexion.

Clinically, this may be important because sustained contraction of the finger flexors greater than 50% or repetitive finger flexion exercises/activities may increase the hydrostatic pressure that the median nerve experiences as a result of crowding in the carpal canal by the lumbricals. The

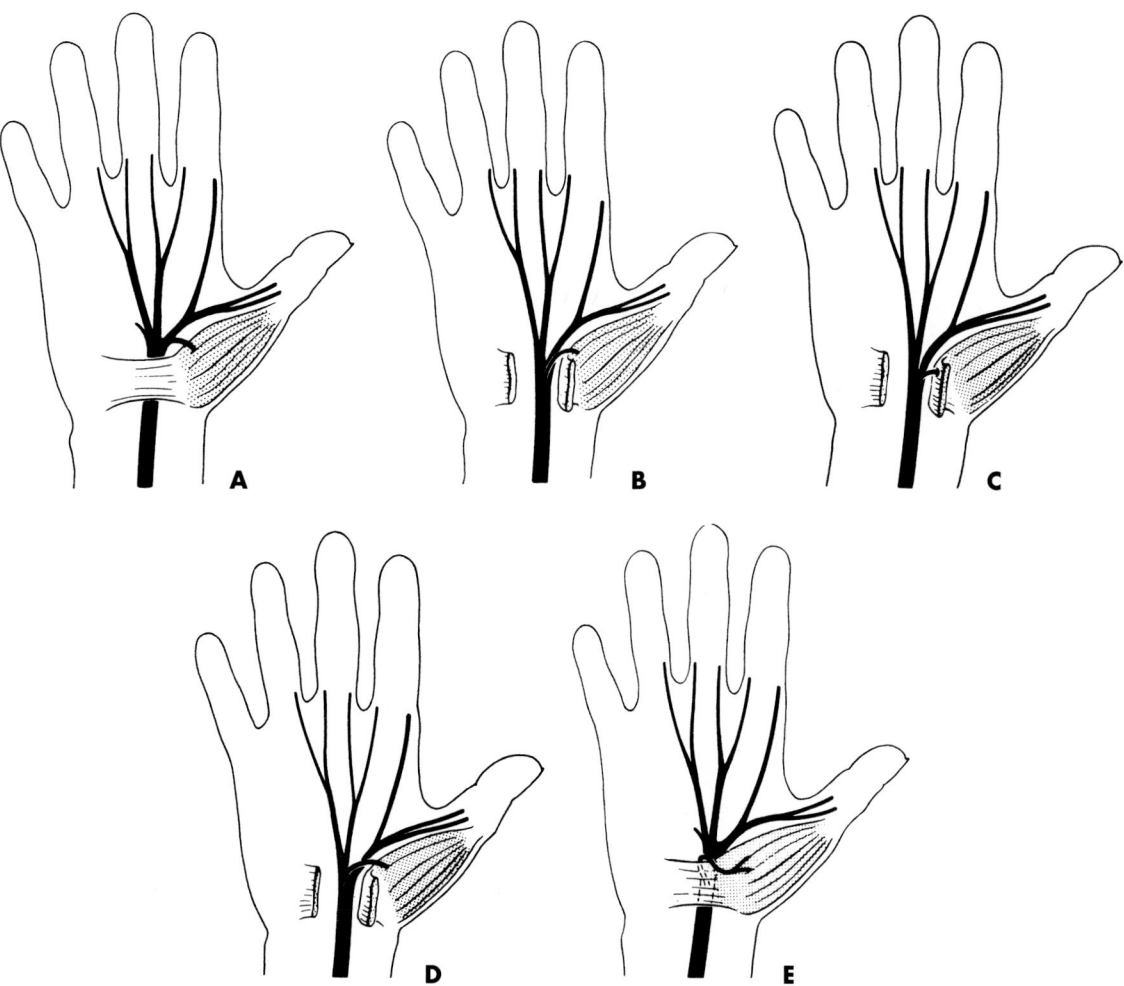

Fig. 36-2. Variations in median nerve anatomy in the carpal tunnel. **A,** The most common pattern of the motor branch is extraligamentous and recurrent. **B,** Subligamentous branching of a recurrent median nerve. **C,** Transligamentous course of the recurrent branch of the median nerve. **D,** The motor branch can uncommonly originate from the ulner border of the median nerve. **E,** The motor branch can lie on top of the transverse carpal ligament. (From Green D: *Green's operative hand surgery,* ed 4, Philadelphia, 1999, Churchill Livingstone.)

method of splinting for patients with CTS may be important, especially for those with hypertrophied lumbricals, those who have synovitis, or those who tend to overwork their hands in an effort to relieve the numbness.[39] Splinting the metacarpophalangeal (MP) joints in extension, in addition to the standard neutral wrist splint, extends the lumbricals distal to the most constrictive area and may decrease the pressure within the canal.

External pressure

Intracarpal tunnel pressure may be affected by external pressure to the palm.[28] Gelberman et al.[47] found that the average intracarpal canal pressure in patients with CTS was 32 mm Hg. Cobb et al.[26] demonstrated that when a 1-kg external force was applied over the flexor retinaculum, the pressure in the carpal canal increased to 103 mm Hg. Force

over the thenar area increased the pressure to 75 mm Hg, and force over the hypothenar area increased the pressure to 37 mm Hg. These findings are clinically significant in a number of areas. With tight fisting, the finger force on the palm may actually increase carpal tunnel pressure, as could the use of many tools, hand grippers, Thera-Putty, dynamic splints that exert force over these areas, and poorly fitted casts. A custom-molded splint, which can provide a more even pressure distribution over the carpal tunnel, may be preferred to a commercial splint with a poorly fitting insert adjusted to neutral.

PRESENTATION

The classic clinical presentation of a patient with CTS is a complaint of pain and paresthesias in the median-nerve distribution of the hand. These symptoms are characteristi-

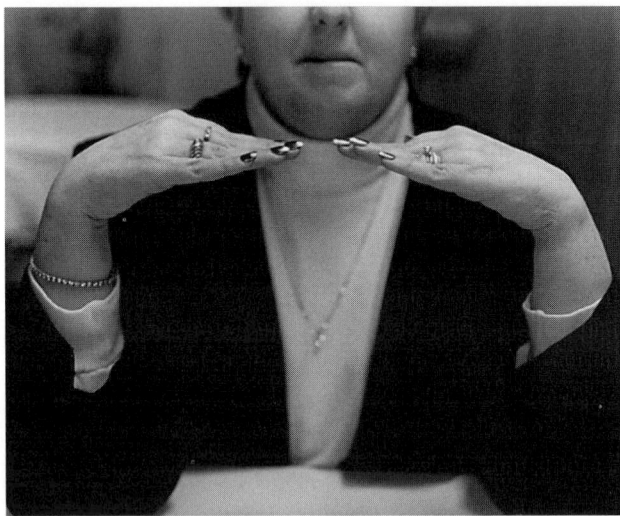

Fig. 36-3. Physical examination of a patient performing Phalen's test.

cally experienced or exaggerated at night or are worsened by repetitive forceful hand motion. Patients may report hand clumsiness or weakness. Improvement in symptoms after shaking or straightening the affected hand is common.

Objective findings in CTS include the limitation of paresthesias to the distribution of the median nerve (the radial 3.5 digits). A positive Tinel's sign, defined as tingling or paresthesias produced in the fingers with tapping over the median nerve at the wrist, is helpful in the diagnosis but has not shown excellent sensitivity in clinical studies.[48] The wrist flexion test, or Phalen's test (Fig. 36-3), is performed by flexing the wrist maximally for 60 seconds to see if this produces or exaggerates numbness and tingling in the affected fingers.[48,101] Thenar atrophy may be observed, indicating more chronic median-nerve compression. When these signs are combined with supporting symptoms, the diagnosis of CTS should be considered.

SUPPORTING STUDIES/TESTS

Electrodiagnostic testing remains the best known supporting study for confirmation of CTS. Other objective tests include Semmes-Weinstein monofilament testing, digital vibrometry, and carpal compression testing.

Semmes-Weinstein monofilament testing, which assesses light-touch discrimination, has been shown to be highly sensitive (91% in Gellman's investigation) but not highly specific.[95] The direct compression test described by Durkan is performed either by using a device that applies a known pressure externally over the median nerve at the wrist or by the examiner exerting even pressure on the carpal tunnel with both thumbs. Compression test using a commercial device has been shown to have a sensitivity of 87% and a specificity of 90% in the diagnosis of CTS.[35]

Electrodiagnostic testing remains the most common form of objective evidence of median-nerve compression. Normal values vary, but general standards include abnormal values for distal motor latency of more than 4.5 msec and distal sensory latency of more than 3.5 msec.[123] Electromyography (EMG) that reveals positive waves or fibrillations in the thenar musculature indicates the severity and chronicity of nerve injury.[8] A recent meta-analysis of the literature regarding the use of electrophysiologic testing and its sensitivity and specificity found median-nerve EMG and nerve conduction velocity (NCV) studies to be valid, reproducible, and highly sensitive and specific.[60] However, it has been shown that 10% to 15% of patients with normal electrodiagnostic results have clinically evident and surgically relieved median-nerve compression. Grundberg demonstrated that in a group of 292 patients with symptoms of CTS who were tested, 33 (or 11.3%) had normal electrodiagnostic results.[51] All of these patients underwent carpal tunnel release, with resolution of their symptoms in nearly all cases. EMG and nerve conduction studies are valuable additions to the diagnostic armamentarium, but negative testing should not be considered as absolute in the exclusion of the diagnosis of CTS.

CARPAL TUNNEL SYNDROME: PREDICTORS OF OUTCOME (PRETREATMENT)

Predictors of outcome after the nonoperative and operative treatment of CTS have been identified. Numerous studies support the importance of the clinical evaluation in the accurate diagnosis of CTS. Patients who can preoperatively identify on a hand symptom diagram an anatomically appropriate pattern of pain and paresthesias are more likely to have a satisfactory outcome after carpal tunnel release.[11] In the general patient population, the results of electrodiagnostic studies have little predictive value on the outcomes after carpal tunnel release.[13,29,50] However, among two groups of patients—diabetics and the worker's compensation population—those reporting poor results after carpal tunnel release tend to have normal or only minimally abnormal preoperative electrodiagnostic studies.[4,55]

In a prospective study of patients with CTS treated with steroid injections and wrist orthoses, women younger than 40 were the least likely to have resolution of symptoms.[129] Among operatively treated patients, those who have a prolonged (ranging in studies from 3 to 5 years) duration of symptoms before surgery are much less likely to have complete symptom resolution than patients treated more expeditiously.[19,34]

Economic and psychosocial variables have a well-documented effect on the return to work and the extent of symptom relief for both surgically and nonoperatively managed patients with CTS.[65,66] Residual symptoms, prolonged absence from work, and the need to change jobs are significantly more common after carpal tunnel release in patients with physically strenuous jobs, especially among worker's compensation recipients. Palmar pain, in particular, contributes to the prolonged postoperative recovery.[4,54,91,133] The management of occupation-associated CTS is challenging and mandates close communication and cooperation among the patient, physician, therapist, and employer.[79]

CONSERVATIVE MANAGEMENT OF CARPAL TUNNEL SYNDROME

The efficacy of nonsurgical management of mild CTS has been well documented. Conservative management is generally not an option for moderate to severe CTS, especially in patients who have signs of muscle atrophy or significant sensory impairment. The diagnosis of CTS should be confirmed with clinical testing, and potential proximal compression sites should be ruled out. Conservative management options that have been described for CTS include splinting, nonsteroidal antiinflammatory drugs (NSAIDs), injection of the carpal tunnel with a corticosteroid, tendon and nerve gliding exercises, vitamins, iontophoresis, ultrasound, and activity or job site modifications. Recent studies evaluating the causes of increased carpal tunnel pressure have led to questions regarding traditional standards of care.[26,28,39,115] The following sections describe various conservative treatment options, including those that may warrant further study and consideration based on current research.

Splinting

Splinting of the wrist is the initial standard of care to treat mild CTS. Traditional cock-up splints and many commercially available splints place the wrist in the functional position of 20 to 30 degrees of extension. However, many scientific studies show that carpal canal pressures increase with increasing wrist flexion *and* extension.[47,70,82,130] Patients with CTS should be splinted with the wrist in a neutral position. Splinting the wrist in a neutral position diminishes intracarpal tunnel pressures, maximizing blood flow to the median nerve.[70] In 1995, Weiss et al.[130] demonstrated that the lowest pressure in the carpal canal was when the wrist was positioned in 2 degress (±9 degrees) of flexion and 1 degree (±9 degrees) of ulnar deviation for patients with CTS, again concluding that a neutral wrist position is most desirable to lower carpal canal pressure.

As described earlier, lumbrical incursion may be a factor in increasing carpal canal pressure.[28] A neutral wrist splint with the MP joints included in extension and the interphalangeal (IP) joints free can potentially decrease intratunnel pressures by pulling the lumbricals distally out of the carpal tunnel.[39] This splint modification may have a significant effect on patients whose lumbricals are contributing to their carpal tunnel symptoms.

Many patients' symptoms are relieved with nighttime splinting. Patients who complain of symptoms constantly or those who experience pain with activity may need to wear a splint full-time, including at work. Rigid thermoplastic splints may not be conducive to the demands of a particular job. Some patients find that commercially available splints with the inserts adjusted to neutral or more flexible splints accommodate job demands and are better tolerated. It is important to remember, however, that external pressure can cause an increase in intracarpal tunnel pressure.[26] A custom-molded splint may provide a more even distribution of pressure over the carpal tunnel as compared with a poorly fitted or adjusted commercial splint. Rempel et al. found that wearing a flexible wrist splint during activity limits range of motion (ROM) but does not decrease the pressure in the carpal canal.[105]

Antiinflammatory drugs

Conservative treatment for CTS has included oral NSAIDs or injection of a corticosteroid into the carpal tunnel. However, NSAIDs have never been shown to be effective in a scientific study. The purpose of the cortisone injection is to decrease the mass of the thickened flexor tendon synovium by decreasing the inflammatory process.[71] After the injection, each patient is placed in a wrist splint for 3 to 4 weeks, and then at night for an additional 3 weeks. Studies show that injection and splinting initially provide relief in approximately 40% to 80% of patients.[45] However, 18 months after injection, this number decreased to 22%.[45] There is value in steroid injection, even if symptoms return, in that improvement in symptoms confirms the diagnosis and is indicative of a favorable outcome if surgery is required. However, poor relief after injection does not predict a poor surgical result.

Iontophoresis using dexamethasone sodium phosphate has been used by many health care providers to treat inflammatory disorders. Some studies support the use of iontophoresis as an alternative to injection. Banta used iontophoresis in conjunction with splinting and NSAIDs and reported a success rate of 17% for patients with mild CTS.[10] This study favorably compares with an 18.4% success rate reported by Kaplan et al. in 1990.[62] Further research in this area is indicated to validate iontophoresis as an alternative to injection.

Ultrasound has not proven to be significantly effective in the conservative treatment of CTS to date. Ebinbichler et al.[36] looked at "sham" versus therapeutic ultrasound as a treatment for CTS. Their initial findings indicate satisfying short- to medium-term effects. These findings need to be confirmed and compared with standard treatment options. Otzas et al.[97] found that both therapeutic ultrasound *and* placebo ultrasound provided symptomatic relief in those studied. They attributed this to the superficial massage effect on the tissues. Because of these inconclusive findings, the unknown efficacy and safety of ultrasound, and its yet-to-be-determined, thermal effects on motor nerve conduction,[97]

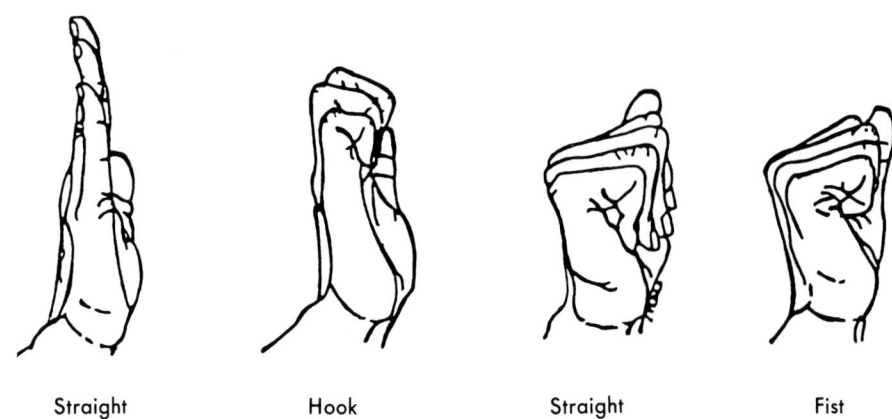

Straight   Hook   Straight   Fist

Fig. 36-4. Three different positions of tendon gliding exercises: hook fist, straight fist, and full fist.

more research is indicated to determine the therapeutic effects of ultrasound with CTS.

The role of exercise in conservative management

The role of exercise in conservative management of CTS is not well documented and somewhat controversial as to its effectiveness. However, patient education about exercises and positions to avoid is essential.

Seradge et al.[112] found that a significant rise in pressure was recorded in the carpal tunnel not only with wrist flexion but also with wrist extension; while making a fist or holding objects; and with isometric flexion of a finger against resistance. The increased pressures during the functional positioning suggest that nonsurgical treatment should include patient education to reduce fisting, gripping, holding of objects, and isolated finger use against resistance, as in typing. Seradge proceeded to measure carpal pressures after 1 minute of active wrist and finger flexion and extension exercise. He noted a decrease in intratunnel pressure, suggesting that brief intermittent exercise of the digits and wrist may be beneficial in relieving symptoms. This may explain the resolution of nighttime numbness when patients wake and briefly exercise their hands in an attempt to "wake them up."

Differential tendon gliding exercises as described by Totten and Hunter[125] (Fig. 36-4) can help facilitate isolated FDS and FDP excursion as they course through the carpal canal. In 1998, Rozmaryn et al.[110] retrospectively looked at conservative treatment of CTS with and without tendon and nerve gliding exercises. The exercises, designed to maximize the excursion of the digital flexors and the median nerve through the carpal tunnel, were performed in five repetitions, three to five sessions per day (Fig. 36-5). The results of this study indicated a significant improvement in patients' carpal tunnel symptoms when tendon and nerve gliding exercises were performed in conjunction with

traditional treatment. Further research to support this study is warranted.

Nerve gliding is described mostly for postoperative management to minimize adhesion formation. As seen in the study by Rozmaryn et al.,[110] it is sometimes advocated for conservative management as well. It is prudent to keep in mind that "nerve gliding is an extremely powerful treatment technique that easily can increase symptoms and irritability if not used very carefully and with a good understanding of the goal."[18] Chronic nerve irritation or compression may result in edema and fibrosis around the nerve. Forced nerve gliding in this instance may cause microscopic stretching tears, bleeding, and increased inflammation.[125] When performing these exercises, patients should not experience increased symptoms.

Work or activity modification/patient education

Whether a patient has CTS that may be related to work, pregnancy, an avocational activity, or other cause, it is important to discuss overall lifestyle with the patient. If the compression is attributed to job duties or other activities of daily living (ADLs), education regarding provocative positions and modification of the method of performing the action may help resolve symptoms with little effort. Patient education is important because it allows the patient to take responsibility for his or her own situation. Splinting schedules should be explained to the patient, not just be prescribed. Precautions include avoidance of repetitive motion or prolonged positioning involving wrist flexion, extension, and ulnar deviation, particularly when combined with application of force to a tool. Patients should be cautioned against tight fisting activities or repetitive finger flexion. If particular activities aggravate the symptoms, analysis of the method of performance and modification of the activity should be attempted. Options include decreasing the duration of the activity, taking rest periods, or if job

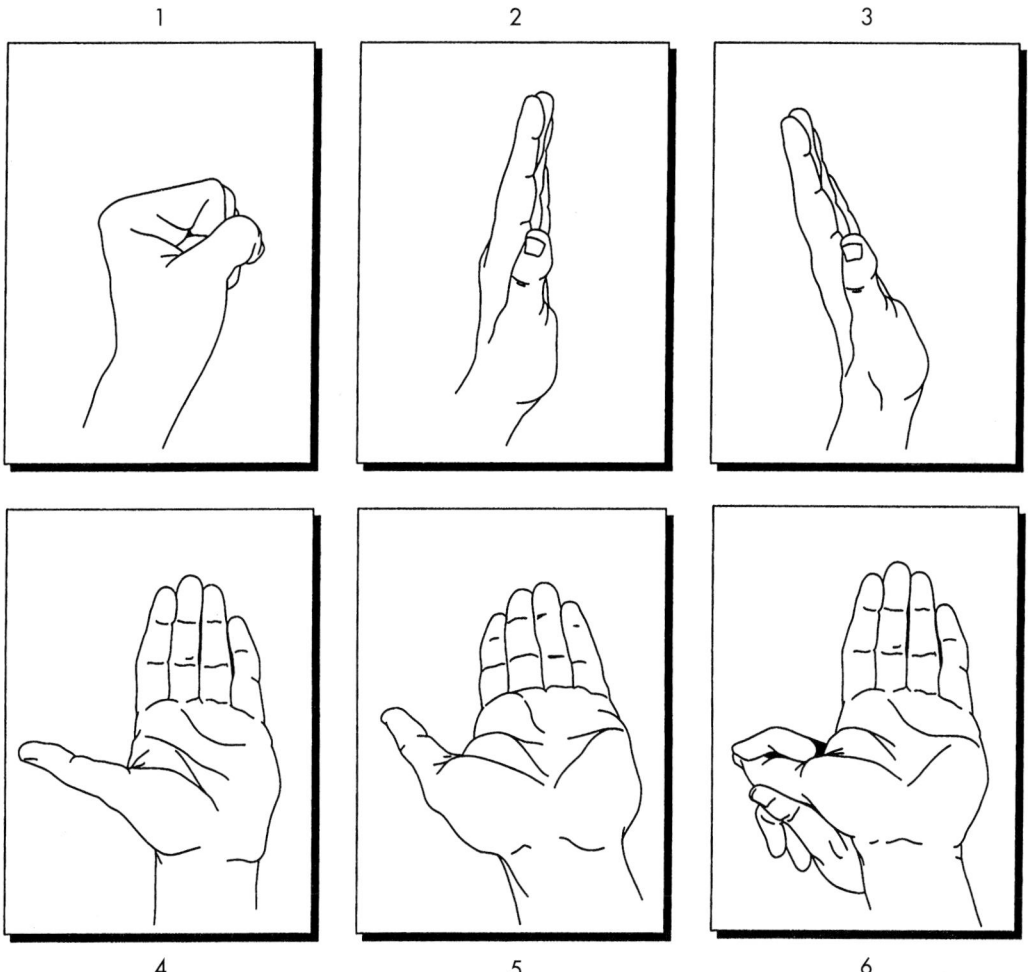

Fig. 36-5. The median nerve gliding program: *position 1,* wrist in neutral, fingers and thumb in flexion; *position 2,* wrist in neutral, thumb in neutral, fingers extended; *position 3,* wrist and fingers extended, thumb in neutral; *position 4,* wrist, fingers, and thumb in neutral; *position 5,* forearm in supination; and *position 6,* the opposite hand applies a gentle stretch to the thumb. (Redrawn from Totten PA, Hunter JM: *Hand Clin* 7:505, 1991.)

related, rotating work assignments between employees. Tools should be assessed, and handles and grips can be modified, keeping in mind not just position but also external forces on the hand. Workstations may be assessed and modified to ensure that symptoms are not aggravated by poor body mechanics or other ergonomic factors such as chair height, workstation keyboard angle and position, or tool design. The previously described conservative treatment measures may be initiated as appropriate in conjunction with the activity modification.

Vitamin B$_6$ treatment

In the 1970s, Ellis et al. proposed that a deficiency in pyridoxine (vitamin B$_6$) may cause CTS. Current literature has conflicting reports and conclusions with regard to vitamin B$_6$ for CTS. Although adding vitamin B$_6$ to the diet is still occasionally advocated in the literature and the press, no controlled, randomized, prospective study has shown

vitamin B$_6$ to be clearly efficacious over other conservative treatments for CTS.[6,61,120]

SURGICAL MANAGEMENT OF CARPAL TUNNEL SYNDROME
Indications

Wrist trauma, as well as infections and systemic rheumatologic and hematologic diseases, can acutely increase the carpal canal pressure, threatening median-nerve viability. Acute CTS requires prompt recognition and early open carpal tunnel release.[121] For idiopathic CTS, a relative indication for surgical release is clinical or electrodiagnostic evidence of denervation of the median nerve–innervated muscles. The functional motor recovery of the median nerve after carpal tunnel release is difficult to predict; therefore carpal tunnel release is preferred in the face of ongoing denervation. In the absence of significant clinical or electrodiagnostic denervation changes, several months of nonsurgical treatment, with particular emphasis on activity modification, is prudent.

The usual indication for surgical treatment of idiopathic CTS is the lack of symptomatic relief with nonoperative modalities. A large retrospective follow-up study of idiopathic CTS patients showed that among those treated nonoperatively, the average duration of symptoms was between 6 and 9 months. However, 22% of nonoperatively treated patients had symptoms for 8 years or longer. Patients who had carpal tunnel release were six times more likely than patients who did not have surgery to have resolution of their symptoms.[34] Particularly among patients who must continue in a manual labor occupation, prolonged nonsurgical treatment without symptomatic improvement does not appear to be fruitful.[88]

Procedures

Open carpal tunnel release. Herbert Galloway is credited with the first open carpal tunnel release, performed in 1924.[6] Sectioning the transverse carpal ligament has been shown to consistently increase the anteroposterior dimension of the carpal canal, changing the normally oval shape to a more circular cross section. Imaging studies have demonstrated a mean 24% increase in carpal canal volume.[106] With the relatively high incidence of anomalies of the median nerve[73] and the ulnar neurovascular structures,[103] in the vicinity of the transverse carpal ligament, open carpal tunnel release remains the preferred method of many surgeons for decompression of the median nerve at the wrist. This technique affords full inspection of the transverse carpal ligament and the contents of the carpal canal.[123]

Local, regional, or general anesthesia may be used. We prefer local infiltration of the tissues with a lidocaine and buspivacaine (Marcaine) mixture in combination with conscious sedation. Others state that a local anesthetic can obscure tissue planes and prefer axillary or intravenous regional block of the extremity.[117] Tourniquet control is used. A palmar incision is made ulnar to the depression between the thenar and hypothenar eminences to minimize damage to branches of the palmar cutaneous branch of the median nerve. Staying radial to the hook of the hamate minimizes risk to the ulnar neurovascular bundle. The incision is extended from Kaplan's cardinal line along the axis of the third web space proximally (Fig. 36-6). Extension proximal to the wrist crease is generally not required. In the subcutaneous tissues overlying the transverse carpal ligament, an effort is made to preserve the larger branches of the palmar cutaneous branch of the median nerve, the nerve of Henle, and cutaneous branches of the ulnar nerve. The superficial palmar fascia is divided in line with the skin incision. The underlying transverse carpal ligament is divided longitudinally along its ulnar aspect. At the distal end of the incision, the superficial palmar arterial arch is identified in its bed of adipose tissue and protected.

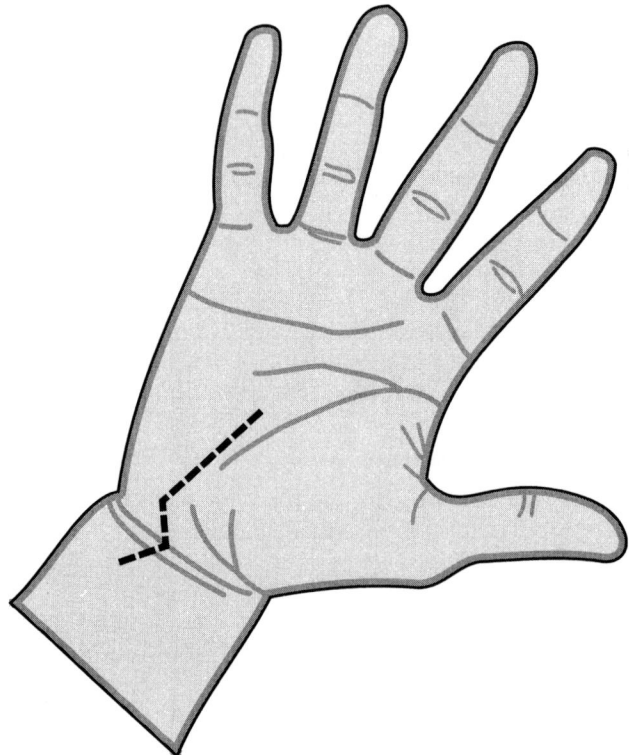

Fig. 36-6. The open carpal tunnel release incision is curved and longitudinal along the axis of the ring finger. (From Green D: *Green's operative hand surgery,* ed 4, Philadelphia, 1999, Churchill Livingstone.)

Proximally, the transverse carpal ligament is incised under direct vision to the level of its junction with the antebrachial fascia at the proximal wrist crease. Releasing the antebrachial fascia may not be necessary in all cases, but thickened antebrachial fascia has been identified as a possible source of compression in patients with collagen vascular disease.[68] After hemostasis is achieved, the wound is irrigated and closed with nonabsorbable suture.[123]

Open decompression of the median nerve has stood the test of time, providing reliable symptom relief in patients. A number of retrospective studies of open carpal tunnel release document patient satisfaction and symptom improvement ranging from 86% to 96%. Nocturnal pain improves to a greater extent than any other symptom.[53,91,96] The resolution of symptoms and functional limitations follows a temporal course with nocturnal pain, tingling, and subjective numbness that improve within 6 weeks after surgery. However, two-point discrimination may remain abnormal in more than half of patients after 2 years. Weakness and functional status improve more gradually. Grip and pinch strength worsens initially and returns to preoperative levels after about 2 or 3 months, with maximum improvement at approximately 10 months.[64,74,91] In a series of 44 patients with mean follow-up of 35 months after open carpal tunnel release,

Osterman reported a 96% rate of patient satisfaction and symptom improvement, with 84% of patients returning to their preoperative jobs after surgery.[96]

Carpal tunnel release is performed frequently, and there has appropriately been focus on improving patient outcome factors. Aside from the relatively rare complications of incomplete transverse carpal ligament release, neurovascular injury, and infection,[57,99] there has been ample documentation of problems with longstanding palmar pain following open carpal tunnel release.[15] Povlsen and Tegnell[104] confirmed that open carpal tunnel decompression has a high success rate, with complete relief of all clinical symptoms of median-nerve compression in 51 patients at 3-month follow-up. However, they found that 41% of patients experienced allodynia over the thenar and hypothenar eminences at 1 month after surgery, 25% at 3 months, and 6% at 12 months.[104] Postoperative palmar pain may contribute to delayed return to work, particularly among manual laborers and worker's compensation patients.[91] Palmar pain has been described after all techniques of carpal tunnel release, whether open, miniopen, or endoscopic (see following discussion), and may be a significant impediment to patients' functional recovery.

Pillar pain is localized to the thenar or hypothenar areas and is to be distinguished from palmar incisional or scar tenderness. The relevant anatomy appears to be the osseous and muscular attachments of the transverse carpal ligament, which originates from the scaphoid tubercle and the pisiform proximally and the tubercle of the trapezium and the hook of the hamate distally. The ligament serves as origin to the three thenar and three hypothenar muscles. Additional functions of the transverse carpal ligament appear to be maintenance of the volar carpal arch and the prevention of flexor tendon bowstringing. Although the exact cause of pillar pain remains elusive, the various theories have been organized as ligamentous or muscular, alterations of the carpal arch, edematous, and neurogenic.[81]

It has been suggested that sectioning the transverse carpal ligament allows the thenar and hypothenar muscles to fall apart from each other. Alterations of the origin of these muscles as well as the swollen, raw edges of the cut transverse carpal ligament are potential sources of pillar pain. The transverse carpal ligament has been postulated to be a stabilizer of the transverse carpal arch, and a variety of anatomic and radiographic studies have documented an increase in the carpal canal volume after all techniques of carpal tunnel release. The anteroposterior dimension increases the most; however, small increases in the mediolateral dimension, presumably from widening of the bony arch, likely occur and may contribute to pillar pain. For the ligamentous, muscular, and skeletal etiologies, pillar pain should occur with all techniques of carpal tunnel release, whether open or endoscopic and whether the incision is large or small.[16,23,58,93]

The edematous and neurogenic etiologies for palmar pain are a consequence of violation of the skin, palmar fascia, and cutaneous nerves superficial to the transverse carpal ligament. This incisional pain may be an important source of morbidity after traditional open carpal tunnel release and could theoretically be ameliorated with endoscopic techniques and miniopen methods using smaller incisions removed from the high-contact midpalm of the hand.[40,87,131]

Endoscopic and miniopen carpal tunnel release. A variety of less invasive techniques such as endoscopic and miniopen carpal tunnel release have been proposed to lessen the morbidity of carpal tunnel release by selectively transecting the transverse carpal ligament through small incisions, often placed outside the palm or at least away from the high-contact midpalm of the hand. Pillar pain, by strict definition, is probably the same regardless of technique because all methods have at their basis transection of the transverse carpal ligament. However, proponents of alternative techniques state that less incisional tenderness and earlier return of grip and pinch strength permit the patient to return earlier to work and ADLs. Morphologic studies confirm that, despite a relatively high incidence of incomplete release of the transverse carpal ligament, endoscopic techniques consistently increase the carpal canal volume in a manner similar to that reported for open carpal tunnel releases.[1,63,75,111] Endoscopic release techniques of the transverse carpal ligament all involve an incision approximately 1 cm proximal to the volar wrist flexion crease. The one-portal releases[2,3,84,95] employ only this proximal incision (Fig. 36-7), whereas the two-portal techniques[20,21] use this proximal incision and a small distal palmar incision. The one- and two-portal releases use a variety of specially designed devices to release the transverse carpal ligament.

Discussion. Endoscopic techniques have similar reliability and temporal course of relief of hallmark CTS symptoms as open decompression of the median nerve at the wrist.* Some series[9,49] were unable to demonstrate any statistically significant difference between patients who underwent open versus endoscopic carpal tunnel release in terms of return to work, return to ADLs, or on a symptom severity scale. However, the majority of randomized, prospective studies support the idea that patients treated endoscopically may have less midpalm tenderness and faster return to work than patients treated via the open technique.[2,67,100] Brown et al.[15] performed a prospective, randomized study of two-portal endoscopic and open carpal tunnel release in 169 hands with clinical and electrodiagnostic CTS that had not responded to nonoperative management. At the end of the follow-up period, both the open and endoscopic groups had essentially equal high levels of patient satisfaction and relief of pain and paresthesias. The open technique resulted in more tenderness of the scar than did the endoscopic method at 84 days

*References 2, 21, 22, 84, 85, 90.

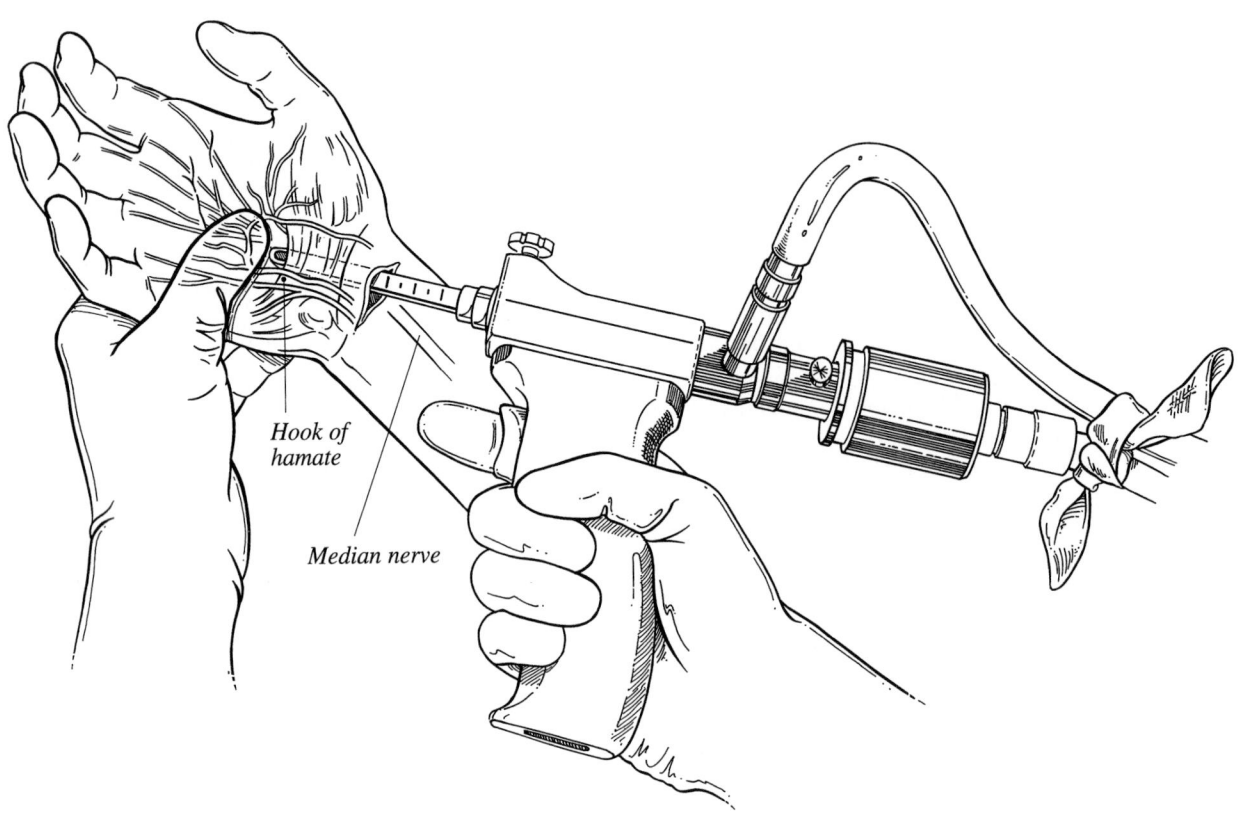

Fig. 36-7. Endoscopic one-portal carpal tunnel release is performed through a transverse incision proximal to the volar wrist crease. (Modified from MicroAire Surgical Instruments, Inc. In Green D: *Green's operative hand surgery,* ed 4, Philadelphia, 1999, Churchill Livingstone.)

postoperatively. The open method resulted in a longer interval until the patient could return to work (28 days) compared with 14 days for the group that had endoscopic release. However, four complications occurred in the endoscopic carpal tunnel release group, and no complications occurred in the open release group.

There is controversy when complication rates of endoscopic release are compared with traditional open techniques. Cadaveric endoscopic release studies[108,109,126] and clinical case reports of endoscopic releases* cite significant risks to and documented injuries of the median nerve, the deep motor branch of the ulnar nerve, the digital nerves, the superficial palmar arterial arch, the ulnar artery, and flexor tendons. In addition, cadaveric studies using different endoscopic techniques of carpal tunnel release have found up to a 50% incidence of incomplete release of the transverse carpal ligament,[75,111,126] a finding that may account for the apparently higher rate of recurrence of CTS symptoms after endoscopic release.[56]

Overall, the literature supports somewhat less palmar pain and scar tenderness, quicker recovery of strength, and in non–worker's compensation patients, earlier return to work using endoscopic carpal tunnel release compared with conventional open methods. The benefits of a mildly accelerated rehabilitative course with endoscopic methods must be weighed against the increased procedural costs and, more importantly, the higher risks of catastrophic complications and recurrence. Vasen et al.,[127] using estimates of the costs of medical procedures, complications, and lost wages, performed a decision analysis to compare the total costs of open versus endoscopic carpal tunnel releases. They found the endoscopic approach is more costly from a societal perspective if the complication rate of endoscopic surgery exceeds 6.2%, if the average work absence following a complication exceeds 15.5 months, and if the difference between the two techniques in mean time to return to work is less than 21 days. Further application of decision analysis models will help define whether the increased risks of endoscopic release outweigh the benefits of faster functional recovery.

Open techniques using small incisions placed away from the midpalm have been developed for carpal tunnel release. The proponents of these techniques claim that the small incisions lessen postoperative palmar pain but still afford the necessary visualization to minimize neurovascular injury and incomplete ligament release. Claims that endoscopic

*References 7, 15, 33, 38, 41, 80, 89, 92, 99, 116.

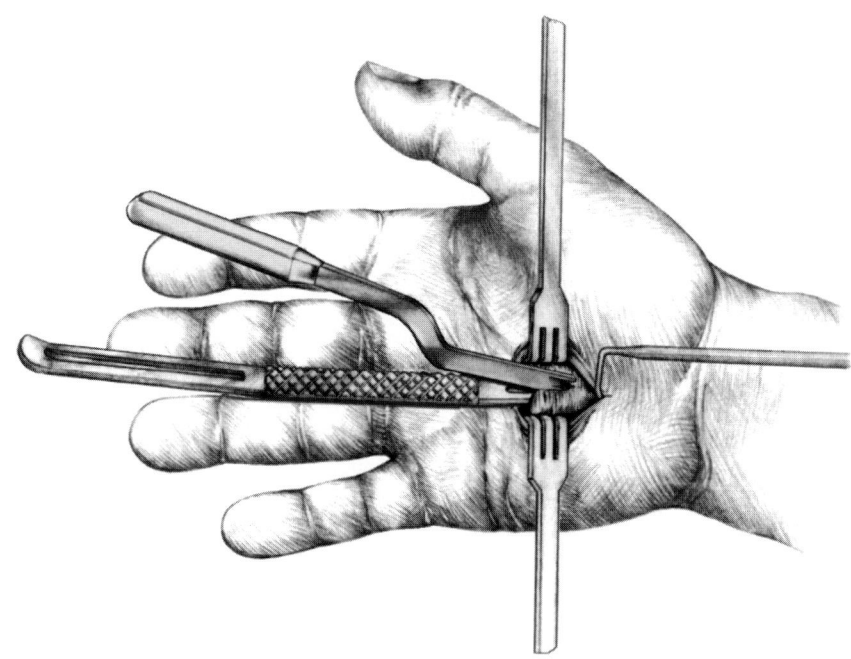

Fig. 36-8. Miniopen carpal tunnel release can be performed with a specially designed cutting guide through a small palmar incision. (Courtesy Kinetikos Medical Incorporated, 4115 Sorrento Valley Blvd., San Diego, CA 92121.)

carpal tunnel release is a less invasive surgery that allows a more rapid functional recovery compared with open methods may be flawed because an open method using the most minimal possible incision was not necessarily used in the comparisons. Miniopen techniques both with and without specially designed tomes and cutting guides have clinical efficacy and functional recovery comparable to those of the most favorable reports of endoscopic and traditional open carpal tunnel release[14,44,76,77,114] (Fig. 36-8).

Hallock and Lutz[52] performed a prospective, consecutive series of 96 patients with CTS and concluded that, regardless of whether a miniopen or endoscopic procedure had been performed, the scar length, rate of complications, length of time before resuming routine activities, and length of time before return to work were not statistically different. A subgroup of 15 patients with bilateral CTS who had decompressions using the opposing methods had no significant difference in preference.[52]

RECURRENT OR UNRELIEVED CARPAL TUNNEL SYNDROME

Primary carpal tunnel release is usually successful; nonetheless, the need for reoperation for persistent or recurrent symptoms ranges in studies from 1.7%[72] to 3.1%[24] of cases. Although most patients improve after reoperation, persistent symptoms to some degree are likely, and failure occurs more frequently than after primary carpal tunnel surgery. Careful patient selection before reoperation is paramount.

In the evaluation of the patient with recurrent or unrelieved symptoms after carpal tunnel release, consideration must be given to both organic and nonorganic etiologies. A detailed history of current symptoms and preoperative symptoms before the initial carpal tunnel release is mandatory. Multiple examinations may be necessary, with attention to reproducibility of abnormal findings. There is the possibility of an inaccurate original diagnosis of CTS or an unrecognized concurrent cervical radiculopathy or pronator syndrome. Patient motivation and the possibility of secondary gain must also be considered. Objective tools such as the Minnesota Multiphasic Personality Inventory may be useful in the evaluation of possible nonorganic reasons for persistent or unrelieved symptoms. Electrodiagnostic tests have an important role in this patient group.[24]

Seror[113] studied 33 patients with electrodiagnostically confirmed CTS who underwent surgical release of the median nerve. Postoperative electrodiagnostic studies showed consistently obvious and often rapid improvement, which was sustained for at least 1 year after surgery. Unresolved electrodiagnostic abnormalities with clinical findings of median neuropathy after carpal tunnel release warrant a diagnosis of persistent or recurrent CTS.[113]

Patients with persistent or early recurrence of symptoms are more likely to have incomplete release of the transverse carpal ligament than those with delayed recurrent symptoms. The distal portion of the flexor retinaculum extends approximately 1 cm distal to the hook of the hamate and is the portion most commonly missed in cases of incomplete release, particularly in endoscopic techniques.[43,72] Patients with delayed recurrent symptoms after primary carpal tunnel release are more likely to have intraneural scarring of the median nerve, adherence of the median nerve with traction dysesthesias, regrowth of the flexor retinaculum, or median-nerve subluxation from the carpal canal.[24]

Nonsurgical treatment should be attempted before revision carpal tunnel release. Patients with repetitive, high-demand occupations should have a trial of activity modification. The same demands that may have precipitated the original CTS can certainly contribute to postoperative recurrence. Occupations associated with repetitive hand movements or vibrating tools in one series were associated with poor employment outcomes after secondary carpal tunnel surgery.[119] Therapy modalities include scar desensitization, nerve gliding exercises, and splinting. Local steroid injections are appropriate.[24]

The outcome of revision open carpal tunnel release is significantly better in patients following a previous endoscopic carpal tunnel release compared with patients who had previous open carpal tunnel surgery. Operative findings in one study included a higher prevalence of incomplete release of the carpal tunnel with prior endoscopic surgery than with previous open release.[56] In a series of 131 patients with reoperation for CTS, many reported residual symptoms. In addition to the 15 patients who required a third operation, 20 patients were dissatisfied with the final result. Risk factors for failure following reoperation include the presence of an active worker's compensation claim, pain in the ulnar-nerve distribution, and the absence of abnormality on preoperative electrodiagnostic studies.[25]

CARPAL TUNNEL SYNDROME IN PREGNANCY

CTS severe enough to warrant treatment rarely occurs during pregnancy (0.34% incidence in a retrospective series of 10,873 pregnant patients),[118] is usually diagnosed during the third trimester, and is associated with generalized edema. The symptoms, most commonly paresthesias, generally respond to conservative treatment or resolve spontaneously postpartum. Splinting, with or without steroid injections, has been found to be effective for decreasing the uncomfortable symptoms. The health care team treating CTS in the pregnant or lactating woman should coordinate all aspects of the treatment plan with the patient's obstetrician and/or pediatrician.[31]

In one large series, 7 of the 50 pregnant patients with the diagnosis of CTS failed conservative treatment. These patients underwent surgery in the postpartum period and had resolution of symptoms postoperatively.[118] Some postpartum patients with mild residual hand symptoms due to CTS may initially respond to conservative treatment, but years later, symptoms may become severe enough to warrant surgical release. Patients with residual postpartum hand symptoms require long-term follow-up.[5]

POSTOPERATIVE REHABILITATION

Progression of postoperative therapy following carpal tunnel release is guided by wound healing principles and tissue response to stress. Individualized factors such as preoperative status, surgical procedure, hand dominance, bilateral symptoms, associated conditions, psychosocial variables, insurance coverage, and job requirements will also influence symptom resolution and rates of return to avocational/vocational activities. Treatment is directed toward patient education, edema control, scar modification, restoration of ROM, improvement of strength, and full return of hand function.

Typically, only a few follow-ups are required to ensure uncomplicated recovery; however, more intensive therapy is indicated for some patients. In the presence of persistent pain, sensory complaints, and ongoing physical limitations, astute clinical reasoning will lead to appropriate interventions that maximize functional return in the complex patient.

Evaluation

Components of a thorough assessment and techniques for measurement are discussed in previous chapters. The following areas are of particular relevance to management of postoperative carpal tunnel release. A history of the preoperative course (prior injury, presenting symptoms and their duration, provocative activities, bilaterality of symptoms, and prior treatment) and the presence of coexisting medical conditions, upper extremity musculoskeletal disorders, and proximal compression sites will direct decisions regarding appropriate treatment. Critical areas of examination include posture, quality of movement patterns, spontaneous hand use, extent of edema, scar characteristics, patterns of tissue tightness that restrict ROM, sensory threshold levels, thenar atrophy, and patient reports of pain level and functional capabilities. Grip and pinch strength are tested when inflammation has subsided.

Provocative maneuvers that detect proximal entrapment and associated neuropathies are performed when the patient complains of new or persistent symptoms. Chronic regional pain syndrome (reflex sympathetic dystrophy [RSD]) is an uncommon complication following carpal tunnel release. Early recognition and treatment of symptoms consistent with this diagnosis will improve outcomes in this otherwise challenging patient population.

Patient education

Beginning with the initial contact, patient education addresses the underlying rationale for treatment procedures and recommendations for appropriate activity level. Educating the patient facilitates compliance, which will lead to optimal recovery while minimizing setbacks attributable to recurrent inflammation. Expectations for symptom resolution and return to function are also addressed. This is especially helpful when patients experience worsening scar tenderness in the first few weeks. Often, patients develop concerns regarding a perceived lack of progress based on reports of acquaintances who have also had carpal tunnel surgery. Understanding that there are individual factors that influence rate of recovery will help promote a positive outlook in these patients.

Edema control

Initial treatment for edema consists of compressive dressings, elevation, icing, and intermittent overhead fisting to stimulate venous and lymphatic flow. When edema is significant and persists longer than 2 or 3 weeks, additional measures are required as edema reduction becomes a paramount goal. Persistent edema is associated with soft tissue fibrosis that results in stiff joints and the development of adhesions that interfere with the normal gliding of the flexor tendons and the median nerve. Movements and positions that put these structures under tension then become painful. Resolution of edema may help to relieve the pillar pain experienced by some patients.[40]

Additional edema management techniques for subacute and chronic edema include active ROM, manual edema mobilization, compression wraps/gloves, contrast baths, and high-voltage galvanic stimulation (HVGS). Pressures generated by these techniques must be low to prevent obstruction of lymphatic flow, which plays a primary role in the absorption of larger plasma proteins associated with chronic edema and fibrosis.

During all phases of wound healing, stress applied to healing tissue must be monitored to prevent inflammatory responses. Patient education regarding activity levels that will exacerbate or reduce edema is of primary importance.

Scar management

Scar discomfort often persists after carpal tunnel release. Tender, unyielding scars in the palm diminish the capacity to handle static and shearing forces during ADLs and work tasks. Patients complain of difficulty performing activities such as brushing their teeth, holding onto a steering wheel, pushing off a chair, and opening jars.

Postoperative management of scar begins immediately with the application of an appropriate compressive dressing that minimizes edema and, subsequently, scar tissue formation. Light scar massage and myofascial release can be initiated 2 to 3 days after suture removal. More vigorous soft tissue mobilization is introduced as tolerated. Pressure inserts and silicone gel sheeting produce clinically observed improvements in scar quality. Conformability of these materials is critical given the concave shape of the palm and the undesirability of excessive pressure over the healing median nerve. Wraps that contain gel pads provide a cushioning effect, allowing function despite hypersensitive scars. Simultaneously, a program of desensitization with graded textures is carried out to minimize discomfort and allow weaning from these protective devices.

The use of therapeutic levels of ultrasound for elevating pain thresholds and achieving scar modification (when followed by stretching) are well established.[86] However, ultrasound use after carpal tunnel release should be approached with caution because the ramifications of its use over a regenerating nerve are not clearly understood. Temperature changes produce alterations in nerve conduction velocity that may be specific to fiber type and intensity levels.[97] Further clinical trials addressing safe and effective dosage levels in the presence of neuropathy are needed.

Splinting

Postoperatively, the use of a supportive dressing that maintains the wrist in extension and avoidance of simultaneous wrist and digit flexion will minimize discomfort and bowstringing.[30] Most patients do not require postoperative wrist immobilization. However, approaches to splinting must be individualized. Traditionally, splinting in slight extension has been advocated for the first 2 to 3 weeks postoperatively to avoid the potential complications associated with wound dehiscence and anterior displacement of the median nerve and flexor tendons.[30] Displacement of these structures may lead to entrapment of the median nerve in newly forming scar at the radial edge of the transverse carpal ligament, resulting in increased nerve irritability and ultimately symptom recurrence.[46] Bowstringing of flexor tendons is postulated to limit full tendon excursion, thereby altering grip strength.[94]

Recently, the trend has been to move away from splinting because the deleterious effects of immobilization on joint mobility and muscle length may outweigh the rare incidence of complications. Results of recent studies support this trend. Cook et al.[30] found that unsplinted patients demonstrated a decreased incidence of scar tenderness and pillar pain as well as more rapid return to work. Wound complications and tendon bowstringing were not observed. Bury, Akelman, and Weiss[17] found no significant difference in grip and pinch strength, bowstringing, complication rates, and patient satisfaction when comparing a group splinted for 2 weeks with an unsplinted group. Similarly, Finsen, Anderson, and Russwurm[42] compared 4 weeks of immobilization with no immobilization and found no significant difference between the two groups for scar discomfort, pillar pain, grip and pinch strength, and time out of work.

Splinting is appropriate for patients who experience nighttime pain associated with flexed postures of the wrist and can also be used to provide rest to persistently inflamed tissues.

Mobilization

Active exercise is begun in the postoperative dressing to ensure adequate glide of the median nerve and flexor tendons during scar formation. At the initial postoperative visit, patients are instructed in specific exercises to achieve differential tendon gliding (see Fig. 36-4) and thumb ROM. Seven to ten repetitions are completed three to five times daily. Exercise technique includes end-range hold to maximize joint mobility and full active extension to achieve maximum tendon excursion. Wrist ROM is initially completed with the digits relaxed during flexion to minimize

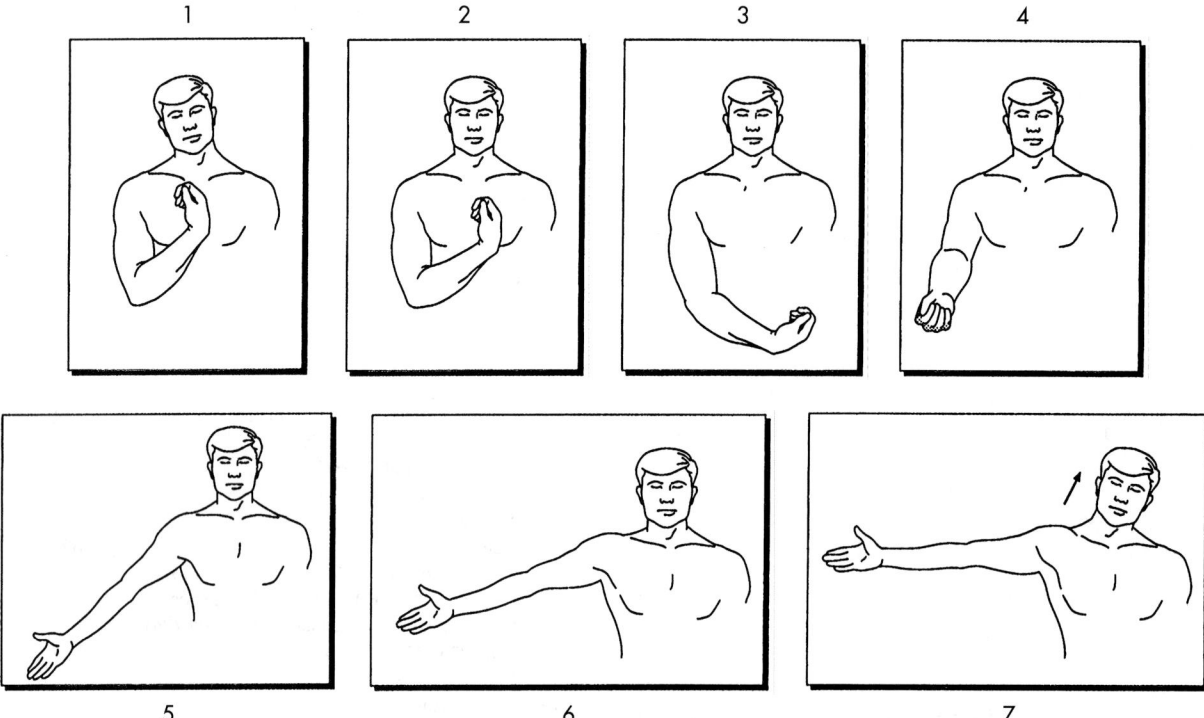

Fig. 36-9. The brachial plexus gliding program begins in *position 1* with the head laterally flexed to the affected side and with the fingers, wrist, and elbow flexed. In *position 2,* the head comes to neutral. By *position 3,* the hand has moved across the chest and down to hip level. The arm gradually abducts as the patient comes to *position 4* and progresses through to *position 6.* Lateral cervical flexion to the opposite side is the final component of this glide, added in position 7. (Redrawn from Totten PA, Hunter JM: *Hand Clin* 7:505, 1991.)

compressive forces exerted on the median nerve. Passive ROM is indicated for mobilization of stiff joints and to elongate tendon adhesions. Median nerve gliding exercises (see Fig. 36-5) are also initiated and progressed according to patient tolerance. If more proximal sites of compression are present, a brachial plexus gliding program (Fig. 36-9) will maximize nerve excursion.

Pillar pain

The nature and possible etiologies of pillar pain were previously described in this chapter. Patients experiencing this phenomenon have difficulty with grip and palmar weight-bearing activities. Return to work is often delayed. References to pillar pain in the literature seldom address interventions. Treatment strategies, including modalities used to decrease inflammation, may control the magnitude and/or duration of symptoms.[81] Steroid injections may reduce symptoms for an extended period.

Strengthening

Light hand use is encouraged immediately after surgery, with resumption of full ADLs, as tolerated, usually within 2 to 4 weeks. Strengthening is initiated at 3 to 4 weeks as wounds heal and inflammation resolves. Exercise progres-

sion depends on pain level and may initially involve isometric muscle contractions and low repetitions. Measurement of grip and pinch strength at this time may reflect pain thresholds and alterations in sensation rather than muscle fiber recruitment. Strengthening activities are chosen to address specific areas of limitations, such as thenar and hypothenar weakness, forearm muscle imbalance, and overall upper extremity conditioning. Repetitive, forceful gripping tasks that increase compression on the median nerve should be used with caution.[39] Aerobic exercise is encouraged for patients with a sedentary lifestyle.

Therapy visits are usually minimal at this time, with emphasis directed at upgrading home exercise programs. More intensive strengthening and/or work hardening programs are indicated for patients with significant out-of-work time as well as for those returning to jobs with heavy physical demands.

Return to work

The time interval between surgery and return to work depends on symptom duration, incision length, scar tenderness, pillar pain, patient motivation, insurance coverage, and specific work requirements. Return to work involving sedentary or light nonrepetitive activity usually occurs at 2 to 4 weeks. Longer return-to-work times can be expected for patients who return to jobs that require repetitive motions of the wrist and digits, forceful gripping, simultaneous wrist and digit flexion, frequent direct impact to the palm, vibration, and/or heavy manual labor. These motions and static postures are associated with increased carpal tunnel pressure and may be responsible for symptom recurrence. Crucial therapeutic interventions for these patients include education regarding body mechanics and appropriate stretching exercises, work simulation, and job site analysis. Recommendations are made for activity modifications and assistive devices (e.g., antivibration gloves, ergonomic tools, adjustable keyboards) that minimize provocative positions and repetitive motions and that redistribute forces away from the palm.

SUMMARY IDEAS FOR CONSERVATIVE MANAGEMENT

The current standard of care in the conservative management of CTS continues to be splinting in the wrist in a neutral position. The potential cause of the increased pressure in the canal must be considered when developing a conservative treatment plan. Patient education, a simple change in splint design, or analysis and modification of the patients' activity or workstation can frequently be effective in decreasing the symptoms in some patients.

More research is needed to validate the use of exercise and/or modalities in the conservative management of CTS.

Postoperative management of carpal tunnel release, when based on sound hand therapy principles, generally follow an uneventful course. Patient education and early identification of problem areas play pivitol roles in minimizing potential complications. Pillar pain, when present, can significantly delay return of normal hand use. Finding treatment approaches that promote resolution of these symptoms remains a challenge to even the astute hand therapist.

REFERENCES

1. Ablove RH, et al: Morphologic changes following endoscopic and two-portal subcutaneous carpal tunnel release, *J Hand Surg* 19A:821, 1994.
2. Agee JM, McCarroll HR, North ER: Endoscopic carpal tunnel release using the single proximal incision technique, *Hand Clin* 10:647, 1994.
3. Agee JM, et al: Endoscopic release of the carpal tunnel: a randomized prospective multicenter study, *J Hand Surg* 17A:987, 1992.
4. al-Qattan MM, Bowen V, Manktelow RT: Factors associated with poor outcome following primary carpal tunnel release in non-diabetic patients, *J Hand Surg* 19B:622, 1994.
5. al-Qattan MM, Manktelow RT, Bowen CV: Pregnancy-induced carpal tunnel syndrome requiring surgical release longer than 2 years after delivery, *Obstet Gynecol* 84:249, 1994.
6. Amadio PC: The first carpal tunnel release? *J Hand Surg* 20B:40, 1995.
7. Arner M, Hagberg L, Rosen B: Sensory disturbances after two-portal endoscopic carpal tunnel release: a preliminary report, *J Hand Surg* 19A:548, 1994.
8. Aulisa L, et al: Carpal tunnel syndrome: indication for surgical treatment based on electrophysiologic study, *J Hand Surg* 23A:687, 1998.
9. Bande S, De Smet L, Fabry G: The results of carpal tunnel release: open versus endoscopic technique, *J Hand Surg* 19B:14, 1994.
10. Banta CA: A prospective, nonrandomized study of iontophoresis, wrist splinting, and anti-inflammatory medication in the treatment of early-mild carpal tunnel syndrome, *J Occup Med* 36:166, 1994.
11. Bessette L, et al: Prognostic value of a hand symptom diagram in surgery for carpal tunnel syndrome, *J Rheumatol* 24:726, 1997.
12. Biyani A, et al: Distribution of nerve fibers in the standard incision for carpal tunnel decompression, *J Hand Surg* 21A:855, 1996.
13. Braun RM, Jackson WJ: Electrical studies as a prognostic factor in the surgical treatment of carpal tunnel syndrome, *J Hand Surg* 19A:893, 1994.
14. Bromley GS: Minimal-incision open carpal tunnel decompression, *J Hand Surg* 19A:119, 1994.
15. Brown RA, et al: Carpal tunnel release: a prospective, randomized assessment of open and endoscopic methods, *J Bone Joint Surg* 75A:1265, 1993.
16. Buchanan RT, et al: Method, education and therapy of carpal tunnel patients, *Hand Surg Q* Summer: 10, 1995.
17. Bury TF, Akelman E, Weiss APC: Prospective randomized trial of splinting after carpal tunnel release, *Ann Plast Surg* 35:19, 1995.
18. Butler DS: *Mobilization of the nervous system*, Melbourne, 1991, Churchill Livingstone.
19. Choi SJ, Ahn DS: Correlation of clinical history and electrodiagnostic abnormalities with outcome after surgery for carpal tunnel syndrome, *Plast Reconstr Surg* 102:2374, 1998.
20. Chow JC: Endoscopic release of the carpal ligament: a new technique for carpal tunnel syndrome, *Arthroscopy* 5:19, 1989.
21. Chow JC: Endoscopic carpal tunnel release: two-portal technique, *Hand Clin* 10:637, 1994.
22. Chow JC: Endoscopic release of the carpal ligament for carpal tunnel syndrome: long-term results using the Chow technique, *Arthroscopy* 15:417, 1999.
23. Citron ND, Bendall SP: Local symptoms after open carpal tunnel release: a randomized prospective trial of two incisions, *J Hand Surg* 22B:317, 1997.
24. Cobb TK, Amadio PC: Reoperation for carpal tunnel syndrome, *Hand Clin* 12:313, 1996.
25. Cobb TK, Amadio PC, Leatherwood DF: Outcome of reoperation for carpal tunnel syndrome, *J Hand Surg* 21A:347, 1996.
26. Cobb TK, An K, Cooney W: Externally applied forces to the palm increase carpal tunnel pressure, *J Hand Surg* 20A:181, 1995.
27. Cobb TR, et al: Anatomy of the flexor retinaculum, *Hand Surg* 18A:91, 1993.
28. Cobb TK, et al: Lumbrical muscle incursion into the carpal tunnel during finger flexion, *J Hand Surg* 19B:434, 1994.
29. Concannon MJ, et al: The predictive value of electrodiagnostic studies in carpal tunnel syndrome, *Plast Reconstr Surg* 100:1452, 1997.
30. Cook AC, et al: Early mobilization following carpal tunnel release, *J Hand Surg* 20B:228, 1995.
31. Courts RB: Splinting for symptoms of carpal tunnel syndrome during pregnancy, *J Hand Ther* 8:31, 1995.
32. DaSilva M, et al: Anatomy of the palmar cutaneous branch of the median nerve: clinical significance, *J Hand Surg* 21A:639, 1996.
33. DeSmet L, Fabry G: Transection of the motor branch of the ulnar nerve as a complication of two-portal endoscopic carpal tunnel release: a case report, *J Hand Surg* 20A:18, 1995.
34. DeStefano F, Nordstrom DL, Vierkant RA: Long-term symptom outcomes of carpal tunnel syndrome and its treatment, *J Hand Surg* 22A:200, 1997.

35. Durkan JA: A new diagnostic test for carpal tunnel syndrome, *J Bone Joint Surg* 73A:535, 1991.

36. Ebenbichler FR, et al: Ultrasound treatment for treating the carpal tunnel syndrome: randomised "sham" controlled trial, *BMJ* 316:731, 1998.

37. Einhor N, Leddy JP: Pitfalls of endoscopic carpal tunnel release, *Orthop Clin North Am* 27:373, 1996.

38. Erdmann MW: Endoscopic carpal tunnel decompression, *J Hand Surg* 19B:5, 1994.

39. Evans RB: Eleventh Natalie Barr lecture: the source of our strength, *J Hand Ther* 10:14, 1997.

40. Eversmann WW Jr: Entrapment and compression neuropathies. In Green DP, editor: *Green's operative hand surgery,* vol 2 and 3, New York, 1993, Churchill Livingstone.

41. Feinstein PA: Endoscopic carpal tunnel release in a community-based series, *J Hand Surg* 18A:451, 1993.

42. Finsen V, Andersen K, Russwurm H: No advantage from splinting the wrist after open carpal tunnel release: a randomized study of 82 wrists, *Acta Orthop Scand* 70:288, 1999.

43. Forman DL, et al: Persistent or recurrent carpal tunnel syndrome following prior endoscopic carpal tunnel release, *J Hand Surg* 23A:1010, 1998.

44. Frank CE: "Two stitch" carpal tunnel surgery: a mini-incision technique, *Am J Orthop* 25:650, 1996.

45. Gelberman RH, Aronson D, Weisman MH: Carpal tunnel syndrome: results of a prospective trial of steroid infection and splinting, *J Bone Joint Surg* 62A:1181, 1980.

46. Gelberman RH, Eaton R, Urabaniak J: Peripheral nerve compression, *J Bone Joint Surg* 75A:1854, 1993.

47. Gelberman RH, et al: The carpal tunnel syndrome: a study of carpal canal pressures, *J Bone Joint Surg* 63A:380, 1981.

48. Gellman H, et al: Carpal tunnel syndrome: an evaluation of the provocative tests, *J Bone Joint Surg* 68A:735, 1986.

49. Gibbs KE, Rand W, Ruby LK: Open versus endoscopic carpal tunnel release, *Orthopedics* 19:1025, 1996.

50. Glowacki KA, et al: Electrodiagnostic testing and carpal tunnel release outcome, *J Hand Surg* 21A:117, 1996.

51. Grundberg AB: Carpal tunnel decompression in spite of normal electromyography, *J Hand Surg* 8A:348, 1983.

52. Hallock GG, Lutz DA: Prospective comparison of minimal incision "open" and two-portal endoscopic carpal tunnel release, *Plast Reconstr Surg* 96:941, 1995.

53. Haupt WF, Wintzer G, Schop A: Long-term results of carpal tunnel decompression: assessment of 60 cases, *J Hand Surg* 18B:471, 1993.

54. Higgs PE, et al: Carpal tunnel surgery outcomes in workers: effect of workers' compensation status, *J Hand Surg* 20A:354, 1995.

55. Higgs PE, et al: Relation of preoperative nerve-conduction values to outcome in workers with surgically treated carpal tunnel syndrome, *J Hand Surg* 22A:216, 1997.

56. Hulsizer DL, et al: The results of revision carpal tunnel release following previous open versus endoscopic surgery, *J Hand Surg* 23A:865, 1998.

57. Hunt TR, Osterman AL: Complications of the treatment of carpal tunnel syndrome, *Hand Clin* 10:63, 1994.

58. Hunter JM: Recurrent carpal tunnel syndrome, epineural fibrous fixation, and traction neuropathy, *Hand Clin* 7:491, 1991.

59. Hybbinette C-H, Mannerfelt L: The carpal tunnel syndrome: a retrospective study of 400 operated patients, *Acta Orthop Scand* 46:610, 1975.

60. Jablecki CK, et al: Literature review of the usefulness of nerve conduction studies and electromyography for the evaluation of patients with carpal tunnel syndrome, *Muscle Nerve* 16:1392, 1993.

61. Jacobson M, Plancher K, Kleinman W: Vitamin B6 (pyridone) therapy for carpal tunnel syndrome, *Hand Clin* 12:253, 1996.

62. Kaplan SL, Glickel SZ, Eaton RG: Predictive factors in the nonsurgical treatment of carpal tunnel syndrome, *J Hand Surg* 15B:106, 1990.

63. Kato T, et al: Effects of endoscopic release of the transverse carpal ligament on carpal canal volume, *J Hand Surg* 19A:416, 1994.

64. Katz JN, et al: Symptoms, functional status, and neuromuscular impairment following carpal tunnel release, *J Hand Surg* 20A:549, 1995.

65. Katz JN, et al: Predictors of return to work following carpal tunnel release, *Am J Int Med* 31:85, 1997.

66. Katz JN, et al: Maine Carpal Tunnel Study: outcomes of operative and nonoperative therapy for carpal tunnel syndrome in a community-based cohort, *J Hand Surg* 23A:697, 1998.

67. Kerr CD, Gittins ME, Sybert DR: Endoscopic versus open carpal tunnel release: clinical results, *Arthroscopy* 10:266, 1994.

68. Ko CY, Jones NF, Steen VD: Compression of the median nerve proximal to the carpal tunnel in scleroderma, *J Hand Surg* 21A:363, 1996.

69. Koris M, et al: Carpal tunnel syndrome: evaluation of a quantitative provocational diagnostic test, *Clin Orthop* 251:157, 1990.

70. Kruger VL, et al: Carpal tunnel syndrome: objective measures and splint use, *Arch Phys Med Rehabil* 72:517, 1991.

71. Kulick RG: Carpal tunnel syndrome, *Orthop Clin North Am* 27:345, 1996.

72. Langloh NH, Linscheid RL: Recurrent and unrelieved carpal tunnel syndrome, *Clin Orthop* 83:41, 1972.

73. Lanz U: Anatomic variations of the median nerve in the carpal tunnel, *J Hand Surg* 2A:44, 1977.

74. Leach WJ, Esler C, Scott TD: Grip strength following carpal tunnel decompression, *J Hand Surg* 18B:750, 1993.

75. Lee DH, et al: Endoscopic carpal tunnel release: a cadaveric study, *J Hand Surg* 17A:1003, 1992.

76. Lee WP, Plancher KD, Strickland JW: Carpal tunnel release with a small palmar incision, *Hand Clin* 12:271, 1996.

77. Lee WP, Strickland JW: Safe carpal tunnel release via a limited palmar incision, *Plast Reconstr Surg* 101:418, 1998.

78. Levine DW, et al: A self-administered questionnaire for the assessment of severity of symptoms and functional status in carpal tunnel syndrome, *J Bone Joint Surg* 75A:1585, 1993.

79. Louis DS, Calkins ER, Harris PG: Carpal tunnel syndrome in the work place, *Hand Clin* 12:305, 1996.

80. Luallin SR, Toby EB: Incidental Guyon's canal release during attempted endoscopic carpal tunnel release: an anatomical study and report of two cases, *Arthroscopy* 9:382, 1993.

81. Ludlow KS, et al: Pillar pain as a postoperative complication of carpal tunnel release: a review of the literature, *J Hand Ther* 10:277, 1997.

82. Lundborg G, et al: Median nerve compression in the carpal tunnel: functional response to experimentally induced controlled pressure, *J Hand Surg* 7:252, 1982.

83. Marie P, Foix C: Atrophie isolee de l'eminence thenar d'origine neuritique: role du ligament annuleur anterieur du cape dans la pathogenie de la lesion, *Rev Neurol* 26:647, 1913.

84. Menon J: Endoscopic carpal tunnel release: a single-portal technique, *Contemp Orthop* 26:109, 1993.

85. Menon J: Endoscopic carpal tunnel release: preliminary report, *Arthroscopy* 10:31, 1994.

86. Michlovitz SL: Therapeutic ultrasound. In *Thermal agents in rehabilitation,* ed 3, Philadelphia, 1996, FA Davis.

87. Mirza MA, King ET, Tanveer S: Palmar uniportal extrabursal endoscopic carpal tunnel release, *Arthroscopy* 11:82, 1995.

88. Monsivais JJ, Bucher PA, Monsivais DB: Nonsurgically treated carpal tunnel syndrome in the manual worker, *Plast Reconstr Surg* 94:695, 1994.

89. Murphy RX Jr, Jennings JF, Wukich DK: Major neurovascular complications of endoscopic carpal tunnel release, *J Hand Surg* 19A:114, 1994.

90. Nagle D, Harris G, Foley M: Prospective review of 278 endoscopic carpal tunnel releases using the modified chow technique, *Arthroscopy* 10:259, 1994.

91. Nancollas MP, et al: Long-term results of carpal tunnel release, *J Hand Surg* 20B:470, 1995.

92. Nath RK, MacKinnon SE, Weeks PM: Ulnar nerve transection as a complication of two portal endoscopic carpal tunnel release: a case report, *J Hand Surg* 18A:896, 1993.

93. Nathan PA, Meadows KD, Keniston RC: Rehabilitation of carpal tunnel surgery patients using short surgical incision and an early program of physical therapy, *J Hand Surg* 18A:1044, 1993.

94. Netscher D, et al: Temporal changes in grip and pinch strength after open carpal tunnel release and the effect of ligament reconstruction, *J Hand Surg* 23A:48, 1998.

95. Okutsui I, et al: Endoscopic management of carpal tunnel syndrome, *Arthroscopy* 5:11, 1989.

96. Osterman AL: The double crush syndrome, *Orthop Clin North Am* 19:147, 1988.

97. Oztas O, et al: Ultrasound therapy effect in carpal tunnel syndrome, *Arch Phys Med Rehabil* 79:1540, 1998.

98. Paget J: *Lectures on surgical pathology,* ed 2, Philadelphia, 1854, Lindsay and Blakiston.

99. Palmer AK, Toivonen DA: Complications of endoscopic and open carpal tunnel release, *J Hand Surg* 24A:561, 1999.

100. Palmer DH, et al: Endoscopic carpal tunnel release: a comparison of two techniques with open release, *Arthroscopy* 9:498, 1993.

101. Phalen GS: The carpal tunnel syndrome: seventeen years' experience in diagnosis and treatment of six hundred fifty-four hands, *J Bone Joint Surg* 48A:211, 1966.

102. Phalen GS: The carpal-tunnel syndrome: clinical evaluation of 598 hands, *Clin Orthop* 83:29, 1972.

103. Polsen C, Netscher D, Thornby J: Anatomical delineation of the ulnar nerve and artery in relation to the carpal tunnel (abstract SS-52). Abstracts of the 49th Annual meeting of American Society for Surgery of the Hand, Cincinnati, 1994.

104. Povlsen B, Tegnell I: Incidence and natural history of touch allodynia after open carpal tunnel release, *Scand J Plast Reconstr Surg Hand Surg* 30:221, 1996.

105. Rempel D, et al: The effect of wearing a flexible wrist splint on carpal tunnel pressure during repetitive hand activity, *J Hand Surg* 19A:106, 1994.

106. Richman JA, et al: Carpal tunnel syndrome: morphologic changes after release of the transverse carpal ligament, *J Hand Surg* 14A:852, 1989.

107. Robbins H: Anatomical study of the median nerve in the carpal tunnel and etiologies of the carpal-tunnel syndrome, *J Bone Joint Surg* 45A:953, 1963.

108. Rotman MB, Manske PR: Anatomic relationships of an endoscopic carpal tunnel device to surrounding structures, *J Hand Surg* 18A:442, 1993.

109. Rowland EB, Kleinert JM: Endoscopic carpal-tunnel release in cadavera: an investigation of the results of twelve surgeons with this training model, *J Bone Joint Surg* 76A:266, 1994.

110. Rozmaryn LM, et al: Nerve and tendon gliding exercises and the conservative management of carpal tunnel syndrome, *J Hand Ther* 11:171, 1998.

111. Schwartz JT, Waters PM, Simmons BP: Endoscopic carpal tunnel release: a cadaveric study, *Arthroscopy* 9:209, 1993.

112. Seradge H, Jia Y, Owens W: In vivo measurement of carpal tunnel pressure in the functioning hand, *J Hand Surg* 20A:855, 1995.

113. Seror P: Nerve conduction studies after treatment for carpal tunnel syndrome, *J Hand Surg* 17B:641, 1992.

114. Serra JM, Benito JR, Monner J: Carpal tunnel release with short incision, *Plast Reconstr Surg* 99:129, 1997.

115. Siegel DB, Kuzma G, Eakins D: Anatomic investigation of the role of the lumbrical muscles in carpal tunnel syndrome, *J Hand Surg* 20A:860, 1995.

116. Stark RH: Ulnar nerve transection as a complication of two-portal endoscopic carpal tunnel release, *J Hand Surg* 19A:522, 1994.

117. Steinberg DR, Szabo RM: Anatomy of the median nerve at the wrist: open carpal tunnel release—classic, *Hand Clin* 12:259, 1996.

118. Stolp-Smith KA, Pascoe MK, Ogburn PL: Carpal tunnel syndrome in pregnancy: frequency, severity, and prognosis, *Arch Phys Med Rehabil* 79:1285, 1998.

119. Strasberg SR, et al: Subjective and employment outcome following secondary carpal tunnel surgery, *Ann Plast Surg* 32:485, 1994.

120. Szabo RM: Carpal tunnel syndrome—general. In Gelberman RG, editor: *Operative nerve repair and reconstruction,* Philadelphia, 1991, JB Lippincott.

121. Szabo RM: Acute carpal tunnel syndrome, *Hand Clin* 14:419, 1998 (review).

122. Szabo RM: Carpal tunnel syndrome as a repetitive motion disorder, *Clin Orthop* 351:78, 1998.

123. Szabo RM: Entrapment and compression neuropathies. In Green DP, editor: *Green's operative hand surgery,* ed 4, Philadelphia, 1999, Churchill Livingstone.

124. Tanaka S, et al: The US prevalence of self-reported carpal tunnel syndrome: 1988 national health interview survey data, *Am J Pub Health* 84:1846, 1994.

125. Totten PA, Hunter JM: Therapeutic techniques to enhance nerve gliding in thoracic outlet syndrome and carpal tunnel syndrome, *Hand Clin* 7:505, 1991.

126. Van Heest A, et al: A cadaveric study of the single-portal endoscopic carpal tunnel release, *J Hand Surg* 20A:363, 1995.

127. Vasen AP, et al: Open versus endoscopic carpal tunnel release: a decision analysis, *J Hand Surg* 24A:1109, 1999.

128. Wehbe M, Hunter JM: Differential tendon gliding in the hand. Annual Meeting of ASSH, Atlanta, 1984.

129. Weiss AP, Sachar K, Gendreau M: Conservative management of carpal tunnel syndrome: a reexamination of steroid injection and splinting, *J Hand Surg* 19A:410, 1994.

130. Weiss ND, et al: Position of the wrist associated with the lowest carpal-tunnel pressure: implications for splint design, *J Bone Joint Surg* 77A:1695, 1995.

131. Wilson KM: Double incision open technique for carpal tunnel release: an alternative to endoscopic release, *J Hand Surg* 19A:907, 1994.

132. Wintman BI: Carpal tunnel release: correlations with preoperative symptomatology, *Clin Orthop* 326:135, 1996.

133. Yu GZ, Firrell JC, Tsai TM: Pre-operative factors and treatment outcome following carpal tunnel release, *J Hand Surg* 17B:646, 1992.

Chapter 37

THERAPIST'S MANAGEMENT OF CARPAL TUNNEL SYNDROME

Roslyn B. Evans

Carpal tunnel syndrome (CTS) or median-nerve compression at the wrist level is one of the most common diagnoses treated in hand surgery[10,80] and hand therapy.[14] In the United States, it is currently among the most commonly performed surgical procedures on the hand and has a profound economic impact associated with the economics of ergonomics and litigation.[94] CTS is credited, along with hearing loss, as being responsible for more morbidity measured in cases and days lost from work than any other illness treated in the United States.[56,57] Chronic work disability statistics associated with this diagnosis are similar to those of low back pain,[31] with costs to industry estimated to exceed $2 billion per year.[75]

Despite its frequency, many issues concerning this symptom complex are in question.[28] Controversy exists in the literature regarding the cause,[26,55,96] techniques of evaluation,* results with conservative care,† technique of surgery,[7,45,75,106] and the value of postoperative care.[32,79,88] A passionate debate wages concerning the effect of occupation on carpal tunnel (CT) and other injuries that may be a result of cumulative-type injuries, with many questions concerning this common and debilitating problem having no clear-cut answer.[40,43,101,105,109,110,120]

The vast number of articles in the literature testifies to the controversial nature of this diagnosis, with more than 4300 articles published on the subject in juried journals as of the writing of this chapter.

The introduction of managed care, with changes in referral patterns to therapy, has increased the number of inappropriate referrals and the number of patients referred with either no diagnosis or an incorrect diagnosis, increasing the demands of clinical evaluation and treatment skills for therapists. Upper extremity therapists must be able to perform a clinical examination equal to that of a hand surgeon to provide appropriate treatment and appropriate recommendations to the patient and primary care physician in the case of nonspecialist referral, and they must be able to provide acceptable outcomes[64] within treatment parameters set by third-party payers. These pressures can best be met by correct diagnosis and treatment procedures that are based on current medical science.

Conservative mismanagement of CTS by the therapist is most commonly related to the inability to diagnose CTS or to identify associated problems that have been missed or misdiagnosed, inappropriate splint geometry, and exercise regimens that increase rather than decrease carpal tunnel pressures (CTPs).

The purpose of this chapter is not to review the obvious or to repeat what is elsewhere in this text, but rather to focus the attention of the hand clinician and physicians from other specialty areas on the variables that affect intratunnel pressures in the carpal canal and that can be influenced with conservative therapeutic management. A few points on postoperative management that may prevent complications and decrease the expense of treatment and lost time from work are made. The preceding chapters on this subject cover in more depth the anatomy, physiology, evaluation, and surgical management of CTS.

---

*References 1, 9, 30, 32, 33, 38, 39, 63, 65-67, 72, 85, 100, 102.
†References 25, 31, 60, 74, 111, 114.

OVERVIEW OF ANATOMY AND PHYSIOLOGY

The CT as described by Kerwin et al.[52] is a "relatively inelastic conduit in the proximal palm which contains 9 flexor tendons, the median nerve and a varying amount of synovium which, in certain cases, may represent a significant space occupying lesion in the carpal canal. The floor of the canal is a concave arch of carpal bones covered by extrinsic palmar ligaments, the roof of the canal is formed by the transverse carpal ligament (TCL) which radially attaches to the scaphoid tuberosity and crest of the trapezium and ulnarly attaches to the pisiform and hook of the hamate. The antebrachial fascia of the distal forearm is confluent with the TCL proximally and further extends the semi-rigid compartment over the distal radius." The palmaris longus (PL) inserts into the palmar aponeurosis (which should be considered the distal portion of the flexor retinaculum) and thus may pull on the retinaculum when the wrist is extended altering CT shape.[19]

The median nerve lies superficially in the CT and in line with the longitudinal axis of the long finger. The anterior position of the median nerve, directly under the rigid transverse carpal ligament (TCL), makes it vulnerable to direct pressure from the flexor tendons, especially with positions of wrist flexion.[26]

Nerve tissue is vulnerable to changes in vascular supply. Interference with intraneural microcirculation of the median nerve in the CT will initially result in sensory disturbances and if untreated may progress to loss of median-innervated motors. These clinical changes of nerve compression can be related to changes in intraneural microcirculation and nerve fiber structure. Alterations in vascular permeability and tissue nutrition with subsequent formation of edema will lead to nerve function deterioration and restricted tissue gliding.[61]

CTS symptoms are related to a change in the ratio of cross-sectional area of the tunnel and the volume of its contents, which may elevate normal tissue pressures above a critical level, interfering with median-nerve nutrition. Tissue fluid pressures in the CT have been measured at 2.5 mm Hg in normal subjects, as compared with 32 mm Hg in patients diagnosed with CTS.[36] Hydrostatic pressures greater than a threshold pressure of 30 mm Hg are known to induce nerve damage when chronically applied.[42] It has been demonstrated experimentally that when intracarpal pressures are increased to 50 to 60 mm Hg, a complete block of sensory and motor conduction in the median nerve will occur, with sensory dysfunction occurring 10 to 30 minutes before motor dysfunction.[62] It has been found that 50 mm Hg represents a critical pressure level for nerve viability in normotensive patients, whereas hypertensive patients require a higher pressure, around 60 to 70 mm Hg before a total ischemic block in the nerve occurs.[99]

A change in the ratio of contents to space may elevate tissue pressure above critical levels, which may impair blood supply to the tissues or may restrict gliding potential between the tissues and the space.[61]

CAUSES OF INTRATUNNEL PRESSURE CHANGES

The CT is relatively unyielding and unable to accommodate the changes in volume that occur with a change in the cross-sectional area or a change in volume of its contents.[21]

There are many causes of median-nerve compression syndrome at the wrist. The causes of elevated intracarpal tissue pressures can be categorized[26] as (1) an *anatomic compression,* which can occur with fracture, carpal dislocation, or osteophytes or may result from space-occupying lesions such as tumors, cysts, or hypertrophic synovium; (2) a *neuropathic* or *inflammatory condition,* such as diabetes, alcoholism, changes in fluid balance as with pregnancy, menopause, or thyroid disorders; or (3) *mechanical forces* caused by changes in joint position, tendon load, external forces, or vibration and from (4) *obesity.*[3,55,96,117]

Of these causes, conservative intervention by the hand therapist might have potential influence on pressures in the CT by altering posture, tendon load, muscle activity, external forces, and exposure to vibration with alterations of forces applied through work or avocational activity and splinting. The other causes require medical or surgical management or weight reduction.

CONSERVATIVE MANAGEMENT
Clinical evaluation

Early and accurate diagnosis is important to ensure the correct or appropriate conservative treatment, to identify the correct surgical candidate, and to minimize potential disability.[35] The duration of symptoms is a key determinant in estimating the predictive factors of recovery[44] and postsurgical outcomes.[25] Conservative treatment is of most value when instituted in the earliest stages of compression. It is critical to identify and treat this compression syndrome before there is axonal loss in the median nerve.[78] Splinting has been found to be the most effective if applied within 3 months of symptom onset.[54] Even with early detection, the value of conservative treatment has not been proven.[31] Many patients experience symptom relief with splinting, injection, antiinflammatory medications, and changes in applied forces but eventually require surgical decompression of the median nerve. DeStafano et al.[25] investigated CTS patients treated operatively and nonoperatively and found those treated surgically to be six times more likely to have resolution of symptoms over those treated conservatively.

Patients referred to hand therapy by the nonspecialist are often misdiagnosed with CTS because of complaints of "hand pain," making a complete clinical evaluation of the upper extremity critical to the delivery of appropriate care. The evaluation should include a directed history to identify any systemic or metabolic problems that could be contributory, assessment of mechanical forces imposed on the extremity in the course of work or avocational activity, a review of symptoms, and treatment to date. The initial interview usually includes questioning the patient about pain, paresthesias, and motor weakness. Patient complaints of pain, numbness, and tingling in the median nerve and complaints of hand swelling[9] followed by a few provocative tests often simplifies the diagnosis. Complaints of increased symptoms at night are a good diagnostic predictor for CTS.[44] The initial stages of CTS will usually occur at night, as revealed by serial overnight recordings of intracarpal tunnel pressure in patients with CTS.[60] There is a redistribution of tissue fluid in the arms at night when there is no active muscle pump, and both intraneural blood pressure and systemic blood pressure are decreased during sleep.[61] Wrist flexion position during sleep may also contribute to median-nerve ischemia.

My approach in an extremely busy clinical practice is to follow history taking with a clinical examination, beginning with Semmes-Weinstein monofilament testing (Semmes-Weinstein Pressure Aesthesiometer Kit, North Coast Medical, Campbell, California) to determine light-touch and deep-pressure thresholds[2,5,13,37] of both median- and ulnar-nerve distribution. Testing is performed both with the upper extremity joints in neutral and also following Phalen's[77] (testing that positions the wrist in flexion for 60 seconds).[53] A quick screen includes a Tinel's test (percussion over the CT)[1,104]; lumbrical incursion, or the Berger test (the patient holds a full fist position with the wrist at neutral for 30 to 40 seconds, which creates lumbrical incursion into the carpal canal)[6,20]; Durkan's test (external pressure applied over the transverse carpal ligament using a calibrated piston (Gorge Medical, Hood River, Oregon)[27,100]; and observation of soft edema.[9] Paresthesias with the first three provocative tests indicate a positive result.

Tests specific to CT are then supplemented with a screen, including provocative tests for proximal compression (distal to proximal) in the fibrous bridge between the heads of the flexor digitorum superficialis (FDS); between the humeral and ulnar heads of the pronator teres; and beneath the lacertus fibrosis, thoracic outlet, and C6 radiculopathy.[37,107] A quick screen for commonly seen associated problems of first carpal metacarpal (CMC) arthritis, de Quervain's tendonitis, stenosing tenosynovitis (trigger fingers), wrist or digital tendonitis, epicondylitis, or ulnar-nerve compression is performed.

A detailed description of sensibility testing and functional testing is included in this text (see Chapters 13, 14, and 16). Provocative testing is described in sources dedicated to clinical evaluation.[12,23,76,107]

A number of studies have recently focused on the value of clinical diagnostic testing. It is known that electrodiagnostic tests for CTS may yield incorrect diagnosis[22] and significant false-positive and false-negative results.[102] MacDermid[63] has made the point that electrodiagnostic tests are not completely accurate nor significantly related to the degree of nerve compression. Other researchers[83] have determined that at this time there is no gold standard for the evaluation of CTS.

Although some authors conclude that there is little scientific evidence regarding the reliability and validity for comprehensive upper extremity clinical examination[66] and that sensitivity and specificity vary greatly with comparison subjects within the various studies,[38] others have demonstrated the value of clinical diagnostic testing for CTS.[9,30,39,65,85,100,102]

Szabo et al.[100] have concluded that if a patient has (in descending order for sensitivity) a positive Durkan's test, abnormal sensibility by Semmes-Weinstein testing, an abnormal hand diagram (patient mapping of discomfort and quality of symptoms), and nocturnal pain, the probability that CT will be correctly diagnosed is 0.86. If all four of these conditions are normal, the probability that the patient has CTS is 0.0068. They found that the addition of electrodiagnostic tests did not increase the diagnostic power of the four clinical tests.[100] Their work is supported by others.[85]

Tetro et al.[102] have demonstrated that wrist flexion combined with the median-nerve compression test (manual pressure applied over the median nerve in the CT) produces a higher sensitivity (82%) than other provocative tests (i.e., Phalen's wrist flexion test, Tinel's test, and the carpal compression test). The serial application of the median-nerve compression test and Phalen's test has been found to be useful in the diagnosis of CTS and can improve decisions for referral to electrodiagnostic studies.[30]

Ghavani and Haghighat[39] have evaluated five clinical provocative tests (Tinel's, Phalen's, reverse Phalen's, carpal compression, and vibration) as an adjunct to electrodiagnostic testing. Other studies have introduced the complaint of subjective swelling of the affected hand as an important diagnostic and prognostic factor with CTS[9] and the distal metacarpal compression maneuver as being helpful in diagnosis and splint design.[65]

Berger[6] suggested that provocative testing to produce lumbrical incursion may be as sensitive and specific as Phalen's test for CTS. The test is performed by asking the patient to make a fist with the wrist in the neutral position. The test is positive if pain and paresthesia occur within 30 to 40 seconds. A full fist results in approximately 3 cm of lumbrical muscle incursion into the CT and can increase the CT contents, possibly contributing to median-nerve compression.[20]

Although opinions and results vary from study to study, most agree that clinical evaluation of CTS has value in itself or as adjunct to electrodiagnostic testing and that early diagnosis is critical to good outcomes in the treatment of CTS.[10,25,44,74]

The effect of posture, load, and external pressure on carpal tunnel pressures

A review of experimental work on CTP may offer some insight into reducing these mechanical pressures with splinting, alterations in work or avocational postures, and load applied to the structures that sit within the CT. CTPs are

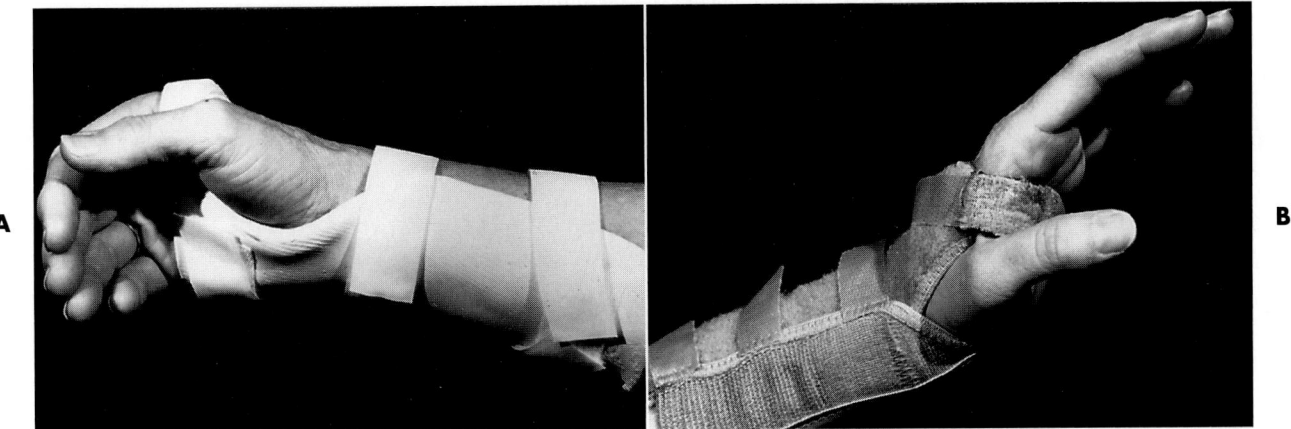

Fig. 37-1. A, The proper position for wrist control splinting to minimize carpal tunnel pressures is neutral with the wrist postured at 2 degrees flexion and 3 degrees ulnar deviation.[8] **B,** Improper splint position may elevate carpal tunnel pressure by 30 to 40 mm Hg.[36,47,51]

affected by changes in posture of the wrist, fingers, thumb, and forearm; by loads applied to the palmaris longus (PL), flexor digitorum profundus (FDP), FDS, flexor pollicis longus (FPL), and the lumbrical muscles; by externally applied forces to the palm and wrist area; and with exposure to vibration.

The effect of wrist posture. We observe clinically that wrist position with CT splinting is critical and that changes in position by as much as 20 degrees can alter nerve compression symptoms. Prefabricated splints with metal bar inserts often increase paresthesias and pain if the wrist is positioned in too much extension.

The shape of the CT changes with wrist posture.[26,34,95,119] A posture of wrist flexion decreases the cross-sectional area in the region of the pisiform and hamate, whereas extension decreases the cross-sectional area at the level of the pisiform.[119] The PL, by virtue of its insertion into the palmar aponeurosis (i.e., the distal portion of the flexor retinaculum), may alter the shape of the CT as it applies tension to the retinaculum when the wrist is extended.[19]

Intratunnel pressures have been measured at 2.5 mm Hg with the wrist in neutral, 31 mm Hg with normal wrist flexion, and 30 mm Hg in maximal wrist extension in normal subjects.[36] Burke et al.[8] also found that wrist position had a significant effect on CTP and demonstrated that intratunnel pressures are the lowest with the wrist near neutral, most specifically at 2 degrees of wrist flexion and 3 degrees of ulnar deviation. They recommended this position for wrist control splinting. Weiss et al.[115] determined that the average position of the wrist associated with the lowest pressure was 2 ± 9 degrees of extension and 2 ± 6 degrees of ulnar deviation; they recommend a splint position similar to that of Burke.[115]

CTPs are dependent on tendon load through the CT and wrist position. Regardless of the loading condition, catheter pressures have been found to be higher with wrist extension than with wrist flexion.[47,51] This has been shown previously

for wrist postures associated with unloaded conditions.* Changes in flexor tendon trajectories due to wrist posture may also increase contact forces on the median nerve, subjecting the median nerve to shear pressure.[50]

Keir and Bach[47] explored the hypothesis that the extrinsic finger flexor muscles have the potential to move into the proximal end of the CT with wrist extension. Muscle excursions of the FDP and FDS were measured relative to the pisiform during wrist extension in cadaveric specimens. They found that the extrinsic finger flexor muscles have the potential to enter the CT during wrist extension, possibly contributing to elevated CTPs during this activity. They conclude that the use of finger flexors when the wrist and fingers are extended should be avoided.[47]

Clinical implications. The proper position for wrist control splinting is neutral, with the wrist postured at 2 degrees flexion and 3 degrees ulnar deviation (Fig. 37-1). Prefabricated splints that often position the wrist in extension may increase CTP (Fig. 37-2). A working posture of the wrist in neutral to slight flexion when digital load is required may minimize intratunnel pressures.

The effect of finger position. We observe clinically that limiting finger motion is sometimes required to decrease the symptoms and pain associated with CT syndrome and that in a number of cases wrist control splinting alone does not offer relief of pain. This is especially true in our manual laborers with well-developed lumbricals or with anxious and often elderly patients who attempt to improve their symptoms by continually flexing their digits (the "compulsive gripper"). These same patients will find relief of symptoms if the metacarpophalangeal (MP) joints are splinted in moderate extension.

With the wrist in neutral, intratunnel pressures are further relieved by finger positions that pull the lumbricals up out of the CT. Several studies published in the last several years

*References 36, 73, 87, 98, 103, 116.

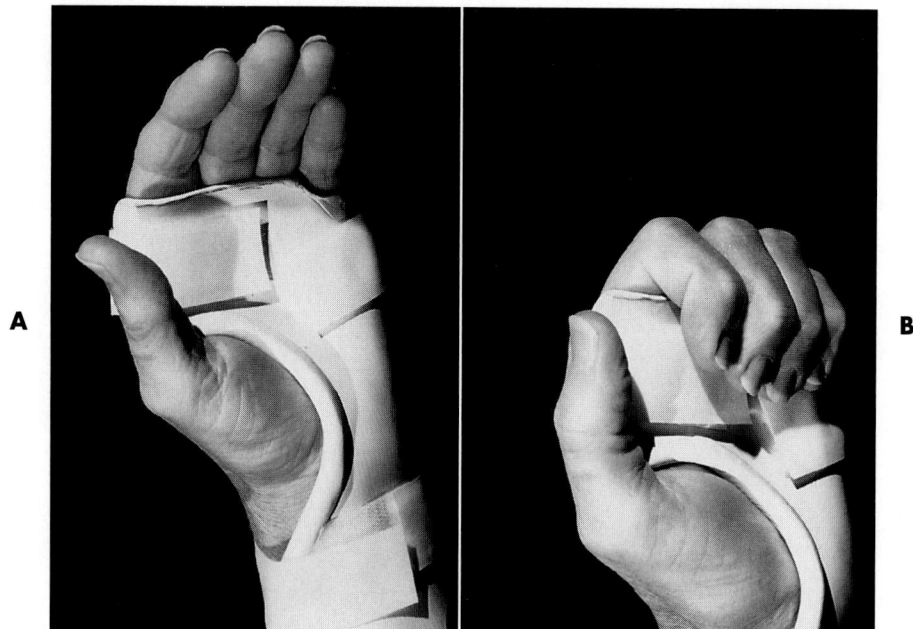

Fig. 37-2. A, Patients with well-developed lumbricals, a positive Berger test, or associated flexor or extensor synovitis, or those who tend to constantly flex the digits to relieve symptoms, should be splinted with the wrist neutral and metacarpophalangeal joints blocked at 20 to 40 degrees flexion to prevent lumbrical incursion and decrease flexor and extensor excursion. **B,** This splint position decreases pressure at the A_1 pulley as well as in the carpal tunnel by forcing a hook fist position, which creates differential excursion between the flexor digitorum profundus and flexor digitorum superficialis tendons.[29,112,113]

examine the dynamic relationship of the lumbrical muscles and the CT.* Lumbrical incursion into the CT that is associated with finger flexion movements increases intra-tunnel pressures by increasing the contents of the carpal canal.

The four lumbricals take their origin from the FDP tendons as the latter cross the palm.[68,108] Anatomic studies have demonstrated that the lumbrical muscles originate distal to the CT with the fingers held in extension but that all four lumbrical muscles lie within the carpal canal when the fingers are actively flexed.[20,68,93,118] As a composite fist is made, the FDP tendons pull the proximal portion of the lumbricals into the carpal canal.

Lumbrical incursion has been studied in four finger positions.[20] The lumbrical muscle origins were found to be an average of 7.8 mm distal to the CT with full finger extension, 14 mm into the tunnel with 50% finger flexion, 25.5 mm with 75% finger flexion, and 30 mm with 100% finger flexion. The lumbrical muscles were distal to the proximal aspect of the hook of the hamate only for the position of full digital extension and 50% finger flexion.[20]

This information is important clinically because the hook of the hamate has been found to be the most constrictive portion of the carpal canal[18,19]; therefore lumbrical incursion to this level could likely have the greatest effect on

*References 16, 18, 20, 21, 26, 41, 68, 93, 118, 121.

median-nerve compression.[16] Others[86] have demonstrated that the median nerve is compressed and flattened to the greatest degree at the level of the hook of the hamate. Therefore, with finger flexion greater than 50%, this already crowded area becomes even more crowded as the lumbricals move in to take up more space and apply more pressure to the median nerve.

CTPs in the same four finger positions as noted earlier were measured.[16] These same investigators found that a progressive and linear increase in CTP was noted for each degree of finger flexion if the lumbricals were intact but that pressures did not change if the lumbricals were excised in any finger position. A greater amount of change in pressure was recorded between the 75% (326 mm Hg) and 100% (361 mm Hg) flexed positions.[16]

Ham et al.[41] have also studied the effect of finger flexion on lumbrical incursion and the median nerve. Successive cross-sectional areas of the CT were measured with the fingers in both full extension and full flexion in 12 healthy volunteers using magnetic resonance imaging (MRI). In this study, the presence, amount, shape, and size of the lumbrical muscles influenced the alignment and shape of the median nerve in the CT. Other changes that were noted in this study during finger flexion were fat compression, flattening and displacement of the median nerve in the presence of lumbrical muscles, and pressure from the superficial and deep flexor tendons.[41]

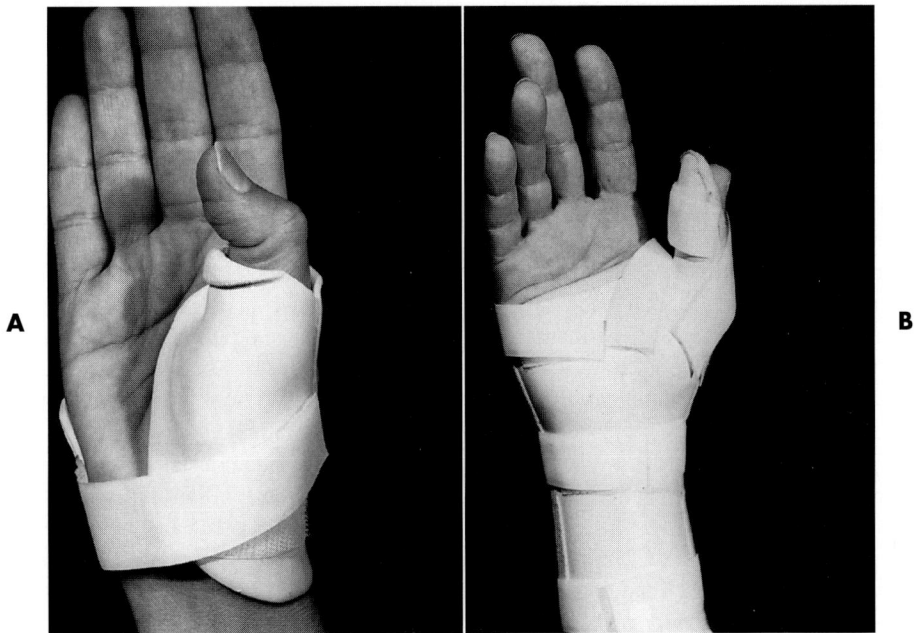

Fig. 37-3. A, Carpal tunnel patients with first carpal metacarpal (CMC) joint inflammation or painful arthritis should be fitted with a short opponens splint for daytime wear. This splint will prevent CMC dislocation and adduction forces with pinching activities and may decrease joint inflammation and edema where the flexor retinaculum attaches to the trapezium. **B,** Night splinting for these patients should include control for both the wrist and thumb kinetic chain.

Ditmars and Houin[26] make the point that the lumbricals retract into the CT with MP flexion and actually contract further during active interphalangeal (IP) joint extension, causing further median-nerve compression within the distal end of the CT. They state that this mechanism can be suspected when the patient complains of intermittent numbness that occurs while writing, holding books, or carrying objects (as with an intrinsic-plus position) for a prolonged time.[26]

A study on the effects of finger posture on CTP as it relates to wrist position demonstrated that 45 degrees of flexion at the MP joint may be optimal when designing splints or work postures.[48]

Clinical significance. The clinical implication from review of these studies and from clinical experience is that in some cases, wrist control splinting alone may be insufficient to decrease intratunnel pressures. A lumbrical block added to the wrist control splint to hold the MP joints at 20 to 40 degrees of flexion will decrease finger flexion by 50% and decrease intratunnel pressures.[16,20,93,118]

In patients with well-developed lumbricals; a positive Berger test[6,20]; or swelling at the volar wrist, indicating flexor synovitis, or for the "compulsive gripper," the MP joints should be blocked in moderate extension to decrease the effects of lumbrical incursion (Fig. 37-3). Limiting flexor tendon excursion in cases with flexor synovitis or hypertrophic synovium[58] is critical to decreasing pain and inflammation and will prevent triggering of digits with stenosing tenosynovitis,[29] often seen in association with CTS by

forcing the patient to work the digits in a hook fist position. Work postures that require repetitive gripping in patients with CTS should be altered, as should postures that require sustained grip or pinch with an intrinsic-plus position. The use of therapy aids that encourage repetitive gripping such as therapeutic putty or hand grippers should be avoided as a part of a strengthening program for any person whose hand is inflamed or edematous as a result of other injury and for those with the diagnosis of CTS. Repetitive flexion exercise increases intratunnel pressures and can contribute to CTS and trigger fingers.[26] A better option is to strengthen with isometric-type exercise that allows less than 50% finger flexion. Strengthening should not be a part of a conservative management program for CTS.

The effects of combined tendon load and posture. Wrist and finger posture, combined with load, as with gripping and pinching, have been found to elevate CTPs.[51,59,82,92] Active-resistant flexion of the fingers creates ulnar sliding of the median nerve beneath the flexor retinaculum.[69]

The combined effects of posture and tendon load have been studied in cadaveric wrists.[51] It has been demonstrated that CTPs are dependent on wrist posture and the loading of tendons passing through the CT. CTPs were measured in eight cadaveric wrists under four muscle-loading conditions with the thumb, index, and long finger in a pinch-grip posture; pressures were measured with both zero load and a 1-kg mass to the flexor tendons of the index and long fingers, the PL, and the FPL. This study demonstrated that muscle load elevated pressure in the CT above the critical pressure. The effect of muscle loading from greatest to lowest was loading of the PL, the finger flexors, the FPL, and no load. The PL created the highest pressure with the wrist extended and only moderate pressure with the wrist in flexion. The authors speculate that the insertion of the PL into the flexor retinaculum may change the shape of the tunnel when the tendon is under pressure. Loading the finger flexors with the wrist flexed increases median nerve pressure to 2.5 times that of loading the flexor tendons in neutral. Tendon load with the wrist in either 45 degrees of extension or flexion increased intratunnel pressure by 30 mm Hg. Loading the FPL in the wrist in flexion or extension induced pressures no different than zero-load conditions, but when the FPL was loaded with the wrist in ulnar deviation, the pressure was twice that of the unloaded state. A forceful grip in ulnar deviation provided high compression for the median nerve.[51]

Pressure has been measured within the CT during nine functional positions of the hand and wrist,[92] adding support to earlier work by Cobb et al.[16] Intratunnel pressures exceed normal pressures[62,89,90] by more than 200 mm Hg upon making a strong fist in normal subjects, and in fact, making a fist increased the intratunnel pressure significantly more than variations of either wrist flexion or extension in normal subjects.[92] Power grip was found to elevate intratunnel pressures to 223 mm Hg, isometric flexion of a finger against resistance to 41 mm Hg, wrist flexion to 56 mm Hg, and wrist extension to 77 mm Hg.[92]

Luchetti et al.[59] investigated intratunnel pressures at 1-cm intervals along the CT in 39 patients with CTS and in 12 control patients. Pressures were measured with the fingers relaxed and with the fingers gripping in combination with three wrist positions (neutral, wrist extension, and wrist flexion). They found that pressures were typically greater with the wrist in extension than in flexion and that gripping hand pressures in the tunnel were the lowest with the wrist flexed.[59]

Remple et al.[82] examined the relationship between CTP and fingertip force and found that (1) fingertip loading increased CTP for all 10 wrist postures tested, (2) fingertip loading elevated CTPs independent of wrist posture, and (3) relatively small fingertip loads have a large effect on CTP. They concluded that sustained pinch and grasp aggravate median-nerve neuropathy at the wrist.[82]

Clinical implication. These measurements of intracarpal pressures vary some from study to study depending on the method of study, but all demonstrate that CTP changes with posture and load. The implication from these studies is that work postures should avoid the positions of forceful grip, pinching with the wrist ulnarly deviated, strong gripping with the wrist in more than 10 to 15 degrees of flexion, and positions of wrist extension. Isolated fingertip pressures and sustained grasp should be avoided in working situations. Again, the point is made for working with the wrist and fingers in a neutral posture. We should be cautious as we ask

patients with other diagnoses that contribute to inflamed or swollen tissues to exercise with Thera-Band, work-simulation tools, work samples, exercise putty, and hand grippers.

The effect of thumb position. Clinically, we observe that some patients with inflammation at the first CMC joint also experience median nerve symptoms and that patients, if questioned carefully, will point out that median-nerve paresthesias worsen with sustained pinch, as when holding the newspaper or a pen. The effect of first CMC joint inflammation, the pull of the opponens muscle on the flexor retinaculum, and sustained intrinsic contraction as when holding a heavy book have been implicated as a source of increased intratunnel pressures.[26]

It has been demonstrated that loading the FPL in wrist flexion or extension does not increase intracarpal pressures more than an unloaded state but that FPL load with the wrist ulnarly deviated increases pressures twice that of the unloaded state.[51] Keir et al.[51] allude to the possibility of the thenar muscle applying traction to the flexor retinaculum, much as the PL does, with load to the index finger in opposition.

Clinical implication. All patients with median nerve symptoms should be evaluated for first CMC joint inflammation or arthritis (see Chapter 100), and if symptomatic, should be fitted with a short opponens splints for daytime (see Fig. 37-3, *A*) and a long opponens splinting for night (see Fig. 37-3, *B*) and should avoid work postures that combine pinch and wrist ulnar deviation. Patients should avoid repetitive gripping and pinching during work and avocational activities. Adduction forces to the first CMC can be minimized by increasing the size of the writing pen, applying arthritic grips to golf clubs, or increasing grip size on other tools.

The effect of forearm position. Rempel et al.[84] have demonstrated that CTP is affected by MP joint motion and forearm positions in a complex way. They measured CTP in 17 normal subjects with relation to pronation and supination position and MP joint angles. The highest mean pressures (55 mm Hg) were recorded with full supination and with the MP joints at 90 degrees of flexion. The lowest mean pressures (12 mm Hg) were recorded with 45 degrees of pronation and 45 degrees of MP flexion.[84] MP joint angle (90 degrees of flexion) increased CTP to 60% above the minimum and pronation/supination (90 degrees of supination) to 225% above the minimum.

Clinical significance. Based on the results of this study, a working position near 45 degrees of pronation and modest flexion for the MP joint may minimize CTP. If CTP plays a role in the etiology of activity related to CTS, then redesigning tools and tasks to minimize CTP will decrease the risk of developing CTS. Isometric forearm strengthening in a neutral position following musculoskeletal injury may be more appropriate in some cases than concentric or eccentric strengthening. This study may cause us to rethink the recommended technique for sensibility testing with the Semmes-Weinstein monofilaments in which the patient's forearm rests supinated while the wrist and digits are supported against a mold of Thera-Putty for testing. This supinated position may increase median nerve pressures not only in the CT but at the flexor-pronator level as well.

The effect of externally applied pressure. We make the observation that some therapy techniques designed for strengthening the hand or for stretching connective tissues appear to increase median nerve symptoms. The application of externally applied forces to the palm in cadaver hands increases CTP and the magnitude of that pressure change is dependent on the location of the applied force.[17] It has been demonstrated that 1 kg of external force will increase CTP by 103 mm Hg if applied over the flexor retinaculum, 37 mm Hg if over the hypothenar region, and 75 mm Hg if over the thenar area adjacent to the distal aspect of the CT. The highest pressures are generated by pressure adjacent to the hook of the hamate (mean, 136 mm Hg).[17]

Clinical significance. Perhaps we should take a closer look at the use of hand grippers, some work-simulation tools, Dynasplints and progressive static splinting for the wrist, and the effects of cast pressures on median nerve symptoms to ensure that our treatments are not contributing to median-nerve compression.

The effect of work tasks

Specific work tasks have been evaluated as risk factors for CTS. Examples are keying on a computer[24]; operating a mouse[49]; using excessive strength, incongruous postures, and movements of wrist hand and elbow; sustaining constant pressure on the palm; engaging in tearing motions; and using gloves.[120] Viikari-Juntura and Silverstein,[110] in a review article on effect of role of postural factors, high handgrip and pinch forces, repetitive hand and wrist movements, external pressure, and vibration in the occurrence of CTS, conclude that there is enough evidence from experimental studies to suggest that both the incidence and severity of CTS could be improved with changes in work patterns, that is, reducing duration, frequency or intensity of forceful repetitive work, extreme wrist postures, and vibration.

However, the current position of the Industrial Injuries and Prevention Committee of the American Society for Surgery of the Hand is that "current medical literature does not provide the information necessary to establish a causal relationship between specific work activities and the development of well-recognized disease entities."[109] The Australian court system does not recognize that repetitive strain injury exists at all as a physical disorder.[43]

OTHER CONSIDERATIONS FOR CONSERVATIVE MANAGEMENT

Conservative treatment other than splinting and alterations of applied forces and postures may include antiinflammatory medications, steroid injections around the mouth of the CT, metabolic control of other medical problems, and weight loss.[10,35,114] Increased weight or body mass index (BMI) have been identified as risk factors for CTS. Individuals classified as obese (BMI greater than 29) are 2.5 times more likely than slender individuals (BMI less than 20) to be diagnosed with CTS.[117] Other studies[3,55,96] have found statistically significant correlations between BMI and CTS. The importance of aerobic activity and overall fitness should be stressed, especially for those with sedentary occupations and weight problems.

Beyond evaluation and splinting, conservative management of CTS in therapy is mostly instructional. Once instructed in activity modification, ergonomic changes, and proximal postural changes, the patient should be discharged to a home program and rechecked informally to screen for sensory changes or change in symptoms.

CONCLUSIONS FOR CONSERVATIVE MANAGEMENT

Intratunnel pressures can be relieved with alterations in posture, muscle activity, and tendon load and through reduction of external forces. Wrist position for splinting is optimal at 0 to 2 degrees of flexion and 3 degrees ulnar deviation to decrease pressure on the median nerve.[8,115] The MP joints should be splinted at 20 to 40 degrees flexion when the lumbrical incursion or full fist test is positive, if the flexor tendons are inflamed or wrist flexor synovitis is present, if the A_1 pulley region is tender or triggering is present with any digit,[29] or for the inadvertent or compulsive gripper. However, although splints and analgesics may be appropriate for mild cases, failure to control symptoms, a prolonged history, or severe CTS will require surgical decompression.[74] Although some have reported successful conservative treatment in a significant number of patients who followed a regimen of preoperative tendon and nerve gliding,[88] this has not been my experience. It is my observation that patients who will respond to conservative management will find immediate relief with night splinting and that those who continue to have pain and paresthesias with splinting will most likely require CT release. Walker et al.,[111] in a study comparing full-time versus part-time splint wear with the wrist in neutral position, found that physiologic improvement occurred with full-time wear; however, others[60] have found no significant alterations in intratunnel pressures with or without use of splints. Patients with more advanced CTS and severe nocturnal pain will usually get some relief with a full resting pan splint that positions the wrist at the predescribed angle: MP joints at 20 degrees flexion, IP joints neutral, and the thumb kinetic chain in neutral to slight abduction to minimize the effects of all joint positions on intracarpal pressures until surgical decompression can be scheduled.

POSTOPERATIVE MANAGEMENT

The literature confirms that CT decompression is effective and the preferred treatment for CTS but that surgical management is not without a small percentage of residual problems.[10,25,44,74] Postoperative problems have been defined as incomplete relief of pain, poor recovery of sensory and motor function, symptom recurrence, perineural scarring with associated symptoms, scar tenderness, pillar pain, laceration to flexor tendon or nerve, and neuroma-in-continuity.[106] Other problems can include postoperative wound infection, wound dehiscence from early suture removal, suture abscess, trigger fingers that were not picked up preoperatively and limit patient's willingness to exercise, PL inflammation, incomplete tendon glide, and reflex sympathetic dystrophy. These complications exist and are reported by hand surgeons with both open and endoscopic release.[75]

It is my experience that scar tenderness is the most common postoperative management problem seen after open CT release and that this complication is most often seen with incisions that cross the wrist and in patients whose sutures are taken out before the wound has gained adequate tensile strength.

In a study of predictors of return to work after CT release, Katz et al.[46] demonstrated that persistent symptoms and scar tenderness most strongly correlated with failure to return to work. Other demographic predictors were defined in this study, but the authors concluded that the work disability at 6 months after CT release is 29% and the principal predictor is clinical outcome of symptom relief and scar tenderness.[46]

Cassidy et al.[15] have suggested that there is an anatomic basis for the increased tenderness of incisions that traverse the area from 5 mm proximal to the wrist flexion crease to 10 mm distal to this crease. In a cadaver study of 10 hands, nerve density was measured within the dermis, between the epidermis and superficial fascia, and between the superficial fascia and the TCL to assess whether a variation in nerve density exists in the region of standard CT release. The results of this study indicate that subcutaneous nerve density peaks in the region extending from 5 mm proximal to the wrist crease to 10 mm distal to the wrist crease, averaging twice the number of nerves seen proximally or distally.[15]

Early suture removal after open CT release resulting in even minor dehiscence often results in the formation of hypertrophic scar, increased scar tenderness, and lengthened therapy. A point so simple as this, which violates the most basic principles of wound biology and tissue healing, costs the employer and patient time and money and results in poorer outcomes for the physician and therapist.

Scar tenderness can be minimized with incisions that do not cross the wrist,[15,70] with detailed attention to wound healing, and with a wrist control splint to prevent tension at the wound site.

In my clinical experience, the most effective scar management techniques are a carefully planned surgical incision that does not cross the wrist crease; benign wound healing, with suture removal around 16 to 17 days postop-

eratively; and wrist control splinting that prevents wound site tension the first few weeks after open CT release. Paper tape applied longitudinally over the incision 2 weeks postoperatively to 2 months postoperatively will help prevent hypertrophic scarring by minimizing wound tension,[71,81,91] especially for incisions that cross the wrist. Topical silicone occlusive gel sheeting can also be used to pad painful scars and to improve hypertrophic scar[97]; however, it has been demonstrated in a bilateral breast-reduction model that when Micropore tape is applied to scars, significantly less scar develops than with scars treated with silicone occlusive sheeting (SIL-K) or silicone gel Epiderm.[71]

Occasionally, wrist pain is related to inflammation of the PL tendon (positive if the patient experiences pain along the PL tendon with applied manual resistance). I have treated two cases in which the PL tendon was nicked during CT release. Patients with PL inflammation are tender with deep pressure at the insertion and have pain with resistive flexion and stretch into extension. These patients are treated with splinting the wrist in 5 degrees of flexion for 3 weeks, with avoidance of stretch into extension and flexion loads, and also with a series of iontophoresis.

In my clinic, we see most postoperative CT release patients 24 hours postoperatively for wound care and splinting. The postoperative dressings are taken down, and the hand is cleansed, massaged, redressed lightly with a contact layer of Xeroform and sterile dressings, and then splinted with a wrist control splint in a position of about 25 degrees of extension.

The patients are instructed to begin working on a gentle composite fist for the first few days, progressing to differential tendon gliding exercises[112,113] and nerve gliding exercises[12] by the fourth postoperative day. Specific written instructions to the patient will decrease the postoperative problems associated with overexercise, underexercise, overuse, and wound problems associated with moisture or infection, especially in elderly, diabetic, and athletic patients.

The value of postoperative splinting is debated. Finsen et al.[32] found that there was no difference in complication rate or function with regard to scar pain, pillar pain, grip, or pinch in CT release patients splinted versus those not splinted for 4 weeks. Others[11] support their findings; however I find that splinting is helpful to control overuse and to prevent incisional line wound tension. Splinting does not appear to contribute to problems with tendon or nerve gliding because patients remove the splint for controlled wrist extension and finger exercise.

Trigger fingers that were not diagnosed before CT release can complicate the postoperative course. Pain at the A_1 pulley with deep pressure, uneven glide, or frank locking can be addressed by altering flexor tendon excursions at the A_1 level. These cases are best splinted with combined wrist control and lumbrical block, which positions the MP joints at about 20 degrees of flexion (see Fig. 37-2). This position, which forces the patient to work the digits in the hook fist position, creates maximal differential gliding of 10 to 11 mm of the FDS and FDP[112] and forces the swollen portion of the tendons to glide at different levels through the A$_1$ pulley, thus preventing the painful locking that occurs with a full composite fist.[29] This position also decreases pressures at the A$_1$ pulley, allowing the pulley and tendons to rest and thus decreasing inflammation. Azar et al.,[4] in a study of the dynamic pressures of the flexor tendon pulley system in cadavers, have demonstrated that a resting position pressure between the annular pulley and flexor tendon of 0 to 50 mm Hg is increased to 500 to 700 mm Hg with flexion of the fingers into the distal palmar crease. If locking persists with this splint design, splinting the distal joint with a one-joint dorsal splint that includes the middle and distal phalanx, allowing only motion at the proximal interphalangeal (PIP) joint, will prevent locking. This splint can be hand based if wrist control splinting is not indicated. Thumb triggers can be splinted with a one-joint dorsal splint that includes the proximal and distal phalanx.

In most cases, minimal therapy is needed after CT release, and in some cases, no therapy is needed. Postoperative care, as with all hand surgeries, includes standard techniques of edema control, wound care, motion for both uninvolved and involved joints, and early intervention for inflammatory or sympathetic problems. I do not attempt to strengthen patients postoperatively except for light isometric exercises for the intrinsic muscles. Patients are advised to allow the operated hand to slowly strengthen with normal use; to avoid repetitive gripping and pinching exercises (with exercise putty or handgrippers), which may contribute to inflammation at the A$_1$ pulley and may aggravate the first CMC joint; if joint changes exist, to avoid the use of vibratory tools for 3 months; and to manage the scar with paper tape for 2 months postoperatively. Strategies for return to work include communication with work supervisors regarding minimizing stresses and repetitive motions, instituting ergonomic changes, avoiding vibratory tools, and using padded work gloves in some cases. The point has been made that although there are several opinions regarding effective treatment for CT release, there is very little scientific support for the range of options currently used in practice (e.g., surgery, physical therapy, drug therapy, chiropractic treatment, biobehavioral intervention, occupational medicine).[31]

The value of postoperative care is debated.[32,79,88] It has been demonstrated that rehabilitation after surgery facilitates a faster return to work but has no effect on functional recovery or symptom reoccurrence.[79] Obviously, therapy will not influence nerve that is still mechanically compressed nor will it affect the rate of regeneration of recovering nerve; however, patients who have complications of wound problems, painful scar, incomplete flexor tendon glide, stiff joints from associated osteoarthritis, painful first CMC joint

arthritis, undiagnosed trigger fingers, inflamed PL, or pillar pain will benefit from supervised therapy.

Most patients, if followed early with the precautions noted earlier, do not require much therapy. The greatest contributions made in therapy preoperatively are proper clinical examination of the extremity with recommendations to the primary care physician regarding treatment or referral to a surgeon, proper instruction to the patient for techniques to decrease pressures in the CT, and proper splint geometry. The most important contribution postoperatively is the proper management of wound healing to help prevent scar problems, proper patient instruction regarding exercise techniques that will prevent inflammation and maximize recovery of tissue gliding, and communication with concerned parties regarding reentry into the workplace.

REFERENCES

1. Alfonso MI, Dzwierzynski W: Hoffman-Tinel sign: the realities, *Phys Med Rehabil Clin North Am* 9:721, 1998.
2. American Society of Hand Therapists: *Clinical assessment recommendations,* ed 2, Chicago, 1992, ASHT.
3. Atroshi I, et al: Prevalence for clinically proved carpal tunnel syndrome is 4 percent, *Lakartidningen* 97:1668, 2000.
4. Azar CA, Fleegler EJ, Culver JE: Dynamic anatomy of the flexor pulley system of the fingers and thumb. Second International Meeting, International Federation of Societies for Surgery of the Hand. Paper #5, Boston, October 1983.
5. Bell-Krotoski JA: Sensibility testing: current concepts. In Hunter JM, Mackin EJ, Callahan AD, editors: *Rehabilitation of the hand,* ed 4, St Louis, 1995, Mosby.
6. Berger R: A new clinical test for carpal tunnel syndrome. Presented American Association for Hand Surgery, Cancun, Mexico, December 1-5, 1993.
7. Boeckstyns MEH, Sorenson AI: Does endoscopic carpal tunnel release have a higher rate of complications than open carpal tunnel release? An analysis of published series, *J Hand Surg* 24B:9, 1999.
8. Burke DT, et al: Splinting for carpal tunnel syndrome: in search of the optimal angle, *Arch Phys Med Rehabil* 75:1241, 1994.
9. Burke DT, et al: Subjective swelling: a new sign for carpal tunnel syndrome, *Am J Phys Med Rehabil* 78:504, 1999.
10. Burke FD: Carpal tunnel syndrome: reconciling "demand management" with clinical need, *J Hand Surg* 25B:121, 2000.
11. Bury TF, Akelman E, Weiss AP: Prospective, randomized trial of splinting after carpal tunnel release, *Ann Plast Surg* 35:19, 1995.
12. Butler DS: *Mobilization of the nervous system,* New York, 1991, Churchill Livingstone.
13. Callahan AD: Sensibility assessment: Prerequisites and techniques for nerve lesions in continuity and nerve lacerations. In Hunter JM, Mackin EJ, Callahan AD, editors: *Rehabilitation of the hand,* ed 4, St Louis, 1995, Mosby.
14. Casanova J:UE Net Project, American Society of Hand Therapists Data Base, Chicago.
15. Cassidy C, Khurana J, Feldon P: Nerve density in the palm: implications for carpal tunnel release. Research session, paper-06. Proceedings American Society for Surgery of the Hand. San Francisco, September 14, 1995.
16. Cobb TK, An KN, Cooney WP: Effect of lumbrical incursion within the carpal tunnel on carpal tunnel pressure: a cadaveric study, *J Hand Surg* 20A:186, 1995.
17. Cobb TK, An KN, Cooney WP: Externally applied forces to the palm increase carpal tunnel pressure, *J Hand Surg* 20A:181, 1995.

18. Cobb TK, et al: Establishment of carpal contents/canal ration by means of magnetic resonance imaging, *J Hand Surg* 17A:843, 1992.

19. Cobb TK, et al: Anatomy of the flexor retinaculum, *J Hand Surg* 18A:91, 1993.

20. Cobb TK, et al: Lumbrical muscle incursion into the carpal tunnel during finger flexion, *J Hand Surg* 19B:434, 1994.

21. Cobb TK, et al: Assessment of the ratio of carpal contents to carpal tunnel volume in patients with carpal tunnel syndrome: a preliminary report, *J Hand Surg* 22A:635, 1997.

22. Corwin HM, Kasdan ML: Electrodiagnostic reports of median neuropathy at the wrist, *J Hand Surg* 23A:55, 1998.

23. Dawson DM, Hallet M, Millender LH: *Entrapment neuropathies,* ed 2, Boston, 1990, Little, Brown.

24. Dennerlein JT, et al: In vivo finger flexor tendon force while tapping on a keyswitch, *J Orthop Res* 17:178, 1999.

25. DeStefano F, Nordstrom DL, Vierkant RA: Long-term symptom outcomes of carpal tunnel syndrome and its treatment, *J Hand Surg* 22A:200, 1997.

26. Ditmars DM Jr, Houin HP: Carpal tunnel syndrome, *Hand Clin* 2:525, 1986.

27. Durkan JA: A new diagnostic test for carpal tunnel syndrome, *J Bone Joint Surg* 73A:4535, 1991.

28. Erhard L, Foucher G: What's new concerning carpal tunnel syndrome? *Ann Chir Plast Esthet* 43:600, 1998.

29. Evans RB, Hunter JM, Burkhalter WE: Conservative management of the trigger finger: a new approach, *J Hand Ther* 1:59, 1988.

30. Fertl E, Wober C, Zeitlhofer J: The serial use of two provocative tests in the clinical diagnosis of carpal tunnel syndrome, *Acta Neurol Scand* 98:328, 1998.

31. Feuerstein M, et al: Clinical management of carpal tunnel syndrome: a 12 year review of outcomes, *Am J Ind Med* 35:232, 1999.

32. Finsen V, Anderson K, Russwurm H: No advantage from splinting the wrist after open carpal tunnel release: a randomized study of 82 wrists, *Acta Orthop Scand* 70:288, 1999.

33. Foye PM, Stitik TP: Diagnostic testing in carpal tunnel syndrome, *J Hand Surg* 25A:183, 2000.

34. Garcia-Elias M, et al: Dynamic changes of the transverse carpal arch during flexion-extension of the wrist: effects of sectioning the transverse carpal ligament, *J Hand Surg* 17A:1017, 1992.

35. Gelberman RH, Aronson D, Weisman MH: Carpal tunnel syndrome: results of a prospective trial of steroid injection and splinting, *J Bone Joint Surg* 62A:1181, 1980.

36. Gelberman RH, et al: The carpal tunnel syndrome: a study of carpal canal pressure, *J Bone Joint Surg* 63A:380, 1981.

37. Gelberman RH, et al: Sensibility testing in peripheral-nerve compression syndromes: an experimental study in humans, *J Bone Joint Surg* 65A:632, 1983.

38. Gerr F, Letz R: The sensitivity and specificity of tests for carpal tunnel syndrome vary with comparison subjects, *J Hand Surg* 23B:151, 1998.

39. Ghavanini MR, Haghighat M: Carpal tunnel syndrome: reappraisal of five clinical tests, *Electromyogr Clin Neurophysiol* 38:437, 1998.

40. Grieco A, et al: Epidemiology of musculoskeletal disorders due to biomechanical overload, *Ergonomics* 41:1253, 1998.

41. Ham SJ, et al: Changes in the carpal tunnel due to action of the flexor tendons: visualization with magnetic resonance imaging, *J Hand Surg* 21A:997, 1996.

42. Hargens AR, et al: Peripheral nerve-conduction block by high muscle-compartment pressure, *J Bone Joint Surg* 61A:192, 1979.

43. Ireland DCR: Strain injury: the Australian experience—1992 update, *J Hand Surg* 20A:S53, 1995.

44. Kaplan SJ, Glickel SZ, Eaton RG: Predictive factors in the non-surgical treatment of carpal tunnel syndrome, *J Hand Surg* 15B:106, 1990.

45. Kasdan ML: Complications of endoscopic and open carpal tunnel release, *J Hand Surg* 25A:185, 2000.

46. Katz JN, et al: Predictors of return to work following carpal tunnel release, *Am J Ind Med* 31:85, 1997.

47. Keir PJ, Bach JM: Flexor muscle incursion into the carpal tunnel: a mechanism for increased carpal tunnel pressure? *Clin Biomech* 15:301, 2000.

48. Keir PJ, Bach JM, Rempel DM: Effects of finger posture on carpal tunnel pressure during wrist motion, *J Hand Surg* 23:1004, 1998.

49. Keir PJ, Bach JM, Rempel D: Effects of computer mouse design and task on carpal tunnel pressure, *Ergonomics* 42:1350, 1999.

50. Keir PJ, Wells RP: Changes in geometry of the finger flexor tendons in the carpal tunnel with wrist posture and tendon load: an MRI study on normal wrists, *Clin Biomech* 14:635, 1999.

51. Keir PJ, Wells RP, Lavery W: The effects of tendon load and posture on carpal tunnel pressure, *J Hand Surg* 22A:628, 1997.

52. Kerwin G, Williams CS, Seiler JG: The pathophysiology of carpal tunnel syndrome, *Hand Clin* 12:243, 1996.

53. Koris M, et al: Carpal tunnel syndrome: evaluation of a quantitative provocational diagnostic test, *Clin Orthop Rel Res* 251:157, 1990.

54. Kruger VL, et al: Carpal tunnel syndrome: objective measures and splint use, *Arch Phys Med Rehabil* 72:517, 1991.

55. Lam N, Thurston A: Association of obesity, gender, age, and occupation with carpal tunnel syndrome, *Aust NZ J Surg* 68:190, 1998.

56. Leigh JP, Miller TR: Occupational illnesses within two national data sets, *Int J Occup Environ Health* 4:99, 1998.

57. Liss GM, et al: Use of provincial health insurance plan billing data to estimate carpal tunnel syndrome morbidity and surgery rates, *Am J Ind Med* 22:395, 1992.

58. Lluch AL: Thickening of the synovium of the digital flexor tendons: cause or consequence of the carpal tunnel syndrome, *J Hand Surg* 17B:209, 1992.

59. Luchetti R, Schoenhuber R, Nathan P: Correlation of segmental carpal tunnel pressures with changes in hand and wrist positions in patients with carpal tunnel syndrome and controls, *J Hand Surg* 23B:598, 1998.

60. Luchetti R, et al: Serial overnight recordings of intracarpal canal pressures in carpal tunnel syndrome patients with and without wrist splinting, *J Hand Surg* 19B:35, 1994.

61. Lundborg G, Dahlin LB: Anatomy, function, and pathophysiology of peripheral nerves and nerve compression, *Hand Clin* 12:185, 1996.

62. Lundborg G, et al: Median nerve compression in the carpal tunnel: functional response to experimentally induced controlled pressure, *J Hand Surg* 7:252, 1982.

63. MacDermid J: Accuracy of clinical tests used in the detection of carpal tunnel syndrome: a literature review, *J Hand Ther* 4:169, 1991.

64. Macey AC, Burke FD: Outcomes in hand surgery, *J Hand Surg* 20B:841, 1995.

65. Manente G, et al: A relief maneuver in carpal tunnel syndrome, *Muscle Nerve* 22:1587, 1999.

66. Marx RG, Bombardier C, Wright JG: What do we know about the reliability and validity of physical examination tests used to examine the upper extremity? *J Hand Surg* 24A:185, 1999.

67. Massy-Westropp N, Grimmer K, Bain G: A systemic review of the clinical diagnostic tests for carpal tunnel syndrome, *J Hand Surg* 25A:120, 2000.

68. Mehta HJ, Gardner WU: A study of the lumbrical muscles in the human hand, *Am J Anat* 109:227, 1961.

69. Nakamichi K, Tachibana S: Transverse sliding of the median nerve beneath the flexor retinaculum, *J Hand Surg* 17B:213, 1992.

70. Nathan PA, Meadows KD, Keniston RC: Rehabilitation of carpal tunnel surgery patients using a short surgical incision and an early program of physical therapy, *J Hand Surg* 18A:1044, 1993.

71. Niessen FB, et al: The use of silicone sheeting (Sil-K) and silicone occlusive gel (Epiderm) in the prevention of hypertropic scar formation, *Plast Reconstr Surg* 102:1962, 1998.

72. Novak CB, et al: Provocative sensory testing in carpal tunnel syndrome, *J Hand Surg* 17B(2):204, 1992.

73. Okutsu I, et al: Measurement of pressure in the carpal canal before and after endoscopic management of carpal tunnel syndrome, *J Bone Joint Surg* 71A:679, 1989.

74. Pal B, et al: Management of idiopathic carpal tunnel syndrome (ICTS): a survey of rheumatologists' practice and proposed guidelines, *Br J Rheum* 36:1328, 1997.

75. Palmer AK, Toivonen DA: Complications of endoscopic and open carpal tunnel release, *J Hand Surg* 24A:561, 1999.

76. Pecina MM, Krmpotic-Nemanic, Markiewitz AD: *Tunnel syndromes,* Boca Raton, 1991, CRC Press.

77. Phalen GS: The carpal tunnel syndrome: 17 year's experience in diagnosis and treatment of 654 hands, *J Bone Joint Surg* 48A:211, 1966.

78. Preston DC: Distal median neuropathies, *Neurol Clin* 17:407, 1999.

79. Provinciali L, et al: Usefulness of hand rehabilitation after carpal tunnel surgery, *Muscle Nerve* 23:211, 2000.

80. Rayan GM: Carpal tunnel syndrome between two centuries, *J Okla State Med Assoc* 92:493, 1999.

81. Reiffel RS: Prevention of hypertrophic scars by long term paper tape application, *Plast Reconstr Surg* 96:1715, 1995.

82. Rempel D, et al: Effects of static fingertip loading on carpal tunnel pressure, *J Orthop Res* 15:422, 1997.

83. Rempel D, et al: Consensus criteria for the classification of carpal tunnel syndrome in epidemiological studies, *Am J Public Health* 88:1447, 1998

84. Rempel D, et al: Effects of forearm pronation/supination on carpal tunnel pressure, *J Hand Surg* 23A:38, 1998.

85. Richter M, Bruser P: Value of clinical diagnosis in carpal tunnel syndrome, *Handchir Mikrochir Plast* 31:373, 1999.

86. Robbins H: Anatomical study of the median nerve in the carpal tunnel and etiologies of the carpal tunnel syndrome, *J Bone Joint Surg* 45A:953, 1963.

87. Rojviroj S, et al: Pressures in the carpal tunnel: a comparison between patients with carpal tunnel and normal subjects, *J Bone Joint Surg* 72B:516, 1990.

88. Rozmaryn LM, et al: Nerve and tendon gliding exercises and the conservative management of carpal tunnel syndrome, *J Hand Ther* 11:171, 1998.

89. Rydevik B, Lundborg G: Permeability of intraneural microvessels and perineurium following acute, graded experimental nerve compression, *Scand J Plast Reconstr Surg* 11:179, 1977.

90. Rydevik B, Lundborg G, Bagge U: Effects of graded compression on intraneural blood flow: an in vitro study on rabbit tibial nerve, *J Hand Surg* 6A:3, 1981.

91. Sawada Y, Urushidate S, Nihei Y: Hydration and occlusive treatment of a sutured wound, *Ann Plast Surg* 41:508, 1998.

92. Seradge H, Jia Y-C, Owens W: In vivo measurement of carpal tunnel in the functioning hand, *J Hand Surg* 20A:855, 1995.

93. Siegel DB, Kuzman G, Eakins D: Anatomic investigation of the role of the lumbrical muscles in carpal tunnel syndrome, *J Hand Surg* 20A:860, 1995.

94. Silverstein B, et al: Claims incidence of work-related disorders of the upper extremities: Washington state, 1987 through 1995, *Am J Public Health* 88:1827, 1998.

95. Skie M, et al: Carpal tunnel changes and median nerve compression during wrist flexion and extension seen by magnetic resonance imaging, *J Hand Surg* 15A:934, 1990.

96. Stallings SP, et al: A case-controlled study of obesity as a risk factor for carpal tunnel syndrome in a population of 600 patients presenting for independent evaluation, *J Hand Surg* 22:211, 1997.

97. Su CW, et al: The problem scar, *Clin Plast Surg* 25:451, 1998.

98. Szabo RM, Chidgey LK: Stress carpal tunnel pressures in patients with carpal tunnel syndrome and normal patients, *J Hand Surg* 14A:624, 1989.

99. Szabo R, et al: Effects of increased systemic blood pressure on the tissue fluid pressure: threshold of peripheral nerve, *J Orthop Res* 1:172, 1983.

100. Szabo RM, et al: The value of diagnostic testing in carpal tunnel syndrome, *J Hand Surg* 24A:704, 1999.

101. Terrano AL, Millender LH: Management of work related upper extremity nerve entrapments, *Orthop Clin North Am* 4:783, 1996.

102. Tetro AM, et al: A new provocative test for carpal tunnel syndrome: assessment of wrist flexion and nerve compression, *J Bone Joint Surg* 80B:493, 1998.

103. Thurston AJ, Krause BL: The possible role of vascular congestion in carpal tunnel syndrome, *J Hand Surg* 13B:397, 1988.

104. Tinel J: Le signe du "fourmillement" dans les l'esions des nerfs periphe'riques, *Presse Me'dicale* 47:388, 1915.

105. Tittiranonda P, Burastero S, Rempel D: Risk factors for musculoskeletal disorders among computer users, *Occup Med* 14:17, 1999.

106. Tomaino MM, Plakseychuk A: Identification and preservation of palmar cutaneous nerves during open carpal tunnel release, *J Hand Surg* 23B:607, 1998.

107. Tubiana R, Thomine JM, Mackin EJ: *Examination of the hand and wrist,* London, 1996, Martin Dunitz.

108. Valentine P: The interossei and the lumbricals. In Tubiana R, editor: *The hand,* vol 1, Philadelphia, 1981, WB Saunders.

109. Vender MI, Kasdan ML, Truppa KL: Upper extremity disorders: a literature review to determine work-relatedness, *J Hand Surg* 20A:534, 1995.

110. Viikari-Juntura E, Silverstein B: Role of physical load factors in carpal tunnel syndrome, *Scand J Work Environ Health* 25:163, 1999.

111. Walker WC, et al: Neutral wrist splinting in carpal tunnel syndrome: a comparison of part-time versus full-time wear instructions, *Arch Phys Med Rehabil* 81:424, 2000.

112. Wehbe' MA, Hunter JM: Flexor tendon gliding in the hand. I: In vivo excursions, *J Hand Surg* 10A:570, 1985.

113. Wehbe' MA, Hunter JM: Flexor tendon gliding in the hand. II: Differential gliding, *J Hand Surg* 10A:575, 1985.

114. Weiss AP, Sachar K, Gendreau M: Conservative management of carpal tunnel syndrome: a reexamination of steroid injection and splinting, *J Hand Surg* 19A(3):410, 1994.

115. Weiss ND, et al: Position of the wrist associated with the lowest carpal-tunnel pressure: implications for splint design, *J Bone Joint Surg* 77A:1695, 1995.

116. Werner C-O, Elmqvist D, Ohlin P: Pressure and nerve lesion in the carpal tunnel, *Acta Orthop Scand* 54:312, 1983.

117. Werner RA, et al: The relationship between body mass index and the diagnosis of carpal tunnel syndrome, *Muscle Nerve* 17:632, 1994.

118. Yii NW, Elliot D: A study of the dynamic relationship of the lumbrical muscles and the carpal tunnel, *J Hand Surg* 19B:439, 1994.

119. Yoskioka S, et al: Changes in carpal tunnel shape during wrist motion: MRI evaluation of normal volunteers, *J Hand Surg* 18B:620, 1993.

120. Zecchi G, Venturi G: Repetitive movements of the upper extremities: the results of assessing exposure to biomechanical overload and of a clinical study in a group of workers employed in the production of plywood and veneer panels, *Med Law* 89:412, 1998.

121. Zeiss J, et al: Anatomic relations between the median nerve and flexor tendons in the carpal tunnel: MR evaluation in normal volunteers, *AJR Am J Roentgen* 153:533, 1989.

Chapter 38

DIAGNOSIS AND MANAGEMENT OF CUBITAL TUNNEL SYNDROME*

George E. Omer

The cubital tunnel syndrome, or *tardy ulnar palsy,* was defined in 1958 by Feindel and Stratford,[14,15] although the ability of the anatomic structures near the elbow joint to produce external pressure on the ulnar nerve was known more than a century ago.[49] It is the most common entrapment of the ulnar nerve.[33]

ANATOMY

The ulnar nerve arises as the extension of the medial cord of the brachial plexus and lies medial to the brachial artery as far as the middle third of the arm. The ulnar nerve then pierces the medial intermuscular septum and descends subfascially on the medial side of the triceps muscle. At the elbow, the ulnar nerve is accompanied by the superior ulnar collateral artery[14,49] as the nerve passes through the cubital tunnel during its course from the arm to the forearm.

The ulnar nerve can be compressed by the arcade of Struthers or the ligament of Struthers in the distal portion of the arm.[43] The arcade of Struthers is formed by fascial attachments between the internal brachial ligament, the medial head of the triceps muscle, and the medial intermuscular septum (Fig. 38-1). In an anatomic study, Spinner[43] found the arcade of Struthers to be present in 14 of 20 upper extremities. The ligament of Struthers arises from a supracondylar process and attaches to the junction of the medial epicondyle and the humeral metaphysis. The liga-

ment of Struthers is found in only 1% of all upper extremities.[43]

The cubital tunnel begins at the condylar groove between the medial epicondyle of the humerus and the olecranon of the ulna. In this area, a condensation of connective tissue has been reported to extend from the nerve to the subcutaneous fascia and skin.[22,43] The floor of the cubital tunnel is the medial collateral ligament (ulnar lateral ligament) of the elbow joint, and the sides are formed by the two heads of the flexor carpi ulnaris muscle. The roof is formed by the triangular arcuate ligament (aponeurotic band) that bridges from the medial epicondyle of the humerus to the medial aspect of the olecranon.[2,38,43,48] In the cubital tunnel the ulnar nerve can be palpated in its course behind and beneath the humeral medial epicondyle until the nerve passes between the two heads of the flexor carpi ulnaris muscle.

The capacity of the cubital tunnel is greatest when the elbow is in extension, because the triangular arcuate ligament (aponeurotic band) is slack. Measurements in cadaveric material demonstrate that the distance between the humeral and ulnar attachments of the triangular arcuate ligament lengthens 5 mm for each 45 degrees of flexion.[47] During flexion the medial head of the triceps pushes the ulnar nerve anteromedially 0.73 cm.[43] At 90 degrees of elbow flexion, the proximal edge of the triangular arcuate ligament is rigidly taut. In addition, the floor of the tunnel is elevated during flexion by the bulging medial collateral ligament.[25]

After the ulnar nerve passes through the cubital tunnel, it remains in the interval between the humeral and ulnar heads of the flexor carpi ulnaris muscle. Fibrous bands have been

---

*Reproduced in its entirety from Omer GE: The cubital tunnel syndrome. In Szabo RM: *Nerve compression syndromes: diagnosis and treatment,* Thorofare, NJ, 1989, Slack.

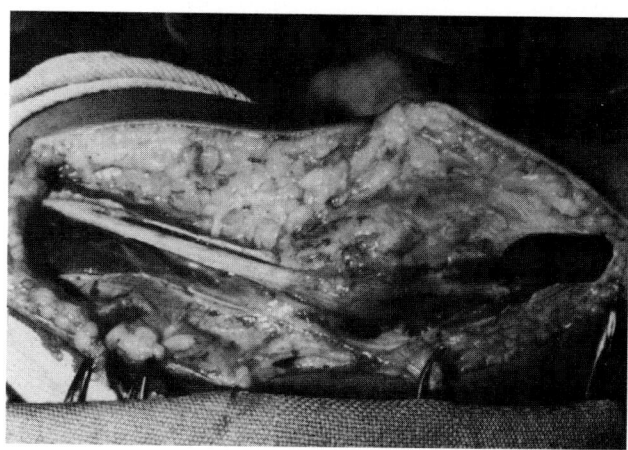

Fig. 38-1. The medial intermuscular septum is a taut fibrotic ridge just anterior (superior in this view) to the ulnar nerve proximal to the medial epicondyle. The nerve is fixed in fibrous tissue in the condylar groove. (From Omer GE Jr: The ulnar nerve at the elbow. In Strickland JW, Steichen JB, editors: *Difficult problems in hand surgery,* St Louis, 1982, Mosby.)

described that compress the ulnar nerve distal to the cubital tunnel.[22]

PATHOPHYSIOLOGY

Pressure may be applied to the ulnar nerve in three ways: compression, stretch, and friction.[43] Low pressure applied to a nerve trunk initially affects the endoneural microcirculation. The nocturnal paresthesias seen in the first phases of compression are based on edema within the nerve secondary to a nocturnal increase in tissue pressure in the cubital tunnel. A critical pressure level has been reported to be 30 mm Hg within the tunnel.[29] Functional loss caused by acute compression is a result of ischemia and not of mechanical deformation.[29] Pechan and Julis[40] have measured intraneural pressure in the ulnar nerve at the cubital tunnel in cadaver experiments: The pressure was 7 mm Hg with full elbow extension and 11 to 24 mm Hg at 90 degrees of flexion. Experimental studies[30] have demonstrated a progressive thickening of the external and internal epineurium as well as thickening of the perineurium. A progressive thinning of the myelin in large myelinated fibers was noted. This change was more pronounced in the peripheral than in the central fascicles of the nerve. This suggests a basis for the patient who presents with marked symptoms but normal electrodiagnostic studies. The abnormal morphometric findings in the worst fascicles account for the symptoms, while the normal myelinated fibers in the best fascicles account for the normal electrodiagnostic findings. Persistent paresthesias are related to chronic alterations in the blood flow resulting from intraneural fibrosis.[29,30] The muscle wasting and loss of two-point discrimination found in advanced nerve compression are related to loss of nerve-fiber function.

ETIOLOGY

Wadsworth[48,49] classifies the cubital tunnel syndrome on an etiologic basis: (1) acute and subacute external compression, and (2) chronic internal compression caused by space-occupying lesions or lateral shift of the ulna (injury of the capitular epiphyses in childhood). Acute ulnar compression neuropathy can follow a single episode of blunt trauma such as fracture or dislocation of the elbow. Tardy ulnar palsy present in the adult as a consequence of injury about the elbow joint in childhood has been well documented.[17,21] However, tardy ulnar palsy in the child is an infrequent occurrence.[21] Congenital cubitus valgus deformity will result in chronic compression and dysfunction.[4] Childress[7] studied 2000 ulnar nerves in 1000 normal subjects and found an incidence of 16% with subluxation of the ulnar nerve from the humeral epicondylar groove during elbow flexion. Childress[7] defined two types of subluxation: (A) the nerve moves onto the tip of the epicondyle when the elbow is flexed to or beyond 90 degrees; and (B) the nerve passes completely across and anterior to the epicondyle when the elbow is completely flexed. Approximately 75% of ulnar nerves with recurring subluxation are type A. Excursion of the ulnar nerve across the epicondyle makes it more accessible to trauma from direct pressure.[27]

Compression of the ulnar nerve can result from fascial bands or from lesions within the cubital tunnel, such as arthritic spurs,[20] rheumatoid synovitis, muscle anomalies,[42,43] ganglia, lipomata, and other soft tissue tumors.

Cubital tunnel syndrome has followed elective surgery or confinement to bed for a variety of reasons.[48] Certain extremity positions, such as marked elbow flexion, put the ulnar nerve within the cubital tunnel at risk during operations. A prolonged period of extreme elbow flexion should be avoided in all chair-bound or bedridden patients. During a surgical procedure, the nerve should be protected by appropriate positioning of soft pads. Sleep position may account for some cases in which the patient observes that symptoms are present when the elbow is acutely flexed during sleep, but relieved by extending the elbow.

Diabetes, chronic alcoholism, and renal disease may increase the sensitivity of the ulnar nerve to compression. Hansen's disease should be considered if there is obvious thickening of the nerve.[33]

DIAGNOSIS

The first symptom of compression of the ulnar nerve near the elbow joint is sharp or aching pain on the medial side of the proximal forearm.[12,13] The pain may radiate proximally or distally and may be accompanied by paresthesias, dysesthesias, or anesthesia in the ring and little fingers. The exact distribution of sensory loss should be determined, because involvement of the dorsal cutaneous branch of the ulnar nerve establishes the lesion proximal to the wrist. The numbness, tingling, or "falling asleep" often is related to repetitive exercises or work involving the elbow. Severe pain

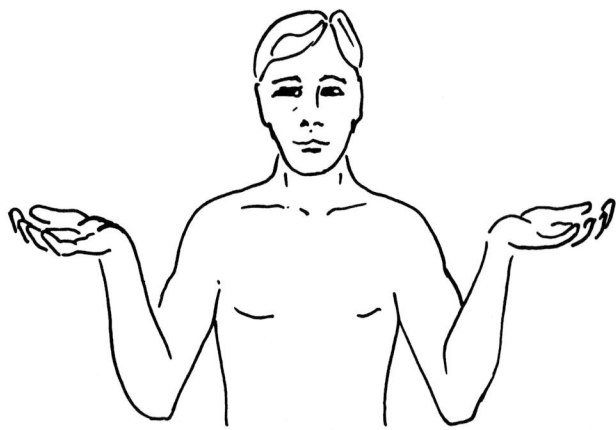

Fig. 38-2. The elbow flexion test, which increases pressure within the cubital canal similar to the wrist flexion test of Phalen. Note that the wrists are held in extension. (From Omer GE: The cubital tunnel syndrome. In Szabo RM: *Nerve compression syndromes: diagnosis and treatment,* Thorofare, NJ, 1989, Slack.)

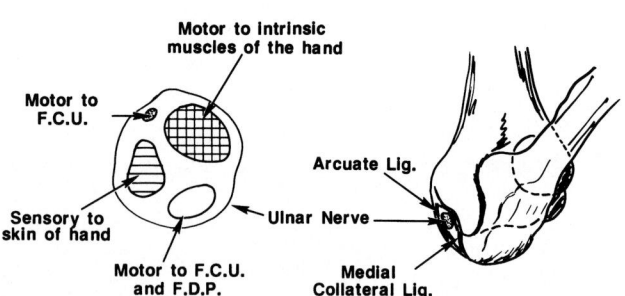

Fig. 38-3. Topography of the ulnar nerve in the cubital tunnel. The intrinsic muscle fibers and cutaneous sensory fibers lie superficially under the arcuate ligament and are very vulnerable to external compressive force. *F.C.U.,* Flexor carpi ulnaris; *F.D.P.,* flexor digitorum profundus. (From Omer GE: The cubital tunnel syndrome. In Szabo RM: *Nerve compression syndromes: diagnosis and treatment,* Thorofare, NJ, 1989, Slack.)

in the hand is not as common as in carpal tunnel syndrome.[16] Localizing physical findings are a positive percussion test over the ulnar nerve at the elbow, abnormal mobility of the ulnar nerve over the medial epicondyle of the humerus, or a positive elbow flexion test of Wadsworth[48] (Fig. 38-2).

Patients complain of weakness and loss of dexterity for handling objects. A more recognizable clinical feature is atrophy of the intrinsic muscles with clawing of the ring and little fingers. When weakness of the extrinsic flexor carpi ulnaris muscle and the flexor digitorum profundus muscle to the little finger is demonstrated, the ulnar neuropathy can be localized at the elbow. Sunderland's studies[46] of the intraneural topography of the ulnar nerve show that the sensory axons and the intrinsic motor axons lie in a more vulnerable superficial position within the ulnar nerve at the elbow, while the motor axons to the flexor carpi ulnaris and flexor digitorum profundus muscles are deep within the nerve and relatively protected from pressure (Fig. 38-3).

A nerve conduction velocity study is usually expressed in meters per second.[18,39] The loss of the evoked sensory potential is a very sensitive indicator of altered conduction.[1] Reduced velocities of less than 25% are probably not significant, but greater than 33% are always significant.[12,13] Electromyographic studies may show denervation potentials in the ulnar-innervated muscles and are consistent with cubital tunnel syndrome when nerve conduction velocity is less than 41 mm per second or the conduction latency across the elbow is greater than 9 or 10 mm per second.[11] It is important to remember that a peripheral nerve can be entrapped simultaneously at two levels.[36,37] Degenerative disc disease, with C8 root ra-

diculopathy, is more likely to involve the radial aspect of the ring finger than more distal lesions at the elbow.[6] Roentgenographic studies should be done to determine the degree of cubitus valgus or evaluate bony lesions compromising the cubital tunnel. Wadsworth[48] described a cubital tunnel view as a slightly oblique anteroposterior view with the elbow in full flexion and the arm externally rotated about 20 degrees.

McGowan[34] developed a clinical classification of ulnar neuropathy: Grade I has no detectable motor weakness in the hand; grade II has weakness of the interosseoi and the ulnar-innervated lumbricals, and grade III demonstrates paralysis of one or more of the ulnar intrinsic muscles.

TREATMENT
Conservative treatment

In the early case, management includes education of the patient regarding sleep positions and protection of the nerves from the edges of furniture and other potentially sharp objects. The patient should avoid repetitive flexion and extension of the elbow, such as occurs when a carpenter uses a hammer. In hospitalized patients with instructions for strict bed rest, lamb's wool elbow pads are useful, and the overhead "monkey bar" should be used to move about the bed.[25] The arms should be extended during the recovery period as well as during an operation. Local heat and ultrasound may be applied, while antiinflammatory agents could be prescribed.[10,33] Once an ulnar nerve becomes symptomatic, either spontaneously or secondary to identified trauma, the symptoms persist. The accepted treatment of an established cubital tunnel syndrome is surgical.

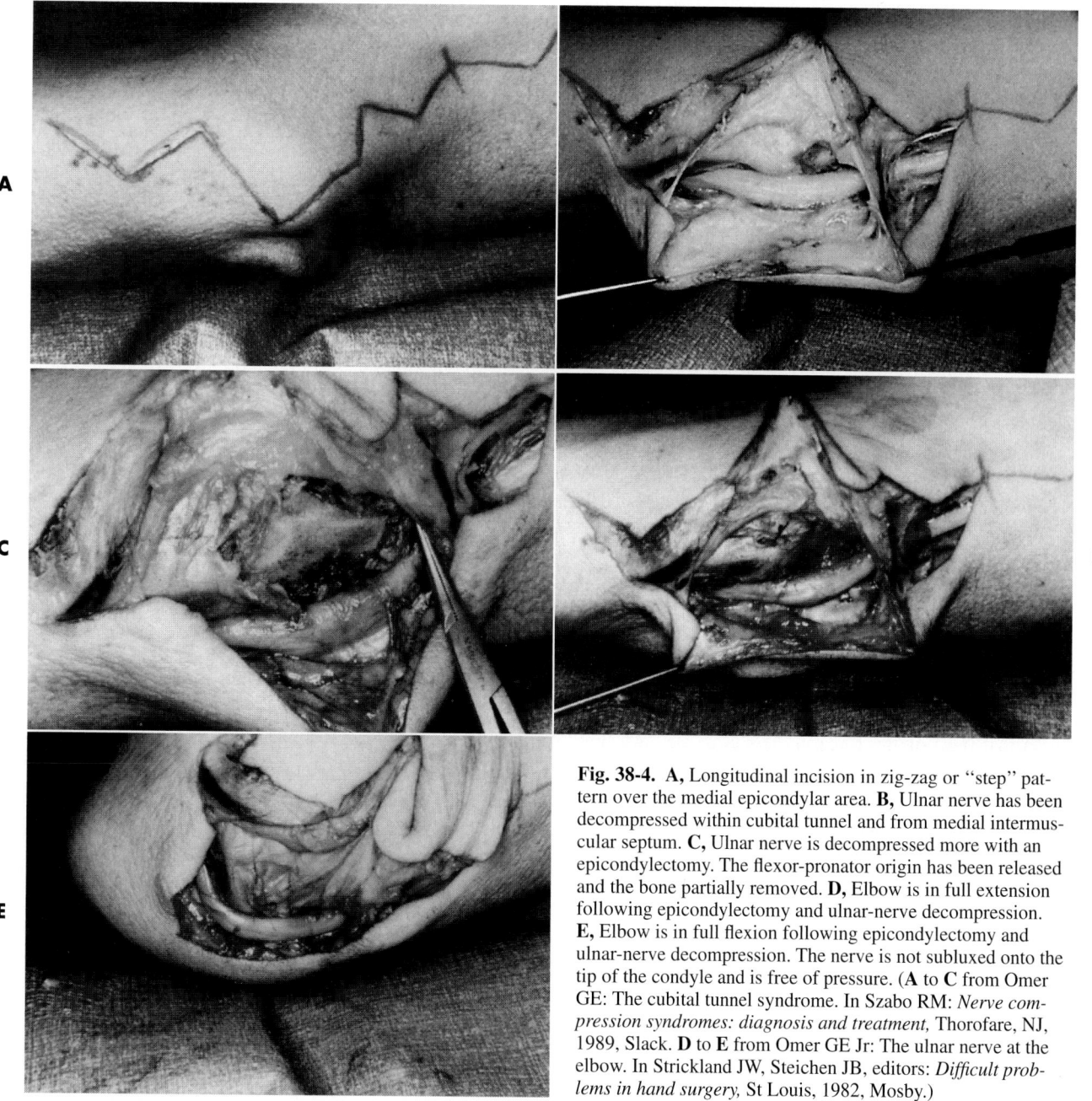

Fig. 38-4. **A,** Longitudinal incision in zig-zag or "step" pattern over the medial epicondylar area. **B,** Ulnar nerve has been decompressed within cubital tunnel and from medial intermuscular septum. **C,** Ulnar nerve is decompressed more with an epicondylectomy. The flexor-pronator origin has been released and the bone partially removed. **D,** Elbow is in full extension following epicondylectomy and ulnar-nerve decompression. **E,** Elbow is in full flexion following epicondylectomy and ulnar-nerve decompression. The nerve is not subluxed onto the tip of the condyle and is free of pressure. (**A** to **C** from Omer GE: The cubital tunnel syndrome. In Szabo RM: *Nerve compression syndromes: diagnosis and treatment,* Thorofare, NJ, 1989, Slack. **D** to **E** from Omer GE Jr: The ulnar nerve at the elbow. In Strickland JW, Steichen JB, editors: *Difficult problems in hand surgery,* St Louis, 1982, Mosby.)

Nerve decompression

The surgical approach is a posteromedial longitudinal incision that is a series of 60-degree "steps" or turns (Fig. 38-4, *A*). The incision should extend 8 to 10 cm proximal to the medial epicondyle and an equal distal distance to the flexor carpi ulnaris muscle. The purpose of this procedure is to decompress the nerve, but also to retain the vincula-like deep attachments that contain the segmental blood supply to the nerve. The nerve should not sublux from the humeral epicondylar groove when the elbow is flexed.

In every case, the ulnar nerve must be released from tight fibrous bands. Proximal to the medial epicondyle, the medial intermuscular septum forms a taut fibrous ridge. A section of this fascial septum must be excised to prevent kinking of the nerve.[27] The ulnar nerve should be freed for at least 8 cm proximal to the medial epicondyle to determine if the nerve is entrapped in the arcade of Struthers[44,45] or entrapped on the medial intermuscular septum. Failure to release the nerve proximally will lead to continued ulnar neuropathy (see Fig. 38-4, *B*).

The aponeurotic roof of the cubital tunnel should be incised and the area inspected. An hourglass compression of the ulnar nerve at the proximal edge of the aponeurotic roof suggests an epineurotomy or an internal neurolysis. My experience has been that epineurotomy is useful in restoring a circulatory blush across a compressed segment, but there is no direct relationship between intraneural neurolysis and improved sensory or motor function of the ulnar nerve. A saline neurolysis is never indicated. A more reliable prognostic indicator is the duration of clinical symptoms, and a McGowan[34] Grade III lesion does not recover function following intraneural neurolysis.

Fixation of the ulnar nerve at the level of the medial epicondylar groove can result in traction neuritis.[2,22,50] Condensation of connective tissue and aponeurotic bands should be released. Bone fragments must be removed. The groove should be carefully inspected, because friction neuritis can develop with repeated movement of the ulnar nerve against osteophytes or bony spurs of the distal aspect of the humerus. The aponeurotic roof of the cubital tunnel may be utilized as a fasciodermal sling[10] or excised. The superior ulnar collateral artery, which accompanies the ulnar nerve in the condylar groove, should not be injured.

I prefer to leave the ulnar nerve attached to the soft tissue in the depth of the groove and within the cubital tunnel, provided this vincula-like tissue is elastic and not fibrotic. The fibrous arcade over the flexor carpi ulnaris is incised, and the ulnar nerve should be explored to the midportion of the proximal third of the forearm. The ulnar nerve is not disturbed in its bed. After the nerve is decompressed, the elbow should be extended and flexed to observe the excursion of the nerve trunk. If the nerve is compressed against the posterior aspect of the medial epicondyle, but is not subluxing across the medial epicondyle, an epicondylectomy is indicated (Fig. 38-4, C).

Epicondylectomy

Removal of the medial epicondyle permits the ulnar nerve to be under minimal tension during extension and flexion of the elbow.[8,16,23,24,35] The ulnar nerve is decompressed without releasing it from the condylar groove, as previously described. The humeral medial epicondyle is exposed by sharp subperiosteal dissection, reflecting the common origin of the flexor-pronator muscles. After the medial epicondyle and the adjacent supracondylar ridge are exposed, both are removed with a bone saw or osteotomes (Fig. 38-4, D). The ulnar nerve is protected with a broad-blade retractor. The medial collateral ligament and its bony attachments must remain intact. Bony spurs are removed with a rongeur. The flexor-pronator muscle flap is reattached to the redundant periosteal flaps, leaving a smooth buttress for the ulnar nerve, which should not be compressed by the remaining medial epicondyle during flexion. I deflate the tourniquet and ensure hemostasis before subcutaneous and skin closure (Fig. 38-4, E).

Subcutaneous transposition

If there is subluxation of the ulnar nerve across the medial epicondyle with flexion of the elbow after decompression, anterior subcutaneous transposition is indicated. Curtis is reported[3,10] to have described in 1898 a technique for subcutaneous anterior transposition of the ulnar nerve, and the procedure was standardized by Platt.[41] After the ulnar nerve is exposed from at least 8 cm above the medial epicondyle to between the heads of the flexor carpi ulnaris muscle in the proximal forearm, the nerve is mobilized as a neurovascular bundle that includes both the arteries and veins that accompany the nerve. The neurovascular bundle is transposed anteriorly beneath the elevated skin flap. Eaton, Crowe, and Parkes[10] have described a fasciodermal sling to support the transposed ulnar nerve. A flap of antebrachial fascial 1 cm wide and 1 cm long, based on the medial epicondyle, is raised and reflected medially. The fascial flap is passed posterior to the transposed ulnar nerve and is sutured to the subcutaneous tissue anterior to the medial epicondyle, preventing the ulnar nerve from returning to its original position. Subcutaneous slings have been reported to result in constriction or kinking of the ulnar nerve,[3,28] and these procedures are not indicated unless there has been symptomatic subluxation prior to surgery.

Submuscular transposition

Submuscular transposition of the ulnar nerve is indicated for a Childress[7] type B subluxation, where the nerve passes completely across and anterior to the medial epicondyle when the elbow is flexed. In addition, submuscular transposition should be considered in cases with severe hypertrophic osteoarthritis.[47]

Learmonth[26] decompresses the ulnar nerve from the point where it penetrates the medial intermuscular septum to beyond the cubital tunnel. The flexor-pronator muscle mass is detached from the medial epicondyle and turned distally and radially to expose the median nerve. The ulnar nerve is transposed to lie alongside the median nerve on the brachialis muscle. The flexor-pronator muscle origin is then reattached to the medial epicondyle. This procedure permits arthrotomy of the elbow joint and inspection of the medial collateral ligament.[9] The technique has been modified by performing an osteotomy of the medial epicondyle with the attached flexor-pronator muscles and then reattaching the epicondyle with screw fixation.[27,32] Fibrous constriction of the ulnar nerve has been observed following submuscular transposition.[16] Campbell, Morantz, and Post[5] have recommended encasing the ulnar nerve in a silastic sleeve to halt progressive fibrosis.

POSTOPERATIVE CARE

A bulky soft dressing is used for 24 to 48 hours after nerve decompression. If an epicondylectomy has been done, the soft dressing is replaced with a posterior plaster splint with the elbow in 90 degrees of flexion for 2 weeks. If the nerve has been transposed, the elbow is immobilized in 90 degrees of flexion and the forearm fully pronated. The initial bulky dressing is replaced by a long arm plaster dressing for 3 weeks. Active range-of-motion exercises are then initiated, with emphasis on regaining full extension at the elbow.

RESULTS

Treatment by in situ decompression, anterior subcutaneous transposition, and submuscular transposition have all been reported to produce satisfactory results.[1,27,34,47] Pain is usually relieved, and other sensory symptoms show consistent improvement. Improvement of the evoked sensory potential correlates well with improvement in clinical symptoms.[1] However, weakness tends to persist, and intrinsic muscular atrophy is the least likely to improve.[1,16,19,31] There is little prognostic difference between successful surgical procedures, but a guarded prognosis always should be given with secondary transposition.[3] The potential for full motor recovery after operation is greatly reduced in those patients in whom preoperative symptoms have been present for more than 1 year or who have intrinsic muscle atrophy before surgery.

REFERENCES

1. Adelaar RS, Foster WC, McDowell C: The treatment of the cubital tunnel syndrome, *J Hand Surg* 9A:90, 1984.
2. Apfelbert DB, Larson SJ: Dynamic anatomy of the ulnar nerve at the elbow, *Plast Reconstr Surg* 51:76, 1973.
3. Broudy AS, Leffert RD, Smith RJ: Technical problems with ulnar nerve transposition at the elbow: findings and results of reoperation, *J Hand Surg* 3:85, 1978.
4. Burman MS, Sutro CJ: Recurrent luxation of the ulnar nerve by congenital posterior position of the medial epicondyle of the humerus, *J Bone Joint Surg* 21:958, 1939.
5. Campbell JB, Morantz RA, Post KD: A technique for relief of motor and sensory deficits occurring after anterior ulnar transposition, *J Neurosurg* 40:405, 1974.
6. Chaplin E, Kasdan ML, Corwin HM: Occupational neurology and the hand: differential diagnosis, *Hand Clin* 2:513, 1986.
7. Childress HM: Recurrent ulnar-nerve dislocation at the elbow, *Clin Orthop* 108:168, 1975.
8. Craven PR, Green DP: Cubital tunnel syndrome: treatment by epicondylectomy, *J Bone Joint Surg* 62A:986, 1980.
9. Del Pizzo W, Jobe FW, Norwood L: Ulnar nerve entrapment syndrome in baseball players, *Am J Sports Med* 5:182, 1977.
10. Eaton RG, Crowe JF, Parkes JC III: Anterior transposition of the ulnar nerve using a non-compressing fasciodermal sling, *J Bone Joint Surg* 62A:820, 1980.
11. Eisen A, Danon J: The mild cubital tunnel syndrome: its natural history and indications for surgical intervention, *Neurol* 24:608, 1974.
12. Eversmann WW Jr: Entrapment and compression neuropathies. In Green DP, editor: *Operative hand surgery,* New York, 1982, Churchill Livingstone.
13. Eversmann WW Jr: Compression and entrapment neuropathies of the upper extremity, *J Hand Surg* 8:759, 1983.
14. Feindel W, Stratford J: Cubital tunnel compression in tardy ulnar palsy, *Can Med Assoc J* 78:351, 1958.
15. Feindel W, Stratford J: Cubital tunnel palsy in tardy ulnar palsy, *Can J Surg* 1:287, 1958.
16. Froimson AI, Zahrawi F: Treatment of compression neuropathy of the ulnar nerve at the elbow by epicondylectomy and neurolysis, *J Hand Surg* 5:391, 1980.
17. Gay JR, Love JG: Diagnosis and treatment of tardy paralysis of the ulnar nerve, *J Bone Joint Surg* 29A:1087, 1947.
18. Gilliatt RW, Thomas PK: Changes in nerve conduction with ulnar nerve lesions at the elbow, *J Neurol Neurosurg Psychiatry* 23:312, 1960.
19. Harrison MJG, Nurick S: Results of anterior transposition of the ulnar nerve for ulnar neuritis, *Br Med J* 1:27, 1970.
20. Hecht O, Lipsher E: Median and ulnar nerve entrapment caused by ectopic calcification, *J Hand Surg* 5:30, 1980.
21. Holmes JC, Hall JE: Tardy ulnar nerve palsy in children, *Clin Orthop* 135:128, 1978.
22. Inglis AE, Kinnett G: Ulnar neuropathy at the elbow: Proceedings of the American Society for Surgery of the Hand, *J Hand Surg* 3:290, 1978.
23. Jones RE, Gauntt C: Medial epicondylectomy for ulnar nerve compression syndrome at the elbow, *Clin Orthop* 139:174, 1979.
24. King T, Morgan F: The treatment of traumatic ulnar neuritis, *Aust NZ J Surg* 20:33, 1950.
25. Lazaro L III: Ulnar nerve instability: ulnar nerve injury due to elbow flexion, *South Med J* 70:36, 1977.
26. Learmonth JR: A technique for transplanting the ulnar nerve, *Surg Gynecol Obstet* 75:792, 1943.
27. Levy DM, Apfelberg DB: Results of anterior transposition for ulnar neuropathy at the elbow, *Am J Surg* 123:304, 1972.
28. Lulch AL: Ulnar nerve entrapment after anterior transposition at the elbow, *NY State J* 75:75, 1975.
29. Lundborg G, et al.: Median nerve compression in the carpal tunnel: functional response to experimentally induced controlled pressure, *J Hand Surg* 7:252, 1982.
30. Mackinnon SE, Dellon AL: Experimental study of chronic nerve compression, *Hand Clin* 2:639, 1986.
31. Macnicol MF: The results of operation for ulnar neuritis, *J Bone Joint Surg* 61B:159, 1979.
32. Mass DP, Silverberg B: Cubital tunnel syndrome: anterior transposition with epicondylar osteotomy, *Orthopaedics* 9:711, 1986.
33. McFarland GB: Entrapment syndromes. In McEvarts C, Burton RI, editors: *Surgery of the musculoskeletal system,* New York, 1983, Churchill Livingstone.
34. McGowan AJ: The results of transposition of the ulnar nerve for traumatic ulnar neuritis, *J Bone Joint Surg* 32B:293, 1950.
35. Neblett C, Ehni G: Medial epicondylectomy for ulnar palsy, *J Neurosurg* 32:55, 1970.
36. Omer GE Jr: Pitfalls in the management of peripheral nerve injuries, *Bull NY Acad Med* 55:829, 1979.
37. Omer GE Jr: The ulnar nerve at the elbow. In Strickland JW, Steichen JB, editors: *Difficult problems in hand surgery,* St Louis, 1982, Mosby.
38. Osborne GV: Compression neuritis of the ulnar nerve at the elbow, *Hand* 2:10, 1970.
39. Payan J: Electrophysiological localization of ulnar nerve lesions, *J Neurol Neurosurg Psychiatry* 32:208, 1969.
40. Pechan J, Julis I: The pressure measurement in the ulnar nerve: a contribution to the pathophysiology of the cubital tunnel syndrome, *J Biomechanics* 8:75, 1975.
41. Platt H: The operative treatment of traumatic neuritis at the elbow, *Surg Gynecol Obstet* 47:822, 1928.
42. Rolfsen L: Snapping triceps tendon with ulnar neuritis, *Acta Orthop Scand* 41:74, 1970.
43. Spinner M: *Injuries to the major branches of peripheral nerves in the forearm,* ed 2, Philadelphia, 1978, WB Saunders.
44. Spinner M: Management of nerve compression lesions of the upper extremity. In Omer GE Jr, Spinner M, editors: *Management of peripheral nerve problems,* Philadelphia, 1980, WB Saunders.

45. Spinner M: Management of nerve compression lesions. *Instr Course Lect* 33:498, 1984.
46. Sunderland S: The intraneural topography of the radial, median, and ulnar nerves, *Brain* 68:243, 1945.
47. Vanderpool DW, et al., Peripheral compression lesions of the ulnar nerve, *J Bone Joint Surg* 50B:792, 1968.
48. Wadsworth TG: The external compression syndrome of the ulnar nerve at the cubital tunnel, *Clin Orthop* 124:189, 1977.
49. Wadsworth TG: *The elbow,* Edinburgh, 1982, Churchill Livingstone.
50. Wilson DH, Krout R: Surgery of ulnar neuropathy at the elbow: 16 cases treated by decompression without transposition: technical note, *J Neurosurg* 38:780, 1973.

Chapter 39

THERAPIST'S MANAGEMENT OF ULNAR NERVE NEUROPATHY AT THE ELBOW

Susan M. Blackmore

Neuropathy of the ulnar nerve at the elbow is caused by compression or traction on the nerve.[55] The terms used in the literature to describe ulnar neuropathy at the elbow include *compressive ulnar neuropathy,*[33,55] *ulnar-nerve entrapment syndrome,*[18] *traumatic ulnar neuritis,*[9,34,37,55] *tardy ulnar-nerve palsy,*[10,23,26,48,51] and more recently, *cubital tunnel syndrome.*[40] The term *cubital tunnel syndrome* is used in this chapter.

Cubital tunnel syndrome is the second most common nerve entrapment syndrome in the upper extremity after carpal tunnel syndrome.[47,49,55] The five potential sites for nerve entrapment at the elbow are the arcade of Struthers, the medial intramuscular septum, the medial epicondyle, the cubital tunnel, and the deep aponeurosis of the flexor carpi ulnaris (FCU)[1,22,57] (Fig. 39-1).

The purpose of this chapter is to describe the clinical presentation, related diagnoses, nonoperative management, and postoperative management of cubital tunnel syndrome. The anatomy, physician's evaluation, diagnostic criteria, and surgical management are described in Chapter 38. The therapist's clinical decision making for the management of cubital tunnel syndrome requires a thorough understanding of anatomy and the possible pathophysiologic mechanisms involved in nerve compression. The therapist's clinical decision making requires consideration of objective findings of sensory motor function, consideration of the patient's subjective report of symptoms, and ongoing assessment of the patient's response to treatment.

CLINICAL PRESENTATION

The symptoms of cubital tunnel syndrome include sensory and motor dysfunction. Symptoms can include pain that is sharp or aching in nature and that is located primarily on the medial side of the proximal forearm.* Pain for some patients can be diffuse and radiate proximally and distally in the arm. Paresthesias, dysesthesias, anesthesia, or a feeling of coldness may be present in the ulnar-nerve distribution. The sensory symptoms often begin at night because the elbow tends to be maintained in flexion during sleep.

Muscle weakness or atrophy may be observed in the ulnar-innervated muscles in the hand. Clawing of the hand may be seen if the ulnar intrinsic muscles are weak. Clawing is more pronounced when ulnar neuropathy occurs at Guyon's canal, when the ulnar intrinsic muscles are weak and the flexor digitorum profundus (FDP) is intact.[34,55] When the ulnar neuropathy occurs at the elbow, the FDP may also be weak, so clawing is less pronounced. The strength of the ring and small FDP can be an important diagnostic tool to help determine the level of compression of the ulnar nerve.[34] A positive Wartenberg's sign is present if the fifth finger is held abducted from the fourth because of interosseous weakness.[62] Froment's sign is present if the patient attempts to perform powerful lateral pinch and the interphalangeal (IP) joint of the thumb flexes because of reliance on the flexor pollicis longus (FPL). This sign indicates weakness or paralysis of the adductor pollicis (AP) and the deep head of the flexor pollicis brevis (FPB)[34,40] (see Chapter 8). Functional limitations for the patient with weakness or paralysis of ulnar-innervated muscles include weakness of pinch, decreased gross grasp strength, and dropping of objects out of the hand. The symptoms often are aggravated by repetitive elbow use and maintained elbow flexion.

*References 15, 17, 18, 34, 40, 47, 55.

679

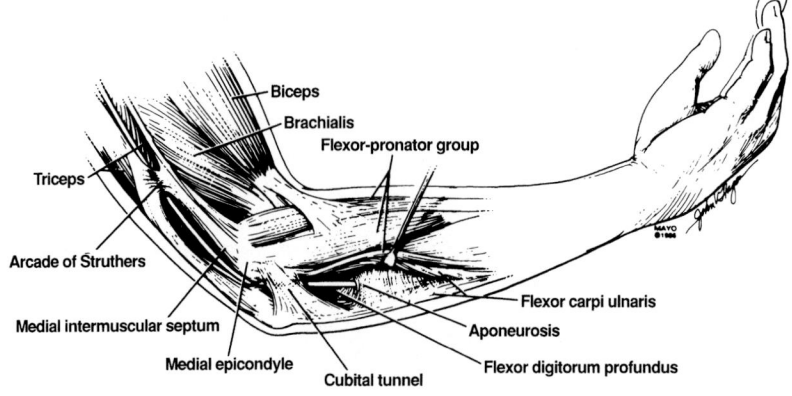

Fig. 39-1. Anatomy of the ulnar nerve at the elbow, which illustrates the five potential sites for nerve entrapment. (Copyright The Mayo Foundation. From Amadio PC: *Surg Radiol Anat* 8:155, 1986.)

Symptoms may be diminished with the elbow held in extension.[40,55]

The patient's pertinent medical history assists the physician with diagnosis, choices for either operative or nonoperative management, and prognosis. In addition to a standard history intake interview, a patient is asked about the following: (1) the description, history, duration, and irritability of the symptoms; (2) previous elbow trauma or event that led to the symptoms; (3) other orthopedic or neurologic history; (4) similar symptoms in other locations; (5) history of systemic problems; and (6) the types of activities, postures, or positions that increase or decrease the symptoms.[3,7,40]

RELATED DIAGNOSES

Localization of ulnar neuropathy to the cubital tunnel requires other potential diagnoses to be ruled out. Most commonly, differential diagnosis involves ruling out alternative sites of compression, including Guyon's canal, thoracic outlet, the cervical spine, and a double crush lesion.[18,27,40,55] Other diagnoses that mimic the symptoms of ulnar neuropathy include Pancoast tumor at the apex of the lung, intraspinal pathology, amyotrophic lateral sclerosis, diabetes, Hansen's disease, chronic alcoholism, hemophilia, and renal disease.[4,27,34,40,47,59,61]

NONOPERATIVE MANAGEMENT

If a patient presents with early and mild sensory symptoms, no motor changes, and no impinging pathology noted, a trial of nonoperative management is considered.[4,21,27,50,61] Nonoperative management may not be appropriate for patients with space-occupying lesions, recent trauma, systemic disease,[15] nerve subluxation,[47] or any condition in which the anatomy of the structures around the elbow contribute to the nerve compression.[50] If nonoperative management is prescribed, the therapist performs a thorough evaluation including subjective and objective testing.[3] Objective testing particular to the ulnar nerve is described in the following sections.

Evaluation

The physician's physical examination usually includes many of the following tests (see Chapter 38). However, in some cases, a generalist refers the patient for a nonoperative program, so these tests may not have been performed. In other instances, the therapist may be the first to see the signs of developing cubital tunnel syndrome, even if the patient is being treated for another limitation (e.g., following a fracture to the olecranon, the ulnar nerve can become fixed in scar). The information is described in this chapter to ensure that the therapist has this information available or performs the tests personally. After a thorough history is performed and subjective information has been obtained, the evaluation begins with upper extremity active range-of-motion (AROM) measurements. The upper quarter is assessed to rule out proximal nerve compression (see Chapter 7). The arm is then inspected for masses or deformities. The nerve is palpated at the cubital tunnel with the elbow in flexion to assess for anterior subluxation and irritability of the nerve. A percussion (Tinel's) test is performed by gently tapping just proximal to the cubital tunnel and at Guyon's canal to assess for nerve irritability.

The elbow flexion test is a provocative maneuver used to assist with localization of compressive neuropathy to the elbow. Apfelberg and Larson[2] demonstrated a narrowing of the cubital tunnel with maximal elbow flexion. Classically, the test is performed by fully passively flexing the patient's elbow, with the forearm in supination and the shoulder and wrist in neutral for 1 minute.[2,56,57] A more recent modification of the test position by Buehler is with "the arm in the anatomical position, the elbow actively but not forcefully flexed, and full extension of the wrist to maximize compressive and tensile forces at the nerve."[6] This position is maintained for 3 minutes. However, Buehler's modification also compresses the ulnar nerve at Guyon's canal and the median nerve at the carpal tunnel. A positive test result for either the classic or modified positions results in pain and paresthesia or numbness in the ulnar-nerve distribution. Rayan et al.[56] performed the classic elbow flexion test on a

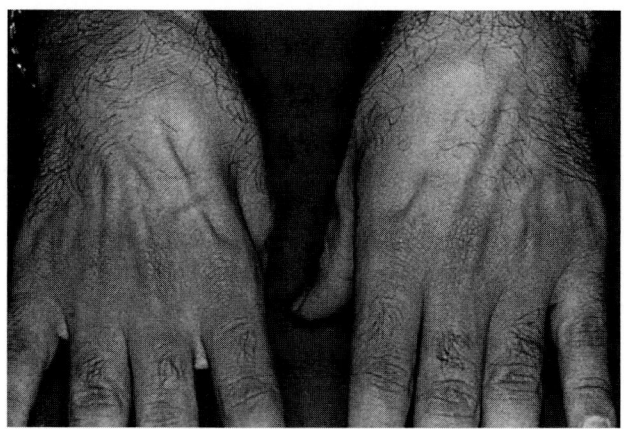

Fig. 39-2. Significant adductor pollicis wasting indicating severe ulnar-nerve neuropathy.

normal, nonsymptomatic population and found 10% to 13% with a positive test result. Novak et al.[45] compared three provocative tests for cubital tunnel on both normal subjects and those with a diagnosis of cubital tunnel syndrome. The provocative tests performed included Tinel's test, elbow flexion test,[2] and combined elbow flexion test and pressure applied just proximal to the cubital tunnel. If the nerve was subluxed, pressure was applied over the nerve in its subluxed position. The authors determined that the combined elbow flexion test with pressure provocation had the highest sensitivity, specificity and positive prediction values within 30 seconds.[45] Other provocative tests are the base nerve tension tests as described by Butler.[7] These tests can be performed to further assess the site and nature of ulnar-nerve compression (see Chapter 45).

The physician usually examines roentgenographic studies as a part of the routine evaluation to assess for any degree of cubitus valgus, skeletal abnormalities, or bony lesions in the cubital tunnel.[24,34,40]

The physician often orders electrodiagnostic testing, including nerve conduction velocities and electromyographic (EMG) testing. Many authors caution against the sole use of nerve conduction tests as an indication for surgery. The patient must have accompanying signs and symptoms.[15,18,27,40,59]

The muscular system is assessed by noting any atrophy in the hypothenar, first web space, and medial forearm (Fig. 39-2). A manual muscle test[31] is performed to determine whether the pattern of muscle weakness correlates with ulnar-nerve innervation. Grip strength and pinch strength measurements may be diminished because of involvement of the interossei, ulnar lumbricals, FPB, AP, and FDP.[40,55]

Sensibility is evaluated with the Semmes-Weinstein monofilaments, static two-point discrimination, and moving two-point discrimination[60] (see Chapters 13 and 14). Decreased sensibility associated with cubital tunnel syndrome is noted on the volar and dorsal surfaces of the ulnar side of the palm, the fifth digit, and ulnar half of the fourth digit. It is important to test sensation for the dorsal cutaneous branch of the ulnar nerve, which innervates the dorsal ulnar side of the hand. This nerve branches proximal to Guyon's canal, so sensory impairment on the dorsum of the hand indicates a lesion proximal to Guyon's canal.[40,47]

Pain assessments can offer some valuable subjective information to help determine the effectiveness of the nonoperative management program. These assessments should be performed throughout treatment (see Chapter 106).

Treatment program

The components of a nonoperative program can include rest; patient education; modification of work, leisure activities, and activities of daily living (ADLs); edema control, use of physical agents, pain control, and strengthening. In addition, some therapists subscribe to nerve mobilization techniques[7] (see Chapter 45). It is not unusual to have a patient referred for a splint and home program rather than a full therapy program. In some instances, the physician will prescribe antiinflammatory medication.[59,61] Generally, local corticosteroid injections are avoided at the cubital tunnel.[25,54] There is little reference to use of injections at the cubital tunnel, and the reasons for the lack of use of injections are not well documented in the literature.[24,54]

Rest can range from avoidance of provocative activities[29,54] and use of pillows or soft supports wrapped around the elbow at night[54,59,61] to splinting throughout the day and night.[13,54,58] The intensity and duration of symptoms will guide the treatment choice. However, the patient who is symptomatic enough to seek medical advice will often require splinting. The purpose of splinting or the use of soft supports is to limit elbow flexion to no more than 90 degrees. The cubital tunnel is at its narrowest in full flexion, which contributes to nerve compression.[2,37] The position of full elbow extension allows for the least amount of nerve compression at the cubital tunnel. However, most patients do not tolerate full elbow extension splinting, so a position of 30 to 60 degrees of flexion is suggested.[12,27,58,61] A long-arm splint can be fabricated either anteriorly or posteriorly (Fig. 39-3). The wrist is included for patient comfort and to relax the FCU.[13] If a posterior splint is used, the elbow must be well padded or pressure must be relieved during fabrication of the splint to prevent placing surface pressure over the cubital tunnel.

Generally, at least a 3-week trial of nonoperative management with nighttime pads/splint is suggested for patients with intermittent or mild symptoms. If the symptoms do not improve with night pads/splint use, the splint also is worn during the day. Full-time splinting is suggested for patients with persistent symptoms. If symptoms improve, nonoperative management can continue as long as symptoms do not worsen. Generally, the physician follows the patient every 4 to 12 weeks to ensure compliance with the program and to monitor for any progression of the compression.[27]

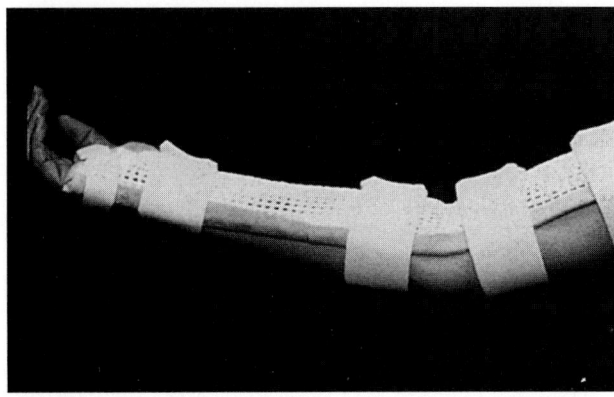

Fig. 39-3. A static splint that rests the elbow at 30 degrees and the wrist in neutral.

Patient education provides an opportunity to increase patient compliance with the program and to increase awareness of changes in symptoms. The anatomy, process of inflammation, nerve compression symptoms, activities and positions to avoid or modify, length of treatment for nonoperative management, and what to do if symptoms or weakness increase are reviewed in understandable terms. Activities and positions to avoid include repetitive elbow flexion and extension (e.g., hammering), maintained elbow flexion (e.g., holding the phone), traction on the arm (e.g., pulling a heavy cart), direct pressure on the nerve (e.g., resting the arm on the table), repetitive forearm rotation (e.g., turning pages), gripping with the elbow flexed and combined shoulder elevation, and elbow flexion with wrist extension (e.g., resting the hand on the top of the head).[54,58,61] For the patient with a double crush injury, general postural education can be useful. It is helpful to have the information in writing so that the patient can refer to the handouts later.

If the patient must perform a particular activity that places the nerve in a compromised position, the patient is given an alternative technique using ergonomic principles. Some ideas include using a phone headset, an elbow pad to disperse pressure on the elbow, and pushing rather than pulling a cart.[30,58] Tools may need to be modified to decrease elbow postures as well as to limit wrist flexion and forearm pronation. Overuse of the flexor-pronator muscle group may contribute to compression of the ulnar nerve at the elbow because the ulnar nerve lies between the two heads of the FCU.

Rest through splinting, activity modification, and ergonomic changes can help control the amount of edema contained in the osseous tunnel and around the nerve. Nerve irritation can occur for many reasons. The factors include inflammation around the nerve, neural ischemia, and/or scar tissue restricting the movement of the nerve as the patient changes positions from elbow extension to flexion. If the edema remains, the ulnar nerve and its blood supply become compromised as the contents of the tunnel increase. A prolonged inflammatory response may lead to extraneural adhesion formation or possibly neural ischemia[27,35,59] (see Chapter 38). In the future, we may be able to evaluate the cause for nerve irritation so that we can plan the appropriate nonoperative management program based on the condition of the nerve (see Chapter 45).

Cryotherapy for the purpose of decreasing inflammation can be applied for no longer than 15 minutes. Cold application when applied for longer periods can decrease motor and sensory nerve conduction velocity[41,42] (see Chapter 32). Other physical agents such as pulsed ultrasound, phonophoresis, or iontophoresis theoretically can help decrease inflammation (see Chapter 107). In the author's clinical experience, iontophoresis is poorly tolerated with this patient population. Edema control through use of compression wraps and massage directly over the cubital tunnel is not suggested. These two treatments apply pressure on the cubital tunnel, and this area does not tolerate pressure well.

Transcutaneous electrical nerve stimulation (TENS) may give some patients relief of discomfort from the sensory symptoms.[42] However, TENS should not be used to mask symptoms that may require surgical intervention. Some patients with cubital tunnel syndrome demonstrate muscular co-contraction around the elbow, and EMG biofeedback can be used for muscular relaxation. If hypersensitivity is present, desensitization techniques are explained and the patient performs the techniques frequently throughout the day.

Once symptoms are reduced, strengthening may be indicated for patients who perform lifting activities or maintain elbow postures throughout the day. With increased shoulder girdle strength and the use of proper body mechanics, effort for lifting can be transferred proximally. Wrist extensor strengthening can assist the patient in maintaining a neutral wrist position when lifting and may prevent overuse of the flexor-pronator muscle group. If muscle weakness is evident in the ulnar-innervated muscles, muscle reeducation and strengthening may be helpful to regain hand function if motor recovery is evident. In some cases, neuromuscular electrical nerve stimulation (NMES) may be helpful to isolate and reeducate the ulnar-innervated muscles.[52]

Nerve mobilization techniques[7,8] can be used in the nonoperative management program. However, the evidence for the effectiveness of these techniques has not yet been researched thoroughly. Positive clinical results will most likely drive the efforts for research. The understanding of the microanatomy of the nerve, pathophysiologic mechanisms involved in neuropathies, and clinical neurobiomechanics helps guide the therapist regarding treatment. The reader is referred to Chapter 45 and other references as guidelines.[7,8,16,36,37] Concepts of clinical neurobiomechanics involve understanding the movement and tension occurring in the nervous system. Structures such as muscle, ligament, and joints (i.e., extraneural structures) lie adjacent to the nerves and move independently of them.[7,16] The nervous system adapts to movement by (1) developing tension, (2) moving through extraneural structures (e.g., the ulnar nerve moving through the cubital tunnel), and (3) intrafascicular movement (i.e., nerve fibers unwinding or moving in relation to the endoneurium).[7,36,37,39,43]

Nerve mobilization techniques can be performed in therapy and as a part of a home program. This treatment approach may help decrease the symptoms and may help maintain improvements gained through nonoperative management. However, a nerve that is severely fixed in scar will not respond to nerve gliding and symptoms may actually worsen. There are three basic treatment approaches with nerve mobilization: (1) mobilization through tension tests and nerve palpation, (2) treatment via related tissues (muscles, joints), and (3) postural advice and ergonomic adaptations.[7] I suggest that the therapist desiring to use these evaluations and techniques consult additional references and attend practical course sessions to ensure appropriate application (see Chapter 45).

Conclusions for nonoperative management

In general, if nonoperative management is chosen, a decrease in the symptoms should be noted within 3 weeks. The decrease in symptoms should be apparent both subjectively and through physical examination.[27,54] Nonoperative management can then continue until symptoms are resolved or stop improving. During this time, the physician follows up on the patient to ensure continued improvement is occurring. Patients may require intermittent splinting and a maintenance home program to ensure resolution of symptoms. Reported successful results from a nonoperative program vary from 50%,[11] 86%,[13] to 90%.[15] Dellon et al.[12] performed a prospective study to determine factors that would identify patients who would most positively respond to nonoperative treatment. Of patients with mild disease, 21% responded initially and then required surgery within the next 6 years. Dellon et al. found those patients who had a history of elbow trauma and/or diabetes did less favorably in a nonoperative treatment program. Limitations of the studies include the lack of a full description of the nonoperative program and unclear staging of the nerve compression.

Bednar et al.[5] identified the following as possible contributing factors when nonoperative management is unsuccessful: treatment of patients with moderate or severe disease with a nonoperative program, patient noncompliance, and failure to follow the patient for signs of progression. If conservative management is unsuccessful, the patient is reevaluated by the physician. If the patient's history, physical examination, and testing indicate a localized nerve lesion, surgery may be recommended.[34,54,61]

OPERATIVE TREATMENT

Several surgical options are available for the management of cubital tunnel syndrome. The support and limitations for each type of procedure are documented in the surgical literature and in Chapter 38. There are several explanations for the fact that there are six surgical options remaining after more than 100 years of critical review in the literature. There are different grading systems for the degree of nerve compression and postoperative results, so it is difficult to compare results among studies.[11] The techniques involved in the surgical procedures have been adapted over the years, such that medial epicondylectomy in one report[20] may not be like another medial epicondylectomy in another report.[24] Finally, many factors contribute to cubital tunnel syndrome, and all of these factors play a role in the recovery of the patient.

The therapist must understand (and in the best case observe) the types of surgical procedures performed to relieve ulnar-nerve compression at the elbow. The therapist should discuss with the surgeon which type of procedure was performed or obtain an operative report before treating the patient. Some surgeons will choose to perform a combination of procedures. For example, decompression is performed along with a release of additional sites of tissue restriction. Chapter 38 provides an overview of the various procedures to enable the therapist to understand why and what structures require protection or early mobilization.

POSTOPERATIVE REHABILITATION

Postoperative rehabilitation is divided into three progressive stages: protection, active motion, and strengthening. The protective stage varies from postoperative day 1 and may last until week 3. The active-motion stage varies from beginning on day 1 to week 3 and lasts until week 5 or 6. The strengthening stage may begin as early as week 5 or 7 and continues as needed. These time frames serve as only a guideline to discuss the progression of treatment with the referring physician. However, these time frames vary widely in the literature. The timetables for treatment are more often based on personal preference than data from clinical trials. The timetable must be adapted to the patient's level of symptoms and wound healing response after surgery. Indications for modification of the treatment progression include excessive edema, significantly limited motion, and rapid scar formation. If edema increases, the patient is maintained on an active-motion program until the edema reduces. If range of motion (ROM) is limited and there is rapid scar formation, the patient may be advanced earlier to active-assisted range of motion (AAROM). Generally, if the flexor-pronator muscle origin has been reflected and reattached in surgery, the initiation of AROM for the elbow, forearm, and wrist may be delayed for up to 3 weeks to allow the reattachment to be secure enough to withstand motion.

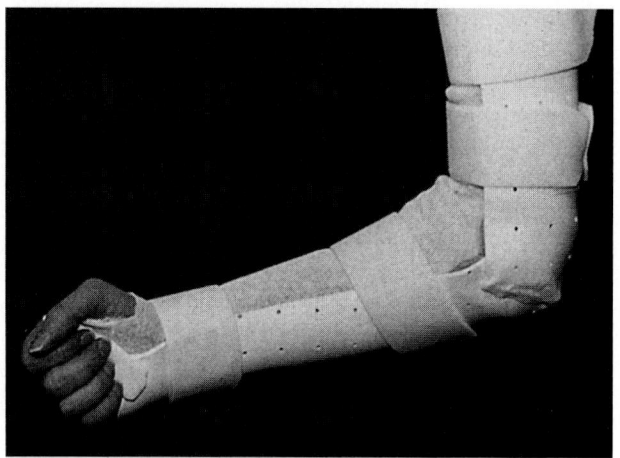

Fig. 39-4. A long-arm static splint rests the elbow at 70 degrees of flexion, neutral forearm rotation, and neutral wrist.

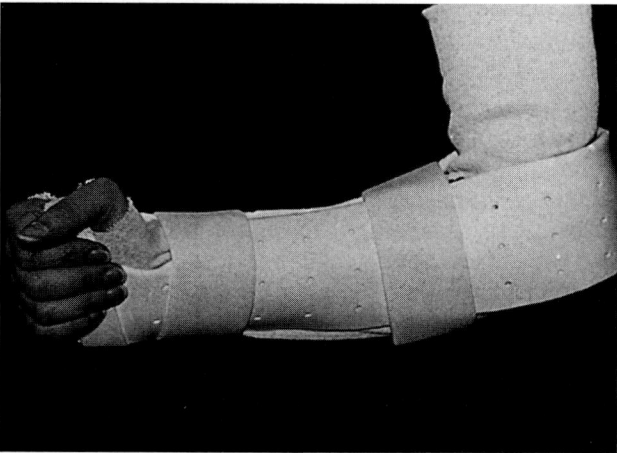

Fig. 39-5. A sugar-tong splint rests the forearm and wrist in neutral and allows for minimal elbow movement.

At the time of initial referral, the following information is obtained: (1) precautions, (2) type of surgery, (3) findings at surgery (e.g., condition of the nerve), (4) type of splint, and (5) timing for stages of treatment. After gathering the necessary information, the therapist initiates evaluation and treatment. Treatment may involve instructions and a follow-up visit for a home program, or the patient may attend therapy regularly.

Stage I: protection (day 1 through week 3)

Evaluation. The evaluation during this stage of treatment is limited by postoperative precautions. A medical and symptom history is taken.[3] Other concomitant diseases, conditions, or injuries may also affect the treatment plan (e.g., a carpal tunnel release performed at the same time). The wound is inspected, and edema can be assessed visually and circumferentially. Edema within the joint capsule presents as a fullness in the infracondylar recesses on the posterior side of the elbow. Pain is assessed through standard pain assessment tools (see Chapter 106). ADLs are assessed because the patient is often using one-handed techniques. AROM measurements are taken for the shoulder and hand. If there are no restrictions on AROM for the elbow, forearm, and wrist (per physician prescription), these measurements also are documented. Depending on the surgery performed, the protective stage may last for only a few days.

Splinting. Postoperative protection varies considerably at this stage. The defining factor is whether the flexor-pronator muscle mass was reflected and surgically reattached to its origin during the operation. In most of these cases (anterior submuscular, anterior intramuscular, and in some medial epicondylectomies), a splint or posterior cast is used to limit elbow, wrist, and forearm motion to protect the reattachment and rest the elbow for 2 to 3 weeks.[18,29,32,40,55] Traditionally, a long-arm splint is fabricated, placing the elbow in 70 to 90 degrees of flexion and the forearm and wrist in neutral (Fig. 39-4). Several authors[32,53] recommend

30 degrees of forearm pronation and 30 degrees of wrist flexion to provide further protection for the reattachment. This flexed wrist position is not used if a carpal tunnel release had been performed at the same time. I believe that the position of forearm pronation and wrist flexion may lead to unnecessary muscle-tendon unit shortening. Another splint alternative is a sugar-tong, which immobilizes forearm and wrist motion but allows a short arc of elbow motion (Fig. 39-5). In any case, the splint must be well padded or pressure must be relieved at the surgical site to prevent irritation. In other cases, a sling may be used. More recently, even if the flexor-pronator muscle mass was reattached, some physicians advocate the use of a bulky dressing and no splint beginning day 5 postoperatively.[59] The rationale is to avoid complications such as flexion contractures and a tethered nerve in a new location. The patient should be cautioned against overuse to prevent increased edema and rupture of the reattachment.

In the other surgical options (decompression, subcutaneous transposition with or without a fasciodermal sling, and some medial epicondylectomies), the flexor-pronator muscle origin is not disturbed. A bulky dressing for the first postoperative week can provide enough protection.[40,59] Some other authors[14,38] recommend a sling or long-arm splint for patient comfort and to prevent stress to the surgical site for 2 weeks.

Treatment program. In stage I, the therapeutic interventions are directed toward ensuring full wound closure, decreasing edema, decreasing or controlling pain, improving one-handed ADLs, and improving AROM of uninvolved joints.

Wound care involves inspection and dressing changes with the use of nonadherent contact dressings and gauze. If edema is significant, cold is applied for 15 minutes or less as tolerated. Massage is performed, with care taken to avoid firm pressure over the surgical area after sutures are removed and the incision is healed. Compression wraps around the elbow are not indicated because the nerve does not tolerate pressure well at this time.[32]

Pain control includes providing the needed soft protection at the surgical site and ensuring that bandages are not too constrictive. Often, the reduction of edema will result in decreased pain. ADL instruction, including one-handed techniques or adaptive equipment, is provided to the patient if needed. The ADL limitations exist for only a short time; provision of equipment may not be needed, especially if the patient has help at home.

All patients are instructed in AROM of the shoulder and digits. If the flexor-pronator origin has not been repaired, gentle active elbow, wrist, and forearm motion can begin out of the splint within the first few days.[44,64] Traditionally, when the flexor-pronator origin has been repaired, strict immobilization of the elbow, forearm, and wrist has been recommended for 3 weeks to allow healing of the origin.[19,32] In more recent literature, early isolated and gentle active/active assistive/passive elbow (with the wrist and forearm in neutral), wrist, and/or forearm motion within patient comfort is suggested beginning anywhere from 5 days to 2 weeks postoperatively.[40,58,60] This early motion program does not appear to stress the surgical reattachment, limits postoperative elbow flexion contractures, and may decrease adhesion formation around the newly transposed nerve.[58] I suggest careful patient selection if all joints are allowed to move during this phase because this program may allow the very active patient an opportunity to rupture the flexor-pronator muscle reattachment.

I find the following third option for ROM provides the benefit of preventing flexion contractures and decreasing adhesion formation and certainly does not stress the surgical reattachment of the flexor-pronator muscle group. In this program, the patient is allowed to perform gentle active assistive/passive elbow flexion and extension beginning 1 to 2 weeks postoperatively. The wrist and forearm are held in neutral while performing the elbow motion. For more protection, the forearm is held with the patient's other hand in midposition pronation and wrist flexion while the elbow is moved. Elbow, wrist, and forearm active motion begin 3 weeks after surgery.

Warwick and Seradge[63] performed a prospective study of 57 cases following medial epicondylectomy and compared early ROM (day 1 postoperatively) with delayed ROM (day 14 postoperatively). The outcomes of improved ROM and earlier return to work were statistically significant for the early ROM group. The study had several limitations, including no discussion of the percentage of worker's compensation between groups, no comparison of staging of the disease, pain scale measures that were not a reliable tool, and no mention of sensibility, hypersensitivity, or muscle function. Also, it is unclear when forearm and wrist ROM was performed.

Weirich et al.[64] performed a retrospective study of patients who underwent anterior subcutaneous ulnar-nerve transposition followed by early versus delayed ROM. A physical examination was performed, and the patients completed an outcomes questionnaire. The early ROM group performed full elbow flexion and limited the last 30 degrees of elbow extension for 8 to 10 days. The delayed ROM group wore a long-arm splint for 7 to 30 days (mean, 14 days) before beginning ROM. Follow-up was performed at 6 to 66 months postoperatively (mean, 22 months). No significant difference at follow-up was found for grip, pinch, two-point discrimination, pain rating, or patient satisfaction. Improvement was noted for both groups in ulnar-innervated musculature. ROM was not evaluated. The early ROM group had an earlier return to work and ADLs. However, the early ROM group had 25% worker's compensation versus 43% in the delayed ROM group. The type of work the patients returned to was not presented. The authors concluded that this type of surgery provides a high degree of patient satisfaction and relief of symptoms, regardless of when mobilization was initiated. I question the need for this study because there is no anatomic reason to limit elbow extension following anterior subcutaneous ulnar-nerve transposition.

Precautions/considerations. The precautions are specific to the surgical procedure performed. The amount of motion and which joints are allowed to move must be discussed with the referring physician. If motion is allowed for the elbow, end-range is not emphasized for any patient during this stage of treatment. If the flexor-pronator muscle origin was reattached, passive forearm supination with wrist and finger extension is prohibited because this motion stresses the repair site. Strong gripping and any lifting are contraindicated. The medial side of the elbow is well padded after any of these surgeries because tenderness is expected.

Stage II: active motion (day 1 to week 3 through 5 or 6)

Evaluation. The therapist's evaluation progresses to include scar mobility, AROM (for all joints because restrictions previously mentioned are now discontinued), passive range of motion (PROM), upper quarter examination (to rule out undiagnosed proximal sites of compression), neural tension (as ROM nears normal), a baseline sensibility test, and assessment for hypersensitivity. Areas previously assessed in stage I continue to be reassessed.

Splinting. Protective splints are generally discontinued after 2 weeks, or after 3 weeks if an anterior submuscular transposition was performed. Continued splinting may be needed for protection when the patient is sleeping or traveling, for rest from overuse, or if the patient could stress the flexor-pronator reattachment. If the surgical site remains tender, the patient can use an elbow pad. Splints to facilitate elbow motion are not recommended because they may place prolonged stretch on neural tissue, which tolerates this stretch poorly.[36]

An anticlaw splint can be used to improve function if the patient has a claw hand deformity secondary to muscle

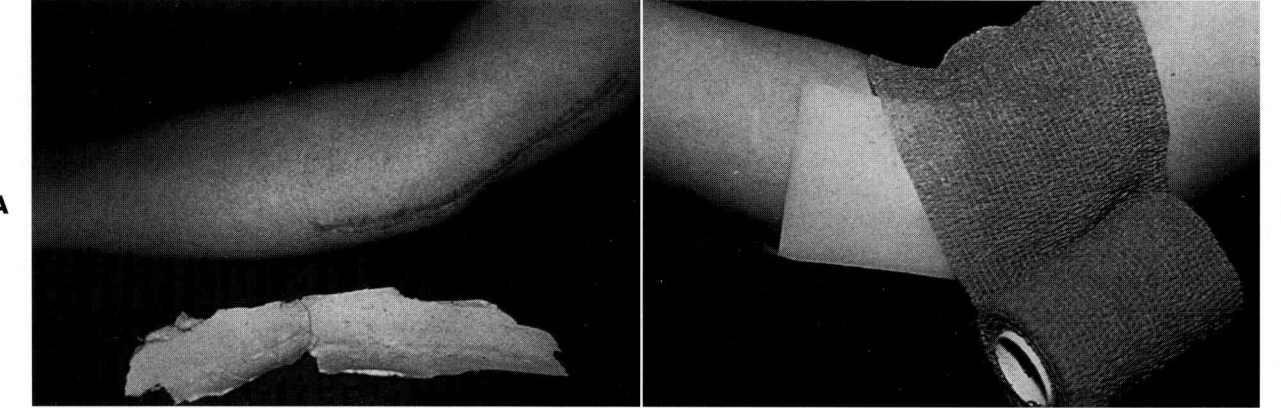

Fig. 39-6. A, Elastomer is used for scar management. **B,** A ½-inch dermal pad can be used for scar management or to provide a cushion at the surgical site.

weakness (see Chapter 34). If fixed-joint or soft tissue contractures are present in the hand because of previous muscle paralysis, additional splinting and PROM can begin to address those limitations (see Chapter 112).

Treatment program. Scar management can begin with elastomer molds or silicone gel sheeting applied to the incisional scar after the wound is healed (Fig. 39-6, *A*). The elastomer products may tear with elbow motion, so a ½-inch dermal pad can be an alternative that also provides good surface contact and padding to the medial side of the elbow (Fig. 39-6, *B*). Edema control continues as stated in stage I. Edema generally resolves as ROM improves.

Pain and neurologic symptoms (e.g., paresthesias) normally diminish over time after release of the nerve. This process can take more than a year. If axonal regeneration is occurring, the patient may experience an increase in discomfort because pain fibers regenerate the fastest.[40] If surgical-site pain persists, the patient is given a dermal pad or a soft elbow pad and is instructed to avoid resting the arm on firm surfaces. Desensitization can help reduce hypersensitivity (see Chapter 33). Often, the hypersensitivity is localized at the medial epicondyle, where the medial antebrachial cutaneous nerve may be caught in scar or may have been injured.[5] Pain control techniques described in the section on nonoperative management may be used. Occasionally, the patient can develop medial epicondylitis following surgery to release the ulnar nerve. Pain control and treatment for this problem are described in Chapters 78 and 79. When active range of the elbow returns, participation in nonresistive ADLs is permitted. Restrictions continue for lifting, carrying, and engaging in resistive activities.

Active motion progresses now to include the elbow, wrist, and forearm if the motion was previously restricted. The restoration of this motion is usually uncomplicated. All exercises emphasize isolated joint motion before composite motion.[32] The end-range of elbow extension may be more difficult to obtain. There are many techniques that can assist

in restoring elbow motion (Box 39-1). The goal during this stage is to restore active motion within the limits of patient discomfort.

Active assistive and passive motion is started if active range is not within normal limits. When assisting the motion, care is taken to limit stretching if paresthesias increase and stretching is performed for short periods. If the patient has other sites of nerve compression, release of the ulnar nerve might help decrease these symptoms. It is important to have the patient continue with the home program for the other sites of nerve compression. When working with the patient with multiple sites of nerve compression, the therapist must identify whether the symptoms are related to release of the ulnar nerve or problems with the other sites of nerve compression.

Patients often experience hypersensitivity at the surgical site. Desensitization techniques help decrease this problem (see Chapter 33). Protective sensory reeducation instructions are given to the patient if anesthesia remains in the ulnar-nerve distribution. Discriminative sensory reeducation is delayed until the patient can perceive touch perception on the fingertips (see Chapter 35).

If prescribed, nerve mobilization techniques may begin as active motion progresses. The cause of nerve restriction should have been eliminated by the surgery. Nerve mobilization proceeds if there is no increase in symptoms. An anteriorly transposed ulnar nerve now lies anterior to the joint axis. The end-range of nerve mobilization after these surgeries should be adapted to a position of cervical contralateral flexion, scapular depression, shoulder abduction, external rotation, elbow extension, forearm supination, and wrist and finger extension. Restriction of motion because of muscle tightness, periarticular joint stiffness, or pain at the surgical site must be differentiated from neurologic symptoms obtained with nerve mobilization. The adapted end-range position for nerve mobilization involves composite elbow extension, forearm supination, and wrist extension,

---

Box 39-1 Techniques to restore elbow range of motion

Thermal agents
Soft tissue massage
Gentle contract-relax exercises for elbow flexion and extension
Elbow extension with the forearm pronated to relax the repaired muscle group
Lying in a prone position to isolate the triceps muscle
Bilateral wand exercises
Proprioceptive neuromuscular facilitation without resistance
Electromyographic biofeedback for muscular co-contraction
Activities that require reaching

---

which places stress on a reattached flexor-pronator origin. Achieving the end-range nerve gliding position may take several weeks because of muscular limitations, not nerve gliding restrictions.

Precautions/considerations. During this stage, achieving the end-range of elbow motion is encouraged but strong stretching is not performed. If neurologic symptoms increase with active motion at the end-ranges or with nerve mobilization, the therapist can suspect several things. There may be an undiagnosed double crush injury. Increased discomfort may be caused by nerve regeneration, incomplete release of all the structures that were compressing the nerve, or scar fixation around the nerve after surgery.

The surgical literature has both identified and disputed potential complications of all the surgical techniques previously listed.* The more commonly cited complications are as follows. Some authors[1,11,18,22] have argued that decompression, medial epicondylectomy, subcutaneous transpositions, and intramuscular transpositions do not allow for inspection and full release of all potential sites of compression for cubital tunnel syndrome. Submuscular transposition can address all potential sites of compression but may lead to a painful neuroma[5,28] or increased scar fixation after surgery if the elbow is not moved early; it may also lead to an elbow flexion contracture.[20,28,29] There also has been concern that this surgery negatively affects the blood supply to the ulnar nerve[24]; however, the clinical relevance of this information is disputed in the literature.[35] After epicondylectomy, pain or tenderness may persist at the medial elbow and elbow instability may result.[18,24,28,29] After decompression, the nerve may sublux onto the medial epicondyle.[18,28] Medial epicondylitis occurs very rarely.[28] The therapist should be aware of the potential limitations of the procedures so that he or she can explain the normal course of therapy to the patient and can assist with treatment planning when the patient does not progress as expected. The

*References 1, 4, 5, 11, 22, 24, 28, 29, 46, 57.

therapist is often the first one to hear of these complications and, when significant, informs the physician so that the treatment plan may be modified.

Stage III: strengthening (week 5 to 7, to continue as needed)

Evaluation. Grip and pinch strength can now be assessed. A manual muscle test[31] is performed if distal muscle weakness is present. A job analysis can be performed at the work site at this time to begin planning for return to work (see Chapter 123). Some patients may have returned to work by this time because their jobs do not involve resistive or repetitive tasks. As the patient nears the end of rehabilitation, a functional capacity evaluation can be performed to determine physical abilities and limitations and the ability to return to former employment (see Chapters 123 and 124). Reevaluation of other limitations continues as described in stages I and II.

Splinting. Splints for the elbow are discontinued except for padding of the elbow if the area remains tender (particularly after a medial epicondylectomy). If the patient develops medial epicondylitis, a wrist splint or a long-arm splint can help provide rest to decrease inflammation. Hand splints continue as indicated.

Treatment program. Edema and ROM now should be within normal limits at the elbow. The focus on PROM increases if motion has not been restored. After anterior submuscular transposition, it has been reported that some patients may not achieve full motion.[32] This may be because of the delayed initiation of AROM or because submuscular transposition is a more extensive surgical procedure than the other procedures. Lack of full elbow motion may be the result of muscle tendon tightness of the flexor-pronator muscle group. Treatment for hypersensitivity, sensory reeducation, and nerve mobilization continue if therapeutic goals have not been met.

When necessary, the patient begins the strengthening program with general warm-ups and stretches. If weakness has been identified, muscle reeducation and strengthening for ulnar-innervated muscles begins as evidence of reinnervation occurs. Isolated strengthening for shoulder, elbow, wrist, and finger musculature begins with isometrics and advances to composite strengthening when tolerated. When evaluation indicates no significant loss of strength, no specific strengthening is recommended. I believe some patients are often subjected to too much repetition when performing a strengthening program. Exercises and activities that require prolonged or repetitive elbow motion are not recommended. If the patient is deconditioned, an aerobic program may be suggested. Functional tasks and work conditioning are included in the final stage of rehabilitation if needed (see Chapter 125). If the patient is a manual laborer, this stage may take as long as 6 to 12 additional weeks.

In some cases, compensatory strategies or adaptive equipment is provided if permanent limitations persist.

Precautions/considerations. If ulnar-innervated musculature remains weak or nonfunctioning in the hand because of permanent nerve damage, functional limitations in grip strength and coordination will remain. If protective sensory function does not return, the patient will always need to adhere to sensory precautions and should not perform work in which he or she cannot see the hand. If neurologic symptoms remain, the nerve might have sustained permanent damage while it was compressed and may not improve. If the damage to the nerve occurring preoperatively was not considered severe enough to warrant the remaining symptoms or if nerve compression symptoms become worse throughout the postoperative period, additional diagnostic testing and surgical reexploration may be indicated.

SUMMARY

The components of clinical decision making for the management of cubital tunnel syndrome have been presented. A trial of nonoperative management may be used if nerve compression symptoms are not severe. If this fails, surgery may be indicated. Recovery may be limited if permanent nerve damage has occurred. This information should be discussed with the patient before surgery. The treatment choices a therapist makes during the nonoperative and postoperative management of cubital tunnel syndrome require a knowledge of anatomy, pathophysiology, diagnostic testing, and the changing clinical presentation of cubital tunnel syndrome. Our daily objective measures of response to therapy for neuropathies are limited. Therefore much of the expertise in managing these patients in therapy lies in our ability to link the patients' subjective symptoms with possible physiologic responses of the nerve.

REFERENCES

1. Amadio PC: Anatomical basis for a technique of ulnar nerve transposition, *Surg Radiol Anat* 8:155, 1986.
2. Apfelberg DB, Larson SJ: Dynamic anatomy of the ulnar nerve at the elbow, *Plast Reconstr Surg* 51:76, 1973.
3. Barbis JM, Wallace KA: Therapist's management of brachioplexopathy. In Hunter JM, Mackin EJ, Callahan AD, editors: *Rehabilitation of the hand: surgery and therapy,* vol 1, ed 4, St Louis, 1995, Mosby.
4. Barrios C, et al: Posttraumatic ulnar neuropathy versus non-traumatic cubital tunnel syndrome: clinical features and response to surgery, *Acta Neurochir* 110:44, 1991.
5. Bednar MS, Blair SJ, Light TR: Complications of cubital tunnel syndrome, *Hand Clin* 10:83, 1994.
6. Buehler MJ, Thayer DT: The elbow flexion test: a clinical test for cubital tunnel syndrome, *Clin Orthop* 233:213, 1988.
7. Butler D: *Mobilization of the nervous system,* Edinburgh, 1991, Churchill Livingstone.
8. Byron PM: Upper extremity nerve gliding: programs used at the Philadelphia Hand Center. In Hunter JM, Mackin EJ, Callahan AD, editors: *Rehabilitation of the hand: surgery and therapy,* vol 1, ed 4, St Louis, 1995, Mosby.
9. Curtis BF: Traumatic ulnar neuritis-transplantation of the nerve, *J Nerve Ment Dis* 25:480, 1898.
10. Davidson AJ, Horowitz MT: Late or tardy ulnar nerve paralysis, *J Bone Joint Surg* 17:844, 1935.
11. Dellon AL: Review of treatment results for ulnar nerve entrapment at the elbow, *J Hand Surg* 14A:688, 1989.
12. Dellon AL, Hament W, Gittelshon A: Nonoperative management of cubital tunnel syndrome, *Neurology* 43:1673, 1993.
13. Diamond ML, Lister GD: Cubital tunnel syndrome treated by long arm splintage, *J Hand Surg* 10A:430, 1985 (abstract).
14. Eaton RG, Crowe JF, Parkes JC: Anterior transposition of the ulnar nerve using a non-compressing fasciodermal sling, *J Bone Joint Surg* 62A:820, 1980.
15. Eisen A, Danon J: The mild cubital tunnel syndrome: its natural history and indications for surgical intervention, *Neurology* 24:608, 1974.
16. Elvey RL: Painful restriction of shoulder movement: a clinical observational study. In *Proceedings of disorders of the knee, ankle and shoulder,* Perth, Australia, 1979.
17. Eversmann WW: Compression and entrapment neuropathies of the upper extremity, *J Hand Surg* 8:759, 1983.
18. Eversmann WW: Complications of compression or entrapment neuropathies. In Boswick JA, editor: *Complications in hand surgery,* Philadelphia, 1986, WB Saunders.
19. Foster RJ, Edshage S: Factors related to the outcome of surgically managed compressive ulnar neuropathy at the elbow, *J Hand Surg* 6:181, 1981.
20. Froimson AI, Zahawi F: Treatment of compression neuropathy of the ulnar nerve at the elbow by epicondylectomy and neurolysis, *J Hand Surg* 5:391, 1980.
21. Froimson AI, et al: Ulnar nerve decompression with medial epicondylectomy for neuropathy at the elbow, *Clin Orthop* 256:200, 1991.
22. Gabel GT, Amadio PC: Re-operation for failed decompression of the ulnar nerve in the region of the elbow, *J Bone Joint Surg* 72A:213, 1990.
23. Gay J, Love J: Diagnosis and treatment of tardy paralysis of the ulnar nerve, *J Bone Joint Surg* 29B:1087, 1947.
24. Heithoff SJ, et al: Medial epicondylectomy for the treatment of ulnar nerve compression at the elbow, *J Hand Surg* 15A:22, 1990.
25. Hong C-Z, et al: Splinting and local steroid injection for the treatment of ulnar neuropathy at the elbow: clinical and electrophysiological evaluation, *Arch Phys Med Rehab* 77:573, 1996.
26. Hunt JR: Tardy or late paralysis of the ulnar nerve, a form of chronic progressive neuritis developing many years after fracture dislocation of the elbow joint, *JAMA* 6:11, 1916.
27. Idler RS: General principles of patient evaluation and nonoperative management of cubital tunnel syndrome, *Hand Clin* 12:397, 1996.
28. Jackson LC, Hotchkiss RN: Cubital tunnel surgery: complications and treatment of failures, *Hand Clin* 12:449, 1996.
29. Jones JA: Pitfalls in the management of cubital tunnel syndrome, *Orthop Rev* 18:36, 1989.
30. Kasch MC: Therapist's evaluation and treatment of upper extremity cumulative trauma disorders. In: Hunter JM, Mackin EJ, Callahan AD, editors: *Rehabilitation of the hand: surgery and therapy,* vol 1, ed 4, St Louis, 1995, Mosby.
31. Kendall FP, McCreary K, Provance P: *Muscles: testing and function,* ed 4, Philadelphia, 1993, Lippincott Williams & Wilkins.
32. King PB, Aulicino PL: The postoperative rehabilitation of the Learmonth submuscular transposition of the ulnar nerve at the elbow, *J Hand Ther* 3:149, 1990.
33. Leffert RD: Anterior submuscular transposition of the ulnar nerve by the Learmonth technique, *J Hand Surg* 7:147, 1982.
34. Lister GD: *The hand: diagnosis and indications,* ed 3, Edinburgh, 1993, Churchill Livingstone.
35. Lundborg G, Dahlin LB: Pathophysiology of nerve compression. In Lundborg G, editor: *Nerve injury and repair,* New York, 1988, Churchill Livingstone.
36. Lundborg G, Rydevik LB: Effects of stretching the tibial nerve of the rabbit, *J Bone Joint Surg* 55B:390, 1973.

37. Macnicol MF: Mechanics of the ulnar nerve at the elbow, *J Bone Joint Surg* 62B:531, 1980.

38. Manske PR, et al: Ulnar nerve decompression at the cubital tunnel, *Clin Orthop* 274:231, 1992.

39. McLellan DL, Swash M: Longitudinal sliding of the median nerve during movement of the upper limb, *J Neurol Neurosurg Psychiatry* 39:566, 1976.

40. McPherson SA, Meals RA: Cubital tunnel syndrome, *Orthop Clin North Am* 23:111, 1992.

41. Michlovitz SL: *Thermal agents in rehabilitation,* ed 3, Philadelphia, 1995, FA Davis.

42. Michlovitz SL, Segal RL: Physical agents and electrotherapy techniques in hand rehabilitation. In Stanley B, Tribuzi S, editors: *Concepts in hand rehabilitation,* Philadelphia, 1992, FA Davis.

43. Millesi H: The nerve gap: theory and practice, *Hand Clin* 2:651, 1986.

44. Nathan PA, Keniston RC, Meadows KD: Outcome study of ulnar nerve compression at the elbow treated with simple decompression and an early programme of physical therapy, *J Hand Surg* 20B:628, 1995.

45. Novak CB, Lee GW, Mackinnon SE, Lay L: Provocative testing for cubital tunnel syndrome, *J Hand Surg* 19A:817, 1994.

46. Ogata K, Manske PR, Lesker PA: The effect of surgical dissection on regional blood flow to the ulnar nerve in the cubital tunnel, *Clin Orthop* 193:195, 1985.

47. Omer GE: The cubital tunnel syndrome. In Szabo RM, editor: *Nerve compression syndromes: diagnosis and treatment,* Thorofare, NJ, 1989, Slack.

48. Osborne GV: The surgical treatment of tardy ulnar neuritis, *J Bone Joint Surg* 39B:782, 1957.

49. Osborne GV: Compressive neuritis of the ulnar nerve at the elbow, *Hand* 2:10, 1970.

50. Osterman AL, Davis CA: Subcutaneous transfer of the ulnar nerve for treatment of cubital tunnel syndrome, *Hand Clin* 12:421, 1996.

51. Paine EW: Tardy ulnar palsy, *Can J Surg* 13:255, 1970.

52. Petterson T, et al: The use of patterned neuromuscular stimulation to improve hand function following surgery for ulnar neuropathy, *J Hand Surg* 19B:430, 1994.

53. Plancher K: Intramuscular transposition of the ulnar nerve, *Hand Clin* 12:435, 1996.

54. Posner MA: Compressive ulnar neuropathies at the elbow: II. Treatment, *J Am Acad Orthop Surg* 6:289, 1998.

55. Rayan GM: Proximal ulnar nerve compression: cubital tunnel syndrome, *Hand Clin* 8:325, 1992.

56. Rayan GM, Jensen C, Duke J: Elbow flexion test in the normal population, *J Hand Surg* 17A:86, 1992.

57. Rogers MR, Bergfield TG, Aulicino PL: The failed ulnar nerve transposition: etiology and treatment, *Clin Orthop* 269:193, 1991.

58. Sailer SM: The role of splinting and rehabilitation in the treatment of carpal and cubital tunnel syndrome, *Hand Clin* 12:223, 1996.

59. Szabo RM: Nerve compressions. In Green DP, Hotchkiss RN, Pederson WC, editors: *Green's operative hand surgery,* vol 2, New York, 1999, Churchill Livingstone.

60. Szabo RM, Gelberman RH: The pathophysiology of nerve compressions, *J Hand Surg* 12A:880, 1987.

61. Tetro AM, Pichora DR: Cubital tunnel syndrome and the painful upper extremity, *Hand Clin* 12:665, 1996.

62. Wartenberg R: A sign of ulnar palsy, *JAMA* 112:1688, 1939.

63. Warwick L, Seradge H: Early versus late range of motion following cubital tunnel syndrome, *J Hand Ther* 8:245, 1995.

64. Weirich SD, et al: Rehabilitation after subcutaneous transposition of the ulnar nerve: immediate versus delayed mobilization, *J Shoulder Elbow Surg* 7:224, 1998.

Chapter 40

RADIAL TUNNEL SYNDROME

Erich E. Hornbach
Randall W. Culp

HISTORY

Radial tunnel syndrome was first described as a distinct clinical entity in 1956 when Michele and Krueger[15] described the "radial pronator syndrome." They presented a pain syndrome distinct from lateral epicondylitis, and proposed an anatomic basis for compression of the posterior interosseous nerve (PIN) that could cause refractory lateral elbow pain. In a summary of the 1960 Annual Meeting of the British Medical Association, Capener became the first to report operative release of the supinator for refractory tennis elbow.[2] In 1972, Roles and Maudsley[19] coined the term *radial tunnel syndrome* and proposed that entrapment of the PIN could cause lateral elbow and forearm pain.

ANATOMY

The anatomy of the radial nerve and its branches about the elbow is variable. A theoretical space,[21] the radial tunnel originates near the level of the radiocapitellar joint where the nerve lies on the capsule of the radiocapitellar joint.[19] The medial border of the tunnel is formed by the brachialis muscle proximally and the biceps tendon more distally. The roof and lateral border of the tunnel begin as the brachioradialis and extensor carpi radialis longus (ECRL) muscles, and more distally are represented by the deep surface of the extensor carpi radialis brevis (ECRB). The radial tunnel was originally described as terminating at the entrance of the nerve into the proximal border of the supinator; other investigators[17] have suggested that the radial tunnel continues to the distal border of the supinator. Five potential areas of entrapment have been described (Box 40-1 and Fig. 40-1).

At the level of the elbow, the nerve is covered by fibrofatty connective tissue. Thickened bands of fascia from the capsule course around the nerve and anchor the surrounding musculature to the elbow capsule. The first potential area of compression of the radial nerve or its branches can occur here.[13,19] The roof of the tunnel begins as a collection of fascial interconnections between the brachialis and the brachioradialis. The structures of the roof continue distally, the biceps tendon becomes the medial border of the tunnel, and the proximal portion of the ECRB becomes the lateral border of the tunnel. At this level, the deep surface of the ECRB may contain thickened fibrous bands from its tendinous origin[13] and contribute to the second possible area of compression of the nerve.

The third potential area of compression is a group of vessels which have an intimate association with the radial nerve and its branches.[19] These vessels have been referred to as the *leash of Henry* and usually are branches of the proximal radial artery. They course laterally across the biceps tendon and proximally into the radial tunnel. These branches may impinge upon the nerve throughout the proximal portion of the radial tunnel.[14]

At the proximal border of the supinator, the radial nerve has divided into its superficial branch and its deep branch, the PIN. The PIN continues, penetrating the supinator muscle on the proximal radius. As it penetrates, a fibrous band on the leading edge of the supinator, the *arcade of Frohse,* may impinge upon the nerve.[23] This represents the most common region where the PIN is compressed. In a series of 90 patients, 83 had distinct compression at this site.[28] The arcade arises as a semicircular structure from the tip of the lateral epicondyle and the medial aspect of the lateral epicondyle. Anatomic variations in the composition of these origins have been reported by Spinner.[23] The lateral origin of the arcade is always firm and tendinous in nature, whereas the medial half of the arcade is firm and tendinous in 30% of specimens. In his 1979 report, Werner[28] described the arcade as fibrous in 78 of 90 cases. In addition, Prasartritha[17] reported that the arcade was tendinous in 57% of dissections performed on 30 Thai cadavers. The nerve then continues distally within the supinator muscle and emerges as its distal aspect giving branches to the superficial extensors. The final potential area of compression of the PIN is the distal border of the supinator muscle.[17,24] Fibrous or tendinous bands present in this region of the supinator were reported to occur in 65% of dissections performed on 30 Thai cadavers.[17]

CLINICAL FEATURES

The patient with radial tunnel syndrome usually complains of pain in the dorsal forearm. It is localized to the mobile wad musculature: the ECRL, ECRB, and brachioradialis (BR), and over the course of the radial nerve in the proximal forearm. The pain is usually 4 to 5 cm distal to the lateral epicondyle and may radiate proximally and distally over the forearm. The pain is characterized as a deep burning or aching, worse after activity involving forearm pronation and wrist flexion.[14] Rest pain and night pain are also features of radial tunnel syndrome.[6,12,22,28] Sensory complaints and muscular weakness have been reported but are not characteristic of the syndrome.[16,18]

Characteristic physical examination findings have been described. The first is resisted extension of the long finger with the elbow in full extension, forearm in pronation, and the wrist in neutral (Fig. 40-2). The test is positive when pain is produced in the ECRB or BR over the course of the radial

nerve. The second provocative maneuver is resisted supination of the forearm, with the elbow in extension (Fig. 40-3). This maneuver is painful when patients with radial tunnel have compression of the PIN at the arcade of Frohse.[10] A third characteristic finding with palpation is a point of maximal tenderness within extensor musculature 4 to 5 cm distal to the lateral epicondyle (Fig. 40-4).[6,10]

The differential diagnosis of radial tunnel syndrome includes intraarticular elbow pathology, PIN compression, cervical radiculopathy, lateral epicondylitis, and other entities (Box 40-2). An important distinction to be made is between radial tunnel syndrome and lateral epicondylitis. These two entities have been reported to coexist in 5% percent of the patients[28] Differentiation between the two syndromes can be difficult because of the overlap in symptoms and difficulty with physical examination. The areas of maximal tenderness are separated by several centimeters at best. Classically, the pain in lateral epicondylitis occurs at or just distal to the lateral epicondyle over

---

Box 40-1 Differential Diagnosis

Brachial plexopathy
Cervical radiculopathy
Chronic extensor compartment syndrome
Chronic anconeus compartment syndrome
Lateral antebrachial neuritis
Lateral epicondylitis
Posterior interosseous nerve syndrome
Radiocapitellar articular pathology

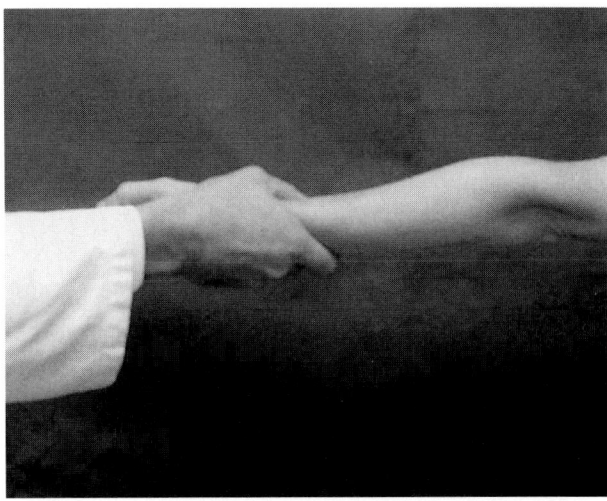

Fig. 40-2. Resisted supination.

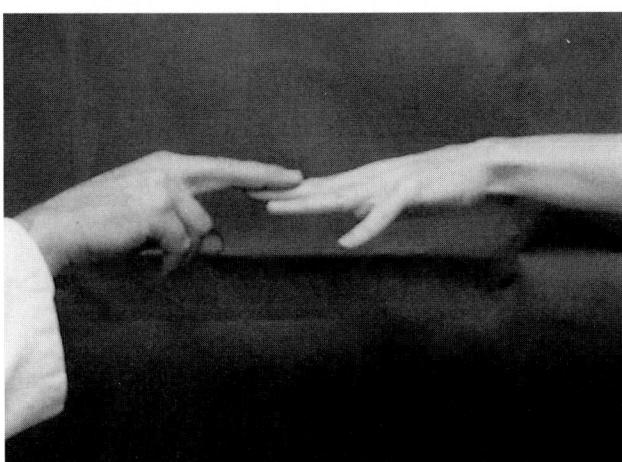

Fig. 40-1. Resisted middle finger extension.

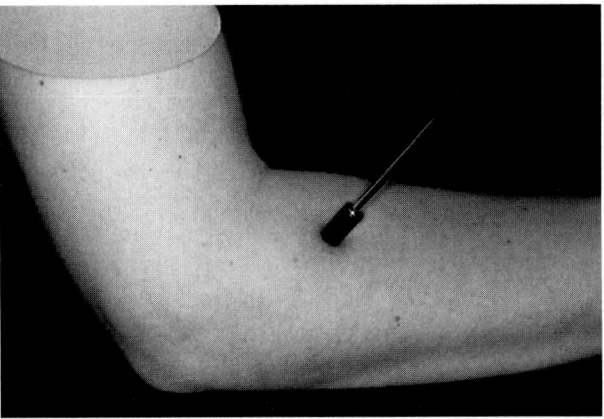

Fig. 40-3. Point of maximal tenderness in radial tunnel syndrome.

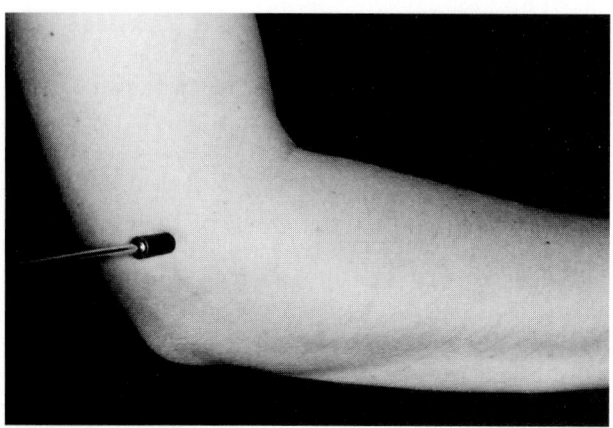

Fig. 40-4. Point of maximal tenderness in lateral epicondylitis.

Box 40-2   Potential Areas of Compression

Thickened fascial tissue superficial to radiocapitellar joint
Radial recurrent vessels—leash of Henry
Fibrous origin of ECRB or fibrous bands within the ECRB
Proximal border of supinator—arcade of Frohse
Distal edge of supinator

ECRB, Extensor carpi radialis brevis.

the ECRB portion of the common extensor origin (Fig. 40-5).[3] The pain in radial tunnel syndrome is located between 4 and 5 cm distal to the epicondyle within the extensor musculature, either laterally between the brachioradialis and ECRB muscles or medially between the mobile wad and the brachialis muscle.[5] Provocative tests for radial tunnel syndrome as listed earlier can be, but usually are not, positive in lateral epicondylitis.[14] Passive stretch of the ECRB muscle and common extensor muscle origin are more likely to be painful in lateral epicondylitis. Passive stretch of the common extensor origin can be performed by extending the elbow and flexing the wrist and fingers.[4] Also, lateral elbow pain is increased with resisted wrist extension in patients with lateral epicondylitis, but not for radial tunnel syndrome.

Diagnostic injection can also be performed to help in the diagnosis of radial tunnel syndrome and to differentiate lateral epicondylitis from radial tunnel syndrome. An injection between the brachialis and brachioradialis within the radial tunnel has been reported to help confirm the diagnosis of radial tunnel syndrome.[18] To help confirm the diagnosis, the injection should produce some degree of motor block and transient relief of symptoms.[18] In patients with possible coexistent radial tunnel and lateral epicondylitis, an injection over the lateral epicondyle common extensor origin that results in incomplete relief of pain favors the diagnosis of radial tunnel syndrome.

PIN compression is differentiated from radial tunnel syndrome by the presence of motor abnormalities. These

abnormalities can range from partial weakness to complete loss of function and may be preceded by pain over the course of the radial and posterior interosseous nerves. Radiocapitellar pathology can be differentiated from radial tunnel syndrome with a history of antecedent trauma or chronic overuse syndrome, magnetic resonance imaging or plain radiography, and mechanical abnormalities on physical examination.

ELECTROPHYSIOLOGIC DIAGNOSIS

The presence of abnormalities on electrophysiologic examination of patients with a clinical diagnosis of radial tunnel syndrome remains controversial. Many believe that radial tunnel syndrome may be present despite normal electrophysiologic studies. Abnormalities have been reported by multiple investigators, but there is no consensus on what abnormalities are uniformly present or diagnostic. In their initial report, Roles and Modsley[19] reported increased motor latencies in 8 of 10 patients. Electromyographic (EMG) abnormalities have been reported in the presence of normal nerve conduction velocities (NCVs) by Jebsen et al.[9] Lister[14] and Ritts[18] and their associates have also reported EMG abnormalities.

In 1980, Rosen and Werner[20] reported on 28 patients with a clinical diagnosis of radial tunnel syndrome. They performed preoperative and postoperative testing, which included motor conduction velocity at rest, motor conduction velocity with active supination, and EMGs. They found no differences in motor conduction velocity at rest between controls and study subjects, nor did they find any differences between sides on subjects. They did demonstrate significant differences in NCV with active supination, as well as EMG differences between controls and subjects. They concluded that a dynamic compression of the PIN at the level of the supinator could produce lateral elbow pain and local tenderness where the nerve passes through the supinator.

In 1991, Verhaar and Spaans[27] concluded that the signs and symptoms present in patients with radial tunnel syndrome are not caused by compression of the PIN. They based their report on 16 patients with radial tunnel who underwent EMGs and NCVs, as well as NCV testing while performing resisted supination. They reported no EMG abnormality in any of the patients. They reported one patient with an increased motor latency, which returned to normal on follow-up examination without operative treatment.

In 1998, Kupfer et al.[11] reported a series of 25 patients who underwent preoperative and postoperative electrodiagnostic evaluation. They recorded radial nerve motor latency with the forearm in neutral, passive supination, and passive pronation. They demonstrated that an increased latency could occur in all three positions. Statistically significant increases in latency were demonstrated with respect to the control group. They also demonstrated a statistically significant decrease in motor latency postoperatively. They concluded that the differential motor latency of the radial

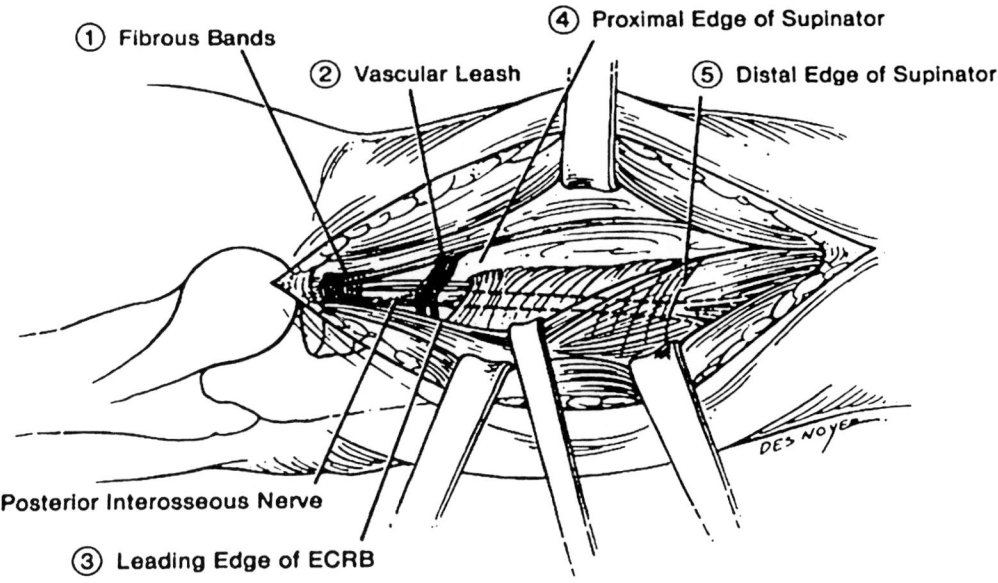

① Fibrous Bands ④ Proximal Edge of Supinator
② Vascular Leash ⑤ Distal Edge of Supinator
Posterior Interosseous Nerve
③ Leading Edge of ECRB

Fig. 40-5. Five compression sites of the posterior interosseous nerve. *ECRB,* Extensor carpi radialis brevis. (From Steichen JB: Radial tunnel compression sites. In Gelberman RH, editor: *Operative nerve repair and reconstruction,* Philadelphia, 1991, JB Lippincott.)

nerve was a sensitive diagnostic tool in patients with radial tunnel syndrome.

OPERATIVE TREATMENT

Operative treatment of radial tunnel syndrome is indicated after failure of nonoperative management. Before operative treatment is considered, all other potential causes for pain should be ruled out. Coexistent lateral epicondylitis and intraarticular pathology of the radiocapitellar joint should be identified and treated if possible. There are four common approaches to surgical decompression of the radial nerve and its branches. Pertinent features of each approach are presented.

Anterior (modified) Henry approach[8]

In the anterior (modified) Henry approach, a curvilinear incision is made beginning approximately 5 cm proximal to the lateral epicondyle extending distally along the anterior portion of the brachioradialis muscle. The incision is then carried obliquely across the elbow flexion crease near the medial border of the brachioradialis muscle. Proximally, the fascia is divided between the biceps/brachialis and the brachioradialis. Distally, the fascia is opened medial to the brachioradialis.

Next, the interval between the brachialis and brachioradialis is developed, and the radial nerve is identified. The brachioradialis is retracted gently with the radial nerve, and the interval with radial nerve is developed distally. At the level of the lateral epicondyle, the superficial branch of the radial nerve is identified and protected. Moving from proximal to distal, the nerve is mobilized by freeing it from the capsule of the radiocapitellar joint and any constricting

fascial bands. The ECRB is then lifted off the nerve, and its deep origin divided if it contains any potentially compressing fibrous bands. Next, the branches of the recurrent radial artery are identified and ligated. The PIN is dissected free and the proximal border of the supinator muscle, the arcade of Frohse, is identified and carefully divided. Moving distally, the supinator muscle is divided, and the PIN is dissected out as it proceeds through the supinator. Care is taken to preserve any branches of the nerve to the supinator. At the distal border of the supinator, branches of the nerve may take acute angles to innervate the superficial extensor muscles, and caution is warranted. The PIN should be freed from any fibrous bands in the distal portion of the supinator.

Posterior approach of Thompson[26]

In Thompson's posterior approach, a curvilinear incision is made from several centimeters proximal to the lateral epicondyle on the supracondylar ridge, anterior to the lateral epicondyle, and distally to the ulnar side of Lister's tubercle. The interval between ECRB and EDC is identified, and the fascia is incised. If difficulty is encountered in entering this interval, distal palpation of the abductor pollicis longus (APL) and extensor pollicis brevis can be used to identify the plane between the ECRB and the extensor digitorum communis (EDC), and the dissection is carried from distal to proximal, mobilizing the ECRB and EDC to reveal the supinator muscle covering the proximal radius.

At this point, the PIN can be identified proximally or distally in the supinator muscle. From proximal to distal, the origin of the ECRB and ECRL are detached from the lateral epicondyle and retracted. The PIN is identified at the proximal border of the supinator, and the arcade of Frohse is identified. The dissection of the PIN and release from potential sites of compression proceeds as previously described.

Another approach is to identify the PIN distally and trace it proximally through the supinator muscle. The dissection is then carried proximally, the leash of Henry is identified, and muscular branches are ligated. The PIN or the proper radial nerve is dissected free from fascial and muscular adhesions on the joint capsule up to the level of the lateral epicondyle.

Transmuscular brachioradialis-splitting approach[13]

Multiple skin incisions have been described for the transmuscular brachioradialis-splitting approach. Straight longitudinal,[19] S-shaped curvilinear,[25] and transverse incisions have been recommended.[13] The subcutaneous tissue is divided, and the lateral antebrachial cutaneous nerve identified and protected if present. The brachioradialis is identified by palpation, and the fascia covering it is split longitudinally. With use of blunt dissection, the brachioradialis is divided by the surgeon while two retractors are used to maintain the interval created. The dissection proceeds until a layer of fat is visualized. The dorsal sensory branch of the radial nerve is identified in the fat, and beneath that the PIN and the proximal border of the supinator muscle are identified. After the branches of the radial nerve are identified, the exposure is extended by further distal and proximal splitting of the brachioradialis. Potential compressing structures can now be identified and released from proximal to distal within the window of the brachioradialis muscle.

Approach through the brachioradialis–extensor carpi radialis longus interval[7]

A lazy S-shaped incision is made over the BR-ECRL interval. The subcutaneous tissues are divided, and the interval between the brachioradialis and ECRL is identified. Care is taken to identify and protect the lateral antebrachial cutaneous nerve. The interval between the brachioradialis and ECRL is developed from their origins on the lateral epicondyle to the middle of the supinator. The dorsal sensory branch of the radial nerve is identified and traced proximally. The PIN is identified. Proximal dissection will also reveal motor branches from the radial or PIN to the ECRB. Retraction of the ECRL and ECRB laterally will allow exposure of the distal border of the supinator muscle, and release of the remainder of the supinator muscle.

The operative approach used should be individualized and will depend on the expected location of pathology and the surgeon's experience. The advantage the anterior approach has over the other surgical approaches that it is extensile. It allows easy access to the proximal portion of the radial tunnel and can be extended above the elbow if necessary. Distally, it can be used to expose the entire radius. With respect to the posterior approach, visualization of the distal border of the supinator muscle through the anterior

approach is more difficult. The main disadvantage with the anterior approach is the potential for extensive scarring.[12,14,16] When this approach is used, particular emphasis is placed on scar minimization modalities during postoperative therapy. Although hypertrophic scar formation is possible with any surgery, it is less likely to occur with the other approaches because they remain more dorsal and avoid the flexion crease of the elbow. The posterior approach through the ECRB-EDC interval provides excellent exposure distally, but identifying the muscular interval and proximal exposure can be difficult.[25] The posterior approach can be used in combination with an anterior approach or BR-ECRL interval exposure to visualize the proximal portion of the radial tunnel. Its main disadvantages are the possibility of a second incision to expose the proximal portion of the radial tunnel and the potential for traction injury to nerve branches during exposure.[13] The brachioradialis-splitting approach provides direct access to the arcade of Frohse. The scar produced using a transverse incision is more aesthetically appealing than the other approaches. The major disadvantage of this approach is that it is not extensile and is limited by the length of the brachioradialis muscle. Both proximal and distal exposure can be difficult.[25] Advantages of exposure of the radial tunnel through the BR-ECRL interval are that it provides similar access to the radial tunnel as the brachioradialis-splitting approach, provides better proximal exposure, and does not result in damage to the brachioradialis muscle.[25]

RESULTS OF SURGICAL TREATMENT

Initial reports of operative treatment for radial tunnel syndrome were favorable. In their study, Roles and Maudsley[19] reported good to excellent results in 35 of 38 patients. Lister et al.[14] reported complete relief of pain in 19 of 20 procedures performed on 18 patients. They also described the relief of pain as being almost immediate, occurring within 1 to 2 weeks. Further promising results were reported by Moss and Switzer[16] when they observed significant or excellent relief of pain in 14 of 15 patients. Their patients reported multiple abnormalities, including radial sensory paresthesias, motor weakness, and crepitation.

Recent reports of surgical treatment for radial tunnel syndrome have been less favorable. Based on their observation that patients treated operatively for radial tunnel syndrome have persistent pain and disability, Ritts et al.[18] reviewed their series of patients treated surgically for radial tunnel syndrome. They reported 74% of patients had improvement in pain. However, 19 of 39 patients had persistent moderate or severe discomfort. Only 51% of the patients were able to return to preoperative activity levels.

In 1991, Verhaar and Spaans[27] reported one good and three fair results after surgical treatment on 10 patients. Jebsen and Engber[9] reported good to excellent results in 16 of 24 extremities, and Atroshi et al.[1] reported complete relief of pain or marked improvement in only 13 of 37 patients;

both groups concluded that outcome is less predictable than in earlier reports. Finally, Sotereanos et al.[22] reported good or excellent results in 11 of 28 patients using the same criteria as Roles and Maudsley.[19] Subjectively, 64% of patients stated they had a good or excellent result. They concluded that operative intervention in patients with radial tunnel syndrome should be done with caution.

COMPLICATIONS OF SURGICAL TREATMENT

Postoperative problems resulting from surgical decompression of the radial tunnel are variable. Hypertrophic scarring requiring steroid injection, and even excision or Z-plasty has been reported.[12,14,16] Recurrence of symptoms because of ECRB scarring has been identified during revision surgery.[14] Superficial radial neuropraxia has also been reported by multiple authors and usually resolves without complication.[12,16,22] Complete PIN palsy has been reported[12] and resolved with conservative treatment. The development of reflex sympathetic dystrophy (RSD) has also been reported but is not common.[9,14] Treatment with stellate ganglion blocks and hand therapy resulted in resolution of the RSD. With strict adherence to operative technique, other complications, including infection, hematoma, and elbow stiffness, are rare.

SUMMARY

Radial tunnel syndrome is an uncommon nerve compression syndrome; its existence has been questioned.[21] Careful history and physical examination, as well as appropriate diagnostic studies, are mandatory to rule out other pathologic conditions causing lateral elbow pain. After diagnosis, nonoperative treatment modalities, described in Chapter 41, should be exhausted before surgical intervention. Patients should be counseled that recent reports of surgical treatment for radial tunnel syndrome suggest that surgery does not give as reliable relief of pain as once thought. The selection of an operative approach should be made individually, based on the suspected area of compression, presence of other existing pathology, and the surgeon's experience. All five potential areas of compression should be identified and explored.

REFERENCES

1. Atroshi I, Johnsson R, Ornstein E: Radial tunnel release: unpredictable outcome in 37 consecutive cases with a 1-5 year follow-up, *Acta Orthop Scand* 66:255, 1995.
2. Capener N: Summary of the proceedings of the British Medical Association, *Br Med J* 2:130, 1960.
3. Coonrad RW, Hooper WR: Tennis elbow: its course, natural history, conservative and surgical management, *J Bone Joint Surg* 55A:1177, 1973.
4. Dawson DM, Hallett M, Wilbourn AJ, editors: Radial nerve entrapment. In *Entrapment neuropathies,* ed 3, Philadelphia, 1999, Lippincott-Raven.
5. Eaton CJ, Lister GD: Radial nerve compression, *Hand Clin* 8:345 1992.
6. Hagert CG, Lundborg G, Hansen T: Entrapment of the posterior interosseous nerve, *Scand J Plast Reconstr Surg* 11:205, 1977.
7. Hall HC, MacKinnon SE, Gilbert RW: An approach to the posterior interosseous nerve, *Plast Reconstr Surg* 74:435, 1984.
8. Hoppenfeld S, deBoer P: The forearm. In *Surgical exposures in orthopaedics: the anatomic approach,* ed 2, Philadelphia, 1984, JB Lippincott.
9. Jebson PJL, Engber WD: Radial tunnel syndrome: long-term results of surgical decompression, *J Hand Surg* 22A:889, 1997.
10. Kleinert MJ, Mehta S: Radial nerve entrapment, *Orthop Clin North Am* 27:30, 1996.
11. Kupfer DM, et al: Differential latency testing: a more sensitive test for radial tunnel syndrome, *J Hand Surg* 23A:859, 1998.
12. Lawrence T, et al: Radial tunnel syndrome: a retrospective review of 30 decompressions of the radial nerve, *J Hand Surg* 20B:454, 1995.
13. Lister GD: Radial tunnel syndrome. In Gelberman RH, editor: *Operative nerve repair and reconstruction,* Philadelphia, 1991, JB Lippincott.
14. Lister GD, Belsole RB, Kleinert HE: The radial tunnel syndrome, *J Hand Surg* 4:52, 1979.
15. Michele AA, Krueger, FJ: Lateral epicondylitis of the elbow treated by fasciotomy, *Surgery* 39:277, 1956.
16. Moss SH, Switzer HE: Radial tunnel syndrome: a spectrum of clinical presentations, *J Hand Surg* 8A:414, 1983.
17. Prasartritha T, Liupolvanish P, Rojanakit A: A study of the posterior interosseous nerve (PIN) and the radial tunnel in 30 Thai cadavers, *J Hand Surg* 18A:107, 1993.
18. Ritts GD, Wood MB, Linscheid RL: Radial tunnel syndrome: a ten-year surgical experience, *Clin Orthop* 219:201, 1987.
19. Roles NC, Maudsley RH: Radial tunnel syndrome: resistant tennis elbow as a nerve entrapment, *J Bone Joint Surg* 54B:499, 1972.
20. Rosen I, Werner CO: Neurophysiological investigation of posterior interosseous nerve entrapment causing lateral elbow pain, *Electro-encephalogr Clin Neurophysiol* 50:125, 1980.
21. Rosenbaum R: Disputed radial tunnel syndrome, *Muscle Nerve* 22:960, 1999.
22. Sotereanos DG, et al: Results of surgical treatment for radial tunnel syndrome, *J Hand Surg* 24A:566, 1999.
23. Spinner M: The arcade of Frohse and its relationship to the posterior interosseous nerve paralysis, *J Bone Joint Surg* 50B:809, 1968.
24. Sponseller PD, Engber, WD: Double-entrapment radial tunnel syndrome, *J Hand Surg* 8A:420, 1983.
25. Szabo RM: Entrapment and compression neuropathies. In Green DP, editor: *Green's operative hand surgery,* ed 4, New York, 1999, Churchill-Livingstone.
26. Thompson JE: Anatomical methods of approach in operation on the long bones of the extremities, *Ann Surg* 68:309, 1918.
27. Verhaar J, Spanns F: Radial tunnel syndrome: an investigation of compression neuropathy as a possible cause, *J Bone Joint Surg* 73A:539, 1991.
28. Werner CO: Lateral elbow pain and posterior interosseous nerve entrapment, *Acta Ortho Scand* 174(suppl):1, 1979.

Chapter 41

THERAPIST'S MANAGEMENT OF RADIAL TUNNEL SYNDROME

Christina D. Alba

Entrapment of the radial nerve may occur about the elbow in the anatomically defined space known as the *radial tunnel*. Compression of the posterior interosseous nerve in this area by various soft tissue structures can result in complaints of significant forearm pain with no sensory disturbance or motor weakness noted. Repetitive forearm rotation and prolonged static posturing have been implicated in the perpetuation of this problem, termed *radial tunnel syndrome*. Patients with this compression neuropathy must be educated on the cause, medical treatment options, and self-management techniques to help them attain successful results and avoid further or repeat provocation of their symptoms. The anatomy, cause, and differential diagnostic techniques were discussed in Chapter 40; this chapter focuses on the rehabilitation techniques for nonoperative and postoperative management of radial tunnel syndrome.

CONSERVATIVE MANAGEMENT
Evaluation

History. Therapeutic intervention for the conservative treatment of radial tunnel syndrome can be a challenging task for the therapist. Several factors must be considered when developing a treatment plan. A detailed history that outlines the causes of the patient's symptoms is of utmost importance. The clinician must gain a clear understanding of the physical demands that are placed on the patient at work, rest, and home, and with avocational activities. This will identify exacerbating and relieving factors so that behavior modification can be implemented, as is discussed later in this chapter.

Observation. As the patient enters the therapy clinic, the therapist can ascertain much information purely through observation. Posturing, transitional movements such as taking off a coat or pulling out a chair, general conditioning, and affect can be noted at this time and observed throughout the evaluation. One must keep in mind that each patient's presentation will vary because of the underlying neural histopathologic changes.[16]

Provocative activities and posturing. The clinician should elicit information regarding work-related and activity-related conditions so that exacerbating postures can be identified. Location, duration, and cause of the patient's pain are noted.[3,22] Static and repetitive postures assumed by the patient must then be analyzed. Not only may these positions contribute to nerve compression, they may also affect the musculoskeletal system through prolonged positioning, which in turn will result in adaptive soft tissue shortening and consequently perpetuate postural faults. The result, according to Novak and MacKinnon,[16] is (1) increased pressure on the nerve at the site of entrapment; (2) adaptive muscle shortening, which in turn may secondarily compress the nerve; and (3) muscles placed in elongated and weakened positions, which will result in adjacent muscle compensation and overuse and create a cycle of muscle imbalance.

Pain. In addition to defining activities that cause pain, the therapist can quantify the complaint of pain using a pain analog scale, such as the Visual Analog Scale (VAS) or the McGill pain questionnaire. Because radial tunnel syndrome is primarily a pain syndrome resulting from the compression of a motor nerve, one would not expect the patient to complain of paresthesias or muscle weakness in the radial nerve distribution. If grip weakness is present, it is most likely because a strong power grasp requires some amount of wrist extension, which can be painful to the patient.[11] The pain is likened to that of a muscle cramp or deep ache located in the extensor mass just below the elbow. It can radiate proximally and/or distally, is often nocturnal, is exacerbated by exercise or repetitive postures involving forearm pronation and supination with wrist extension, and is relieved with rest.[1,5,7,9,11,19]

Clinical tests. By the completion of the subjective evaluation, the therapist, through a solid understanding of upper extremity anatomy and biomechanics, should have developed a strong clinical picture and confirmation of the patient's diagnosis. Objective testing, including definitive palpation, range of motion (ROM), strength of the forearm extrinsic musculature, and specific provocative maneuvers (see Chapter 40), will provide further understanding of the patient's condition and will enable a differential diagnosis between radial tunnel syndrome and lateral epicondylitis. A general cervical and upper quarter screening must also be performed to rule out any concomitant or proximal nerve conditions.

Treatment

Once the evaluation has been completed and radial nerve compression has been determined to be within the radial tunnel, conservative therapeutic treatment techniques may be implemented to target the acute problem areas identified during the evaluation.[3] The primary goal in this phase is to reduce the patient's pain and inflammation. Techniques include rest via splinting, avoidance of exacerbating posturing or activities, pain control and edema reduction through the use of nonsteroidal antiinflammatory agents and therapeutic modalities, ROM exercises, and activity modification with work and all activities of daily living (ADLs).[1,7,9,16,22] This intervention must continue until the patient reports a decreased pain level at rest and with activities. Once the acute phase has subsided, a gradual rehabilitation program including progressive strengthening and modified work-simulated tasks may be implemented.[5] In this phase, the goal is to reintroduce dynamic forces across the forearm in a gentle, controlled manner to build endurance, strength, and postural awareness. Conservative treatment may last from 3 to 6 months.[7,18]

Rest. The primary means of therapeutic rest is to avoid the repetitive and excessive activities that initially caused the nerve irritation and/or compression. When a nerve is compressed or adherent, joint motion will produce a "minitraction" lesion, which will result in further epineural compromise. Consequently, a cycle of compression and irritation will ensue, and this cycle continues to produce adhesions, which, again, result in increased internal compression within the nerve.[24] Exacerbating postures, which were defined dur-

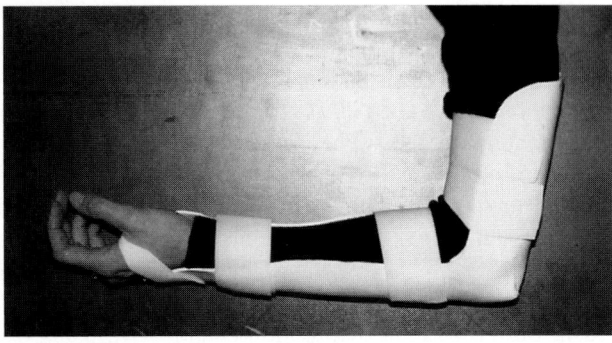

Fig. 41-1. Long-arm splint positioning the elbow in flexion, the forearm in supination, and the wrist in neutral.

ing the subjective evaluation, must be revisited at this point and activity modification implemented to decrease the neural and soft tissue stresses and to prevent further symptom provocation.

Another method of "resting" the inflamed nerve uses positional thermoplastic splinting for several weeks to facilitate the resolution of the inflammatory response about the nerve and surrounding soft tissue.[20] According to Gelberman et al.,[9] the optimal position for radial nerve decompression is elbow flexion, forearm supination, and wrist extension (Fig. 41-1). When the forearm is supinated, the nerve migrates toward the posterolateral portion of the joint line of the elbow, as opposed to being compromised and further compressed by the radial head when the forearm is pronated.[12] Therefore a long-arm splint that positions the elbow in 90 degrees flexion, full supination, and slight wrist extension (20 to 30 degrees) is indicated when treating radial tunnel syndrome; the patient is advised to wear it as much as possible with activities and at rest but is able to remove the splint for hygiene and gentle ROM exercises (see following discussion).

Modalities. Besides therapeutic rest, management of pain, edema, and inflammation can be addressed through the use of oral antiinflammatory medications and various therapeutic modalities, such as ultrasound, phonophoresis, electrical stimulation, and cryotherapy.

In the acute phase, pulsed ultrasound may be applied for its mechanical effects of increasing intercellular metabolism and microcirculation for edema and pain reduction and to enhance tissue healing. In the subacute and chronic stages, which generally is the most commonly seen patient presentation, continuous-wave ultrasound is used for its thermal effects, which among other factors, aids in increasing tissue extensibility, altering blood flow, and increasing the pain threshold.[25] Phonophoresis, which requires the thermal effects of ultrasound to drive topically applied antiinflammatory and/or analgesic medication into underlying tissues, may be applied to reduce the inflammatory process with consequent reductions in pain and edema.

Electrical modalities used in the clinic for pain and edema reduction may include high-voltage pulsed current (HVPC), iontophoresis, and transcutaneous electrical nerve stimulation (TENS). HVPC is one method of treating either acute or chronic edema. For acute edema reduction, a high-frequency electrical current is applied to repel negatively charged proteins resulting from the inflammatory process out of the interstitial space and into the lymphatic system. For chronic edema, a low-frequency current is applied to induce a "muscle pump" action to increase blood flow and aid in the flow of the lymphatic system.[14,15] Modulation of acute and chronic pain can also be accomplished using HVPC, with a higher frequency applied to treat acute pain and a lower frequency applied for chronic pain.[14] Several research reports on HVPC exist, and the literature states that pain modulation can occur through many different combinations of waveform parameters. Therefore trial periods to determine which parameters produce the greatest reduction in pain for each individual patient must be conducted.

Iontophoresis is the use of direct electrical current for the introduction of topically applied ions into the underlying tissue. Antiinflammatory medication, usually dexamethasone, can be delivered by an identically charged electrode applied over the most tender point along the radial tunnel, as identified through palpation and the patient's subjective report. Although the depth of penetration is relatively superficial, approximately 1 mm, deeper absorption into the subcutaneous tissue can occur through membranous transport and may offer the patient some pain relief.[14]

TENS can be an effective treatment modality for managing both acute and chronic pain, the primary component/complaint of patients with radial tunnel syndrome. There are many theories of electroanalgesia that form the basis for pain reduction with the use of TENS, the two most common being that of the gate control theory of pain (by Melzack and Wall) and the relationship between TENS and the production of endogenous opiates (most recently substantiated by Mayer and Price).[2] The stimulus parameters and electrode placements chosen can effectively provide symptomatic relief of the patient's pain through the attainment of analgesia.

Finally, cryotherapy techniques may be used to decrease the patient's pain, edema, inflammation, and muscle-guarding spasms. Studies show that cold alters the conduction velocity and synaptic activity of peripheral nerves. If the nerve temperature is decreased, the motor and sensory nerve conduction velocities will subsequently decrease. Therefore cooling the skin can reduce pain by acting as a counterirritant as well as by elevating the pain threshold. In addition to reducing pain, cold agents also reduce edema by decreasing the infiltration of interstitial fluids into the affected area and reduce muscle spasms by lowering the muscle's motor nerve conduction velocity.[13]

Range of motion. Active, active-assistive, and gentle passive ROM exercises can be performed in the initial therapy evaluation and continued daily at home. The patient should be instructed in general cervical and upper quarter stretching to correct proximal muscle imbalances, which in turn allows for improved posture and proximal flexibility. More concentrated stretching of the supinator and extrinsic extensor muscle complex must also be performed, always within the patient's tolerance. Intensive stretching, using contract-relax techniques, may be implemented as the patient's irritability decreases and must be continued to maintain the achieved muscle length.[16] If the arm has been placed in a long-arm splint, isolated joint motion of the wrist, forearm, and elbow should also be conducted at regular intervals to avoid joint stiffness resulting from immobilization.

Strengthening. When the patient's symptoms of radial nerve compression have significantly decreased, strengthening to correct proximal weakness and muscle imbalance should be commenced. Generally, isometric exercises can be used earlier in the course of rehabilitation because they allow for strengthening while minimizing the stresses placed on soft tissue and joints.[21] Progressive resistive exercises that target the strengthening of functional muscle groups rather than isolated muscles can be added once the patient is able to perform the exercise using the correct muscles; here, the emphasis is on endurance, not power.[16,21]

Activity modification. Perhaps the most important aspects of conservative treatment of radial tunnel syndrome are patient education and behavior modification. The therapist must educate the patient about the pathology/etiology of radial nerve compression; aggravating and pain-relieving postures, tasks, and positions; and sleep patterns. Without a clear understanding of the problem, the patient will not be able to successfully manage his or her symptoms through the avoidance of provocative activities or positions.[16] In particular, the patient must understand that this syndrome is dynamic in nature, exacerbated by repetitive forearm rotation and wrist extension. Studies have shown that neural pressures with active supination are five times greater than with passive pronation, thus strongly suggesting dynamic compression by the fibrous edge of the supinator as a cause of radial nerve irritation and compression.[17]

An ergonomic evaluation should be performed so that the appropriate job modifications may be implemented. When possible, tool grips can be built up to lessen the effects of a tight power grasp. Tasks that involve repetitive forearm rotation must be analyzed and body mechanics altered to decrease the involved stresses and to avoid overuse and consequent reinjury. With patient knowledge of the cause and effect of radial nerve compression, methods of prevention or early recognition can be perpetuated.

POSTOPERATIVE MANAGEMENT

Following decompression of the radial nerve, Eversmann[8] noted that the postoperative recovery is generally

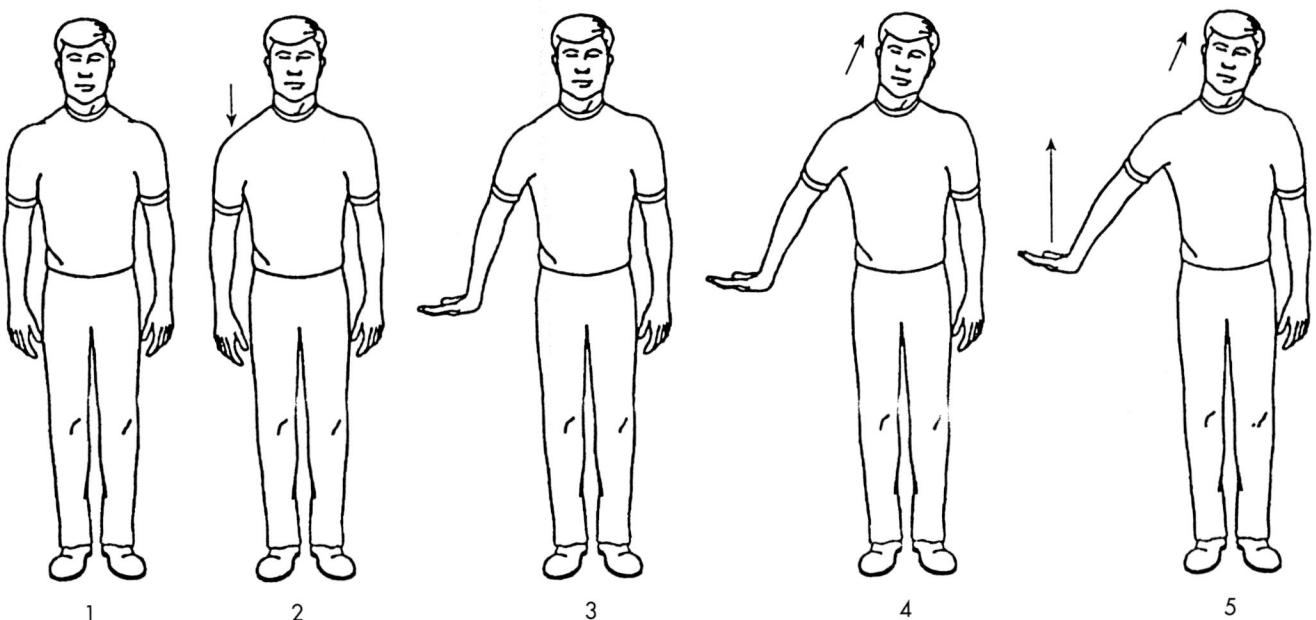

Fig. 41-2. Radial nerve gliding program. Position 1 begins with the patient standing and the body in a relaxed posture. Position 2 adds shoulder decompression. In position 3, the arm is internally rotated and the wrist flexed. Position 4 adds lateral cervical flexion. In position 5, the wrist is flexed as the shoulder is extended. (Redrawn from a home program form used by Spectrum Health Rehabilitation and Sports Medicine Services.)

prolonged over 3 to 4 months compared with the other peripheral neuropathies of the upper extremity. Relief of the epicondylar pain generally occurs within days, but full resolution of the muscular ache may take several months or up to a year.[17]

Generally, the patient is seen in the therapy clinic after the postsurgical splint and dressings have been removed, which is typically within the first week. At this time, a comprehensive evaluation must be conducted. Pathologic and significant medical history and current level of pain and dysfunction or difficulties with ADLs can be obtained subjectively. Objectively, the surgical incision, edema, and active ROM values can be assessed to provide a baseline of measurements for treatment guidelines. Although early ROM exercises are critical, a volar wrist splint that places the patient in wrist extension may be fabricated to promote healing and patient comfort. This splint may be worn for an additional 10 to 14 days between therapy and home exercise sessions if needed.[8,9]

Treatment for postsurgical pain, inflammation, and edema uses the same modalities that are afforded for the conservative treatment of radial tunnel syndrome. Oral antiinflammatory medications and any one modality or combination of therapeutic modalities, including pulsed ultrasound, high-frequency electrical stimulation, TENS, and cryotherapy, can be implemented in accordance with the patient's clinical presentation, as was presented earlier in this chapter.

Scar management is an important component of the postoperative treatments. Peimer and Wheeler[17] believe that

any surgery about the elbow may lead to a hypertrophic, widened scar, which they observed to be the most common postoperative problem. Once the wound has completely closed, massage and other mediums such as elastomer molds and/or silicone gel sheets may be used to provide pressure to the scar region to aid in preventing hypertrophic scar tissue from forming. Desensitization exercises may also be initiated upon full wound closure and progressed as tolerated.

Under normal physiologic conditions, longitudinal gliding of the peripheral nerve occurs with upper extremity motion. If the nerve is tethered by adhesions or a compressive anatomic structure, these normal movements can increase stress and strain at the site. Once the radial nerve is decompressed, therapeutic techniques must be implemented so as to maintain the longitudinal excursion of the nerve.[24] As soon as the postoperative dressings are removed, ROM exercises at the joints crossed by the released nerve and nerve gliding exercises must be implemented to prevent restrictive adhesions from forming between the nerve and adjacent soft tissue. Dellon[6] emphasizes the importance of *not* immobilizing the nerve for more than a week (i.e., allow gliding after nerve release for chronic compression).

When instructing the patient in the radial nerve gliding exercise, the therapist must emphasize the fact that involvement of this level of the radial nerve does not include a sensory component. Therefore, when the patient is performing these exercises, no feeling of dysesthesia or paresthesia will originate that will alert the patient that the nerve is beginning to be elongated and/or stressed. Therefore, according to Butler,[4] the patient should progress only to the point where soft tissue tension is increased in the involved upper extremity, and then it is "backed off a notch." This will alleviate any increased nerve irritability, which can easily be produced by nerve gliding exercises.[4]

As ROM and longitudinal nerve gliding improve, the patient can move further through the sequence of radial nerve glides, as shown in Fig. 41-2.

Treatment emphasizing normal physiologic function is more effective in achieving adaptive muscle length changes than passive exercises.[23] At 5 to 6 weeks postoperatively, the patient may begin resistance exercises in functional movement patterns to strengthen forearm extrinsic and proximal upper quarter musculature, as well as to increase grip strength. Isometric and concentric exercises will be better tolerated by the patient during the early strengthening stage because less force output is required of the targeted muscles.[10] Progression to eccentric exercises against resistance can then occur as strength and endurance increase, provided the patient's pain and edema remain insignificant. Once the "exercise dosage" has been established, an ergonomic evaluation can be conducted, and work-simulated tasks and modifications may be implemented. The patient now has all of the information needed to continue an independent exercise program for the maintenance of normal strength and endurance, and he or she may also begin a full, functional return to work.

CONCLUSION

As with most cumulative trauma disorders, the real key to treatment of radial tunnel syndrome is patient education. Aggravating postures and repetitive tasks and activities, once defined, can be modified or eliminated to discourage neural and soft tissue inflammation and to allow anatomic decompression of the nerve. Therapeutic modalities can also be implemented to further enhance soft tissue extensibility and remediate a reduction in pain and inflammation. Should conservative management fail to provide pain relief for the patient, a surgical approach may be indicated. Postoperative management should focus on maintaining neural and soft tissue mobility to discourage restrictive, compressive adhesions from reforming. General upper quarter conditioning and ergonomic changes must take place, and patient compliance is of the utmost importance for successful management and relief of radial nerve compression symptoms.

REFERENCES

1. Barnum M, et al: Radial tunnel syndrome, *Hand Clin* 12:679, 1996.
2. Barr JO: Transcutaneous electrical nerve stimulation for pain management. In Nelson RM, Currier DP, editors: *Clinical electrotherapy*, ed 2, Stamford, Conn, 1991, Appleton & Lange.
3. Baxter-Petralia P, Penney V: Cumulative trauma. In Stanley BG, Tribuzi SM, editors: *Concepts in hand rehabilitation*, Philadelphia, 1992, FA Davis.
4. Butler DS: *Mobilisation of the nervous system*, Edinburgh, 1991, Churchill Livingstone.
5. Dawson DM, Hallett M, Millender LH: *Entrapment neuropathies*, Boston, 1990, Little, Brown.
6. Dellon AL: Patient evaluation and management considerations in nerve compression, *Hand Clin* 8:229, 1992.
7. Eaton CJ, Lister GD: Radial nerve compression, *Hand Clin* 8:345, 1992.
8. Eversmann WW: Entrapment and compression neuropathies. In Green DP, editor: *Operative hand surgery*, ed 3, New York, 1993, Churchill Livingstone.
9. Gelberman RH, Eaton R, Urbaniak JR: Peripheral nerve compression, *J Bone Joint Surg* 75A:1854, 1993.
10. Kisner C, Colby L: *Therapeutic exercise: foundations and techniques*, ed 2, Philadelphia, 1990, FA Davis.
11. Lister GD, Belsole RB, Kleinert HE: The radial tunnel syndrome, *J Hand Surg* 4:52, 1979.
12. Maffulli N, Maffulli F: Transient entrapment neuropathy of the posterior interosseous nerve in violin players, *J Neurol Neurosurg Psychiatry* 54:65, 1991.
13. Michlovitz SL: Cryotherapy: the use of cold as a therapeutic agent. In Michlovitz SL, editor: *Thermal agents in rehabilitation*, ed 2, Philadelphia, 1990, FA Davis.
14. Mullins PA: Use of therapeutic modalities in upper extremity rehabilitation. In Hunter JM, Mackin EJ, Callahan AD, editors: *Rehabilitation of the hand: surgery and therapy*, ed 4, St Louis, 1995, Mosby.
15. Newton R: High-voltage pulsed current: theoretical bases and clinical applications. In Nelson RM, Currier DP, editors: *Clinical electrotherapy*, ed 2, Stamford, Conn, 1991, Appleton & Lange.
16. Novak CB, Mackinnon SE: Repetitive use and static postures: a source of nerve compression and pain, *J Hand Ther* 10:151, 1997.
17. Peimer CA, Wheeler DR: Radial tunnel syndrome/posterior interosseous nerve compression. In Szabo RM, editor: *Nerve compression syndromes*, Thorofare, NJ, 1989, Slack.
18. Plancher KD, Peterson RK, Steichen JB: Compressive neuropathies and tendinopathies in the athletic elbow and wrist, *Clin Sports Med* 15:331, 1996.
19. Schwartzman RJ, Maleki J: Postinjury neuropathic pain syndromes, *Med Clin North Am* 83:597, 1999.
20. Skirven T: Nerve injuries. In Stanley BG, Tribuzi SM, editors: *Concepts in hand rehabilitation*, Philadelphia, 1992, FA Davis.
21. Stanley BG: Therapeutic exercise: maintaining and restoring mobility in the hand. In Stanley BG, Tribuzi SM, editors: *Concepts in hand rehabilitation*, Philadelphia, 1992, FA Davis.
22. Terrono AL, Millender LH: Management of work-related upper-extremity nerve entrapments, *Orthop Clin North Am* 27:783, 1996.
23. Tomberlin JP, Saunders HD: *Evaluation, treatment and prevention of musculoskeletal disorders*, ed 3, Chaska, Minn, 1994, The Saunders Group.
24. Wilgis EF: Clinical aspects of nerve gliding in the upper extremity. In Hunter JM, Schneider LH, Mackin EJ, editors: *Tendon and nerve surgery in the hand: a third decade*, St Louis, 1997, Mosby.
25. Ziskin MC, McDiarmid T, Michlovitz SL: Therapeutic ultrasound. In Michlovitz SL, editor: *Thermal agents in rehabilitation*, ed 2, Philadelphia, 1990, FA Davis.

Part IX

BRACHIAL PLEXOPATHIES

Chapter 42

THORACIC OUTLET SYNDROME: A BRACHIAL PLEXOPATHY

Stephan H. Whitenack
James M. Hunter
Richard L. Read

Thoracic outlet syndrome (TOS) is a term that encompasses a variety of clinical entities involving structures about the shoulder girdle. Symptoms can include pain, numbness, paresthesias, headaches, weakness of the arm and hand, and arm swelling. *TOS* is a term that engenders a great deal of controversy in the literature (especially neurology) because of the difficulty in defining the very term. The syndrome may be viewed as a clinical complex that includes four parts: (1) neuropathy of the brachial plexus, (2) compression vasculopathy of the subclavian vessels, (3) reflex sympathetic dystrophy (RSD), and (4) cervicothoracic and brachial myofasciitis. Conversely, some would choose to limit the use of the term *TOS* to problems involving only the lower portions of the plexus—the C8 and T1 nerve roots, lower trunk, and medial cord.

There are distinct manifestations of compromise of the lower versus the upper plexus. For this reason, we have chosen to separate the discussion of the neurologic manifestations somewhat differently than it is usually presented. However, because the term *TOS* is so well entrenched in the literature, in this chapter we attempt to broaden the understanding of the various manifestations of TOS rather than to use an entirely new nomenclature. This should improve both the diagnosis and treatment of this difficult entity.

The variability in presentation, which causes great debate and misunderstanding, can be explained rationally if time is taken to fully comprehend the complex anatomy of the thoracic outlet region. The variation in mechanism of injury and in anatomy of the structures surrounding the brachial plexus causes the lack of a typical clinical profile desired by many neurologists.[116] Many typical profiles can be both explained and understood thoroughly when these anatomic variations are studied. TOS is also a dynamic entity. Alterations in posture and activity can profoundly affect the clinical picture.

Everyone who deals with the type of patients who are discussed in this chapter suffers from the narrow vision of those who persistently attack the use of the term *TOS* to include patients who do not have intrinsic muscle atrophy from lower trunk compression. We have sometimes used terms such as *posttraumatic brachial plexus neuropathy* to categorize these patients, but this only added confusion when dealing with outside agencies. *TOS* is a term that is with us; onward to better understanding.

HISTORICAL BACKGROUND

Many different and distinct entities have been grouped together under the term *TOS*. Rob and Standeven[79] generally are credited with coining the term *thoracic outlet compression syndrome*. Peet et al.[72] first grouped cervical rib syndrome, scalenus anticus syndrome, subcoracoid-pectoralis minor syndrome, costoclavicular syndrome, and first thoracic rib syndrome into the TOS. Others have added the scalenus medius syndrome, Paget-Schroetter syndrome (i.e., effort thrombosis of subclavian vein), rucksack palsy, droopy shoulder syndrome, and hyperabduction syndrome. Although including these separate etiologies under one heading can obscure the important differences in diagnosis and treatment, such a grouping is more likely to aid in understanding TOS.

The history of TOS has been well documented in many prior excellent reviews. The first recognition of cervical ribs dates to Galen and Vesalius. Sir Astley Cooper was said to have treated cervical ribs medically with some success. Willshire[118] generally is credited as the first to make the diagnosis of *cervical rib syndrome.* Coote reported the first successful cervical rib resection in 1861. Kean[36] and Halsted[29] wrote extensive reviews and described surgical results.

Ultimately, patients were described with similar or identical symptoms in the absence of a cervical rib. Murphy,[61] in 1910, was the first to resect a normal first rib with relief of symptoms. In 1927, Brickner[7] was the first to describe resection of the normal first rib in the American literature. In that same year, Adson and Coffey[2] began a shift in thinking with their belief that the symptoms were related to the relationship of the anterior scalene to the cervical rib and not to the rib itself. Adson was "convinced that it was not necessary to remove cervical ribs routinely, and that the chief etiologic element was the scalenus anticus muscle."[1] This belief was based on operative findings, surgical results, and the fact that most cervical ribs were asymptomatic. Adson's operative procedure consisted of sectioning of the anterior scalene, removal of any tendonous bands, and occasionally, removal of the cervical rib. Adson's sign was described at that time.

The next step in surgical thinking led to the resection of the anterior scalene in the absence of a cervical rib. *Scalenus anticus syndrome,* as credited to Naffziger[62] by Ochsner et al.,[66] became a relatively common diagnosis, and scalenotomy became a common procedure. However, over time the failures in treatment in patients with Naffziger's syndrome led to disenchantment with scalenotomy. It is important to remember that other upper extremity pain syndromes had not yet been described, and that many failures may have been in diagnosis rather than in procedure. Semmes and Murphy[93] described cervical radiculopathy in 1943. It was not until 1950 that Phalen et al.[73] described carpal tunnel syndrome, or until 1952 that Kremer et al.[40] defined the nerve conduction abnormalities at the carpal tunnel.

Other etiologic factors were also described to explain the symptoms being attributed to scalenus anticus syndrome. Lewis and Pickering[44] in 1934, and subsequently Eden[18] in 1939, implicated compression of the neurovascular bundle between the clavicle and the first rib as the cause of the symptoms. This was later termed *the costoclavicular compression syndrome* by Falconer and Weddell.[23] Eden[18] also further defined abnormalities of the first rib contributing

to the syndrome. In 1945, Wright[98,120] added the concept that hyperabduction of the arms caused neurovascular compression at two levels. In addition to the similarly described costoclavicular compression, he added the concept of compression by the posterior border of the pectoralis minor against the anterior border of the upper ribs. Wright's test was also described at that time.

In 1953, Lord[46] added the concept of resection of the clavicle for relief of the costoclavicular compression syndrome. Scalenotomy remained the preferred procedure, but because of disenchantment with results as described by Raaf,[76] scalenotomy fell into disfavor. Falconer and Li[22] were the first to support direct attack on the first rib in 1962. Later that same year, during the presidential address before the American Association of Thoracic Surgery, Clagett[10] solidified the importance of the first rib as the common denominator in the pathophysiology of TOS. His approach was a posterior, thoracoplasty-type resection of the first rib, befitting a thoracic surgeon trained in tuberculosis surgery.

A major advancement in the surgical approach to TOS was reported by Roos[81] in 1966. The transaxillary first rib resection that he described rapidly became the standard procedure for patients with TOS. Roos' 93% improvement rate was reaffirmed by others, including Urschel et al.[112] and Sanders and Pierce.[87] Roos[82-84] also has been primarily responsible for redirecting attention away from the vascular compression and toward the brachial plexus compression. Roos[82] also has carefully classified the many different types of congenital bands that contribute to TOS.

Nerve compression has remained the central concept for the cause of symptoms of TOS by most authors. Scar fixation of the nerves causing traction and fixation of the brachial plexus, rather than compression as the primary pathologic process, has been the latest concept to aid understanding of this complex problem. Sunderland[102] has attempted to help define the difference between nerve compressive problems and nerve entrapment and has written, "the key to the pathogenesis of the entrapment nerve lesion is the local inflammatory reaction that occurs in response to repeated mechanical irritation during limb movements." Thus simple decompressive procedures may be inadequate to relieve the pathologic process found in many of these complex cases.

VASCULAR SYNDROMES

Vascular manifestations of TOS are uncommon. Of the reported cases of TOS, 3% to 5% are vascular, with only 1% being arterial. These percentages probably are overstated because the recognition of neurogenic TOS involving the upper plexus has increased. In our series, vascular TOS represents less than 0.5% of the cases. The misunderstanding of the relationship between the vascular diagnostic signs and the neurologic manifestations of TOS is one of the many aspects of this problem, which creates the controversy that surrounds this diagnosis. Vascular syndromes are divided into arterial and venous types. Pure lymphatic disorders have not been described. There are aspects of the picture of RSD that undertake an apparent vascular component. This is discussed in the section, Reflex sympathetic dystrophy.

Arterial

Symptomatic arterial manifestations of TOS are representative of either acute or chronic compression. Chronic compression of the subclavian artery can cause both occlusive and aneurysmal disease. Both aneurysms and arterial occlusive disease are relatively rare. Dense fascial bands running forward and inferiorly from a cervical rib or elongated transverse process of C7 are the usual structural anomalies that predispose to arterial manifestations of TOS. These bands may create positional compression with motion of the arm. Adson's, Wright's, and Halsted's maneuvers are used to demonstrate arterial compression. However, presence of the capacity to obliterate the pulse at the wrist with arm motion does not in itself define TOS. Many completely asymptomatic individuals are able to shut off their pulse, particularly at the extremes of range of motion (ROM) of the shoulder.

The symptoms of arterial compression are generally described as having a "dead arm" or fatigue with use. The symptoms may be positional and thus may interfere with occupations requiring overhead arm use. Absence of pulses with a completely abducted arm will likely cause fatigue when trying to perform tasks such as ceiling painting. With appropriate accommodation, many of these types of activities may be continued without creating undue risk of repetitive trauma to the artery. Use of extension devices, for example, can allow continued productive work to be accomplished.

The sequelae of repetitive trauma to the artery are intimal damage to the vessel, leading to either thrombosis or occlusive disease, and damage to the full thickness of the artery wall, leading to aneurysm formation.[29] The initial symptoms of subclavian artery occlusion depend on the rapidity of the occlusion. A slowly progressive occlusion may allow time for adequate collateral circulation to develop. In this situation, the patient may have complaints only when the arm is used excessively. A more rapid occlusion, representing acute thrombosis, will cause the patient to have symptoms of arm claudication, with muscle cramping after minimal use or even at rest. Before complete occlusion, examination will reveal diminished to absent pulses in the involved arm and a bruit in the infraclavicular space.

The presenting symptoms of aneurysmal disease[69] are usually related to distal embolization to the arm, hand, or fingers. This is caused by fragments of the clotted material within the aneurysm breaking loose and lodging in the distal vessels. The symptoms may vary from acute ischemia of the arm with pain, pallor, paresthesias, and pulselessness to fingertip necrosis suggestive of Raynaud's phenomenon. Presence of a pulsatile mass in the supraclavicular fossa should raise the question of a subclavian aneurysm. Neurogenic symptoms may be caused less frequently by pressure from the aneurysm. An ultrasound study usually can confirm the presence of an aneurysm. An arteriogram or magnetic resonance (MR) angiogram is needed to complete the documentation of an aneurysm. Color Plate 5 shows the relational anatomy of the plexus and a subclavian artery aneurysm. An aneurysm may be found as an incidental finding on arteriography of the upper extremity being performed for other indications. In the absence of cardiac sources of emboli to the upper extremity (e.g., atrial fibrillation, recent myocardial infarction, valvular heart disease), the possibility of a subclavian source associated with TOS should be considered.

Venous

Acute venous occlusion of the subclavian vein results in sudden painful swelling of the arm, often with a bluish discoloration. Most commonly, this subclavian venous thrombosis (SVT) is the result of sudden maximal arm use, and thus is known as *effort thrombosis* or *Paget-Schroetter syndrome*. If the thrombosis is more insidious in onset, the sudden painful swelling will not occur, but rather swelling will occur with significant use.

Other etiologies of intravascular thrombosis must be considered; for example, factor VIII, antithrombin III, anticardiolipin antibodies, or protein C and protein S abnormalities. Spontaneous development of any venous thrombosis without obvious cause should also raise the question of occult malignancy. Subclavian venous catheters for intravenous access and, particularly, dialysis are the most common cause of SVT at present.

Treatment of vascular thoracic outlet syndrome

The treatment of vascular manifestations of TOS can be divided into immediate and long-term therapy. In the presence of distal arterial embolization, heparin therapy is instituted rapidly. If the embolus is in the larger vessels, embolectomy is indicated. Subsequent thoracic outlet decompression and repair of the arterial pathologic condition with a vein graft or patch should soon follow.[13]

Venous thrombectomy can be effective if performed in the first few days after the onset of symptoms. Thrombolysis with streptokinase or urokinase infusion is more likely to be of benefit if the diagnosis is delayed.[41] When operative thrombectomy is performed, rib resection, resection of abnormal bands, and possibly, scalenectomy should be done at the same time. Rib resection can be delayed 2 to 3 months after thrombolysis is performed, maintaining the patient on anticoagulation therapy until surgery. A residual stricture in the vein after resection of the compressive bands sometimes responds to balloon dilation. The failure rate is high if the angioplasty of the vein is performed before decompression. The practice of intraluminal stenting should be avoided if the cause of the venous occlusion is external compression.

Short-term anticoagulation therapy should be considered for all forms of vascular TOS. Warfarin therapy for a minimum of 3 months provides a lower incidence of postthrombotic complications in cases of SVT, and thus should be used unless there is clear contraindication (e.g., bleeding diathesis, active ulcer disease).

NEUROLOGIC SYNDROMES

Until recently, most thinking on TOS centered on lower plexus pathology, which results in ulnar-mediated complaints in the arm and hand. These symptoms are generally more clear cut and easily defined than with other varieties and consequently have been more accepted over time. Most patients now seen with TOS have been involved in some type of significant trauma, particularly with a flexion/extension component. The delayed onset of symptoms 1 to 3 months after this type of injury should be expected if the natural consequences of scar contraction and fibrosis are considered and the anatomic abnormalities described later in this chapter are understood. The use of the term *whiplash* carries many of the same negative connotations as does TOS, a position it does not deserve. Recent observations will perhaps elevate the understanding of both of these complex problems.[8,21]

The neurology literature recently has been filled with an aggressive attack on thoracic outlet diagnoses.[9,116] The neurologists' bias has been made clear by using the terms *true neurogenic* and *disputed* to differentiate types of TOS. One can also consider the more commonly accepted definitions of TOS in the surgical literature as *classic TOS.*

True neurogenic thoracic outlet syndrome

The most clearly defined subset of TOS has been labeled by Wilbourn[117] as *true neurogenic TOS.* Patients with true neurogenic TOS have atrophy of the ulnar intrinsic hand muscles (particularly the thenar eminence and first dorsal interosseus), numbness and paresthesias in the ulnar distribution, and clear peripheral electromyographic evidence of neuron loss, always associated with the presence of a cervical rib. The rib itself or a tight musculotendinous band emanating from the end of the rib causes the compressive neuropathy. Pain is often remarkably absent in this variation of TOS, perhaps as a result of the selective compression of only the C8 nerve root. We have only a few patients without a prominent pain component to the upper extremity associated with intrinsic atrophy. This syndrome variety also is called *motor type neurogenic TOS;* because it was first electrically defined accurately by Gilliat[25] in 1970, this type of TOS also is called *Gilliat's disease.*

Because of the symptoms of hand weakness, the mistaken diagnosis of carpal tunnel syndrome is commonly made in these cases. Any time the diagnosis of carpal tunnel

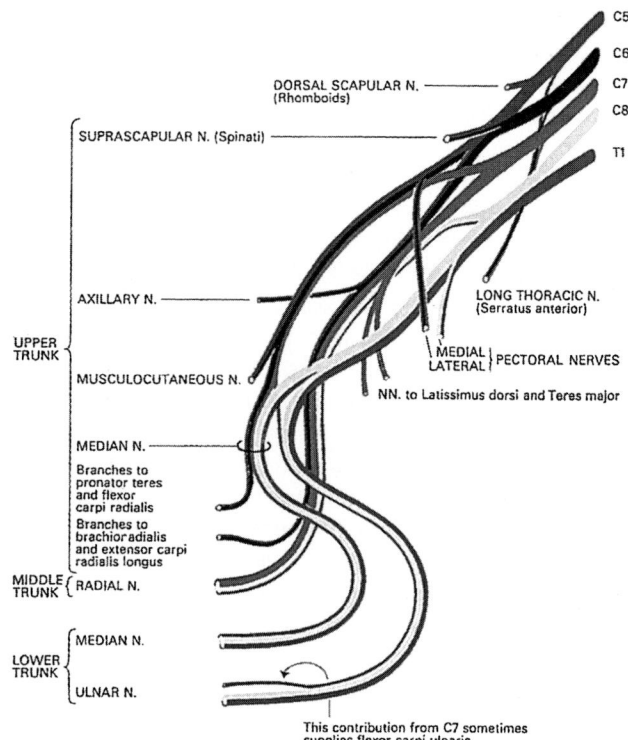

Fig. 42-1. Branches of the brachial plexus. The distribution of symptoms of proximal compression can be manifest in any of the branches and is not limited to the radial, median, or ulnar nerves. (From Seddon H: *Surgical disorders of the peripheral nerves,* Baltimore, 1975, Williams & Wilkins.)

syndrome is made in a teen who has thenar wasting, it is imperative to rule out TOS (usually related to a cervical rib) before proceeding with carpal tunnel surgery. It must be reemphasized that the fine motor intrinsic function of the hand is mediated more via the ulnar nerve than the median.

The true neurogenic variation of TOS is uncommon in its most narrow form in most reported series, as well as in our own. In our experience, the C8 nerve root compression has been extreme in these cases, to the point that the nerve has a gelatinous appearance from demyelination when observed at surgery. The onset of symptoms usually occurs in the late teens or early twenties, presumably resulting from the decreasing bony flexibility and angulation of the cervical rib.

"Classic" thoracic outlet syndrome

Those cases of TOS that do not fulfill the restrictive criteria of some neurologists have been labeled *disputed TOS.* The central issue in these arguments is the variability in symptoms in those patients who do not fit precisely into the "true neurogenic" category. A corollary argument centers on the lack of uniform criteria for the physical examination. When a full understanding of the anatomic basis for TOS is reached, the concerns of the detractors can be put aside. There is no dispute if the pathophysiology is understood. Fig. 42-1 shows the full distribution of the nerves that ultimately derive from the brachial plexus. Compromise at any level of the plexus will create a symptom complex in the anatomic distribution of the involved nerve. Descriptions of symptoms being on a "nonanatomic" basis usually indicate a lack of understanding of the brachial plexus anatomy.

The extensive anatomic studies of Roos[82] and others[63] have documented the variety of muscle anomalies and fibrous bands found in these patients. The nearly infinite minor variations in the location, path, severity of compression, and density of these muscles and bands are responsible for the differences in symptoms from one patient to another. Fascial bands leading from the C7 transverse process to the pleura and first rib may compress the C8 or T1 nerve roots either separately or together and anywhere from immediately distal to the foramen to the junction of the anterior and posterior divisions. Thus the symptoms will mirror the point of entrapment and the expression of the upper extremity complaints can be manifest in any of the peripheral nerves of the shoulder girdle and arm that ultimately arise from these nerves.

Mackinnnon and Dellon[51] have continued the work of Sunderland[102] and have shown that the response of nerves to compression passes through many stages. Initially, there is periodic ischemia related to interruption of local blood flow. Microscopically, there is subperineural edema. More chronic ischemia results in reactive thickening of the perineural tissues. Initially, the most external nerve fascicles alone show degeneration, whereas the central fibers remain intact. The implications of these findings are not to be underestimated. Clearly, there can be variation in the peripheral manifestations of more proximal nerve compression based on local anatomic factors.

The arguments of Wilbourn,[116] requiring a fixed set of criteria in all patients that can be uniformly reproduced, indicate a lack of appreciation for clinical evaluation of patients. In entities such as appendicitis, it is well recognized that the entire picture of the patient including history, physical, and laboratory studies must be put together to establish a diagnosis. Not all patients with appendicitis have identical presentations. It seems unrealistic to expect all patients with TOS to have fixed criteria for diagnosis. Nelems[48] has developed a set of subjective criteria that are divided into "must have, may have, and can't have" criteria. This is a useful methodology when approaching nearly all pain-mediated syndromes.

Patient complaints in cases of TOS can be broadly grouped into upper and lower plexus components. They have become clearly separable in our evaluations, along with other secondarily associated manifestations brought about by misuse of the arm and shoulder girdle. The anatomy of the brachial plexus must be studied repeatedly to comprehend the variety of nerve symptoms that are possible. The distribution of symptoms can follow any of the nerves derived from all branches of the brachial plexus. It is most important to understand that the symptoms caused by proximal plexus compression and entrapment therefore can be distributed to multiple sites distally.

Lower brachial plexus syndromes (lower TOS)

The symptoms of lower trunk plexus involvement include varying combinations of pain and other sensory disturbances in the arm and hand and mild weakness of the hand and arm. In the so-called true neurogenic variety, pain is remarkably absent and motor symptoms predominate. Pain is the central feature of the remainder of TOS cases that involve the lower plexus.

The pain of lower plexus TOS is often described as beginning at the base of the neck and supraclavicular fossa and heading to the area just inferomedial to the deltopectoral groove, which is the path of the nerve after passing under the acromion. The pain then extends variably down the arm in the ulnar distribution. More prominent distally are usually numbness and paresthesias extending into the fourth and fifth fingers. Elevation of the arm laterally and above the head places traction on the lower plexus and almost always reproduces the patient's symptoms. Careful history and sensory testing shows that the numbness generally involves the ulnar aspect of the middle finger.[90] This is helpful in differentiating TOS from pure ulnar-nerve compression.

Sunderland[103] believed that the usual descriptions of the peripheral sensory distribution of the nerve roots of the brachial plexus were misrepresented in the forearm. Fig. 42-2 represents the usual presentation of nerve root sensory distribution, with C6 supplying the index finger and thumb. In Fig. 42-3, Sunderland's view shows C6 to have almost no sensory distribution distal to the wrist, with C7 supplying the index finger and thumb. Notice also that the distribution in the radial forearm is described as C5-C6 (upper trunk) and the ulnar forearm and hand as C8-T1 (lower trunk), rather than as separate nerve roots. This more clearly fits the distribution of sensory complaints in these patients. In our experience, the lower trunk seems to split the long finger in patients with lower trunk sensory complaints[90] rather than involve the whole finger as described by Sunderland.[103]

Variations in the ulnar and median nerves must be understood when differentiating plexus-level neuropathies from distal neuropathies.[15,16] Absence of thenar wasting with a distal injury to the median nerve at the wrist can occur if both a Martin-Gruber and a Riche-Cannieu anastomosis are present. These communications generally contain motor neurons only. The Martin-Gruber anastomosis occurs distal to the elbow. The sensory findings in the hand should still correlate appropriately with the other findings of plexus-level pathology.

The motor complaints of lower trunk TOS usually are described as fatigue of the hand and loss of penmanship or the ability to write for lengthy periods. Wasting of the ulnar intrinsic and thenar muscles seldom occurs but must be watched for carefully in patients who are being followed in

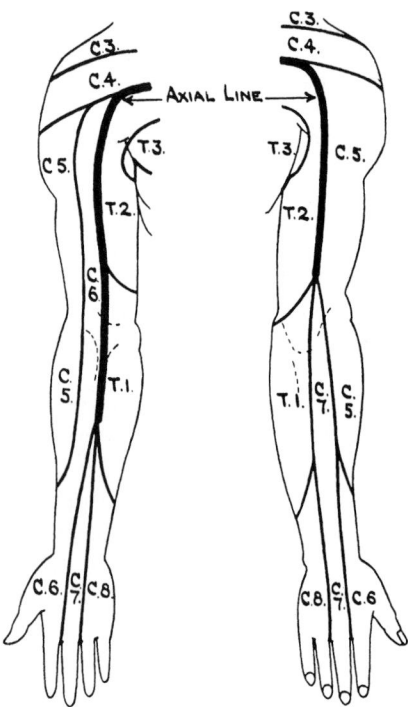

Fig. 42-2. "Classic" description of the peripheral sensory distribution of the roots of the brachial plexus. (From Seddon H: *Surgical disorders of the peripheral nerves,* Baltimore, 1975, Williams & Wilkins.)

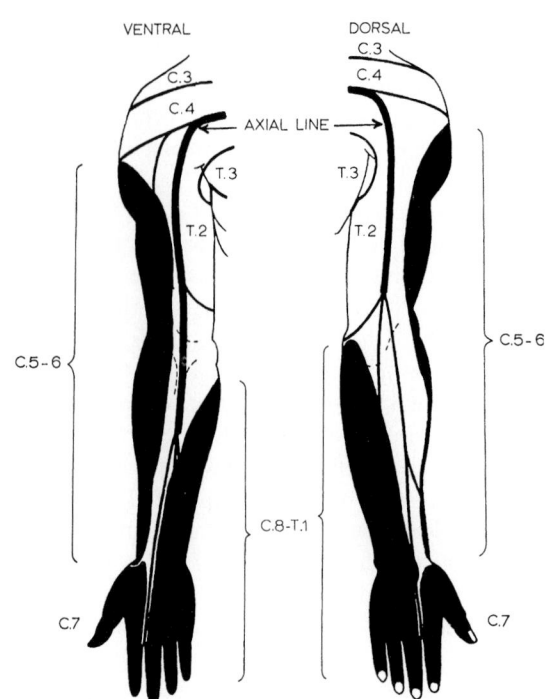

Fig. 42-3. Sunderland's depiction of the peripheral sensory distribution of the plexus. Note that the C6 is believed not to cross the wrist. (From Seddon H: *Surgical disorders of the peripheral nerves,* Baltimore, 1975, Williams & Wilkins.)

a therapy program. Development of atrophy is an indication for immediate surgical intervention.

Upper brachial plexus syndromes (upper TOS)

There are many recognizable forms of upper plexus involvement with TOS, which fall into repeatable patterns of complaint. To decipher these complaints, one must evaluate all aspects of the history, including the exact mechanism of injury, history of prior injuries, the precise nature of prior treatment and therapy, details of the conditions of the workplace, and other similar details.

The most common constellation of complaints in upper plexus cases involves pain along the trapezius ridge, into the suprascapular notch, and along the medial scapular border. There is also pain running posterior up the back of the neck to the occipital protuberance, and headaches that pass from the back of the skull forward toward the eye. Also commonly found is pain into the pectoral region, which often has a burning quality. Pain along the distribution of the long thoracic nerve, with winging of the scapula, is seen less often.

In many longstanding cases, patients will have facial pain, which is interpreted as symptoms of temporomandibular joint dysfunction. They may also develop what appear to be sympathetic-mediated swelling of the unilateral face, occasional lid droop, and eye pain. These groups of patients also commonly complain of difficulty with night vision.

To the skeptics of upper plexus–type TOS, these multiple manifestations of nerve compromise are ignored, discarded, and placed into diagnostic categories such as fibromyositis, migraine equivalent, and any variety of shoulder pathologic conditions. If one clearly and dispassionately reviews the anatomy of the brachial plexus, it becomes apparent that all of the aforementioned complaints are in the ultimate distribution of C5, C6, and the upper trunk or portions of the cervical plexus involved by scalene spasm and scarring. The pectoral symptoms come from the medial and lateral pectoral nerves, the periscapular symptoms from the suprascapular and long thoracic nerves, and more obviously, the radial sensory and first through third finger symptoms from the final peripheral-nerve distribution of the lateral cord.

The occipital pain is mediated through the irritation of the greater occipital nerve as it passes through the posterior musculature of the neck, which may be secondarily in spasm.[77] Although often called *migraine headaches,* there is usually no aura preceding the headache, and seldom nausea and vomiting. In Britain, these types of posttraumatic headaches have been labeled *footballer's migraine.*[55] There also appears to be a referred pain aspect to these complaints mediated through communications with the cervical plexus. Subcortical crossover pathways are known to exist, which may explain the origin of contralateral pain in some instances. These spinal and midbrain-level pathways also may explain the complaints of ipsilateral pain or numbness in equivalent fingers and toes that are found occasionally. In the teaching of acupressure techniques for relief of these posterior headaches, pressure is placed alternately over the occipital protuberance and the web space of the thumb with excellent results.

Mixed plexus syndromes

As understanding of the complexities of the brachial plexus improves, it becomes increasingly evident that the upper and lower plexus symptoms become intertwined. Patients with diffuse arm and shoulder symptoms must not be written off as having "nonanatomic" complaints. The anatomic abnormalities described by Roos,[82] which are repeatedly confirmed at surgery, make it clear that the distribution of complaints depends on the mixture of anomalies found in any given individual. There is marked variability in the involvement of C7 and the middle trunk with either the upper or lower trunk, symptomatically as well as anatomically. Considering that injury is usually the basis of modern plexopathy, it is wise to consider that with lower plexus injury, C7 may be involved in dense scar fixation to the lower trunk. A "sausage-casing" type of material can envelope the middle and lower trunk. Thus the symptoms may overlap in the median-nerve distribution.

In upper plexus injuries, C5 and C6 may be bound with C7 or the middle trunk to create symptoms and findings overlapping the median nerve with the upper plexus–lateral cord distribution. It should be remembered that the prefixed plexus has contribution from C4 and the postfixed plexus, which has contribution from T2, creating further variability in the usual manifestations of TOS.[53] The nerve roots and trunks will not conform to the same ultimate distribution and thus the symptoms may be variable.

Reflex sympathetic dystrophy

RSD is a poorly understood symptom complex that affects a small but important group of patients who have had some type of trauma to the upper extremity. Two of the more commonly used terms that are used interchangeably with RSD are *shoulder-hand syndrome* and *causalgia*.[42,98,99] The term *causalgia* is derived from the Greek words *causos,* meaning "heat," and *algos,* meaning "pain." The term *causalgia* was coined by and the first full description was written by Weir Mitchell during the Civil War.[78] Many other terms have been used, which further enforces the misunderstanding (Box 42-1). The International Association for the Study of Pain proposed a new term, *complex regional pain syndrome* (CRPS).[96]

CRPS is further divided into two types. Type 1 represents those cases classically referred to as RSD. Type 2 corresponds to causalgia. The essential differentiating feature between the two types using this nomenclature is that causalgia is associated with a major nerve injury. The trauma believed to be associated with RSD is often considered

---

Box 42-1 Terms used for reflex sympathetic dystrophy

Posttraumatic sympathetic dystrophy
Sudeck's atrophy
Sudeck-Leriche syndrome
Causalgia
Shoulder-hand syndrome
Sympathetic dystrophy
Complex regional pain syndrome
Vasomotor instability
Posttraumatic osteoporosis
Reflex dystrophy
Posttraumatic dystrophy
Posttraumatic neuralgia
Neurovascular dystrophy

"trivial." There remains no definitive test for RSD, causalgia, or CRPS.

It is common for patients to be labeled with the diagnosis of RSD or CRPS because of slight mottling of the hand, unexplained pain, pain with arm motion, edema, sweating, or similar complaints that may be associated with RSD. RSD should be excluded if a more definitive diagnosis can be made, and a diligent search for other causes should be undertaken before allowing this diagnosis of exclusion to be made.

Drucker et al.[17] divided RSD into three stages based on clinical presentation. Stage 1 is a reversible state characterized by hyperhidrosis, warmth, erythema, rapid nail growth, and edema of the hand. Resolution of symptoms may occur after treatment or spontaneously. In stage 2, mottling and coldness of the skin, associated with brittle nails and increased pain, is present. Osteoporosis is always present. Spontaneous resolution is rare, and response blocks or sympathectomy is less likely to be of benefit. Stage 3 shows a fixed atrophic hand with severe osteoporosis. There is seldom any response to therapy. Clearly, some overlap exists between the various stages, but this framework serves to reasonably divide the syndrome to allow appropriate expectations from interventions to be forwarded. Schwartzman and McLellan[91] authored an excellent review in 1987.

In our view, RSD remains a series of symptom-complex descriptions, not a freestanding diagnosis in most patients. A patient presenting with RSD-type symptoms should be evaluated thoroughly for evidence of a plexus-level condition. The relationship between plexus injuries and the development of RSD was recognized in the past, but has been understated in the recent literature. To quote from Barnes' 1952 manuscript on causalgia in Seddon's text,[4] "Multiple nerve injuries are commonly present and causalgia may be associated with all. In the upper limb there is always an incomplete lesion of the lower trunk or medial cord of the brachial plexus or the median nerve." Although our practice may see a skewed population, in all cases of "true RSD" that we have studied, there has been evidence of significant plexus conduction deficits. The findings at surgery in this group of patients uniformly show extensive fixation of the plexus to the surrounding tissues, particularly at the level of the lower trunk secondary to presence of a Roos band or scalene minimums type of anomaly. This fits the type of injury usually seen.

The most confusing aspect of RSD is that the development and severity of the RSD has not been directly correlated with the severity of the injury. Classically, development of RSD follows a traumatic injury to peripheral nerve.[39] The injury often is caused by the hand being caught in some type of machinery such as a punch press or roller. A neuroma or peripheral-nerve entrapment may precede the development of the RSD symptoms.[97] Careful history of the injury may show that the injury resulted in traction to the brachial plexus as the patient attempted to extract the hand from the machinery. The weight of a cast on the arm may cause traction to the plexus.

Fixation of the C7 nerve root (middle trunk) to the C8 nerve root or lower trunk is also found almost universally in these patients. The traction-fixation signs, which are elicited by the provocative postures on examination, have profound implications. It is probably safe to say that these signs will not develop unless the patient has more than one point of traction and fixation along the length of the nerve (i.e., the "double crush" phenomenon).

Others have clinically implicated sympathetic dysfunction as a significant problem in patients with TOS. Urschel[113] now performs a sympathectomy in all patients during transaxillary rib resection. This adjunct to surgery was found to be of limited value early in our experience and was ended in 1983. In most cases, the residual neurologic complaints after transaxillary rib resection appear to be related more to incomplete decompression and failure to release the traction-fixation at higher levels of the plexus than to the presence of sympathetic dystrophy.

Several issues remain confusing to those who study sympathetic-mediated syndromes: the severity of injury is not clearly related to the severity of the RSD; the response to therapy is extremely variable; untreated RSD usually "burns out" after several years; and the pain ultimately begins to subside, although the hand may remain nearly functionless.

ASSOCIATED MUSCULOSKELETAL PROBLEMS

Numerous musculoskeletal complaints are common in TOS patients and require further elucidation. The importance of understanding the interrelationship between TOS and these other associated problems cannot be understated. Major orthopedic texts[11] do not have even cursory mention of TOS, which further adds to the lack of understanding and recognition of the patient with TOS.

Impingement syndrome (rotator cuff tear)

The diagnosis of rotator cuff tear has been made and surgery has been performed in a large number of patients who eventually are referred for unrelenting arm and hand symptoms.[32] The suprascapular nerve, as it comes off the upper trunk, is the site of significant fibrous fixation in patients with upper plexus TOS. This can clearly lead to dysfunction of the supraspinatus and infraspinatus muscles and thus laxity of the rotator cuff. The sensory branches supply the articular surfaces of the shoulder joint. Impingement also occurs in patients with TOS because of the forward displacement of the scapulothoracic articulation at the shoulder. As a result of this forward displacement, the structures in the suprahumeral space (e.g., the tendon of the long head of the biceps, the supraspinatus tendon, the subacromial bursa, the superior aspect of the joint capsule) may become impinged between the greater tuberosity of the humerus and the acromion as the arm is abducted. Typically, the signs of impingement include pain referred within the C5 dermatome, a classic "painful arc," and loss of ROM at the glenohumeral joint.[11]

Appropriate shoulder posture and strengthening of the rotator cuff muscle group, particularly the supraspinatus muscle, can rapidly improve this entity. Certainly, multiple causes of rotator cuff injuries are not related to TOS. Those who do have TOS must be recognized because surgery on the rotator cuff will not be successful in most cases until the underlying upper plexus condition is treated appropriately.

Trapezius spasm

The trapezius is innervated by the cranial nerve XI (spinal accessory) nerve, and thus plexus pathology cannot be directly implicated in the sometimes severe pain in the trapezial ridge. The forward-sloping shoulder causes an imbalance in the shoulder girdle muscles. When the shoulder is elevated in a shrugging motion, the trapezius works alone if the shoulder is forward. The rhomboids and levator scapulae do not adequately assist the trapezius. Therefore the trapezius fatigues and tends to spasm. Appropriate posture, massage, and deep heat will often relieve this problem over time.

Biceps tendonitis

Similar to the previous discussion, biceps tendonitis occurs as the tendon partially subluxes out of the groove when the arms are used laterally and the shoulder is again positioned forward. This responds quickly to antiinflammatory agents in concert with proper shoulder positioning. In severe cases, steroids may be used, but repetitive injections should be avoided. The more proximal biceps tendon also can be involved in shoulder impingement.

Trigger points

Patients who have the other ancillary manifestations almost always have painful areas along the medial scapular border, along the posterior neck, and in the trapezial insertion into the scapula. These points of irritation are areas of periosteal inflammation at muscle insertions or areas of chronic muscle tension from either spasm or improper use of the muscle caused by poor posturing of the shoulder girdle. This may also be manifest as motor endplate sensitivity that becomes involved in a circular reflex within the spinal column. With improvement in the overall position of the shoulder girdle, the tender areas will gradually improve.[108] Moist heat, ultrasound, and massage may be beneficial. Resistant areas can be injected with local anesthetic and steroids, but this should not be repeated often.

Lateral epicondylitis

Symptoms at the lateral elbow are commonly associated with TOS. Chronic use of the extremity in abnormal posture, with the shoulders forward, causes the patient to inappropriately use the extensor muscles of the forearm. The chronic improper use of these muscles causes irritation at the muscle insertion into the lateral epicondyle. Treatment consists of retraining of shoulder posture and appropriate use of the arms in lifting and with repetitive use. Antiinflammatory agents and local modalities will sometimes be needed. Surgery should be avoidable with proper preventive measures. Symptoms referable to radial-nerve entrapment in the proximal forearm often are confused with lateral epicondylitis. The radial nerve is exquisitely tender at the border of the extensor carpi radialis. Careful examination should differentiate between the two entities.

PATHOPHYSIOLOGY

To understand TOS is to understand the variety of anatomic abnormalities as well as the pathophysiologic changes that are a consequence of these abnormalities. Sanders and Roos collaborated in a study of the thoracic outlet that compared the anatomy of cadaver specimens with the anatomy at surgery in patients with TOS. This study helps define the multitude of findings at surgery. If anything, however, their study and others underestimate the abnormalities found at surgery, particularly at the level of the upper plexus. The interdigitating fibers of the anterior scalene between the C5, C6, and C7 nerve roots found in the upper plexus TOS cases that we have explored have been severely underestimated.

A number of structures are at risk of compromise in the thoracic outlet: the brachial plexus, the subclavian artery, and the subclavian vein. The etiology of the resultant brachial plexus compression neuropathies is multifactorial, but certain risk factors predispose persons to this entity. Three broad categories of risk factors are (1) congenital structural, (2) posttraumatic structural, and (3) posttraumatic postural. When an inciting event occurs, a clinically significant compromise of the brachial plexus can result. The degree of congenital predisposition and the nature of the

inciting event will determine the severity and the clinical course of the neuropathy and or vasculopathy.

When the neck has sustained a significant trauma, particularly a flexion/hyperextension type, resulting in tearing of the scalene muscle bundles, two potential problems occur that directly affect the nerves of the plexus. First, contraction and fibrosis of the muscle bundles can increasingly compress the nerve roots and trunks. Because scar is an active tissue and undergoes progressive contraction for as much as 18 to 24 months, it is understandable that symptom progression often begins and continues many months after an injury.

Second, and even more poorly understood, is the fixation of the nerves to the muscle fascia of the scalene anomalies. This fixation is extremely common and occurs at all levels of the plexus. It most likely is caused by bleeding from the torn muscle and epineural connective tissue, causing adherence of the muscle fascia to the epineural tissues. This interferes with the basic need for the roots and trunks to have separate and free mobility with arm-shoulder and neck motion that allows the shoulder to function in a 360-degree arc. Repetitive traction injury causes anatomic deformity of the plexus and results in inflammatory repair, adhesion, and progression of the painful neuropathy. This scarring also is likely to progress over time.

Machleder et al.[50] have reported significant abnormal histologic patterns of the anterior and middle scalene in patients with traumatic TOS. Sanders et al.[89] found atrophy of type II fibers, and an increase in the average number of type I fibers has been demonstrated. In addition, the amount of connective tissue was increased by a mean of 36%. The importance of these findings should not be underestimated. The fibrous tissue content of the scalene muscles is often clinically apparent at the time of surgery as the muscle is transected.

Embryology

During the embryonic development of the upper extremity, a number of changes occur as the limb bud forms, which ultimately may become manifest in the problems encountered in patients with TOS. The scalene muscles form as one confluent muscle mass. This scalene muscle mass becomes separated into specific muscles only as the neurovascular structures penetrate it. Some argument remains regarding whether the scalene minimus variant arises from this original scalene mass. The muscle abnormalities found at surgery represent the variable fragmentation of the scalene mass as the structures of the limb bud pass through it.[53]

A C7 rib also forms in the early embryo, then regresses variably. Thus the residual cervical rib may vary from a complete rib to an elongated C7 transverse process. A dense fibrous band may be left in the place of the supernumerary rib. Some think that the presence of a cervical rib also signals the presence of a prefixed type of plexus (small T1 nerve and

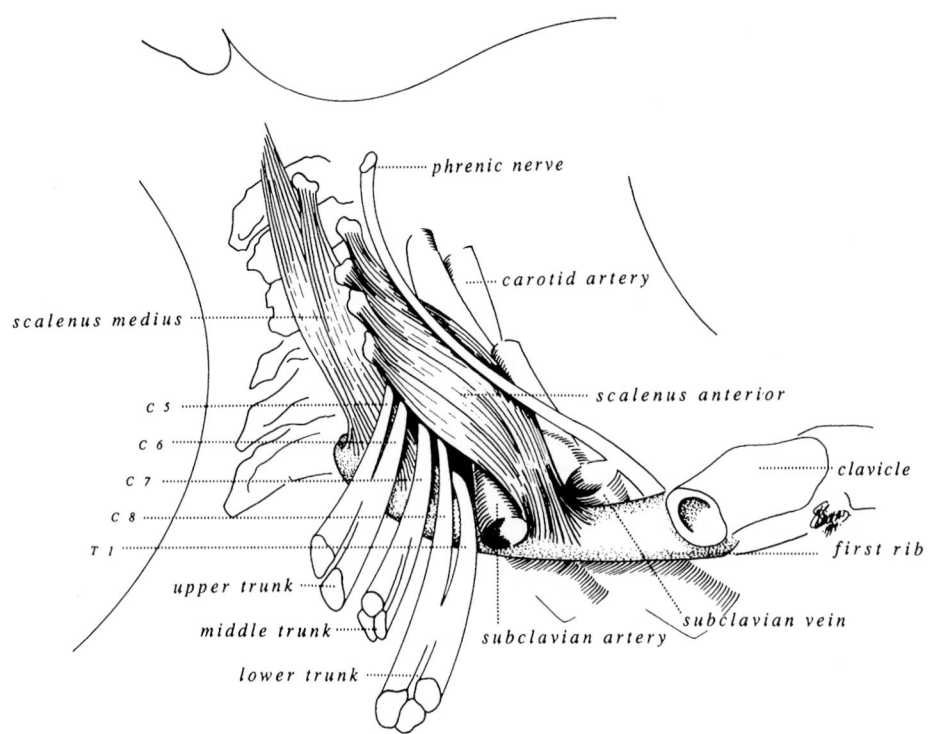

Fig. 42-4. Normal anatomy of the thoracic outlet. The brachial plexus and the subclavian artery exit between the anterior and middle scalene. The phrenic nerve arises from C4 and lies anteromedial to the anterior scalene.

major contribution top the plexus from C4). Our operative findings support this finding only on occasion.

Anterior scalene anomalies

The many abnormal origins and insertions of the anterior scalene muscle are the "lynch-pin" upon which the remainder of the plexus anomalies are built. In every textbook of anatomy, the anterior scalene is described to take origin from the anterior tubercles of the third through sixth cervical vertebrae, and thus lies in its entirety anterior to the plexus. The insertion is on the scalene tubercle of the first rib. The scalene muscles assist in flexion and lateral flexion of the neck. The function of the scalene as an accessory muscle of respiration has been questioned. The nerve supply to the scalene muscles is from the cervical plexus.

Abnormalities of the anterior scalene can affect the low plexus or the high plexus. The low plexus anomalies have been well described since the beginning of the understanding of TOS.[2,62] The importance of the upper plexus muscle anomalies has only recently been recognized as has the variability of symptoms related to minor variations in the exact nature of the compression.

The insertion of the anterior scalene may be anomalously attached posteriorly and laterally on the first rib, or onto the pleura (really Sibson's fascia). This serves to fix the lower plexus posteriorly and is more of an inciting factor when other structures posterior to the plexus force

it anteriorly. The insertion may be split, with a portion of the muscle posterior to the artery, which also fixes the plexus posteriorly.

Anomalies of the muscle origin superiorly are extremely common. The most common anomaly is a splitting of fibers around the C5 nerve root. This can vary from a tiny slip of tendonous tissue to a large mass of muscle. The muscle origins also may pass beneath C6 (Figs. 42-4 and 42-5) and thus affect the proximal C5, C6, or C7 nerve roots. The fibrous fixation of these proximal anomalies also may extend superiorly and create fixation to the nerves of the cervical plexus. The fusion of the muscle bundles to the C5 and C6 nerve roots may be on a congenital basis or may be related to injury with scar fixation. The fibrous tethering restricts nerve gliding. The layer of fascia that invests the anterior scalene extends upward in the neck and may tether portions of the cervical plexus to create the neck and facial symptoms often found with upper plexus TOS cases. Sanders and Roos[89] found this type of abnormality in 76% of dissections in patients with TOS.

Perhaps the most important anomaly to recognize is the complete posterior position (Fig. 42-6) of the anterior scalene, which places the C5 and C6 nerve roots in jeopardy for injury by the inexperienced surgeon during anterior approaches to the plexus. We have seen a number of cases in which nerve roots were transected when this anatomic variation was not recognized by the prior surgeon.

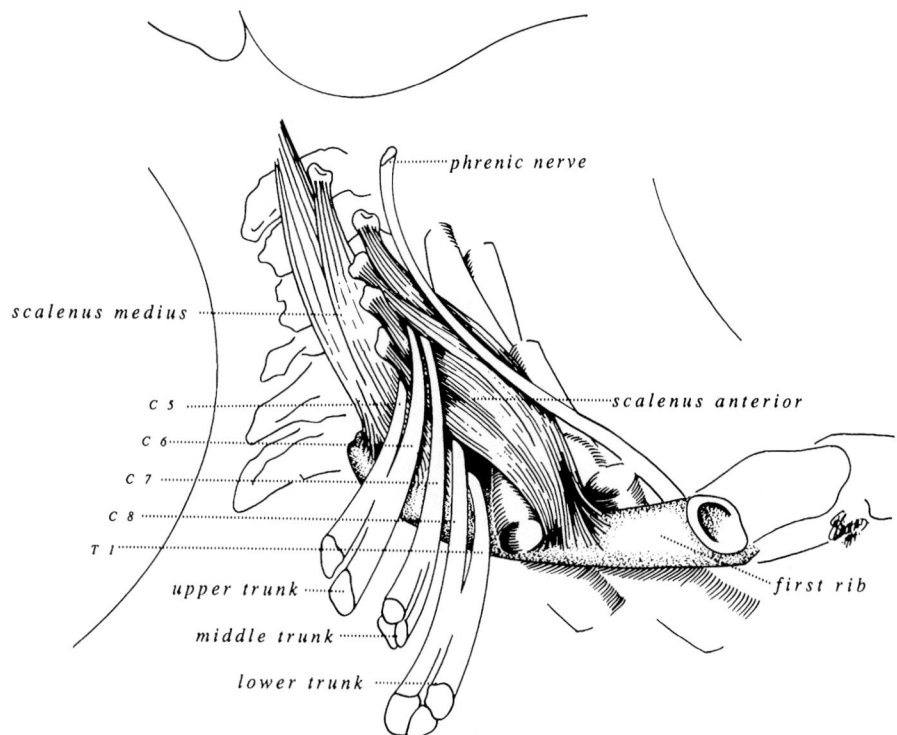

Fig. 42-5. Roots of the brachial plexus passing through the anterior scalene muscle. Here, C5 and C6 lie between slips of muscle that are originating from the transverse processes rather than the anterior tubercles. In the most common variation, a portion of the anterior scalene passes between C5 and C6.

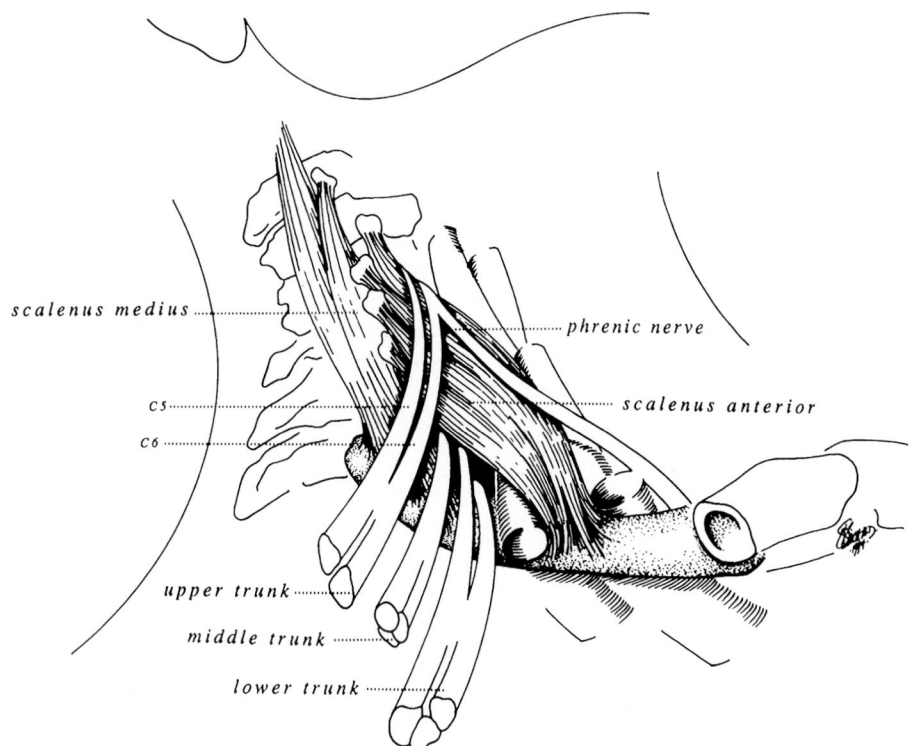

Fig. 42-6. Anterior displacement of the C5 and C6 nerve roots and low origin of the phrenic nerve. The phrenic nerve may arise anywhere along the upper trunk and thus may be more susceptible to injury during supraclavicular scalenectomy.

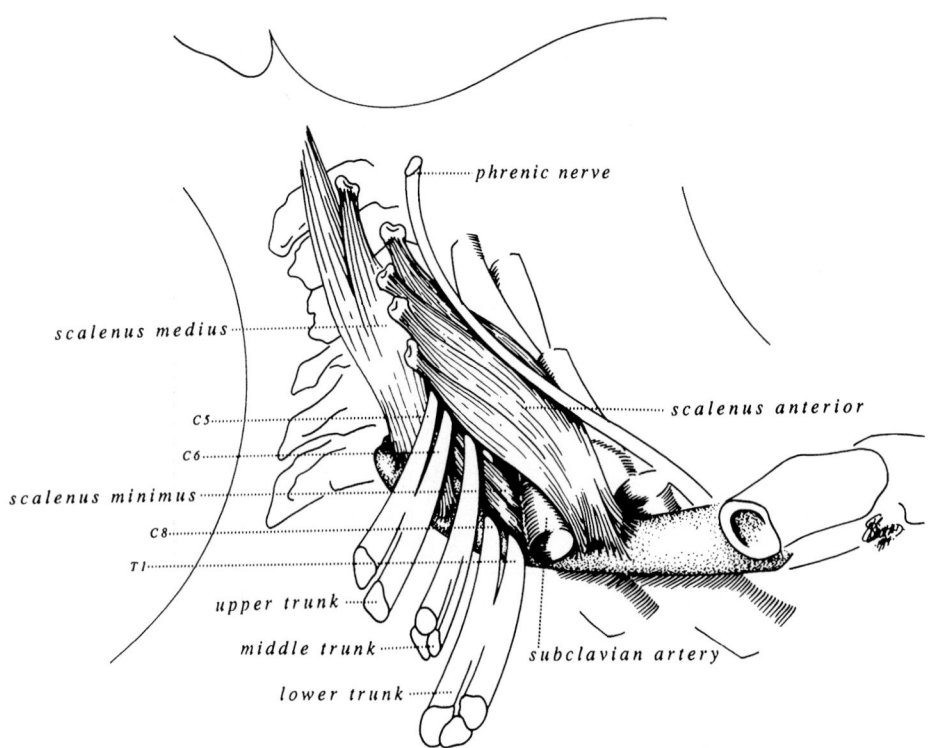

Fig. 42-7. Scalene minimus muscle causing lower trunk compression. This muscle may pass between the C8 and T1 nerve roots, causing only T1 compression.

There are occasionally unusual medial origins of the anterior scalene. The most inferior of these may compress the subclavian artery.

Middle scalene anomalies

Middle scalene anomalies are less well recognized than are anterior, but they are equally important.[106] The insertion commonly extends well forward on the first rib, occasionally forward of the anterior scalene insertion. This may throw the entire plexus forward, into anterior scalene abnormalities, and even against the clavicle. With the arms abducted and supinated, any motion of the arms in a plane posterior to the midline causes the nerves of the plexus to be stretched taut over the forward-placed middle scalene. These abnormalities are particularly important when the anterior border of the muscle is fibrous and sharply demarcated; this is the so-called middle scalene band. Slips of the middle scalene origin may arise anterior to the plane of the lower portions of the plexus and thus trap the lower plexus against the anterior scalene.

Congenital fibromuscular bands

Roos[82] has described and categorized 10 types of tissue bands that contribute to the compromise of the nerves of the brachial plexus. Type 1 passes from the tip of a short cervical rib to the first rib. Type 2 is a dense band that passes in the position of a cervical rib from the tip of an elongated transverse process of C7. Type 3 is a rib-to-rib band that

passes from the posterior to the anterior first rib, elevating the lower trunk or T1 nerve root. Roos believes that this is the most common anomaly he encounters. Type 4 is the aforementioned forward abnormal middle scalene attachment to the first rib. Types 5 and 6 are the scalene minimus anomalies. Type 7 is a thin tendonous band that passes from the middle scalene muscle to the sternum under the subclavian vessels. Type 8 is similar to type 7, and arises from the anterior scalene. Type 9 is a dense broad band of tissue, which is like a drum head through which the T1 nerve root must pass. This is what Sunderland[103] thinks is the extension of Sibson's fascia. Type 10 is similar to type 3, but extends to the back of the sternum or costal cartilage.

Scalene minimus and pleuralis

Scalene minimus and scalene pleuralis are muscles that arise from the anterior transverse processes of C7 and occasionally C6 and insert onto either the first rib (Fig. 42-7) or pleura. These muscles, also known as *Albinus' muscles,* are variously present, unrelated to the presence of any of the other described anomalies. The scalene minimus muscle then passes anterior to the lower trunk or the C8 and T1 nerve roots to insert onto the first rib. A scalene pleuralis variation may be identical except for inserting onto the pleura anteriorly. Occasionally, there is a double insertion onto rib and pleura. Uncommonly, the scalene pleuralis variant may pass between the C8 and T1 nerve roots, in which case the lower trunk is not formed until the roots pass beyond the first rib. These muscles vary greatly in their mass, angle of origin and insertion, and fibrous content. Thus the exact nature and position of the lower plexus entrapment may vary significantly.

Axillary arch muscles

The axillary arch muscle of Langer and the sternalis muscle are two muscles of the lateral chest that can cause peripheral-nerve compression lateral to "thoracic outlet." The muscle of Langer is a broad, flat muscle that originates from the tendon of the latissimus and passes anteriorly to insert anterior to the bicipital groove next to the pectoralis major insertion. It may trap the ulnar and median nerves high in the axilla just distal to the plexus and thus cause symptoms similar to lower trunk or medial cord entrapment. Supposedly present in 2% to 3% of the population, the muscle of Langer has been found only twice in our series and has seldom been described in modern texts. The presence of this anomaly should be considered in patients who are immediate failures after supraclavicular plexus dissections.

Radiation fibrosis

Radiation therapy is a well-known cause of scarring and fibrosis. The plexus may be included in the radiation field in cases of breast cancer and in the treatment of the mediastinum in lung cancer and lymphomas. Acute radiation injury to the plexus is relatively uncommon in the modern era. The delayed scarring that occurs after radiation therapy progresses slowly over time. Dissection of the plexus can be dangerous after radiation therapy from interference with the blood supply within the nerves.

Other fibrous anomalies

Fixation of C7 and C8 in a dense fibrous sheath, which appears almost like sausage casing, is found often. This type of anomaly may extend well out to fuse the entire middle and lower trunks. Similarly, the upper plexus can be entrapped in this dense matting. Based on its location, we have labeled this tissue mesoepineural fibrosis. This mesoepineural fixation represents the result of trauma, whereas hemorrhage and oxidative reaction results in fixed scarring. These types of fixation are extremely important in patients with symptoms associated with arm motion. When the arm is abducted, the nerves of the lower plexus are required to move differential distances, similar to the reins of a team of horses. When the nerve roots and trunks are fixed together, significant traction on the nerves occurs with motion. These fibrous sheaths also create significant compression when placed under traction, similar to the tightening of a Chinese finger trap.

Clavicle abnormalities

Clavicle fractures may heal with exuberant callus, or may heal improperly with posterior angulation. This can easily cause pressure on the brachial plexus with entrapment against the first rib.[48] First rib resection rather than clavicle resection generally is recommended to relieve the plexus-level compression.

Cervical rib anomalies

Cervical ribs are the most easily understood congenital anomaly and the most easily documented. Anteroposterior and oblique cervical radiographs are the best way to document a cervical rib. However, caution must be taken to view the radiographs personally, rather than to accept the radiologist's report of a "normal cervical spine." While looking for more serious acute pathologic conditions, one may not notice the rib. A chest radiograph is not optimal for evaluation of cervical rib anomalies because the standard posteroanterior view throws the shoulders forward and thus may hide the extra rib behind the first rib.

Cervical spine radiographs are much more sensitive at this time for rib anomalies than are studies such as computed tomographic (CT) and magnetic resonance imaging (MRI) scans. The "slices" viewed on both MR and CT images make it difficult to mentally reconstruct the presence of these types of rib anomalies in three dimensions. The radiographs of the spine should be obtained in at least four views. The oblique views of the spine are enlightening and often give a much better idea of how far the rib may be angled forward to interfere with the nerves of the plexus (Fig. 42-8). The cervical rib may occasionally be entirely within the substance of the middle scalene and not directly causative of any pathologic conditions.

The length of cervical ribs is often discussed relative to their likelihood of causing symptoms. Interestingly, a short rib that is angled forward is more likely to cause severe deficits than a long rib, which may even be fused to the first rib. Fig. 42-9 is an excellent example of this point, with the short, forward-directed left cervical rib being the symptomatic side. The few cases of "true neurogenic" TOS that we have seen have had sharp, forward-pointing ribs that indent the C8 nerve root from behind. All rib anomalies must be considered a significant predisposition to the development of TOS after some type of inciting event.

Elongated C7 transverse process

Cervical spine films should always be inspected carefully for the presence of an elongated transverse process of the C7 vertebra. This is defined as a projection beyond the plane of the transverse process of T1 and is easily visualized and measured. The importance lies in the anomalous attachments of scalene minimus, scalene pleuralis, and fibrous bands that are commonly associated with these elongated processes. In the angled cervical spine films, the space-occupying nature of this anomaly can be appreciated.

First rib anomalies

Deformity of the first rib is much less common than the presence of a cervical rib. A surprising number of first rib

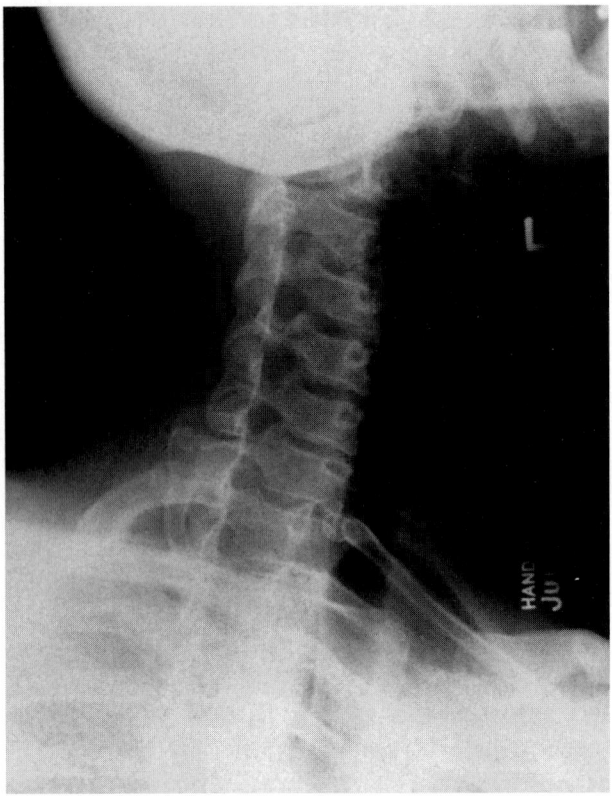

Fig. 42-8. Oblique cervical radiograph showing the forward angulation of the cervical rib (same patient as in Fig. 42-2). There was lower trunk compression and fixation caused by the anomalous muscles attached to the tip of the rib and direct trauma to the C7 nerve root as the nerve was displaced anteriorly.

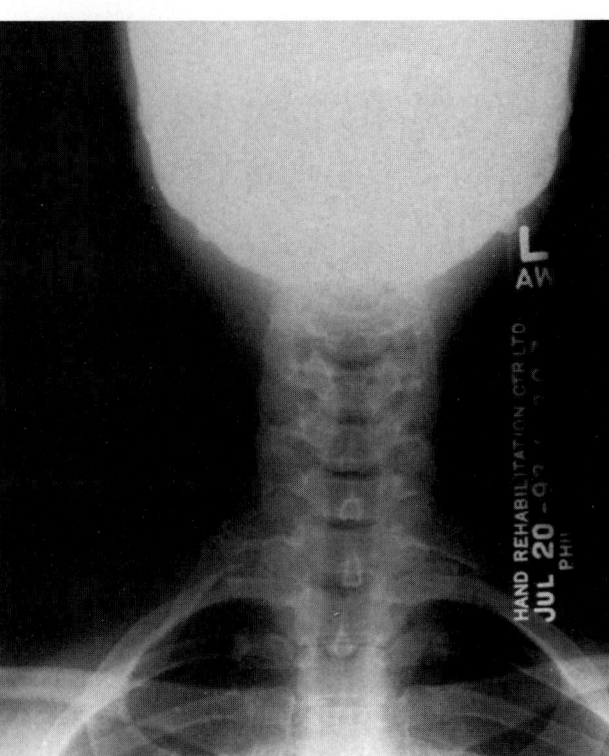

Fig. 42-9. Cervical spine radiograph showing bilateral cervical ribs. The left rib, although much smaller, is the more symptomatic.

deformities exist, however. Fusion of the first to the second rib at a point even with the location of the scalene tubercle (Fig. 42-10) occurs most commonly. The insertion of the anterior scalene may be displaced most obviously, but the middle scalene may be displaced significantly as well, and thus the possibility of pressure on the plexus (particularly the lower) may occur. The first rib also may be displaced superiorly, which lessens the already compromised space at the thoracic inlet (outlet). This particularly predisposes the lower plexus to the effects of downward traction of the arm.

Tumors of the first rib as a cause of TOS have been described by Melliere et al.[57] Fracture of the first rib may heal with protuberant callus, which may also compromise the thoracic outlet. First rib fractures usually are associated with severe trauma, and thus injury to the scalene muscles as well as direct plexus injury can occur easily.

Postural abnormalities

Postural abnormalities can contribute significantly to the development of TOS. Most clinicians recognize the concept of the "droopy shoulder syndrome."[105] When the angle of the clavicle is below parallel from the junction with the sternum, the entire shoulder girdle causes traction on the plexus. When there is an underlying congenital structural

abnormality, the malpositioned shoulder may in and of itself create the onset of symptoms. Distal injuries in the arm can also contribute greatly to the development of new-onset TOS symptoms. The weight of a heavy forearm cast can create downward forces on the arm.

Fatigue of the scapular elevator muscles in large-breasted women eventually may create drag on the plexus over the first rib. Breast reduction surgery may be warranted in some cases if a trial of physical therapy is unsuccessful at improving the posture and the symptoms. Pregnancy may similarly initiate symptoms in susceptible individuals as the breasts enlarge. Breast reconstructive surgery can also lead to compromise of the plexus by altering the space at the distal plexus, behind the pectoralis minor.[86]

Unusual positioning for long periods can also cause severe problems at the plexus level. There have been many descriptions of lower plexus neurogenic and acute arterial occlusive events occurring after coronary bypass surgery and lateral thoracotomy incisions. The commonly accepted wisdom has been to implicate improper positioning and overzealous sternal retraction causing direct clavicle–to–first rib compression. It is more reasonable to think that the problems arise in those individuals who have an anatomic predisposition from one of the many types of tissue bands.

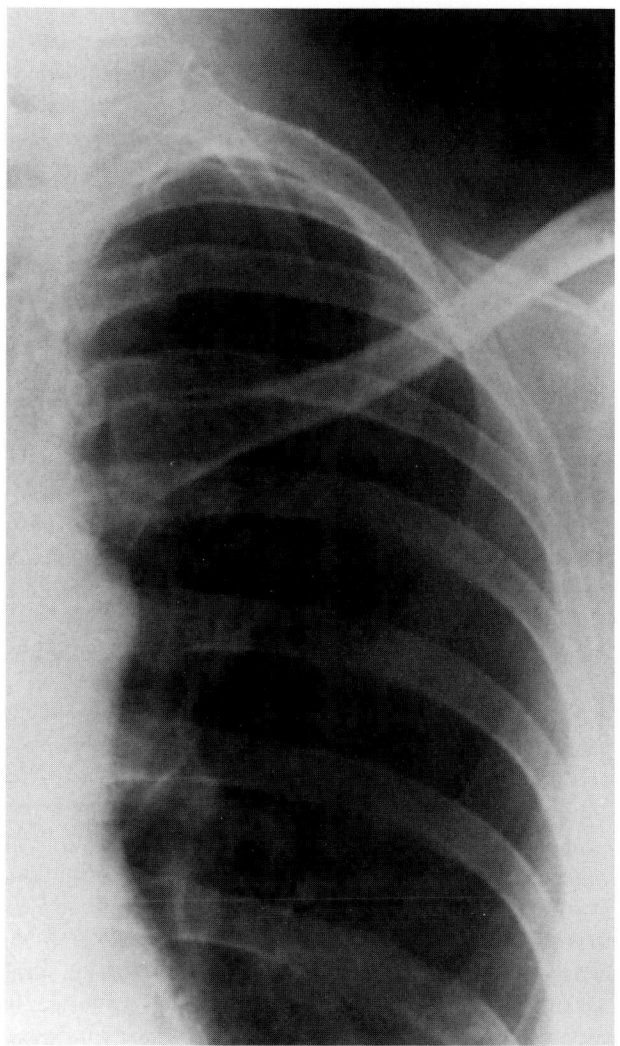

Fig. 42-10. Chest radiograph showing an anomalous first rib.

History

As with any evaluation of complaints by a patient, the evaluation of a patient with TOS begins by taking a thorough history. It is always best to begin by listening to the patient's complaints in his or her own words to avoid any bias based on misinformation in his or her records. Only after hearing the patient's description of complaints should one review the accompanying records.

We have developed a worksheet that aids in obtaining complete information. In addition to the history, the worksheet includes areas for documentation of prior studies, radiographs, the physical examination, and recommendations for care and follow-up. This has been valuable on many occasions, particularly because there often are legal aspects to these cases.

A full recording of the variety of complaints that have been described under manifestations begins the evaluation. With appropriate questioning, the clinician often can then bring out other complaints that the patient had not associated with the TOS symptoms. The exact mechanism of injury needs to be documented, including details such as the position of the arm, shoulder, and head as the injury occurred, and the type of machinery used. In automobile accidents, the use of seat belts and location and speed of impact must be documented. Box 42-2 lists the specific questions that must be answered.

The history also should include information concerning other medical problems that could influence peripheral neuropathies. The presence of diabetes, heavy metal or other toxic exposures, and thyroid disease should be questioned. Charcot-Marie-Tooth syndrome should be eliminated in patients with peripheral wasting; the lower extremity is initially involved before there is significant hand wasting. In endemic areas, leprosy should be considered in the differential diagnosis. There is usually profound sensory loss to localized areas of skin in cases of leprosy, followed later, if at all, by motor dysfunction as the enlarging nerve creates pressure on the motor nerves.

Particularly in the lateral thoracotomy position, an axillary roll or beanbag to elevate the chest wall away from the operating table is imperative.

The pivotal concept that unites these various etiologies of TOS is that TOS is often a dynamic problem. Until an event, or series of events, occurs that causes an alteration in the microanatomy of the tissues surrounding the plexus, patients may have no symptoms of any kind.

COMPREHENSIVE EVALUATION

The evaluation of a patient always begins with a thorough history and physical examination. In these complicated patients, it is best to request complete old records to understand prior treatments, nerve conduction studies, therapies, and surgical procedures. Many patients have been so thoroughly confused by the results of prior consultations that the history may be biased by their partial understanding of the problem. Thus the appropriate background information may be necessary to understand the entire picture.

Psychologic considerations

Chronic neurogenic pain syndromes such as the TOS complex can cause severe psychologic disturbances, and preexisting psychologic disturbances can contribute to the cause of chronic pain syndromes. Effective treatment of these syndromes requires the physician and therapist to be aware of the psychologic factors that often complicate the management of these patients.

The clinician should always remember what the patient has been through, in terms of the injury, the pain, the sometimes inappropriate treatments he or she has received previously, and not least important, the often-repeated statements made to him or her that "there is nothing wrong." We see many patients 2 or 3 years after injury, sometimes with several failed procedures predating our evaluation.

Because of the lack of reliable, objective pain evaluation techniques, difficulty is encountered in determining the relative importance of the psychologic factors and their relationship as either a cause or an effect of the chronic pain syndrome. Our inability to objectively assess the degree of psychologic contribution to the management of chronic pain presents an additional obstacle to the treatment of these patients.

The physician-patient relationship can be undermined by conflict of interest issues, which can insidiously interfere with the success of the treatment regimen. Impending worker's compensation claims and liability litigation can have a significant effect on the patient's response to any therapeutic measures. The treating physicians and therapists should not assume too readily that the failure of treatment in these patients is caused by psychologic illness, malingering, or motivation of secondary gain.

Proper consideration of these issues as impediments to successful treatment is important, but care must be taken to ensure that misconceptions are not allowed to interfere with good medical judgment and the quality of care. An approach must be adopted that will accept and integrate both the neurologic and the psychologic factors in the management program.

Because many of the symptoms of TOS are subjective, attempts to develop a reliable and repetitive measurement tool continue. These measurement tools also should be helpful in the long-term follow-up of patients as well as in providing a mechanism for reporting results. These measurement tools use the patient as the observer rather than the surgeon or therapist and thus can remove some unintentional inherent biases that occur because of the subjective nature of the complaints.

The Nottingham Health Profile is presently the most reliable measuring tool. To be used appropriately, it must be given preoperatively and followed for a minimum of 6 months after initiation of treatment to avoid the placebo effect. Placebo effect can show improvement in 20%; thus results of treatment must clearly exceed this effect. Other studies such as the Hendler Screening Test and the McGill Pain Scale are used by some to exclude candidates for surgery because it is believed that the degree of functional overlay would make a good surgical response unlikely.

Physical examination

The physical examination requires a thorough evaluation of the entire patient, especially of the entire upper extremity. The clinician must be sure that other diagnoses are not overlooked and that all coexisting diagnoses are made so that an appropriate treatment program can be initiated. The evaluation for carpal tunnel, cubital tunnel, and radial neuropathies is covered elsewhere in this text and should not be overlooked because multiple neuropathies are quite common.

Examination begins with the hands, looking for evidence of prior surgery or injuries, any changes in color, warmth, moisture, excessive nail or hair growth, and muscle atrophy. The skin and color changes of patients who are classified as having RSD are easily recognized. The skin is thin and glistening and hair and nail growth are excessive. The hand is held in a protective posture, and the patient usually tries to avoid any contact by the examiner.

Pulses at the wrist and capillary refill of the fingers are documented, as is any evidence of embolic disease or gangrene of the fingers. Arterial conditions are rare but must never be missed.

The atrophy of intrinsic muscles of the hand is best seen when viewed tangential with the fingers extended. The "true neurogenic" type of TOS involves both ulnar and median nerve fibers that originate in the lower plexus. Thus the thenar atrophy seen in this type of TOS can result from median-nerve or lower trunk compression. It must be remembered that the first dorsal interosseus muscle can sometimes be innervated by the median rather than the ulnar nerve. However, the involvement of the remaining intrinsic muscles should immediately alert the examiner that the patient has a problem other than carpal tunnel syndrome.

Neurologic examination of the upper extremity is performed, including sensory testing, deep tendon reflexes, and motor function. Motor strength is tested, first of the intrinsic muscles and thenar muscles, then progressively up the arm. The pinch test and resistance testing of the fingers and thumb are performed as measures of intrinsic muscle strength. The radial nerve (extensor) muscles of the hand, forearm, and wrist are then tested, followed by triceps and biceps testing. The triceps is supplied partially by C8, and thus may be weak in cases of lower trunk TOS. Biceps weakness is found in C5 disc disease.

Phalen's test is specific for carpal tunnel syndrome if performed properly. If the patient's shoulders are abducted to allow the dorsum of the hands to oppose, the resultant paresthesias may not be specific for carpal tunnel syndrome, but rather a reflection of upper plexus traction. Historically, Tinel's sign has been a reflection of nerve regeneration. More recently, it has been used to determine points of nerve fixation and irritability. An "electric shock" down the arm or into the hand with percussion over the nerve follows the nerve distribution. Division of positive Tinel's sign into upper plexus and lower plexus pathologic process significantly aids in localizing the areas of plexus involved. The shocks go to variable areas of the arm depending on the areas of the plexus involved. Palpation tenderness is equally important because no symptoms other than slight discomfort should be present. Upper plexus TOS symptoms can involve the entire distribution of the branches of the upper plexus. Thus symptoms commonly are noted into the pectoral muscle via the lateral pectoral nerve and into the suprascapular notch via the suprascapular nerve. Atrophy of the supraspinatus and deltoid muscles can occur following a severe traction injury to the upper plexus.

Inspection of the shoulder both anteriorly and posteriorly begins the proximal evaluation. Severe drooping of the shoulders with the clavicle well beneath horizontal is suggestive of droopy shoulder syndrome.[105] The drag on the upper plexus caused by this posture is not well recognized. The lower trunk can also be further tented over the first rib, or portions of the plexus may be compressed between the first rib and clavicle if the shoulders are held posteriorly. The clinician also should observe for abnormal posturing of the neck, laterally or forward in a swan-neck position, which often is seen after chronic scalene shortening. From the posterior view, inspection for scapular winging, supraspinatus or infraspinatus atrophy, and trapezius spasm is performed.

Evaluation of the neck is then undertaken to rule out cervical disc disease. Full ROM needs to be documented, both laterally and in flexion/extension. Compression of the cervical spine by pressure on the head is indicative of disc disease and should not be present in TOS.

The supraclavicular fossa is palpated to feel for masses, lymphadenopathy, and even cervical ribs, which are sometimes palpable. The muscles about the shoulder girdle are palpated for evidence of chronic spasm or myofasciitis. The sinewy areas of a muscle in constant use are tender and easily demonstrated.

Provocative maneuvers

A series of provocative maneuvers is then performed, which is very important in the diagnosis of TOS and should be documented clearly. It is important to understand what these tests represent and why there is variability from series to series.

The presence or absence of a positive Adson's, Halsted's, Wright's, or Roos' test neither confirms nor eliminates the diagnosis of TOS. It is only one piece of the puzzle. The presence of paresthesias in any of the provocative maneuvers is of more clinical importance in the diagnosis of TOS than is loss of pulse. Symptoms produced by these maneuvers represent the added compression or traction effects on the nerves of the plexus with motion of the arm and neck. This places the anomalous structures under increased stretch. Depending on the precise nature and orientation of the anomalous structure, variable compromise of the nerves is created.

The only situation in which arterial obliteration is believed to be of equal clinical significance to the nerve symptoms produced is when the pulse obliterates by simply turning of the head in Adson's maneuver or by elevation of the arm to less than approximately 70 degrees. This appears to represent compressive bands that put the artery at risk for development of later compromise. They also are so dense that attempts at therapy are unlikely to achieve any significant alteration in the degree of compression.

Pressure provocative test (Spurling maneuver). The brachial plexus lies much more superficial in the neck than is generally appreciated and can be palpated easily except in very robust individuals. Direct pressure applied to a nerve at the point of nerve irritation is quite tender. This phenomenon has been described in detail by McKinnon and Dellon.[51] Sanders[88] believes that this is the most reliable sign of TOS and that scalene tenderness is equally part of the cause of the tenderness to palpation.

Tinel's sign. The electric shocks that pass down the arm and even into the hand with percussion of a nerve are evidence of a positive Tinel's sign. This classically was used to follow the progress of a healing nerve as the regenerating axons produce tingling progressively down the arm.[107] It has become clear over time that nerves that are significantly irritated by either traction or compression also demonstrate a Tinel's sign. Tinel's sign at the plexus level can often show upper or lower plexus involvement as the position of the percussion is changed. The distribution of the signal down the arm is evidence of the areas of involvement of the plexus. Tinel[107] also described painful axon irritation when the injured nerve is tapped. Both types of Tinel's signs may be present in the compromised plexus.

The nerves of the arm should be tested at all levels for evidence of Tinel's sign. Multiple neuropathies of the upper extremity are much more common than appreciated previously, and thus Tinel's sign may be positive in the ulnar nerve at the cubital tunnel, the radial nerve at the radial tunnel, the median nerve at the wrist, or the plexus. The traction tests for the plexus may cause these signs to be acutely positive, and thus identify additional sites of peripheral-nerve entrapment.

Adson's test. The importance of the Adson's test in the diagnosis of TOS has been poorly understood. There are misconceptions that a positive test is essential for the diagnosis. It has also been stated that the pulse obliteration is so common that it is irrelevant. Adson's test originally was described in 1927 by placing the arm held at the side, with the head turned toward the affected side, and with a deep inspiration.[2] A positive test was considered to show paresthesias in the ulnar fingers and loss of radial pulse. Later, the presence of paresthesias as necessary for a positive test were eliminated by Adson. Currently, most examiners consider a positive test to be loss of radial pulse with the head turned to *either* side with the arm at the side and slightly hyperextended. The variability in the anterior scalene origins both anterior and posterior to the plexus may explain positional variation of pulse loss and nerve symptoms. Having the patient take a deep breath adds significantly to the percentage of positive tests. The clinician should also note which head position creates pulse loss.

Halsted's test. Halsted's maneuver places the arm at the midaxial point with the elbow at 90 degrees and the palms forward. The arm is then raised toward horizontal. Loss of pulse at any point as the arm is elevated is noted, as is the point at which the pulse is lost. Loss of pulse at 45 to 50 degrees of elevation is considered extremely positive and is indicative of a very tight Roos band, a muscle originating from the tip of a cervical rib, or scalene minimus muscle.

Wright's test. Wright's test[120] was described in 1945, and consists of progressive hyperabduction of the arm while palpating the radial pulse. Later, motion of the head away from the affected side was added to the provocative posture. Depending largely on the amount of shoulder mobility, compression of the subclavian artery by the clavicle can easily occur in this position.

Roos' (elevated arm stress) test. Roos originally described the Elevated Arm Stress Test (EAST) in 1976.[82] He believes that this is the most reliable test for TOS. The patient places both arms in Halsted's position, but with the arms braced behind the frontal plane. The patient then opens and closes the hands slowly for 3 minutes. A normal patient can perform this task with only mild fatigue. In a TOS patient, the patient's usual symptoms will appear. Most patients will notice distress very quickly and drop their arms into their lap. If the symptoms are confined to numbness of the thumb, index finger, or long finger after fisting the hand for this amount of time, the patient may have carpal tunnel syndrome.

Our experience has found the EAST to be valuable when the symptoms of numbness, pain, or paresthesias begin rapidly after arm elevation. Patients who have late symptoms most likely can benefit from a comprehensive program of physical therapy.

Costoclavicular compression test. The costoclavicular test of Falconer and Weddell[23] places the patient in exaggerated military posture with the shoulders braced firmly backward. As with the hyperabduction test, many normal subjects will obliterate the radial pulse.

Hunter's test (brachial plexus tension test). The concept of recreating symptoms by creating brachial plexus tension has been described by Elvey.[20] This concept has been modified by Hunter to include very specific arm motions that isolate the various roots and trunks. The additive effect of distal arm motion alters the tension at various portions of the plexus, which becomes more significant in the presence of a second distal area of entrapment. As we have become

increasingly aware of the traction neuropathy component in the patient with TOS, the effect of arm and neck motion has become clearer. Particularly in patients who are considered to have a double crush neuropathy, the additive effect of traction at two separate points over the length of the nerve creates symptoms as the nerve is placed under increasing traction.

The lower plexus is placed under maximum tension when the arm is placed at 90 degrees, with the elbow straightened, the palm upward, and wrist extended. When the lower trunk is fixed, the additive effect of this traction is to cause shooting pain and paresthesias down the arm in the ultimate distribution of the lower trunk (largely ulnar nerve). Thus most patients will complain of pain along the medial arm at the elbow with numbness and paresthesias into the fourth and fifth fingers.

The middle trunk or C7 nerve root will be under maximum stretch when the arm is held posterior to the midline and the arm is abducted to 40 degrees. Wrist extension adds further traction.

The upper plexus comes under maximum stretch with the arm placed in the exaggerated "waiter's tip" position. This will then send signals down the lateral arm and along the sensory paths of lateral cord/radial nerve and into the base of the thumb (as per Sunderland's nerve distribution in Fig. 42-3).

Our concept of double crush neuropathy is related more to traction than to compression. Just as the Chinese finger trap tightens as it is pulled taut, so does the dense mesoepineural fibrous fixation tissue about the plexus or distal nerves. This then can cause the transient ischemia that underlies the creation of nerve symptoms. A foreshortened nerve is at even more risk of entrapment (compression) by these traction effects.

Radiologic studies

Cervical spine roentgenography. Roentgenograms of the cervical spine are an essential part of the evaluation of TOS. Cervical spondylosis can simulate the syndrome; however, the presence of degenerative changes need not exclude the diagnosis of TOS. Cervical ribs (see Figs. 42-8 and 42-9), malunited fractures of the clavicle, and evidence of masses can be noted on cervical spine films. The length of the C7 transverse process should be noted because elongated processes commonly serve as the site of origin of muscle or tendonous anomalies that underlie the development of TOS.

Chest roentgenography. Roentgenograms of the chest in the posteroanterior and lateral projections should not be overlooked. The presence of cervical ribs or first rib anomalies (see Fig. 42-4) may be noted but can easily be missed because the angles of projection may obscure the extra rib. Entities such as superior sulcus lung carcinoma, myeloma of ribs, and intercostal artery aneurysms can be found on plain film radiographs of the chest. Superior sulcus (Pancoast) tumors with invasion of the T1 nerve root or the lower trunk of the plexus can mimic a lower plexus TOS, with pain in the lower trunk distribution being particularly prominent.

Angiography. Arteriography is necessary in the evaluation of vascular manifestations of TOS but is rarely needed when the neurologic manifestations are prominent. Documentation of a positive Adson's or Halsted's sign with an arteriogram is completely unnecessary because of the potential morbidity. When there is a question of aneurysm or occlusion of the subclavian artery or evidence of distal emboli, arteriography should be performed. Standard trans-femoral arteriography now usually can be replaced with digital arteriography or MR angiography.

Venography of the upper extremity is needed to evaluate venous occlusion in patients suspected of having subclavian thrombosis. Therapeutic clot lysis can be instituted immediately at the same sitting.

Magnetic resonance imaging. MRI is considered by most neurologists and neurosurgeons as the best study to evaluate discogenic disease of the cervical spine and nerve roots. As such, it is often done to eliminate central pathology as a cause of symptoms in a patient being evaluated for the possibility of TOS. In clear-cut cases of TOS, the additional cost of MRI cannot be justified. When other long-tract signs are present, such as Horner's syndrome or loss of bladder control, MRI should be performed to detect entities such as syringomyelia, gliomas of the spinal cord, and intradural metastasis.

At present, MRI, being a two-dimensional study, has not been helpful in demonstrating the abnormal structures that are often the underlying cause of TOS. High-resolution MRI with computerized three-dimensional reconstruction capability may lead soon to the ability to more easily demonstrate the anomalies that cause nerve compression.

Computed tomography. Presently, CT scan has limited use in the evaluation of patients with TOS, although CT scanning is considered superior for bony abnormalities. If there is any question of rib or pulmonary lesions as a causative factor, CT scanning is clearly indicated. Computerized three-dimensional rendition of the plexus, as with MRI, may be helpful in the future.

Nerve conduction studies

The use of a variety of nerve conduction studies to document the presence of TOS depends on the ability and interest of the examiner to thoroughly study the plexus. "Negative" studies commonly accompany patients with severe TOS because of the restrictive concepts of some neurologists. If deterioration of nerve function that is severe enough to cause loss of muscle mass is the only accepted end point in evaluation, quite clearly, few patients will be properly evaluated and helped. We have developed complete

confidence in the ability of our examiners to complement the workup with helpful nerve conduction studies.

Electromyography and motor nerve conduction studies. Electromyography (EMG) and nerve conduction velocity studies have been two of the traditional methods of evaluating patients with suspected TOS. Classic measurement has been to calculate the motor conduction velocity of the ulnar nerve across the supraclavicular transaxillary segment of the ulnar-nerve component of the medial cord of the lower brachial plexus. To accomplish this, a surface recording electrode is usually placed distally on the abductor digiti quinti muscle and super maximal-level stimulation is applied at the level of the axilla and at the supraclavicular space just proximal to the clavicle. To calculate reliable and accurate conduction velocities for this nerve segment, caliper measurements of interelectrode distance between the axilla and supraclavicular fossa are an absolute necessity. Normal conduction values for this segment have been calculated at 72 m/sec, with a normal and acceptable range of conduction being higher than 60 m/sec.[113] Because of the differences in cutaneous distribution between the lower and upper brachial plexus as they present in patients with suspected TOS, conduction across the lateral cord of the upper brachial plexus have been performed in much the same manner as the lower plexus cord components. Surface recording electrodes are used over the biceps muscle as the terminal muscle innervated by the musculocutaneous nerve component of the lateral cord and super maximal stimulation applied at the axilla and in the supraclavicular space just proximal to the clavicle. In this instance as well, accurate caliper interelectrode distance measurements are critical for valid conduction velocity calculations.

This technique has been challenged in the past,[25] partially because of technical considerations and partially because of the relative normalcy of conduction studies in patients who would appear to have clinically positive signs for TOS. The apparent paradox in that statement may be explained in part because the site of supraclavicular stimulation may be distal to the site of acute nerve compromise; that is to say that the compromise may be in the proximal component of the brachial plexus involving the upper, middle, and/or lower trunk segments. Because of this, normal conduction values across the more distal lateral, medial, and posterior cords of the brachial plexus can result in an erroneous ruling out of a thoracic outlet neuropathy.

In an attempt to evaluate more accurately the probability of injury or compromise to the proximal region of the thoracic inlet at the levels of the upper, middle, and lower trunks of the brachial plexus, techniques of cervical nerve root stimulation as described by McLean and Taylor,[56] later by Johnson,[34] and still more recently by Pavot et al.[71] have been used. This technique involves the use of stimulation with intramuscular needle electrodes at the level of the C8 nerve root for the lower trunk, the C7 root for the middle trunk, and the C5-C6 roots for the upper trunk and allows for calculations of the conduction time across the respective trunks of the more proximal plexus and components. When this technique is used in conjunction with traditional methods of supraclavicular-level stimulation of the lateral, medial, and posterior cords of the more distal brachial plexus, they collectively present a way of objectively evaluating the more distal cord components as well as the more proximal trunk components of the upper, middle, and lower brachial plexus. When interpreting the results of these nerve conduction studies, the clinician may look to find local slowing of conduction velocity across the cords or conduction time across the trunks as an indication of local segmental demyelinating-type neuropathy, or he or she may look at changes in the evoked motor amplitudes of response between those responses evoked with supraclavicular, cord-level stimulation versus cervical nerve root stimulation for the trunks of the plexus. The normal values for conduction across the cord components of the brachial plexus should be at least greater than 60 m/sec for the medial and posterior cord and greater than 70 m/sec for the lateral cord on a side-to-side comparison. Conduction times across the upper and lower trunks of the brachial plexus should be less than 1.0 m/sec on a side-to-side comparison. It is believed that the changes in either the amplitude or the conduction time and velocity of the responses across the respective components of the brachial plexus are indicators of local neuropathic compromise within the respective segments of the brachial plexus. These findings would then need to be correlated with the clinical signs and symptoms to facilitate a more comprehensive diagnosis of brachial plexus neuropathy and then further need to be integrated with the peripheral-nerve conduction studies to differentially identify multiple compartment neuropathies within the upper extremity as described later in this chapter.

When possible and when within a patient's tolerance, these studies should be performed bilaterally. This affords the opportunity of comparison with the "normal" or uninvolved nerve segments. Occasionally, slowed conduction will be recorded across segmental components of either brachial plexus, but the patient will exhibit or complain of little or no signs and symptoms. These findings can be used to call attention to potential clinical problems and afford the opportunity to provide prophylactic education, posturing job-site task modification and appropriate exercise instruction in an attempt to avoid or minimize the clinically acute situation from developing.

Sensory nerve conduction studies. Sensory nerve conduction studies (S-NCS) are performed during the evaluation of brachial plexus lesions and are concerned with the differential assessment of preganglionic versus postganglionic (dorsal root) disorders or injuries to the brachial plexus and between complete and incomplete brachial plexus lesions.*

Sensory nerve action potential (SNAP) amplitudes are usually reduced in postganglionic, incomplete lesions and are preserved and normal in preganglionic (complete/root avulsion) lesions. Traditional S-NCS in the evaluation of brachial plexus lesions have involved the use of "routine" studies (i.e., median curve stimulating at the wrist and recording from digit 2; ulnar-nerve stimulation at the wrist and recording from digit 5).[14,26] Some authors have discussed the importance of performing atypical S-NCS for more optimal assessment of focal lesions within the postganglionic brachial plexus.* Because none of the distal sensory nerve fibers traditionally studied traverses all of the proximal components of the brachial plexus, it is not possible for any single distal sensory nerve response to assess all components of the brachial plexus. Ferrante and Wilbourn[24] sought to more definitively evaluate specific distal sensory nerve conduction responses as indicators of more proximal, axonal loss–type postganglionic brachial plexus lesions. They reported on 53 lesions confined to a confirmed single trunk element of the brachial plexus and in the process described the optimal "route" taken by these respective nerves through the brachial plexus. They reported the following:

Upper plexus: In confirmed upper trunk lesions, 25 of 26 (96%) abnormalities were recorded from the lateral antebrachial cutaneous (LABC) and median digit 1 nerve responses traveling through the lateral cord, upper trunk, and C5-C6 nerve roots, and 15 of 26 (58%) were recorded from the radial digit 1 response traveling through the posterior cord, upper trunk, and C6 nerve root

Middle plexus: In a single confirmed middle trunk lesion, the abnormal recording was made from median digit 3 traveling through the lateral cord, posterior division of the middle trunk, and C7 nerve root.

Lower plexus: In confirmed lower plexus lesions, 25 of 26 (96%) abnormalities were recorded from the ulnar digit 5, 22 of 23 (96%) were recorded from the dorsal ulnar cutaneous (DUC) and 11 of 17 (65%) were recorded from the medial antebrachial cutaneous (MABC) sensory nerves, all traveling through the medial cord, lower trunk, and C8 nerve root. Thus, in suspected focal postganglionic lesions or with comprehensive screening of the postganglionic sensory components of the brachial plexus, it would be prudent and relatively simple to perform S-NCS of the LABC, median, and radial digit 1 sensory responses for suspected upper plexus lesions; median digit 3 for suspected middle plexus lesions; and ulnar digit 5, DUC, and MABC sensory responses for suspected lower plexus lesions.

Somatosensory evoked potential. Somatosensory evoked potential (SSEP) examination is an effective tool[33] to aid in measurement of brachial plexus conduction deficits.

*References 5, 37, 45, 67, 68, 103, 114.

*References 3, 19, 24, 49, 85, 100, 115, 117.

Machleder et al.[50] have shown the study to be helpful during evaluations and have shown intraoperative improvement in SSEP conduction after release of constricting bands or scalene anomalies. SSEP studies measure sensory conduction in the peripheral nerve and cord/trunk distribution of the brachial plexus, the cervical roots/posterior cervical cord, and the subcortical sensory pathways. All recording electrodes are in fixed positions along the somatosensory pathway (i.e., elbow, axilla, supraclavicular, second cervical spinous process, and scalp locations). Assessment of peripheral, proximal, and central sensory lesions could be performed from median-, ulnar-, and radial-nerve stimulation at the wrist.

Summary. A group of electrophysiologic studies is recommended for evaluating suspected brachial plexus neuropathies. This group includes motor nerve conduction studies (M-NCS) of the respective cords (lateral, posterior, and medial) and trunks (upper, middle, and lower) of the brachial plexus; S-NCS involving the respective upper plexus (MABC, median, and radial digit 1), middle plexus (median digit 3), and lower plexus (ulnar digit 5, DUC, and MABC) distributed sensory nerves; SSEP testing of respective sensory afferent nerves; and needle EMG studies of the respective myotomal distribution musculature. These tests can be a powerful complement of objective measures that can be used collectively in the differential documentation of postganglionic brachial plexus (traction and incomplete avulsion) injuries. All M-NCS and S-NCS responses should be recorded and compared bilaterally. Conservatively, a side-to-side focal SNAP amplitude difference greater than 50%[24] is considered suspect for a postganglionic brachial plexus, axonal loss–type neuropathy. The specificity of focal nerve involvement, correlated with the clinical signs and symptoms, will assist in localizing and quantifying the involved brachial plexus segments.

Sensory testing. Objective measurement of sensory nerve function has classically consisted of two-point discrimination testing and monofilament pressure testing. Vibration thresholds have been described, which might prove to be a very important addition to the armamentarium. The use of vibration thresholds includes the concept of provocative positioning. Clearly, many patients' symptoms are worsened by altered positions of the extremity. Electrical studies under stress positioning have technical difficulties that can render the studies unreliable and poorly reproducible. A reproducible, easily performed, painless study is a significant addition to the evaluation of the nerve-injured extremity.

Semmes-Weinstein monofilament testing is the most commonly used pressure test. By using graded fine monofilaments, a pattern of sensibility in the hand can be established. This is a time-intensive study to perform. Two-point discrimination can be measured with both static and moving techniques. Plexus-level pathology has been poorly correlated to either method of two-point study.

It is well known that loss of response to vibration is one of the earliest manifestations of peripheral neuropathies. Vibration threshold measures the smallest threshold of the quickly adapting nerve fibers to stimulation by a fixed-frequency, variable amplitude device. After baseline measurements, the symptoms are provoked by elevation of both arms overhead for 30 seconds, with pressure applied to the plexus. Novak, Mackinnon, and Patterson[65] reported accurate correlation with TOS symptomatology.

Noninvasive vascular laboratory studies

The presence of vascular occlusive signs does not directly correlate with the presence of neurologic types of TOS. Therefore the usefulness of these studies is somewhat limited. A vascular laboratory evaluation that shows no arterial compression does not eliminate the diagnosis of neurogenic TOS. The diagnosis of TOS is missed in many patients because of the continuing misconception that a positive Adson's sign or diminished pulse volume recordings in stress positions is necessary to make the diagnosis of TOS.

Hard-copy documentation of positive postural arterial occlusive signs is easily done with pulse volume recordings or plethysmography. Duplex ultrasound also can show flow disturbances and is indicated in all cases in which there is evidence of arterial pathologic involvement (e.g., embolic disease, unilateral decrease in blood pressure, pulsatile supraclavicular mass). Differentiation of fixed small-vessel arterial occlusions such as Buerger's disease from vasospastic disorders can be accomplished, which may assist in the decision whether to consider sympathectomy.

THERAPY FOR THORACIC OUTLET SYNDROME

A trial of physical therapy is initiated in all patients before considering surgical decompression. Even in patients in whom surgery is recommended at the initial visit because of evidence of atrophy of intrinsic muscles, the presence of cervical ribs, or vascular complication, therapy will be of benefit in the postoperative period. The therapy program must be performed faithfully and appropriately to achieve satisfactory results. If there is dissatisfaction about the treatment plan that has been administered previously, renewed efforts at a proper therapy program should be undertaken.

After surgery, therapy has an equally important role in achieving the ultimate results. Roos[84] believes that "active physical therapy should be avoided—and offers no particular benefit." On this point we disagree completely. Certainly, inappropriate forceful exercises, particularly those performed on some types of passive motion machines, may injure the patient. To achieve maximal benefit from nerve release, nerve gliding must be maintained to prevent delayed scar fixation and contraction. Proper posture, stretching, and later, strengthening exercises must be completed daily for at least 1 year postoperatively. Some patients will require close supervision. If therapy is unlikely to be completed because of compliance problems, insurance denial, or nonavailability, surgery is best avoided in complex cases because the results will not be satisfactory. For details on the therapy, refer to Chapter 44.

TREATMENT OF REFLEX SYMPATHETIC DYSTROPHY

The initial evaluation should include a complete upper extremity examination. Clear-cut etiologies for initiation of RSD, such as fracture fragments irritating the median nerve, should be addressed immediately. The use of a stellate or sympathetic block then becomes both a diagnostic and a therapeutic tool. A proper block requires a limited volume of local anesthetic properly placed. There should be no local anesthetic "leakage" to the nerve roots. If the response to sympathetic blockade is good and prolonged, repeat injections may be performed. If the response to sympathetic blockade is good but is of limited duration, early sympathectomy should be considered. The results of sympathetic blockade in cases approaching stage 3 usually are disappointing, as are the results of surgical sympathectomy. The intermediate levels of severity are associated with variable results from treatment. Intravenous phentolamine, bretylium, reserpine,[6] and guanethedine[30,56] can sometimes achieve a more long-lasting effect.

What is clear to all investigators is that severe symptoms of long duration will result in disappointing results from treatment. Patients must not be allowed to progress into stages 2 and 3 without intervention. After diagnostic blockade confirms the diagnosis, further treatment with analgesics as well as nontraumatic physical therapy is undertaken. In some instances, α-blockers will have benefit, but in the absence of significant hypertension, may not be well tolerated. Combinations of calcium channel blockers and nonsteroidal and narcotic medication offer a modest chance of relief.[32] The use of a Bier block of local anesthetic and steroids has been popularized by Poplawski et al.[74]

Physical therapy is undertaken to aid in diminishing the edema and joint contractures. Wrapping techniques, elevation, intermittent compression, and careful joint mobilization is begun. A transcutaneous electrical nerve stimulation unit may be of some benefit.[101] Postural exercises and mobilization of the lower plexus with appropriate therapy is done. If improvement is short-lived and symptoms recur rapidly, surgery should be performed. In stage 1 RSD, sympathectomy alone may be considered if there is no evidence of significant plexus pathology.[70] With newer thoracoscopic techniques, video-assisted transthoracic sympathectomy is accomplished with minimal risk or discomfort.

However, sympathectomy alone is unlikely to yield optimal benefit in stage 2 disease. Without relief of the severe traction and fixation of the lower plexus, recovery will be limited. Surgery should also be directed at relief of other associated lesions such as painful neuromas or nerves trapped in a suture. The results of our honest attempts to ameliorate the pain of severe stage 3 RSD have been nearly uniform in their failure. Despite finding significant pathologic conditions at the time of surgery, which accounts for the symptoms, once stage 3 disease is reached, treatment has had little impact. At this time, we do not recommend surgery on patients with stage 3 RSD.

SURGERY

Failure of conservative therapy is indication for surgery if the symptoms are severe enough to warrant intervention. In a few instances, surgery should be undertaken rapidly, sometimes without a trial of physical therapy. Development of muscle atrophy is indication for immediate intervention before further loss of motor units ensues rapidly. Immediate surgery is indicated in cases of venous and arterial thrombosis. In these instances, decompression of the vessels should commence soon after clot removal or lysis. We also believe that extremely positive vascular occlusive signs with minimal arm motion should prompt early intervention because of the risk of arterial complications.

The type of procedure recommended is based on a number of factors. Presently, the two major approaches to surgical decompression of the thoracic outlet are transaxillary first rib resection and comprehensive supraclavicular plexus decompression with scalenectomy. Other procedures such as scalenotomy are of historical interest only.

In cases of lower trunk compression only, without history of significant trauma, the transaxillary approach described by Roos[81] is the approach of choice. When there has been significant whiplash-type trauma or direct trauma to the neck at the level of the plexus, the likelihood of fibrous fixation of the upper plexus makes transaxillary resection of the first rib a poor choice. In this instance, we prefer a supraclavicular approach. A small number of surgeons prefer performing first rib resections via a posterior approach. These procedures should be performed only by those with specific interest in this field. The complication rate of surgery reported by some authors is excessive. Leather[43] has reported that thoracic outlet operations are the number one cause of payment in malpractice claims in the state of New York.

Transaxillary first rib resection

Roos[81] described the transaxillary approach for resecting the first rib in 1966. Before that time, the posterior thoracotomy approach was favored, similar to rib resection for thoracoplasty for tuberculosis. The transaxillary approach proved to be much easier technically and came into favor by most chest and vascular surgeons. The theory for first rib resection lies in the concept that TOS is a disease of the lower trunk and medial cord of the plexus, caused by a number of anomalous structures that attach to the first rib or pleura, and are accessible through this approach.

Roos[81-83] has described this approach in great detail in many publications and recently made a videotape of the procedure, which should be reviewed by anyone who plans to use this technique. The written description in Rutherford's text, *Vascular Surgery,*[84] is very clearly presented and is recommended for the many technical details of the procedure. Urschel[111] has suggested using a video scope to assist visualization of the nerves and vessels at the apex.

In the hands of experienced surgeons like Roos, the transaxillary approach is indeed safe and the risk of nerve injury or vascular injury is minimal. However, for the occasional operator, the risks are quite high. Thus it is common to see on follow-up cervical spine films that a long length of first rib has been left in place posteriorly. When this type of radiologic evidence is found, one can be sure that an inadequate decompression of the lower plexus has been performed. Other problems encountered with the transaxillary approach are inadequate removal of the myofascial bands and intercostobrachial nerve neuralgia, which is very annoying to the patient.

Patients with fixed adhesions of the upper plexus (traction fixation injury) may have increased symptoms after transaxillary first rib resections as the scalene muscle retracts superiorly. If this does occur, an early supraclavicular resection of residual scalene muscle is indicated.

Scalenotomy and scalenectomy

Division of the anterior scalene or partial resection, as practiced for many years as first described by Adson,[1,2] will relieve symptoms in a moderate number of patients. Which patients with isolated lower trunk symptoms will respond to scalenectomy alone is difficult to predict. As has been well documented by a number of anatomic studies, many other structures exist that can create lower plexus symptoms other than anomalous attachments of the anterior scalene. In patients with only posterior displacement of the scalene attachments to the first rib or pleura, the resection of the scalene should relieve lower plexus compression.

When combined with resection of other anomalous bands, scalenectomy will increase the likelihood of satisfactory decompression of the lower plexus. Other problems will not be resolved by partial lower anterior scalenectomy, which has resulted in development of the concept of total plexus decompression.

Total brachial plexus decompression

Limitations of the transaxillary first rib resection led to reevaluation of scalenectomy. Naffziger and Grant's original scalenotomy procedure[62] consisted simply of division of the anterior scalene above its attachment to the first rib. When scalenectomy was performed in the past, it was divided from the first rib and then resected above the C7 level. Recurrences, particularly at the level of the upper plexus, were common enough to cause continuing reevaluation of the procedure. The concept of compression and fixation of the lower plexus was clearly understood; however, continuing symptoms from the upper plexus remained an issue. Scarring

and fixation caused by the interdigitating bundles of anterior scalene between the C5, C6, and C7 roots eventually received the attention they deserved.

The patient is placed supine on the operating table. Nonparalyzing general endotracheal anesthetic is given so that nerves can be tested throughout the procedure. The endotracheal tube should be brought out of the nonoperative side of the mouth to avoid kinking and to provide access for the anesthesiologist. The head is tilted away from the operative side approximately 20 degrees, and the chin is elevated. We use a vacuum beanbag to hold the head in place. The entire neck, anterior chest, and arm are prepped and draped. The impervious stockinet that has been placed on the arm is clipped to the chest wall to keep it in place throughout the procedure. Slight downward traction is placed on the arm by clipping a Kling that has been wrapped about the stockinet to the drapes.

The incision, which splits the lateral border of the sternocleidomastoid, is made in the skin line 2 to 3 cm above the clavicle, depending on the size of the patient. The incision is taken through the platysma muscle. Hemostasis is obtained with electrocautery. The lateral border of the sternocleidomastoid is mobilized extensively and the dissection is carried down to the deep cervical investing fascia. The fascia is opened superior to the omohyoid muscle and is widely separated. This exposes the scalene fat pad. An avascular plane is developed either medially or laterally around the fat pad to avoid both venous and lymphatic vessels.

The fat pad is retracted with a small self-retaining retractor. The anterior scalene can now be seen. Careful note of the position of the phrenic nerve is immediately made. At this time, the upper trunk of the plexus can be encountered lying anterior to the scalene, which must be recognized (see Fig. 42-6). When the phrenic lies on the anterolateral aspect of the scalene, it must be mobilized with its surrounding fascia over its full length so that it can be carefully kept medial out of harm's way throughout the procedure. When the phrenic originates directly off the upper trunk, it is quite short and the dissection must tediously work around it because it cannot be retracted.

The medial and lateral aspects of the lower anterior scalene are freed, exposing the subclavian artery. A plane is developed between the artery and the muscle with a large right-angled clamp. A Kocher clamp is placed across the muscle, carefully observing the phrenic nerve. A bipolar cautery is used to detach the anterior scalene from the first rib and the muscle is retracted superiorly.

Numerous small vessels are usually found along the medial aspect of the muscle; these are also divided with the bipolar cautery. Any aberrant portions of the muscle distally are removed with the specimen. As the dissection continues superiorly, the anterior scalene origins from the transverse processes of C4, C5, and C6 split and pass between the C5, C6, and C7 nerve roots in a variety of patterns. These anomalies occur in almost every case of upper plexus TOS. With use of blunt and sharp dissection as appropriate, these slips of muscle are dissected away from the upper nerve roots and divided at the origins from the transverse processes. The use of bipolar electrocautery makes this dissection safe and hemostatic. Care is taken to avoid the branches to the long thoracic nerve, which emanate variably from the posterior aspect of C5, C6, and C7.

After the anterior scalene is totally removed, the C7 nerve root/middle trunk is identified and encircled with a vessel loop. Sometimes, C7 is fused to C8 with a dense matted epineural fixation that must be dissected away to free the nerves completely. The subclavian artery is encircled with a vessel loop. If there are any branches of the subclavian passing through the lower plexus, they are divided with small silk ties.

If a scalene minimus muscle is present, it will be encountered at this time and is resected. Any other anterior Roos bands are resected. The lower trunk is thus exposed and is also encircled with a vessel loop. Any anomalies of the middle scalene are resected at this time. When the middle scalene has a firm fibrous anterior border or inserts well forward on the first rib, it is partially resected. Portions of the origins of the middle scalene superiorly also quite commonly pass forward to lie in a plane anterior to the nerve roots. These slips of muscle are also resected.

When present, a cervical rib is now resected along with any muscle attachments. The periosteum is removed with the rib to avoid the possibility of regrowth of the rib. Angled Kerrison rongeurs are used to remove the rib proximally so that the nerves can be fully visualized as the rib is removed.

Once all of the muscle anomalies have been resected, attention is directed to the nerves themselves. The fusion of C7 to either the upper or lower trunk is common. The mesoepineural fixation of the various trunks must be separated to allow the nerves of the plexus to move through the full ranges of shoulder motion. The need to release this fixation is apparent when the arm is moved during surgery. At different positions during motion, the tension on the various trunks is assessed. Nerves that are significantly taut either require further mobilization and relief of the mesoepineural fixation or are fixed at other levels distally. The root trunks and divisions of the plexus can be mobilized without fear of devascularization. There is never any bleeding from the nerves when the dense scar is removed, indicating that the blood supply of the nerves is internal at this level. Equally important is the complete lack of any nerve functional loss when this type of dissection is performed. It must be understood that this is not an internal neurolysis.

Assessment of the need for a first rib resection is then made. If there is compression of the plexus between the first rib and clavicle or if there is evidence of the lower trunk being pulled tight over the rib with arm motion, a first rib resection is done. First rib resection can be accomplished safely via this same incision, except in extremely muscular individuals. The middle scalene attachments to the first rib are cleared from the superior surface of rib. Care must be taken to be sure of the position of the long thoracic nerve, which often passes through the substance of the middle scalene. The most posterior aspect of the first rib is transected serially with Kerrison rongeurs. The intercostal muscle is then separated from the first rib by either blunt or sharp scissors dissection. By forward displacement of the shoulder, a good view of the anterior rib can be obtained. Using angled duckbill or Kerrison rongeurs, the rib is transected anteriorly and removed. In some cases, piecemeal resection is necessary.

A sympathectomy is easily done from this approach, if required. The pleura is bluntly separated from the ribs at the posteromedial rib and retracted forward. Finger palpation easily identifies the sympathetic chain at the level of the second rib. The sympathetic chain is elevated on a right-angle clamp and grasped with the right angle. Dissection is then taken distally at least to the fourth rib and the chain is divided. Through this approach, the stellate ganglion is easily seen. The efferent branch to the T1 nerve root can be seen, and the chain is divided at this level. In theory, there should never be a Horner's syndrome if the sympathetic chain is divided at this level. We have seen several cases in which no eye symptoms have been present, but there is absence of facial sweating on the operated side, as well as two cases of permanent Horner's syndrome despite carefully dividing the sympathetic chain at a level that is clearly below the stellate ganglion.

The wound is drained with a 7-mm silicone drain, which is brought out lateral to the external jugular vein. The scalene fat pad is tacked back in place over the plexus. The platysma is closed with 3-0 absorbable polygalactin suture. The skin is then closed with a 4-0 pull-out polypropylene.

The drain is left in place until there is minimal drainage over a 24-hour period. Therapy is begun on the first postoperative day. The initial direction of therapy is to maintain full ROM and proper posture.

Combined anterior and transaxillary procedure

Because of dissatisfaction with the completeness of plexus decompression that was accomplished with the transaxillary and the anterior approach, the concept of a combined procedure was introduced. Roos[84] continues to recommend the combined procedure, largely because of comfort with the transaxillary approach to rib resection. The first rib can be removed from the anterior approach but is technically difficult in heavy-set or muscular individuals. When rib resection is deemed necessary, it should be performed by whatever technique with which the surgeon is most comfortable.

Complications

A number of postsurgical complications can occur; however, most can be avoided with careful attention to surgical detail. Careful hemostasis will prevent significant hematoma formation, which increases the likelihood of recurrent scar fixation. Permanent silk ties should be used for ligatures rather than surgical clips. Clips can get caught in the surgical drain and can be pulled out when the drain is removed. An infected pseudoaneurysm of the subclavian artery resulted in one such case and prompted conversion to ties for all vessels. The thoracic duct on the left and the accessory duct on the right must be avoided at the inferomedial end of the scalene fat pad. If a significant amount of chyle is seen in the drainage after surgery, the incision should be reexplored. The proteinaceous fluid of a chylous leak will leave extremely dense scar around the plexus if not repaired immediately.

Phrenic nerve injury occurs in a small number of cases despite careful attention to detail and attempts to avoid undue traction by the small handheld retractors. Our series mimics Sanders et al.'s 7% temporary diaphragmatic palsy, which usually recovers over several months.[88] There are only 4 cases of permanent palsy in our series of nearly 1000 patients.

Two cases of permanent plexus injury have been associated with primary surgery in our series. Both occurred in patients who had prior radiation therapy for carcinoma of the breast. Thus supraclavicular brachial plexus dissection should be undertaken with extreme caution on patients who have undergone prior radiation therapy near the plexus. If possible, radiation therapy ports should be adjusted to avoid the plexus in patients who carry a diagnosis of TOS.

Temporary motor dysfunction occurs occasionally, more likely involving the upper trunk from traction on the nerves as they are dissected from the dense scar tissue. Injury to the long thoracic nerve can occur easily if the nerve is displaced anteriorly within the substance of the middle scalene. Care must be taken to serially section the muscle over a right-angle clamp or similar technique to prevent winging of the scapula.

Mild numbness and paresthesias are common from manipulation of the plexus early after plexus decompression, but recovery is rapid. There is sometimes hypersensitivity in the peripheral-nerve distribution as the distal signals return.

Pneumothorax from pleural entry should not be problematic if a Jackson-Pratt–type drain that has a one-way valve at the bulb is used. At the time of drain removal, the drain site must be treated like a chest tube and covered with an occlusive dressing.

Horner's syndrome may occur after sympathectomy, even if the division of the sympathetic chain is done carefully below the efferent nerve to the T1 nerve root. Also of interest is the incidence of absence of unilateral facial sweating without miosis or lid droop. According to anatomic descrip-tions, this should not occur. Thus it is clear that there is more variation in the level of the fibers involved in the development of a Horner's syndrome than has been appreciated.

Vascular injury is uncommon but is potentially hazardous. If the artery has been severely entrapped by anomalous bands or muscles, it may become somewhat fragile to manipulation as in Adson's original description of scalenotomy.[2] This has occurred once in our series, and occurred before the dissection near the artery had commenced. Some slight subintimal dissection occurs infrequently and has presented no significant sequelae. Manipulation of the artery should be kept to a minimum. Venous injury will most commonly occur as the anterior scalene is being removed from the first rib in the anterior approach. During transaxillary rib resection, the subclavian vein is at greatest risk during resection of the anterior rib. Control of the vein when injured during an anterior approach usually will require a subclavicular counterincision. There has been only one significant venous injury in our series.

Reoperative surgery has a more significant likelihood of serious neurologic complication. Partial nerve palsy is more common, and permanent palsy occurs unavoidably in a small percentage of cases. This is precisely why initial surgery should not be undertaken lightly. It is not at all clear from the findings at surgery what places some nerves at greater risk for permanent injury than others. This makes the risk of permanent injury somewhat unavoidable. Reasons for failure at the initial procedure should be evaluated carefully and objectively before recommending reoperation on the brachial plexus.

Results

The success of surgical procedures for TOS can be divided into short- and long-term results. The success rate has been shown to deteriorate over time through the first 2 years because of a number of factors. Recurrent injury and failure to conform to the therapy program lead the causes of failure. Rear-end automobile collisions are a frighteningly familiar problem in our society and will continue to be the leading cause of TOS as well as the leading cause of treatment failure. Although the concept that postoperative therapy is equally important to the surgery is stressed from the initial consultation, one of the most frustrating problems we see is patients who stop the daily exercise program after 3, 4, or 5 months because they are "feeling fine."

Successful surgical results depend on the definition used for determination of success. Several points must be stressed. Complete relief of symptoms is unlikely except in nontraumatic cases limited to the lower plexus. In this instance, a transaxillary rib resection can achieve superior results that are likely to be permanent. Recurrent scarring about the upper plexus is unlikely, and the likelihood of new onset upper plexus symptoms secondary to muscle abnor-malities is low. When there are upper plexus symptoms, muscle abnormalities are present. These cases in which transaxillary rib resection is recommended present in a more straightforward manner and tend to have less of the ancillary manifestations described in this chapter. Cases related to posttraumatic and repetitive injuries are more likely to have other associated problems, be of a more chronic nature, and have more significant perineural traction and fixation.

If return to prior levels of activity is demanded to require inclusion as a good or excellent result, a large number of patients will be eliminated from consideration. Demands that patients resume such occupations as assembly-line work, heavy construction, and repetitive and overhead activities often cannot be met without significant likelihood of recurrence. When there is willingness on the part of insurance agencies, businesses, and patients to help the patient return to the workplace with appropriate accommodation rather than limit the patient to the preinjury status, the entire workman's compensation process would be improved. It is also incumbent on the patient to accept some of the responsibility for his or her future by avoiding avocations that would be likely to cause reinjury.

A small number of injuries will recur despite careful follow-up and compliance. In Sanders et al.'s series,[88] the delayed poor results occurred equally with transaxillary rib resection, anterior scalenectomy, and supraclavicular rib resection. The immediate improved results showed a 93% cumulative success rate at 3 months, 81% at 1 year, and 74% at 5 years. Our data mirror Sanders et al.'s report if limited to TOS procedures only. We believe that some of the 1-year failures reported by both Roos[84] and Sanders[88] represent less a failure of the primary TOS surgery than a failure to recognize the significant associated peripheral neuropathy (double crush). However, we have concluded that transaxillary rib resection has a significantly higher failure rate when used in patients who have upper plexus symptoms. Thus we would recommend that the supraclavicular approach be used in cases of traumatic TOS.

Early in our experience, the number of immediate failures from transaxillary rib resection despite a technically satisfactory procedure caused a reevaluation of the approach. It became apparent after study that the upper plexus involvement was found in posttraumatic cases and that transaxillary rib resection alone worsened the upper plexus symptoms in a surprisingly large number of patients. The nearly constant anterior scalene anomalies at the upper plexus level had not been recognized previously. Significant relief of the upper plexus symptoms, headache, and facial pain can be achieved only if completed decompression of the upper plexus is performed.

PREVENTION
Posttraumatic

Perhaps the most unrecognized and underutilized tool in the management of patients with TOS is prevention. Acceptance of the aforementioned concepts leads to rec-

ognition that a significant percentage of patients have a problem that was potentially preventable with appropriate early intervention. Flexion/extension (whiplash) injuries have occurred in ever-increasing numbers because of high-velocity-impact motor vehicle accidents. Accidents that may have left individuals with severe permanent injuries (or death) 20 years ago now often result in only "soft tissue" injuries because of seat belt restraints and air bags. The resultant injuries now commonly take their toll on the neck. In 1989, more than 12 million automobile accidents occurred, of which 25% were rear-end collisions. It seems clear why there is an epidemic of TOS in the United States.

Standard care after a flexion/extension injury includes placement of a cervical collar until there is absence of cervical muscle spasm. In the presence of anatomic anomalies described previously, 2 to 4 weeks of immobility may be all that is necessary to create the fibrous fixation of the plexus to and within these injured muscles. The history will nearly always confirm that the patient's complaints began in a delayed manner 6 weeks to 3 months after injury and then slowly progressed thereafter. The symptoms also may become manifest only when the patient returns to work with a significantly higher demand. Rather than castigate the patient as is so common with the workman's compensation physician mentality, a reasoned approach toward avoidance through early mobility would much better serve the patient.

Head restraints are now mandatory in cars sold in the United States. Appropriate positioning of the head restraints most likely would significantly reduce the incidence of whiplash injury.

A remarkable number of our patients are health care workers who have been injured when attempting to lift an overweight or stroke-injured patient. Most of these injuries appear to be preventable either by using appropriate mechanical assist devices, or avoidance of such situations. The patient usually describes a sudden sharp neck pain, which can be associated with immediate or delayed onset of pain and paresthesias. The acute process is generally caused by a tearing of an anomalous scalene anterior of minimus.

Repetitive stress disorder

TOS often is totally overlooked as a repetitive stress disorder, for reasons that are not clear. Carpal tunnel, cubital tunnel, and radial tunnel disorders are well recognized, perhaps because of the more easily documented nerve conduction changes. The ergonomics of the workplace are receiving appropriate amounts of attention in attempts to decrease the near-epidemic rise in carpal tunnel syndrome. Jaeger et al.[32] recently developed an easily repeated nerve conduction apparatus and has shown that by early night splinting of those patients at risk (from diabetes, job description), the development of and days lost because of carpal tunnel syndrome can be reduced dramatically.

Using similar reasoning, the prevention of TOS is perhaps possible if those patients at great risk could be identified. Patients who demonstrate significant pulse obliteration or a positive EAST might be best served by avoiding certain types of employment that require activities such as overhead use of the arms.

Postoperative recurrence

Surgical results are satisfactory. Longitudinal studies show a decline in the good and excellent outcomes over time. Failure to satisfactorily complete the prescribed therapy program accounts for most problems after surgery. Reinjury from repeat motor vehicle or lifting accidents account for the majority of the remainder of recurrent problems. Scar fixation to the surrounding tissues with progressive contraction of the scar underlies the cases of spontaneous recurrence.

It seems logical that if the scar formation around the dissected plexus could be inhibited, the risk of both spontaneous and posttraumatic recurrence would be reduced significantly. Active research is underway using a variety of techniques for scar reduction.

SUMMARY

TOS, particularly the neurogenic type, is a complex problem that can be understood only by comprehensive study of the anatomy, embryology, pathomechanics, and neurophysiology of the brachial plexus and by thorough evaluation of the patient.

REFERENCES

1. Adson AW: Surgical treatment for symptoms produced by cervical ribs and the scalenus anticus muscle, *Surg Gynecol Obstet* 85:687, 1947.
2. Adson AW, Coffey JR: Cervical rib: a method of anterior approach for relief of symptoms by division of the scalene anticus, *Ann Surg* 85:839, 1927.
3. Aminoff M, et al: Relative utility of different electrophysiologic techniques in the evaluation of brachial plexopathies, *Neurology* 38:546, 1988.
4. Barnes R: Causalgia: a review of 48 cases. In Seddon HJ, editor: *Peripheral nerve injuries,* London, 1954, HM Stationery Office.
5. Benecke R, Conrad B: The distal sensory nerve action potential as a diagnostic tool for the differentiation of lesions in the dorsal roots and peripheral nerves, *J Neurol* 223:231, 1980.
6. Benzon HT, Chomka CM, Brunner EA: Treatment of reflex sympathetic dystrophy with regional intravenous reserpine, *Anesth Analg* 59:500, 1980.
7. Brickner WM. Brachial plexus pressure by the normal first rib, *Ann Surg* 85:858, 1927.
8. Capistrant TR: Thoracic outlet syndrome in whiplash injury, *Ann Surg* 185:175, 1977.
9. Cherington M, et al: Surgery for thoracic outlet syndrome may be hazardous to your health, *Muscle Nerve* 9: 632, 1986.
10. Clagett OT: Research and prosearch, *J Thorac Cardiovasc Surg* 44:153, 1962 (presidential address).
11. Crenshaw AH, editor: *Campbell's operative orthopaedics,* ed 8, St Louis, 1992, Mosby.
12. Dale WA: Thoracic outlet compression syndrome, *Arch Surg* 117:143, 1982.
13. Dale WA, Lewis MR: Management of thoracic outlet syndrome, *Ann Surg* 181:575, 1975.
14. Daube J: Nerve conduction studies. In Aminoff M, editor: *Electrodiagnosis in clinical neurology,* ed 2, New York, 1986, Churchill Livingstone.
15. Davlin LB, Bergfield T, Aulcino PL: Variations of the median nerve at the wrist: a surgical perspective, *Orthop Rev* 21:955, 1992.
16. Davlin LB, Bergfield TG, Aulcino PL: Variations of the ulnar nerve: a surgical perspective, *Orthop Rev* 22:33, 1993.
17. Drucker W, et al: Pathogenesis of post traumatic sympathetic dystrophy, *Am J Surg* 97:454, 1959.
18. Eden KC: The vascular complications of cervical ribs and thoracic rib abnormalities, *Br J Surg* 27:111, 1939-40.
19. Eisen A: The electrodiagnosis of plexopathies. In Brown W, Bolton C, editors: *Clinical electromyography,* Boston, 1993, Butterworth-Heinemann.
20. Elvey RL: Brachial plexus tension test and the pathoanatomical origin of arm pain. In Glasgow EF, et al, editors: *Aspects of manipulative therapy,* ed 2, Melbourne, 1986, Churchill Livingstone.
21. Evans RW: Some observations in whiplash injuries, *Neurol Clin* 10:975, 1992.
22. Falconer MA, Li FWP: Resection of the first rib in costoclavicular compression of the brachial plexus, *Lancet* 1:59, 1962.
23. Falconer MA, Weddell G: Costoclavicular compression of the subclavian artery and vein: relation to the scalenus anticus syndrome, *Lancet* 2:539, 1943.
24. Ferrante M, Wilbourn A: The utility of various sensory nerve conduction responses in assessing brachial plexopathies, *Muscle Nerve* 18:879, 1995.
25. Gilliat R: Thoracic outlet syndromes. In Dyck PJ, Thomas PK, Lambert EH, editors: *Peripheral neurology,* Philadelphia, 1984, WB Saunders.
26. Gilliat R, Sears T: Sensory nerve action potentials in patients with peripheral nerve lesions, *J Neurol Neurosurg Psychiatry* 21:109, 1958.
27. Graham GG, Lincoln BM: Anterior resection of the first rib for thoracic outlet syndrome, *Am J Surg* 126:803, 1973.
28. Greep JM, et al, editors: *Pain in the shoulder and arm,* The Hague, 1979, Martinus Nijhoff.
29. Halsted W: An experimental study of circumscribed dilatation of an artery immediately distal to a partially occluding band, and its bearing on the dilatation of the subclavian artery observed in certain cases of cervical rib, *J Exp Med* 24:271, 1916.
30. Hanningtonkiff JG: Intravenous regional sympathetic block with guanethidine, *Lancet* 1:10, 1974.
31. Hawkins RJ, Abrams JS: Impingement syndrome in the absence of rotator cuff tears (stages 1 and 2), *Orthop Clin North Am* 18:373, 1987.
32. Jaeger SH, et al: Mid-latency somatosensory evoked potential abnormalities in proximal sensory neuropathies, *Muscle Nerve* 8:618, 1985.
33. Jaeger SH, et al: Nerve injury complications: management of neurogenic pain syndromes, *Hand Clin* 2:217, 1986.
34. Johnson EW: *Practical electromyography,* Baltimore, 1980, Williams & Wilkins.
35. Kaye BL: Neurologic changes with excessively large breasts, *South Med J* 65:177, 1972.
36. Kean WW: The symptomatology, diagnosis, and surgical treatment of cervical ribs, *Am J Med Sci* 133:173, 1907.
37. Kimura J: *Assessment of individual nerves: electrodiagnosis in diseases of nerve and muscle,* Philadelphia, 1989, FA Davis.
38. Kleinert HE, Southwick G: *Reflex sympathetic dystrophy: difficult problems in hand surgery,* St Louis, 1982, Mosby.
39. Kleinert HE, et al: Post traumatic sympathetic dystrophy, *Orthop Clin North Am* 4:917, 1973.
40. Kremer M, et al: Acroparesthesia in the carpal tunnel syndrome, *Lancet* 2:590, 1953.

41. Kunkel JM, Machleder HI: Treatment of Paget-Schroetter syndrome: a staged multidisciplinary approach, *Arch Surg* 124:1153, 1989.

42. Lankford L, Thompson J: Reflex sympathetic dystrophy, upper and lower extremity: diagnosis and management. In *AAOS instructional course lectures,* vol 26, St Louis, 1977, Mosby.

43. Leather RP: *Surgical symposium,* Philadelphia, 1989, Thomas Jefferson University.

44. Lewis T, Pickering G: Observations on maladies in which the blood supply to the digits ceases intermittently or permanently, *Clin Sci* 9:327, 1934.

45. Liveson J, Ma D: *Laboratory references for clinical neurophysiology,* Philadelphia, 1992, FA Davis.

46. Lord JW: Surgical management of shoulder girdle syndromes, *Arch Surg* 66:69, 1953.

47. Lord JW: Thoracic outlet syndrome: real or imaginary?, *NY State J Med* 45:1488, 1981.

48. Luoma A, Nelems B: Thoracic outlet syndrome: thoracic surgical perspective, *Neurosurg Clin North Am* 2:187, 1991.

49. Ma D, Wilbourn A, Kraft G: *Unusual sensory conduction studies: American Association of Electrodiagnostic Medicine Workshop,* ed 2, Rochester, Minn, 1992, AAEM.

50. Machleder HI, et al: Somatosensory evoked potentials in the assessment of thoracic outlet compression syndrome, *J Vasc Surg* 6:177, 1987.

51. Mackinnon SE, Dellon AL: *Surgery of the peripheral nerve,* New York, 1988, Thieme Medical.

52. Mackinnon SE, Holder LE: The use of three-phase radionucleotide bone scanning in the diagnosis of reflex sympathetic dystrophy, *J Hand Surg* 9A:556, 1984.

53. Makhoul RG, Machleder HI: Developmental anomalies at the thoracic outlet: an analysis of 200 consecutive cases, *J Vasc Surg* 16:534, 1992.

54. Mass DP: Treatment of painful neuromas by their transfer into bone, *Plast Reconstr Surg* 74:182, 1984.

55. Matthews WB: Footballer's migraine, *Br Med J* 2:326, 1972.

56. McLean I, Taylor R: *Nerve root stimulation to evaluate brachial plexus conduction.* Abstracts and communications of the Fifth International Congress of Electromyography, Rochester, Minn, 1975.

57. Melliere D, et al: Thoracic outlet syndrome caused by a tumor of the first rib, *J Vasc Surg* 14:235, 1991.

58. Melzak R, Wall P: Pain mechanisms: a new theory, *Science* 150:971, 1965.

59. Meyer RA, et al: Neural activity originating from a neuroma in a baboon, *Brain Res* 325:255, 1985.

60. Miller RG: Acute vs. chronic compressive neuropathy, *Muscle Nerve* 7:427, 1984.

61. Murphy T: Brachial neuritis caused by pressure of first rib, *Aust Med J* 15:582, 1910.

62. Naffziger HC, Grant WT: Neuritis of the brachial plexus mechanical in origin: the scalenus syndrome, *Surg Gynecol Obstet* 67:722, 1938.

63. Nelson RM, Davis RW: Thoracic outlet compression syndrome: collective review, *Ann Thorac Surg* 8:437, 1969.

64. Nichols HM: Anatomic structures of the thoracic outlet, *Clin Orthop* 207:13, 1986.

65. Novak CB, Mackinnon SE, Patterson GA: Evaluation of patients with thoracic outlet syndrome, *J Hand Surg* 18A:282, 1993.

66. Ochsner A, Gage M, DeBakey M: Scalenus anticus (Naffziger) syndrome, *Am J Surg* 28:699, 1935.

67. Oh S: *Anatomical guide for common nerve conduction studies: clinical electromyography nerve conduction studies,* ed 2, Baltimore, 1993, Williams & Wilkins.

68. Olney R, Wilbourn A: *Sensory nerve conduction study workshop,* course 150, American Academy of Neurology Annual Meeting, 1993.

69. Pairolero PC, et al: Subclavian-axillary artery aneurysms, *Surgery* 90:757, 1981.

70. Palumbo L: Upper dorsal sympathectomies without Horner's syndrome, *Arch Surg* 83:717, 1955.

71. Pavot A, Ignacio D, Gagour G: *Diagnosis of thoracic outlet syndrome by assessment of conduction time from C8 root supraclavicular fossa in the lower trunk of the brachial plexus,* Proceedings of the American Academy of Physical Medicine and Rehabilitation, 1981.

72. Peet PM, et al: Thoracic outlet syndrome: evaluation of a therapeutic exercise program: staff meetings, *Mayo Clin* 281, 1956.

73. Phalen GS, Gardner WJ, LaLonde AA: Neuropathy of median nerve due to compression beneath transverse carpal ligament, *J Bone Joint Surg* 32:109, 1950.

74. Poplawski ZJ, Wiley A, Murray JF: Post traumatic dystrophy of the extremities: a clinical review and trial treatment, *J Bone Joint Surg* 65A:642, 1983.

75. Qvarfordt PG, Ehrenfeld WK, Stoney RJ: Supraclavicular radical scalenectomy and transaxillary first rib resection for the thoracic outlet syndrome: a combined approach, *Am J Surg* 148:111, 1984.

76. Raaf J: Surgery for cervical rib and scalenus anticus syndrome, *JAMA* 157:219, 1955.

77. Raskin NH, Howard MW, Ehrenfeld WK: Headache as the leading symptom of thoracic outlet syndrome, *Headache* 25:208, 1985.

78. Richards R: Causalgia: a centennial review, *Arch Neurol* 16:339, 1967.

79. Rob CG, Standeven A: Arterial occlusion complicating thoracic outlet compression syndrome, *Br Med J* 2:709, 1958.

80. Roeder DK, et al: First rib resection in the treatment of thoracic outlet syndrome: transaxillary and posterior thoracoplasty approaches, *Ann Surg* 178:49, 1973.

81. Roos DB: Transaxillary approach for first rib resection to relieve thoracic outlet syndrome, *Ann Surg* 163:354, 1966.

82. Roos DB: Congenital anomalies associated with thoracic outlet syndrome, *Am J Surg* 132:771, 1976.

83. Roos DB: The place for scalenectomy and first rib resection in thoracic outlet syndrome, *Surgery* 92:1077, 1982.

84. Roos DB: Thoracic outlet nerve compression. In Rutherford RB, editor: *Vascular surgery,* ed 3, Philadelphia, 1989, WB Saunders.

85. Rubin M, Lange D: Sensory nerve abnormalities in brachial plexopathy, *Eur Neurol* 32:245, 1992.

86. Rubio PA, Rose FA: Thoracic outlet syndrome caused by a latissimus dorsi flap for breast reconstruction, *Chest* 97:494,1990.

87. Sanders RJ, Pierce WH: The treatment of thoracic outlet syndrome: a comparison of different operations, *J Vasc Surg* 10:626, 1989.

88. Sanders RJ, et al: Scalenectomy versus first rib resection for treatment of the thoracic outlet syndrome, *Surgery* 85:109, 1979.

89. Sanders RJ, et al: Scalene muscle abnormalities in traumatic thoracic outlet syndrome, *Am J Surg* 159:231, 1990.

90. Schwartzman RJ: Brachial plexus traction injuries, *Hand Clin* 7:547, 1991.

91. Schwartzman RJ, McLellan TL: Reflex sympathetic dystrophy: a review, *Arch Neurol* 44:555, 1987.

92. Seiler WA, et al: Double crush syndrome: experimental model in the rat, *Surg Forum* 34:59, 1983.

93. Semmes RE, Murphy F: The syndrome of unilateral rupture of the sixth cervical intervertebral disc with compression of the seventh cervical nerve root, *JAMA* 121:1209, 1943.

94. Sendzischew H, Hempel GK: Anterior approach for resection of the first rib and total scalenotomy, *Surg Gynecol Obstet* 160:272, 1985.

95. Smith JR, Gomez NH: Local injection of neuromata of the hand with triamcinolone acetonide: a preliminary study of twenty-two patients, *J Bone Joint Surg* 52A:71, 1970.

96. Stanton-Hicks M, et al: Reflex sympathetic dystrophy: changing concepts and taxonomy, *Pain* 63:127, 1995.

97. Steinbrocker O: The shoulder-hand syndrome: present perspective, *Arch Phys Med Rehab* 49:388, 1968.

98. Steinbrocker O, Argyrose TG: The shoulder hand syndrome: present status as a diagnostic and therapeutic entity, *Med Clin North Am* 42:1533, 1958.

99. Steinbrocker O, Spitzer N, Friedman HH: The shoulder hand syndrome in reflex dystrophy of the upper extremity, *Ann Intern Med* 29:22, 1947.

100. Stewart J: *Focal peripheral neuropathies,* New York, 1987, Elsevier.

101. Stilz R, Conn H, Sanders DB: Reflex sympathetic dystrophy in a 6 year old successful treatment by transcutaneous nerve stimulation, *Anesth Analg* 56:438, 1977.

102. Sunderland S: The connective tissues of peripheral nerves, *Brain* 88:841, 1965.

103. Sunderland S: *Nerve and nerve injuries,* ed 2, New York 1978, Churchill Livingstone.

104. Swanson AB, Bover NR, Biddulph S: Silicone rubber capping of amputation neuromas investigation and clinical experience, *Interclass Inf Bull* 11:1, 1972.

105. Swift TR, Nicholas FT: The droopy shoulder syndrome, *Neurology* 34:212, 1984.

106. Thomas GI, et al: The middle scalene muscle and its contribution to the thoracic outlet syndrome, *Am J Surg* 145:589, 1983.

107. Tinel J: Le Signe du "Fourmillement" dans le lesions des nervis peripheriques, *Press Med* 47:388, 1915.

108. Totten PA, Hunter JM: Therapeutic techniques to enhance nerve gliding in thoracic outlet syndrome and carpal tunnel syndrome, *Hand Clin* 7:505, 1991.

109. Tufa JW, Boothe PN: Treatment of painful neuromas of the sensory nerves in the hand for comparison of tradition and newer methods, *J Hand Surg* 1:44, 1976.

110. Upton AR, McComas AJ: The double crush syndrome in nerve entrapment syndromes, *Lancet* 2:359, 1973.

111. Urschel H: *Thoracic outlet syndrome,* Gibbon Lecture, Society of Thoracic Surgery, San Antonio, January 1993.

112. Urschel HC, Paulson DL, McNamara JJ: Thoracic outlet syndrome, *Ann Thorac Surg* 6:1, 1968.

113. Urschel HC, Razzuk MA: Management of the thoracic-outlet syndrome, *New Engl J Med* 286:1140, 1972.

114. Wilbourn A: Electrodiagnosis of plexopathies, *Neurol Clin* 3:511, 1985.

115. Wilbourn A: *Iatrogenic brachial plexopathies: clinical and EMG features: American Association of Electrodiagnostic Medicine, Course D—electrodiagnosis of iatrogenic neuropathies,* Rochester, Minn, 1990, AAEM.

116. Wilbourn A: Thoracic outlet syndromes: a plea for conservatism, *Neurosurg Clin North Am,* 2:235, 1991.

117. Wilbourn A: Brachial plexus disorders. In Dyck P, Thomas P, editors: *Peripheral neuropathy,* ed 3, Philadelphia, 1993, WB Saunders.

118. Willshire WH: Supernumerary first rib: clinical records, *Lancet* 2:633, 1860.

119. Wood VE, Biondi J: Double-crush nerve compression in thoracic outlet syndrome, *J Bone Joint Surg* 72:85, 1990.

120. Wright IS: The neurovascular syndrome produced by hyperabduction of the arm, *Am Heart J* 29:1, 1945.

Chapter 43

ENTRAPMENT NEUROPATHIES OF THE BRACHIAL PLEXUS AND ITS TERMINAL NERVES: HUNTER TRACTION TESTS FOR DIFFERENTIAL DIAGNOSIS

James M. Hunter
Stephan H. Whitenack

Posttraumatic peripheral nerve lesions in the upper extremity often result from traction injury (a straight-line pull) to the brachial plexus and its terminal branches. In these patients, painful nerves and muscles promote altered shoulder posture with functional imbalance in the arm, forearm, and hand. With time and eventual entrapment, these painful nerve lesions become traction neuropathies. Because they may be difficult to diagnose, they often result in faulty treatment programs and chronic disability.

Reviewing the results of treatment for the nerve disabilities that follow injuries of the brachial plexus and terminal peripheral nerves, we learned that diagnosis and treatment were clouded by misconceptions about the etiology of the problem. The concept that gradual scarring and entrapment of the nerves of the brachial plexus could occur after injury is rarely considered, and physicians develop their opinions based on painful symptoms, such as those caused by fibromyalgia, reflex sympathetic dystrophy, shoulder-hand syndrome, and psychogenic causalgia. When the diagnosis is unclear, treatment programs often involve long therapy sessions and multiple operative procedures, and the result is often the failure to return to work. The larger number of clinical cases of brachial plexus injury studied by Stevens was important in con-

firming the mechanism of injury and the location of injury. It becomes easier to understand where the acme of stress is most likely to fall in those less severe and much more common cases in which injury has occurred without actual loss of continuity in any part of the plexus. The anatomy of the brachial plexus and the large number of clinical cases reported by Dr. James H. Stevens, published in *The Shoulder* by Codman, 1934,[1] significantly influenced our understanding of the brachial traction injury that has become so common in this millenium.[5]

Stevens laid down three important rules for us to remember as we try to make a correct diagnosis of the nerve-injured patient.

1. The brachial plexus is injured either at its roots beyond their exit from the spine and before they join with other roots to form the plexus (trunks), or
2. In the terminal branches of the arm, but
3. Not in the plexiform part of the brachial plexus (the fascia-wrapped and integrated trunk and roots), which is never injured, except by cuts or wounds, but nevertheless may be involved secondarily by hemorrhage and exudate between the nerve bundles. (We now understand that this is the beginning of scar and

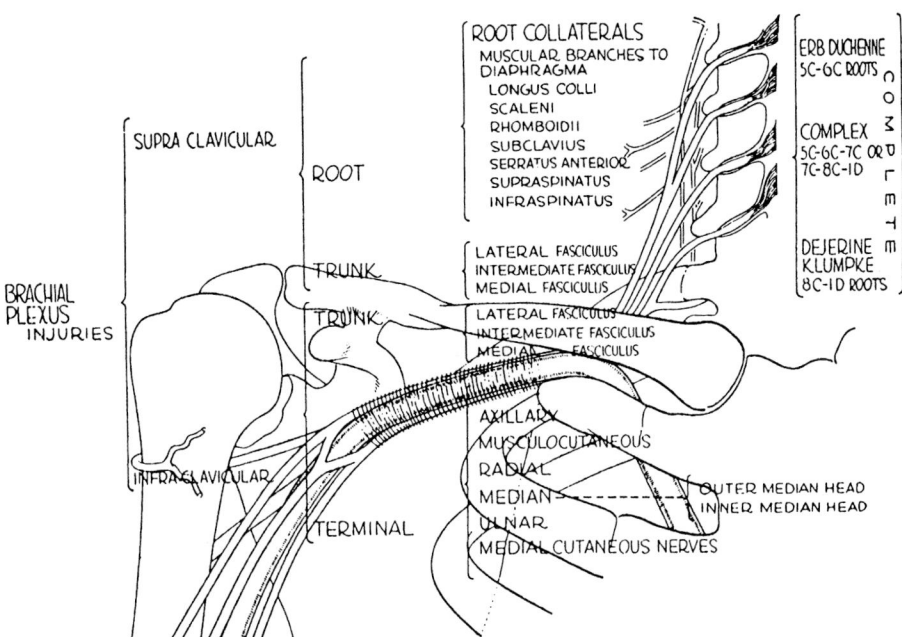

Fig. 43-1. Brachial plexus injuries. Editor's note: Anatomic term *cord* now replaces *fascicular.* (From Stevens JH: Brachial plexus paralysis. In Codman EA, editor: *The shoulder,* Malabar, Fla, 1934, Robert E Krieger.)

entrapment of the plexiform portion of the brachial plexus.)

ANATOMY OF BRACHIAL PLEXUS INJURY

In our discussion we will often refer to the part of the brachial plexus between the junction of the roots and the origin of the great terminal branches as the *trunk.* Trunks, when dissected, are in the upper plexiform part and cords are in the lower plexiform part of the brachial plexus. The engineering term *cord* refers to the plexiform length of the brachial plexus. Because, in most of its extent, the "plexiform part" forms a compact bundle about the axillary artery, we also speak of it as the *neurovascular cord* or the *integrated cord.* The fascial wrappings of the clavipectoral and axillary fascia bind the trunks together as a single neurovascular cord.

Although this fascia-bound structure, the neurovascular cord (Fig. 43-1), is a real anatomic entity, its limits are somewhat vague, because each structure that enters or leaves it contributes or carries away accompanying strands of fascia. It is a single cord axillary sheath, closely integrated by deep fascia investment from just beyond the interscalene segments to well below the shoulder. The great terminal branches occur here in varying lengths—the axillary, musculocutaneous, median, radial, and ulnar nerves. This single cord flares at the bases (proximally) into five roots of varying sizes and, far below the apex of the axilla, flares again into its terminal branches.

Rupture of the brachial plexus is a rare condition, although temporary palsy and pain are common. The reason for this is that the stresses do not fall entirely on the brachial plexus, as noted in the theoretic traction apparatus (Fig. 43-2). After the bones and ligaments are separated by injury, stresses are distributed to all the fascial investments of the axilla and neck and thus disseminated (e.g., rupture of the long head of the biceps, dislocations and fractures of the upper end of the humerus) (see Fig. 43-1).

Following a traction injury, there always seem to be small tears and injuries of the fascia about the nerves and vessels, and probably also far removed along the fascial planes. There are petechial hemorrhages and exudate that surround not only the roots and trunks but also the cords of the plexus in both the supraclavicular and axillary regions. The trunks may be swollen by pressure of the exudate within the fascia surrounding it. (In 400 documented cases of supraclavicular exploration with a comprehensive mobilization of the brachial plexus,[8] the upper plexiform level [trunks] is the principal site of epineural fibrous fixation resulting in entrapment and painful traction neuropathies in the brachial plexus.)

THE PATHOMECHANICS OF BRACHIAL PLEXUS INJURY
Theories of the mechanism of brachial plexus injuries

For a cord to be broken in tension, whether by a blow on its side transmitting the *stress* to both ends, or by direct pull, it must be held firmly at the ends or there will be no tension. All cases of plexus injury of the type under discussion are

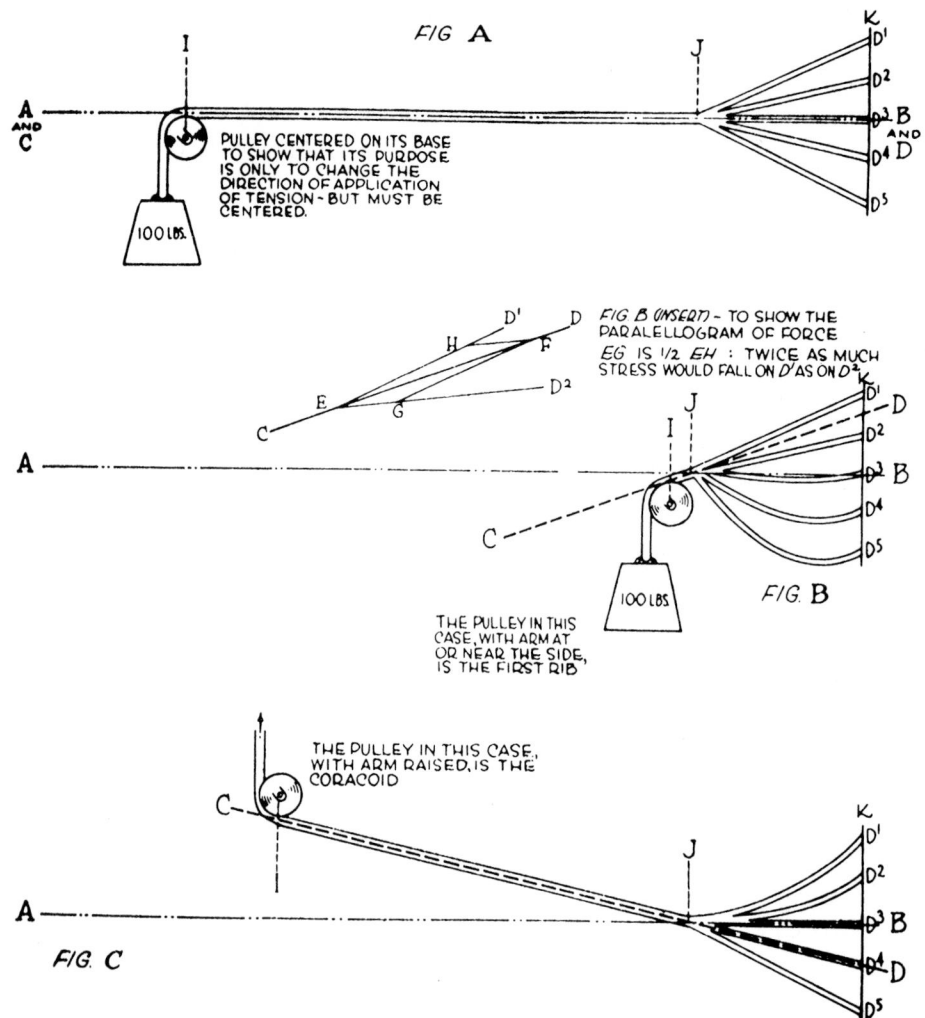

Fig. 43-2. Stress on nerve roots. Brachial plexus paralysis. Traction apparatus formed on the lines of the brachial plexus. (From Stevens JH: Brachial plexus paralysis. In Codman EA, editor: *The shoulder,* Malabar, Fla, 1934, Robert E Krieger.)

caused by tension, that is, traction (Fig. 43-3). If a mechanical stress is exerted on the integrated plexus, it creates tension. This is true whether the source of the stress is slipping while carrying a heavy load; being struck by a blow, depressing the shoulder; exerting straight traction forces on the arm; or having the head forced away from the shoulder, the face rotated away from or toward the side undergoing stress, the arm pulled in abduction and in external rotation, or the arm raised, lowered, supinated, or pronated. However, the different varieties of stress and the relative position of the arm and head at the time of stress make tremendous differences in the kind of lesion sustained, the locations of the lesions, and the prognosis. The nature, location, and seriousness of the injury depend on whether the stress is received from above or is transmitted from below, whether the arm is above or below horizontal, and whether the arm is externally or internally rotated (see Fig. 43-3). These factors, together with velocity and magnitude of

stress, usually determine the severity and location of the injury. Nevertheless, in all cases the stresses are of the same nature.

RATIONALE FOR HUNTER DIAGNOSTIC TESTS FOR TRACTION NEUROPATHY OF THE BRACHIAL PLEXUS AND MEDIAN, ULNAR, AND RADIAL NERVES

Think of the brachial plexus as a traction apparatus with its normal axis as a mechanical appliance on the C7 vertebra, with the arm at the horizontal (i.e., a single cord with five separate points of attachment firmly snubbed at the transverse processes). In the clinical situation, the upper brachial plexus C5-C6-C7 is slanted laterally and downward from the spinous processes so that C7, or the axis of mechanical appliance, is 40 degrees lateral from the thigh with external rotation of the arm and extension of the elbow. A provocative clinical test (the low lateral abduction arm test) evolved that

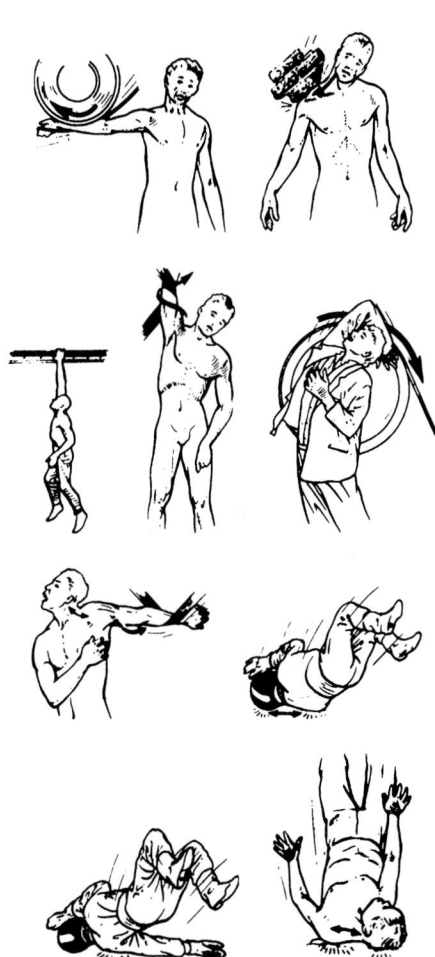

Fig. 43-3. Some examples of injury to the brachial plexus. The acme of stress can be focused on different levels of the plexus. (From Coene LN: Pathomechanical aspects of brachial plexus injuries and in particular axillary nerve injuries. In Holland, de Kempenaer, editors: *Axillary nerve lesions and associated injuries,* Oegstgeest, Holland, 1985.)

Box 43-1   Hunter low abduction arm test

Testing

Spinal nerves: C6, C7
Terminal nerve: median nerve wrist and proximal forearm entrapment

Position

Trunk and head are firm, looking straight ahead (no tilt)
Arm: to side 40 degrees of abduction from knee, external rotation, wrist and elbow neutral

Pulley

Neck: first rib, clavipectoral fascia
Wrist: volar surface of carpal bones on hyperextension of wrist

Nerve traction

BP proximal: C6, C7, spinal nerve, median trunk, medial and lateral cord
Terminal nerve: median nerve, tender on arm abduction and traction, painful on hyperextension of wrist proximal to wrist
Entrapment: middle trunk cords, median nerve to the flexor fibrous sheath in carpal canal

Hand symptoms

Numbness and paresthesia of palmar surface of thumb and index finger, radial side of middle finger

Signs

Protects arm in internal rotation, wearing a wrist splint, sloping shoulder forward, atrophy, weak median grip

BP, Brachial plexus.

---

placed the C7 spinal nerve, the middle trunk, the lateral cord of the brachial plexus, and the terminal trunk of the median nerve under longitudinal traction; it requires abduction of the arm 40 degrees from the thigh, external rotation of the arm, elbow extension, and head possibly slightly tilted. Simultaneous fingertip pressure over the C7 root completes the circuit (the Hunter Low Abduction Arm Test, Box 43-1). The thumb, index, and proximal palm will register paresthesia. The sensory decrease will be on the radial side of the middle finger (Shwartzman's sign), index finger, and thumb, aggravated by wrist entrapment of the median nerve.

When tension is applied to its structure (the integrated cord), it falls on the offset roots (see Figs. 43-1 and 43-2). An arrangement of this kind will rarely transmit stress through five cords equally. If the force of the pull could fall exactly through the neutral axis at the exact center and at an exact right angle to the base or plane of the structure to be lifted, the size of the cords being the same, it might be possible to lift a weight evenly; however, stress always tends to travel in straight lines, and depending on the position of the application of stress, the acme will usually fall to one side or the other of the neutral axis of such a structure.

A suspension apparatus is governed by much the same laws as a traction apparatus (see Fig. 43-2). A three-point suspension is more reliable than a suspension from a greater number of points. Perhaps this is the reason three roots are injured in so many cases of brachial-plexus paralysis, because either the two upper roots or the two lower ones may combine with the median root (C5-C6-C7 or C7-C8-T1).

A traction apparatus must have a neutral axis and a line of resistance, and when the force of traction falls through this neutral center or axis, the traction is equally borne by all parts of the apparatus. Even a slight deviation from this neutral axis makes an offset pull to one side or the other. In a structure of this kind, the entire force is transferred from that neutral axis; all tension is released on the cords on the other side, and a new neutral axis is instantly formed about the components that are now bearing the stress to conform to the new line of resistance. All other components are out of the structure; they are lax and their influence is nil.

A pulley inserted as part of a traction apparatus is not placed to change the degree of pull on the structure to be lifted or moved, but rather to change the direction of the application of the force to make it more convenient or effectual (i.e., to keep the neutral axis in the desired direction). The pulley must be placed so that a line from the pulley to the center of the structure to be raised or moved falls through the neutral axis and the line of resistance (see Fig. 43-2). If this is not so, the force applied falls to one or the other side of the axis and the entire force of the pull may therefore fall to one side. If the pulley is elevated, the lines of tension and resistance will come below the first neutral axis and the acme of stress will be below the original axis. If the pulley is lowered, the acme of stress will be above the original axis. Because the scapula is movable and the integrated plexus passes under the arch formed by the coracoid and the pectoralis minor, a condition similar to a movable pulley exists in the shoulder (see Fig. 43-2 C). As the arm externally rotates in the Hunter Low Abduction Arm Test, the integrated cord is traction-compressed over the first rib pulley. Likewise, if the externally rotated arm is abducted to 90 degrees with the elbow extended, the coracoid pulley directs the acme of stress to the lower plexus or T1-C8-C7 spinal nerves (the Hunter High Abduction Arm Test, Box 43-2).

There is no real pulley, but the cords of the plexus are held in this arch, and as the arm is raised and the clavicle and the coracoid rise, the coracoid acts much like a pulley because it changes the direction of any force applied distal to it. In raising the arm, when the coracoid rises above the horizontal, the acme of stress is on the lower roots. Lowering the arm lowers the coracoid, and the acme of stress is on the upper roots. This mechanism could explain why some patients who have had only transaxillary first-rib resection complain of more upper-plexus symptoms (C5-C6-C7) after surgery. Trunks of the upper plexus fixed together in posttraumatic scar cause biologic gliding to be eliminated, and the irritated plexus becomes painful with traction from shoulder arm movements. Similarly, a completely mobilized upper plexus (root and trunk) may still produce traction symptoms if the lower-plexus cords remain scarred to the first rib or the clavipectoral fascia.

With the arm at the side and pulled downward, the pulley is not the coracoid but the place where the plexus comes over the rib anteriorly (see Fig. 43-2, B). Because of the obliquity of C5-C6-C7, upper trunk, and middle trunk, tension is set by erect posture and aggravated quickly with the arm weighted and with the shoulder sloped forward and downward. There is a protection built into the spinal nerves of C5-C6-C7 as they leave the transverse processes. They are protected by arachnoid and epineural connections, prevent-

ing rupture (see Fig. 43-1). This slight change of direction of the force would relieve, to some extent, the strain on the upper roots in a downward pull. Combined with this would be help from the clavipectoral fascia. The upper-plexopathy patient may complain of tingling, aching, and swelling in the hands with the arms hanging by the sides; thus the preferred posture of the arm flexed in front of the chest provides plexus relaxation and patient comfort. We might call this position *plexus O*.

A breaking strain expended on the brachial plexus from above, such as from a blow on the shoulder or from slipping while carrying a weight, usually causes a lesion of the C5 root. Five cords divided will not stand the strain as well as five combined in one.

If the apparatus breaks under supraclavicular stress, it will break at the weakest point (i.e., at one of the roots between the point where it is snubbed on the transverse process and the junction of that root with others). If it does not break, the acme of stress is, nevertheless, at the same point.

Box 43-2   Hunter high abduction arm test

Testing

Spinal nerves: C7, C8, T1
Terminal nerve: ulnar-nerve entrapment
Medial elbow: olecranon canal and cubital canal
Occasionally at arcade of Struthers of arm

Position

Trunk and neck: firm, looking straight ahead
Arm: high abduction of arm at 90 degrees at shoulder, external rotation
Elbow: extension, wrist neutral; may not tolerate full extension because of pain

Pulley

Scapular coracoid process and pectoralis minor muscle, cervical rib, Roos bands may be present in the neck

Nerve traction

Spinal roots C7, C8, T1: medial nerve trunk and medial cord very sensitive to traction; true causalgia may occur here
Terminal nerves: entrapment of ulnar nerve may cause pain on shoulder abduction 90 degrees with extension of elbow; examiner should monitor elbow extension in external rotation of arm, palm up = pain in forearm, muscles

Hand symptoms

Numbness and paresthesia, hypothenar level, volar and dorsal, fingers: middle, ring, small, pain at medial elbow

Hand signs

Atrophy of intrinsic muscles, thenar atrophy with cervical rib, Roos bands, weak grip ulnar side of hand

Impact is infinitely greater than static load. When a person carrying 100 pounds on the shoulder slips or makes a false step and falls even as little as 4 to 6 inches, the static load (which was carried with ease) instantly causes an impact trauma. For example, a person carrying a small box with 60 pounds of metal bolts sustains injury because the concentrated weight is supported by a shoulder fully abducted so that the hand can balance the box. The weight is jolted by walking but remains fixed by the abducted elbow and flexed arm. Misjudging a step down in poor light, this person will hit the second step with impact now greater than the static load, thus sustaining a traction injury to the lower and middle trunks (T1-C8-C7) because the cord (in this instance, the medial cord) is turned around the movable pulley, that is, the coracoid of the scapula (see Fig. 43-2).

The mechanical stress sustained here is exactly the same as if struck on the shoulder by a 100-pound hammer falling 4 to 6 inches and depressing the clavicle and coracoid. The brachial plexus is instantly stretched between its two firm points of attachment: (1) the transverse processes above and (2) at the clavipectoral fascial snubbing below in the upper axilla. Again, the stress in tension is exactly the same as if

the cords themselves received a side blow. Impact causes a remarkable increase in stress over a static load. This concept of disseminated stress explains how the seemingly small injury can damage by tearing the epineural sleeves system, resulting in fibrosis fixation and nerve irritability from traction stress.

When surgeons contend that rupture of the roots would be impossible in the ordinary trauma or in that caused by dislocation, they fail to consider the manner in which mechanical stresses may be magnified at the point of final application. The roots do not always break because, in many cases, the stress does not fall on these limited structures alone but is disseminated (see Fig. 43-1). In both cases cited previously, the stress is transmitted to both points of attachment; half is referred back to the roots, and the other half falls on the place below, where the cords are held firmly by the clavipectoral fascia and the integrated cord.

Sometimes we have an accompanying rupture or injury to the artery because the fascial snubbing surrounding the cords gives way and the vessel is torn. Stress coming through the arm from below as pure tension is probably a more common cause of injury to the artery than stress exerted by blows

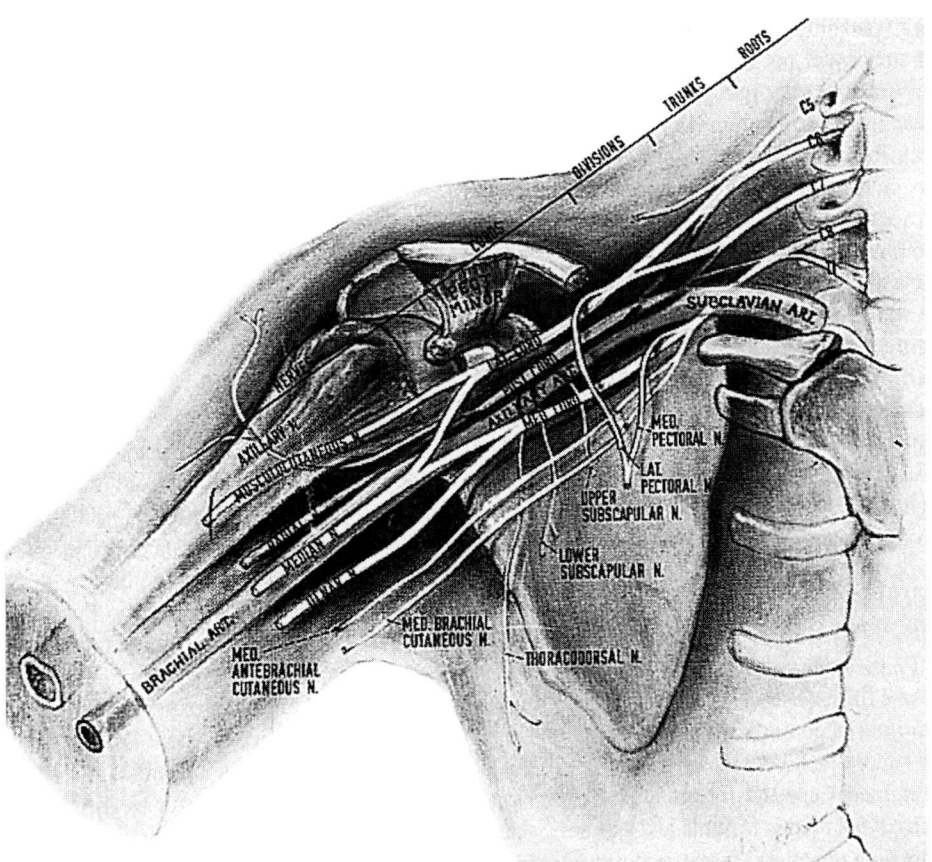

Fig. 43-4. Illustration of the open plexus vulnerable to traction of the lateral and medial cords. The arm is rotated externally with muscle and fascia removed. Traction injury and the fibrous reaction of repair seals or tethers the trunks of the plexus. The plexus cannot open on external rotation. A traction neuropathy and pain develop. (From Clemente C: *Anatomy,* Philadelphia, 1975, Lea & Febiger. Copyright Urban & Fischer Verlag.)

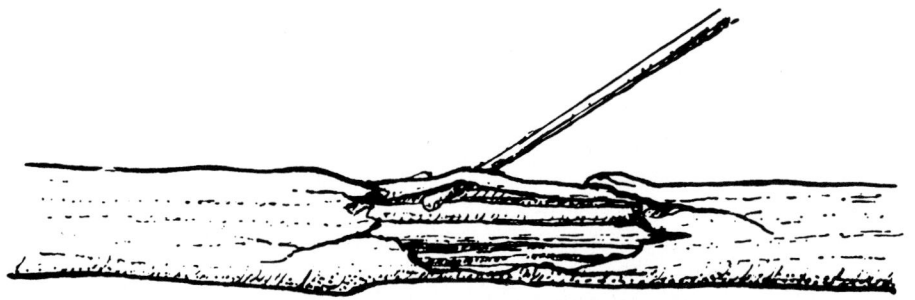

Fig. 43-5. The state of a peripheral nerve in a case of neuropraxia. The external epineurium is torn by traction, exposing the internal fasciculus and internal epineurium. A peripheral nerve injured this way, if it remains functional, will likely become scar-fixed and locally painful to pressure or traction. (From Seddon H: *Surgical disorders of the peripheral nerves,* Baltimore, 1972, Williams & Wilkins.)

from above because stress from tension is not dissipated. It falls first on the clavipectoral fascial snubbing and is then transmitted back to the pulley at the first rib and the roots, but not until the fascial snubbing in the axilla has been injured. A traumatic aneurysm without rupture of the roots is possible because the stress might be disseminated after the fascia and the vessels have been injured and then be too weak to break the roots. Here also could be an instance where the terminal plexus, the median or ulnar nerves, could sustain injuries. The plexus nerves are opened with external rotation of the arm (open plexus effect). The entire length of the median nerve, from the neck (C7) to the carpal tunnel, is vulnerable to traction injury (Fig. 43-4).

ENTRAPMENT OF THE BRACHIAL PLEXUS

Stevens[5] was unable to find a single case of rupture in the plexiform part of the plexus, although the artery itself may be torn. In reading the accounts of his operations, on the other hand, one usually finds such statements as "the plexus seemed a mass of scar tissue," "the cords were welded together in an inflammatory mass," and "on account of the scar tissue, nothing could be made out as to the exact location of the injury." In our clinical experience of more than 400 supraclavicular explorations in the brachial plexus in a recent 4-year period, we have found these to be typical pathologic findings in traction injuries to the brachial plexus. We have been able to reaffirm the conclusion of Stevens that these findings represent epineural fibrous fixations; that is, entrapment neuropathies with tethering of the upper, middle, and lower trunks of the brachial plexus with layers of dense fibrous tissue. In the main, this represents the late phases of traction injury, inflammatory abrasion, and finally, fibrous fixation with traction neuropathy. This nervous system is now prone to causalgia. However, many such patients have recovered in whole or in part, indicating that no real rupture had occurred in the nerve fibers and that the gross appearance was the result of the graded process of a healing injury, including ecchymoses, exudate, and scar tissue among the fascial envelopes and fibrous septa in the nerve trunks. In this region, as in others, intensive anatomic study of the

mechanics of the structures reveals marvelous examples of architectural and mechanical designs (e.g., the integrated cord when dissected is shown to be "plexiform," after the fashion of a complex design of parallelograms of forces) (see Fig. 43-2). This is an admirable arrangement to disseminate stresses because if the cord were pulled at both ends before rupturing the longitudinal strands, the force must break the little lateral bands of tissue, which are cut during dissections of the plexus.

It is probable that many small local hemorrhages about, among, and within the individual trunks cause the appearance so often described (epineural fibrous fixation of the trunk of the plexus) (Figs. 43-5 and 43-6). Subsequent exudate of epineurium followed by scar tissue complicates the picture and chokes the nerve fibers.

Undiagnosed patients, subjected to overuse by lifting at work or a "no pain, no gain" therapy program, may present in the clinic with a weak shoulder or hand with causalgia-like pain. The picture is worsened with ulnar- and median-nerve entrapment. (Some have called this the *double crush syndrome.*) In such patients, the stage has been set for the later stages of epineural fibrosis and scar-fixed nerve sleeves that limit excursion by tethering the trunks and cords of the brachial plexus together so that, with the shoulder depressed and the arm abducted, traction causes the nerves to explode into a painful phenomenon described by some patients as "burning that I can't stand." The limb movement is producing compressive ischemia because of scar entrapment in the plexus, resulting in pain.[6] This same process can be seen around a single nerve trunk beyond the brachial plexus level (e.g., the median nerve in the carpal tunnel, the ulnar nerve in the cubital tunnel, and the radial nerve in the radial tunnel). Causalgia seems to result from recurrent traction/fixation in patients with no true diagnosis. These patients, subjected to continued work stress, slowly develop major causalgia.

Consider the stresses that often result in terminal-branch lesions. Imagine an arm in abduction and external rotation subjected to still greater backward stress (see Figs. 43-3 and 43-4). In this position, the terminal branches tend to separate

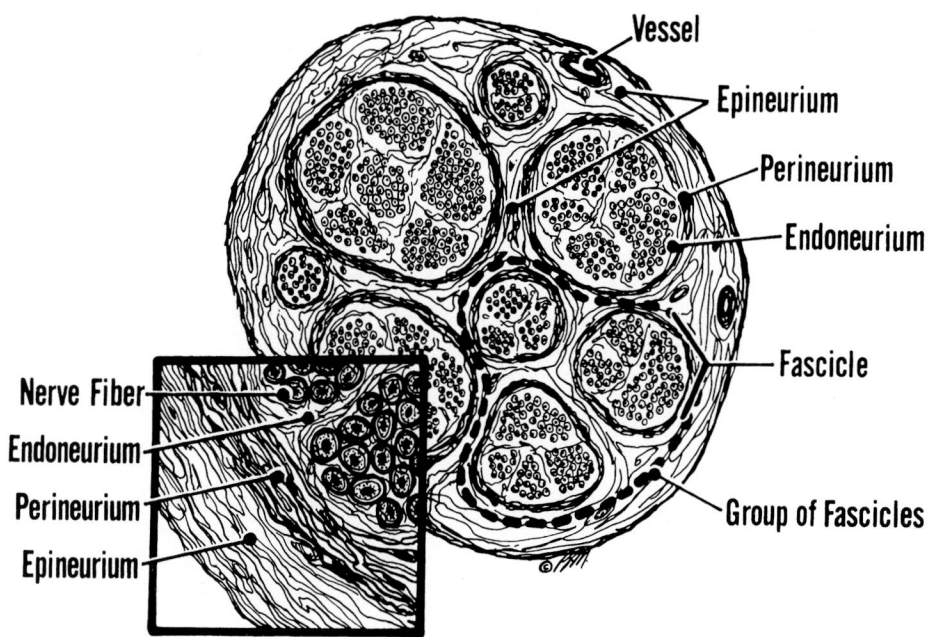

Fig. 43-6. Cross section of normal peripheral nerve. The reaction of peripheral nerve fibrosis of the epineurium constricts the nerve anatomy and metabolism of the axion flow, resulting in altered functional and sensory patterns. (Copyright, Elizabeth Roselius, 1993. From Wilgris EFS, Brushart TM: Nerve repair and grafting. In Green DP, Hotchkiss RN, editors: *Operative hand surgery,* vol 2, ed 3, New York, 1993, Churchill Livingstone.)

from one another, and in the opposite position (internal rotation with the arm at the side), they continue their course almost side by side. Likewise, the arm in pronation and abduction gives severe radial nerve stress from entrapment at the elbow level.

In other words, the patient has added other factors to the mechanics. Offset may now fall, not alone on the roots, but at the other end of the apparatus. If offset falls on any terminal branch that is smaller or weaker than any part of the integrated cord or roots above, it will break that terminal branch below its point of insertion into the integrated plexiform part.

If the traction stress falls through the *radial nerve,* which is greater in strength and size than most of the roots, it probably would be transmitted back to the roots at the weaker points. Force applied to the radial nerve would be transmitted through the integrated cord back to C5 and C6 to a greater degree than to C7, from which its motor portion arises originally.

The weaker points of the brachial plexus in the upper extremity are in the terminal nerves and at the roots. This is why there have been ruptures reported of the musculocutaneous, median, and ulnar nerves at their origins in the axilla. We have many reports of injury involving each of these nerves in the axilla, but rupture of the radial nerve alone is rare because it is stronger than the clavipectoral fascia. The radial nerve tends to predominate with entrapment pain at the elbow level.

The "waiter's tip," or *Erb, position* is the provocative test for the C5-C6 roots and radial nerve entrapment. This is the Hunter Low Abduction Internal Rotation Arm Test (Box 43-3), which produces symptoms on the lateral border of the elbow to the thumb and the posterior shoulder ridge. If traction positive, this test renders the entire radial nerve—at the lateral border of the wrist, dorsum of elbow, muscles of the triceps, teres major, suprascapular, and subscapular—tender to palpation. The muscles supplied by the radial nerve are usually inflamed and are pressure sensitive during internal rotation and radial nerve traction with the arm by the side. This is the Hunter test for high brachial plexus neuropathy (C-5, C-6, C-7).

ENTRAPMENT NEUROPATHY OF THE BRACHIAL PLEXUS

Traction injuries seem to be the mechanism that can set the stage for entrapment of the brachial plexus and peripheral nerves.[2] Entrapment usually occurs at specific active locations where gliding motion is essential for normal nutrition and comfortable function. When gliding is lost because of mesoepineural and epineural injury to the peripheral nerves, repair and fibrous adhesions cause nerve adhesion entrapment and fixation.[3,7] Fortunately, in most instances, remodeling of the epineural and mesoepineural tissues form mesothelial planes for gliding motion. When this type of repair fails, however, fibrous scar takes over and eventually entrapment occurs. This concept of traction injury was

---

Box 43-3   Hunter low abduction, internal rotation arm test

Test

Spinal nerves: C5, C6, (C7)
Terminal nerve: radial-nerve entrapment at humeral and suprascapular level, and radial tunnel

Position

Best standing, no tilting, looking straight ahead; arm held by therapist in internal rotation, wrist hyperflexion (waiter tip position)

Pulley

First rib, clavipectoral fascia, posterior shoulder = teres major and triceps
Elbow: lateral humeral condyle, BR, and ECRL fascial bed
Wrist: radial styloid level

Nerve traction

Spinal nerve: C5, C6, posterior division of brachial plexus— all roots, posterior cord
Terminal nerves: axillary, radial
Entrapment: C5, C6, upper trunk and radial nerve at brachial radialis, extensor carpi radialis tunnel at elbow, and dorsal interosseous tunnel and motor sensory radial in radial tunnel in forearm

Hand symptoms

Radial styloid level of wrist, dorsal forearm, dorsum of hand and fingers, base of thumb, thenar muscle

Hand signs

Dry skin, weak extrinsic extensor muscles of thumb and index finger, wrist weakness

Elbow signs

Pseudocontracture as a result of triceps weakness and supracondylar radial nerve entrapment

Shoulder signs

Posterior shoulder girdle muscle inflammation and pain

BR, Brachioradialis; *ECRL,* extensor carpi radialis longus.

---

emphasized by Sir Sydney Sunderland in 1991[6] and J.H. Stevens in 1934.[5]

No root or cord breaks until after its sheath has given way. No nerve can be stressed until its surrounding fascia gives. Tension or traction injuries to the brachial plexus have their most damaging effect on the epineural sheath and the perineural connective tissue (see Fig. 43-5). Normally, joint movements can be freely carried out over a wide range, both actively and passively, during which nerves are subjected to stresses and strains that are tolerated without pain or any disturbance of neurologic function. However, there is always a point at which a traumatic incident is sufficient to overcome these

protective devices in and around the nerve trunk, and when this occurs, traction injuries of nerves are the result.

The key to the pathogenesis of the entrapped peripheral nerve lesion is the local inflammatory reaction that occurs in response to repeated mechanical irritation during limb movements. This reaction culminates in the development of local areas of constrictive nerve fibrosis and the formation of adhesions that attach to the nerve in the entrapment site. It is the fixation of the nerve in this way that justifies the term *entrapment.*

Frictional fibrosis followed by entrapment therefore imperils the peripheral nerve by resulting in the following:

1. Constriction of the nerve structure, causing nerve obstruction to axonal nerve flow
2. Impairment of the blood supply
3. Formation of adhesions that fix the nerve to surrounding structures at the involved site

Traction on an entrapped peripheral nerve, caused by limb movement, may deform the nerve between two fixed points, causing a hypersensitive nocigenic focus resulting in pain. The cardinal symptoms of the entrapment lesion, pain or dull aching after prolonged muscle effort, occur particularly with overuse of those muscles whose contractions are known to contribute directly to nerve entrapment. Pressure over the entrapment site, providing the nerve is accessible, elicits a painful response. Evidence of sensory involvement appears only in late stages.

It is important to recognize that the delayed diagnosis of traction neuropathy is a classic problem. "The symptom complex surrounding entrapment separates this nerve disease very clearly from a compression neuropathy."[6] Because entrapment takes time to become established, it may be caused by situations in which motion of the extremity creates repetitive stress at certain points of fixation. The symptoms of pain and weakness may become profound in patients during cumulative injury at work and in daily activities, resulting in chronic disability. Accurate diagnosis can be difficult for many reasons. The symptoms and physical examination may be altered by the protective pattern each patient acquires to become comfortable. If the nerve release operation fails to provide the expected benefits, the patient's condition will worsen.

Other factors contribute to the delay in diagnosis often encountered in these patients. Scar tissue by its very nature has a tendency to contract. This contraction occurs progressively over a period of up to 2 years. Thus a combination of recurrent stresses, overuse syndromes that create further frictional fibrosis, and the intrinsic contraction of scar tissue is responsible for the natural history of slow progression of symptoms. Electromyography and other nerve conduction studies may be normal initially. Later, these studies may be positive only with stress testing, until ultimately the electrical testing is clearly abnormal and the diagnosis is obvious.

There are several factors that separate patients who develop traction neuropathies of the brachial plexus (neurogenic thoracic outlet syndrome) from patients who have sustained similar injury or perform similar repetitive activities but have no nerve symptoms. The "upper plexiform plexus" (roots and trunks) is the site of traction neuropathy that follows traction injury in nearly all cases. This fixation to the surrounding structures occurs in this portion of the plexus because the anatomic abnormalities are found at this level (see Chapter 42). Cervical ribs cause direct trauma to the C8 nerve root or the lower trunk. The muscle abnormalities associated with cervical ribs may affect the lower or middle trunks or the C7, C8, or T1 nerve roots. The bands described well by Roos[4] affect largely the lower plexus. Abnormalities of the anterior scalene origin are universally found in patients with traction neuropathies of the upper plexus.

Patients with traction injury to the brachial plexus also commonly develop other peripheral nerve neuropathies in that extremity; this represents the double crush injury. This has created delay in diagnosis in many patients. Sometimes the diagnosis of brachial plexopathy is one of exclusion when other peripheral neuropathies in the same extremity fail to respond to conservative and surgical treatment. A study completed at the Hand Rehabilitation Center showed that 32% of patients with recurrent median-nerve symptoms after carpal tunnel release actually had brachial plexopathy upon testing. This study recommends that a brachial plexus screening test be part of the routine evaluation for peripheral neuropathy in the upper extremity.

As the concept of traction neuropathy developed in this chapter has become clearer to us, so has the explanation for the interplay between brachial plexus and peripheral neuropathies. The peripheral nerves of the extremity are a single, continuous structure that is not intended to be fixed at any point after it leaves the neural foramen. Fixation of the nerve structure at the plexus, elbow, or carpal tunnel shortens the potential distance over which the nerves are capable of traveling as the arm passes through its full range of motion. This then places additional tension on the already troubled nerves, particularly when the patient is placed in untenable work situations or "no pain, no gain" types of therapy.

REFERENCES

1. Codman EA: *The shoulder,* Malabar, Fla, 1934, Robert E Krieger.
2. Hunter JM: Recurrent carpal tunnel syndrome, epineural fibrous fixation, and traction neuropathy, *Hand Clin* 7:491, 1991.
3. Hunter JM, Read RL, Gray R: Carpal tunnel neuropathy caused by injury: reconstruction of the transverse carpal ligament for the complex carpal tunnel syndromes, *J Hand Ther* 6:145, 1993.
4. Roos DB: Congenital anomalies associated with thoracic outlet syndrome, *Am J Surg* 132:771, 1976.
5. Stevens JH: Brachial plexus paralysis. In Codman EA, editor: *The shoulder,* Malabar, Fla, 1934, Robert E. Krieger.
6. Sunderland S: *Nerve injuries and their repair: a critical appraisal,* Edinburgh, 1991, Churchill Livingstone.
7. Totten PA, Hunter JM: Therapeutic techniques to enhance nerve gliding in thoracic outlet syndrome and carpal tunnel syndrome, *Hand Clin* 7:505, 1991.
8. Whitenack SH, et al: Thoracic outlet syndrome complex: a brachial plexopathy. In Hunter JM, Mackin EJ, Callahan AC, editors: *Rehabilitation of the hand: surgery and therapy,* ed 4, St Louis, 1995, Mosby.

BIBLIOGRAPHY

Coene LN: Mechanisms of brachial plexus lesions, *Clin Neurol Neurosurg* 95(suppl):24, 1993.

Delbert P, Cauchoix A: Les paralysies dans les luxations de l'epaule, *Revue de Chirurgie* 41:327, 1910.

Duval P, Guillain G: Pathogenie des accidents nerveux consecutifs aux luxations et traumatismes de l'epaule, *Arch Gen Med* 8:143, 1898.

Erb W: Diseases of the peripheral cerebro-spinal nerves. In von Ziemmsen H, editor: *Cyclopedia of the practice of medicine,* London, 1876, Samson Low, Marston, Searle and Rivington.

Horsley V: On injuries to peripheral nerves, *Practitioner* 63:131, 1899.

Malgaigne JF: *Traite des fractures et des luxations,* Paris, 1847-1855, JB Bailliere.

Nerve injuries committee of the Medical Research Council, Seddon HJ, editor: Peripheral nerve injuries, Medical Research Council Special Report Series, no 282, London, Her Majesty's Stationery Office, 1954.

Secrétan H: *Contribution a l'etude des paralysies radiculaires du plexus brachial* (thesis), no 205, Paris, 1885.

Seddon HJ: *Surgical disorders of the peripheral nerves,* Baltimore, 1972, Williams & Wilkins.

Chapter 44

THERAPIST'S MANAGEMENT OF BRACHIAL PLEXOPATHIES

Mark T. Walsh

Brachial plexus neuropathy (BPN) is a common upper extremity pain syndrome. Peripheral neuropathies of the involved upper extremity and cervical spine pathology complicate the diagnosis. The existence of the type of BPN often referred to as *thoracic outlet syndrome* (TOS) remains controversial.[48,72] As this pain syndrome becomes more ingrained within the central nervous system, accompanying alterations in the neural biomechanics of the brachial plexus and peripheral nerves occur, making diagnosis and treatment more difficult. It is the intent of this chapter to communicate a clearer understanding of brachial plexopathy and its varied manifestations, allowing the clinician to develop a logical sequence of evaluation, assessment, and treatment.

Two major types of brachial plexopathy are discussed. The first, compressive brachial plexus neuropathy (CBPN), is the type classically described as TOS. This implies compression is occurring on the neurovascular structures as they pass through the thoracic inlet as a result of a reduction in the diameter of this potential space. The mechanism for this compression could be anatomic anomalies,[2,22,74] muscular hypertrophy or adaptive shortening of surrounding fascia, or space-occupying lesions.[74] Postural dysfunction is a major component of both types of brachial plexopathies.[29,56] Alterations in posture, especially longstanding ones, may result in the narrowing of spaces necessary for the neurovascular structures to freely traverse the thoracic inlet. Longstanding forward head posture can potentially create space limitations in shape and size secondary to adaptive shortening of tissues of the scalene triangle, costoclavicular, or axillary interval. The second type of brachial plexopathy, brachial plexus traction injury (BPTI), is less understood. A result of a traction injury to the brachial plexus,[16,17] BPTI impairs neural tissue gliding and the ability to tolerate tension, possibly as a result of intraneural or extraneural fibrosis from direct trauma,[10] local pathology within the cervical or thoracic spine,[70] or longstanding compression or over use. This limitation in the nerve's adaptability is called *adverse mechanical tension* (AMT).[9,52] AMT occurs each time the individual uses the affected upper extremity and places traction on the involved nerve and its surrounding tissue bed.

ANATOMIC RELATIONSHIPS

Several anatomic relationships are important to the therapist's evaluation and management of BPN. The first relationship is at the level of the cervical spine between the exiting nerve roots of the brachial plexus and the prevertebral fascia.[43] The trunks of the brachial plexus enter the thoracic inlet through the scalene triangle. An important distinguishing feature at this level is the relationship of the subclavian artery as it accompanies the trunks of the brachial plexus through the scalene triangle. In comparison, the subclavian vein enters the thoracic inlet anterior to the scalene triangle. Clinically this may explain why patients present with neurogenic and classic arterial symptoms without venous symptoms (Fig. 44-1).

Moving laterally, the neurovascular bundles converge and traverse the costoclavicular interval, inferior to the clavicle and superior to the first rib. Continuing laterally, the neurovascular bundle enters the upper extremity through the axilla. At the costoclavicular interval, the patient may present with neurologic symptoms related to the anterior and posterior divisions of the brachial plexus. At the axilla the symptoms may follow a cord distribution. Fig. 44-1 further illustrates these relationships. Clinically, each of these could present with differing neurologic complaints and pain

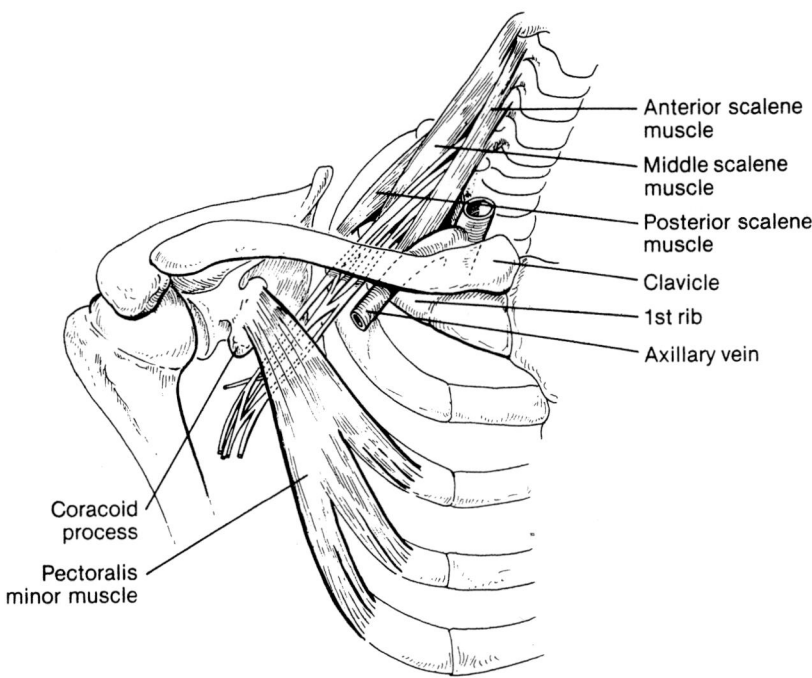

Fig. 44-1. Illustration of the anatomic relationships of the thoracic inlet. (From Pratt N: *Clinical musculoskeletal anatomy,* Philadelphia, 1991, JB Lippincott.)

distribution. The final relationship to consider is muscular. Machleder et al.[34] and Sanders et al.[51] described histologic changes of the scalene muscles in patients presenting with a diagnosis of BPN. These changes include an increase in type I collagen fiber and type II muscle fiber atrophy within the scalene muscles. These histologic changes support the theory that longstanding cervicobrachial pain may be an underlying etiology and pathology for BPN. The increased percentage of connective tissue within the scalene muscles compared with normal muscle tissue may indicate a "stiffening" of the scalene triangle, resulting in a decrease in compliance of these muscles placing the neurovascular structures at greater risk.

Potential spaces of involvement

There are three potential spaces for CBPN or the development of BPTI within the thoracic inlet. The first and most medial space is the interscalene triangle located within the boundaries of the posterior cervical triangle. The presence of a prefixed or postfixed brachial plexus along with other anatomic anomalies may add to poor neurovascular mobility and tension attenuation. Injury to the shoulder girdle or repetitive trauma may lead to symptoms and pathology. As previously discussed, the second potential space is the costoclavicular interval. The third potential space moving laterally is the axillary interval. In this area of the anterior structures, the deltopectoral fascia, pectoralis minor, and coracoid have all been implicated as potential sources of compression of the neurovascular structures.[76]

INCIDENCE OF BRACHIAL PLEXOPATHY

BPN occurs more often in women, usually between the fourth and the sixth decades of life.[60] Brachial plexopathies have also been associated with a history of cervical, thoracic, or shoulder trauma,[37,70] arthritis,[70] bad posture, and repetitive motion disorders.[39] Brachial plexopathies can include symptoms that are related to the venous, arterial, neurologic, or autonomic systems. Because symptoms of multiple-system involvement can be extremely variable, the diagnosis of CBPN or BPTI is predominantly a clinical diagnosis made by a process of exclusion rather than specific objective signs or diagnostic tests. Therefore careful and meticulous evaluation, assessment, and hypothesis formulation are necessary to identify the potential causes of the multiple problems that may coexist in many of these patients.

DIAGNOSIS AND CLASSIFICATION

The diagnosis and classification of these patients continues to remain controversial. Arguments have been put forth to support and refute the existence of brachial plexopathy, especially those labeled as TOS.[48,72] The classification and diagnosis of brachial plexopathy centers around four types, based on symptoms: vascular-arterial, vascular-venous, true (specific) neurogenic, and false (nonspecific) neurogenic TOS.[13] The problem is that the term *TOS* is often used as a diagnosis for other neuropathologies that include the brachial plexus. This confused classification makes it difficult for the treating clinician to develop a treatment strategy. Either way, the brachial plexopathy patient needs to be considered an upper-quarter pain patient. This requires the therapist to have a clear understanding of pain mediation (see Chapter 106).

Cuetter and Bartoszek[13] attempted to classify thoracic outlet and brachial plexopathy patients into four categories. They identified two vascular components, arterial and venous, and believed that these were undisputed because diagnostic tests are available to confirm occlusion or changes of either vascular system. In addition, specific clinical examination techniques, discussed later in this chapter, may further support the presence of vascular involvement. The remaining two classification categories are neurogenic.[13] These have been identified as true (nondisputed) or false (disputed) neurogenic TOS or BPTI.[31,64] Four criteria for true neurogenic TOS are the presence of a cervical rib on radiograph, intrinsic wasting of the hand, sensory changes, and pain/paresthesia over the lower trunk distribution.[31,64] LeForestier et al.[31] also included a fifth criterion—positive electrodiagnostic findings. Approximately 5% of patients with neurovasculopathies within the thoracic inlet are true neurogenic or vascular.[54,64] The remaining 95% are classified as false neurogenic TOS.[54,64] Within this classification, false neurogenic TOS symptoms are identical to those found in true neurogenic TOS; however; there are no appropriate diagnostic signs. Ribbe et al.[47] developed a TOS index of signs and symptoms in an attempt to establish clear criteria for the diagnosis of TOS. The index included positive symptoms provoked by arm elevation, paresthesia over the ulnar nerve or lower trunk distribution, tenderness of the brachial plexus over the supraclavicular fossa, and a positive Roos' test. (These tests are subjective in that they require the patient's report of symptoms and therefore should be interpreted with caution.) The lack of a standardized classification system clouds the identification or diagnosis BPN and hinders the development of a logical treatment approach.

Proposed therapist's classification

As a result of this lack of consensus, I found it necessary to develop a clinical classification dividing brachial plexopathies into two major types. The contrast between these two types is found in Box 44-1. The first type of brachial plexopathy is classic TOS, a compressive vasculopathy and/or neuropathy of the brachial plexus. Classic TOS, as described in the literature, has six identifiable components (see Box 44-1). Posture appears to play a role in the patient's symptoms. The onset of discomfort is usually described as insidious with transient symptoms. These symptoms are usually associated with extremity position, posture, and/or particular motions described by the patient. Extended periods of static positioning or activities that require the arms to be in the elevated position for an extended period are two examples. After the offending posture or activity is corrected, symptoms usually subside. These same symptoms may be provoked during treatment. Provocative tests,

---

Box 44-1   Proposed clinical classification for TOS and BPTI

TOS	*BPTI*
Postural relationship	Trauma related: shoulder, cervical spine
Insidious onset	
Transient symptoms pain/paresthesia	Delayed onset
	Intractable pain/paresthesia
Provocation tests more reliable	Provocation tests not reliable
	Positive upper limb tension
Adson: scalene triangle	Traction on plexus
Costoclavicular: retro-clavicular space	Treatment provokes symptoms, delayed response
Wright's: axillary space	Irritable
Treatment provokes transient symptoms	
Nonirritable	

BPTI, Brachial plexus traction injury; *TOS,* thoracic outlet syndrome.

---

discussed later, may be more reliable in identifying the potential location of the compression. Finally, most of these patients are *nonirritable*. This means they have minimal resting pain; minimal sleep disturbance; low pain scores (verbal reporting or visual analog pain scales); rapid recovery when symptoms are provoked; less mechanical tissue sensitivity to physical examination, with rapid resolution of symptoms once the offending clinical examination is terminated; and the knowledge needed to relieve their symptoms.

The second type of brachial plexopathy is BPTI, often associated with trauma at the onset.[16,17] The trauma involves either a traction injury directly to the brachial plexus or local soft tissue inflammation resulting in a compromise of adequate blood flow to the brachial plexus and the development of intraneural or extraneural fibrosis. This compromises neural excursion and the brachial plexus' ability to attenuate tensile forces placed across it from upper limb and/or combined cervical motion. These patients usually report delayed onset of their intractable pain that can occur several days, weeks, or months after their injury. It is theorized that the delay in onset of the symptoms is explained by the normal course of biologic healing. Mature scar formation eventually compresses the neurovascular structures and/or limits brachial plexus mobility, creating adverse neural tension. Under these conditions, upper-quarter motion results in repetitive traction to the neural tissues and development of symptoms. In these patients, the reliability of provocative tests for determining the level or location of involvement is poor. Provocative tests can provoke symptoms by placing traction on the neural or surrounding tissues, creating a false-positive result. Treatment that might be used for the classic TOS patient may provoke symptoms in BPTI patients at the time of treatment, or the response may be delayed by several hours to a day.

Box 44-2   Therapist differential diagnosis considerations

Myofascial trigger points
GH joint pathology
Double/multiple crush
Cervical dysfunction/pathology
Visceral pathology

GH, Glenohumeral.

Table 44-1. Common myofascial trigger points that may mimic TOS of BPTI

Muscle	Area of referral
Trapezius	Face and interscapular region
Scalene	Posterolateral arm/radial three digits
Supraspinatus	Lateral arm/forearm
Infraspinatus	Lateral arm/forearm and radial half of hand
Latissimus dorsi	Posteromedial arm, forearm, and ulnar half of hand
Pectoralis	Anterior shoulder, medial arm, and ulnar two digits
Subscapularis	Posteromedial arm and wrist
Serratus	Medial arm, forearm, and ulnar half of hand and digits

BPTI, Brachial plexus traction injury; *TOS*, thoracic outlet syndrome.

These patients report a significant increase in symptoms at the next follow-up appointment. Finally, the tissue response of BPTI patients tends to show much more irritability. Symptoms are easily provoked with minimal movement of the upper quarter, and patients often report spontaneous bursts of pain that may be the result of an ectopic (abnormal) pain generator within the peripheral nervous system.[4] In addition, there may be additional concomitant dysfunction accompanying the brachial plexus symptoms.

The pain experienced in the BPTI group can be categorized into two different types. *Nerve trunk pain* results from increased activity in the normal nociceptive endings in the nerve sheaths, called *nervi nervorum*. In contrast, *dysesthetic pain* arises from impulses in damaged or regenerating afferent fibers.[4] The pain could also be nonneurogenic, a result of connective tissue damage causing the release of endogenous chemicals such as bradykinins, serotonin, histamine, acetylcholine, prostaglandin, and leukotrienes. These chemicals have been shown to affect nociceptive afferents. In contrast, the pain may be neurogenically mediated by neuropeptides such as substance P, calcitonin gene–related peptide, vasoactive intestinal peptide, and enkephalins. These substances are released by primary afferent neurons as a result of damaging chemical or physical stimulation of peripheral nociceptive afferents.[71]

Differential therapy diagnosis

In addition to classifying these patients, it is also essential for the therapist to consider differential diagnoses of other potential conditions that may mimic the symptoms associated with brachial plexopathy. Major ones are listed in Box 44-2. Myofascial trigger points as indicated by Travell and Simons[62] can mimic the distribution of brachial plexopathy involvement. Table 44-1 contains common myofascial trigger points that may mimic brachial plexopathy symptomatology.[62] Glenohumeral joint pathology or dysfunction may also provoke symptoms that are similar in nature to the brachial plexopathies referred to as the *Dead arm syndrome*.[30] As reported by Upton and McComas[63] and others,[63,67] the presence of double or multiple crush syndromes may also disguise the involvement of the brachial plexus. Eurroll et al.[18] and MacKinnon[35] reported that these associated double crushes could include carpal tunnel syndrome or ulnar-nerve involvement. The presence of these

disorders and others may help explain treatment failure. Therapists must also be mindful to consider visceral causes such as an apical lung tumor encroaching on the brachial plexus or coronary pathology.

THERAPIST SOLUTION-EVALUATION
History

To classify a patient presenting with a brachial plexopathy, a careful and thorough evaluation performed by the therapist is essential. This evaluation starts with a detailed inquiry as to the mechanism of the problem and the specific distribution and qualitative attributes of the patient's symptoms. As previously discussed, the distribution of symptoms can be extremely variable. The history also provides insightful information about particular positions, postures, or activities that relieve, accentuate, or aggravate the symptoms. This helps the therapist determine the tissue or anatomic space involved. Fig. 44-2 is an example of the presentation of symptoms related to the upper and lower trunks of the brachial plexus. The neurogenic symptoms are classically distributed over the lower trunk[26,50] but may also include the upper trunk,[50] middle trunk,[73,74] and cords of the brachial plexus.[76] With upper trunk plexopathies (C5-C6 distribution), the pain may tend to be more proximal in nature. This proximal pain may be distributed over the anterior and lateral aspect of the cervical region, portions of the face, and the scapular and interscapular region of the involved side.[25] Distal paresthesia and pain may be distributed over what appears to be the median- and/or ulnar-nerve distribution or the C5-C6 dermatomal region. In contrast, lower trunk (C8-T1) plexopathy symptoms of pain and paresthesia are distributed mostly distal. The paresthesia may be located over the medial aspect of the arm, the forearm, and the ulnar aspect of the hand, appearing to be ulnar nerve related. If involvement of the brachial plexus occurs at a more lateral position, such as the division or cord level, the variability of the symptom distribution may be even more pronounced. The use of a body diagram to represent symptom distribution may provide further insight.

Taking the patient history also includes investigating past injuries or medical problems to determine prior upper-quarter trauma or symptoms (e.g., a previous motor vehicle accident with cervical spine injury, or blunt trauma directly over the superior aspect of the shoulder and upper trapezius region). Prior injury might suggest preexisting mobility problems of the plexus. The medical history will also provide valuable information regarding medical conditions such as diabetes mellitus, hyperthyroidism or hypothyroidism, arthritis, or other systemic neurologic disease. It is also important to note the length of time the symptoms have been present. There is a tendency for secondary tissue dysfunctions to develop as the duration of the symptoms increases; knowing the duration of symptoms helps in developing an accurate prognosis. In general, symptoms that have persisted for a longer time require extended therapy and are not as likely to completely resolve.[7] Specific questioning with regard to occupational or avocational activities that could compromise the neurovascular structures within the thoracic inlet is also essential.

Symptoms

Information regarding symptom distribution and previous history leads to more specific questions regarding the qualitative nature of the symptoms. Symptoms with neurogenic features involve the motor, sensory, or autonomic nervous system, such as specific muscle performance deficits, alterations in sensibility, and vasomotor instability. These may be intertwined in the pain as associated sensory disturbances of paresthesia and numbness over the same distribution. Accompanying these early neurologic symptoms may be autonomic nervous system complaints such as hyperhidrosis and burning pain over the same distribution.[1] Raskin et al.[45] reported that headache was present in 26 of 30 patients diagnosed with TOS. Validation of the diagnosis was based on relief of symptoms after first rib resection.

Late neurogenic symptoms can include complaints of pain; sensory changes; and paresthesia distributed over the posterolateral cervical region, anterior shoulder, and posterolateral aspects of the humerus.[26,48,50] More evident intrinsic muscular weakness of the hand with lower trunk involvement, reflex changes, and actual sensory loss[29] may be present. These sensory changes may also present with pencil pointing of the digits for the involved nerve distribution.

Vascular symptoms

Venous symptoms include reports of distal edema, especially after activity and pain described as a dull ache over a nonspecific distribution. The patient may also report a sensation of heaviness in the involved extremity.[26,50] With more significant venous involvement, cyanosis may also be present. Arterial symptoms can include descriptions of fatigue, ischemia-like pain, coldness in the distal part of the extremity, and Raynaud's phenomenon.[26,50] The complaint of ischemia pain may be diffuse or specific to a localized area over the distal extremity. Although rarely seen, late arterial signs could include distal thrombosis or embolization with ischemia changes. Clinical signs of vascular involvement would include loss or a decrease in the quality of distal pulses when performing provocative stress tests; vascular involvement may also be detected with an arteriogram.

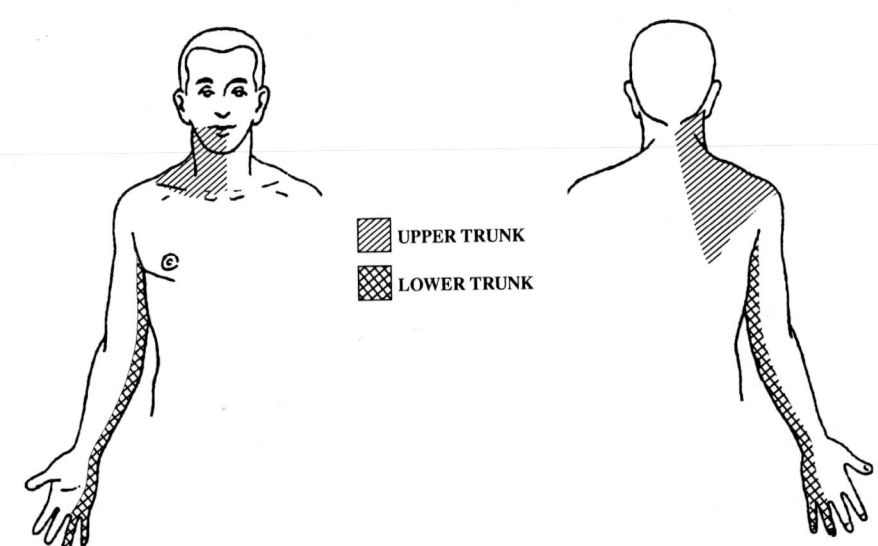

Fig. 44-2. Illustration of the distribution of symptoms that may involve the upper trunk or lower trunk of the brachial plexus.

Diagnostic tests

Diagnostic tests can also be of assistance. Radiographs may indicate the presence of a possible cervical rib, other bony conditions, or a prominent C7 transverse process, which may suggest the presence of a rudimentary fibrous band that has the potential of occupying space in the scalene triangle. Arteriograms may indicate a possible blockage of subclavian or axillary vessels. The use of somatosensory evoked potentials,[28,45] nerve conduction velocities of the medial antibrachial cutaneous nerve, and electromyographic studies are also helpful.[28,31,77] All of these tests may provide additional information as to the location and degree of the neuropathology and determine the presence of double or multiple crush syndromes.

Observation

While obtaining the history from the patient, the therapist can make general observations regarding the patient's standing and sitting postures. The therapist should look for any cervical asymmetry, thoracic kyphosis changes, or accessory breathing patterns. Examples of cervical postures are demonstrated in Fig. 44-3. As is evident from these photos, observing the posture strictly in the sagittal plane may result in obtaining insufficient information. As illustrated by Fig. 44-3, observation of posture in the sagittal plane demonstrates the classic forward-head and rounded-shoulder posture, with a flattened upper thoracic

kyphosis. In the frontal plane (Fig. 44-3, *B*) cervical asymmetry is evident with rotation and lateral flexion of the cervical spine toward the affected side, accompanied by increased upper trapezius muscle tone. Through this observation alone, the therapist is able to hypothesize the patient's level of irritability. This demonstrates the patient's effort to decrease the tension on the brachial plexus by elevating the scapula via contraction of the upper trapezius and levator scapulae and rotating and laterally flexing the cervical spine towards the involved side. At the same time, the therapist must evaluate for edema in the supraclavicular fossa and any atrophy, trophic, temperature, or color changes in the extremity. The position of the upper extremity should also be noted to determine whether the patient is using distal joints to reduce neural tension by maintaining the elbow in flexion, the forearm in neutral, and the wrist and digits in flexion.[42,44] These components may exist separately or in combination, and each may vary in the amount it contributes to the patient's position and pain.

Upper-quarter screening

The therapist performs an upper-quarter screen (see Chapter 7). The cervical spine's active range of motion (ROM) is examined to determine the presence of mechanical spine pain. Special tests, including Spurling's test for foraminal encroachment[55] and the vertebral artery test, are executed to determine nerve root or vascular involvement.[23]

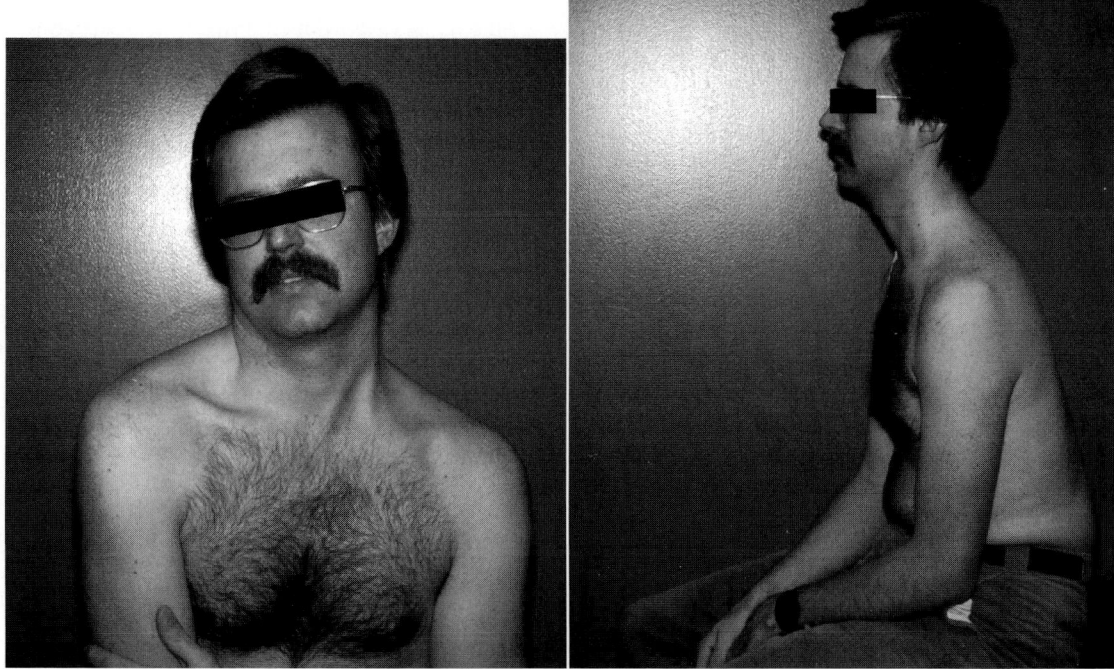

Fig. 44-3. Photograph of common cervical posture seen in patients with BPN. **A,** Frontal plane. **B,** Sagittal plane. Note how examining in one plane only may not give the therapist the complete picture.

Myotomal scanning and reflex testing will provide further information on neural conduction. Tinel's test in the supraclavicular fossa, in the axilla, and along the peripheral nerves allows identification of neural hyperalgesia or other peripheral nerve pathology in the upper extremity. Finally, the supraclavicular fossa and axilla should be auscultated for the presence of a bruit.

Careful sensory evaluation is undertaken using vibrometry and monofilament cutaneous pressure sensation testing. These threshold tests have been reported to be more sensitive than other forms of sensibility testing for early detection of peripheral neuropathies.[58,59] Sensory evaluation should be carried out to investigate (1) dermatomal distribution, to rule out possible cervical root involvement; (2) peripheral nerve distribution, to rule out the possible local peripheral nerve entrapment neuropathies; and (3) sensory disturbance related to the brachial plexus and its divisions. Upon completion of the general upper-quarter screen, assessment for active motion dysfunction is undertaken. This process is explained in Chapter 45. Its purpose is to determine whether imparting tension on the peripheral nervous system in various locations alters active motion of the cervical spine or upper extremity. The presence of active motion dysfunction will assist the therapist in identifying the nervous system's role in the presenting complaints.

Specific tests

Specific provocative tests, described later in this chapter, are carried out only after the therapist has completed an adequate history and upper-quarter screening to develop an initial hypothesis regarding the level of irritability. These provocative positions can potentially place adverse tension on the peripheral nervous system or brachial plexus, exacerbating the patient's symptoms and creating false-positive results. These special tests were originally designed to examine the integrity of the vascular system and the brachial plexus.

Numerous authors have questioned the specificity, sensitivity, and reliability of these tests.* Most of these studies examined asymptomatic subjects as to the frequency of positive tests. A positive test is defined as diminished or lost pulse. None of these studies compared normal subjects with a patient population or considered provocation of symptoms. Falconer and Weddell[19] examined the specificity and sensitivity of the costoclavicular maneuver. In four case studies, three vascular and one neurogenic, they confirmed the involvement of the costoclavicular interval surgically. In 100 normal subjects, 50 males and 50 females 19 to 47 years of age, the costoclavicular maneuver was positive in 25 males and 29 females. In 50% of the males and 60% of the females, there was either a positive Adson's or costoclavicular maneuver.[19] In contrast, Adson[1] found 9 males

*References 11, 19, 20, 39, 41, 46, 61, 69.

and 11 females had a decrease or obliteration of pulse performing his provocative maneuver. In 1980, Gergoudis and Barnes[20] investigated the reliability and validity of the provocative maneuvers. The authors used photoplethysmography to measure the changes in vascular status that occurred with Adson's, costoclavicular, and Wright's test in 130 normal subjects. They determined that 60% had an abnormal finding with at least one test, 27% with two tests, and less than 7% had an abnormal finding when all three tests were performed. It should be noted that the provocation of any kind of symptoms from a neurogenic standpoint was not measured. In 1987, Warrens and Heaton[69] examined the validity of these provocative maneuvers by determining the frequency of false-positive results and the role of photoplethysmography. In 64 normal volunteers, they found 17% were reporting some symptoms. They determined that complete obliteration of the pulse occurred in 58% of the population with at least one test, and 30% had bilateral findings. The incidence of positive findings was 27% for the costoclavicular maneuver, 15% for Adson's test, and 14% for Wright's test. Using photoplethysmography, at least one test was positive in 39% of the subjects. In only 2% of the population were all three tests positive.

In determining the prevalence of a positive elevated arm stress test (EAST) or Wright's maneuver, Costigan and Wilbourn[11] used two groups, 24 normal subjects and 65 patients diagnosed with carpal tunnel syndrome (CTS). They determined that the EAST was positive for 92% of the CTS patients and 74% of the controls. Novak et al.[39] reported that in 65 of 115 patients with possible TOS, the EAST was positive in 94% of the 65 patients and in 100% of the 65 patients with confirmed TOS when direct pressure over the supraclavicular region was combined with the EAST. A positive result was symptom production, but not necessarily the exact symptoms reported by the patient. In 1995, Rayan and Jansen[46] studied the prevalence of a positive response for three provocative maneuvers in a typical patient population of 100. The subjects were divided into two groups: those younger than 40 and those older than 40. They reported that 87 of 100 subjects had at least one positive test for vascular signs and that 41 of 100 had at least one positive test for a neurogenic response. Plewa and Dillinger[41] examined 50 healthy subjects and reported changes in pulse in 11% for both Adson's and costoclavicular maneuver, 62% for Wright's test, and 21% for supraclavicular pressure. Provocation of symptoms (pain or paresthesia) was positive for 11% with Adson's maneuver, 15% with costoclavicular maneuver, and 36% with Wright's test. They concluded that as the number of positive maneuvers increased in each subject, the specificity improved because only six subjects had all three tests positive. Finally, in 1999, Toomingas et al.[61] examined the position of abduction/external rotation among male industrial and office workers. They determined the positive prevalence value was 24% of the population in 1987 and 15% in 1992. Distal symptoms were positive in 12% to 20% of the population, whereas proximal symptoms were present in 5% to 6%. It was their opinion that the symptoms of numbness in the hands had the highest specificity and sensitivity associated with decreased sensitivity to touch.

Provocative test performance

The original proponents of provocative tests used them to delineate the location of compression of the neurovascular structures in the thoracic inlet. Adson proposed that his test implicated compromise at the scalene triangle. This test, described by Adson and Coffey in 1927,[2] involves cervical rotation and extension to the tested side with the upper extremities supported in the patient's lap. This is followed by a deep inspirational breath, which is held for 30 seconds while the examiner palpates for changes in the radial pulse. Obliteration or diminution of the pulse is a positive test. As discussed previously, the importance of the pulse remains in question.[20] Of equal or greater importance is symptom provocation reported by the patient.[29] The clinician is also reminded that this position may stress the contralateral scalene triangle and indirectly provoke symptoms.

The stress hyperabduction test (Wright's test) described by Wright[76] in 1945 implicates the axillary interval. This test is performed in two steps as the patient sits comfortably positioned with the cervical spine in neutral. The arm is passively positioned in 90 degrees of adduction and 90 degrees of external rotation for up to 1 minute while the clinician monitors the patient's symptoms and the quality of the radial pulse. The maneuver may implicate the subclavian vessels and plexus as it is stressed across the coracoid process. A positive test is loss of pulse and implicates the axillary interval. When this test was performed on 150 normal young adults, 83.3% had obliteration of their radial pulse on the right and 82% on the left.[76]

Falconer and Weddell[19] described the costoclavicular maneuver or military brace position for stressing the costoclavicular interval. This test is performed with the patient in the sitting position while the clinician helps position the patient into scapular protraction, elevation, retraction, and depression. The patient holds this position for 30 seconds. The patient's arms remain comfortably supported on the thighs while the examiner simultaneously monitors for any pulse changes. The test is positive when radial pulse changes occur or symptoms are provoked.

In 1966, Roos and Owens[50] described a provocative maneuver that uses exercise stress and positioning. No specific anatomic interval is tested. The patient sits in a neutral position, humerus abducted to 90 degrees, full external rotation, and elbows flexed to 90 degrees. The patient then performs repetitive finger flexion/extension that can be continued for up to 3 minutes. The examiner monitors

for any evidence of dropping of the extremities indicating possible fatigue and arterial compromise. The therapist also observes the color of the distal extremity, comparing left to right. According to Roos, this test stresses all three intervals and places the arterial, venous, and nervous system in tension. The test is considered positive when the patient is unable to maintain the elevation for 3 minutes because of fatigue or pain. Examples of these four maneuvers are depicted in Fig. 44-4.

Smith,[53] Lindgren,[33] Elvey,[16] and Butler[9] hypothesized three additional tests to stress the neurovascular structures through the thoracic inlet. Smith described the stress hyperextension position[53] (Fig. 44-4), which potentially implicates all three intervals and is nonspecific for vascular or neural involvement. A positive test is a change in pulse and provocation of symptoms. In 1992, Lindgren et al.[33] described the cervical rotation/lateral flexion test, designed to assess the elevated position of the first rib in patients presenting with brachialgia (TOS). They examined the reproducibility of this test by comparing it with the cineradiography for first rib position. In 23 symptomatic patients, the test was positive for restricted cervical motion. First described by Elvey[16] and refined by Butler,[6,9] the upper limb tension test systematically places the neurovascular structures of the upper extremities into segmental tension. A positive response is when the patient's symptoms and motion limitations occur. The test should be performed on the noninvolved side first to determine each patient's normal response. See Chapter 45 for further definitions and an explanation of the correct application of this test.

Tissue mobility and palpation

The pectoralis minor and the deltopectoral fascia should be observed for tightness with the patient in a supine position, noting shoulder height and symmetry in the frontal plane. The therapist can also examine for pectoralis minor tightness. Standing at the patient's side facing toward the patient's head, the therapist places the inside hand on the inferior angle of the thoracic cavity and then passively forward flexes the shoulder on the same side. The therapist palpates the inferior costal angle to determine whether any anterior and superior movement occurs. This movement is the result of pectoralis minor tightness as the coracoid process translates superiorly and posteriorly. This test is illustrated in Fig. 44-5. An examination for active myofascial trigger points as described by Travell and Simon[62] is performed to ascertain whether the pain or symptoms are related to the myofascial trigger points mimicking brachial plexus pathology. The most common myofascial trigger points capable of this are listed in Table 44-1. Finally, examination for any evidence of sternoclavicular joint tenderness or muscle spasm of the cervical and shoulder girdle region should be undertaken. This is done to differentiate tissue involvement of the cervical region and

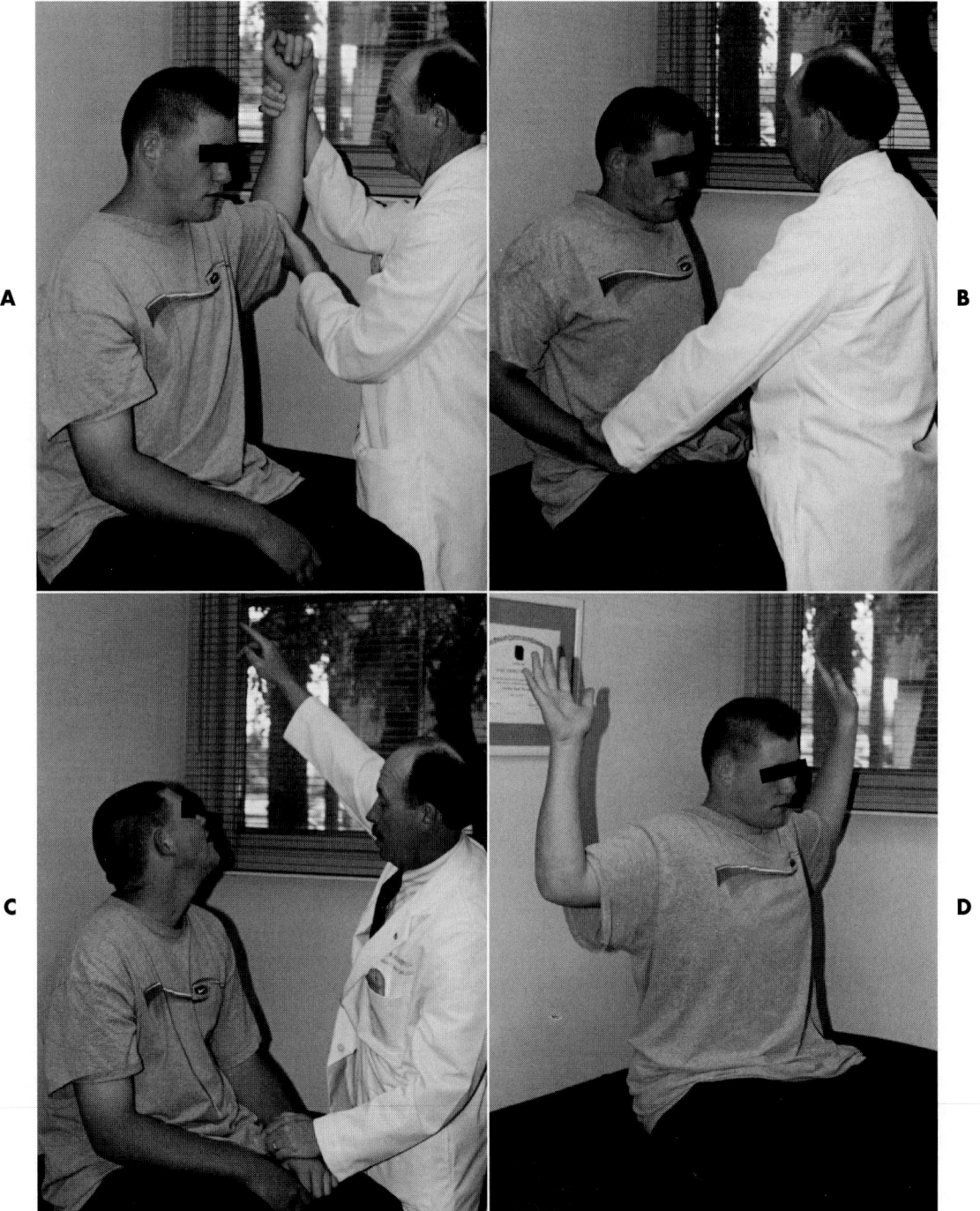

Fig. 44-4. The four commonly applied tests for thoracic outlet syndrome: **A,** Wright's. **B,** Costoclavicular. **C,** Adson's. **D,** Roos'. The breath is held only for the Adson's test.

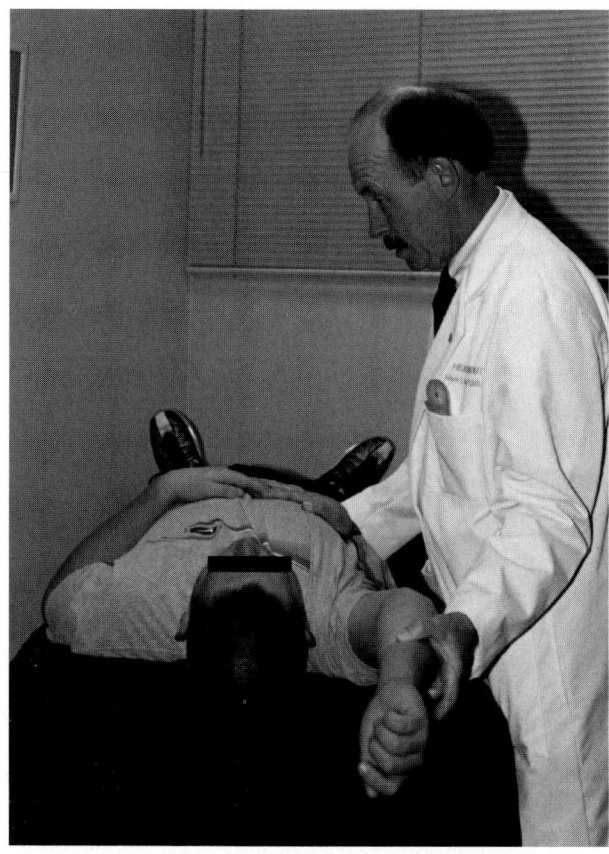

Fig. 44-5. Photograph of testing for pectoralis minor tightness. If the pectoralis is tight the costal inferior angle will translate anteriorly into the examiner's palpating hand.

upper quarter, which may help support or refute the hypothesis of BPN.

TREATMENT
History of conservative management

The therapist is likely to encounter different opinions regarding the role of conservative care for the management of TOS or BPTI. Much of the discrepancy that surrounds the implementation of conservative care is related to controversies regarding the existence of this entity and the criteria used to verify the diagnosis. Peet et al.[40] reported one of the first descriptions for conservative management for TOS in 1956. Treatment techniques for the 55 patients in their study included moist heat, massage, shoulder elevator strengthening, pectoralis strengthening, and postural correction exercises. They reported improvement in 70.9% of the patients; 20 patients improved in 3 to 28 days, and 13 patients improved in 4 to 12 weeks. In 1968, Urschel et al.,[65] using a conservative approach of moist heat, active motion, shoulder elevation strengthening, and cervical traction, reported their treatment was "effective" for 50% of the 120 patients in the study. Treatment duration varied from 3 months to several years.[65] In 1974, Dale and Lewis[14]

described a conservative treatment program consisting of shoulder girdle strengthening and medication. They stated that 63% of the 150 extremities "did well."[14] McGough et al.[36] studied a large population of 1300 patients. Treatment consisted of shoulder girdle strengthening, postural correction, moist heat, massage, and medication; only 9.4% required surgery. The average treatment time was 7.2 months, ranging from 2 months to 2 years.[36] Woods[75] described a treatment program including medication, exercise, and transcutaneous electrical nerve stimulation (TENS). Of the 109 patients in the study, 50% obtained relief within 9 months mean treatment time; TENS was found effective in 40 of the 109 patients. The major weaknesses with each of these studies was a lack of consistent criteria for the diagnosis and that only descriptive outcomes were reported.

In 1979, Smith[53] described a treatment protocol composed of orthopedic manual techniques to increase flexibility of the thoracic inlet, flexibility exercises, and behavioral and postural modification. A significant decrease in symptoms was obtained in 75% of the 20 patients. The mean treatment time was 10 visits, with a range of 1 to 14. In 1984, Walsh[68] re-created this treatment approach using inclusion criteria of insidious onset of symptoms, no history of trauma, and two or more of the provocative maneuvers positive for pulse changes and symptom provocation. Symptoms were predominantly transient paresthesia and pain. Asymptomatic relief was obtained in 68.5% of 16 patients involving 19 extremities; 10.5% reported moderate relief, 5.2% reported temporary relief, and 15.8% reported no relief. Surgery was performed in three of the six patients with moderate or no relief. There was one reoccurrence that was relieved after 14 additional visits.

Other conservative approaches have been tested. Ingesson et al.[24] described a physiotherapeutic method of treatment for CBPN (TOS). Treatment included general and specific components. General components were patient education, avoidance of provocative postures and activities, and ergonomic intervention. Specific components were relaxation for involved muscles; breathing exercises and training; stretching of shortened muscles; postural training, including coordination for anterior and posterior postural muscles; specific mobilization of the cervical and thoracic spine; and a home exercise program. A "positive effect" was achieved in 50% of the patients (63 of 125); 45 of the remaining 62 patients required surgery. In 1990, Sucher[57] presented four case studies in which patients were treated with myofascial release techniques as the primary tactic. In all four cases symptoms were "markedly improved." The particular techniques were not described in detail. However, it appears that contract-relax, spray and stretch, and vigorous stretching of involved musculature or surrounding fascia were discussed. In 1995, Novak et al.[38] reported on 42 patients treated conservatively for TOS. Treatment included education regarding pathophysiology, avoidance of offending positions, and postural awareness. Therapy treatment incorporated postural correction, pain control, stretching and therapeutic exercise, aerobic conditioning, and a home exercise program. Symptomatic improvement was obtained in 25 patients, 10 were unchanged, and 7 worsened. Poor overall outcome was related to obesity, worker's compensation, and concomitant double crush injury (carpal or cubital tunnel syndrome). Arm and hand pain was significantly improved in patients who did not have these concomitant problems. In 1997, Lindgren[32] reported on 139 patients treated with a therapeutic model of scapula ROM, upper cervical spine normalizing exercises (chin tucks while standing against the wall), resisted cervical forward flexion, rotation and extension to normalize first rib function, and stretching the anterior cervical spine and levator muscles. At the time of discharge from the hospital, 88.1% of the patients were satisfied with the outcome and improved impairment.

Cramer[12] described a reconditioning program for athletes to decrease the rate of recurrence of injury-induced brachial plexus neuropraxia. The program included 4 weeks of conservative management and 8 weeks of progressive reconditioning consisting of cervical strengthening three times per week and cervical mobilization and modified shoulder strengthening two times per week. No specific patient data was presented to support this approach.

Numerous other authors* have also described conservative approaches. The concept of adverse neural tension (ANT)[9,52] provides additional etiologies and treatment approaches to be considered in the treatment of BPN patients. The recent theory of ANT has lead to the development of my approach to classifying CBPN and BPTI patients.

Variability in the duration of the various conservative treatment plans relates to the lack of diagnostic criteria and specific treatment approaches. Guidelines for treatment duration are based on patient symptom response and the therapist's physical examination. In general, (1) the longer the duration of symptoms, the longer conservative care may be necessary; (2) multiple-system involvement such as glenohumeral joint pathology, myofascial trigger points, or double crush syndromes may necessitate longer-term conservative measures; (3) conservative care may take longer for the patient with BPTI than for those that have the classically described TOS; (4) social, medical, emotional and occupational factors play an important role in the patient's response to conservative care; and (5) the presence of multiple or double crush syndrome may require treatment to address the cervical spine, distal pathology, and BPN.

Treatment considerations

General. Multisystem involvement is often present in TOS and BPTI patients. Treatment programs are developed

*References 3, 5, 15, 27, 37, 42, 57, 66, 67, 74.

from information obtained from the evaluation and assessment. There is no recipe or cookbook approach to treating these patients, especially when their conditions are highly complex. Whether the problem is compressive TOS or BPTI, the purpose of stage I treatment is to decrease and control the patient's symptoms. In the more complex patient, it may be useful to formulate a problem list for each system and/or tissue involved. This list may include bursitis or specific tendonitis of the shoulder; adhesive capsulitis; active myofascial trigger points; mechanical, cervical, or thoracic spine pain; double or multiple crushes; and other soft tissue conditions. The therapist must keep in mind that a double or multiple crush syndrome involvement may necessitate treatment for a more distal peripheral neuropathy.[18,60,63] The problem list should be prioritized based on the overall goal of stage I. Therefore the brachial plexus component of the patient's symptomatology may in fact be the last issue addressed in the treatment program. Initially, attempting to manage the brachial plexus component may only exacerbate the patient's symptoms and result in failure. Also imperative in stage I is identifying activities, positions, and treatments that exacerbate or relieve the patient's symptoms. The therapist's understanding of the level of tissue irritability and methods of relief is essential for progressing to stage II.

Stage II conservative management commences only after control and comfort have been achieved. The patient should have a minimal level of resting pain and no sleep disturbance. During this stage, treatment of tissues that create structural limitations to motion directly related to the compression or traction of the brachial plexus and its accompanying neurovascular structures may be initiated. Treatment may transiently exacerbate the patient's complaints; however, this should not last beyond the treatment session. To ensure that it does not, the therapist must have command of the methods necessary to regain symptom control. Postural awareness and correction are also being initiated during this stage.

Stage III, or the *restorative phase,* involves conditioning and strengthening the muscles necessary to maintain postural correction. Postural correction is carried over into activities of daily living and occupational situations that may lead to adverse neural tension situations. Functional and occupational activities are addressed via patient education and ergonomic intervention.

Stage I: symptom control phase. In general, the treatment approach for classic compressive TOS and the more complex BPTI patient can be combined based on the goal of symptom control and relief. Although the duration of treatment is extremely variable for each type of patient, the BPTI patient is likely to require more time. Stage I treatment centers around behavior modification, postural correction and awareness, and the development of a diaphragmatic breathing pattern. Behavior modification addresses factors contributing to symptoms, quality of life,

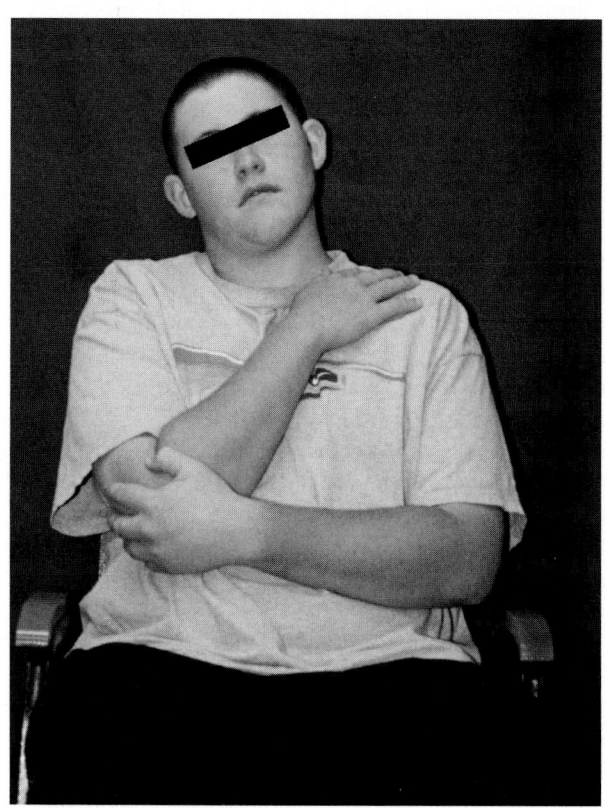

Fig. 44-6. Brachial plexus slack position; note the posture of the head and cervical spine favoring the involved side.

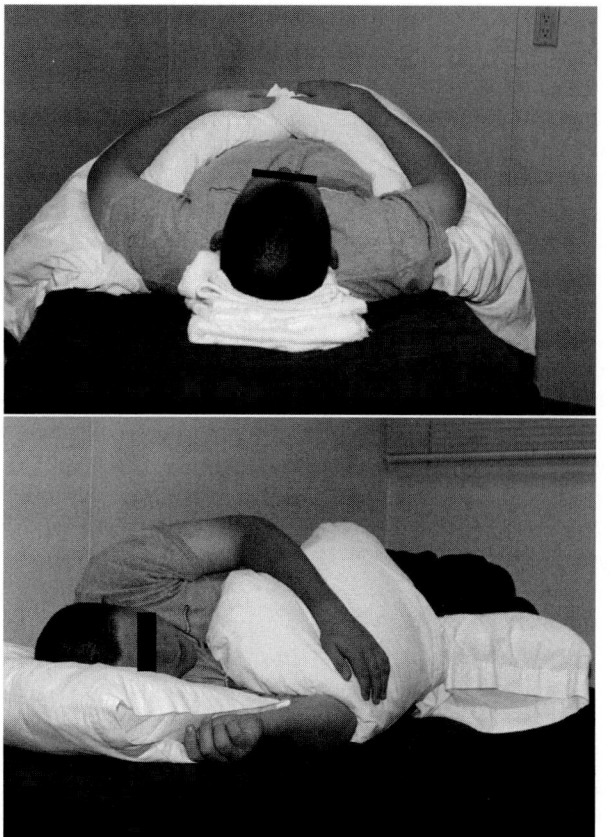

Fig. 44-7. Examples of sleep positions. **A,** Supine. **B,** Side lying.

and occupational or avocational activities. Behavior modification may include instructing the patient in appropriate positioning of the upper extremity at rest to avoid placing tension across the brachial plexus and accompanying vascular structures. Passive shoulder elevation corrects the depressive traction component on the brachial plexus and has been beneficial in decreasing symptoms. Positioning suggestions include using the opposite, noninvolved extremity to support the involved extremity in the brachial plexus slack position, as demonstrated in Fig. 44-6, or resting the affected extremity on the armrest of a chair or a pillow on the lap. Further relief from tension while standing can be accomplished by having the patient place his or her hand in a coat pocket or by supporting it on a belt. When symptoms are exacerbated, resting the affected arm on the armrest of a chair or pillow for 30 minutes before bedtime may also decrease symptoms before sleeping. Obtaining adequate rest after strenuous activities is important for relaxation of any muscular components involved. It is beneficial during the initial stages of treatment to have the patient refrain from engaging in strenuous aerobic activities, which may create exertional breathing. This increases accessory muscle activity and potentially compromises the neurovascular structures throughout the thoracic inlet.

Activities that aggravate the patient's symptoms are identified during history taking. Many times, the patient is unaware of similar activities that require the same component movements. The patient should be educated to avoid all activities and motions that tend to exacerbate symptoms during the initial treatment phase. This educational process continues throughout the course of care. The patient should avoid any pressure over the thoracic inlet. Additional padding that increases the surface area can diminish pressure from automobile shoulder-restraint straps. Women should wear a strapless bra or use additional padding to increase the strap surface area. Finally, the patient should avoid carrying heavy objects, including handbags with the affected extremity. These activities increase shoulder depression and traction on the neurovascular structures.

Proper sleep positioning is often important to obtain symptom control and avoid sleep disturbance. Sleep positions should place the affected upper extremity in a position that minimizes tension on the brachial plexus and its neurovascular structures, the cervical spine, and distal peripheral nerve tissues. Examples of sleep positions are demonstrated in Fig. 44-7. The position should maintain the spine in neutral and support the upper extremity in a posture without tension. Finding a helpful sleep position may require nothing more than changing sides of the bed. The postures and activities that contribute to the patient's symptoms should be discussed. Eliminating offending resting postures during work, such as the forward-head and rounded-shoulder posture, or upper extremity over head positions, is an important component of this education. Modifications in the workplace may be necessary to achieve these goals. It is important to respect longstanding offending posture and lengthening or shortening adaptations. Changes will not occur overnight. The patient takes postural awareness and correction seriously only when the therapist presents these concepts appropriately. It is necessary to spend time at each treatment session discussing and working on posture and breathing. A proper balance of stretching and strengthening exercises is necessary to obtain posture correction. The therapist must be aware of any fixed deformities that may preclude achieving corrected posture. Overcorrecting to an established "textbook" posture often leads to further exacerbation of symptoms. Because most of these patients are 40 years of age or older, these posture abnormalities result in longstanding adaptive tissue changes. These soft tissue adaptations occur within the fascia, muscle, articular structures, and neurovascular structures. Postural correction should respect the nervous system to avoid additional adverse neural tension on the plexus and its accompanying nerve roots and peripheral nerves. It may also be helpful to involve family members in the postural correction process and teach them to recognize abnormal breathing patterns to increase patient awareness. A low-impact, tolerable aerobic program to encourage large segmental and muscle group activity is implemented during this stage as well. As reported by Novak and MacKinnon,[38] many of these patients have body weight issues and compromised fitness status.

Altered breathing patterns at rest and during activity are common in patients with BPN. Accessory breathing patterns using the scalene, intercostal, and pectoralis minor muscles often occurs when patients are focused and statically postured. All of these structures affect the path of the neurovascular structures as they progress laterally through the thoracic inlet. This accessory breathing pattern is identified by shallow breaths with increased cephalic excursion and a decrease in circumferential expansion of the thoracic cavity. This same breathing pattern may be evident during activities such as playing an instrument, working at a computer, reading, or writing. Patient education and instruction regarding these aberrant breathing patterns is essential in developing a diaphragmatic breathing pattern. Diaphragmatic breathing requires instruction by the therapist to help the patient reestablish the diaphragm as the major muscle responsible for breathing. Diaphragmatic breathing allows for accessory muscle relaxation and improved excursion of the thoracic cavity. Patient command of this will be beneficial when progressing into the latter stages of treatment that incorporate diaphragmatic breathing into manual treatment techniques and the home program.

Stage I treatment of BPTI patients involves two additional considerations. First, the therapist must identify which of the five clinical pain patterns described by Gifford and Butler[21]— peripheral nociceptive, peripheral neurogenic, central nervous system related, sympathetic nervous system related, and affective/motivational—are present. Although one or two of these may dominate the patient's complaints, all five may be present, adding complexity to the problem. Through identification of these different pain patterns, a more direct treatment approach is established and the prognosis is improved. Patients with predominant central nervous system, sympathetic nervous system, or affective/motivational pain patterns are more difficult to treat, and their outcomes are often less successful. Often, it is necessary for a therapist to accept that complete resolution of a patient's symptoms is unrealistic. The goal in this particular group of patients may be to improve the quality of the patient's life by controlling symptoms and providing a greater pain-free ROM, thus allowing the patient to use the upper extremity in a more functional and comfortable manner.

During this time, identified secondary problems may be treated directly, for example, addressing active myofascial trigger points that are referring symptoms, providing pain modulation through modalities and exercise, or treating double or multiple crush situations. It is also appropriate to implement large-amplitude motions using all extremities through a low-impact aerobic program or using general nerve mobilization techniques via the spine and lower extremities. See Chapter 45 for further information and direction regarding this issue.

Stage II: restoration. I refer to stage II as the restorative phase because treatment of the soft tissue dysfunction identified during the evaluation is initiated. Stage II treatment is initiated only after comfort and symptom control have been achieved. In classic compressive TOS, soft tissue mobilization described by Smith[53] may be instituted. The goals of these manual techniques are to improve flexibility of the associated tissues, restore normal tissue resting lengths, and assist in restoring normal posture. Addressing these problems may increase the size of the potential compression intervals and minimizes neurovascular compression.[56] Soft tissue mobilization includes addressing joint and soft tissue mobility of the acromioclavicular and sternoclavicular joints and scapulothoracic articulation as necessary. In addition, it is appropriate to improve first rib position,[32] mobility, and cervical spine function. These techniques also address adaptively shortened muscles such as the pectoralis group and the scalene muscles via deep massage and stretch while avoiding brachial plexus tension. Brachial plexus gliding and/or peripheral-nerve mobilization as described by Butler and Elvey may be instituted. Examples of these techniques are demonstrated in Fig. 44-8.

It is beyond the scope of this chapter to discuss the specifics of peripheral-nerve mobilization. See Chapter 45

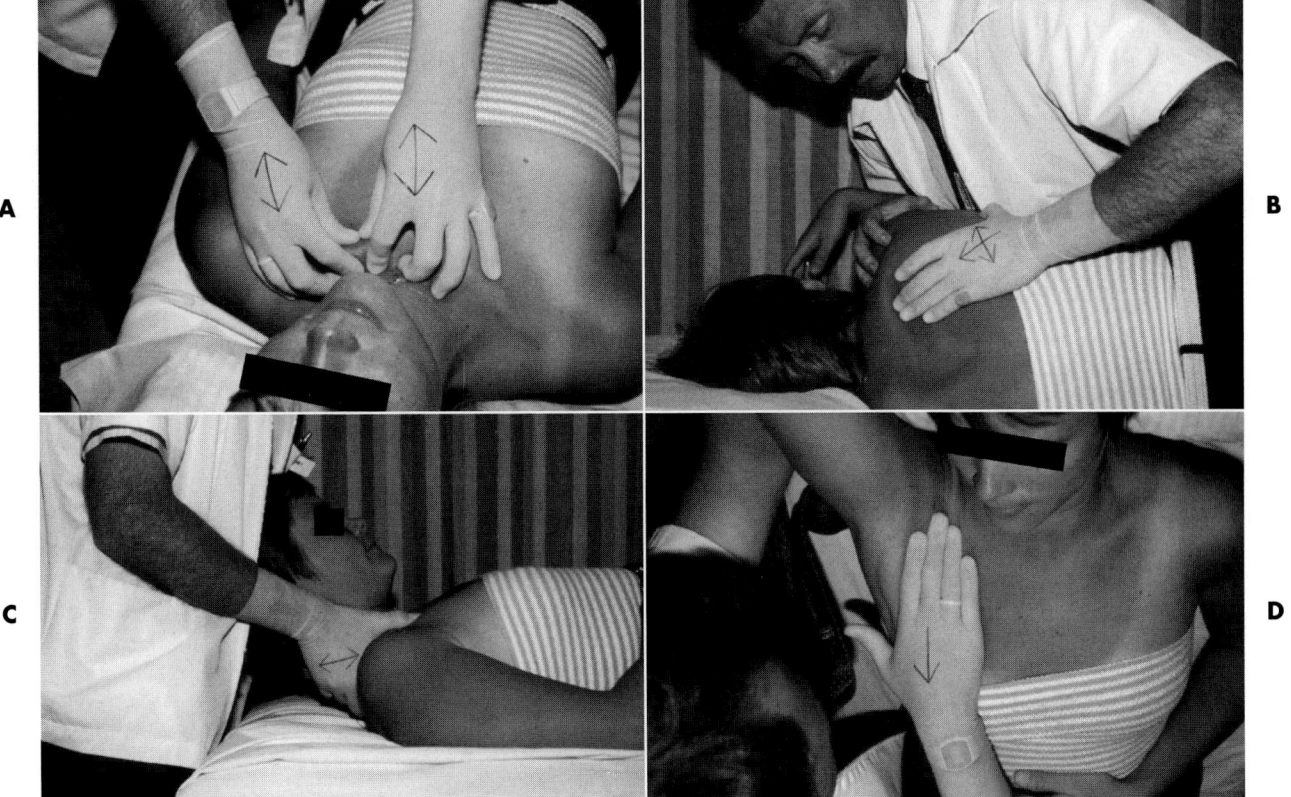

Fig. 44-8. Manual techniques that can be used to improve the flexibility of the thoracic inlet.
A, Sternoclavicular joint. **B,** Scapular-thoracic articulation. **C,** First rib. **D,** Pectoralis minor tightness.

for additional information. In general, the purpose of peripheral-nerve mobilization is to restore normal neurophysiology and neurobiomechanics, thereby improving tension tolerance and intraneural and extraneural excursion.[7] It is theorized that alleviating intraneural and extraneural compression results in improved vascular function and axoplasmic flow.[8,9] This is accomplished by using components of the upper and lower limb tension tests to restore neural mobility. However, therapists are advised to obtain further information regarding these techniques and their appropriate use before proceeding with peripheral-nerve mobilization. *Use of these techniques, especially during the early portions of stage II, without symptom control could result in significantly exacerbating the patient's symptoms.*

A home exercise program is instituted during stage II treatment. Originally described by Peet et al.[40] and subsequently modified by numerous other authors, the home program aims to improve the flexibility of the entire thoracic inlet region and its accompanying neurovascular structures. The following examples are not intended to be all-inclusive; other exercises may be more appropriate for a particular patient. Scalene stretching is preferably done in a supine position to minimize cervical muscle activity while maximizing stretch. Cervical protraction and retraction or "axial extension" exercises[7] help eliminate the forward-head and

rounded-shoulder posture and reestablish proprioceptive input for proper cervical spine positioning. The therapist is reminded to correct any occipital rotation and restore lumbar posture. Incorporating diaphragmatic breathing into the exercise program assists the patient in habituating diaphragmatic breathing and is a gentle way of adding restorative forces to the involved tissues. Diaphragmatic breathing can be combined with scalene, deltopectoral fascia, and pectoralis stretching. The patient performs shoulder forward flexion to a position of tolerance. The patient then uses diaphragmatic breathing to stretch the pectoralis minor by using the diminishing circumference of the lower thoracic cavity on exhalation to stretch the pectoralis minor. Pectoralis stretching can also be accomplished with a corner stretch or while the patient stands with arms elevated at 90 degrees in a doorway. Scapulothoracic flexibility exercises can be performed to improve flexibility and motor control. In addition, scapulothoracic stabilization techniques such as quadruped positioning or using a therapeutic ball may help restore optimal scapulothoracic motor control. Cervical spine flexibility may be improved with active ROM, contract-relax, and a host of other techniques. Appropriate nerve gliding exercises may be instituted in conjunction with these techniques or as separate exercises. Examples of some home exercises are demonstrated in Fig. 44-9.

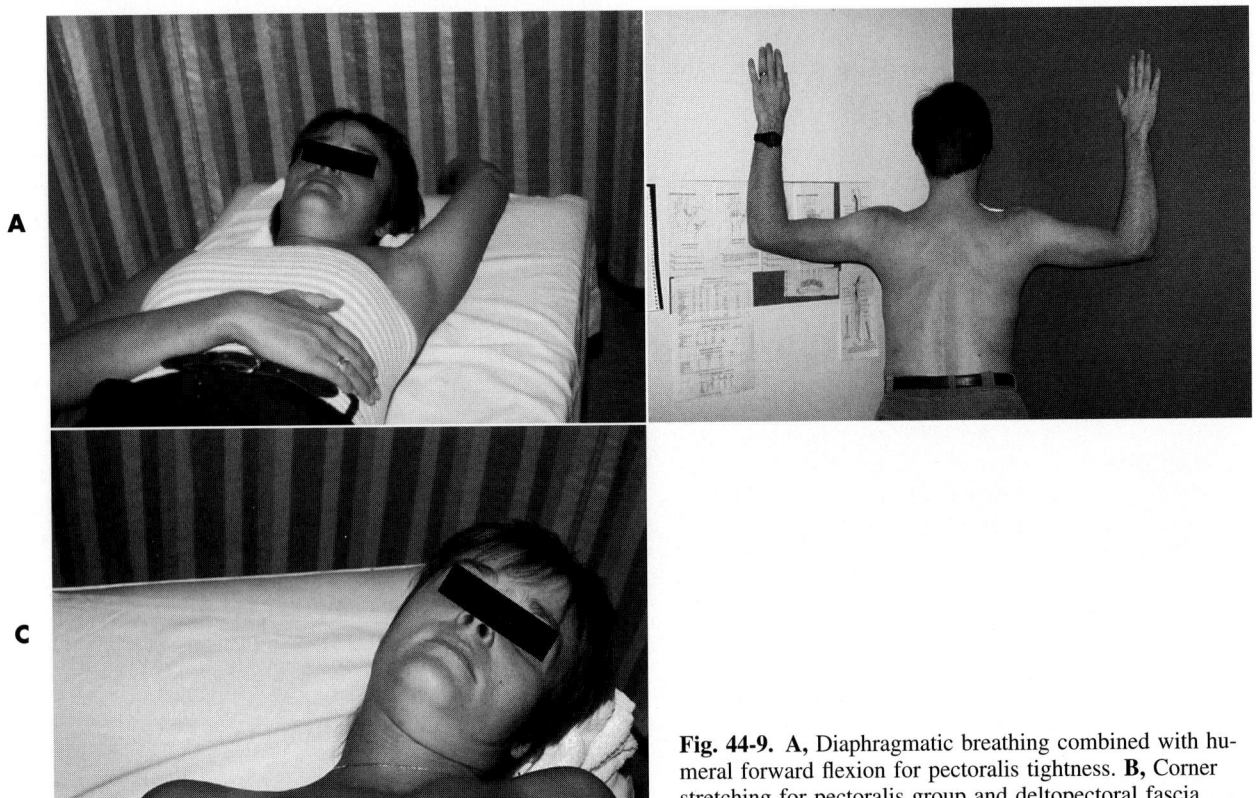

Fig. 44-9. A, Diaphragmatic breathing combined with humeral forward flexion for pectoralis tightness. **B,** Corner stretching for pectoralis group and deltopectoral fascia tightness. **C,** Scalene stretching.

In BPTI patients, these exercises may need to be modified to avoid placing tension on the brachial plexus and its vascular structures and the peripheral nerves. Treatment for previously identified secondary problems continues. During this stage, the therapist must be mindful of any active motion dysfunction resulting from neurogenic involvement to avoid the end-ranges of motion, which may lead to adverse tension and exacerbation of pain. If symptom control has been achieved, specific nerve gliding techniques for the brachial plexus may be instituted. Because of the longstanding nature of the problems faced by this patient population, a home program is imperative and may be more important than specific hands-on techniques performed in the clinic. It is only over an extended period that the adaptive tissue changes can be corrected and balances between the soft tissues and the neurovascular structures can be restored. At no time during this phase should any treatment or home exercise program provoke more than mild transient symptoms. As previously alluded to, most of these patients present with chronic pain and too aggressive handling or too rapid a progression in therapy may result only in restoring their initial level of tissue irritability.

Stage III: rehabilitative. Stage III treatment strategies for compressive BPN are intended to increase overall aerobic capacity and fitness, restore postural muscle imbalances, and institute workplace modifications, while continuing to emphasize posture awareness and breathing. In addition, a balanced nutritional program is encouraged to assist overweight patients; excess weight is a problem because obesity has been associated with TOS. Strengthening of postural muscles and incorporating these into postural correction continues to support the emphasis on postural awareness. It is sometimes unrealistic to expect that a longstanding postural fault or habit can be totally overcome through strengthening and awareness. It is realistic to expect the patient to reverse the offending posture as often as possible throughout the day. Rehabilitation exercises should also address work conditioning, be work task specific, and include modifications that will help avoid inappropriate stresses across the brachial plexus region. In conjunction with this, the continued application of posture and diaphragmatic breathing in the workplace should continue to be addressed. The patient's awareness of these latter two components often begins to fail, resulting in continuance or recurrence of symptoms. Finally, during stage III treatment of compressive BPN patients, reassessment of their subjective, objective, functional, and vocational status should be performed to address any final issues before discharge.

These same strategies may also be instituted in patients with BPTI. In addition, specific nerve gliding or "tensioning" exercises for localized and secondary involvement of the peripheral nervous system should be implemented and previous nerve mobilization techniques continued as needed. This may require periodic visits to the clinic to appropriately adjust the exercise prescription. The patient's subjective, objective, functional, and vocational status should be reassessed to apply more specific exercises and/or nerve mobilization techniques. It is also important during this stage for the therapist to reevaluate expectations for the patient. It has been my unfortunate experience on several occasions, upon achieving a 60% to 70% improvement; that further attempts to improve upper extremity conditioning resulted in exacerbation of the patient's initial complaints. This necessitated a return to the stage I level of treatment to gain control before progressing again through the remaining two stages. The goals and expected outcome established by the therapist and patient may have to be tempered by the reality that 100% alleviation of symptoms may not be possible. Therefore educating patients about the levels of activity they can tolerate and the positions that exacerbate their symptoms becomes extremely important in allowing continued daily activities and occupational tasks.

CASE EXAMPLE

The following case example may help exemplify the treatment approach for brachial plexus neuropathy patients:

A 29-year-old woman was involved in a motor vehicle accident 18 months before she was referred to our clinic with the diagnosis of "brachial plexus neuropathy." Three physicians and two physical therapists provided previous treatment without any significant improvement. Previous therapy included palliative modalities and a rigorous conditioning program. Despite this intervention, her symptoms progressively became worse. Objectively, the patient presented with three active myofascial trigger points, restricted cervical spine motion, glenohumeral joint limitations, and evidence of brachial plexus involvement. The patient also had active and passive motion dysfunction of the involved extremity indicating possible adverse neural tension.

Stage I treatment was directed toward the patient's myofascial trigger points and used appropriate modalities to deactivate the trigger points, used passive stretching of involved muscles, and sought to eliminate tension on the neurovascular structures. This was achieved by placing the patient in the brachial plexus slack position (see Fig. 44-6). From this position, localized stretching of the involved trigger points was performed, minimizing stimulation of the sensitized peripheral nervous system. Restricted cervical ROM was managed with an active ROM program and manual mobilization techniques. At this point,

the BPN components of her problem were not specifically addressed.

Progression into stage II was initiated once the active myofascial trigger points were deactivated and cervical spine motion improved. Treatment now included soft tissue mobilization and peripheral-nerve mobilization (gliding). These techniques continued until the patient no longer demonstrated evidence of adverse neural tension signs, negative provocative TOS maneuvers, inactive myofascial trigger points, and symmetrical cervical motion. Although complete subjective relief was not attained, the patient returned to work and functional activities she had been avoiding before treatment. During stage III, she was instructed in additional postural strengthening exercises. Postural and breathing awareness and symptom avoidance education continued. Fig. 44-10 contrasts the pretreatment and posttreatment findings for this patient.

SUMMARY

The treatment of brachial plexus neuropathy patients, especially those presenting with long-term pain, can be a complex and challenging problem for the occupational or physical therapist. Literature supports the use of conservative care as the preferred initial approach with these patients. Many of these patients present with additional secondary system complaints, including active myofascial trigger points, primary or secondary glenohumeral pathology, cervical pathology, and more distal peripheral neuropathies in the form of double or multiple crush. For this reason, treatment of these patients is rarely straightforward and is usually complex.

Treatment requires that the therapist understand the pathologic mechanism contributing to the patient's complaints. This understanding, which is obtained only through a thorough evaluation performed by the therapist, is extremely important in classifying these patients. Treatment should initially address the issues of comfort and symptom control. Gradual progression through the three stages of treatment requires that the therapist be responsive to the patient's symptom responses throughout the course of care. The therapist must also appreciate that tissue adaptations occur over a number of years, especially when there was a strong postural and concomitant repetitive nature to their symptoms. In these particular cases, treatment requires patience and understanding that this is an ongoing process, best addressed through compliance with the home exercise prescription, postural awareness, and correction of abnormal breathing patterns. Finally, treatment progression requires the therapist to proceed in a very gentle manner with minimal symptom response. Proper education of the patient for behavior modification, exercise compliance, symptom control, and postural awareness is requisite for optimal results.

SUBJECTIVE

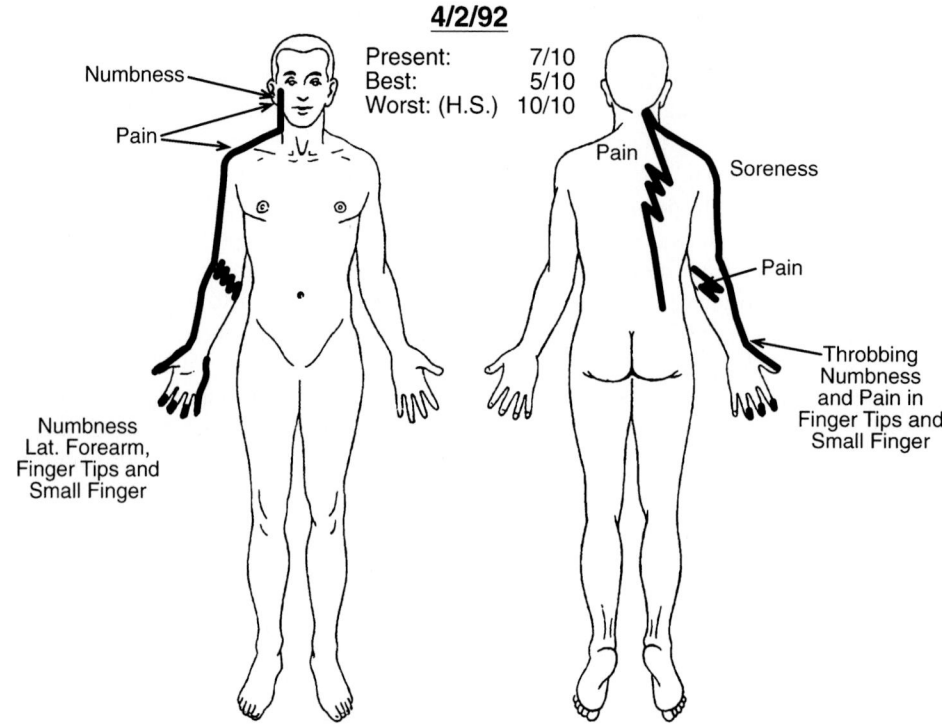

OBJECTIVE FINDINGS

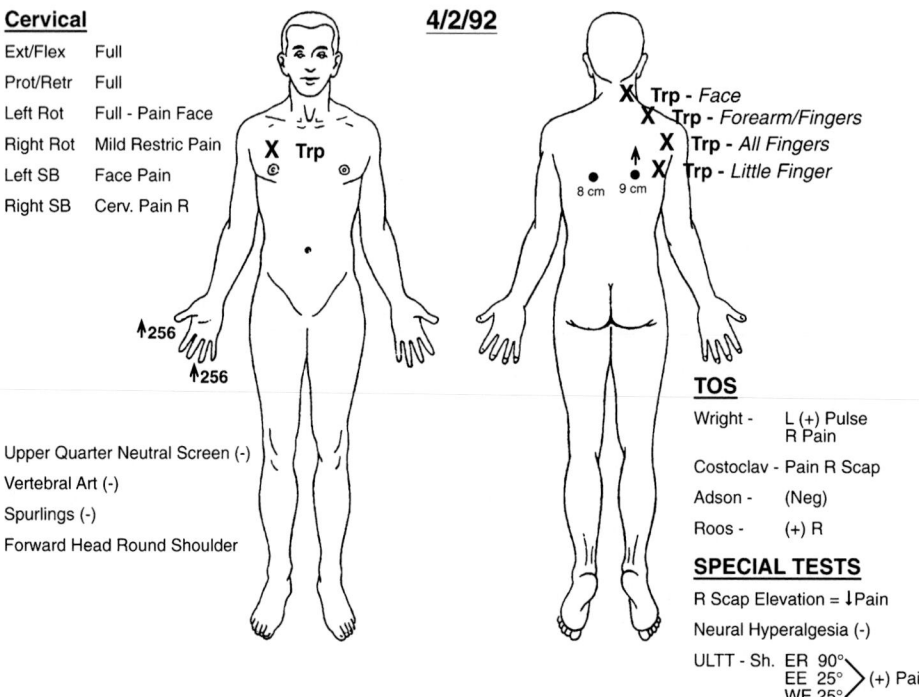

Fig. 44-10. Actual patient diagrams of pretreatment and posttreatment findings for the patient in the case example. **A,** Pretreatment subjective pain diagram. *Continued*

SUBJECTIVE

6/4/92

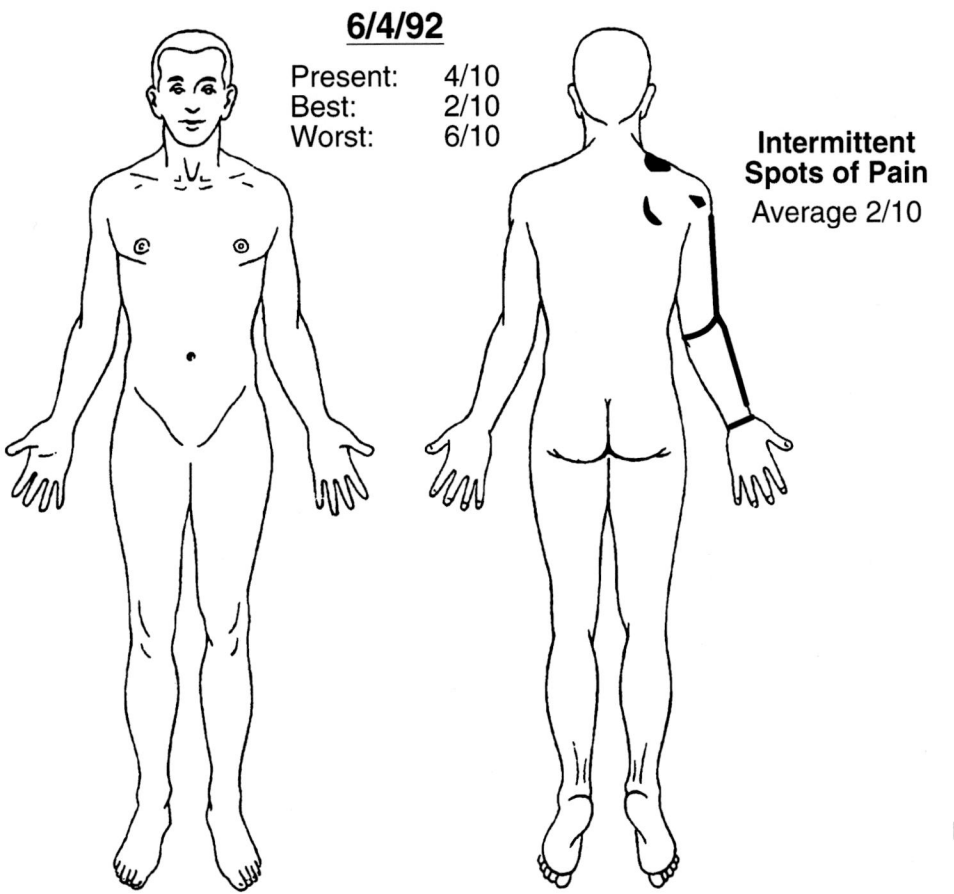

Present: 4/10
Best: 2/10
Worst: 6/10

**Intermittent
Spots of Pain**
Average 2/10

B

OBJECTIVE FINDINGS

Cervical

Left Rot	Min. Face Pain
Left SB	Min. Face Pain
Right SB	Min. Restriction (-) Pain
All Others	Full - Pain Free

5/5/92

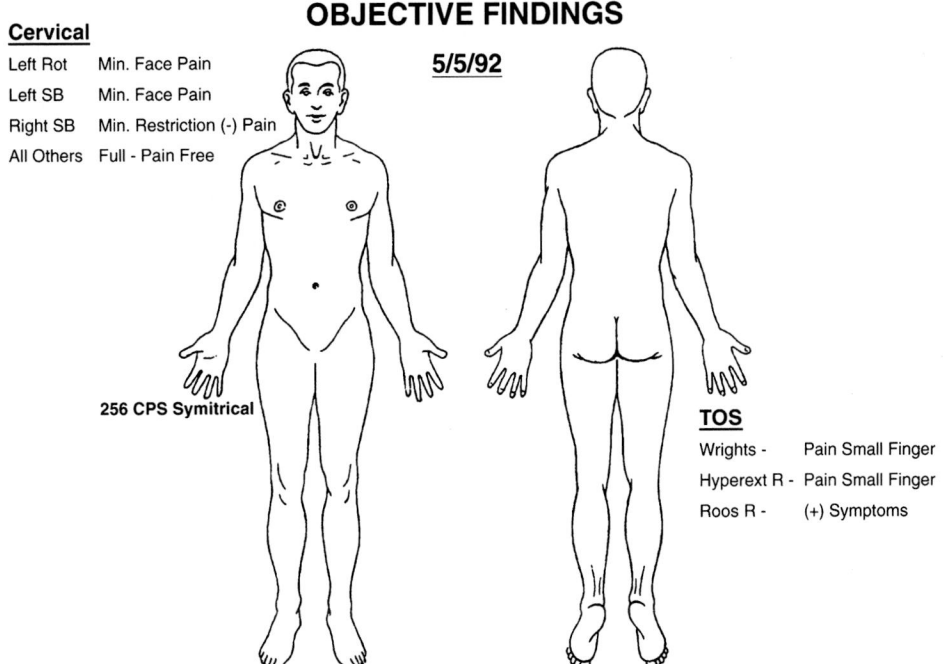

256 CPS Symitrical

TOS

Wrights -	Pain Small Finger
Hyperext R -	Pain Small Finger
Roos R -	(+) Symptoms

6/4/92

No Objective Findings Noted

Fig. 44-10, cont'd. B, Posttreatment subjective pain diagram.

REFERENCES

1. Adson AW: Cervical ribs: symptoms, differential diagnosis, and indications for section of the insertion of the scalenus anticus muscle, *J Int Coll Surg* 14:546, 1951.

2. Adson A, Coffey JR: Cervical rib: a method of anterior approach for relief of symptoms by division of the scalenus anticus, *Ann Surg* 85:839, 1927.

3. Aligne C, Barral X: Rehabilitation of patients with thoracic outlet syndrome, *Ann Vasc Surg* 6:381, 1992.

4. Asbury A, Fields H: Pain due to peripheral nerve damage: an hypothesis, *Neurology* 34:1587, 1984.

5. Britt L: Nonoperative treatment of thoracic outlet syndrome, *Clin Orthop* 51:45, 1967.

6. Butler D: Adverse mechanical tension in the nervous system: a model for assessment and treatment, *Aust J Physiother* 35:27, 1989.

7. Butler D: *Mobilization of the nervous system,* London, 1991, Churchill Livingstone.

8. Butler D, Gifford L: The concept of adverse mechanical tension in the nervous system part 1: testing for "dural tension," *Physiotherapy* 75:622, 1989.

9. Butler D, Gifford L: The concept of adverse mechanical tension in the nervous system: Part 2 Examination and treatment, *Physiotherapy* 75:629, 1989.

10. Capistrant T: Thoracic outlet syndrome in whiplash injury, *Ann Surg* 185:175, 1977.

11. Costigan DA, Wilbourn AJ: The elevated arm stress test: specificity in the diagnosis of thoracic outlet syndrome, *Neurology* 35(suppl 1):74, 1985 (abstract).

12. Cramer C: A reconditioning program to lower the recurrence rate of brachial plexus neuropraxia in collegiate football players, *J Athletic Training* 34:390, 1999.

13. Cuetter AC, Bartoszek DM: The thoracic outlet syndrome: controversies, overdiagnosis, overtreatment, and recommendations for management, *Muscle Nerve* 12:410, 1989.

14. Dale W, Lewis M: Management of thoracic outlet syndrome, *Ann Surg* 181:575, 1989.

15. Derkash R, et al: The results of first rib resection in thoracic outlet syndrome, *Orthopedics* 4:1025, 1981.

16. Elvey R: Brachial plexus tension test and the pathoanatomical origin of arm pain. In Glasgow E, Tavomey L, editors: *Aspects of manipulative therapy,* Melbourne, Australia, 1979, Lincoln Institute of Health Sciences.

17. Elvey R: Treatment of arm pain associated with abnormal brachial plexus tension, *Aust J Physiother* 32:225, 1986.

18. Eurroll R, Hurst L: The relationship of thoracic outlet syndrome and carpal tunnel syndrome, *Clin Orthop* 164:149, 1982.

19. Falconer MA, Weddell G: Costoclavicular compression of the subclavian artery and vein: relation to the scalenus anticus syndrome, *Lancet* 2:539, 1943.

20. Gergoudis R, Barnes R: Thoracic outlet arterial compression: prevalence in normals, *Angiology* 31:538, 1980.

21. Gifford L, Butler D: The integration of pain sciences into clinical practice, *J Hand Ther* 10:86, 1997.

22. Halsted WS: An experimental study of circumscribed dilation of an artery immediately distal to a partially occluding band and its bearing on the dilation of the subclavian artery observed in certain cases of cervical rib, *J Exp Med* 24:271, 1916.

23. Hopenfield S, editor: *Physical examination of the spine and extremities,* New York, 1976, Appleton-Century-Crofts.

24. Ingesson E, Ribbe E, Norgren L: Thoracic outlet syndrome: evaluation of a physiotherapeutical method, *Manual Med* 2:86, 1986.

25. Jamieson, WG, Chinnick B: Thoracic outlet syndrome: fact or fancy? A review of 409 consecutive patients who underwent operation, *Can J Surg* 39:321, 1996.

26. Kelly T: Thoracic outlet syndrome current concepts of treatment, *Ann Surg* 190:657, 1979.

27. Kenny R, et al: Thoracic outlet syndrome: a useful exercise treatment option, *Am J Surg* 165:282, 1993.

28. Komanetsky RM, et al: Somatosensory evoked potentials fail to diagnose thoracic outlet syndrome, *J Hand Surg* 21A:662, 1996.

29. Leffert R: Thoracic outlet syndrome, *Hand Clin* 8:285, 1992.

30. Leffert R, Cumley G: The relationship between dead arm syndrome and thoracic outlet syndrome, *Clin Orthop* 223:20, 1987.

31. LeForestier N, et al: True neurogenic thoracic outlet syndrome: electrophysiological diagnosis in six cases, *Muscle Nerve* 21:1129, 1998.

32. Lindgren KA: Conservative treatment of thoracic outlet syndrome: a 2-year follow-up, *Arch Phys Med Rehabil* 78:373, 1997.

33. Lindgren KA, Leino E, Manninen H: Cervical rotation lateral flexion test in brachialgia, *Arch Phys Med Rehabil* 73:735, 1992.

34. Machleder H, Moll F, Verity A: The anterior scalene muscle in thoracic outlet compression syndrome: histochemical and morphometric studies, *Arch Surg* 121:1141, 1986.

35. MacKinnon S: Double and multiple "crush" syndromes: double and multiple entrapment neuropathies, *Hand Clin* 8:369, 1992.

36. McGough E, Pearce M, Byme J: Management of thoracic outlet syndrome, *J Cardiovasc Surg (Torino)* 77:169, 1979.

37. Mulder D, Greenwood F, Brooks C: Posttraumatic thoracic outlet syndrome, *J Trauma* 13:706, 1981.

38. Novak C, Collins D, Mackinnon S: Outcome following conservative management of thoracic outlet syndrome, *J Hand Surg* 20A:542, 1995.

39. Novak CB, Mackinnon SE, Patterson GA: Evaluation of patients with thoracic outlet syndrome, *J Hand Surg* 18A:292, 1993.

40. Peet RM, et al: Thoracic outlet syndrome: evaluation of a therapeutic exercise program (in-staff meeting), Rochester, Minn, 1956, The Mayo Clinic.

41. Plewa M, Delinger M: The false-positive rate of thoracic outlet syndrome shoulder maneuvers in healthy subjects, *Acad Emerg Med* 5:337, 1998.

42. Pollach W: Surgical anatomy of the thoracic outlet syndrome, *Surg Gynecol Obstet* 150:97, 1980.

43. Pratt N: *Clinical musculoskeletal anatomy,* Philadelphia, 1991, JB Lippincott.

44. Quinter J: Stretch induced cervicobrachial pain syndrome, *Aust Physiother* 36:99, 1990.

45. Raskin NH, Howard MW, Ehrenfeld WK: Headache as the leading symptom of the thoracic outlet syndrome, *Headache* 25:208, 1985.

46. Rayan G, Jensen C: Thoracic outlet syndrome: provocative examination maneuvers in a typical population, *J Shoulder Elbow Surg* 4:113, 1995.

47. Ribbe EB, Lindgren SHS, Norgren LEH: Clinical diagnosis of thoracic outlet syndrome: evaluation of patients with cervico-brachial symptoms, *Manual Med* 2:282, 1986. 47:327, 1990.

48. Roos DB: Thoracic outlet syndrome is under diagnosed (comment), *Muscle Nerve* 22:126, 1999.

49. Reference deleted in proofs.

50. Roos D, Owens C: Thoracic outlet syndrome, *Arch Surg* 93:71, 1966.

51. Sanders RJ, et al: Scalene muscle abnormalities in traumatic thoracic outlet syndrome, *Am J Surg* 159:231, 1990.

52. Shacklock M: Positive upper limb tension test in a case of surgically proven neuropathy: analysis and validity, *Manual Ther* 1:154, 1996.

53. Smith K: The thoracic outlet syndrome: a protocol of treatment, *J Orthop Sports Phys Ther* 1:89, 1979.

54. Sobey A, et al: Investigation of non specific thoracic outlet syndrome, *J Cardiovasc Surg (Torino)* 34:343, 1993.

55. Spurling RG, Scoville WB: Lateral rupture of the cervical intervertebral discs: a common cause of shoulder and arm pain, *Surg Gynecol Obstet* 78:350, 1944.

56. Sucher BM: Thoracic outlet syndrome—a myofascial variant: Part 1. Pathology and diagnosis, *J Am Osteopath Assoc* 90:686, 1990.

57. Sucher BM: Thoracic outlet syndrome—a myofascial variant: Part 2. Treatment, *J Am Osteopath Assoc* 90:810, 1990.

58. Szabo R, Gelberman R, Dimick M: Sensibility testing in patients with carpal tunnel syndrome, *J Bone Joint Surg* 66A:60, 1984.

59. Szabo R, et al: Vibratory sensory testing in acute peripheral nerve compression, *J Hand Surg* 9A:1104, 1984.

60. Thomas G, et al: Thoracic outlet syndrome, *Am Surg* 78:483, 1978.

61. Toomingas A, et al: Predictive aspects of the abduction external rotation test among male industrial and office workers, *Am J Ind Med* 35:32, 1999.

62. Travell J, Simmons D: *Myofascial pain and dysfunction, the trigger-point manual,* Baltimore, 1983, Williams & Wilkins.

63. Upton A, McComas A: The double crush in nerve entrapment syndrome, *Lancet* 2:359, 1973.

64. Urschel J, Hamred SM, Grewal R: Neurogenic thoracic outlet syndrome, *Postgrad Med J* 70:785, 1994.

65. Urschel H, Paulson B, McNamara J: Thoracic outlet syndrome, *Ann Surg* 6:1, 1968.

66. Urschel H, Razzuk M: Management of thoracic outlet syndrome, *N Engl J Med* 286:1140, 1972.

67. Urschel H, et al: Objective diagnosis (ulnar nerve conduction velocity) and current therapy of the thoracic outlet syndrome, *Ann Thoracic Surg* 12:608, 1979.

68. Walsh MT: Therapist management of thoracic outlet syndrome, *J Hand Ther* 7:131, 1994.

69. Warrens A, Heaton J: Thoracic outlet compression syndrome: the lack of reliability of its clinical assessment, *Ann R Coll Surg Engl* 69:203, 1987.

70. Weinberg H, et al: Arthritis of the first costovertebral joint as a cause of thoracic outlet syndrome, *Clin Orthop* 86:159, 1972.

71. Weinstein J: Neurogenic and nonneurogenic pain and inflammatory mediators, *Orthop Clin North Am* 22:235, 1991.

72. Wilbourn AJ: Thoracic outlet syndrome is overdiagnosed, *Muscle Nerve* 22:130, 1999 (comment).

73. Williams H, Carpenter N: Surgical treatment of the thoracic outlet compression syndrome, *Arch Surg* 113:850, 1978.

74. Willshire WH: Supernumerary first rib clinical records, *Lancet* 2:633, 1860.

75. Woods S: Thoracic outlet syndrome, *West J Med* 128:9, 1978.

76. Wright I: The neurovascular syndrome produced by hyperabduction of the arms, *Am Heart J* 29:1, 1945.

77. Yiannikas C, Walsh J: Somatosensory evoked potentials fail to diagnose thoracic outlet syndrome, *J Hand Surg* 21:662, 1996.

Chapter 45

RATIONALE AND INDICATIONS FOR THE USE OF NERVE MOBILIZATION AND NERVE GLIDING AS A TREATMENT APPROACH

Mark T. Walsh

The use of nerve mobilization or gliding as a treatment approach requires an understanding of the general principles of the nervous system neuropathology and its consequences of pain and movement dysfunction. Knowledge of treatment principles, guidelines, progression, precautions, and contraindications are essential for executing a safe and effective treatment strategy. This can be summed up by the concept of *neurodynamics,* developed by Shacklock.[41] Neurodynamics combines mechanical and physiologic properties of the peripheral nervous system (PNS) that are dynamically interdependent and correlates the effects of tension and excursion on the PNS. Attempting to separate these features clinically is nearly impossible. Movement of the nervous system ultimately results in changes in the internal nerve physiology by altering neural tension. These changes in neural physiology may result in the development of the patient's symptoms of pain and/or other sensory disturbances. This same concept is also used as a treatment approach to alter abnormal physiology or pain originating in the nervous system.

GENERAL PRINCIPLES OF THE PERIPHERAL NERVOUS SYSTEM

Using nerve mobilization (i.e., gliding) mandates that clinicians understand that most of the patients they may be treating have pain as a primary feature. For successful use of

these techniques, therapists must recognize the interaction between the patient's pain and accompanying limitations in motion. These findings may relate directly to increased mechanosensitivity of the nervous system for a number of reasons. Pain originating from the nervous system may be caused by a number of potential sources (Box 45-1).

A person with pain of the PNS can have *nerve trunk pain,*[1] which may result from increased activity in nociceptive endings in the nerve connective tissues, called *nervi nervorum.*[1,32] Asbury[1] theorizes that nociceptive activity causing nerve trunk pain is created by a chemically mediated increased mechanosensitivity of the nerve tissue. Applying an adequate stimulus such as tension or compression will produce a noxious response. A second form of pain, which may be related directly to the PNS, has been described as *dysesthetic pain.*[1] This pain arises from impulses in demyelinated, damaged, or regenerating afferent fibers.

It is possible to clinically distinguish these two forms of neuropathic pain. Nerve trunk pain has been described as an ache, as knifelike, or as similar to toothache pain, and is deep in nature and overlying a specific peripheral nerve trunk or distribution. It usually improves with rest or by placing the extremity in the optimal position to decrease tension along the path of the peripheral nerve. Moving the extremity or mechanically altering the nerve through joint position or direct compression can exacerbate nerve trunk pain. Nerve

---

Box 45-1   Nervous system as a source of pain

Nerve trunk
Dysesthetic
Nonneurogenic
Neurogenic

---

root or brachial plexus neuritis are two examples of nerve trunk pain. In contrast, dysesthetic pain often is described as burning or tingling, accompanied by sensory loss or disturbance (paresthesia). Often, the patient is unable to localize the pain but may report it to be superficial, covering a particular cutaneous area innervated by the nerve involved. Usually, no particular position or activity improves the symptoms, and the pain often is exacerbated after activities. Causalgia and diabetic neuropathic pain[1] are examples of dysesthetic pain.

Two additional sources of pain attributed to the nervous system are related to chemical sensitization of the PNS. The pain may be nonneurogenic in origin as a result of connective tissue damage or breakdown. Endogenous chemicals such as bradykinins, serotonin, histamine, prostaglandin, and leukotrienes are released. These chemicals have been shown to affect the nociceptive afferents.[49] In contrast, chemicals of neurogenic origin also have been shown to mediate pain via the use of neuropeptides such as substance P, calcitonin gene–related peptide, vasoactive intestinal peptide, and enkephalins. Released by primary afferent neurons, these substances result from damaging chemical or physical stimulation of the peripheral nociceptive afferent. These two forms of chemical mediation of pain result in increasing the mechanosensitivity of the nervous system.[49]

A second principle is the nervous system as a continuum.[22,35] The peripheral, central, and autonomic nervous systems all combine to form one system that interacts as a unit of input and output. This concept of a continuum is achieved mechanically, electrically, and chemically, and is visually demonstrated in Fig. 45-1. This black and white photograph, entitled "Harriet," is an anatomic preparation dissected by Rufus Weaver, MD of Hahnemann Medical College in 1887, and was exhibited at The North Columbian Exhibition in 1893. It illustrates how placing tension or strain on either the PNS or the central nervous system (CNS) could have a potential affect on the nervous system in another location. For example, the straight leg raise (SLR) or the upper limb tension test (ULTT) alters neuroaxial or meningeal tension. These techniques provide the clinician with screening maneuvers used to examine the irritability of the patient's nervous system and its accompanying surrounding tissues.[5,6]

As a continuum, the nervous system must have a mechanism for tolerance of elongation and tension. Sunderland and Bradley[44-46] examined the mechanical properties of the peripheral nerve and the nerve root to investigate strain failure

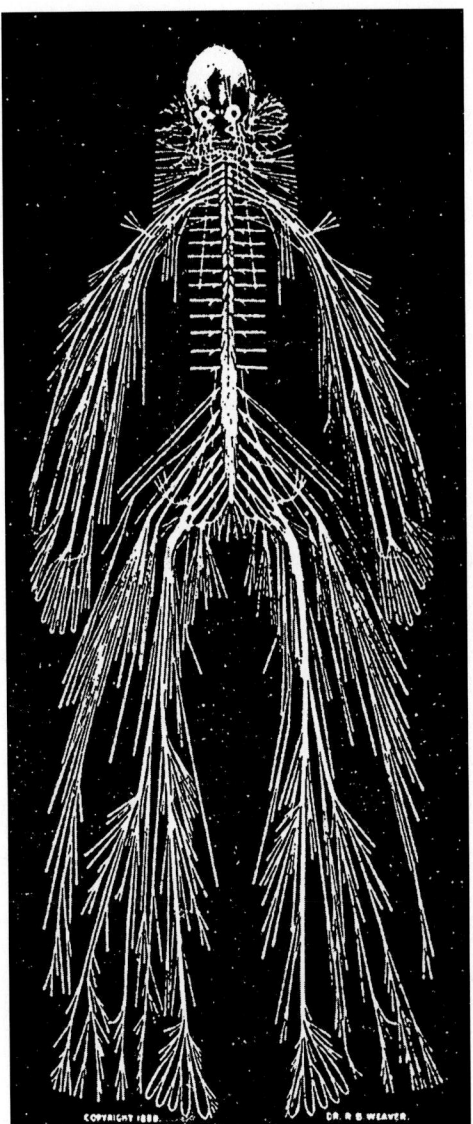

Fig. 45-1. Photograph of the dissected nervous system demonstrating the continuum. (Courtesy MCP/Hahnemann University, Philadelphia.)

rate. They reported that the elastic limit in the peripheral nerve varied 7% to 20% and failure strain varied 7% to 30%. For the nerve root, the maximal elastic limit was less than 15% and failure strain occurred at 25%, indicating the nerve root failed at lower loads than the peripheral nerve.[45,46] Hafteck[15] investigated the effect of slow and quick stretch on albino rat tibial nerves. He reported that the initial process of elongation did not affect the nerve fiber but was physiologic in nature, described as *unfolding*. Progressive strain to failure loads histologically demonstrated that rupture of the epineurium occurs first. Before epineural rupture, damage in the form of neuropraxia or axonotmesis occurs.[15] These strain levels are much higher than a clinician would want to impart when performing nerve gliding or mobilization.

Tension within the nerve can also affect intraneural blood flow and nerve function.[15,21,25,36,38] Lundborg and Rydevik[25] determined that lower limits of strain (5% to 10%) demonstrated the first signs of changes in blood flow in the epineural and perineurial vessels. The upper stretch limit was 11% to 18%, causing complete occlusion that resolved after relaxation of the nerve. Using rabbit sciatic nerve, Ogata and Naito[36] found that strain limits greater than 15.7% resulted in complete ablation of blood flow to the nerve. Complete ablation of blood flow also occurred when external compression was 50 to 70 mm Hg. Studying the effect of strain on rat tibial-nerve function, Kwan et al.[21] reported that strains of 6% or greater resulted in a 60% decrease in compound nerve action potential (CNAP) after 20 minutes. They concluded that longstanding low stress could affect the functional properties of the nerve.

In 1992, using rabbit tibial nerves and measuring nerve conduction, Wall et al.[48] also determined that strain rates of 6% or greater resulted in a 70% decrease in CNAP after 20 minutes. Recovery occurred to within 10% of prestretch values when the load was removed. At 12% strain, CNAP was reduced rapidly, with complete conduction block after 50 minutes. Once the load was removed, only a 40% recovery was achieved. It is the opinion of Wall et al.[48] that mechanical deformation contributed to decreased nerve conduction, as does ischemia. Wall et al.[48] concluded that the response to stretch may not be immediate; however, prolonged stretch may cause irrecoverable damage. Finally, Porter and Wharton[38] examined the effect of nerve function by occluding the nerve's blood supply and measuring the irritability of a muscle innervated by that nerve. They discovered that irritability in muscle increased within 2 to 11 minutes after the blood flow was occluded. This information supports that maximal strain rates should be less than 6% during treatment.

The nervous system's ability to tolerate tension associated with movement results from an intraneural (within the nerve) and an extraneural (outside the nerve) anatomic design. Internally, the nerve has designed undulations of a tortuous nature.[42] The nerve's ability to unfold as length increases was described by Clarke and Bearn[7] when investigating the presence of the spiral bands of Fontana. Although present in the relaxed state of the nerve, the spiral bands of Fontana disappear as tension is applied. These oblique spiral bands found within the course of the nerve support this theory of unfolding as the nerve lengthens. The second mechanism by which the nerve is able to tolerate elongation is through *intraneural gliding.*[26,32,42] This unique makeup of the nerve's connective tissue allows for intraneural excursion between individual nerve fibers and their surrounding endoneurium and the endoneurium surrounding each nerve fiber. The epineurium allows excursion to occur between it and the perineurium of each fascicle. Finally, the nerve's internal ability to tolerate tension and to permit elongation results from an intrafunicular plexus formation described by Sunderland.[43]

Extraneural gliding provides for attenuation of tension via a gliding surface between the paraneurium and the epineurium.[32] Extraneural excursion or gliding has been demonstrated in the CNS[3,39] and in the PNS.[32,42,43] In the CNS, Reid[39] demonstrated that 1.8 cm of excursion occurred in the spinal cord when performing movements of cervical and lumbar spine flexion and extension. He reported that 11.3% strain occurred in the cervical spine, with the greatest amount of strain between C2 and C5 levels. This increased to 17.6% when C2 to T1 levels were combined. Movement of the nerve root was transmitted via the dural sheath and dentate ligaments, and not directly to the rootlets. In 1946, O'Connell[35] demonstrated that cervical flexion caused excursion of the cord in the cephalad direction with increased nerve root tension, whereas cervical extension caused movement in the opposite direction and decreased nerve root tension. Cervical spine flexion caused 5 mm of excursion in the cervical region, 4 mm in the thoracic region, and 1 mm in the lumbar region. Straight leg raising and prone knee bend created caudal excursion of the spinal cord and increased nerve root tension at the lumbar level. Finally, Lew et al.,[22] examining baboon cadavers, also reported that cervical flexion caused cephalad movement of the spinal cord. Combined hip and cervical spine flexion increased excursion further.

This same phenomenon also has been demonstrated to occur in the PNS. McLellan and Swash[30] demonstrated that the median nerve underwent an excursion of 7.4 mm distally and 4.3 mm proximally with wrist and finger motion and elbow flexion/extension. In 1986, Wilgis and Murphy[50] measured excursion of the brachial plexus and the median, ulnar, and radial nerves in 15 cadaver arms. The greatest excursions occurred at the brachial plexus level (15.3 mm) with movement of the shoulder, in the median nerve at the wrist (proximal 14.5 mm and distal 6.8 mm), in the ulnar nerve at the wrist (13.8 mm), and 6.8 mm distal excursion of the ulnar nerve with elbow extension to flexion. Using five fresh frozen cadaver specimens, Wright[51] examined excursion of the median nerve. He and his associates demonstrated that the average distal excursion measured at the wrist was 24 mm and occurred when the upper extremity was positioned with the shoulder in abduction of 30 degrees, the elbow at 90 degrees, and the wrist and fingers in extension. The average proximal excursion measured at the wrist was 12 mm with the shoulder abducted 110 degrees, the elbow in 10-degree extension, and the wrist and fingers in flexion. Excursion of the median nerve measured at the elbow revealed an average distance of 14.7 mm occurred distally with 30-degree shoulder abduction, 10-degree elbow flexion, and wrist and finger extension. Proximal excursion averaged 15.4 mm with 110-degree shoulder abduction, 90-degree elbow flexion, and combined wrist/finger flexion. Table 45-1

Table 45-1. Summary of Wright et al.'s work on median nerve excursion at the wrist and the elbow and the position of each of the joints when measured

	Wrist			Elbow		
Direction	**Average Distance**	**Joint**	**Motion**	**Average Distance**	**Joint**	**Motion**
Distal	24 mm	Shoulder	ABD 30 degrees	15 mm	Shoulder	ABD 30 degrees
		Elbow	EF 90 degrees		Elbow	EF 10 degrees
		Forearm	EXT 60 degrees		Forearm	Pron 60 degrees
		Wrist	EXT 35 degrees		Wrist	EXT 60 degrees
		Finger			Finger	EXT 35 degrees
Proximal	12 mm	Shoulder	ABD 110 degrees	15 mm	Shoulder	ABD 110 degrees
		Elbow	EF 10 degrees		Elbow	EF 90 degrees
		Forearm	FLEX 60 degrees		Forearm	FLEX 60 degrees
		Wrist	FLEX 35 degrees		Wrist	FLEX 35 degrees
		Finger			Finger	

ABD, Abduction; *EF,* external flexion; *EXT,* extension; *FLEX,* flexion.

summarizes these results. From these data, it can be seen that changing the position of the shoulder, elbow, wrist, and fingers can result in median-nerve excursion distally or proximally. In general, it can be stated that movements in one direction at the wrist and elbow will result in excursion of the nerve in the same direction and is influenced by the position of other upper extremity joints. These CNS and PNS studies support the continuum theory and play a role in nerve tensioning and gliding.

An integral component to peripheral nerve gliding is appreciating that the interfacing tissues surrounding the nerve along its entire course are required to have the ability to adapt in length in relationship to joint motion. Millesi et al.[31,32] reported that the median-nerve bed must adapt to as much as a 20% increase in length at the elbow and wrist to accommodate motion. Zoech et al.[54] specifically investigated the difference in the length of the median-nerve bed in positions of maximal flexion and extension of the upper extremity. They demonstrated that maximal extension required a 4.3% change in length and that flexion resulted in as much as a 14.9% decrease in overall length. Therefore not only must the peripheral nerve be able to adapt to elongation and tension, but the surrounding interfacing tissues that form the nerve bed also must adapt independently to changes in length resulting from joint motion. This same adaptation of the nerve bed occurs within the CNS.[22,35,39]

One final biomechanical principle of the PNS to consider is the property of strain and/or stress that occurs along the course of the nerve as a result of upper extremity joint motion. *Strain* is the change in length that occurs in a nerve as a result of unfolding and gliding as the extremity moves. Millesi et al.,[33] Zoech et al.,[54] and most recently, Wright et al.[52] and Kleinrensink et al.[19,20] have demonstrated that motion of the upper extremity results in stress being

imparted along the entire course of the nervous system as measured by strain. Studying the effect of the ULTT on strain in the peripheral nerves, Kleinrensink et al.[19,20] determined that motion at the wrist increased the strain at the cord level of the brachial plexus. In addition, contralateral lateral flexion of the cervical spine increased strain in the cords of the brachial plexus and in the arm for each of the three major nerves. Finally, the ULTT for the median nerve was the most sensitive for the three major nerves and the most specific for the median nerve than the other ULTTs were for their respective nerves. Research performed in animal, cadaver, and limited human models verifies that the nervous system has multiple mechanisms to attenuate strain, tension, and elongation, and upper extremity and spinal motion can affect tension throughout the nervous system.

In addition to the ability of the PNS to accommodate movement, its physiology and function also depend on its vascularity and the maintenance of a pressure gradient system. This system allows for the maintenance of vascular perfusion and physiology and is best depicted by Sunderland's[43] model as shown in Fig. 45-2. This model requires arterial pressure to be greater than capillary pressure, which is greater than fascicular pressure that exceeds venous return pressure and ultimately is greater than tunnel pressure. Alterations of any one of these five pressures have the potential to affect circulation[43] and axoplasmic flow[23,47] throughout the nerve. Alterations in tunnel pressure often result in the more common peripheral-nerve entrapments in the upper extremity, such as cubital tunnel or carpal tunnel syndrome. Pechan and Julis[37] examined ulnar-nerve pressures at the elbow. They demonstrated a twofold increase in cubital tunnel pressure with cervical spine and shoulder motion and a sixfold increase with ulnar-nerve provocative testing (elbow flexion, wrist extension, and the

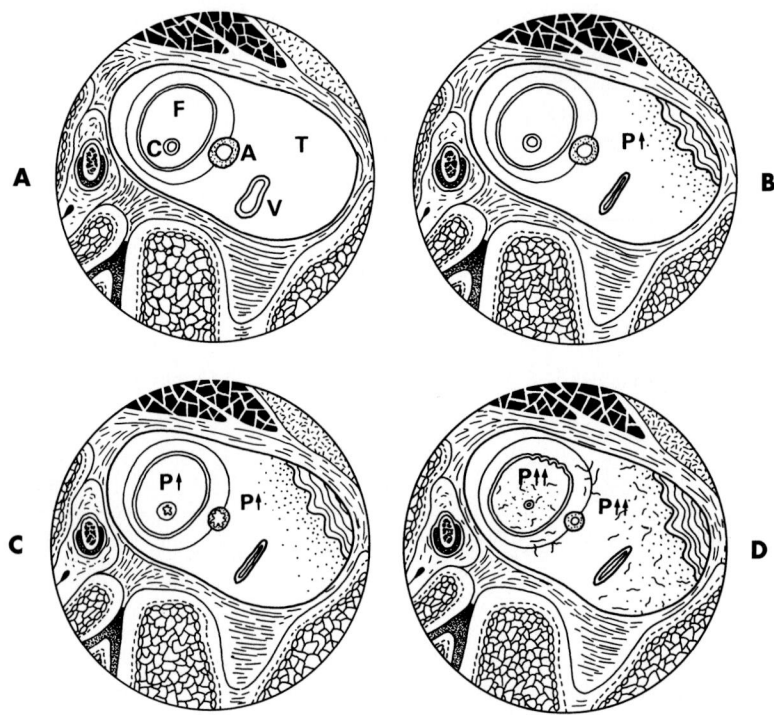

Fig. 45-2. Illustration demonstrating Sunderland's model of compression. Representation of the pressure gradients in the carpal tunnel and the stages that follow alteration of the pressure gradients. For simplicity, one nerve fiber in a fascicle is represented. **A,** Normal tunnel. For adequate nerve fiber nutrition, the pressure gradient must be PA > PC > PF > PV > PT. **B,** Hypoxia. Increased tunnel pressure → Venule collapses. Venous stasis → Hypoxic axons. **C,** Edema. Venous stasis → Deterioration of capillary endothelium → Edema→ ↑ Intrafascicular pressure. **D,** Fibrosis. Intrafascicular fibroblastic activity →Scar tissue → ↑ Pressure, ↑ Hypoxia → Segment of nerve becomes fibrous cord → Cycle of irritation. *A,* Arteriole; *C,* capillary; *F,* fascicle; *P,* pressure; *T,* tunnel; *V,* venule. (From Butler D: *Mobilisation of the nervous system,* London, 1991, Churchill Livingstone. Adapted from the work of Sunderland S: *J Neurol Neurosurg Psychiatry* 39:615, 1976.)

arm above the head). Studying the rabbit vagus nerves, Dahlin and McClean[9] verified that a conduction block with 30 and 50 mm of external compression sustained for 2 hours was reversible within 24 hours. At 200 mm of external compression for 2 hours, reversal took as long as 3 days, and at 400 mm, reversal took 7 days. Nemoto et al.[34] clamped dog sciatic nerves at one of two locations proximal and distal to an experimental compression site. Their work established that two low-grade compressions along the nerve trunk created greater damage than a single compression. This supports the theory of double crush described by Upton and McComas.[47] In addition to affecting vascular flow, axoplasmic flow also is altered with less external pressure than occurs with minor carpal tunnel syndrome.[23]

Collectively, these general principles (summarized in Box 45-2) emphasize the following key point: The nervous system is designed for movement. As with any other soft tissue structure, when the nervous system is in a diseased and hyperirritable state, mechanical stresses such as compression or tension may provoke pain syndromes and movement dysfunction associated with the nervous system

Box 45-2 General nervous system principles	
Source of pain	Excursion or gliding
Continuum	Pressure gradient model
Tolerance to tension	Vascularity
and strain	Designed for movement

and its interfacing tissues. The clinician should maintain awareness that, not only is direct and local tissue affected, but other tissues innervated by the involved nerves may also be the source of the patient's pain and movement dysfunction.

NEUROPATHOLOGY AND ITS MANIFESTATIONS

Although it is not the purpose of this chapter to discuss the neural pathology of compression in detail, several clinical considerations must be considered before using nerve mobilization (i.e., gliding or tensioning) techniques for treatment. The clinician must consider the neuropathologic

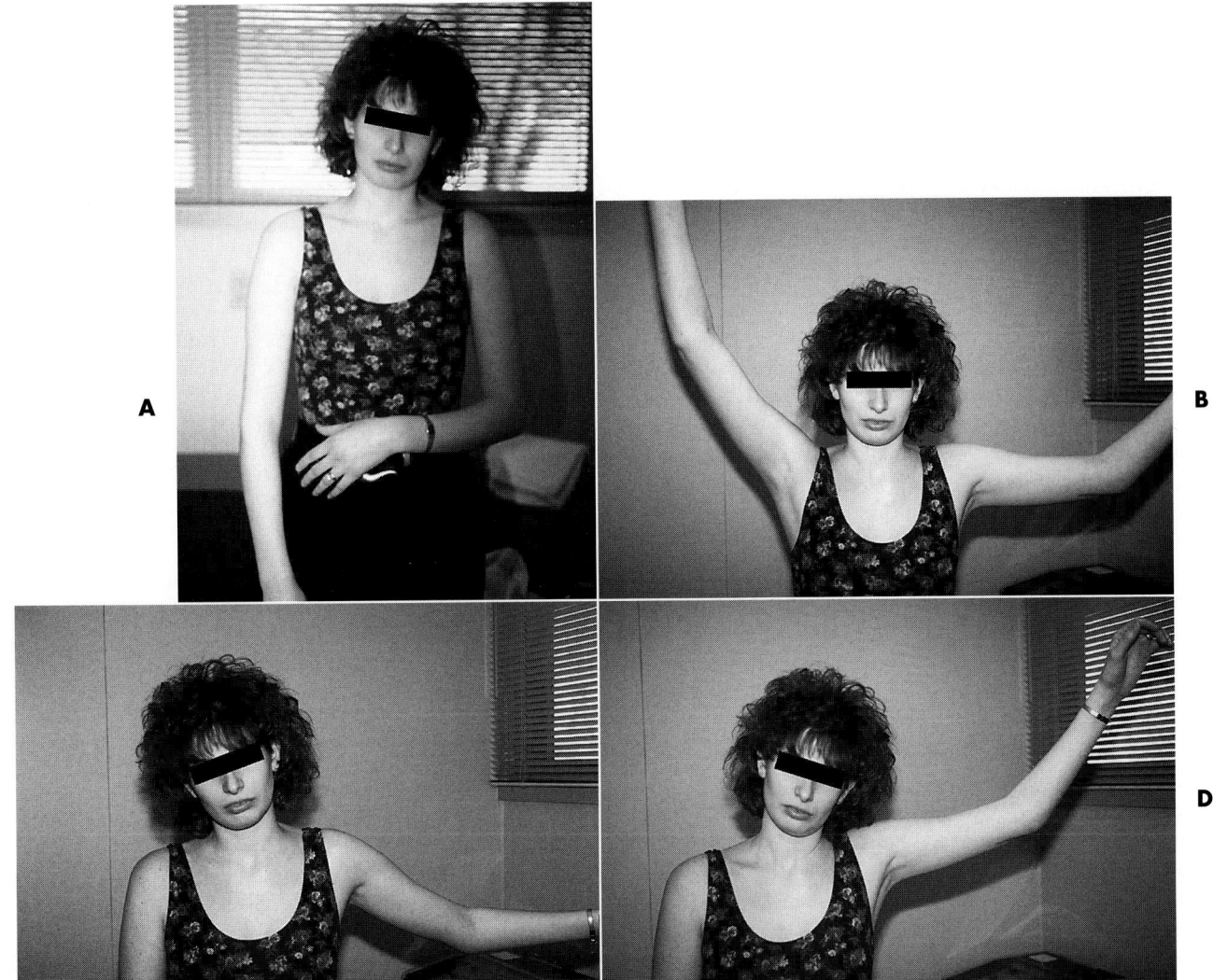

Fig. 45-3. Photographs of active motion dysfunction in a patient after anterior submuscular ulnar nerve transposition. **A,** Resting posture. **B,** Active shoulder elevation. **C,** Coronal plane abduction with contralateral cervical lateral flexion. **D,** Coronal plane shoulder abduction with ipsilateral cervical lateral flexion. Note the change in shoulder abduction with the change in cervical position.

consequences on the mechanical, vascular, and axoplasmic aspects of the nerve. These three factors contribute to the hyperirritability of the PNS and its interfacing tissues. The vascular system may be compromised by external compression or adverse tension. Adverse tension may be the result of adaptive shortening from positioning or external scarring of the nerve. Compromise of a nerve's vascularity can lead to the release of chemical mediators such as histamine or bradykinins, potentially creating a state of inflammation in or around the connective tissues of the nerve, increasing its level of irritability.[23,28] Vascular changes may also lead to alterations in neurovascular dynamics and intraneural fibrosis as an end result.[23,32,43] As previously described, external compression can lead to compromise in axoplasmic flow.

This compromise reduces the transport of neural filaments, microtubules, and neurotransmitters along the axon to its terminal ending as well as the return of metabolic byproducts, potentially altering the nerve's physiology and function. As a result of this chemically mediated inflammatory process and/or the loss of intraneural or extraneural gliding capabilities, mechanical irritability of the nerve will occur, resulting in repetitive forces placed across the fixed (i.e., adherent) nerve segment. This loss in neural motion tolerance in one segment requires force attenuation to be achieved over a shorter segment of the nerve, exposing it to further damage or injury.

This neuropathologic process increases the nerve's vulnerability throughout the upper extremity such as in a confined space like the cubital or carpal tunnel. The soft tissues that surround the nerve along its entire course also create these spaces or tunnels. Two examples of these are the median nerve passing through the pronator or the radial nerve passing through the supinator. Nerves are also more vulnerable at relatively fixed points where motion introduced at these levels minimizes the nerve's capability of tolerating elongation forces. This frequently occurs where the nerve branches or is relatively fixed such as passing through fascia. Finally, the nerve is vulnerable to external compression whenever it rests across a hard surface such as the radial sensory nerve as it passes across the radius.

The final consequence of peripheral neuropathology is fibrosis.[24,27,28,43] Intraneural and extraneural fibrosis removes the nerve's inherent ability to elongate and reduces the gliding that occurs between the connective tissue layers of the nerve and its interfacing tissues. Intraneural fibrosis causes the loss of the tortuous course of the nerve or its undulations.[42] This results in loss of internal glide and the unfolding that occurs as the nerve elongates. Extraneural fibrosis limits the nervous system's ability to move within its nerve bed or between the interfacing tissues creating mechanical interference. This results in mechanical interference with external gliding. In either scenario, the lack of nerve mobility results in increased stress or strain delivered to a shorter nerve segment as joint motion occurs.[54] As discussed, this fibrosis may ultimately lead to the onset of pain. A pain syndrome could indirectly lead to adaptive shortening of the nervous system, altering joint movement and extremity function.

Elvey,[10,12] Butler,[4,5,14] and Gifford[14] all have described the clinical manifestations of this pathologic process and resulting fibrosis. These manifestations are pathophysiologic (symptoms reported by the patient such as paresthesia or pain) and pathomechanic (alterations in neuromechanics that limit isolated or multisegmented motion of the upper extremity). Elvey[12] also has described the clinical response observed through a series of clinical examination techniques, discussed in the next section. These techniques result in provocation of the patient's symptoms and identification of motion dysfunction or limitations of the involved extremity, spinal segment, or both. Elvey[12] and Butler[4,5] describe a resistance encountered with passive extremity motion resulting from altered neuromechanics. Butler[4,5] refers to the resistance as *tissue barriers* encountered while performing a ULTT. Elvey[12] theorizes that the resistance encountered results from hyperirritability of nervous tissue, causing a protective reflexive muscle contraction.

THERAPIST ASSESSMENT OF NEURAL TISSUES

Using nerve mobilization and gliding techniques requires the careful assessment of the patient to establish the presence of a neurogenic component of the patient's complaints. The assessment may identify active motion dysfunction, an

---

Box 45-3 Upper extremity neural tension testing components

Median nerve: Shoulder abduction
Shoulder external rotation
Forearm supination
Wrist/finger extension
Elbow extension
Shoulder depression
Cervical contralateral lateral flexion
Ulnar nerve: Shoulder abduction
Shoulder external rotation
Pronation or supination
Wrist/small finger extension
Elbow flexion
Shoulder depression
Cervical contralateral lateral flexion
Radial nerve: Shoulder abduction
Shoulder internal rotation
Pronation
Wrist/thumb-index flexion
Elbow extension
Shoulder depression
Cervical contralateral lateral flexion

---

example of which is presented in the four photographs in Fig. 45-3. From this series of photographs of a patient with postoperative anterior submuscular transposition for cubital tunnel syndrome, it can be noted how the patient is attempting to reduce adverse tension in her nervous system by positioning. The cervical spine is in lateral flexion and rotation, the shoulder in adduction and internal rotation, the elbow flexed, and the forearm in slight pronation (Fig. 45-3, A). The presence of active dysfunction can especially be observed when monitoring the position of the shoulder as the patient moves her extremity through coronal plane abduction within a comfortable range (Fig. 45-3, B). With the cervical spine in contralateral rotation and lateral flexion (Fig. 45-3, C) away from the affected side, shoulder abduction decreases compared with ipsilateral cervical rotation and lateral flexion toward the affected side, resulting in increased shoulder abduction.

Following active motion assessment, passive motion is evaluated using the ULTT. The base component motions for the three major nerves in the upper extremity are outlined in Box 45-3. As each successive sequence of motion is applied, the previous positions are maintained to successively apply tension to the nervous system. The therapist must pay close attention to the presence of encountered resistance (e.g., reflexive muscle contraction) and the level of irritability (e.g., through patient response), to avoid progressing beyond the end point of resistance and symptoms. Movement beyond this point may result in exacerbation of the patient's symptoms. An example of the sequence of this motion for the

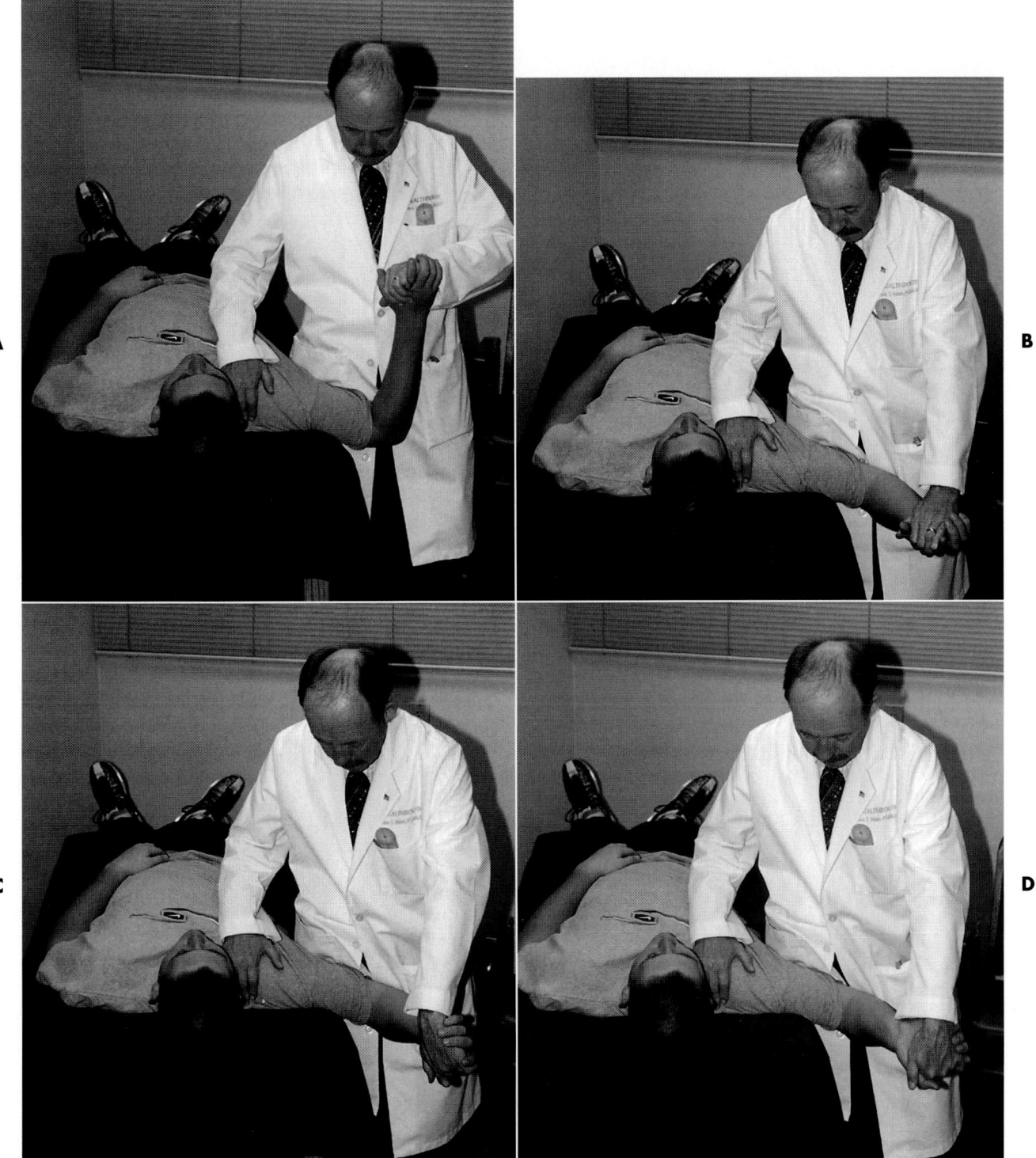

Fig. 45-4. Photographs of the successive application of the median-nerve (base) upper limb tension. **A,** Shoulder abduction. **B,** Shoulder external rotation. **C,** Forearm supination. **D,** Wrist/hand extension.
                                                                                            Continued

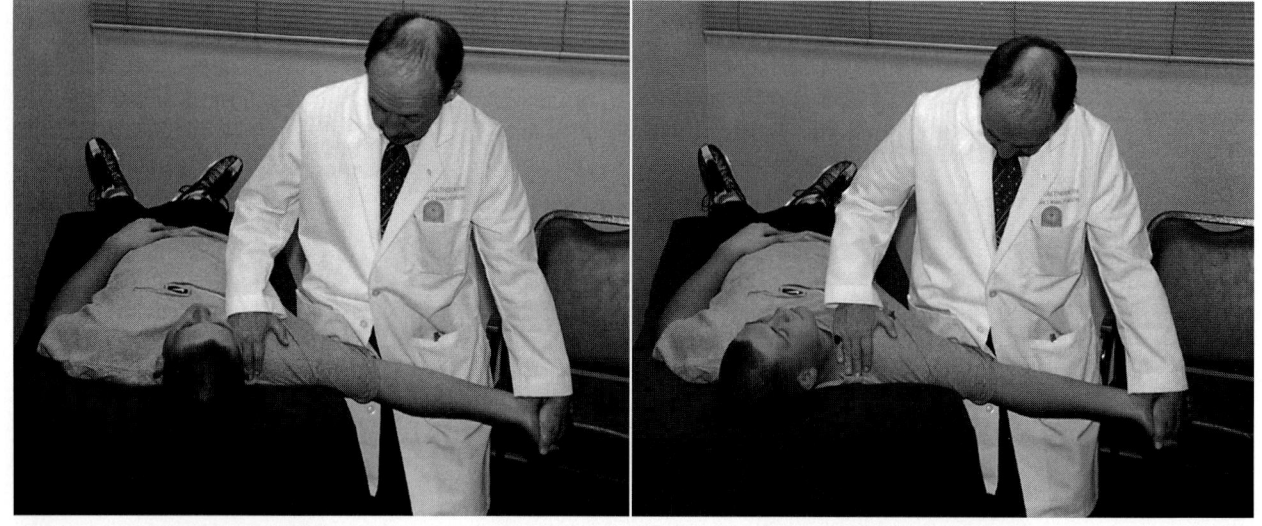

Fig. 45-4, cont'd. E, Elbow extension. **F,** Additional sensitizing motions of contralateral cervical flexion and scapular depression.

<table>
<tr><td>

Box 45-4 Evaluation components

Active dysfunction

Active abduction/forward flexion
  Observe:
    Cervical spine and extremity joint positioning
    Patient's willingness to move
Specific motions
  Observe:
    Joint position changes in upper quarter
    Coronal plane shoulder abduction with elbow extended
    Coronal plane shoulder abduction with proximal (cervical spine) component
      Ipsilateral rotation (IR)
      Ipsilateral lateral flexion (ILF) or side-bending
      Contralateral rotation (CR)
      Contralateral lateral flexion (CLF)
    Coronal plane shoulder abduction with distal component
      Wrist flexion
      Wrist extension
      Variation with elbow/forearm position

Passive motion limitation

Upper limb tension test (ULTT)

Nerve trunk hyperalgesia

Local peripheral nerves

Tender spots

Local tissues

Local dysfunction

Cervical spine segments

</td></tr>
</table>

ULTT is demonstrated in Fig. 45-4. The therapist can vary the order in which each component motion is applied; however, it is recommended that the test for each nerve first be applied in a standard manner. The final position of each joint and the patient response is recorded for baseline purposes to monitor progress. In addition to active and passive motion dysfunction, the therapist should be able to demonstrate palpable neural hyperalgesia along the suspected involved nerves. In addition, Elvey[12] describes the presence of local tender points in tissues innervated by the hypothesized peripheral nerve or nerve root segment, and the presence of local dysfunction within the cervical segment(s) contributing to the peripheral nerve involved.

The normal responses to upper limb tension testing have been reported by Kenneally et al.[17,18] and others.[2,8,53] An alternative interpretation for a positive ULTT is reproduction of the patient's symptoms and motion limitations determined by patient tolerance or encountered resistance. Altering a distal or proximal component (joint) motion should change the baseline results of the ULTT. For example, placing the wrist in neutral may increase elbow extension, or cervical contralateral lateral flexion may decrease elbow extension when performing a particular ULTT.[20,40] These changes in motion or response are then documented for comparison with the baseline test performed. A positive test also may be confirmed by identifying a difference in response or movement by comparing the involved with the noninvolved side. The components of neural assessment of the upper extremity are outlined in Box 45-4. It is beyond the scope of this chapter to explain in detail the principles of ULTT examinations and their findings. The reader is referred to the additional sources in the reference list and is urged to pursue further study to gain a more in-depth understanding.

TREATMENT
Treatment principles

Once the therapist has determined the presence of a neural component of the patient's problem, the development of a logical treatment approach using neural tensioning and gliding techniques can be guided by three basic principles: First is education of the patient and knowledge of the therapist. It is imperative that the patient understand the role that the nervous system plays in his or her complaints, the concept of neural mechanics, and how this alters movement and function. The patient must comprehend the concepts of neural tension and gliding to prevent exacerbation and assist with progression. Equally important is clinician knowledge and understanding of neural mechanics and pathology contributing to the patient's problem. Sound clinical reasoning that formulates a working hypothesis is required. These hypotheses must include the source of the symptoms or dysfunction; contributing factors; precautions and contraindications to evaluation; and treatment, management, and prognosis.[16]

The second treatment principle is the application and prescription. In most cases, the therapist is presented with a patient whose pathologic process has occurred over an extended period, resulting in pain and movement dysfunction. These adaptive changes may take months to alter. Although neural mobilization techniques are used in the clinic, the restoration of movement and elimination of pain require the diligent use of a home program that is adjusted periodically based on reassessment and response of the patient. Finally, the therapist plays a major role in empowering the patient in the performance and follow-through of the exercise program. This is achieved through assisting the patient in observing and appreciating changes in his or her symptoms, improvements in impairments such as specific joint or multisegment motion limitations, and ability to use the upper extremity for functional activities.

Treatment guidelines

Multiple considerations in guiding treatment must be considered. No clear-cut protocol for the development and implementation of treatment exists. Therefore a thorough working knowledge of the nervous system and the ULTT components is required. The ULTT components are transformed into mobilization techniques and exercises for treatment. The symptoms of a patient with adverse neural tension vary daily; therefore evaluation and ongoing reevaluation will continuously guide treatment progression and implementation.

The next concept to consider is nerve tension (stress and strain) and glide (excursion). Clinically, tension creates length changes within the nerve. The strain created by simultaneously pulling on both ends of the nerve causes the nerve to unfold.[20,52] This will have a profound effect on the nerves' neurophysiology because of alterations in vascular and axoplasmic flow, as discussed previously. In

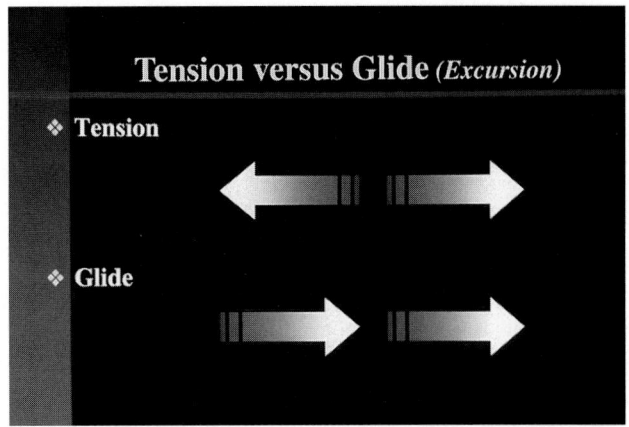

Fig. 45-5. Illustration of tension versus glide.

contrast, glide refers to placing tension on the nerve at one point while releasing it at another. In theory, the overall resting tension and strain remains unchanged. Gliding can occur within the nerve itself[33] or between the nerve and its interfacing tissue.[20,30,50,52] Fig. 45-5 is an example of tension versus glide. An oversimplification of this concept would be simultaneously pulling on both ends of dental floss creating tension as compared with gliding the floss back and forth.

The presenting level of patient irritability guides the use of tension and/or glide. In the irritable patient, glide may be the most appropriate approach. When using gliding techniques, the therapist needs to be aware of the tissue barriers (reflexive muscle contraction)[5,6,10-12] encountered. Treatment is kept within the pain- and tension-free range of motion (ROM) below stimulus threshold. It may be necessary to begin at remote sites away from the hypothesized location, progressing toward the site as tolerated. The nonirritable patient may be able to tolerate tension when symptoms are mild and are absent at rest and when recovery from exacerbation is rapid. In this case, it may be appropriate to tension the involved nerve directly or at a more remote site, progressing toward the hypothesized location. Restoring mobility or improving tolerance to tension at a remote location may assist the nerve in attenuating tension throughout its course, thereby decreasing symptoms. As irritability decreases, the therapist can begin to work through the tissue barriers to restore movement to the extremity and increase function.

Treatment is also guided by the tissue hypothesized to be involved, neural or nonneural. The treatment of nonneural tissues initially may require that the nervous system be placed in a position of antitension or slack. This would allow for direct treatment of the nonneural tissues while minimizing stimulation of the sensitized nerve and avoiding further risk of adverse tension. For example, if the clinician is attempting to improve glenohumeral (GH) motion, the

---

Box 45-5   Treatment guidelines

Working knowledge/understanding of the ULTT components
    Evaluation/reevaluation
      Response to treatment change
      Hypothesis of location and tissues at fault
    Tension versus glide (excursion)
      Tension: lengthens the nerve, stresses vascular supply
      Glide: tension in one location and release in another
    Irritable versus nonirritable
      Irritable: gliding (tissue barriers), selected component distal to site (lower extremity or trunk), pain-free range tension free
      Nonirritable: tension, (+) symptoms (mild) rapid recovery, select component/nerve directly involved
    Neural versus nonneural
      Treat nonneural tissues directly with neural tension eliminated (brachial plexus slack position)
      Treat nonneural tissues under neural tension (nonirritable)
    Intraneural versus extraneural fibrosis
      Intraneural: attempt to increase mobility away from site
      Extraneural: treat interfacing tissue in conjunction with glide/tension

ULTT, Upper limb tension test.

---

combination of ipsilateral cervical flexion and scapular elevation may minimize the additional tension created by GH motion. In contrast, the treatment of nonneural tissue may be desirable with the nerve under tension to benefit both systems in the less irritable patient. The clinician may want to mobilize the GH joint to recover abduction with the elbow extended or the cervical spine laterally flexed to the contralateral side.

Finally, the therapist should have a working hypothesis regarding the existence of any intraneural or extraneural fibrosis.[4,33] If intraneural fibrosis is suspected, it may be more appropriate to attempt to increase the nerve's tolerance to tension and mobility at a location that is remote from the hypothesized site of the lesion. It is my opinion that these therapeutic techniques are unlikely to improve the internal structure of the nerve. However, if it is hypothesized that the nerve's ability to glide within its tissue bed is compromised (extraneural fibrosis), treatment of the interfacing tissues at the site(s) hypothesized may be indicated. This may be performed in conjunction with glide or tension of the nerve in question, depending on the level of irritability. Box 45-5 summarizes the guidelines the treating practitioner should consider when developing a treatment strategy.

Augmenting nerve mobilization

Using other treatment techniques can augment nerve mobilization exercises or techniques. Superficial and deep heating modalities may be used to precondition the tissues, keeping in mind this may alter the stimulus threshold for provoking symptoms. This could result in a delayed response (1 to 24 hours) of exacerbation. Performing massage, joint mobilization, or other manual techniques could be applied to assist in restoring mobility and decreasing interfacing tissue adherence with the nerve under tension or in a slackened (antitension) position. Postural education and awareness and the use of physiologic ROM exercises to improve soft tissue mobility and strength can be used in conjunction with nerve mobilization techniques. The list of combining and augmenting treatments is exhaustive, as long as the clinical state of the nerve and its interfacing tissues are respected. The therapist is limited only by his or her imagination.

Progression of nerve mobilization techniques

The progression of nerve mobilization techniques is dictated by the patient's response and requires continual clinical reasoning to avoid further injury or exacerbation. In the clinic, the use of Maitland's gradation[29] for joint mobilization has been advocated.[4-6] This concept divides the total range of available motion into four parts for any given joint. These are then applied clinically using motion in the first half of available range for symptom control and motion in the last half of available motion for restoring mobility. An alternative way to look at this is that the first half of the available range is the pain-free or *through range*[29] within a given total available range; the last half of the range includes the tissue barriers or end-ranges[4-6] that eventually must be overcome to restore lost motion. This is an oversimplification of the concept, but the most important aspect is its consideration for the level of irritability of the tissues involved.

Presently, no clear guidelines or research support the most effective amplitude, dosage, or duration necessary to achieve the desired result. Therefore sound clinical reasoning regarding these three parameters is necessary to progress nerve mobilization techniques and exercises. In general, Elvey[13] recommends that end-range grades should not be used and the duration should be less than that used for joint mobilization. In contrast, Butler[4] recommends that, for an irritable disorder, pain-free midrange (through range) mobilizations and end-range mobilizations may be used for an initial treatment lasting 20 to 30 seconds This progression can be based only on the patient's response to the treatment, while keeping in mind the biomechanical and pathologic aspects of nerve and connective tissue.

The use of additional components of the ULTT, using additional joints, will result in increased tension within the nervous system. As irritability decreases and mobility improves, additional component motion may be appropriate and necessary. Working from a remote site and progressing toward the hypothesized involved site or nerve is another way to progress nerve mobilization. For example, if the ulnar

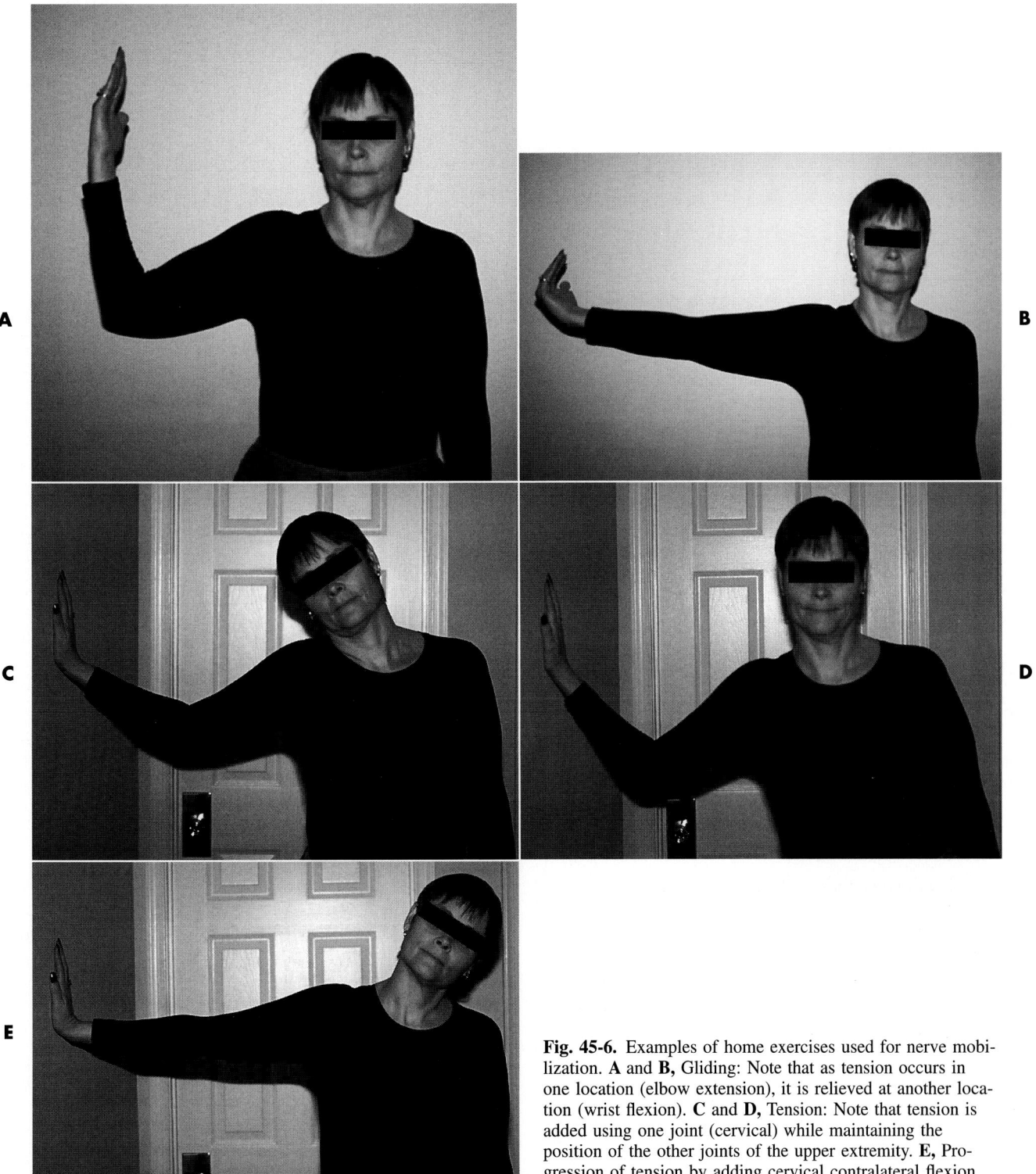

Fig. 45-6. Examples of home exercises used for nerve mobilization. **A** and **B,** Gliding: Note that as tension occurs in one location (elbow extension), it is relieved at another location (wrist flexion). **C** and **D,** Tension: Note that tension is added using one joint (cervical) while maintaining the position of the other joints of the upper extremity. **E,** Progression of tension by adding cervical contralateral flexion and elbow extension.

---

nerve is involved at the level of the elbow, it may be more appropriate, because of high irritability, to initiate nerve gliding at the wrist, cervical spine, or even the lumbar spine before using the elbow joint itself for mobilizing the nerve. In the end, however, it is the patient's response that dictates the progression. If the clinician appreciates that adaptive length changes occur in the connective tissues of the nerve and that structural, chemical, mechanical, and electrical changes occur within the nervous system over time, he or she will recognize that reversal of these changes will also take time. Therefore, in longstanding cases, these principles are best applied in conjunction with a home program, with periodic visits to adjust the exercise prescription. Fig. 45-6 illustrates examples of the application of ULTT components used actively and passively for a home program.

Contraindications and precautions

The contraindications and precautions for the use of ULTT and nerve mobilization are listed in Box 45-6. The clinician is reminded that these are to be used for treatment and evaluation. As previously discussed, the application of the ULTT or nerve mobilization techniques can easily result in significant exacerbation and prolonged recovery of the patient's symptoms when applied incorrectly, especially in the irritable patient. Cord and nerve root signs, especially in the presence of hard neurologic signs (e.g., reflex changes, motor weakness, sensory changes), may indicate the presence of adverse neural tension within the CNS. The clinician must approach these patients with care. Unremitting night pain that is not associated with a mechanical stimulus or is undiagnosed may indicate referred pain of visceral origin. For example, cardiac, hepatic, diaphragmatic, and upper gastrointestinal structures can refer pain into the upper quadrant. Recent sensory changes could indicate that a systemic neurologic or inflammatory disease such as multiple sclerosis or rheumatoid arthritis may be the cause of the

patient's symptoms. This also may be indicative of a recent CNS condition, such as nerve root compression, or a peripheral lesion with neuropraxia or a higher level of nerve injury. Complex regional pain syndrome may be an underlying component of the patient's pain, and aggressive handling may contribute to further exacerbation of the patient's symptoms. Pain originating from cervical spine structures may also be referring pain into the upper extremity. In all of these cases, the clinician must exercise caution in the application of the ULTT and nerve mobilization techniques. Mechanical mobilization of the nervous system is definitely contraindicated in the case of a recently repaired nerve, malignancy (primary or metastatic) involving a nerve or its surrounding tissues, and active neurologic or inflammatory diseases.

SUMMARY

The judicious use of nerve mobilization as a treatment approach requires the therapist to have a sound knowledge of the nervous system's histology, vascularity, gross anatomy, biomechanics, and pathology. Only through the application of this knowledge is it possible to effectively evaluate and treat the PNS. Clinically recognizing how nervous system pathology may manifest itself is a required building block for proceeding with an evaluation to confirm or exclude its involvement in the patient presenting with upper extremity symptoms. The evaluation should include examination of active and passive movement dysfunction and its correlation with the presenting complaints, neural hyperalgesia, tender points, and accompanying local dysfunction. Application of neural mobilization is guided by the principles of education, exercise, and encouragement. Nerve mobilization as a treatment rarely is used alone, and it is augmented by the other treatment techniques used each day. Treatment progression is based on continuous reassessment of the patient's response to the treatment tactics used. Nerve mobilization is not a cure-all; it is another tool available to clinicians and their patients presenting with difficult and complicated diagnoses in the upper extremity.

REFERENCES

1. Asbury A, Fields H: Pain due to peripheral nerve damage: an hypothesis, *Neurology* 34:1587, 1984.
2. Balster SM, Jull GA: Upper trapezius muscle activity during the brachial plexus tension test in asymptomatic subjects, *Manual Ther* 2:144, 1997.
3. Breig A, Troup JDG: Biomechanical considerations in the straight-leg-raising test: cadaveric and clinical studies of the effects of medial hip rotation, *Spine* 4:242, 1979.
4. Butler D: Adverse mechanical tension in the nervous system: a model for assessment and treatment, *Aust J Physiother* 35:27, 1989.
5. Butler D: *Mobilisation of the nervous system,* London, 1991, Churchill Livingstone.
6. Butler D, Gifford L: The concept of adverse mechanical tension in the nervous system: part 2 examination and treatment, *Physiotherapy* 75:629, 1989.
7. Clarke E, Bearn JG: The spiral bands of Fontana, *Brain* 95:1, 1972.

8. Coppieters MW, et al: A qualitative assessment of shoulder girdle elevation during upper limb tension test 1, *Manual Ther* 4:33, 1999.

9. Dahlin L, McLean G: Effects of graded experimental compression on slow and fast axonal transport in rabbit vagus nerve, *J Neurosci* 72:19, 1986.

10. Elvey R: Brachial plexus tension test and the pathoanatomical origin of arm pain. In Glasgow E, Tavomey L, editors: *Aspects of manipulative therapy,* Melbourne, Australia, 1979, Lincoln Institute of Health Sciences.

11. Elvey R: Treatment of arm pain associated with abnormal brachial plexus tension, *Aust J Physiother* 32:225, 1986.

12. Elvey R: Physical evaluation of the peripheral nervous system in disorders of pain and dysfunction, *J Hand Ther* 10:122, 1997.

13. Elvey R, Quinter J, Thomas A: A clinical study of RSI, *Aust Fam Physician* 15:1314, 1986.

14. Gifford L, Butler D: The integration of pain sciences into clinical practice, *J Hand Ther* 10:86, 1997.

15. Haftek J: Stretch injury of peripheral nerve: acute effects of stretching on rabbit nerve, *J Bone Joint Surg* 52B:354, 1970.

16. Jones M: Clinical reasoning in manual therapy, *Phys Ther* 72:875, 1992.

17. Kenneally M: The upper limb tension test. In the Proceedings of the Fourth Biennial Conference of the Manipulative Therapists Association of Australia, 1983, Melbourne, Australia.

18. Kenneally M, Rubenach H, Elvey R: The upper limb tension test: the SLR test of the arm. In Grant R, editor: *Physical therapy of the cervical and thoracic spine,* New York, 1988, Churchill Livingstone.

19. Kleinrensink GJ, et al: Mechanical tension in the median nerve: the effects of joint positions, *Clin Biomech* 10:240, 1995.

20. Kleinrensink GJ, et al: Upper limb tension tests as tools in the diagnosis of nerve and plexus lesions: anatomical and biomechanical aspects, *Clin Biomech* 15:9, 2000.

21. Kwan M, et al: Strain, stress, and stretch of peripheral nerve: rabbit experiments in vitro and in vivo, *Acta Orthop Scand* 63:267, 1992.

22. Lew PC, Morrow CJ, Lew AM: The effect of neck and leg flexion and their sequence on the lumbar spinal cord, *Spine* 19:2421, 1994.

23. Lundborg G: Intraneural microcirculation, *Orthop Clin North Am* 19:1, 1988.

24. Lundborg G, Dahlin L: The pathophysiology of nerve compression, *Hand Clin* 8:215, 1992.

25. Lundborg G, Rydevik B: Effects of stretching the tibial nerve of the rabbit: a preliminary study of the intraneural circulation and the barrier function of the perineurium, *J Bone Joint Surg* 55B:390, 1973.

26. Lundborg G, et al: Peripheral nerve: the physiology of injury and repair. In Woo S, Buckwalter J, editors: American Academy of Orthopedic Surgeons Symposium: injury and repair of the musculoskeletal soft tissues. Park Ridge, Ill, 1998.

27. Mackinnon SE: Double and multiple "crush" syndromes: double and multiple entrapment neuropathies, *Hand Clin* 8:369, 1992.

28. Mackinnon SE, Dellon AL: Experimental study of chronic nerve compression clinical implications, *Hand Clin* 2:639, 1986.

29. Maitland GD: Treatment of the glenohumeral joint by passive movement, *Physiotherapy* 60:3, 1983.

30. McLellan DL, Swash M: Longitudinal sliding of the median nerve during movements of the upper limb, *J Neurol Neurosurg Psychiatry* 39:566, 1976.

31. Millesi H: The nerve gap: theory and clinical practice, *Hand Clin* 2:651, 1986.

32. Millesi H, Zoch G, Rath T: The gliding apparatus of peripheral nerve and its clinical significance, *Ann Chir Main Memb Super* 9:87, 1990.

33. Millesi H, Zoch G, Reihsner R: Mechanical properties of peripheral nerves, *Clin Orthop* 314:76, 1995.

34. Nemoto K, et al: An experimental study of the "double crush" hypothesis, *J Hand Surg* 12A:552, 1987.

35. O'Connell JE: The clinical signs of meningeal irritation, *Brain* 69:9, 1946.

36. Ogata K, Naito M: Blood flow of peripheral nerve effects of dissection, stretching and compression, *J Hand Surg* 11B:10, 1986.

37. Pechan J, Julis I: The pressure measurement in the ulnar nerve: a contribution to the pathophysiology of the cubital tunnel syndrome, *J Biomech* 8:75, 1975.

38. Porter EL, Wharton PS: Irritability of mammalian nerve following ischemia, *J Neurophysiol* 12:109, 1949.

39. Reid JD: Effects of flexion-extension movements of the head and spine upon the spinal cord and nerve roots, *J Neurol Neurosurg Psychiatry* 23:214, 1960.

40. Selvaratnam PJ, Matyas TA, Glasgow EF: Noninvasive discrimination of brachial plexus involvement in upper limb pain, *Spine* 19:26, 1994.

41. Shacklock M: Positive upper limb tension test in a case of surgically proven neuropathy: analysis and validity, *Manual Ther* 1:154, 1996.

42. Sunderland S: The connective tissues of peripheral nerves, *Brain* 88:841, 1965.

43. Sunderland S: *Nerve and nerve injuries,* ed 2, Edinburgh; New York, 1978, Churchill Livingstone.

44. Sunderland S, Bradley K: Stress-strain phenomena in denervated peripheral nerve trunks, *Brain* 64:125, 1961.

45. Sunderland S, Bradley K: Stress-strain phenomena in human peripheral nerve trunks, *Brain* 64:102, 1961.

46. Sunderland S, Bradley K: Stress-strain phenomena in human spinal nerve roots, *Brain* 64:102, 1961.

47. Upton A, McComas A: The double crush in nerve entrapment syndrome, *Lancet* 2:359, 1973.

48. Wall E, et al: Experimental stretch neuropathy: changes in nerve conduction under tension, *J Bone Joint Surg* 74B:126, 1992.

49. Weinstein J: Neurogenic and non-neurogenic pain and inflammatory mediators, *Orthop Clin North Am* 22:235, 1991.

50. Wilgis EF, Murphy R: The significance of longitudinal excursion in peripheral nerves, *Hand Clin* 2:761, 1986.

51. Wright IS: The neurovascular syndrome produced by hyperabduction of the arms, *Am Heart J* 29:1, 1945.

52. Wright T, et al: Excursion and strain of the median nerve, *J Bone Joint Surg* 78A:1897, 1996.

53. Yaxley G, Jull G: A modified upper limb tension test: an investigation of responses in normal subjects, *Aust Physiotherapy* 37:143, 1991.

54. Zoech G, et al: Stress strain in peripheral nerves, *Neuro-Orthop* 10:73, 1991.

Part X

SURGICAL RECONSTRUCTION FOR NERVE INJURIES

Chapter 46

MECHANICS OF
TENDON TRANSFERS

Paul W. Brand

The goal of tendon transfer operations is to restore balance to a hand after one or more of its muscles have been paralyzed or destroyed. In so doing, the surgeon must compare the usefulness of the action of the lost muscle with that of the muscle that will have to be transferred, leaving a defect in the place where the muscle was before.

It is not enough to consider the function and usefulness of these muscles in a qualitative sense. One also has to make an attempt to quantify the gains and losses at each joint, so that one does not overbalance a hand in an attempt to restore balance.

In this process of planning tendon transfers it is useful to think about those mechanical qualities that are transferred with a tendon and those that remain in the distal part of the limb as passive structures that have to be moved and that sometimes resist movement.

FACTORS TRANSFERRED WITH A MUSCLE

When a muscle-tendon unit is transferred, it carries with it some but not all of the qualities it had in its original situation.

Strength

In this context, *strength* refers to the ability to generate tension in the tendon. The tension capability of a muscle depends on the number of muscle fibers that it has and on the total cross-sectional area of all its fibers. Its ability to sustain its tension over time and over a number of repeated contractions depends also on the adequacy of its blood supply; however, the act of transferring a tendon should not change the vascular supply or the nerve supply of its muscle. There used to be a widely quoted rule that said when a muscle-tendon unit was transferred, its strength dropped one

level in the scale of 0 to 5 by which muscles were graded.[5,10,12,13,16] This rule was worked out when polio was the most common cause of paralysis demanding tendon transfers and surgeons had to grade muscles carefully, not only in terms of paralyzed versus unparalyzed but also in various grades of paralysis. We were warned not to use a grade 3 muscle without realizing that after transfer it would only work as grade 2. Any truth in this generalization must have resulted from factors other than muscle strength, such as "drag," which is discussed later. The actual strength of a muscle is unchanged by transfer.

Just within the last two decades surgeons have started to transplant muscles by microvascular and nerve anastomosis. This is quite a different thing from simple transfer; it involves removing a muscle from another limb, with its major artery, vein, and nerve, and placing it in a new situation, using locally available vessels and the motor nerve of the muscle that it is to replace. This is a new challenge, and one for which some of the rules have not yet been worked out. The fascicular patterns of the grafted nerve and the recipient stump may be very different, and even with the highest skill there is no chance that every nerve fiber will get through to a muscle unit. The published reports[4,11] so far have indicated that the successful cases are those in which the transplanted muscles are bigger and bulkier than the muscles they are to replace, presumably to allow for considerable loss of muscle units and yet allow for adequate survival. How much discrepancy to allow between the strength of the donor and the required strength after transplant has not yet been estimated. I suspect that a ratio of 2:1 would be a conservative estimate.

For transfer, however, the task is simpler. Here the muscle keeps its nerve supply. The muscle is only redirected, or "transferred." We choose one that is about the right size to restore the balance of the hand that has been disturbed by paralysis. This is not the same as choosing a muscle of the same size as the one it is to replace. In most cases of paralysis, the sum of the strengths of all the muscles that remain will be substantially less than the original total. Therefore, to obtain a new balance for the hand, the surgeon should be content to replace only part of the strength of the muscles that have been paralyzed.

Fortunately, there is a good deal of flexibility in this choice because muscles fairly quickly adapt their tension output to the demand. A strong muscle will become weaker if it is not used, and a weak muscle will become stronger, up to a point, as long as it is used to its maximum tension capability. However, it will become stronger only if it is used, and used in phase. A muscle will not become stronger just by being placed in a situation that demands strength. It must be used daily and hourly to its maximum by active contraction. Passive lengthening may result from the activity of other muscles, but active contraction results from the patient's recognition of the new function of the muscle. Here the therapist may be a great help. As an aid in the selection of a muscle of the right strength, the tables published by Brand, Beach, and Thompson[3] may be used. At operation the relative diameters of exposed tendons serve as a good approximation. If one muscle is twice as strong as another, then the cross-sectional area of all its muscle fibers will be double that of the other, and the cross-sectional area of its tendon also will be about double that of the other tendon.[3] This is true only of the preparalysis strength. The extent to which tendon diameters change after periods of paralysis or of hypertrophy of the muscle is not known.

Excursion

Another feature of a muscle that is transferred with it is its potential range of excursion. However, this statement needs to be qualified by defining terms. We may recognize three kinds of excursion: potential, required, and available.

If a muscle is freed from all its connective tissue attachments and the naked muscle is stimulated from its fully stretched position, it should contract through a distance that is approximately equal to the resting length of its individual muscle fibers. This is a basic quality of muscle fibers, depending on the number of sarcomeres they contain. We have called this the *potential excursion of the muscle.* However, in the intact limb, very few muscles are able to achieve their full potential range of excursion, either because of restrictions imposed by surrounding connective tissue or because the joints they control do not have the range of motion (ROM) that requires that much excursion.

Required excursion is determined more by joints than by muscles. It is the excursion that is needed to put the joints through their whole ROM. The extensor carpi radialis brevis, for example, has fibers that are about 6 cm long and therefore

could potentially contract through 6 cm. However, the full ROM of the average wrist can be accomplished with about 3.5 cm. Thus, in the average hand, this muscle never uses more than 3.5 cm of excursion. Previously published lists of tendon excursions have been mostly estimates of what we now call *required* excursion.[3]

Perhaps the most significant information needed by the surgeon is the *available* excursion, as Freehafer[6] calls it. Freehafer measures this at operation after cutting the tendon distally. We think that excursion is permitted by the investing connective tissue. This available excursion varies from case to case and probably largely depends on the extent to which the patient has actually used the joints and muscles during the previous months. Connective tissue is responsive to the pattern of use. For example, people who have not previously done jogging or ballet dancing find that they cannot stretch their calf muscles far enough to run or dance effectively. By persistent stretching exercises, they finally obtain a larger range. They probably have not actually lengthened their muscle fibers; they have merely lengthened the connective tissue of the paratenon and perimysium. After such activity, their available excursion would have increased.

Available excursion may be measured at operation after the tendon to be transferred has been divided. It may be held at its end by a hemostat or stitch and pulled out to its full stretch. At this point, the muscle is stimulated by a tetanizing current while the movement of the tendon is measured. If the patient is awake, he or she may make the contraction voluntarily. The figure should be recorded for reference after surgery. Available excursion is transferred to the new site at operation only if the transfer involves minimal change of position and minimal dissection. Sometimes, a long-fibered (long potential excursion) muscle is transferred from a site where it had a short required excursion to a site where it has a long required excursion. In such a case, it will take time and active use to lengthen the connective tissue in and around the muscle and tendon so that the available excursion increases to match the new required excursion. If a tendon is to be widely rerouted and if the transfer is done through open wounds, the normal compliant connective tissue and paratenon are divided and will be replaced by scar. In many operations for tendon transfer, the final success or failure is determined more by the mechanical qualities of the para-tendinous scar than by any other single factor. It is difficult enough for the patient to have to learn to use a muscle for a new action in an unfamiliar situation, but if that action cannot be accomplished until scar has been mobilized and lengthened, it may never be accomplished at all.

There is wide variation in the mechanical qualities of various types of connective tissue. Paratenon typically is easily stretchable. It has a long, low length-tension curve. This means that a great deal of lengthening results from very little tension. This situation permits nearly free tendon movement over a wide range of excursion. The common fatty areolar connective tissue that serves to fill spaces between structures in the body is not quite as compliant, but it also will lengthen with moderate tension and then, with repeated movement, will become modified into a kind of paratenon.

Fascia and retinaculum, fibrous septa, and scar all tend to have steep length-tension curves, lengthening only about 10% even under considerable tension. Thus, if a tendon comes to lie on a ligament that has been cut or scarified at surgery, the tendon may become united to the ligament through a collagen scar whose short fibers become parallel oriented by the pull of the tendon. Such fibers, only 1 or 2 mm long, would allow almost no tendon movement. If, instead, the transferred tendon is passed through a tunnel in loose fat and connective tissue, the scar that forms around the tendon will attach it only to the soft and compliant tissues through which the tendon tunneler has found its way. When traction is applied to that tendon, the new scar may not stretch but the surrounding fat and areolar tissue will stretch and move with the tendon through several millimeters. This early movement will allow the patient to sense the new action and use it. Thus the patient will continue to stimulate further muscle contraction and movement and further stretch and then lengthening and remodeling of the new paratendinous tissue.

Thus the concept of excursion of a tendon is complex and involves many factors. The true potential excursion, dependent only on the number of sarcomeres in each fiber, is not responsive to movement or active use; it is responsive to the tension in the resting fiber. Tarbary et al.[14,15] have shown in experimental animals that if a muscle fiber is immobilized in a slack position it becomes shorter by loss of sarcomeres, and if it is immobilized in a stretched position, it becomes longer by the addition of sarcomeres, until neutral tension is achieved.

Thus there is no way that a patient or a therapist can make a permanent change in the length of a muscle fiber. If a hand is kept at rest (splinted) in a posture that keeps some muscles slack and others stretched, every muscle fiber will undergo cell activity, with whole sarcomeres being added to the stretched fibers and removed from the slack fibers until all are returned to their normal tension. When the hand is released and allowed movement again, the patient will find that it is difficult to return to the normal position of rest. It will take time until a reverse process of sarcomere adjustment restores fiber lengths to what they were.

If, while transferring a tendon, a surgeon makes the new attachment at a high tension, he or she might assume that the result will be a stronger muscle action. This is not so. As soon as the muscle is at a high resting tension, more sarcomeres will be added in series to each fiber until the resting tension is the same as all other muscles. The fibers will be longer but not stronger.

MECHANICAL FACTORS AT DISTAL END OF TRANSFER
Leverage

All that a muscle can give to a joint is tension and excursion of the tendon. At the joint, this is turned into action according to the leverage. The actual movement of a joint around an axis is accomplished by "torque," or "moment." These two terms mean the same thing and are the product of force times leverage, or tension times moment arm. We all know that a lever enables a small force to move heavy objects (Fig. 46-1). We also know that a heavy weight can be moved most easily by a small force if the force is applied

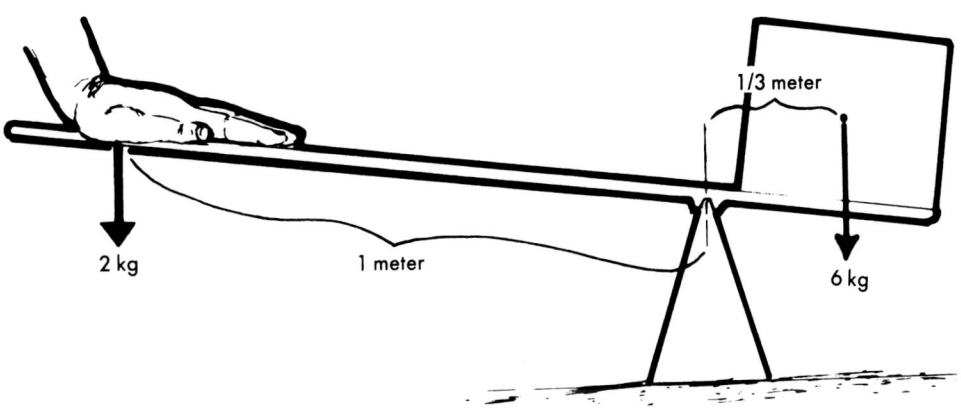

Mechanical advantage of arm = 3:1
Moment of hand = 2 kg-m
Moment of weight = 2 kg-m

Fig. 46-1. Equilibrium in lever system.

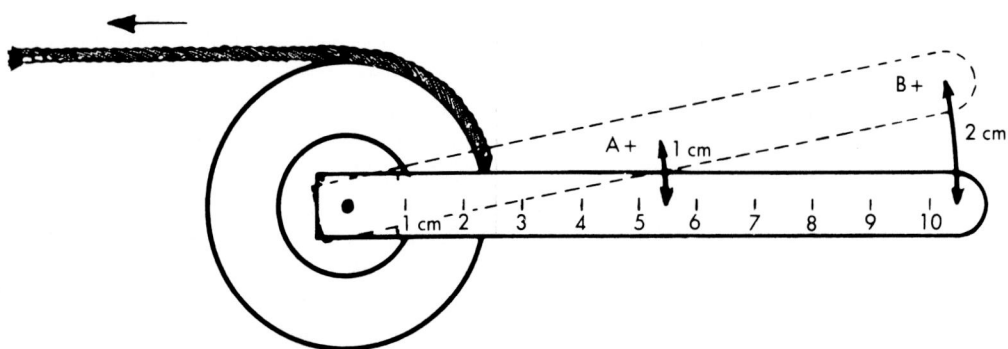

Fig. 46-2. Pulley-wheel axis and lever (tendon and bone at joint). Every point on lever (bone) moves through distance proportional to distance from axis.

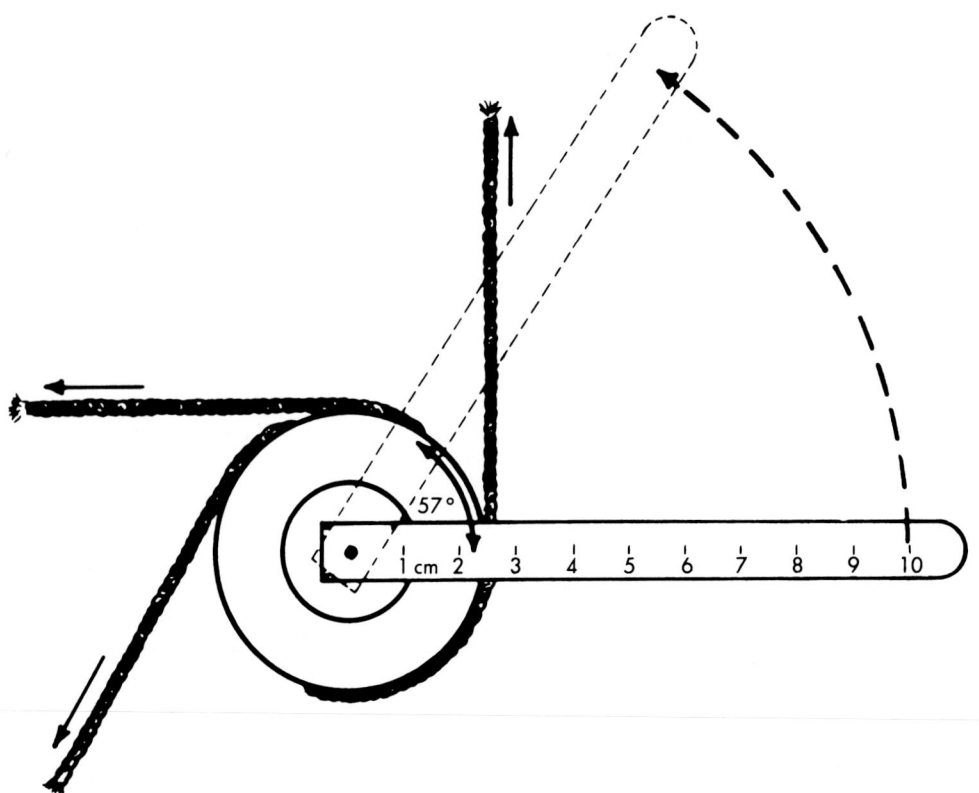

Fig. 46-3. Rope moving off pulley has same moment arm in many directions and will move same distance for same angular movement of lever.

far up the lever, away from the axis, or if the load is close to the axis. This increases the mechanical advantage. (Mechanical advantage is equal to the moment arm of the force divided by the moment arm of the load.) What we often forget is that the force has to move farther if its lever arm is long and that the load will move very little if its lever arm is short.

Now this concept must be translated into the terminology of tendons and joints. The leverage that a tendon has at a joint is the perpendicular distance between the joint axis and the tendon as it crosses the joint. The lever arm beyond that is the length of the bone or digit distal to the joint axis. Thus, in the body, almost all levers work with the force at the short end of the lever and the load at the long end. We are using a system of muscles that can produce enormous forces over rather short distances. The lever and pulley systems around joints are designed to take big forces with short ranges and make them effective over bigger ranges, with reduced force.

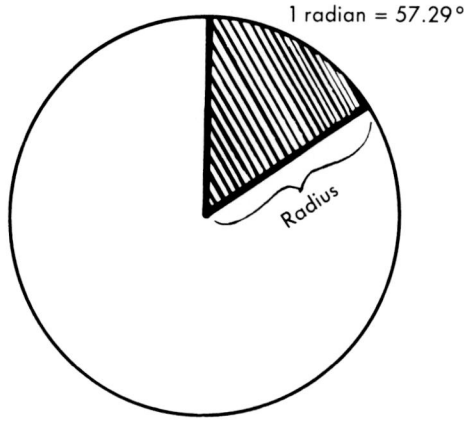

Fig. 46-4. Radius along circumference of circle subtends radian at center.

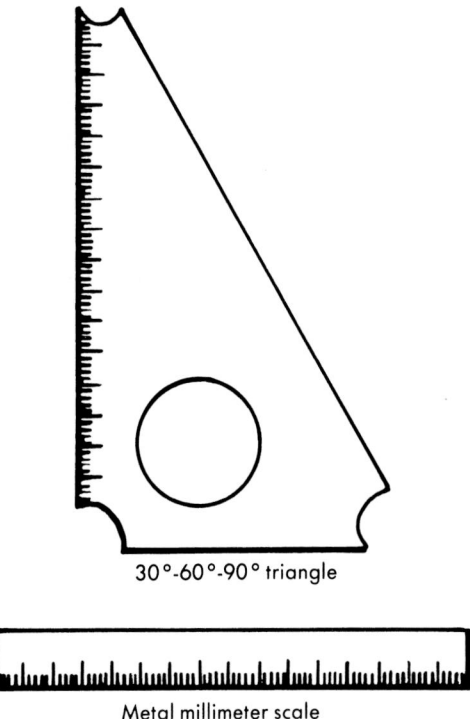

30°-60°-90° triangle

Metal millimeter scale

Fig. 46-5. Corners of triangle are cut out to allow it to fit between fingers over webs with edges intersecting at metacarpophalangeal joint axis.

There is no way to beat this system. The price of increased power is reduced range. I often hear surgeons say that they have found a way to increase the "strength" of a transfer at a joint. I rarely hear them mention the amount of excursion that has been used up, leaving less "strength" for other joints in the same sequence, or the fact that the transfer will now be effective over a smaller range.

One reason that surgeons usually do not try to work out the moments or leverages of the tendons they transfer is that they know it is so difficult to identify exactly where the axis of a joint is located. Therefore it is not possible at surgery to measure the perpendicular distance between the axis and the tendon.

However, there is a simple and practical method of estimating the moment arms of tendons at joints that will enable surgeons to know exactly how effective each tendon will be at each joint it crosses. The method is based on two rules of geometry (Fig. 46-2). The first is that when a lever (bone) moves around an axis (joint), every point on the lever moves through a distance proportional to its own distance from the axis. The second rule grows out of the first and is an example of it (Fig. 46-3). If a lever moves around an axis through an angle of 57.29 degrees, then every point on the lever moves a distance equal to its own distance from the axis. If a length of a radius is marked on the circumference of a circle and the two ends of that radius are joined to the center, the angle between them is called a *radian* and measures about 57.29 degrees (Fig. 46-4). As a lever moves around an axis, a number of points on its length may be thought of as marking out a number of arcs of concentric circles. When the lever has moved a radian, every arc that has been described is the same length as the distance (radius) of that point on the lever from the axis. This becomes a way to relate angles to distances; angles of joint movement can be related to excursions of the tendons that cause the movement or are affected by it.

In the stressful, time-dominated atmosphere of the operating room, nobody is going to measure tenths of a degree, or even single degrees. I find it useful to have in the operating room a metal triangle with angles of 30, 60, and 90 degrees (Fig. 46-5). I also have a metal millimeter scale. Keeping a little tension on a tendon, I move a joint through 60 degrees, while my assistant measures exactly how far the tendon has moved. The excursion of the tendon that matches 60 degrees of joint movement is the same as the moment arm or leverage of that tendon at that joint. I often use 90 degrees of joint movement because I find it is easier to guess a right angle. In that case, the tendon excursion will be 1.5 times the moment arm (Fig. 46-6). If I use only 30 degrees of joint motion, the tendon will move half the moment arm.

Engineers have objected that this becomes imprecise when there is a variable axis (instant center) or when the bowstringing of a tendon results in a changing moment arm. It is in just these situations that this system is so valuable. What is the use of knowing the exact moment arm at which a tendon ought to be? I need to know just how effective my tendon is going to be in the place I have put it, even if it is wrong—in fact, especially if it is wrong. In the case of a bowstringing tendon, the measured tendon excursion will give the mean moment arm. In such a case, it is useful to take two readings (Figs. 46-7 and 46-8): one of the first 30 degrees of motion and the other of the last 30 degrees of motion. In the case of a flexor tendon graft that has no sheath at the metacarpophalangeal (MP) joint and that has had a new pulley reconstruction, the surgeon may measure the tendon excursion that matches 0 to 30 degrees, and then 60 to 90 degrees, of MP joint motion (Fig. 46-9). A normal finger might give readings of 5 and 6 mm, indicating a moment arm of 10 mm (near-extension) and 12 mm (near-flexion). The measured excursion has been doubled to obtain the moment arm because the joint has been moved only 30 degrees at a time rather than 60 degrees. With a well-reconstructed pulley, a surgeon might find readings of 5 and 7 mm, showing just a little increase in bowstringing. However, if the surgeon gets readings of 5 and 10 mm, he or she will

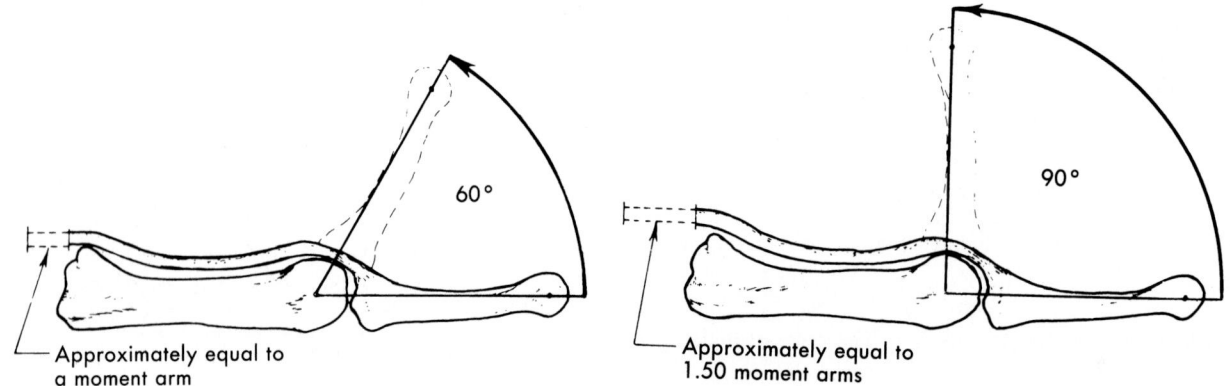

Fig. 46-6. Tendon excursion that matches 60 degrees is approximately equal to moment arm of that tendon at that joint.

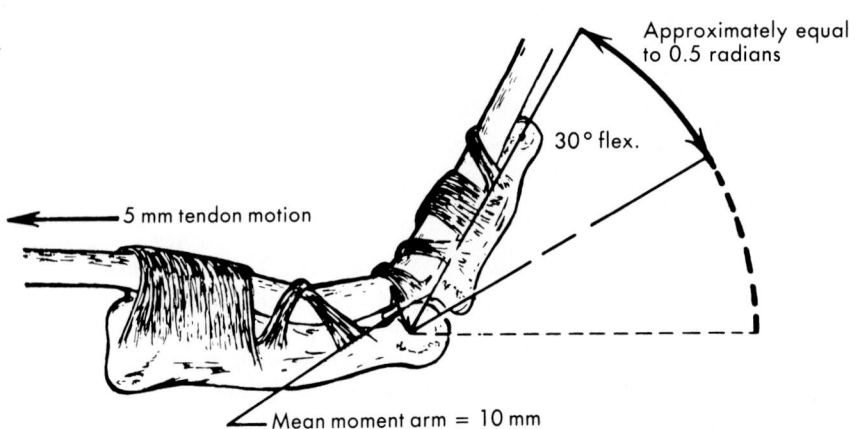

Fig. 46-7. Tendon excursion that matches 30 degrees of joint motion is approximately equal to half the moment arm of that tendon at that joint.

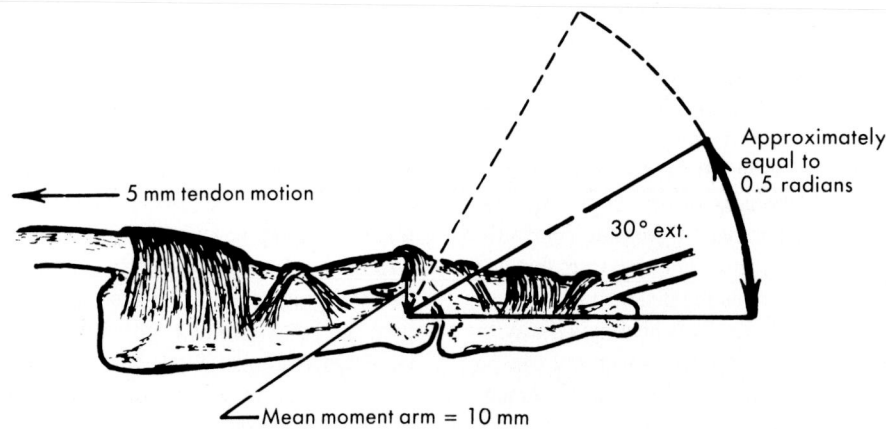

Fig. 46-8. When joint is nearly straight, tendon hugs skeletal plane. Moment arm measured through 30 degrees of flexion is 5 mm.

know that there is severe bowstringing. The new pulley is either too loose or too far up the finger away from the axis. If the surgeon accepts that result, some poor patient will struggle vainly to obtain flexion of the proximal interphalangeal (PIP) joint while the MP joint flexes too strongly, using up the best of the available excursion.

Two axes

In placing a tendon transfer, the surgeon must consider all of the possible directions in which the joint may move in response to the transferred tendon. In many cases, there will be an axis for flexion and extension and another axis for abduction and adduction. The tendon may cross the joint in an oblique direction, so the surgeon may be uncertain exactly how the joint will respond. Here I suggest a quick test. Keep tension on the tendon by a stitch marker while the joint is moved first through 60 degrees of flexion/extension and then through 30 degrees of abduction/adduction. I suggest 30 degrees because few joints can do a full 60 degrees of lateral movement. It is important not to forget to double the 30-degree reading to obtain the abduction/adduction moment arm. Now the two vector moment arms can be plotted on a graph to give the real or resultant moment arm as the diagonal of the rectangle so formed (Fig. 46-10).

The third axis—rotation

The third movement is rotation, and the axis is longitudinal, at right angles to both the other axes. Many joints, such as MP joints, do not have much active rotation in normal strong hands but may develop significant rotation if the finger either is hypermobile or has damaged stabilizing ligaments, as in rheumatoid arthritis. This becomes a more severe problem if a tendon transfer is added that is unopposed in a rotational sense.

Hollister et al.[8,9] have pointed out that this concept of three axes at right angles to each other is often an oversimplification of reality. This is because frequently what appears to be a simple hinge joint of flexion/extension, such as the distal interphalangeal (DIP) joint of the thumb, is actually offset in relation to the natural planes of flexion/extension and abduction/adduction. This means that it is impossible to flex that joint without also involving some degree of abduction and even a little rotation.[1,8,9]

A full analysis of this important subject is beyond the scope of this chapter. It is well developed in the chapter,

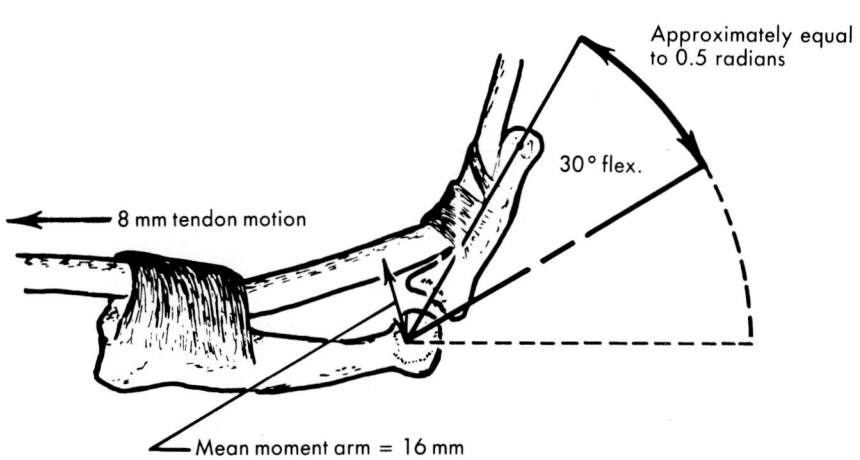

Fig. 46-9. Demonstration of increasing moment arm. As joint flexes, with excised flexor sheath, tendon bowstrings. Next 30 degrees of flexion takes 8 mm of tendon excursion.

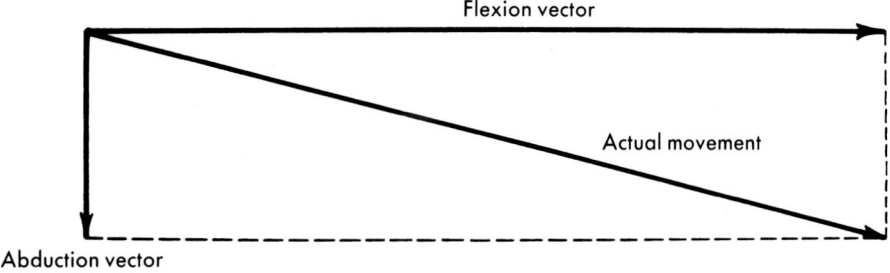

Fig. 46-10. Vector diagram of motion at joint in two planes. There is also a rotational vector, with axis at right angles to the plane of this page.

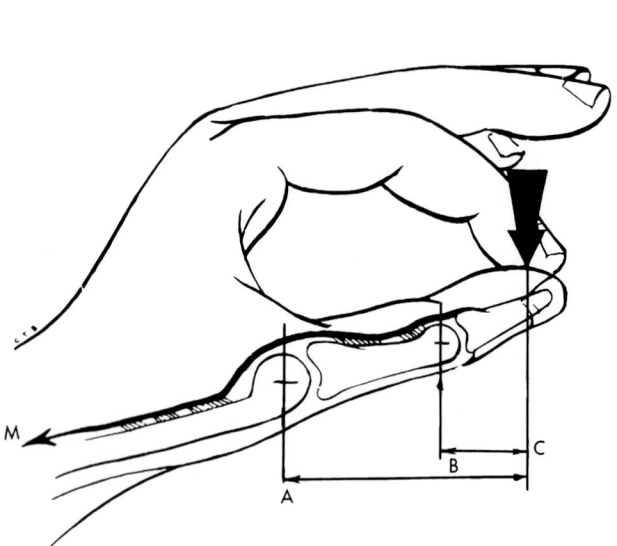

Fig. 46-11. Diagram of a tendon that crosses more than one joint. External force of pinch, *arrow* at *C,* has a tendency to force joints *A* and *B* into extension. Turning moment at *A* is proportional to *A-C,* whereas that at *B* is proportional to *B-C*. (From Brand PW: Tendon transfers in the forearm. In Flynn JE: *Hand surgery,* ed 3, Baltimore, 1982, Williams & Wilkins.)

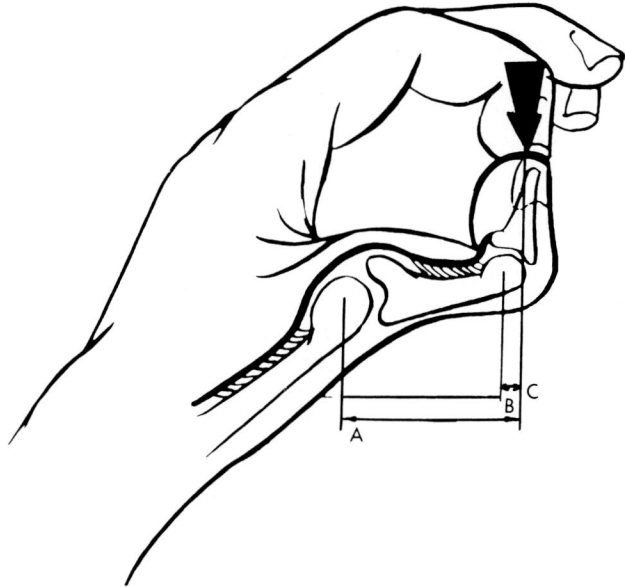

Fig. 46-12. Deformity that results from having only one flexor tendon crossing two joints. (From Brand PW: Tendon transfers in the forearm. In Flynn JE: *Hand surgery,* ed 3, Baltimore, 1982, Williams & Wilkins.)

"How joints move" by Hollister in *Clinical Mechanics of the Hand.*

Joints in series

In severe paralysis, a single tendon is sometimes placed across a series of joints, without the support of other muscles at the proximal joints. This might be satisfactory if each segment of a digit were always supported by external opposing forces as it is when one grasps a cylinder. However, if the distal segment alone is opposed by a force, as in pinch, the proximal segments may buckle. The surgeon must remember the following: (1) A tendon crossing several joints exerts equal force at each. There is no way a person can instruct his muscle to apply more force at one joint than at another. The actual moment or torque that is exerted at each joint varies only according to the moment arms of that tendon at each joint. (2) The distal external force or load at the tip of the digit exerts an opposing moment or torque at each joint, and this also varies according to the moment arm of the external force, at that joint. The moment arms of tendons in the hand are usually small because tendons are held close to the skeleton and are only a little larger at proximal joints as the skeleton becomes thicker. However, the moment arms of the external force or load are based on the length of the bones and the length of the digit and thus become enormously greater at proximal joints. Thus an unopposed digit may be flexed by a single muscle-tendon unit acting on all of the joints. The flexor profundus, unaided by other muscles, produces a full sweep from extended finger to clenched fist. As soon as the fingertip is opposed by a load or external force, it becomes necessary to recruit the flexor superficialis for the PIP and MP joints and the intrinsic muscles for the MP joints, or the fingers will flex distally and hyperextend proximally.[2]

Consider the mechanism of the well-known Froment sign in the thumb. When the short flexors and adductor muscles are paralyzed, the long flexor will have equal tension along its length and will exert flexion moment at the MP and interphalangeal (IP) joints in proportion to the moment arms at each joint, which are only marginally different from each other. When a firm pinch is used, the index finger (Fig. 46-11) may push the thumb toward extension. The long flexor, though, immediately increases its tension to oppose the index finger and stabilize the pinch. However, the extension moment resulting from the index finger is far greater at the MP joint of the thumb, where it has more than double the moment arm that it has at the IP joint.

The long flexor increases its tension to prevent hyperextension at the MP joint and thereby unavoidably flexes the IP joint, at which less moment is needed. In flexing the IP joint, the terminal phalanx is brought to a position end-on to the index finger so that the force from the index is applied still closer to the axis, or even at the axis (Fig. 46-12). Thus the Z-shaped buckling of the thumb becomes irreversible. Many surgeons, noting the flexed tip of the thumb, have assumed that it can be corrected by adding extra power to the extensor. This is not so. The problem can be corrected only by adding an extra flexor to the MP joint so that the long flexor can relax at this joint and avoid overflexing the IP joint. Because it is so difficult to balance a series of joints against a distal load, it is often wise to arthrodese one or more joints in the chain so that the few remaining muscles may effectively control the joints that remain. In the previous example, arthrodesis of the MP joint of the thumb will allow a strong pinch without the Froment flexion of the tip.

Drag

In any operation for tendon transfer, we consider first the capability of the motor, the muscle-tendon unit, that we transfer. Then we consider the geometry and mechanics by which the tension of the motor is transformed into the torque at each joint and thus into effective movement of segments of limbs. Finally, we have to realize that at each stage of this process we shall encounter internal resistance in the form of friction and the need to stretch passive soft tissues. This we may collectively call *drag,* which we must recognize as an obstacle that may frustrate all of our endeavors, unless we plan a way to minimize its effect and work to overcome its unavoidable residue.

Friction. Friction occurs whenever two objects move against each other. It is minimized when their surfaces are congruous and smooth and when the materials have a low coefficient of friction. This is not discussed in detail here because true independent movement of surfaces over each other occurs only in joints and in synovial tendon sheaths. All of the features of the architecture, the selection of low-friction materials for joint surfaces, and the lubrication systems involved are so amazingly well designed and work so efficiently that it is hard to imitate or match them. There is little we can do to restore them if they are lost. In the case of transferred tendons, true gliding may occur in a sheath if it was there before we interfered and if the transferred tendon has a blood supply. If true gliding is needed after transfer in a place where it was not present before, the only thing we can do is to restore movement of the tendon, which is accomplished by stretching and relaxing the investing connective tissue, and wait for the synovial space to open up in its own good time. Such synovial spaces usually develop on the concave side of a curving tendon, but it takes months to happen.

Lengthening of soft tissue. Except in the limited areas where synovial spaces occur, all movement within limbs is permitted by the lengthening and shortening of connective tissue. We often use the word *gliding* in referring to tendon movement, but it is not real gliding in most cases. A tendon does not move over the tissue next to it. It is attached to the paratenon that surrounds it. That tissue is usually relaxed when the tendon is at its midpoint of motion. It stretches and lengthens when the tendon needs to move. Peritendinous tissues are made of collagen and elastin and of some interesting structureless ground substance that is semifluid and that has gel-like qualities. When this composite soft tissue is subjected to tension, it becomes longer. When

relaxed, it shortens back to where it was before. When the tissue is pulled, it takes energy to make it longer. When it is allowed to shorten, it gives up energy.

The application of this simple concept is very straightforward. Every time a tendon is placed in a new situation, it becomes attached there by soft tissue. Therefore every time it moves, it takes energy to lengthen that soft tissue, and it tends to get pulled back to its original position of attachment when it is no longer under tension. The amount of force that it takes to lengthen that soft tissue and the distance through which it has to be lengthened are absolutely critical to the success of any tendon transfer. Yet they are the least studied aspect of tendon transfer. I have simplified this so that you may be willing to follow me into a step or two of complexity so that we may be in a position to understand and control this most important aspect of tendon transfer operations and postoperative rehabilitation.

Most studies on the mechanical qualities of soft tissues have been done on excised tissue.[7,17] A piece of skin, ligament, tendon, or connective tissue is removed, placed in a machine, and tested under various levels of stress and varying rates of stretch. From these studies we are able to identify the elasticity of a tissue and its viscosity. We may note that there is a hysteresis, in that when a tissue is stretched it lengthens, but when it is relaxed, it comes back to its resting state by a different curve and takes longer in the process. We also may note a "creep," which means that when it is overstretched it does not come back to its first length, but rather remains a little longer (Figs. 46-13 and 46-14). This type of study gives a good background for understanding soft tissue mechanics, but it may give a false impression of what happens in living tissue. For example, if living soft tissue is overstretched, it also will exhibit creep, but this may be accompanied by an inflammatory reaction that occurs in response to the violence that has been done to some elements of the tissue fabric. That inflammation may result in the exudation of some tissue fluid containing fibrinogen, and there may be an incursion of inflammatory cells. The final result may be the laying down of some new interstitial collagen scar that will make the tissue more contracted and less compliant in the future.

We have to study the qualities of living soft tissue in response to mechanical force. This must include its ability to remodel or to be remodeled. It is this remodeling that is the basis for the gradual increase in ROM at a joint that is limited by a soft tissue contracture. It does not improve simply by passive stretching or by creep but by growing in length, or remodeling of the shortened tissue. This is the basis by which a transferred tendon gradually becomes free to move. The adhesions have not just been stretched; they have been remodeled or have grown to accommodate to new requirements. Now some of this remodeling may be just a change in the bonding of collagen, but it is accomplished by living cells, by fibroblasts that act in response to mechanical and biomechanical orders that they understand. Our duty is to

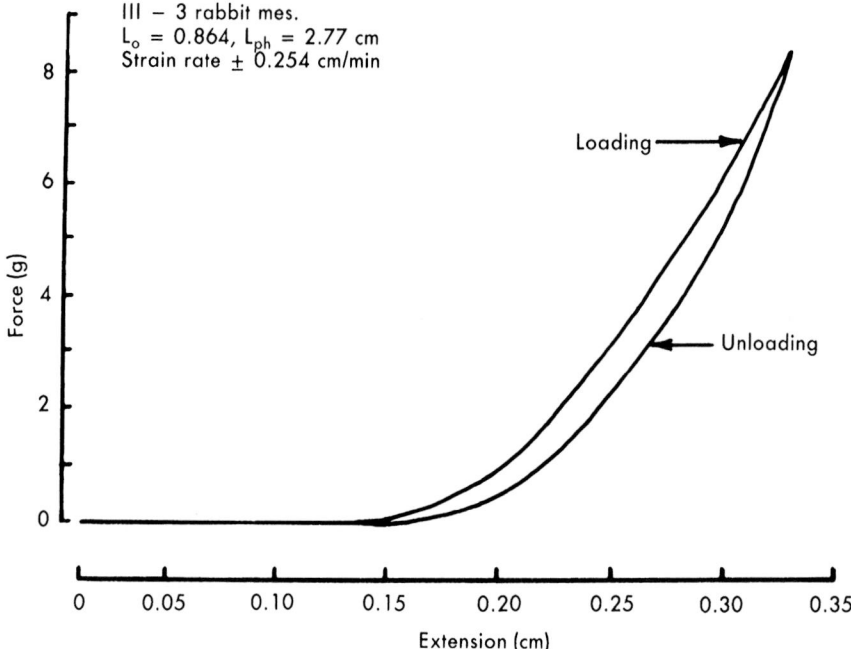

Fig. 46-13. Hysteresis curve. Rabbit mesentery. Loading and unloading curves after Y.C.B. Fung. Note that the stretched length of this tissue is more than three times the relaxed length. This curve shows only the end part of the length-tension curve of a piece of mesentery. The full curve is five times as long and is all flat; that is, the tension needed to lengthen or stretch the mesentery is so small that it is not measurable until the mesentery is nearly fully stretched. This is very much like the behavior of paratenon tissue, for which we do not yet have a precise curve. (From Fung YCB: *Am J Physiol* 213:1532, 1967.)

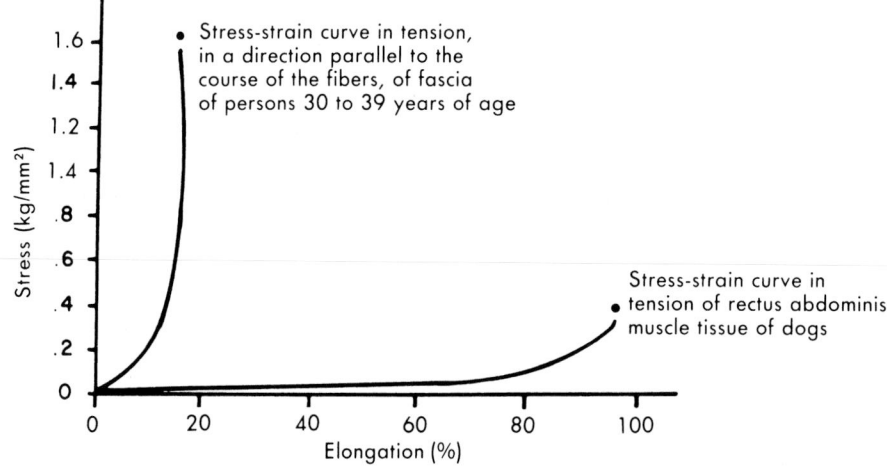

Fig. 46-14. Length-tension curves for fascia *(left)* and muscle (passive stretch only). Note that even fascia and tendon are lengthened 10% to 20% under tension and that muscle fiber is lengthened nearly 60% to 80% before it offers increasing resistance. This is from the fully relaxed length, not the physiologic resting length in situ. (Composite of curves after Evans FG. In Yamada H, editor: *Strength of biological materials,* Baltimore, 1970, Williams & Wilkins.)

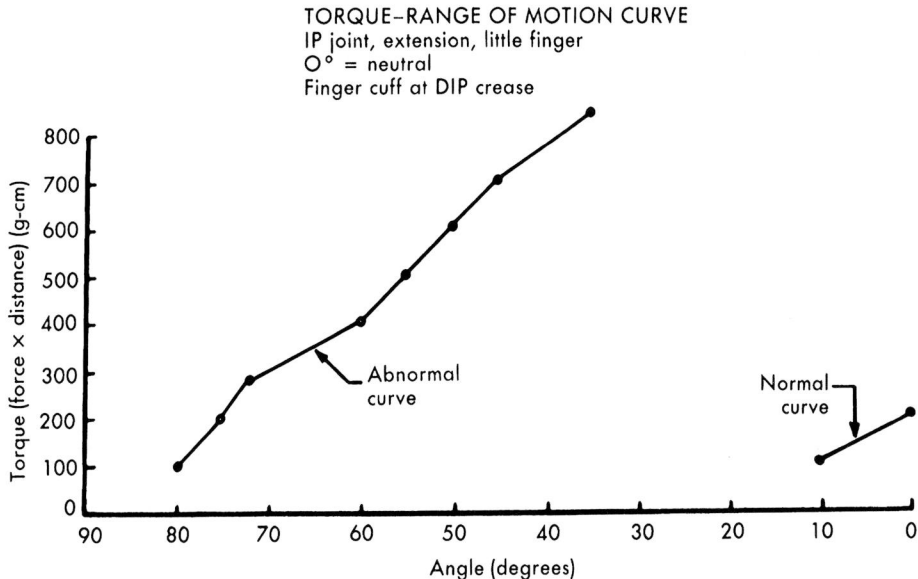

Fig. 46-15. Torque-angle curve of a stiff interphalangeal joint moving into extension. The segment of curve on the right shows that a normal proximal interphalangeal joint would need only a small torque to achieve 0 degrees (full extension). The curve of a stiff finger shows a gradually increasing angle with gradually increasing torque. This indicates that the stiffness is "soft"; that is, the resistance is caused by tissues that can be progressively stretched and that therefore may be expected to grow longer with sustained therapy.

learn the type of mechanical stimulus to which these cells respond and to use these stimuli as our instruments to change the pattern of adhesions and scar.

It is difficult to study the behavior of collagen and elastin and connective tissue complexes in the intact hand because, as we open the tissues to look, it ceases to be an intact hand. However, even without knowing exactly how these tissues respond, at a molecular level, we may study total tissue response to a known input of mechanical stress.

This involves the discipline of the measurement of stress input, recorded against ROM output. Our present methods of prescribing the forces that are intended to lengthen adhesions are usually completely nonquantitative ("use gentle passive movement"), and even our measurements of ROM are partly subjective in that we tend to pull or press a little harder when we measure the range of passive motion if we are expecting or hoping that it has improved.

I suggest therefore that all serious hand surgeons and therapists adopt a "torque–range of motion" (T-ROM) principle in monitoring the progress of tendon movement or joint stiffness preoperatively and postoperatively.

The principle of T-ROM is based on the recognition that although we can rarely measure the actual lengthening of any tissue or any adhesion without cutting the skin, their lengthening can be monitored by measuring the angular movement of the joint against the torque applied to it because

all the tissues that concern us have an effect on a joint. Thus we need to have a repeatable way to apply known force at a known distance from the axis while we measure the range of joint motion in response to it.

The key word, for most of us, is *repeatable.* For research workers, the actual moment arms and exact forces are very important, but for understanding a given case and for following the progress of scar lengthening, it is enough if we use repeatable criteria.

For the measurement of torque, I suggest that we apply a known force—say 1 kg—at a standard position, such as at a skin crease, at right angles to a segment of the digit. We measure the joint angle while the torque is being applied. A day later, or a week later, the same force is applied at the same skin crease so that the torque is the same, and then we know for sure that any change in angle represents a change in the tissue restraints at the joint (or around the tendon).

There are three ways to increase the usefulness (and the complexity) of this measurement, each of which will teach us something different.

1. Use a series of forces to vary the torque. This results in a T-ROM curve (Fig. 46-15). We often use 200, 400, 600, 800, and 1000 g, applied by a spring scale at the same distance from the joint axis. We measure the joint angle at each level of torque. In general, we find that

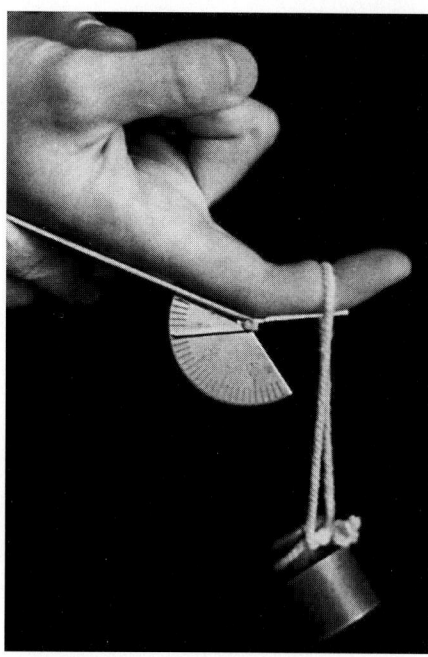

Fig. 46-16. A simple way to obtain a torque-angle measurement is for a hand to be positioned so that a hanging weight, of, say, 250 g is pulling at right angles to a segment of a finger and at a finger crease. Alternatively, the weight may hang over a pulley wheel, so that the string is horizontal and the hand is more easily positioned. (From Brand PW, Hollister A: *Clinical mechanics of the hand,* ed 2, St Louis, 1993, Mosby.)

the shape of the curve gives some idea of the quality of the restricting adhesions. A shallow curve shows a compliant tissue. A steep curve means a more rigid tissue, or a tissue with shorter fibers and therefore poor prognosis for great increase in length.

2. Repeat the T-ROM measurement on the finger joint with different positions of the proximal joints (wrist). This gives a good idea of the relative role played by proximal tendon and muscle restrictions as compared with distal joint stiffness.

3. Repeat the T-ROM measurement in a time sequence, such as early morning, before exercise, after exercise, or if the hand is swollen, before and after hand elevation.

Although a T-ROM curve is based on a sequence of angles, it may be interpreted in terms of the length of the soft tissue restraints that cross the joint and those that limit the excursion of the tendon that crosses the joint.

I recognize that surgeons and therapists will find, at first, that these measurements are time-consuming and that it requires manual dexterity to manipulate a joint, a protractor, and a spring at the same time with only one pair of hands (Fig. 46-16). This will become easier with practice, and there are a couple of tricks that make it simple.

One trick is to have a voice-activated tape recorder and to speak out the angles and the figures for tension (for torque). This eliminates the need to release the hand and protractor to record the readings. When all measurements are finished, the angle readings and tension readings are plotted on graph paper while the tape is played back. It is a waste of time to record numbers and then make a graph. Record the graph directly with dots or crosses. It is the graph that gets looked at—nobody reads numbers!

With such a monitoring system, it will be possible to be quite precise about relating the therapy program to the changes that result from it. For example, it will be possible to compare the results of intermittent high-torque exercises with the results of continuous immobilization in low-torque extension (or flexion).

In general, it will be found that where restraints to joint movement have a viscous element to them, it is best to prescribe a great deal of movement and exercise. Where the restraint is mainly elastic, there may be more benefit from continuous low-torque stretching (for a digit, this torque may be as low as 250 g-cm). To distinguish viscous from elastic resistance, one needs only to measure ROM before and after a short period of active movement. Because viscous damping of ROM is mostly caused by movement of fluids in tissues, there would be marked changes in ROM at the same torque after just minutes of exercise or of elevation of the hand.

SUMMARY

In this chapter on mechanics of tendon transfers, I have written mostly about methods of measurement and methods of monitoring change rather than giving instructions about methods of treatment. This is because there is little available quantitative information on the relative merits of different types of transfer and of different methods of mobilizing stiff joints or adherent tendons. Rather than giving my opinions to rival opinions of others, I want to stress the fact that we need to develop disciplines of measurement so that we can each find out for ourselves whether procedure A is more effective than procedure B. It is numbers that we need, not more theories.

Finally, we have to keep in mind that whenever we direct therapy with the object of changing just one tissue, we will always have some effect on the whole hand and often on the whole person. If we want to lengthen a contracture on the flexor side of a hand and if we use long-term low-torque extension, by splinting, we may achieve that goal. At the same time, we may produce loss of length in dorsal structures and limit flexion. Other fingers in the same hand may lose ROM just by disuse. Any form of immobilization will tend to cause loss of compliance in capsular tissues and loss of fluid components of hyaline cartilage. Thus, when possible, we should avoid single-minded mechanical approaches to any deformity. If long-term tension is called for, at least 1 hour per day should be reserved for free, active exercise and purposeful movement to keep tissue fluids moving, to move collagen fiber on collagen fiber, and to encourage the restoration of normal balance between the fluids and gels in cartilage and in paratenon tissues. Then with restored homeostasis, relaxed fibroblasts, and contented fat cells, we may return to the discipline of tension and torque to accomplish a specific objective.

REFERENCES

1. Agee J, Hollister AM, King F: The longitudinal axis of rotation of the metacarpophalangeal joint of the finger, *J Hand Surg* 11:767, 1986.
2. Brand PW: Tendon transfers in the forearm. In Flynn JE, editor: *Hand surgery,* ed 2, Baltimore, 1975, Williams & Wilkins.
3. Brand PW, Beach RB, Thompson DE: Relative tension and potential excursion of muscles in the forearm and hand, *J Hand Surg* 6:209, 1981.
4. Buncke HJ: The role of microsurgery in hand surgery (presidential address, American Society for Surgery of the Hand), *J Hand Surg* 6:553, 1981.
5. Daniels L, Williams M, Worthingham C: *Muscle testing: techniques of manual examination,* ed 2, Philadelphia, 1956, WB Saunders.
6. Freehafer AA, Pecham H, Keith MW: Determination of muscle-tendon unit properties during tendon transfer, *J Hand Surg* 4:331, 1979.
7. Fung YCB: Elasticity of soft tissues in simple elongation, *Am J Physiol* 213:1532, 1967.
8. Hollister A, et al: The axes of rotation of the thumb carpometacarpal joint, *J Orthop Res* 10:454, 1992.
9. Hollister A, et al: The axes of rotation of the thumb interphalangeal and metacarpophalangeal joints, *Clin Orthop* Nov:188, 1995.
10. Legg AT, Merrill JB: Physical therapy in infantile paralysis. Reprinted from Mock HE, Pemberton R, Coulter JS, editors: *Principles and practices of physical therapy,* Hagerstown, Md, 1932, WF Prior.
11. Manktelow RT, Zuker RM, McKee NH: Functioning free muscle transplantation. Presented at the thirty-seventh annual meeting of the American Society for Surgery of the Hand, New Orleans, Jan 18-20, 1982, *J Hand Surg* 9A:32, 1984.
12. Nelson N: Factors to be considered in evaluating effect of treatment in anterior poliomyelitis, *Arch Phys Med* 28:358, 1947.
13. Sharrard WJW: Muscle recovery in poliomyelitis, *J Bone Joint Surg* 37B:63, 1955.
14. Tabary JC, et al: Physiological and structural changes in the cat's soleus muscle due to immobilization at different lengths by plaster casts, *J Physiol* 224:231, 1972.
15. Tabary JC, et al: Functional adaptation of sarcomere number of normal cat muscle, *J Physiol (Paris)* 72:277, 1976.
16. Wright WG: Muscle training in the treatment of infantile paralysis, *Boston Med Surg* 167:567, 1912.
17. Yamada H: In Evans FG, editor: *Strength of biological materials,* Baltimore, 1970, Williams & Wilkins.

Chapter 47

TENDON TRANSFERS: AN OVERVIEW

Lawrence H. Schneider

The goal of a tendon transfer is to restore to the extremity a needed motor function that has been lost secondary to paralysis from nerve injury or disease or by muscle or tendon loss. To be considered is the effect that the transfer will have on the extremity and whether the function of the transferred motor can be spared. This technique in which the motor power of one muscle is transferred to a deficient muscle is now well established, with most of the procedures standardized. Until recently, only the tendinous portion of the musculotendinous unit was transferred, but today there is also a capability to transplant a complete muscle with its origin and insertion to a new location. This latter technique, free muscle transfer,[15] is now a potentially useful tool when simpler techniques are not available. The gracilis, latissimus dorsi, and pectoralis major have been used as free muscle transfers on neurovascular pedicles into the upper extremity. Manktelow et al.[15] have presented a series of patients with severe problems in whom these techniques were used to recover finger and thumb flexion.

HISTORY

Study of the evolution of these tendon transfer techniques takes one through an exciting period in the history of reconstructive extremity surgery. Excellent reviews have summarized the early efforts of workers in this field.[1,30,31] Based on the work of these early surgeons, the modern principles of tendon transfer were developed. Although many of the original procedures were developed for use in patients having deficits caused by poliomyelitis,[31] today most transfers are applied in patients with peripheral nerve injury[13,14] or traumatic muscle loss.[25] Patients with central nervous system disorders are probably a third group in whom tendon transfers are done today. The more recent refiners of the work of the masters include Brand,[3,4] Brand et al,[5] Riordan,[22] Curtis,[10] Littler,[13] Omer,[20,21] White,[32] and Zancolli.[33] Students who plan to work in this field should familiarize themselves with their work.

INDICATIONS FOR TENDON TRANSFER

The absence of a particular needed function after irreparable nerve injury, nerve disease, or muscle loss should bring up a consideration for tendon transfer. Time is allowed for wound healing to occur and for recovery of function, either spontaneously in the case of neuropraxia or axonotmesis or for reinnervation after a nerve repair. This usually requires a delay of 4 to 6 months.[21] Although there are some who have advocated tendon transfer while awaiting recovery, I do not believe that there are many indications for early transfers if nerve regeneration is expected. During this waiting period, it is important that the physician, therapist, and patient work to maintain passive mobility in the involved joints. This would be achieved through passive motion exercises and by the use of splints when indicated. Nerve damage in itself is not always an indication for tendon transfer surgery because patients can sometimes perform unexpectedly through substitutive or adaptive methods or can function through dual-innervated musculature and/or variations in innervation. For example, solitary median nerve injury at the wrist may not result in loss of true thumb opposition in many patients because this action may be performed through the use of thenar eminence muscles partially or completely ulnar nerve innervated.[23] The point here is that each problem must be individualized in terms of the loss of function, its severity, the reconstructive possibilities, and the patient's needs and desires. Also to be stressed is the fact that tendon transfer is a palliative procedure that does not restore full and normal function. It is a redistribution of available power in an attempt to reduce a functional impairment.

When tendon transfer is being considered for the treatment of a particular patient's problem, certain basic conditions should be satisfied, including joint mobility and adequate soft tissue coverage. There must also be available motor tendons for the transfer.

BASIC CONDITIONS FOR TENDON TRANSFER
Joint mobility

The participating joints in the motor function in question should be freely capable of passive motion if the transfer is to succeed. Hand therapy using physical modalities, including dynamic splinting, may be needed to keep the joints mobile. This therapy can be taught to the patient and carried out by himself or herself, but the supervision and guidance of trained therapists are often necessary and are the ideal. At times, if joints have contracted and do not respond to therapy, the surgeon will do preliminary surgical releases to restore passive mobility.

Adequate soft tissue coverage

Well-healed and pliable soft tissues must be present to provide gliding planes through which the transfer can function. This may require the shifting of skin and the use of local, distant, or free vascularized skin flaps before the actual tendon transfer.

Available motor tendons

A donor muscle must be available in the extremity. In single-nerve injury in the upper extremity, there may be a choice of motor tendons available for transfer and suitable for the function needed to be restored. If two of the major nerves in the extremity are involved and irreparably damaged, choices become more limited and the prognosis in terms of function will be greatly reduced. Tendons available in the upper extremity vary with the injury or disease and may include wrist flexors, wrist extensors, flexor digitorum superficialis (FDS), proprius extensors (extensor indicis proprius and extensor digiti minimi, and brachioradialis.

SELECTION OF A MOTOR TENDON FOR TRANSFER

Although most of the transfers performed today have been well described for particular needs, it is useful to understand the decision-making processes that led to the development of specific tendon transfers that are most commonly applied. Boyes, in 1962, discussed those factors involved in the selection of a motor tendon. Amplitude of the donor tendon and power are the prime factors in tendon selection.[2]

Amplitude

The distance that a muscle can shorten from its maximum length is the excursion or amplitude.[5] A muscle contracts to

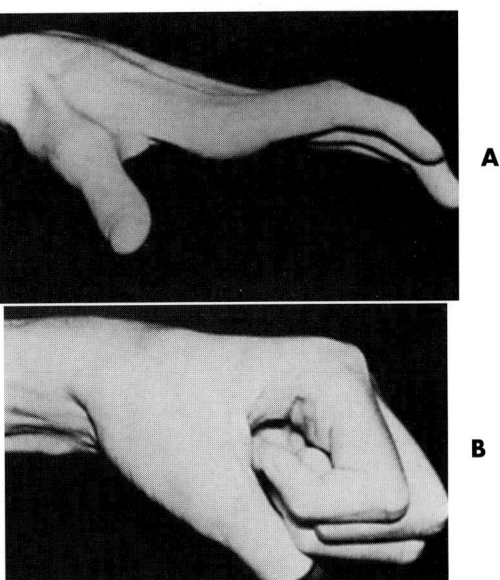

Fig. 47-1. Postoperative photos of a patient with severe injury to median and ulnar nerves in the proximal forearm who had undergone transfer of the extensor carpi radialis longus into the flexor profundi in an attempt to restore finger flexion. **A,** Extension of the fingers. **B,** Flexion through the transfer is surprisingly good.

approximately 40% of its resting length. Average amplitude of the wrist flexors and extensors is about 3.5 cm. Full finger extension at the metacarpophalangeal (MP) joints requires 5 cm and the flexor digitorum profundus (FDP) group needs an amplitude of 7 cm for full flexor function. As motor tendons, the FDS group, which provide an amplitude of about 6 cm, is the only group of available tendons that can approach the necessary amplitude to replace the profundus. Therefore, when the extensor carpi radialis longus is used to power the FDP, some sacrifice in range of motion (ROM) must be accepted (Fig. 47-1). This deficit is partially overcome by the additional amplitude provided to the system by the tenodesis effect of the mobile wrist joint. Restoration of the long extensor system by transfer of a wrist flexor is a better matched situation as far as their respective amplitudes of motion are concerned.

Power

Power ability of a muscle to perform work is directly proportional to its cross-sectional diameter. Examples of the power of muscles relative to each other in the forearm are as follows[10]:

Pronator teres, 1.2 m/kg
Brachioradialis, 1.9 m/kg
Flexor carpi ulnaris, 2.0 m/kg
Flexor carpi radialis, 0.8 m/kg
Extensor carpi radialis longus, 1.1 m/kg
Extensor carpi ulnaris, 1.1 m/kg

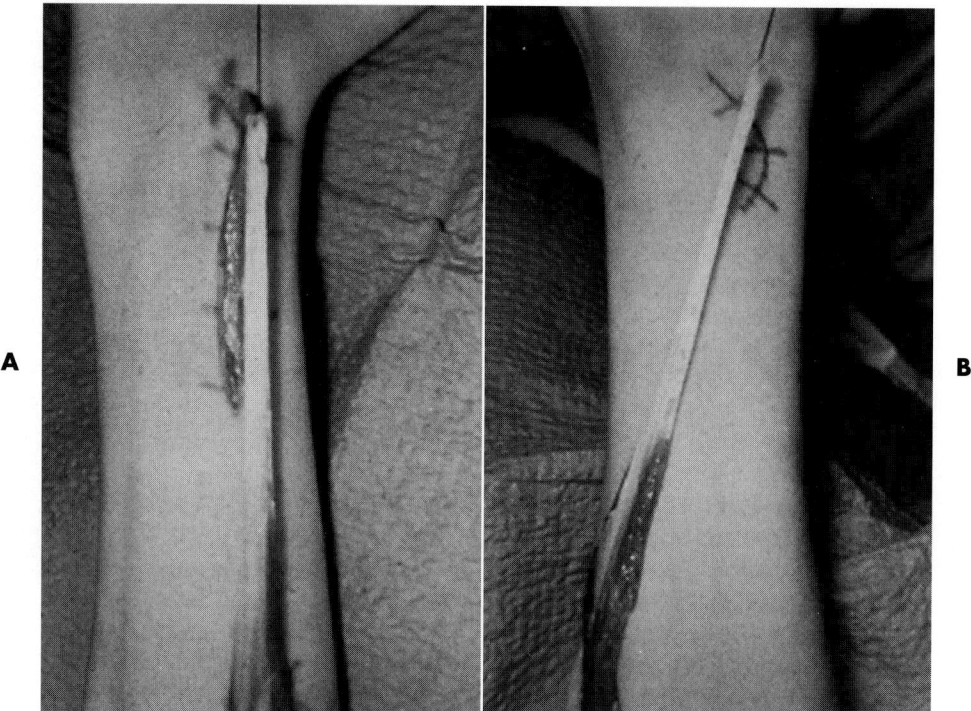

Fig. 47-2. Direction of the tendon transfer should be as straight as possible in its route to its new insertion. **A,** Flexor carpi ulnaris is freed from its insertion and taken back into the proximal forearm. **B,** The tendon is as straight as possible in its route to its new insertion at the radial wrist extensors in this patient with spastic paralysis.

In the preoperative period, accurate muscle testing is essential in the evaluation of a potential motor tendon. Each available muscle must be graded to ensure adequate strength for the transfer. The rating system 0 to 5 is used:

0   Total paralysis
1   Flicker of muscle action
2   Muscle contracts and moves joint with gravity eliminated
3   Muscle moves joint through full ROM against gravity
4   Muscle moves joint through full ROM against resistance
5   Normal muscle

It is widely believed that a transferred muscle loses one grade in strength, but this is questioned by Brand, who believes that the loss of effectiveness experienced after transfer is probably brought about by adhesions and drag rather than by actual loss of muscle strength.[4] Whatever the reason, a four-power muscle may be inadequate for transfer and should be used with caution.

Direction (Fig. 47-2)

The pathway of the transferred muscle should be as straight as possible to its new insertion, which may require extensive proximal mobilization of the muscle. This rule is occasionally violated in redirecting a tendon by the use of a pulley, such as in the flexor superficialis opponensplasty.[6,7] Care must be taken to prevent injury to the nerve and vascular supply of the muscle when extensive mobilization is carried out.

Phase

Wrist extensors and digital flexors perform synergistically and are said to function in phase. The same applies for the activities of wrist flexors and digital extensors. Although it may be true that transfers within the phasic groupings are easier to train, the phasic action of a transfer is no longer regarded as a major factor in the selection of a motor tendon for transfer. In fact, muscles 180 degrees out of phase are not uncommonly used, an example being the use of the FDS as a motor for the extensor digitorum communis in radial nerve paralysis.

TECHNICAL ASPECTS OF TENDON TRANSFERS

When one is setting up a transfer procedure, it is helpful to have a plan of action in which available assets are listed against functional needs. Then, an attempt is made to rebalance the situation providing power for lost functions while, if possible, only minimally affecting present function. The importance of a stable functioning wrist is important for success in many transfers, and wrist fusion is often contraindicated except in extreme situations. For the same reason, it is necessary to preserve at least one wrist extensor and one wrist flexor when these tendons are used as transfers.

The general rules of tendon surgery have to be observed.[17,18] Gentle handling of the tendon to prevent damage to its surface is recommended. When possible, the tendon is passed through soft gliding planes. Appropriate incisions are planned that cross transversely to the planned direction of the transfer, thereby reducing the area of potential adhesion formation. Tendon junctures can be carried out end-to-end, side-to-side, or by interweaving techniques. The junctures should be strong, and nonabsorbable, low-reactive, 3-0 or 2-0 suture material is used. In general, the transfers are put in so as to err on the tight side. This especially applies when transfers are done into the extensor system, where failures are likely to occur if the transfer is too loose.

Plaster immobilization is used for 3 to 4 weeks before removal for exercises. Splint protection is usually added for an additional 3 weeks while the muscle is educated in its new role. If the rules are obeyed, this usually is a rapid relearning process but may at times tax the ingenuity of both surgeon and therapist.

Tendon transfers have proven useful in various paralytic conditions. Many of these procedures were developed in the era of poliomyelitis. With the elimination of this once widespread source of paralyzed patients, these same transfers now serve in the treatment of those with peripheral nerve injury or nervous system disease. At this time, patients with irremediable injuries to the peripheral nerves serve as the largest group to benefit from the application of these same techniques. Other conditions for which these procedures are helpful in the upper extremity include tetraplegia, rheumatoid arthritis,[12,16] traumatic tendon or muscle loss,[26-29] and cerebral palsy. To study these techniques, one very common indication that presents itself for tendon transfer is illustrated.

RESTORATION OF OPPOSITION TO THE PARALYZED THUMB
Opposition transfer[11,19]

The application of the tip of the thumb to the fingers is essential for the performance of most fine manipulative functions and also in heavy gripping. When the thumb is in true opposition, its pad is opposite the pad of the finger.[8,33] This complex positioning action is accomplished through the activity of the thenar muscles, mainly the abductor pollicis brevis, but the opponens as well as the flexor pollicis brevis also contribute. As power is added, the flexor pollicis longus and the abductor pollicis brevis come into play. The motion, occurring mainly at the basilar joint of the thumb, the trapezial-metacarpal joint, starts with abduction, then pronation, and finally flexion in a complex maneuver.[9] It should be stressed that this transfer is palliative, and in severe paralysis, the transfer of one motor cannot restore all elements of this complex action.

Loss of ability to oppose the thumb to the fingers is a devastating loss to the hand. Patients with this deficiency will have median nerve injuries at some level, which has led to the paralysis of the thenar group muscles. Not all patients with median nerve damage need surgery to restore opposition because some hands function quite well through ulnar-innervated muscles in the thenar eminence.[23] Careful preoperative evaluation is therefore essential. When both the median and the ulnar nerves are irretrievably injured, the need for oppositionplasty is more clear cut.

General principles for opponensplasty

Bunnell[6] told us that any tendon that pulls subcutaneously from the general area of the pisiform bone and inserts into the dorsal ulnar corner of the base of the proximal phalanx of the thumb would help restore lost opposition. This means that many different tendons could be used in the restoration of this function.[8,24] Minkow[19] and Herrick and Lister[11] undertook reviews of the literature on this subject and came up with many different techniques and scores of references on this topic.

Preoperative evaluation

The therapist and surgeon should attempt to learn what the patient needs and expects from the procedure. Because most patients with loss of opposition also have decreased sensation in the thumb, this latter deficit may, in fact, be the primary functional problem. The preoperative period should be occupied with restoration and maintenance of passive opposition and, if necessary, loosening the basilar joint of the thumb using therapy measures. Pretransfer surgery, such as joint release, may be necessary if therapy cannot return a useful range of passive motion. At times, surgical manipulation of skin in the form of skin grafts and scar revisions may be necessary to provide a satisfactory gliding bed for the transfer. To illustrate the application of the tendon transfer to the restoration of opposition, see Figs. 47-3 and 47-4.

CAUSES FOR DISAPPOINTMENT IN TENDON TRANSFERS

Suboptimal results do occur in tendon transfer, and this is a more likely event when an overly ambitious program is attempted in severe functional loss. This can be avoided if realistic attainable goals are established. Although the reinstitution of active motion through transfer is desirable, the treating surgeon should not lose sight of the place for tenodeses and arthrodeses in the reconstructive program.

When patients whose results were found to be less than expected were analyzed, the following issues were seen to have been a factor.

1. Acceptance of less than full passive motion before transfer

A   **B**   **C**

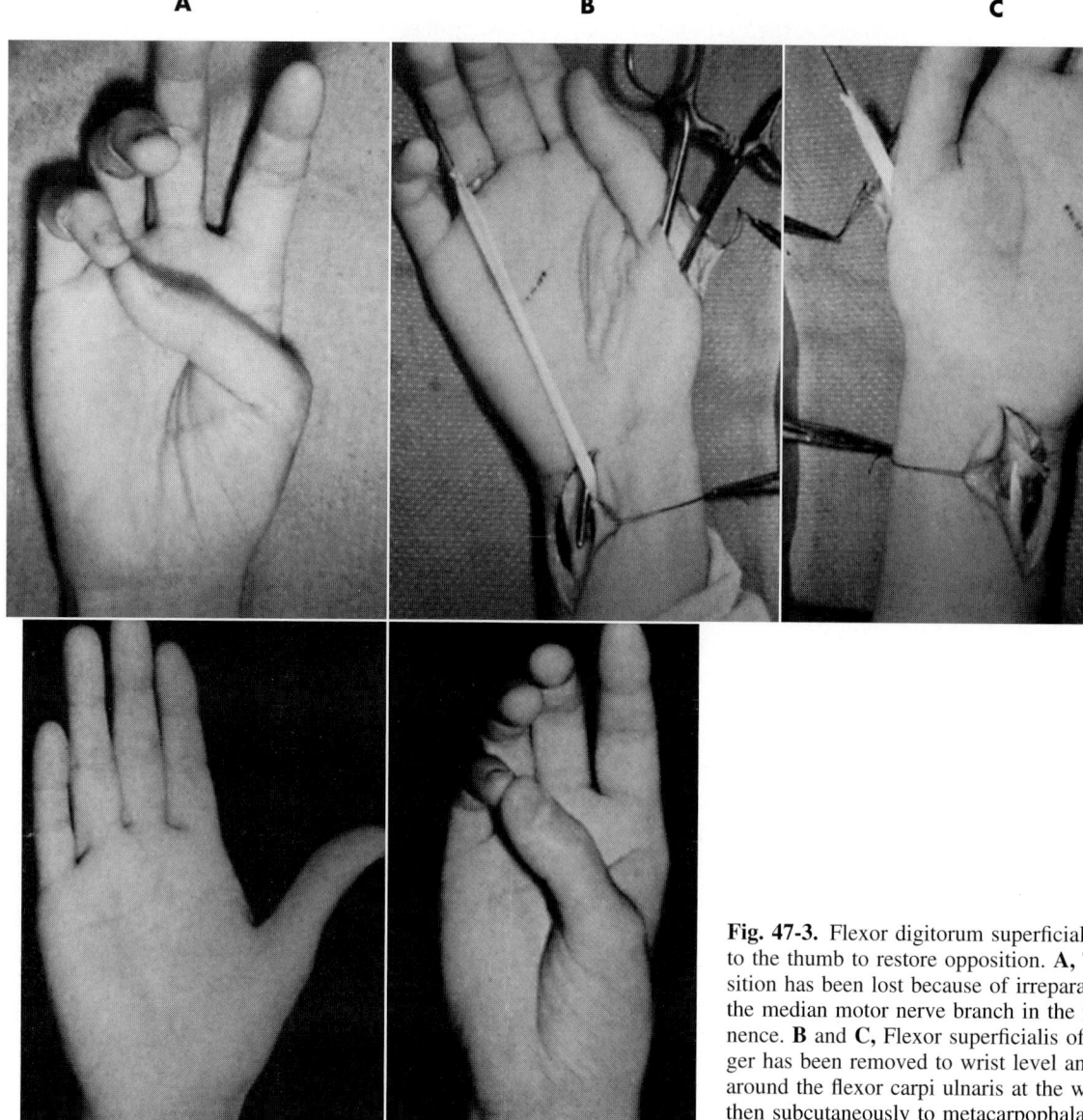

D   **E**

Fig. 47-3. Flexor digitorum superficialis transferred to the thumb to restore opposition. **A,** True opposition has been lost because of irreparable injury to the median motor nerve branch in the thenar eminence. **B** and **C,** Flexor superficialis of ring finger has been removed to wrist level and passed around the flexor carpi ulnaris at the wrist and then subcutaneously to metacarpophalangeal joint region of the thumb. **D** and **E,** The range of motion into opposition is shown.

2. Overestimation of the strength of the donor muscle (careful here, especially when transferring a reinnervated muscle)
3. Adhesions along the course of transfer
4. Technical failures
   - Breakdown of the juncture
   - Transfer put in too tight or too loose

The solutions to these problems include careful attention to the details of evaluation and surgery. It should be remembered that tendon transfer is a palliative procedure, and although great gains in function can be accomplished, normal function is not expected.

SUMMARY

The dynamic procedure that involves the transfer of the action of a muscle from its usual function to a different one is still an exciting and challenging area of reconstructive extremity surgery. Although the guidelines discussed here have been well established, they are nonetheless guidelines and at times may have to be modified in individual difficult cases with the understanding that prognosis may be affected. For example, the absence of some of the preoperative criteria may not contraindicate surgery if it is done with the foreknowledge that there will be a reduced prognosis. Careful planning and preoperative patient evaluation, along

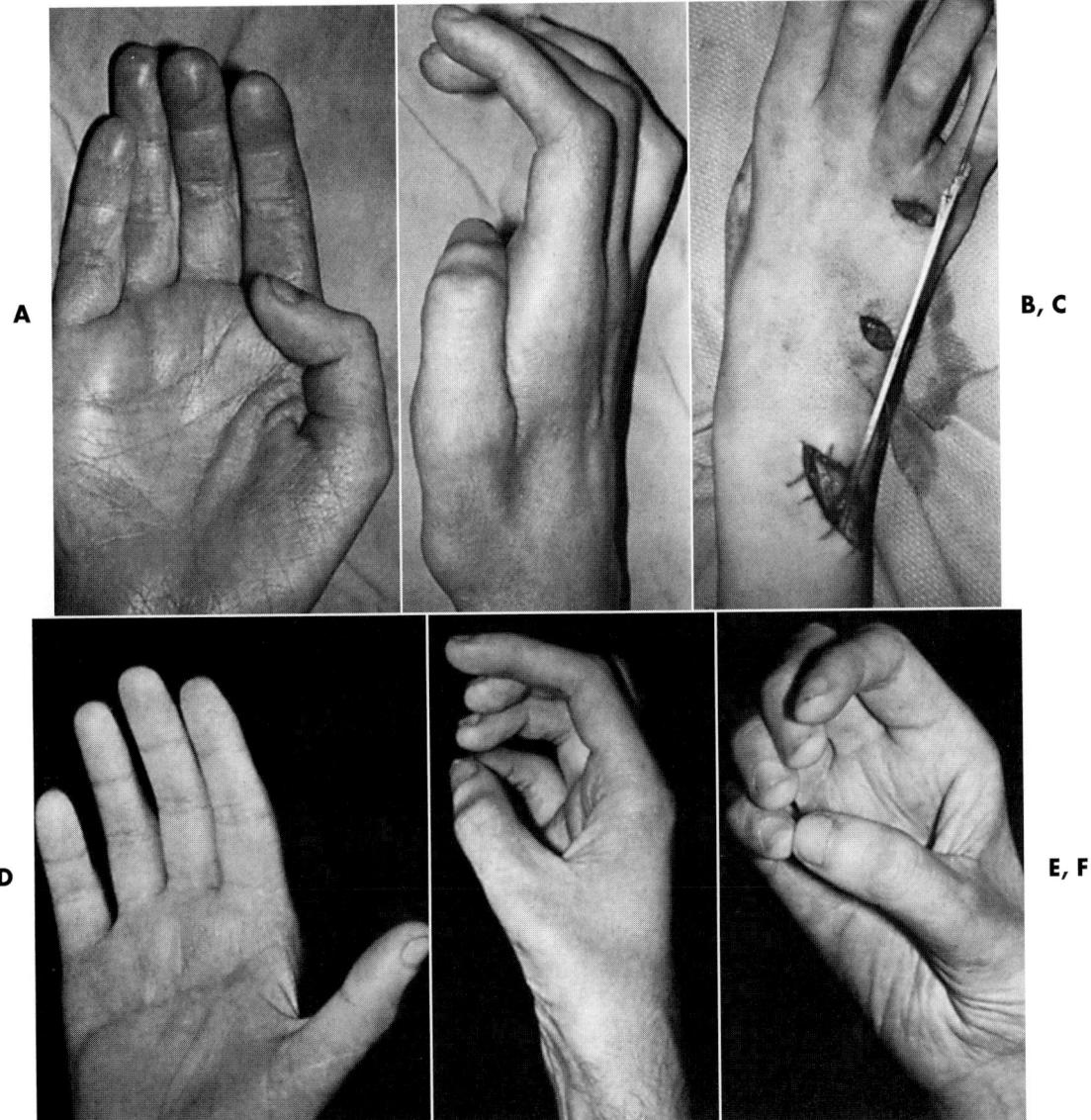

Fig. 47-4. Restoration of opposition using the extensor digiti minimi.[24] Brachial plexus injury had left this 20-year-old man with a loss of opposition and shortage of available motors for opponensplasty. The extensor digiti minimi was normal and available. **A,** Preoperative attempt at opposition shows the thumb to be ineffective. **B,** Preoperative radial view. The thumb cannot be brought out of the plane of the palm. **C,** The extensor digiti minimi is mobilized through three incisions and then will be passed subcutaneously around the border of the ulna to be inserted into the abductor pollicis brevis. **D, E,** and **F,** Result of the transfer at 6 months. Excellent opposition has been restored.

with attention to the details of the procedure, can benefit the patient, therapist, and surgeon.

REFERENCES

1. Adamson J, Wilson JN: The history of flexor tendon grafting, *J Bone Joint Surg* 43A:709, 1961.
2. Boyes JH: Selection of a donor motor for tendon transfer, *Bull Hosp Joint Dis* 23:1, 1962.
3. Brand PW: Biomechanics of tendon transfer, *Orthop Clin North Am* 5:205, 1974.
4. Brand PW: *Clinical mechanics of the hand,* St Louis, 1985, Mosby.
5. Brand PW, Beach RB, Thompson DE: Relative tension and potential excursion of muscles in the forearm and hand, *J Hand Surg* 553, 1981.
6. Bunnell S: Opposition of the thumb, *J Bone Joint Surg* 20:269, 1938.
7. Bunnell S: Tendon transfer in the hand and forearm. In American Academy of Orthopaedic Surgeons: *Instructional course lectures 6:106,* Ann Arbor, Mich, 1949, JW Edwards.
8. Burkhalter WE: Median nerve palsy. In Green DP, editor: *Operative hand surgery,* New York, 1988, Churchill Livingstone.

9. Cooney WP, Linscheid RL, An KN: Opposition of the thumb: An anatomic and biomechanical study of tendon transfers, *J Hand Surg* 9:777, 1984.

10. Curtis RM: Fundamental principles of tendon transfer, *Orthop Clin North Am* 5:231, 1974.

11. Herrick RT, Lister GD: Control of first web space contracture, *The Hand* 9:253, 1977.

12. Kwon ST, Schneider LH: Extensor tendon ruptures in rheumatoid arthritis. In Hunter JM, Schneider LH, Mackin EJ, editors: *Tendon and nerve surgery in the hand: a third decade.* St Louis, 1997, Mosby.

13. Littler JW: Tendon transfers and arthrodeses in combined median and ulnar palsies, *J Bone Joint Surg* 31A:225, 1949.

14. Littler JW: Restoration of power and stability in the partially paralyzed hand. In Converse J, editor: *Reconstructive plastic surgery,* vol 4, Philadelphia, 1964, WB Saunders.

15. Manktelow RT, Zuherf RM, McKee NH: Functioning free muscle transplantation, *J Hand Surg* 9:32, 1984.

16. Mannerfelt LG: Tendon transfers in surgery of the rheumatoid hand, *Hand Clin North Am* 4:309, 1988.

17. Mayer L: The physiological method of tendon transplantation, *Surg Gynecol Obstet* 22:182, 1916.

18. Mayer L: The physiological method of tendon transplants renewed after forty years. In American Academy of Orthopaedic Surgeons: *Instructional course lectures 12:116,* Ann Arbor, Mich, 1955, JW Edwards.

19. Minkow FV: Operations to restore thumb opposition: a historical review. In *AAOS symposium on tendon surgery in the hand,* St Louis, 1975, Mosby.

20. Omer GE: Evaluation and reconstruction of the forearm and hand after acute traumatic peripheral nerve injuries, *J Bone Surg* 50A:1454, 1968.

21. Omer GE: The technique and timing of tendon transfers, *Orthop Clin North Am* 5:243, 1974.

22. Riordan DC: Surgery of the paralytic hand. In American Academy of Orthopaedic Surgeons: *Instructional course lectures 16:79,* St Louis, 3959, Mosby.

23. Rowntree T: Anomalous innervations of the hand muscles, *J Bone Joint Surg* 44: 26O, 1949.

24. Schneider LH: Opponensplasty using the extensor digiti minimi, *J Bone Joint Surg* 51A:1297, 1969.

25. Schneider LH: Tendon transfers in muscle and tendon loss, *Hand Clin North Am* 4:267, 1988.

26. Schneider LH: Tendon transfers for radial nerve palsy. In Gelberman RH, editor: *Operative nerve repair and reconstruction.* Philadelphia, 1991, JB Lippincott.

27. Schneider LH, Rosenstein R: Restoration of extensor pollucis longus function by tendon transfer, *Plast Reconstr Surg* 71:533, 1983.

28. Schneider LH, Wehbe MA: Delayed repair of flexor profundus tendon in the palm (zone 3) with superficialis transfer, *J Hand Surg* 13A:227, 1988.

29. Schneider LH, Whiltshire D: Restoration of flexor pollucis longus function by flexor digitorum superficialis transfer, *J Hand Surg* 8:98, 1983.

30. Smith RI: *Tendon transfers of the hand and forearm,* Boston, 1987, Little, Brown.

31. Waterman JH: Tendon transplantation: its history, indications and technique, *Med News* 32:54, 1902.

32. White WL: Restoration of function and balance of the wrist and hand by tendon transfers, *Surg Clin North Am* 40:427, 1960.

33. Zancolli E: *Structural and dynamic bases of hand surgery,* Philadelphia, 1968, JB Lippincott.

Chapter 48

PREOPERATIVE AND POSTOPERATIVE MANAGEMENT OF TENDON TRANSFERS AFTER MEDIAN- AND ULNAR-NERVE INJURY

Judith A. Bell-Krotoski

THE ROLE OF THERAPY IN TENDON TRANSFER SURGERY

If surgical repairs were perfect and tissue healing occurred in predictable and precise order and timing, little might be required of therapists in the preoperative and postoperative management of tendon transfers. The surgeon would have to concentrate only on his or her surgical technique, and the patient would need to cooperate with immobilization only for the necessary healing period. In the imperfect world of reality, surgery is sometimes more an art than a science. Results of tendon transfers, in large part, depend on the deft hands of skilled surgeons, and anticipated healing can follow any course.

Results of surgery can be enhanced greatly either by the surgeon extending his or her fingers and acting as a therapist or by developing a close, interactive relationship with a therapist who works in concert with the surgeon and the patient. Therapy cannot improve every surgical case and, in some cases, is not needed nor warranted in view of cost versus potential benefits. However, therapy often can make the difference between a marginal result and a good one, and therapy intervention at appropriate points in patient treatment can ward off potential disasters. Regardless of who assumes the therapist role, he or she must know specific guidelines and, even more important, must be able to determine when those guidelines apply and when exceptions are appropriate and safely made.

The therapist, who often is in a position to augment or improve surgical results, also is in a position to affect adversely the surgical results. Unless it is established that the therapist knows when to consult about problems and changes in treatment, he or she will never gain the confidence of the surgeon, which is necessary for early and innovative hand therapy. The surgeon-therapist-patient interaction is different with different surgeons, and the treating therapist is well advised to exercise the old adage "when in doubt, check it out."

When an interactive relationship is established between the surgeon and therapist, the background is set for a program of postoperative follow-up that is determined by the needs of the patient. In an uncomplicated postoperative period, for example, (1) significant swelling or adhesion formation that could limit excursion of tendons is absent and (2) new transfers can be identified and mobilized throughout most range of motion (ROM). The therapist's job is simplified to one of overseeing, protecting, and implementing the patient's return to hand function in a safe and timely manner.

Not all postoperative hand cases progress smoothly, and the therapist often finds it necessary to become more aggressive in treatment and in implementation of treatment changes. For example, if a patient is developing abnormal postoperative swelling, it immediately becomes necessary to monitor that swelling and to implement remediation techniques.

Elevation of the surgical hand, patient education about the need to elevate the surgical hand, and a plan to check postoperative swelling exemplify the first type of protective/educational therapy. The therapist consulting with the surgeon and releasing a constricting area of the cast or finding a way to ensure that a noncompliant patient will elevate the hand exemplify the second type of therapy—interventive therapy.

THERAPIST IN THE OPERATING ROOM

The importance of the therapist's understanding of the surgical procedure cannot be overstated. The therapist should know the specific muscle-tendon units transferred,[24,33,36,37] including their origin and insertion (normal and transferred insertions), through what route, to what surface, through what pulley (or other structure), and into what structure for attachment.[11,42] The site or level of tendon suture is also important. If tendon grafts are used, the donor tendon, type of graft, and site or level of attachment also should be known. The timing of the surgery or stage of surgery is important to the projection of expected results. Fortunately, this information is usually on the operative report in the patient's medical record. A copy of this report can be included in therapy records.

What is not readily available is the subtle information not found in the medical chart. This information includes the surgeon's "feeling" about the success or failure of the surgery, his or her opinion of the appearance or feel of a tendon, the strength of the anastomosis, the intended tension for the tendon, and the potential the surgeon sees for a tendon scarring down or rupturing. This information can be gained only by communication between surgeon and therapist. To foster this communication, the therapist's initial presence in the operating room is advantageous. The therapist's observation of surgery, as normal and poor-quality tendons are found, problems are encountered, solutions are worked out, alternative plans are made, and results are anticipated, gives the therapist an understanding that is difficult to obtain otherwise. For example, the therapist develops an understanding of how much force can be used safely in mobilizing a newly transferred tendon by watching the surgeon retract on the tendon in surgery to check the strength of the anastomosis.

Perhaps most important, the therapist's presence in the operating room gives the surgeon an appreciation of the depth of understanding of the surgical procedure that the therapist is willing to seek. The therapist's presence provides opportunity for the surgeon to teach his or her specific techniques and idiosyncrasies to the therapist. The surgeon then views the therapist as "hand taught." This interaction

pays tenfold as the surgeon entrusts to the therapist with his or her cases, in all of whom the surgeon has made an investment, has ultimate responsibility, and has the highest hopes for success. The surgeon then appreciates and considers the therapist's comments and suggestions regarding possible surgical procedures, alternative ways of treatment, and new approaches.

In addition, the therapist in the operating room has an opportunity to take photographs. While observing surgery, many therapists photograph difficult or unusual cases. The photographs are most appreciated after a particularly good result from a difficult case. They become invaluable records for teaching and training and in the monitoring of results from the surgery/therapy program.

TENDON TRANSFERS AS REBALANCING PROCEDURES

Bunnell[3] first described tendon transfers as *rebalancing procedures*. Time has added to the understanding of this approach. The hand is a delicate but durable balance of flexors and extensors, stabilizers and positioners that quickly interchange in balance and on command for performing 72 operational tasks.[13] With few arguable exceptions, all of the muscles of the hand are needed for operational balance, and one muscle cannot be transferred without having a direct biomechanical effect on others.[7,17,38,41,42] Thus tendon transfer surgery is the attempt to rebalance internally what has become imbalanced as a result of disease or injury, which causes the loss of certain muscles in the system. Therefore tendon transfers must be considered within their functional relationship with other muscle-tendon units.[5,9]

The therapist can best appreciate and augment the balance that has been restored to a hand that has undergone tendon rebalancing surgery by seeing and measuring the hand before surgery. At that time, the hand exhibits its biomechanical imbalance in a number of ways that can be recorded and with which postoperative balance can be compared.

BIOMECHANICS OF DEFORMITY

In ulnar-nerve injuries, the power grip functions of the hand are diminished or lost (the more diminished, the higher the level of injury). This loss compromises hand function.[12,25] Normally, the ulnarmost two fingers, the ring and little fingers, supply the power flexion aspect of the hand, whereas the most radial two fingers, the index and middle fingers, are freed for manipulation with the thumb. When the power function of the ulnar two fingers is lost because of nerve injury, the radial two fingers must assume this function on hand grasp, and freedom for manipulation during grasp is lost. Power grasp is weakened further by the selective loss of intrinsic muscles of the thumb and hypothenar eminence, reducing hand grasp and the thumb's mechanical stabilization against the fingers during hand use. The lack of intrinsic stabilization of the hypothenar muscles leads to a flattened or reversed metacarpal arch, changing the whole structural

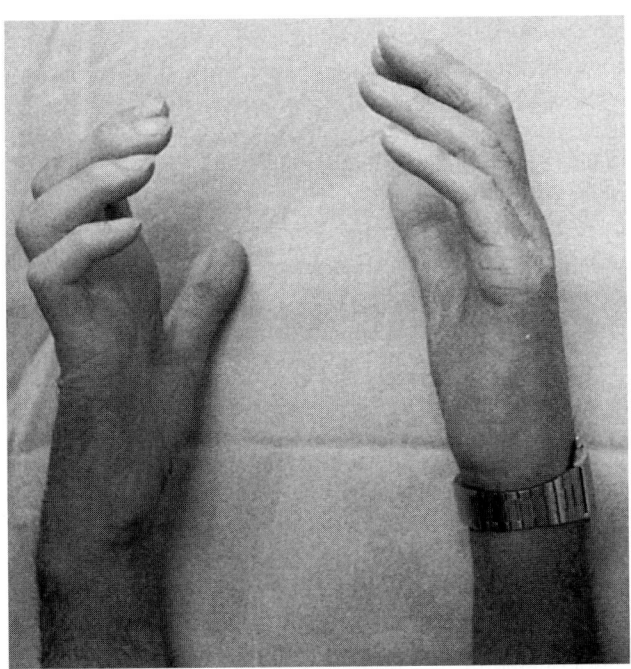

Fig. 48-1. Patient with bilateral ulnar- and median-nerve loss. Hand on the left is uncorrected; hand on the right has been surgically corrected by intrinsic replacement transfers. Intrinsic muscles of the hand supply balance to the finger flexor and extensor systems, without which the fingers collapse on use.

arrangement of the thumb and the fourth and fifth metacarpals, which normally rotate around the keystone second and third metacarpals during grasp.

Low nerve injury

Fingers. Power grip is specifically diminished in low ulnar-nerve injuries by the inability of the fingers (most ulnar two and sometimes middle and index) to assume lumbrical positions and gradations of lumbrical positions. In median- or ulnar-nerve injuries, the fingers biomechanically collapse on attempts at extension and flexion.[14,18] On attempts at finger extension, the metacarpophalangeal (MP) joints that have lost their intrinsic support in flexion hyperextend by unopposed overpull of the extrinsic finger extensor (extensor digitorum communis [EDC]), mechanically limiting full gliding and extension of the dorsal hood and thus full extension of the fingers at the interphalangeal (IP) joints[23] (Fig. 48-1). When the proximal interphalangeal (PIP) joints can fully extend, they do not until the MP joints are fully extended.[20] On patient attempts at finger flexion, the absence of the intrinsics as primary flexors at the MP joint and extenders on the opposite surface at the IP finger joint results in the unopposed out-of-sequence overpull of the extrinsic finger flexors (flexor digitorum superficialis [FDS] and flexor digitorum profundus [FDP]) into flexion. The distal interphalangeal (DIP) and PIP joints must fully flex before excursion of the extrinsic finger flexors can flex the MP joints.

The intrinsic muscles then supply the balance to the flexor and extensor systems, without which the fingers lose their selective positioning and support in selective positions. The power that normally would be available from the extrinsic finger flexors and extensors is lost because their power is wasted either fully flexing or fully extending their specific finger joints, beginning with the points of their insertions; there is no in-between. This imbalance and collapse of the fingers is seen as the fingers attempt to assume full flexion, extension, and lumbrical positions. The collapse is demonstrated even more significantly by any load that is applied to the fingers, such as when the patient attempts to pick up objects. Objects cannot be held by the involved fingers unless the fingers are fully flexed at the IP joints (to the size limits of the object).

In low median-nerve injuries, the radial two fingers, the index and middle, can be compromised severely in their ability to provide fine manipulation necessary for dexterity. In some cases, little change in function of the index and middle fingers is apparent with injury of the median nerve.

Although the median nerve usually innervates the lumbricals to the radial two fingers (the index and middle) and the ulnar nerve innervates the ulnar two fingers and the dorsal and palmar interossei to all the fingers, there can be overlap of intrinsic innervation between the ulnar and median nerves. The ulnar nerve sometimes innervates all of the intrinsic muscles to the index and middle fingers. The variations in ulnar-nerve innervation must be considered in tendon transfer rebalancing. If the intrinsics to the index and middle fingers are innervated only partially, or are only weak versus absent, these fingers may not show as much imbalance as the ulnar two fingers and may sometimes be considered normal. It is important that the fingers be loaded with some force resistance for testing. They can be tested in the lumbrical position with resistance at the proximal phalanx (Fig. 48-2, *A*). If they collapse with resistance, as in Fig. 48-2, *B,* they are imbalanced for hand use and should be included in surgical rebalancing procedures.

The ulnar-nerve–innervated hypothenar muscle mass, and in particular the opponens digiti quinti, flexes, stabilizes, and brings into opposition the fourth and fifth metacarpals and ulnar two fingers and, with the thumb, enables the hand to cup the palm securely and grasp around objects. Loss to the intrinsic hypothenar muscles and resultant flattened or reversed metacarpal arch disrupts the grasping and securing power functions of the hand, leaving the patient to experience weakness and clumsiness in handling large objects.

Some hands with intrinsic losses from nerve injuries may not appear to claw enough to warrant surgery. Surgery may not be indicated when cosmesis of the hand is the major consideration or in a few instances when the structure of the hand permits the patient to compensate without deforming imbalance. Biomechanically, the median- or ulnar-nerve–injured hand is imbalanced and greatly limited in function in

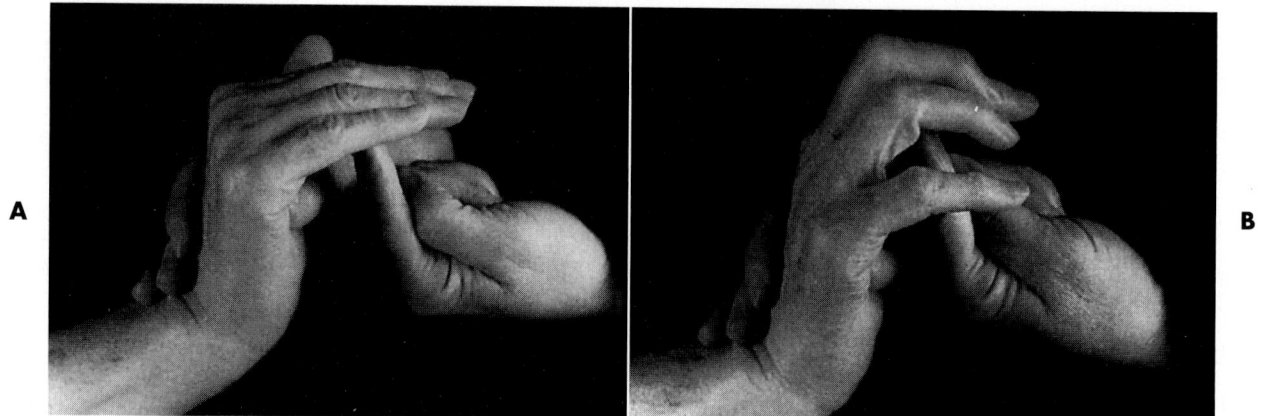

Fig. 48-2. **A,** Intrinsic balance of fingers may appear normal, and the patient may be able to assume a lumbrical position, until loaded with external force. **B,** In ulnar-nerve injuries, it is important to also test the middle and index fingers for collapse.

the previously described ways. Even when cosmesis is the major concern, the appearance of the hand may be deceptive because the imbalance usually becomes more exaggerated and more deforming over time.

In the imbalanced hand caused by nerve weakness or loss, remodeling of the skin and joints usually occurs as the hand is used in abnormal patterns with abnormal forces. The MP joints lose their soft tissue retention and overstretch into hyperextension, sometimes even rupturing volar plates and elongating other soft tissue restraints at this joint by the enormous overpower of the imbalanced extrinsic finger extensor as the patient tries unsuccessfully to fully extend his or her fingers. As the IP joints remodel, the skin over their dorsal surface grows, whereas skin is lost on the volar surface. Joint stiffness occurs when the joints do not operate in their full ROM. The extensor tendons eventually become attenuated. All in all, the imbalance is progressive into deformity, and when these changes have occurred, results of tendon transfer surgery are likewise progressively compromised. The amount the surgery is compromised is directly proportional to the extent and duration of secondary changes and tissue remodeling.[8] Therefore tendon transfer surgery is best performed while the hands appear not to claw enough to warrant surgery, before secondary remodeling changes have become established and have worsened.

Remodeling and progressive deformity take time but are accelerated by the force with which the patient uses the hand and the patient's lack of passive extension of the involved joints. The muscle imbalance that occurs when the fingers collapse into flexion causes abnormal force concentrated at the tips of the involved fingers and distal palm as the hand grips and manipulates objects in abnormal positions. In addition to soft tissue damage caused by excessive concentration of force, abnormal forces on joints can add to or cause joint stiffness and cause joint structural damage.[4,39]

Remodeling and progressive deformity also are accelerated by reduced or absent sensory feedback. The sensory portion of the ulnar nerve is often involved if the motor portion is involved. If the sensory portion of the nerve is compromised in addition to the motor part of the ulnar nerve, the patient has lost the feedback system that reports how much force he or she is using with the fingers, and enormous force can be concentrated in small areas of skin, such as at the tips of the fingers. The skin was never intended to be subjected to such force on a repetitive basis,[27,40] and the result is injury, scarring, and callus formation, with compromised skin nutrition. In imbalanced hands that are heavily used, bony and soft tissue reabsorption can occur, leading to deformity and shortening of the fingers.

Minimal use of the hand does not prevent deformity. Remodeling of the hand will occur in the biomechanically imbalanced hand that is used or in one that is not used. In some cases, the greatest tendon attenuation, skin contractures, and joint stiffness will occur in the hand that is not used in preference to a good "other" extremity. This is because some mechanical stress (force X area) on the skin in moderate amounts, as produced in a balanced hand, is normal and is beneficial in maintaining healthy skin. Skin of hands that either cannot be or are not used becomes thin and shiny and tears easily. Joints that are not used lose their normal synovial gliding surfaces.[35]

Attenuation of the finger extensor tendons from remodeling that has occurred can be shown by the examiner fully flexing the patient's MP joints, blocking these in flexion, and asking the patient to extend the IP joints with the extrinsic finger extensor (EDC) (Fig. 48-3). The intrinsic-minus hand with no tendon attenuation can extend the IP joints fully when the MP joints are flexed because the extrinsic finger extensor is positioned where it can extend the IP joints. If extension of the joints is limited or absent (and the joints will

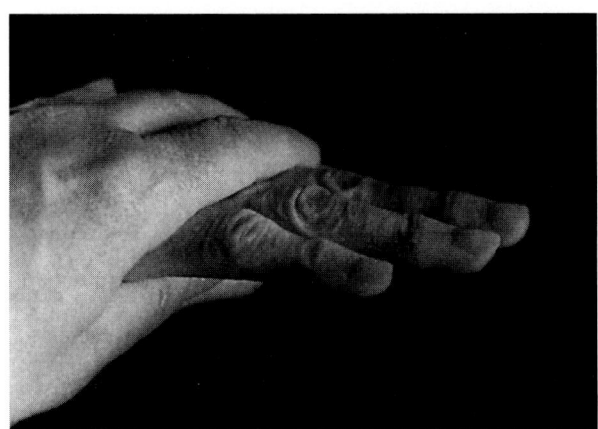

Fig. 48-3. Unless the extensor tendons are attenuated, the intrinsic-minus fingers should extend fully at the interphalangeal joint by the extrinsic finger extensor (extensor digitorum communis) when the metacarpophalangeal joint is supported in flexion or kept from hyperextending.

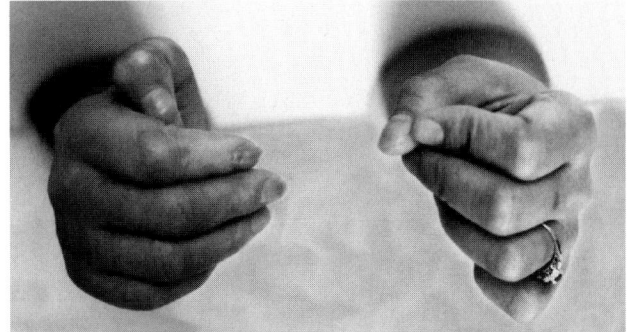

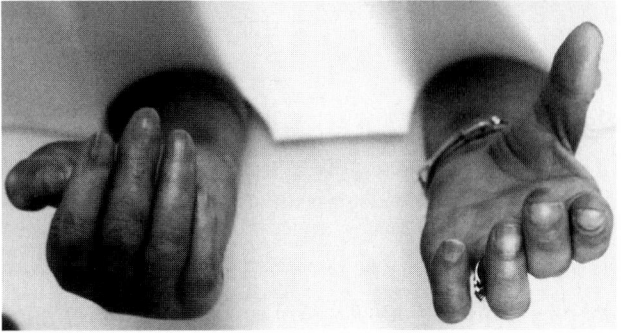

Fig. 48-4. In median-nerve injuries, the ability to abduct and bring the thumb into opposition with the fingers is lost **(A),** and the thumb is rotated out of the palm by the unopposed action of the muscles that extend, adduct, and externally rotate the thumb **(B).**

otherwise passively extend), attenuation of the extensor tendons is probable. In checking for attenuation, one must ascertain that the extrinsic extensor has the strength to extend the fingers; for example, no radial-nerve involvement is present.

Another remodeling problem can limit or reduce active extension of the IP joints. After a hand has been positioned and used in an intrinsic-minus position (i.e., claw hand position), the short extrinsic flexor (FDS) muscle-tendon units often shorten through loss of muscle sarcomeres. The short extrinsic flexor tends to become shortened more than the long extrinsic flexor (FDP) because of the usually more severe flexion-contracture of the fingers at the PIP joint. The long extrinsic flexor can contract also. The initiating cause is the intrinsic-minus imbalance: The muscle-tendon units of the extrinsic flexors respond by readjusting to their reduced tension requirement when the fingers are maintained in a claw position.[28] This contracture can be checked first by passively extending the fingers fully with the wrist flexed, then passively extending the fingers fully with the wrist in extension. Tightness of the extrinsic superficialis will limit the full passive or active extension of the IP joints with the wrist in extension much more than with the wrist in flexion.

Thumb. Mechanically, because the thumb must operate by itself in space unsupported by any other digit, it depends on at least three muscles in proper alignment to support its position.[20,21] To translate directional force across joints, it depends on at least one muscle to hold a joint position and another muscle to supply force in that position. The extrinsic and intrinsic muscles position the thumb. Then the intrinsic muscles supply the power to hold that position for force to be translated by the extrinsic muscles for use. (The whole system is like a fishing rod: The wrist holding the rod is supplying the intrinsic power to stabilize the line, and the

winding of the reel is supplying the extrinsic power to bring in the fish. If the intrinsic wrist support is lost, so is the extrinsic power. The hand that was supplying the external power by winding the reel must now support and stabilize the rod, thus the reel cannot be wound.)

In median-nerve injuries, the ability to abduct and bring the thumb into opposition with the fingers is lost, and the thumb is rotated out of the palm by the unopposed action of the muscles that extend, adduct, and externally rotate the thumb (Fig. 48-4). It has been said that what makes the difference between the hand function of humans versus that of the ape is the opposable thumb in humans. Manipulation of the hand in median-nerve injury is greatly affected by the inability to assume the position for best prehension, and a decrease in selective positioning of the thumb and sometimes index and middle fingers. Grip is reduced by the inability of the thumb to make a wide opening out of the palm to close around objects, and the inability of the thumb to stabilize around objects for a secure and locking grasp.

In median-nerve injury, there is a flattening of thenar muscle mass but its mass is innervated both by the ulnar and median nerves. It is fortunate that for a function as critical as the thumb, that if one nerve is lost, total use of the thumb is not lost. However, where there is median and ulnar involvement, the combined results is total loss of thenar musculature, and the thumb is operated (in low nerve injury)

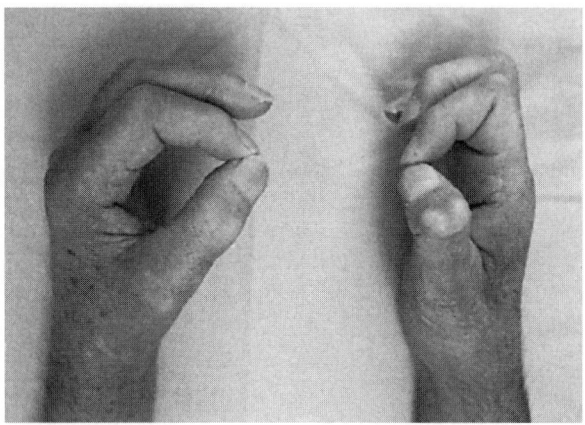

Fig. 48-5. Partial weakness or loss of thumb intrinsic muscles in the ulnar-nerve–injured hand also results in a collapsing instability and weakened pinch in normal positions. Hand on the left has been surgically corrected by a ring superficialis transfer to the thumb; on the right, contralateral hand with ulnar-nerve injury is uncorrected.

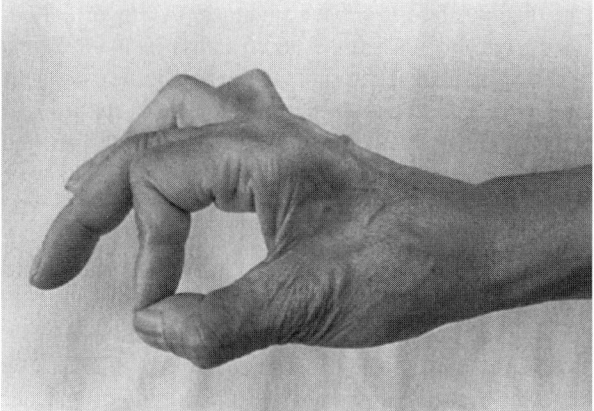

Fig. 48-6. Froment's sign. When used in this position, the thumb must flex at the interphalangeal joint before the strength of the extrinsic flexor (flexor pollicis longus) can be used to pick up objects. The skin and tendons at the interphalangeal joint eventually become attenuated. Note hyperextension of index interphalangeal in thumb pinch.

only by extrinsic muscles without their stabilizers and positioners.

In the low median-nerve injury, some of the intrinsics of the thumb are disrupted, whereas the extrinsic muscles acting on the thumb remain intact. Usually lost are the abductor pollicis brevis, the opponens pollicis, and the superficial head of the flexor pollicis brevis (FPB). Reconstruction of the thumb for function requires transfer procedures that both rotate the thumb back into the palm and stabilize it for function. This is hard to accomplish by one tendon transfer only unless it is given more than one point of insertion (splits into two insertion points that will help stabilize prehension).

In the low ulnar-nerve injury, some of the intrinsics of the thumb are disrupted, whereas the extrinsic muscles acting on the thumb remain intact. The lateral half of the intrinsic flexor of the thumb, the first dorsal interosseous, and the adductor (adductor pollicis brevis) usually are lost. Some overlap of innervation with the median nerve can occur, particularly in an anatomic Martin-Gruber anastomosis of the nerves.[10] Any disruption of a muscle around the thumb or finger metacarpals causes an instability (flexible torque tube of Agee[1]). The partial weakness or loss of the thumb intrinsics in the ulnar-nerve–injured hand causes a collapsing instability of the thumb and a weakened pinch in normal positions (Fig. 48-5).

Without all or part of the intrinsic flexor of the thumb (FPB), its stabilization, and the stabilization provided by the adductor at the thumb MP joint, the extrinsic flexor (flexor pollicis longus) overpulls into hyperflexion at the IP joint, as in Fig. 48-6 (Froment's sign).[8] As with the fingers, the thumb must fully flex before full strength of the extrinsic flexor can be used to pick up objects. Thus the thumb, when used, collapses into flexion.

The patient may attempt to stabilize the thumb also by extending the thumb IP joint (positioning the thumb so the force of the index against the thumb on pinch will fully extend the thumb IP joint) and flexing the MP joint as in Fig. 48-7 (reverse Froment's sign).[8] In this case, the patient uses the soft tissue restraint of the dorsal MP joint to block further flexion and the volar IP joint to block further IP joint extension.

Either way the thumb is used, it is unstable and usually progresses into deformity as the soft tissue restraints tend to remodel and elongate from excessive stress. Abnormal excessive force, which can be deforming, is concentrated in the MP and IP joints of the thumb and at the tip of the thumb. Secondary joint stiffness and contracture are common, particularly in flexion of the thumb at the IP joint.

The loss of the first dorsal interosseous muscle in the ulnar-nerve–injured hand adds an additional problem to the thumb and also to the index finger because this muscle is in large part responsible for stabilizing the thumb metacarpal and providing stability for lateral pinch against the index. One head of the muscle originates from the thumb metacarpal and inserts on the base of the index proximal phalanx, and one head originates from the index metacarpal and inserts on the base of the index proximal phalanx. Both provide adduction of the index against the thumb and index stability against ulnar rotation. The first dorsal interosseous has a larger tension fraction than most of the flexor profundus and flexor superficialis muscles.[8] Without this muscle, the thumb loses stability against the index finger, and with the additional adductor muscle loss, the thumb and index tend to rotate in opposite directions on pinch, further adding to instability of the thumb and pinch.

The patient may substitute for loss of the adductor and first dorsal interosseous by pinching to the side of the thumb,

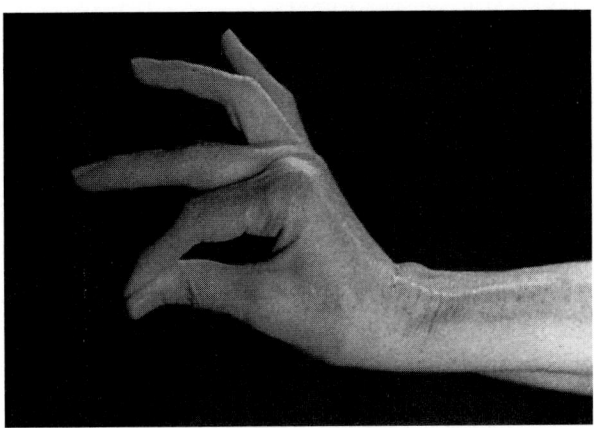

Fig. 48-7. Reverse Froment's sign. The patient attempts to stabilize the thumb by extending the thumb interphalangeal joint, positioning the thumb so the force of the index finger will fully extend the interphalangeal joint and fully flex the metacarpophalangeal joint. In addition to loss of selective thumb positioning except at extremes of joint range, excessive stress produced in joints can be deforming.

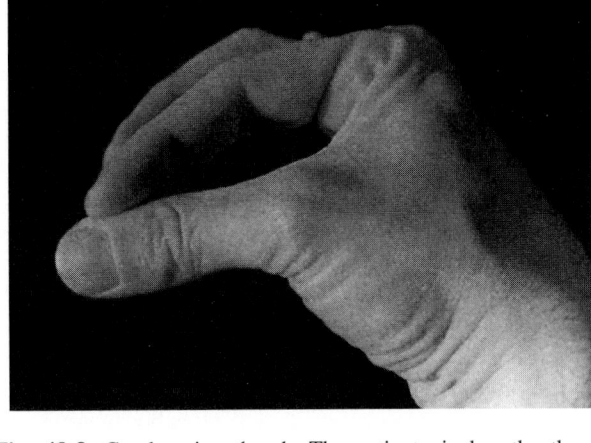

Fig. 48-8. Crank-action thumb. The patient pinches the thumb from the side and uses the limits of soft tissue restraints to stabilize the thumb in pinch. Once the ulnar collateral ligaments have become deformed by excessive stress or the thumb joints are used in flexion, any additional external force on the tip of the thumb rotates the thumb and progressively increases the deformity.

using the restraints of the thumb ulnar collateral ligament (MP and IP) and the thumb web to limit abduction and external rotation of the thumb. (The extensor pollicis longus [EPL] muscle also has a small moment for adduction at the MP joint and a large moment for adduction of the metacarpal, but this is combined with external rotation of the thumb.[8]) The ligamentous soft tissue restraints can be abnormally stressed by lack of their normal muscle support. The ulnar collateral ligament at the MP joint is the most commonly deformed by excessive force. After this has begun and if uncorrected, a "crank-action thumb" can result[8] and is similar to the mechanics of any mechanical crank, in that any further pinch (force) at the tip or side of the thumb rotates its entire length into external rotation, as in Fig. 48-8.

Occasionally, the web of the thumb will increase, either with or without the crank-action thumb, to the point that any pinch is ineffective because the index can no longer meet against any restraint of the thumb. Alternatively, the patient may use his or her EPL to adduct and externally rotate the thumb, where it can be used for pinch on the back of the index finger. In Fig. 48-9, thumb abduction, extension, and external rotation moments of the EPL are shown.

The patient may attempt to substitute for the first dorsal interosseous at the index finger and stabilize index ulnar rotation on pinch against the thumb by hyperextending the index DIP joint, thus supporting this finger by bracing it along the side of the other fingers. This abnormal positioning of the joint to translate force for prehension also causes progressive deformity in that the DIP joint extension tends to increase over time. In Fig. 48-6, hyperextension of the index can be seen as the patient pinches against the thumb.

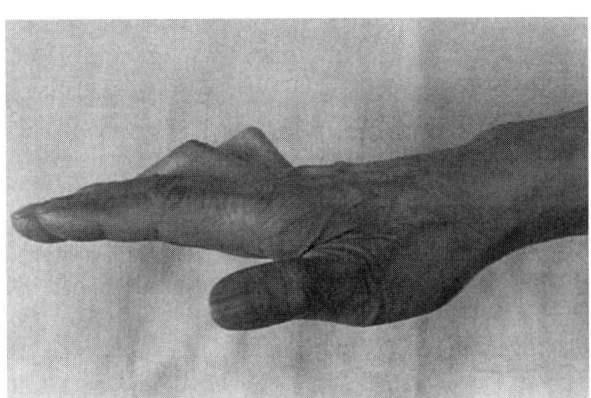

Fig. 48-9. Extensor pollicis longus pinch. The thumb is positioned in the adduction and external rotation to be pinched against the index finger and, in extreme cases, against the back of the index finger. The extensor pollicis longus muscle–tendon unit has moments for positioning in adduction, extension, and external rotation.

These considerations make it clear that if the hand is to be functional and useful, tendon transfer surgery to rebalance the hand is not a luxury but a necessity, and tendon transfer surgery, although not an emergency, should be planned early before joint stiffness and remodeling occur.

High nerve injury

A high ulnar-nerve injury takes the same course as the low ulnar-nerve injury in intrinsic muscle involvement and imbalance. In addition to the long extrinsic finger flexor (FDP) to the little finger, the ring finger usually is involved (and sometimes other fingers) as well as the ulnar wrist flexor (flexor carpi ulnaris [FCU]).

As with the low nerve injuries, if the hand is not used, the skin becomes thin, shiny, or macerated where joints are contracted, and can tear easily. If the hand is used, the skin becomes thickened and calloused anywhere it must assume abnormal contact pressure stemming from mechanically imbalanced muscle-tendon units. In Fig. 48-10, callus can be seen on the ring finger of a patient who has lost the FDP and the ulnar intrinsic muscles. The area of pressure results from the unaided use of the FDS. The distal tip of the finger is unable to flex because of the loss of the FDP. The area of skin taking the pressure of hand use was never intended to sustain such repetitive pressure, and it will probably break down with continual use. The problem in this case can be corrected by suture of the profundus tendon of the little finger to the profundus tendon of the middle finger, which has a working FDP muscle-tendon unit.[4]

In high ulnar-nerve injury, the patient has even less finger function for power grip than in the low nerve injury and cannot support the wrist in flexion on the ulnar side. The FCU is a powerful muscle and is the strongest muscle that crosses the wrist. Its loss to hand function greatly limits the use of the hand, because architecturally, the more proximal wrist needs stability for force to be translated to the digits.

A high median-nerve injury takes the same course as the low median-nerve injury in intrinsic muscle involvement and imbalance. Depending on the level of the injury, the long extrinsic finger flexors (FDP) to the index, middle, and sometimes, ring fingers; palmaris longus; FDS; flexor pollicis longus; and radial wrist flexor (flexor carpi radialis) also can be involved.

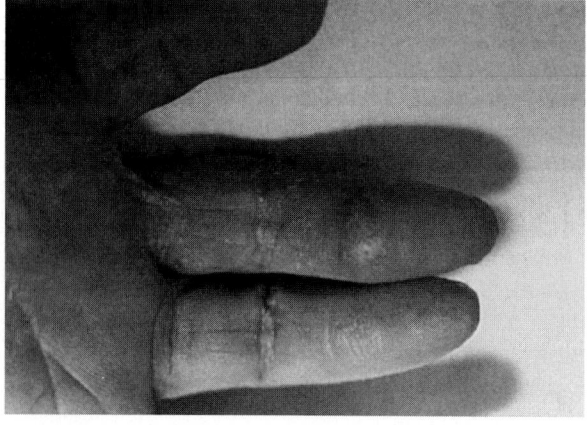

Fig. 48-10. Callus on the ring finger of a patient who has lost the flexor digitorum profundus in a high ulnar injury. The area of callus results from the use of the short extrinsic flexor in the absence of the long extrinsic flexor.

OBJECTIVE MEASUREMENT AND PREOPERATIVE TREATMENT
Need for objective measurement

Objective measurements that quantify the type and extent of involvement and imbalance are important in preoperative and postoperative records. In this way, changes by surgery and changes by therapy can be demonstrated and documented. Adjustments can be made that will improve the overall surgical and therapeutic program.

The postoperative treatment can be dictated by the preoperative measurements. For example, if a hand is hypermobile, a reversing of the metacarpal arch can be much more of a problem after tendon transfers. A wrist extensor transferred in a Brand many-tailed procedure[8] to flex the MP joint and to extend the IP joint of the fingers may unavoidably become an active extender of the fifth metacarpal and lose any ability to function effectively, as intended at the other joints. For such a hypermobile hand, the time the hand is casted or splinted to support the metacarpal arch and the time of limitation of full extension of the metacarpal joints may be anticipated to be extended several weeks. As an alternative, an additional transfer may be included in the surgical rebalancing plan to stabilize the fifth metacarpal in supination, such as a transfer of the extensor digiti minimi in a radial route to the fifth metacarpal.[32]

Need for preoperative treatment

Preoperative recommendations can be made at the time of measurement for therapy that can upgrade the hand status before surgery and increase the chance for success postoperatively. The most obvious treatment indicated is cylinder casting of IP joints to reduce contractures and mobilize these joints before surgery (see Chapter 114). Joint contractures that remain uncorrected before surgery can seriously compromise surgical results by mechanically limiting joint extension and reducing intended tension of transferred tendons. If one IP joint is stiff and the others are supple, tendon transfers from the same motor to all fingers can result in the excursion of the transfer taken up differentially by different fingers. Most of the transferred tendon excursion can be taken up by the finger with a stiff joint, rendering ineffective the transfer slips to the other joints.[8]

Any scar decreases the chances of mobility for small joints, and because excessive or unwanted scar formation after tendon transfer is already a potential problem, surgical correction for joint contractures before tendon transfers is usually contraindicated if the contractures can be reduced in any other way. An exception is when correction cannot be achieved by therapy, such as a superficialis "check-rein" contracture that has developed at the scarred ends from where the superficialis tendon slips. After this contracture has become longstanding, no or little improvement in joint angle is achieved with progressive increases in force, and contracture remodeling attempts usually fail.

Other therapy may be indicated if it can improve the presurgical hand and increase possibilities of successful surgical outcome. Contracted web spaces may respond to massage and serial splinting. Stiff fingers may be exercised to reduce the amount of viscoelastic tissue resistance they will give to newly transferred tendons. Contracted scar tissue may be softened and relaxed by gentle massage and positive-pressure bandaging and splinting. Mobilization and strengthening of the intended transfers may be desirable before surgery.

A not-so-obvious recommendation for therapy before tendon transfer surgery is correction of a hand that has developed superficialis tightness (FDS). Failures have been encountered in tendon transfer surgeries in which these muscle-tendon units have been tight, because the tension provided by intrinsic transfers to the fingers to flex the MP joints and extend the IP joints is rendered ineffective by the abnormal flexion tension on the IP joints by the superficialis muscle-tendon units.

The amount of superficialis tightness can be deceiving because the fingers often will extend fully when the wrist is in degrees of flexion. The extent of tightness is often made apparent by a patient's intolerance of attempts to correct the tightness by splinting the wrist in neutral and the fingers fully extended. If the splint is left on overnight, patients insist on removing the splint or, in the presence of insensitivity, develop distal fingertip skin blisters. Therapists find they must begin by splinting the fingers in extension with the wrist in some flexion or by cylinder casting the IP joints and gradually including the wrist. Gradually, approximately every other day, the splint can be remolded progressively into extension, as the hand remodels and allows more extension of the muscle-tendon units. *It is important to realize that superficialis tightness cannot be corrected after surgery by therapy because the necessary position to reduce the superficialis tightness is the exact position to affect adversely the desired tension of the new intrinsic transfers.*

Another serious consideration is the tendon transfer selection in a hand with superficialis tightness. If a superficialis tendon is transferred from the ring or middle finger to the thumb, and the remaining superficialis muscle-tendon units are tight, a marked finger imbalance can occur. The fingers will flex out of phase with the donor finger lagging behind. If the IP joint from the donor tendon is in any way hypermobile, the reduced tension at the volar IP joint results in the finger hyperextending on extension while the other finger IP joints remain in flexion. If intrinsic transfers are made to the fingers, the out-of-phase extension of the donor tendon becomes exaggerated and can become progressively deformed in hyperextension. Therapy can do little or nothing to assist or correct this amount of imbalance after surgery, and further corrective surgery is needed. With care, this problem can be

handled by reducing the muscle-tendon unit contractures before surgery or perhaps by routing the intrinsic transfers to all except the superficialis donor finger. This will increase IP extension tension at the other fingers to counterbalance the flexor muscle–tendon tightness and will result in less extension tension translated to the extension of the donor finger.

The profundus muscle–tendon units also may become shortened, and when this is combined with superficialis tightness, it is sometimes hard to tell how much is profundus and how much is superficialis. The profundus also can affect the tendon transfer tension but is not as critical to the individual finger balance because it is not usually a donor for transfer. The profundus responds to preoperative remodeling therapy.

Patients are more trusting of a therapist who sees their hand before surgery because they see this therapist as someone they know and someone who is familiar with their hand and particular problems.

A therapist who sees a hand before surgery has opportunities to augment and improve the postoperative treatment. Therapists can work with patients who have had hand surgery, referred postoperatively, but often not as effectively or without guesswork. There is benefit to the therapist's first becoming familiar with the extent of mechanical imbalance that the surgeon is attempting to improve. Therapists often attend, refer to, or are available for medical/surgical hand clinics to make therapy recommendations and become familiar with planned surgical cases.

Where to begin

Patients often feel confined and pressed for time in surgical clinic situations. They later explain to the therapist considerations that may affect their surgical and rehabilitation plans, such as a death in the family or a need to return to work in a time frame that is insufficient for follow-up care such as therapy. Most surgeons appreciate feedback about patient problems.

The patient is told by the surgeon and the therapist what he or she should anticipate as a result of the surgery and that, although the surgeon has had much experience, surgery is different in each case. The patient is told the length of time for immobilization, the anticipated length of time for therapy if no complications develop, and the length of time that might be necessary if problems such as infection or tendon adhesions develop. Possible complications are explained, including that if complications occur, the team is prepared to resolve them early, so that they are minimized and results are maximized. In this way the patient develops the understanding that, although surgery is not always 100% successful, every effort is made for him or her, and that he or she will be watched and counseled through the surgery to maximize the benefit. This helps minimize the patient's fear of pain and surprises. Sometimes the patient's greatest discomfort comes from (1) fear of the unknown, (2) concern that having

HAND SURGERY ASSESSMENT—PREOPERATIVE

Date_____   Patient no._____
Hand: Right or Left   Hand dominance_____
Name_____Birth date_____Sex_____
HD class_____Date dx'd_____Physician_____
Occupation_____Last time reaction/Neuritis_____
Condition of other hand_____
Other information_____

_____

A. Related Problems

Arch reversal angle_____   Superficial tightness   I_____ M_____ R_____ L_____
Scar/callous   I   M   R   L   Cont ret lig   I   M   R   L
Bone absorption   I   M   R   L   PIP Hyperextension   I   M   R   L
Guttered ext mech   I   M   R   L   Attenuated ext mech   I   M   R   L
Sensory loss: Median_____ Ulnar_____ Radial_____
     (3.61 MN [.21 g] or heavier)
Wrist flexion pattern (describe)_____

B. Muscle Status (5-4-3-2-1)

	Right	Left		Right	Left		Right	Left		Right	Left
ADM	_____		APB	_____		FDS M/R	/	/	ECRL-B	_____	
1st DI	_____		OP	_____		FCR	_____		EPL	_____	
Intr pos I/M	/	/	FPB	_____		FCU	_____		ECU	_____	
Intr pos R/L	/	/	FPL	_____		Pr T	_____		Br Rad	_____	
FDP R/L	/	/				PL	_____				

C. Grip & Pinch

Grip strength	Jamar	Right	Left		Pinch strength	Right	Left
Level_____	A	/	/		Pulp to pulp	_____	_____
Level_____	B	/	/		Key (lat)	_____	_____
Level_____	C	/	/		Three-point	_____	_____
Level_____	D	/	/				
Level_____	E	/	/				

Describe: Grip_____Pinch_____

Finger closure sequence_____

Grip contact holding cylinder   Th   I   M   R   L = T

1					
2					
3					

Comments_____

D. Preoperative therapy

Hand exercise _____weeks   Casting_____weeks   Overall duration_____weeks

Type: Wound care   Casting   Splinting
      I M R L   I M R L   I M R L

Fig. 48-11. Sample surgical evaluation form.

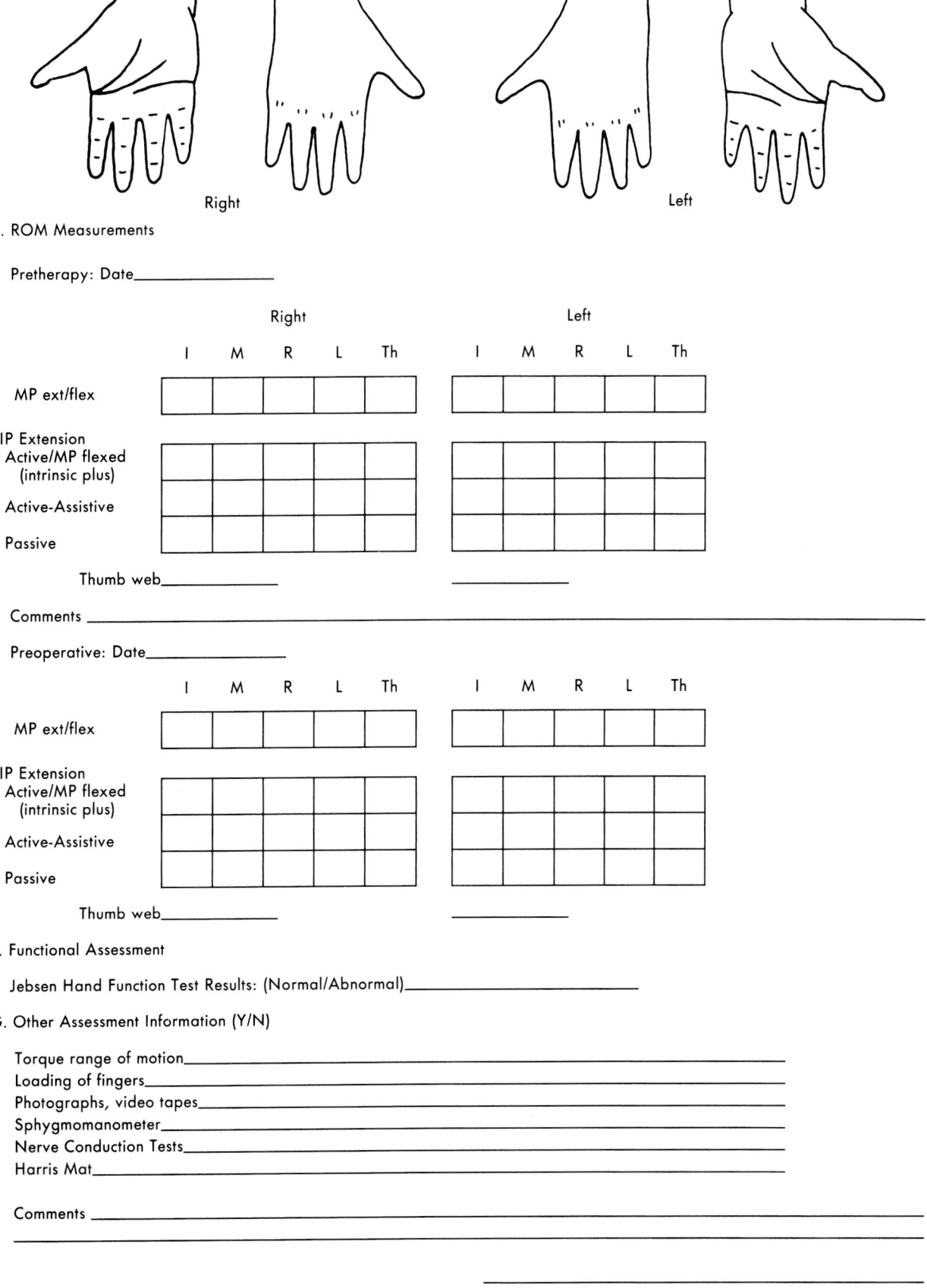

Palm   Dorsum   Dorsum   Palm

Right   Left

E. ROM Measurements

Pretherapy: Date_____

Right   Left

	I	M	R	L	Th		I	M	R	L	Th
MP ext/flex											

PIP Extension
Active/MP flexed
(intrinsic plus)

Active-Assistive

Passive

Thumb web_____   _____

Comments _____

Preoperative: Date_____

Right   Left

	I	M	R	L	Th		I	M	R	L	Th
MP ext/flex											

PIP Extension
Active/MP flexed
(intrinsic plus)

Active-Assistive

Passive

Thumb web_____   _____

F. Functional Assessment

Jebsen Hand Function Test Results: (Normal/Abnormal)_____

G. Other Assessment Information (Y/N)

Torque range of motion_____
Loading of fingers_____
Photographs, video tapes_____
Sphygmomanometer_____
Nerve Conduction Tests_____
Harris Mat_____

Comments _____
_____

_____
Therapist

Fig. 48-11—cont'd.

surgery is not in his or her best interest, or (3) that he or she will be in a dependent role without assistance.

History taking and initial examination

During the history intake, the therapist has the opportunity to observe the patient's use of hands while he or she is not under obvious scrutiny. Much of the examination can be accomplished while shaking the patient's hand, asking for a signature, and watching the patient remove a piece of paper from a wallet or purse to take notes. A functional observation of the patient using the hand sometimes is better made in this way before the focus is turned to the hands.

The therapist examines the hand by noting anything abnormal. Often, the patient has a normal other extremity with which to compare. All skin contractures, joint contractures, wounds, scars, and general condition of the skin should be noted. These can be recorded easily on a form that has a drawing of the hands to identify locations and problems

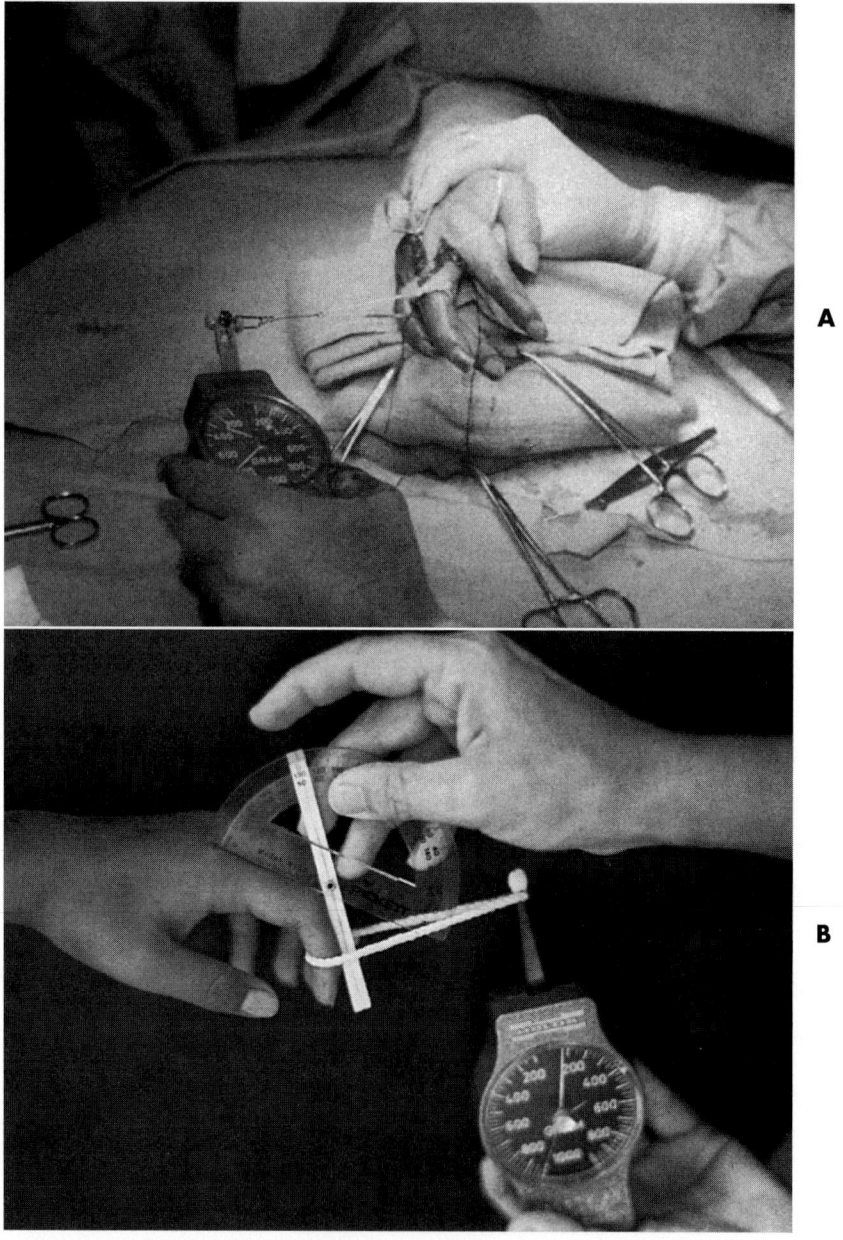

Fig. 48-12. Torque range of motion, described by Brand, can help assess objectively the balance of joint and muscle-tendon unit tension before and after tendon transfers. **A,** Surgeon measurement of passive resistance to metacarpophalangeal extension before and after tendon transfer surgery to assess transfer-tendon tension. **B,** Therapist measurement of resistance to finger interphalangeal joint extension before and after surgery (after resistance is possible) to assess superficialis tightness before and after surgery.

(Fig. 48-11). Previous surgeries and dates should be recorded briefly for easy reference, or copies of operative reports and referrals can be attached to therapy forms.

Routine measurements

A voluntary muscle examination is performed using standard muscle-grading procedures, noting absences and weaknesses. Particular attention is given to muscles found in specific nerve groups—ulnar, median, and radial—so the extent of nerve involvement is well recognized. Nerve problems often are bilateral and can involve more than one nerve.

A sensory examination is performed using standard measurement technique. Sensory function is measured with regard to function of different nerve groups (ulnar, median, and radial). Screening or mapping with Semmes-Weinstein monofilaments (see Chapter 13) and nerve conduction is recommended.

Special measurements

In ROM measurements for the nerve-injured hand, particular attention is given to the extension of the IP joints with flexion of the MP joints. The patient is asked to assume a lumbrical position (MP joints flexed and IP joints extended) as in Fig. 48-2, *A*. In this position, measurements are taken for joint passive, active, and active-assistive extension angles at the IP joints. For measurement of the active-assistive joint angles, the examiner flexes the MP joint for the patient and blocks extension of this joint, while allowing extension of the IP joints as in Fig. 48-3. The difference between this measurement and the passive joint measurement determines the amount of extension lag that would be present at the IP joint were intrinsic replacement surgery performed. (Unless attenuated, the EDC will fully extend the IP joints of the fingers when blocked in this position, provided the joint is not limited by stiffness, volar skin contracture, or muscle-tendon unit contracture.)

Because the joint-angle measurements of the fingers may change when the hand is placed in different wrist positions, the extension measurements at the IP joints are taken first with the wrist in 45 degrees of extension, then again with the wrist in 45 degrees of flexion. The difference in these two measurements represents the limitation introduced by the extrinsic muscle–tendon units. If extrinsic tightness is present, a difference in the measurements with wrist flexion and extension will occur. IP joint extension measurements are taken with the MP joints in neutral position.

Torque ROM has been described by Brand[8] and is used in some hand treatment programs to objectively assess the balance of joint and muscle-tendon tension before and after tendon transfers.[2] It is particularly useful in assessing the amount of FDS tightness when present. The torque (force × distance from the joint) necessary to achieve full IP joint extension with the wrist in 45 degrees of extension and MP

joints in neutral gives an understanding of the amount of resistance the tendon transfers must overcome to be successful. Torque measurements of the force necessary to extend MP joints before surgery give an understanding of the amount of tension provided by the transfers when measurements are repeated at the MP joint after surgery (Fig. 48-12). It is important that the therapist recognize the postoperative tension of transfers because the therapist can optimize or reduce the tension, as needed, by the soft tissue mobilization or restricted mobilization around the tendon in the early postoperative phase.

In the thumb the web space should be measured, because this often changes after ulnar-nerve injury. The web often contracts or elongates. If contracted, the web greatly limits the grasp of the hand around objects. Thumb web space contractures can require special releases and/or grafts to restore function for successful tendon transfers. ROM of the thumb should include abduction out of the palm (Figs. 48-4 and 48-13) as well as active and passive flexion and extension angles of its joints. An active assistive measurement can be made of the IP joint of the thumb by the examiner's flexing and supporting the MP joint while the patient extends the IP joint.

If noted from the aforementioned measurements and examination, specific problems should be recorded including superficialis tightness, Froment's sign, reverse Froment's sign, ligament tightness, hypermobility, arch reversal, guttered extension mechanism (i.e., ulnarly decentralized extensor mechanism toward or into interosseous space), ligament laxity, attenuated extensor mechanism, bone absorption, bone deformity, pulley disruption, abnormal sequence of finger flexion/extension, collapse of lumbrical position on resistance at the proximal phalanx, and necessity of wrist to flex for successful finger extension.

Photographic positions

As indicated in the preceding measurement, the positioning of the fingers and joints is critical in producing the balance of the hand. For this reason, photographic records of the most important positions are useful to augment the descriptive information. These photographs should reproduce the ROM measurement positions and should be repeated after surgical correction. The following positions are suggested:

   I. Ulnar view (elbows on table)
     A. Lumbrical position
     B. Full finger extension
     C. Active-assistive extension (Fig. 48-3)
     D. Full finger flexion
     E. Pinch
   II. Radial view
     A. Tip pinch
       1. Soft
       2. Hard

B. Key pinch
   1. Soft
   2. Hard
III. Front midline view (palms up)
  A. Thumb
    1. Adduction
    2. Abduction
    3. Pinch
      a. Index
      b. Middle
      c. Ring
      d. Little

Note in particular the front midline view taken from the fingertips (Fig. 48-12). This view allows record of thumb abduction and adduction. Other views can be taken as desired, but it is important to have standard views that are repeated for every patient.

Functional test

Many functional hand skill tests are available. The optimal functional test is one suited to the requirement of individual patients for work or leisure, because the real disability of the injury is a combination of its physical and psychologic impairment parameters. Most functional tests depend on elements that are repeatable for measurements of change. Of available tests, only a few are standardized,[15] leaving the therapist to select tests and test elements that are best suited to individual patients and programs.

For the ulnar-nerve–injured hand, functional tests should include those that will otherwise demonstrate normal pinch and grasp and release patterns. In this way, mechanical imbalances can be seen and measured in severity, and substitution patterns can be identified. The Moberg pickup test[29] or a similar one, is a good beginning. This test was designed originally to demonstrate altered sensibility, but it is good for demonstrating prehension patterns of small objects, and the objects are commonly found in any clinic or office. The same series of objects can be used on all patients, and other small objects can be added to those available. How patients pick up the objects with thumb and fingers collectively and individually can be observed and timed. Omer[30] has suggested adding soft chalk to the objects because the chalk will rub off on the fingers and show contact areas. Normally the fingers should not show any collapse, such as clawing of the fingers or thumb, when picking up the objects. Graded fishing weights (50 to 200 g) are important objects to add because imbalanced fingers often will not collapse or show imbalance until loaded with some force. Small blocks attached to a board with Velcro are helpful additions because these give resistance to patients' fingers and thumb when they are pinched and lifted. The turning of a key in a lock or doorknob can demonstrate key pinch: first positional, as the patient picks up the key; then resistive, as the patient turns the key.

Clear plastic cylinders of three sizes (1½-, 2-, and 3-inch diameters) are useful to demonstrate abnormal grasp patterns. Because the normal fingers and thumb will make total

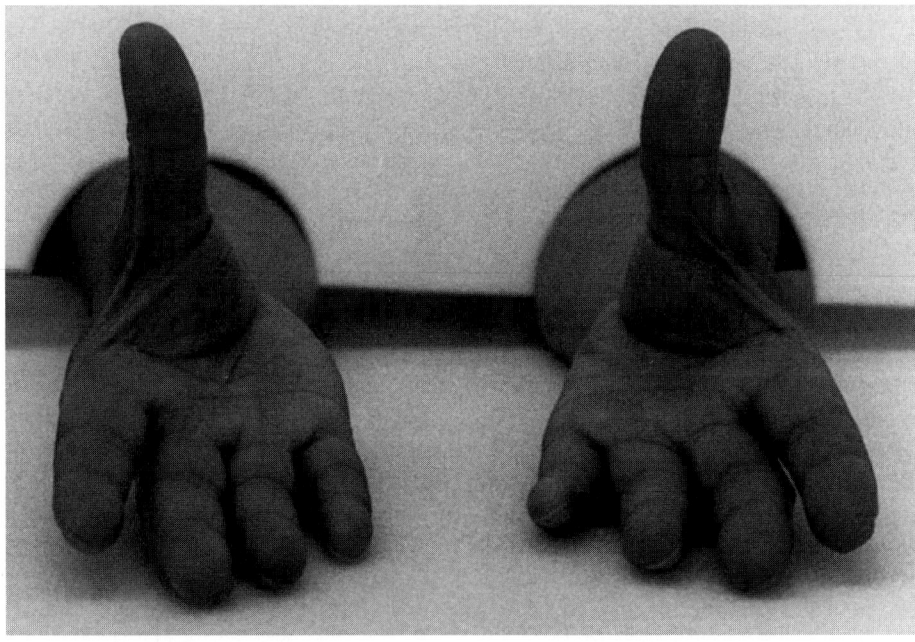

Fig. 48-13. Photographic view from fingertips taken with thumb in full abduction (followed with photo in adduction) to show muscle imbalance. With loss of the median-nerve abductor pollicis brevis and opponens muscles, the thumb cannnot be abducted out of the palm and rotated into a position in which it can oppose the little finger.

contact on a cylinder, they can be graded regarding which segments make contact on the test cylinders.[22] In the event of clawing of the ulnar two fingers and Froment's sign of the thumb, as often happens in ulnar-nerve injuries, only the tips of the fingers and thumb will show contact on one or another of the cylinders.

Other large objects can be included to demonstrate gross grasp and manipulation, such as turning the lid of a jar and picking up a glass with one hand. Writing a name with a pencil can be used to demonstrate dexterity.

Splinting

Splints can be used to restore balance externally for what has become imbalanced internally in the hand. If the hand is not to undergo surgery for a while, an intrinsic splint is recommended for the fingers to help prevent remodeling of tissue into deformity. Just as the examiner can allow the patient to fully extend the IP joints of an intrinsic-minus hand by flexing the MP joint, a splint can be made to support the MP joints in flexion. This splint is relatively difficult to fit without pressure points and must be checked carefully. The patient can use the strong power of the extrinsic extensor (EDC) to overcome the splint and can receive damaging pressure on the dorsum of the IP joints at the proximal phalanx. The patient should be taught to extend the fingers with only the minimum extension force necessary. If the patient has developed a pattern of dropping the wrist to achieve finger extension, this problem should be corrected by either instruction or splint immobilization (Fig. 48-14).

The splint should always be padded where it supplies a "lumbrical bar" to hold the finger MP joints in flexion. It has been calculated that, as the patient extends his or her fingers,

for every gram of force that is used to extend the fingers, at least twice that force is exerted on the dorsum of the finger proximal phalanges.[8] To allow for this high concentration of pressure, padding of the splint and securing of the hand in the splint by a palmar support that will curve and support the metacarpal arch is important. Usually the lumbrical bar extends across all of the fingers at the proximal phalanx to help disperse force that would concentrate more in the ring and little fingers if splinted separately. Occasionally, the ring and little fingers can be splinted alone if pressure problems are controlled. The thumb should be free to move where it does not press against the splint on pinch and cause shear stress. Fig. 48-14 is an example of one such splint. Other designs are available.[16]

The thumb is harder to support externally than the fingers and thus is often left unsplinted. The patient is given corrective exercise instructions, such as therapist or patient blocking of extension of the MP joint with patient active extension of the IP joint. Splints also can be made to accomplish this purpose if blocking of the MP joint results in extension of the thumb IP joint.

Additional splinting is possible to improve thumb positioning and encourage pulp rather than deforming side pinch. The thumb can be strapped in a 1½- to 2-inch-wide figure-of-eight strap made of adhesive stockinette that is wrapped from the forearm around the thumb to supply positioning support,[6] as in Fig. 48-15. Care should be taken that the strapping is proximal to the MP joint and therefore does not increase stress on the ulnar collateral ligament. One advantage of this type of strapping to achieve thumb positioning is that the support on the thumb will be increased when the patient extends the wrist for pinch and will be decreased as the wrist is flexed.

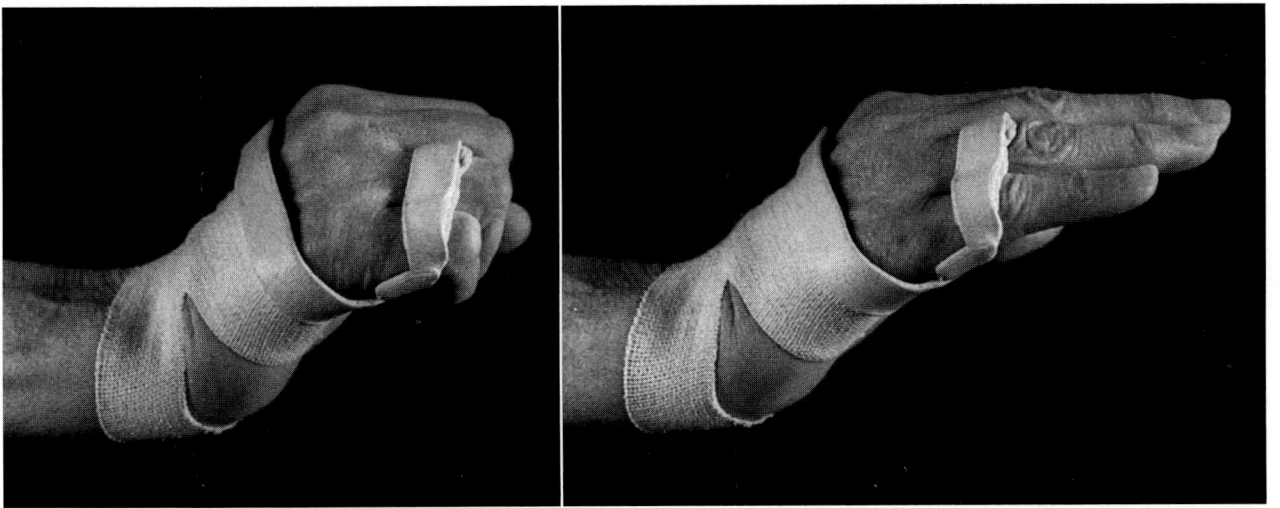

A   **B**

Fig. 48-14. Splinting of ulnar-nerve–injured hand to provide external support of finger metacarpophalangeal joints to facilitate interphalangeal (IP) extension. **A,** IP flexion. **B,** IP extension. The same splint can incorporate the index and middle fingers when needed for a median- or ulnar-nerve–injured hand.

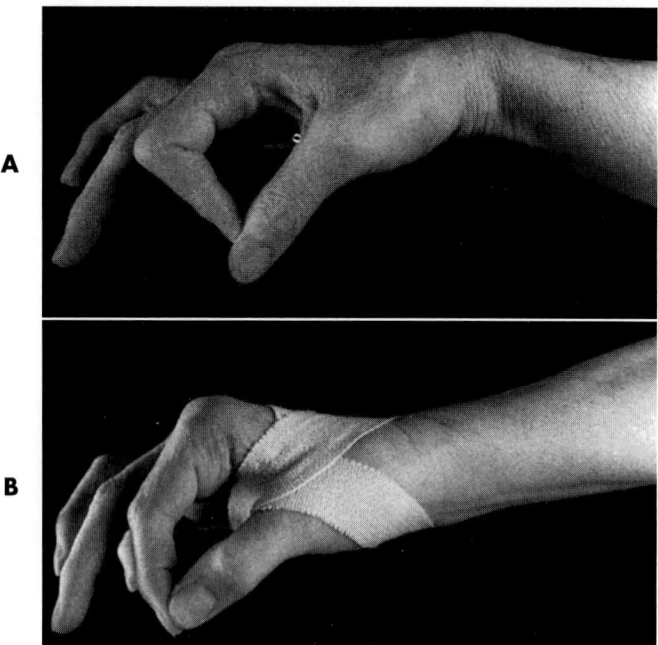

A

B

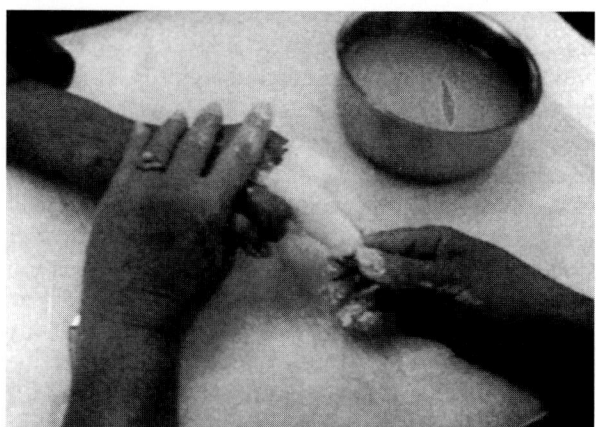

Fig. 48-16. Plaster cylinder casting of the fingers or thumb can be used several ways; (1) to serially correct contractures by progressive remodeling or (2) as an alternative ulnar-nerve splint to support the interphalangeal (IP) joints of the fingers or thumb in extension and transfer the force of the extrinsic flexors to the metacarpophalangeal (MP) joints. (The fingers usually will not continue to hyperextend at the MP joints when IP joints are casted; but if they do, a dorsal block splint to prevent the MP joints from hyperextending also must be used.)

Fig. 48-15. Thumb strapping of thumb with adhesive elastic to support thumb in position for functional pulp pinch. Active wrist extension increases strap support tension and pinch stability. Strapping can be used in conjunction with other splinting. **A,** Pinch without thumb support. **B,** Pinch with thumb support.

Cylinder casting can be used preoperatively or postoperatively to support the IP joints of the fingers and transfer the force of the extrinsic flexors to the MP joints as in Fig. 48-16. This allows active flexion of the MP joints in those fingers that are intrinsic minus. The cast fabrication is the same as that used for cylinder casts for joint remodeling. The casts can be removed (e.g., for handwashing) and then replaced.

The thumb also can be cylinder casted at the IP joints, but like fusion of this joint, casting must be done with caution. A stabilized thumb IP joint can increase rotation of a crank-action thumb[8] as well as provide increased strain on the thumb metacarpal ulnar collateral ligament.

POSTOPERATIVE MANAGEMENT

Additions and changes are made to the treatment plan in the operating room when the final intricacies of the surgery have unveiled. At this point, the surgeon has formulated how he or she perceives the surgery and is developing a plan of follow-up. The therapist should talk with the surgeon soon after surgery while the details of the surgery are still fresh. If the therapist routinely talks with the surgeon after surgery, the surgeon is prepared to offer quick, precise reports of successes and difficulties in the operating room that may affect the course of patient treatment, and he or she conveys clear concerns and specific requests.

In contrast with this surgeon-therapist interaction is the therapist who waits for therapy referrals. The success of the

surgery is the surgeon's first concern, after which mobilization and patient return to work are desired. If surgeons must contact therapists and details have become less clear, the surgeons are much more likely to do early movement themselves or let the patients do so with instructions, and refer when problems occur or late in follow-up, when chances for successful therapy are reduced.

First days after surgery

The hand should be elevated after surgery or otherwise kept from a dependent position, which encourages swelling. The therapist can check the patient's compliance with elevation and, if necessary, fashion one of many possible elevation devices. It is helpful to tell the patient that the hand must always be above heart level. A sling of stockinette with the side cut for the cast and hand and the remaining part tied to an IV tree works satisfactorily. Other methods are available.

When the hand is checked postsurgically, the therapist can examine the hand for areas of constricting cast, friction areas causing abrasion, poor circulation of the hand, or evidence of infection.

The success of the mechanical rebalancing by tendon transfers is often in direct relationship to the maintenance of correct positioning of the hand during healing. The tension of an otherwise successful surgery can be ruined by inadvertent changes in positioning or unsatisfactory positions. It is not uncommon after a long surgical procedure for positioning in the surgical cast to be less than desired. For example, it is not uncommon for the MP joints after intrinsic replacement of the fingers to be in less flexion than desired, or the thumb after an adductor replacement to be in too much extension. The position should be readjusted at first opportunity, which is usually at the first cast change.

One week after surgery

The postoperative cast is often guardedly removed by the surgeon 1 week after surgery and the hand recasted to improve position and to accommodate the loss of postoperative swelling; resolution of swelling can allow too much hand movement in the cast and cause the digits to shift into positions that may adversely affect tendon tension. Removal of the cast at this time also allows the hand to be checked for infection, sutures to be removed, and the hand to be otherwise inspected for healing of surgical wounds. Tendon transfers can be examined for continuity, and the patient is occasionally asked to move them slightly to check their operation. Much movement of the tendons is risky at this point because too much force could result in elongation of a tendon anastomosis or rupture at the site of suture. The hand is usually recasted for 2 more weeks.

Early movement is not as necessary for tendon transfers as for tendon repairs because transfers usually are not routed through areas of massive scar or at the time of accompanying injury. The routing of tendon transfers often is chosen specifically to avoid areas of previous scar. The advantages of early movement versus later movement of tendon repairs have been debated in surgical lectures and literature.[19] Far more repairs seem to scar down and to have limited movement than to rupture, and strong arguments can be made for early movement of any tendon that is sutured, to maintain tendon gliding while limiting the amount of adhesions through which a newly repaired tendon must glide. However, scar adhesions in ulnar-nerve tendon transfers do not often limit the transferred tendon's function if the hand is held for 3 weeks in a cast. In addition, the cast provides less opportunity for tendon rupture. Tendon grafts also may be a part of the transfer surgery, and grafts are believed to require more immobilization for nutrition for healing, although this too has been debated. Some studies indicate that the tendon, while gliding, will be able to derive enough nutrition from surrounding synovial tissue rather than depend on intrinsic tendon healing alone.[26]

More important determinants for late or early movement may be the strength of the tendon suture, the quality of the transfer including graft, and the strength of the tendon attachment during different stages of healing.[31] In any case, it is the surgeon who is in the best position to determine any possibility of early movement. The therapist must work closely with the surgeon and receive the surgeon's concurrence if attempts at early movement are made. Many hands with ulnar-nerve transfers will also have sensory involvements, and the patient, because of impaired sensory feedback, is in danger of pulling too hard on the transfers too soon, particularly in low ulnar-nerve injuries where ulnar-nerve extrinsic muscle function remains intact. The patient may even rupture in the cast if he or she attempts to use the hand while casted, and specific instructions for the patient to not use the hand even though it is casted are prudent.

Exceptions do occur that necessitate the early movement of tendon transfers when the transfer must be routed through an area of old scar, and occasionally surgeons simply elect to move the tendon transfer earlier than 3 weeks. This certainly can be done, but risks are obvious and early movement requires the availability, supervision, and close interaction of the surgery-therapy team in a controlled environment with patient cooperation. Therapists in programs in which patients may not return as instructed for follow-up or are unavailable for follow-up are advised to leave the cast for 3 weeks.

Early mobilization period

When the postoperative cast is removed, it is weaned away, not totally removed. Often, removal of the cast will result in a little swelling of the hand over the next day because of the release of soft compression that the cast has provided to the hand. This swelling should be minimal and is more controlled if the hand is removed from the cast for a relatively short period (15 to 30 minutes) and then replaced. A half cast secured with a circular plaster or elastic bandage can be used as a splint for this purpose, or a new one can be made, as in Fig. 48-17. The surgeon, therapist, or technician who removes the cast can do so in such a way that the volar portion (or dorsal if desired) can be used as a holding splint. Brand[6] would be quick to say that a new cast is desirable because the hand does not always fit into the cast in quite the same position. However, to disturb the hand as little as possible when it is first removed from the cast for mobilization of transfers, a half cast can be used safely if the therapist will carefully check and relieve any pressure points of the cast that might cause local skin damage. If functioning well, the half cast can continue to be used as the hand is taken out for progressively more time for mobilization of transfers and restoration of hand function, or a new plaster cast or thermoplastic splint can be made at any desirable point.

Plaster serves as a good material for postoperative cast splints because the material is inexpensive, allows air access to wounds, can be made quickly, and can be remade frequently as needed for optimal positioning and changes as the hand recovers function. The therapist is not as likely to discard an ill-fitting thermoplastic splint as a plaster splint because of the time and cost involved. (The splint should be fitted to the hand, not the hand to the splint.)

The position maintained during tendon transfer mobilization at first is the same as in the postsurgical cast. Any movement of the hand and new tendons adds to the amount of swelling the patient will have in the first few days. This is because any movement causes rupture of adhesions that have been formed around the entire length of the transferred tendons, in particular at sites of their anastomosis, at incision and dissection sites, and anywhere else proteinaceous

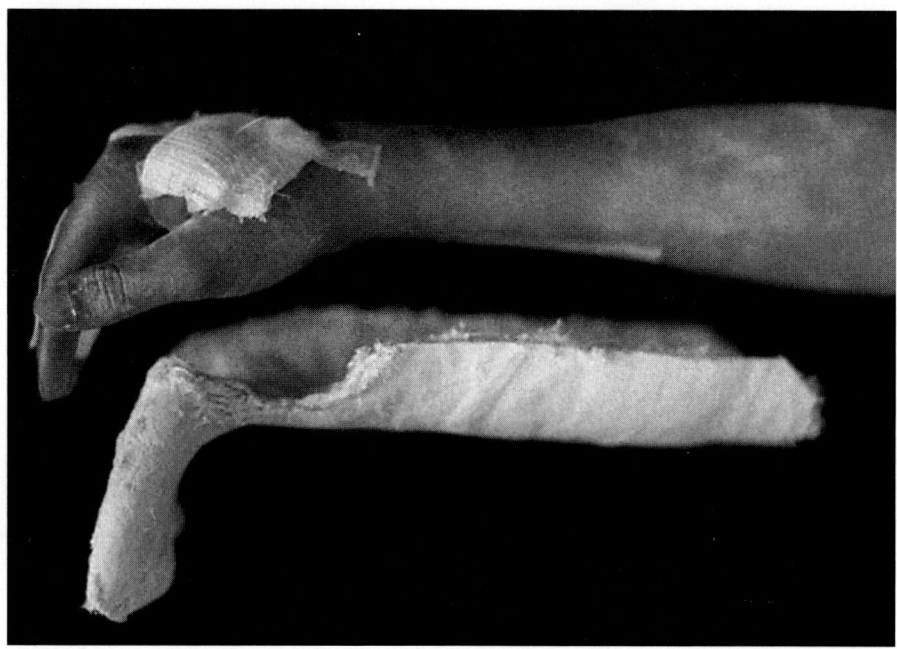

Fig. 48-17. Early postoperative cast splint. A half cast secured with a circular plaster or elastic bandage can be used as a first postoperative splint in the early mobilization period. Areas of cast likely to cause pressure should be relieved, not just padded.

fibrinous material has been formed. As adhesion ruptures occur, more protein material is released, encouraging more scar to form. Therefore the objective on day one is one of only beginning to mobilize the tendon transfers with a gentle loosening that will cause minimal swelling and additional scar formation. On the first postsurgical day, it usually is sufficient to ask the patient to attempt flexion and extension of the fingers, thumb, and wrist gently through possible ROM without undue stress. Attempts can be made to identify the tendon transfers by eliciting their slight active pull by the patient. The hand is then wrapped for another day.

The first day out of the cast is the most exciting for the surgeon, therapist, and patient. Here one sees the evidence of the success or failure of the tendon transfer surgery, and the treatment plan unfolds accordingly. If the transfers can be identified and can support their intended joint(s) and if they appear to glide freely even within a small ROM, the therapist's job is easy. The treatment plan becomes one of protection for further healing while progressively mobilizing the transfers over the next 3 weeks, until moderate resistance can be given to the transferred muscles and other muscles of the hand for strengthening and augmentation of rebalancing.

Positioning again is critical, and the therapist must be sure, by whatever means are necessary (e.g., supervision, splinting), that the desired position is maintained at all joints during the patient's hand use until the tendon transfers are strong enough to support their intended function. The patient cannot just be released to use the hand because he or she will quickly return to former disuse habits and, by doing so, can render the transfers ineffective. For example, a patient who

has had an intrinsic-minus hand becomes used to the habitus of wrist flexion and of depending on his or her extrinsic finger extensor (EDC) to extend the fingers. This muscle can be powerful. If after intrinsic replacement surgery the patient is not protected from using this extrinsic finger extensor, the muscle can overcome any tension in the intrinsic transfers and continue to pull the MP joints into hyperextension. By repetitively doing so, the patient remodels the healing tissue to adjust to this position. The intrinsic transfers may actually rupture. However, even if they do not rupture, the overpull of the extrinsic extensor causes a loosening of the fibrous adhesions and soft tissue around and throughout the length of the transferred tendons, which has the effect of reducing their mechanical tension for correction (of the MP joints in flexion and the IP joints in extension).

Scar tissue is necessary for healing and is not always bad. It becomes bad only when it inhibits function, such as intended tendon gliding. The fact that scar will form along the bed of the transferred tendon can be used to an advantage, such as in augmenting the support of the intrinsic transfers in the previously cited case. If the positioning of the fingers is supported and maintained throughout tendon healing, some of the adhesions around the tendon and within the surrounding soft tissue will actually aid in supporting the tendons in their new position and in maintaining desired tissue remodeling. Brand[4] often uses the example of the over-corrected intrinsic-minus hand that is now in an intrinsic-plus position with limitation of extension at the finger MP joints and progressive hyperextension (because of mechanical imbalance and tension overpull) at the IP joints. He maintains that the transferred tendons can actually be released in these cases, and the MP joints will never return to hyperextension. This is because the tissue surrounding the tendon transfers and along the length of the tendon transfers has scarred and remodeled in a position to support the MP joints in flexion and can continue to do so even without the transferred tendons. The tension exhibited by the transfers and their corrective positions of the fingers is very important when the hand begins to move and gives clear evidence of where the correction balance is falling. If the tension of intrinsic transfers is a little less than desired, the MP joint can be protected from full extension by a splint or supervised instruction and, it is hoped, the forming adhesions will help adjust for the minimal tension.

In the reverse then, if the tension is a little too tight, more freedom is given for full flexion and extension of the transferred tendons so they will be freed as much as necessary from their surrounding tissue restraints.

Most of the balance that results from surgery will be seen in the first 3 weeks of therapy. The patient first learns to identify the transfers on command. The tendon tension can change drastically during this period and should be watched closely. Use of the hand for activities other than identifying the transfers and finger positioning can significantly affect the tendon balance as the patient reverts to old habits. This should be controlled, and the surgical and immobilization period should be used to break old use patterns. The patient can be told that he or she will never use the hand the same way as before surgery because this could waste the surgery. The patient is told that he or she must first move the hand by assuming the positions requested and that when these are mastered, he or she will progress to other movements.

For intrinsic transfers, the position of movement is the lumbrical position. The patient flexes the fingers at the MP joints and then extends at the MP joints to three-fourths extension, as in Fig. 48-18. Full extension at the MP joints is avoided, particularly in the first 3 weeks. If exercised to three-fourths extension, the fingers with the transfers will later loosen naturally as the hand is used, and it is far better that the transfers remain somewhat tight than eventually becoming too loose. If too tight, increased exercises and splinting slightly into the opposite direction 3 to 6 weeks after beginning movement can achieve the required tension. If the transfers become too loose, attempts can be made to splint the fingers at the MP joints into flexion for extended periods and to limit greatly extension of the finger MP joints in extension. However, if not successful, the therapist can do nothing more, and the tension can be readjusted only by another surgery.

The balance is checked immediately upon cast removal, and sometimes the patient can move the fingers with the transfer only 15 to 20 degrees. This is gently increased over the first week, with the hand out of the splint once daily. The ROM of the fingers with the transfer should loosen to 75 to 80 degrees of flexion actively at the MP joint to minus 30

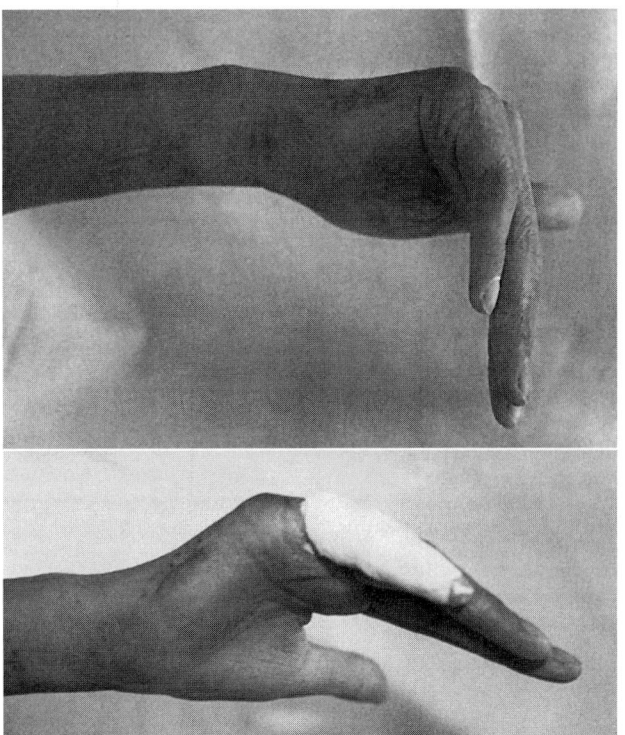

Fig. 48-18. Early postoperative mobilization of intrinsic replacement transfers. **A,** The patient is asked to keep the interphalangeal (IP) joints in extension and flex the fingers at the metacarpophalangeal (MP) joints. **B,** The patient is asked to keep the IP joints in extension and extend the MP joints. The tension of the transferred tendons should be apparent in the amount of MP flexion maintained. Extension at the MP joints is increased gradually, but never past neutral or to hyperextension. A full fist is avoided for several weeks.

degrees extension with the IP joints of the fingers straight in a neutral position. Then the patient can be asked to flex the IP joints slightly and to move the thumb to restore joint gliding.

The patient is instructed to avoid making a full fist in the first few weeks because this puts undue stress on the new intrinsic replacement tendon transfers. The flexors of the hand are mechanically stronger than the extensors and rarely will have a problem eventually returning the fingers to a full fist. The patient will appear to be limited in flexion for the first few weeks that he or she moves because the tension of the transfers initially limits full finger flexion. This is acceptable and even good. If desired, after approximately 2 weeks, when the transfers can be easily identified and the patient can move the fingers in lumbrical positioning, the patient can flex the fingers slightly from the fingertips after other exercises.

Once the patient correctly identifies the transfers on command and can assume the lumbrical positioning, he or she is transferred to light pickup activities with cotton balls. The patient must continue to exhibit lumbrical positioning upon grasp and release of the cotton and should be supervised. This is when he or she is most likely to assume old patterns and needs counseling. If the patient is unable to pick up in a lumbrical position, splinting to assist this should be considered or the patient should spend more time extending and flexing the finger in a lumbrical position on command.

At the beginning of the 3-week early mobilization period, the hand should be removed from the cast for supervised activity and then replaced in the cast that maintains its lumbrical position of the fingers and abduction of the thumb. The time out of the cast is increased gradually until the hand is out most of the day, but the retainer cast or splint is worn overnight. ROM is gradually increased, but unsupervised full ROM is not allowed, nor is motion against resistance. Any overloading of the tendon junctures before 8 weeks after surgery can result in stretching or rupture/avulsion.[34]

Accessory splinting can be done to help support positioning and to achieve a little more correction. If flexion-contractures persist at the IP joints, cylinder casts can be placed on the fingers to encourage IP extension. Cylinder casts can be placed on the fingers while the fingers are either in or out of the retainer splint, to encourage more MP flexion. In most cases, when cylinder casts are placed on the fingers, the fingers will not extend into hyperextension at the MP joints. If the fingers do completely straighten or hyperextend at the MP joint, they should be protected from hyperextension.

At this point, other pickup activities are introduced, omitting those that require resistive exercise, such as turning a key or opening a jar. Small objects of various shapes are helpful, particularly those that can be stacked and thus encourage shoulder movement. In all cases of pickup activities, the patient should use lumbrical positioning, extending to less than full ROM at the MP joints. Graded fishing weights are helpful, as are Velcro checkers.

The procedure for mobilization of adductor or opponens replacements follows the same principles as for intrinsic replacement surgery, except that the thumb is maintained in an abducted position in the postsurgical cast. If the thumb rests in too much extension, it is harder for the patient to identify the transfer and to use it in sequence of prehension with the fingers. If it rests in too much flexion, the transfer can become a little too tight and the skin at the thenar crease may macerate at the suture site. Optimal is abduction out of the palm in a position where the patient will place a little tension on the transfer when the thumb is extended. This helps give the patient some internal feedback from the new transfer.

Sometimes a thumb intrinsic replacement is done before finger intrinsic replacement, sometimes vice versa, and sometimes both surgeries are performed together. For retraining, it is easier if both surgeries are performed together. For rebalancing, it is better if one surgery is done

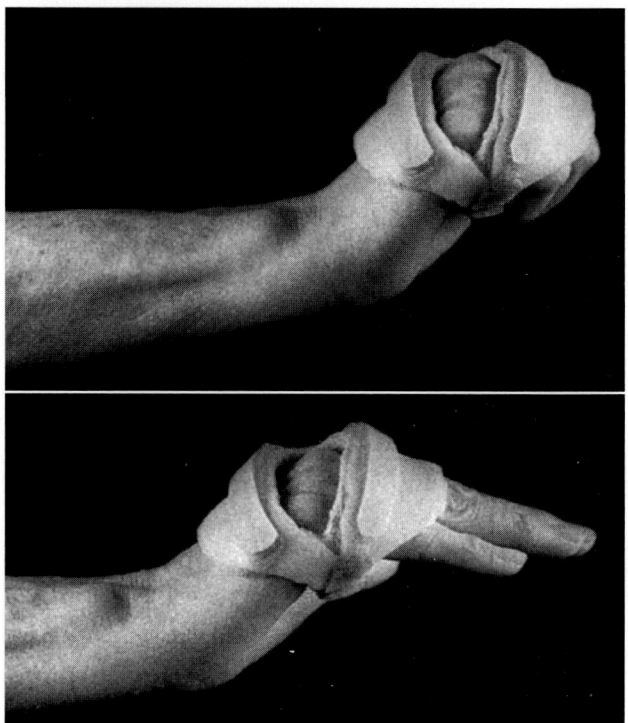

Fig. 48-19. Postoperative ulnar splint used in the late mobilization period. This splint is padded liberally and includes all of the fingers to minimize point pressure. **A,** Gentle interphalangeal (IP) flexion. **B,** IP extension with support of the metacarpophalangeal (MP) joints in flexion to augment new intrinsic tendon transfers while the hand is used and to prevent inadvertent MP hyperextension.

first so the second can be adjusted slightly to the first surgery to provide optimal contact surfaces and pinch of the thumb to the fingers.

Late mobilization period

At the end of the first 3-week mobilization period, unless the transfers have become looser in tension than desired, the cast should be removed for the day and be worn at night for another 3 weeks or longer. An MP flexion splint can be made to continue to support the fingers and to help the patient maintain this position if necessary. The splint can be of the same design as the ulnar-nerve splint worn before surgery but is best made to include all of the fingers to minimize pressure points, as in Fig. 48-19. However, one caution is needed, because the IP joints will extend by the extrinsic extensor when the MP joints are supported in flexion. The therapist must be sure the patient is actually using the transfers. This can be accomplished by frequent removal of the splint for exercise. A splint that prevents only full extension of the MP joints but allows almost full movement otherwise is preferred, to allow full use of the transfers and a gradual return of full finger flexion.

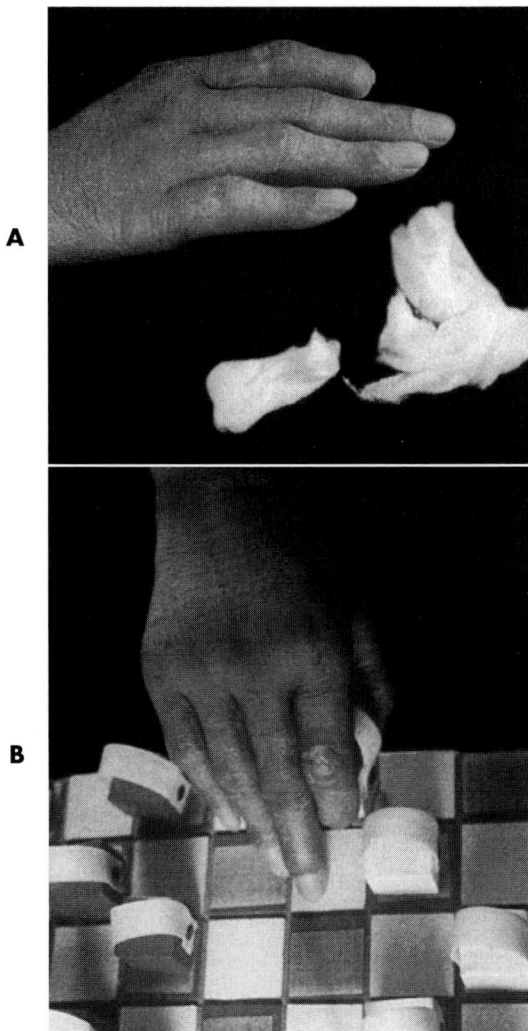

Fig. 48-20. Supervised functional hand use. Essential in early hand use is the transfer to use of corrected positioning. Old habit patterns (e.g., wrist drop to achieve finger extension, forceful extension of the fingers into metacarpophalangeal extension, or full fist too early) are hard to break and can ruin tendon transfer correction. As patients are able to maintain correct positioning and resistance to tendon transfers is safe, they are allowed to assume normal hand skills. Assistive splinting may be necessary to achieve maximum results. Retainer splints can be helpful until no longer necessary. **A,** Light pickup exercise with cotton. **B,** Velcro resistive checkers.

The patient is gradually encouraged to resume normal skill activities (Fig. 48-20), omitting those that offer heavy resistance to the tendons. Gradually full ROM is encouraged, and mild resistance is allowed. The transferred tendons are protected from heavy use for as long as 3 months. Ruptures have been noted as late as 3 months, such as when the patient believes it is possible to use the hand normally and falls, grabs a steering wheel, or pulls on a refrigerator. It is explained to the patient that if balance of the hand is achieved, strength will come later and he or she will have function of the hand for a long time, but if the tendons rupture or if deformity recurs, the hand can be corrected only by another surgery and recovery period.

Other surgical needs

Not all tendon tension can be readjusted or augmented by positioning of the fingers and mobilization of tendon transfers. Sometimes adjustments must be made in surgery. This is particularly true when one muscle is made to go to more than one finger by more than one tendon slip. The muscle will pull hardest on the tendon with the shortest excursion. All or most of the tension of the muscle may be translated to this shortest tendon, rendering further pull of the other tendon ineffective or impossible. For example, if the superficialis of the ring finger has been transferred as an intrinsic replacement of the little and ring fingers, the flexion tension on one is likely to be tighter than on the other. Sometimes this is not enough to cause a problem, and in fact, the tension to the little finger is often made a little tighter because it seems often to have the least tension after surgery (possibly because of the hyperextension of the fifth metacarpal). For the appearance and function of the hand, it is even desirable for the little finger to be a little tighter than the ring. However, in the instance the tension to the little finger is such that most of the transferred motor power acts on the little finger, the unsupported ring finger may return to clawing (with the MP joint in hyperextension and the IP joint in flexion). This can easily result in a progressive deformity of both fingers, because not only will the ring finger continue to claw, but the little finger, if it has a very mobile IP joint, will begin to hyperextend at the IP joint and possibly progressively "swan-neck" from the mechanical overpull of the tendon transfer force.

SUMMARY

Tendon transfer procedures are muscle-rebalancing procedures and biomechanically serve to rebalance what has become imbalanced in the hand from disease or injury. Therefore the therapeutic management of tendon transfers after ulnar- or median-nerve injuries must (1) replace externally, by splinting and/or exercising, the imbalance caused by weak or missing muscles; (2) correct secondary problems that have occurred, such as skin and joint contractures; or (3) augment what has been corrected through surgical transfers by corrective positioning and by mobilizing surgical hands in a way that maintains, increases, or decreases transferred tendon tension.

REFERENCES
1. Agee JA, Guidern M: The functional significance of the juncturae tendineae in dynamic stabilization of the metacarpophalangeal joints of the fingers. Paper presented at the Annual Conference of the American Society for Surgery of the Hand, Atlanta, 1980.

2. Bell JA: Rehabilitation: tendon transfers panel discussion, Richard Smith, moderator. In Hunter JM, Schneider LH, Mackin EJ, editors: *Tendon surgery in the hand,* St Louis, 1987, Mosby.

3. Boyes JH: *Bunnell's surgery of the hand,* ed 5, Philadelphia, 1970, JB Lippincott.

4. Brand PW: Paralytic claw hand, *J Bone Joint Surg* 40B:618, 1958.

5. Brand PW: Tendon transfers for median and ulnar nerve paralysis, *Orthop Clin North Am* 1:447, 1970.

6. Brand PW: Personal communications, 1978.

7. Brand PW: Biomechanics of tendon transfers. In Hunter JM, Schneider LH, Mackin EJ, editors: *Tendon surgery in the hand,* St Louis, 1987, Mosby.

8. Brand PW: *Clinical mechanics of the hand,* ed 2, St Louis, 1992, Mosby.

9. Brand PW, et al: Relative tension and potential excursion of muscles in the forearm and hand, *J Hand Surg* 6:209, 1981.

10. Brandsma JW, Birke JA, Sims D Jr: The Martin-Gruber innervated hand, *J Hand Surg* 11A:536, 1986.

11. Brooks AL: A new intrinsic tendon transfer for the paralytic hand, *J Bone Joint Surg* 57A:730, 1975.

12. Burkhalter WE: Restoration of power grip in ulnar nerve paralysis, *Orthop Clin North Am* 2:289, 1974.

13. Casanova JS, Grunert BK: Adult prehension: patterns and nomenclature, ASHT Annual Conference, Sept. 13, 1987.

14. Cochran GVB: *A primer of orthopedic biomechanics,* New York, 1982, Churchill Livingstone.

15. Fess EE: The need for reliability and validity in hand assessment instruments, *J Hand Surg* 11A:621, 1986.

16. Fess EE, Phillips C: *Hand splinting principles and methods,* ed 2, St Louis, 1987, Mosby.

17. Flatt AE: *The care of the rheumatoid hand,* ed 4, St Louis, 1983, Mosby.

18. Frost HM: *An introduction to biomechanics,* Springfield, Ill, 1967, Charles C Thomas.

19. Gelberman RH, Manske PR: Effects of early motion on the tendon healing process: experimental studies. In Hunter JM, Schneider LH, Mackin EJ, editors: *Tendon surgery in the hand,* St Louis, 1987, Mosby.

20. Harris EC Jr: Intrinsic balance of the extensor system. In Hunter JM, Schneider LH, Mackin EJ, editors: *Tendon surgery in the hand,* St Louis, 1987, Mosby.

21. Kapandji IA: Biomechanics of the thumb. In Tubiana R, editor: *The hand,* Philadelphia, 1981, WB Saunders.

22. Kumar RP, Brandsma JW: A method to determine pressure distribution of the hand, *Lepr Rev* 57:39, 1986.

23. Landsmeer JMF: The anatomy of the dorsal aponeurosis of the human finger and its functional significance, *Anat Rec* 104:31, 1949.

24. Littler JW: Tendon transfers and arthrodeses in combined median and ulnar nerve paralysis, *J Bone Joint Surg* 31A:225, 1949.

25. Long C, et al: Intrinsic-extrinsic muscle control of the hand in power grip and precision handling: an electromyographic study, *J Bone Joint Surg* 52A:853, 1970.

26. Manske PR, Lesker PA: Diffusion as a nutrient pathway to the flexor tendon. In Hunter JM, Schneider LH, Mackin EJ, editors: *Tendon surgery in the hand,* St Louis, 1987, Mosby.

27. Marks R, Payne PA: *Bioengineering and the skin,* Lancaster, England, 1979, MTP Press United International Medical Publishers.

28. Mathews R: Personal communications, Rat studies, 1979.

29. Moberg E: Objective methods for determining the functional value of sensibility of the hand, *J Bone Joint Surg* 40B:454, 1958.

30. Omer GE Jr: Tendon transfers as early internal splints following peripheral nerve injury in the upper extremity. In Hunter JM, Schneider LH, Mackin EJ, editors: *Tendon surgery in the hand,* St Louis, 1987, Mosby.

31. Peacock EE Jr: Collagen metabolism during healing of long tendons. In Hunter JM, Schneider LH, Mackin EJ, editors: *Tendon surgery in the hand,* St Louis, 1987, Mosby.

32. Ranney DA: Reconstruction of the transverse metacarpal arc in ulnar palsy by transfer of the extensor digiti minimi, *Plast Reconstr Surg* 52:406, 1973.

33. Riordan DC: Tendon transplantation in median-nerve and ulnar-nerve paralysis, *J Bone Joint Surg* 35A:312, 1953.

34. Riordan DC: Principles of tendon transfers. In Hunter JM, Schneider LH, Mackin EJ, editors: *Tendon surgery in the hand,* St Louis, 1987, Mosby.

35. Salter RB, et al: The biological effect of continuous passive motion on the healing of full-thickness defects in articular cartilage: an experimental investigation in the rabbit, *J Bone Joint Surg* 62A:1232, 1980.

36. Stiles HJ, Forrester-Brown MF: *Treatment of injuries of the peripheral spinal nerves,* London, 1922, Henry Frowde Hudder and Stoughten.

37. Thompson TC: Modified operation for opponens paralysis, *J Bone Joint Surg* 24:623, 1972.

38. Van der Meulen JC: Causes of prolapse and collapse of the proximal interphalangeal joint of the hand, *Hand* 4:147, 1972.

39. Wright V: Stiffness: a review of its measurement and physiological importance, *Physiotherapy* 59:107, 1973.

40. Yamada H: *Strength of biological materials,* Baltimore, 1970, Williams & Wilkins.

41. Zancolli EA: *Structural and dynamic bases of hand surgery,* ed 2, Philadelphia, 1979, JB Lippincott.

42. Zancolli EA: Claw hand caused by paralysis of the intrinsic muscles: a simplified surgical procedure for its correction, *J Bone Joint Surg* 39A:1076, 1957.

Chapter 49

PREOPERATIVE AND POSTOPERATIVE MANAGEMENT OF TENDON TRANSFERS AFTER RADIAL NERVE INJURY

C. Christopher Reynolds

Peripheral nerve injuries in the upper extremity are caused by laceration, compression, perforation, traction, and occasionally the toxic effects of injected drugs. The radial nerve is particularly susceptible to damage because it courses along the shaft of the humerus. Perforating injuries are common from fragments of fractured bone, although typically the nerve is injured by direct external compression. Sustained pressure under the axilla from crutches may result in significant damage to nerve fibers. Prolonged pressure at the midhumeral level results in paralysis of muscles innervated by the radial nerve; this paralysis is often referred to as *Saturday night palsy* or *drunkard's palsy.*[1,4]

A familiar clinical picture emerges with radial nerve paralysis. The forearm is pronated and the classic "wrist drop" position is assumed (Fig. 49-1). Grip strength is substantially reduced because inactive wrist extensors create an unstable wrist and minimize the power of the long finger flexors. The inability to extend the fingers at the metacarpophalangeal (MP) joints prevents satisfactory grasp and release of large objects. Paralysis of the forearm supinator does not pose an additional problem. Supination is still possible through the action of the musculocutaneous innervated biceps brachii.[11]

Several tendon transfer procedures are used to restore function after radial nerve injuries.[9,10,12] Muscles commonly used for the radial nerve transfers include the pronator teres (PT) for wrist extension; flexor carpi ulnaris (FCU), flexor carpi radialis (FCR), or flexor digitorum superficialis (FDS) for finger extension; and palmaris longus (PL) or FDS for thumb extension (Table 49-1). Transfer procedures affecting wrist and digital extension are among the most favorable and predictable in hand surgery. However, without a comprehensive preoperative and postoperative hand therapy program, success is much more difficult to obtain.

PREOPERATIVE HAND THERAPY PROGRAM

Preoperatively, the goals of the hand therapist are to obtain a baseline motor evaluation, maintain function without allowing bad habits to develop, prevent contractures of the hand and forearm, and strengthen muscles that are to be used for transfer.[2,8]

Motor evaluation

An early motor evaluation helps determine the level of injury and defines a baseline from which progress can be measured if regeneration occurs. Typically, with a high radial nerve palsy, the muscles innervated distal to the branches of the triceps are involved. These include the brachioradialis (BR), supinator, and all wrist and extrinsic digital extensors. The radial nerve divides into two branches at or about the level of the elbow as it passes deep to the BR. The superficial radial nerve, a sensory branch, provides sensation to the

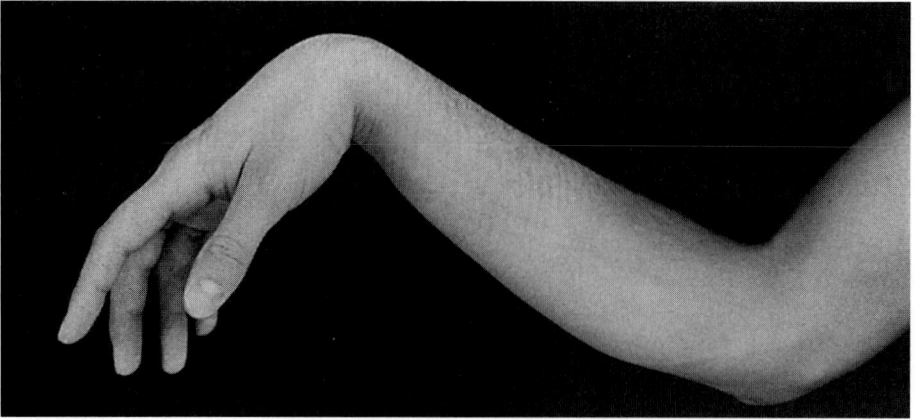

Fig. 49-1. Paralysis of the supinator muscle and all wrist and digital extensors creates the classic wrist-drop posture of the hand and forearm.

Table 49-1. Commonly used tendon transfers for radial nerve paralysis

Muscle	Action
Pronator teres	Wrist extension (extensor carpi radialis brevis, longus)
Flexor carpi ulnaris or flexor digitorum sublimus	Finger extension (extensor digitorum communis)
Palmaris longus or flexor digitorum sublimus	Thumb extension (extensor pollicis longus)

dorsal radial aspect of the hand. Because sensory distribution is usually confined to a small dorsal area, sensory loss will have little affect on patient function. The posterior interosseous nerve, the motor branch, has variable innervation. Characteristically, the posterior interosseous nerve innervates at least one radial wrist extensor, the supinator, the extensor carpi ulnaris (ECU), and the digital extensors.

Injury to this branch of the radial nerve does not result in wrist drop because one innervated wrist extensor remains. However, with posterior interosseous nerve injury, wrist extension is radially deviated because the ECU is not functioning to centralize the wrist unit.

A baseline muscle test evaluates the power of individual muscles innervated by the radial nerve. Several methods of manual muscle testing are currently used.[7] In addition to these tests, a comparison can be made between the injured and uninjured sides. The BR, an elbow flexor, is a superficial muscle that stands out readily with resistance to the flexed elbow. To observe a contraction, the forearm is positioned in a neutral position and resistance is applied at the wrist (Fig. 49-2). If the muscle is weak, the contraction will not be as prominent as the muscle on the contralateral side. Elbow flexion is rarely affected by the absence of the BR because of the strength of the biceps brachii. Careful observation and palpation of the contraction of the BR indicate functional regeneration or return. Radial wrist extension is

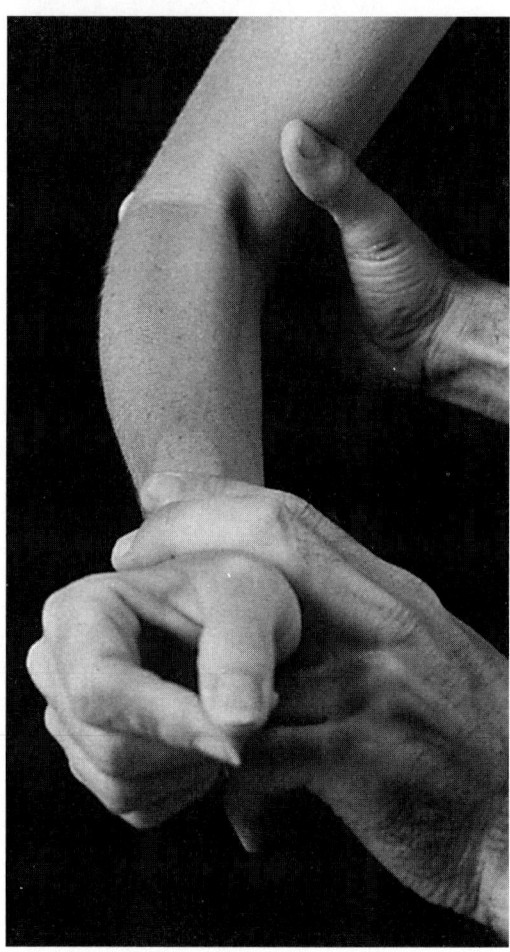

Fig. 49-2. An intact brachioradialis stands out readily when resistance is applied to the flexed elbow.

accomplished by the extensor carpi radialis longus (ECRL) and extensor carpi radialis brevis (ECRB) muscles. These muscles are tested with the forearm pronated and the wrist positioned over the edge of a table or towel roll. Finger and thumb extensors may substitute for the action of the wrist

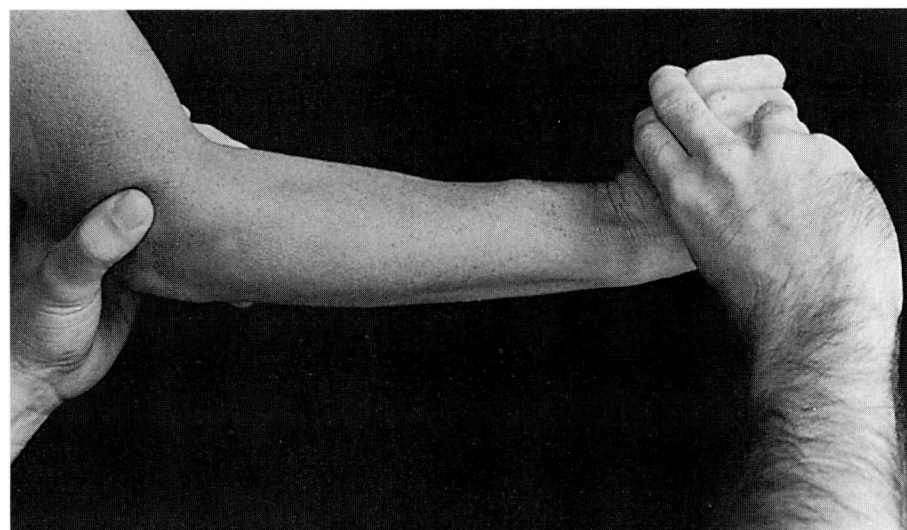

Fig. 49-3. To test the extensor carpi radialis longus and brevis, resistance is applied to the dorsoradial aspect of the hand in the direction of flexion and ulnar deviation.

extensor muscles. Flexing the fingers and the thumb in the palm helps prevent substitution and isolate wrist extensor power. Resistance is applied on the dorsum of the second and third metacarpals as the patient holds the position of extension and radial deviation (Fig. 49-3). A second wrist position is used if the patient cannot extend the wrist against gravity. The forearm is supinated to midline or neutral while the ulnar side of the hand is resting on the table.

The ECU extends the wrist in an ulnar direction. This muscle is tested in the same fashion as the radial wrist extensors. However, resistance is applied to the dorsum of the fifth metacarpal in the direction of flexion and radial deviation. Careful palpation of the prominent ECU tendon, distal to the ulnar head, is helpful in determining the activity of the muscle when there is significant weakness (Fig. 49-4).

Supination of the forearm is possible through the action of both the biceps brachii and the supinator muscles. The biceps muscle is not the primary supinator of the forearm; however, its influence is significant. As the biceps flexes the elbow, supination occurs. To eliminate biceps activity, the elbow is extended completely and supination power can be measured. As the patient pronates and then supinates the forearm, resistance is applied at the extreme of supination and then compared with that of the opposite side (Fig. 49-5).

The extensor digitorum communis (EDC), extensor indicis proprius (EIP), and extensor digiti minimi (EDM) extend the fingers at the MP joints of the second through fifth digits. The proper muscle test position is with the wrist in a neutral position and the interphalangeal (IP) joints flexed (Fig. 49-6). A neutral wrist prevents extensor tenodesis of the fingers, and the IP joints are flexed to inhibit the activity of the lumbrical and interossei. In this test position, the patient attempts to extend the MP joints against gravity while resistance is applied to the proximal phalanges. If the patient is unable to extend the MP joints against gravity, the hand is repositioned to eliminate gravity's effects. The forearm is placed in neutral while the ulnar side of the hand rests on the

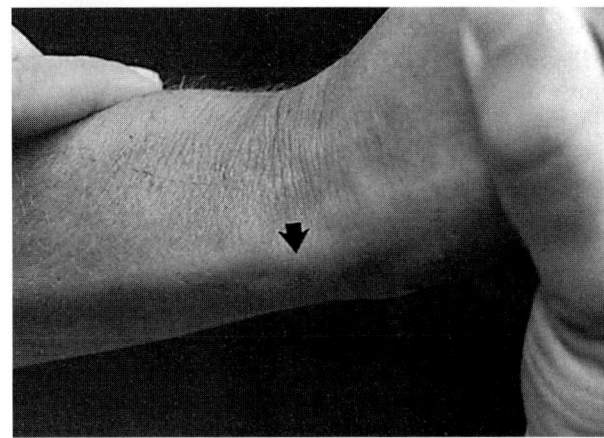

Fig. 49-4. The extensor carpi ulnaris tendon *(arrow)* is visible and palpable distal to the ulnar styloid.

table; the patient is then retested. With extreme weakness, observing and palpating tendon movement over the metacarpals is helpful. The EIP and EDM can be isolated by having the patient extend the MP joint of the index finger for the EIP and the little finger MP joint for the EDM.

Muscles of the first extensor compartment, abductor pollicis longus (APL), and extensor pollicis brevis (EPB) are true radial abductors of the thumb. The APL is the primary radial abductor of the first metacarpal. The EPB performs the same task in addition to extending the MP joint of the thumb. These muscles are the most difficult of the radial nerve muscles to isolate and measure. The extensor pollicis longus (EPL) can substitute for the action of both muscles. Its function can be minimized during testing by flexing the IP joint of the thumb (Fig. 49-7). Careful palpation of the tendons of the first extensor compartment is necessary as the patient radially abducts the thumb and extends the MP joint.

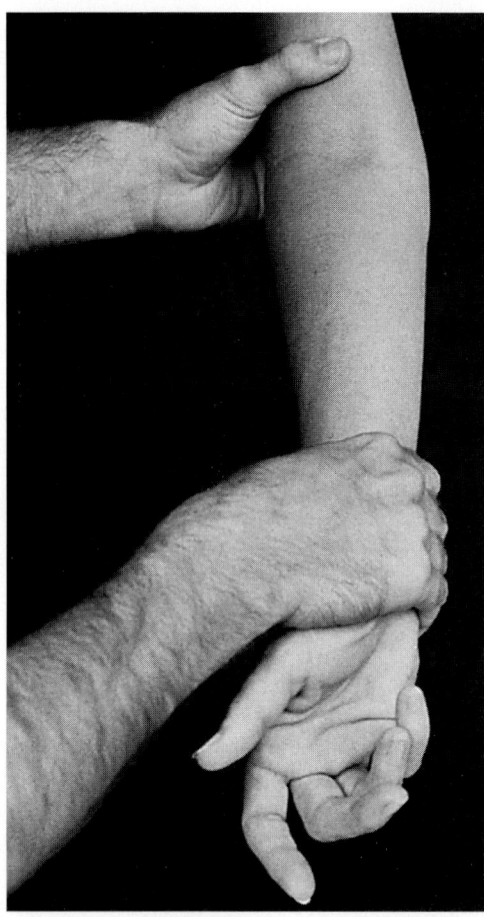

Fig. 49-5. Resisted supination is tested with the elbow extended to eliminate biceps brachia activity.

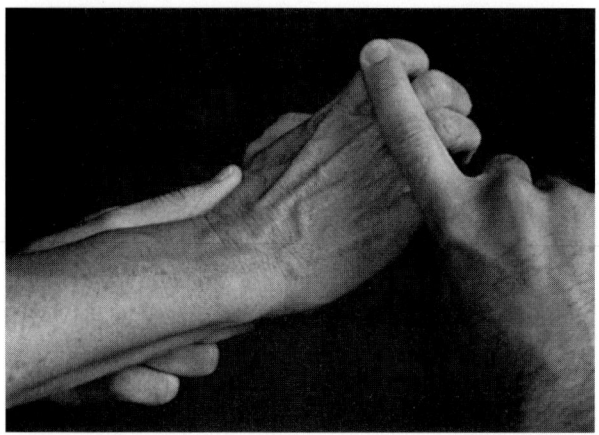

Fig. 49-6. To test extensor digitorum, resistance is applied to the proximal phalanges while the patient maintains the fingers in a claw position.

Extension of the distal phalanx of the thumb is accomplished by three muscles. The primary extensor is the EPL. The accessory pull from slips of the abductor pollicis brevis (APB) and flexor pollicis brevis (FPB), which are innervated by the median nerve, assists in extending the IP joint of the

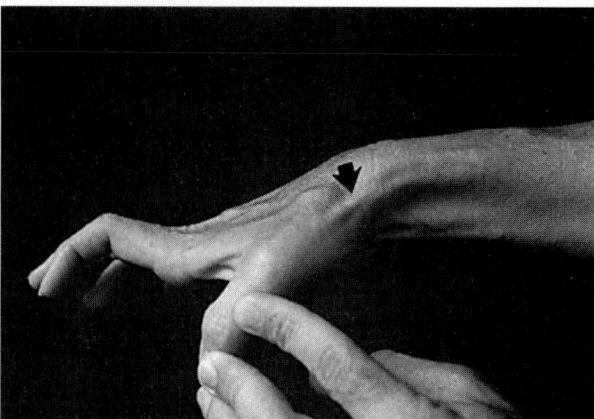

Fig. 49-7. Palpation of the first extensor compartment tendons *(arrow)* is necessary to determine their level of activity.

thumb. To prevent APB and FPB activity, the thumb is placed in extreme passive extension. In this position the EPL can extend the IP joint of the thumb. A strong EPL maintains the IP joint in hyperextension against maximum resistance. If the EPL is weak, hyperextension of the joint will not occur and palpation or observation of the tendon on the dorsal radial aspect of the wrist is necessary (Fig. 49-8).

If tendon transfers are expected for weak or absent radial innervated muscles, it is important to test the strength of the muscles to be transferred. Isolating and testing the strength of the PT, FCU, FCR, FDS, and PL muscles is an important component of the preoperative evaluation.

Prevention of contractures and maintenance of function

Preventing or avoiding contractures is the second goal of the preoperative program. Maintaining a supple wrist and hand is generally not difficult after radial nerve injuries. However, if the wrist and digits remain flexed for a prolonged period, the long flexors of the fingers become tight, whereas the extrinsic extensors stretch out. Tight finger flexors prevent simultaneous wrist and finger extension. Serial splinting is helpful in overcoming tightness of the long finger flexors. Anteroposterior plaster splints that are changed frequently will gradually stretch the tight tendons. However, because of managed care constraints on patient visits and on the manufacturing of multiple splints, other innovative dynamic splints can accomplish the same goal of stretching tight finger flexors (Fig. 49-9).

More commonly, bad habits occur that lead to functional problems after tendon transfer surgery. For instance, if the patient allows the wrist to flex during functional activities preoperatively, even after wrist extensor transfers, he or she may habitually flex the wrist during grasp-and-release activities. Similarly, habitual finger extension using intrinsic muscles preoperatively continues after tendon transfers. The patient may ''forget'' how to extend the fingers at the MP

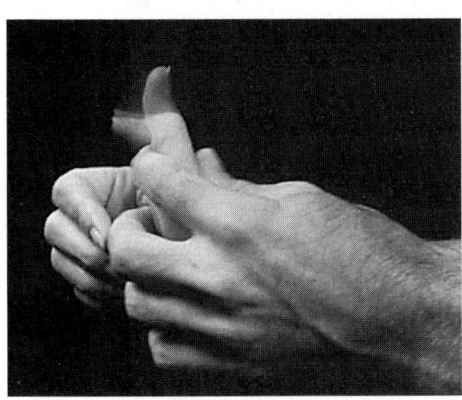

Fig. 49-8. The extensor pollicis longus is the sole extensor of the interphalangeal joint of the thumb when abductor pollicis longus and flexor pollicis brevis activity is eliminated.

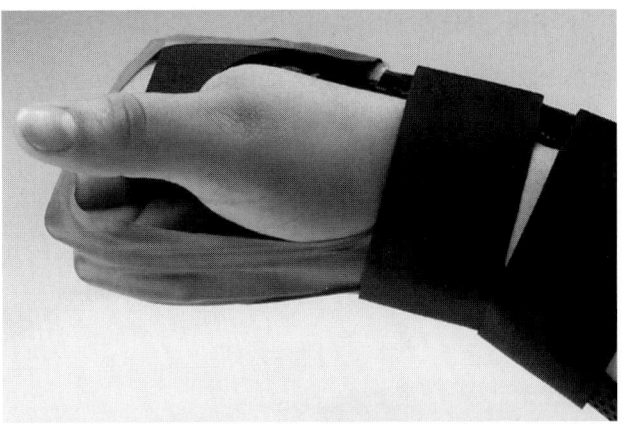

Fig. 49-9. A dynamic splint is used to stretch tight finger flexors, which may result from longstanding radial nerve paralysis. (© 2000 Stephen G. Dreiseszun/Viewpoint Photographers, 9034 N. 23rd Ave., Suite 11, Phoenix, Ariz 85021.)

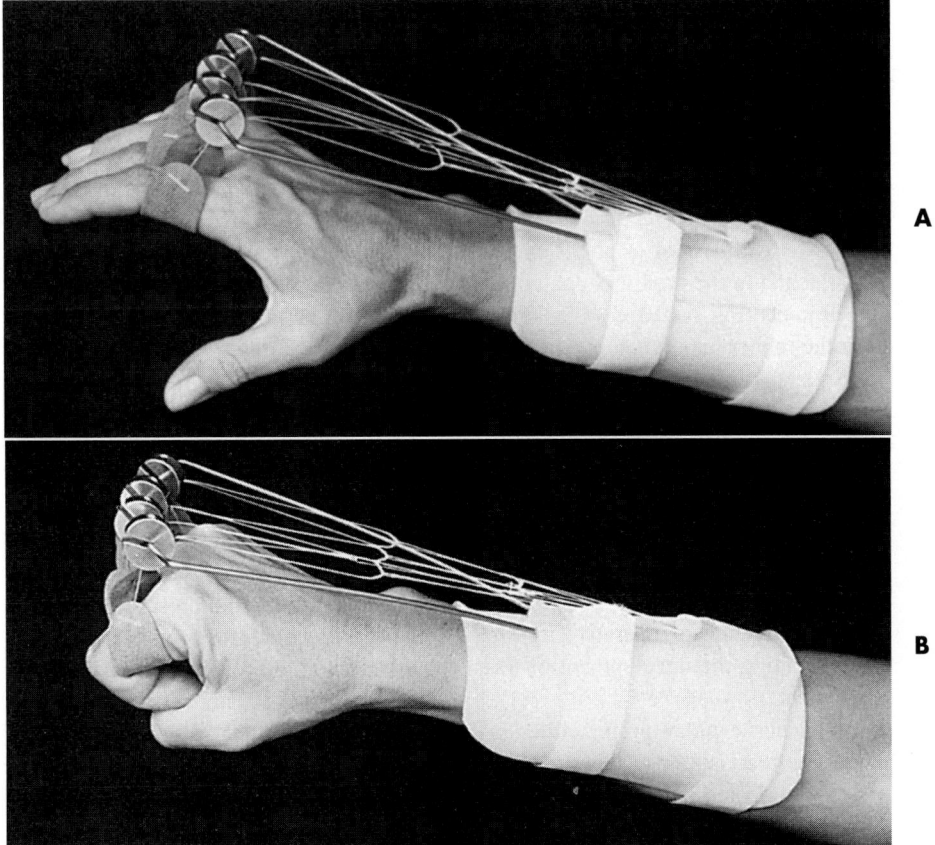

Fig. 49-10. The improved Hollis-type splint prevents wrist drop while allowing finger extension (**A**) and flexion (**B**).

joints even after transfers. For these reasons, preoperative splinting and reeducation exercises are necessary.

To maintain function and prevent the establishment of bad habits, the wrist and digits are splinted to support the wrist in neutral or slight extension and recreate extensor power of the digits. One splint option is based on a design illustrated by Hollis in 1978 and Colditz in 1987[3,5,6] (Fig. 49-10). It allows finger flexion with wrist extension and finger extension with wrist flexion. Slings or loops placed at the proximal phalanges are attached to

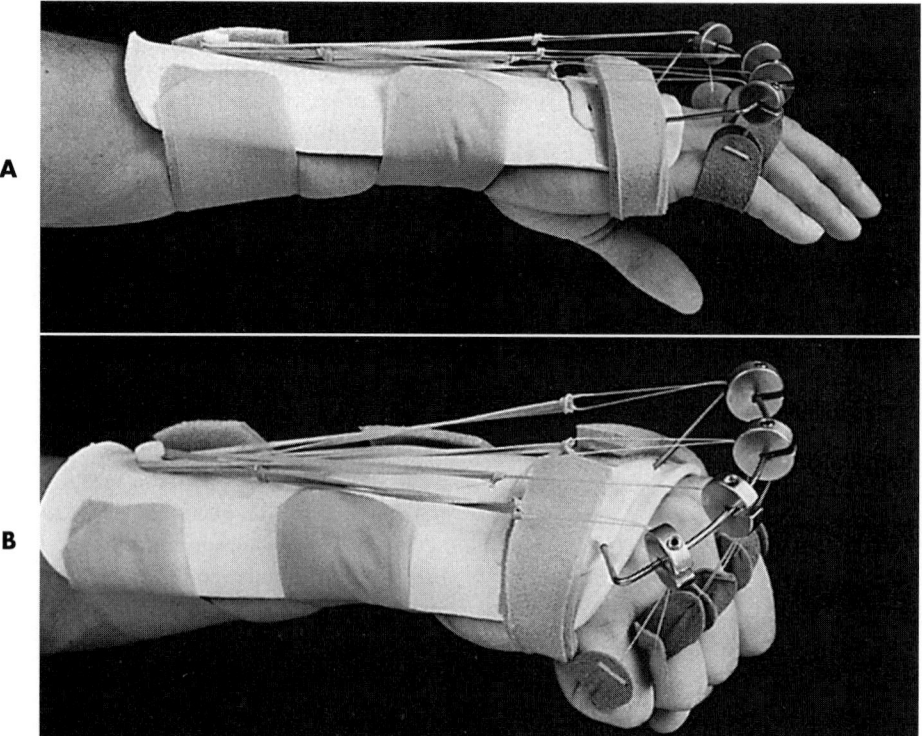

Fig. 49-11. A, Another radial nerve splint supports the wrist while rubber-band tension extends the metacarpophalangeal joints. **B,** The wrist is maintained in an extended position with flexion of the fingers.

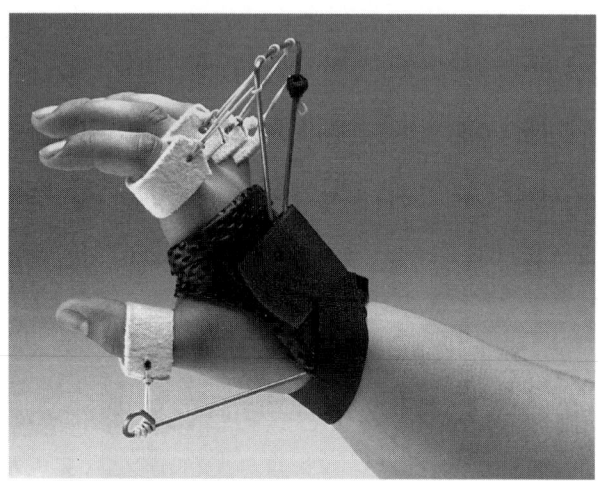

Fig. 49-12. A splint for a patient with posterior interosseous nerve paralysis or partial radial nerve return. In this case, wrist extension is available but digital extensors are paralyzed. The hand-based splint assists digital extension. (© 2000 Stephen G. Dreiseszun/ Viewpoint Photographers, 9034 N. 23rd Ave., Suite 11, Phoenix, Ariz 85021.)

the forearm by a static, taut line. As the wrist flexes to neutral, the loops support the MP joints in extension, permitting intrinsic muscles to extend the IP joints. As the patient flexes the fingers, support at the proximal phalanges through the loops maintains the wrist in extension. A

second splint option statically supports the wrist in neutral or slight extension while rubber bands attached to the proximal phalanges dynamically extend the MP joints (Fig. 49-11, *A*). Flexion of the fingers occurs against the rubber band traction while the wrist is maintained in an extended position (Fig. 49-11, *B*). Thumb slings may be used but are not always necessary to position the thumb. Most patients can substitute extension of the thumb with palmar abduction.

There are advantages to both splint designs. The Hollis splint has less bulk and enhances function by allowing wrist motion. However, many patients prefer the wrist support afforded by the more rigid and distally based dynamic splint. Both designs offer an effective preoperative tool to improve function while preventing the development of undesirable patterns of movement.

Most patients with radial nerve palsy prefer either of these splints in addition to one that supports the wrist only, such as a custom-made or prefabricated wrist cock-up. These splints provide simple wrist support when finger extension is not necessary. The wrist cock-up is useful when the patient is sleeping or engaged in activities requiring sustained grip.

If wrist extensors remain intact or are innervated yet the patient has weak digital extensors, a "hand-based" digital extension splint may be helpful (Fig. 49-12).

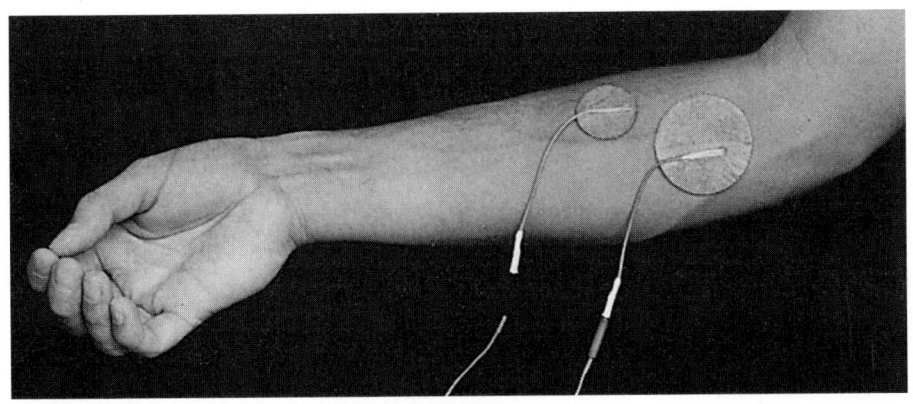

Fig. 49-13. Electrical stimulation is used in conjunction with exercise to increase the strength of muscles to be used for transfer. The pronator teres muscle is stimulated before transfer to the wrist extensors.

Strengthening muscles selected for transfers

The final preoperative therapy goal is to strengthen muscles that will be used for transfer. Because a tendon is potentially weaker when it is transferred, a strengthening program helps maximize its effectiveness. Strengthening can be accomplished by a graded, progressive resistive exercise program and may include electrical stimulation (Fig. 49-13). Isolating muscles for strengthening preoperatively facilitates a postoperative program as well. The patient is more likely to know how to use the tendon transfer after surgery if the muscle has been isolated and activated preoperatively.

POSTOPERATIVE HAND THERAPY PROGRAM
General principles of postoperative therapy management

There are several basic, yet key, principles each hand therapist must consider when given the task of rehabilitating radial nerve tendon transfers (or for that matter, all tendon transfers of the hand). The most important concept is to avoid early tension on the newly transferred tendon until the appropriate time (usually 5 to 6 weeks postoperatively). Early tension can either tear out the sutured transfer or stretch the transfer, thus rendering it less effective. Early postoperative splinting to protect the tendon transfers in a "slackened" position is paramount. Generally, this period of splinting is 4 weeks. Once motion is initiated, tension on the tendon transfer can be prevented by avoiding composite joint motions. For example, if the pathway of the PT to ECRB is considered, the therapist should avoid combined elbow extension and wrist flexion until 5 to 6 weeks after surgery because the PT originates above the elbow and the ECRB inserts distal to the wrist joint. Therefore extending the elbow and flexing the wrist will stretch the transfer. Similarly, the FCU-to-EDC or FCR-to-EDC transfer pathway dictates that tension can be avoided if the elbow is not extended with wrist/finger flexion for a full 5 to 6 weeks. This is because the FCU and FCR originate just proximal to the elbow joint at the medial epicondyle, whereas the distal insertion of the transfer is distal to the MP joint. Finally, the PL-to-EPL transfer pathway extends from the medial epicondyle of the elbow to the distal phalanx of the thumb.

Avoiding combined elbow extension, wrist flexion, ulnar deviation, and thumb flexion/adduction is necessary for the first 5 to 6 weeks to prevent tension on this transfer.

A second principle is to maximize individual joint motions to prevent contractures, starting at 4 weeks after the tendon transfer. Mobilization of the elbow, forearm, wrist, and individual joints of the fingers is necessary to achieve a supple quality to each joint. This period lasts from the fourth to sixth weeks. Patients must be given specific instructions at this time to maximize each joint's potential.

A third principle is to initiate reeducation of the patient regarding the specific tendon transfers at the appropriate time, as determined by the surgeon (usually at 5 weeks). A discussion of reeducation techniques for each transfer can be found in the next section.

Finally, strengthening techniques begin 8 weeks after surgery. At the same time, general precautions regarding "overstretching" the transfer are dismissed and the patient should be trying to resume more normal activities.

Specific postoperative splinting and rehabilitation techniques

Hand therapists do not always get the opportunity to see tendon transfer patients before surgery. Often, the therapist will see the patient 1 to 2 weeks postoperatively in a postoperative bulky dressing or a posterior protective slab applied by the surgeon. At that time, the therapist is asked to fabricate a thermoplastic splint to protect the transferred structures (Fig. 49-14). Three to five weeks of complete immobilization (as determined by the surgeon) following surgery is necessary to protect the transferred tendons. When the PT is used for wrist extension, the elbow must be immobilized in 90 degrees of flexion with the forearm maximally pronated and the wrist extended from 30 to 45 degrees. When the FCU is used for finger extension, the MP joints of the fingers are extended to neutral. If the PL is transferred for thumb extension or abduction, the thumb must be immobilized as well, with the IP and MP joints extended completely and the thumb maximally abducted at the carpometacarpal (CMC) joint. In this postoperative splint, only the IP joints of the fingers remain free and are

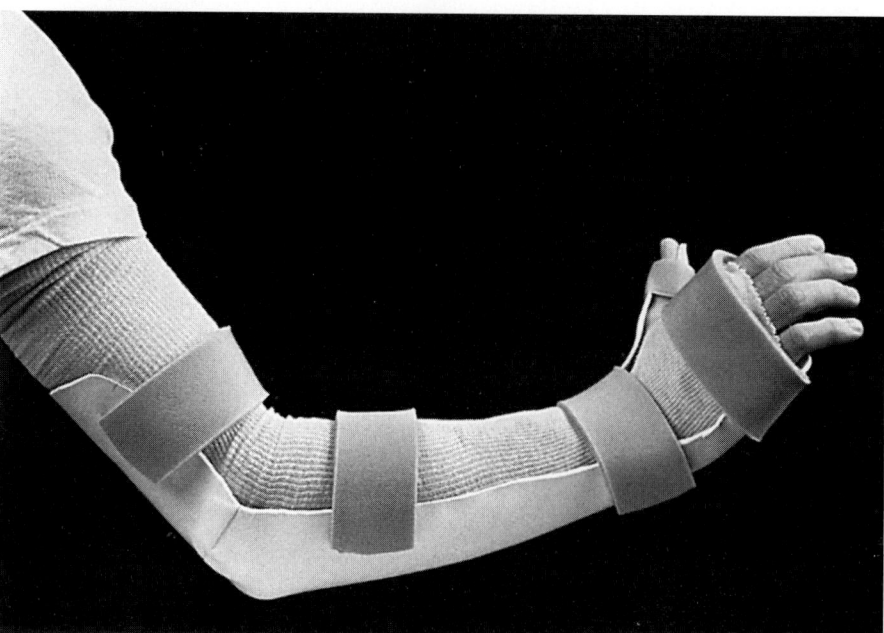

Fig. 49-14. A thermoplastic splint is constructed at 4 weeks after surgery to protect the transfer, but it can be removed for exercises.

exercised. With the other joints immobilized, tension is taken off the tendon transfer junctions and healing takes place without overstretching or rupturing of the transfers. During the immobilization period, shoulder motion is maintained with flexion/extension, abduction/adduction, and rotation exercises. In addition, IP joint flexion and extension exercises are performed for each of the fingers.

Mobilization and reeducation

Mobilization and tendon transfer reeducation exercises begin 4 weeks after surgery. Protective splinting is necessary for another 3 to 4 weeks, for a total of 7 to 8 weeks after surgery. The thermoplastic splint continues to protect the patient when he or she is sleeping or riding in a car or during situations in which the arm may be forced into an overstretched position. Initially, the splint is removed during the exercise periods and when the patient is bathing or dressing. It is removed more frequently as light activities are incorporated into the exercise and therapy program.

Individual joint range-of-motion (ROM) exercises are performed in the first week of mobilization (Fig. 49-15). This is a very tedious and mundane part of the program, but it is vital to the success of the transfers. Exercising individual joints that were immobilized for 4 weeks will not overstretch tendon transfers. Attention is focused at the MP joints of the fingers. These joints are most susceptible to debilitating extension contractures after postoperative immobilization. The MP joints are exercised with the wrist and the IP joints of the fingers extended. In this manner, flexion and extension of the MP joints are maximized with the least amount of tension on the tendon transfers. In addition to the MP joint exercises, other joints are isolated and ROM exercises are carried out. For example, elbow flexion and extension

exercises are performed while the forearm is maintained in pronation and the wrist and fingers are held in extension. Exercises for forearm rotation are performed with the elbow flexed and the wrist and fingers maintained in extension. Gentle, active-assisted wrist flexion and extension exercises are performed while the elbow is held flexed, the forearm is pronated, and the fingers are positioned in extension. Assistance is needed with extension of the wrist because the tendon transfer does not function well at this early stage of the mobilization process. Other exercises include gentle, active-assisted ROM for thumb IP, MP, and CMC joints. Care is taken to mobilize individual joints of the thumb and avoid composite IP and MP flexion and abduction to the fifth metacarpal head. Composite motion stretches the thumb transfers too vigorously.

Exercises are performed in the clinic by the therapist and also by the patient at home. A home exercise program is outlined in both written and verbal form. The patient is told to remove the splint six to eight times daily and to practice the individual joint ROM exercises 10 times.

During the first week of mobilization, attention is also given to the various forearm and hand scars, which may be hypersensitive but most often are just thick and attenuated to the skin and deeper soft tissue structures. Friction massages with a lubricating cream or lotion are performed to soften the scar and mobilize adjacent skin and subcutaneous tissues. Hypersensitive scars are desensitized by rubbing progressively coarser fabrics and materials over the scars or using a handheld vibrator (see Chapter 33). Transcutaneous electrical nerve stimulation is necessary if conventional desensitization techniques are not effective.

An important component of any stretching or mobilization program is the use of gentle therapeutic heat (from

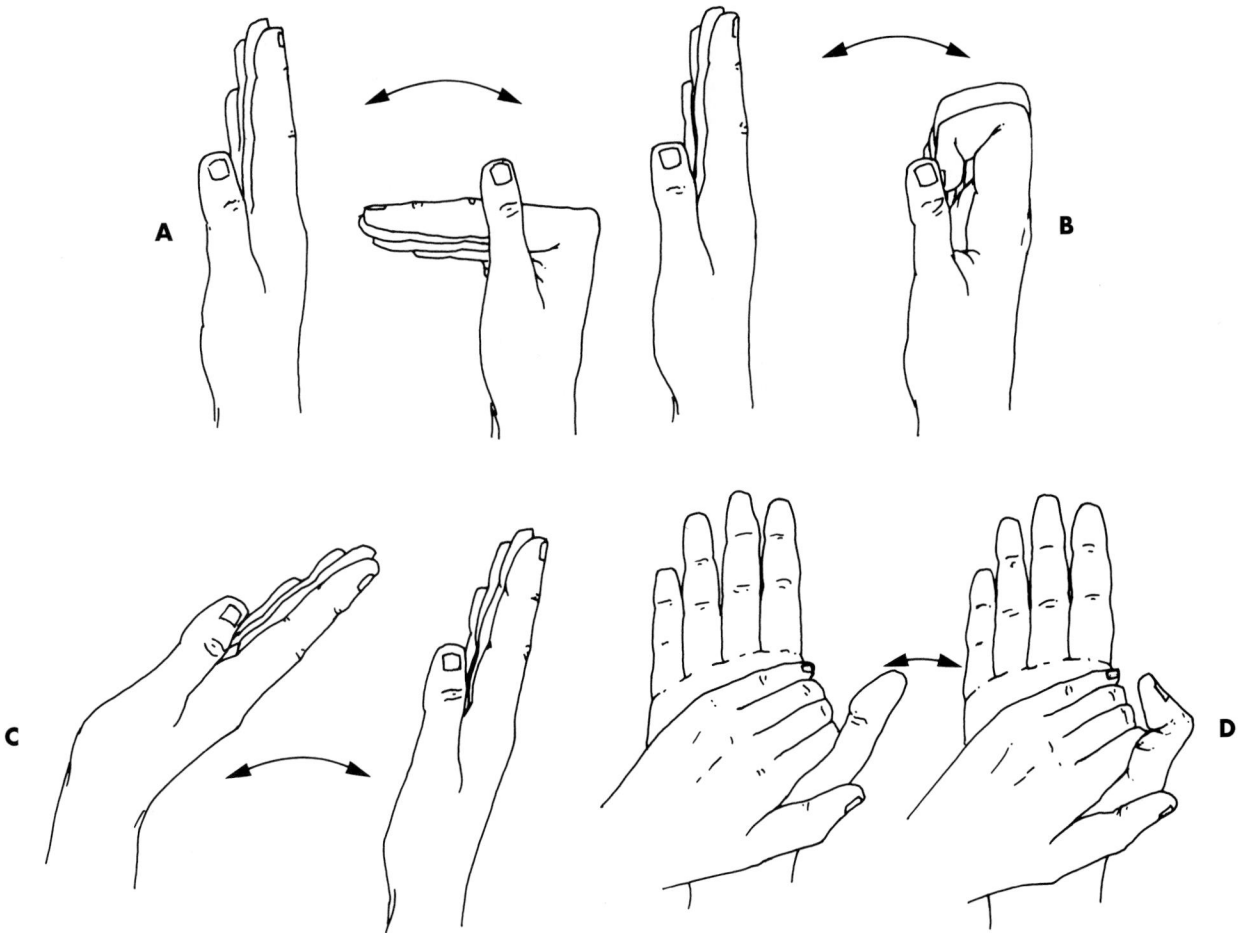

Fig. 49-15. Gentle exercises are performed initially to improve range of motion of individual joints. The metacarpophalangeal joints of the fingers are most susceptible to contracture after tendon transfer surgery. **A,** Gentle metacarpophalangeal flexion and extension with the interphalangeals extended. **B,** Interphalangeal joint flexion and extension with the metacarpophalangeals extended as much as possible. **C,** Gentle wrist flexion to neutral position. **D,** Thumb interphalangeal joint flexion and extension.

40° to 45° C) applied in the form of hot packs, paraffin, or fluidotherapy. These superficial heating methods are helpful in increasing elasticity to the tissue as well as reducing joint stiffness and improving blood flow. The patient is instructed to use moist heat at home two or three times daily for 20 minutes.

In the second week of mobilization or the sixth postoperative week, attention is turned to the tendon transfers themselves. Activating the appropriate muscle for a certain task is difficult or easy, depending on the muscles used for transfer and the preoperative training used. Muscles used for normal tenodesing patterns of wrist flexion with digital extension are fairly easy to reeducate. For example, if the FCU is used for finger extension, the patient is asked to gently flex the wrist in an ulnar direction while extending the fingers. Performing this motion on the uninjured hand first helps the patient visualize and understand what the therapist is trying to accomplish. After the patient understands the

concept, the motion is attempted on the reconstructed hand. As the patient slowly flexes the wrist, extension of the fingers occurs at the MP joints. The tendons of the EDC muscle across the metacarpals stand out slightly, indicating activation of the transfer. Care is taken to avoid wrist flexion past neutral because this promotes extensor tendon tightness or tenodesis, not pure tendon transfer activity. Therefore the patient should maintain some wrist extension position while attempting to extend the MP joints. Early training attempts result in rapid muscle fatigue. It is not uncommon for the patient to perform only a few repetitions before the transfer tires. The patient must be encouraged to stop exercising when this happens and to not force the muscles to perform. Slow, controlled, and precise contractions are practiced to promote and develop good patterns of motion.

When the PL is used for thumb extension, the same tenodesing pattern of wrist flexion with digital extension is practiced. The patient palpates and observes contraction of

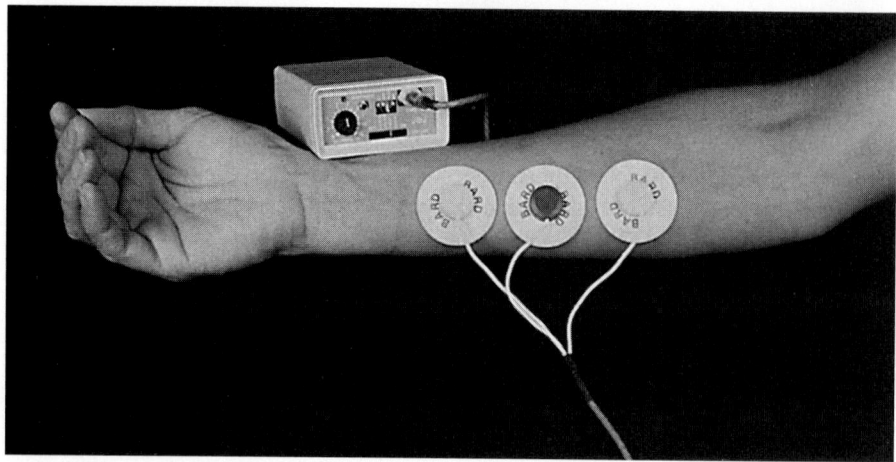

Fig. 49-16. Visual and auditory biofeedback techniques help patients become aware of muscles used for transfer procedures.

the EPL tendon above the anatomic snuffbox when the appropriate muscle is activated.

A reeducation challenge occurs when the finger flexors are transferred to digital extensors. Transfers of the FDS to the EDC or to the EPL are prime examples. Greater patient concentration and cooperation are required to achieve extension of the digits with the FDS transfer.

For MP joint extension of the fingers, the patient is taught to extend these joints while flexing the IP joints of the fingers. In this "claw" position, all long flexors are activated, including the one used for the extensor transfer. For the thumb, the patient can perform the same claw movement with the fingers while attempting to abduct and extend the thumb.

A tendon transfer that has excellent reeducation potential is the PT-to-ECRB transfer. The PT is a strong muscle and is the primary pronator of the forearm. Therefore substitution patterns do not threaten the reeducation process. The patient is asked to pronate the forearm while the elbow is extended to achieve wrist extension. Extension occurs in a radial direction only because of the absence of the ulnar wrist extensors, but nonetheless it is adequate for functional grasp.

During the retraining sessions, special care must be taken to keep the wrist and digital extension transfers from overstretching. Simultaneous wrist flexion and composite finger flexion are avoided for 7 weeks after surgery. Wrist flexion is limited to 10 to 30 degrees past neutral until this time.

In addition to specific muscle retraining exercises, other light activities are incorporated into the treatment and exercise program as the patient begins to activate transfers more effectively. This usually takes place late in the second week of mobilization. Light pickup activities, such as manipulating checkers, taking lids off large and small containers, and picking up cotton balls or small foam rubber pieces, offer excellent training techniques for normal tenodesing. Other repetitive grasp-and-release exercises are included to provide visual feedback and ensure normal patterns of motion. For thumb transfers, twisting activities,

such as nut-and-bolt assembly, promote extension and abduction.

Mechanical facilitation techniques using electrical stimulation, vibration, or tapping provide additional feedback to help the patient identify the appropriate muscles for the new task. Biofeedback exercises are an integral part of the therapy program, especially when antagonistic muscles are used for tendon transfers. A biofeedback machine with auditory or visual signals helps the patient relax or contract the appropriate muscles during reeducation (Fig. 49-16). For example, if the FDS of the middle finger is used for extension of the fingers, an electrode is placed over its muscle belly in the forearm. A loud tone indicates contraction of the correct muscle on attempted extension of the fingers. Auditory feedback is especially helpful in the early phases of training when there is little visual evidence of the transfer working. Similarly, biofeedback can be used to relax antagonistic flexors that may be cocontracting as the patient tries to extend the fingers too vigorously. Electrodes are placed on adjacent flexor muscle bellies, and the patient attempts to keep the auditory tone to a minimum.

At 7 weeks after surgery, dynamic splinting is initiated if extrinsic extensor tightness is apparent, but even with dynamic splinting, it is rarely possible to get full composite wrist and digital flexion (Fig. 49-17). If the patient can flex the wrist to 20 degrees past neutral with the fingers fully flexed, functional problems are not significant.

A proximal IP joint flexion contracture may develop in a finger if its superficialis is used for transfer. Exercises and dynamic splints are incorporated at this time to return the joint to its supple nature.

Strengthening

Resistive exercises are introduced at 8 weeks and protective splinting discontinued. By this time, the patient should be capable of using the transfer unconsciously. Manual resistance for wrist and finger extension begins by applying gentle resistance to the dorsum of the wrist and

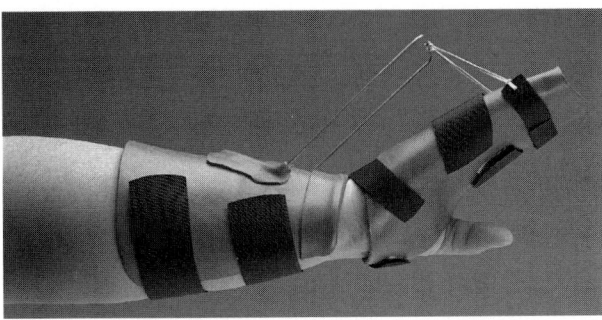

Fig. 49-17. A dynamic splint for stretching tight extrinsic extensors using elastic band material attached dorsally to the ulnar gutter splint, and stretching over the digits to the volar wrist area. (© 2000 Stephen G. Dreiseszun/Viewpoint Photographers, 9034 N. 23rd Ave., Suite 11, Phoenix, Ariz 85021.)

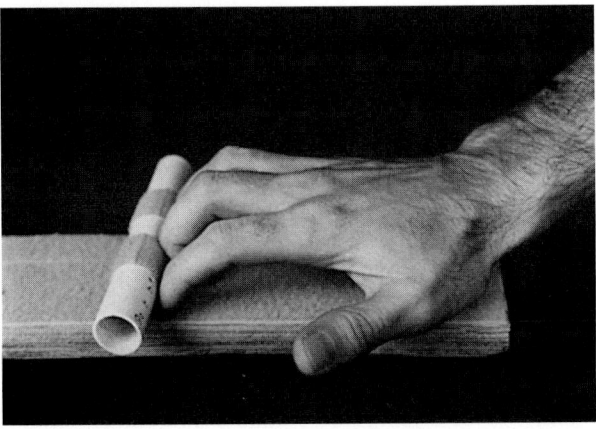

Fig. 49-18. Pushing Velcro dowels on a board exercises the extensor mechanism and strengthens transferred muscle.

fingers, progressing to light weights for wrist extension and a Velcro dowel board for finger extension (Fig. 49-18).

Resistance can be increased by using various tools on the BTE work simulator for forearm rotation, wrist extension, and grip strengthening. A hand-gripper is issued for home exercises, along with therapy putty for resistive finger and thumb extension. An additional 2 to 4 months of this type of strengthening may be needed before the patient maximizes potential of the transferred tendon. During this period, all other activities of daily living and recreational activities are encouraged.

SUMMARY

A preoperative program for radial nerve transfers includes obtaining a baseline motor evaluation, maintaining joint and tissue pliability, strengthening muscles involved in transfer procedures, and providing functional bracing. Postoperatively, the transfers are protected completely for the first 4 weeks while maintaining flexibility in the IP joints, elbow, and shoulder. After 4 weeks, a specific therapist-guided ROM program is initiated, with additional protection until 7 or 8 weeks. From 4 to 8 weeks, it is imperative that joint flexibility be recovered and transfers exercised without overstretching the transferred tendons. After 8 weeks, there are no precautions as strengthening is carried out and more normal function returns.

The results of tendon transfer for radial nerve injuries are generally very good. With a conscientious preoperative and postoperative therapy program, maximum potential can be achieved.

REFERENCES

1. Boyes JH: *Bunnell's surgery of the hand,* ed 4, Philadelphia, 1964, JB Lippincott.
2. Brown AP: Tendon transfers for radial nerve palsy. In Clark GL, et al, editors: *Hand rehabilitation,* New York, 1998, Churchill Livingstone.
3. Colditz JC: Splinting for radial nerve palsy, *Hand Ther* 1:1, 1987.
4. Green DP: Radial nerve palsy. In Green DP, editor: *Operative hand surgery,* New York, 1993, Churchill Livingstone.
5. Hollis I: Innovative splinting ideas. In Hunter JM, et al, editors: *Rehabilitation of the hand,* St Louis, 1978, Mosby.
6. Irani KD: Wrist and hand orthosis: state of the art reviews, *Phys Med Rehab* 154, 1987.
7. Kendall H, Kendall F, Wadsworth G: *Muscles: testing and function,* ed 2, Baltimore, 1971, Williams & Wilkins.
8. Laseter GF, et al: Rehabilitation: tendon transfers. In Hunter JM, Schneider LH, Mackin EJ, editors: *Tendon surgery in the hand,* St Louis, 1987, Mosby.
9. Omer GE: Tendon transfers in radial paralysis. In Hunter JM, Schneider LH, Mackin EJ, editors: *Tendon surgery in the hand,* St Louis, 1987, Mosby.
10. Riordon DC: Principles of tendon transfers. In Hunter JM, Schneider LH, Mackin EJ, editors: *Tendon surgery in the hand,* St Louis, 1987, Mosby.
11. Spinner M: *Injuries to the major branches of the peripheral nerves of the forearm,* Philadelphia, 1978, WB Saunders.
12. Tajima T: Tendon transfers in radial nerve palsy: recommended choices based on retrospective analysis of methods used and their follow-up results. In Hunter JM, Schneider LH, Mackin EJ, editors: *Tendon surgery in the hand,* St Louis, 1987, Mosby.

Chapter 50

TENDON TRANSFERS FOR BRACHIAL PLEXUS PALSY

Scott H. Kozin
Roberta Ciocco
Terry Speakman

Children and adults are of brachial plexus injuries, which can occur from various causes. The principal etiology is traction across the brachial plexus that results in differential strain (i.e., stretch) across the roots or trunks.[41] The upper and middle trunks course from superior to inferior and possess a slight baseline tension. The inferior trunk traverses over the first rib and is slightly lax. This anatomic arrangement predisposes the upper and middle nerve segments to a traction injury when compared with the lower brachial plexus.[29] However, excessive or prolonged traction can disrupt all parts of the brachial plexus as force is dispersed throughout the nerve elements. The amount of damage caused by the traction is variable and can range from a temporary disruption in nerve conduction (i.e., neuropraxia) to complete nerve discontinuity (i.e., neurotmesis).

Traction can be applied via multiple mechanisms such as a motor vehicle accident, an athletic endeavor, or passage through the birth canal. Motorcycle accident victims are particularly prone to brachial plexus injuries (approximate incidence of 2%) via direct depression of the shoulder or forceful neck lateral flexion during impact. Therefore brachial plexus injuries are more prevalent when motor-cycles are the principal mode of transportation.[7,29] Sporting injuries usually cause minor stretch injuries across the brachial plexus known as *burners* or *stingers,* which occur when the shoulder is forcefully depressed or the neck is vigorously flexed away from the shoulder.[19] Burners are usually temporary, although permanent sequelae are possible and a concomitant spinal cord injury can occur at the time of contact. Obstetric palsies have a reported incidence between 0.4 and 2.5 palsies per 1000 live births.[10,18] The

mechanism of injury is secondary to lateral flexion of the neck against a fixed shoulder or longitudinal traction on the arm, which results in preferential traction across the upper portion of the brachial plexus.[14,15] Brachial plexus injuries have been recreated in stillborns by traction applied to a restrained shoulder.[33] Breech presentation or caesarean section does not preclude brachial plexus injury because stretch can occur during hyperabduction of the arm, which tends to stretch the lower brachial plexus (Fig. 50-1).[29,31]

Additional causes of brachial plexus injury include penetrating trauma, infection, and compressive neuropathy. These causes represent a direct insult to the brachial plexus and their distribution is more variable and dependent on the trajectory of the bullet or knife, site of infection, or location of compression. For example, a viral infection (Parsonage-Turner syndrome) commonly affects the supra-scapular or long thoracic nerve and presents with weak abduction or scapular winging, whereas brachial plexus compression (thoracic outlet syndrome) usually involves the lower cord and presents with ulnar nerve signs or symptoms.[29,34]

Regardless of the source of the brachial plexus injury or age of the patient, similar treatment principles are applied to reconstructive surgery. Early management (within the first year) focuses on exploration and nerve reconstruction via interposition grafting or nerve transfer. Delayed treatment concentrates on improving limb function via tendon transfers about the shoulder, elbow, wrist, and hand. In addition, arthrodesis and corrective osteotomy are additional tech-niques employed to improve limb stability and position. This chapter discusses the evaluation and treatment of brachial

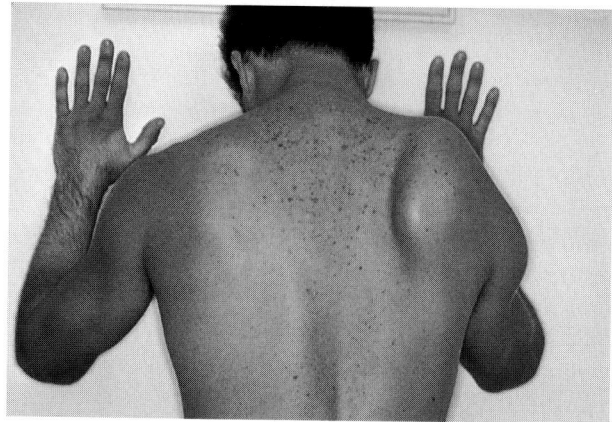

Fig. 50-1. Twenty-year-old man with Parsonage-Turner syndrome and marked lateral scapular winging from involvement of the long thoracic nerve.

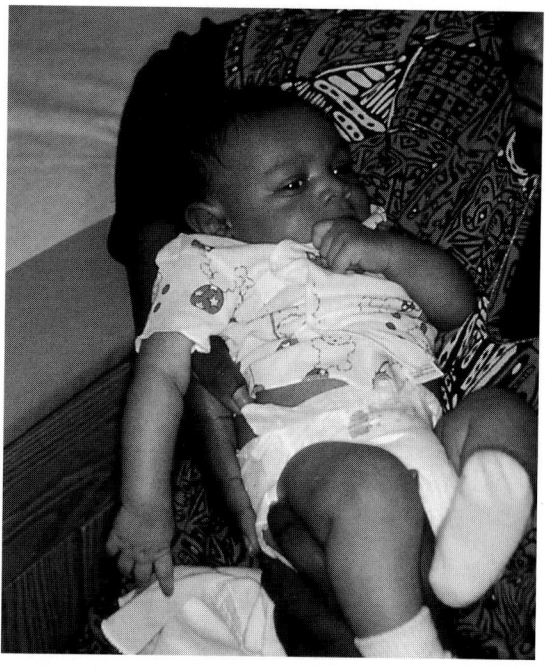

Fig. 50-2. Three-month-old male product of difficult vaginal delivery with right shoulder internally rotated and elbow extended indicative of upper brachial plexus palsy.

plexus injuries that are not amenable to nerve reconstruction or have undergone nerve surgery with incomplete recovery. Subtle differences between children and adults are highlighted throughout this chapter.

PATIENT EVALUATION

The initial evaluation includes the history, physical examination, and imaging studies. The history should include the details of the initial injury with a focus on the amount and extent of trauma incurred. The use of the extremity after the initial insult and subsequent return of function are important facts. Treatment of the injury and its effect on extremity function also are valuable. Associated systemic and local injuries that occurred are essential factors to consider while planning reconstructive surgery. For example, the evaluation of a child with an obstetric brachial plexus injury should include the following: details about the labor (duration of delivery, weight of the child, forceps or vacuum extraction), inquiries into shoulder dystocia, questions about associated injuries (i.e., fractures of the clavicle or Horner's syndrome), queries about initial extremity function, and particulars about timing and extent of motor return.

A basic knowledge of brachial plexus anatomy and concomitant muscle innervation is a prerequisite to adequate patient assessment. A thorough physical examination is the foundation that dictates surgical reconstruction and must include the entire extremity, from neck to hand. Observation of the patient and posture of the extremity provides valuable information about the underlying injury. For example, an upper plexus injury (Erb's palsy) results in a limb positioned with the shoulder adducted and internally rotated, whereas a global lesion presents with a flaccid extremity (Fig. 50-2). The physical examination must assess the muscle strength, sensory status, and joint motion. The range of active and passive joint motion and the corresponding muscle strength are critical elements during formulation of a treatment

strategy. A uniform appraisal system for muscle strength grading and documentation is mandatory when evaluating a patient for surgical reconstruction. A brachial plexus tabulation sheet is the most efficient manner to record manual muscle strength and prevent inadvertent omission of important data (Table 50-1). Muscle strength is graded from 0 to 5, enhanced by the use of a minus modifier to denote incomplete range (Table 50-2). This documentation also allows serial examinations by different individuals. The sensibility of the extremity is assessed by standard measures, including light-touch and two-point discrimination. A peripheral vascular examination with palpation of the radial and ulnar pulses is required because damage to the axillary or subclavian vessels can occur at the time of initial injury.

Children are more difficult to examine because of their limited attention span, poor ability to follow commands, and lack of cooperation. Extreme patience, diligence, and repeated examinations are required to obtain an adequate evaluation. Children often are unable to follow instructions for assessment of manual muscle testing. Interactive play is used to assess the functional use of the extremity. Various toys, props, and games are used to accomplish this task and the assessment of particular function often is graded as absent (−) or present (+) (Fig. 50-3). The sophistication of the interactive modality varies with the age, development, and intellect of the child. Sensory function also is difficult to assess because the only reaction may be to pain, which will preclude any subsequent examination. Children are unable to participate in object recognition until they are 4 to 5 years of age. Common objects can be used for identification; two sets of objects are required so that the child does not have to name the object but rather can point to the one that matches the object in his or her hand. Occlusion of vision is best accomplished by using a shield. Children older than 5 also can be evaluated by graphesthesia or the ability to recognize numbers or letters written in the palm with a dull-pointed object. Children older than 9 years of age can participate in a standard two-point discrimination examination. Historical information gained from the parents in regard to the child's reaction to painful stimuli or frequency of injuries to the involved extremity is indicative of sensory status.

A functional assessment via a questionnaire and examination is a fundamental component in the formulation of a treatment plan. The questionnaire should concentrate on the ability to perform activities of daily living (ADLs). The

examination should focus on the mannerisms used to perform such tasks. For example, a patient with deficient finger extension may indicate that he or she is able to grasp and release simple objects. However, observation of this task will reveal that passive wrist flexion and tenodesis of the extensor digitorum communis to extend the fingers is used for release of objects. Therefore any surgical reconstruction must be cognizant of this maneuver and either avoid limitation of wrist flexion or restore active finger extension to maintain object release.

A consideration of the patient's expectations is another important element of the preoperative evaluation. Careful counseling of the benefits and disadvantages is essential before surgical reconstruction. Realistic goals will prevent disappointment and foster a better doctor-therapist-patient

Table 50-1. Brachial plexus examination form

Muscle	Date		Date		Date	
	L	R	L	R	L	R
Rhomboids (C4, C5)						
Levator scapulae (C3, C4, C5)						
Supraspinatus (C5, C6)						
Infraspinatus (C5,C6)						
Serratus anterior (C5, C6, C7)						
Teres major (C5, C6)						
Latissimus dorsi (C6, C7, C8)						
Subscapularis (C5, C6)						
Pectoralis major (C5-T1)						
Biceps (C5, C6)						
Brachialis (C5, C6)						
Deltoid (C5, C6)						
Triceps (C6, C7, C8)						
Pronator teres (C6, C7)						
Supinator (C5, C6)						
Brachioradialis (C5, C6)						
Extensor carpi radialis longus (C6, C7)						
Extensor carpi radialis brevis (C6, C7, C8)						
Extensor carpi ulnaris (C7, C8)						
Flexor carpi radialis (C6, C7)						
Flexor carpi ulnaris (C7, C8, T1)						
Flexor digitorum profundus (C7, C8, T1)						
Flexor digitorum superficialis (C7, C8, T1)						
Flexor pollicis longus (C7, C8, T1)						
Extensor digitorum comminus (C7, C8)						
Extensor digitorum minimi (C7, C8)						
Extensor indicis (C7, C8)						
Extensor pollicis longus (C6, C7)						
Extensor pollicis brevis (C6,C7)						
Pronator quadratus (C7, C8, T1)						
Abductor pollicis longus (C6, C7)						
Abductor pollicis brevis (C6, C7, C8, T1)						
Opponens pollicis (C8, T1)						
Abductor digiti minimi (C8, T1)						
Abductor pollicis brevis (C8, T1)						
Opponens digiti (C8, T1)						
Interossei (C8, T1)						
Lumbricals (C8, T1)						

Note: Underline denotes principal level of innervation.

relationship. In children, the developmental level has to be carefully considered when planning surgical intervention to ensure compliance with postoperative regimens.

A baseline outcome measurement is also part of the initial patient evaluation even though the exact outcome tool appropriate for brachial plexus injuries remains unclear and outcome measurements are notoriously difficult in children. Currently, most of the standardized tests are designed to look at dominant hand function and do not consider unilateral

Table 50-2. Manual muscle grading scale

Grade*	Terminology	Description
5	Normal	Full ROM and full strength
4	Good	Full ROM against gravity with some resistance
3	Fair	Full ROM against gravity
2	Poor	Full ROM with gravity eliminated
1	Trace	Slight contraction without joint movement
0	None	No evidence of contraction

ROM, Range of motion.

*A minus modifier can be used to indicate incomplete range. For example, a triceps muscle that can extend the elbow against gravity but lacks terminal extension is graded a 3−.

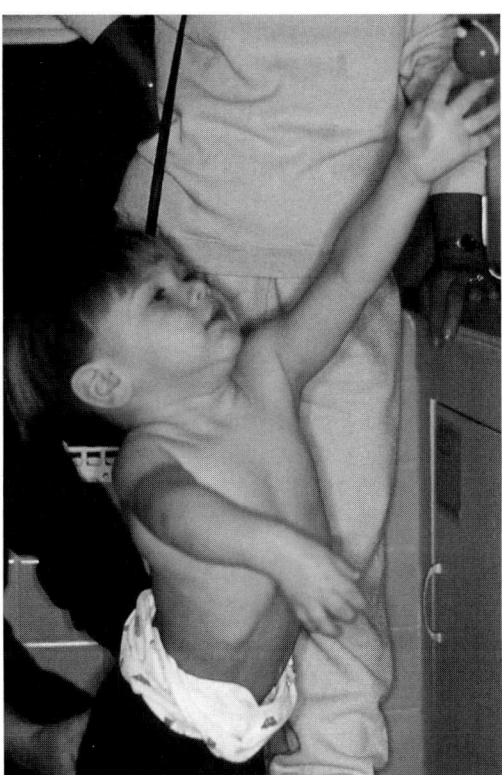

Fig. 50-3. Three-year-old with right global obstetric brachial palsy having difficulty elevating right arm for ball.

dysfunction, such as after a brachial plexus injury. Many times, the involved extremity will be delegated to serve as an assist during activity, which is difficult to measure by an outcome tool. Nonetheless, a critical examination of the results is necessary to improve future care in patients with this complicated disorder. This task requires faithful documentation of the preoperative state and postoperative change from a subjective and objective standpoint.

Adults should at least complete a DASH (disability of the arm, shoulder, and hand questionnaire) or SF-36 form before surgical intervention.[1,23] In children, the Mallet classification provides a gross evaluation and score of shoulder motion with categories for global abduction, global external rotation, hand to neck, hand on spine, and hand-to-mouth function.[42,43] This functional classification can serve as an outcome guide with respect to changes in score following surgical intervention.[42] Several tests that are used for assessing pediatric brachial plexus patients include the Jebsen-Taylor hand function test, Moberg pick-up test, Melborne assessment of unilateral upper extremity function (designed for cerebral palsy population), and a nonstandardized bimanual task assessment.[25,26] In addition, a videotape analysis of the child performing various tasks before and after brachial plexus reconstruction is informative.

ANCILLARY STUDIES

Imaging and electrodiagnostic studies provide supplemental information that can be helpful at the time of patient evaluation and during the formulation of a treatment plan. Radiographs of the injured extremity are used to assess for previous fractures and to evaluate bony development in children. Limited passive motion may be secondary to soft tissue contracture or bony abnormalities and requires x-ray examination. For the shoulder, anteroposterior and axillary views are adequate in the adolescent or adult patient (Fig. 50-4). However, children that are skeletally immature may require

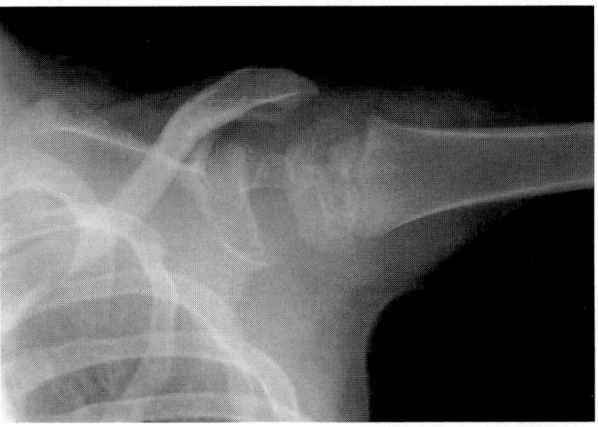

Fig. 50-4. Axillary radiograph of 10-year-old with obstetric brachial plexus palsy and deficient external rotation. Loss of glenoid anteversion and irregular shape of the humeral head is evident.

Table 50-3. Classification of glenohumeral deformity

Type	Glenohumeral deformity
I	Normal glenoid (<5 degrees retroversion compared with contralateral normal)
II	Minimal deformity (<5 degrees retroversion compared with contralateral normal)
III	Moderate deformity (posterior humeral head subluxation)
IV	Severe deformity (posterior humeral head subluxation with false glenoid)
V	Severe flattening of humeral head ± complete dislocation
VI	Infantile glenohumeral dislocation
VII	Proximal humeral growth arrest

Table 50-4. Patterns of brachial plexus injuries

Pattern	Nerve roots involved	Primary deficiency
Erb-Duchenne lesion	C5 and C6	Shoulder abduction and external rotation
Upper brachial plexus		Elbow flexion
Extended Erb's lesion	C5 through C7	Above plus
Upper and middle plexus		Elbow and finger extension
Dejerine-Klumpke lesion	C8 and T1	Hand intrinsic muscles
Lower brachial plexus		Finger flexors
Total or global lesion	C5 through T1	Entire extremity
Entire brachial plexus		

advanced imaging modalities (e.g., magnetic resonance imaging, glenohumeral arthrography) to truly depict the contour of the glenohumeral joint.[35,44] Waters and Jaramillo[44] have classified glenohumeral deformity into seven types of increasing severity based on the status of the humeral head and glenoid (Table 50-3). In the immature skeleton, additional joints (e.g., elbow, wrist) also can develop abnormally after brachial plexus injury, and x-ray examination is routinely performed before reconstruction.

Electrodiagnostic tests are subdivided into two different components: the nerve conduction part and the electromyography section.[4,11] The nerve conduction test assesses the continuity of nerve fibers while the electromyogram (EMG) evaluates the properties of the muscle. EMG characteristics provide useful data when considering tendon transfer because reinnervated muscle demonstrates an abnormal EMG signal with decreased amplitude and polyphasic waveforms. These findings indicate a previously paralyzed muscle with inherent weakness and altered contractile properties, which often precludes use of that muscle as a suitable donor for tendon transfer. However, the EMG is not truly quantitative with regard to muscle strength and does not substitute for an astute physical examination coupled with manual muscle testing.

CLASSIFICATION

Brachial plexus injuries can be classified according to the level of involvement (Table 50-4). Upper plexus lesions are most common and typically involve the fifth and sixth cervical roots or upper trunk. These injuries are referred to as either an Erb-Duchenne or Erb's palsy and are characterized by loss of elbow flexion and weakness of shoulder abduction and external rotation.[12,29] The lack of elbow flexion prohibits hand-to-mouth activity while the deficient shoulder motion diminishes the available workspace, especially with overhead activities. The seventh cervical root or middle trunk also can be included (extended Erb's palsy), which compromises elbow and finger extension and further limits the available workspace. Lower

plexus lesions (eight cervical and first thoracic or lower trunk) are termed a *Dejerine-Klumpke* or *Klumpke's palsy* and affect the finger flexors and hand intrinsic muscles.[28] Deficient finger flexion limits grasp while lack of intrinsic muscle function impairs fine motor function (i.e., dexterity). Isolated lower plexus lesions are exceedingly uncommon and are usually part of a global injury that affects the entire brachial plexus.

APPROACH TO TENDON TRANSFERS

The formulation of a treatment plan requires careful consideration of numerous factors including the patient (general health, goals, expectations), joint motion (active and passive), sensibility, and manual muscle testing. The manual muscle testing provides the baseline data when planning tendon transfer. The muscles and their respective function are grouped into four general categories entitled "what's in," "what's out," "what's needed," and "what's available." Each category has certain inclusion criteria that require elucidation. The "what's in" collection lists all muscles that are detected by manual muscle testing along with their respective grades. The "what's out" category records all muscles not detected by testing. The "what's needed" list identifies all deficient movements that would enhance function if restored. The "what's available" register includes all muscles that have been graded 4 or 5 by manual muscle testing and their respective availability. Muscles graded 3 or less are not suitable for transfer because strength tends to diminish by one grade after transfer, which would result in only gravity-eliminated motion and no improvement in function. The "what's available" list also must consider the availability and expendability of the muscle. A prerequisite to transfer is that the function of a donor muscle must be preserved after transfer for it to be considered expendable. For example, a grade 4 extensor carpi radialis longus (ECRL) muscle is a viable donor as long as the extensor carpi radialis brevis (ECRB) muscle is intact.

The functional needs list (i.e., "what's needed") may exceed the number of available donors; therefore alternative procedures (e.g., arthrodesis, capsulodesis, tenodesis) must be considered. The final decision also must take into account the inherent properties of the muscle, including its excursion and line of pull. The excursion is the distance a muscle can contract and is proportional to the length of the individual muscle fibers. Tendon transfers should attempt to match the donor and recipient muscle excursion to allow full range of motion (ROM) after transfer. For example, the flexor digitorum superficialis muscle possesses a considerable amount of excursion (approximately 5 to 7 cm) and makes an excellent donor for finger extension as long as the flexor digitorum profundus is functioning. The *line of pull* refers to the direction of force applied after transfer, which should attempt to replicate the muscle being replaced. This vector can be altered during transfer by rerouting the muscle or tendon.

The treatment algorithm also must incorporate the rehabilitation program, which requires communication between the surgeon and therapist. The reconstruction plan must consider the postoperative immobilization and therapeutic paradigm. When different positions of immobilization are required, a staged surgical plan is required to protect the tendon transfer. This approach is most applicable when tendon transfers are performed for both flexion and extension about the elbow, wrist, or digits.

Example of planning for tendon transfer

A 17-year-old boy sustained a right brachial plexus injury from a motorcycle accident 3 years ago involving C5, C6, and C7 (extended Erb's palsy). Early nerve grafting was performed on the upper and middle trunks with some return of function. The patient presents for additional reconstructive options.

1. What's in? What muscles are working and what is their respective manual muscle grade?
    Deltoid 3/5
    Supraspinatus 3/5
    Infraspinatus 3/5
    Pectoralis major 4/5
    Serratus anterior 4/5
    Latissimus dorsi 4/5
    Teres major 4/5
    Triceps 3/5
    Flexor carpi radialis 3/5
    Flexor carpi ulnaris 5/5
    Flexor pollicis longus 5/5
    Extensor carpi ulnaris 2/5
    ECRL 3/5
    ECRB 3/5
    Abductor pollicis longus 3/5

Flexor digitorum profundus 5/5
Flexor digitorum superficialis 5/5
Pronator teres 4/5
Pronator quadratus 5/5
Supinator 4/5
Intrinsics (interossei, thenar, and hypothenar muscles) 5/5

2. What's out? What muscles are not working?
    Biceps/ brachialis 0/5
    Brachioradialis 0/5
    Extensor pollicis longus 0/5
    Extensor pollicis brevis 0/5
    Extensor digitorum comminus 0/5
    Extensor digiti minimi 0/5
    Extensor indicis 0/5
    Extensor pollicis brevis 0/5

3. What's needed? What movements will improve function?
    Shoulder motion is weak, but suitable with good function. Intrinsic hand function is relatively unaffected because the inferior cord and ulnar nerve were uninjured. The primary action lacking is elbow, which is a major deterrent to function (e.g., hand-to-mouth activities). Function also would be enhanced by restoration of finger extension.

4. What's available? What muscles are expendable and can be transferred?
    Latissimus dorsi
    Pectoralis major muscle (unipolar versus bipolar)
    Flexor digitorum superficialis (flexor digitorum profundus is intact)
    Pronator teres (pronator quadratus is intact)
    Flexor carpi ulnaris (flexor carpi radialis is 3/5)
    Triceps muscle is not available because of its grade (3/5) and reinnervation following nerve grafting.

5. Tendon transfer options? What are realistic tendon transfer options?
    Elbow flexion
        Latissimus dorsi → Biceps
        Pectoralis major → Biceps
    Finger extension
        Flexor digitorum superficialis → Extensor digitorum ± extensor pollicis longus
        Pronator teres → Extensor digitorum ± extensor pollicis longus
        Flexor carpi ulnaris → Extensor digitorum ± extensor pollicis longus
    Proposed surgical plan? Definitive surgical and rehabilitation plan?
        Latissimus dorsi → Biceps
        Flexor digitorum superficialis → Extensor digitorum ± extensor pollicis longus
    This option was chosen because latissimus dorsi transfer is a favored elbow flexorplasty with considerable excursion (approximately 11 cm) and a suitable

line of pull for elbow flexion when transferred using the bipolar technique. In addition, transfer of the flexor digitorum superficialis for finger extension provides similar excursion for finger extension. One or two flexor digitorum superficialis tendons can be transferred either through the interosseus membrane or around the forearm bones to create a good vector for finger extension. The rehabilitation program (position of immobilization and subsequent therapy) following both transfers does not conflict and both transfers can be performed during a single stage.

PRINCIPLES OF POSTOPERATIVE MANAGEMENT

There are essentially four main areas of concentration in the postoperative management of tendon transfers: immobilization, scar management, muscle reeducation, and functional performance.

In all tendon transfers, there is an initial period of casting, followed by protective splinting with a removable splint. The initial period of cast immobilization usually continues for approximately 3 to 6 weeks, depending on the specific muscle transferred and the method used to connect the tendon transfer. It is important to remember that the initial tendon transfer site is fairly strong, but the repair gradually decreases in strength and is weakest 2 weeks after surgery. At that time, the transfer is most vulnerable to disruption and should be carefully protected.

After the initial immobilization, a removable splint is fabricated for full time use. During this period, the splint may be removed for bathing and therapy. The position of splinting usually replicates the position of casting; however, splinting is usually lower profile and may be less restrictive. For example, transfer of the brachioradialis to the ECRB for wrist extension initially requires a long-arm cast. At the time of splint fabrication, only a forearm-based splint is required without inclusion of the elbow. The duration of splint use is usually 2 to 6 weeks, with adjustments in splint position dependent on the specific procedure and the patient's progress. For example, elbow extension transfers require weekly splint changes to allow progressive flexion at a rate of 15 degrees per week. However, if the patient is not able to adequately activate the transfer by the end of the week, progression is delayed until sufficient firing is demonstrated. The last period of splint use is for protection at night, which continues for 3 to 6 months after surgery.

An important part of the rehabilitation process is scar management, which begins after cast removal, as long as there are no open wounds. Therapists should address both the superficial (incision) and deeper scar, which can be motion limiting. The superficial (incisional) scar can be managed with massage for soft tissue mobilization. Topical lotions or creams can be used as lubricants to facilitate massage, although it is important to consider patient skin sensitivity and allergies. The use of silicone gel sheets and/or elastomer products are valuable adjuncts to scar massage, especially if the patient is prone to hypertrophic scarring or keloid formation.[17,46] These products usually are used in combination with an elasticized stockinette or wrap to provide pressure to the scar. Vibration or suction also can enhance scar mobilization and may mobilize some of the deeper layers of scar.

The primary goal of deep scar management is to reduce excessive scar tissue formation around the tendon transfer(s), which would negatively affect the ability of the transfer to glide and succeed. Scar massage applied with greater pressure can affect the deeper tissues; however, early tendon gliding is the most efficacious method to prevent adhesion formation (motion limiting scar). These exercises yield tendon excursion, which will limit the number of adhesions that can form around the tendon and/or transfer site. Ultrasound is another modality that may encourage deeper tissue mobilization, although this technique should be delayed until tendon healing has occurred.

The therapist must bear in mind that scar management can be perceived as uncomfortable (especially to younger children), and the use of distraction or other pain management techniques can be helpful. Scar management should be taught to patients and/or caretakers early in the rehabilitation process so that it can be performed several times a day.

Muscle reeducation is one of the most important considerations in the postoperative management of tendon transfers. Patients vary greatly in the ease with which they learn to use their transfers. Use of verbal cues to perform the previous action before transfer is an effective prompt. For example, children who undergo a latissimus dorsi to supraspinatus transfer may be cued to pretend they are squeezing a large rubber ball between their body and arm, which activates the latissimus dorsi muscle. During this maneuver, stabilization of the arm prevents interference from surrounding muscles and provides resistance to adduction, which allows better recruitment of the transferred muscle for shoulder movement. Use of tapping and/or vibration over the muscle belly also can assist the patient to elicit a muscle contraction. When isolated muscle contraction is a problem, biofeedback can sometimes be helpful. In problematic situations, neuromuscular electrical stimulation may be warranted but should not be considered before 6 weeks after surgery.

Once the muscle transfer can be isolated and active range of motion (AROM) is reasonable, functional activities should be incorporated to increase the strength of the tendon transfer. Activities used should be motivating and relevant to the patient, and when possible, they should address the preoperative goals for improved function. The therapist's creativity is sometimes challenged at this stage for some of the transfers. For example, finding activities that are specific for external rotation following transfer can be difficult. Playing zip ball is an activity that requires external rotation and works well with children (Fig. 50-5).

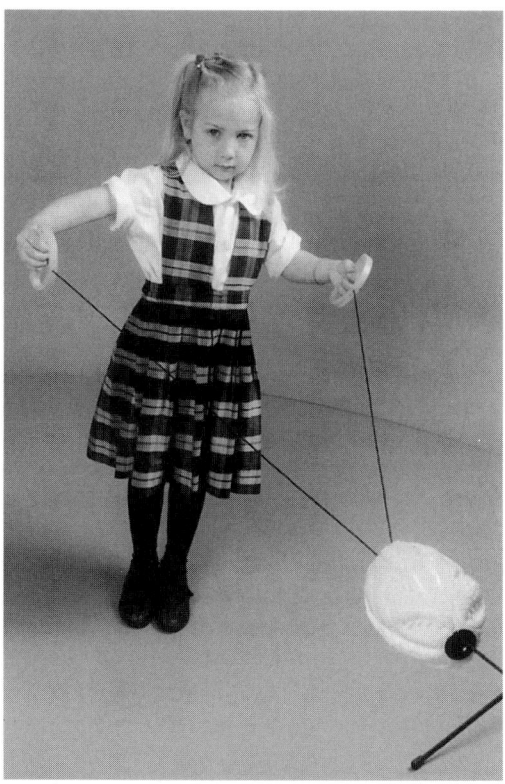

Fig. 50-5. Six-year-old status after latissimus dorsi transfer for external rotation playing zip ball to strengthen the transfer.

The amount and intensity of formal therapy following tendon transfer varies, depending on the procedure and patient factors such as age, motivation, and complications. Involvement and education of the patient and family in the postoperative care is the key to success of the tendon transfer.

SHOULDER

Shoulder impairment is common after brachial plexus injury because its primary motors are innervated by the upper plexus. The confluence of rotator cuff muscles acts to move the glenohumeral joint and depress the humeral head, which maintains the concentric relationship between the humeral head and glenoid. This function allows the deltoid muscle to move the shoulder through multiple planes of motion. The function and precise synchrony between the rotator cuff and deltoid muscles is distorted after brachial plexus injury. Loss of abduction and deficient external rotation are the most common problems. Internal rotation is usually not affected because multiple muscles (pectoralis major, latissimus dorsi, and subscapularis muscles) provide this motion.

This resultant imbalance and unopposed muscle forces create a propensity for an internal rotation contracture over time. This contracture is especially problematic in the pediatric population after obstetric brachial plexus palsy. Therefore, at the time of initial evaluation of an infant after

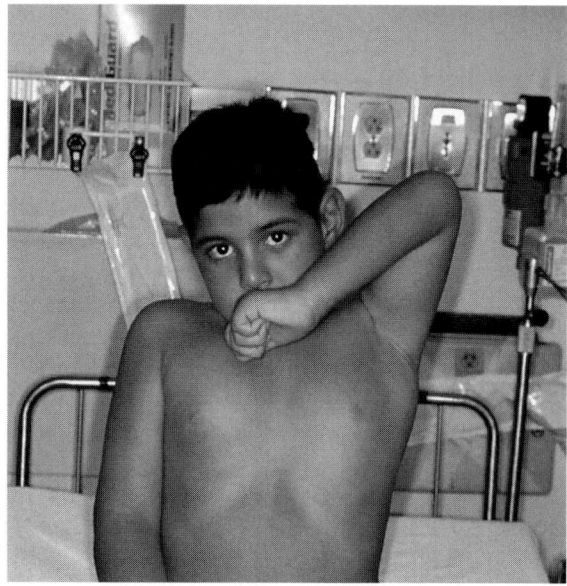

Fig. 50-6. Eight-year-old with positive trumpet sign during attempted hand-to-mouth function.

obstetric brachial plexus palsy, the family is instructed to perform passive external rotation exercises. These passive maneuvers are performed at each diaper change to maintain a mobile shoulder joint. The status of the glenohumeral joint must be monitored carefully. Early detection of a diminution in passive external rotation requires a referral for formal therapy aimed at glenohumeral rotation. An established internal rotation contracture (i.e., no external rotation) that is recalcitrant to therapy requires surgical release. Failure to regain and maintain external rotation will cause distorted development of the glenohumeral joint with an irregularly shaped humeral head and corresponding deficient glenoid cavity[35,42] (see Fig. 50-4). In addition, a fixed internal rotation posture prohibits hand-to-mouth function without compensatory shoulder or scapulothoracic abduction (positive trumpet sign) (Fig. 50-6). An internal rotation contracture greater than 45 degrees combined with abduction less than 80 degrees negates hand-to-mouth function entirely.[45] Surgical release of the tightened structures is recommended between 2 to 5 years of age and can be combined with tendon transfer to restore active external rotation.[21,22,36,37] Older children with advanced glenohumeral dysplasia are not candidates for tendon transfer, but are treated with external rotational osteotomy of the humerus to provide a better limb position for hand-to-mouth function.[16]

Surgery for shoulder rotation

Release of internal rotation contracture. The child is placed supine or lateral on the operating room table. An anterior approach between the deltoid and pectoralis muscle is performed. If the pectoralis muscle is tight, a portion of the tendon is released at its insertion into the humerus. The subscapularis muscle is isolated and released from the underlying anterior capsule (Fig. 50-7). The capsule is not violated because capsular release can create anterior shoulder instability. The arm is positioned in 45 degrees of abduction and as much external rotation as possible, which is maintained by a long-arm cast attached to an abdominal component.

This procedure also can be performed via an axillary incision and release of the subscapularis muscle from its scapular origin, which allows the entire muscle to slide. A similar immobilization and postoperative management is employed. Release of the internal rotation contracture also can be combined with tendon transfer to restore external rotation at the same setting or as a staged procedure after supple passive motion has been restored.

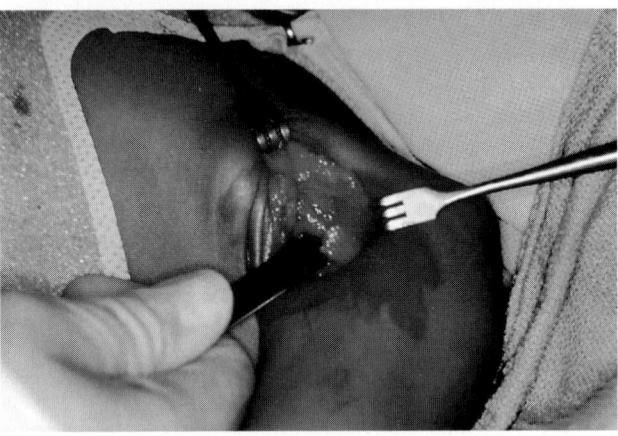

Fig. 50-7. Isolation of subscapularis muscle from anterior capsule during release of internal rotation contracture.

Postoperative management. Postoperative cast immobilization is continued for 4 weeks. On occasion, the weight or comfort of the cast is an issue and the trunk portion of the cast can be exchanged for a lightweight, low temperature splint material. The trunk portion is attached to the abduction bar, which is incorporated into the long-arm fiberglass cast. This fabricated trunk portion can be reused when the removable splint is fabricated 4 weeks after surgery (Fig. 50-8). This splint replicates the casted position and is worn uninterrupted for 2 to 4 weeks, except for bathing and therapy. Subsequently, the splint is worn only at night until 12 weeks after surgery (Fig. 50-9).

Daily gentle passive range of motion (PROM) is initiated 4 to 5 weeks after the procedure and can usually be accomplished through a home program with a care provider. The therapist/caregiver must be sure to stabilize the scapula by placing one hand on the lateral border of the scapula to stabilize it while rotating the humerus within the glenohumeral joint in an antigravity plane. The rotation should be throughout the available range with emphasis on external rotation.

PROM should continue two to three times a day for 6 to 8 weeks following surgery. It is pertinent that the patient and family understand that they must maintain this glenohumeral range until active external rotation is adequate to balance the joint or until the external rotation is restored by tendon transfer.

External rotation transfer. The child is positioned in the lateral decubitus or prone position on the operating room table. A longitudinal incision is made beginning in the posterior axillary fold. The latissimus dorsi muscle is

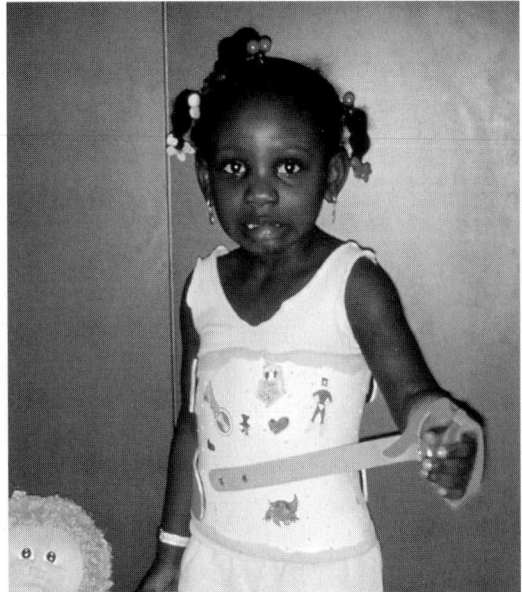

Fig. 50-8. Removable splint applied 4 weeks after anterior shoulder release and latissimus dorsi transfer for external rotation.

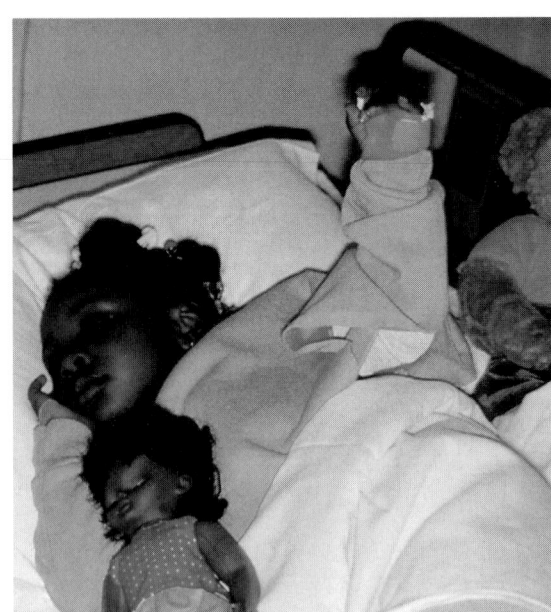

Fig. 50-9. Child adapts to sleeping with splint, which is continued until 12 weeks after surgery.

identified and traced to its insertion into the humerus. The insertion of the infraspinatus muscle is isolated by cephalad retraction of the deltoid muscle. The latissimus dorsi tendon is released from the humerus and transferred to the infraspinatus insertion site (Fig. 50-10). The tendon can be sutured further superiorly (supraspinatus insertion site) to enhance shoulder abduction (Fig. 50-11). The arm is positioned in 45 to 60 degrees of abduction and external rotation using a long-arm cast attached to an abdominal component via an abduction bar.

This procedure also can be performed by transfer of both the latissimus dorsi and teres major muscles to the rotator cuff. Similar immobilization and postoperative management is followed.

Postoperative management. The cast is exchanged for a removable splint 4 weeks after surgery. The splint is fabricated to replicate the position of casting using an abdominal portion attached to a forearm splint by means of an abduction bar (Fig. 50-12). General guidelines for splint fabrication are 60 degrees of shoulder abduction and 70 degrees of external rotation. At this time, therapy is initiated with the focus on scar management and teaching the patient to activate the transferred muscle consistently.

Scar massage should be performed twice daily with use of a lotion to decrease the friction over the surgical site. The superficial (incision) and deeper scar (where adhesion to the transfer occurs) should be addressed. If the patient appears to have signs of hypertrophy, the therapist may consider use

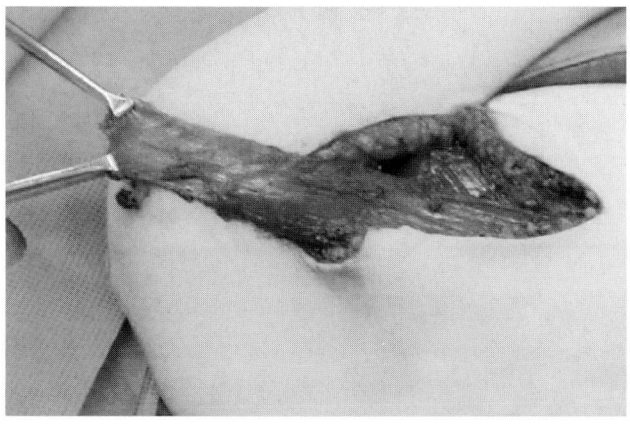

Fig. 50-10. Six-year-old child positioned in the left lateral decubitus position (i.e., left side down) and right latissimus dorsi muscle harvested for transfer.

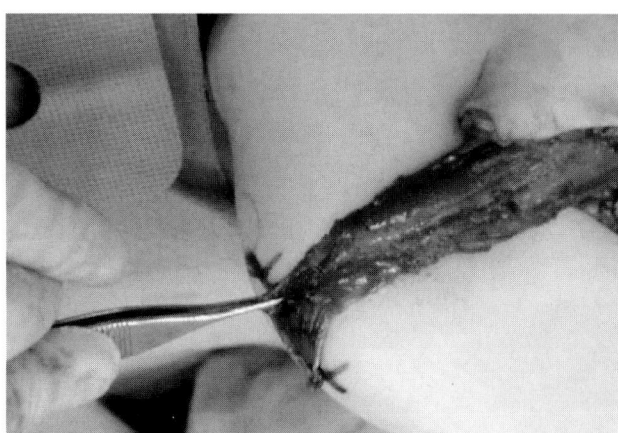

Fig. 50-11. Latissimus dorsi muscle can be advanced to the supraspinatus insertion site to enhance shoulder abduction.

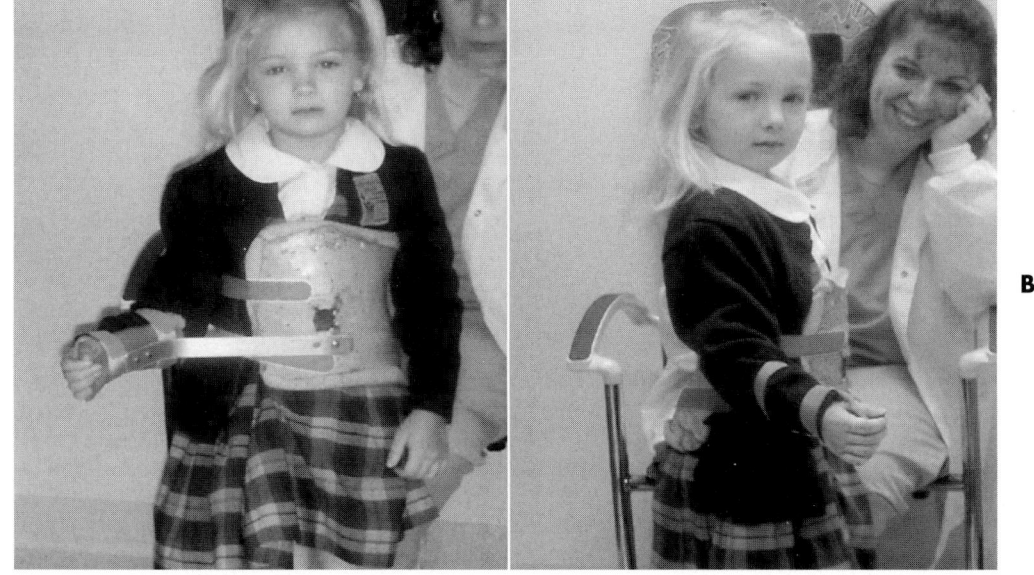

A   **B**

Fig. 50-12. Front **(A)** and side **(B)** view of splint fabricated after latissimus dorsi transfer for external rotation depicted in Fig. 50-11.

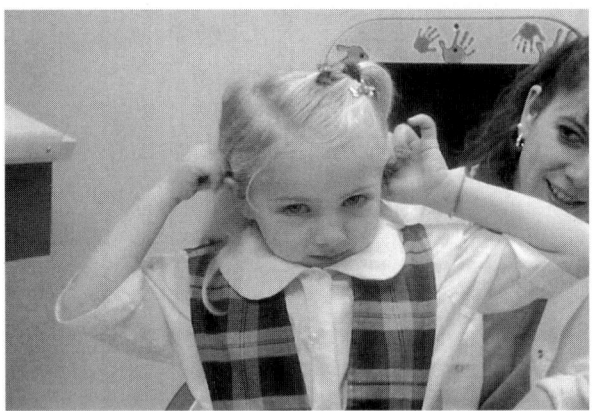

Fig. 50-13. Child can activate external rotation transfers by pushing hair behind ear.

of supplemental products such as a silicone gel or elastomer pad in conjunction with elastic stockinet. This will provide prolonged pressure and may facilitate better organization of collagen, which will decrease the risk of adhesion formation.[17,46] In addition, vibration and/or suction can be used to prevent dense incisional scar formation. Ultrasound is another modality that can encourage tissue mobilization, although this technique usually is reserved for recalcitrant scar formation and should be delayed until tendon healing is complete (6 to 7 weeks postoperatively).

Early tendon gliding is the most efficacious method to prevent deep scar formation (motion-limiting scar). It is pertinent that the patient learns to fire the transferred muscle consistently, with minimal to no compensation from other proximal musculature. During the first several days, the therapist attempts to palpate an isolated contraction of the transfer in an antigravity plane. The connection is often taught by having the patient complete the original function of the transferred muscle isometrically. For example, children who undergo a latissimus dorsi to infraspinatus transfer may be cued to pretend they are squeezing a large rubber ball between their body and their arm. This should activate the latissimus dorsi muscle, thus resulting in external rotation. During this maneuver, stabilization of the shoulder and the trunk prevents interference from surrounding muscles and provides resistance to adduction, which allows better recruitment of the transferred muscle for shoulder movement. If the patient has difficulty activating the transfer, use of tapping and/or vibration over the muscle belly of the latissimus dorsi can assist the patient to elicit a muscle contraction. If the patient is unable to isolate the transfer, biofeedback may be helpful in the reeducation process. As the patient achieves a consistent contraction, therapy may progress to functional activities using the restored external rotation (Fig. 50-13).

During week 6, the patient may engage in some light resistive strengthening as long as he or she is gaining active range without compensatory movement. Children may engage in zip ball (see Fig. 50-5) in which they must pull rope handles apart to send a ball to the other player at the end of the rope. Adults may use low resistance Thera-Band for external rotation exercises. As more isolated control is gained and range improves, they also may begin external rotation against gravity (e.g., overhead external rotation). Again, if the patient is isolating the transfer, the splint may be removed during the day except during activities that put the patient at risk for falls or passive stretch to the transfer. At this time, more aggressive PROM may be initiated to isolate glenohumeral movement from scapulothoracic motion. Firm stabilization of the scapula allows passive motion to be concentrated at the glenohumeral joint. The therapist should always consult the surgeon regarding the development of the glenoid cavity. Children may have a hypoplastic glenoid cavity, which prevents full glenohumeral motion.

During weeks 7 and 8, more resistance may be added to the strengthening program. This may be instituted by grading the earlier example of the forward pass game to include ROM in a plane of gravity, or by placing the adult patient on a weighted pulley system or Cybex equipment for progressive resistive external rotation exercises. In addition, functional activities such as hair brushing or ball throwing that facilitate spontaneous inclusion of the restored motion are encouraged.

Twelve weeks after surgery, the splint is discontinued and unrestricted activity is allowed.

Tendon transfer for shoulder abduction. Lack of abduction from paralysis or paresis of deltoid and supraspinatus muscle function is common in both adult and child after upper brachial plexus injuries. In addition, decreased scapulothoracic motion (e.g., scapular winging from long thoracic nerve deficit) compounds the reduction of shoulder abduction. Restoration of abduction is a difficult task because of the inherent properties of the intact deltoid and rotator cuff muscles that provide exceptional strength and coordination. During external rotation transfer, passage of the latissimus dorsi tendon superiorly to the supraspinatus insertion site can enhance shoulder abduction. Transfers of the trapezius muscle to the lateral aspect of the humeral head or latissimus dorsi transfer are viable options to improve abduction.[13,15,24] The use of a bipolar latissimus transfer is more complicated but has been reported with encouraging results.[24]

Trapezius transfer. The patient is placed in the beach-chair position on the operating room table. A saber-cut or transverse incision is made about the acromioclavicular joint (Fig. 50-14). The trapezius muscle is identified via skin flap elevation. The trapezius insertion into the acromion is isolated in preparation for transfer. The lateral trapezius muscle is harvested along with a piece of acromion for transfer to the humerus (Fig. 50-15).

The deltoid muscle is split longitudinally to expose the lateral aspect of the proximal humerus. The trapezius and attached acromion are advanced to the lateral humerus and secured with a screw with the arm held in abduction.

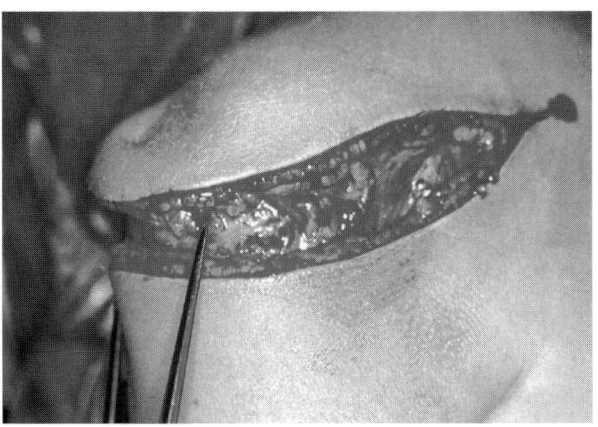

Fig. 50-14. Transverse incision and approach for trapezius transfer to lateral humerus to enhance shoulder abduction.

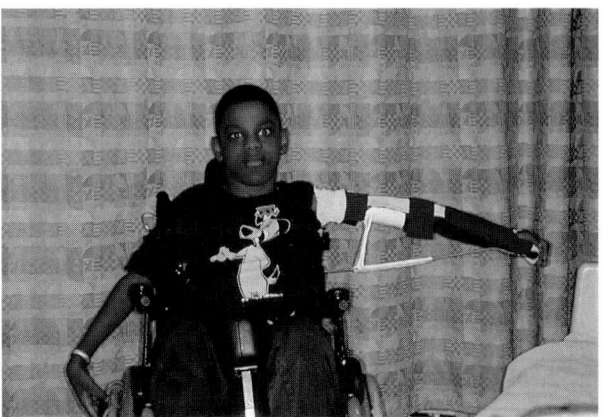

Fig. 50-16. Frontal view of fabricated splint following trapezius transfer for shoulder abduction. Elbow placed in full extension to protect concomitant elbow extension transfer.

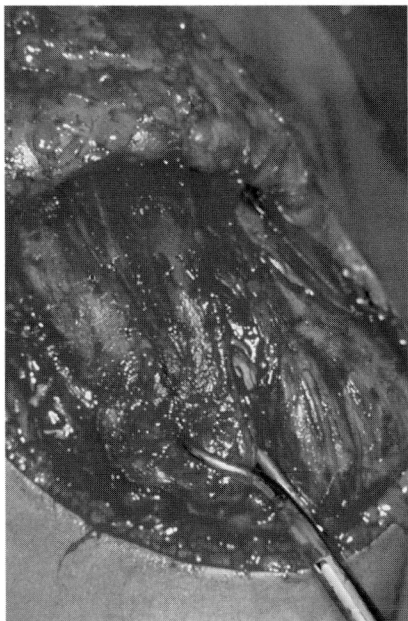

Fig. 50-15. Trapezius muscle harvested with piece of acromion in preparation for transfer (towel clip into bone).

Latissimus dorsi transfer. Bipolar transfer of the latissimus dorsi muscle moves the humeral insertion to the deltoid attachment and the thoracolumbar origin to the acromion/clavicle. The patient is placed in the lateral decubitus position, and a longitudinal incision is made from the posterior axillary fold to the inferior aspect of the latissimus dorsi muscle. The entire muscle is mobilized, including a strip of thoracolumbar fascia and the tendinous insertion into the humerus. The thoracodorsal nerve and vascular pedicle are isolated and protected.

Additional incisions are made along the acromioclavicular area and at the deltoid insertion. A superficial tunnel is prepared connecting these incisions. The entire latissimus dorsi muscle is raised on its neurovascular pedicle and

rotated such that its undersurface is superficial. The latissimus origin and thoracolumbar fascia is passed to the acromioclavicular insertion and secured to bone. The humeral insertion is placed through the subcutaneous tunnel and fixed to the deltoid muscle attachment into the humerus. The position of the neurovascular bundle must be carefully monitored to prevent excessive rotation or kinking, which could result in vascular thrombosis and muscle necrosis.

Postoperative management. The arm is abducted 90 degrees and immobilized in this position using a long-arm cast attached to an abdominal segment via an abduction bar. At 6 weeks after surgery, the cast is removed and a splint is fabricated with the arm maintained in abduction. This is accomplished with an abduction bar secured between a fabricated body segment and a long-arm splint (Fig. 50-16). At this time, therapy is initiated and consists of scar management and muscle reeducation.

Scar management is recommended twice a day until the patient is consistently firing the transfer and there is little chance of adhesion formation. The superficial incision can be managed with massage for soft tissue mobilization combined with topical lotions or creams as lubricants. If hypertrophy is evident, silicone gel sheets or elastomer products can be applied to the scar tissue to aid in the prevention of hypertrophic tissue.[17,46] Deep scarring is best managed by early tendon gliding to produce tendon excursion, which limits the formation of motion limiting adhesions. If adhesions are evident, ultrasound may be used to encourage deep tissue mobilization. Use of this modality should be delayed until tendon healing has occurred, around 6 to 7 weeks postoperatively.

Muscle reeducation is variable with respect to the patient's ease in learning to activate the transfer. Verbal cues to perform the previous action of the muscle before the transfer are effective in helping initiate firing of the muscle. The patient may be placed in a position to perform shoulder abduction in an antigravity plane. It is important that the

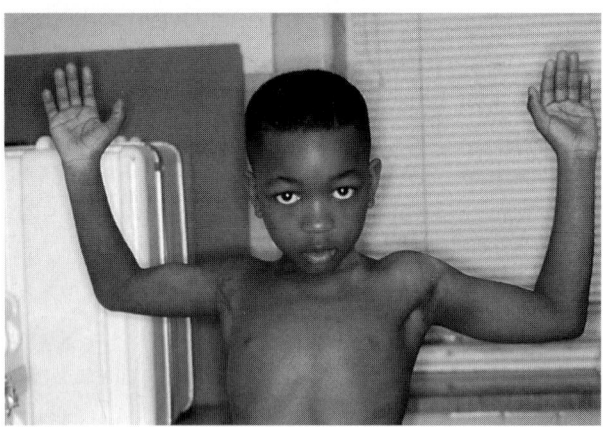

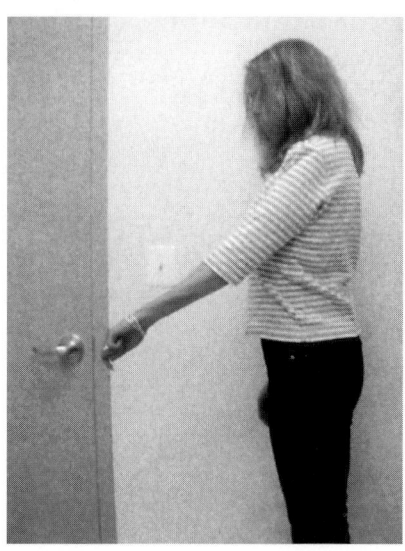

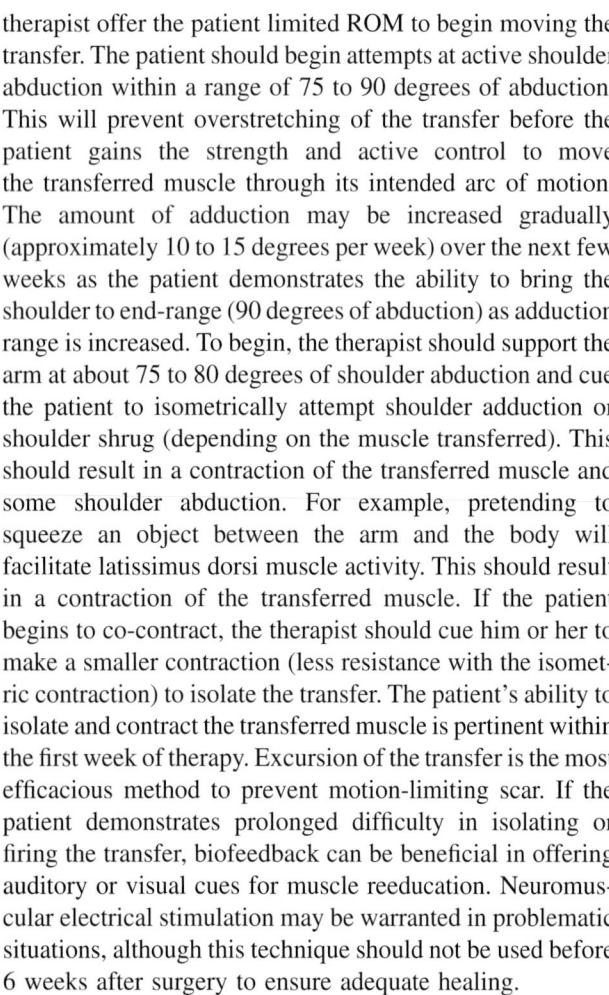

Fig. 50-17. Eleven-year-old boy who underwent left anterior shoulder release and latissimus transfer for external rotation 3 years ago.

Fig. 50-18. Forward elevation in a 25-year-old woman with global left traumatic brachial plexus palsy and persistent shoulder instability treated with glenohumeral fusion.

therapist offer the patient limited ROM to begin moving the transfer. The patient should begin attempts at active shoulder abduction within a range of 75 to 90 degrees of abduction. This will prevent overstretching of the transfer before the patient gains the strength and active control to move the transferred muscle through its intended arc of motion. The amount of adduction may be increased gradually (approximately 10 to 15 degrees per week) over the next few weeks as the patient demonstrates the ability to bring the shoulder to end-range (90 degrees of abduction) as adduction range is increased. To begin, the therapist should support the arm at about 75 to 80 degrees of shoulder abduction and cue the patient to isometrically attempt shoulder adduction or shoulder shrug (depending on the muscle transferred). This should result in a contraction of the transferred muscle and some shoulder abduction. For example, pretending to squeeze an object between the arm and the body will facilitate latissimus dorsi muscle activity. This should result in a contraction of the transferred muscle. If the patient begins to co-contract, the therapist should cue him or her to make a smaller contraction (less resistance with the isometric contraction) to isolate the transfer. The patient's ability to isolate and contract the transferred muscle is pertinent within the first week of therapy. Excursion of the transfer is the most efficacious method to prevent motion-limiting scar. If the patient demonstrates prolonged difficulty in isolating or firing the transfer, biofeedback can be beneficial in offering auditory or visual cues for muscle reeducation. Neuromuscular electrical stimulation may be warranted in problematic situations, although this technique should not be used before 6 weeks after surgery to ensure adequate healing.

At 7 weeks after surgery, the patient is allowed to work through a greater arc of motion. Exercises against gravity can be initiated. However, AROM in an antigravity plane must be continued to ensure contraction and excursion of the muscle. Once the muscle transfer can be isolated and AROM is reasonable, functional activities are incorporated to increase the strength of the tendon transfer. Restriction to adduction is continued to prevent stretching of the transfer.

At 8 to 10 weeks after surgery, provided the patient has progressed appropriately, the splint is discontinued during the day. Treatment foci are to strengthen the transfer and to assist the patient in meeting his or her functional goals. Nighttime splinting is continued for an additional 4 to 8 weeks.

Results. The results after tendon transfers about the shoulder vary with the particular transfer and expected outcome. External rotation transfers are very successful, with restoration of motion and improved ability to perform hand-to-mouth function with the arm at the side (Fig. 50-17).[15,22,36,37] In contrast, abduction transfers are less predictable and have a variable success rate.[13,24]

Arthrodesis

Severe shoulder involvement without available donors for transfers precludes reconstruction. Persistent pain, instability, or arthritis can be remedied only by glenohumeral fusion[38] (Fig. 50-18). However, functioning scapular muscles are required to prevent progressive scapulothoracic winging and instability after shoulder arthrodesis. A stable shoulder can actually enhance extremity function by alleviating pain, maximizing scapulothoracic motion, and provid-

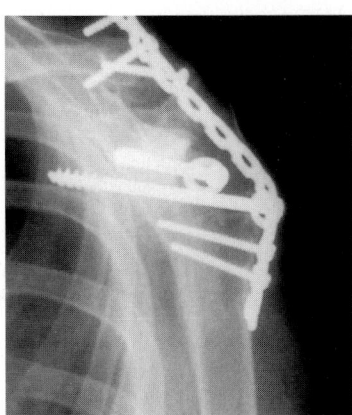

Fig. 50-19. Radiograph demonstrates solid glenohumeral arthrodesis and internal fixation construct.

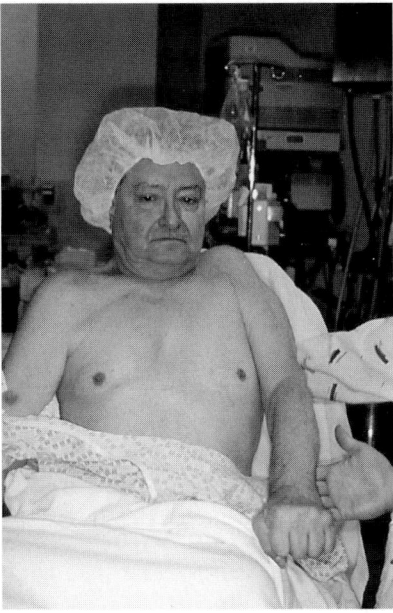

Fig. 50-20. Sixty-year-old man with traumatic right upper brachial plexus injury and inability to flex the elbow.

ing a stable construct for tendon transfers about the elbow (Fig. 50-19).

ELBOW

The elbow is often impaired after brachial plexus injuries, especially elbow flexion secondary to loss of the biceps and brachialis muscles. Inability to flex the elbow is a severe functional handicap because hand-to-mouth function is impossible. The restoration of active elbow flexion through a functional arc of motion (30 to 130 degrees) is a high

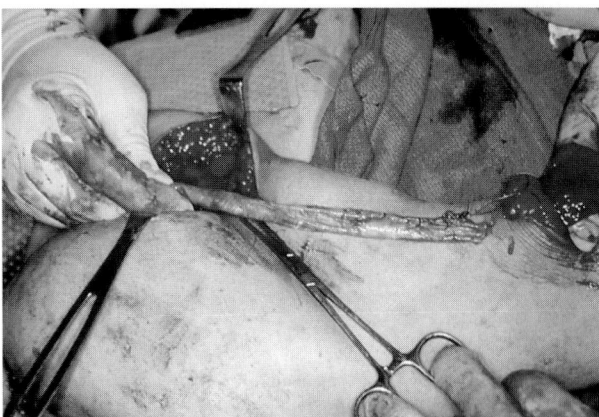

Fig. 50-21. Unipolar transfer of pectoralis major insertion using fascia lata as an intervening graft.

priority during brachial plexus reconstruction.[29] The assessment of potential muscles for transfer is performed via inventory of available donors. Multiple donor muscles are described for elbow flexorplasty, including the latissimus dorsi, pectoralis major, triceps, and flexor-pronator muscles.* The latissimus dorsi or pectoralis major muscle can be transferred using a unipolar or bipolar method. In the unipolar technique, the pectoralis major humeral insertion or sternocostal origin is transferred to the biceps tendon (Figs. 50-20 and 50-21).[3,9] Similarly, the unipolar latissimus transfer redirects the thoracolumbar origin to the biceps tendon. Fascia lata can be used to reinforce the transfer site or as an intervening graft (see Fig. 50-21). The bipolar technique requires both the origin and insertion sites and transfer of the entire muscle (pectoralis major or latissimus dorsi) into the anterior compartment of the arm.[6,47] The muscle origin is attached to the coracoid process or acromion and the insertion is transferred into the biceps tendon. The bipolar transfer is preferred over the unipolar method because it provides a better line of pull, increased muscle mass (cross-sectional area), and superior restoration of muscle fiber length. The bipolar technique also reinforces the anterior support of the flail shoulder and may obviate the need for arthrodesis.

When multiple donor muscles are available, the latissimus dorsi is the preferred donor for elbow flexorplasty as long as it is not required for an alternative transfer (e.g., external rotation). This muscle is expendable, possesses adequate strength (large cross-sectional area), and provides sufficient excursion for elbow flexion.[47] The drawbacks are related to the magnitude of the operation and difficulty in determination of muscle strength because of its substantial

*References 2, 3, 5, 6, 32, 40, 47.

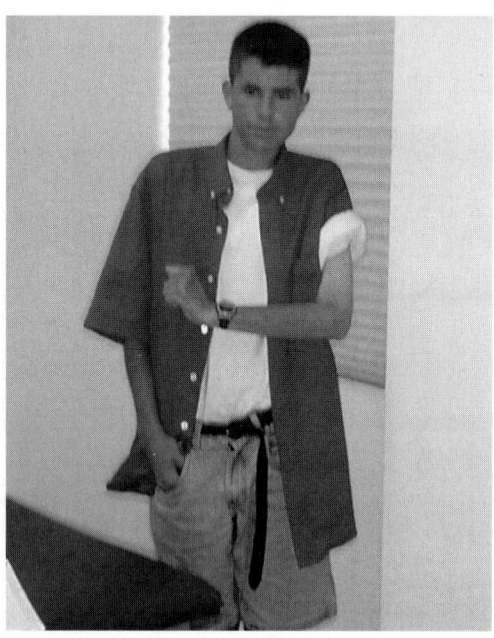

Fig. 50-22. Sixteen-year-old boy following left Steindler transfer with 90 degrees of active elbow flexion and concomitant fist formation.

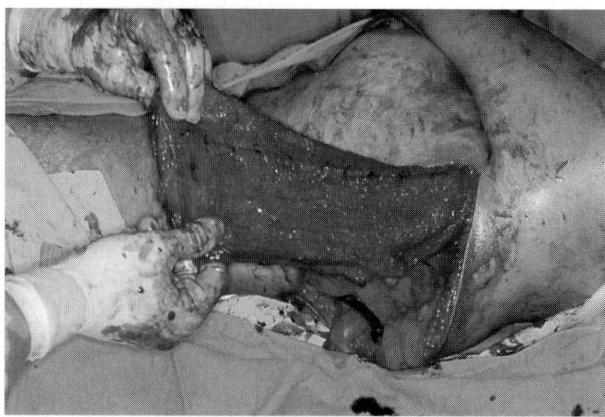

Fig. 50-23. Twenty-five-year-old woman with traumatic left brachial palsy and lack of elbow flexion. Bipolar latissimus dorsi muscle harvested after isolation of thoracodorsal neurovascular pedicle.

bulk. In addition, the latissimus dorsi is innervated by the upper brachial plexus (primarily C5 through C6) and may not be available for transfer.[39] The pectoralis major muscle is another workable donor for elbow flexorplasty, although cosmetic concerns limit its use.[6] The pectoralis major muscle is supplied by C5 through T1 and is transferable in the majority of brachial plexus injuries.[39] The triceps muscle is also a viable option because it has similar inherent properties (i.e., muscle fiber length and excursion) when compared with the biceps muscle.[20] Actually, the triceps muscle is double the strength of the biceps and can provide sufficient elbow extension.[39] However, loss of active extension is a disadvantage and limits the use of the triceps to biceps transfer. In fact, triceps muscle transfer is contraindicated in patients that require forceful extension for upper limb weight bearing (e.g., transfer) or crutches for ambulation.[20] The transfer or proximal advancement of the flexor-pronator muscle group (Steindler procedure) is less commonly used for restoration of elbow flexion. This technique is disadvantaged by the limited motion and strength following transfer and the unwanted forearm pronation and fist formation that occurs with attempted elbow flexion (Fig. 50-22). A Steindler transfer rarely results in the ability to lift greater than 1 kg. This transfer can be used to augment weak elbow flexion (e.g., grade 2) following nerve surgery or elbow flexorplasty transfer.[7,20]

Elbow flexorplasty

Latissimus dorsi transfer (bipolar technique). The patient is placed in a lateral position for harvest of the latissimus dorsi muscle and rotated into the supine position

during transfer of the muscle into the anterior arm. A longitudinal incision is made from the posterior axillary fold to the inferior aspect of the latissimus dorsi muscle. The entire muscle is mobilized, including a strip of thoracodorsal fascia and the tendinous insertion into the humerus (Fig. 50-23). The thoracodorsal nerve and vascular pedicle are isolated and protected.

An anterior deltopectoral approach is performed to create a passageway for the bipolar transfer. A portion of the pectoralis major insertion is released to ease access for the transfer. The latissimus dorsi muscle is passed from posterior to anterior with the tendinous insertion proximal and the fascial origin distal (Fig. 50-24). The thoracodorsal nerve and vessels are protected and prevented from twisting.

The latissimus dorsi muscle is passed into the arm through a subcutaneous tunnel. The tendon of origin is secured to the clavicle or acromion via drill holes and the thoracodorsal fascia is woven into the biceps tendon, which can be reinforced by fascia lata graft. The transfer is placed in enough tension to create a 30-degree tenodesis effect (i.e., tension in the transfer prevents the last 30 degrees of elbow extension). The wounds are closed, with drains placed in the posterior wound. A long-arm splint that maintains 100 to 110 degrees of flexion and a Velpeau dressing is applied. This dressing secures the arm against the body by wrapping an elastic bandage around the torso and arm.

A unipolar latissimus transfer can be performed, although it is not preferred. A similar approach is used for harvest of the latissimus dorsi muscle. However, the insertion site is not released and the origin is passed into the arm, along with a strip of thoracodorsal fascia. The origin is sutured to the biceps tendon using the attached thoracodorsal fascia to complete the unipolar transfer.

Pectoralis major transfer (bipolar technique). The patient is placed in the supine position on the operating room table. The pectoralis muscle is harvested via an incision that

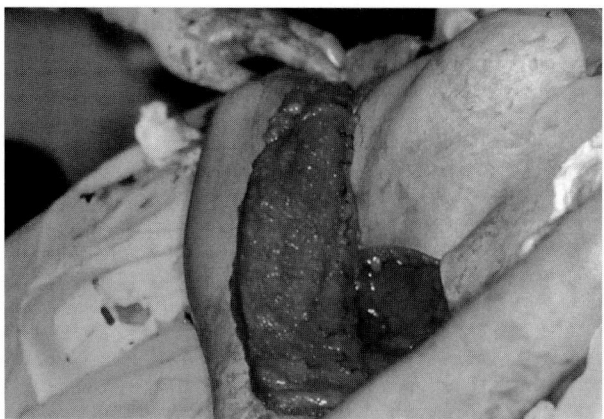

Fig. 50-24. Entire latissimus dorsi muscle passed from posterior to anterior to achieve active elbow flexion.

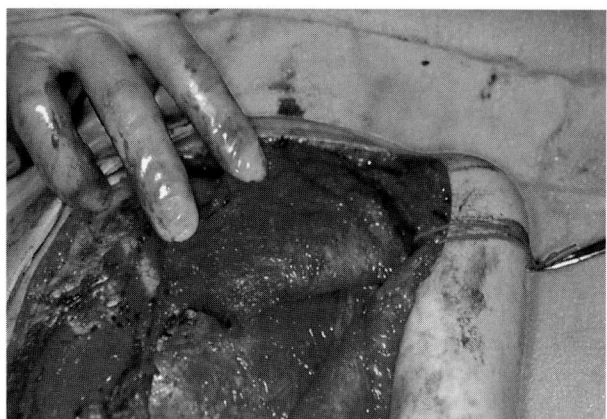

Fig. 50-25. Pectoralis major muscle isolated in an 8-year-old boy in preparation for bipolar transfer to restore active elbow flexion.

runs longitudinally along the medial border of the sternum and curves laterally inferior to the clavicle (Fig. 50-25). The sternocostal origin is released with a strip of rectus abdominus fascia. The clavicular origin is freed while the underlying neurovascular pedicles (medial and lateral pectoral nerves and arteries) are identified and preserved. The pectoralis major tendon of insertion into the humerus is released in preparation for transfer.

The entire pectoralis muscle is mobilized into the arm and passed through a subcutaneous tunnel. The insertion site is oriented proximal and the sternocostal origin distal. The tendon of origin is secured to the clavicle or acromion via drill holes and the rectus abdominus fascia is woven into the biceps tendon, which can be reinforced by a fascia lata graft (Fig. 50-26). The transfer is placed in enough tension to create a 30-degree tenodesis effect (i.e., tension in the transfer prevents the last 30 degrees of elbow extension). The wounds are closed and a long-arm splint is applied that maintains the elbow in 100 to 110 degrees of flexion. A Velpeau dressing is applied with an elastic bandage, which secures the arm to the thorax.

Various additional techniques are available for transfer of the pectoralis major muscle. A unipolar or bipolar transfer of only the sternocostal part of the pectoralis major muscle without disturbing the clavicular portion is an option, which preserves the function of the clavicular component.[3,10] Last, elongation of the humeral insertion with a tendon graft and attachment to the biceps tendon can be performed (see Figs. 50-20 and 21).

Triceps transfer. The patient is placed in a supine position, and the distal half of the triceps is exposed via a posterior incision. The triceps tendon is elevated from the olecranon and elongated with a strip of periosteum. The radial nerve is identified and protected as it traverses around the humerus from posterior to anterior. The biceps tendon is exposed using an anterior zigzag or transverse antecubital incision. The triceps tendon is passed laterally through a subcutaneous tunnel and secured to the biceps tendon

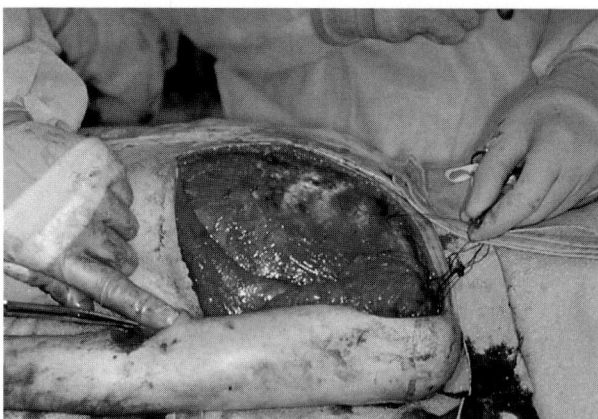

Fig. 50-26. Pectoralis major humeral insertion attached to acromion and passage of muscle origin through subcutaneous tunnel to elbow.

(Fig. 50-27). The transfer is placed in enough tension to create a 30-degree tenodesis effect (i.e., tension in the transfer prevents the last 30 degrees of elbow extension). The wounds are closed and a long-arm splint is applied that maintains 100 to 110 degrees of elbow flexion. The arm is secured to the thorax by a Velpeau dressing.

The triceps tendon and strip of periosteum can be anchored to the ulna just distal to the coronoid process instead of the biceps tendon. This is accomplished using a bone tunnel passed through the ulna from anterior to posterior. The tendon is secured within the tunnel, which provides firm fixation. This transfer supplies elbow flexion without forearm concomitant supination.

Flexor-pronator transfer (Steindler procedure). A medial incision is performed beginning in the arm, traveling across the elbow, and extending into the forearm. The flexor-pronator muscle group is isolated at its origin from the medial epicondyle (Fig. 50-28). The ulnar nerve is identified within the cubital tunnel and transposed anteriorly. The median nerve also is isolated as it passes through the

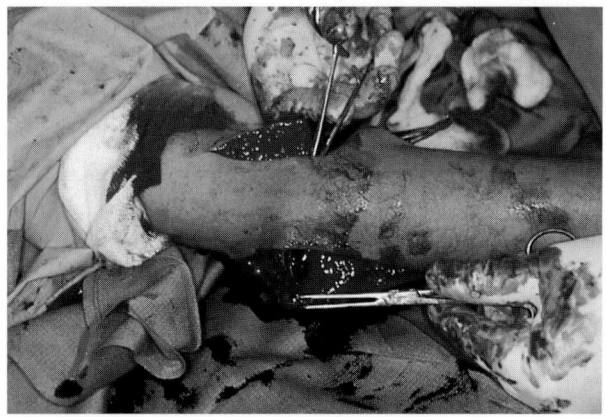

Fig. 50-27. Transfer of triceps muscle from posterior to anterior during elbow flexorplasty in a 10-year-old without active elbow flexion.

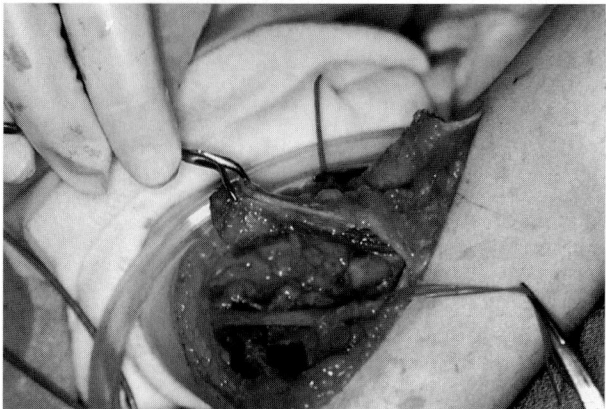

Fig. 50-29. Flexor-pronator muscle group and piece of medial epicondyle elevated and transferred to humerus.

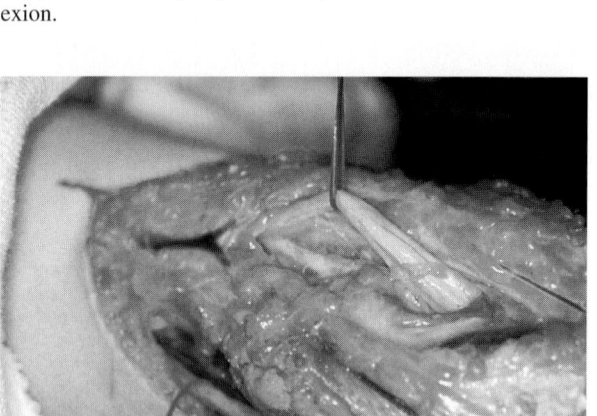

Fig. 50-28. Exposure of left medial epicondyle and flexor-pronator muscle group in 16-year-old depicted in Fig. 50-22. Median nerve isolated anteriorly and ulnar nerve protected posteriorly.

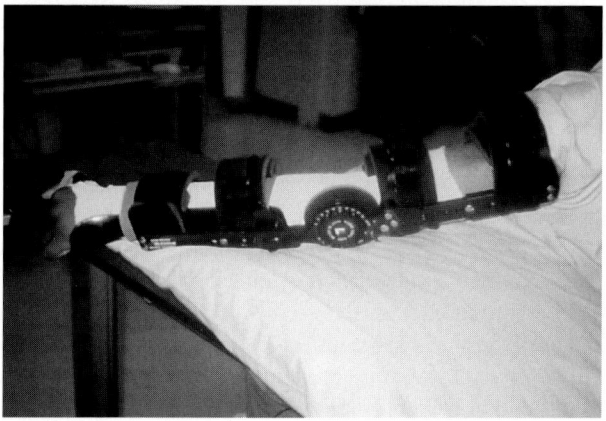

Fig. 50-30. Adjustable variable lock hinge brace used to adjust the amount of available flexion and/or extension.

pronator muscle. The flexor-pronator muscle group is elevated with a piece of medial epicondyle in preparation for transfer (Fig. 50-29).

The entire muscle group is transferred 4 to 5 cm proximal and anterior to increase its ability to flex the elbow. The elbow is flexed and the muscles secured to the humerus via a screw placed across the piece of transferred bone and into the humerus. This creates an immediate tenodesis effect that prevents full extension. The arm is positioned in an arm splint that maintains 100 to 110 degrees of flexion and supination.

Postoperative management. Regardless of the muscle transfer for elbow flexion, the initial postoperative regimen is similar. The arm is splinted or casted for 4 to 6 weeks time, depending on the status and effectiveness of the proximal and distal transfer sites. At the time of cast removal, the patient is placed in a long-arm splint with an adjustable elbow hinge that can variably lock the degree of flexion and

extension (Fig. 50-30). Initial positioning in the splint is approximately 110 degrees of elbow flexion. A separate static night splint that maintains the elbow at 110 degrees of flexion should be fabricated. Early therapy goals include scar management and muscle reeducation.

Scar massage is performed two times a day until the patient is actively firing the transfer and shows no indications of hypertrophy of the incision or adhesions around the tendon transfer. Scar massage should be performed with lotion, which will aid in decreasing friction and prevent shearing to newly healed skin. The therapist may use silicone gel sheets or elastomer products as a supplement to scar management if hypertrophy is evident.[17,46] These products may minimize hypertrophy through prolonged pressure. Ultrasound is another modality that can encourage tissue mobilization, although this technique usually is reserved for recalcitrant scar formation and should be delayed until tendon healing is completed (6 to 7 weeks after surgery).

Muscle reeducation begins with active elbow flexion from a flexed position. Incremental elbow extension is allowed as long as the patient can demonstrate the ability to fire the transfer to end-range of elbow flexion (expected end-range depends on the surgery completed). The therapist can aid the patient in learning to fire the muscle by cueing them to complete the original motion of the transferred muscle. For example, if the patient underwent a Steindler flexorplasty, the therapist would place the arm on a table to facilitate elbow flexion in an antigravity plane. Subsequently, support of the patient's wrist and forearm is provided, and the patient is encouraged to contract the flexor-pronator musculature. The therapist can palpate the flexor-pronator muscles for contraction while cueing the patient to flex the wrist and pronate the forearm. This maneuver is completed until the patient can consistently fire the transfer. When the patient is successful at isolating the transfer and can work the transfer against its antagonist, the splint may be progressed into extension at a rate of 15 degrees per week. When this control is evident, functional activities that require elbow flexion should be added to the therapy sessions. Although these activities will vary according to the patient's goals, some examples of antigravity flexion activities are games that require the patient to support his or her extremity on a table and progress game pieces via active elbow flexion or a tabletop craft activity that requires sustained elbow flexion and reaching within the allowed range (following postoperative precautions). Activities may progress to hand-to-mouth tasks or activities such as buttoning or other basic ADLs.

Light resistive activities (AROM against gravity) may begin when the patient demonstrates a 30-degree arc of range (from 90 to 120 degrees of elbow flexion). At this time, upgrading functional tabletop activities will assist the patient in incorporating the transfer into normal movement patterns. Formal strengthening may begin when the transfer is not at risk for passive overstretching (approximately 10 weeks) and sufficient tendon excursion has been obtained. Passive manipulation to increase elbow extension is not allowed for 3 months. Tendon transfers may actually function better in those patients who lack full extension (improved lever arm of the transfer); therefore the goal for terminal extension is 20 to 30 degrees.

When the patient gains active elbow flexion against gravity, from an arc of 90 degrees to end-range, the day splint may be discontinued. Twelve weeks after surgery, the night splint is discontinued and unrestricted activity is allowed.

Results. The results of tendon transfer for elbow flexion are generally good, with a return of flexion against gravity (i.e., muscle strength grade 3).[2,5,6,32,47] This affords a considerable improvement in function when compared with the paralyzed elbow, although lifting power is limited. The outcome is directly related to the strength and integrity of the donor muscle. The presence of poor shoulder control will

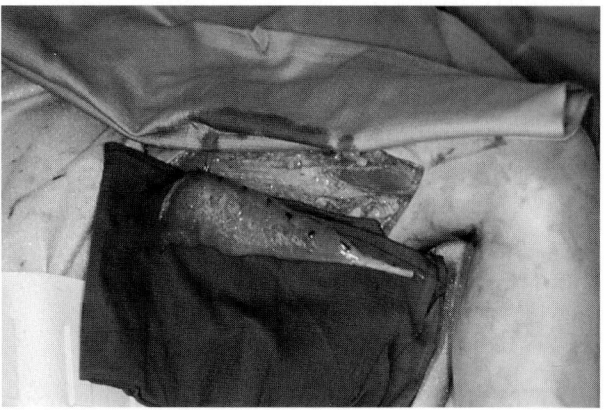

Fig. 50-31. Harvest of a left gracilis muscle in a 6-year-old boy with right obstetric brachial plexus palsy, no active elbow flexion, and no local muscle available for transfer.

create proximal instability and diminish the effectiveness of the elbow flexorplasty.

Free muscle transfer

Free muscle transfer is a microneurovascular transplantation of an entire muscle-tendon unit with neurorrhaphy and revascularization. This technique is indicated when no local muscles are available for transfer. Free muscle transfer is a demanding procedure that requires proficiency in microvascular surgery. The gracilis muscle is the most common donor muscle because of its availability, expendability, and lengthy excursion.[7,8,30] The gracilis muscle is reinnervated via multiple intercostal nerves or the spinal accessory nerve.

Microvascular gracilis transfer. A two-team approach often is used for free tissue transfer surgery. One team harvests the gracilis muscle while the second team prepares the arm and recipient neurovascular structures. The gracilis is harvested via a medial thigh incision, and the underlying medial femoral circumflex artery and vein are isolated as the vascular pedicle (Fig. 50-31). The anterior division of the obturator nerve is the nerve supply to the gracilis muscle and is also carefully dissected. Sutures are placed along the muscle at regular intervals to allow recreation of proper length after transfer. The origin and insertion of the muscle are released in preparation for transfer.

Concurrently, the arm is prepared using deltopectoral and antecubital incisions. A subcutaneous tunnel is created between these incisions for passage of the gracilis muscle. When using intercostal nerves, a transverse incision is made over the fourth rib for exposure of the ribs. The third through fifth intercostal nerves are isolated from beneath their respective ribs via meticulous dissection to avoid a pneumothorax. The intercostal nerves are dissected from anterior axillary line to the sternocostal junction for adequate length.

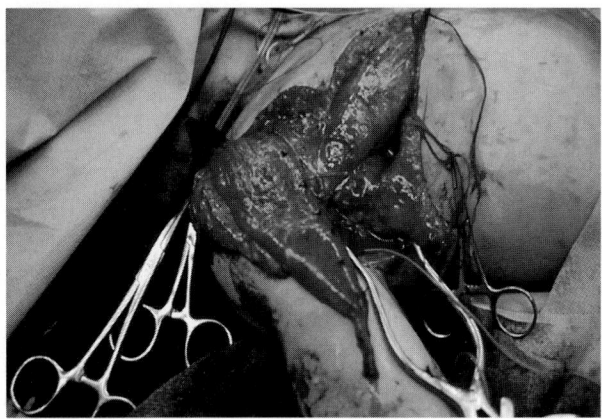

Fig. 50-32. Free gracilis muscle secured to acromion during revascularization and transfer of intercostal nerves.

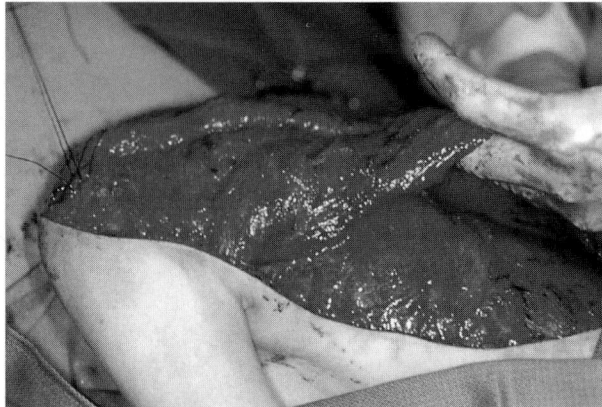

Fig. 50-33. Ten-year-old girl positioned prone for harvest of left latissimus dorsi muscle for elbow extension.

The brachial artery and cephalic vein are identified in preparation for vascular anastomosis.

The gracilis is disconnected from the thigh and secured to the acromion and clavicle using drill holes (Fig. 50-32). The microneurovascular connection between the recipient structures within the gracilis muscle and the donor artery, vein, and nerve is performed using a microscope. The muscle is placed through the subcutaneous tunnel within the arm and secured to the biceps tendon.

The spinal accessory nerve also can be used to reinnervate the gracilis muscle. A supraclavicular exposure of the brachial plexus is required to isolate the spinal accessory nerve within the posterior triangle of the neck. The nerve is harvested distal to the innervation of the upper trapezius muscle to preserve shoulder shrugs function. An interposition nerve graft may be necessary to reach the obturator nerve to the gracilis muscle.

Postoperative management. The elbow is positioned in 100 to 110 degrees of flexion and fastened to the torso using a Velpeau dressing. Complete immobilization is continued for 5 to 6 weeks. Scar management and gentle passive motion can then be instituted with avoidance of terminal extension. A resting splint with the elbow at 90 degrees is worn until reinnervation of the biceps, which requires nerve regeneration and time (usually 6 to 12 months). Initial excitation of the muscle occurs with coughing or sneezing before voluntary control.

Results. The outcome after free muscle transplantation for elbow flexion is impressive. Approximately 75% to 80% of patients regain elbow flexion against gravity.[8,30]

Elbow extension transfer

A deficiency in elbow extension can result from brachial plexus injuries that involve the middle portion of the plexus. Surgical reconstruction is less commonly performed because elbow flexion is a greater priority and elbow extension can be accomplished by gravity.[27] In certain cases, elbow flexion is adequate and the lack of elbow extension is disabling.

Deficient elbow extension will decrease the patient's available workspace, limit the ability to perform overhead tasks, and impair transfers in wheelchair-constrained patients.

Evaluation of the patient for elbow extension transfer requires an inventory of the available muscles. The preferred donor is the latissimus dorsi muscle transferred using a bipolar technique. Another option is the posterior deltoid or biceps muscle transferred to the triceps. When transferring the biceps, a stringent prerequisite is intact brachialis and supinator muscles to maintain elbow flexion and supination, respectively. The identification and strength grading of the brachialis and supinator muscles is difficult and a supplemental EMG may be necessary to evaluate their function and inherent properties.

Latissimus dorsi transfer (bipolar technique). The patient is placed in a lateral position for harvest of the latissimus dorsi muscle. A longitudinal incision is made from the posterior axillary fold to the inferior aspect of the latissimus dorsi muscle. The entire muscle is mobilized, including a strip of thoracodorsal fascia and the tendinous insertion into the humerus. The thoracodorsal nerve and vascular pedicle are isolated and protected.

The latissimus dorsi muscle tendon of origin is secured to the clavicle or acromion via drill holes. The remaining muscle is passed through a subcutaneous tunnel, and the thoracodorsal fascia is woven into the triceps tendon, which can be reinforced by fascia lata graft (Figs. 50-33 and 50-34). The transfer is sutured in place with the arm positioned full extension. The wounds are closed and the arm is placed in a long-arm splint in complete extension.

Biceps transfer. The patient is placed supine, and the biceps muscle and tendon are exposed via an incision that parallels the medial arm and traverses across the antecubital fossa (Fig. 50-35). The biceps tendon is released from its insertion into the radial tuberosity. A second longitudinal incision is performed to identify the triceps tendon and its insertion into the olecranon. The biceps tendon is passed medially through a subcutaneous tunnel and into the

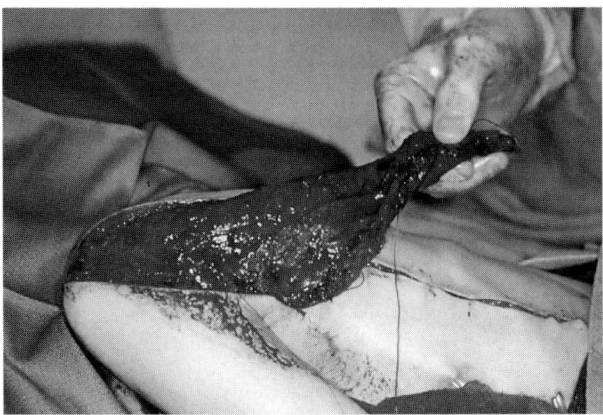

Fig. 50-34. Latissimus dorsi humeral insertion transferred to posterior acromion and origin prepared for transfer into the arm and attachment to triceps tendon.

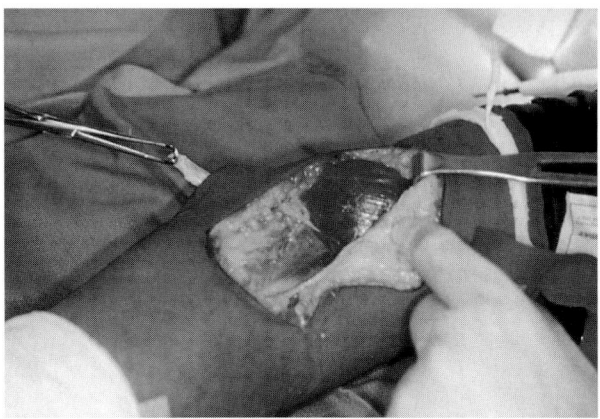

Fig. 50-36. Biceps transferred medially through a subcutaneous tunnel to triceps tendon.

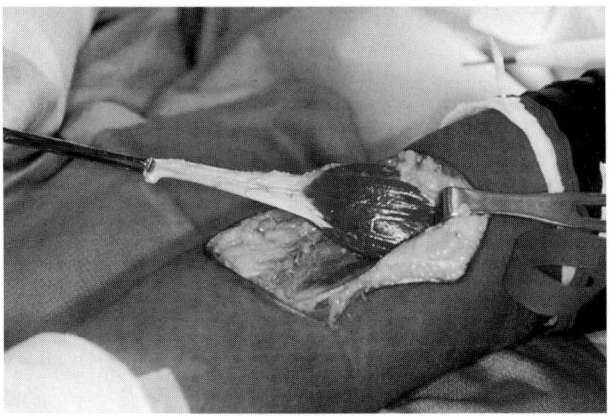

Fig. 50-35. Anterior elbow incision and isolation of biceps tendon during transfer in a 16-year-old with intact elbow flexion but deficient elbow extension.

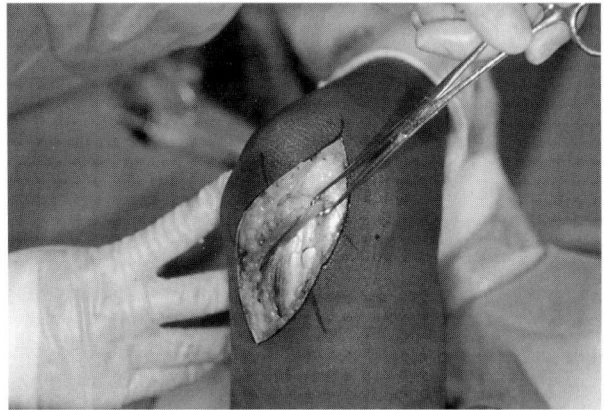

Fig. 50-37. Biceps tendon within posterior incision in preparation for attachment to triceps tendon.

posterior incision (Fig. 50-36). The tendon is woven through the triceps tendon and passed into an olecranon bone tunnel with the arm in extension (Fig. 50-37). The transfer is sutured in place with the arm positioned full extension. The wounds are closed and the arm is placed in a long-arm splint in complete extension.

Postoperative management. Regardless of the muscle transfer for elbow extension, the initial postoperative regimen is similar. The arm is splinted or casted for 4 to 6 weeks, depending on the effectiveness of the proximal and distal transfer attachment sites.

At 4 to 6 weeks, the patient is placed in a removable long-arm splint with an adjustable variable-lock elbow hinge that can regulate the amount of flexion and extension (see Fig. 50-30). The splint is locked at 0 degrees of elbow extension during the first week of therapy. Treatment goals during the first week of therapy include scar management and muscle reeducation.

Scar massage is completed two times a day until the patient is actively firing the transfer and shows no indications

of hypertrophy of the incision or adhesion around the transfer. Scar massage should be completed with lotion, which will aid in decreasing friction and prevent shearing to recently healed skin. The therapist may use silicone gel sheets or elastomer products as a supplement to scar management if hypertrophy is evident. Ultrasound is another modality that can encourage tissue mobilization, although this technique is usually reserved for dense scar formation and should be delayed until tendon healing is completed (6 to 7 weeks after surgery).

To begin activating the transfer, the therapist should support the patient's arm at 90 degrees of shoulder flexion or abduction (whichever posture places the transfer on slack) and passively flex the elbow 5 to 10 degrees. The therapist will then cue the patient to attempt to complete the original motion, or in some cases the secondary motion, that the transferred muscle completed. For example, if the patient has undergone a biceps to triceps transfer, the therapist would position the patient elbow in slight (5 to 10 degrees) elbow flexion (with the shoulder forward flexed) and cue the patient to supinate the forearm to palpate a contraction from the biceps transfer. An early goal is to achieve consistent and isolated contraction of the transfer.

During the second week of therapy, the day splint may be advanced to allow the patient 15 degrees of active extension. A night splint is fabricated to maintain the elbow in full extension. This places the transfer in its relaxed position without tension to prevent overstretching. As the patient continues to master firing of the transfer, the goals change to accomplish an isolated and consistent movement. If the patient has achieved this goal, advancement of the splint may continue at 15 degrees of elbow flexion each week as long as active terminal extension is maintained. Functional activities that require use of elbow extension should be included into treatment. If the patient is delayed in his or her ability to consistently fire the transfer, biofeedback should be implemented.

Light resistive strengthening, in the form of isolated ROM against gravity, may begin when the patient reaches a 45-degree arc of range (from 45 to 0 degrees). Desktop-type functional activities will challenge the patient to maintain varying degrees of elbow extension while using his or her hand in space. This is a good activity to encourage use of the elbow extension transfer and will improve endurance.

In general, the daytime splint is worn until the patient regains 90 degrees of active flexion and can actively extend from 90 to 0 degrees. At this time, the patient may begin higher-level resistive exercises (use of hand weights) targeting the transfer and surrounding musculature that may be deconditioned secondary to postoperative precautions. The addition of functional reaching tasks will further challenge the patient while improving the endurance of the transfer.

Three months after the surgery, the patient may resume higher-level performance tasks, such as sports, and the night extension splint can be discontinued.

WRIST AND HAND

Wrist and hand involvement is less predictable after brachial plexus injury. Upper brachial plexus lesions have a minimal effect on hand use, while global plexus injuries can severely hamper hand function. A definitive treatment algorithm is more difficult to recommend because of the variable clinical presentation. A detailed functional evaluation and manual muscle testing is the foundation for the development of a treatment paradigm. The formulation of a list of what's in, what's out, what's available, and what's needed is the basis for the decision-making process. Individualized treatment is required and many of the principles of radial, median, and ulnar nerve transfers are applied. The principles and techniques of these tendon transfers are covered in other chapters of this text.

REFERENCES

1. Amadio PC: Outcomes assessment in hand surgery: what's new? *Clin Plast Surg* 24:191, 1997.
2. Beaton DE, et al: Steindler and pectoralis major flexorplasty: a comparative analysis, *J Hand Surg* 20A:747, 1995.
3. Brooks DM, Seddon HJ: Pectoral transplantation for paralysis of the flexors of the elbow, *J Bone Joint Surg* 41B:36, 1959.
4. Campion D: Electrodiagnostic testing in hand surgery, *J Hand Surg* 21A:947, 1996.
5. Carroll RE, Hill NA: Triceps transfer to restore elbow flexion: a study of fifteen patients with paralytic lesions and arthrogryposis, *J Bone Joint Surg* 52A:239, 1970.
6. Carroll RE, Kleinman WB: Pectoralis major transplantation to restore elbow flexion to the paralytic limb, *J Hand Surg* 4A:501, 1979.
7. Chuang DC, et al: Functional restoration of elbow flexion in brachial plexus injuries: results in 167 patients (excluding obstetric brachial plexus injury), *J Hand Surg* 18A:285, 1993.
8. Chung DC, Carver N, Wei FC: Results of functioning free muscle transplantation for elbow flexion, *J Hand Surg* 21A:1071, 1996.
9. Clark JMP: Reconstruction of the biceps brachii by pectoral muscle transplantation, *Br J Surg* 34:180, 1946.
10. Clarke HM, Curtis CG: An approach to obstetrical brachial plexus injuries, *Hand Clin* 11:563, 1995 (review).
11. Deletis V, Morota N, Abbott IR: Electrodiagnosis in the management of brachial plexus surgery, *Hand Clin* 11:555, 1995.
12. Duchenne GB: Studies on pseudohypertrophic muscular paralysis or myosclerotic paralysis, *Arch Neurol* 19:629, 1968.
13. Egloff DV, et al: Palliative surgical procedures to restore shoulder function in obstetric brachial palsy: critical analysis of Narakas' series, *Hand Clin* 11:597, 1995.
14. Gilbert A: Long-term evaluation of brachial plexus surgery in obstetrical palsy, *Hand Clin* 11:583, 1995.
15. Gilbert A, Romana C, Ayatti R: Tendon transfers for shoulder paralysis in children, *Hand Clin* 4:633, 1988.
16. Goddard NJ, Fixsen JA: Rotation osteotomy of the humerus for birth injuries of the brachial plexus, *Arch Neurol* 66:257, 1984.
17. Gold MH: Topical silicone gel sheeting in the treatment of hypertrophic scars and keloids: a dermatologic experience (see comments), *J Dermatol Surg Oncol* 19:912, 1993.
18. Greenwald AG, Schute PC, Shiveley JL: Brachial plexus birth palsy: a 10-year report on the incidence and prognosis, *J Pediatr Orthop* 4:689, 1984.
19. Hershman EB: Brachial plexus injuries, *Clin Sports Med* 9:311, 1990.
20. Hoang PH, Mills C: Triceps to biceps transfer for established brachial plexus palsy, *J Bone Joint Surg* 71B:268, 1989.
21. Hoffer MM: Closed reduction and tendon transfer for treatment of dislocation of the glenohumeral joint secondary to brachial plexus birth palsy, *J Bone Joint Surg* 80A:997, 1998.
22. Hoffer MM, Wickenden R, Roper B: Brachial plexus birth palsies: results of tendon transfers to the rotator cuff, *J Bone Joint Surg* 60A:691, 1978.
23. Hudak PL, Amadio PC, Bombardier C: Development of an upper extremity outcome measure: the DASH (disabilities of the arm, shoulder and hand) [corrected]. The Upper Extremity Collaborative Group, *Am J Ind Med* 29:602, 1996.
24. Itoh Y, et al: Transfer of latissimus dorsi to replace a paralysed anterior deltoid: a new technique using an inverted pedicled graft, *J Bone Joint Surg* 69B:647, 1987.
25. Jebsen RH, Taylor N: An objective and standardized test of hand function, *Arch Phys Med Rehabil* 50:311, 1969.
26. Johnson LM, et al: Development of a clinical assessment of quality of movement for unilateral upper-limb function, *Dev Med Child Neurol* 36:965, 1994.

27. Jones BN, et al: Latissimus dorsi transfer to restore elbow extension in obstetrical palsy, *J Pediatr Orthop* 5:287, 1985.
28. Klumpke A: Klumpke's paralysis: 1885 [classical article], *Clin Orthop Rel Res* 368:3, 1999.
29. Kozin SH: Injuries of the brachial plexus. In Iannotti JP, Williams GR, editors: *Disorders of the shoulder: diagnosis and management,* Philadelphia, 1999, Lippincott Williams & Wilkins.
30. Krakauer JD, Wood MB: Intercostal nerve transfer for brachial plexopathy, *J Hand Surg* 19A:829, 1994.
31. Laurent JP, et al: Neurosurgical correction of upper brachial plexus birth injuries, *J Neurosurg* 79:197, 1993.
32. Marshall RW, et al: Operations to restore elbow flexion after brachial plexus injuries, *J Bone Joint Surg* 70B:577, 1988.
33. Metaizeau JP, Gayet C, Plenat F: Brachial plexus birth injuries. An experimental study (author's transl) (French), *Chir Pediatr* 20:159, 1979.
34. Misamore GW, Lehman DE: Parsonage-Turner syndrome (acute brachial neuritis), *J Bone Joint Surg* 78A:1405, 1996.
35. Pearl ML, Edgerton BW: Glenoid deformity secondary to brachial plexus birth palsy, *J Bone Joint Surg* 80A:659, 1998.
36. Phipps GJ, Hoffer MM: Latissimus dorsi and teres major transfer to rotator cuff for Erb's palsy, *J Shoulder Elbow Surg* 4:124, 1995.
37. Price AE, Grossman JA: A management approach for secondary shoulder and forearm deformities following obstetrical brachial plexus injury, *Hand Clin* 11:607, 1995.
38. Richards RR, Waddell JP, Hudson AR: Shoulder arthrodesis for the treatment of brachial plexus palsy, *Clin Orthop Rel Res* 250, 1985.
39. Rostoucher P, et al: Tendon transfers to restore elbow flexion after traumatic paralysis of the brachial plexus in adults, *Int Orthop* 22:255, 1998.
40. Stern PJ, Caudle RJ: Tendon transfers for elbow flexion, *Hand Clin* 4:297, 1988.
41. Stevens JH: Brachial plexus paralysis. From Stevens JH, 1934 [classical article], *Clin Orthop Rel Res* 237:4, 1988.
42. Waters PM: Comparison of the natural history, the outcome of microsurgical repair, and the outcome of operative reconstruction in brachial plexus birth palsy, *J Bone Joint Surg* 81A:649, 1999.
43. Waters PM, Peljovich AE: Shoulder reconstruction in patients with chronic brachial plexus birth palsy: a case control study, *Clin Orthop* 364:144, 1999.
44. Waters PM, Smith GR, Jaramillo D: Glenohumeral deformity secondary to brachial plexus birth palsy, *J Bone Joint Surg* 80A:668, 1998.
45. Wickstrom J: Birth palsies of the brachial plexus: treatment of defects in the shoulder, *Clin Orthop* 23:187, 1962.
46. Widgerow AD, et al: New innovations in scar management, *Aesthetic Plast Surg* 24:227, 2000.
47. Zancolli E, Mitre H: Latissimus dorsi transfer to restore elbow flexion: an appraisal of eight cases, *J Bone Joint Surg* 55A:1265, 1973.

REHABILITATION OF THE HAND AND UPPER EXTREMITY IN TETRAPLEGIA

Allan E. Peljovich
Kevin A. Kucera
Eduardo Gonzalez-Hernandez
Michael W. Keith

Among the most disabling aspects of traumatic tetraplegia is the loss of useful hand function. During the acute phase of a patient's injury, the focus of treatment concerns the survival of the patient. In the subacute phase, care is often shifted into the rehabilitation environment, where the long road to recovery, both mentally and physically, begins. The focus of this chapter is aimed toward the long-term phase, where the patient's medical and psychologic systems are maintained, and he or she becomes reintegrated into society. In this final phase, patients are hopefully discharged from a full-term care facility into a more personal environment and, just as important, into an environment that provides them with purpose and gain. During this entire process, a large, multidisciplinary team including physicians, nurses, therapists, and social workers cares for the patient. Since the inception of the first specialized Spinal Cord Center, established in England in 1944, and the emergence of Model Spinal Cord Injury Systems in the United States in 1970, knowledge has accrued considerably concerning the care of these patients, and has become so specialized in its own right that there are journals devoted exclusively to this subject.[96] It is our opinion that, despite the tremendous research and effort devoted to improving the care of tetraplegic patients, rehabilitating the hand all too often is given a lower priority. This is unfortunate considering that research has documented the loss of hand function in tetraplegic patients to be among the most disabling features of their injury and that they often regard the hope for restoration of hand function to be of paramount importance.[36]

As knowledge of spinal cord injury (SCI) care has improved, so too has that of hand and upper extremity restoration. Since the late 1940s, a body of research has devoted itself to the restoration of tetraplegic hands and has vastly improved patients' levels of independence.* This research, from a variety of different disciplines, has provided us with a vast armamentarium to treat the patient. Conceptually, we believe that, to aid the patient in the long run, treatment directed to the hand and upper extremity should begin early in the acute phase of care and that this treatment extends beyond traditional concepts of exercise, splinting, and braces. In fact, true rehabilitation of the tetraplegic hand should be thought of as the judicious application of nonoperative and operative interventions that are tailor-made to the particular patient to maximize his or her function, bearing in mind the patient's global psychosocial and medical state. This chapter introduces concepts of pathophysiology of SCI in tetraplegia as they apply to hand and upper extremity function, reviews the functional deficits the patients suffer, and describes a comprehensive approach to rehabilitation

*References 8, 18, 23, 29, 62, 81, 97, 102, 104, 105.

based on the former that involves both nonoperative and operative modalities.

THE SCOPE OF THE PROBLEM

Critical to the understanding of the magnitude of the problem related to the tetraplegic hand is first understanding the epidemiology of SCI.[79] Data gathered from the National SCI Database, and recently updated in 2000, indicate that the annual incidence of SCI is approximately 40 per million people, or approximately 10,000 new cases per year. It is also estimated that approximately 183,000 to 230,000 Americans currently live with an SCI (721 to 906 per million). Just more than half of the patients (51.9%) are tetraplegic. The average age of a person who sustains an SCI is 31.8 years, and if the person is in his or her twenties at the time of injury and receives modern standards of care and rehabilitation, he or she will live, on average, an additional 51.6 years for all levels of injury, and 39.4 additional years with low-level tetraplegia (C5 to C8). If the patient is in his or her forties, he or she will live 38.4 additional years for all levels of injury, and 23 additional years if he or she has low-level tetraplegia (C5 to C8). This means that a patient who sustains low-level tetraplegia can expect to live a fairly long life. To this end, estimates of direct costs of SCI have been compiled, and for low-level tetraplegia, the estimated cost of the first year of injury is $342,041, each subsequent year is $38,865, and the lifetime costs for a young patient is $950,257. These figures do not include indirect costs of injury, such as lost income, nor do they estimate the true impact of the injury on the patient or his or her family and friends.

Although tetraplegia is defined as the impairment from an injury to any of the cervical segments of the spine, the extent of disability is determined primarily from the specific functional level of the injury.[2] The fifth cervical spinal cord segment not only is the most common injured level in tetraplegia, it also is the most common level injured in all SCIs (15.8%).[79,85] The next two most commonly injured levels are also in the cervical spine, namely the C4 and C6 segments, with each totaling approximately 12% of all SCIs. The remaining cervical segments comprise approximately 13% of all SCIs. Most tetraplegic patients retain at least the ability to flex their elbows, and some can extend their wrists; however, most do not retain the voluntarily elbow extension, wrist flexion, or finger control. It is the rare patient who retains voluntary finger control or lacks complete volitional use of his or her upper limb. Factors that influence functional ability include whether the injury is "complete," whether any cognitive impairment exists (i.e., brain injury), the age of the patient, any other upper extremity injury, the presence of uncontrolled spasticity, contractures that limit mobility, and depression.[11]

Intuitively, the level of function and independence improves as the patient retains more function.[2,11] Patients with high-level tetraplegia, with functional levels from C2 to C4, generally have no movement of the arms, short of some shoulder elevation. They have some control of their neck muscles and may be ventilatory support dependent, depending on the actual functional level of injury. Patients who retain voluntary innervation in the C5 myotome can flex their elbows, and they retain functional deltoid control. They are able to feed themselves and perhaps even groom themselves with the aid of special adaptive equipment attached to their wrists and hands. At the C6 level, patients can voluntarily extend their wrists, and as such, with the aid of adaptive equipment, they can be independent in activities of daily living (ADLs) such as grooming, bathing, driving, and preparing a simple meal. At the C7 level, patients retain use of their triceps and perhaps the ability to extend their fingers. These patients may be able to perform all the aforementioned activities and be fairly efficient in daily living tasks. Importantly, if the triceps is of sufficient strength, they may be able to independently transfer themselves, provided they have voluntary control of most of their shoulder musculature, and therefore can live alone with the aid of special hand and environmental adaptive equipment. With the exception of this latter patient, all patients require an able-bodied attendant most of the time to help them with their daily activities. Although this is an oversimplified and generalized view of function based on level of injury, it should be readily apparent that any treatment or intervention that improves a level of function, for example, C5 to C6, would result in a dramatic improvement in both function and independence.[21,58,105,106,108]

The severity of the impairments that patients with SCI experience is truly great. The spinal cord not only serves as the conduit for transmission of efferent and afferent information between the limbs and the brain but is also an important neural conduit for the bowel, bladder, respiration, temperature regulation, cardiovascular integrity, and sexual function.[96] All of these important physiologic systems are affected by the injury and, until recently, served as a common and serious cause of morbidity. Sir Ludwig Guttmann, one of the pioneers of SCI management declared in 1976, "of the many forms of disability which can beset mankind, a severe injury or disease of the spinal cord undoubtedly constitutes one of the most devastating calamities in human life. . . ."[96] The affected people are young, are usually otherwise healthy, and might otherwise have expected to live a long and productive life. At the time of injury, approximately 60% are employed and 20% are in school.[96] The impact of injury extends well into their personal lives, with sound data indicating lower rates of marriage and higher rates of divorce among patients with SCIs.[96] The results of modern SCI care and management have dramatically improved the quantity of life, in terms of long-term survival, to a level near able-bodied individuals. Similar care has dramatically improved the quality of their lives as well, but any intervention that can improve a patient's functional ability will have a tremendous positive effect that will extend beyond activities he or she can perform. To this end, Hanson

Table 51-1. Characteristic clinical patterns of motor neuron disease and injury

	Upper motor neuron	Lower motor neuron
Muscles involved	Groups (myotomes) are affected	Individual muscles may be affected
Atrophy	Slight and secondary to disuse	Pronounced, up to 70%-80% of normal bulk
Muscle tone	Spasticity, hyperactive tendon reflexes, Babinski sign present	Flaccidity, hypotonia, loss of deep tendon reflexes
Fascicular twitches	Absent	May be present
EMG/NCS	Normal NCS, no denervation on EMG	Abnormal NCS, denervation present on EMG

From Adams R, Victor M, Ropper A: *Principles of neurology*, ed 6, New York, 1997, McGraw-Hill.
EMG, Electromyelogram; *NCS*, nerve conduction study.

and Franklin[36] studied patients with SCIs to determine what they perceived as their greatest functional losses. Among both tetraplegic patients (76%) and caregivers (64%), the restoration of hand and upper extremity function was considered the most important function to be restored. Waters et al.[101] noted that "the greatest potential for improvement of quality of life lies in rehabilitation and maximal restoration of upper extremity function." Clearly, attention should be directed to rehabilitating the hand and upper extremity as part of a more global approach to treating patients with tetraplegia.

PATHOPHYSIOLOGY

Traumatic SCI disrupts the neural communication that exists between the central and peripheral nervous systems at the level of the spinal cord. Traditional simplified patterns of nerve injury have been used to explain the resulting pathophysiology—SCI represents loss of upper motor/sensory neurons as opposed to peripheral nerve injuries, which affect lower motor/sensory neurons. Table 51-1 displays the common clinical patterns associated with these two different injury patterns. Both careful examination of a spinal cord–injured patient and clinical research have documented that a spectrum of nerve loss is associated with the injury.[50,51,85,86] It is more appropriate to think in terms of a "zone of injury" to the nervous system centered around, but not exclusively confined to, the spinal cord. This is a three-dimensional zone, extending in a proximal/distal plane and a central/peripheral or mediolateral/anteroposterior plane. This is because most SCIs result from a high-energy, blunt trauma injury (e.g., motor vehicle accident, diving) where energy is transferred to the affected bones and soft tissues in a global pattern. This is in contrast to a sharp, penetrating injury (e.g., gunshot wound, laceration) where the energy is transmitted to a more specific area of tissue. Because the zone of injury can include both the cord and the peripheral nervous system around the neck, varying patterns of nerve injury are manifest. Above the zone of injury, the central and peripheral systems and their interconnections are intact and fully functional. Below this zone, nerve physiol-

ogy is generally an upper motor neuron lesion with hyperreflexia. Within the zone of injury, which can extend from the spinal cord to the level of the dorsal sensory ganglia and nerve roots, the pattern of nerve loss is a combination of pure upper motor neuron and lower motor neuron and sensory involvement. For example, the nerve-root injury at the level of the intervertebral foramen from cervical fracture-dislocation, or a nerve-root avulsion from the stretch of the initial trauma, can result in a pure lower motor/sensory neuron injury. Conversely, injury at the level of the anterior horn cell may result in a variable upper/lower motor/sensory neuron pattern of injury. Many muscles in the upper extremity receive innervation from multiple cervical roots, and these peripheral nerves may have been separately injured at the same time that the cervical spine sustained an injury. All of the aforementioned are often the reasons that two patients with two seemingly similar injuries at the same cervical spine injury level can have different degrees of paralysis, spasticity, and neural loss.

To transfer the concepts of pathophysiology into the realm of the clinically relevant, several classification systems have been formulated to group and characterize the patterns of injury.* Classification systems based on the anatomic level of injury results in too much uncertainty. The zone of cord injury and the functional consequences are not precisely concordant with the skeletal anatomic level of the injury. Health care providers discovered that gross motor functions conferred important prognostic information. This is because the innervation of the hand and upper extremity, from spinal roots C4 through T1, proceeds in a fairly ordered and segmental pattern from proximal to distal (Fig. 51-1), making predictions of functional loss and retention fairly reliable once the functional level of the injury is apparent. The classification system most commonly used, devised by the American Spinal Injury Association (ASIA), is based on this functional level and distinguishes the completeness of the injury and the motor and sensory integrity between the extremities.[2] In this system, the most distal myotome with

*References 2, 22, 25, 26, 59, 68, 69, 77, 106, 108.

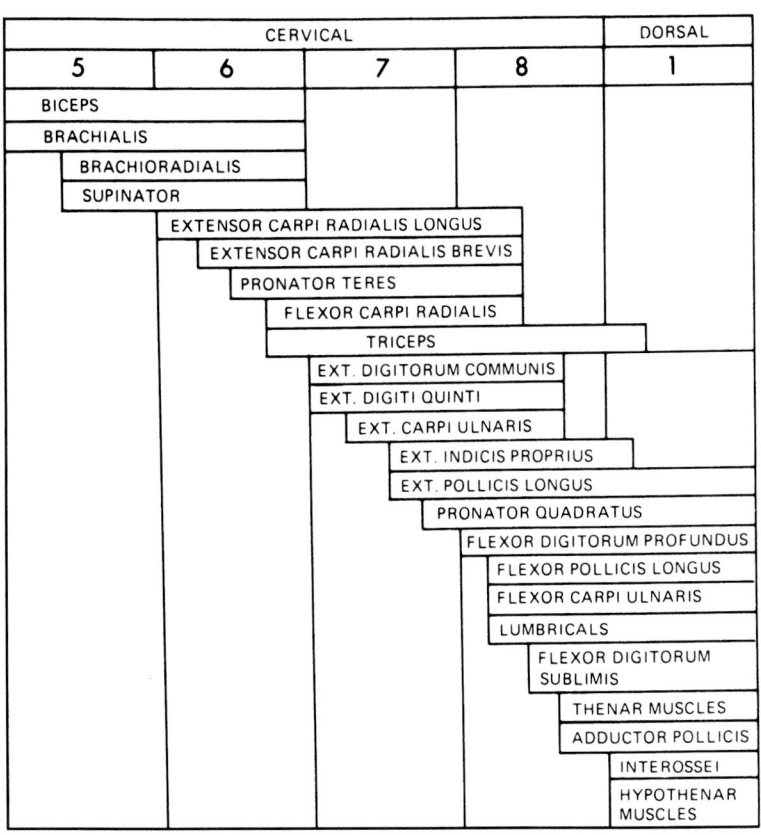

CERVICAL				DORSAL
5	6	7	8	1

BICEPS
BRACHIALIS
BRACHIORADIALIS
SUPINATOR
EXTENSOR CARPI RADIALIS LONGUS
EXTENSOR CARPI RADIALIS BREVIS
PRONATOR TERES
FLEXOR CARPI RADIALIS
TRICEPS
EXT. DIGITORUM COMMUNIS
EXT. DIGITI QUINTI
EXT. CARPI ULNARIS
EXT. INDICIS PROPRIUS
EXT. POLLICIS LONGUS
PRONATOR QUADRATUS
FLEXOR DIGITORUM PROFUNDUS
FLEXOR POLLICIS LONGUS
FLEXOR CARPI ULNARIS
LUMBRICALS
FLEXOR DIGITORUM SUBLIMIS
THENAR MUSCLES
ADDUCTOR POLLICIS
INTEROSSEI
HYPOTHENAR MUSCLES

Fig. 51-1. Segmental innervation of muscles of the elbow, forearm, and hand. (From Zancolli E: *Clin Orthop* 112:101, 1975.)

British Medical Research Council (BMRC) strength of at least 3 is the motor level, and similarly, the most distal dermatome with sensation is the sensory level. Motor grade 3 was chosen because it is unambiguous, whereas motor grades 4 and 5 cannot be differentiated when examiners of varying strength confront persons with varying strength. Despite the simplicity and general usefulness of the system, it is not precise enough from the standpoint of hand surgical rehabilitation. Patients with preserved myotomes can still vary in terms of the motors with voluntary innervation. For example, a C5 patient, defined by at least grade 3 elbow flexion, may or may not have a strong, voluntary brachioradialis, and a C6 patient, defined by at least grade 3 wrist extension, may or may not have a strong, voluntary extensor carpi radialis brevis (ECRB). From the standpoint of surgical restoration, these differences are significant and were the impetus for the International Classification of Tetraplegia (ICT), created in 1984 by a group of hand surgeons devoted to the care of tetraplegic patients.[69] Since that time, the classification system has undergone some modification, and its present form is shown in Table 51-2.[59] The basis for the classification is the segmental innervation of the hand and because tendon transfers typically are considered only in muscles with at least grade 4 strength, the system supplies the physician with the potential transferable motors. This is

Table 51-2. Classifications

American Spinal Injury Association (ASIA) Classification

Spinal cord root level	Functional group at grade 3 strength
C5	Elbow flexors
C6	Wrist extensors
C7	Elbow extensors
C8	Finger flexors
T1	Fifth finger abduction

International Classification for Surgery of the Hand in Tetraplegia

Group	Muscle at grade 4 strength
1	Brachioradialis (BR)
2	Extensor carpi radialis longus (ECRL)
3	Extensor carpi radialis brevis (ECRB)
4	Pronator teres (PT)
5	Flexor carpi radialis (FCR)
6	EDC and finger extensors
7	EPL and thumb extensors
8	Finger flexors
9	All except intrinsics
X	Exceptions
T+ or T–	Triceps at grade 4

Revised in Cleveland, 1998 at the 6th International Conference on Surgical Rehabilitation of the Upper Limb in Tetraplegia, Cleveland.
Cu, 10-mm static two-point discrimination of the index finger (C6 dermatome); *O,* ocular feedback.

currently the accepted classification used by most surgeons performing tetraplegic hand surgery.

PATIENT EVALUATION

Only through thorough evaluation of the patient at various points in time can the practitioner determine the appropriate goals of rehabilitation and reconstruction for that particular patient.* The health care provider must develop a relationship with the patient that provides the practitioner with insight into the patient's own goals and desires. Consideration for rehabilitation, especially surgical intervention, requires that the patient and primary caregivers understand the reconstructive options and their risks and benefits. For example, surgery means that, for a period of time, the patient will be more disabled than normal as his or her arm is temporarily immobilized and he or she goes through a period of rehabilitation. Patients must have good support and aid systems in place to assist them through what is a trying time for the patient and his or her family and caregivers. A patient must be motivated to improve and must remain cooperative throughout the postoperative phase of rehabilitation. Similarly, the patient's general medical condition and cognition must be stable enough to undergo a potentially lengthy surgery and to not interfere with the postoperative rehabilitation program. The success of restorations requires continual effort on the part of the patient both physically and mentally; otherwise, he or she may lose the benefits of any surgical reconstruction. Then, too, if the patient or surgeon is too overly optimistic about the results of surgery, patients will lose the motivation to continue rehabilitation and may be worse off for it. Clearly, the decision to undergo surgical restoration must not be taken lightly.

Other considerations must be taken into account as practical to the success of any restorative program.† Patients should be easily transferable to a wheelchair and have good trunk support and adequate seating so that they can stay seated in order to take full advantage of any use of their upper extremities. Any restorative program should be delayed until it is apparent that no further motor recovery is predicted. This may take as long as 1 year from the time of a complete cord injury, or even longer in the case of incomplete injury. In some cases where the lesion is well defined and severe and where there is no progression, early intervention is justified. Because many of the restorative procedures involve the transfer of voluntary muscles to more effective insertions (tendon transfers), the prerequisites to successful procedures must be met, including supple joints and sufficient strength of the donor muscle. A patient who is allowed to develop joint contractures in his or her hands,

*References 15, 24, 33, 40, 45, 50, 52, 57, 58, 73, 85, 86, 101, 103, 105, 106, 108.
†References 15, 24, 33, 40, 45, 50, 52, 57, 58, 73, 85, 86, 101, 103, 105, 106, 108.

wrists, forearms, elbows, and shoulders will be a poor candidate for a complete restorative program that includes surgical reconstruction or even a splinting program. A muscle that is spastic and difficult to control with therapy or medication cannot serve as a useful donor. These criteria have been established through years of experience and remain a useful tool in guiding surgeons to distinguish which patients will have a good chance of success through surgical restoration. The addition of medications that selectively weaken spastic muscles, such as botulinum toxin type A (Botox), and reduce contractures is an essential part of early management.

Physical examination

Although the relationship and understanding between the patient and his or her providers help formulate the achievable goals of any hand rehabilitation program, it is the physical examination of the patient upon which the actual plans are founded. The integrity and function of both the motor and sensory systems in the upper extremity must be understood. The motor system must be evaluated in its entirety, from the proximal muscles in the shoulder to the intrinsic muscles in the hand, to determine which muscles are voluntary, which are spastic, and which are flaccid. Each muscle must be evaluated independently in order to classify the patient, and the examiner should not discontinue the examination with what appears to correspond to the most distal functional myotome. All muscles should be examined because voluntary innervation may skip myotomes depending on whether the injury is complete, or on that particular patient's neural system and zone of injury. We use the BMRC grading system that is well accepted (strength graded from 0 to 5).[2] If patients do have spastic muscles, they should be assessed for the degree of spasticity and whether the muscle is functional.[16,68,69,101,108] For example, a patient who develops spasticity of the flexor pollicis longus (FPL) muscle on voluntary wrist extension may have a strong lateral pinch that should neither be sacrificed nor necessarily augmented.[105] At the same time, if the spasticity on the FPL is constant and severe, it cannot be used in a tendon transfer as an electrically stimulated muscle, nor can useful lateral pinch occur without chemical or surgical release of that muscle. Uncontrolled, global spasticity is considered a contraindication to restorative surgery and fortunately is rare. Sensory examination stresses the two-point discrimination in the digits, particularly the thumb. Much has been written concerning the presence of two-point discrimination in the thumb as a means of both classifying the patient under the international system and understanding the outcomes of surgical restoration. Many authors have stressed that goals should be limited in patients who require direct visualization of grasp because they lack meaningful sensation; however, others, including ourselves, have found that patients adapt well and prefer increased function even in the face of poor sensation.* The motion of the joints, both passive and active, must be ascertained. A final aspect of our motor assessment involves determining the muscles that are electrically excitable using transcutaneous electrical stimulation (TES).[85] This is because previous study has documented that up to 50% of ASIA C5 patients and 13% of C6 patients have important muscle groups that are not electrically excitable.[53,89]

Evaluation of the upper extremity in the patient with a new injury should begin within 48 hours of admission, within the limits of precautions.[99] The evaluation should consist of a brief social and functional history. The patient's physical appearance should be documented, identifying incisions, edema, scars, and apparent atrophy of the muscles. Examination of strength, sensation, and motion should be completed as indicated previously. Reevaluation of the upper extremity should then take place regularly, typically every 4 weeks; specific areas showing improvement should be evaluated weekly.

PRINCIPLES OF NONOPERATIVE MANAGEMENT

One of the recurring themes of this chapter is that the choice of a rehabilitation strategy must be individualized to suit the patient's general condition. Forethought is critical during the early phases of injury recovery to ensure that a patient can even become a candidate for reliable, but sophisticated, reconstructions. This means that joints should be kept supple, and consideration should be given to an early program of TES to maintain muscle strength and metabolism to innervated motor groups. The relationship between the patient and his or her care providers cannot be overemphasized. This relationship helps the health care provider choose among therapy, orthotics, and surgery. The usage rate of orthotics can be as low as 39%, and poor patient selection is probably the primary reason patients fail splinting programs and surgical reconstruction.[103] Moberg[73,74] believed that as many as 60% of tetraplegic patients could benefit from traditional surgical restoration, whereas Wuolle et al.[103] found that 13% of all cervical cord injuries at one center met the rigid criteria for functional electrical stimulation. Careful patient evaluation addresses these issues.[33,101]

Therapeutic intervention should begin as soon as the spine has been deemed stable clinically and radiographically, and it should continue throughout the individual's life. The main goals of therapy include maintaining the normal appearance of the upper extremity, maintaining joint integrity, and maximizing function. These goals need to be addressed for successful management of the upper extremity in tetraplegia.

With the patient's motor and sensory functioning understood, therapy can be directed toward maintaining or

*References 16, 38, 40, 57, 68, 69, 73, 75, 101.

restoring range of motion (ROM) and strength.[99] Passive range of motion (PROM) and stretching of the muscles should be completed twice daily. The patient should assist with these exercises when volitional movement is present. Stretching should be done slowly, and joints should not be forced. Stretching the wrist and fingers in the natural tenodesis pattern should be emphasized to take advantage of the functional nature of this synergistic motion complex. The fingers should be extended when the wrist is flexed and the fingers flexed when the wrist is extended. Metacarpophalangeal (MCP) joint hyperextension should be avoided to prevent clawing and loss of the important palmar supports needed in grasp. Edema in the upper extremity is one important cause of limited ROM and is minimized through daily active and passive ROM exercises. Retrograde massage is another useful tool, as well as proper positioning of the upper extremity in the wheelchair and in bed.

Because the strength of a muscle contraction increases as more motor units are recruited, increasing the load requirements of voluntary movements is an important component of the therapy. Weight training and endurance training, with particular emphasis on functional motions and activities, are effective in strengthening muscles. Another modality that has been shown to improve muscle strength and endurance is TES.[88] The role of TES in the therapy program is discussed later in this chapter. When establishing a strengthening program, it is important to begin thinking about possible surgical procedures and tendon transfers that could be performed to increase functional independence. These muscles, if voluntary, should be incorporated into the strengthening program. Muscles that should be focused on include the posterior deltoid (PD) (Fig. 51-2) for elbow extension transfer; the brachioradialis (BR), for wrist extension, thumb flexion, and finger extension transfers; and the extensor carpi radialis longus (ECRL), for finger flexion transfer.

Splinting

Splinting is an important means of preventing deformity, promoting function, and promoting a normal appearance of the hand. Two schools of thought have emerged regarding the management of the upper extremity with splints.[14] One thought is to maximize function by encouraging contractures in a tenodesis posture that may provide sufficient lateral pinch to pick up light objects. The fingers and thumb essentially are made to resemble the tongs of pliers; they are controlled by the wrist through stiffening of the interphalangeal (IP) and MP joints. The other school of thought emphasizes the supple hand as its goal. By keeping the fingers supple, more options can be used, including universal cuff orthoses and flexor hinge splints. Contractures present after intentional development of a stiff hand are almost impossible to overcome by conservative methods in a reasonable amount of time. These contractures must be released surgically, both delaying other procedures and

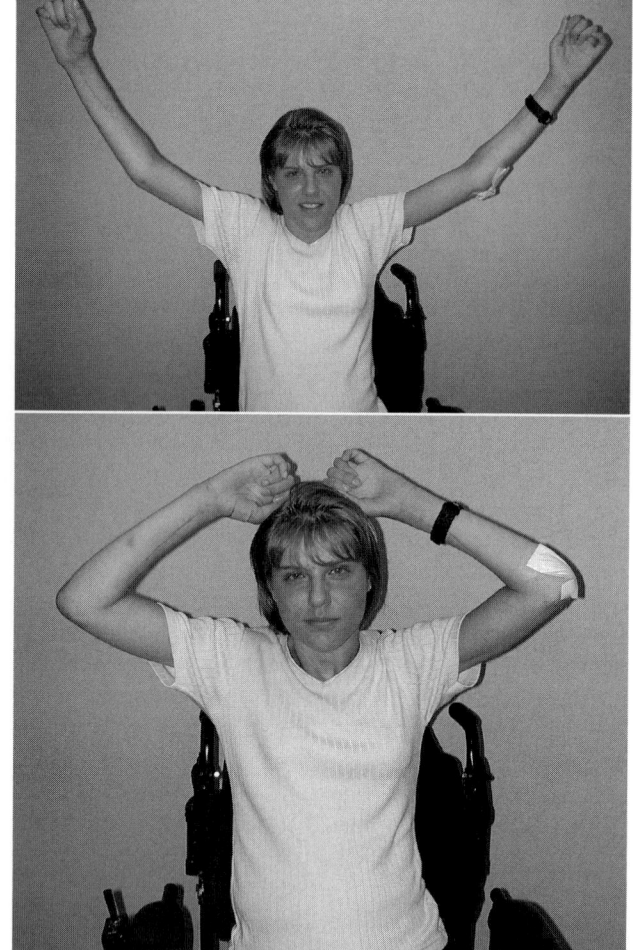

A

B

Fig. 51-2. A, Posterior deltoid to triceps tendon transfer (PDT) showing full elbow extension and radial pronation osteotomy. **B,** Elbow flexion range of motion after PDT tendon transfer.

limiting the surgical alternatives for restoration.[98] We have found that a person has better functional outcomes with the use of functional electrical stimulation (FES) and/or tendon transfers when his or her hand is supple. A supple hand without contractures is also more pleasant and acceptable to patients, a feature the patients themselves are all too aware of.[72] We recommend that contractures be avoided and patients be educated and encouraged to use functional splints during early rehabilitation. We have found it more efficient to create tenodesis posture later, when final planning is done and all options can be considered.

It is important to establish clear goals, with the patient involved with regards to splints and orthoses. Different splints provide different functional advantages, and understanding the individual patient's needs is critical to providing him or her with the most effective splints (Table 51-3). Splints should be incorporated early in the recovery from injury because patients who begin to use splints early following their injury and those who realize functional gains

are more likely to continue to use them. We have found certain splints to be more useful in promoting functional hand positions and diminishing the degree of contractures (see Table 51-3). Individuals with C5 and C6 motor levels have been the most challenging population to establish a successful splinting protocol. Patients with a C5 motor level (no voluntary wrist control) benefit from a dorsal wrist support with a universal cuff when performing ADLs and a splint at night for better hand position. Those with C6 motor levels (voluntary wrist extension) benefit from the use of a flexor hinge splint on the dominant hand and a short opponens splint on the opposite hand. Occasionally, patients prefer flexor hinge splints bilaterally. Despite a carefully chosen program, however, the rate of splint use among tetraplegic patients varies from as low as 39% to as high as 89%.[103] We have found that becoming brace free and more able bodied in appearance is among the major goals of patients who desire surgical reconstruction, even if the sole reason for a wrist arthrodesis is cosmetic.

Role of electrical stimulation

TES is a technique that applies electrical pulses to peripheral nerve fibers through the skin surface causing paralyzed, but innervated, muscles to contract. FES involves the stimulation of the motor unit and control of useful patterns with an electrical impulse, usually applied by implanted electrodes. Although the nerves remain functional, the muscles they innervate do undergo atrophy and develop type II glycolytic metabolism. These changes can be reversed by electrical stimulation of the intact peripheral nerve branch in a conditioning and exercise program. A suprathreshold stimulus applied directly to the nerve and muscle at a frequency of 12 Hz for 8 hours a day has been effective in changing the contractile properties of the muscle to a slow oxidative metabolic state, rendering them more fatigue resistant.[89] Over time, consistent exercise will yield softening of joint capsular contracture and reduction in spasticity during the stimulation. Increasing the strength of weak, but innervated, muscle groups; decreasing the effects of muscle atrophy; and increasing the ROM of tight tendons before contractures develop are among the positive effects of a TES program. Several studies clinically confirm that a stimulation-induced contracture of BMRC grade 2 or higher could be strengthened by electrical stimulation to functional levels of force.[48,53,55,88] Strengthening innervated, but paralyzed, muscles improves the efficacy of splinting programs, tendon transfers, and FES systems.

We have found TES to be beneficial when also applied early in the rehabilitation process. We believe that such a program is especially useful in patients under consideration for FES implantation because their muscles are properly conditioned for maximal efficiency and the optimal positioning for electrical stimulation on the muscle surface is realized. We start patients with as little as 20 minutes of stimulation per day per muscle group, and advance slowly to

Table 51-3. Available hand splints based on level of injury in tetraplegia

Level of injury	Splint	Purpose	Wearing schedule
C1-C4	Resting hand splint	Maintains the hand in a functional position, prevents deformity, maintains aesthetically pleasing hand	When in bed, complete PROM regularly
C5	Long opponens splint	Provides a stable post against which index finger can pinch; positions thumb in a functional key-pinch position	As needed to increase function
	Dorsal wrist support	Protects integrity of wrist joint; acts as a universal cuff to increase function	As needed to increase function
	Modified resting hand splint	Protects the integrity of wrist and fingers; splint should allow wrist flexion with MCP, PIP, DIP extension and thumb extension	
	Elbow extension splint	Prevents biceps contraction	When in bed
C6	Short opponens	Provides a stable post against which index finger can grasp; thumb in key pinch based on preference of patient	As needed to increase function
	Wrist drive flexor hinge splint	Augments natural tenodesis and alignment of fingers	As needed to increase function
	Elbow extension splint	Prevents biceps contraction	When in bed
	Modified resting hand splint	Protects the integrity of wrist and fingers; splint should allow wrist flexion with MCP, PIP, DIP extension and thumb extension	When in bed
C7	MCP block splint	Prevents hyperextension deformity of the MCP joints	As needed to increase function and decrease deformity

DIP, Distal interphalangeal; *MCP,* metacarpophalangeal; *PIP,* proximal interphalangeal; *PROM,* passive range of motion.

a total of 4 to 6 hours per day. Patients tolerate the program quite well and are compliant if properly motivated. Improved strength and endurance of involuntary, innervated functional muscle groups is the goal of a TES program. Muscle groups emphasized include finger flexors (median/ulnar nerve), thumb flexors/abductors (median nerve), and thumb/finger extensors (radial nerve). Thus far, TES programs have been implemented primarily as part of the pre-FES implantation therapy protocol; however, based on our experience, we believe that its role is valid as part of a therapy protocol that seeks to maintain motion, prevent contractures, and prevent atrophy.

PRINCIPLES OF SURGICAL RECONSTRUCTION

The ultimate goal of upper extremity rehabilitation is to provide patients with the ability to manipulate objects in space efficiently and effectively (i.e., create an "able-bodied" person's arm and hand). We must strike a balance with what is achievable (this requires an understanding of what minimal functions will confer improvements in ability) and what the reasonable goals are for a particular patient. In general, surgical restoration improves a patient by one or two levels on the ASIA scale. Not all patients meet our strict criteria for surgical reconstruction. Dedicated and experienced multidisciplinary teams in regional referral centers are continuously working to improve current methods and, in the end, restore the patients to independence, social integration,

and occupation. Our current bias is that surgical restoration, as outlined subsequently, should be undertaken by surgeons skilled and experienced in taking care of patients with tetraplegia and should be performed in concert with similarly experienced teams of physiatrists, nurses, and therapists.

The fundamental functions we seek to restore, in order of priority, include elbow extension, wrist extension, lateral pinch and release, and palmar grasp and release.* Current surgical techniques and technology do not yet allow us to reliably restore shoulder function, and therefore patients with ASIA motor levels proximal to C5 are rarely candidates for surgery. The combination of shoulder function and elbow extension allows patients to effectively "reach out" to manipulate objects in space in front of them and above them. Without this ability, a patient's effective workspace is limited. Wrist extension activates the natural tenodesis grasp pattern and serves as the foundation upon which finger function is activated and restored. Regarding finger function, although it would be ideal to restore all the different grasp patterns we apply subconsciously in our daily activities, previous study has demonstrated that lateral pinch, not opposition, and palmar grasp, not tip pinch, are used most commonly.[50] Planning the reconstruction begins with a balance of the remaining voluntary, nonspastic function. In addition, as previously discussed, reconstruction is best

*References 17, 24, 25, 50, 57, 58, 68, 73, 74, 76, 101, 105.

suited for patients whose hands and arms are supple and are not contracted; this is because when we superimpose joint stiffness on the goals of the reconstructive efforts, our results can be severely curtailed.

However, too much surgical restoration can be attempted, and experience and research have taught us that there is occasion to "downsize" a surgical plan under certain conditions. Too much may be needed when patients fail to meet the criteria for surgery. We have also learned that patients occasionally will require later secondary surgery to modify loosened transfers, to augment weak transfers, to surgically immobilize a joint that becomes unstable, and so forth. Patients also must continuously use and exercise the hand and arm to maintain the muscle tone and endurance qualities necessary for successful transfers and FES systems. Patients who do not have easy access to their therapists and physicians, because of physical distance or insufficient family infrastructure, likely will experience poor outcomes if the restorative regimen is complex and sophisticated. In these instances, it may better serve the patient to limit the goals of surgery to what he or she will be able to take advantage of, although a motivated, intelligent, and well-adjusted patient will be unsatisfied with a restorative program that undercuts his or her true rehabilitative potential. Finally, the surgical program should seek to accomplish as much as possible as efficiently as possible. Prolonged postoperative periods of overburdening dependency generally will lead a patient and his or her family to postpone or cancel future staged procedures, which in turn will reduce the likelihood of success. Paul et al.[83] have previously demonstrated that combining multiple procedures in one stage is efficacious.

Goals

We previously discussed the hierarchic order of surgical goals: elbow extension, wrist extension, key pinch, palmar grasp, and then finger/thumb extension. The ability to achieve this depends on the patient's functional level (i.e., his or her ICT. If FES systems are part of the reconstructive protocol, we typically will combine neuroprosthesis implantation in one arm and proceed with tendon transfer reconstruction in the opposite arm as part of a comprehensive, staged reconstruction. The arm we select for the FES system typically is the dominant arm and has no compromising denervation. In the future, we believe we will be able to implant both arms of a patient as systems and their controls improve. In these situations, both arms will have elbow extension transfers performed at the same time as other ipsilateral procedures or in a staged fashion. The surgery on the contralateral arm can take place within 1 to 2 weeks to minimize postoperative disability, or in a longer interval depending on the patient's needs and desires. We have found that some patients need or want only one arm to be reconstructed. Table 51-4 outlines the specific procedures performed by level; however, we follow a few generaliza-

tions in planning reconstructions. These are described in the following sections.

Treating each patient individually

The sequelae of the initial trauma is so varied and multifactorial that patients truly are unique in their presentations. Surgical protocols that are rigidly set to the level of injury will fail in a number of patients if certain issues are not considered early in the surgical planning. In particular, spasticity and the patient's goals and desires are two specific examples of where surgical planning must be both flexible and creative. To accommodate variations in patient presentations and goals, surgeons should be aware of the various described techniques in achieving similar reconstructive goals.

Because different patterns of upper and lower motor neuron injury are manifest clinically in patients, the degree to which muscle spasticity varies is considerable. Clearly, any spasticity must be controlled for a patient to be a candidate for surgery. Typically, this is achieved through therapy and pharmacy. Control at a plateau of tolerance and efficacy is the goal. The problem lies in striking a balance between the benefits and side effects of the medication. Higher levels of effective spasmolytic agents, such as diazepam, may produce muscle weakness. Side effects such as drowsiness or blunting of affect are a common reason patients reduce intake of or discontinue use of these agents. Concerns about habituation or abuse have also led to fewer prescriptions being written for spasmolytic agents. Use of implantable baclofen pumps may lead to steady-state suppression of spasticity. Unfortunately, sudden withdrawal of these medications, as in the case of a pump failure, is an emergency because seizures and vasomotor instability may occur with fatal consequences. Since the U.S. Food and Drug Administration's (FDA) approval of botulinum toxin in 1989, its role in the management of spastic paralysis, including tetraplegia, is increasing. Recent clinical trials combining electrical stimulation and dynamic splinting in spastic cerebral palsy appear effective and may obviate the need for repeated botulinum or phenol injections.

It is believed that uncontrollable spastic muscles should not be transferred, and they often need to be released to prevent severe contractures.[50,58,68,69] However, mildly spastic muscles can be useful transfers.[70,101,105] In addition, certain "functional" spasticity, such as contraction of the FPL with wrist extension, may be desirable and probably should not be altered.[105] Because each patient presents with unique patterns of spasticity and the ability to control it, surgical protocols must be flexible to accommodate the patient.

The surgical planning must be tailored to the patient's own needs for it to be successful. Patients, especially those whose initial injury occurred many years previously, develop a number of substitution maneuvers that allow them to function, sometimes with surprising independence. Some

Table 51-4. Surgical protocol by the International Classification Group

Level	Goals of surgery
O/Cu:0 No muscles for transfer	**Elbow extension** *Our approach* Posterior deltoid-to-triceps transfer[1a,1b,6a,9a,15,17,20,21,24,25,28,40,55a,56a,57,69a,72-76,78,83,92a,92b,99a,101] *Option* Biceps-to-triceps transfer[17,29,40,56,93,107] FES to triceps[9,13,35,71] (Fig. 51-3) **Hand grasp** *Our approach* FES neuroprosthesis[24,32,35,48,50-55,84-87,90]
O/Cu:1 BR	**Elbow extension** As for O/Cu:0 **Forearm pronation** *Our approach* Pronation osteotomy of radius[4,63,91] *Option* Biceps pronatorplasty[31,65,82,94,104] FES to pronator quadratus[60] **Lateral pinch and release** Key-pinch procedure is modified because wrist extension is not present[8,16,17,21,23,25,27,40,45,50,58,66,68,69,72,75,76,78,83,97,101,102,105,106,108] *Our approach* Wrist extension through transfer of BR Natural tenodesis of fingers with wrist extension provides lateral pinch (extension and flexion augmentation if necessary) Thumb stabilization for pinch strength (CMC arthrodesis and FPL bridle transfer to IP) *Option* FES neuroprosthesis
O/Cu:2 ERCL	**Elbow extension and forearm pronation** As previous **Grasp and release** Standard key-pinch procedure for lateral pinch (wrist extension transfer not needed, and brachioradialis used as a donor motor)[16,40,42-46,50,57,66,69,77,78,83,100,101,105,108] *Our approach* FES neuroprosthesis *or* FPL powered by BR Thumb stabilized by CMC arthrodesis and split FPL tenodesis Finger/thumb extension and flexion natural tenodesis augmented as necessary *Option* Restore palmar grasp with BR to FDP transfer[21,25-27] Restore palmar and lateral grasp with Zancolli two-stage reconstruction[108] Restore weak palmar grasp with ECRB to FDP via interosseous membrane[37] Intrinsic balance[47,108]
O/Cu:3 ECRB	**Elbow extension and forearm pronation** As previous **Grip, pinch, and release** As for previous, exception is now two motors; BR and ECRL are available for transfer *Our approach* FES neuroprosthesis *or* Zancolli two-staged reconstruction with flexor/extensor stages[107,109] (Fig. 51-4) *Options* Standard key pinch *plus*[10,58,106] ECRL to FDP[17,45,46,57,58,101,106] ECRL to FDP and FDS[40] Restore thumb opposition and adduction with BR[21,25,45] Intrinsic balance as previous

Continued

Table 51-4. Surgical protocol by the International Classification Group—cont'd

Level	Goals of surgery
O/Cu:4 PT	**Elbow extension** As previous **Grip, pinch, and release** These patients can undergo transfers to power finger/thumb extension *Our approach* FES neuroprosthesis *or* two-stage extensor/flexor reconstruction via Zancolli (PT powers FCR) or House (PT powers FPL) methods; we prefer this method of reconstruction for groups 4-8, differences based on references 43-46, 101, 105, 106, and 108
O/Cu:5 FCR	**Elbow extension** As previous only if triceps power is not present because these patients may have useful voluntary elbow extension **Grasp, pinch, and release** As previous *Our approach* Leave FCR as a powerful wrist flexor that also augments finger extension via tenodesis effect *Option* Use FCR for opponensplasty, keep FPL powered by BR, and FDP powered by ECRL as single stage[58]
O/Cu:6 EDC	**Grasp, pinch, and release** As previous These patients may be less functional than level 5 because they may lose the finger flexion effect from wrist extension because they have voluntary finger extensors (same with group 7); this must be taken into account in planning transfers (i.e., through finger flexion and intrinsic reconstruction)[101]; radial-sided intrinsics can be powered via EIP[107] *Option* Single-stage grasp and pinch procedure[66]
O/Cu:7 EPL	**Grasp, pinch, and release** As previous Both ulnar- and radial-sided intrinsics can be powered[107] *Option* Thumb adduction-opponensplasty[67]
O/Cu:8 Finger flexors (usually stronger on ulnar side)	**Grasp, pinch, and release** As previous Standard opponensplasty should be performed; intrinsic reconstruction more likely is necessary because extrinsic flexors and extensors are present to create an intrinsic-minus imbalance Powered intrinsic reconstruction via ECRL or BR[107] Standard opponensplasty using EIP or EDQM[107]
O/Cu:9 Lack intrinsics	**Grasp, pinch, and release** As previous As with group 8, intrinsic reconstruction and opponensplasty may be required

BR, Brachioradialis; *CMC*, carpometacarpal; *ECRB*, extensor carpi radialis brevis; *ECRL*, extensor carpi radialis longus; *EDC*, extensor digitorum communis; *EDQM*, extensor digiti quinti minimi; *EIP*, extensor indicis proprius; *EPL*, extensor pollicis longus; *FCR*, flexor carpi radialis; *FDP*, flexor digitorum profundus; *FDS*, flexor digitorum superficialis; *FES*, functional electrical stimulation; *FPL*, flexor pollicis longus; *IP*, interphalangeal; *PT*, pronator teres.

C5 (ICT 0 to 1) patients use their biceps to help propel a manual wheelchair or to help with weight shifts critical to preventing pressure sores. The surgeon who chooses to restore elbow extension using the biceps as a donor motor should take caution and explain to the patient that such a procedure may result in the loss of important functions that he or she had before surgery, especially supination and elbow flexion.

Finally, the surgeon and patient must be cognizant of the duration of postoperative rehabilitation. During the initial period of immobilization, which may last from 3 weeks to 3 months (deltoid to triceps transfer), patients become totally

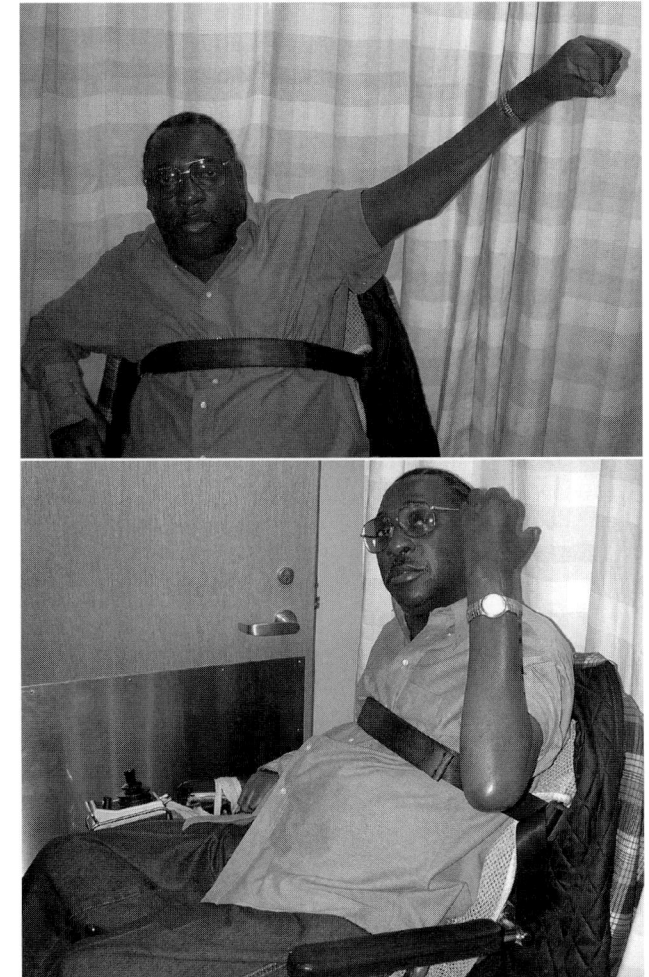

Fig. 51-3. A, Biceps to triceps tendon transfer shows full elbow extension. Also seen are the radial pronation osteotomy, wrist arthrodesis, and Freehand neuroprosthesis. **B,** Elbow flexion preserved after biceps to triceps tendon transfer.

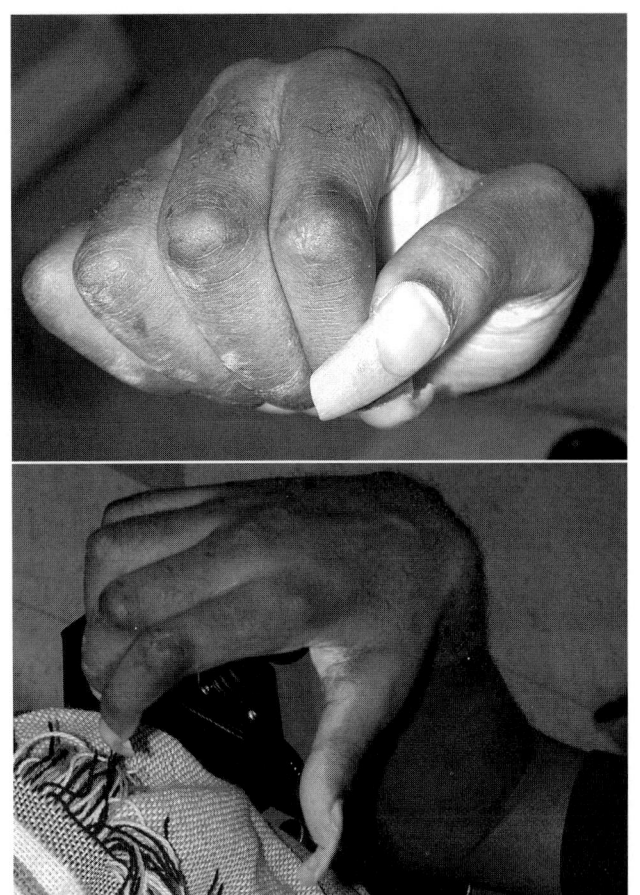

Fig. 51-4. A, Two-stage reconstruction of grasp and release, shown in grasp position. **B,** Two-stage reconstruction of grasp and release, shown in release position.

dependent on attendant care. This places great personal stress on the patient and his or her support group, especially if family is the primary source of help. Arrangements must be secure before surgery.

Special considerations for children and adolescents. Children with an SCI have special needs and considerations. New SCI centers, especially within the Shriners Hospitals, have developed special protocols and focus on this group of patients. The textbook by Betz and Mulcahey[3] is devoted to these patients and is the foundation for their management. Successful rehabilitation requires extra attention to developmental status, family support, and reaction to the surgical process. Explanation and agreement is needed for the time and personal investment during periods of physical dependency, loss of mobility, and loss of personal freedom.

Children may be less tolerant of failure than adults. Children are compelled to be trusting in a complex process that they may not fully understand or consent to. Their

parents can be educated to understand the reconstruction and technology, but children may not fully understand the mechanisms. They are sharp critics and good observers of true progress. They are hard to satisfy. Many children expect miracles or immediate gratification and lack tolerance for months of rehabilitation. Younger children have short attention spans and need reinforcement and repetition in their training. Older children and adolescents are distracted by their social needs and are conscious of cosmetic appearance, incisions, braces, and hardware. They want to be normal both physically and visibly. Reconstruction that incorporates correction of paralytic posture, removes wrist braces, or improves social contact is well received.

Many children dread the return to the "sick role" and many have bad memories of the time they spent in the hospital for the acute injury. Overcoming their physical loss and restoring hand function must also minimize the stress of reentry to the hospital. Performing procedures in combination, as an outpatient, or in rehabilitation rather than acute care sites all contribute to better acceptance. The therapist often has the key role in preparing, guiding, and befriending the child, contributing the subjective support and continuity to recovery.

Preoperative assessment often can be accomplished in the context of play or ADLs. The functional emphasis for children often will be on accomplishments at school using pencils, artistic materials, computer access, and reading. Self-care activities are the same as for adults.

Postoperative care follows the same protocols as for adults, except that longer-term monitoring is required to assess the effects of growth and development.

Children are harder on hardware, braces, wheelchairs, and electronic components compared with adults. They have a sense that they will heal themselves and that someone else can repair broken things. Careful instruction is important because reconstructed limbs are not normal in their tolerance for injury, weight bearing, or use as tools.

The results of surgical reconstruction in children can be very rewarding, both for the automatic way they adjust to new capabilities, the generally good results they experience with surgery, and the joy toward the health care team for changing their lives.

Concepts

Stability, mobility, and power are all required to create movements, which in turn provide functional ability. This section focuses on the principles and concepts involved and dwells less on the actual described procedures. Table 51-4 is a list of the surgical procedures we recommend based on classification. We refer the reader to the references provided to further explore the history, details, and development of these procedures and their alternatives. Case studies are provided, which summarize outcomes that can reasonably be expected.

Joint balance. For the best functional results, procedures that mobilize a joint, such as a tendon transfer, require balance to prevent subsequent deformity.[5] It has been our observation, for example, that patients with ASIA motor level C6 (ICT 2 and 3) who have voluntary wrist extension develop a slight extension contracture over time. The extent of the contracture is limited by gravity because most functional activities are performed with the forearm pronated and the flexion moment produced by the weight of the hand counterbalances the active wrist extensors. Conversely, bedridden or poorly rehabilitated patients and those who are C5 or ICT 0 to 1 can develop severe elbow flexion/supination contractures because of the lack of an elbow extension/pronation moment to overcome a powerful or spastic biceps.[5,19,25,50,105] Other contractures that can develop include shoulder adduction, internal rotation contractures, and finger contractures (flexion, clawing, and/or extension).[25,98] These contractures are best prevented but can be

treated by a staged surgical release.* In a similar fashion, if tendon transfers or FES systems are used to power a particular joint(s) that becomes imbalanced as a result of surgery, contractures can also develop. Procedures that restore grasp through transfer of the ECRL or BR to the flexor digitorum profundus (FDP) without the creation of an extensor moment may result in tighter fingers[10,30,57,78,100] or the development of finger flexion contractures. This extensor can be a static force like a tenodesis, or a dynamic force like an "antagonist" tendon transfer. Both Zancolli[105,106,108,109] and House[43,45-47] have written extensively about such principles as they apply to achieving finger function with tendon transfers. With regards to FES systems, Keith et al.[49] described wrist imbalance in patients caused by the strong flexor moments provided by activation of the FDP, flexor digitorum superficialis (FDS), and FPL insufficiently counterbalanced by voluntary wrist extension through the ECRB. An improperly balanced joint will lose function over time. The treating surgeon must bear this principle in mind to optimize results of surgery. The transfer for finger flexion should not be set too tight. A grade 3 flexion force over a full ROM is the intraoperative goal, modeled by temporary stimulation.

Bone and joint procedures

Joint releases. Mobility and function are mutually inclusive. Whether a joint is under voluntary control or will be mobilized through surgical restoration, suppleness and ROM is critical to ability. Stiffness occasionally develops despite appropriate nonoperative care, and when contractures develop and inhibit function, the joint must be released and rebalanced.[16,25,40,77] Wrist flexion contractures are uncommon except in patients with spasticity of the extrinsic wrist flexors who may develop a flexion contracture. Finger and thumb contractures are usually a result of a therapeutic philosophy that creates key pinch using stiffened thumbs and fingers as a "claw." Treanor et al.[98] described surgical releases of severely contracted fingers with the result in improved function. We believe that stiff fingers preclude a successful restorative program, and should be avoided instead of treated.

One relatively common example of a contracture in tetraplegia is the forearm supination deformity that can develop in patients with ICT 0 to 2. The deformity develops from an imbalance between voluntary or spastic elbow flexors/supinators and weak elbow extenders/pronators. Poor bed positioning, neglect of the person, therapy, and/or a highly spastic muscle can lead to the development of a chronically supinated forearm and flexed elbow. Because most functional activities are performed with the hand and wrist pronated, this contracture is disabling. Concomitant mild to moderate elbow flexion contractures and forearm supination deformities in tetraplegia often respond to

---

*References 19, 25, 40, 58, 98, 105.

conservative measures with serial casting in extension and pronation at weekly intervals.[19] Residual contractures must be released surgically.

Our management algorithm proceeds from conservative measures such as the use of botulinum toxin type A (Botox), serial cast correction, and stretching for mild to moderate flexion supination contractures to a radial pronation osteotomy.[91] If an elbow flexion deformity also is present, we will perform anterior capsular release with associated biceps and brachialis fractional lengthening. We have found the osteotomy to be a particularly effective procedure because a functional arc of rotation is restored and maintained, the procedure is technically straightforward, and it is well suited as part of a comprehensive single-stage surgical reconstruction because no rehabilitation is required to learn it.[91] The biceps pronatorplasty, originally described by Zancolli,[104] is an alternative procedure that both releases the deformity and rebalances the forearm by creating an active pronator.[82]

Joint stabilization. The individual digital rays of the hand are, in effect, a series of intercalated segments normally controlled by muscles that have multiple attachments throughout these segments to create a finely balanced and coordinated mechanism for motion. In tetraplegic patients with few voluntary motors for transfer, and only a finite number that can be electrically activated with currently available implantable systems, the able-bodied finger cannot yet be recreated. Because the goals of surgery are limited to providing the fewest functions that provide the greatest abilities, joint stabilization becomes an integrated part of reconstruction. Restoring thumb flexion to create key pinch, for example, is impossible without stabilizing one or more of the three joints of the thumb ray because control of the hypermobile carpal metacarpal (CMC) joint, in addition to the MCP and IP joints, is impossible with one or two donor motors. A common strategy that has developed is to power effective key pinch using one motor that flexes the thumb through the scaphotrapezium and MCP joint, positioned in space by stabilizing the CMC joint in opposition and transferring the power of flexion to the thumb pulp via a stabilized IP joint (Fig. 51-5). Various techniques are available to "hold" joints for balance and stability.

Arthrodesis. Stabilizing a joint in series through arthrodesis reduces the dissipation of torque exerted by an active motor or tendon transfer, prevents deformity from torque and subsequent joint imbalance, and aids in placing a joint or finger/thumb ray in a more functional position. In effect, arthrodeses can increase the efficiency and efficacy of voluntary, transferred, or activated motors, which is a beneficial situation in the tetraplegic patient. The tradeoff, of course, is lost motion and stiffness. In 1956, Nickel et al.[81] described the creation of a functional grasping hand by fusing the digital joints and creating a stiff "plierslike" claw powered through the tenodesis effect of wrist extension. Although it produced function, there were the undesirable

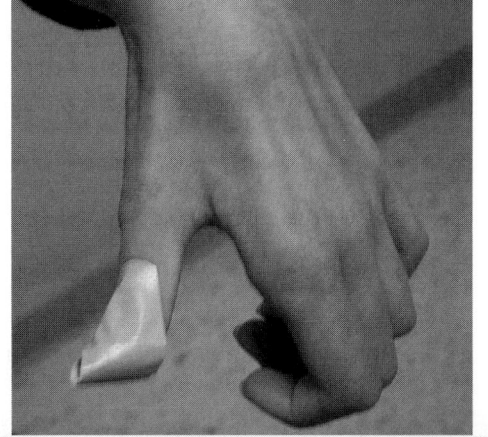

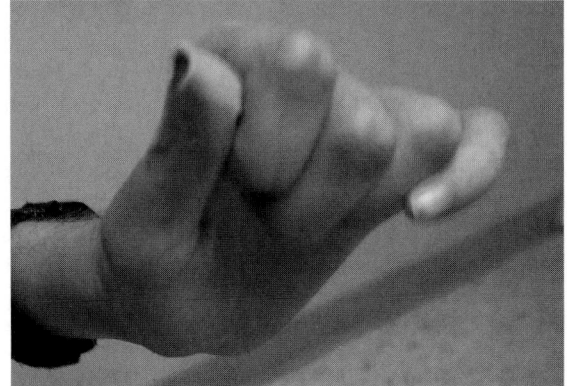

Fig. 51-5. A, Modified key-grip reconstruction with single-stage carpal metacarpal arthrodesis, extensor pollicis longus tenodesis, brachioradialis to flexor pollicis longus tendon transfer. Hand opening is shown. **B,** Modified key-grip reconstruction with hand closure.

effects of irreversibility and a stiff hand. Today, through the teachings of Moberg,[72] we seek to create supple hands that are more reconstructible and, importantly, more appealing to patients reintegrating themselves into their community. Therefore arthrodesis should be applied judiciously and sparingly.

Thumb CMC arthrodesis is one of the most useful operations in tetraplegia hand reconstruction. By positioning the thumb in opposition, a flexion moment provided through the FPL by transfer creates a stable and effective key pinch. This procedure has been applied extensively in tetraplegic reconstruction, with reliable results.[40,43,46,47] In select patients with low-level tetraplegia (ICG in excess of 4), House[43,46] has written extensively on an alternative to CMC arthrodesis whereby an adduction-opponensplasty is constructed through two donor motors, the pronator teres (PT) and the BR. Wrist arthrodesis is rarely indicated because the important tenodesis effect is lost. It is indicated to replace an external splint or, if insufficient motors are available, for wrist extension. Some patients select the procedure for cosmetic qualities and the strong desire to be free of a brace.

A patient with weak ASIA C5 motor strength (ICT 0) who has some voluntary BR function with a BMRC grade less than 4, which is unsuited for transfer into ECRB, may benefit from BR into FPL transfer, wrist fusion, and FDP, extensor pollicis longus (EPL) tenodesis. However, when possible, we prefer to reconstruct such patients with a Freehand FES System (NeuroControl Corp., Cleveland, Ohio) because of the possibility of controlling eight new muscles in the hand.

Split transfers. As an alternative to arthrodesis, the split transfer technique has been described in the reconstruction of tetraplegic hands to stabilize select joints. The premise of this transfer is to balance a functionally single-axis joint with one motor, thereby converting a moment force into a balanced compressive force. Specifically, the IP joint of the thumb traditionally has been stabilized by arthrodesis or pinning when performing key-pinch procedures.* This improves the efficiency and efficacy of an FPL transfer, because its moment is transferred primarily to mobilizing the MCP and CMC joints (or just the MCP if the CMC is fused). The irreversibility of arthrodesis and problems associated with permanent pins or screws across the joint in order to stabilize it, however, led to the creation of a split transfer described by Mohammed et al.[78,95] The radial half of the FPL at the level of the oblique pulley is transferred dorsally into the EPL proximal to the IP joint. In the passive state, the joint remains supple. In the activated state, as through FPL activation during key pinch, the IP joint is held stable on both sides of the joint. This procedure is now our standard method of IP stabilization.

Capsulodesis. In the capsulodesis technique of joint stabilization, static balance is achieved by tightening one of the axes of any particular joint. This technique has been described in key-pinch procedures where the volar plate of the thumb MCP is tightened if hypermobile because there is the risk for the development of volar plate laxity over time.[105] In this scenario, the pinch force produced by the thumb becomes steadily weaker as force that should be applied through the thumb pulp is lost through a hyperextensible MCP joint. PIP volar capsulodesis is indicated in the hyperlax patient who develops swan-neck posturing preventing functional grip. These procedures can both be performed primarily when dysfunctional laxity is already present or secondarily if the same laxity develops from use or chronic joint imbalance from a previous reconstruction.

Dynamic stabilization. Mobilization procedures such as tendon transfers and tenodesis provide joint stability when they serve as an antagonist to an agonist motor. For example, the BR is a more powerful donor when an extension transfer stabilizes the elbow, whether through a PD or biceps donor.[7,27,57,73,74] The reason is that in the absence of an elbow extension moment, the force of the BR contraction is distributed between elbow flexion and whatever tendon it has been transferred to. In the presence of an active elbow extension moment, this same force is distributed primarily to the tendon to which it has been transferred. A tenodesis, the static equivalent of a tendon transfer, can perform a similar function. The finger extension moment provided through a tenodesis described by Zancolli[106,108] or House,[45,46] in which the intrinsic muscles are mimicked by a slip of the FDS tendon, can similarly empower grasp strength when the finger flexors are motorized or activated.

The basis for surgical restoration of the tetraplegic hand lies in mobilizing paralyzed joints. The next sections concerning soft tissue procedures and neuroprostheses discuss the fundamental principles.

Soft tissue procedures

Tenodeses. Tenodesis is a technique of creating a static tethering effect of a tendon by stabilizing it proximal to its site of insertion. As a result of this "anchoring," the muscle-tendon unit loses elasticity, and when the joint is mobilized in an eccentric direction or motion, the tendon behaves as a tether, restricting continued motion depending on the tension it was set in. In the hand, tenodesis procedures can take advantage of the intercalated segments where tendons cross multiple joints before inserting on bone. As a result, instead of limiting motion, they produce it. The normal wrist tenodesis effect is the foundation for motion produced by tenodesis in tetraplegia hand reconstruction. For example, in high-level patients (ICT 1), no motors are available to transfer once the BR is transferred to the ECRB to create wrist extension; however, by anchoring the FPL tendon on the distal radius in appropriate tension, wrist extension now produces a flexion moment to the thumb ray. In concert with appropriate thumb-joint and finger-joint balancing, and perhaps extensor tenodesis, the basis for the key-pinch procedure originally described by Moberg[72-74] becomes apparent.* The problem is that tenodeses tend to stretch over time; therefore they currently are used in high-level tetraplegia when no other option is available and when the patient is not a candidate for a neuroprosthesis or an antagonist-balancing procedure as discussed previously.

Tendon transfers. Tendon transfers permit relocation of available motors for loss of function. Together with tenodeses, these procedures represent the core of traditional reconstruction of the upper extremity in tetraplegia. The basic principles for transfers continue to apply[5,34]:

1. Supple joints free of contractures are necessary for mobility.
2. Comparable excursion and force of contraction between the transfer with the muscle it is to replace should be present or provided.[6,61]
3. Synergy, when possible, will facilitate reeducation. Transferring the ECRB to the FDP takes advantage of synergy.

---

*References 40, 42, 57, 72, 100, 101.

*References 16, 39, 50, 100, 101, 108.

4. The transfer should traverse a healthy bed of tissue to minimize scarring.

5. Stabilization of a joint, whenever a transfer spans across multiple joints, increases its efficacy and efficiency, as has been clearly demonstrated with BR transfers.[7,24,25]

6. A straight line of pull from the donor motor to the recipient tendon will minimize lost strength from the transfer.

7. Side-to-side transfers allow a single motor to effect motion across several joints. The entire FDP can be activated by one donor motor.

8. The morbidity from loss of the donor motor should be none or minimal.

There is an important technical caveat with regards to setting the transfer in the appropriate degree of tension. The technique of tendon weaving described by Pulvertaft[92] (three to four weaves) greatly enhances the strength of the transfer and allows early motion. When the weave is held with a hemostat before securing it with sutures, the tension can be tested by activating the tenodesis effect intraoperatively or by using intraoperative electric stimulation. This allows the surgeon to loosen or tighten the transfer until the desired affect is achieved.

Neuroprostheses. High-level SCI leaves few opportunities for reconstruction of the hand. At ASIA levels C5 and C6, the most common levels, only key pinch can be created using traditional tendon transfer and rehabilitation tools. With the FDA approval in 1997 of the NeuroControl Freehand FES neuroprosthesis, eight additional muscles become available for control.[12,51-53,55,85] This system, its application, and its outcomes have been well described in the literature. The currently commercially available system consists of an implantable stimulator that controls eight separate channels or leads that activate eight different muscles (or one lead for cutaneous sensory feedback). The leads are attached to the epimysium of the desired muscle near the motor point such that a dose-dependent relationship between electrical stimulation intensity and the strength of contraction exists. A radiofrequency receiver that interprets protraction/retraction and elevation/depression signals from a removable joystick secured to the patient's shoulder sends signals to activate appropriate muscles through the implanted system in a preprogrammed fashion. A combination of eight muscles and tendon transfers are used to restore/activate wrist extension, finger flexion and extension, thumb adduction/abduction/flexion, and extension. Separate key-pinch and palmar grasp patterns are created based on these activated functions and provide patients with as much function as patients whose ICT is in excess of 5.

When neuroprostheses should be considered. Our current indications for neuroprosthesis are in candidates who are ICT 4 or less. (Criteria is discussed in section on patient evaluation.[85,86,103]) This translates to patients with ASIA motor levels C5 and C6. As the technology expands and more channels are added and as clinical experience confirms utility, patients with ASIA level 4 or higher may benefit from FES implantation. Although this has not been studied specifically, we believe that patients who have ASIA C7 motor strength or greater (ICT greater than or equal to 5/6) are either very functional as is or have very satisfactory results through more traditional surgical restoration. Most of these patients have strong voluntary triceps function and may have voluntary finger/thumb function.

FES neuroprosthesis: technique.[48,51,52,85] The surgical procedure for implantation of the neuroprosthesis requires a general anesthetic without depolarizing blockers, temperature control of the operating room, and the administration of preoperative antibiotics and careful anatomic study of the muscles to be stimulated. Surgical incisions are made on the volar and dorsal aspects of the forearm and flexor and extensor muscles are identified. Fig. 51-6 shows the muscles in the grasp patterns typically used. Intraoperative electrical stimulation and mapping to an optimum force is achieved using a portable stimulator. After a brief period of electrode encapsulation and stabilization of other tendon transfers performed simultaneously, the neuromuscular stimulator is activated and exercises are resumed. Typically, at approximately the twelfth week, the patient has recovered control of grasp and release in eight muscles of the forearm and wrist.

FES tendon transfers. Tendon transfers powered by FES-stimulated muscles play an important role in the situation where critical muscles are electrically inexcitable because of denervation from the trauma. We have previously reviewed the use and advantages of FES-powered tendon transfers in the restoration of the tetraplegic hand during FES implantation.[53] For example, to achieve balanced torque of the wrist under the influence of a strong electrically activated FDS, strong wrist extension is needed. Typically, a voluntary transfer, BR to ECRB, can provide some wrist extension of grade 3 strength. However, this is not sufficient, and wrist flexion deformities can develop. A stimulated transfer of extensor carpi ulnaris (ECU) to ECRB increases the force sufficiently to balance the wrist flexion torque provided by strong stimulation of finger flexors. Tendon transfers of this type expand the usefulness of paralyzed muscles and overcome the deficit of denervated functional groups.

Which motors should be preserved

Wrist extensors. Because wrist extension is critical to restoration, a wrist extensor is not a suitable donor motor unless at least two are under voluntary control and of sufficient strength. This means patients must be of ICT 3 or more. In addition, biomechanical studies have demonstrated that the different force vectors of the ECRL and ECRB confer different motions.[5] The ECRL, with its insertion radial to the center of the wrist on the base of the index metacarpal, produces untoward radial deviation along with wrist extension. With a full cadre of voluntary motors as

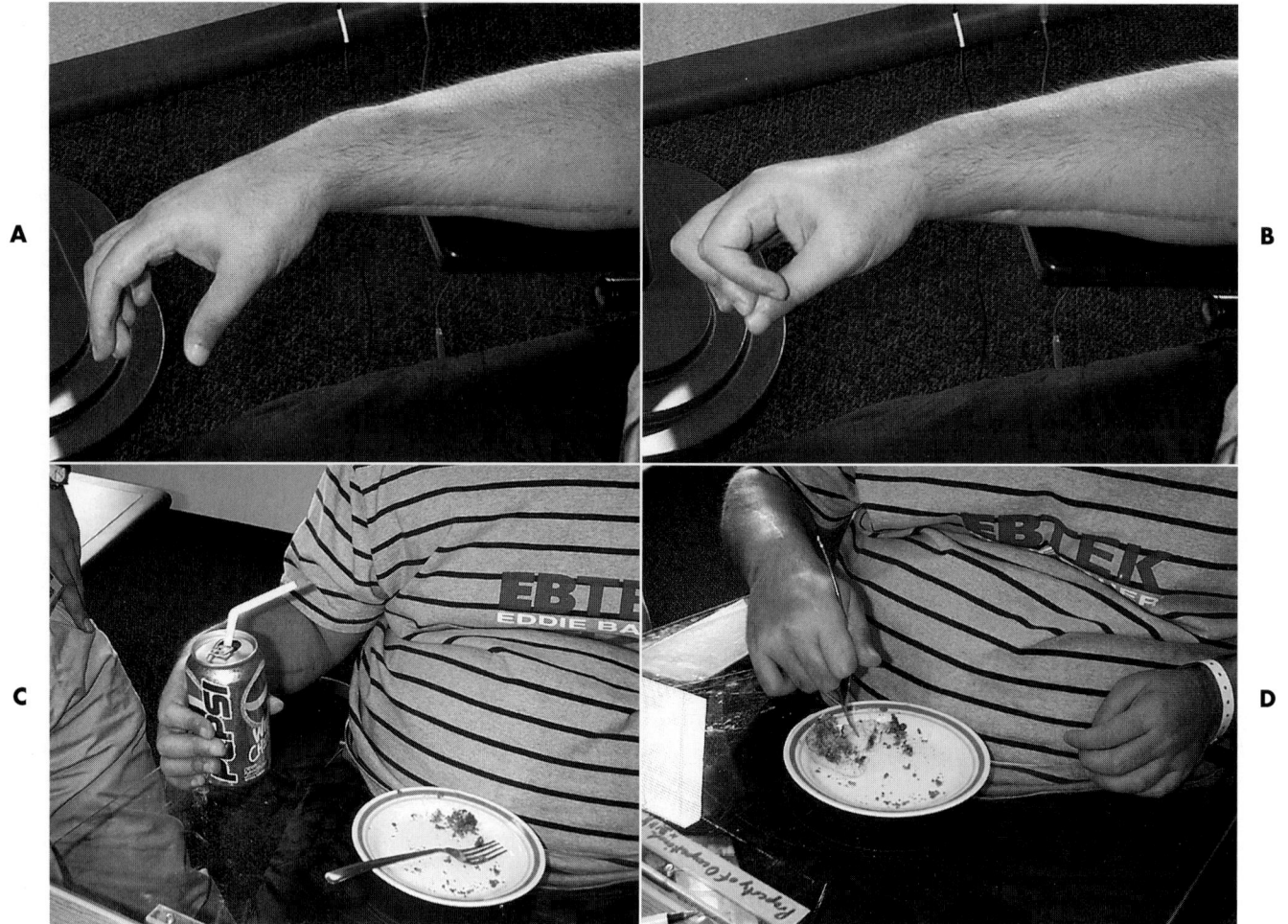

Fig. 51-6. A, Freehand System neuroprosthesis function in C6 tetraplegic patient, showing finger and thumb extension in palmar prehension. **B,** Freehand neuroprosthesis function in electronically programmed three jaw chuck pinch. **C,** Example of Freehand neuroprosthesis palmar grasp of can. **D,** Freehand neuroprosthesis key pinch used for grasping fork and feeding.

exists in able-bodied individuals, this fine-tuning of wrist motion allows for the full range of hand function; however, in the tetraplegic patient who has no voluntary hand function, radial deviation with wrist extension is an unbalanced situation. The ECRB, on the other hand, with its central insertion on the base of the long finger metacarpal, produces wrist extension with minimal radial/ulnar deviation, a more balanced and desirable motion. As such, when one of two strong and voluntary wrist extensors are transferred, the ECRL is chosen either to restore lateral pinch or palmar grasp depending on the patient's ICT. Similarly, when wrist extension is restored, the ECRB is the preferred recipient.[21,24,25,101] When implanting a neuroprosthesis, we demonstrated previously that insufficient wrist extension moments can result in flexion deformities from the overpowering activated finger flexors. In this latter situation, patients of ICT greater than or equal to 3 should not have either wrist extensor donated in a transfer unless the ECU or

flexor carpi ulnaris is to be activated as a wrist extensor. The corollary is that in patients less than grade 3, wrist extension should be augmented with an electrically activated muscle, typically the ECU, either primarily or as an FES transfers to the ECRB.[49]

We have found one situation in which transfer of the ECRB is useful. In a patient undergoing surgical restoration without the use of a neuroprosthesis and with weak grade 3/5 or less ECRB, transfer with a straight line of pull to the FDP via a window in the interosseous membrane provides some finger flexion without sacrificing critical wrist extension. The operation was performed originally to act as a superior passive tenodesis in patients with weak ECRB. Haque et al.[37] reviewed our series of seven patients undergoing this transfer. The total active finger flexion averaged 122 degrees per digit, and lateral pinch and palmar grasp strength were improved. The patients did experience a variable loss of wrist extension motion but not of wrist extension strength, we believe, as a result of the wrist flexion moment created by the transfer.

The key to performing a transfer involving the wrist extensors is determining that a patient is, in fact, ICG 2 versus 3. Clinical examination of the wrist extensors is not always reliable, and several authors have described means of assessing the presence of a sufficiently strong ECRB in the patient who has voluntary wrist extension.[16,75,77,78] As described in Mohammed et al., Bean found that a groove forms between the ECRL and ECRB in the proximal lateral forearm with the elbow in 90 degrees of flexion and resisted wrist extension when both are grade 5/5 strength.[78] Moberg[75] recommended that the ECRB be surgically exposed under local anesthesia to assess its independent function and to grade its strength.

Wrist flexors. In patients with ICT in excess of 5, the flexor carpi radialis (FCR) is of sufficient strength to be considered a potential donor motor. With an increasing number of available donor motors, significant gains in function through tendon transfers could be realized.[58] However, Zancolli[105,108] and House[43,45,46] advocate preservation of the FCR. They believe that the presence of an active, voluntary wrist flexor improves the finger tenodesis extension and prevents wrist extension contractures by improving wrist balance. Voluntary wrist flexion is also helpful in patients who use a manual wheelchair (most use motorized wheelchairs), in weight shifts to prevent pressure sores, and in weight transfers. We do not currently use the FCR as a donor motor when presented with the uncommon patient with an ICT in excess of 5 desiring surgical restoration.

Which motors are transferable

Brachioradialis. The BR is the most readily available and versatile muscle for reconstructive transfers in tetraplegia. Because it functions primarily as an elbow flexor and because most patients have an active and strong biceps or brachialis, the BR is commonly sacrificed with minimal deficit to the patient. It is truly the workhorse muscle in tetraplegia surgery. In fact, a variety of tendon transfers using the BR have been described: BR to ECRB for wrist extension, BR via tendon graft to FDP for palmar grasp, BR to FPL for lateral pinch, BR for adduction opponensplasty, and BR to extensor digitorum communis (EDC)/EPL for finger and thumb extension.* The muscle characteristics of the BR have been studied extensively while performing tendon transfers in tetraplegic patients.[27] The BR has a broad origin along the lateral epicondylar ridge, and its proximal muscle belly has significant fibrofascial tethers that limit its potential excursion. The average excursion demonstrated surgically is 41.7 mm. Typically, finger and thumb extensors require 40 to 60 mm of excursion, and finger flexors require up to 60 to 70 mm.[6,61] By releasing the proximal muscle belly from the surrounding connective tissue without

*References 8, 23, 26, 45, 62, 100, 108.

detaching its origin, its excursion can be increased to 77.9 mm, making it a suitable donor for these latter functions. The length-tension characteristics of the BR also have been investigated intraoperatively.[27] The active force produced by the BR was found to be more than 90% of maximal over a range of 1.5 to 2 cm centered around its resting length. Therefore transfers of the BR should be tensioned at its resting length with the recipient joint mobilized in a balanced position. Intraoperative muscle stimulation is a great aid to the surgeon in making this decision.

Some surgeons and therapists believe that the BR is difficult to train, especially in the absence of elbow stabilization. In the absence of elbow stabilization, the BR is effectively a two-joint muscle and will be a weak transfer as would be predicted under the general principles of tendon transfer surgery. Studies have shown that when the elbow is stabilized either by a brace or an elbow extension transfer, the BR becomes a more effective distal transfer.[7,25,100] We currently perform an elbow extension transfer as a first-stage procedure or combined with transfers, including the BR.

Extensor carpi radialis longus. The ECRL is available for transfer whenever there is a strong ECRB (ICT greater than or equal to 3). We commonly transfer the ECRL to a synchronized FDP to restore palmar grasp. We initially create a reverse cascade such that all fingers flex simultaneously and equally as advocated by Hentz.[38-41] The transfer is synergistic for wrist extension and finger flexion, although the line of pull around the radial border of radius is not ideal. Other common uses that have been described for the ECRL include transfer to the FPL for lateral grasp and to the EDC/EPL for finger extension and for intrinsic reconstruction.[17,21,24,25,44-46,57,58,78,101,108]

Pronator teres. We previously discussed the occurrence of supination contractures that limit the functional capacity of the patient's hand. It would seem that the presence of an active, voluntary PT would prevent these latter contractures and would be useful as an active pronator to position the hand for use. Indeed, just as for the FCR, one would tend to advocate preservation of the PT in patients of ICT in excess of 4. However, experience has proven otherwise. House has had favorable experience with transfer of the PT into the FPL since the early 1970s without adverse effects on pronation.[67] Zancolli[106,108,109] also favors transfer of the PT, especially to the FCR, placing emphasis on the restoration of active wrist flexion to stabilize the wrist in patients with strong wrist extension, and to improve the finger tenodesis effect. In addition, we have not observed, nor have we seen reported, cases of supination contractures occurring in patients with ICT greater than or equal to 2.

Postoperative therapy

After surgery, it is important not to damage the electrodes for the Freehand System and rupture the tendon transfers. Certain precautions should be followed. The arm should be elevated in bed when initially splinted, until the swelling decreases. The patient, being unable to weight bear on the affected upper extremity, will be dependent for weight shifts in the wheelchair and should not propel a manual wheelchair. The operated extremity should not be pulled on and, for posterior deltoid to triceps transfer, the arm should not be flexed past 90 degrees nor abducted past 0 degrees. Positioning at the side is recommended and shown by Friden[28] to reduce elongation of the posterior deltoid tendon graft. These precautions should be followed for 10 to 12 weeks postoperatively or until cleared by the hand surgeon. Because the hand and wrist generally are immobilized, no specific precautions are warranted regarding protection of the distal tendon transfers.

General tendon transfer management. We immobilize the hand and wrist for approximately 3 weeks after surgery. During this period, treatment should be focused on educating the patient and family regarding signs of infection, proper positioning, and precautions to be taken. Information should be given on techniques for functional transfers while the patient is dependent, and adaptations that need to be made for ADLs, wheelchair mobility, and weight shifts should be in place.

Protective splints are applied once the cast is removed and are worn, except during therapy, until cleared by the operating surgeon. Active range of motion (AROM), active-assisted ROM exercises, edema control, soft tissue mobilization, and scar management techniques form the crux of the early therapy program. Facilitation techniques, including biofeedback, taping, and vibration, are then progressively added. The patient may begin performing light functional activities such as tenodesis activity with light objects. Typically, a patient will have more than one procedure performed on the same extremity at a time; therefore more than one protocol may need to be followed. Any evidence of weakening of a transfer during the first 3 to 6 weeks warrants temporary immobilization of the transfer because this indicates stretching of the repair site; however, we have found that with regards to the hand and wrist, such occurrences are rare provided the patient is compliant. Certain tendon transfers that we commonly perform require separate discussion subsequently.

Posterior deltoid to triceps tendon transfer (see Fig. 51-2). Unfortunately, stretching and weakness are an all too common problem with the posterior deltoid to triceps transfer, and therapy must be precise and deliberate to minimize these problems. We place the patient in a hinged elbow extension splint set to a range between 0 and 15 degrees elbow flexion as soon as the postoperative extension splint is removed (1 to 2 weeks postoperatively). The brace is worn during the day, except for supervised exercise, and an elbow extension splint is worn at night. We start active elbow flexion and extension within the preset motion limits in a gravity-eliminated plane isolating the PD for extension. The

brace typically is adjusted weekly, increasing elbow flexion by 15 degrees. This is continued until 90-degree elbow flexion is achieved and active elbow extension continues to be 0 degrees. If the patient is unable to extend the elbow to 0 degrees, the brace is not advanced. The elbow extension splint is worn for 12 weeks following surgery, and then is discontinued as long as the elbow is maintaining 0-degree extension.

The PD transfer should be strengthened in all planes of space. Light resistive exercises may be incorporated into the exercise program as long as the individual is maintaining the precautions and is not substituting. The patient should begin ADLs and functional activities as AROM becomes available in the elbow. At week 12, the patient may begin functional transfer training and manual wheelchair propulsion. This transfer will continue to strengthen and become more useful for a year or more after surgery, and patients should not be discouraged with early weakness.

FPL split and BR to ECRB. A modified wrist cock-up splint incorporating the thumb IP joint is constructed with the wrist in 50-degree wrist extension. This protects both the wrist extension transfer and the thumb IP stabilization procedure. The splints should be worn at all times, except for exercise, until 6 to 8 weeks postoperatively. At that time, the splints may be discontinued except when performing strenuous activities. Passive motion is not initiated in the hand until week 6. Strengthening of this transfer begins at approximately 3 weeks. A patient may have difficulty activating this transfer, and if this is the case, we hold the elbow at 90 degrees of flexion and ask the patient to flex the elbow and observe for wrist motion. Too much resistance may cause rupture of the transfer. Progress to light-object activities such as using a fork is effective in providing the feedback to learn the transfer. The patient may begin functional transfer training and pushing the wheelchair without splints at 12 weeks.

TES and Freehand system training. As discussed previously, preoperative TES is a part of the preparation for implantation of FES to strengthen and condition the muscles of the forearm and hand. This program usually begins 3 to 4 weeks before surgery with the individual applying surface electrical stimulation using a neuromuscular electrical stimulation (NMES) unit. An evaluation using NMES determines the optimal placement for the surface electrodes, which is where the most muscle fiber recruitment and strongest muscle contraction is achieved for a specific muscle or muscle group. We start by stimulating the radial, median, and ulnar nerves and instructing the patient on electrode placement and a protocol whereby the intensity and duration of stimulation are increased gradually at home. Patients generally begin exercising for 1 hour, then 2 hours, and finally up to 6 hours as tolerated. Our NMES unit affords two separate channels to allow for two muscle groups to be exercised alternately during one session.

After surgery, the patient's arm is immobilized for approximately 3 weeks. After removal of the cast, a baseline profile of the electrodes and their recruitment properties is established. An exercise protocol similar to the preoperative protocol is designed, except that grasp patterns instead of muscle groups are stimulated. Palmar grasp and release and lateral grasp and release become the exercise motions. When tendon transfers are completed with FES implantation, strong stimulation is avoided for at least 6 to 8 weeks after surgery. As with the preoperative protocol, patients start modestly and build to a total of 8 hours of exercise per day. The muscles usually will be stimulated for a total of 6 hours, with intermittent rest for 2 hours. The patient will exercise the hand for 10 to 12 weeks after surgery. Patients are observed carefully by the therapist at regular intervals to help maintain joint mobility, prevent contractures, prevent adhesions, and aid in tailoring the exercise program. The therapist should be aware of the location of the electrodes, including the implanted stimulator in the chest wall, to avoid damage from external pressure. The electrodes also are profiled at regular intervals, approximately every 3 to 4 weeks, to account for changes in electrode (muscle) properties. Muscles generally become stronger and more fatigue resistant, and electrode settings and grasp profiles need to be adjusted appropriately.

OUTCOMES

A well-selected, comprehensive program of hand and upper extremity rehabilitation will have a reliably beneficial impact on patients' lives. These benefits can and have been measured in terms of improved strength of grasp and pinch; increased number of different ADLs that can be performed independently and brace free, including bowel and bladder care; and decreased need for orthotics/braces and full-time assistive care. The impact that these improvements confer onto the patients' quality of life have been inferred by the high rates of satisfaction; their improved comfort level in the community; and the number of patients who develop personal interests including vocations, education, and hobbies. The greatest benefit may be on patients' psyche, with dramatic improvements in their self-image, confidence, and overall quality of life. As stated by Sterling Bunnell many years ago, "... if you have nothing, a little is a lot. ..."[74]

As early as 1972, authors reported results from surgical restoration that extended beyond simply measuring voluntary motion that was not available previously.[58] House[45,46] found that patients improved in their ability to function, including bowel and bladder care. In 1983, Lamb and Chan[57] reported that of the 41 patients with greater than 7-year follow-up, 83% experienced good to excellent results with regards to improved function. They noted a change from being completely dependent, especially with regards to bowel and bladder care, and that hand restoration facilitated the development of personal interests and hobbies. In

Freehafer et al.'s experience with treating 68 patients, none were worse, and only 4 remained unimproved.[21] Ejeskar and Dahllof[17] noted improvements in 35 of 43 patients. In 1992, Mohammed et al.[78] presented their results of surgical restoration using tendon transfers in a heterogeneous group of 57 patients, with 84% reporting an improved quality of life. Approximately two thirds noted independence in eating, writing and typing, and using a telephone, as well as improvements in self-care. In 1998, Lo et al.[64] found that, of 9 patients with C6 motor level tetraplegia, all benefited from surgical reconstruction both objectively and subjectively, and would have the surgery again. Paul et al.[83] reported that, in addition to improvements in ADLs, many were able to become brace free.

Results from the application of FES reveal similar successes. Among the earliest studies, patients who were ASIA C5 functioned at the level of C6 or higher without the need for adaptive tools and equipment.[51] Kilgore et al.[55] reported that the neuroprosthesis not only improved on the ability to perform functional tasks, but also allowed patients to perform many activities without adaptive equipment. All five patients evaluated used the system at home, with four doing so on a regular basis. In a separate follow-up study, patients were able to pinch and grasp objects with more strength than required for most ADLs, experienced improved abilities especially with heavy objects, and were less dependent on braces, assistive devices, and attendants.[48] In 1999, results of subjective outcomes on 34 patients with an average 5.2-year follow-up were reported[103]; these results included high rates of general satisfaction (87%), life improvements (88%), improved ADLs (87%), and increased independence (81%) and confidence (67%). Motor level correlated with success, with the best subjective outcomes noted in C5 or C5/6 patients.

CONCLUSION

Rehabilitating a person who sustains traumatic tetraplegia from the time of injury to "reintegration" into the community involves focused and dedicated care and effort on the part of a multitude of health care providers. This process seeks to both improve and maximize the quantity and quality of the individuals' life. Rehabilitation of the hand and upper extremity is an integral part of this process and ideally should begin at the inception of care. With use of techniques such as splinting, therapy, medicine, and surgery, function can be maximized and often restored or reconstructed. The effect on a patient's life is generally beneficial and lifelong.

REFERENCES

1. Adams R, Victor M, Ropper A: *Principles of neurology,* ed 6, New York, 1997, McGraw-Hill.
1a. Allieu Y, et al: Restoration of elbow extension in the tetraplegic by transplantation of the posterior deltoid: study of 21 cases, *Rev Chir Orthop* 71:195, 1985.

1b. Allieu Y, et al: Restoration of elbow extension in tetraplegic patients. In Vastamäki M, editor: *Current trends in hand surgery,* New York, 1995, Elsevier.

2. American Spinal Injury Association: *Standards for neurological and functional classification of spinal cord injury,* rev ed, Chicago, 1992, American Spinal Injury Association.

3. Betz RR, Mulcahey MJ, Shriners Hospitals for Crippled Children: *The child with a spinal cord injury: symposium, Phoenix, Arizona, December 8-11, 1994,* Rosemont, Ill, 1996, American Academy of Orthopaedic Surgeons.

4. Blount W: Osteoclasis for supination deformities in children, *J Bone Joint Surg* 22A:300, 1948.

5. Brand P: *Clinical mechanics of the hand,* St Louis, 1985, Mosby.

6. Brand P, Beach R, Thompson D: Relative tension and potential excursion of the muscles in the forearm and the hand, *J Hand Surg* 6A:209, 1981.

6a. Bryan RS: The Moberg deltoid-triceps replacement and key-pinch operations in quadriplegia: preliminary experiences, *Hand* 9:207, 1977.

7. Brys D, Waters RL: Effect of triceps function on the brachioradialis transfer in quadriplegia, *J Hand Surg* 12A:237, 1987.

8. Bunnell S: Instructional course lectures: American Academy of Orthopaedic Surgeons. In Blount WP, Banks SW, editors: *Tendon transfers in the hand and forearm,* vol VI, Ann Arbor, Mich, 1949, JW Edwards.

9. Carroll S, et al: Electrical activation of triceps brachii using the Freehand System: a case report. In *Proceedings of the 2nd Annual IFESS Conference,* Vancouver, 1997, IFESS.

9a. Castro-Sierra A, Lopez-Pita A: A new surgical technique to correct triceps paralysis, *Hand* 15:42, 1983.

10. Colyer RA, Kappelman B: Flexor pollicis longus tenodesis in tetraplegia at the sixth cervical level: a prospective evaluation of functional gain, *J Bone Joint Surg* 63A:376, 1981.

11. Consortium for Spinal Cord Medicine, Paralyzed Veterans of America: *Outcomes following traumatic spinal cord injury: clinical practice guidelines for health-care professionals,* Washington, DC, 1999, Paralyzed Veterans of America.

12. Crago PE, Peckham PH, Thrope GB: Modulation of muscle force by recruitment during intramuscular stimulation, *IEEE Trans Biomed Eng* 27:679, 1980.

13. Crago PE, et al: An elbow extension neuroprosthesis for individuals with tetraplegia, *IEEE Trans Rehabil Eng* 6:1, 1998.

14. Creasey G, Keith M: Principles of upper extremity surgery in tetraplegia. In Peimer C, editor: *Surgery of the hand and upper extremity,* New York, 1996, McGraw-Hill.

15. DeBenedetti M: Restoration of elbow extension in the tetraplegic patient using the Moberg technique, *J Hand Surg* 4A:86, 1979.

16. Ejeskar A: Upper limb surgical rehabilitation in high-level tetraplegia, *Hand Clin* 4:585, 1988.

17. Ejeskar A, Dahllof A: Results of reconstructive surgery in the upper limb of tetraplegic patients, *Paraplegia* 26:204, 1988.

18. Flatt A: An indication for shortening of the thumb: description of technique and brief report of five cases, *J Bone Joint Surg* 46A:1534, 1964.

19. Freehafer A: Flexion and supination deformities of the elbow in tetraplegics, *Paraplegia* 15:221, 1977.

20. Freehafer AA: Tendon transfers in tetraplegic patients: the Cleveland experience, *Spinal Cord* 36:315, 1998.

21. Freehafer AA, Kelly, Peckham PH: Tendon transfer for the restoration of upper limb function after a cervical spinal cord injury, *J Hand Surg* 9A:887, 1984.

22. Freehafer AA, Kelly CM, Peckham PH: Planning tendon transfers in tetraplegia: Cleveland technique. In Hunter J, Schneider L, Mackin E, editors: *Tendon surgery in the hand,* St Louis, 1987, Mosby.

23. Freehafer A, Mast W: Transfer of the brachioradialis to improve wrist extension in high spinal cord injury, *J Bone Joint Surg* 44A:648, 1967.

24. Freehafer AA, Peckham PH, Keith MW: New concepts on treatment of the upper limb in the tetraplegic: surgical restoration and functional neuromuscular stimulation, *Hand Clin* 4:563, 1988.

25. Freehafer AA, Peckham PH, Keith MW: Surgical treatment for tetraplegia: upper limb. In Chapman M, editor: *Operative orthopaedics,* Philadelphia, 1988 JB Lippincott.

26. Freehafer AA, Vonhaam V: Tendon transfer to improve grasp after injuries of the cervical spinal cord, *J Bone Joint Surg* 56A:951, 1974.

27. Freehafer AA, et al: The brachioradialis: anatomy, properties, and value for tendon transfer in the tetraplegic, *J Hand Surg* 13A:99, 1988.

28. Friden J, et al: Protection of the deltoid-to-triceps tendon transfer repair sites. In Proceedings of the 17th International Society of Biomechanics, Calgary, 1999.

29. Friedenberg Z: Transposition of the biceps brachii for triceps weakness, *J Bone Joint Surg* 36A:656, 1954.

30. Gansel J, Waters R, Gellman H: Transfer of the pronator teres tendon to the tendons of the flexor digitorum profundus in tetraplegia, *J Bone Joint Surg* 72A:427, 1990.

31. Gellman H, et al: Rerouting of the biceps brachii for paralytic supination contracture of the forearm in tetraplegia due to trauma, *J Bone Joint Surg* 76A:398, 1994.

32. Gorman P, Peckham P: Upper extremity functional neuromuscular stimulation, *J Neurol Rehab* 5:3, 1991.

33. Gorman PH, et al: Patient selection for an upper extremity neuroprosthesis in tetraplegic individuals, *Spinal Cord* 35:569, 1997.

34. Green D: Radial nerve palsy. In Green D, Hotchkiss R, Pederson W, editors: *Green's operative hand surgery,* New York, 1999, Churchill Livingstone.

35. Grill JH, Peckham PH: Functional neuromuscular stimulation for combined control of elbow extension and hand grasp in C5 and C6 quadriplegics, *IEEE Trans Rehabil Eng* 6:190, 1998.

36. Hanson RW, Franklin MR: Sexual loss in relation to other functional losses for spinal cord injured males, *Arch Phys Med Rehabil* 57:291, 1976.

37. Haque M, et al: Clinical results of ECRB to FDP transfer through the interosseous membrane to restore finger flexion. In Proceedings of the 6th International Conference on Surgical Rehabilitation for Tetraplegia, Cleveland, 1998.

38. Hentz VR: Historical background and changing perspectives in surgical reconstruction of the upper limb in quadriplegia, *J Am Paraplegia Soc* 7:36, 1984.

39. Hentz VR, Brown M, Keoshian LA: Upper limb reconstruction in quadriplegia: functional assessment and proposed treatment modifications, *J Hand Surg* 8A:119, 1983.

40. Hentz VR, Hamlin C, Keoshian LA: Surgical reconstruction in tetraplegia, *Hand Clin* 4:601, 1988.

41. Hentz V, et al: Rehabilitation and surgical reconstruction of the upper limb in tetraplegia: an update, *J Hand Surg* 17A:964, 1992.

42. Hiersche DL, Waters RL: Interphalangeal fixation of the thumb in Moberg's key grip procedure, *J Hand Surg* 10A:30, 1985.

43. House JH: Reconstruction of the thumb in tetraplegia following spinal cord injury, *Clin Orthop* 195:117, 1985.

44. House JH, Comadoll J, Dahl AL: One-stage key pinch and release with thumb carpal-metacarpal fusion in tetraplegia, *J Hand Surg* 17A:530, 1992.

45. House JH, Gwathmey FW, Lundsgaard DK: Restoration of strong grasp and lateral pinch in tetraplegia due to cervical spinal cord injury, *J Hand Surg* 1A:152, 1976.

46. House JH, Shannon MA: Restoration of strong grasp and lateral pinch in tetraplegia: a comparison of two methods of thumb control in each patient, *J Hand Surg* 10A:22, 1985.

47. House J, et al: Intrinsic balancing in reconstruction of the tetraplegic hand. In Vastamäki M, editor: *Current trends in hand surgery,* New York, 1995, Elsevier.

48. Keith MW: Restoration of tetraplegic hand function using an FES neuroprosthesis. In Hunter J, Schneider L, Mackin E, editors: *Tendon and nerve surgery in the hand: a third decade,* St Louis, 1997, Mosby.

49. Keith MW, Kilgore K: The provision of wrist extension for C5 level spinal cord injury through tendon transfers of voluntary and paralyzed muscles. In Proceedings of the 53rd meeting of the American Society for Surgery of the Hand, Minneapolis, Minn, 1998.

50. Keith M, Lacey S: Surgical rehabilitation of the tetraplegic upper extremity, *J Neuro Rehabil* 5:75, 1991.

51. Keith MW, et al: Functional neuromuscular stimulation neuroprostheses for the tetraplegic hand, *Clin Orthop* 233:25, 1988.

52. Keith MW, et al: Implantable functional neuromuscular stimulation in the tetraplegic hand, *J Hand Surg* 14A:524, 1989.

53. Keith MW, et al: Tendon transfers and functional electrical stimulation for restoration of hand function in spinal cord injury, *J Hand Surg* 21A:89, 1996.

54. Kilgore K, et al: Synthesis of hand grasp using functional neuromuscular stimulation, *IEEE Trans Biomed Eng* 36:761, 1989.

55. Kilgore KL, et al: An implanted upper-extremity neuroprosthesis: follow-up of five patients, *J Bone Joint Surg* 79A:533, 1997.

55a. Kirsch R, et al: Measurement of isometric elbow and shoulder moments: position-dependent strength of posterior deltoid-to-triceps muscle tendon transfer in tetraplegia, *IEEE Trans Rehab Eng* 4:403, 1996.

56. Kuz J, Van Heest A, House J: Biceps-to-triceps transfer in tetraplegic patients: report of the medial routing technique and follow-up of three cases, *J Hand Surg* 24A:161, 1999.

56a. Lacey S, et al: The posterior deltoid to triceps transfer: a clinical and biomechanical assessment, *J Hand Surg* 11A:542, 1986.

57. Lamb DW, Chan KM: Surgical reconstruction of the upper limb in traumatic tetraplegia: a review of 41 patients, *J Bone Joint Surg* 65B:291, 1983.

58. Lamb DW, Landry RM: The hand in quadriplegia, *Paraplegia* 9:204, 1972.

59. Leclercq C, McDowell C: Fourth international conference on surgical rehabilitation of the upper limb in tetraplegia, *Ann Chir Main Memb Super* 10:258, 1991.

60. LeMay M, Crago P, Keith MW: Restoration of pronosupination control by FNS in tetraplegia: experimental and biomechanical evaluation of feasibility, *J Biomech* 29:435, 1996.

61. Lieber R, et al: Architecture of selected muscles of the arm and forearm: anatomy and implications for tendon transfer, *J Hand Surg* 17A:787, 1992.

62. Lipscomb P, Elkins EC, Henderson ED: Tendon transfers to restore function of hands in tetraplegia, especially after fracture-dislocation of the sixth cervical vertebra on the seventh, *J Bone Joint Surg* 40A:1071, 1958.

63. Lipskeir E, Weizenbluth M: Derotation osteotomy of the forearm in management of paralytic supination deformity, *J Hand Surg* 18A:1069, 1993.

64. Lo IK, et al: The outcome of tendon transfers for C6-spared quadriplegics, *J Hand Surg* 23B:156, 1998.

65. Manske P, McCarroll H, Hale R: Biceps tendon rerouting and percutaneous osteoclasis in the treatment of supination deformity in obstetric palsy, *J Hand Surg* 5A:153, 1980.

66. McCarthy CK, et al: Intrinsic balancing in reconstruction of the tetraplegic hand, *J Hand Surg* 22A:596, 1997.

67. McDowell C, House J: Tetraplegia. In Green D, Hochkiss R, Pederson W, editors: *Green's operative hand surgery,* New York, 1999, Churchill Livingstone.

68. McDowell C, Moberg E, House J: The second international conference on surgical rehabilitation of the upper limb in tetraplegia (quadriplegia), *J Hand Surg* 11A:604, 1986.

69. McDowell CL, Moberg EA, Smith AG: International conference on surgical rehabilitation of the upper limb in tetraplegia, *J Hand Surg* 4A:387, 1979.

69a. Mennen V, Boonzaier A: An improved technique of posterior deltoid to triceps transfer in tetraplegia, *J Hand Surg* 16B:197, 1991.

70. Merle d'Aubigne R, et al. In *symposium on reconstructive surgery of the Royal Society of Medicine,* 1949.

71. Miller L, Peckham P, Keith M: Elbow extension in the C5 quadriplegic using functional neuromuscular stimulation, *IEEE Trans Biomed Eng* 36:771, 1989.

72. Moberg E: Surgical treatment for absent single-hand grip and elbow extension in quadriplegia: principles and preliminary experience, *J Bone Joint Surg* 57A:196, 1975.

73. Moberg E: Helpful upper limb surgery in tetraplegia. In Hunter J, et al, editors: *Rehabilitation of the hand,* St Louis, 1978, Mosby.

74. Moberg E: *The upper limb in tetraplegia: a new approach to surgical rehabilitation,* Stuttgart, 1978, Thieme.

75. Moberg E: Current treatment program using tendon surgery in tetraplegia. In Hunter J, Schneider L, Mackin E, editors: *Tendon surgery in the hand,* St Louis, 1987, Mosby.

76. Moberg E: The present state of surgical rehabilitation of the upper limb in tetraplegia, *Paraplegia* 25:351, 1987.

77. Moberg E, McDowell C, House J: Proceedings of the third international conference on surgical rehabilitation of the upper limb in tetraplegia (quadriplegia), *J Hand Surg* 14A:1064, 1989.

78. Mohammed K, et al: Upper limb surgery for tetraplegia, *J Bone Joint Surg* 74B:873, 1992.

79. National Spinal Cord Injury Statistical Center: *Spinal cord injury: facts and figures at a glance—May 2001.* Birmingham, 2001, The University of Alabama at Birmingham, National Spinal Cord Injury Statistical Center. Accessed at http://www.spinalcord.uab.edu/show.asp?durki=21446.

80. Newman JH: The use of the key grip procedure in improving hand function in quadriplegia, *Hand* 9:215, 1977.

81. Nickel V, Perry J, Garret AL: Development of useful function in the severely paralyzed hand, *J Bone Joint Surg* 45A:933, 1963.

82. Owings R, et al: Biceps brachii rerouting in treatment of paralytic supination contracture of the forearm, *J Bone Joint Surg* 53A:137, 1971.

83. Paul SD, et al: Single-stage reconstruction of key pinch and extension of the elbow in tetraplegic patients, *J Bone Joint Surg* 76A:1451, 1994 (comments).

84. Peckham P: Functional electrical stimulation: current status and future prospects of applications to the neuromuscular system in spinal cord injury, *Paraplegia* 25:279, 1987.

85. Peckham PH, Creasey GH: Neural prostheses: clinical applications of functional electrical stimulation in spinal cord injury, *Paraplegia* 30:96, 1992.

86. Peckham P, Keith M, Freehafer A: Restoration of functional control by electrical stimulation in the upper extremity of the quadriplegic patient, *J Bone Joint Surg* 70A:144, 1988.

87. Peckham P, Marsolais E, Moritimer J: Restoration of key grip and release in the C6 tetraplegic patient through functional electrical stimulation, *J Hand Surg* 5:462, 1980.

88. Peckham P, Mortimer J, Marsolais E: Alteration in the force and fatigability of skeletal muscle in quadriplegic humans following exercise induced by chronic electrical stimulation, *Clin Orthop* 114:326, 1976.

89. Peckham PH, Mortimer JT, Marsolais EA Upper and lower motor neuron lesions in the upper extremity muscles of tetraplegics, *Paraplegia* 14:115, 1976.

90. Peckham P, Mortimer J, Marsolais E: Controlled prehension and release in the C5 quadriplegic elicited by functional electrical stimulation of the paralyzed forearm musculature, *Ann Biomed Eng* 8:369, 1980.

91. Peljovich A, et al: The treatment of paralytic forearm supination contracture in tetraplegic patients with a rotational osteotomy and rigid internal fixation. In the proceedings of the 6th international conference on surgical rehabilitation for tetraplegia, Cleveland, 1998.

92. Pulvertaft R: Tendon grafting for the isolated injury of flexor digitorum profundus, *Bull Hosp Joint Dis* 44:424, 1984.

92a. Rabischong E, et al: Length-tension relationship of the posterior deltoid to triceps transfer in C6 tetraplegia, *Paraplegia* 31:33, 1993.

92b. Raczka R, Braun R, Waters R: Posterior deltoid-to-triceps transfer in quadriplegia, *Clin Orthop* 187:163, 1984.

93. Revol M, Briand E, Servant J: Biceps-to-triceps transfer in tetraplegia: the medial route, *J Hand Surg* 24B:235, 1999.

94. Schottstaedt E, Larsen L, Bost F: The surgical reconstruction of the upper extremity paralyzed by poliomyelitis, *J Bone Joint Surg* 40A:633, 1958.

95. Smith AG: Early complications of key grip hand surgery for tetraplegia, *Paraplegia* 19:123, 1981.

96. Stover SL, Fine PR: *Spinal cord injury: the facts & figures,* Birmingham, 1986, The University of Alabama at Birmingham.

97. Street D: Finger flexor tenodesis, *Clin Orthop* 13:155, 1989.

98. Treanor WJ, Moberg E, Buncke HJ: The hyperflexed seemingly useless tetraplegic hand: a method of surgical amelioration, *Paraplegia,* 30:457, 1992.

99. Trombly C: *Occupational therapy for physical dysfunction,* ed 4, Baltimore, 1995, Williams & Wilkins.

99a. Vastamäki M, Brummer H, Solonen K: Deltoid-to-triceps transfer and key-pinch operations in tetraplegia. In Vastamäki M, editor: *Current trends in hand surgery,* New York, 1995, Elsevier.

100. Waters R, et al: Brachioradialis to flexor pollicis longus tendon transfer for active lateral pinch in the tetraplegic, *J Hand Surg* 10A:385, 1985.

101. Waters RL, et al: Functional hand surgery following tetraplegia, *Arch Phys Med Rehabil* 77:86, 1996.

102. Wilson J: Providing automatic grasp by flexor tenodesis, *J Bone Joint Surg* 38A:1019, 1956.

103. Wuolle KS, et al: Satisfaction with and usage of a hand neuroprosthesis, *Arch Phys Med Rehabil* 80:206, 1999.

104. Zancolli E: Paralytic supination contracture of the forearm, *J Bone Joint Surg* 49A:1275, 1967.

105. Zancolli E: *Structural and dynamic basis of hand surgery,* Philadelphia, 1968, JB Lippincott.

106. Zancolli E: Surgery for the quadriplegic hand with active, strong wrist extension preserved: a study of 97 cases, *Clin Orthop* 112:101, 1975.

107. Zancolli E: Functional restoration of the upper limb in traumatic quadriplegia. In *Structural and dynamic bases of hand surgery,* ed 2, Philadelphia, 1979, JB Lippincott.

108. Zancolli E: *Structural and dynamic basis of hand surgery,* ed 2, Philadelphia, 1979, JB Lippincott.

109. Zancolli E, Zancolli EJ: Surgical reconstruction of the upper limb in middle-level tetraplegia. In Tubiana R, editor: *The hand,* vol 4, Philadelphia, 1993, WB Saunders.

Part **XI**

VASCULAR
AND LYMPHATIC
DISORDERS

Chapter 52

VASCULAR DISORDERS
OF THE UPPER EXTREMITY

John S. Taras
Mark S. Lemel
Ross Nathan

Vascular disorders of the upper extremity make up only 5% of all vascular disease,[38] but their infrequency is contrasted by their potential range of presentation. The clinical picture can be as dramatic as a life-threatening hemorrhage that requires immediate surgery, but more typically, the patient is prompted to seek care as a result of experiencing subtle symptoms of pain with activity, noticing color changes, or discovering a mass. Vascular disorders are often misdiagnosed, and it is not unusual for a patient to consult several physicians over the course of 6 to 12 months before his or her problem is recognized.

This chapter provides a sequential guide to the evaluation of the patient with a suspected vascular disorder. It reviews the pertinent anatomy; presents a specialized workup consisting of a guided history, physical examination, and diagnostic tests; and describes the most common vascular disorders along with their treatment protocols.

VASCULAR ANATOMY
Embryology

Between the third and fourth weeks of gestation, the heart develops out of the splanchnic mesoderm and the developing limb bud becomes visible as a swelling on the lateral aspect of the cervical somites. By the fourth week, primitive vascular channels form within the limb, and the seventh dorsal segmental vessel, located along the central axis of the limb bud, is destined to become the axial artery—the major inflow vessel to the upper extremity. Developing as a branch of this vessel is the interosseous artery, which perfuses the primitive hand. This vessel may persist into adult life as the interosseous artery of the forearm with a diminished but occasionally important contribution to the hand's blood supply. As the interosseous artery regresses, the median artery becomes the dominant vessel to the upper extremity. This vessel also may persist into maturity in association with the median nerve, and it has been implicated as an etiologic factor in carpal tunnel syndrome after thrombosis.[51]

The factors that control the sequence of vessel formation and regression are not known. According to one theory, hemodynamically selected capillaries enlarge to form the final vascular pattern—a mechanism that would explain the persistence of fetal vessels as well as the common anomalous vessel origins. As the vascular system develops, the radial and ulnar arteries provide the final inflow channels to the distal upper extremity. These vessels originate from the brachial artery, but they also may arise from anomalous areas.

Anatomy

Adult vascular anatomy consists of arteries, veins, lymphatic vessels, and sympathetic nerves. This chapter provides a standard view of vascular anatomy and describes the more common normal variations. A comprehensive treatment of this subject can be found in specialized texts of anatomy.[1,7,25,44,83]

Arterial system. (Fig. 52-1) The brachial artery is the major inflow vessel to the forearm and hand. It arises from the axillary artery at the lower border of the teres major muscle[35] and courses distally along the medial aspect of the arm with the triceps posteriorly, the median nerve in close approximation medially, and the biceps and brachialis laterally. At the level of the antecubital fossa, it dives below

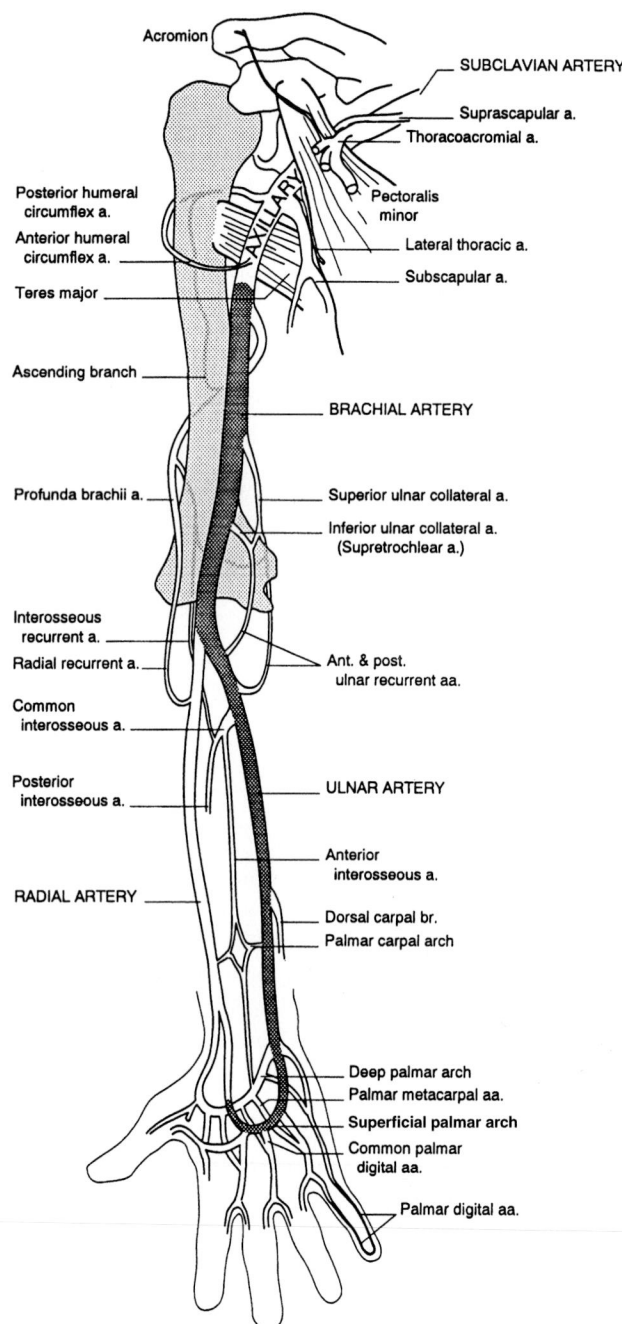

Fig. 52-1. The vascular anatomy of the upper extremity.

the lacertus fibrosus and divides into the two principal vessels of the forearm—the radial and ulnar arteries. Before this division, it gives off important branches that serve as collateral vessels for the shoulder and elbow. The profunda brachii artery anastomoses proximally with the posterior humeral circumflex beneath the deltoid, and distally with the recurrent branches of the radial and interosseous arteries. Two other branches of the brachial artery—the superficial and inferior ulnar collateral arteries—anastomose with the recurrent branch of the ulnar artery. Despite this extensive

collateral network around the elbow, interruption or thrombosis of the brachial artery is associated with acute ischemia of the distal limb in approximately 10% of cases.[10]

In the forearm, the radial and ulnar arteries take divergent paths to the wrist. The radial artery remains relatively superficial beneath the brachioradialis muscle in association with the sensory branch of the radial nerve. Its major branch is the radial recurrent artery. Distally, it passes more superficially, just lateral to the flexor carpi radialis tendon. At the level of the wrist, it subdivides into a smaller superficial palmar branch, which passes volarly through the thenar musculature and classically joins the superficial palmar arch. The larger branch passes to the dorsum of the wrist through the anatomic snuffbox and head of the first dorsal interosseous muscle. It then dives deeply to form the major contribution to the deep palmar arch.

The ulnar artery takes a deeper course to the hand. This vessel passes deep to the pronator teres and flexor digitorum superficialis before passing medially to lie deep to the flexor carpi ulnaris muscle and tendon in the distal forearm. From this point, it enters the hand via the canal of Guyon accompanied by the ulnar nerve laterally. The ulnar artery provides approximately 60% of the supply to the hand, the majority of which is through the superficial palmar arch. One of its branches at the level of the pisiform contributes to the deep palmar arch.

Unlike the radial artery, the ulnar artery has two important branches in the forearm. The ulnar recurrent artery anastomoses with the ulnar collateral branches of the brachial artery. The common interosseous artery, which eventually divides to form the anterior and posterior interosseous arteries, arises in the proximal forearm. The latter two vessels travel distally along with the anterior and posterior interosseous nerves. In the wrist, three dorsal and three volar arches form an anastomotic network joined on the medial and lateral sides by the ulnar and radial arteries, respectively. The most distal volar carpal arch is the deep palmar arch. The anterior interosseous artery contributes to the volar arches in approximately 87% of the population.[26]

The majority of blood flow to the hand comes by way of the palmar arches. The median artery provides accessory flow in 10% to 20% of patients. The superficial arch, which lies distal to the deep arch at the same level as the abducted thumb tip, is in close proximity to the transverse carpal ligament and may be injured during carpal tunnel release. This arch is "complete" in 78.5% of specimens, either by the ulnar artery alone (37%) or from an anastomosis of the ulnar with the radial or interosseous artery (41.5%). An incomplete arch occurs when vessels other than the ulnar artery provide total flow to one or more digits. The thumb is the most common autonomous digit in hands with incomplete arches.[16] According to Coleman and Anson,[16] the deep palmar arch is less variable; they found complete arches in 98% of their specimens, but a more recent study by Ikeda et al.[37] found this pattern in only 77%.

The superficial palmar arch gives off the common digital vessels, which divide to form the proper digital arteries to the fingers. The deep arch gives rise to the princeps pollicis artery, which provides the majority of flow to the thumb via an ulnar volar vessel; this vessel is the one that is most frequently repaired in thumb revascularization. The branches of the deep arch—the deep palmar metacarpal arteries—terminate in the common palmar metacarpal arteries and supply the metacarpophalangeal joint and the interosseous musculature. These vessels frequently join the common digital arteries and provide important collateral flow to the digits in trauma. The dorsal circulation to the hand is often overlooked, but it too provides alternative flow to the digits. Vessels that contribute to the dorsal circulation arise from dorsal branches of the radial and ulnar arteries as well as from the digital dorsal carpal arch. Perforating vessels from the deep palmar arch also contribute to the dorsal metacarpal and digital arteries.

Blood flow to the digits comes predominantly through the common and proper digital arteries branching from the superficial palmar arch.[72] These vessels, which lie in close proximity to the digital nerves, form a ladderlike branching pattern that supplies the bones, joints, and flexor tendons. A corresponding but smaller dorsal network is the vascular supply to the extensor tendons. The digital arteries are larger on the ulnar side of the thumb, index, and long fingers, averaging 1.8 mm at the base of the proximal phalanges and 0.95 mm in the distal phalanges.[45]

There are many variations of the arterial anatomy of the forearm and hand. These anomalies have no particular significance in the normal state, but they may affect the diagnostic picture after injury and alter classic surgical anatomy. Significant variations occur in up to one third of specimens. For example, the radial artery may originate proximal to the antecubital fossa in 15% of the population.[56] This vessel may be cannulated accidentally during venipuncture or lacerated during a surgical approach to the elbow and distal humerus. A vessel often confused with the radial artery is the superficial brachial artery, which divides distally into the radial and ulnar arteries, whereas the proper brachial artery supplies the distal interosseous artery.[30] A superficial brachial artery exists in 2% of specimens. Finally, a persistent median artery makes a contribution to the palmar arch in 15% of specimens.[8]

Venous system. Venous anatomy is best understood by proceeding from distal to proximal, in the direction of flow. Identifiable veins have been found distal to the nail fold in the lateral and volar positions.[48] These vessels are generally small, measuring 0.5 to 0.8 mm in diameter.[60] The first identifiable dorsal vessel is the terminal vein just proximal to the nail fold. Proximally, dorsal and volar networks known as *ladders* provide drainage in the digit. The dorsal system is somewhat larger than the volar system, and these are the vessels used in replantation. These two systems are connected via oblique anastomotic veins. The digital vessels have no discernible venae comitantes. However, these are not the dominant drainage system to the digit.

Dorsal and volar veins in the hand drain into the superficial cephalic and basilic veins as well as the deep venae comitantes of the radial and ulnar arteries. The radial and ulnar veins drain into the deep brachial vein, which combines with the basilic vein to form the axillary vein. The cephalic vein does not enter the deep system until just proximal to the clavicle, and it provides collateral circulation when the deep circulation is disrupted. The venous system of the upper extremity has more extensive variations than does the arterial system. However, these vessels usually are not significant unless proximal obstruction of the central venous system causes dilation of the superficial vessels.

Lymphatic system. The lymphatic system is often overlooked in studies of vascular anatomy and does not become clinically important unless obstruction causes swelling and edema of the extremity. Generally, the lymphatic drainage of the hand runs parallel to the superficial venous anatomy and arterial structures of the arm.[28] These two systems join at the level of the axillary lymph nodes, which become engorged and painful when the hand is infected.

Nervous system. Knowledge of the sympathetic nervous system completes one's understanding of the vascular anatomy. Fibers from the lower cervical and upper thoracic ganglia pass into the peripheral nervous system mainly by way of the median and ulnar nerves. However, all nerves that cross the wrist contribute sympathetic fibers to the hand and digits. These fibers control vessel constriction and dilation in response to physiologic stimuli such as cold or stress. They also may participate in pathologic processes such as reflex sympathetic dystrophy (RSD) and Raynaud's phenomenon.

THE MEDICAL WORKUP
History and physical examination

Most vascular disorders of the upper extremity can be diagnosed with an appropriate history and physical examination. The examination must be tailored to the clinical situation. An acute, life-threatening arterial injury with pulsatile bleeding is easily recognized. However, even in an emergent situation, an assessment of the distal peripheral pulses and the patient's vascular status is mandatory. In addition, a brief but comprehensive neurologic examination distal to the traumatic injuries will reveal deficits that require exploration of nearby nerves at the time of vascular repair.

A more detailed history and physical examination are needed when evaluating an individual with nonacute symptoms. Questions and diagnostic tests are involved that are not part of the routine evaluation of a hand surgery patient. For this reason, the examiner is advised to use a comprehensive and organized data worksheet, which will ensure a complete evaluation as well as aid in diagnosis.

The most common presenting complaints in patients with vascular disorders are pain, color changes, cold intolerance, and skin changes. Before detailed questioning, it is important to determine whether the symptoms are unilateral or bilateral. In addition, the patient's age, handedness, occupation, and work history should be noted.[49]

Pain is present in two thirds of patients with upper extremity vascular disease. Callow[14] notes that sudden arterial occlusion causes pain that is severe and abrupt in onset, but vasospasm may produce only mild paresthesias and marked pallor. Pain with exertion that is relieved by rest is most indicative of an obstructive arterial problem. In contrast, pain at rest may indicate severe arterial insufficiency, although it also could be symptomatic of a neurologic, bony, or bursal pathologic condition.

Color changes may be part of the "triple response" or Raynaud's phenomenon. Ischemic pallor usually is followed by cyanotic coloring, and a reactive erythema marks the return of flow. Cyanotic coloring also may occur in longstanding venous obstruction or insufficiency. Cold intolerance can manifest as a heightened sensitivity to cold climates, the winter months, or even the refrigerated sections of the grocery store. The patient may complain of mild to severe pain that is relieved when the extremity is warmed. Digital stiffness after exposure to cold also can indicate vascular disease. Thus it is important to obtain a history of the patient's response to cold exposure. Skin complaints include changes in nail shape (clubbing) or quality (pitting). Skin atrophy often occurs in patients with scleroderma and may result in ulcerations either at the tips of the digits or over the extensor surfaces of the interphalangeal joints.

The examiner should establish whether the patient has a history of limb trauma, swelling, a mass, associated lower extremity symptoms, or nonspecific symptoms of numbness and paresthesias. Significant medical conditions such as diabetes, renal failure, inflammatory arthritis, or collagen-vascular disease should be noted, because they may be associated with vascular problems. Cigarette smoking, alcohol intake, and illicit injection of recreational drugs also may have a bearing on the patient's condition. Often, the patient will be too embarrassed or unwilling to respond to inquiries about lifestyle choices that may explain otherwise puzzling symptoms. The patient should be assured that the information will not be used to prosecute him or her and that it is vital in reaching the correct diagnosis and choosing the appropriate treatment. Finally, questions about family history often will reveal that relatives have experienced similar symptoms, especially when Raynaud's phenomenon is suspected. Additional history may be obtained during the physical examination.

Physical examination for suspected vascular disease should follow the general principles of inspection, palpation, auscultation, and special testing. Again, the patient with acute ischemia may require a comprehensive but abbreviated examination before emergency radiologic or surgical procedures are performed. Chronic symptoms allow an examination that is more complete and detailed.

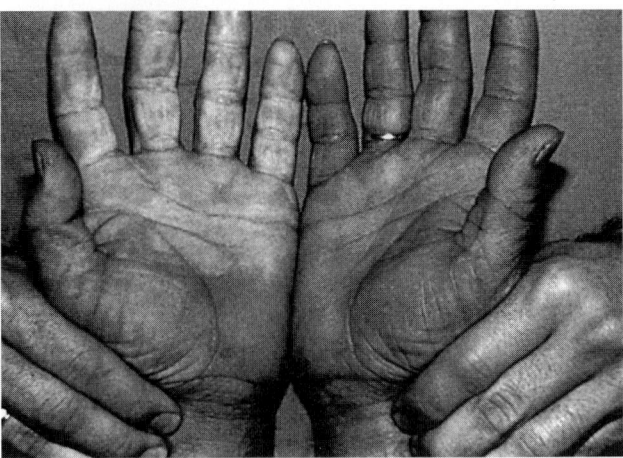

Fig. 52-2. When the Allen's test was performed in this patient with artery thrombosis, the hand remained pale when compression on the ulnar artery was released.

The complete vascular examination should be performed in a warm room to prevent inadvertent vasospasm, and the patient should wear a gown that allows access to both upper extremities. The examination should be performed on both extremities, even if the symptoms are unilateral. Gross inspection will demonstrate skin texture changes as well as frank ulcerations and tissue necrosis. Color changes consistent with cyanosis may indicate chronic venous insufficiency, and dilated distal veins in an edematous extremity may indicate proximal obstruction. Cold stimulation may trigger the color changes of Raynaud's phenomenon. The axillary, brachial, radial, and ulnar pulses should be palpated throughout the entire extremity. The carotid pulse may be affected in proximal arterial disease. Masses are palpated for thrills, pulsations, or tenderness. Auscultation of vessels and masses may demonstrate bruits.

One important and relatively simple test to perform is the Allen's test. First described by Allen[1] in 1929, this test has many variations. The most common one involves simultaneous compression of the ulnar and radial arteries while the hand is exsanguinated by opening and closing the fist. Pressure over the radial artery is released, and the return of flow to the palm and digits is observed. Compression of the ulnar artery is then released, and further changes are noted. The test is then repeated, releasing pressure on the ulnar artery first (Fig. 52-2). The test results are considered abnormal when reflow to all or part of the hand takes more than 7 seconds; this indicates inadequate flow secondary to obstruction or vascular anomaly. Allen's test of the digital arteries may be useful in evaluating digital vessel flow, in which case palpation can be supplemented with various objective methods such as laser Doppler flowmetry and pressure manometry to measure return of flow.[46]

During the initial evaluation, physical examination of the extremity should be supplemented by segmental pressure measurements and Doppler studies. Proximal obstruction

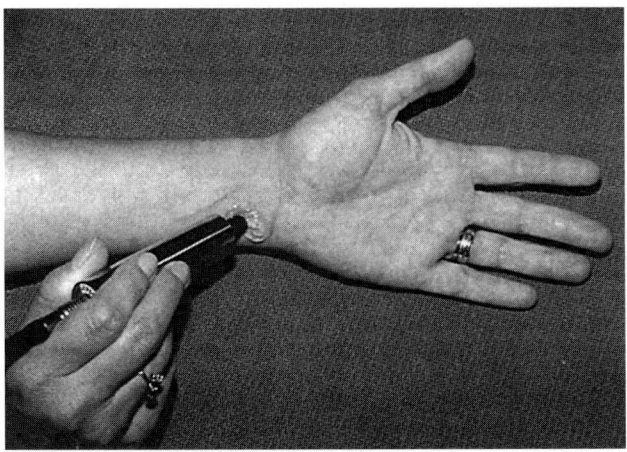

Fig. 52-3. Doppler examination allows quick and accurate mapping of the major arteries.

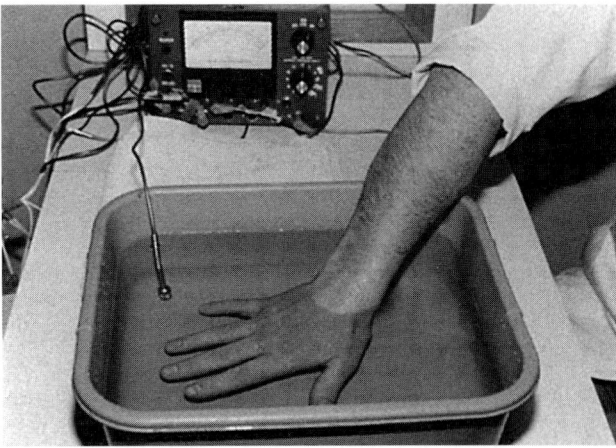

Fig. 52-4. Cold stress testing is useful in evaluating patients with vasospastic disorders.

may be detected by the use of a simple blood pressure cuff. Systolic blood pressure is measured in both arms at the antecubital level. A side-to-side difference of more than 15 mm Hg or a ratio of less than 0.96 is considered abnormal and indicates obstruction proximally.[73] Cuffs may be placed on the upper arm, forearm, and digits to identify obstruction as low as the palmar arch.

Perhaps the most useful supplement to the physical examination is Doppler ultrasonography (Fig. 52-3).[71] A special probe is used that transmits high-frequency ultrasonic signals (10 MHz for upper extremity testing), which are reflected off the patient's blood; the movement of fluid and cells causes a change in the frequency of the transmitted signal known as the Doppler effect. After the reflected signal is processed, it is projected as an audible signal or visible waveform. To administer the examination, special conducting gel is applied to the skin followed by the probe, which is positioned at a 45- to 60-degree angle and manipulated until the strongest signal is obtained. Normal arterial signals consist of a triphasic sound: a high-pitched peak during systole, a fall in pitch during diastole, and then a short increase in pitch before the next systole. Venous sounds are lower in pitch and vary with respirations. Abnormal signals have characteristic audible and waveform changes and can be used to identify the location and nature of the problem. For example, a stenotic arterial segment has relatively fast flow with a resultant high-pitched Doppler signal. The Doppler also may be used to map the location of normal or variant arterial anatomy before surgery and as an adjunct to the Allen's test in patients in whom pulses are difficult to palpate.

Noninvasive testing

Noninvasive testing in the vascular laboratory is the most significant development in the screening and evaluation of patients with vascular disorders. Initially developed to evaluate lower extremity problems, the vascular laboratory

has been applied only recently to disorders of the upper extremity.

One of the most common tests performed in the vascular laboratory is segmental pressure monitoring. As mentioned previously, segmental pressures can be obtained at the level of the arm, forearm, or digit. Serial measurements can be obtained quickly with serial pressure cuffs and accurate ratios can then be calculated to screen for obstructive disease.[13] It is also possible to recalculate segmental pressures after exercise stress testing; this may reveal subclinical obstructive disease that causes symptoms only after activity.

Digital plethysmography, or pulse volume recording (PVR), uses a strain gauge or photo sensor that measures changes in the volume of the digit with each pulse. Normally, this change is expressed as a linear tracing that defines the relative difference in volume between pulse waves. Normal tracings show a sharp systolic upslope followed by a dip that has been termed the *dicrotic notch,* and then the sequence is terminated with a less sharp downslope.[74] In the tracing of an obstructed pulse, the normal upsweep is delayed and has a less acute slope; the peak is often rounded, and the downslope is longer and away from the baseline. PVRs may be obtained under stress conditions.

PVR has been shown to correlate well with arteriographic findings.[5,20] It does not localize lesions or provide absolute values that enable comparison of results between patients. Thus it may be most useful as a screening tool or for monitoring a patient to evaluate the results of treatment. Most studies agree that PVR should be used in conjunction with other noninvasive modalities.

Cold stress testing was developed by Koman et al.[44] to evaluate the upper extremity in patients who suffer from cold intolerance or possible vasospasm (Fig. 52-4). In this test, skin temperature probes that have been placed on each digit are monitored before, during, and after brief exposure to a cold stress, usually an ice-water bath. The baseline measurements provide an index of resting blood flow, and the temperature change after exposure is a measurement of the vascular response to the stress. The temperature curve after the stress is withdrawn reflects the return of blood flow. Patients with a vasospastic disorder may demonstrate lower baseline temperatures, more dramatic temperature decreases after exposure, and prolonged recovery periods. Cold stress testing after sympathetic blockade has been used to predict the outcome of surgical sympathectomy for relief of vasospasm.[83] Laser Doppler flowmetry,[65] capillaroscopy,[34] and transcutaneous oxygen–tension monitoring are among other noninvasive techniques that have been used to evaluate blood flow in the upper extremity. All of these methods are safe and effective screening tools for vascular disorders and can be performed in a short amount of time.

Diagnostic imaging

The radiographic evaluation of patients with suspected vascular problems includes plain films and arteriography.[78] New modalities such as radionuclide imaging,[54] duplex ultrasonography,[19] and magnetic resonance (MR) imaging[33] also are used and represent some noninvasive alternatives to angiography.

All evaluations of vascular problems should include plain film radiographs of the hand (Fig. 52-5). In cases of suspected vascular compression in the neck, films of the cervical spine also are obtained. Radiographs of all masses should be obtained and assessed for the presence of calcifications, which often accompany vascular tumors. Radiographs also will delineate the extent of bony involvement before resection of invasive arteriovenous malformations.

Until recently, contrast studies have been the primary radiographic means of evaluating vascular disorders of the upper extremity. Most often, arteriography is performed via cannulation of the femoral artery. The catheter is threaded retrograde to the level of the subclavian or axillary artery, depending on the desired level of study. Contrast material— usually an iodine-containing radiopaque liquid—is injected proximally, and serial radiographs of the extremity are then taken. This technique allows complete evaluation of the vascular tree (Fig. 52-6, *A*). Digital subtraction arteriography is a newer technique that eliminates background tissues to enhance visualization of the vessels. Venography is performed after catheterization of a peripheral vessel to the superior vena cava.

Angiography is a very sensitive and specific means of detecting most vascular disorders of the upper extremity. Atherosclerotic, embolic, aneurysmal, and inflammatory diseases are well visualized with this modality. Traumatic injuries, including lacerations and intimal damage, also can be detected by angiography. Feeder vessels in arteriovenous malformations can be localized for surgical excision. Angiography also has been used to establish the vascular supply to injured and donor tissue when a free tissue transfer (Fig. 52-6, *B*) or tumor excision (Fig. 52-6, *C* and *D*) is planned.

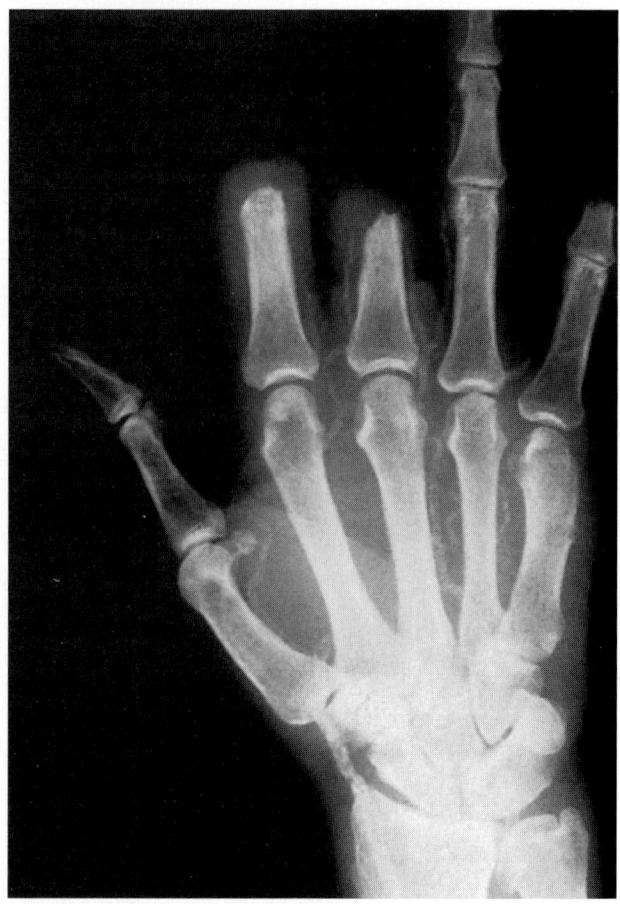

Fig. 52-5. Radiograph demonstrating calcification of the arterial system in a patient receiving renal dialysis. The patient developed gangrene in multiple digits secondary to inadequate perfusion.

Contrast angiography is not without complications.[32] The catheter itself must be placed in a relatively large vessel, from which significant hemorrhage may occur. Likewise, the catheter may injure the vessel lumen and cause postangiographic ischemia. Injection of iodinated contrast material has been associated with refractory vasospasm, thus vasodilators often are given before contrast injection. The contrast material itself has been implicated in postangiographic renal failure and, in some cases, anaphylactic reaction.

Newer angiographic technology has lowered the complication rate. The use of contrast agents that have low toxicity or are nontoxic has reduced reactions; also, less of the agent is needed when digital subtraction arteriography is performed, because this technique does not require as much contrast agent to produce an acceptable image.[12] Interventional angiography also has become popular as a therapeutic application of technology that once was used for diagnosis only. The best-known intervention is balloon angioplasty. Originally developed for coronary artery dilation, this technique has been successfully applied to the upper extremity.[82] Transcatheter infusions of thrombolytic agents for acute thrombotic and embolic disease of the upper extremity have

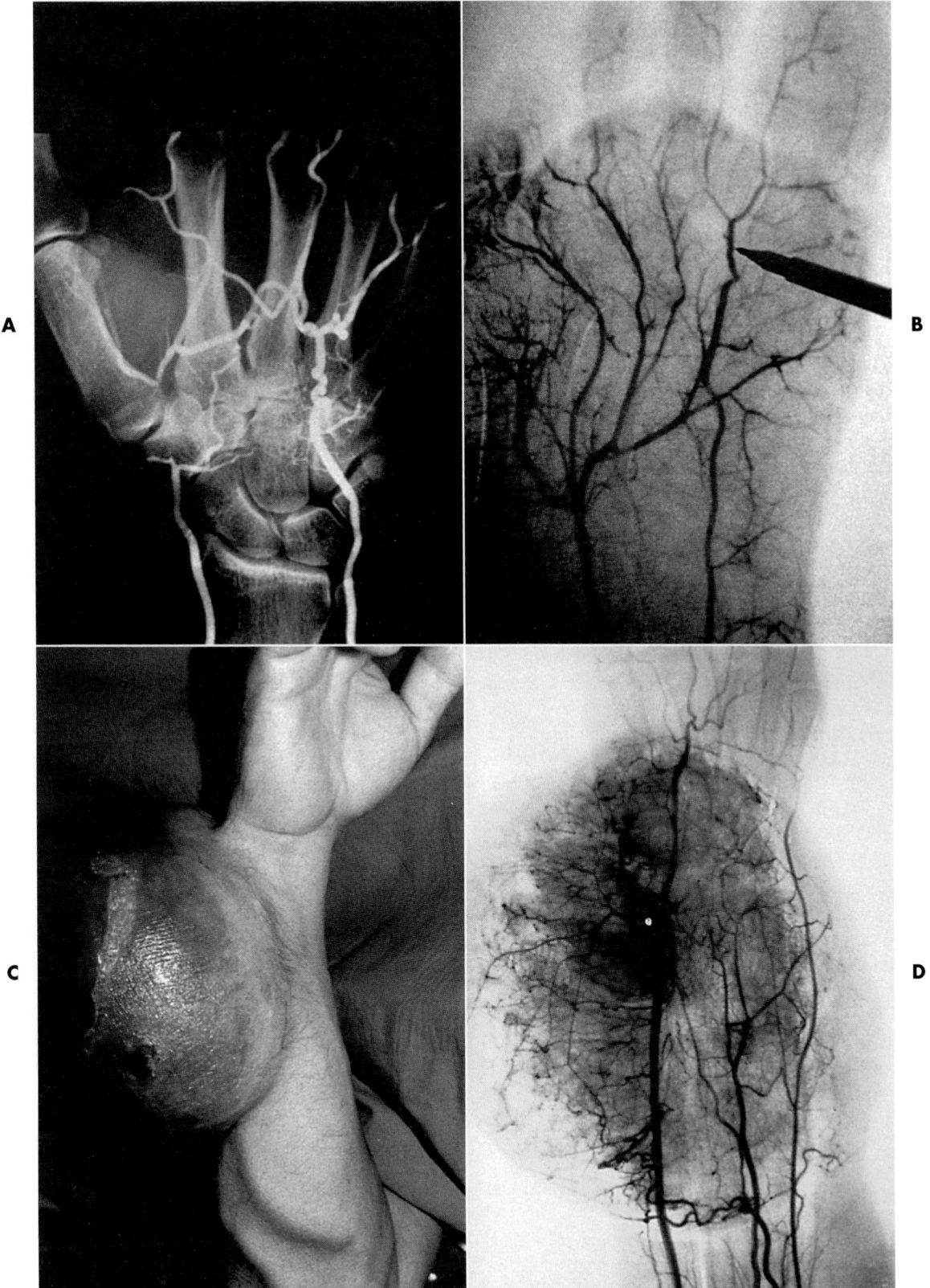

Fig. 52-6. The vascular anatomy can be visualized using angiography. **A,** Normal appearance of the hand and wrist. **B,** The vascular supply to the foot is seen before toe-to-hand transfer. **C** and **D,** Gross and angiographic appearance of a large forearm mass. The latter was used to determine the surgical margin necessary for resection.

been performed.[84] Finally, selective embolization of feeder vessels in arteriovenous malformations has been performed as a definitive preoperative treatment for the reduction of intraoperative blood loss during planned definitive excision.

Radionuclide imaging, commonly called *bone scan,* is another traditional method of evaluating suspected vascular conditions. Injection of a small amount of contrast material, usually ^{99m}Tc-labeled diphosphonate-1, is followed by three separate scans that provide dynamic information about perfusion of the extremity. Immediate scanning provides both arterial and venous angiograms, and delayed scanning provides information on the overall metabolic activity of the limb. Scanning is especially useful in cases in which sensitivity is required but fine resolution is not. Circumstances of this kind are encountered when determining the level of tissue viability after replantation or after an insult such as frostbite.[58] Perhaps the best-known use of three-phase scanning in hand surgery is in the assessment of RSD. Although this condition is not entirely a vascular disorder, it can demonstrate characteristic changes on three-phase scanning, such as diffusely increased uptake on delayed imaging.[57]

Duplex ultrasonography is a newer technique that uses traditional ultrasound technology to provide a detailed assessment of the upper extremity vasculature. It has the ability to provide images comparable in detail with those obtained in angiography. This method has several advantages. The procedure is noninvasive, inexpensive, and portable; requires minimal setup; and can be performed quickly. However, it lacks the invasive advantages of angiography. The procedure uses B-mode imaging, which is a more complex ultrasound technique. This application of Doppler ultrasound technology produces detailed images of the vascular tree in real time with color coding for different flow directions and velocities. The vessels may be scanned in cross section or longitudinally. The technique is applicable to both intraluminal and vessel-wall pathologic conditions. Newer contrast agents are being tested to enable this technique to be applied to microvascular procedures. Currently, vessels as small as 0.5 mm can be visualized.

MR arteriography, a new application of MR technology, is a noninvasive means of imaging vascular disorders that was made possible by improvements in imaging sequences and in the coils used to enhance contrast. In addition, gadolinium intravenous (IV) contrast has been used to enhance the resolution of small vessels. One great advantage of MR arteriography is that it enables the perivascular tissues to be examined for abnormalities—a capability that is especially useful when evaluating vascular masses. It is also the only modality that can view the image from any projection after it has been recorded. Its disadvantages include the amount of time required to perform the study, the claustrophobic environment of the scanner, separation of the patient from the medical team in cases of life-threatening trauma, and its expense.

COMMON VASCULAR DISORDERS OF THE UPPER EXTREMITY
Penetrating and blunt injuries

Critical traumatic injuries of the upper extremity that involve the arterial system are those in which distal flow is disrupted completely with resultant limb-threatening ischemia. In patients with such damage, treatment consists of emergent exploration and repair of the injured vessels. In contrast, noncritical injuries can remain asymptomatic or manifest subtly, presenting as upper limb claudication with prolonged exercise or overhead activity. Penetrating injury is one of the most obvious types of traumatic damage and typically is encountered as a knife or gunshot wound or a wound suffered in an industrial or motor vehicle accident. In patients with such injuries, the following seven features indicate a possible vascular injury that requires evaluation or exploration: (1) loss of distal pulses, (2) pulsatile or profuse bleeding from the wound, (3) a large hematoma at the entrance or exit wound, (4) hypotension, (5) the presence of a bruit near the wound, (6) injury to a nerve in proximity to a known vessel, and (7) proximity of the wound to vascular structures.[67] Patients with any of these seven features require evaluation with Doppler ultrasonography, angiography, or surgical exploration. Recent studies comparing ultrasonic and angiographic imaging have shown that these two methods are comparable in diagnostic sensitivity and specificity.[4] Emergent surgical exploration is indicated if distal ischemia is present.

In cases of penetrating injury to the subclavian, axillary, or brachial artery, limb-threatening ischemia usually results despite the presence of collateral vessels. Early exploration and repair is indicated (Fig. 52-7). An interposition vein graft is necessary when vessels have retracted or when a wide zone of injury precludes primary repair. Injury to the peripheral nerves may accompany the vessel damage; therefore the surgeon should be prepared to repair these structures. Some controversy exists over the repair of "noncritical" arterial injuries in the forearm and hand. Several studies have attempted to predict the outcome based on repair of single-vessel lacerations in the forearm.[24,25,66] Current microvascular repair techniques achieve patency rates of 50% to 75%. The role of these repairs in preventing late claudication and cold intolerance is unknown. Results appear to be poorer in the presence of injury to a peripheral nerve.[24]

Blunt trauma also may produce vascular injury. Shoulder dislocations and proximal humeral fractures may interrupt the axillary artery, and fractures of the clavicle or first rib may injure the subclavian artery. In children, supracondylar humeral fractures may compress or lacerate the brachial artery. These injuries may be avulsions of the vessels with subsequent loss of distal perfusion. Intimal injuries lacking gross vessel disruption also may result in decreased distal perfusion. In all cases of combined proximal vascular and orthopedic injury, diagnosis of the vascular injury may be overlooked because of the more obvious bony or even

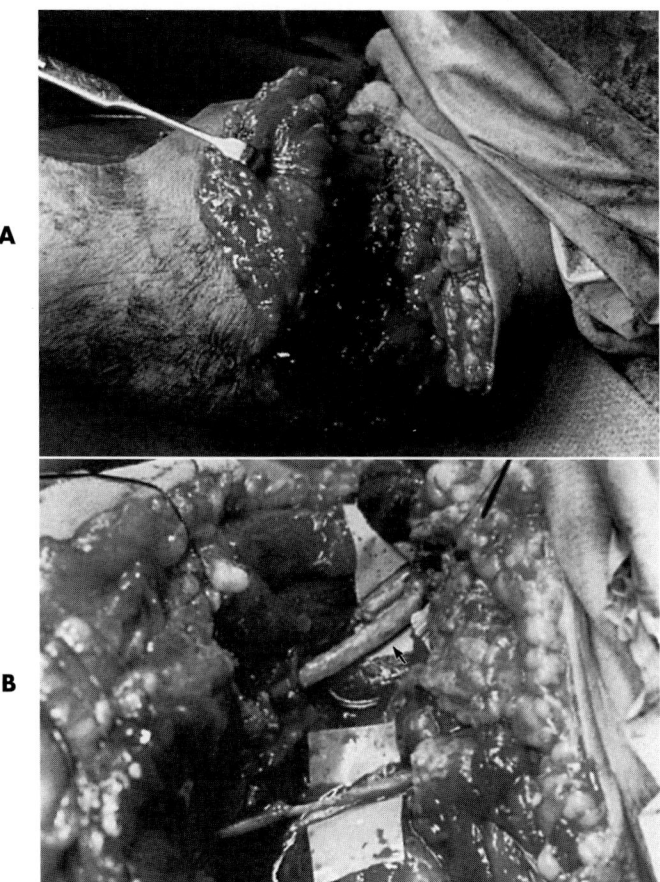

Fig. 52-7. A, This limb-threatening brachial artery laceration was sustained in a machete attack. **B,** Repair was accomplished using a reversed saphenous vein graft *(arrow).*

neurologic injury. Prompt assessment and treatment of the vascular injury may prevent limb loss, late aneurysm, or arteriovenous fistula formation. Stabilization of fractures should be performed at the same time as vessel repair to prevent further injury.

Compartment syndrome

Classically, compartment syndrome of the upper extremity is not defined by injury of the vascular system. However, it does involve a loss of perfusion of the forearm and muscles of the hand that can have potentially devastating results. Compartment syndromes result from a variety of traumatic insults, either blunt or penetrating. Crush injuries of the upper extremity are especially prone to develop this condition. Compartment syndrome also occurs after post-ischemic reperfusion of the upper extremity. Endothelial cell retraction during ischemia allows extravasation of large amounts of fluid within the enclosed fascial space, elevating interstitial pressure beyond tolerable limits.

Compartment syndrome is a clinical diagnosis that should be considered when swelling and pain in an extremity appear to exceed the amplitude of the initial injury. A well-known diagnosis mnemonic of compartment syndrome is the four P's: (1) *p*ain with passive muscle stretch, (2) *p*aresthesias, (3) *p*allor, and (4) *p*ulselessness. Pain and paresthesias are the most reliable indicators because excellent distal pulses and tissue color may exist with full-blown forearm compartment syndromes; however, the presence of these symptoms may be particularly difficult to determine in the patient who has a head injury or is intoxicated.

Several devices have been designed to measure tissue pressures. The classic construct by Whitesides et al.[81] is simple and can be made from readily available materials, but there are also newer and compact devices with digital readouts. Care must be taken to measure tissue pressures in all potentially involved parts of the upper extremity. There are 3 compartments in the forearm (the dorsal, volar, and mobile wad) and 10 in the hand. Each interosseous muscle, as well as the thenar, hypothenar, and adductor musculature, may be involved.

The tissue pressure above which compartment release should be considered is controversial. Normal tissue pressure is between 8 and 10 mm Hg. Critical pressures have been noted at levels 30 mm Hg below diastolic,[81] which translates into absolute values of 30 mm Hg[47] to 45 mm Hg.[53] Serial measurements or monitoring with indwelling wick catheters[61] have been advocated in borderline situations where clinical examination may be difficult. However, even though they are convenient, tissue pressure monitors should be used only in an adjunctive role in diagnosis because clinical suspicion and examination are the keys to proper treatment.

Compartment syndrome is treated by decompression (Fig. 52-8, *A* and *B*). Incisions should be extensive and provide for complete release of the involved muscle. Skin and fascia are incised along the entire length of the compartment. Often, the muscle will bulge into the open wound as a dusky mass, resuming normal color as it is allowed to escape from the restricted compartment. Release of the volar forearm—the most commonly involved compartment—should include the carpal tunnel and the proximal antebrachial fascia. After decompression, the wound is left open and covered with a sterile dressing.

The patient may require several inspections under general anesthesia to debride nonviable tissue and gain skin closure. As the swelling decreases, skin approximation may be facilitated by interweaving elastic vessel loops stapled to the skin edges and drawing the skin edges together without tension (Fig. 52-8, *C*). Skin grafting may be required for large defects. Return of function after decompression is excellent if surgery is performed early. However, if the condition goes unrecognized, severe fibrosis and contracture may result. If this is the case, then release, tendon transfers,[77] or perhaps free muscle transfer will be needed to restore minimal hand and forearm function.[52]

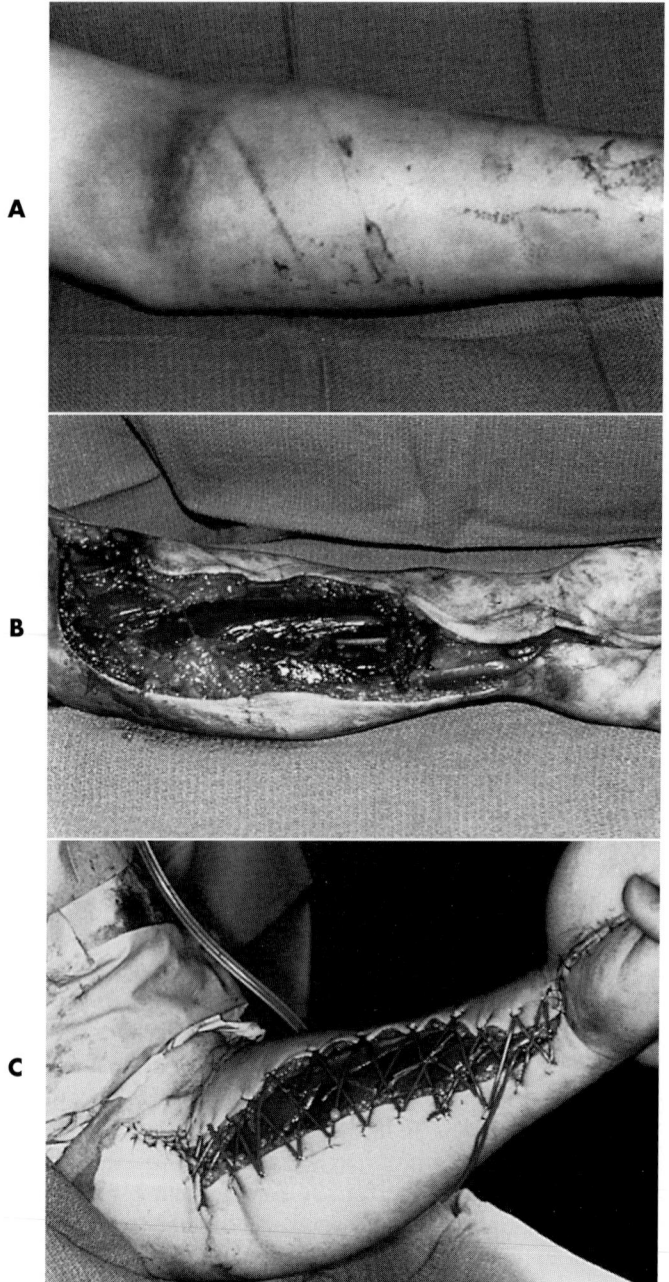

Fig. 52-8. A, This young woman developed compartment syndrome after an accident in which her car rolled over and pinned her forearm. **B,** Fasciotomy was performed. **C,** After the swelling receded, the wound was approximated using vessel loops stapled to the skin edges.

Cannulation injuries

Cannulation of upper extremity arteries is performed for diagnostic and monitoring purposes. For example, the brachial artery is often the site of catheter introduction for coronary angiography. Passage of the cannula may injure the vessel lumen and cause the formation of a clot or internal flap that intermittently obstructs distal flow. Complications of the brachial artery cannulation occur at rates of 1.0% to 1.5%[50]

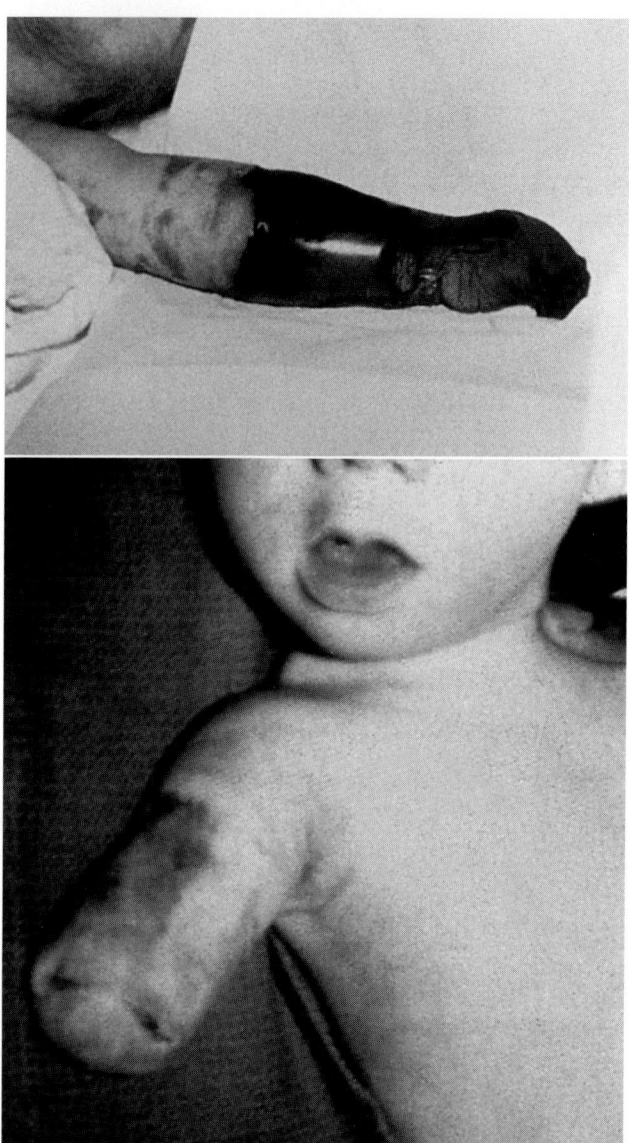

Fig. 52-9. A, After cannulation of the brachial artery, this child's arm became ischemic. **B,** Amputation above the elbow was necessary.

and may consist of acute ischemia distal to the catheter site (Fig. 52-9), fingertip embolization and gangrene, or even vague claudicatory pain. The diagnosis may be confirmed by Doppler examination as well as by alteration in segmental arterial pressures with a significant drop at the level of the injury.

Cannulation of the distal radial artery is the most common invasive arterial procedure because radial artery catheters are used for pressure monitoring and blood gas analysis. The

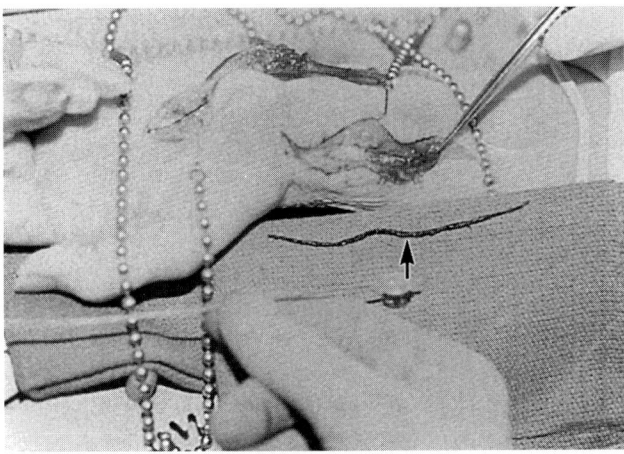

Fig. 52-10. Thrombosis of the radial and ulnar arteries occurred in this patient after multiple arterial cannulations, necessitating emergent exploration, thrombectomy *(arrow),* and vein grafting of the damaged arterial segments.

complications of radial artery cannulation include thrombosis (Fig. 52-10), infection, and aneurysm formation.[49] Thrombosis may lead to distal ischemia and possible thumb loss, but it usually can be prevented by the use of small-gauge Teflon catheters. Before the insertion of any catheter, an Allen's test must be performed to identify digits that may be at risk for ischemia. A positive test contraindicates catheter placement.

If ischemia develops after insertion of a radial artery catheter, the catheter should be removed immediately; this alone may restore flow. However, if flow is not improved, there are two options. Arteriography may reveal a thrombosed or vasospastic artery, and salvage of the digits with intraarterial thrombolytics or vasodilators may be achieved via the angiography catheter. Alternatively, surgical exploration of the vessel with embolectomy or resection and vein grafting may restore normal vascularity. Regardless, the patient should be administered anticoagulants after the procedure; heparin should be used for the first 5 to 7 days, followed by oral antibiotics or aspirin for approximately 1 month. If the patient's condition does not permit anticoagulation therapy, then axillary or peripheral catheters may be inserted for infusion of vasodilating agents. Infections or aneurysms of the radial artery may be asymptomatic. However, they also may be a source of distal emboli to the digits, which lead to digital ischemia and necrosis. Treatment involves resection of the affected vessel with direct anastomosis or vein graft interposition.

Cannulation of peripheral veins is less subject to complications. Peripheral IV infusions may lead to either a chemical or infectious thrombophlebitis that usually responds to symptomatic treatment with heat, moist wraps, and perhaps, antibiotics. Occasionally, surgical excision is required for a painful vessel that does not respond to supportive measures. Central venous cannulation also is

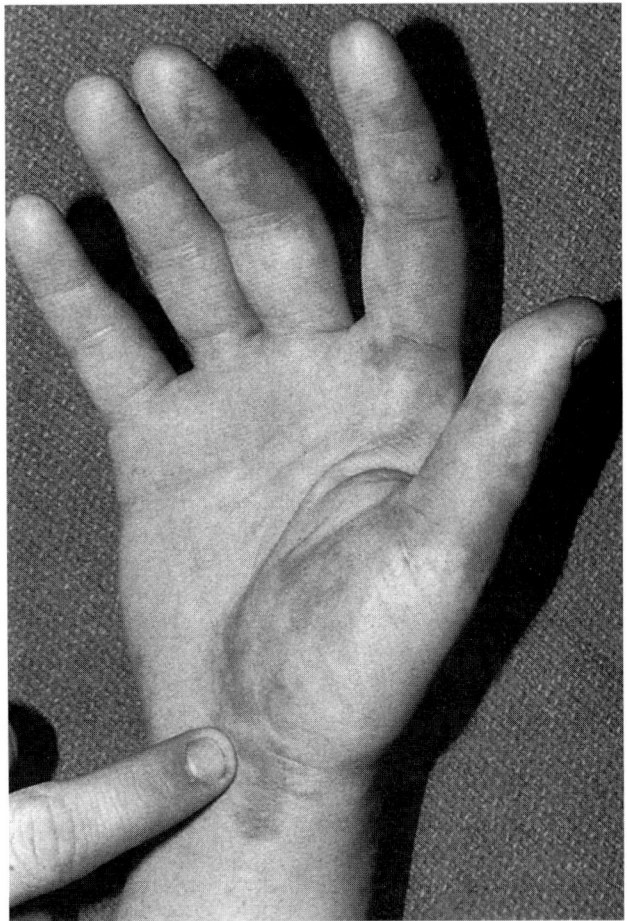

Fig. 52-11. In this patient, intraarterial injection of heroin led to digital skin loss in the region supplied by the radial artery.

performed routinely for monitoring or infusion and can lead to subclavian vein thrombosis. These thromboses may occasionally require heparin or thrombolytic drugs if severe upper extremity swelling or pulmonary embolism occurs. More often, withdrawal of the catheter allows for cannulation of the central veins and resolution of symptoms. Treatment is based on acuteness of the symptoms. Systemic heparinization, thrombolysis, thrombectomy, and even resection and grafting may be required to alleviate the symptoms.

Intraarterial injection

Accidental arterial injection commonly occurs during attempted IV administration of recreational drugs (Fig. 52-11), and it also may occur after inadvertent cannulation of an anomalous artery in the antecubital region. The hospitalized patient who presents with acute distal ischemia after injection must be suspected of accidental intraarterial injection.[22] After this event, a severe reaction develops whose pathophysiology is not completely understood. Three factors have been implicated. First, the particulate matter serves as an intraarterial embolism as it travels through and blocks the smaller arteries. Second, many drugs generate a chemical arteritis, which leads to arterial thrombosis. Finally, venous spasm and inflammation are caused by material passing through the capillary bed, resulting in proximal sludging and loss of digital inflow. The differential diagnosis includes other causes of acute ischemia, trauma, embolic disease, and Raynaud's phenomenon.

The symptoms of the outpatient who comes to the emergency department soon after the intraarterial injection may include severe burning pain, cyanosis, and tissue swelling, all of acute onset. A concise history may be difficult to obtain because of the patient's obtundance or unwillingness to admit drug use.[15] Charney and Stern[15] recently reported on five young patients with digital ischemia and gangrene who did not have the "appearance" of the typical IV drug user. These patients initially denied attempted self-injection despite their severe symptoms. Patients admitted the injections only after repeated questioning.

The treatment of acute intraarterial injection is somewhat controversial. Traditionally, supportive measures, including sympathetic blocks, intraarterial vasodilation, administration of thrombolytics, and anticoagulation, have been the mainstay of treatment. Arteriography and surgery are much less proven. However, during the acute period, it seems reasonable to perform arteriography, especially for localized areas of injury. If obstructive lesions are noted, attempts at thrombolysis or microarterial reconstruction are indicated. Diffuse injury carries a less favorable prognosis. In such cases, further supportive treatment is best and includes pain control, prevention of infection, and ultimately, amputation.

The patient who seeks treatment days to months after intraarterial injection presents a different clinical picture. In the most severe cases, the injection will result in irreversible ischemic changes, especially at the digital level. Again, supportive measures alone are indicated. Patients who have more proximal injection injuries of the brachial or forearm arterial structures and signs and symptoms of chronic ischemia, including cold intolerance, Raynaud's phenomenon, or claudication, should undergo noninvasive and arteriographic workup and microsurgical reconstruction if necessary.

Ulnar artery thrombosis

The patient who presents with ulnar wrist pain and paresthesias commonly has an entrapment neuropathy of the ulnar nerve at the wrist or elbow. Vascular disorders must be considered in cases where a palmar mass, symptoms of cold intolerance, or unilateral Raynaud's phenomenon are present. Ulnar artery thrombosis, also known as *hypothenar hammer syndrome*,[17] occurs most often in males who engage in manual labor where the palmar aspect of either hand is exposed to repetitive trauma (Fig. 52-12, *A*). This entity was first described by Von Rosen[79] in 1934, yet it is often overlooked in the differential diagnosis. Koman and Urbaniak[43] reviewed 28 patients with proven ulnar artery thrombosis and found that the correct diagnosis was made on initial examination in only half of the patients.

The diagnosis is missed primarily because of the nonspecific presenting symptoms, which usually consist of pain on the ulnar side of the hand. This pain is worsened by pressure over the course of the ulnar artery. It may be intermittent and dull, but it also may progress to severe pain at rest if the arterial thrombosis decreases digital blood flow to a significant degree. Digital ulcers or frank gangrene may develop if the thrombosis is left untreated at this stage. Cold intolerance with symptoms of Raynaud's phenomenon occurs routinely. Of the patients in the study by Koman and Urbaniak,[43] 80% experienced discomfort in cold weather or while holding a cold object.

Symptoms of ulnar-nerve compression commonly occur in hypothenar hammer syndrome. The ulnar nerve may be compressed either by the expansion of the arterial wall caused by the clot or by a small aneurysm in the arterial wall. Usually, there are sensory symptoms of numbness in the ulnar digits without motor involvement. However, other types of deficits also have been reported.[9]

Physical diagnostic maneuvers focus on evaluating the patency of flow to the hand as well as locating the thrombosis. In the study by Koman and Urbaniak,[43] all patients had a positive Allen's test at the wrist and delayed or nonexistent flow when pressure over the ulnar artery was released. Doppler examination demonstrates a decreased signal in the area of Guyon's canal and obliteration of the signal at the level of the superficial arch with compression of the radial artery. Digital plethysmography is abnormal in the ulnar digits, and transcutaneous oxygen measurements are decreased, especially in the presence of digital ulcers. Arteriography is usually unnecessary, because excellent real-time ultrasonic evaluation is now possible. Arteriography of the proximal arterial tree can be used to visualize a possible embolic cause and is helpful in cases where distal embolism of the fingers is suspected and microvascular reconstruction is planned (Fig. 52-12, *B*).

The treatment of ulnar artery thrombosis may be purely supportive in patients who have no digital ischemia or signs of nerve compression and can avoid further trauma to the ulnar side of the wrist. In contrast, severe pain and digit-threatening ischemia should be treated urgently with stellate ganglion blocks, vasodilators, or surgical exploration and reconstruction. Intraarterial thrombolytic therapy has been performed successfully in patients with acute extension of the clot into the palmar arch. However, the chances of recurring thrombosis are high, and the patient may require surgery if that occurs.[39]

In most patients with chronic symptomatic ulnar artery thrombosis, resection of the involved vessel may relieve local pain and decompress the ulnar nerve. If poor backflow occurs with release of the distal arterial segment, microvascular reconstruction with a vein graft is indicated (Fig. 52-12, *C* and *D*). According to Koman and Urbaniak,[43] if the

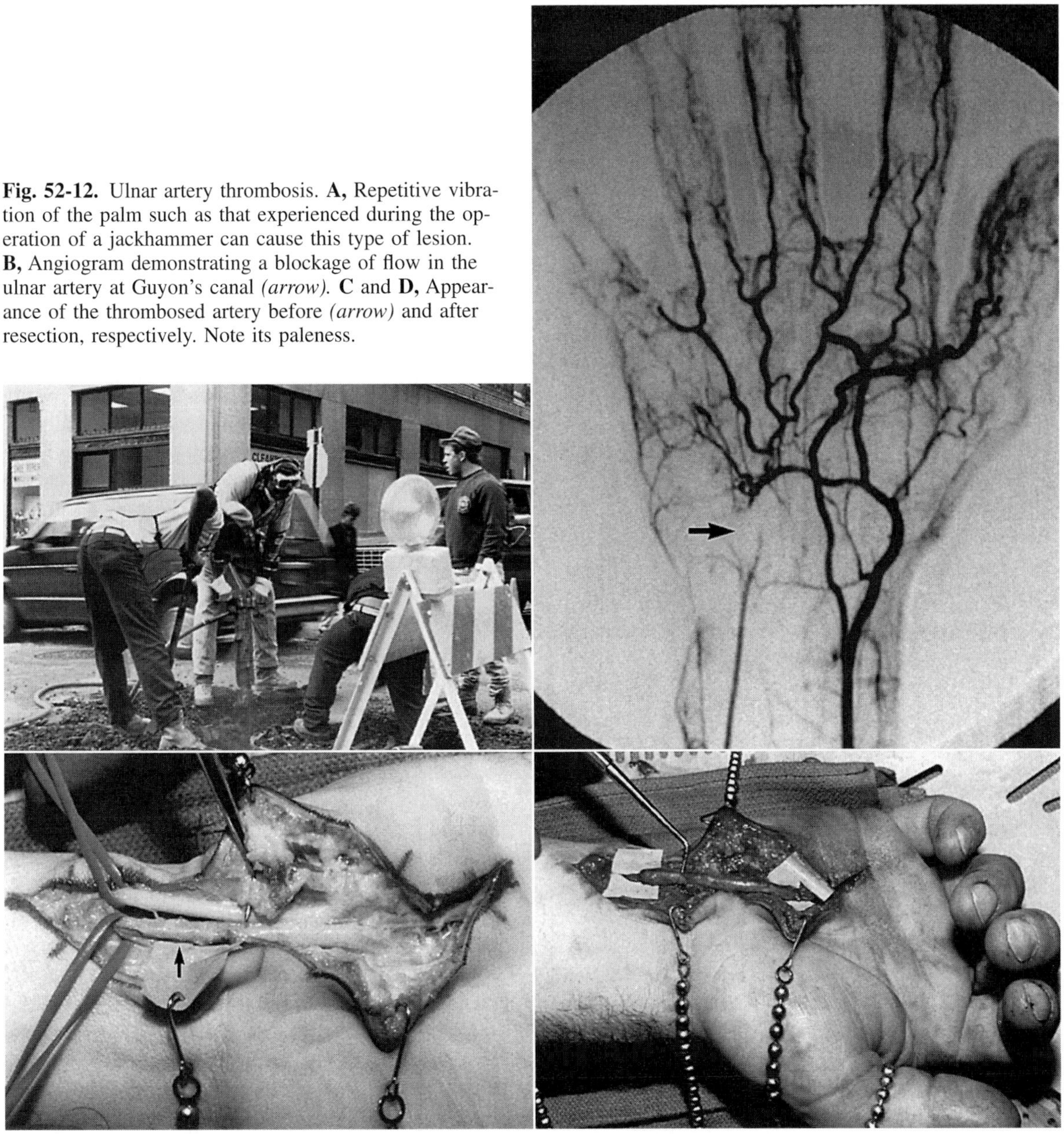

Fig. 52-12. Ulnar artery thrombosis. **A,** Repetitive vibration of the palm such as that experienced during the operation of a jackhammer can cause this type of lesion. **B,** Angiogram demonstrating a blockage of flow in the ulnar artery at Guyon's canal *(arrow)*. **C** and **D,** Appearance of the thrombosed artery before *(arrow)* and after resection, respectively. Note its paleness.

patient smokes, he or she must agree to quit smoking before reconstruction. The results of resection with or without reconstruction are generally good. Most patients resume normal activity, although they may retain some cold intolerance.

Vascular thoracic outlet syndrome

Vascular compression at the thoracic outlet represents only 3% of all thoracic outlet problems and may be arterial (1%) or venous (2%) in origin.[70] It can have a variety of causes ranging from congenital fibromuscular bands to fracture callus. Claudication, especially with overhead activity, is the primary symptom. Distal embolization and unilateral Raynaud's phenomenon also may occur and lead

to digital ischemia and gangrene. Venous obstruction may cause intermittent or persistent extremity edema. Both arterial and venous compression may be accompanied by symptoms of neurologic compression. These symptoms may be vague, so problems of the cervical spine or shoulder and peripheral-nerve compression must be considered in the differential diagnosis.

Provocative testing for vascular compromise includes the elevated arm stress test, wherein the patient holds his or her arms elevated, abducted, and externally rotated to narrow the thoracic outlet (Fig. 52-13). Overhead activity is simulated by rapidly opening and closing the hands. Vascular compression may be evidenced by muscular aching, which signifies inadequate arterial inflow. Paradoxically, venous

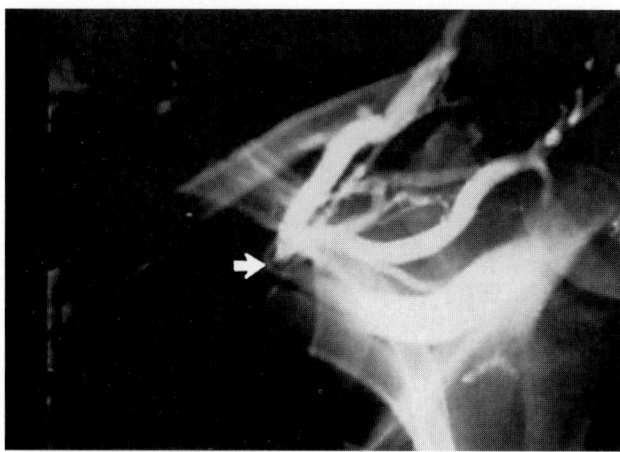

Fig. 52-13. Venogram of the abducted shoulder in a patient with vascular thoracic outlet syndrome. Occlusion of the subclavian vein is evident *(arrow)*.

obstruction may result in dilation of the venous vasculature with elevation of the arm. Other tests, such as the Adson test, are less reliable because normal subjects may exhibit pulse diminution. Conversely, decreased pulse characteristics may be absent in patients with angiographic evidence of vascular occlusion. Ultrasonography and contrast angiography can help confirm the diagnosis if they show significant flow decreases when the arm is elevated from the dependent position.

The treatment of vascular compression parallels that of neurogenic thoracic outlet syndrome. Posture and stretching exercises may alleviate mild symptoms. For more severe symptoms, especially those stemming from distal embolization, operative excision, thrombolysis, and possible vessel grafting are indicated. The technique of thoracic-outlet decompression is well described by Whitenack et al.[80] (see Chapter 42).

Vasospastic diseases

Unlike vascular trauma or thromboembolic problems, vasospastic diseases of the upper extremity have many different etiologies linked by common symptoms, Raynaud's phenomenon. The clinical signs of classic Raynaud's phenomenon consist of a triad of cutaneous skin color changes in response to cold stimulation or stress: one or more fingers turn black or white, indicating complete lack of arterial inflow to the digit; then, the fingers gradually turn dusky blue or purple as deoxygenated blood pools in the affected digits; finally, as flow is restored, a red flush occurs that is characteristic of reactive hyperemia. Although this pattern is typical of Raynaud's phenomenon, not all patients will manifest the triphasic color changes, and any patient with complaints of "white fingers" or "cold sensitivity" should be evaluated for a vasospastic condition. Pain, especially severe pain, is not as common as are the color changes. Most patients who report pain

with Raynaud's changes describe a dull aching feeling during the "attack" and/or "pins and needles" as flow is reestablished.

Interestingly, Raynaud's phenomenon is not a purely vasospastic problem. In 1862, the French physician Raynaud described this condition in 25 patients and attributed its cause to overactivity of the then recently described sympathetic nervous system.[68] In fact, most cases involve constriction of the digital arteries. Conditions in which proximal obstruction exists may reduce baseline flow to the point at which normal physiologic vasoconstrictive responses to cold produce the symptoms of Raynaud's phenomenon. Likewise, an increase in blood viscosity may decrease flow rates and result in digital pallor after a normal sympathetic response to stress. Thus the scope of Raynaud's attacks is broadened to include not only sympathetic overdrive but also the complex interplay between local factors and general sympathetic tone.

Raynaud's phenomenon is the term used to describe the pathophysiologic event of loss of arterial inflow to the digits. If a diagnostic workup reveals any of the myriad conditions associated with vasospasm, the patient has Raynaud's phenomenon. If no other problems are found, the patient has Raynaud's disease. Raynaud's disease, therefore, is idiopathic Raynaud's phenomenon. In 1932, Allen and Brown[2,3] established minimal criteria for diagnosing Raynaud's disease: bilaterality of symptoms; absence of gangrene; absence of other primary disease, especially collagen-vascular diseases; and symptoms of at least 2 years' duration. Fingertip gangrene was later added to this list.[1]

Epidemiologic study of Raynaud's disease reveals that it most often affects women between the ages of 20 and 40 years, and it is more prevalent in colder climates. General population surveys in Scandinavia and northern Europe have found that as many as 20% to 30% of healthy people complain of cold intolerance and color changes.[76] Patients who initially present with Raynaud's disease may later develop symptoms of collagen-vascular disease. Likewise, any patient with unilateral Raynaud's attacks or digital ulceration proximal to the finger tip should be suspected of having a mechanical obstruction rather than Raynaud's disease.[11]

Raynaud's phenomenon has been associated with a multitude of primary causes, including inflammatory diseases such as rheumatoid arthritis. Ingestion of drugs such as ergot, which is used to treat migraine headaches, also may cause peripheral vasospasm. More recently, vibratory occupational trauma to the digits has been associated with Raynaud's phenomenon.[36] Indeed, 50% of people in occupations such as those involving jackhammer operation will report symptoms of Raynaud's phenomenon.[31] Similarly, vibration white finger disease is associated with 125-Hz vibrations.[36] Occlusive disorders that may result in reduced digital arterial pressure (e.g., atherosclerosis, thrombosis) should be considered in the differential diagnosis.

Classically, Raynaud's phenomenon is associated with collagen-vascular disease, particularly scleroderma. Of patients with scleroderma, 85% will manifest symptoms of Raynaud's phenomenon, and the attacks may be the presenting symptom in up to 50% of individuals with this diagnosis.[27] Scleroderma is associated with a constellation of problems, of which hand symptoms make up only a part. Thorough evaluation of the patient by an internist or rheumatologist should be performed after the diagnosis has been made.

The diagnostic evaluation of the patient with Raynaud's phenomenon should begin with a thorough history and physical examination. The stimuli of the attacks, the mechanisms by which they are relieved, and whether the symptoms are unilateral or bilateral should be ascertained during questioning. Smoking, drug, and family histories may suggest an alternative primary diagnosis. Physical examination begins with observation for skin and nail changes as well as skin ulcers. All pulses should be palpated for integrity. Pulse variations may occur with positional changes of the arm. Neurologic evaluation is needed to identify signs of peripheral-nerve compression. Doppler studies and the Allen's test may reveal proximal obstruction. Provocative tests, such as placing the hands under cold running water, are rarely indicated.

Laboratory studies should include a complete blood count, erythrocyte sedimentation rate, and tests for rheumatologic abnormality, such as the presence of rheumatoid factor and antinuclear antibodies. Other tests, such as complement level determination and protein electrophoresis, also may be needed for diagnosis. Radiographic evaluation should include bilateral plain films of the hand; in addition, any other films that are prompted by clinical suspicion should be obtained. Ultrasonography is a noninvasive technique that provides excellent visualization of the arterial tree. However, arteriography is still the most commonly used means of evaluating peripheral obstruction. Noninvasive cold testing is helpful in diagnosing Raynaud's attacks and in evaluating the effectiveness of treatment. Patients with Raynaud's symptoms experience an abnormal drop in digital temperature in response to cold stimulus and a prolonged recovery to baseline after the stimulus is removed.[42,44]

After a diagnosis has been made, treatment of the underlying problem may alleviate the Raynaud's symptoms. For example, removing a proximal obstruction may restore distal flow to a level that allows normal sympathetic function. If symptoms persist, three levels of intervention can be instituted. Behavioral therapy is the first level. Abstaining from vasoconstrictive medications, caffeine, and cigarette smoking may be difficult for the patient, but it can reduce symptoms by approximately 50%. Biofeedback training also has reduced Raynaud's attacks, especially in Raynaud's disease.[59] Medical treatment is based on the oral administration of vasodilatory medications. Currently, nifedipine is used most often to prevent vasospastic events.[69]

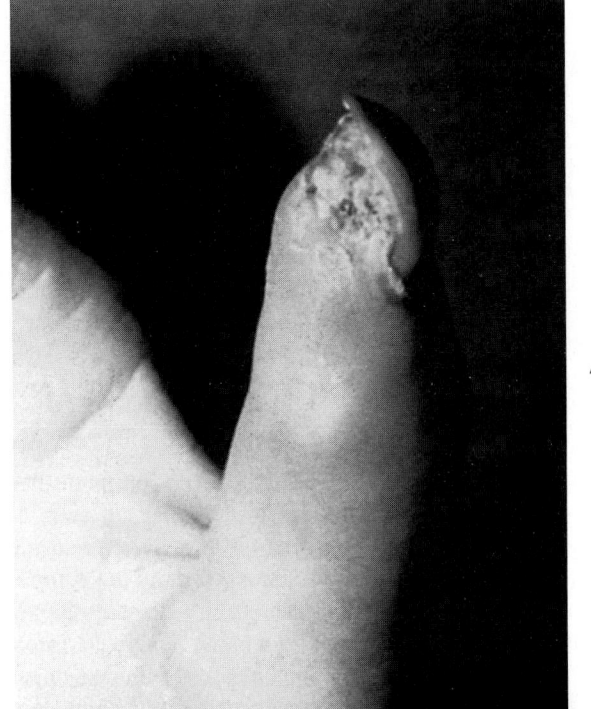

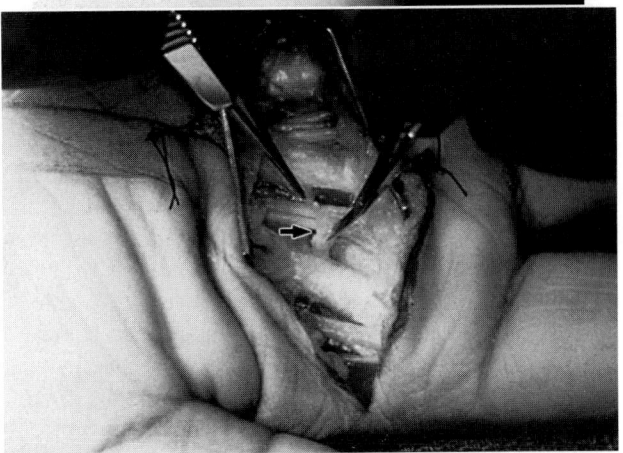

Fig. 52-14. A, This digital ulcer in a patient with Raynaud's syndrome healed after the administration of oral vasodilatory medications. **B,** Peripheral sympathectomy is achieved by excising the fine network of sympathetic nerves from the digital arteries *(arrow),* thus blunting the sympathetic vasospastic constriction of the vessels.

This medication is a calcium channel blocker and operates by inhibiting smooth muscle contraction in response to sympathetic stimulation. Nifedipine causes significant systemic side effects, the most common one being postural hypotension.

Digital ulcers will usually heal with conservative care (Fig. 52-14, *A*). Such care includes whirlpool use, gentle dressing changes, and the avoidance of provocative situations. Medical therapy with topical or systemic vasodilators also may aid healing. Debridements are limited to frankly

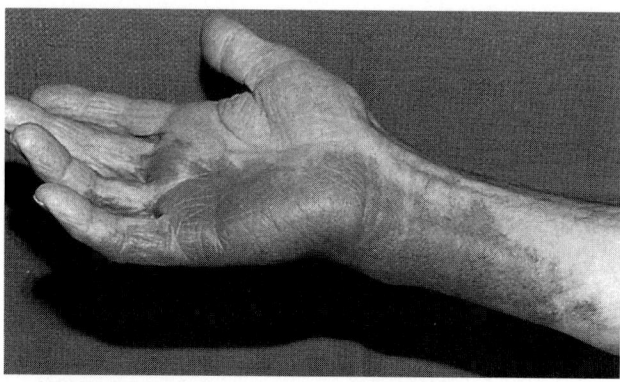

Fig. 52-15. Appearance of the capillary hemangioma, or "port wine stain."

necrotic segments to preserve as much digital length as possible. Appropriate antibiotics are given for localized infection. Occasionally, recalcitrant digital ulcers require sympathectomy or microvascular reconstruction. Ultimately, pain and necrosis may result in subtotal or total amputation.

When conservative treatments fail, surgical intervention is considered. Surgical management consists of sympathectomy or microvascular reconstruction. In the past, the standard procedure consisted of sympathectomy just peripheral to the spinal cord at the level of the cervical ganglia. However, the results were usually poor or transient, probably because of the alternative sympathetic pathways to the extremity. Digital sympathectomy has gained popularity since it was reported by Flatt in 1980.[21,59,83] Adventitial stripping of the common and digital vessels with separation of the connections between the nerve and artery have shown good results (Fig. 52-14, *B*). Postoperatively, patients experience relief of pain, ulcer healing, and an increased feeling of "warmth" in their fingers.[29] Currently, sympathectomy is indicated if local sympathetic blockade improves the response to stress such as exposure to cold. Microvascular reconstruction has become more popular since microsurgical techniques have improved.[40] Reconstruction is effective, especially in patients with localized disease at the level of the superficial arch or more proximally. Diffuse disease at the level of the distal arteries is not likely to be remedied by vein grafting.

Hemangiomas and vascular malformations

Vascular conditions that are found predominantly in children range from the relatively benign hemangioma to the debilitating high-flow arterial venous malformation. Traditionally used terms such as *port wine stain* (Fig. 52-15) and *cavernous hemangioma* are descriptive but do not reflect the true endothelial nature of the lesions. Current reports divide congenital vascular anomalies into two categories: hemangiomas and arteriovenous malformations.[62]

In 30% of cases, hemangiomas are present as red spots at birth; however, they grow rapidly, and 90% are visible by age

4 weeks. Their growth rate is initially worrisome but usually slows with time, and they eventually involute without treatment. Seventy percent fade, many of these completely resolving by age 7. Females are affected up to five times more often than males. Historically, the lesion demonstrates a hypertrophic endothelium with an increased number of mast cells. A mixture of fibrous and fatty tissue with minimal vasculature remains with involution.

Symptomatic treatment is recommended. Ulcerations are uncommon and are treated with supportive wound care. The size of the lesion also may be controlled by compressive garments. Large hemangiomas that are unresponsive to local measures may lead to high-output cardiac failure. For this type of lesion, locally injected corticosteroids may hasten involution. No clear mechanism has been delineated, but lowering of circulating serum estrogens has been proposed as a trigger for resorption. Occasionally, a large hemangioma must be excised surgically in infancy (Fig. 52-16).[55]

According to Mulliken and Glowacki,[62] vascular malformations that contain normal endothelial cells also are present at birth as hemangiomas. As these normal vessels in abnormal locations grow with the child, they become more apparent and manifest in either a high- or low-flow state. Low-flow malformations consist of superficial capillary disorders; these have previously been referred to as *port wine stains*. Other low-flow malformations include the venous malformation, or cavernous hemangioma; lymphatic malformations; and mixed vascular malformations. These lesions are slow growing and may either localize superficially in the dermis or be deep and diffuse. Both bony and soft tissue limb hypertrophy occurs and is more noticeable when the limb is in the dependent position. If the lesions are localized and small, supportive care may be sufficient. Larger, more diffuse lesions may be treated with compression, but surgical excision may be required if they are painful, and extensive debridement may be necessary. Preoperative evaluation with venography, color duplex ultrasonography, or MR angiography may be used to define the lesion. Prognosis in these cases is good.

Arterial or high-flow malformations are rare but potentially devastating congenital vascular problems. Patients have tissue hypertrophy with palpable thrills and audible bruits. Severe pain as a result of distal ischemia from shunting or compression neuropathy occurs in most cases. Ulceration and frank gangrene may develop (Fig. 52-17). Patients may experience high-output cardiac failure and manifest a significant decrease in pulse with compression of the feeder arteries (the Branham-Nicoladoni sign).[64]

Surgical management is the recommended treatment for large painful lesions. Preoperative arteriography with possible embolization of feeder arteries is required before surgery. Surgical excision, often in multiple stages with free tissue or skin grafts, may successfully eradicate the malformation. Simple ligation of the inflow vessels usually will not remedy the problem. Recurrence after an apparently suc-

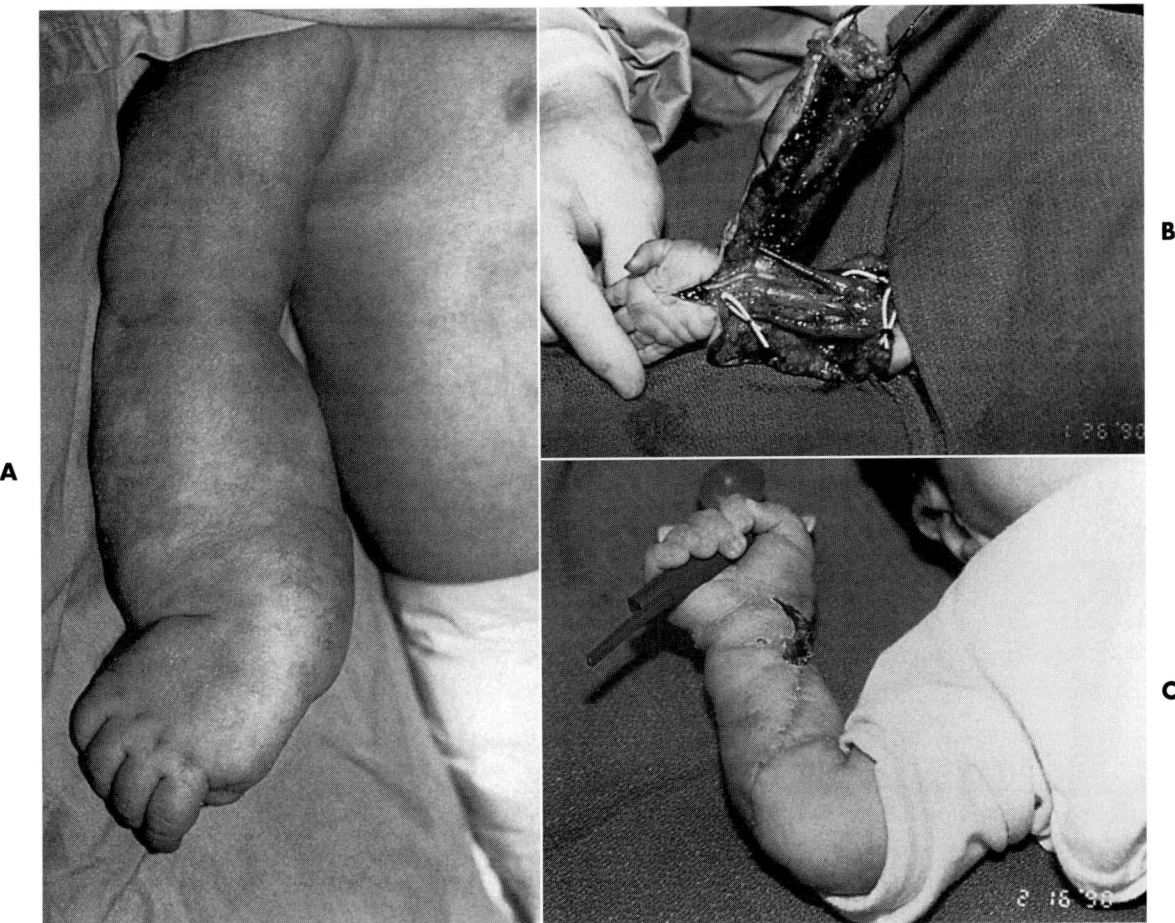

Fig. 52-16. This large hemangioma of the forearm in a 6-week-old infant led to high-output cardiac failure. **A,** Preoperative appearance of the lesion. **B,** Resection and skin grafting was performed. Postoperatively, the cardiac failure resolved and the patient had normal hand function. **C,** Postoperative appearance.

cessful extirpation also may occur. Ultimately, amputation of the extremity because of pain or severe ischemia may be necessary.[23]

Acquired arteriovenous fistulas

Acquired arteriovenous fistulas of the hand occur most often after a penetrating trauma. In contrast with pseudoaneurysm formation, where only arterial injury occurs, arteriovenous fistulas form after trauma to arterial and venous vessels that are in close proximity. An anomalous lumen forms between the vessels, creating a shunt proximal to the capillary bed; the result is distal ischemia or claudication and proximal venous dilation. Physical examination reveals a thrill or bruit. Ischemic pain may decrease with occlusion of either the arterial or venous feeder vessels. Diagnostic workup with color duplex ultrasonography or MR angiography will delineate the condition. Early excision allows vascular repair. Care must be taken to ligate all communicating vessels; otherwise, the fistula may recur.

Iatrogenic fistulas in the forearm and antecubital fossa used for access to renal dialysis have led to distal ischemia and tissue loss as well as compression neuropathy of the median and ulnar nerves. Early treatment, with either bending to reduce flow or revision to another site, alleviates this problem.[18,63]

Aneurysmal disease

Aneurysms of the upper extremity are rare and have been classified according to pathologic origin (trauma, infection, or atherosclerosis), wall consistency (true or false), and location (subclavian, ulnar, or digital artery). Traumatic aneurysms (Fig. 52-18, *A*) are the most common form of the disease; these lesions usually lack vessel-wall elements and, for that reason, are called *false aneurysms.*[47] True aneurysms (Fig. 52-18, *B*) have vessel walls with normal intima, media, and adventitia[6] and usually result from blunt trauma, atherosclerosis, or collagen diseases such as Marten's syndrome.

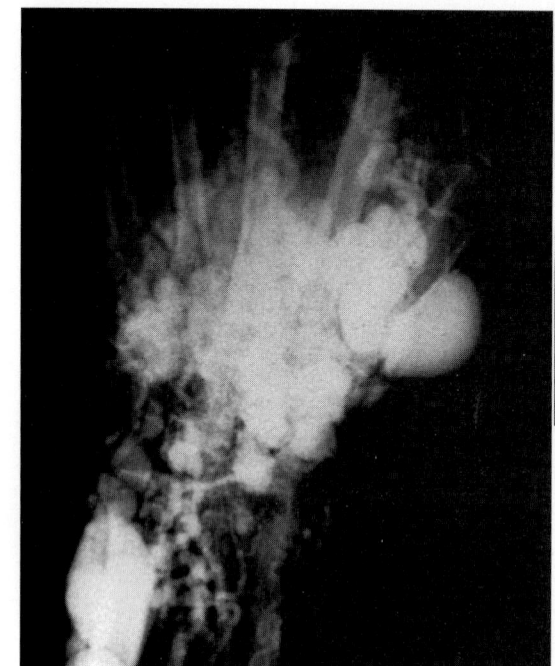

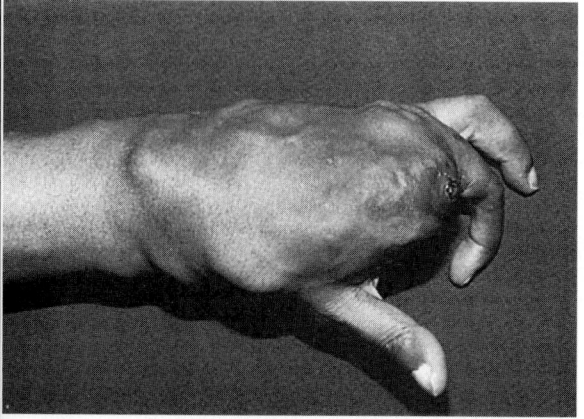

Fig. 52-17. A, Angiogram of an advanced arterial malformation. **B,** Progression of the malformation led to digital ischemia requiring amputation.

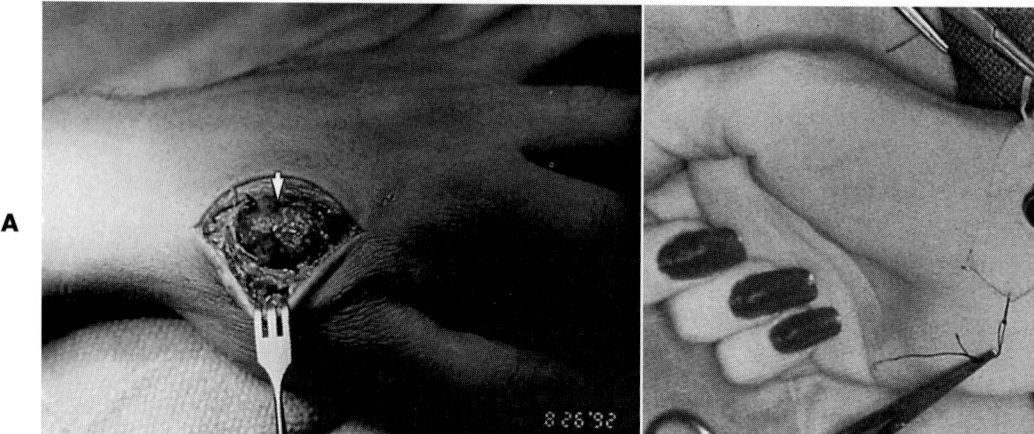

Fig. 52-18. A, This traumatic aneurysm *(arrow)* developed after a stabbing that injured the radial artery in the first web space. **B,** This true aneurysm of the radial artery developed after a blunt trauma.

An aneurysm presents most often as a mass. As such, all masses of the forearm must be palpated for thrills and auscultated for bruits. Doppler studies will improve the evaluation. Symptoms of distal embolization or nerve compression may be present, especially when the ulnar artery is involved.[41] The differential diagnosis of these masses includes ganglia, giant cell tumors, vascular tumors, and nerve tumors. Arteriography has been the traditional radiographic modality of choice for evaluating these masses, but noninvasive assessment has been possible since the advent of duplex ultrasonography.[55]

Asymptomatic masses are simply observed, especially when they occur at the digital level. More often, though, the aneurysm will cause local pain or shower distal emboli, in which case resection and vessel ligation are performed to relieve the symptoms.[75] Before ligation, the presence of adequate collateral flow must be confirmed by either preoperative Allen's testing or intraoperative plethysmography and backflow. Microvascular reconstruction with vein grafting is necessary when adequate collateral flow is not present.

REFERENCES

1. Allen EV: Thromboangiitis obliterans: methods of diagnosis of chronic occlusive arterial lesions distal to the wrist with illustrative cases, *Am J Med Sci* 178:237, 1929.
2. Allen EV, Brown GE: Raynaud's disease: a critical review of minimal requisites for diagnosis, *Am J Med Sci* 132:187, 1932.

3. Allen EV, Brown GE: Raynaud's disease affecting man, *Ann Intern Med* 5:1384, 1932.

4. Anderson RJ, et al: Reduced dependency on arteriography for penetrating extremity trauma: influence of location and noninvasive studies, *J Trauma* 30:1059, 1990.

5. Archic JP, Larson BO: Noninvasive laboratory evaluation of subclavian artery occlusion, *South Med J* 71:482, 1978.

6. Aulicino PL, Blatton PMI, DuPuy TEL: True palmar aneurysms: a case report and review of the literature, *J Hand Surg* 71A:613, 1982.

7. Backhouse KM: The blood supply of the arm and hand. In Tubiana R, editor: *The hand,* vol 1, Philadelphia, 1981, WB Saunders.

8. Barfred T, et al: Median artery in carpal tunnel syndrome, *J Hand Surg* 10A:246, 1985.

9. Benedict J, et al: The hypothenar hammer syndrome, *Radiology* 111:57, 1974.

10. Biasi F, et al: Arterial injuries of the upper extremities, *Cardiovasc Surg* 20:165, 1979.

11. Bonhoutsos J, et al: Unilateral Raynaud's phenomenon in the hand and its significance, *Surgery* 82:547, 1977.

12. Brady WR, et al: Intravenous arteriography using digital subtraction techniques, *JAMA* 48:671, 1982.

13. Bushner JW, Koontz CL: The examination in the vascular laboratory, *Hand Clin* 9:5, 1993.

14. Callow A: Vascular disorders of the upper extremity. In Jupiter J, editor: *Flynn's hand surgery,* Baltimore, 1991, Williams and Wilkins.

15. Charney MA, Stern PJ: Digital ischemia in clandestine intravenous drug users, *J Hand Surg* 16A:308, 1991.

16. Coleman SS, Anson BJ: Arterial patterns in the hand based on the study of 650 specimens, *Surg Gynecol Obstet* 113:409, 1961.

17. Conn JR, et al: Hypothenar hammer syndrome, *Surgery* 33:73, 1964.

18. Conolly JE, et al: Complications of dialysis access procedures, *Arch Surg* 119:325, 1984.

19. Dooley TW, Walsh CF, Puckett CL: Noninvasive assessment of microvessels with the duplex scanner, *J Hand Surg* 14A:670, 1989.

20. Downs AR, et al: Assessment of arterial obstruction in vessels supplying the fingers by measurements of local pressures and skin temperature response test: correlation with angiographic evidence, *Surgery* 77:530, 1975.

21. Flatt AE: Digital artery sympathectomy, *J Hand Surg* 5:550, 1980.

22. Gaspar MR: Acute arterial lesions due to drug abuse. In Haimo JH, editor: *Vascular emergencies,* New York, 1982, Appleton-Century.

23. Gelberman RH, Goldner JL: Congenital arteriovenous fistulas of the hand, *J Hand Surg* 3A:451, 1978.

24. Gelberman RH, et al: Forearm arterial injuries, *J Hand Surg* 5:401, 1979.

25. Gelberman RH, et al: The results of radial and ulnar arterial repair in the forearm, *J Bone Joint Surg* 64A:383, 1982.

26. Gelberman R, et al: The arterial anatomy of the human carpus. Part I: the extraosseous vascularity, *J Hand Surg* 8A:367, 1983.

27. Gifford RW Jr: Arteriospastic disorders of the extremities, *Circulation* 27:970, 1963.

28. Gilbert A: Anatomy of the lymphatics of the upper limb. In Tubiana R, editor: *The hand,* vol 1, Philadelphia, 1981, WB Saunders.

29. Gomis R: Segmental arterial sympathectomies in the fingers, *Ann Chir Main* 10:30, 1991.

30. Gonzales-Compta X: Origin of the radial artery from the axillary artery and associated hand vascular anomalies, *J Hand Surg* 16A:293, 1991.

31. Greenstein D, et al: Raynaud's phenomenon of occupational origin, *J Hand Surg* 16B:370, 1991.

32. Hassell SJ, Adams DF, Abrams HL: Complications of angiography, *Radiology* 138:273, 1981.

33. Holder LE, Marine DS, Yang A: Nuclear medicine, contrast angiography, and magnetic resonance imaging for evaluating vascular problems in the hand, *Hand Clin* 9:88, 1983.

34. Houtman PM, Wonde AA, Kellenberg CGM: The diagnostic role of nailfold microscopy, *Vasa* 5:21, 1987.

35. Huelke D: Variations in the origin of the axillary artery, *Anat Rec* 135:33, 1959.

36. Hywarianan J, Pyyleko I, Sundberg S: Vibration frequencies and amplitudes in the etiology of vasospastic diseases, *Lancet* 1:791, 1973.

37. Ikeda A, et al: Arterial patterns of the hand based on a three dimensional analysis of 220 hands, *J Hand Surg* 13A:501, 1988.

38. Jarrett F, Hirsch SA: Current diagnosis and management of upper extremity ischemia, *Surg Ann* 15:20, 1983.

39. Jelalien C, et al: Streptokinase in the treatment of acute arterial occlusion of the hand, *J Hand Surg* 10A:534, 1985.

40. Jones NF, et al: Microsurgical revascularization of the hand in scleroderma, *Br J Plast Surg* 40:264, 1987.

41. Kalisman M, Leborde IL, Wolff TW: Ulnar nerve compression secondary to ulnar artery false aneurysm at Guyon's canal, *J Hand Surg* 7:137, 1982.

42. Koman LA, Smith BP, Smith TL: Stress testing in the evaluation of upper extremity perfusion, *Hand Clin* 9:59, 1993.

43. Koman LA, Urbaniak JR: Ulnar artery insufficiency: a guide to treatment, *J Hand Surg* 6A:16, 1981.

44. Koman LA, et al: Isolated cold stress testing in the assessment of symptoms in the upper extremities. Preliminary communication, *J Hand Surg* 9A:305, 1984.

45. Leslie BM, et al: Digital artery diameters: an anatomic and clinical study, *J Hand Surg* 12A:740, 1987.

46. Levinsohn D, Gordon L, Sessler DI: The Allen's test, analysis of four methods, *J Hand Surg* 16A:279, 1991.

47. Louis DA, Simon MA: Traumatic false aneurysms of the upper extremity, *J Bone Joint Surg* 56A:176, 1979.

48. Lucas GL: The patterns of venous drainage in the digits, *J Hand Surg* 9A:448, 1984.

49. Machleder HI: Vasoocclusive disorders of the upper extremity, *Curr Probl Surg* 4:1, 1988.

50. Machleder HI, et al: Pulseless arm after brachial artery and catheterization, *J Hand Surg* 16A:166, 1990.

51. Malek R: Embryology of the hand. In Tubiana R, editor: *The hand,* vol 1, Philadelphia, 1981, WB Saunders.

52. Mantkelow RT: Functioning free muscle transfers. In Green DP, editor: *Operative hand surgery,* ed 3, vol 1, New York, 1993, Churchill Livingstone.

53. Matsen FA, Wilquist RA, Krugmir RB: Diagnosis and management of compartment syndromes, *J Bone Joint Surg* 62A:286, 1988.

54. Maurer AH: Nuclear medicine in the evaluation of the hand and wrist, *Hand Clin* 7:183, 1991.

55. McClinton MH: Tumors and aneurysms of the upper extremity, *Hand Clin* 9:115, 1993.

56. McCormack LJ, et al: Brachial and antebrachial arterial patterns, *Surg Gynecol Obstet* 96:43, 1953.

57. McKinnon SE, Holder LE: The use of three phase bone scanning in the diagnosis of reflex sympathetic dystrophy, *J Hand Surg* 9A:556, 1984.

58. Meahta RC, Wilson MA: Frostbite injury: prediction of tissue viability with triple phase bone scanning, *Radiology* 170:511, 1989.

59. Miller LM, Morgan RP: Vasospastic disorders, *Hand Clin* 9:171, 1993.

60. Moss SH, et al: Digital venous anatomy, *J Hand Surg* 10A:73, 1985.

61. Mubarek SJ, et al: The wick catheter technique for measurement of intramuscular pressure, *J Bone Joint Surg* 55A:1016, 1976.

62. Mulliken JB, Glowacki J: Hemangiomas and vascular malformations in infants and children: a classification based on endothelial characteristics, *Plast Reconstr Surg* 69:412, 1982.

63. Newmeyer WJ: Vascular disorders. In Green DP, editor: *Operative hand surgery,* ed 3, vol 2, New York, 1993, Churchill Livingstone.

64. Nisbat NW: Congenital arteriovenous fistulas in the extremities, *Br J Surg* 41:658, 1954.

65. Oberg PA, Tenland T, Wilson GE: Laser Doppler flowmetry: a noninvasive and continuous method for blood flow evaluation in microvascular studies, *Acta Med Scand (Suppl)* 687:17, 1984.

66. O'Shaunessy M, et al: Consequences of radial and ulnar artery ligation following trauma, *Br J Surg* 78:735, 1991.

67. Perry MO, Thal ER, Shires GT: Management of arterial injuries, *Ann Surg* 173:403, 1971.

68. Raynaud M: *On local asphyxia and symmetrical gangrene of the extremities:* selected monographs translated by T Barlow, London, 1888, New Sydenham Society.

69. Rodehoffer RF, et al: Controlled double blind trial of nifedipine in the treatment of Raynaud's phenomenon, *N Engl J Med* 308:880, 1983.

70. Roos DB: Overview of thoracic outlet syndromes. In Machleder HI, editor: *Vascular disorders of the upper extremity,* ed 2, Mt Kisco, NY, 1989, Futura Publishing.

71. Strandness DE Jr, McCutcheon EP, Rushmer RF: Application of transcutaneous Doppler flowmeter in evaluation of occlusive arterial disease, *Surg Gynecol Obstet* 122:1039, 1966.

72. Strauch B, de Moura W: Arterial system of the fingers, *J Hand Surg* 15A:148, 1990.

73. Sumner DS: Noninvasive vascular laboratory assessment. In Machleder HI, editor: *Vascular disorders of the upper extremity,* Mt Kisco, NY, 1989, Futura Publishing.

74. Sumner DS, Strandness DE: An abnormal finger pulse associated with cold sensitivity, *Ann Surg* 175:294, 1972.

75. Swanson E, et al: Radial artery infections and aneurysms after catheterization, *J Hand Surg* 16A:166, 1990.

76. Thulesius O: Primary and secondary Raynaud's phenomenon, *Acta Chir Scand* 465:5, 1976.

77. Tsuge K: Management of established Volkmann's contracture. In Green DP, editor: *Operative hand surgery,* ed 3, vol 1, New York, 1993, Churchill-Livingstone.

78. Vogelzang RL: Arteriography of the hand and wrist, *Hand Clin* 7:63, 1991.

79. Von Rosen S: Ein fall von thrombose in der arteria ulnaris nech einwirling von stumpfer genalt, *Acta Chir Scan* 73:50, 1934.

80. Whitenack SH, et al: Thoracic outlet syndrome complex: diagnosis and treatment. In Hunter JM, editor: *Rehabilitation of the hand: surgery and therapy,* ed 3, St Louis, 1990, Mosby.

81. Whitesides TE, et al: Tissue pressure measurements as a determinant for the need of fasciotomy, *Clin Orthop* 113:43, 1975.

82. Wildulus DM, et al: Fibrinolytic therapy for upper extremity arterial occlusion, *Radiology* 175:393, 1990.

83. Wilgis EFS: Digital sympathectomy for vascular insufficiency, *Hand Clin* 1:361, 1985.

84. Yakes WR, et al: Alcohol embolotherapy of vascular malformations, *Radiology* 170:1960, 1989.

Chapter 53

MANUAL EDEMA MOBILIZATION: TREATMENT FOR EDEMA IN THE SUBACUTE HAND

Sandra M. Artzberger

Manual edema mobilization (MEM) is not indicated for all hand patients but can be highly effective in cases of recalcitrant subacute or chronic edema. "Oedema is glue," a phrase popularized by Watson-Jones in 1941, sums up the importance of reducing edema in swollen hands.[46] Many edema treatment techniques were developed with the rationale that they "stimulated the venous and lymphatic systems."[22,34,43] This rationale gave the impression that one technique would affect each system with equal effectiveness. Clinically, however, some edemas seemed to reduce with little effort, whereas others progressed into a gellike and fibrotic state regardless of the intensity of therapy. The purpose of this chapter is to present the physiologic rationale and clinical application of MEM, developed by Artzberger in 1995.[1] MEM is used to prevent or reduce subacute or chronic high-protein edema as seen in postsurgical, trauma, or post–cerebrovascular accident (CVA) hand edema.

REVIEW OF THE LITERATURE

Information specifically about the role of the lymphatic system for reducing edema, or methods to activate lymph uptake from the interstitium, has not been readily addressed in American hand therapy literature. A Medline and CINAHL search going back 20 years using the search terms *hand edema* and *hand edema rehabilitation* listed 32 articles and only 2 specifically discussed lymphatic function and edema reduction.

Burkhardt and Joachim[6] published a one-paragraph description of manual lymph drainage. Faghri[18] acknowledged the role of lymphatics for drainage of protein-rich fluid from the tissues in his research using neuromuscular stimulation on the edematous hands of CVA patients. Numerous animal research studies addressing the effects of electrical stimulation for edema reduction, edema prevention, and lymphatic stimulation for protein uptake have been conducted.[3,13,36]

In Europe, the significance of the lymphatics for reducing edema became widely known from the work begun in the 1930s by Emil Vodder, a massage therapist, who called his therapy *manual lymphatic drainage* (MLD).[24] Initially, the therapy was directed at reducing recurrent nose and throat infections and later involved other conditions.[24] Following Vodder's successes, others began researching lymphatic function, mapping lymphatic pathways, and in recent decades, using the electron microscope to study the lymphatic system.[9] Some of these physicians and researchers developed treatment techniques (e.g., compression bandaging, remedial exercise programs) that continue to be the standard for reducing lymphedema.[9,21,27-29] *Manual lymphedema treatment* (MLT) is a generic term used to describe massage principles common to all schools of lymphatic drainage.[12] The most common application of MLT techniques is for secondary lymphedema that can occur after breast or prostate cancer treatment (i.e., lymphadenectomy and/or lymph node radiation), in filariasis (filarial worm infestation damaging the lymphatic vessels and/or nodes), and in primary lymphedema (congenital, unknown cause).

In the mid-1990s, the use of MLT (drainage) techniques for secondary and primary lymphedema started to become known and gain popularity in the United States through reported outcomes.[4,29] Experts such as the Casley-Smiths from Australia report that this lymph drainage technique works for "other edemas," referring to inflammation and

Table 53-1. Types of edema

Type	Etiology	Clinical description and stages
Inflammatory edema (high-plasma protein edema)	Trauma to tissue as a result of injury, infection, or surgical procedure. The result is high capillary permeability, imbalance in Starling's equilibrium, and an overload of the intact lymph nodes and lymph system as a result of an excess of plasma proteins flowing into the interstitium. There is also a temporary obstruction and/or damage to the surrounding lymphatics that decreases protein uptake.[5,15,39]	Inflammatory edema usually spontaneously decreases within 2 days to 2 weeks. It responds to elevation because this decreases arterial hydrostatic pressure[45] and thus reduces the flowing of fluid into the interstitium. If edema lingers beyond 2 weeks, it is considered subacute. Now there is a decreased lymphatic transport out of the involved area as a result of damage or destruction of the lymphatics resulting from incisional scar, compression from a cast, tissue loss, etc. Fibroblasts are activated by the proteins trapped in the interstitium and produce collagenous tissue.[28] Thus, in the subacute phase, edema progresses from a soft spongy state to a dense gellike state. Edema lasting 3 months and longer is considered chronic and often leads to a fibrotic state.
Lymphedema (high-plasma protein edema)	Often associated with lymphadenectomy and/or lymph node radiation, primary lymphedema, or filariasis. Defined, in part, by the International Lymphology Society as "a progressive condition characterized by four main components: excess tissue protein and edema, chronic inflammation and fibrosis."[11] Foldi et al.[21] describe it as a "low output failure of the lymph vascular system."	Classified by grades. Grade I: pitting that reduces with elevation; no fibrosis. Grade II: does not reduce with elevation, fibrosis; ranges from moderate to severe with elephantiasis as the extreme of this grade.[9] Magnetic resonance imaging and isotopic lymphoscintigraphy show that lymphedema occupies the epifascial compartments.[44] Thus fibrosis of joints rarely occurs.
Stroke edema (complex edema)	Initially a simple low-protein edema from accumulation of fluid in the tissue as a result of loss of muscle pump, dependency positioning, etc. If edema is not reduced, increased tissue hydrostatic pressure compromises lymph flow capacity and then edema can become gellike and indurated.	A simple pitting edema that is perpetuated by loss of motor function (muscle pump) and eventually can become gellike and then fibrotic.
Venous edema (legs) (complex edema)	Excess low-protein fluid in tissue as a result of valve dysfunction or incompetence resulting in venous stasis. In severe cases, tissue hydrostatic pressure increases significantly, causing a leakage of plasma proteins, red blood cells, etc., into the interstitium. Tissue becomes indurated, "leathery," and discolored by hemosiderin (an iron-rich pigment that is a byproduct of red cell breakdown).[33,38]	At first, this is a simple pitting edema of excess fluid in the tissue that will decrease with elevation, compression hose, and retrograde massage because these push low-protein fluid from the periphery into the deep venous system. As venous valve incompetence progresses, tissue becomes hard. Previous treatment has minimal effect because the lymphatic system is compromised from the increased tissue hydrostatic pressure, resulting in eventual leakage of plasma proteins and red blood cells into the tissue.
Edema from kidney or liver disease (decreased plasma proteins)	Caused by decreased plasma proteins in the interstitium (i.e., loss of proteins through the urine as in nephrotic syndrome) or failure to produce plasma proteins (as in liver disease).[23]	This is a pitting edema. MLT or MEM is not appropriate treatment.
Edema resulting from cardiac conditions	Heart failure, etc.[23]	Often seen as bilateral pitting edema around the ankles/feet. However, other conditions can also produce this bilateral swelling. MLT or MEM is not appropriate treatment.

MEM, Manual edema mobilization; *MLT,* manual lymphedema treatment.

sports injuries.[9] However, little information is given regarding specific application or methods to reduce these "other edemas." These "other edemas" have an etiology different than the types of lymphedema described earlier, but the element common to all is an increase in plasma proteins in the interstitium and decreased lymph transport capacity. A high-protein edema has a concentration of plasma proteins greater than 1 g/dl in the tissue fluid.[7] If excess plasma proteins remain in tissue for a prolonged period, they cause chronic inflammation, with the eventual fibrosis of tissue.[7,10] For high-plasma protein edemas, a program of MEM or MLT is necessary to move excess proteins out of the interstitium to break the scenario of chronic inflammation leading to fibrosis. Only lymphatic drainage along with macrophage phagocytic activity removes the excess proteins. Table 53-1 describes common types of high-protein edemas, complex edemas, and low-protein edemas commonly seen by therapists. From reading the table, it becomes evident that as soon as there is some type of compromise of the lymphatic system and excess proteins remain in the interstitium, the gellike edema begins, which can lead to fibrosis.

THE LYMPHATIC SYSTEM
Anatomy of the lymphatic system

A knowledge of the anatomy of the lymphatic system and its function is essential to develop effective edema reduction treatment programs. This understanding begins at the arterial, venous, and lymphatic capillary level. Arteriole hydrostatic pressure of 35 mm Hg is sufficient to cause the escape into the interstitium of electrolytes, nutrients, a few plasma proteins, and other elements needed for continued tissue cell metabolism.[2,16] Ninety percent of the plasma and protein substances not needed by the cells leave the interstitium via the venous system; the remaining 10% leave via the lymphatic system.[23] When fluid and large molecules enter the lymphatic system, it is called *lymph.*[25] Lymph contains large molecules not permeable to the venous system, such as fat cells, hormones, tissue waste products, bacteria, and excess plasma proteins.[14,25,30,41] The lymphatic tissue drainage system consists of three levels of structures. Lymph capillaries, called the *initial lymphatics* and *precollectors,* make up the first level.[9,30] These are finger-shaped, closed at one end, netlike vessels located in the interstitium that directly or indirectly drain every part of the body.[23] The vessels consist of a single layer of overlapping endothelial cells that have connector filaments anchoring them to surrounding connective tissue[9,25] (Fig. 53-1). The flaplike junctions formed by the overlapping endothelial cells open when the local interstitial pressure changes. The junctions open; fluid flows in, changing the internal pressure of the lymphatic from low to high, thus closing the flaplike junctions.[23,25] Lymph then enters into the deeper collector lymphatics that have walls consisting of three layers. The inner layer is called the *intima* or *endothelium.*[47] The media

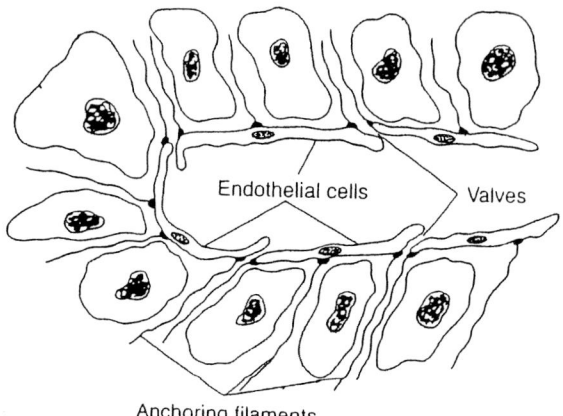

Fig. 53-1. Special structure of the lymphatic capillaries that permits passage of substances of high molecular weight into the lymph. (From Guyton AC, Hall JE: *Textbook of medical physiology,* Philadelphia, 1996, WB Saunders.)

or middle layer consists of smooth muscle and thin strands of collagen fibers[47] that respond to the stretch reflex. The outer layer, called the *adventitia,* is formed by connective tissue.[25] Every 6 to 20 mm within the collectors are valves that prevent the backflow of lymph.[47] These collector segments with a distal and a proximal valve and a space between the valves are called *lymphangions.*[21] As fluid enters a lymphangion, it fills the segment, stimulating a stretch reflex of the medial smooth muscle layer. The ensuing contraction causes the proximal valve to open and propel the lymph to the next proximal lymphangion[19] (Fig. 53-2). At rest, lymphangions pump 6 to 10 times per minute.[47] However, with muscle contraction from exercise, lymphangions can pump 10 times that amount.[9,47]

Collector lymphatics propel lymph to the nodes.[25] The nodes consist of a complex of sinuses that perform immunologic functions. After leaving nodes, lymph either enters the venous system through lymph-venous anastomoses or continues to move into deeper lymphatic trunks and eventually returns to the heart.

Anatomically, the trunk is divided into four lymphatic quadrants, or lymphotomes (drainage territories)[9] (Fig. 53-3). These consist of left and right upper quadrants, called *thoracic lymphotomes,* and left and right lower quadrants, called *abdominal lymphotomes.*[9] The thoracic lymphotomes extend from the anterior midline to the vertebral column on both the left and right sides of the upper trunk. Lymph drains within the lymphotomes from superficial to deeper vessels that connect to nodes (see Fig. 53-3). Between the lymphotomes are watershed areas (i.e., dividing areas) where normal drainage is away from the watershed moving toward the nodes[9] (see Fig. 53-3). There are only a few superficial and deep connecting lymph vessels across watershed areas, but there are superficial collateral vessels.[9] These collateral connections across watersheds are very important because when

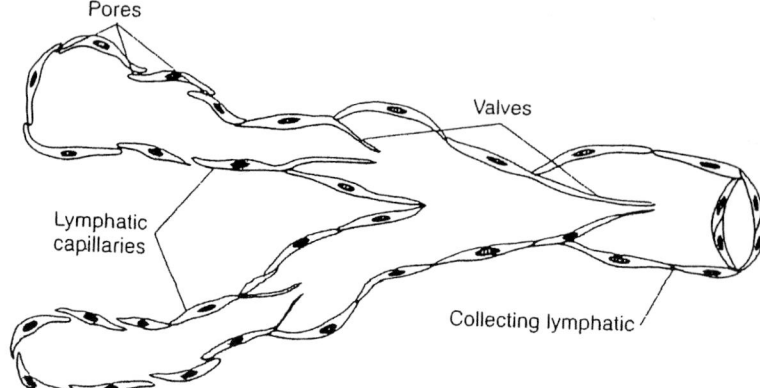

Fig. 53-2. Structure of lymphatic capillaries and a collecting lymphatic, showing also the lymphatic valves. (From Guyton AC, Hall JE: *Textbook of medical physiology,* Philadelphia, 1996, WB Saunders.)

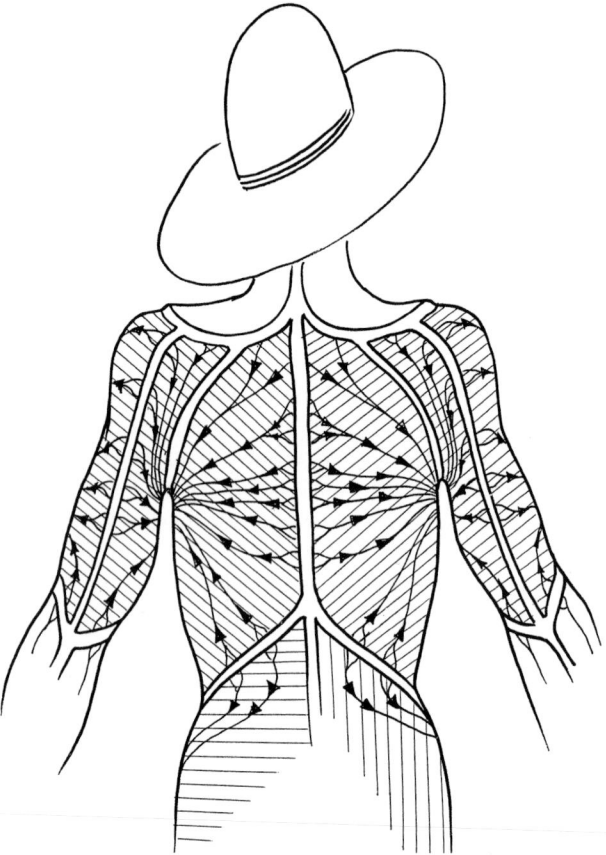

Fig. 53-3. Lymphotomes // = \\ ||, watersheds, and lymph flow direction within the lymphotomes →. (Redrawn and modified from Foldi M, Kubik S: *Lehrbuch der Lymphologie,* Munchen, 1989, Urban & Fischer-Verlag.)

there is lymph congestion, they provide alternative pathways to uncongested lymph vessels. The extremities also have lymphotomes. The upper extremity lymphotomes drain mainly into the axillary nodes. Detail of this information and more extensive drawings can be found in the work of Foldi and Kubik.[20]

Lymph from the right thoracic lymphotome, right upper extremity, and right side of the head drains into trunks that eventually empty into the right lymphatic duct. This duct empties into the right subclavian vein and into the superior vena cava of the heart. Both lower extremities, both abdominal lymphotomes, the left thoracic lymphotome, and the left side of the head drain into the thoracic duct, which is the largest lymphatic vessel in the body and extends from L2 to T4.[47] The thoracic duct empties into the venous system at the juncture of the left subclavian and jugular veins.

Clinical application of lymphatic anatomy and physiology

Success of edema reduction programs and related problem solving depends on clinically applying lymphatic anatomic information. For instance, movement of the large molecules not permeable to the venous system out of the interstitium depends on stimulating the flaplike endothelial cell junctions of the initial lymphatics to open and close.[9,47] Heavy massage or compression will not stimulate, but instead collapse, the initial lymphatics and prevent absorption of lymph. Eliska and Eliskova[17] found that a 10-minute friction massage to the dorsum of feet done with 70 to 100 mm Hg of force caused temporary damage to the endothelial lining of the initial and collector lymphatics. For patients with edema, this damage occurred within 3 to 5 minutes. Miller and Seale[35] found that external pressure facilitates lymph clearance. They also found that a pressure of 60 mm Hg initiated lymphatic closure, with complete closure at 75 mm Hg.[35] With complete closure of the initial lymphatics, there is no uptake of lymph from the interstitium. Thus the clinical treatment approach should be light-compression massage to stimulate, not hinder, absorption at the dermis level. Heavy compression or squeezing collapses the lymphatics, causing the fluid component of lymph to be pushed into the venous system.[9] However, plasma proteins, tissue waste products, fat cells, and so forth, remain in the interstitium. The digit or limb temporarily looks smaller, but the swelling returns. Plasma proteins that remain in the interstitium increase colloid osmotic pressure, attracting more fluid out of the capillaries and into the interstitium,[23] thus refilling occurs.

Light compression of initial lymphatics for absorption of protein can also be accomplished through a multilayered low-stretch bandaging system. Leduc et al.[31,32] demonstrated that multilayered bandages consisting of stockinette, latex foam, and low-stretch bandages placed on the forearm, combined with exercise, had a positive effect of absorbing protein from the interstitium. It has also been shown that temperature affects movement of lymph.[30] The flow of lymph within the vessel is best between 22° and 41° C and sharply slows down or stops before and after those temperatures.[30] Thus bandaging can clinically affect the protein absorption, provide light compression, and provide a buildup of "neutral warmth" to mobilize lymph.

Lymph moves from the collector lymphatics through the lymph nodes. The Casley-Smiths[9] state that congestion of lymph is often present around lymph nodes. They further state that lymph nodes give 100 times the resistance to the flow of fluid as the thoracic duct.[9] Thus nodes can act as "bottlenecks" or "kinks in the hose" to the flow of lymph fluid as it is being filtered through them for immunologic purposes. In clinical treatment, it is seen that massaging the nodes proximal to the edematous site increases the rate of lymph movement out of the area and prevents lymph congestion in the node area. Thus, if the nodes proximal to the edematous area are first massaged (e.g., cubital elbow nodes[37] when there is hand edema), tissue massage and active muscle contraction can more effectively move congested lymph out of an area. Enlarged nodes (e.g., potentially fighting infection) should never be massaged.

All lymph fluid eventually returns to the venous system and enters the heart as part of the venous system. As a result, therapists have to be careful not to quickly return a large volume of fluid back into the heart if there are any preexisting or uncontrolled cardiac or pulmonary problems. MEM classes teach how to safeguard against potential problems.

The division of the trunk into four lymphatic quadrants, or lymphotomes, is significant clinically. When edema is present, it often backs up into the entire quadrant.[21] Pecking et al.[40] showed that in a postmastectomy lymphedema patient, the speed of lymphatic transport increased in the involved hand immediately if the contralateral normal quadrant was treated with MLD. Pecking et al.[40] also reported a 12% to 38% uptake from the involved limb when nodes were massaged in the contralateral axilla. Thus, when possible, MEM techniques begin in the contralateral quadrant. MEM done in the contralateral thoracic lymphotome can facilitate the flow of lymph across the few collateral lymph vessels lying deep and superficial in the watershed areas.

The final feature of the lymphatics to be addressed is effect of exercise on lymph uptake. Weissleder and Schuch-

hardt[47] state that lymphatic uptake is increased by up to 10 times with exercise because muscle contraction increases the rate of lymphangion contraction. Exercise also increases the pumping speed of the thoracic duct.[47] Thus exercise facilitates the movement of lymph fluid. It has been theorized that stretching and range-of-motion (ROM) exercises started proximally will have the effect of moving the most central lymph further in the direction of the heart and kidneys, and more peripheral fluid will move centrally.[9] Vodder believed that changes in the intrathoracic pressure that occur during exercise and diaphragmatic breathing will stimulate lymph to flow more proximally in the thoracic duct.[30] For these reasons, MEM includes a program that begins with diaphragmatic breathing, followed by exercises that begin at the trunk and proceed distally to the digits. In some cases, I have seen that this intervention alone will move lymph out of an area, for example, out of an edematous upper arm.

Table 53-2 summarizes some of the unique features of the lymphatic system with clinical application.

DEFINITION AND PRINCIPLES OF MANUAL EDEMA MOBILIZATION

Casley-Smith and Gaffney[10] found that when they injected excess native proteins into rat tissue, it caused chronic inflammation within 64 days. The Casley-Smiths[8] also state, "If edema lasts several weeks, this promotes chronic inflammation with its aftermath of excess fibroblasts and collagen deposition in the tissue." Thus the goal of therapy should be to reduce the excess plasma proteins in the interstitium. This will potentially reduce or eliminate chronic inflammation and eventual fibrosis of tissue.

MEM is a method of edema reduction based on methods to activate the lymphatic system (Box 53-1). These methods include the principles of MLT massage, medical compression bandaging, exercise, and external compression adapted to meet the specific needs of subacute and chronic postsurgical and poststroke upper extremity edema. The goals are to stimulate the initial lymphatics to absorb excessive fluid and large molecules from the interstitium and to move this lymph centrally. See Fig. 53-4 for direction of lymph flow in the arm.

Contraindications for manual edema mobilization

Precautions and contraindications are those universal to most massage programs and specific to the impact of moving large volumes of fluid through the system (Box 53-2). A physician should always be consulted if the therapist is concerned about the patient's present or past cardiac or pulmonary status. For instance, if there is an 80-ml volumetric difference between the two extremities, a therapist should inform the physician that there is the potential to move that much fluid through the heart and lungs. The physician should be asked whether this would compromise the patient's cardiac status.

Box 53-1   Principles and concepts of manual edema mobilization

- Light massage, ranging from 20 to 30 mm Hg pressure, is used to prevent collapse of the lymphatic pathways or arterial capillary reflux.
- Where protocol allows, preexercises and postexercises are performed in a specific sequence, starting proximal to the edematous area or in the contralateral quadrant, if possible.
- Massage is performed in segments, proximal to distal, then distal to proximal. The direction of the massage ends proximal, meaning toward the trunk.
- When possible, treatment includes exercises specific to muscles in the segment being massaged.
- Massage follows the flow of lymphatic pathways.
- Massage reroutes around scar areas.
- This provides a method of massage and type of exercise that does not cause further inflammation of the involved tissue.
- Treatment includes a patient home self-massage treatment program specific to the hand condition.
- Adaptations to various diagnoses and stages of high-plasma protein edema are available.
- Guidelines are available for incorporating traditional edema control, soft tissue mobilization, and strengthening exercises without causing an increase in edema.
- Specific precautions are followed.
- When necessary, low-stretch compression bandaging or other compression techniques are incorporated.

Box 53-2   When not to perform manual edema mobilization (MEM)

- If infection is present because there is the potential to spread the infection
- Over areas of inflammation because of the potential of increasing the inflammation and pain (Do MEM proximal to the inflammation to decrease congested fluid.)
- If there is a blood clot or hematoma in the area because there is the opportunity to activate (move) the clot
- If there is active cancer (A controversial theory notes the potential to spread cancer. Absolutely never do MEM if the cancer is not being medically treated. Always seek a physician's advice.)
- If the patient has congestive heart failure, severe cardiac problems, or pulmonary problems because there is the potential to overload the cardiac and pulmonary systems
- In the inflammation stage of acute wound healing because theoretically there is the possibility to disrupt the "clean-up" process and the invasion of fibroblasts
- If renal failure or severe kidney disease problems exist (This is not a high-protein edema. There is the potential for overloading the renal system and/or moving the fluid elsewhere.)
- If the patient has primary lymphedema or postmastectomy lymphedema (To successfully treat this condition involves knowing how to reroute lymph to other parts of the body and how to perform specific treatment techniques that are beyond the scope of this chapter.)

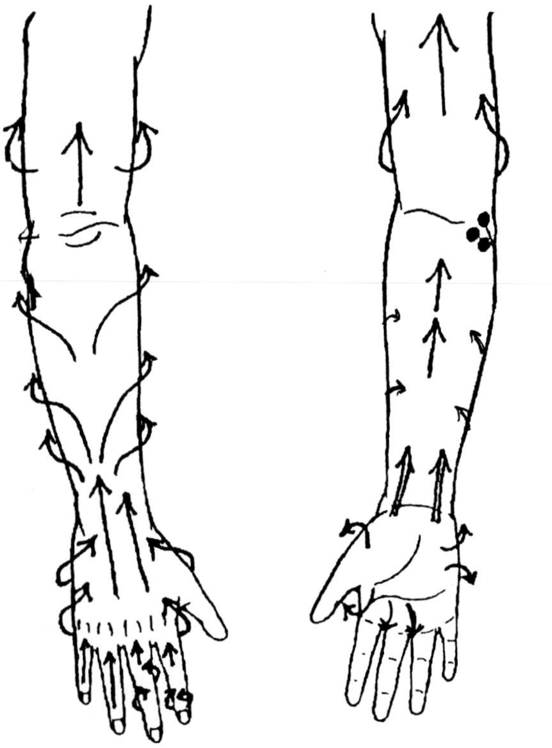

Fig. 53-4. Generalized pattern of superficial lymphatic flow in arm.

OVERVIEW OF THREE MANUAL EDEMA MOBILIZATION TREATMENT CONCEPTS

The following is an overview of three MEM treatment concepts: "clear" and "flow" exercises, MEM drainage terms, and incorporation of traditional treatment techniques. It is not intended as treatment instruction. Only an MEM course can fully teach the concepts needed for safe application. The biologic and scientific rationale for many of these concepts is found in Table 53-2.

Concept I: "clear" and "flow" exercises

Every session starts with active or passive exercise beginning proximal to the edema, if not contraindicated for the specific diagnosis. Best results are obtained if the exercises begin at the trunk. These are called *clear exercises;* these exercises facilitate first the proximal fluid to move deeper into the trunk and the more distal fluid to move proximally. After the massage or drainage part of MEM treatment, the patient is asked to do "flow exercises." Because of the sequence, these exercises facilitate distal fluid and lymph to move proximal by the muscle pump action. Critical to effective edema reduction is active muscle contraction (if not contraindicated by the diagnosis) following the lymphatic and node stimulation in the particular

Table 53-2. Activating lymph uptake

7 whys	Rationale	Clinical application
Why keep pressures light?	Initial and precollector lymphatics have to be stimulated to open and close to uptake lymph[23]; it is not a passive filtration/osmosis system.	Keep compression light to avoid collapse of the dermis layer lymphatics.[17,35]
Why are stimuli needed to facilitate lymphatic pumping?	Initial lymphatics have no pumping mechanism of their own and have to be stimulated to open and close to uptake the large molecules and fluid from the interstitium. Collector lymphatics are capable of pumping.[19,47]	Initial lymphatic uptake and flow are increased by mild stimulation,[21] such as massage, light compression, and muscle contraction. Collector lymphatic rate of pumping is increased by surrounding muscle contraction.[47]
Why start proximal?	Research by Pecking et al.[40] showed that in a postmastectomy lymphedema case, the speed of lymphatic transport from the involved hand increased immediately if the contralateral normal quadrant was treated by MLD. They also reported a 12% to 38% uptake in the involved limb when the contralateral axillary nodes were massaged.	Start light manipulation (massage) very proximal to the edema. Start stimulation in the noninvolved contralateral quadrant.
Why proximal exercise?	Exercise and diaphragmatic breathing cause changes in the intrathoracic pressure, which draws lymph centrally.[30]	Create a proximal suctioning effect by beginning exercises at the trunk.
Why massage nodes?	Lymph fluid passes through lymph nodes that can give 100 times the resistance to the flow of fluid as the thoracic duct.[7] Nodes can become a "bottle neck" or "kink in the hose" to flow of lymph.	Use heavier manipulation (massage) pressure at the nodes.
Why exercise?	Exercise can increase lymph transport 10 times.[47]	Consider a total body exercise program.
Why low-stretch multilayer bandages?	Leduc et al.[31,32] found that the combination of multilayered bandages on the forearm and exercise increased protein absorption. Optimal temperatures to facilitate lymph movement are between 22° and 41° C.[30]	When induration is present, consider using low-stretch bandages to increase protein absorption during exercise and for the buildup of "neutral warmth" and light compression with prolonged use for increasing lymph mobility.

MLD, Manual lymphatic drainage.

segment that was massaged before proceeding to the next segment.

Clear exercises start with diaphragmatic breathing, which causes a change in thoracic pressure. Next, the patient massages the axillary nodes of the uninvolved and then the involved extremity. Exercises begin at the trunk and progress distally to the digits. These exercises could consist of trunk twists and lateral bends, head and neck rotation, shoulder flexion/extension, shoulder horizontal abduction/adduction, back and forward shoulder rolls, pectoralis stretches, elbow flexion/extension and forearm supination/pronation, wrist flexion/extension and circumduction, and extrinsic and intrinsic finger motion.

Flow exercises are performed at the end of the massage and involve active muscle contraction or passive movement starting at the digits and ending at the trunk. This is a reversed sequence of the same exercises used for the clear exercises.

To cause stretch and compression on the lymph nodes and to achieve good muscle pumping action, these exercises must be taken to full muscle excursion when protocol allows. Choosing appropriate exercises is based on what is allowable within the diagnosis protocol. A home program that incorporates clear and flow exercises is essential to success.

Concept II: MEM massage, drainage, and term description

U's are a pattern of hand movement that involves placing the flat, but relaxed, hand lightly on the skin. The hand gently tractions the skin slightly distal and circles back up and around, ending in the direction of the lymph flow pattern. The movement is consistently a clockwise or counterclockwise motion in a U or teardrop configuration. A very light pressure of 20 mm Hg or less is used to move just the skin, thereby stimulating the initial lymphatics. Clinically, this is taught by having the therapist place the full weight of his or her hand on the patient's arm and then lifting so that only half the hand weight rests on the arm. However, the therapist's entire palm and digits must remain in contact with the patient's skin. The MEM massage proceeds at this very light pressure tractioning and moving, not sliding, the skin.

Clearing U's are a pattern of skin tractioning done in segments starting proximal and moving to the designated distal part of the trunk or arm segment (i.e., the upper arm, forearm, or hand). A minimum of five U's are done in three sections of each segment. The purpose is to create interstitial pressure changes, causing the initial lymphatics to uptake lymph. The direction of "flow" movement follows the lymphatic pathways toward the heart (i.e., flowing proximally, not distally). Active muscle contraction is done in each segment following "clearing" in that segment, if not contraindicated by diagnosis protocol. This increases the rate of lymphangion contraction.

Flowing U's consist of sequential U's (one following another) starting in the distal part of the segment being treated and moving proximally past the nearest set of lymph nodes or slightly beyond them. This could be described as "waltzing" up the arm. This process of moving one U after another from distal to beyond the node is repeated five times. When the final repetition is completed, the flowing U motion is performed all the way to the contralateral upper quadrant. The purpose is to move the softened lymph out of the entire segment and facilitate its eventual return back into the venous system and the heart.

Stimulating U's consist of several light "in-place U's" done to soften thickened or indurated tissue. At the lymph nodes, more pressure (i.e., 30 to 40 mm Hg) is used because of the resistance that nodes give to lymph flow.

Concept III: incorporation of traditional treatment techniques

Clinically, it has been seen that MEM decreases swelling and pain. Traditional treatment techniques are still essential to increase ROM, decrease stiffness if present, and increase strength and so on. It has also been observed that using selected traditional edema control techniques works more effectively and with a consistent edema reduction after initiation of MEM. However, if traditional treatment techniques are done too vigorously, causing even microscopic reinflammation of tissue, then swelling recurs. Thus therapists have to progressively grade advancement of treatment programs and assess whether the traditional technique they are using will collapse the lymphatics.

CASE EXAMPLES

The results of using MEM can be seen in the following brief case examples. The first case example, Mrs. M.G., shows the results of exclusive initial use of MEM and low-stretch bandaging followed by ROM modalities once the edema reduction had begun. The second example, Mr. L.S., demonstrates edema reduction with the exclusive use of MEM after edema was not reduced with traditional techniques.

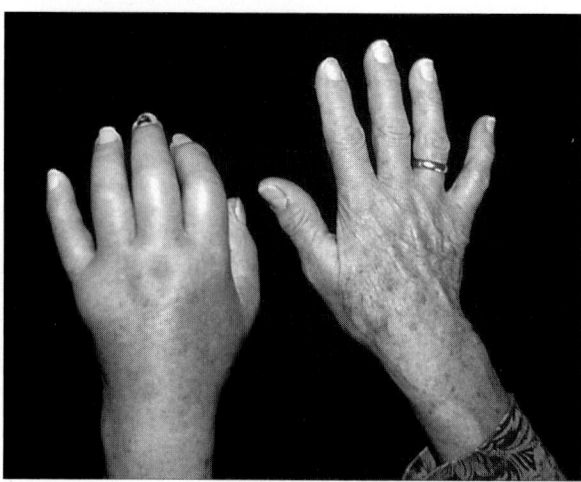

Fig. 53-5. M.G. before manual edema mobilization and therapy. (Courtesy Janine Hareau, PhD, PT, OT.)

Case example: Mrs. M.G.

M.G. is a 75-year-old woman who was referred to hand therapy 8 weeks after a (L) hand infection that had involved the thumb, thenar eminence, and first dorsal interosseous space (Fig. 53-5). Infection was resolved after a series of antibiotics. The exact cause of the infection was never determined but was thought to be related to a (L) thumb nailbed infection. Evaluation revealed severe hand inflammation, severe left hand thenar eminence and dorsal swelling, "spongy pitting" dorsal hand and digit edema, shiny taut tissue on the dorsum of the hand and digits, a pain rating of an 8 on a scale of 1 to 10, active flexion ranging 0 to 20 degrees for each joint of each digit, full active extension to 0 of all digits, pain prohibiting passive flexion, no functional use of the hand, and sensory limitations ranging from decreased to loss of protective sensation throughout the entire hand. Hand pain prevented M.G. from sleeping throughout the night for 8 weeks. Left and right comparison girth measurements were taken at the elbow, palm, wrist, and proximal phalanx of each digit. These girth measurements were totaled up for each upper extremity from elbow to fingertips. The total girth measurement for the left was 102.5 cm, compared with 89 cm on the right, or a 13.5-cm girth difference.

Initial treatment consisted of MEM proximal to the inflammation and low-stretch bandaging to the forearm and hand. After 2 consecutive days of treatment, total edema from the elbow to fingertips reduced 3.5 cm; M.G. had no pain and was able to sleep throughout the night for the first time in 2 months. One month later, the total left lower arm

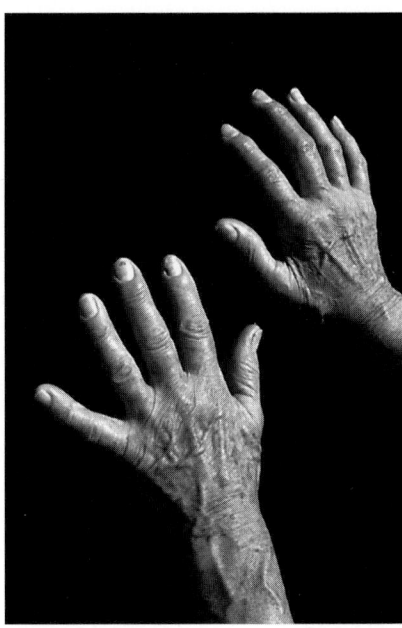

Fig. 53-6. M.G. 2 months later at discharge. (Courtesy Janine Hareau, PhD, PT, OT.)

and hand girth was only 3 cm greater than that of the right. In other words, M.G. lost 10.5 cm of girth from the initial 13.5-cm girth difference between the two extremities. After the 2 days it took to reduce the initial edema, an ROM program was initiated, limited to isometrics and tendon gliding for 1 week. This promoted joint/tendon motion without causing tissue inflammation. Beginning the second week of treatment, a progressive exercise program was started. This included electrical stimulation and use of a continuous passive motion machine. At the end of 2 months of treatment, sensation throughout the hand had improved, ranging from normal light touch to decreased light touch, and the patient had complete active flexion and extension ROM of all digits (Fig. 53-6). At 1-year follow-up, reevaluation revealed that the left hand girth was 1 cm less than that of the right hand.

Case example: Mr. L.S.

L.S., a 28-year-old man, was diagnosed as having a soft tissue crush injury to the extensors on the dorsum of his (L) hand. This occurred at work while L.S. was using a table saw. A piece of wood bounced back, hitting the dorsal aspect of his hand. Two weeks later, he was referred to therapy because of (L) hand pain, swelling, decreased active and passive flexion and extension ROM, and decreased strength. Treatment techniques used included retrograde massage, active range of motion (AROM), blocking exercises, tendon glides, and a metacarpophalangeal (MP) night extension splint when the edema started to

restrict MP extension. After 3 weeks, the edema had not reduced, strength had not increased, and AROM had improved only slightly. Note that the (R) hand became swollen because at work he was compensating for decreased (L) hand function. Thus there was no way to approximate the preinjury size of the (L) hand. Because of the swelling, a rheumatoid factor test was performed, but the results were negative. L.S.'s hand therapy treatment was put on hold. Because swelling was not decreasing and pain was limiting his function at work, L.S. was referred 2 months after the injury to a hand surgeon. The surgeon's evaluation and the magnetic resonance imaging results showed synovitis in and around the MP joints and extensor mechanisms of the (L) index and middle fingers, plus an old traumatic swan-neck deformity of the (L) ring finger. For 6 weeks, the patient was put on a conservative treatment program, but this was unsuccessful in decreasing the tenosynovitis. Subsequently, a tenosynovectomy of the extensor mechanism and the dorsal capsule of the MP joints of the index and middle fingers was performed, as well as a sublimis slip procedure to correct the ring finger swan-neck deformity.

Two weeks after surgery, hand therapy was again initiated because of decreased ROM and increasing edema and pain in the (L) hand. Treatment included an ROM program and traditional edema control methods of elevation, retrograde massage, and an elastic edema glove. By 8½ weeks after the surgery, pain had increased to a constant 4 on a scale of 1 to 10; AROM and strength continued to decrease from preoperative levels, and edema, measured volumetrically, had increased to 704 ml, which was a 108-ml increase from the preoperative level of 596 ml. The initial edema increase occurred because lymphatics had been damaged from the original accident, thus decreasing and blocking lymph flow. Surgery then caused inflammatory edema with more lymphatic overload and edema resulting. At 8½ weeks after the surgery, MEM was instituted and used exclusively for edema management. It consisted of one 45-minute treatment by the therapist and instruction in a 15-minute home MEM program, including tendon gliding performed three times a day by the patient. Six days later, edema had decreased by 120 ml on the (L) to 540 ml. This is 56 ml less than the preoperative measurement, but presurgical edema was present and not reduced since the initial accident. Digit ROM after MEM improved 3 to 5 degrees per digit. (L) grip increased by 17 pounds, and the pain rating reduced from 4 to 0. Without the pain associated with movement, the patient was able to achieve pain-free functional ROM within the next 2 weeks. Only the (L) ring finger proximal interphalangeal joint procedure showed minimal improvement in ROM. L.S. was discharged 2 weeks after MEM, following a generalized progressive work-conditioning program to the (L) hand. L.S. presently reports that edema vacillates with "overuse" but that he can reduce

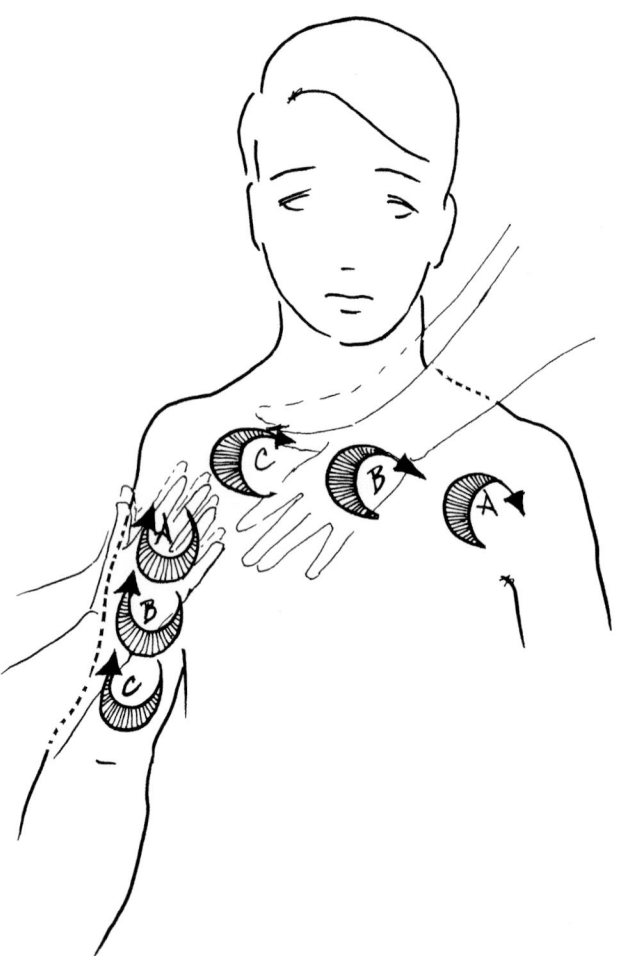

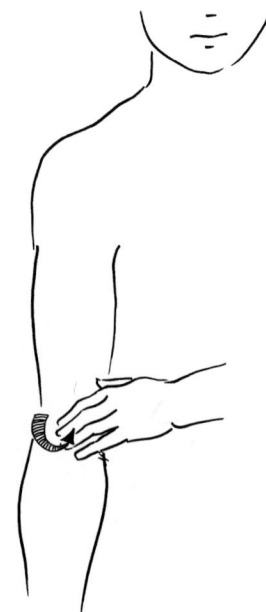

Fig. 53-8. Elbow node: clear 10 to 15 times.

Fig. 53-7. Trunk: clear A, B, C, and flow C, B, A. Upper arm: clear A, B, C tractioning skin from posterior to biceps. Flow C, B, A up to the sternum or to uninvolved quadrant.

it with MEM and has not needed therapy intervention since discharge in September 1997.*

The MEM program initiated at 8½ weeks after the surgery consisted of beginning with diaphragmatic breathing and "clear" exercises at the trunk, progressing distally to the digits. This was followed by MEM massage (drainage) techniques. While L.S. was seated, the therapist began the massage techniques as shown in Fig. 53-7. After completing massage in a segment (i.e., the upper trunk), she asked L.S. to do bilateral active muscle contraction. In this case, it consisted of shoulder flexion/extension, horizontal shoulder abduction/adduction, and shoulder "rolls" forward and backward. Then she proceeded to massage the upper arm as in Fig. 53-7. This consisted of clearing U's as far as the elbow that lightly tractioned the skin from the posterior aspect of the arm directed to the biceps area. This was followed by

*Case Study presented by Artzberger at 1998 American Society of Hand Therapists Annual Meeting. Reprinted with permission by the American Society of Hand Therapists. All rights reserved.

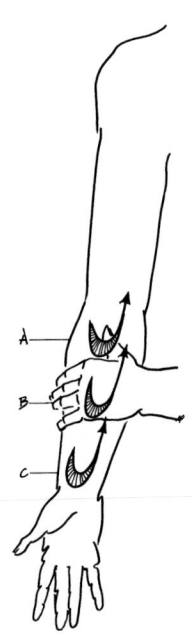

Fig. 53-9. Forearm: clear A, B, C. Flow C, B, A. Clear elbow node five times and continue massage to biceps or head of humerus. Pronate forearm and repeat same sequence on dorsum of arm.

flowing U's from the elbow to the sternum and active muscle contraction of biceps, triceps, and deltoids. The sequence of clear, flow, and active exercise was carried out for the forearm and hand also as in Figs. 53-8 through 53-16. Treatment concluded with flow exercises, starting with active muscle contraction of the digits and ending with total

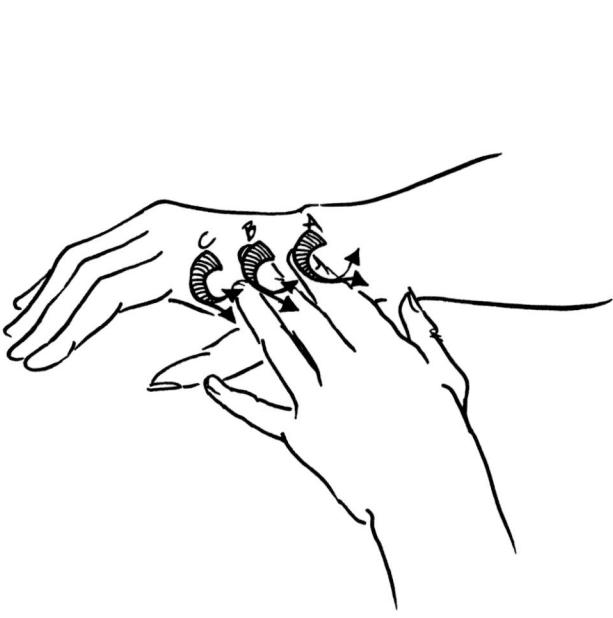

Fig. 53-10. First dorsal interosseous space: clear A, B, C, and flow in one large U to carpal metacarpal joint.

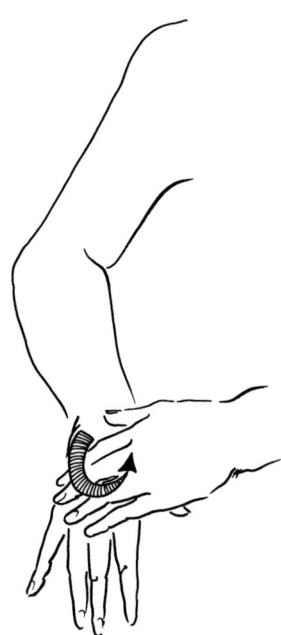

Fig. 53-11. Dorsum of hand: clearing U's flow five times to the elbow node; clear node, and flow to biceps or beyond.

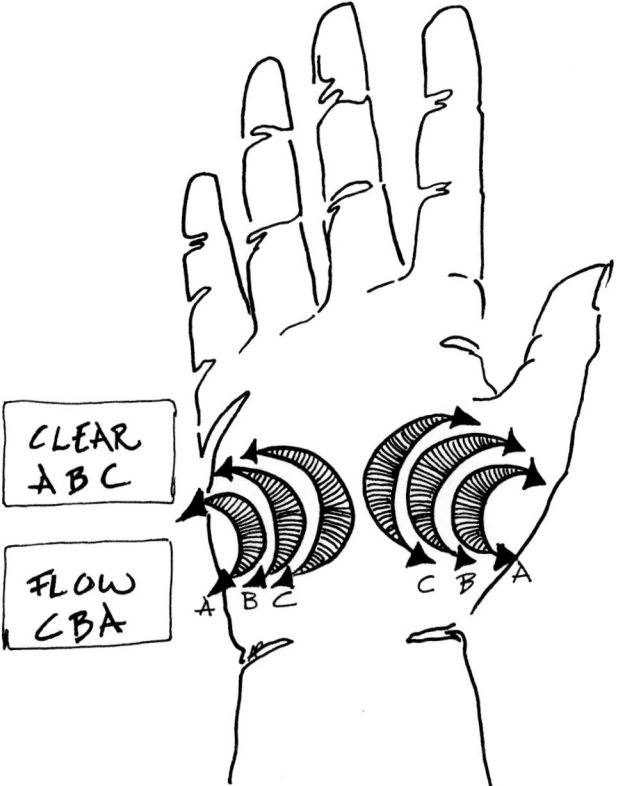

Fig. 53-12. Palm: Lateral side of therapist's thumbs are placed along the lateral sides of the patient's first and fifth metacarpal, and clear A, B, C and flow C, B, A sliding across the flexor retinaculum to the outside edges of the hand. Flow dorsum of hand to midforearm.

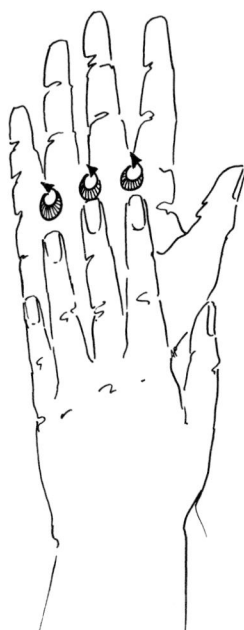

Fig. 53-13. Distal palm: clear and flow.

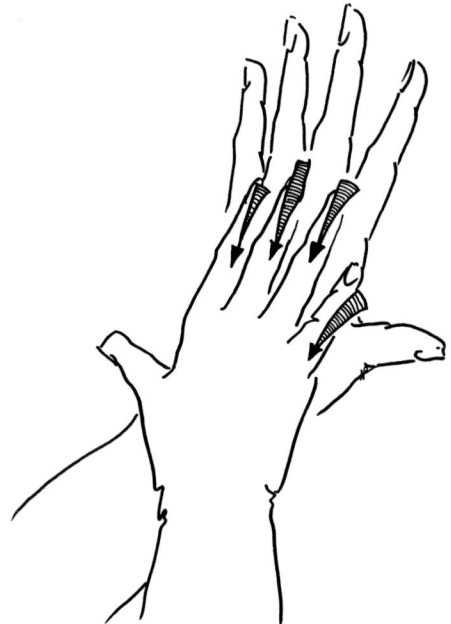

Fig. 53-14. Dorsum of hand: flow to midforearm and/or elbow node and clear node.

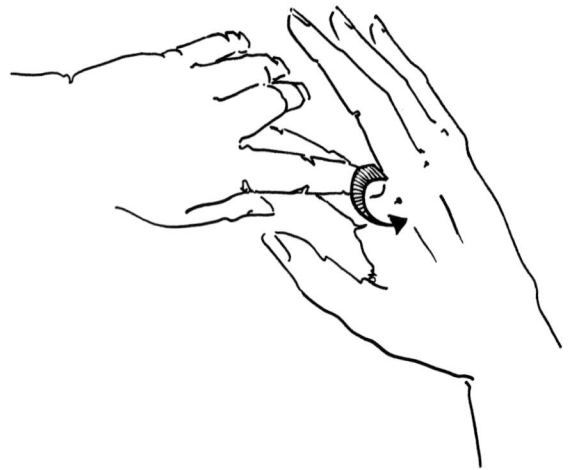

Fig. 53-15. Digits: clear to dorsum of hand.

trunk exercises and diaphragmatic breathing. After this first treatment session, L.S. was given a home program consisting of clear and flow exercises and MEM massage to the upper arm, elbow nodes, forearm, and dorsum of the hand. These were to be performed for 15 minutes three times daily, in addition to an active digit tendon gliding exercise program. L.S. also wore a loosely fitting elastic glove on the (L) hand at all times. At the beginning of the second clinical MEM treatment, some edema remained trapped at the second dorsal interosseous space between the vertical incision scars. The therapist did massage at the pump point shown in Fig. 53-17 and reduced the trapped edema. This is an example of an MEM program designed for L.S. and is not

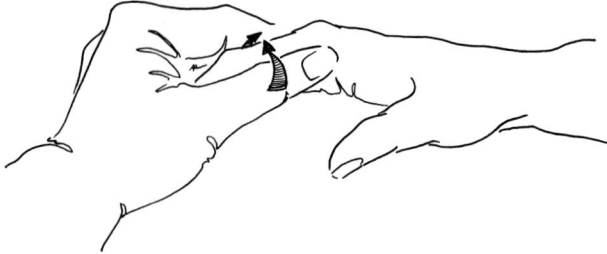

Fig. 53-16. Digits: clear and flow lateral sides of digits to dorsum of hand. Flow to forearm, massage elbow nodes 10 times, and continue flow to sternum.

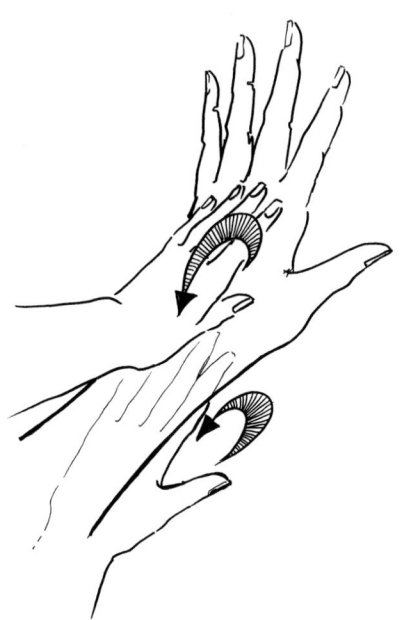

Fig. 53-17. "Pump point."

intended as MEM instruction. It is hoped that these case studies will stimulate additional research.

FREQUENTLY ASKED QUESTIONS ABOUT MEM

1. *Who are candidates for MEM?* Patients who have a stagnate high-protein edema are candidates for MEM. This includes patients who have edema beyond the normal acute phase that is not reducing with the usual acute-phase treatment methods. See Table 53-1. MEM can also be used to prevent edema for the trauma or postsurgical hand problems that are beyond the acute phase, that have barely visible or no edema, but that are being seen for other treatment needs such as ROM. Lymphatics have a safety valve function[30] and can take on considerably more than the usual 10% of interstitial fluid before they become overloaded and edema occurs. Thus doing MEM to the trunk and upper arm and at pump points at the beginning of one or two sessions can unblock congested lymphatics and prevent an overload

resulting in edema. Acute postsurgical edema or trauma edema is also high-protein edema. However, plasma proteins are only temporarily trapped in the interstitium while the phagocytolytic clean-up activity takes place and invasion of fibroblasts at the end of this stage of wound healing occurs. It would be a logical conclusion that massage could disrupt the fibrin blocks in the lymphatics, which confine bacteria for the phagocytolytic activity or disturb the invasion of fibroblasts during this stage. Until biologic research can determine the effect that MEM or any massage has on this clean-up phase, MEM is not recommended for the acute inflammatory phase.

2. *When should MEM begin?* As stated earlier, MEM should not be started until the therapist is certain that the patient is in the fibroplasia stage of wound healing. MEM is not begun on stroke patients until they are medically stable, have had a program of proximal trunk exercises, have consistent good arm positioning, and despite all of this, have edema that is beginning to become gellike.

3. *How can a therapist determine whether the edema is high protein?* An edema that is "spongy" and has slow tissue rebound from being pitted often is a high-plasma protein edema. The best way to determine the type of edema is to look at the cause and also to check out if there are coexisting edemas such as cardiac edema.

4. *Do I begin at the trunk even for a finger fracture?* Yes, because when there is visible or barely visible edema, lymph congestion can often be palpated as proximal as the posterior deltoid. This edema needs to be moved out first so that the more distal edema can move proximally. Sometimes this has to be done only once (i.e., the first treatment session). The next session would begin with proximal trunk exercises, deltoid pump point, and axillary and cubital node massage, and then MEM would begin at the volar forearm.

5. *What are "pump points"?* This is a term Artzberger[1] coined to describe a massage technique that appears to get a faster flow of congested lymph out of an area. The therapist simultaneously places one hand on a watershed area and the other over nodes and/or bundles of lymphatics. The therapist then synchronously massages these areas using the U pattern. For instance, one hand is placed on the deltoid pectoral triangle located over the deltoid pectoral node. The second hand is on the posterior deltoid and teres minor border, where there is a watershed between lymphotomes. A synchronous U motion ending toward the acromion will facilitate drainage of the posterior arm. This occurs because there is both node massage and stimulation of fluid movement over a watershed that results in decongesting a lymph backup in the upper posterior arm. Pump point areas include medial anterior/posterior deltoid borders, posterior deltoid and cubital (elbow) node, cubital node and

triceps insertion, cubital node and volar distal wrist, and dorsum of hand and distal volar wrist.

6. *For a geriatric patient with multiple diagnoses, should I do MEM to the entire extremity in one session?* No, you could easily overload the cardiopulmonary system. Often, this edema moves out of an area quickly because it is a complex edema. Thus it is recommended to treat only one segment the first time and observe whether any complications occur. If none occur, the therapist may decide to gradually include more segments in further treatment. An MEM course is needed to teach how to safely work with this population and how to modify other aspects of MEM.

7. *How long should I do MEM?* The first session may take 20 minutes, consisting of MEM to the trunk and upper arm without massaging the edematous hand. Usually, the hand edema will begin to reduce or soften because of this proximal work. The patient is taught a home program to do several times daily. At the next session, MEM might be done to the entire extremity, and the patient is instructed in an expanded home therapy program. Subsequent treatments might involve the therapist doing MEM at the trunk and at pump points and then beginning MEM proximal to the edema. Care must be taken not to add treatment techniques that could cause reinflammation of tissue (e.g., an overly aggressive strengthening program). A Kinesiotaping program is an excellent addition to MEM in order to have more continuous lymphatic stimulation as the patient performs routine daily tasks (see Chapter 110).

8. *What are low-stretch bandages, and when are they used?* These are 100% cotton bandages with only a 20% stretch. Light compression is obtained from the layering of multiple bandages, not from the applied stretch. Because these bandages have little stretch, they provide a compressive counterforce to an expanding muscle belly. This causes a change in interstitial pressure, which stimulates the lymphatics to absorb fluid and other materials from the interstitium. When the muscle belly relaxes, the bandages do not contract and thus do not give a force that would collapse the initial lymphatics. Bandages might be advised if the indurated tissue remains after a couple of MEM treatments, edema recurs because of the presence of plasma proteins, or decreased motor function is present. Neutral warmth builds under the bandages. This warmth has been seen clinically to help soften the induration and mobilize the lymph.

9. *What are "chip bags," and what is their function?* These are items described by the Casley-Smiths.[9] Chip bags can consist of pieces of ½-inch foam with a variety of densities that are enclosed in a stockinette bag and placed on the skin over indurated areas of edema. The chip bags can be secured with a low-stretch bandage or can be worn under an elastic glove. This gives

light stimulating compression combined with neutral warmth, resulting in further tissue softening.

10. *If the patient previously had lymphedema from a mastectomy, then has a hand injury and/or surgery and the edema gets worse, can I effectively use MEM?* No, MEM does not teach rerouting around areas of node removal or around fibrotic radiated tissue. The therapist must seek the help of a person adequately trained in MLT techniques.

11. *How is rerouting around scar done?* The goal is to reroute congested lymph around areas of tissue damage into adjacent functioning lymph capillaries (lymphatics). This reduces lymph congestion with its negative buildup of plasma proteins. The therapist begins clear and flow massage proximal to the incision or congested site while his or her other hand is lightly massaging (flowing) congested lymph into the "cleared" area.

12. *If excess proteins cause inflammation, should the patient go on a low-protein diet?* No! Reducing food proteins will not reduce congested plasma (blood) proteins.

13. *If present edema control techniques are working, why change to MEM?* The challenge is to reexamine the success of these techniques in light of what stimulates the lymphatics. "Fisting above the head" is often referred to for reducing edema.[26] A closer examination of this technique reveals motion beginning proximal at the trunk and proceeding distal as the scapula rotates along with stretching of the trunk and arm muscles and ending with distal active muscle contraction from "fisting" as the arm is extended above the head. This technique follows the principles that stimulate lymphatic flow. Are elastic gloves effective because they are loose fitting, giving light compression and thus stimulating the lymphatics? Is use of the pneumatic pump effective because the pressure is set at 35 mm Hg or less rather than diastolic pressure, which exceeds the pressure needed to collapse the lymphatics and prevent lymph uptake? Is the retrograde massage effective because it is being used on a low-protein edema such as early stroke edema or on very early stages of subacute edema before stagnation of lymph occurs? Is the use of sponge-type finger wraps effective to soften hard edema and scars because they are providing prolonged light compression and neutral warmth? Possibly all of these techniques would make the more distal edema reduce faster if a couple of sessions included MEM to the trunk, upper arm, and pump points because of the decongesting effect on the proximal nodes and lymphatics.

CONCLUSION

The Casley-Smith and Gaffney experimental findings[10] in an animal model that showed that excess plasma proteins remaining in the interstitium (i.e., induced lymphedema) cause chronic inflammation leading to fibrosis was the first key to understanding why chronic hand edema after injury can lead to fibrosis. Both are high-protein edemas. The second key was to learn the role of the lymphatics for removing these excess plasma proteins and other lymph constituents from the interstitium. The third key was to learn how to specifically stimulate lymphatic uptake. MEM is a technique that adapts lymphatic drainage principles to specific hand diagnoses and incorporates selected traditional edema control methods. The clinical results have been very positive. The next step is to conduct research regarding subacute postsurgical and trauma high-protein edema. Future areas for more in-depth study could include the biologic stages of high-protein edema, the effect of lymph massage on enhancing macrophage proteolysis of excess plasma proteins, the effect of massage and edema reduction on laying down of collagen, the immunologic impact of massaging lymph nodes, the neurologic impact of using light massage in patients with diagnoses such as complex regional pain syndrome, and the effect of prolonged neutral warmth and light compression on indurated tissue. Effective clinical techniques can then be developed on the basis of the biologic research. MEM opens a door to another facet of edema reduction that needs to enter the research arena.

ACKNOWLEDGMENT

I would like to express my gratitude to the following people who contributed their time and material for this chapter: Janine Hareau, PhD, PT, OT, from Clinica de Rehabilitacion de la Mano Montevideo Uruguay for data and photos of M.G.; Joni Westenberger, OTR, from Occupational Therapy and Hand Clinic, West Bend, Wisconsin, for providing the L.S. case study data; Judy Colditz, OTR, CHT, FAOTA, of Raleigh, North Carolina, for drawing Fig. 53-4; to Alice Pollack, teacher and artist, from Colgate, Wisconsin, for all of the MEM sketches; and finally to Cynthia Cooper, MFA, MA, OTR, CHT, and Wendy Camp, OTR, CHT, for their insights and inspirations. A separate special thanks to Anne Callahan and the other editors of this text who are willing to risk bringing new concepts to the hand therapy community and for their challenging questions that mentored me through the development of this chapter and its subsequent effect on MEM. Thanks.

REFERENCES

1. Artzberger S: Edema control: new perspectives, *Phys Disabil Special Interest Section Quarterly* 20:March, 1997.
2. Berne R, Levy M: *Physiology*, ed 4, St Louis, 1998, Mosby.
3. Bettany JA, Fish DR, Mendel FC: Influence of high voltage pulsed direct current on edema formation following impact injury, *Phys Ther* 70:219, 1990.
4. Boris M, et al: Persistence of lymphedema reduction after noninvasive complex lymphedema therapy, *Oncology* 11:99, 1997.
5. Bryant WM: Wound healing, *Clin Symp* 29:1, 1977.
6. Burkhardt A, Joachim L: Clinical options in edema control, *J Hand Ther* 6:337, 1993.
7. Casley-Smith JR: Modern treatment of lymphoedema, *Mod Med* May:70, 1992.
8. Casley-Smith JR, Casley-Smith JR: The pathophysiology of lymphoedema and the action of benzo-pyrones in reducing it, *Lymphology* 21:190, 1988.

9. Casley-Smith JR, Casley-Smith JR: *Modern treatment for lympho-edema,* ed 5, Adelaide, Australia, 1997, The Lymphoedema Association of Australia.

10. Casley-Smith JR, Gaffney RM: Excess plasma proteins as a cause of chronic inflammation and lymphodema: quantitative electron microscopy, *J Pathol* 133:243, 1981.

11. Casley-Smith JR, et al: Lymphedema summary of the 10th international congress of lymphology working group discussions and recommendations, *Lymphology* 10:175, 1985.

12. Consensus Document of the International Society of Lymphology Executive Committee: The diagnosis and treatment of peripheral lymphedema, *Lymphology* 28:113, 1995.

13. Cook HA, et al: Effects of electrical stimulation on lymphatic flow and limb volume in the rat, *Phys Ther* 74:1040, 1994.

14. Cotran R, et al, editors: *Robbins pathologic basis of disease,* ed 6, Philadelphia, 1996, WB Saunders.

15. Crowley L: *Introduction to human disease,* ed 3, Boston, 1992, Jones and Bartlett.

16. Davis B, et al: *Conceptual human physiology,* Columbus, 1985, Charles E Merrill.

17. Eliska O, Eliskova M: Are peripheral lymphatics damaged by high pressure manual massage? *Lymphology* 28:21, 1995.

18. Faghri P: The effects of neuromuscular stimulation-induced muscle contraction versus elevation on hand edema in CVA patients, *J Hand Ther* 10:29, 1997.

19. Földi M, Földi E: *Lymphoedema methods of treatment and control: a guide for patients and therapists,* Victoria, Australia, 1991, Lymphoedema Association of Victoria.

20. Földi M, Kubik S: *Lehrbuch der Lymphologie,* Munchen, 1989, Urban & Fischer-Verlag.

21. Foldi E, et al: The lymphedema chaos: a lancet, *Ann Plast Surg* 22:505, 1989.

22. Griffin J, et al: Reduction of chronic posttraumatic hand edema: a comparison of high voltage pulsed current, intermittent pneumatic compression, and placebo treatments *Phys Ther* 70:279, 1990.

23. Guyton A, Hall J: *Textbook of medical physiology,* ed 9, Philadelphia, 1996, WB Saunders.

24. Harris R: An introduction to manual lymph drainage: the Vodder method, *Massage Ther J* Winter:55, 1992.

25. Hole JW: *Human anatomy and physiology,* ed 4, Dubuque, Iowa, 1987, William C Brown.

26. Hunter J, Mackin E: Edema techniques of evaluation and management. In Hunter J, Mackin E, Callahan A, editors: *Rehabilitation of the hand: surgery and therapy,* vol 1, ed 4, St Louis, 1995, Mosby.

27. Hutzschenreuter PO, et al: Post-mastectomy arm lymphedema: treated by manual lymph drainage and compression bandage therapy, *Eur J Phys Med Rehabil* 1:6, 1991.

28. Kasseroller R: *Compendium of Dr. Vodder's manual lymph drainage,* Heidelberg, 1998, Haug.

29. Ko DS, et al: Effective treatment of lymphedema of the extremities, *Arch Surg* 133:452, 1998.

30. Kurz I: *Textbook of Dr. Vodder's manual lymph drainage,* vol 2, ed 4, Heidelberg, 1997, Haug.

31. Leduc O, et al: The physical treatment of upper limb edema, *Cancer* 15:2835, 1988.

32. Leduc O, et al: Bandages: scintigraphic demonstration of its efficacy on colloidal protein reabsorption during muscle activity, Progress in Lymphology XII, Excerpta Med, *Int Cong Ser* 887:421, 1990.

33. Micheletti G: Ulcers of the lower extremities. In Gogia P, editor: *Clinical wound management,* Thorofare, NJ, 1995, Slack.

34. Miles W: Soft tissue trauma, *Hand Clin* 2:33, 1986.

35. Miller GE, Seale J: Lymphatic clearance during compressive loading, *Lymphology* 14:161, 1981.

36. Mohr T, Akers TK, Landry RG: Effect of high voltage stimulation on edema reduction in the rat hind limb, *Phys Ther* 67:1703, 1987.

37. Netter F: *Atlas of human anatomy,* Summit, NJ., 1995, CIBA.

38. Nunnelee J: Healing venous ulcers, *RN* Nov:39, 1997.

39. Olszewski W: On the pathomechanism of development of postsurgical lymphedema, *Lymphology* 6:35, 1973.

40. Pecking A, et al: Indirect lymphoscintigraphy in patients with limb edema, Progress in Lymphology, Proceedings of the Ninth International Congress of Lymphology, pp. 201-206, 1985.

41. Porth CM: *Pathophysiology concepts of altered health states,* ed 5, Philadelphia, 1998, Lippincott.

42. Romrell L, Bland K: Anatomy and physiology of the normal and lactating breast. In Bland K, Copeland E III, editors: *The breast: comprehensive management of benign and malignant diseases,* Philadelphia, 1991, WB Saunders.

43. Sorenson MK: The edematous hand, *Phys Ther* 69:1059, 1989.

44. Szuba A, Rockson S: Lymphedema: classification, diagnosis and therapy, *Vasc Med* 3:145, 1998.

45. Vasudevan S, Melvin J: Upper extremity edema control: rationale of treatment techniques, *Am J Occup Ther* 33:520, 1979.

46. Watson-Jones R: *Fractures and other bone and joint injuries,* ed 2, Baltimore, 1942, Williams & Wilkins.

47. Weissleder H, Schuchhardt C: *Lymphedema diagnosis and therapy,* ed 2, Bonn, 1997, Kagerer Kommunikation.

Chapter 54

MANAGEMENT OF BREAST CANCER–RELATED EDEMAS

Linda T. Miller

Breast cancer–related edema can be a potentially serious complication of the current treatment for breast cancer. If left untreated, edema may progress from an annoying nuisance to a debilitating functional impairment. Although often considered chronic, breast cancer–related edema can be managed successfully through various treatment modalities, including manual lymphatic therapy (MLT), compression, and exercise. However, like breast cancer itself, the success of edema treatment can depend on its early detection and early intervention.

Breast cancer is the most prevalent cancer among women in the United States and is the second leading cause of death from cancer. It is the leading cause of malignancy-related death among American women 15 to 54 years of age.[46] Currently, it is estimated that 1 of every 8 women has a lifetime risk of developing breast cancer, with an estimated 192,000 women being diagnosed with invasive breast cancer in 2001.[17] It is also estimated that approximately 15% to 20% of women treated for invasive breast cancer will go on to develop some breast cancer–related edema.[40] Given that edema can occur any time after the treatment for invasive breast cancer, at this rate of incidence, even a conservative estimate of 15% may leave more than 28,000 new cases of breast cancer–related edema to be diagnosed each year.

MEDICAL MANAGEMENT OF INVASIVE BREAST CANCER
Surgery

Currently, the standard of care for invasive breast cancer involves removal of the breast tumor, either by *mastectomy* (removal of the entire breast) or *lumpectomy* (removal of the mass with a margin of clean tissue around it).[19] Regardless

of the surgical procedure to the chest wall, some form of *axillary dissection* (removal of lymph nodes in the axilla) is also performed.

The axilla is bordered superiorly by the axillary vein, laterally by the latissimus dorsi, and medially by the serratus anterior (Fig. 54-1). The axillary contents are divided anatomically into three levels. Each level is defined in relation to the pectoralis minor.[13,19] Level I tissue sits medial to the latissimus dorsi and lateral to the pectoralis minor, level II tissue sits directly posterior to the pectoralis minor, and level III tissue lies between the pectoralis minor and the clavicle.

The axillary lymph nodes are the principal site of regional metastases from breast cancer. The presence and number of axillary lymph nodes found to have metastases are important prognostic factors, helping determine the stage of the disease and the course of adjuvant therapy such as chemotherapy. Dissecting the axilla also has been shown to improve local control of the disease.[2] Currently, a dissection that includes levels I and II is the standard procedure for most invasive breast cancers.[2,13] However, a new procedure aimed at decreasing the morbidity of the axillary dissection is under clinical investigation. *Lymphatic mapping,* also called *sentinel lymph node dissection,* is based on the hypothesis that the status of the sentinel lymph node (the first node in the regional axilla that drains a primary breast tumor) will mirror the status of the remainder of the axilla.[12,20] If this theory proves accurate, then only one or two axillary lymph nodes would need to be dissected to stage the disease accurately.

Although an axillary dissection usually is necessary in the management of invasive breast cancers, this surgical procedure may lead to complications such as pain and decreased

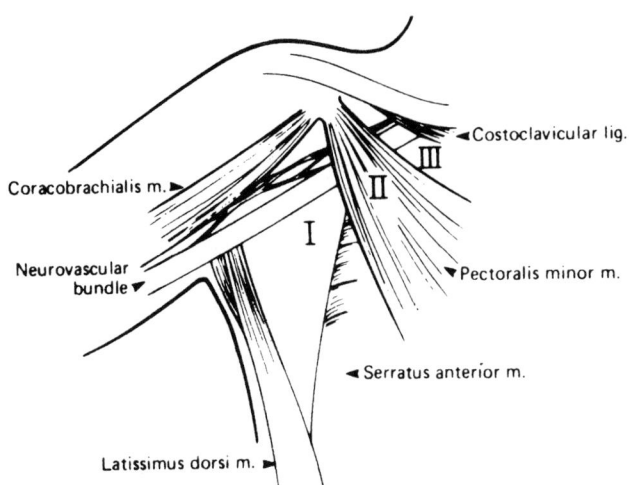

Fig. 54-1. The anatomical levels (I, II, III) of the axillary contents, designated according to their relationship to the pectoralis minor. (From DeMoss, et al: Complete axillary lymph node dissection before radiotherapy for primary breast cancer. In Harris JR, Hellman S, Silen W, editors: *Conservative management of breast cancer*, Philadelphia, 1983, JB Lippincott.)

shoulder mobility. The dissection may also compromise or interrupt lymphatic flow at the site of the lymph node removal and can be a contributing factor to the development of postoperative swelling and chronic edemas.

Radiation therapy

In many cases of invasive breast cancer, the local management of the disease also involves the use of radiation therapy. In an attempt to destroy any remaining cancer cells after surgery, radiation may be applied to the chest wall and, in some cases, to the axilla itself. Radiation works to destroy tumor cells by interrupting cellular division and damaging the DNA of the cell.[5]

However, it has been well documented that radiation therapy also predisposes a patient to chronic edema because of its negative impact on the regeneration of new lymphatic pathways.[29,34] Even when there is no intention to include the axilla in the radiation field, evidence demonstrates that at least level I lymph nodes can be affected by chest wall radiation "scatter."[29]

Chemotherapy

Chemotherapy, a combination of drugs designed to destroy cancer cells by different mechanisms, is used to prevent the systemic spread of the disease. Although the use of chemotherapy itself may not directly cause edema formation, some chemotherapy regimens include the use of corticosteroids such as dexamethasone to help control nausea and glucocorticoids to help control hypersensitivity reactions.[16,35] Because steroids can cause fluid retention throughout the body, a patient may experience short-term edema problems in the arm and trunk on the side where the lymph nodes were removed.

NORMAL PHYSIOLOGY OF TISSUE FLUID BALANCE

Maintaining tissue fluid balance to prevent chronic edema is a dynamic process of microcirculation that involves three interrelated systems working together: blood vessels, protein-lysing cells, and the lymphatics.[8,9] These systems maintain tissue fluid homeostasis by facilitating a dynamic equilibrium between the interstitium and the blood and lymphatic vasculature by transporting proteins and fluid into and out of the interstitial tissue. Protein and fluid levels are being adjusted continually in response to changes in the microenvironment. Physiologic mechanisms such as Starling's law are at work to ensure balance of fluids and proteins in the interstitium with fluids and proteins in the hematologic vasculature.[1,43]

Arterioles and postcapillary venules are the blood vessels of microcirculation. The arteriole carries blood and its nutrients, including oxygen and proteins, into the tissue. Approximately 90% of the fluid that enters the tissue is returned to the heart via the venous system. In addition to resorbing the fluid, the venous system is responsible for returning carbon dioxide; other waste products; and most of the smaller, unused proteins to the blood system. The remaining 10% of the fluid, along with the larger proteins, is returned to the blood system via the lymphatic system.[21,43]

THE LYMPHATIC SYSTEM OF THE UPPER QUARTER

In 1908, the surgeon Lord Moynihan wrote, "The surgery of malignant disease is not the surgery of organs, it is the anatomy of the lymphatic system."[18] This insightful comment helps explain the importance of the current practice of dissecting the axilla in the medical management of breast cancer. It also captures the importance of understanding the anatomy of the lymphatics, especially of the upper quarter, to effectively treat the complication of breast cancer–related edema.

The anatomic arrangement of superficial and deep lymphatic pathways that drain the interstitium of the upper extremity, thorax, and head explain their vulnerability to the axillary dissection and the subsequent swelling that can occur. The superficial lymphatic vessels outnumber the deeper collecting vessels in the limb, but ultimately, most of the vessels converge toward the axilla. Furthermore, approximately 97% of the flow from the deep subcutaneous and intramammary lymphatic vessels makes its way to the axilla.[38] Thus any surgery to the axilla can put the entire upper quarter at risk for edema.

A normal functioning lymphatic system is essential if tissue fluid balance is to be maintained. The *initial lymphatic*, the beginning of the unidirectional lymphatic system, is a vessel made up of a single layer of overlapping endothelial cells. The junctions between the cells can be open or closed. When the local tissue pressure is low, there is no compression of the vessel by the surrounding tissue.

Therefore fluid, protein, and other macromolecules can pass through the open endothelial cell junctions into the lumen of the initial lymphatics. The function of the initial lymphatic is purely mechanical and responds to the changes in total tissue pressure created through movement, muscular contraction, pulsating arteries, and respiration.[8,33,43,44]

The fluid is propelled from the initial lymphatic vessel to the *collecting vessel,* a structure that has valves to ensure unidirectional flow, as well as a layer of smooth muscle. This layer of muscle allows for an intrinsic contraction to propel the lymph.[28] However, because the contraction is fairly weak, the collecting vessel, like the initial lymphatic, requires a change in total tissue pressure to function normally. It responds to the same physiologic mechanisms of tissue pressure change that affect the initial lymphatic.

The collecting lymphatics subsequently merge into larger lymphatic trunks that, although subcutaneous, remain extrafascial and make their way toward regional lymph nodes. These structures serve as filters to remove broken cells, toxins, bacteria, and the like.[8,10] The regional lymph nodes are areas of high impedance because the lymphatic flow must slow to allow for filtration.[10] When lymph nodes are removed, as in the axillary dissection, or damaged by radiation therapy, the impedance is even greater. The lymphatic flow can become sluggish and eventually can lead to an edematous condition.

Although there are multiple lymphovenous anastomoses at various points of both systems, the bulk of the lymphatic fluid reaches the blood system via two major lymphatic ducts. The *thoracic duct,* the largest lymphatic vessel, originates in the cisterna chyli in the abdominal region. It collects the lymphatic fluid from every part of the body except for the right upper quarter and right side of the head and neck. The fluid from these regions reaches the blood system via the right lymphatic duct. The thoracic duct joins with the blood system at the left subclavian-jugular junction, and the right lymphatic duct joins at the right subclavian-jugular junction just before these veins enter the superior vena cava (Fig. 54-2).

The skin is divided into a series of lymphatic drainage regions called *lymphotomes,* which are superficial areas of the body that drain to the deeper lymphatic pathways.[10,15] Fluid from a specific lymphotome will drain in the same direction. Lymphotomes are divided by *watersheds.* A watershed is not an actual anatomic structure. Rather, each watershed marks the change in direction of superficial lymphatic flow between adjacent lymphotomes.[10]

The trunk itself is divided into four lymphotomes or quadrants: left thoracic, right thoracic, left abdominal, and right abdominal. A midline watershed separates the right and left trunk lymphotomes, and a transverse watershed, at approximately the level of the umbilicus, separates the upper and lower trunk lymphotomes.[10,15] The right thoracic lymphotome and the right arm drain mainly via the right axillary lymph nodes. The left thoracic lymphotome and the

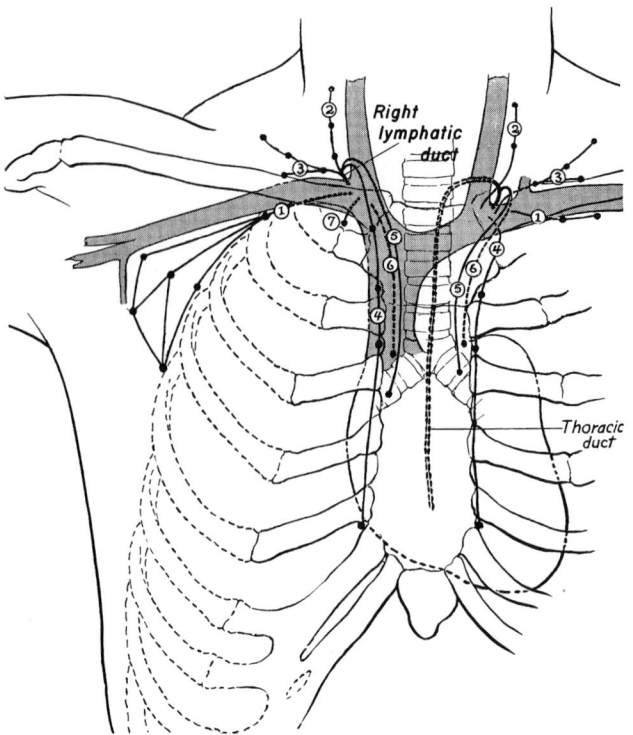

Fig. 54-2. The great lymphatic trunks at the base of the neck. (From Haagensen CD: *Diseases of the breast,* ed 3, Philadelphia, 1986, WB Saunders.)

left arm drain mainly via the left axillary lymph nodes. Because of the specific nature of lymphatic anatomy, what disrupts axillary drainage can go on to disrupt the lymph flow of the entire ipsilateral upper quarter.

Below the umbilical watershed, the trunk and leg drainage is mainly into the superficial inguinal lymph nodes on each side. From there, the fluid drains into the deeper pelvic nodes on its way to the thoracic duct and, eventually, to the left subclavian-jugular junction. Therefore the left subclavian-jugular junction receives lymphatic fluid from the left upper extremity, left thoracic lymphotome, both abdominal lymphotomes, and both lower extremities. The right subclavian-jugular junction receives fluid from only the right upper thoracic and right upper extremity lymphotome (Fig. 54-3).

Although distinct drainage regions, each lymphotome is connected to neighboring lymphotomes via superficial and deep collateral lymphatics that cross over watersheds. These collateral lymphatics are important because they are an avenue by which fluid can be drained through careful manual technique from a congested lymphotome to an uncongested or less congested lymphotome.[10]

In addition to the main drainage pathways taken by the larger collecting vessels of the upper extremity as they converge toward the regional (i.e., axillary) lymph nodes, alternative pathways exist. There is considerable anatomic variance among individuals with respect to these pathways.

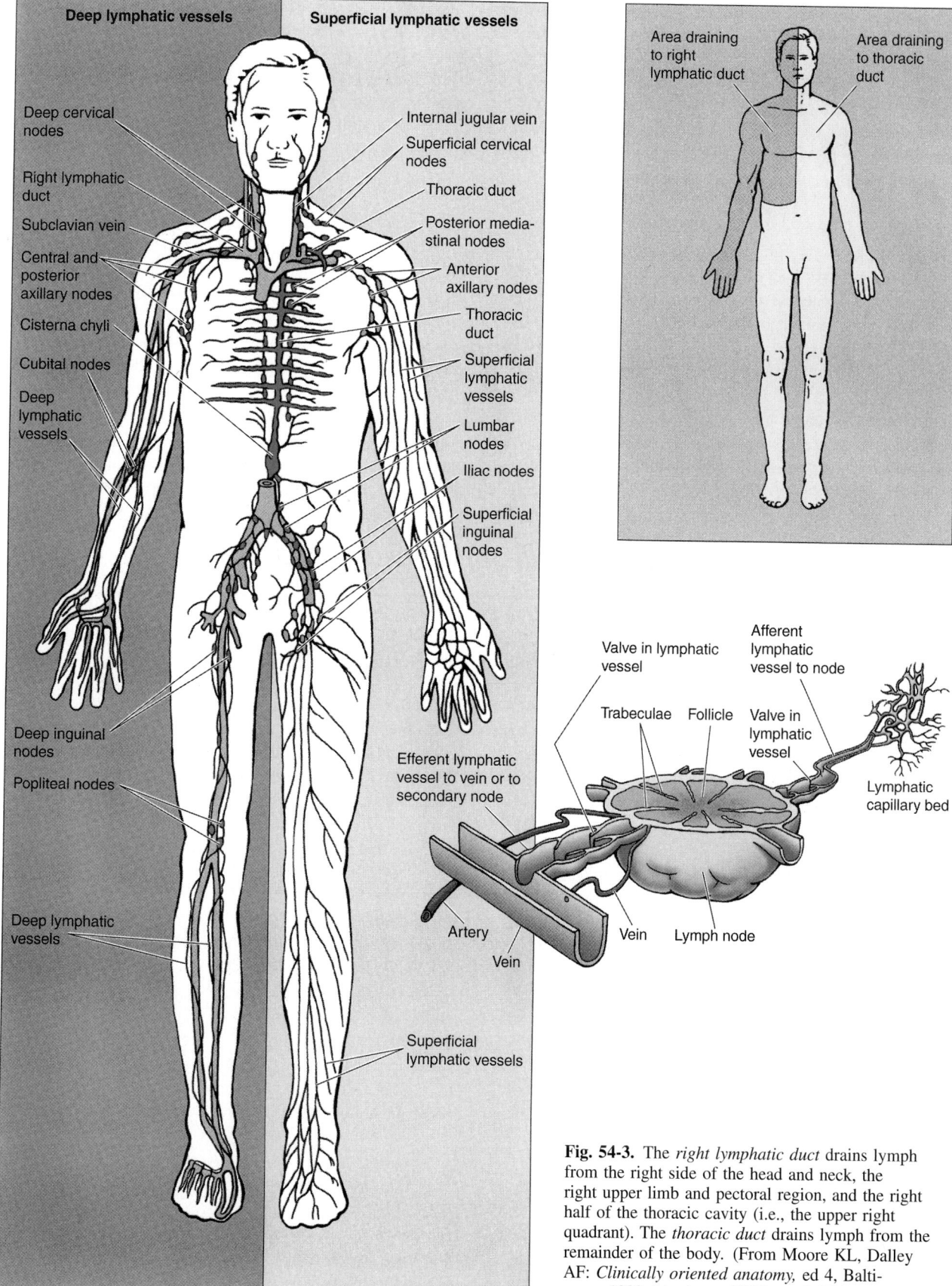

Fig. 54-3. The *right lymphatic duct* drains lymph from the right side of the head and neck, the right upper limb and pectoral region, and the right half of the thoracic cavity (i.e., the upper right quadrant). The *thoracic duct* drains lymph from the remainder of the body. (From Moore KL, Dalley AF: *Clinically oriented anatomy,* ed 4, Baltimore, 1999, Lippincott Williams & Wilkins.)

Leduc[23] has demonstrated that several alternative or substitution pathways exist in the upper limb, and a single individual may have one or more of these substitution pathways available. Most of these interlymphatic anastomoses connect the posterior aspect of the arm and shoulder with the posterior thoracic wall. These alternative pathways eventually drain the lymph into the thoracic duct or the ipsilateral or contralateral axillary lymph nodes.[23]

Recognizing the existence of alternative pathways is critical because it may help explain why some people develop lymphedema after surgical and radiation management of breast cancer and why some do not. Knowledge of the potential existence of these pathways is crucial in the appropriate management of lymphedema, should it occur.

EDEMA FORMATION AFTER BREAST CANCER TREATMENT

Despite considerable focus on the lymphatic system, evidence in the literature demonstrates that there may be two potential sources of breast cancer edema formation. Both lymph drainage failure and blood flow imbalances may cause edema problems after treatment for breast cancer. Although most authors suggest that arm edema primarily results from impaired lymphatic circulation,[14,27] the failure to also acknowledge the possible contribution of documented hemodynamic imbalances[47,48] may lead to a limited view of possible treatment options.[31]

Lymph drainage failure

Secondary lymphedema has been defined as an accumulation of high-protein fluid, which occurs when lymphatic vessels are impaired. As previously discussed, the current medical management of breast cancer predisposes the patient to developing lymphedema. Treatment for breast cancer results in obliteration and obstruction of lymphatics through the surgical removal of axillary lymph nodes and the administration of radiation therapy (if indicated). The resultant scar tissue from these procedures only further complicates matters. When the lymphatic system becomes impaired, it can become sluggish and may have a diminished capacity to transport the residual 10% of fluid from the interstitium that is not removed via the venous system.[33] With longstanding edema, there is an accumulation of excess fibroblasts secondary to induced chronic inflammation. This eventually can result in histologic changes in the tissue, including fibrosis, thickening of the deep fascia, and changes in the skin.[33,42]

Hemodynamic imbalance

Evidence dating back to 1938 has shown that a blood flow imbalance exists in some women who develop edema following treatment for breast cancer.[50] Some more recent data suggest that there is a decreased venous return or venous flow abnormalities in 14% to 70% of the swollen arms assessed.[27,47] These data suggest that venous congestion and impaired venous return may be an important part of the pathophysiology of breast cancer–related edema.

Furthermore, an increase in arterial inflow was seen in 42% to 68% of the swollen arms assessed when compared with the uninvolved limb.[27,48] It is theorized that this increase in limb blood flow causes increased capillary filtration into the tissues. This translates into an increased workload for the already compromised lymphatic and/or venous system and may be a contributor to edema formation.

None of the research concludes what causes these hemodynamic imbalances, merely that they do exist. Although some researchers hypothesize that the blood flow imbalances found in the swollen limbs of women with breast cancer–related edema may contribute to the cause of the swelling,[47,48] others argue that the imbalances are more likely a consequence of the edema precipitated by the compromised lymphatic system.[27] Regardless of which hypothesis is ultimately correct, recognizing the potential contribution of both mechanisms widens the scope of treatments available for successful management of breast cancer–related edema.[31]

EVALUATION OF BREAST CANCER–RELATED EDEMA

Lymphedema has often been called a chronic condition that never resolves. Some breast cancer–related edemas do develop into chronic conditions. Although the threat of chronicity may always exist, not all postoperative edemas go on to become chronic. However, a detailed evaluation including the specific medical management of the breast cancer and the timing of the onset of the swelling will help the skilled clinician accurately define the nature of the edema. Defining a postoperative edema condition accurately will help the clinician develop an appropriate treatment program for the stage of the edema as it presents.

Types of breast cancer–related edemas

Postoperative edema. Although lymphedema can occur at any time after treatment for breast cancer,[39] postoperative edema, often called *acute lymphedema,* occurs within the first 6 weeks after breast cancer surgery. Mild postoperative edema and subtle changes in tissue are expected and often transient, resolving with the healing of the surgical site and lymphatic regeneration.[11] Often, such therapeutic interventions such as simple active range-of-motion (ROM) exercises and appropriate positioning may be all that is necessary to assist in resolving the edema.

Cording-related edema. At approximately 2 to 3 weeks after the axillary dissection, many patients will experience pain along the anteromedial aspect of the involved upper extremity,[52] which appears to follow a neurovascular pattern. Cordlike, superficial, fibrous bands usually develop, which are often visible and palpable, especially through the

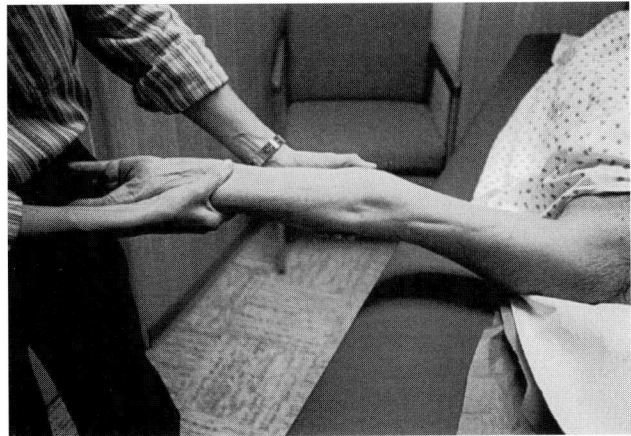

Fig. 54-4. Cordlike structures down arm and over anterior elbow into forearm, following axillary dissection.

anterior elbow and ventral forearm (Fig. 54-4). Pain associated with cording, also known as *sclerosing lymphangitis*,[44,52] is often described as a "drawing" or "pulling" feeling, which extends from the axilla to the fingers. Shoulder flexion with the elbow extended becomes increasingly difficult because of tightness of the cords.

These cordlike bands usually soften and often disappear at approximately 8 to 12 weeks. However, a mild moist heat applied to the outstretched arm, followed by gentle, skillful stretching of the cords and soft tissue, can provide a dramatic decrease in pain and increase in ROM in only a few therapy sessions.

Often, cording-related edema is most noticed initially in the ventral forearm and radial hand and is often described as "painful," fitting the pain pattern as described previously. This edema often presents during the first 3 months postoperatively but can appear with the same symptomology years later and usually corresponds with some traumatic irritation of the sclerosed lymphatic vessels, such as a quick stretch of the arm or an attempt to lift something that is too heavy.

Edema that presents with cording as its underlying cause must be treated concurrently with the cording. Manual therapy, including gentle passive ROM of the shoulder with elbow and wrist extension and mild skin traction, can be followed by the appropriate edema techniques. When caught early and treated appropriately, cording-related edema usually resolves.

Chemotherapy-induced edema. Patients undergoing certain chemotherapy regimens may develop an edema of the arm or adjacent trunk. Corticosteroids such as dexamethasone and glucocorticoids may cause short-term fluid retention throughout the body.[16,35] Because of the axillary dissection, drainage from the ipsilateral lymphotome may be impaired. Any increase in fluid in the compromised area can tip the balance in favor of an edematous condition.

At the first sign of edema, management techniques should be initiated. Treatment success may be hampered as long as the patient continues to receive chemotherapy. However, once chemotherapy is concluded, the edema can resolve with continued treatment.

Emphasis must be placed on early detection and treatment of these acute edemas. They often will resolve with skillful, early intervention. However, if allowed to progress, even these early edemas can go on to become chronic conditions.

Chronic lymphedema. Lymphedema occurs between the deep fascia and the skin. In addition to a decrease in lymphatic transport capacity, there is also a decrease in macrophage activity and an increase in the action of fibroblasts.[34,42] The accumulating protein creates an environment for chronic inflammation and a progressive fibrosis of the tissues. Fibrosis of the initial lymphatic vessels and collectors leads to a failure of the endothelial junctions to close and valvular dysfunction in the deeper collecting vessels. This results in the failure of the vessels to remove proteins from the interstitium.[41] As the condition progresses, protein continues to accumulate, forming a network of fibrosclerotic tissue.

Other histologic changes such as deep fascial thickening also occurs as edema progresses. Changes such as circumference and tissue texture can easily be detected and documented. However, before the development of such obvious symptoms, an increase in the infection rate may indicate an impending lymphedema.[34,42]

CAN LYMPHEDEMA BE PREVENTED?

Currently, there is no way to guarantee anyone who has undergone treatment for invasive breast cancer that lymphedema can be prevented. Once the axillary bed has been damaged, either through surgery or radiation, the patient will be at risk for lymphedema. However, a patient can follow several precautions that can help minimize the risk.

1. *Protect the skin.* Skin protection is important for anyone who has had treatment to the axilla and is critical for the person who already has lymphedema.[10,15,34,45] Any break in the skin of the involved upper quarter, whether from a sterile needle or a thorn of a rose opens the area up to bacteria that can cause infection. The patient should be advised to wash the area thoroughly, apply a topical antibacterial ointment, and monitor the area for any signs of infection.[10] A patient with lymphedema may experience delayed healing of an injury because of a decrease in the transport of oxygen and poor function of tissue cells.[33]

2. *Watch for signs of infection.* Infection is one of the most common causes of lymphedema and is one of the most common complications for those who have the condition.[10,33,39] The excess of stagnant protein in the tissue causes a low-grade inflammation. This, in

Girth (in cm)

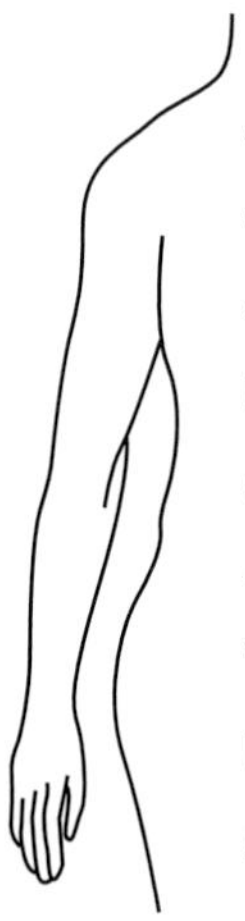

	R	L
Axilla	_____	_____
6″ above elbow	_____	_____
4″ above elbow	_____	_____
Elbow	_____	_____
6″ above wrist	_____	_____
4″ above wrist	_____	_____
Wrist	_____	_____
IP of thumb	_____	_____
Mid palm	_____	_____

Sensation

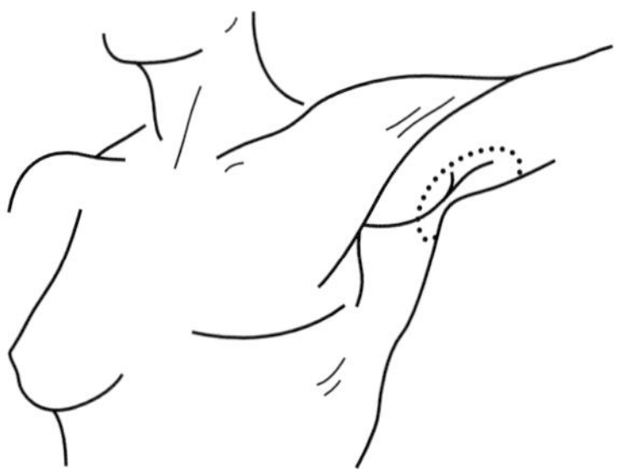

Anterior 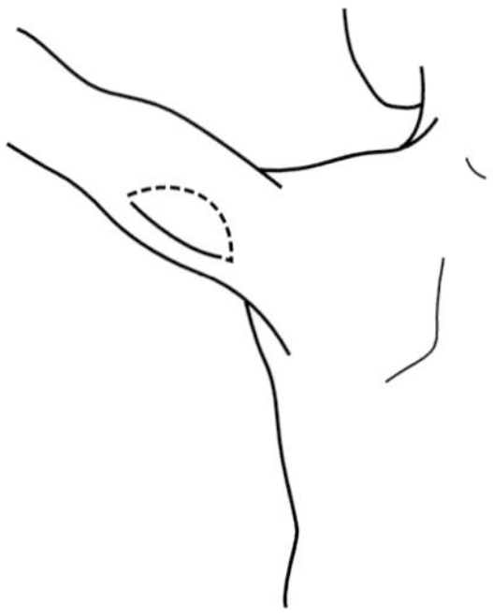   *Posterior*

	AROM	PROM	ENDFEEL
FL	_____	_____	_____
EXT	_____	_____	_____
ABD	_____	_____	_____
IR	_____	_____	_____
ER	_____	_____	_____
Horizon ABD	_____	_____	_____
Horizon ADD	_____	_____	_____

Strength

Contractile Testing: Strong/Painfree _____   Strong/Painful _____

MMT: Glenohumeral joint   FL _____ EXT _____ ABD _____ IR _____ ER _____
(0–5 scale)
                        Horizon ABD _____   Horizon ADD _____

      Scapular   Lower Trapezoids _____   Mid Trapezoids _____   Rhomboid _____

                Serratus _____

Fig. 54-5. Circumferential measurements taken along the extremity.

turn, causes an increase in temperature and, combined with the protein, provides an excellent medium for bacteria to proliferate.[10,33,37]

Signs and symptoms of an infection include redness, warmth, pain, and edema. The patient may feel feverish and report of a general malaise.[10] The patient should be evaluated for an infection when any sudden change in the limb status occurs.

Most cases of cellulitis are caused by *Streptococcus*, which is sensitive to penicillin.[33,37] It usually is recommended that the patient be on antibiotics for 3 to 5 days before treatment of the lymphedema is initiated or resumed.

3. *Restore ROM to the shoulder.* Lymph flow is accelerated by muscle contraction and movement of the limb.[28] The more the functional motion of the limb is available, the more the limb will be used and the less stagnant lymphatic flow will become. Patients should be encouraged to stretch regularly to ensure adequate flexibility of the chest wall and axilla.

4. *Gradually return the patient to activity.* Patients should be able to return to full activity following breast cancer surgery as long as the return is gradual. Baeyens et al.[4] found that no increase in the incidence of lymphedema occurred in those women with breast cancer who returned to full activity, including sports, when compared with those women who did not.

Most patients do not develop lymphedema after breast cancer surgery[40]; however, that does not minimize the importance of instructing all patients who are at risk in how to take care of the involved extremity. Lymphedema precautions should be clear enough to help minimize the risk but practical enough to be followed.

EVALUATION COMPONENTS
Medical history

A comprehensive evaluation of breast cancer–related edema begins with a detailed and thorough medical history. This includes the date and mechanism of onset of the swelling. The earlier an edema is detected and treated, the greater the success in its management. Many edemas can be traced to a precipitating event, such as infection, trauma, or overuse; however, in some cases, lymphedema occurs without any known precipitating event.[45]

A complete medical history also includes documentation of the surgical procedure and follow-up medical treatments such as radiation therapy and/or chemotherapy. If a patient is undergoing adjuvant medical treatment, the status of that treatment also must be documented (e.g., "Patient is currently in week 2 of radiation."). Other medical conditions such as active disease, infection, or cardiac or kidney dysfunction should be noted.

Finally, subjective information provided by the patient, including how the limb feels, pain, and sensation changes,

should be included to complement objective findings.[42] Improvement in subjective data can be equally important as improvement in objective data in determining treatment outcome.

Orthopedic assessment of the shoulder complex

Measuring upper extremity joint ROM and strength of the involved limb, and comparing the data gathered from the uninvolved limb can provide information on other compounding factors related to the lymphedema. The data also will aid in the development of essential components in the treatment plan. For example, if a patient presents with a functional limitation in shoulder motion, flexibility exercises can be used to increase the range of muscular activity.[42,45]

To date, there is no consensus on what measurement differential constitutes a lymphedema or which method is best to use to document arm size and limb volume.[6,40] Circumferential girth measurements taken along the limb can give a quantitative amount of edema at various points when compared with the other side (Fig. 54-5). There is good correlation between circumference measurements and calculated limb volumes and the actual volume of the limb.[10,42] The volume of each segment is calculated using the circumferential measurements and then totaled into a single estimate of the limb's volume (Box 54-1).[10] Changes in circumferential measurements and calculated volumes can be used to demonstrate limb progress.

Tonometry (also called *durometry*) is used to objectively quantify tissue texture changes by measuring tissue compressibility.[41] A tonometer (or durometer) is a plungerlike device that, depending on how depressed it becomes when placed on tissue, will indicate fluid and fibrin changes in the tissue[10,41,42] (Fig. 54-6). It is also an indicator of whether a treatment is working because tissue softening often occurs before a change in circumference or volume can be measured.[41]

Several readings are taken with each use of the tonometer. First, an initial measurement of tissue "hardness" is obtained by reading the tonometer gauge when it is first placed on the area of the limb to be assessed. Subsequent readings are taken at 30 seconds, 1 minute, and every minute thereafter for 5 minutes, for a total of seven readings. The points are then plotted to determine tissue "creep," the slow deformation in response to sustained constant pressure over time[49] (Fig. 54-7). Normal tissue has little creep, whereas edematous tissue has significant creep. As the limb improves, the amount of creep measured should decrease. Tonometry readings that indicate a softening strongly correlate with subjective reports of improvement.[41] Measurement of the normal limb in the same anatomic position as the affected limb is also performed to establish a baseline value.

The inclusion of quantitative and qualitative data in the evaluation process allows for a more holistic understanding of the edematous limb and its impact on the patient. It also provides the clinician with a solid foundation on which to base a comprehensive and an effective treatment program.

TREATMENT TECHNIQUES FOR BREAST CANCER–RELATED EDEMA

The main purpose of a comprehensive edema treatment program should be long-term maintenance of improved arm size and shape. This can be achieved through the combination of various treatment modalities. The application of these modalities must be compatible with the patient's personal goals, lifestyle, overall health status, and insurance or financial resources to be effective long term.[30,45]

Manual lymphatic therapy

MLT is a massage technique that directly affects tissue pressure, thereby facilitating fluid and protein resorption from the tissue.[10,22,45] The various strokes are applied with

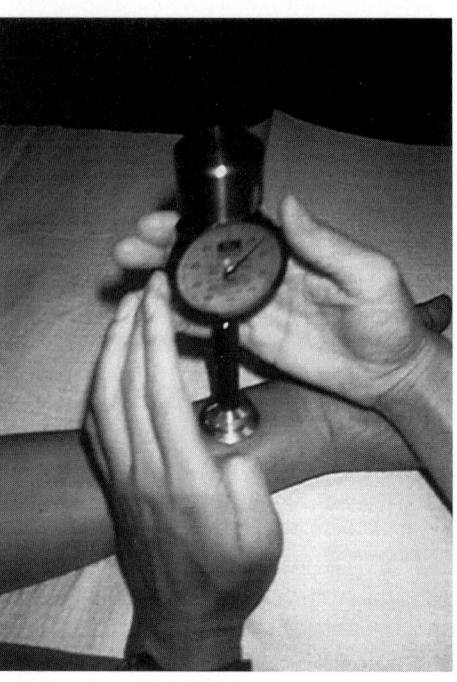

Fig. 54-6. The tonometer (durometer) indicates fluid and fibrin changes in the tissue.

Box 54-1   Equations to calculate limb volume and changes in edema

Estimating volumes from circumferences

$$\text{Volume} = \frac{h \times (C_t \times C_t + C_t \times C_b + C_b \times C_b)}{12 \times \pi}$$

where h = height

C_t = circumference of top of cone

C_b = circumference of base of cone

% Difference of total volume

$$\% \text{ Change in edema} = \frac{(V_f - V_i)}{(V_i - V_n)} \times 100$$

where V_f = final volume

V_i = initial volume

V_n = normal volume

From Casley-Smith JR, Casley-Smith JR: *Modern treatment of lymphedema,* ed 5, Adelaide, SA, 1997, Lymphoedema Association of Australia.

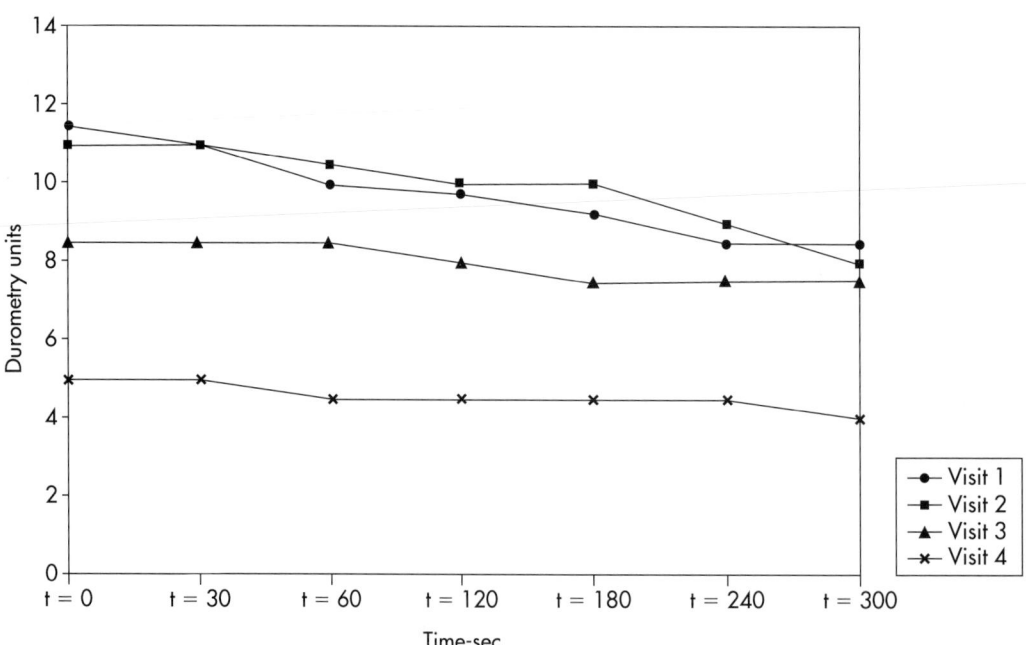

Fig. 54-7. Tonometry readings are taken at one point over a period of 5 minutes. The readings are plotted on a graph to determine initial tissue "hardness" and deformation over time.

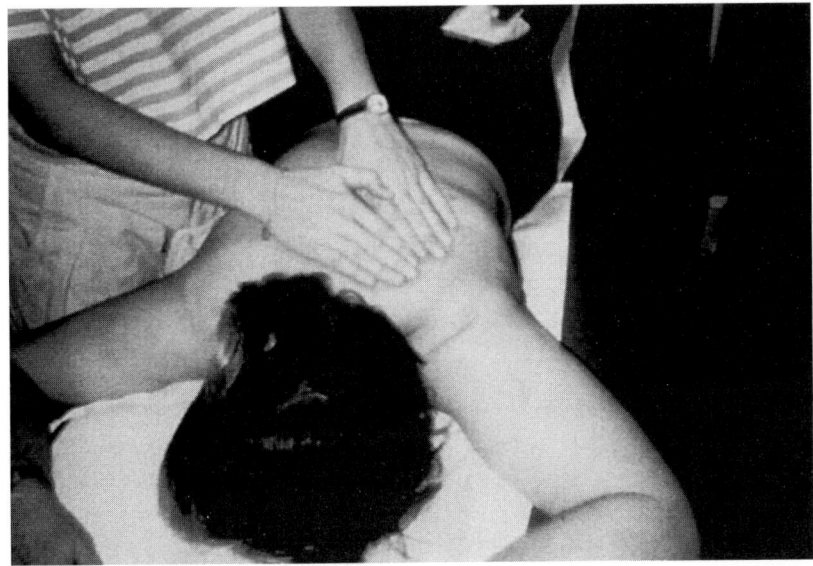

Fig. 54-8. Shunting of lymphatic fluid from a congested lymphotome to a functioning lymphotome during manual lymphatic therapy.

both *intentionality* and *directionality*. The pressure applied will determine the "intention" of the stroke (i.e., lymph transport, fibrous tissue softening) and the use of alternating pressures throughout the stroke will determine the "direction" of lymph movement.

MLT achieves fluid and protein resorption by changing the underlying tissue pressure, a necessary factor if the initial lymphatics are to function properly.[8,9] In cases of chronic edema in which total tissue pressure remains high, the lymph capillaries are not able to operate properly. The application of the appropriate manual strokes provides the variation in tissue pressure that can then facilitate lymphatic function.

The nature of the MLT stroke is also to apply a stretch to the skin, thereby pulling on the filaments that anchor the initial lymphatic to the matrix of the interstitium. This will cause a widening of the gaps between the endothelial cells of the initial lymphatics, allowing fluid and protein to enter the vessel.[36] The stretch of the wall of the lymphangion (i.e., the contractile unit of the collecting lymph vessel) also facilitates lymphatic activity.[15]

An important component of MLT is the shunting of lymphatic fluid from a congested lymphotome to a functioning lymphotome, thus enabling the fluid to be removed.[45] Using the collateral vessels that join one lymphotome to the one adjacent to it allows clearing of the affected lymphotome[10] (Fig. 54-8). Clearing of the throat and trunk are performed first, followed by drainage of the affected extremity.

Compression therapy (bandages and garments)

Low-stretch (inelastic) compression bandages serve two main purposes. First, the external pressure of the bandages on the tissue supports the elasticity of the skin and its underlying vessels. The pressure from longstanding edema reduces skin elasticity and the skin can become lax, even after the edema has been treated. Providing support to the skin during treatment allows the integrity of the skin to be restored.[10,45]

Second, compression therapy facilitates the function of the underlying lymphatic vessels by causing a mild increase in total tissue pressure. The semirigid support created by the bandages also improves the muscle pump by providing the muscle with something to work against. Increased force is then imparted to the underlying lymphatic vessels and veins, enhancing fluid and protein return.[25]

Various forms of padding can be used with compression bandaging. The purpose of the padding is to protect the limb, soften fibrous tissue,[10] and improve the gradiency of the bandage. Graded pressure is achieved by the number of layers applied to the limb. To achieve a properly graded bandage, more layers are applied at the distal portion of the limb. The final product will result in the bandage feeling "firmer" distally than it does proximally.

Compression garments may be used to support compromised skin elasticity after the limb has stabilized. However, they are not interchangeable with compression bandages. When applied appropriately, compression *bandages* serve as a working treatment that facilitates lymphatic flow by improving the muscle pump. Compression *garments* may help maintain the achieved limb reduction but have not been shown to reduce limb circumference.[53]

Exercise

Movement is crucial in maintaining normal lymphatic function. Tissue pressure changes caused by muscular contraction and pulsating arteries facilitate lymphatic flow.[28,36] The changes in intrathoracic pressure that occur with breathing also promote an increase in lymph flow.[28] These physiologic principles seem to indicate that participation in an exercise program that includes flexibility and strengthening activities and an aerobic program may be essential in lymphedema management.[30] In the case of breast

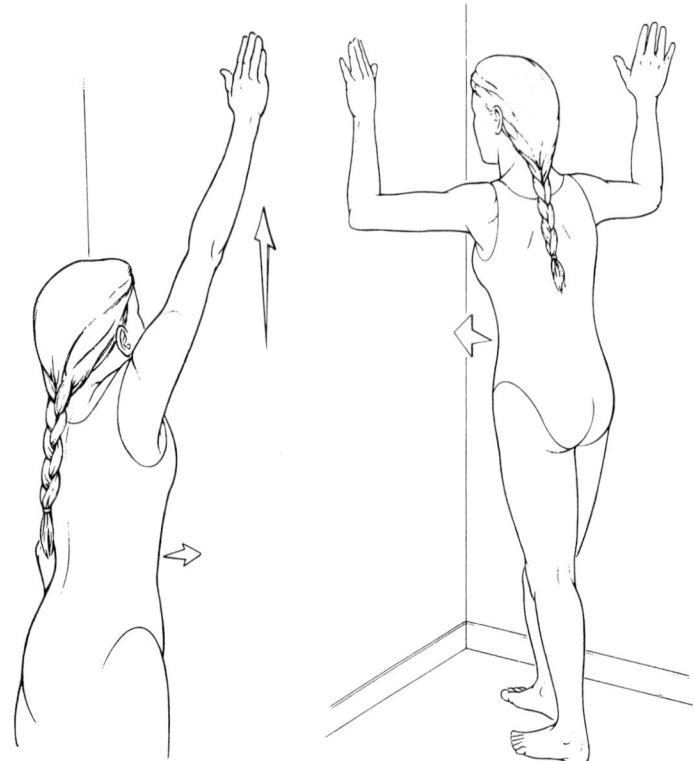

Fig. 54-9. Flexibility exercises performed to decrease axillary and chest wall tightness.

cancer–related edema, these types of exercise can be extremely beneficial because they improve both venous and lymphatic return and therefore can directly affect the well-documented lymphatic and the venous components of the edema.[31]

Currently, no published data look at the intensity at which exercise can be performed safely after lymph node removal. Therefore individual guidelines concerning the return to full activity and exercise should be developed for each patient after nodal dissection.[7] The presence of lymphedema makes it even more critical to do so.

The response of the limb to exercise is an invaluable tool to assess the limb's tolerance for that activity. If the limb size or texture remains relatively unchanged after an activity, it may be concluded that the activity was well tolerated.[7,31,45] If the limb swells or the tissue texture hardens, the duration and the intensity of the exercise must be assessed and the activity adjusted. By using the limb as a barometer of response to exercise and by taking proper steps such as monitoring the activity and wearing compression bandaging while performing the activity, a patient should be able to return to a full and active lifestyle, even after the onset of lymphedema.

A comprehensive exercise program to address breast cancer–related edema should contain shoulder and chest wall flexibility exercises (Fig. 54-9). Minimizing axillary and pectoral tightness after surgery can alleviate compression of

the vessels of the thoracic outlet responsible for normal venous return from the limb. Because women with this condition can have compromised venous outflow[27,47] as well as lymphatic impairment, the edema condition may be complicated further by muscle and soft tissue tightness compromising venous return.[31,45]

A progressive weight-training program can prepare the swollen limb for more functional activities and also can help facilitate limb lymphatic flow. Wearing short-stretch compression bandages while performing active muscle contraction increases protein resorption and enhances lymphatic flow.[25] The progression of a weight-training program is gradual, moving from a very light weight (1 to 2 pounds) at its inception to heavier weights as the limb tolerates.[7] All muscle groups of the arm are used, with emphasis on the larger muscles of the shoulder girdle and elbow complex (Fig. 54-10). Teaching the patient how to monitor the arm and to recognize when an activity is tolerated and when it is not, and how to adjust accordingly, is critical in the carryover from the clinic to everyday life.[25]

Aerobic activities, performed with the limb bandaged, can also be used to enhance venous and lymphatic flow in the patient with breast cancer–related edema. With normal physiologic function, the negative pressure buildup in the thorax with each breath causes an increase in lymphatic uptake at the thoracic duct and an increase in venous return at the venous arch. Increased respiration also accelerates

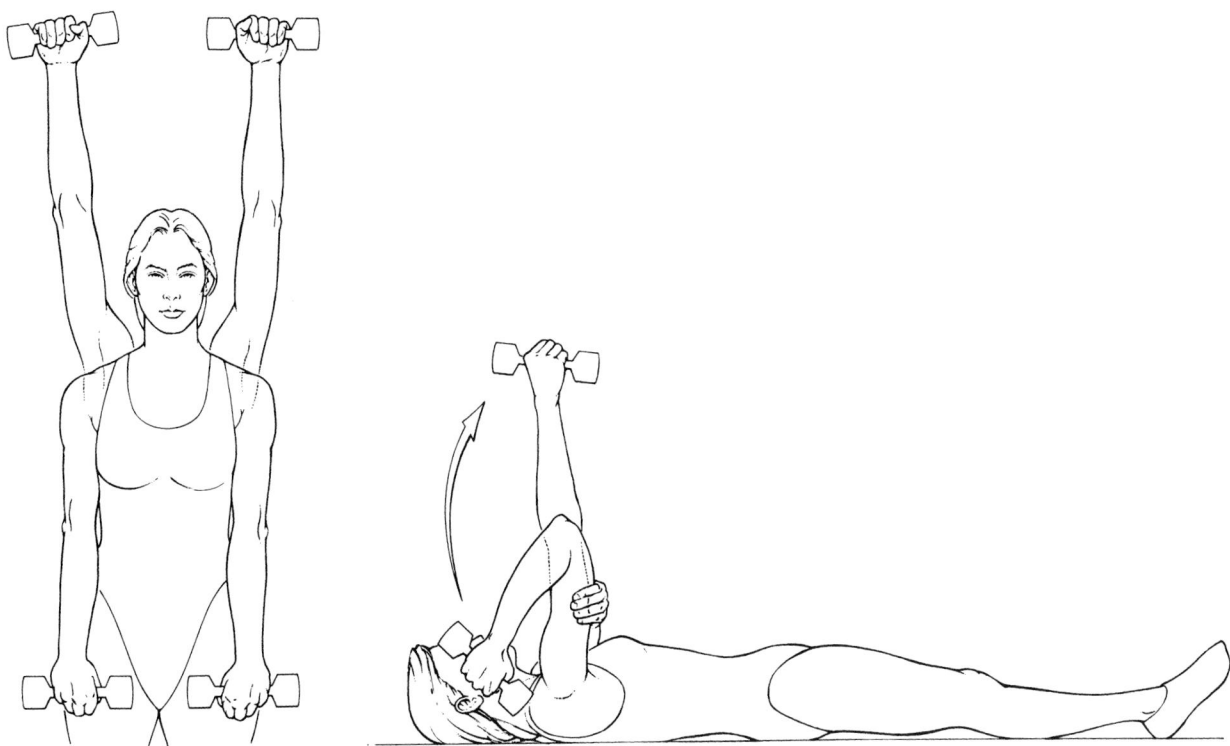

Fig. 54-10. Progressive resistive exercises performed with emphasis on the larger muscles of the shoulder girdle and elbow complex.

lymph flow.[36] Aerobic cross-training can be used to improve the efficiency of the lymphatic system just as it can improve the efficiency of the cardiorespiratory system.

The benefits of aerobic exercise in the patient who has undergone treatment for cancer and has developed edema cannot be underestimated. Fatigue is a common complaint for many cancer patients, and it can persist long after the treatment has ended.[51] It has been shown that cardiorespiratory capacity of the cancer patient greatly diminishes with cancer treatment.[3] However, women with breast cancer who perform aerobic exercise during the months of chemotherapy treatment demonstrate improved cardiorespiratory capacity compared with those who do not.[26] Participation in an individualized and monitored aerobic program after developing breast cancer–related edema not only assists in venous and lymphatic return but also can put the patient on the road to full recovery from the side effects of the cancer treatment itself.

Pneumatic compression pumps

The use of pneumatic compression pumps in the treatment of lymphedema has become a heated debate as more therapists move toward manual techniques and bandaging. However, understanding the mechanism of action of the compression pump may allow for more appropriate screening of patients who might actually benefit from the addition of this modality to their treatment regimen.

The term *lymphedema pump* is clearly a misnomer. The literature does support that compression pumps reduce limb volume.[7] However, very little literature has focused on the mechanism by which the limb volume has been reduced. Leduc and Leduc[24] have demonstrated that compression pumps actually decrease limb volume by enhancing venous return and have little or no effect on the removal of protein from the tissue.[24] This indicates that the "lymphedema pump" has little effect on the lymphatic system.

Given this physiologic explanation of how the compression pump works, it is clear that this modality should not be the only treatment prescribed for a patient with lymphedema. Otherwise, only the fluid component of the edema will be removed, and the protein component will be left behind. Because of the hydrophilic nature of protein, that which is left behind will draw water back into the tissue, leading only to a temporary reduction in edema.[45] However, when combined with other treatment techniques such as MLT, compression bandages, and exercise, there may be a physiologic rationale for using the compression pump with some edema conditions. The venous congestion identified in some breast cancer–related edemas may respond well to the use of the compression pump as part of the comprehensive management program.[45] In this example, MLT and compression bandaging with exercise treat the lymphatic component of the edema, and the compression pump will treat the venous component of the edema. Combining all of these

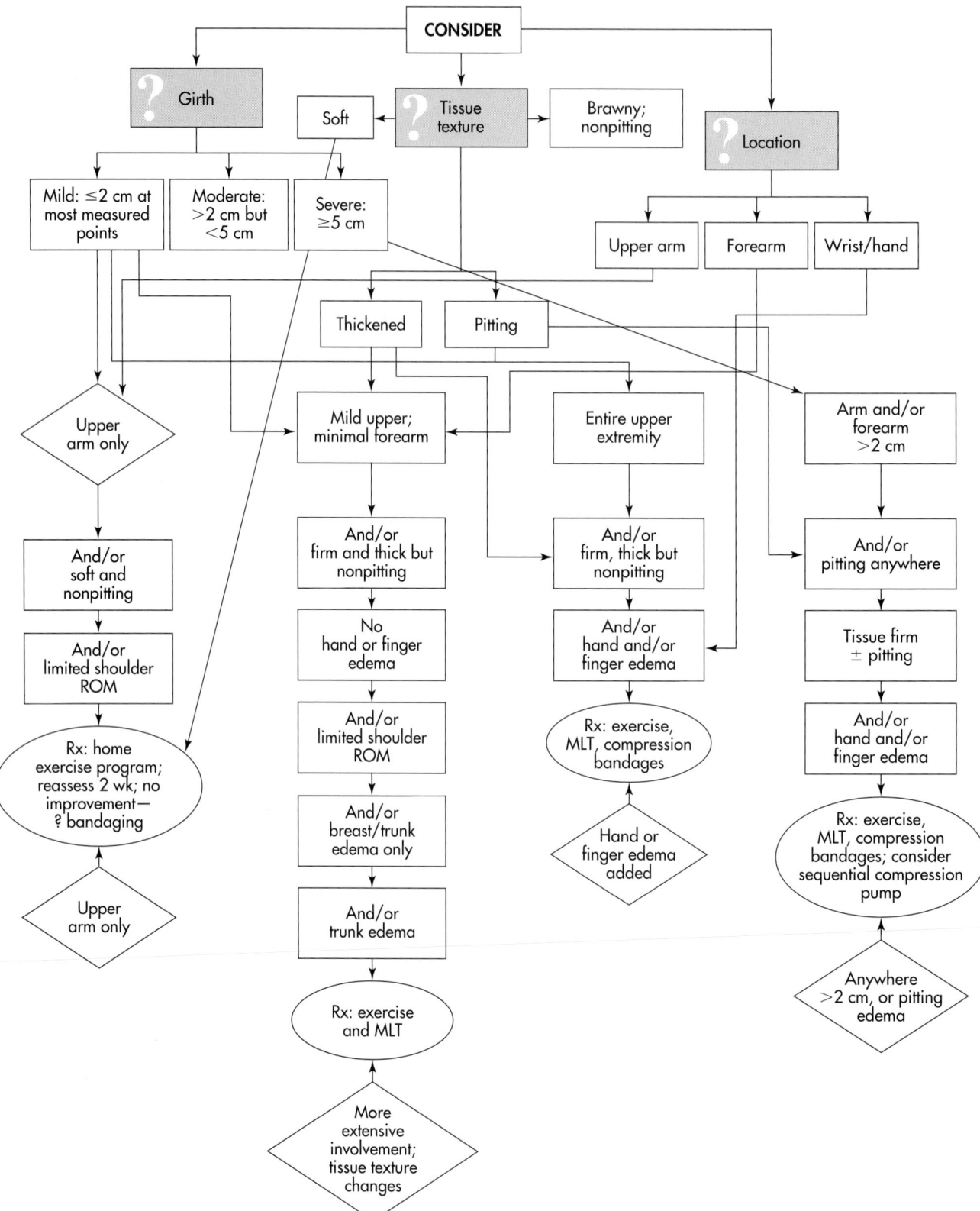

Fig. 54-11. Guidelines for treatment decision making for breast cancer–related lymphedema. *MLT,* Manual lymphatic therapy; *ROM,* range of motion. (Copyright © Linda T. Miller, PT, and Anne D. Callahan, OTR/L, CHT.)

modalities may be the best way to maximize the results obtained with each treatment.

Clearly, the compression pump may not be indicated in all lymphedemas. However, a better understanding of the pathophysiology of breast cancer–related edemas, along with an appreciation for the mechanism of action of the compression pump, may allow for a more safe determination of which patients may be appropriate. If it is determined that the pump would be beneficial, its use should be combined with other treatment techniques to maximize its effectiveness and decrease the incidence of complications.

COMPREHENSIVE LONG-TERM LYMPHEDEMA MANAGEMENT

To achieve treatment goals and to realize long-term outcomes, a comprehensive management approach is necessary. Patient education, individualized programs of self-care, and skilled follow-up, when needed, contribute to a successful intervention that will sustain the patient over time.

Treatment implementation should follow a detailed evaluation and decisions for combining the various treatment modalities are based on the degree of lymphedema (including size and tissue texture), the location of the edema, and arm function (Fig. 54-11). The lifestyle of the patient also must be taken into consideration.

The long-term goal of lymphedema management is reduction and maintenance of a more healthy limb through edema control and normalized tissue texture. An effective program should emphasize achieving this goal while compromising the patient's quality of life as little as possible. This strategy will make short- and long-term management of breast cancer–related edemas a more realistic possibility.

REFERENCES

1. Adair TH, Montani JP: Dynamic of lymph formation and its modification. In Olszweski WL, editor: *Lymph stasis: pathophysiology, diagnosis and treatment,* Boca Raton, Fla, 1991, CRC Press.
2. Ahearne PM, Leach SD, Feig BW: Invasive breast cancer. In Feig BW, Berger DH, Fuhrman GM, editors: *The M.D. Anderson surgical oncology handbook,* Philadelphia, 1999, Lippincott Williams & Wilkins.
3. American College of Sports Medicine: *Guideline for exercise testing and prescription,* Philadelphia, 1991, Lea & Febiger.
4. Baeyens L, Lescrainier JP, Afeich TC: Sporting activity after axillary dissection. XXI Congress of the European Group of Lymphology: Rome, Italy, May, 1996, *Eur J Lymphol* 6:1, 1996.
5. Behrend SW, Slivjak A: Radiation therapy. In Liebman M, Camp-Sorello, editors: *Multimodal therapy in oncology,* St Louis, 1996, Mosby.
6. Box RC, Reul-Hirche HM, Bullock-Saxton JE: Early detection of lymphedema after axillary dissection: a preliminary study investigating the intra- and inter-observer reliability of three measurement methods, *Eur J Lymphol* 7:74, 1999.
7. Brennan MJ, Miller LT: Overview of treatment options and review of the current role and use of compression garments, intermittent pumps, and exercise in the management of lymphedema, *Cancer* 83(suppl): 2821, 1998.
8. Casley-Smith JR, Casley-Smith JR: The structure and functioning of the blood vessels, interstitial tissues, and lymphatics. In Földi M, Casley-Smith JR, editors: *Lymphangiology,* Stuttgart, Germany; New York, 1983, FK Schattauer.
9. Casley-Smith JR, Casley-Smith JR: *High-protein oedemas and the benzo-pyrones: the causes, effects, incidence, and treatment of high-protein oedemas, including lymphoedema, and how these are improved by the benzo-pyrones, including the coumarins and the flavonoids,* Philadelphia, 1986, JB Lippincott.
10. Casley-Smith JR, Casley-Smith JR: *Modern treatment of lymphedema,* ed 5, Adelaide, SA, 1997, Lymphoedema Association of Australia.
11. Cooley ME, Erikson B: Rehabilitation. In Fowble B et al, editors: *Breast cancer treatment: a comprehensive guide to management,* St Louis, 1991, Mosby.
12. Cox CE, et al: Lymphatic mapping in the treatment of breast cancer, *Oncology* 12:1283, 1998.
13. Danforth D, Lippman M: Surgical treatment of breast cancer. In Lippman M et al, editors: *Diagnosis and management of breast cancer,* Philadelphia, 1988, WB Saunders.
14. Földi E, Földi M, Clodius L: The lymphedema chaos: a lancet, *Ann Plastic Surg* 22:505, 1989.
15. Földi M, Földi E: Conservative treatment of lymphedema. In Olszewski WL, editor: *Lymph stasis: pathophysiology, diagnosis, and treatment,* Boca Raton, Fla, 1991, CRC Press.
16. Giani L, Capri G: New chemotherapy drugs. In Bonadonna G, Hortobagyi GN, Gianni AM, editors: *Textbook of breast cancer,* London, 1997, Martin Dunitz.
17. Greenlee RT, et al: Cancer statistics, 2001, *CA Cancer J Clin* 51:15, 2001.
18. Haagensen CD: *Diseases of the breast,* ed 3, Philadelphia, 1986, WB Saunders.
19. Harris JR, Morrow M: Treatment of early-stage breast cancer. In Harris JR, et al, editors: *Diseases of the breast,* Philadelphia, 1996, Lippincott-Raven.
20. Hseuh EC, et al: Intraoperative lymphatic mapping and sentinel lymph node dissection in breast cancer, *CA Cancer J Clin* 50:279, 2000.
21. Jeffs E: Management of lymphedema: putting treatment into context, *J Tissue Viabil* 2:127, 1992.
22. Leduc A, Bourgeois P, Leduc O: Manual lymphatic drainage: scintigraphic demonstration of its efficacy on colloidal protein resorption, *Prog Lymphol* XI:551, 1988.
23. Leduc A, Caplan I, Leduc O: Lymphatic drainage of the upper limb: substitution lymphatic pathways, *Eur J Lymphol* 4:11, 1993.
24. Leduc A, Leduc O: Physical treatment of oedema, *Eur J Lymphol* 1:8, 1990.
25. Leduc O, Peters A, Bourgeois P: Bandages: scintigraphic demonstration of its efficacy on colloidal protein reabsorption during muscle activity, *Prog Lymphol* XII:421, 1990.
26. MacVicar MG, et al: Effects of aerobic interval training on cancer patients' functional capacity, *Nurs Res* 38:348, 1989.
27. Martin KP, Földi E: Are hemodynamic factors important in arm lymphedema after treatment of breast cancer? *Lymphology* 29:155, 1996.
28. McHale NG: Influence of autonomic nerves on lymph flow. In Olszweski WL, editor: *Lymph stasis: pathophysiology, diagnosis and treatment,* Boca Raton, Fla, 1991, CRC Press.
29. Meek AG: Breast radiotherapy and lymphedema, *Cancer* 83(suppl): 2788, 1998.
30. Miller LT: Lymphedema: unlocking the doors to successful treatment, *Innovations in Oncol Nurs* 10:58, 1994.
31. Miller LT: Exercise in the management of breast cancer related lymphedema, *Innovations in Breast Cancer Care* 3:101, 1998.
32. Moore KL, Dalley AF: *Clinically oriented anatomy,* ed 4, Baltimore, 1999, Lippincott Williams & Wilkins.

33. Mortimer PS: Investigation and management of lymphedema, *Vasc Med Rev* 1:1, 1990.
34. Mortimer PS: Managing lymphoedema, *Clin Exp Dermatol* 20:98, 1995.
35. Ogawa M, Ariyoshi Y: Supportive care: chemotherapy-induced emesis and cancer pain. In Bonadonna G, Hortobagyi GN, Gianni AM, editors: *Textbook of breast cancer,* London, 1997, Martin Dunitz.
36. Ohkuma M: Dermal lymph and lymphatics. In Olszweski WL, editor: *Lymph stasis: pathophysiology, diagnosis and treatment,* Boca Raton, Fla, 1991, CRC Press.
37. Olszewski WL: Lymphangitis. In Olszweski WL, editor: *Lymph stasis: pathophysiology, diagnosis and treatment,* Boca Raton, Fla, 1991, CRC Press.
38. Osborne MP: Breast development and anatomy. In Harris JR, et al, editors: *Diseases of the breast,* Philadelphia, 1996, Lippincott-Raven.
39. Petrek JA, Heelan MC: Incidence of breast carcinoma-related lymphedema, *Cancer* 83(suppl):2776, 1998.
40. Petrek JA, et al: Lymphedema: current issues in research and management, *CA Cancer J Clin* 50:292, 2001.
41. Piller NB: Pharmacological treatment of lymph stasis. In Olszweski WL, editor: *Lymph stasis: pathophysiology, diagnosis and treatment,* Boca Raton, Fla, 1991, CRC Press.
42. Piller NB: Gaining an accurate assessment of the stages of lymphedema subsequent to cancer: the role of objective and subjective information when to make measurements and their optimal use, *Eur J Lymphol* 7:1, 1999.
43. Ryan TJ: Structure and function of lymphatics, *J Invest Dermatol* 93:18S, 1989.
44. Ryan TJ, Mortimer PS, Jones RL: Lymphatics of the skin: neglected but important, *Int J Dermatol* 25:411, 1986.
45. Smith JK, Miller LT: Management of patients with cancer-related lymphedema, *Oncol Nurs Updates* 5:1, 1998.
46. Smith RA: Breast cancer screening among women younger than age 50: a current assessment, *CA Cancer J Clin* 50:312, 2000.
47. Svensson WE, et al: Colour doppler demonstrates venous flow abnormalities in breast cancer patients with chronic arm swelling, *Eur J Cancer* 30A:657, 1994.
48. Svensson WE, et al: Increased arterial inflow demonstrated by doppler ultrasound in arm swelling following breast cancer treatment, *Eur J Cancer* 30A:661, 1994.
49. Tillman LJ, Cummings GS: Biologic mechanisms of connective tissue mutability. In Currier DP, Nelson RM, editors: *Dynamics of human biologic tissues,* Philadelphia, 1992, FA Davis.
50. Veal JR: The pathological basis for swelling of the arm following radical amputation of the breast, *Surg Gynecol Obstet* 67:752, 1938.
51. Winningham ML, et al: Fatigue and the cancer experience: the state of the knowledge, *Oncol Nurs Forum* 21:23, 1994.
52. Wood C, Gerber L: Rehabilitation of the patient with breast cancer. In Lippman M, et al, editors: *Diagnosis and management of breast cancer,* Philadelphia, 1988, WB Saunders.
53. Yasuhara H, Shigematsu H, Muto T: A study of the advantages of elastic stockings for leg lymphedema, *Int Angiol* 15:272, 1996.

Part XII

SOFT TISSUE
CONDITIONS

Chapter 55

SURGEON'S AND THERAPIST'S MANAGEMENT OF TENDONOPATHIES IN THE HAND AND WRIST

Marilyn Petersen Lee
Susan Nasser-Sharif
David S. Zelouf

Tendons transmit forces from muscle to bone, and help accomplish the movement and stability required for hand function. Tendons are subjected to tensile stresses as they contract and stretch, and to compressive and shear stresses as they move through the tight fibroosseous tunnels en route to their insertions. These fibroosseous canals maintain the tendon in close proximity to the bones to prevent bowstringing and to maximize tendon excursion.[12] Most wrist and hand tendonopathies occur in these tunnels—specifically, at the first annular (A_1) pulleys in the hand and at the flexor and extensor retinacula in the wrist. These conditions are called *stenosing tendovaginitis.* Less common are insertional tendonopathies that affect tendons at their insertions into bone, for example, the radial wrist extensors as they insert onto the metacarpal bases.

Inflammation and thickening occur in both the tendon and the retinacular sheath. The fibroosseous tunnel then becomes a source of constriction that results in pain and impaired tendon gliding. Systemic conditions that affect connective tissues can aggravate these conditions. For example, patients with diabetes are four to five times more likely to develop carpal tunnel syndrome (CTS) or trigger digits[19] than the nondiabetic population. Patients with rheumatoid arthritis develop a proliferative synovitis that involves the synovial lining and that may invade the tendon itself. Pregnancy and its associated hormonal fluctuations can result in fluid retention, which may increase the pressure in the fibroosseous tunnels.

In this chapter, we have selected *tendonopathy* as the inclusive term for all tendon pathologies, embracing acute and chronic, inflammatory and noninflammatory conditions (i.e., tendonitis and tendonosis). Primary tendonopathies, resulting from local degenerative processes or overuse, are discussed first, followed by those that are secondary to systemic diseases and infection. The chapter concludes with a review of congenital trigger digit.

STENOSING TENDOVAGINITIS
Pathology

Stenosing tendovaginitis describes the condition of the tendon and its overlying retinacular sheath that hypertrophy, causing stenosis and constriction.[16,47,113] The retinacular sheath undergoes fibrocartilaginous metaplasia. The thickness of this sheath can increase up to threefold.[91] Except in some systemic conditions, inflammation of the synovial sheath usually does not occur. In patients with tendovaginitis, biopsies demonstrate that synovial proliferation is uncommon, and that degeneration is limited to the retinacular sheath. In chronic cases, adhesions can develop between the tendons, synovium, and pulleys. Blood flow and nutrition are compromised by both constriction and thickening of tissue layers, which increases the distance for diffusion.[4] Although pain typically is present, it is not a ubiquitous symptom; for example, a patient can experience pronounced but painless triggering. The source of pain is unclear; some authors suggest that it may be the innervated tenosynovium.[58,83]

Demographics and etiology

Tendovaginitis is more common in women than in men. Lapidus[63] reports a female/male ratio of 4:1. Occupational factors may play a role, but the problem usually is multifactorial. Tendonopathies tend to cluster in some individuals. Often, multiple conditions coexist, such as CTS, trigger digits, de Quervain's disease, lateral epicondylitis, and rotator cuff disease. Over the past century, anecdotal reports and research studies have debated the role of trauma and repetitive stress in the development of tendovaginitis.* Burman[16] stated:

The three primary causes of stenosing tendovaginitis are occupational stretching of the tendon, repeated active contraction of the muscle moving the tendon, and direct injury, the stenosis being the residuum of a gross blunt injury (p. 752).

Medl[70] echoed these concerns:

Are our women working too hard? Those with painful hands outnumber the male patients by a ratio of two to one. Housewives, particularly the mothers of small children, lead in being afflicted by Quervain's (sic) disease ... Secretaries, typists, bookkeepers, accountants, electricians, painters, jewelry manufacturers, sedentary workers who overuse ill-trained muscles in weekend activities—all are likely victims, particularly in times of increased work load ... Lesions at these sites occur most frequently in workers who use their hands continuously on various business machines" (pp. 375-376).

More recently, Armstrong et al.[4] stated that the risk of hand and wrist tendonopathy in persons who perform highly repetitive and forceful jobs is 29 times greater according to epidemiologic data. Assemblers, musicians, and meat cutters are vulnerable. Of 100 musicians treated at the Mayo Clinic, onset of symptoms was associated with dramatic increase in practice time; more than half presented with symptoms of tendonopathy.[3] Keyboard players stress multiple tendons at the wrist and digits[69] as they play up to 24 notes per second[13] with pronated forearms; repetitive radial and ulnar deviation of the wrist; hyperabduction of the small finger; and digital flexion, extension, and abduction. Guitarists are prone to multiple tendonopathies affecting both wrist and digital flexors as they assume extreme wrist flexion and sustained finger pulp pressure on the left and sustained pinch or thumb movement on the right.[69] A high incidence of trigger digits has been found in meatpackers.[38] When holding knives with small, slippery handles and wearing work gloves in cold environments, the hand will grip more tightly, thereby increasing stress in the fibroosseous tunnels.

Assessment

Assessment begins with a thorough history, including exploration of aggravating activities and associated medical

conditions that may predispose the patient to tendonopathies. The pain, which is generally localized, can be provoked with direct pressure, stretch, and/or resistance to the affected tendons. Acutely, there may be concomitant swelling and erythema. In subacute or chronic cases, crepitus may be palpable. At the A_1 pulley, triggering or locking may be detected. When the diagnosis is unclear, some physicians recommend auscultation[69] or a transducer[104] on the premise that certain mechanical disorders produce distinctive, reproducible patterns of vibrations. Wallace[104] notes that harsh, high-pitched rubbing sounds often are heard in stenosed, as compared with unaffected, tendon tunnels.

General principles of management

Although often controversial, treatment of these tendonopathies has evolved over the past century. Howard[47] advocated "adequate, complete immobilization of [the] joints . . . moved by the affected . . . tendons [as] the logical and most effective treatment." He stated that "baking, heat, massage, elastic compression or strapping are makeshifts and are utilized without a true understanding of the pathological changes existing." Griffiths[40] concurred that massage, heat, and cold were "useless." In subsequent decades, surgery was advocated most often. Lapidus and Fenton[63] operated on 354 of 423 (84%) patients with wrist or digital tendovaginitis. They stated that, "although spontaneous recovery may occur, operative release is preferable, particularly when symptoms are present more than one month." With the advent of steroid injections in the 1950s, a decrease in the frequency of surgery followed. Lapidus and Guidotti[64] reported a 67% success rate with injection of trigger digits and the first extensor compartment. With the emergence of hand therapy as a specialty over the past 30 years, new and improved rehabilitative equipment and approaches have become available to the hand therapist. Following is a review of goals, strategies, and current techniques used in the management of these tendonopathies in general. More specific interventions are discussed under each condition.

Reduction of pain and inflammation

Rest. In the acute phase, rest of the involved muscle-tendon units is indicated until symptoms subside,[27,40] and pain-producing movement should be eliminated or minimized. A thermoplastic splint can be used initially for complete immobilization; a softer, semiflexible splint is indicated as symptoms subside and/or when rigid immobilization is impractical (Fig. 55-1). Splint use should be tapered gradually according to symptom response.

Cryotherapy. Cold applications can reduce pain and inflammation by delaying microscopic hemorrhage, neutralizing the effect of histamine, and decreasing nerve-conduction velocity. Cold is most appropriate within the first 48 hours of injury or onset of symptoms. A cold pack stored in the freezer can be placed over a moist lukewarm towel to cover multiple sites or a diffuse area of involvement. The

*References 31, 60, 74, 84, 101, 113.

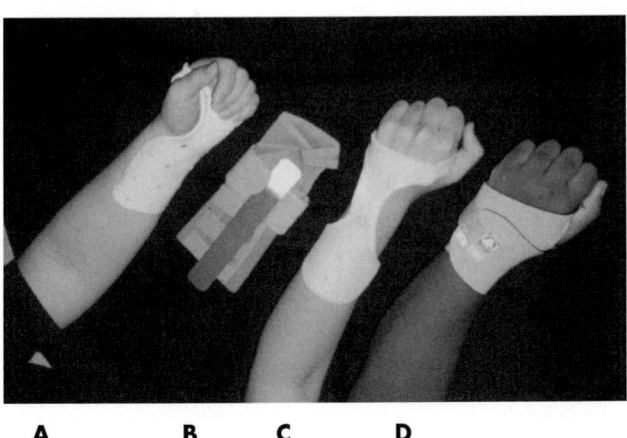

A   B   C   D

Fig. 55-1. Splinting options. **A,** Rigid thermoplastic splint for complete rest. **B,** Prefabricated elastic wrist brace with removable bar. **C,** Semiflexible light thermoplastic dorsal-based design, allowing partial wrist motion and tactile feedback on palm. **D,** Flexible neoprene wrap.

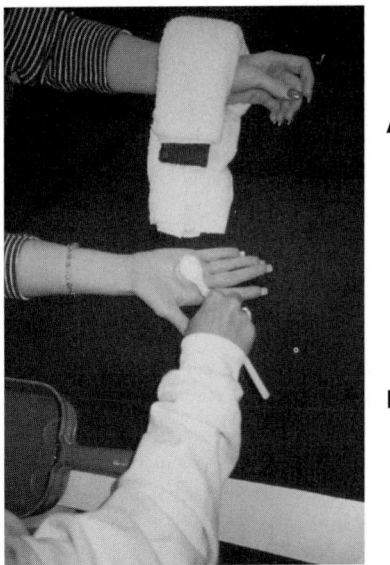

Fig. 55-2. Cold application. **A,** A cold pack for more diffuse area(s) of inflammation. **B,** Ice massage for small area of inflammation.

cold pack can be a commercially available gel pack, a homemade mixture of isopropyl alcohol and water in a 1:3 ratio, or a bag of frozen vegetables. For more localized symptoms, ice massage can be performed with an "ice pop" or water frozen in a paper cup. The ice is rubbed in a circular fashion over the affected tendon for approximately 10 minutes or until analgesia occurs[98] (Fig. 55-2). Because cold can mask pain, patients should be advised about overuse and reinjury following its application.[71] Use of cold should be avoided in individuals with cold hypersensitivity or Raynaud's phenomenon.[43]

Nonsteroidal antiinflammatory drugs. In addition to reducing inflammation, nonsteroidal antiinflammatory drugs (NSAIDs) may promote healing by accelerating the formation of cross-linkages between collagen fibers.[107] NSAIDs include aspirin, ibuprofen, naproxen, and the newer cyclooxygenase-2 agent inhibitors (e.g., celecoxib [Celebrex], rofecoxib [Vioxx]).

Corticosteroids. Corticosteroids inhibit the inflammatory process by inhibiting prostaglandin synthesis and by reducing migration of white blood cells to the injured area.[111] Sampson et al.[90] suggest that corticosteroids may act to reduce the fibrocartilaginous metaplasia that occurs in tendovaginitis. Steroids inhibit collagen synthesis and therefore can weaken tendons, if used in excess.[54] Corticosteroids also should be given with caution in immunocompromised patients because they interfere with the immunologic defense mechanisms.[21] Steroids can be administered orally, transcutaneously, or by injection. Ultrasound or iontophoresis can be used to enhance drug delivery across the skin.

Injection. In general, one or two injections of corticosteroid are offered to the patient. These are given several weeks to months apart. If the tendovaginitis is secondary to a systemic condition such as diabetes mellitus or rheumatoid arthritis, the patient is informed that the chance of success with injection alone is reduced. A mixture of lidocaine (plain with no epinephrine) and a soluble corticosteroid solution are placed in a 3-ml syringe. A small 27- or 25-gauge needle is used for injection. The needle should be placed in close proximity to the tendon or into the sheath, but not into tendon substance. Controversy exists about whether or not the efficacy of the steroid is altered by placement into or outside of the sheath. Complications include nerve injury, depigmentation, skin and subcutaneous atrophy, and infection, especially in the immunosuppressed patient. Patients with diabetes should be warned that there can be a transient elevation in their blood glucose after the injection.[90]

Phonophoresis. The efficacy of ultrasound as an enhancer of transdermal drug delivery is controversial.[30,59,71] Of the studies reviewed by Byl,[17] 75% found positive effects of ultrasound on local subcutaneous drug diffusion. Thermal ultrasound may enhance drug absorption by increasing the kinetic energy of molecules of both the drug and tissues. In their analysis of corticosteroid preparations used in phonophoresis, Cameron and Monroe[18] reported that betamethasone in gel transmitted 88% of ultrasound energy, whereas hydrocortisone powders and creams transmitted less than 30%, relative to water. To maximize absorption of medications, Byl[17] recommends using topical agents that transmit ultrasound, pretreating the skin by warming and/or shaving, and using an occlusive dressing after treatment to maximize drug concentration. Selection of ultrasound intensity should be appropriate for the phase of tissue healing. In acutely inflamed tissues, using a low intensity of 0.1 to 0.2 W/cm^2 (spatial-average temporal-average) will avoid a thermal effect.[78] Recommendations for optimal duty cycle (on/off time) vary in the literature from 20% (pulsed) to 100% (continuous mode). Some authors suggest that a low duty cycle will ensure a nonthermal effect. Others believe that the continuous mode is more efficacious, arguing that the desired treatment effect is diluted when a low duty cycle is combined with the constant movement of the ultrasound head. It should be stressed that the properties of the medicated medium are more important to the treatment outcome than are the ultrasound parameters.[17,78]

Iontophoresis. Iontophoresis is the use of direct current to deliver ionizing medications transdermally, to target structures such as tendons. Research suggests that dexamethasone sodium phosphate administered iontophoretically is effective in controlling pain and inflammation, but more controlled studies are needed.[6,20,21,30,42] Banta[6] reported that, at 6-month follow-up, iontophoresis was efficacious in 11 of 19 (58%) patients with CTS who had failed a 3-week course of NSAIDs and splinting; however, the unique effect of iontophoresis is not known because patients were also splinted during the iontophoresis treatment time period, and there was no control group. Summarizing several clinical studies, Ciccone[20] suggests the following as optimal parameters:

- Amplitude (current intensity): 1.0 to 4.0 milliamperes (mA)
- Duration: 20 to 40 minutes
- Total current dosage: 40 to 80 mA-minutes
- Frequency: not more frequently than every other day to maximize antiinflammatory effects while minimizing potential detrimental effects such as breakdown of collagenous tissues
- Number of treatments: if no benefit is seen after three to four treatments, discontinue; an ideal maximal number is not specified in the literature

Amplitudes and dosages at the higher end of the ranges are recommended by some authors,[20,21] but further study is needed to determine ideal stimulus parameters. Patient tolerance is also a determining factor. Because depth of penetration is at least 1 cm,[21] iontophoresis is a convenient way to administer dexamethasone to superficial hand and wrist structures in the acute inflammatory phase, especially for patients who will not tolerate injections. Although generally safe, iontophoresis is contraindicated for individuals with demand-type cardiac pacemakers, open wounds, or infection (Fig. 55-3).

Enhancement of tendon healing and mobility. Ultrasound, massage, superficial heat, and tendon-specific range-of-motion (ROM) exercises have been used to facilitate tendon healing and glide.

Ultrasound. Ultrasound has been shown to increase collagen synthesis, tissue repair, and tensile strength of

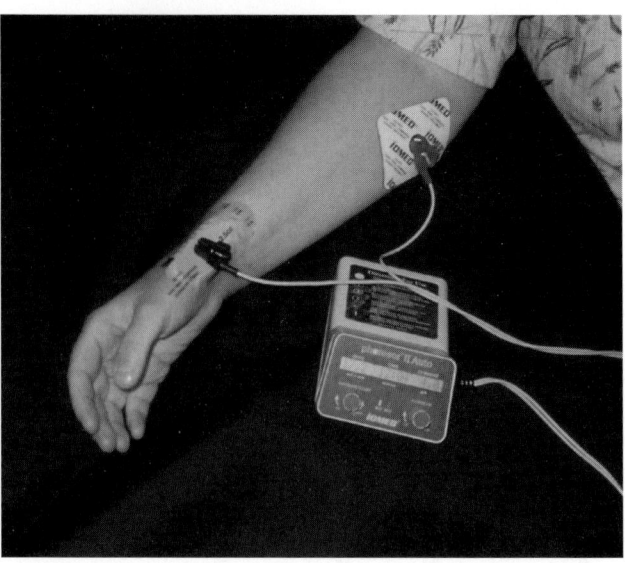

Fig. 55-3. Iontophoresis. Dexamethasone administered iontophoretically to the first dorsal compartment.

tendons.[17,25,45] Via its thermal effects, ultrasound enhances blood flow, increases soft tissue extensibility, and decreases pain.[71] There are few studies on its efficacy in hand and wrist tendonopathies. Klaiman et al.[59] reported a significant short-term decrease in pain in four patients with de Quervain's disease. Intensity and duty cycle should be adjusted according to stage of healing as discussed previously: Lower intensities or pulsed modes in the inflammatory phase can be selected to avoid undesired heating. Treatment time also can be reduced; 30 to 60 seconds per effective radiating area (ERA) is recommended. In cases of recent contracture or soft tissue tightness, and in which inflammation is absent or minimal, intensities of 0.8 W/cm^2 or higher may be administered continuously for a thermal effect. Painful overheating should be avoided; if it occurs, the intensity can be reduced or the transducer head should be moved more rapidly. Because depth of penetration is inversely proportional to frequency, the higher frequency of 3 MHz is appropriate for targeting tissues 1 to 2 cm below the skin surface, such as tendons of the hand and wrist. However, a frequency of 1 MHz also can be used; in fact, at a given intensity the lower frequency may feel more comfortable on the skin because more heat is shifted from the skin to deeper tissues such as tendons and joint structures. Nussbaum[77,78] recommends that when thermal effects are desired, ultrasound should be administered for approximately 8 to 10 minutes to an area twice the size of the ERA of the ultrasound head. There is no safety limit on the number of ultrasound treatments given; however, ultrasound should be discontinued if no measurable benefits such as pain reduction, increased mobility, or improved function are seen, or if the patient's condition plateaus.[77,78]

Massage. Massage is purported to improve tendon function by increasing circulation and tendon nutrition and

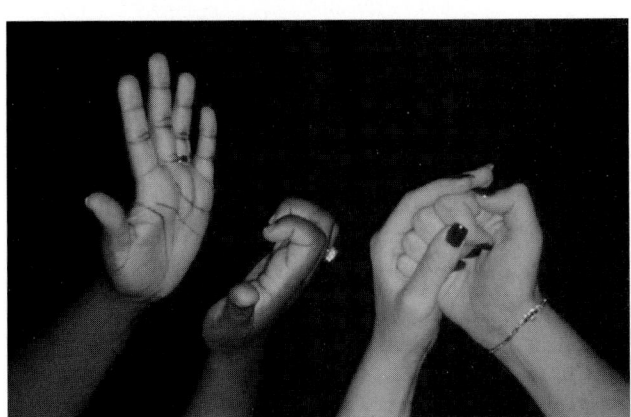

Fig. 55-4. Tendon gliding of extrinsic finger tendons.

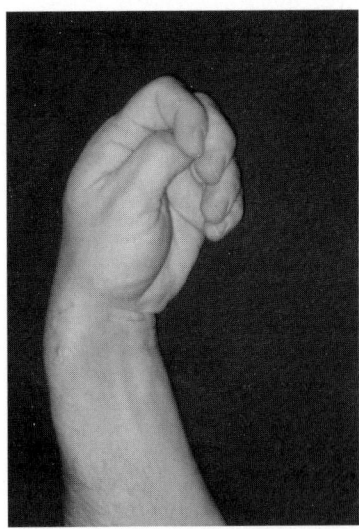

Fig. 55-6. Composite stretch of first dorsal compartment tendons (Finkelstein's test position).

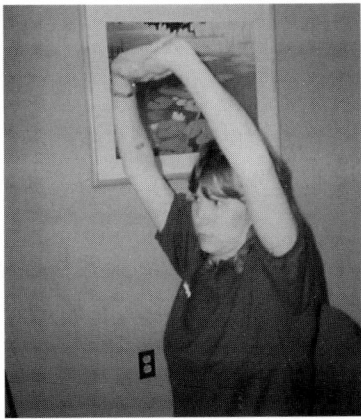

Fig. 55-5. Composite stretch of wrist and digital flexors and extensors.

by "softening" (remodeling) hypertrophic tendons, thus reducing tissue bulk at the pulleys.[22,28,55] Evans et al.[28] advocate massage of the entire tendon sheath and adjacent areas. Cyriax and Cyriax[22] popularized transverse friction massage (TFM), in which the clinician moves the patient's skin over the affected area perpendicular to tendon fiber orientation, with increasing pressure, working up to 15 minutes. If tendon and pulley are involved, they state that the clinician should hold the tendon taut and mobilize perpendicular to the sheath. This technique is described for extensor carpi radialis, extensor carpi ulnaris (ECU), flexor carpi radialis (FCR), flexor carpi ulnaris (FCU), abductor pollicis longus (APL), and extensor pollicis brevis (EPB) tendons. Other than anecdotal reports, no controlled studies prove the efficacy of TFM in the hand and wrist, particularly for stenosing tendovaginitis. TFM is a vigorous technique that is not always well tolerated by the hand of the patient or the clinician who is performing it.

Gliding and stretching. Gliding and stretching of the affected tendons can prevent or reduce adhesions and enhance nutrition by synovial diffusion. When the length of a muscle-tendon unit is increased, strain during joint movement is decreased.[94] Superficial heat such as moist hot packs before, or fluidotherapy in conjunction with, ROM can be used to enhance tissue extensibility. Tendons should be mobilized gently, progressively, and in pain-free ranges. Hook, full, and straight fisting can be used to glide both flexor and extensor tendons of the fingers (Fig. 55-4). Composite elbow, wrist, and digital extension will bring the flexors of the wrist and digits to their full length, whereas elbow extension with composite wrist and digital flexion will stretch the extensors of the wrist and digits (Fig. 55-5). The components of Finkelstein's maneuver can be performed in stages to glide and lengthen the APL and EPB tendons[31] (Fig. 55-6).

Progressive strengthening. Strengthening can be initiated when acute symptoms have subsided. When performed in a graded, symptom-free manner, it can accelerate tenocyte metabolism, speed repair, and prepare the patient to meet the physical demands of daily activities.[52,53] Strengthening may be done in isometric, isotonic, and isokinetic modes. Isometric contractions are initiated at a muscle's resting length (roughly midrange). Lowe[68] recommends starting with brief repetitive isometric exercise for hand and wrist musculature: specifically, five repetitions, six seconds each, performed once daily. When isometrics can be performed at multiple joint angles, isotonic exercise can be added. Isotonic exercise can be performed against gravity (concentric or shortening contraction) or in the direction of gravity (eccentric or lengthening contraction). Eccentric strengthening may be helpful in cases of chronic tendonitis.[52,56,94] In addition, computerized equipment affords yet a third mode

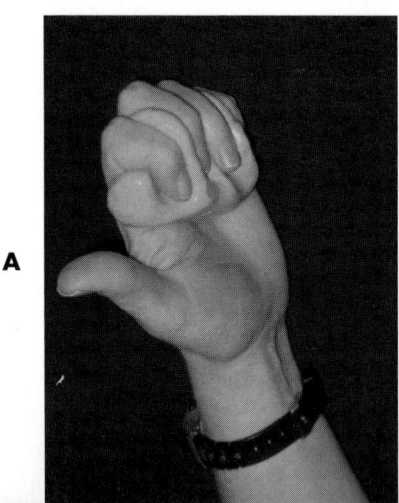

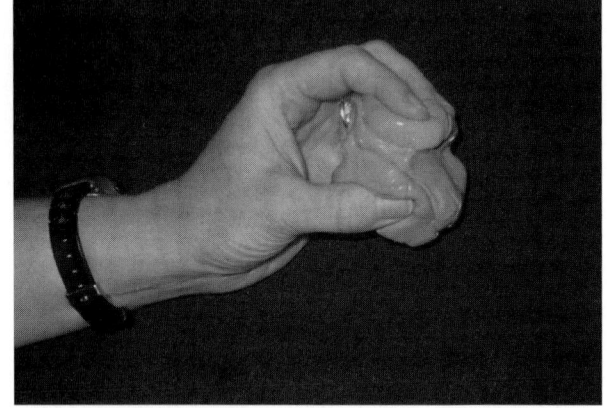

Fig. 55-7. Putty exercises. **A,** Hook fisting can be performed to strengthen extrinsic finger tendons. **B,** Exercise for intrinsic and pinch strengthening.

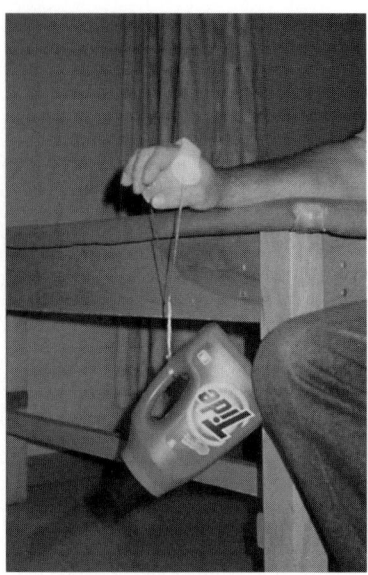

Fig. 55-8. Homemade weight for wrist strengthening (large handle prevents tight fist).

of exercise: during isokinetic strengthening, the speed of motion is constant but the resistance is varied throughout the range to "match" the changing force output of a given muscle group. Thus the resistance of the dynamometer will increase at midrange of a given joint where muscle length is typically optimal for force production, and decrease at the extremes of joint range where muscle forces are usually at their lowest.

Exercise programs should be tailored to an individual's functional needs. For a racquet ball player who requires sudden recruitment of wrist extensors for a backhand stroke, progressive resistive exercises may be most appropriate. For a typist or pianist, more frequent, submaximal repetitions may be indicated. Putty, free weights, and Thera-Band are practical for home use (Figs. 55-7 and 55-8).

Return to activity and lifestyle changes. Activities should be resumed gradually and performed in a pain-free manner. Affected tendons can be protected with rigid splints initially, then progressed to semiflexible supports or taping. Rigid splints should be weaned as symptoms abate because prolonged immobilization causes stiffness and weakness,

and may increase stress at segments proximal or distal to the immobilized area.

Ergonomic modifications and alterations of playing or sports technique may be required to prevent recurrence. These include strategies to reduce the force of grip and pinch such as using friction material on hand tools and utensils, maximizing surface contact with the hand, wearing handle straps to relax grip intermittently, using electrically powered tools to replace a manual stapler or can opener, spreading the force over four rather than one finger on trigger-activated tools, and applying force at the middle rather than distal phalanx to reduce torque at the A_1 pulley. Gloves can be helpful in distributing pressure and reducing shear forces, but they also may cause the wearer to grip harder in attempting to overcome fabric stiffness and compensate for impaired sensory feedback.[92] Working with the forearm in neutral or supination and the wrist in neutral or slight extension optimizes muscle efficiency and takes stress off tendons as they cross the wrist.[51,52] The motto, "bend the tool, not the wrist," has materialized into a variety of adapted equipment ranging from ergonomic keyboards to pistol grips (Figs. 55-9 and 55-10). Other strategies include using larger joints to accomplish the task, reducing task frequency and duration, and diversifying work (see Chapters 59 and 60).

Finally, the clinician should encourage general health and fitness by teaching the patient principles of good nutrition; aerobic conditioning; and how to balance work, leisure, and rest. The effect of lifestyle choices on tissue health should be explained.

Surgical intervention. If conservative measures fail, surgical intervention may be indicated. In general, surgery includes the release of constricting fibrous pulleys and, in some systemic conditions, excision of hypertrophied teno-

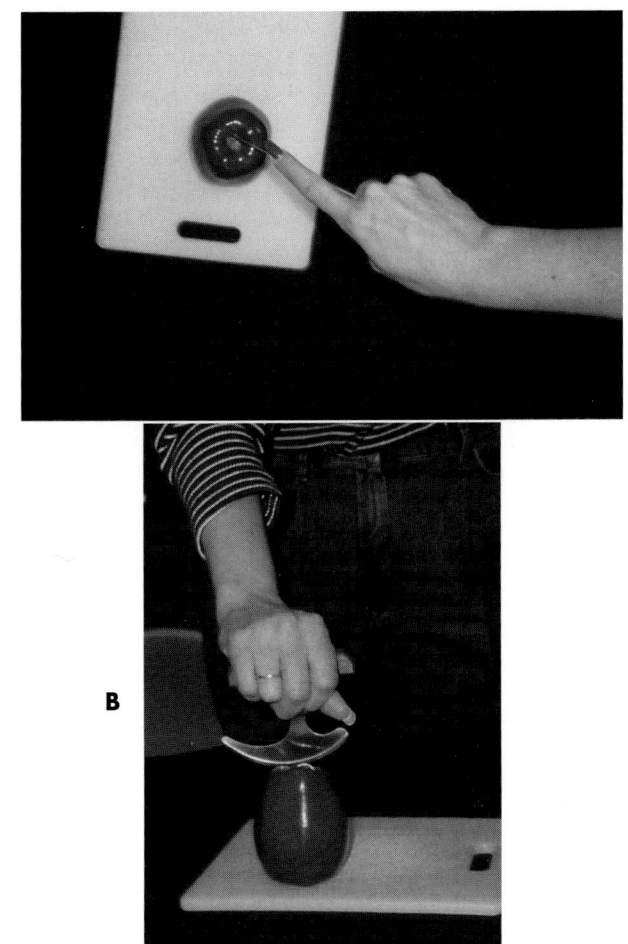

Fig. 55-9. Effect of tools on joint and tendon stresses. **A,** Use of standard knife places wrist in ulnar deviation and focuses forces on thumb and index finger. **B,** Use of T- or L-handled knife places wrist in neutral and distributes forces across entire hand.

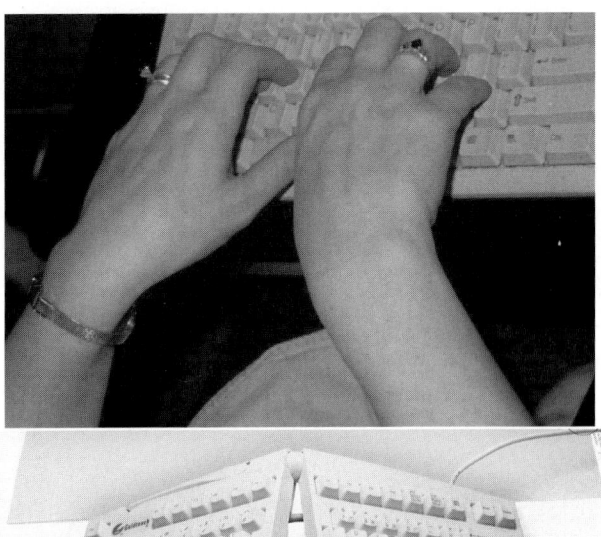

Fig. 55-10. Keyboards. **A,** Standard keyboard on high surface forces wrists into flexion and ulnar deviation. **B,** Ergonomic keyboard facilitates neutral wrist position and reduces extreme forearm pronation. (Photograph courtesy Goldtouch Technologies, Inc., 17300 Redhill, Suite 100, Irvine, CA 92614, www.goldtouch.com.)

synovium. Specific operative procedures are discussed in the following sections under their respective conditions.

Maximizing surgical results postoperatively. After surgery, the wrist and affected digits are usually immobilized in a plaster dressing for up to 1 week postoperatively. Gentle active and passive motion are initiated by the end of the first week with the goal of achieving full joint motion and tendon glide. The clinician should also monitor wound status, edema, and sensation, instituting edema reduction techniques such as elevation, retrograde massage, Coban wrapping, and use of compressive finger sleeves or gloves. Once wounds are closed and edema has resolved, thermal modalities such as fluidotherapy, moist heat packs, and ultrasound can assist with desensitization, scar remodeling, and mobilization. During heating, shortened tissues can be placed on stretch, followed by tendon gliding and additional lengthening[43] (Fig. 55-11). Massage, application of silicone elastomer sheeting or molds, and use of compressive wraps such as Coban are indicated for hypersensitive and hyper-

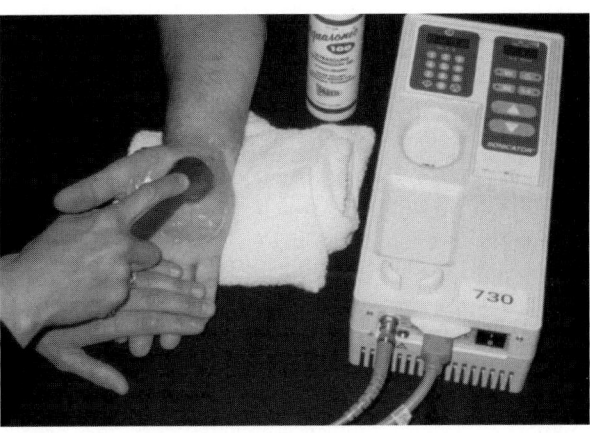

Fig. 55-11. Applying heat (thermal ultrasound) with stretch following carpal tunnel release and flexor tenosynovectomy.

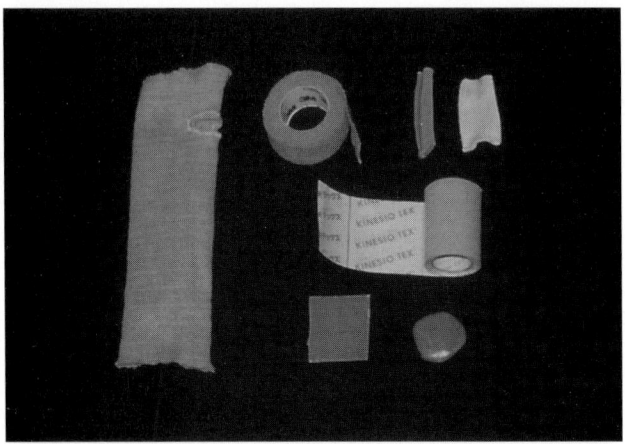

Fig. 55-12. Materials for edema and scar management, clockwise starting at left, items are Tubigrip gauntlet, Coban, prefab finger sleeve, custom-sewn Lycra spandex sleeve, Kinesiotape, Silastic gel sheeting, elastomer custom mold.

trophic scars (Fig. 55-12). Between the third and sixth weeks, strengthening is typically initiated as is gradual resumption of functional activity. Between the sixth and twelfth weeks, the patient may return to work or sports according to his or her progress and the physical demands of the tasks in question.[46a]

Types of stenosing tendovaginitis

Stenosing tendovaginitis can affect any of the 23 extrinsic tendons that power the wrist and hand. The digital flexor tendons are susceptible to compression and shear at the level of the wrist and the metacarpophalangeal (MP) joints where they enter fibroosseous tunnels. The wrist flexors, which also are enveloped in synovial sheaths as they cross the carpus, occasionally are affected. Most extensor tendonopathies occur at the extensor retinaculum of the wrist. The six compartments, formed by tough fibrous septations of the extensor retinaculum and the underlying radius and ulna, collectively contain at least 12 tendons that extend the wrist and/or digits. The compartment containing the APL and EPB tendons is by far the most commonly affected dorsal compartment, followed by the sixth compartment, which contains the ECU tendon. Insertional tendonopathies of wrist extensors and interosseous tendons occur infrequently and are discussed in a separate section.

Digital flexor tendonopathy in the carpal tunnel. CTS, which is discussed in depth in Chapters 36 and 37, results from compression of the median nerve at the wrist. Often, the source of this compression is hypertrophy of the flexor tenosynovium at the carpal tunnel deep to the nerve. Conservative management includes splinting the wrist in neutral, flexor tendon and median-nerve gliding, and activity modification. Steroid injection usually does not provide lasting relief. Success rates reported in the literature are low: 11% to 22%.[37,80] Surgical treatment includes an endoscopic

or open (standard, mini, or two-incision) release of the transverse carpal ligament. When tenosynovial proliferation is the main source of compression, a tenosynovectomy is performed in addition to an open release. In these cases especially, therapy management should include pain, edema, and scar control; flexor tendon gliding; and isolated exercises for flexor digitorum superficialis (FDS) and flexor digitorum profundus (FDP) tendons. These patients may require more prolonged wrist splinting; a soft support can be added at night, which places the digits in relative extension to assist with resolution of digital pain and edema, and to maintain flexor tendon length.

Trigger digits

Anatomy and pathomechanics. Triggering of the digital flexor tendons most commonly occurs at the fibroosseous tunnel formed by the metacarpal neck dorsally and the A_1 pulley volar to the MP joint at the distal palmar crease. In rare cases, triggering also may occur at the A_3 pulley.[86] At the thumb MP joint, the sesamoid bones, on which the flexor pollicis brevis inserts, also may be a site of constriction. The FDS generally is affected because it lies directly underneath the A_1 pulley.[80,91] Other authors implicate the FDP tendon,[39,88] and some speculate that adhesions between the two tendons may contribute to triggering in more advanced cases.[83,97a] During pinch activities in which forces are applied at the distal end of the digits, flexor tendons are subjected to maximal stress at the proximal end of the fibrous sheath (A_1 pulley overlying the MP joint) because the resistance arm is the longest. In addition, as MP flexion increases, so does the tension on the pulley (Fig. 55-13). Direct compression at the A_1 pulley from blunt trauma or sustained tool use also can be a source of injury. The tendon swells and thickens, and its fibers bunch up at the distal end of the pulley in a manner similar to strands of a thread as it is pushed through a needle's eye.[48] As first described by Notta in 1850,[39] a palpable nodule develops with an hourglass restriction adjacent to this bulbous enlargement.[63] In addition, the poor tendon vascularity between the A_1 and A_2 pulleys renders the tendons more susceptible to degenerative changes[2] (Fig. 55-14).

Demographics. Primary trigger digit, which occurs in otherwise healthy individuals, affects women two to six times as frequently as men,[16,29,70,113] with a mean age of 58 years.[88] The thumb is most frequently affected (approximately 50% of the time), followed by the ring and middle fingers (approximately 20% each). The index and small fingers are involved infrequently.[33,63] Secondary trigger digit, which occurs in individuals with connective tissue disorders, is discussed subsequently.

Diagnosis. The quality and ease of digital motion varies with progression of the disease, from sluggish movement upon rising only, to locking and flexion contracture of the proximal interphalangeal (PIP) joint. Pain may or may not accompany the abnormal tendon gliding. When present, pain is typically at the A_1 pulley and sometimes at the PIP joint.

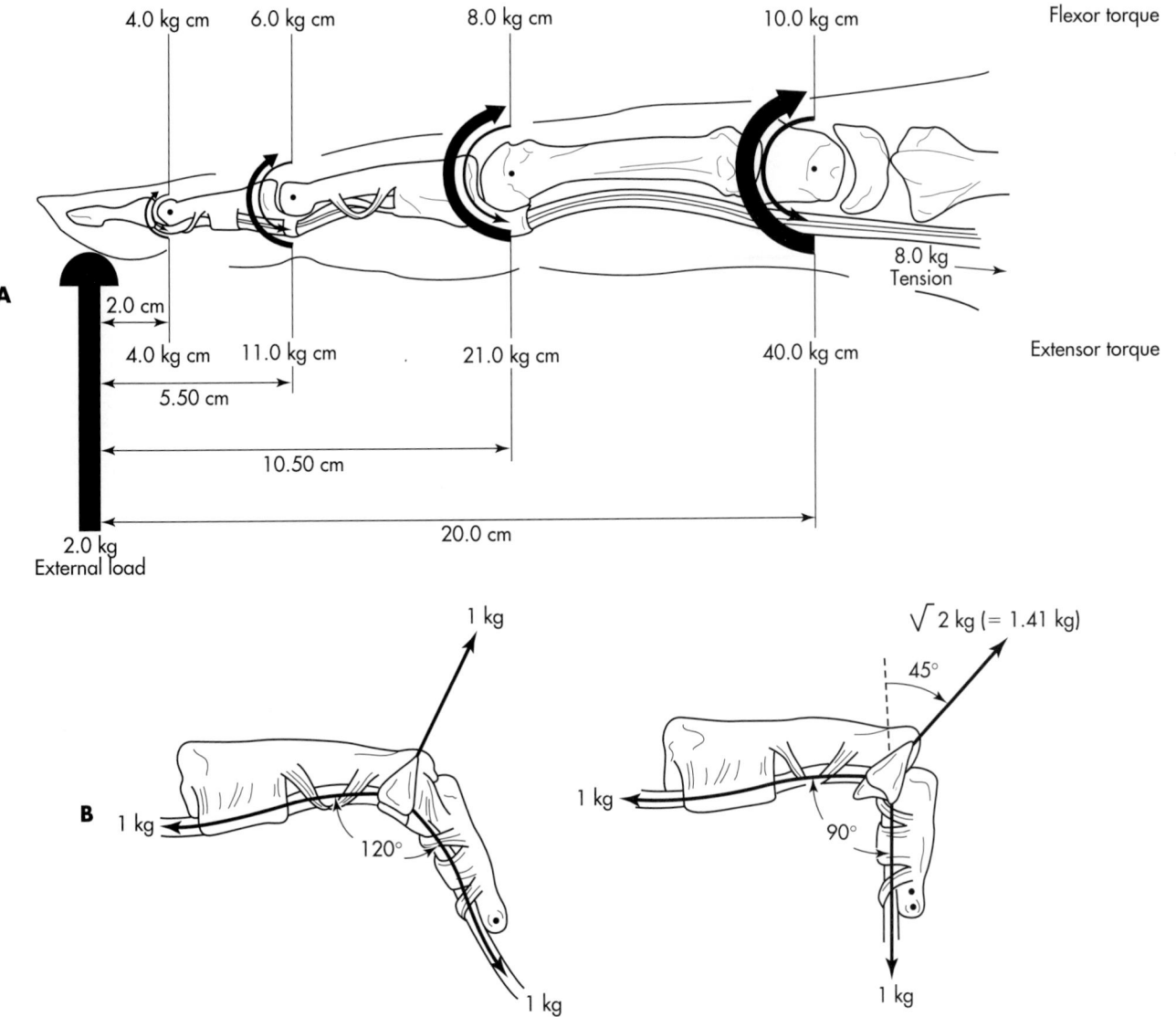

Fig. 55-13. Biomechanics of stresses at the A_1 pulley. **A,** The further away from a joint that force is applied, the higher the torque required to oppose that force. Thus when an extensor force is applied to the fingertip, the flexor torque required to oppose that force is greatest at the wrist and MP joints and is least at the IP joints. **B,** Tension in the flexor pulley system increases with joint flexion. (Modified from Brand P, Hollister A: *Clinical mechanics of the hand,* ed 2, St Louis, 1993, Mosby.)

Dorsally based PIP joint pain may result from extensor overpull.[79a] For more precision in classification, the quality of tendon gliding can be staged as follows[82]:

Stage	Quality of digital movement
1	Normal
2	Uneven
3	Triggering (clicking or catching)
4	Locking of finger in flexion or extension; unlocked by active finger movement
5	Locking of finger in flexion or extension; unlocked by passive finger movement
6	Locked finger in flexion or extension

Differential diagnosis of trigger digit includes loose bodies, anomalies of sesamoid bones,[14] sesamoiditis,[62] and flexor tendon masses (i.e., ganglia, tumors, and lipoma).[108]

Conservative management. A poorer outcome with conservative measures is associated with multiple digit involvement, duration of symptoms greater than 4 to 6 months,[76,87] diffuse tendon thickening versus a discrete nodule,[33] and the presence of significant triggering.[82] Many of these indicators characterize patients with secondary trigger digit related to connective tissue disorders.

Corticosteroid injection

EFFICACY. Success rates reported in the literature vary between 50% and 94%.[33,46a,80,82,113] Success generally is

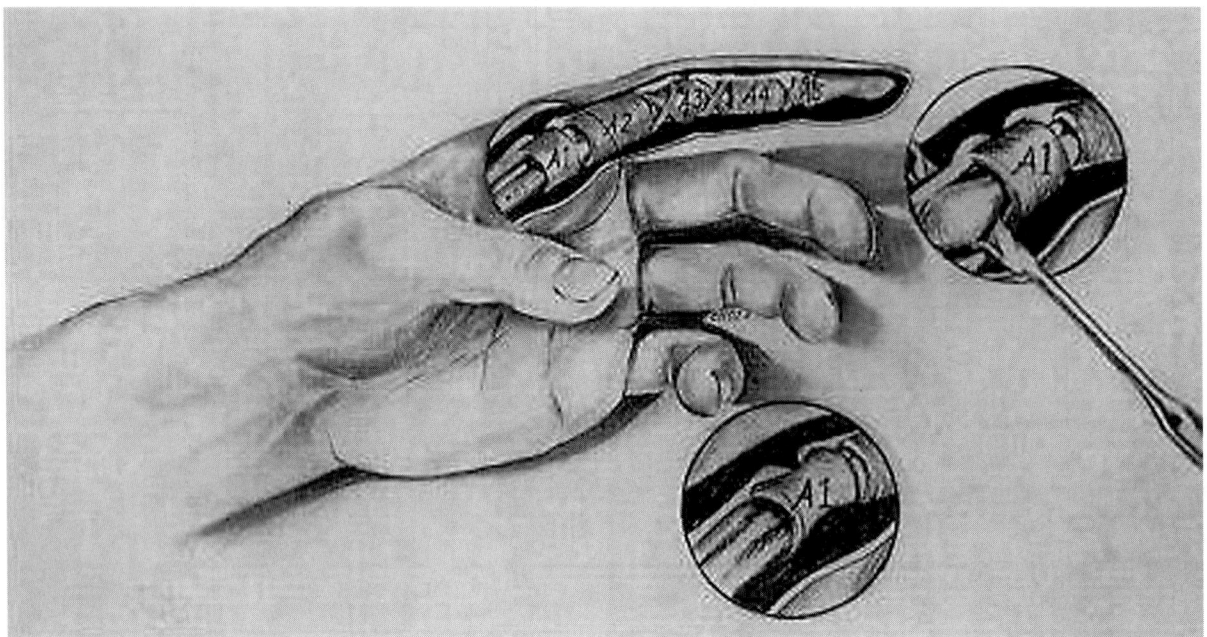

Fig. 55-14. Anatomy of the flexor tendon pulley system. *Top inset,* Flexor digitorum profundus nodular thickening. *Bottom inset,* Flexor digitorum superficialis fraying. (From Taras S, Miskovsky C: *Atlas Hand Clin* 4:1, 1999.)

defined as complete resolution of symptoms, or only minimal and occasional symptoms that do not interfere with function. Some studies do not specify duration of the symptom-free period following the injection or patient characteristics such as coexisting medical conditions. In general, success rates are much lower in individuals with coexisting conditions such as diabetes (50%)[41] as compared with the general population (72% to 93%). In a study of 235 nonrheumatoid patients with 338 trigger digits, Newport et al.[76] reported that 77% resolved or improved after one to three injections. Follow-up time averaged 3 years with no splinting or other treatment given.

TECHNIQUE. Injection techniques vary, but we generally use a combination of 0.2 ml of lidocaine (plain without epinephrine) with 1.0 ml of a soluble corticosteroid (beta-methasone). With the patient's hand prepped and the affected digit slightly extended, the surgeon palpates the metacarpal head and introduces the needle directly into the flexor tendon sheath. If necessary, placement of the needle can be confirmed by asking the patient to flex and extend the digit; it will move if it is properly located. The needle should be withdrawn slowly, and when it emerges from the tendon into the sheath, resistance will be reduced. As the corticosteroid/lidocaine solution is injected, a fluid wave may be palpated proximally or distally to the injection site.

Splinting. There is a dearth of literature on splinting trigger digits. Rhoades et al.[87] reported a 72% success rate with combined splinting and injection; therefore no conclusion could be drawn about the efficacy of splinting alone. The affected digits were splinted with MP and interphalan-

geal (IP) joints in 15 degrees of flexion continuously for 3 weeks. Eaton[27] advocated a similar splint design for night use primarily. He stated that the splint draws the tendons distally, reducing the redundancy and swelling at the pulley entrance, thereby allowing the tendons to glide more easily in the morning. Based on a similar rationale, in 1988 Evans et al.[28] introduced a splint that rests the MP joints at 0 degrees, leaving the IP joints free. They reported a 73% success rate in 55 fingers of 38 nonrheumatoid patients with daily splint use and hook fisting exercises for 3 to 6 weeks. PIP flexion contractures were treated with nighttime PIP extension splinting. Results were best in patients with a symptom duration of less than 4 months. Patel and Bassini[82] used a splint design and extrinsic tendon gliding protocol similar to that of Evans et al.[28] They reported a success rate of 66% in 50 digits treated with a 3- to 9-week course of full-time splinting and exercise alone, as compared with 84% in another 50 digits treated with injection alone. Fingers fared much better with splinting than did thumbs: 70% versus 50% success rates, respectively. The authors did not include information about coexisting medical conditions in their sample. Most recently, Rodgers et al.[88] splinted 31 fingers of 21 meat cutters with symptoms of pain or triggering but no locking. They reported a 55% success rate, with an average of 8 weeks of splinting only the DIP joint in extension. In contrast to other authors, they hypothesized that the FDP is involved in the pathogenesis of trigger finger and by decreasing its excursion, the synovitis or nodule may resolve. In summary, extension of one or more of the digital joints may be necessary to reduce or eliminate symptoms. A

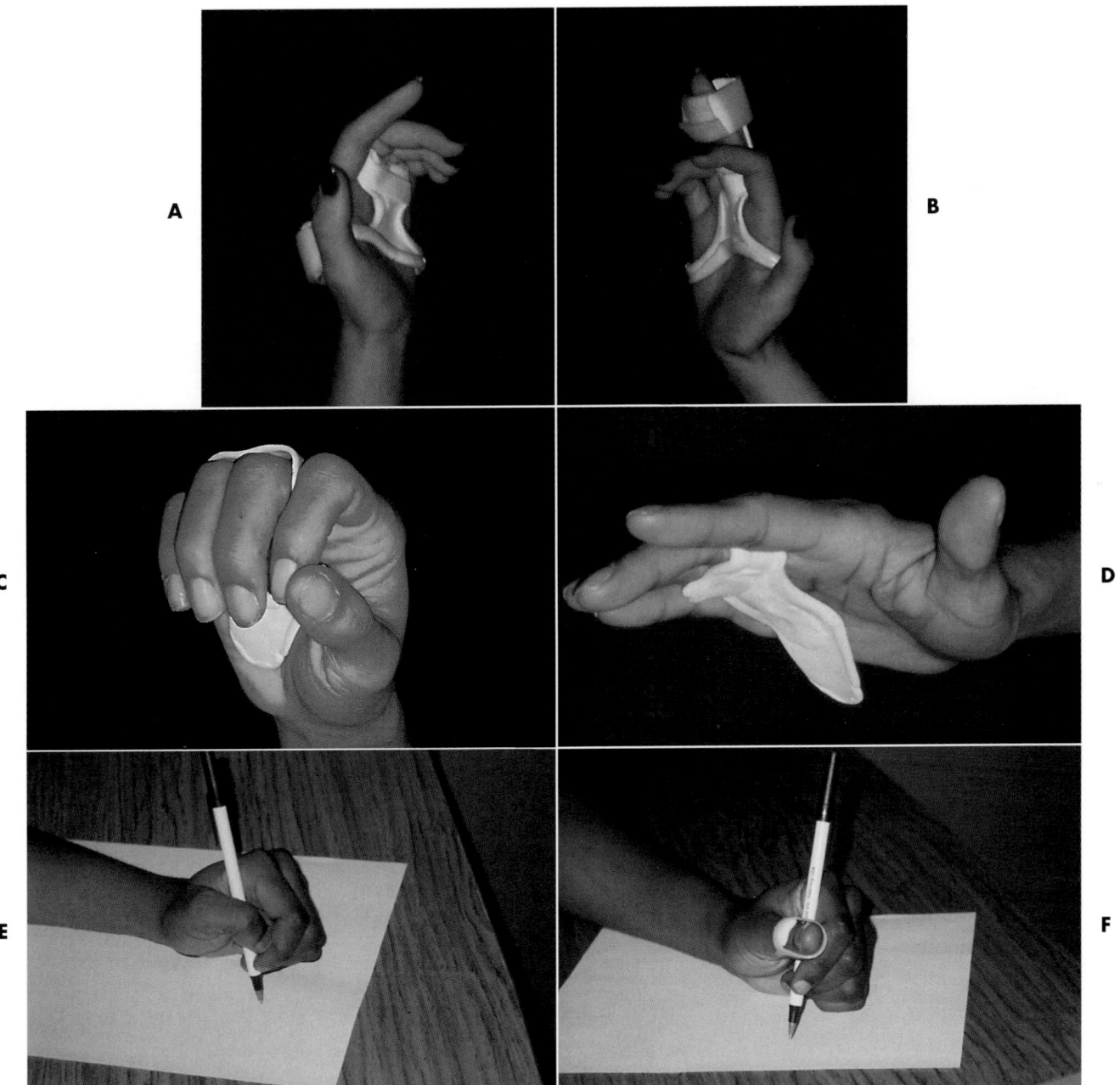

Fig. 55-15. Splinting options for trigger digits. **A,** Hand-based metacarpophalangeal extension splint. **B,** For proximal interphalangeal contracture, dorsal component for static progressive extension. **C** and **D,** Paddle design blocks extreme flexion but allows more freedom in extension, and allows easier donning and doffing. (Based on design by Linder-Tons and Ingell, 1998.) **E,** Excessive thumb interphalangeal (IP) flexion during writing in man with trigger thumb. **F,** Three-point extension splint for thumb IP joint prevents excessive flexion (3-Point Products, Inc., 1610 Pincay Court, Annapolis, Maryland 21401, 410-349-2649, e-mail: the3ptprod@aol.com).

Continued

simple way to guide the clinician's splint selection is to hold a given joint of an involved digit in extension while allowing the other joints to flex, noting the effect of each position on pain and smoothness of tendon glide. The least restrictive splint that accomplishes this goal should be used.[65] For trigger fingers, we generally use an MP joint extension splint with IP joints free; however, for thumbs, a three-point extension splint on the IP joint is most practical for hand function and usually eliminates triggering while being worn (Fig. 55-15).

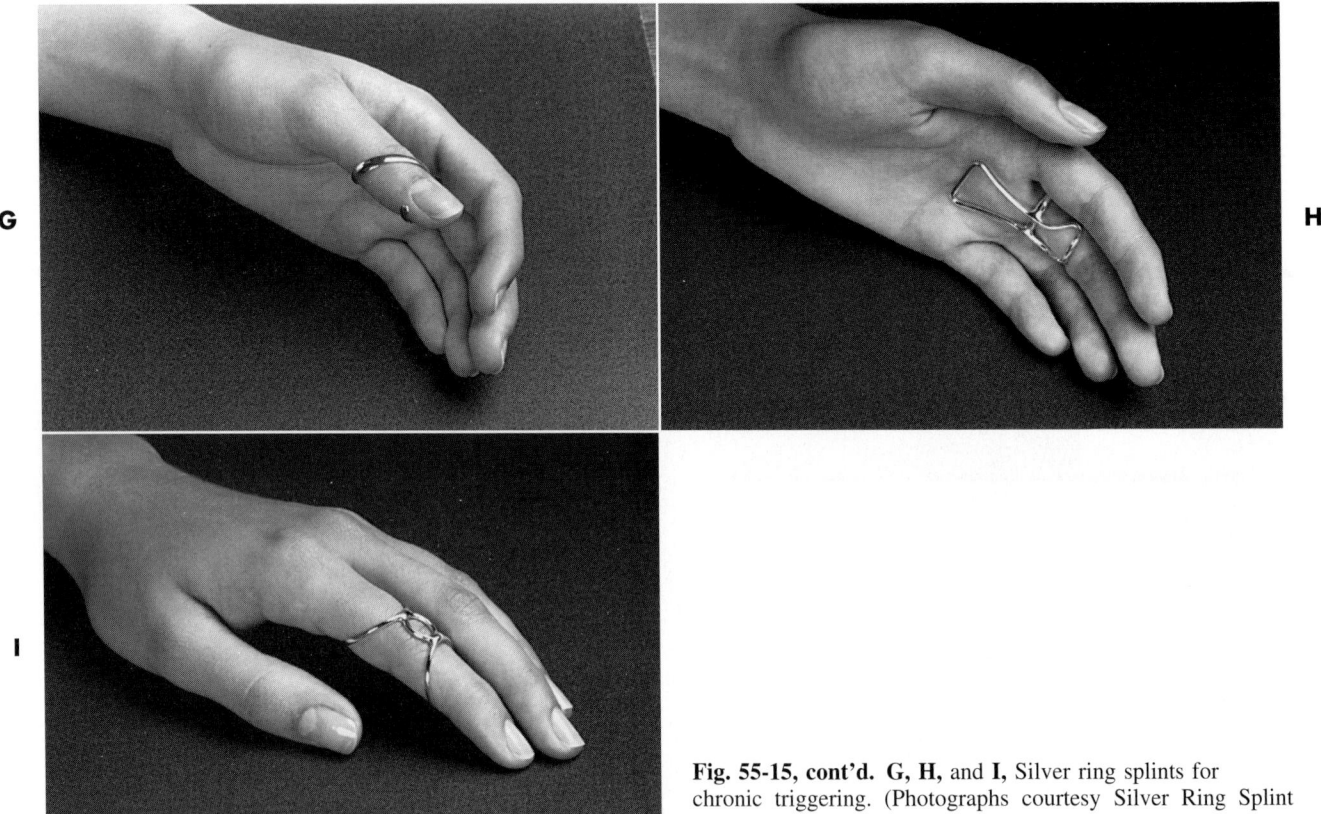

Fig. 55-15, cont'd. G, H, and **I,** Silver ring splints for chronic triggering. (Photographs courtesy Silver Ring Splint Company, P.O. Box 2856, Charlottesville, Virginia 22902-2856, e-mail: cindy@silverringsplint.com, fax: 804-971-8828.)

Exercise and activity. According to Wehbe' and Hunter,[105,106] tendon gliding exercises are helpful in improving tendon nutrition and in resolving nodules and adhesions. In the hook fist position, differential gliding between the FDS and FDP tendons is maximal and triggering usually does not occur. Evans et al.[28] advocate hook fisting 20 times in a splint and place-holding in a full fist every 2 hours while awake (see Fig. 55-4), augmented by massage to the entire digital tendon-sheath unit. As stated previously, full and repetitive fisting should be avoided while symptoms persist. Resistive exercises can be performed in alternative hand positions, such as hook fisting, and a modified intrinsic-plus position (see Figures 55-7 and 55-8). This also is important in patients with CTS both preoperatively and postoperatively; overzealous exercise can precipitate triggering at the A_1 pulley.

Surgery. Surgery may be indicated when conservative treatment has failed, as well as in patients with significant fixed flexion contractures. Cure rates reported in the literature range from 60% to 100% and are usually at least 85%.[7,11,83,100,103]

TECHNIQUE. Trigger digits can be released via open or percutaneous means. The open technique is performed under local anesthesia and with a tourniquet. Some patients require intravenous sedation with the use of a tourniquet. A 1.0- to 1.5-cm transverse or longitudinal incision is made over the metacarpal head of the affected finger. Blunt dissection is carried down through the subcutaneous tissues and the palmar fascia to the flexor sheath. The proximal edge and the entire A_1 pulley is identified. The proximal edge of the A_2 pulley also is identified. The entire A_1 pulley and the palmar aponeurosis pulley are incised. Care is taken not to damage the A_2 pulley. Some surgeons advocate excision of part of the A_1 pulley to prevent recurrent triggering. The patient is asked to actively flex and extend the finger to ensure that the triggering has been eliminated. A small hand dressing is then applied, leaving the fingers free. Percutaneous release has been advocated by some surgeons. This is performed with sterile technique in the office. After a local anesthetic is infiltrated into the region, a 19-gauge needle is placed in the A_1 pulley and, with a sweeping motion, the A_1 pulley is released. The finger must be triggering for this to be performed in the office. Complete release is confirmed by asking the patient to actively flex and extend the digit. This technique is not used for the index finger or the thumb because of the risk of neurovascular injury. It also should not be used in cases of complex trigger digit in which additional procedures, such as debulking of the bulbous nodule (i.e., reduction flexor tenoplasty) and release of adhesions between the FDS and FDP, may be required[79a] (Fig. 55-16).

COMPLICATIONS. Complications include digital nerve injury; inadvertent sectioning of the A_2 pulley, which can result

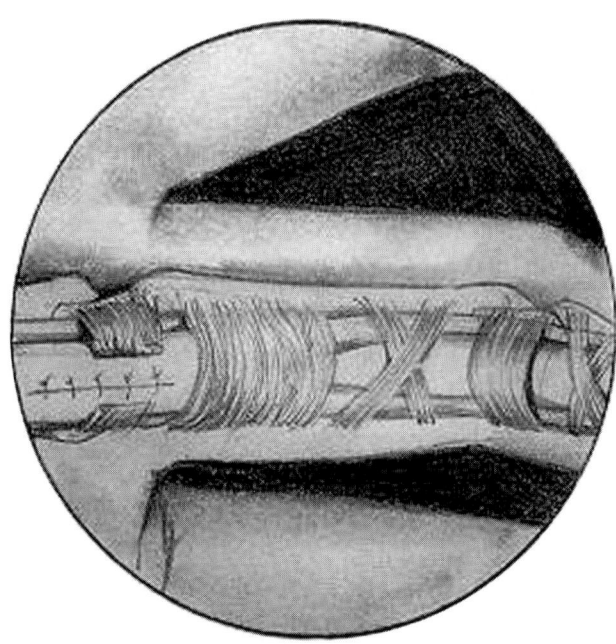

Fig. 55-16. Surgical release of A$_1$ pulley; reduction flexor tenoplasty for complex trigger digit. (From Osterman AL, Sweet S: *Atlas Hand Clin* 4:9, 1999.)

in bowstringing of the tendon; and subsequent loss of full finger flexion. Recurrent triggering and scar hypertrophy has been reported.[24,26,46] If digital nerve injury does occur, the patient should undergo prompt surgical exploration and repair or reconstruction. Individuals with significant preoperative PIP joint flexion contractures often do not regain full motion despite surgical release and postoperative therapy.

POSTOPERATIVE MANAGEMENT. Active motion can be initiated on the day of the procedure.[113] Patients who fail to regain full, smooth ROM by the third postoperative day,[39] those with PIP flexion contractures, or those who develop hypertrophic or hypersensitive scars should undergo formal hand therapy. Initial hand therapy should include wound and edema management and tendon gliding. A splint supporting the MP in extension can protect the incision while allowing IP joint motion. When PIP flexion contractures are present, a dorsal piece can be added for static progressive PIP extension (see Fig. 55-15, *B*). Strengthening usually can be initiated after 3 weeks, but resumption of forceful composite fisting should be delayed or minimized by patients who are prone to triggering in multiple digits.

Flexor carpi radialis tendonopathy

Etiology and pathology. The FCR tendon is prone to both primary stenotic tendovaginitis and injury secondary to degenerative changes or trauma of the carpus. The FCR tendon occupies 90% of its fibroosseous tunnel, which is formed by the ridge of the trapezium and the carpal ligament (Fig. 55-17). The FCR tendon runs a sharply angulated course around the trapezium to its primary insertion on the base of the index metacarpal, also sending slips to the

trapezial tuberosity and the base of the third metacarpal.[8] FCR tendonopathy can be confused with ganglion cysts, basal joint degenerative arthritis, scaphoid fractures and nonunions, and de Quervain's disease. Traumatic or degenerative changes of the carpus, particularly at the scaphotrapezial joint, can coexist with FCR tendonopathy, particularly in older women. Fitton et al.[32] have proposed that underlying degenerative process may be responsible for the attritional changes seen in and around the tendon. These include fraying or rupture of the tendon, hyperemia of synovial tissue, thickening of the sheath, adhesions, and exostosis formation.

Symptoms. Pain over the proximal wrist crease and at the scaphoid tubercle is common. The pain may radiate distally to thenar eminence or proximally into the forearm.[32] Localized swelling may be evident. Pain can be provoked with resisted wrist flexion and radial deviation. Passive wrist extension, which stretches the tendon, also may provoke discomfort.

Management. The initial treatment for FCR tendonopathy consists of nonoperative measures. The options include immobilization with a forearm-based wrist support splint (Figs. 55-1 and 55-18), NSAID use, and corticosteroid injection.[34] Gabel et al.[36] state that conservative treatment usually is effective for primary FCR tendonopathy, but surgery often is necessary for other local lesions. Attritional rupture may occur if the underlying pathologic condition is not addressed. Surgical procedures include release of the sheath, decompression of the tunnel, and excision of a ganglion or exostosis, if present. The tendon usually is approached through a longitudinal incision over the tendon that extends proximally from the wrist crease. Injury to the palmar cutaneous branch of the median nerve and the thenar branches of the radial sensory nerve must be avoided. The sheath is opened proximally and then followed distally beyond the trapezial tunnel. The tendon should be inspected thoroughly. Osteophytes along the trapezial ridge should be removed and the tendon sheath should be left open. A conforming dressing is applied and wrist motion is encouraged postoperatively. In two studies reviewed, success rates postoperatively ranged between 80% and 90%.[32,36]

Flexor carpi ulnaris tendonopathy[34,50]

Symptoms and provocation. Symptoms generally are localized to the FCU insertion into the pisiform and hypothenar fascia. Pain can radiate both proximally to the forearm and medial elbow, and distally to the ulnar side of the hand. The pain can be provoked by resisted wrist flexion and ulnar deviation. Passive stretching of the FCU (e.g., wrist extension and radial deviation) also may provoke discomfort. FCU tendonopathy is often bilateral.[95] Activities that can provoke FCU tendonopathy include golf, racquet sports, and badminton.

Management. Treatment for FCU tendonopathy usually is nonoperative. In the acute phase, NSAIDs and a resting splint in slight wrist flexion are used. Surgery is indicated

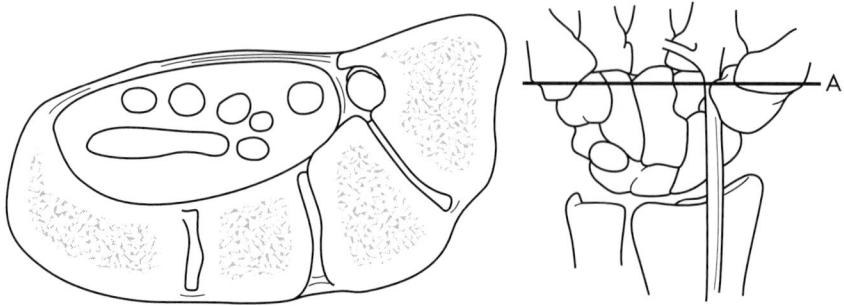

Fig. 55-17. Anatomy of the flexor carpi radialis (FCR) tendon tunnel. **Left,** Cross section of the FCR tunnel at the distal aspect of the trapezium. The FCR tunnel consists of the trapezial crest palmarly, the trapezial body radially, the trapezium-trapezoid joint and trapezoid dorsally, and the retinacular septum ulnarly. The tendon occupies 90% of the available space in the tunnel. **Right,** Insertions of the FCR tendon *(A).* (From Bishop AT, Gabel GT, Carmichael SW: *J Bone Joint Surg* 76A:1011, 1994.)

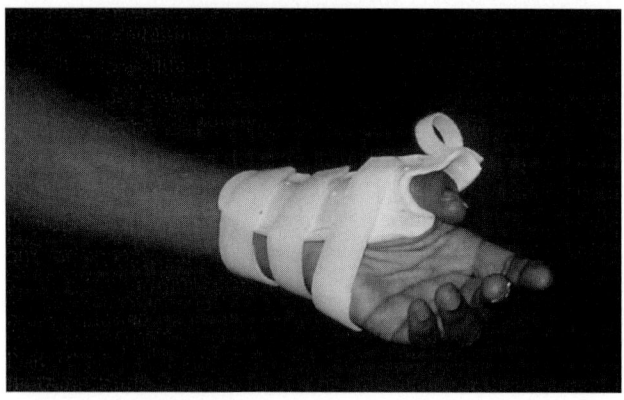

Fig. 55-18. Splint for patient with flexor carpi radialis tendonopathy and trigger thumb; removable thumb strap, allowing interphalangeal motion in trigger-free range.

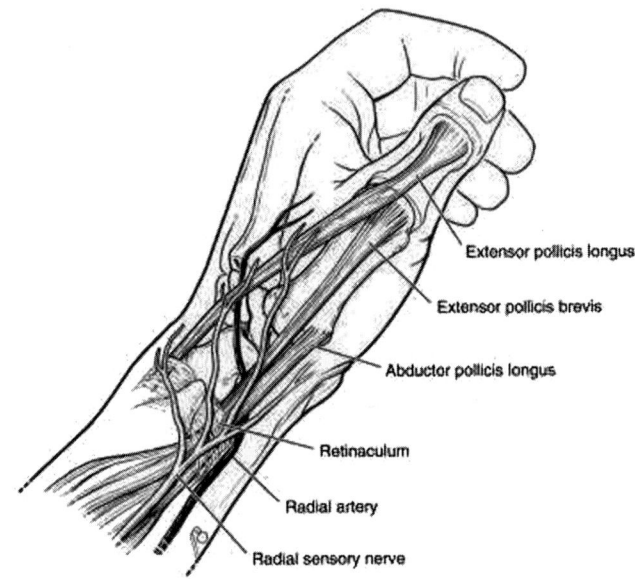

Fig. 55-19. First dorsal compartment, radial nerve, and artery. (From Bednar JM, Santarlasci PR: *Atlas Hand Clin* 4:39, 1999.)

rarely; however, for individuals with chronic FCU tendonopathy, a subperiosteal pisiform excision, which preserves the continuity of the FCU tendon, and a Z-plasty tendon lengthening may provide relief.[81]

de Quervain's disease. Fritz de Quervain, a Swiss surgeon, described stenosing tendovaginitis of the first dorsal compartment in 1895. In the 1893 edition of *Gray's Anatomy,* a similar condition named *washerwoman's sprain* was described.[113] De Quervain's stenosing tenosynovitis is a common condition; in two series reviewed, it made up more than one third of all cases of tendovaginitis affecting the hand and wrist.[63,66]

Anatomy and pathology. The APL and EPB tendons pass through the first dorsal compartment of the extensor retinaculum, which is approximately 2 cm in length (Fig 55-19). However, the synovial sheaths encasing the tendons are of much greater length. There is a great deal of anatomic variation between individuals. In fact, fewer than 20% of individuals may have the "normal" anatomy. The EPB is always thinner than the APL, and may be absent in 5% to 7% of people. The APL often has two, three, or more

tendinous slips that may insert into the base of the first metacarpal, trapezium, volar carpal ligaments, opponens pollicis, or abductor pollicis brevis. The EPB may occupy its own compartment.[73] In a study of 300 cadaveric wrists, 40% had a septation between the APL and the EPB. In contrast, in two studies of surgical patients with de Quervain's syndrome, 67% to 73% had this septation.[49,112] As in other types of tendovaginitis, the fibrous retinaculum hypertrophies. The synovial membrane is thickened except at the point of constriction. The tendons may have an hourglass appearance and can be bound together by fine adhesions.[31,73]

Etiology and associated factors

Cumulative microtrauma. Forceful, sustained, or repetitive thumb abduction and simultaneous wrist ulnar deviation may contribute to the development of de Quervain's tendovaginitis. Opening jars, wringing the hands, cutting with scissors, holding surgical retractors, playing the piano, and doing needlepoint are a few examples of activities that may provoke de Quervain's disease.[13,31,40,85,113] In contrast to Finkelstein et al.,[31] Muckart[73] suggested that radial deviation with pinch is more stressful than thumb abduction with ulnar deviation because the APL and EPB tendons are taut and sharply angulated at the wrist and trapeziometacarpal joints. This results in a "tearing strain" at the distal edge of the pulley. Muckart[73] also argued that friction is not a significant factor, citing Thompson et al.,[99] who studied 419 cases of peritendinitis crepitans in factory workers, of whom only two developed de Quervain's disease.

Sex. As in other conditions of stenosing tendovaginitis, women are more susceptible to de Quervain's disease than men by at least a 4:1 ratio.[73,80,95,112] The incidence is high in persons 35 to 55 years of age. Women in the third trimester of pregnancy and those with young children also are vulnerable.[44,72,73] Increased acute angulation of the tendons in women may be a predisposing factor.[15]

Acute trauma. Although less common, acute injuries to the first dorsal compartment can occur. A sudden wrenching of the wrist and thumb while trying to restrain an object or person or a fall on an outstretched hand can precipitate injury.

Diagnosis and physical examination. The most common complaint of de Quervain's tenovaginitis is radial-sided wrist pain, specifically at the first dorsal compartment over the radial styloid, which can radiate to the thumb or distal forearm. The pain is aggravated with movement of the thumb. Typically, increased tensile load on the EPB or APL (i.e., stretching or contraction) intensifies the pain. Finkelstein's test is pathognomic: with the thumb held in the palm and the wrist ulnarly deviated (see Fig. 55-6), the patient often will experience sharp pain because the tendons are simultaneously stretched and compressed over the radial styloid.[31] Wrist flexion and extension can be added to this maneuver; flexion should intensify the pain and extension should relieve it.[90] Resisted thumb extension also is typically painful and reproduces symptoms. Other symptoms include swelling and, very rarely, pseudotriggering (approximately 1% of cases). Additional sources of radial-sided wrist pain must be considered; these include trapeziometacarpal arthritis, scaphoid fractures, arthritis of the radioscaphoid or scaphotrapeziotrapezoidal joints, scapholunate instability, intersection syndrome, and radial neuritis.[70,113] Some of these conditions can coexist with de Quervain's disease. Radiographic studies should be performed to rule out many of the aforementioned conditions. Magnetic resonance imaging may show increased fluid in the first extensor compartment.

Nonoperative management

Activity modification and splinting. Adapted or alternative equipment that minimizes ulnar deviation at the wrist and substitutes power grip for pinch can be used. Examples include ergonomic keyboards, tools with a pistol grip, and a key holder. Strong evidence in the literature to support the efficacy of splinting is lacking.[73] Stern[95] recommended a 3-week trial of splinting, with the wrist in neutral and the thumb radially abducted. Witt et al.[112] reported a 62% satisfactory outcome with injection and splinting with the wrist positioned in 20 degrees of extension and the thumb MP and IP joints in extension. Weiss et al.[109] reported only a 30% success rate with splinting alone in 37 patients, as compared with a 69% success rate for injection alone and 57% for the injection plus splint. Weiss et al.[109] concluded that splinting provided no additional benefit when combined with cortisone injection. In our clinical experience, judicious splint wearing in the acute phase can assist with symptom control; the splint can be removed for brief periods of movement in pain-free ranges. As pain subsides, the patient can progress from a rigid splint to a flexible support (Fig. 55-20).

Injection. Success rates ranging from 50% to 90% are reported in the literature following one to two injections.[44,80,113] In Medl's series,[70] patients with a symptom duration of less than 2 months had a success rate of 90%.

TECHNIQUE. The area over the radial styloid is prepped. The APL and EPB can be palpated easily as the patient abducts and extends the thumb. The two tendons are bracketed by the gloved index finger and thumb of the examiner proximal to the radial styloid. The needle is introduced into the tendon sheath. Initially, resistance may be felt. The needle is withdrawn slowly while pressure is maintained on the plunger of the syringe. When the resistance lessens, half the corticosteroid and lidocaine solution is injected. A fluid wave should be palpable both proximally and distally to the injection site. The needle then should be redirected more ulnarly in an attempt to infiltrate the sheath of the EPB (which may be in a separate compartment).

Operative management. Surgical release of the first dorsal compartment is indicated after failed conservative management. Patients with pseudotriggering respond poorly to conservative measures and very often require surgical release.[1] Success rates are typically high; most recently, Ta et al.[97] reported that 91% of 43 surgical patients were satisfied and had complete symptom resolution.

Technique. A pneumatic tourniquet is placed on the upper arm. A 2-cm transverse or longitudinal incision is made over the first dorsal compartment approximately 1 cm proximally to the radial styloid. Care is taken to identify and protect the branches of the radial sensory nerve. These branches cross the compartment obliquely and are just deep to the dermal layer. The annular ligament covering the compartment should then be incised. Complete excision of the sheath should be avoided because painful palmar subluxation of the tendons may ensue. It is important to look for separate compartments and to release all intervening septa. Debulking of thickened tenosynovial tissue is recommended. The tendons are explored individually and are lifted

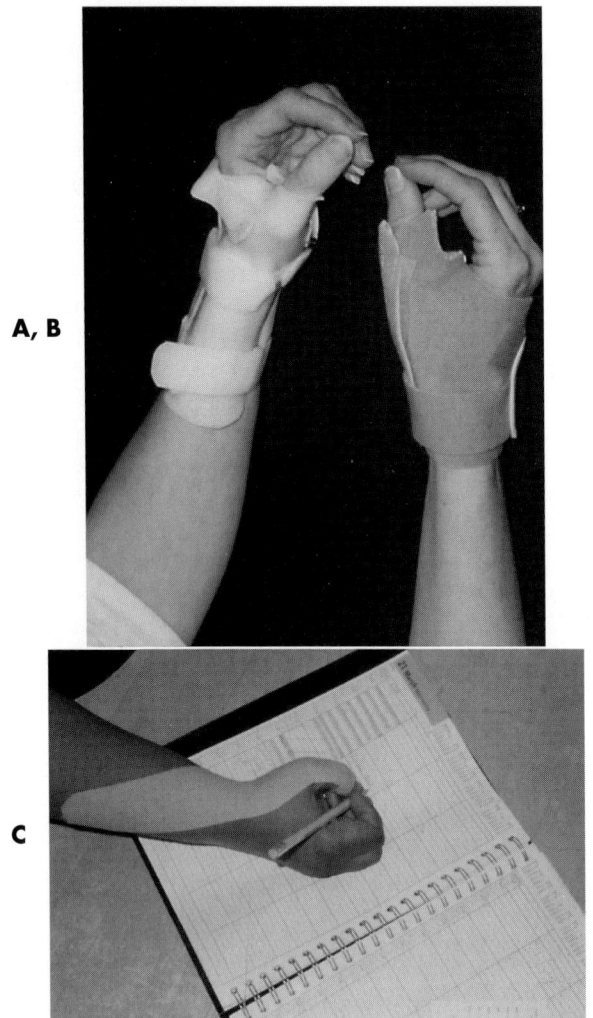

Fig. 55-20. Splinting and taping for de Quervain's syndrome. **A,** Thermoplastic splint. **B,** Semiflexible splint with removable support (3-Point Products, Inc., 1610 Pincay Court, Annapolis, MA 21401, 410-349-2649, e-mail: the3ptprod@aol.com). **C,** Kinesiotape for maximum flexibility.

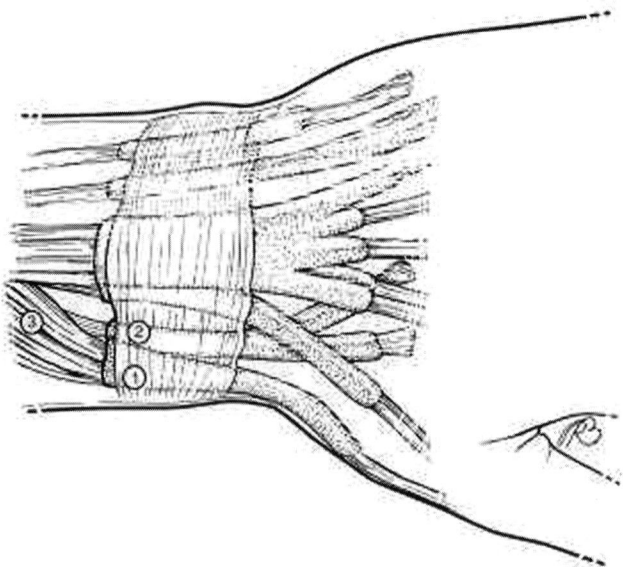

Fig. 55-21. Anatomy of intersection region includes *(1)* the first dorsal compartment, *(2)* the second dorsal compartment, and *(3)* the muscles bellies of the first dorsal compartment tendons (abductor pollicis longus, extensor pollicis brevis) overlying the second dorsal compartment tendons (extensor carpi radialis longus, extensor carpi radialis brevis). (Reproduced with permission from Kirkpatrick WH: *Atlas Hand Clin* 4:55, 1999.)

out of the tunnel to ensure complete decompression from the musculotendinous junction to a point at least 1 cm distally to the retinaculum. Hemostasis is attained after deflation of the tourniquet and the skin is closed. A bulky hand dressing is applied.

Complications. Complications include iatrogenic injury to the radial sensory nerve. This can result in painful neuroma formation. Vigorous retraction of the nerve, with laceration, may produce a neuroma-in-continuity. Other complications include reflex sympathetic dystrophy, scar hypersensitivity or adhesion, incomplete release, and tendon subluxation.[5] Incomplete relief of pain is not uncommon. Other associated diagnoses, including carpometacarpal joint arthritis, should be considered. In cases of persistent pain, the possibility of a separate, unreleased EPB compartment should be ruled out. Louis[67] states that in such cases, pain

can be reproduced by placing the patient's thumb in radial abduction and passively flexing the MP joint: In this maneuver, the EPB is stressed while the APL is placed on slack.

Postoperative management. The hand is maintained in a soft bulky dressing for the first 2 to 3 days, then the dressing is removed. A forearm-based thumb spica splint is then used during the first 2 weeks to control postoperative pain and swelling. Gentle active ROM and tendon gliding should be initiated in the first few days postoperatively. The goal is full, pain-free excursion of the APB and EPB, approximating Finkelstein's test position. Grip and pinch strengthening starting at approximately 2 weeks can be progressed gradually. By 6 weeks, the patient usually is able to resume heavier activities.[10]

Intersection syndrome. As its name suggests, *intersection syndrome* occurs at the intersection of the radial wrist extensor tendons as they pass underneath the muscle bellies of the APL and EPB approximately 4 cm proximally to Lister's tubercle[58] (Fig. 55-21). Intersection syndrome has been described variably as stenosing tenosynovitis of the second dorsal compartment with pain and swelling of the overlying muscle bellies of the APL and EPB,[113] exertional compartment syndrome of the APL and EPB muscles[34] and peritendinous bursal inflammation or "squeaker's wrist."[79] According to Wolfe,[113] it is the synovium of the second dorsal compartment tendons that become inflamed rather than a separate bursa. It is seen frequently among athletes, particularly weightlifters and rowers. Findings include localized pain and swelling 4 cm proximal to wrist, and in more severe cases, redness and painful crepitation with thumb and wrist movements. Grip and pinch are often painful and weak. The patient may report a history of repetitive wrist or thumb activities.[79]

Conservative management is similar to that of de Quervain's syndrome. A steroid injection into the second dorsal compartment; use of a forearm-based wrist or thumb spica splint; and activity modification, including avoidance of repetitive wrist flexion and extension, may relieve symptoms. For recalcitrant cases, the second dorsal compartment can be released surgically and inflamed bursa can be removed, if present.[34,58,113] Postoperatively, a splint supporting the wrist in slight extension can be worn for 1 to 2 weeks, followed by progressive mobilization.

Tendovaginitis of the digital extensors. The long extensor tendon of the thumb (extensor pollicis longus [EPL]), found in the third dorsal compartment, angulates sharply around Lister's tubercle. The EPL tendon can be affected adversely by degenerative or inflammatory conditions of the wrist, distal radius fractures, or a hypertrophied muscle belly extending into the third dorsal compartment.[34,113] Provocative activities, though rarely causative, include repetitive wrist and thumb motions, especially in extreme excursions. Musicians who play drums, accordions, and other keyboards are susceptible as are writers who hold their pens in dorsiflexion and radial deviation.[16] Symptoms include pain, swelling, tenderness, and often, crepitus at Lister's tubercle. Pain may radiate proximally or distally.[16] Both active and passive flexion of the IP joint may elicit pain. Conservative management includes NSAID use and forearm-based thumb splinting, with the IP joint included. Surgical release of the third dorsal compartment often is necessary to prevent attritional rupture of EPL tendon.[50] A 2-cm incision is centered over Lister's tubercle; care is taken to avoid injury to the branches of the radial sensory nerve. The third dorsal compartment is identified and incised. The EPL is displaced radially to Lister's tubercle and the compartment is then closed to prevent resubluxation of the tendon into the groove.[113] Wolfe[113] states that postoperative splinting is unnecessary and the patient can begin using his or her wrist and hand as tolerated.

The extensor tendons of the fingers, which include the extensor indicis proprius (EIP) and the extensor digitorum communis (EDC) found in the fourth dorsal compartment, and the extensor digiti minimi found in the fifth compartment, rarely are involved in primary stenosing tendovaginitis. Of these, the EDC to the index and small fingers are involved most commonly because they angulate more acutely at the distal edge of the extensor retinaculum. Isolated EIP tendovaginitis has been described secondary to the presence of muscle within the retinacular sheath and following a Colles' fracture.[113] Clinically, there is swelling

and tenderness over the affected compartment, and pain may be increased with resisted MP extension of the affected digit with the wrist flexed. Treatment consists mainly of nonoperative measures including rest, ice, NSAIDs, and corticosteroid injections. A splint supporting the wrist in slight extension and the affected MP joints in approximately 60 degrees of flexion may be helpful.

Tendovaginitis of the extensor carpi ulnaris. The sixth dorsal compartment, which contains the ECU, is the second most frequently involved extensor compartment. The floor of the ECU sheath is thick and forms part of the triangular fibrocartilage complex (TFCC), which helps stabilize the distal radioulnar joint (DRUJ). ECU tendonopathy can occur in isolation or with other conditions, such as destabilizing injuries to the TFCC.[57,79] (See Chapter 70 for a discussion of triangular fibrocartilage complex injuries.) Precipitating events can include repetitive snapping motions of the wrist, which can occur while playing tennis, golfing, or weightlifting.[34,57,79] Abrupt twisting injuries, particularly hypersupination with wrist flexion, can result in a tear in the ulnar border of the fibroosseous tunnel overlying the ECU tendon. Symptoms include diffuse ulnar-sided wrist pain with wrist and forearm motions, which is intensified by resistance to ulnar deviation and wrist extension, or by passive stretch into radial deviation and flexion.[35] To rule out instability, the extended, supinated wrist can be moved into flexion and ulnar deviation. If the ECU tendon is unstable, it will subluxate volarly with or without audible snap.

Conservative measures include use of NSAIDs and ice, wrist splinting, and injection, although injection rarely provides lasting relief.[113] Futami and Itoman[35] report a high success rate with nonoperative treatment in patients with a history of repetitive overuse, but not violent trauma, instability, or TFCC involvement: Of 43 patients, 40 were symptom free with use of an elastic bandage or wrist brace, NSAIDs, and/or steroid injections. Activities such as turning a screwdriver or wringing a cloth should be avoided because they require forceful, repetitive wrist and forearm motions in combination.

Surgical management. The need for surgical intervention in tendovaginitis of the ECU is rare. However, when conservative measures fail, the sixth compartment can be released on the radial side. A 3-cm incision is made over the DRUJ, with care taken to protect the branches of the dorsal sensory ulnar nerve. The sixth fibroosseous tunnel then is completely released. Retinacular repair is controversial. Kip and Peimer[57] and Wolfe[113] report that postoperative instability has not been a problem. Complications include injury to the dorsal ulnar sensory nerve. Postoperatively, the wrist should be splinted in neutral for 1 to 2 weeks, after which therapy can be initiated to restore tendon gliding and strength.[57] The patient can work on isolated uniplanar motions first (i.e., wrist flexion/extension, then radial/ulnar deviation, and finally, pronation/supination) before doing them in combination.

INSERTIONAL TENDONOPATHIES
Radial wrist extensors

Activities that subject the radial wrist extensors to sudden, forceful, or sustained exertion can result in microtears of the tendons. Over time, the site of their insertions on the bases of the second and third metacarpals can hypertrophy and undergo degenerative changes, a condition called *carpometacarpal boss.* Provocative activities include forceful gripping; sports in which the wrist is subjected to sudden acceleration or deceleration such as racquetball, tennis, and golf; or sustained hyperextension of the wrist such as with harp playing.[13,79] Management includes rest from, or modification of, activity; wrist support; and use of NSAIDs. Oral intake rather than injection is preferable because injection may result in tendon rupture. Sports equipment, musical instruments, and other tools should be modified when possible, as should body mechanics and playing technique. For a tennis player, adjusting the racquet handle and string tension, taping the wrist, and changing his or her hitting technique may reduce stress to the radial wrist extensors and prevent recurrence.[50] In recalcitrant cases, a portion of the joint can be excised surgically, and some surgeons would advocate fusion.

Interosseous tendons

Sudden, forceful, or repetitive radial or ulnar deviation at the MP joints can stress the interosseous tendons. Symptoms are vague but generally occur at the level of the MP joint and/or intermetacarpal region. Pain may be provoked with a handshake or with pressure at the tubercle of the proximal phalanx, the bony insertion of the interosseous tendon.[50,79] In addition to the usual conservative measures, the involved MP joints can be splinted in approximately 70 degrees of flexion. As symptoms resolve, buddy strapping at the proximal phalanges will allow MP joint flexion and extension while preventing lateral motions.

TENOSYNOVITIS ASSOCIATED WITH SYSTEMIC DISORDERS

Several systemic disorders alter connective tissues and can predispose an individual to stenosing tendovaginitis. Tendons, their synovial sheaths, fibrous retinacula, or local vasculature may be affected adversely, depending on the condition.

Diabetes mellitus

Diabetes mellitus is a disease caused by altered glucose metabolism. This leads to abnormal accumulation of stable endproducts of collagen glycosylation, which are thought to be responsible for increased cross-linking, packing, and stiffening of collagen.[19] The resulting proliferation of fibrous tissue in the tendon sheath is responsible for the stenosis of tendon tunnels. Diabetes also produces a microangiopathy that is believed to be responsible for many of its deleterious effects, including resistance to nonoperative measures.

Because the disease process is diffuse, it is not uncommon for patients with diabetes to have multiple sites of involvement. Patients with diabetes are four to five times more likely to develop stenosing conditions of the tendons, such as CTS and trigger digits, especially if they are insulin dependent.[19] They also are more likely to have multiple digit involvement and bilateral disease.[9] Griggs et al.[41] reported a 59% incidence of multiple digit involvement in patients with insulin-dependent diabetes as opposed to only 28% for patients with non–insulin-dependent diabetes. They suggested that patients with more severe disease might have a diffuse rather than nodular type of tendon hypertrophy, as well as poor microvasculature and a greater fibroblast response. If conservative therapy is chosen as an initial course of treatment, the patients must be advised to carefully monitor glucose levels because these can vary greatly after a corticosteroid injection. For many, surgical release is inevitable, particularly for those who are insulin dependent (56% as opposed to only 28% for patients with non–insulin-dependent diabetes).

Rheumatologic disorders

Rheumatoid arthritis, psoriatic arthritis, and lupus can adversely affect tendons. More than 65% of patients with rheumatoid arthritis will develop tenosynovitis of the hand or wrist, most commonly at the extensor retinaculum.[113] Proliferative tenosynovitis may begin with inflammation of the synovial lining of the tendon sheath, or may invade the tendon from the adjacent joint. The tenosynovium proliferates not only at the tendon-pulley interface but diffusely along the entire sheath (Fig. 55-22, *A*). Because of its increased bulk and destructive enzymes, the tendons and pulleys adjacent to the diseased tenosynovium can become adherent, weakened, or ruptured. Preventing rupture is the most important goal in treating rheumatoid arthritis. Medical management is essential to attempt to control the active disease. Splints that rest the affected tendons and support unstable joints can provide symptomatic relief. For patients with chronic or multiple trigger digits, three-point splints are a practical choice (see Fig. 55-15, *F, G,* and *H*). In addition to pharmacologic management, surgical measures may be necessary, which include extensive tenosynovectomy and tendon transfers in cases of rupture. The A_1 pulley is left intact or released on its radial border only, to prevent ulnar subluxation of the flexor tendons (Fig. 55-22, *B*).

Crystalline tendonopathies

Deposition of crystalline substances in the enclosed space of the tendon sheath can incite an acute inflammatory response characterized by intense pain, swelling, and erythema.

- *Gout* is a disorder of urate metabolism in which the patient has hyperuricemia and hyperuricosuria. Mono-

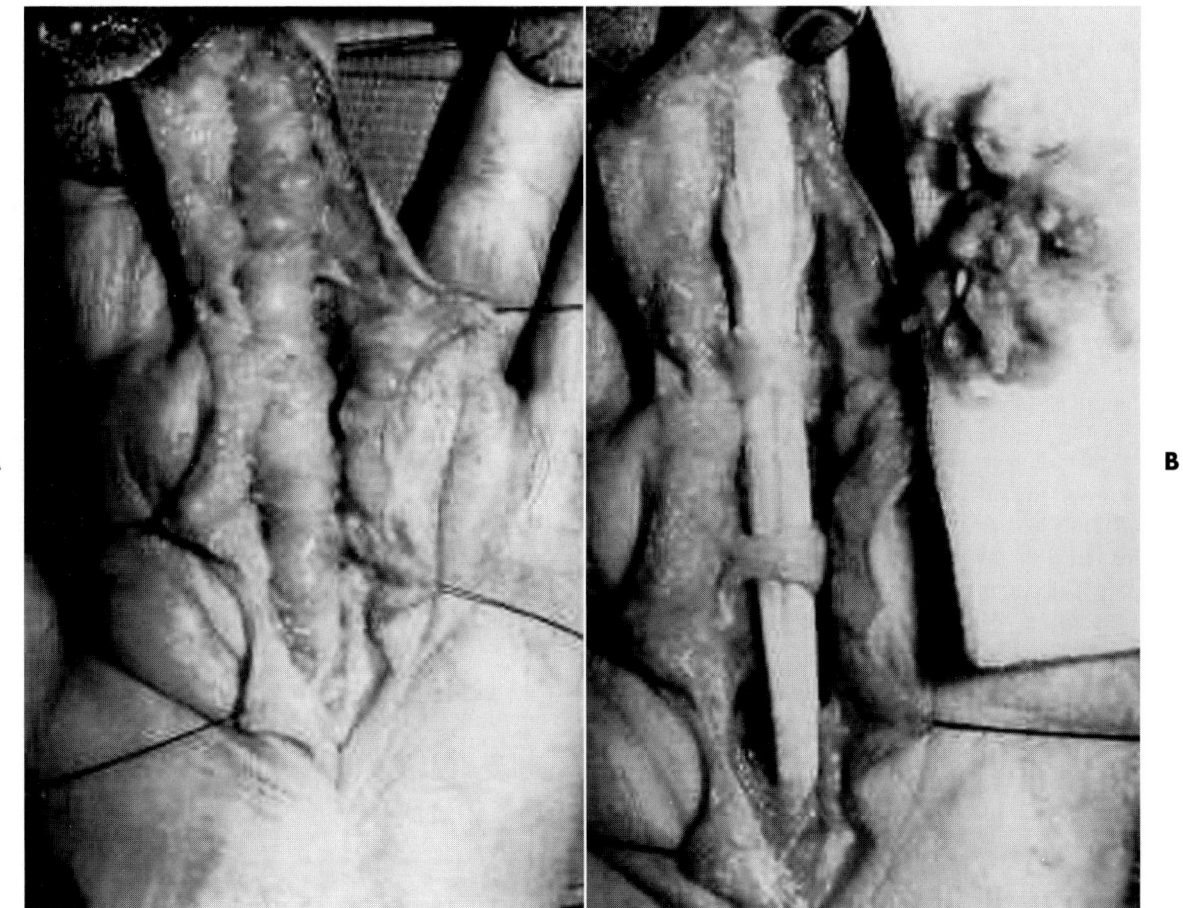

Fig. 55-22. Rheumatoid tenosynovitis. **A,** Digital tenosynovitis: the bulging of the fibroosseous tunnel is resisted by the A_1, A_2, and A_4 pulleys. **B,** Appearance of the tendons following a complete digital tenosynovectomy. The A_1, A_2, and A_4 pulleys have been preserved. Note the amount of tenosynovium that was excised. (From Leslie BM: *Atlas Hand Clin* 4:95, 1999.)

sodium urate crystals are deposited into the joints or tendons, resulting in synovitis. In the treatment of gouty tophi, splinting and pharmacologic management usually suffice. Medications include colchicine and anti-inflammatory agents. In severe or untreated cases, surgical procedures, such as synovectomy, excision of intratendinous tophi, and tendon transfer, may be necessary.

- *Calcific tendonitis* can result from the release of calcium salts. Calcific deposits usually respond to splinting and NSAIDs; rarely are surgical excision and tenolysis required.
- *Calcium pyrophosphate deposition disease* (pseudogout) rarely causes a fulminant tenosynovitis within the carpal tunnel, producing symptoms of median-nerve compression.[113]

Deposition diseases

- *Amyloidosis* is a disorder that results in the deposition of a serum protein, β_2-microglobulin, in bones and soft

tissues. Thick, plaquelike material is deposited on tendons, leading to poor gliding, triggering, and ruptures. The condition occurs as either a primary enzymatic defect or as part of a secondary syndrome in individuals with renal failure on dialysis. Involvement in the hand is usually in the form of cystic lesions in the carpal bones and destructive arthritis. Treatment is surgical; tenosynovectomy is effective in relieving symptoms of CTS and stenosing tenosynovitis.[61]
- *Ochronosis* is a rare genetic defect in tryptophan metabolism. Deposits of homogentisic acid, a darkly pigmented protein, often are found in joints, intervertebral discs, and tendons. Surgical release may relieve cases of stenosing tendovaginitis.[113]

Sarcoidosis

Sarcoidosis is a systemic granulomatous disease that is immune mediated. It primarily affects the lungs, spleen, and lymph nodes. Approximately 25% of cases have bone and joint or tenosynovial involvement. Sarcoidosis may precipitate secondary gout. Treatment options include use of systemic corticosteroids and tenosynovectomy.[113]

Septic tenosynovitis

Infectious agents can spread to the digital flexor tendon sheath from a deep laceration or puncture wound. Needle sticks or animal bites are common causes. Immunocompromised individuals or those with severe diabetes are vulnerable. The affected digit is typically swollen, slightly flexed, tender to palpation over the sheath, and painful with passive extension—Kanavel's four cardinal signs of flexor tendon sheath infection. Management within the first 48 hours of onset includes aspiration of the sheath, followed by appropriate antibiotic coverage. In unresponsive or established cases, surgical drainage is indicated. Postoperatively, the hand should be rested in a splint with the digits in the intrinsic-plus position. The wrist should be included when infection is present more proximally. When the infection is under control, mobilization and tendon gliding can be initiated. In cases of persistent contracture and adhesion, techniques of low-load prolonged stress, such as dynamic, serial static, or static progressive splinting, may be necessary.[110]

CONGENITAL TRIGGER DIGITS

The term *congenital trigger digit* technically is a misnomer because the condition is not diagnosed until after birth and children so affected present with an IP joint flexion contracture of the involved digit, *not triggering*. Rodgers and Waters[89] found no trigger digits in 1046 newborns prospectively examined, and of 73 children with "congenital trigger digit," none presented before 3 months of age. Slakey and Hennrikus[93] also found none in 4719 newborns, prospectively examined; of 15 children with the condition, none presented at less than 3 months of age, 14 of 15 were diagnosed after 1 year of age, and 10 of 15 after 2 years of age. Therefore, acquired flexion contracture is a more accurate description.[93] Incidence in the general population is 0.05%[113] and almost equally divided between males and females. The thumb is involved most frequently; occurrence is rare in the fingers.[23] The cause is unclear; some parents report antecedent trauma or thumb-sucking. Acquired IP joint flexion contracture can occur in association with trisomy.

The pathology of congenital trigger digit also differs somewhat from the adult form. Tendon and synovium are involved, not the fibrous sheath. A firm, nontender nodule is found on the flexor pollicis longus over the MP joint (Notta's node),[113] and the IP joint typically is contractured in 20 to 75 degrees of flexion, although it occasionally is locked in extension.[29] Other conditions that can result in a flexed thumb include cerebral palsy, arthrogryposis, and hypoplasia of thumb extensors.[96] If the IP joint can be extended with the MP joint held flexed, IP joint pathology can be ruled out.[114]

According to Dinham and Meggitt,[23] if the condition is diagnosed early in the first year of life, there is a 30% chance of spontaneous resolution. Therefore their recommendation is to wait a year before deciding to operate. If diagnosed between 6 and 30 months of age, the digit can be watched for 6 months because there is a 12% chance of spontaneous recovery. If there is no resolution, a surgical release is indicated.[23,29,113] Delay in treatment beyond 3 years of age may prolong recovery and result in residual deformity.[96]

Some authors have recommended splinting of the thumb IP joint conservatively. Tsuyuguchi et al.[102] reported that 75% of cases completely resolved with continuous IP extension splinting using a spring-wire coil for an average of 9 months. Nemoto et al.[75] reported only a 56% success rate with static extension splinting worn at night and during nap times for an average of 10 months. Approximately 23% dropped out of treatment. It is our opinion that prolonged splinting is impractical and restrictive, particularly for this young age group.

Following surgical release of the A_1 pulley, parents should be instructed to keep a clean and dry postoperative dressing on for 2 to 3 days, after which time a bandage should be sufficient. Most authors believe that normal activity is sufficient to restore full motion, and that splinting and formal therapy are unnecessary.[113] However, if full active MP and IP thumb extension are not achieved within the first postoperative week, hand therapy and corrective splinting should be provided.

SUMMARY

Tendonopathies of the hand and wrist are a common source of pain and dysfunction. They are often manifestations of aging, systemic disease, and predilection to pathologic fibrosis, although they also can be precipitated by overuse in otherwise healthy individuals. Women are more susceptible than men because of hormonal, anatomic, and occupational factors. In some individuals such as the young child with acquired IP flexion deformity, the cause is not clear. The hand surgeon or therapist should take a thorough history, explore precipitating factors, and assess the nature of the symptoms and their impact on the individual's occupational roles. Intervention will vary according to the duration of symptoms and the patient's age, lifestyle, and comorbidities. In the acute phase, corticosteroids and resting splints can be helpful in reducing pain and inflammation. As symptoms are controlled, pain-free tendon gliding can be initiated with progression to strengthening, if needed. When conservative management fails, surgical release of constricting fibrous pulleys will cure the problem for most patients. Patients with rheumatoid arthritis are an exception; they may require extensive tenosynovectomies and, occasionally, tendon transfers. Finally, the therapist should teach the patient how to modify provocative activities, select appropriate ergonomic equipment, and provide splints or semiflexible supports to minimize the chance of recurrence.

REFERENCES

1. Alberton GM, et al: Extensor triggering in de Quervain's stenosing tenosynovitis, *J Hand Surg* 24A:1311, 1999.
2. Amadio PC, Jaeger SH, Hunter JM: Nutritional aspects of tendon healing. In Hunter JM, et al, editors: *Rehabilitation of the hand,* St Louis, 1995, Mosby.
3. Amadio PC, Russotti GM: Evaluation and treatment of hand and wrist disorders in musicians, *Hand Clin* 6:405, 1990.
4. Armstrong TJ, et al: Ergonomics considerations in hand and wrist tendinitis, *J Hand Surg* 12A:830, 1987.
5. Arons MS: De Quervain's release in working women: a report of failures, complications, and associated diagnoses, *J Hand Surg* 12A:540, 1987.
6. Banta CA: A prospective, nonrandomized study of iontophoresis, wrist splinting, and antiinflammatory medication in the treatment of early-mild carpal tunnel syndrome, *J Occup Med* 36:166, 1994.
7. Benson LS, Ptaszek AJ: Injection versus surgery in the treatment of trigger finger, *J Hand Surg* 22A:138, 1997.
8. Bishop AT, Gabel GT, Carmichael SW: Flexor carpi radialis tendinitis: I. Operative anatomy, *J Bone Joint Surg* 76A:1009, 1994.
9. Blyth MJ, Ross DJ: Diabetes and trigger finger, *J Hand Surg* 21B:244, 1996.
10. Bolger JT: De Quervain's release. In Blair WF, editor: *Techniques in hand surgery,* Baltimore, 1996, Williams & Wilkins.
11. Bonnici AV, Spencer JD: A survey of 'trigger finger' in adults, *J Hand Surg* 13B:202, 1988.
12. Brand P, Hollister A: *Clinical mechanics of the hand,* ed 2, St Louis, 1993, Mosby.
13. Brandfonbrener AG: The epidemiology and prevention of hand and wrist injuries in performing artists, *Hand Clin* 6:365, 1990.
14. Brown M, Manktelow RT: A new cause of trigger thumb, *J Hand Surg* 17A:688, 1992.
15. Bunnell S: *Surgery of the hand,* Philadelphia, 1944, JB Lippincott.
16. Burman M: Stenosing tenovaginitis of the dorsal and volar compartments of the wrist, *Arch Surg* 65:752, 1952.
17. Byl NN: The use of ultrasound as an enhancer for transcutaneous drug delivery: phonophoresis, *Phys Ther* 75:539, 1995.
18. Cameron MH, Monroe LG: Relative transmission of ultrasound by media customarily used for phonophoresis, *Phys Ther* 72:142, 1992.
19. Chammas M, et al: Dupuytren's disease, carpal tunnel syndrome, trigger finger, and diabetes mellitus, *J Hand Surg,* 20A:1, 1995.
20. Ciccone CD: Iontophoresis. In Robinson AJ, Snyder-Mackler L, editors: *Clinical electrophysiology: electrotherapy and electrophysiologic testing,* ed 2, Baltimore, 1995, Williams & Wilkins.
21. Costello CT, Jeske AH. Iontophoresis: applications in transdermal medication delivery, *Phys Ther* 75:554, 1995.
22. Cyriax JH, Cyriax PJ: *Illustrated manual of orthopedic medicine,* London, 1983, Butterworths.
23. Dinham JM, Meggitt BF: Trigger thumbs in children: a review of the natural history and indications for treatment in 105 patients, *J Bone Joint Surg* 56B:153, 1974.
24. Dunn MJ, Pess GM: Percutaneous trigger finger release: a comparison of a new push knife and a 19-guage needle in a cadaveric model, *J Hand Surg* 24A:860, 1999.
25. Dyson M: Non-thermal cellular effects of ultrasound, *Br J Cancer* 45:165, 1982.
26. Eastwood DM, Gupta KJ, Johnson DP: Percutaneous release of trigger finger: an office procedure, *J Hand Surg* 17A:114, 1992.
27. Eaton RG: Entrapment syndromes in musicians, *J Hand Ther* 5:91, 1992.
28. Evans RB, Hunter JM, Burkhalter WE: Conservative management of trigger finger: a new approach, *J Hand Ther* 1:59, 1988.
29. Fahey JJ, Bollinger JA: Trigger finger in adults and children, *J Bone Joint Surg* 36A:1200, 1954.
30. Fedorczyk J: The role of physical agents in modulating pain, *J Hand Ther* 10:110, 1997.
31. Finkelstein, H: Stenosing tendovaginitis at the radial styloid process, *J Bone Joint Surg* 12:509, 1930.
32. Fitton J, Shea F, Goldie W: Lesions of the flexor carpi radialis tendon and sheath causing pain in the wrist, *J Bone Joint Surg* 50:359, 1968.
33. Freiberg A, Mulholland RS, Levine R: Nonoperative treatment of trigger fingers and thumbs, *J Hand Surg* 14A:553, 1989.
34. Fulcher SM, Kiefhaber TR, Stern PJ: Upper extremity tendinitis and overuse syndromes in the athlete, *Clin Sports Med* 17:433,1998.
35. Futami T, Itoman M: Extensor carpi ulnaris syndrome: findings in 43 patients, *Acta Orthop Scand* 66:538, 1995.
36. Gabel GT, Bishop A, Wood MB: Flexor carpi radialis tendinitis: II. Results of operative treatment, *J Bone Joint Surg* 76A:1015, 1994.
37. Gelberman RH, Aronson D, Weisman M: Carpal tunnel syndrome: results of a prospective trial of steroid injection and splinting, *J Bone Joint Surg* 62A:1181, 1980.
38. Gorsche R, et al: Prevalence and incidence of stenosing flexor tenosynovitis (trigger finger) in a meat-packing plant, *J Occup Environ Med* 40:6, 1998.
39. Greider JL: Trigger thumb and finger release. In Blair WF, editor: *Techniques in hand surgery,* Baltimore, 1996, Williams & Wilkins.
40. Griffiths DL: Tenosynovitis and tendovaginitis, *Br Med J* 1:645, 1952.
41. Griggs SM, et al: Treatment of trigger finger in patients with diabetes mellitus, *J Hand Surg* 20A:787, 1995.
42. Gudeman SD, et al: Treatment of plantar fasciitis by iontophoresis of 0.4% dexamethasone: a randomized, double-blind, placebo-controlled study, *Am J Sports Med* 25:312, 1997.
43. Hardy M, Woodall W: Therapeutic effects of heat, cold, and stretch on connective tissue, *J Hand Ther* 11:148, 1998.
44. Harvey FJ, Harvey PM, Horsely MW: De Quervain's disease: surgical or nonsurgical treatment, *J Hand Surg* 15A:83, 1990.
45. Harvey W, et al: The stimulation of protein synthesis in human fibroblasts by therapeutic ultrasound, *Rheumatol Rehab* 14:237, 1975 (abstract).
46. Heithoff SJ, Millender LH, Helman J: Bowstringing as a complication of trigger finger release, *J Hand Surg* 13A:567, 1988.
46a. Hohman L, et al: *Treatment guidelines for conservative and post-operative management of trigger finger,* 1999, ASHT.
47. Howard NJ: Peritendinitis crepitans: a muscle-effort syndrome, *J Bone Joint Surg* 19:447, 1937.
48. Hueston JT, Wilson WF: The aetiology of trigger finger, *Hand* 4:257, 1972.
49. Jackson WT, et al: Anatomical variations in the first extensor compartment of the wrist, *J Bone Joint Surg* 68A:923, 1986.
50. Johnson RK: Soft tissue injuries of the forearm and hand, *Clin Sports Med* 5:701, 1986.
51. Johnson SL: Ergonomic hand tool design, *Hand Clin* 9:299, 1993.
52. Johnson SL: Therapy of the occupationally injured hand and upper extremity, *Hand Clin* 9:289, 1993.
53. Kannus P, et al: Effects of training, immobilization and remobilization on tendons, *Scand J Med Sci Sports* 7:67, 1997.
54. Kapetanos G: The effect of local corticosteroids on the healing and biomechanical properties of the partially injured tendon, *Clin Orthop* 163:170, 1982.
55. Kessler RM, Hertling D: *Management of common musculoskeletal disorders,* Philadelphia, 1983, Harper and Row.
56. Khan KM, et al: Histopathology of common tendonopathies: update and implications for clinical management, *Sports Med* 27:393, 1999.
57. Kip PC, Peimer CA: Release of the sixth dorsal compartment, *J Hand Surg* 19A:599, 1994.

58. Kirkpatrick WH, Lisser S: Soft tissue conditions: trigger fingers and de Quervain's disease. In Hunter JS, Mackin EJ, Callahan AD, editors: *Rehabilitation of the hand: surgery and therapy,* ed 4, St Louis, 1995, Mosby.

59. Klaiman MD, et al: Phonophoresis versus ultrasound in the treatment of common musculoskeletal conditions, *Med Sci Sports Exerc* 30:1349, 1998.

60. Kroemer KHE: Avoiding cumulative trauma disorders in shops and offices, *Am Ind Hyg Assoc J* 53:596, 1992.

61. Kurer MH, Baillod RA, Madgwick JC: Musculoskeletal manifestations of amyloidosis: a review of 83 patients on haemodialysis for at least 10 years, *J Bone Joint Surg* 73B:271, 1991.

62. Lang CJ, Lourie GM: Sesamoiditis of the index finger presenting as acute suppurative flexor tenosynovitis, *J Hand Surg* 24:1327, 1999.

63. Lapidus PW, Fenton R: Stenosing tenovaginitis at the wrist and fingers: report of 423 cases in 369 patients with 354 operations, *Arch Surg* 64:475, 1952.

64. Lapidus PW, Guidotti FP: Stenosing tenovaginitis of the wrist and fingers, *Clin Orthop* 83:87, 1972.

65. Lindner-Tons S, Ingell K: An alternative splint design for trigger finger, *J Hand Ther* 11:206, 1998.

66. Lipscomb PR: Tenosynovitis at the radial styloid process, *Ann Surg* 134:110, 1951.

67. Louis DS: Incomplete release of the first dorsal compartment: a diagnostic test, *J Hand Surg* 12A:87, 1987.

68. Lowe C: Treatment of tendinitis, tenosynovitis, and other cumulative trauma disorders of musicians' forearms, wrists, and hands . . . restoring function with hand therapy, *J Hand Ther* 5:84, 1992.

69. Markison RE: Treatment of musical hands: redesign of the interface, *Hand Clin* 6:525, 1990.

70. Medl WT: Tendonitis, tenosynovitis, trigger finger and Quervain's disease, *Orthop Clin North Am* 1:375, 1970.

71. Michlovitz SL, editor: *Thermal agents in rehabilitation,* Philadelphia, 1996, FA Davis.

72. Moore JS: De Quervain's tenosynovitis: stenosing tenosynovitis of the first dorsal compartment, *J Occup Environ Med* 39:10, 1997.

73. Muckart RD: Stenosing tendovaginitis of abductor pollicis longus and extensor pollicis brevis at the radial styloid (DeQuervain's disease), *Clin Orthop* 33:201, 1964.

74. National Institute of Occupational Safety and Health (NIOSH): Musculoskeletal disorders and workplace factors: a critical review of epidemiologic evidence for work-related musculoskeletal disorders of the neck, upper extremity and low back, Bernard PB, editor, DHHS (NIOSH) Publication 97-141, 1997.

75. Nemoto K, et al: Splint therapy for trigger thumb and finger in children, *J Hand Surg* 21B:3, 1996.

76. Newport ML, Lane LB, Stuchin SA: Treatment of trigger finger by steroid injection, *J Hand Surg* 15A:748, 1990.

77. Nussbaum EL: Therapeutic ultrasound. In Behrens B, Michlovits S, editors: *Physical agents: theory and practice for physical therapy assistants,* Philadelphia, 1996, FA Davis.

78. Nussbaum EL: The influence of ultrasound on healing tissues, *J Hand Ther* 11:140, 1998.

79. Osterman AL, Moskow L, Low DW: Soft-tissue injuries of the hand and wrist in racquet sports, *Clin Sports Med* 7:329, 1988.

79a. Osterman AL, Sweet S: The treatment of complex trigger finger with proximal interphalangeal joint contracture, *Atlas Hand Clin* 4:9, 1999.

80. Otto N, Wehbe' MA: Steroid injections for tenosynovitis in the hand, *Orthop Rev* 15:290, 1986.

81. Palmieri TJ: Pisiform area pain treatment by pisiform excision, *J Hand Surg* 7A:477, 1982.

82. Patel MR, Bassini L: Trigger fingers and thumb: when to splint, inject, or operate, *J Hand Surg* 17:110, 1992.

83. Patel MR, Moradia VJ: Percutaneous release of trigger digit with and without cortisone injection, *J Hand Surg* 22A:150, 1997.

84. Perry GF: Why do some people develop two or more inflammatory conditions (i.e., carpal tunnel syndrome, Dupuytren's contracture, trigger finger, etc.) without any clear-cut etiologic factor(s) being present? *J Occup Med* 36:295, 1994.

85. Putz-Andersen V, editor: *Cumulative trauma disorders: a manual for musculoskeletal diseases of the upper limbs,* New York, 1988, Taylor Francis.

86. Rayan GM: Distal stenosing tenosynovitis, *J Hand Surg* 15A:973, 1990.

87. Rhoades CE, Gelberman RH, Manjarris IF: Stenosing tenosynovitis of the fingers and thumb: results of a prospective trial of steroid injection and splinting, *Clin Orthop* 190:236, 1984.

88. Rodgers JA, McCarthy JA, Tiedeman JJ: Functional distal interphalangeal joint splinting for trigger finger in laborers: a review and cadaver investigation, *Orthopedics* 21:305, 1998.

89. Rodgers WB, Waters PM: Incidence of trigger digits in newborns, *J Hand Surg* 19:364, 1994.

90. Sampson SP, Wixch E, Badalamente MA: Complications of conservative and surgical treatment of DeQuervain's disease and trigger digits, *Hand Clin* 10:73, 1994.

91. Sampson SP, et al: Pathobiology of the human A_1 pulley in trigger finger, *J Hand Surg* 16:714, 1991.

92. Schultz-Johnson K: Upper extremity factors in the evaluation of lifting, *J Hand Ther* 3:72, 1990.

93. Slakey JB, Hennrikus WL: Acquired thumb flexion contracture in children: congenital trigger thumb, *J Bone Joint Surg* 78B:481, 1996.

94. Stanish WD, Rubinovich RM, Curwin S: Eccentric exercise in chronic tendinitis, *Clin Orthop* 208:65, 1986.

95. Stern PJ: Tendinitis, overuse syndromes and tendon injuries, *Hand Clin* 6:467, 1990.

96. Steyers CM: Trigger thumb release. In Blair WF, editor: *Techniques in hand surgery,* Baltimore, 1996, Williams & Wilkins.

97. Ta KT, Eidelman D, Thomson JG: Patient satisfaction and outcomes of surgery for de Quervain's tenosynovitis, *J Hand Surg* 24:1071, 1999.

97a. Taras S, Miskovsky C: Nonoperative management of trigger digits, *Atlas Hand Clin* 4:1, 1999.

98. Taylor Mullins PA: Use of therapeutic modalities in upper extremity rehabilitation. In Hunter JS, Mackin EJ, Callahan AD, editors: *Rehabilitation of the hand: surgery and therapy,* ed 4, St Louis, 1995, Mosby.

99. Thompson AR, et al: Peritendinitis crepitans and simple tenosynovitis: a clinical study of 544 in industry, *Br J Indust Med* 8:150, 1951.

100. Thorpe AP: Results of surgery for trigger finger, *J Hand Surg* 13B:199, 1988.

101. Trezies AJ, et al: Is occupation an aetiological factor in the development of trigger finger? *J Hand Surg* 23B:539, 1998.

102. Tsuyuguchi Y, Tada K, Kawaii H: Splint therapy for trigger finger in children, *Arch Phys Med Rehabil* 64:75, 1983.

103. Turowski GA, Zdankiewicz PD, Thompson JG: The results of surgical treatment of trigger finger, *J Hand Surg* 22A:145, 1997.

104. Wallace RG, Mollan RA, Kernohan WG: Preliminary report on a new technique to aid diagnosis of some disorders found in hands, *J Hand Surg* 10B:269, 1985.

105. Wehbe' MA, Hunter JM: Flexor tendon gliding in the hand. Part I. In vivo excursions, *J Hand Surg* 10:570, 1985.

106. Wehbe' MA, Hunter JM: Flexor tendon gliding in the hand. Part II. Differential gliding, *J Hand Surg* 10:575, 1985.

107. Weiler JM: Medical modifiers of sports injury: the use of nonsteroidal anti-inflammatory drugs (NSAIDs) in sports soft tissue injury, *Clin Sports Med* 11:625, 1992.

108. Weinzweig J, et al: Angiolipoma of the finger masquerading as flexor tenosynovitis, *Plast Reconstr Surg* 104:1052, 1999.

109. Weiss AP, Akelman E, Tabatabai M: Treatment of DeQuervain's disease, *J Hand Surg* 19:595, 1994.

110. Wheeler DR: Suppurative flexor tenosynovitis. In Blair WF, editor: *Techniques in hand surgery,* Baltimore, 1996, Williams & Wilkins.

111. Wingard LB, et al: Glucocorticoids and other adrenal steroids. In Wingard LB, editor: *Human pharmacology: molecular-to-clinical,* St Louis, 1991, Mosby.

112. Witt J, Pess G, Gelberman RH: Treatment of deQuervain tenosynovitis: a prospective study of the results of injection of steroids and immobilization in a splint, *J Bone Joint Surg* 73:219, 1991.

113. Wolfe SW: Tenosynovitis. In Green DP, editor: *Operative hand surgery,* vol II, Philadelphia, 1999, Churchill Livingstone.

114. Yenidunya MO, Tasbas BA: A simple sign for the differential diagnosis of the congenital trigger thumb, *Plast Reconstr Surg* 103:748, 1999 (letter).

Chapter 56

SOFT TISSUE TUMORS
OF THE FOREARM AND HAND

David C. Bush

Soft tissue tumors of the forearm and hand present many challenges to the hand surgeon. Although most are benign, the diagnosis and management of these lesions can be confusing and difficult. Hand tumors can arise from any of the structures of the hand: skin, fat, blood vessels, lymph vessels, nerves, and bone elements. Most series report ganglia to be the most common tumor.* We have reviewed our surgical pathologic diagnoses over the past 15 years (Table 56-1). In our series, inclusion cysts and xanthomas were the most common surgical diagnoses.

Most tumors of the hand present as painless masses. In many instances, when a patient is referred to a hand surgeon for evaluation of a lump, the diagnosis is obvious and no biopsy is indicated. The diagnosis of a ganglion, the most common hand tumor, is usually evident. Gout is another good example. Most cases of gout can be easily diagnosed on examination (Fig. 56-1). A tophus† should rarely be surgically treated because it involves the tendon or joint capsule and excision is impossible without injuring the normal structures. In our series, we have had 19 cases of gout, but only 3 were tophi. The rest were biopsies from the carpal tunnel area during median-nerve decompression.

Occasionally, a solitary rheumatoid nodule can cause confusion, but when multiple nodules are present, the diagnosis is usually obvious (Fig. 56-2). Swelling as a result of arthritis or synovitis secondary to rheumatoid arthritis usually needs no operation for the diagnosis. However, if the synovitis is localized to one joint, a synovectomy may be indicated to treat the joint or to rule

out an infection or granulomatous disease such as tuberculosis[12] (Fig. 56-3).

Early Dupuytren's fibromatosis can be confusing, but the diagnosis usually can be made by examination and follow-up evaluation. If Dupuytren's fibromatosis had been included as a tumor in our series, it would have been the most common pathologic diagnosis. Fibroma of tendon sheath is the only fibrous tumor we have included. We have included calcified lesions. Usually, a calcium deposit presents more like an infection than a tumor.[59] We have excised some calcium deposits in which the diagnosis was not clear. Fig. 56-4 shows a calcium deposit secondary to an infiltrated IV in a cancer patient. A soft tissue chondroma is another tumor that can show some calcium on x-ray examination[3] (Fig. 56-5). One of the two chondromas in our series recurred.

Solid tumors often come to surgery because they tend to slowly enlarge and the diagnosis is usually in doubt. Many patients are referred because of a fear of cancer. Current scientific and public persuasions dictate that most solid soft tissue tumors should be evaluated by an excisional biopsy. Hand tumors are usually asymptomatic unless they cause pressure on a nerve. An exception is a glomus tumor. A history of trauma may be useful in diagnosing a ganglion or an inclusion cyst. A tumor that varies in size is probably a ganglion. A tumor that rapidly increases in size raises the concern of a malignancy. An apparently benign tumor that rapidly recurs after excision also raises this concern and brings the diagnosis into question. It should be kept in mind that any soft tissue tumor of the hand has the very small but real chance that it might be malignant. If it is not clearly a ganglion, an inclusion cyst, or a lipoma, consideration should be given to evaluation and removal.

*References 8, 13, 22, 25, 31, 50, 68.
†See Glossary at end of chapter.

Table 56-1. Tumor location and frequency

TUMOR TYPE	NUMBER
Giant cell tumor or xanthoma	83 (80 hand, 3 arm)
Inclusion cyst	71 (7 recurrent)
Ganglions	58 (24 wrist, 20 mucous cyst, 11 fingers, 3 elbow)
Nerve tumors	27 (23 hand, 4 arm)
Lipomas	37 (26 hand, 11 arm)
Rheumatoid	24 (17 hand, 7 arm)
Vascular	27
Gout	19
Malignant	19 (7 squamous cell, [1 nail bed], 4 aggressive digital papillary adenoma, 2 melanoma, 2 epitheloid sarcoma, 1 Bowen's disease, 1 malignant fibrous histiocytoma, 1 synovial sarcoma (arm), 1 Merkle cell)
Fibroma	15
Calcification	9
Pyogenic granuloma	9
Glomus	8 (2 recurrent)
Soft tissue chondroma (synovial chondromatosis)	7
Dermatofibroma	4
Verruca vulgaris	4
Sweat gland adenoma	3 (1 arm)
Keratoacanthoma	3
Metastatic	3 (lung, stomach, adenocarcinoma ?primary)
Angioma	3
Angiolipoma	2
Nodular hidradenoma	2
Leiomyoma	2
Myxoma	1
Steatocytoma	1

Note: These tumors represent the experience of the author from 1978 through 1999. The numbers of cases were obtained by reviewing the pathology reports of tumors excised during this period. Pathologic reports that were not clearly tumors were excluded. Synovitis is a nonspecific diagnosis. Most synovitis is the result of surgery on a rheumatoid patient or synovitis removed during carpal tunnel surgery. The cases listed here include only those in which the differential diagnosis included a tumor. Rheumatoid nodules were included because often the diagnosis is not clear before surgery and microscopic evaluation. Dupuytren's fibromatosis is a form of tumor but it is not included in this series. If it had, it would have been the most common diagnosis. Some might question the listing of ganglion, but most authors have included this diagnosis in their series.

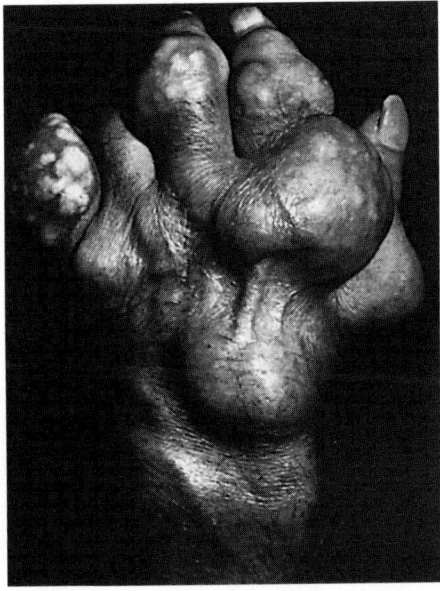

Fig. 56-1. Massive tophaceous gout.

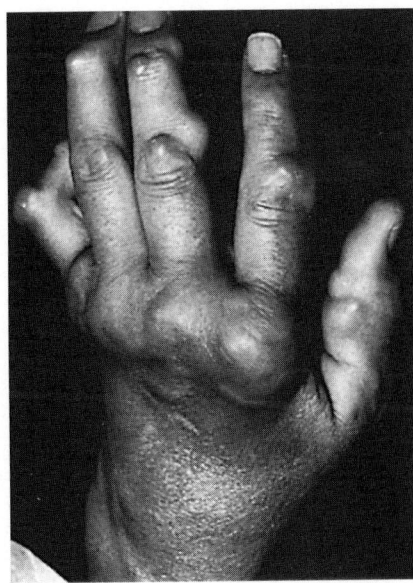

Fig. 56-2. Multiple rheumatoid nodules.

The diagnosis of a hand tumor is made by a detailed history, a precise physical examination, and an excisional biopsy. The examination of the hand should include an x-ray study as a matter of routine. If there is any question about the benignity of a soft tissue tumor, the workup should be more extensive. Such a workup should include a magnetic resonance imaging (MRI) scan and might include computed tomographic (CAT) scan and a bone scan. MRI has become the gold standard in terms of delineating and evaluating hand tumors before biopsy or definitive surgery.[49] Fig. 56-6 shows an MRI of the hand delineating a lipoma of the hypothenar eminence. As Finn et al[32] point out, one has to decide whether to do an open or closed biopsy or whether to do an incisional (only a portion of the tumor is excised) or an excisional (all of the tumor is excised) biopsy. Most biopsies of hand tumors are open excisional. However, when doing a biopsy, one must consider the possibility that the tumor might be malignant and may require radical surgery or reconstruction. As Mankin[53] points out, "an amputation in a live patient is a far better result than a functional restoration of the hand in a dead one."

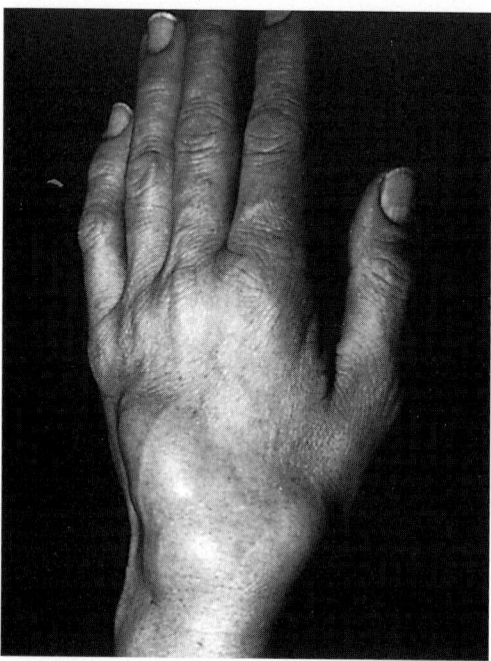

Fig. 56-3. Synovitis localized to one area in an asymptomatic patient with normal radiographs. This is probably rheumatoid, but infection or granulomatous disease must be included in the differential diagnosis.

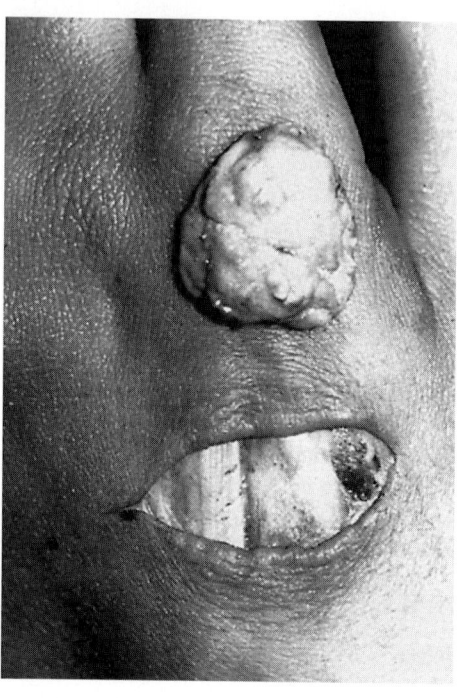

Fig. 56-4. Calcium deposit secondary to an IV infiltration in a cancer patient.

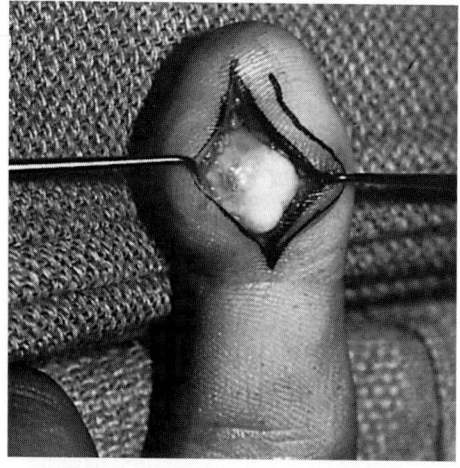

Fig. 56-5. Soft tissue chondroma.

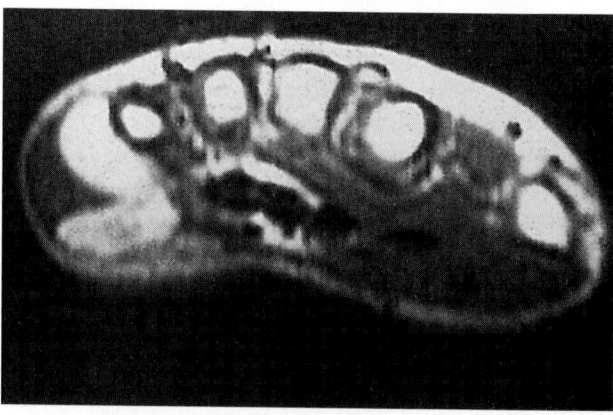

Fig. 56-6. Magnetic resonance imaging scan showing a lipoma in the hypothenar area.

GANGLIA

Ganglion cysts are the most common soft tissue tumors of the hand and wrist. Posch[68] has reported an incidence of 56% of 2113 cases. Butler et al[13] reported an incidence of 33%, and Bogumill et al[8] reported an incidence of 52%. Our incidence of 15% is much lower than that from these series. Our cases are surgical cases proven by pathology and include only a small minority of those seen. We see more problems caused by the excision of ganglions than caused by ganglions themselves. Fig. 56-7 shows a recurrent ganglion and an iatrogenic neuroma. Recurrences are common. Nerve problems, stiffness, and persistent pain are all-too-common sequelae of primary excision of ganglia. Our basic approach is to aspirate, splint, procrastinate, and then reaspirate.

A *ganglion* is a synovial cyst arising from the synovial lining of a tendon sheath or from the synovial lining of a joint. The cause of these tumors is not clear. Trauma, mucoid degeneration, and synovial herniation have all been implicated. Angelides and Wallace[1] have written extensively about the diagnosis and treatment of ganglions. The most common location for a ganglion is on the radial side of the wrist, either dorsal or volar. The usual origin is from the area of the scapholunate ligament. When excising a ganglion, one must excise the joint capsule in this region to prevent recurrence.[20]

Watson et al,[82] however, have reported the development of rotary subluxation of the scaphoid after ganglion excision. We have seen this on several occasions. Kivett et al[46] did not find wrist instability but did find a 25% incidence of persistent wrist symptoms. Perhaps, arthroscopic removal of ganglion cysts will decrease the incidence of instability, symptoms, and recurrence.[62]

When ganglia arise from the small joints, they are the result of a degenerative arthritic process. The most common site is the distal joint. Aspiration with or without a steroid injection into the joint can cure these mucous cysts. Surgical treatment of these cysts involves a complete excision of the stalk and an arthrotomy of the joint with excision of the arthritic osteophytes.[28] On occasion, the skin may be thin enough over the ganglion to require a skin graft. Recurrence can be a problem because of the underlying arthritis. The differential diagnosis of this tumor is a Heberden's node.

The third type of ganglion cyst is the volar retinacular ganglion. This small tumor arises from an apparent defect in the flexor retinaculum of a finger or thumb. The retinaculum of the first dorsal compartment is a less common but possible location. Needle rupture with or without steroid injection can prevent the need for surgery.[10] An eccentric location of the ganglion may preclude an aspiration because of the danger of injury to a digital nerve. In our series, 7 of 32 ganglia were of this type. Most of these were early in the series. We became more conservative as our experience grew. For the most part, these can be treated by needle rupture or aspiration (Fig. 56-8). A ganglion occasionally may protrude into the bone or invade the bone (Fig. 56-9). Most of the reported cases have been in the scapholunate area. Uribu and Levey[78] have reviewed 15 cases of intraosseous ganglions. These were all either in the scaphoid or the lunate. We have had five of these as well as one in the capitate.

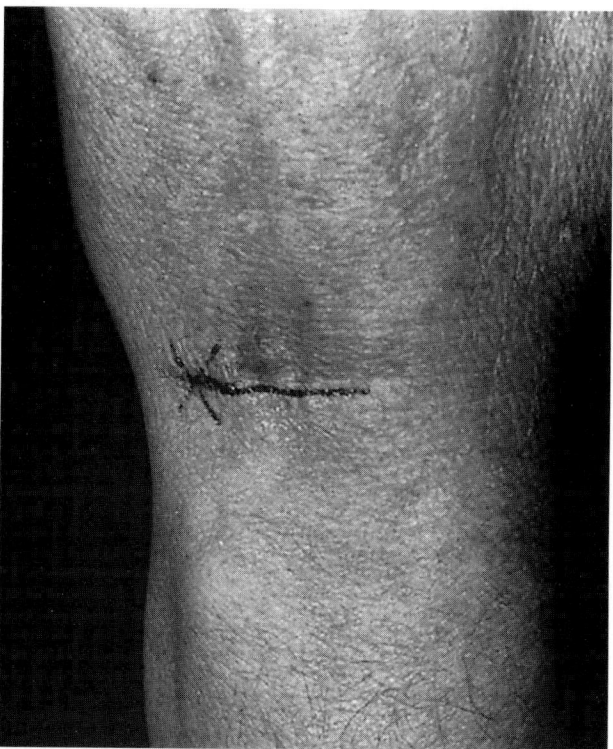

Fig. 56-7. Recurrent ganglion and a painful scar from an ulnar sensory neuroma after a ganglion excision.

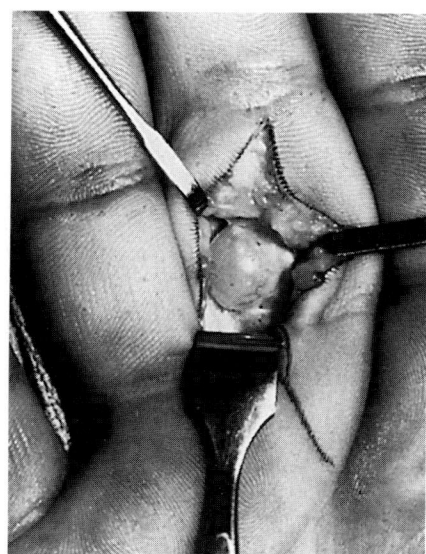

Fig. 56-8. A volar retinacular ganglion. This tumor arose from the area of the A$_2$ pulley and probably should not have been excised.

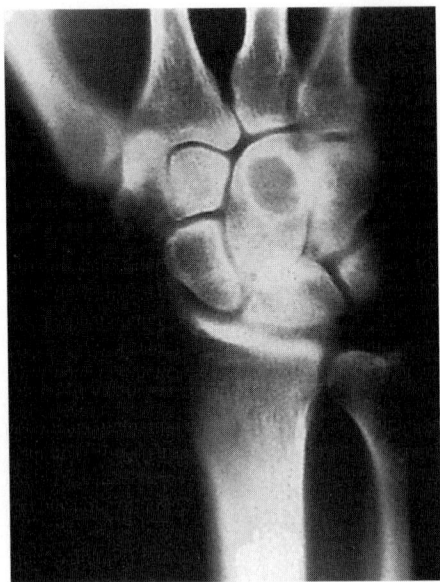

Fig. 56-9. An interosseous ganglion in the capitate.

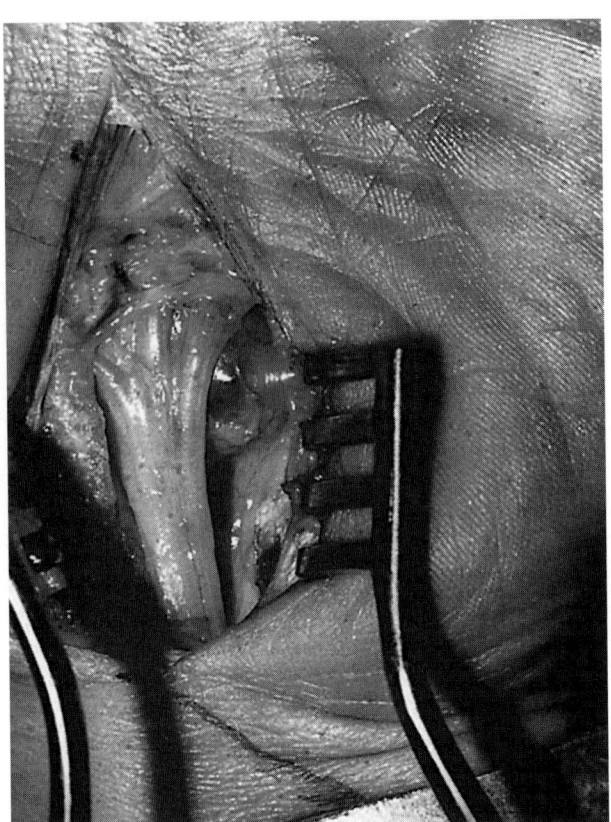

Fig. 56-10. A ganglion compressing the median nerve in the carpal tunnel.

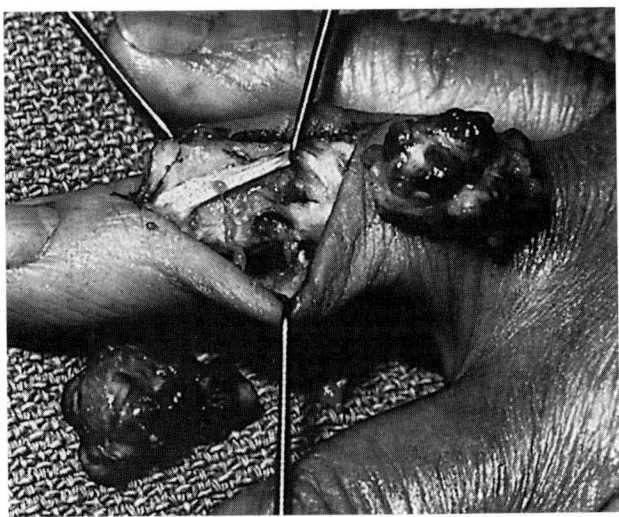

Fig. 56-11. A large xanthoma in both the dorsal and volar aspects of a finger.

Ganglia can be symptomatic, and there may be an occasion when surgery is indicated for the symptomatic tumor. For the most part, we favor aspiration to confirm the diagnosis and then observation. There is certainly little reason to operate on a pediatric ganglion. Rosson[71] recently reported a series of ganglia in pediatric patients where 20 of 29 resolved within 2 years. In adults, we favor multiple aspirations. Zubowicz and Ishii[89] have shown a cure rate of 85% with multiple aspirations. Korman et al[48] reported a 51% success rate with aspiration and no advantage to immobilization. A ganglion compressing a nerve is clearly a reason for surgery rather than observation or aspiration (Fig. 56-10).[45] Our series included five such cases.

XANTHOMA

The most common solid tumor of the hand is the giant cell tumor of tendon sheath, or xanthoma. Jaffe et al[41] termed these lesions *localized pigmented villonodular synovitis*. Moore et al[58] prefers the term *localized nodular tenosynovitis*. These tumors are painless, slow-growing masses that usually arise on the dorsal surface of the hand or finger. They may become quite large (Fig. 56-11). Most occur in the middle decades. It is not clear whether they arise in the joint or invade the joint. In our series, there was one case that clearly arose in the wrist joint (Fig. 56-12). This represents the diffuse type, or pigmented villonodular synovitis. When a giant cell tumor has been present for a long time, it may produce a pressure deformity on the bone[79] (Fig. 56-13).

At the time of resection, these tumors appear to be well-encapsulated, gray-brown neoplasms with patches of yellow pigmentation throughout. Histologically, the tumors contain foam cells with small nuclei and a granular cytoplasm full of lipid granules. This accounts for the yellow color. Hemosiderin deposits produce the brown color.

Although they may appear to be invasive of the bone or tendon, giant cell tumors are well encapsulated. Although tedious, complete excision is technically feasible in most

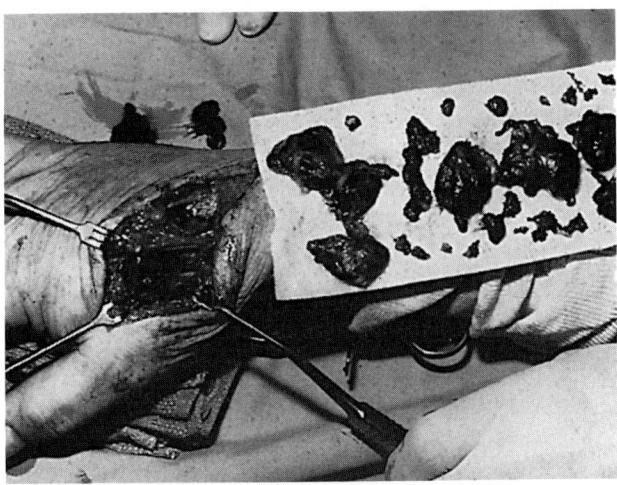

Fig. 56-12. A diffuse xanthoma or pigmented villonodular synovitis arising from the wrist. This tumor recurred.

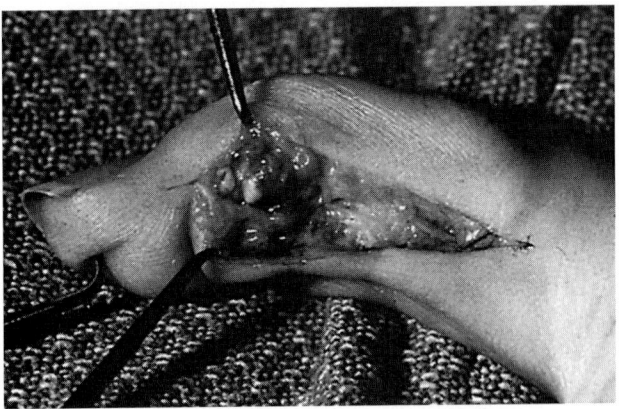

Fig. 56-14. A recurrent xanthoma.

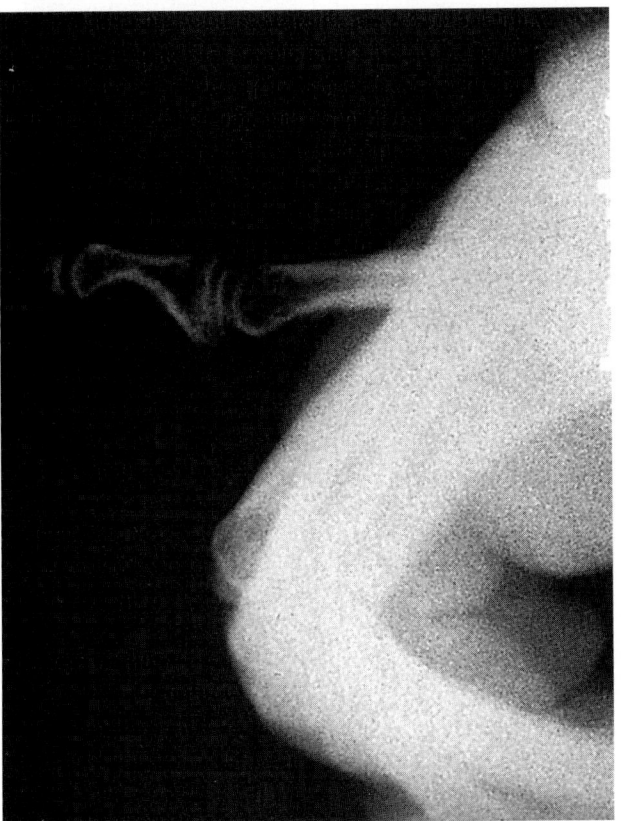

Fig. 56-13. Erosion of bone secondary to a xanthoma.

cases. Some series have reported a recurrence rate of up to 10%.[79] In our series, we have had only two recurrences. This is a case of true pigmented villonodular synovitis of the wrist, and the recurrence clearly is the result of incomplete excision. We have operated on two patients with recurrent giant cell tumors who had their initial operations elsewhere

(Fig. 56-14). Both of these patients clearly had an inadequate excision at the time of the first operation. Recurrence is related to the failure to completely excise the tumor. If the tumor is a diffuse type involving a joint, it may be necessary to do a fusion to prevent recurrence.

A giant cell tumor should be differentiated from xanthoma tuberosum, which occurs in patients with hypercholesterolemia. In this condition, the deposits tend to invade the tendon and excision is nearly impossible without excising some of the normal tissue.

LIPOMAS

Lipomas are relatively common tumors that have a characteristic soft consistency on palpation. These tumors are slow growing and usually asymptomatic; as a result, when they become clinically significant, they may be quite large.[61] Usually, they become symptomatic because they grow large enough to interfere with function or cause nerve compression. Babins and Lubahn[4] have reported a series of five patients who presented with nerve compression. On x-ray examination, there is a characteristic area of radiolucency. A CT scan or MRI may be useful if the diagnosis is in doubt.[85] These tumors differ little in microscopic appearance from the surrounding fat. Usually, the fat cells are mature and the tumors have only a thin capsule. On occasion, there may be an admixture of fibrous connective tissue in the tumor, thus the term *fibrolipoma*. Large tumors are a challenge to excise (Fig. 56-15). The most common site of origin is the deep palmar space; however, they can arise anywhere there is fatty tissue. We have had several cases in fingers. Two thirds of our cases were in the hand and one third in the arm. It is likely that the percentage of upper extremity cases in the arm and forearm is much higher than 50% relative to the hand. Many lipomas proximal to the hand are excised by general surgeons rather than by hand

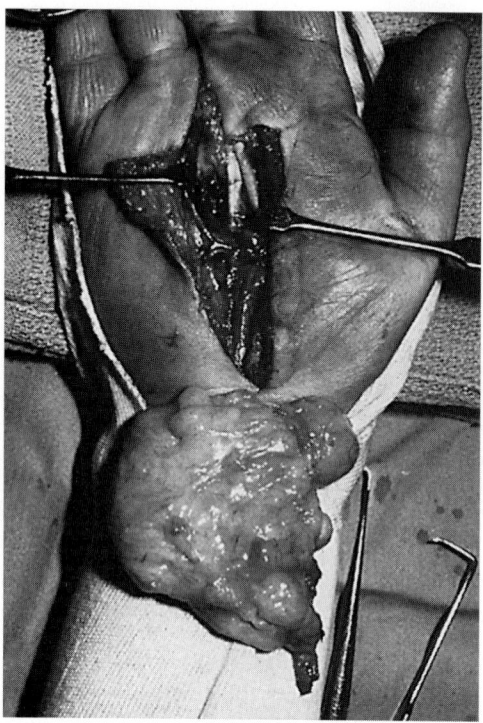

Fig. 56-15. A large lipoma arising from the deep palmar space.

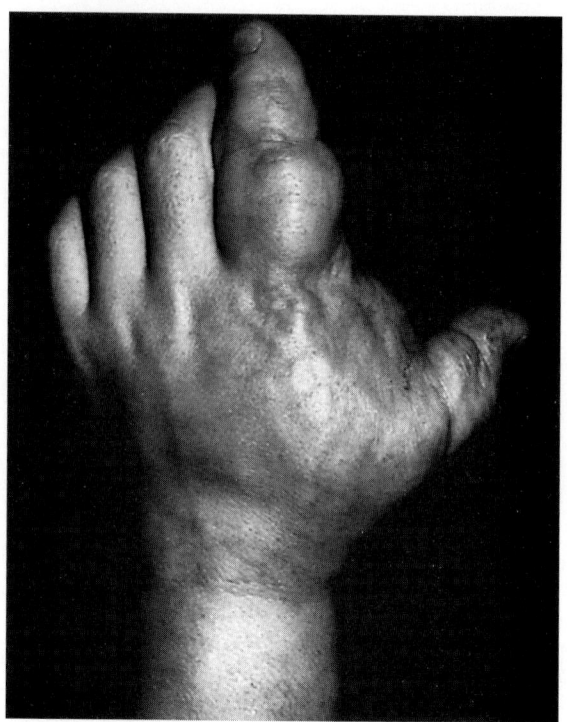

Fig. 56-16. A massive hemangioma.

surgeons. There is a negligible recurrence rate after excision. However, we have had two: one was in a child in whom the diagnosis was a lipoblastosis or an intramuscular lipoma (this may be a different tumor than an adult lipoma) and the other, interestingly enough, was a finger (this one recurred 15 years after the original excision).

VASCULAR TUMORS

Most vascular tumors are congenital and thought to arise as a result of failure of differentiation of common embryonic channels. The result is a hemangioma, lymphangioma, or congenital arteriovenous fistula. There are several approaches to classification. Goidanich and Companacci[37] prefer to call them *hamartoma,* relating their origin to a growth of new blood vessels early in life. Stout and Lattes[75] favor a classification based on microscopic appearance. Blackfield et al[6] after much study, recommended the useful classification of *involuting* and *noninvoluting hemangiomas.* The acquired tumors are aneurysms, arteriovenous fistulas, glomus tumors, and pyogenic granulomas.

The diagnosis of vascular tumors is usually obvious (Fig. 56-16). Most are blue or reddish blue and compressible. Some may be pulsatile. Occasionally, radiographs will show calcification. Isotope scanning may be useful in determining the nature and extent of a vascular lesion.[54] Angiography can be useful. Geiser and Eversmann[36] have described a method of closed-system venography to delineate these lesions. In this method, the radiographic dye and Xylocaine are injected into the exsanguinated limb distal to the tumor. Most

vascular tumors will fill rapidly, delineating the tumor. This is probably safer than arteriography.

Hemangiomas become symptomatic as a result of progressive enlargement or pain. Treatment of hemangiomas must be individualized. Because many involute spontaneously, treatment should be delayed for tumors that appear soon after birth. Many modes of treatment have been proposed, but surgery remains the mainstay. Fig. 56-17 shows a tumor that might easily be excised. Palmeri[65] reported a 98% cure rate with only a 2% recurrence rate. Apfelberg et al[2] have reported success using the argon laser. Injection of the sclerosing agent sodium morrhuate has been used, but it is not recommended because of the possible injury to normal tissues.[64] The author has found some of these tumors to be difficult to treat surgically. The small, localized, thrombosed tumor can be easily excised. However, with a large tumor, separating normal tissue from the tumor can be difficult. The abnormal vessels can invade or be a part of tendon, nerve, or skin, making function-sparing excision impossible. Large tumors usually contain elements of an arteriovenous fistula. The symptoms often are the result of relative avascularity because of shunting through the arteriovenous connections. Ligation of the feeding vessels may lead to further devascularization and result in amputation.[24]

When the diagnosis of hemangioma of the hand is made or suspected, precise anatomic staging is needed before a commitment to surgical excision. The risks of surgical injury or tumor recurrence can outweigh the expected benefits. Careful follow-up is better seen as a prospective choice than

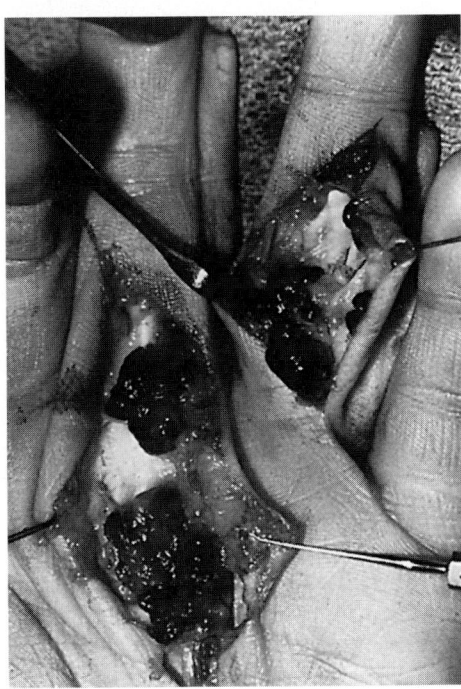

Fig. 56-17. A localized hemangioma that might easily be excised.

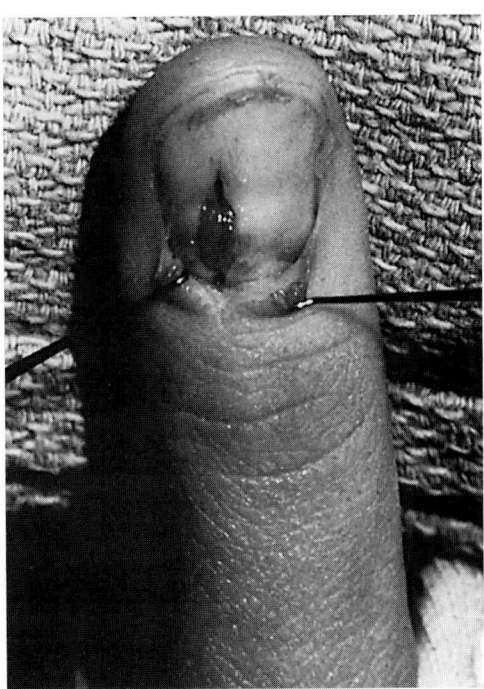

Fig. 56-18. Subungual glomus tumor.

a retrospective wish. The glomus tumor is an unusual but interesting tumor. It arises from the glomus body or neuromyoarterial apparatus. The glomus body is a normal arteriovenous anastomosis that lies in the stratum reticulum of the skin and helps regulate temperature. These tumors are common subungual (Fig. 56-18) and in the distal pads of digits but can exist in other areas of the hands and body (Fig. 56-19). People with glomus tumors present with paroxysms of lancinating pain, tenderness, and cold sensitivity.[16] When this tumor has been present for a long time, it may erode the bone. Clinical suspicion is the key to the diagnosis, especially if the tumor is under the nail. The treatment is excision.

Lymphangiomas, as the name implies, are tumors arising from lymph channels. Like hemangiomas, they usually are present at birth and usually enlarge slowly and become symptomatic. As Blair et al[7] point out, there is no good nonsurgical treatment. In our experience, the excision of these tumors is much like the excision of hemangiomas. It is hard to separate normal from abnormal (Fig. 56-20). However, the problems with distal avascularity are not encountered as with hemangiomas.

The pyogenic granuloma is usually classified as a vascular tumor because of abundant capillary granulation tissue that is present histologically. Most authors believe that these lesions are posttraumatic with a superimposed infectious component.[80] The usual presentation in the hand is that of a polypoid, friable, red mass that bleeds easily (Fig. 56-21). Treatment is excision.

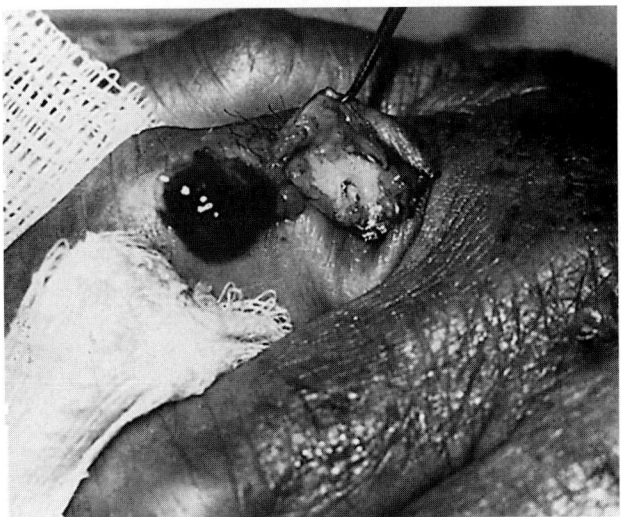

Fig. 56-19. Glomus tumor arising from the dorsal aspect of a finger.

INCLUSION CYSTS

Most of the literature about epidermal cysts in the hand is related to cysts of the hand skeleton.[14] In our series, cysts of the skin occurred nearly as often as giant cell tumors of tendon sheath. They are usually the result of a penetrating injury or a laceration that drives a fragment of keratinizing epithelium into the subcutaneous tissue, where it survives, produces keratin, grows, and produces a tumor. These tumors usually occur on the volar aspect of the hand or finger, although, as in our series, a dorsal location is also

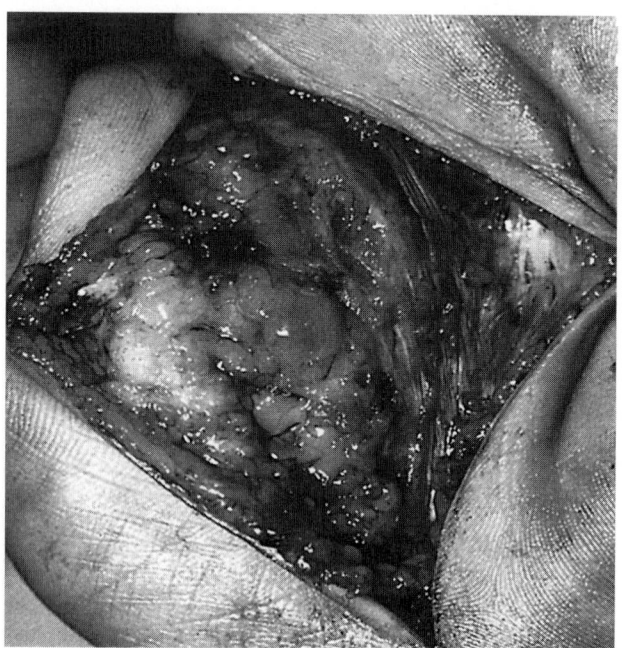

Fig. 56-20. A large lymphangioma arising from the palm.

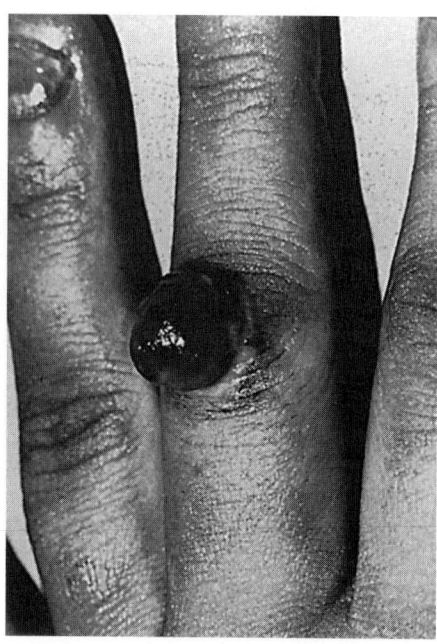

Fig. 56-21. Pyogenic granuloma.

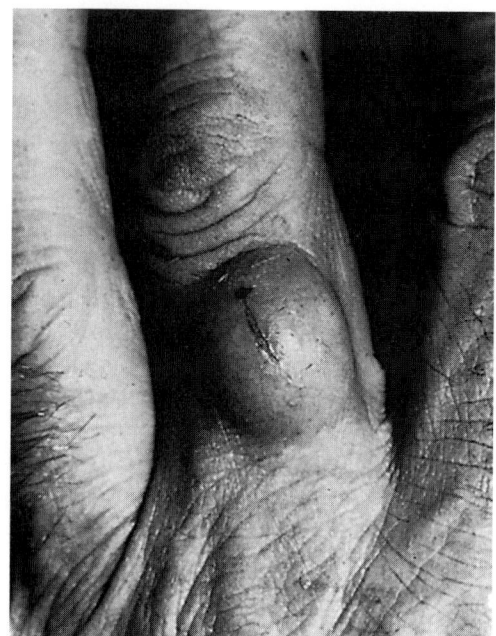

Fig. 56-22. Inclusion cyst.

possible. However, only one third of our cases had a clear history of a penetrating injury. If a penetrating injury is the cause, then why are they not even more common? One wonders if perhaps another mechanism is possible. Ward and Labosky[81] have suggested that embryonic epithelial cell rests can be stimulated by trauma. They then become cystic and produce the characteristic tumors. The treatment of these tumors is excision. Usually, there is a small dimple or scar on the skin that is pathognomonic of these cysts (Figs. 56-22 and 56-23). An elipse of skin should be excised around this entry point to ensure a complete excision. In our series, we have had six recurrences. The assumption is that a few viable epithelial cells were left in the subcutaneous area with the surgery. It is remarkable that inclusion cysts are not a more common result of any type of laceration or surgery.

NERVE TUMORS

Nerve tumors in most series are unusual, occurring at a rate of less than 1% of the tumors of the hand.[13,76] In our series, we had 27, so perhaps the incidence is higher than previously reported. The two common types of nerve tumors are neurilemoma and neurofibroma. A neurilemoma or schwannoma appears to arise from the Schwann's cells that surround the nerve fibers. They usually can be easily excised without injuring the nerve fibers[67] (Fig. 56-24). Histologically, these tumors have two types of nerve tissue. Antoni-A cells are dense, compact, and spindle-shaped. These spindly cells can align themselves in a picket-fence type of arrangement called *Verocay bodies*. Antoni-B cells are loosely arranged retinacular cells with smaller nuclei. Neurilemomas characteristically have alternating areas of Antoni-A and Antoni-B cells. In our series, we had six neurilemomas.

A neurofibroma is the other type of nerve tumor. These tumors also are thought to arise from the Schwann's cells, but unlike the neurilemoma, these are a part of the nerve and excision without destroying the nerve is nearly impossible (Fig. 56-25). These have a more variegated pattern with mucoid material, lymphocytes, mast cells, and xanthoma cells. These tumors are more likely to present with some sort of neurologic symptom. They may be multiple and commonly occur as a part of von Recklinghausen's disease. We have often found the café-au-lait spots in retrospect.

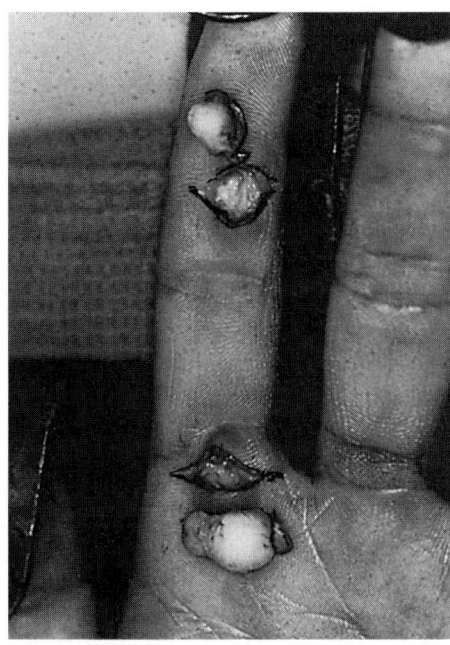

Fig. 56-23. Multiple inclusion cysts in the same finger.

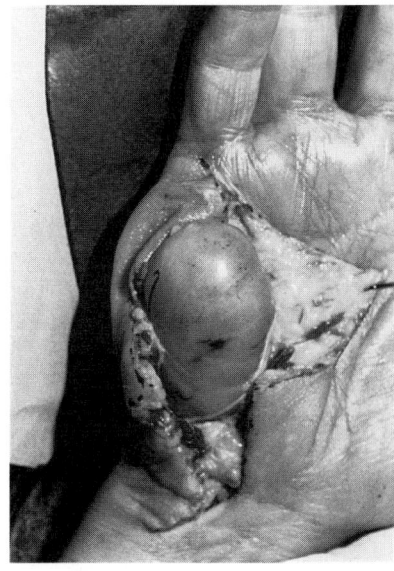

Fig. 56-25. A large neurofibroma in the palm.

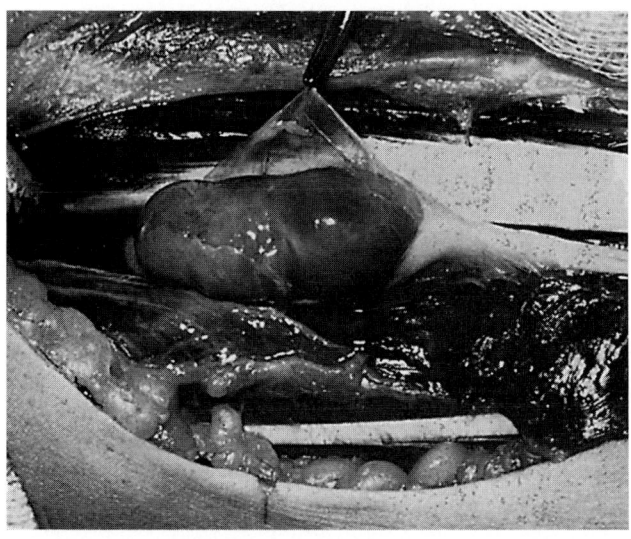

Fig. 56-24. Schwannoma.

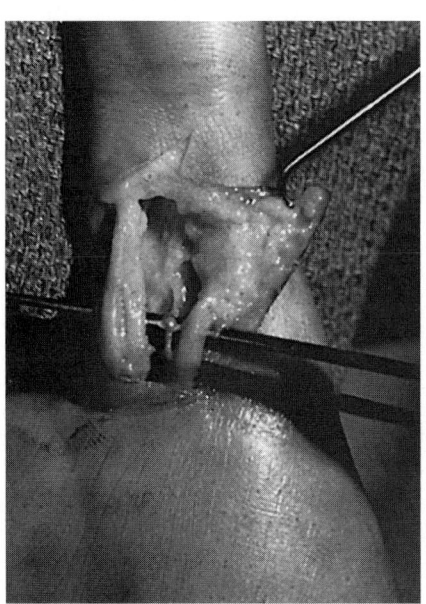

Fig. 56-26. Bowler's thumb.

Holdsworth[39] has reviewed a series of nine neurilemomas and eight solitary neurofibromas. The diagnosis was suspected preoperatively in only five patients. Only two had a positive Tinel's sign. In Phalen's series of 16 neurilemomas, the diagnosis was made preoperatively only five times.[67] In our series, it was also rare to make the diagnosis preoperatively. One would expect a positive Tinel's sign or some manifestation of nerve irritation, but this was not the case.

Various hamartomas can cause neural enlargement and present as a nerve tumor. Ganglions,[5] lipomas,[35] hemangiomas,[47] and lipofibromas[52] have been reported. These tumors usually present as a painful mass. Excision of a lipoma or a ganglion might be possible. However, this is usually impossible in the case of a hemangioma or a lipofibroma of nerve, where decompression might be the only alternative. Repeated trauma will cause fibrous enlargement of a nerve and thus result in a nerve tumor. The bowler's thumb is an example[27] (Fig. 56-26).

FIBROMA OF TENDON SHEATH

Clearly, the most common fibrous tumor seen in any hand practice is the Dupuytren's nodule or cord. In our series, we had 15 fibrous tumors best classified as fibroma of tendon sheath. These lesions may be more common than previously recognized. Millon et al[56] reviewed eight cases in the hand in 1994. Chung and Enzinger[18] reviewed a series of 138 cases in 1982. These tumors present much like xanthomas. They are painless solid tumors associated with tendon sheaths, slowly growing over a number of years. Unlike the giant cell tumors, however, they do not produce any bony erosions and are in general not as lobulated. Histologically, these tumors have scattered benign fibroblasts with abundant amounts of dense intercellular hyalinized collagen. Slitlike vascular spaces often are present. There are no giant cells. They are more difficult to excise than the typical xanthoma (Fig. 56-27). In one case, we had to excise a neurovascular bundle to remove the tumor completely. We have had no recurrences to date, although one might anticipate a rate similar to or slightly greater than that for xanthomas because of the similarity of the lesions.

TUMORS OF THE EPITHELIUM

Tumors of the epithelium often fall into the province of the dermatologist. With the advent of Mohs micrographic surgery, many skin lesions are referred to the skin specialist rather than the hand specialist. This technique has made it possible to completely and accurately excise these skin tumors.[57] These tumors can be difficult to diagnose. Small,

seemingly innocuous lesions may be premalignant or malignant and a threat to the patient's life. The hand surgeon must have a knowledge of the types and behavior of the various skin tumors.

The most common skin tumor is the wart or verruca vulgaris. These benign lesions are caused by a human papillomavirus. They are spread by direct or mediate contact. Trauma may be a precipitating factor.[60] They often regress spontaneously. Surgical excision can result in the production of satellite lesions in the surgical scar. It is preferable to curette and cauterize or use cryotherapy rather than excise a wart.[51]

A *dermatofibroma* or *cutaneous fibrous histiocytoma* (Fig. 56-28) is a small, firm nodule that can appear anywhere on the hand. Histologically, the tumor is primarily made up of short intersecting fascicles of fibroblastic cells with a few scattered round histiocytes. Treatment is excisional biopsy, which is usually done to

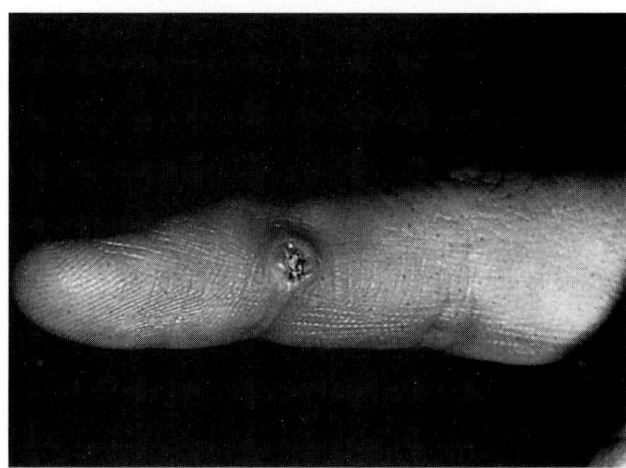

Fig. 56-28. Dermatofibroma.

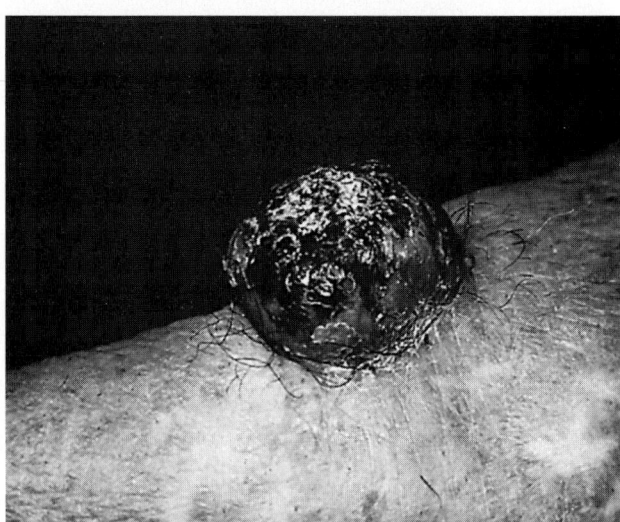

Fig. 56-29. Umbilicated keratoacanthoma.

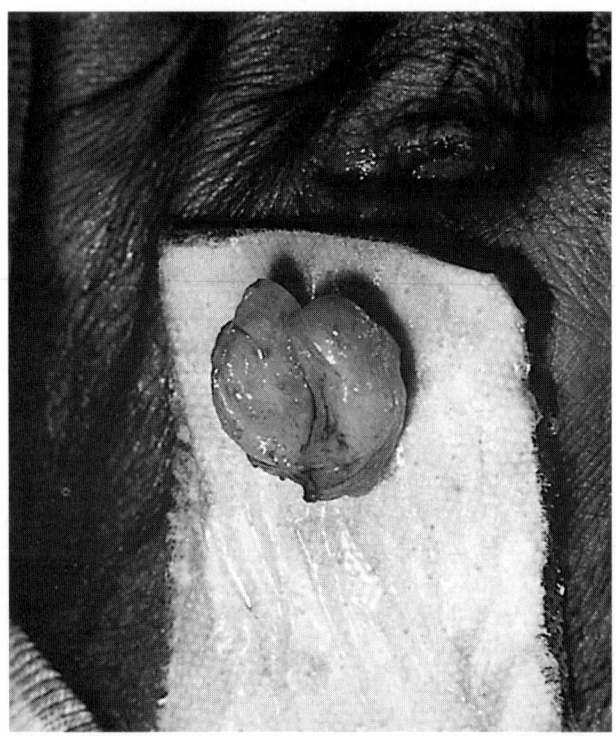

Fig. 56-27. Fibroma of tendon sheath.

differentiate these lesions from their malignant cousins, such as a juvenile aponeurotic fibroma or even a malignant fibrous histiocytoma.[34]

A *keratoacanthoma* is a skin lesion that can be difficult to distinguish from a squamous cell carcinoma.[17] It has a crusty keratotic appearance that is often umbilicated (Fig. 56-29) or sessile (Fig. 56-30) in appearance. Even microscopically, the differentiation is difficult.[33] Although they look ominous, they are not fixed to the underlying tissues and are benign. The treatment is excision. In large cases, a flap or skin graft may be needed. The pathologic diagnosis in Fig. 56-29 was squamous cell carcinoma, low grade, arising in a keratoacanthoma.

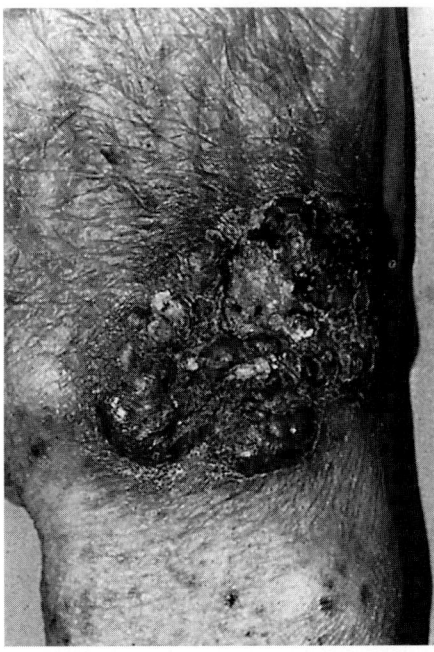

Fig. 56-30. Sessile keratocanthoma.

Bowen's disease is another skin lesion that seems to straddle the line between benign and malignant (Fig. 56-31). It is thought that arsenic compounds may be an important etiologic factor.[77] Sunlight is also a possible factor. This intraepithelial squamous cell tumor usually presents as a scaly and crusty verrucous plaque. The histopathology shows dysplasia. The treatment is complete removal or destruction of the dysplastic tissue by either surgery or cauterization.[42]

Sweat gland tumors are more likely to be confused clinically with giant cell tumors or hemangiomas than with skin tumors; however, their cell of origin makes inclusion in this section appropriate. The most common pathologic term is *eccrine spiradenoma,* although other terms such as *dermal cylindroma, eccrine poroma,* and *hidroacanthoma* are also used (Fig. 56-32). The treatment is excisional biopsy. In their malignant form, these small tumors can be deadly. The term *aggressive digital papillary adenoma* (Fig. 56-33) is used for lesions that require an aggressive clinical approach.[43] Sweat gland carcinoma is the malignant variety of this tumor. These innocent-looking lesions can metastasize and be fatal.[88] There are three basic types of malignant epithelial tumors: basal cell carcinoma, squamous cell carcinoma, and malignant melanoma. The incidence of all three of these tumors is increasing, and all seem to be related to sun exposure. The basal cell is the least common in the hand, although it is very common in other areas of the body, especially the head and neck.[72] It typically presents as a raised lesion with a pearly edge. Treatment is complete excision with tumor-free margins. Again, since the development of Mohs micrographic surgery, most are treated by dermatologists.

Squamous cell carcinoma is the most common skin malignancy in most series. Although these tumors do not metastasize as readily as the sarcomas, they do have the capacity to be fatal. These lesions may vary in size from a small, slow-growing lesion to a large necrotic lesion as seen in Fig. 56-34. If the lesion involves only the skin, complete

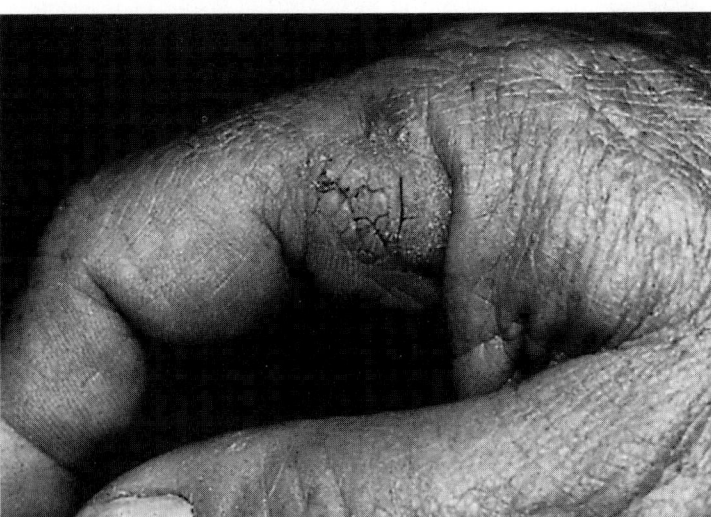

Fig. 56-31. Bowen's disease.

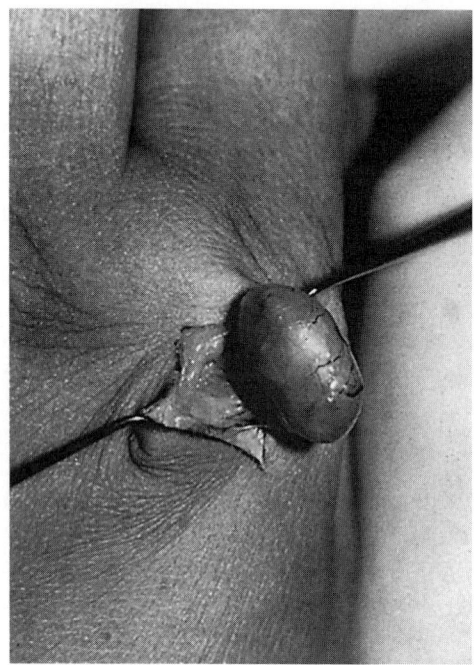

Fig. 56-32. Sweat gland adenoma.

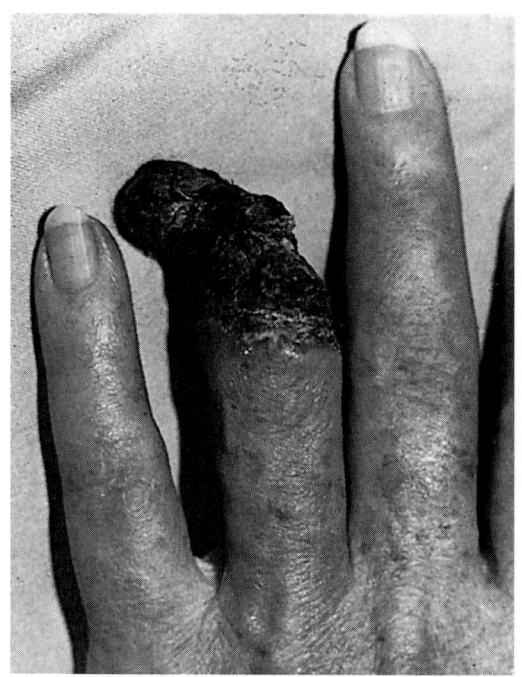

Fig. 56-34. Squamous cell carcinoma.

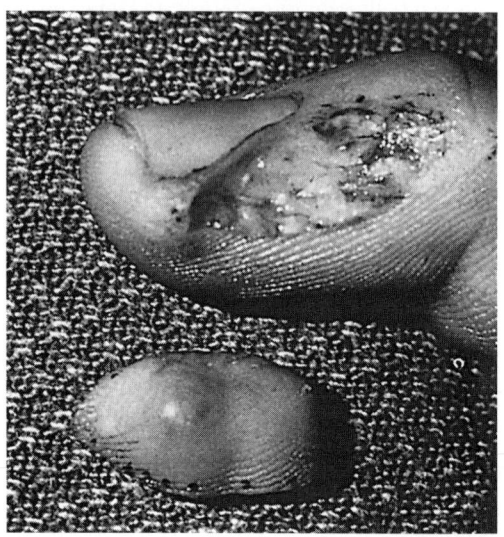

Fig. 56-33. An aggressive digital papillary adenoma.

excision and skin grafting may be appropriate. If the lesion involves the deeper structures, amputation is the procedure of choice. Schiavon et al[73] have reported a 22% recurrence rate and a 28% incidence of metastasis in a series of 55 tumors. In their series, the lymph nodes often were the first site of metastasis, and they thought that lymphadenectomy was indicated in every case of recurrence because it seemed to improve survival. The use of Mohs techniques in surgery for squamous cell carcinoma of the hand should decrease the incidence of recurrence. Amputation is the recommended

treatment for squamous cell tumors of the nail bed.[15] Sentinal node identification and biopsy techniques may also help predict the survival and decrease the morbidity associated with regional lymphadenectomy. A malignant melanoma is a tumor that arises from the epidermal melanocytes. These tumors appear to be related to sun exposure, and their incidence is rapidly rising. The natural history of the tumor is changing, and the cure rate seems to be increasing. Clark et al[19] have described a useful classification that has become the standard. They related the prognosis to the depth of the lesion. It is apparent that aggressive early treatment of localized lesions can be very successful. Cohen et al[21] have reviewed a series of 250 patients in whom there were no deaths or metastases in level I or II lesions over a 14-year period. Again, Mohs surgery is useful in determining the accurate surgical approach to these tumors. We have had only one melanoma in our series because all of the pigmented skin tumors at our institution are evaluated and treated in melanoma clinic by the dermatologists and the oncologic surgeons. Subungual melanoma appears to have a very poor prognosis related to a delay in diagnosis and advanced disease at the time of presentation.[40]

MALIGNANT TUMORS

Cancers that arise from mesodermal tissues, such as muscle, fat, vessels, and fibrous tissue, are called *sarcomas*. Although soft tissue sarcomas are uncommon, they constitute an important category of hand tumors. They are malignant tumors that have the capacity to metastasize. Excisional biopsies should be done with the idea that the tumor may be malignant. The tumors are named according to their cell of origin. Thus they can be called *fibrosarcoma, rhabdomyosarcoma,* or *synovial sarcoma,* relating their origin to fibrous tissue, muscle, or synovium. The classification of these tumors is complex.[29] Most sarcomas are composed of spindle cells—thin cells whose length is twice that of their short axis. Some of the tumors have cells that are more square or cuboidal. These cells are called *epithelioid.* Tumors with both spindle cells and epithelioid cells are called *biphasic.*[70] Sarcomas also are classified by histologic grading. A tumor that resembles its cell of origin is well differentiated. Conversely, a tumor that has little resemblance to its primary tissue is poorly differentiated. In general, the poorly differentiated tumors have a worse prognosis.

Soft tissue sarcomas are rare tumors. We have had only four in our series. In a 24-year period at Memorial Sloan-Kettering, Owens et al[63] reported only 17 cases involving the hand. Creighton et al[23] have reviewed 61 soft tissue sarcomas cases from four major hospitals over a 10-year period. Of these, only seven involved the hand. McPhee et al[55] have reviewed 24 soft tissue sarcomas over 24 years. The most common histologic type was malignant fibrous histiocytoma; the second most common tumor was eiptheloid sarcoma. As expected, smaller tumors had a better prognosis. Brien et al[9] reviewed 23 patients over 26 years. The most common presentation was a small, painless soft tissue mass. The most common diagnosis was synovial sarcoma. They recommended wide excision with preservation of the function of the hand if possible. Surgical tumor-free margins were important. Adjuvant treatment did not seem to influence outcome. Gustafson and Arner[38] reviewed 108 cases over 29 years. Malignant fibrous histeosystoma was the most common type. Small size and a lack of vascular invasion were related to the prognosis. At a follow-up of 3 years, 30% had developed metastatic disease.

The problems associated with these tumors can probably best be demonstrated by an illustrative case (Fig. 56-35). H.U. is a 50-year-old fork-lift operator who presented with swelling on his fourth finger. He related the swelling to irritation of his finger on a steering knob at work. He underwent an excisional biopsy at another hospital. The soft tissue mass was poorly marginated and not entirely excised. The many pathologists who reviewed the tissue slides diagnosed the lesion as a typical fibrohisteocytic proliferation. One month later, he underwent an excisional biopsy of the tumor. After an extensive review, the same pathologic diagnosis was made. One year later, H.U. developed a new nodule on the same finger. An incisional biopsy showed the same pathologic lesion, and he underwent a ray resection of the fourth finger. The tumor extended to one margin on the specimen. This time, again after much review, the diagnosis was changed to myxoid malignant fibrous histiocytoma. One year later, H.U. developed another nodule in the incision

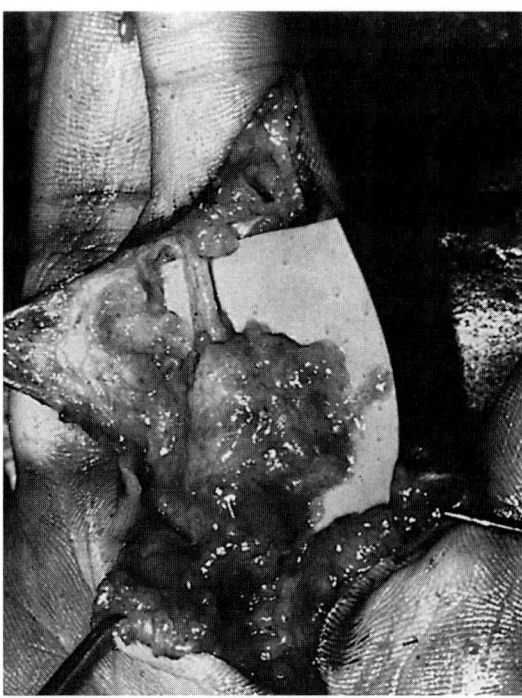

Fig. 56-35. A poorly localized tumor arising from the fourth finger. This was eventually diagnosed as a myxoid malignant fibrous histiocytoma.

line. This time he underwent a resection of the ulnar side of his hand. He has been disease free for 6 years.

This case illustrates many of the teaching points about soft tissue sarcomas. First, if the tumor is not well defined and localized at surgery, the surgeon should be suspicious. Second, if the pathology report returns as atypical, be careful. Third, if the tumor recurs, the possibility of a malignancy must be considered. Fourth, the case points out the reluctance of a hand surgeon to necessarily become a tumor surgeon in such a case. Smith[74] emphasized that the hand surgeon is best qualified to treat tumors of the hand but that he or she must alter the routine when treating an aggressive hand tumor. The possibility that this is a work-related problem suggests another volume of legal letters that is beyond the scope of this chapter.

Epithelioid sarcoma (Fig. 56-36) may be the most common malignant soft tissue tumor of the hand. Unfortunately, it may also be the most deadly. Enzinger[30] first described this tumor in 1970. The pathology is often confusing, leading to a delay in diagnosis. These tumors can resemble a granuloma or a rheumatoid nodule. The principal cell is an epithelioid cell. Spindle cells typical of sarcomas surround these epithelioid cells. Bryan et al[11] reviewed a series of 13 cases. In their cases, the initial diagnosis was misleading and the typical clinical course was one of recurrence and metastasis. They recommended primary en bloc excision and midforearm amputation for recurrent

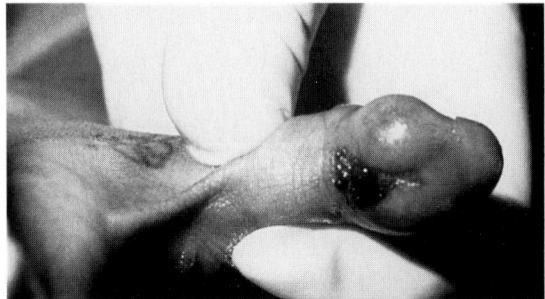

Fig. 56-36. Epithelioid sarcoma of the thumb.

lesions. Peimer et al[66] had a similar experience with six cases. They found the patterns of spread to be inconsistent and recommended early radical surgery. Whitworth et al[84] reviewed a series of 42 extremity epithelioid sarcomas and found that amputation offered no advantage over local resection as long as the pathologic margins were clear.

Rhabdomyosarcomas show a differentiation tending toward skeletal muscle. Although rare in the hand, they are the most common soft tissue sarcoma in children. Three types exist. The alveolar is the most common in the hand. It has characteristic alveolar-like spaces on histologic examination. The other two types are embryonal and pleomorphic. The clinical presentation and difficulties in delayed treatment are similar to those for epithelioid sarcomas. The prognosis of rhabdomyosarcoma has improved markedly over the past few decades.[69] Complete resection and multiagent chemotherapy have improved the survival rates.

The malignant fibrous histiocytoma is so named because it is thought to arise from a monocyte, macrophage type of cell rather than from a fibroblast. This tumor is the most common adult soft tissue sarcoma, but it is still rare in the hand. Dick[26] has reviewed a series of 11 cases of the upper extremity, 5 of which involved the hand. This tumor can arise in bone or spread to bone from the soft tissues. Recommended treatment includes aggressive surgical therapy and adjuvant chemotherapy.[83]

Synovial sarcomas are so named because they tend to arise close to major joints and because, pathologically, they look like synovium. Radiographs can be useful in diagnosing these tumors because of the common presence of focal calcification.[86] Treatment guidelines are not clear because of the small numbers, but again, radical surgery combined with chemotherapy and radiotherapy seems to be favored. Other soft tissue sarcomas such as fibrosarcoma, clear-cell sarcoma (malignant melanoma of soft parts), leiomyosarcoma, malignant schwannoma, angiosarcoma, and alveolar soft-part sarcoma do occur in the forearm and hand, but they are quite rare. As a result, it is difficult to make statements about treatment and prognosis.

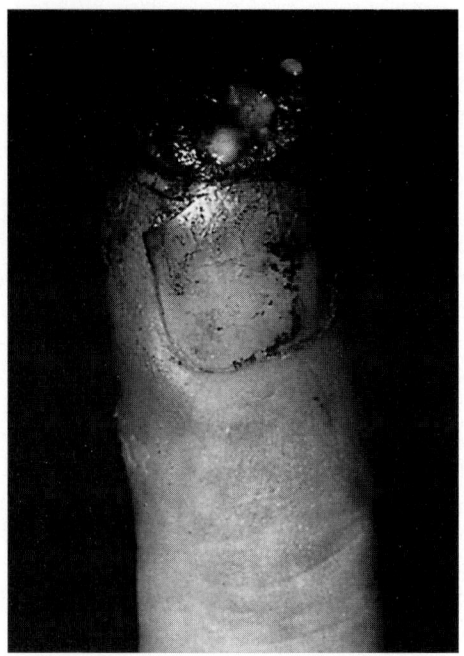

Fig. 56-37. Squamous cell from the lung.

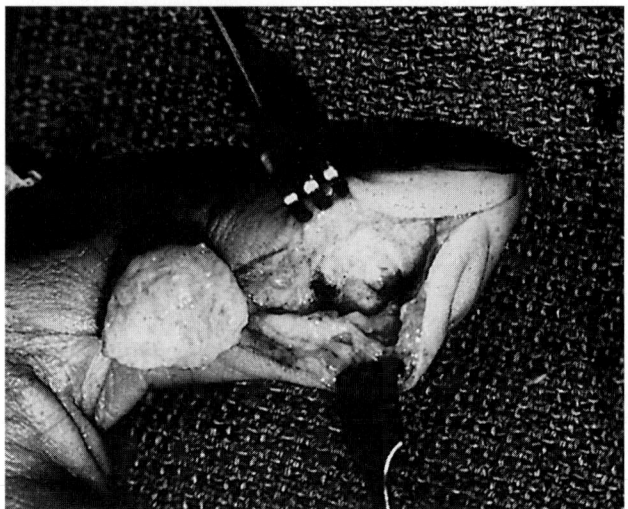

Fig. 56-38. Adenocarcinoma from the stomach.

METASTATIC TUMORS

Metastatic tumors of the hand are unusual, but they do need to be included in the differential diagnosis of any hand tumor.[44,87] We have had three cases. The one to the forearm was the most difficult. This was an adenocarcinoma to bone that was initially treated as an infection. The primary was never identified. Usually, the hand tumor identity is obvious and a part of an ongoing downhill course. The squamous cell case (Fig. 56-37) and the adenocarcinoma of the stomach (Fig. 56-38) both had known primary sources. The treatment of these cases is palliative.

THE ROLE OF THE THERAPIST

It can be difficult for the hand surgeon to understand the concern that a patient may have when he or she develops a hand tumor. Patients with a clear-cut synovitis may be extremely apprehensive until the final pathology report is available. A therapist may recognize such concerns and either reassure the patient or relate these concerns to the physician. In the postoperative period, the therapist assumes a more vital role. The emphasis shifts from one of diagnosis and treatment to one of recovery of motion and function. If the lesion is a malignant tumor, the therapist may be a vital sounding board for fears and concerns that the patient may have.

GLOSSARY

Adenocarcinoma malignant tumor with glandlike pattern

Angiosarcoma malignant tumor arising from the lining of blood vessels

Chondroma benign cartilage tumor

Clear-cell sarcoma a tendosynovial sarcoma with clear cytoplasm in the tumor cells

Fibroma benign tumor arising from fibrous tissue

Fibrosarcoma malignant tumor arising from fibrous tissue

Foam cells cells containing lipid or fatty substance

Giant cell large multinucleated cell

Glomus vascular tumor

Granulomatous inflammatory process

Hamartoma normal tissue in an abnormal location

Hemosiderin byproduct of the breakdown of hemoglobin

Leiomyosarcoma malignant tumor arising from smooth muscle

Lipoma benign tumor composed of fat or lipid cells

Neurilemoma benign tumor arising from nerve tissue

Pyogenic infectious in origin

Malignant schwannoma malignant tumor arising from nerve tissue

Squamous cell tumor type of lung cancer

Tophus gouty deposit

Villonodular part of the tumor pigmented villinodular synovitis

REFERENCES

1. Angelides AC, Wallace PF: The dorsal ganglion of the wrist: its pathogenesis, gross and microscopic anatomy, and surgical treatment, *J Hand Surg* 1:228, 1976.
2. Apfelberg DB, et al: Results of argon laser exposure of capillary hemangiomas of infancy, *Plast Reconstr Surg* 67:188, 1981.
3. Armin A, Blair SJ, Demos TC: Benign soft tissue chondromatous lesion of the hand, *J Hand Surg* 10:895, 1985.
4. Babins DM, Lubahn JD: Palmar lipomas associated with compression of the median nerve, *J Bone Joint Surg* 76A:1360, 1994.
5. Barrett R, Cramer F: Tumors of the peripheral nerves and so-called "ganglia" of the peroneal nerve, *Clin Orthop* 27:135, 1963.
6. Blackfield HM, et al: Visible hemangiomas: a preliminary statistical report of a 10 year study, *Plast Reconstr Surg* 26:326, 1960.
7. Blair WF, et al: Lymphangiomas of the forearm and hand, *J Hand Surg* 8:399, 1983.
8. Bogumill GP, Sullivan DJ, Baker GI: Tumors of the hand, *Clin Orthop* 108:214, 1982.
9. Brien EW, et al: Treatment of soft-tissue sarcomas of the hand, *J Bone Joint Surg* 77A:564, 1995.
10. Bruner JM: Treatment of "sesamoid" synovial ganglia of the hand by needle rupture, *J Bone Joint Surg* 45A:1689, 1963.
11. Bryan RS, et al: Primary epithelioid sarcoma of the hand and forearm, *J Bone Joint Surg* 56A:458, 1974.
12. Bush DC, Schneider LH: Tuberculosis of the hand and wrist, *J Hand Surg* 9:931, 1984.
13. Butler ED, et al: Tumors of the hand: a ten-year survey and report of 437 cases, *Am J Surg* 100:293, 1960.
14. Carroll RE: Epidermal (epithelial) cyst of the hand skeleton, *Am J Surg* 85:327, 1953.
15. Carroll RE: Squamous cell carcinoma of the nail bed, *J Hand Surg* 1:92, 1976.
16. Carroll RE, Berman AT: Glomus tumors of the hand: review of the literature and report of 28 cases, *J Bone Joint Surg* 54A:691, 1972.
17. Carroll RE, Bowers WH: Keratoacanthoma: an unusual hand tumor, *Clin Orthop* 118:173, 1976.
18. Chung EB, Enzinger FM: Fibroma of tendon sheath, *J Clin Pathol* 44:1945, 1982.
19. Clark WH, et al: The histogenesis and biologic behavior of primary human malignant melanomas of the skin, *Cancer Res* 29:705, 1969.
20. Clay NR, Clement DA: The treatment of dorsal wrist ganglia by radical excision, *J Hand Surg [Br]* 13:187, 1988.
21. Cohen MH, et al: Surgical prophylaxis of malignant melanoma, *Ann Surg* 213:308, 1991.
22. Colon F, Upton J: Pediatric hand tumors: a review of 349 cases, *Hand Clin* 11:223, 1995.
23. Creighton JJ Jr, et al: Primary malignant tumors of the upper extremity: retrospective analysis of one hundred twenty-six cases, *J Hand Surg* 10:805, 1985.
24. Curtis RM: Congenital arteriovenous fistulae of the hand, *J Bone Joint Surg* 35A:917, 1953.
25. Diao E, Moy O: Common tumors, *Orthop Clin North Am* 23:187, 1992.
26. Dick HM: Malignant fibrous histeocytoma of the hand, *Hand Clin* 3:263, 1987.
27. Dobyns JH, et al: Bowler's thumb: diagnosis and treatment, *J Bone Joint Surg* 54A:751, 1972.
28. Eaton RG, Dobranski AL, Litler JW: Marginal osteophyte excision in treatment of mucous cysts, *J Bone Joint Surg* 55A:570, 1973.
29. Enzinger FM, Weiss SW: *Soft tissue tumors,* St Louis, 1988, Mosby.
30. Enzinger FM: Epithelioid sarcoma: a sarcoma simulating granuloma or a carcinoma, *Cancer* 26:1029, 1970.
31. Evers B, Klammer HL: Tumors and tumorlike lesions of the hand: analysis of 424 surgically treated cases, *Arch AAOS* 1:34, 1997.
32. Finn HA, Dean LP, Simon MA: Principles of biopsy. In Bogumil GP, Fleeger EJ, editors: *Tumors of the hand and upper limb,* London, 1993, Churchill Livingstone.
33. Fisher ER, McCoy MM II, Weschler HL: Analysis of histopathologic and electron microscopic determinants of keratoacanthoma and squamous cell carcinoma, *Cancer* 29:1387, 1972.
34. Fleegler EJ: Tumors involving the skin of the upper extremity, *Hand Clin* 3:197, 1987.
35. Friedlander HL, Rosenberg NJ, Graubard DJ: Intraneural lipoma of the median nerve, *J Bone Joint Surg* 51A:352, 1969.
36. Geiser JH, Eversmann WW Jr: Closed system venography in the evaluation of upper extremity hemangiomas, *J Hand Surg* 3:173, 1978.
37. Goidanich IF, Companacci M: Vascular hamartoma and infantile osteohyperplasia of the extremities, *J Bone Joint Surg* 44A:815, 1962.
38. Gustafson P, Arner M: Soft tissue sarcoma of the upper extremity: descriptive data and outcome in a population-based series of 108 adult patients, *J Hand Surg* 24A:668, 1999.
39. Holdsworth BJ: Nerve tumours in the upper limb: a clinical review, *J Hand Surg* 10B:236, 1985.
40. Hudson DA, et al: Subungual melanoma of the hand, *J Hand Surg [Br]* 15:288, 1990.

41. Jaffe HL, Lichtenstein HL, Elsutro CJ: Pigmented villonodular synovitis, bursitis and tenosynovitis, *Arch Pathol* 31:731, 1941.

42. Jansen GT, Dillaha CJ, Honeycutt WM: Bowenoid conditions of the skin: treatment with topical 5-fluorouracil, *South Med J* 60:185, 1967.

43. Kao GF, Helwig EB, Graham JH: Aggressive digital papillary adenoma and adenocarcinoma: a clinicopathological study of 57 patients, with histochemical, immunopathological, and ultrastructural observations, *J Cutan Pathol* 14:129, 1987.

44. Kerin R: Metastatic tumors of the hand, *J Bone Joint Surg* 40A:263, 1958.

45. Kerrigan JJ, Bertoni JM, Jaeger SH: Ganglion cysts and carpal tunnel syndrome, *J Hand Surg* 13:763, 1988.

46. Kivett WF, et al: Does ganglionectomy destabilize the wrist over the long-term? *Ann Plast Surg* 36:466, 1996.

47. Kojima T, et al: Hemangioma of the median nerve causing carpal tunnel, *Hand* 8:62, 1976.

48. Korman J, Pearl R, Hentz VR: Efficacy of immobilization following aspiration of carpal and digital ganglions, *J Hand Surg* 17:1097, 1992.

49. Kransdorf MJ, Moser RP, Madewell JE: Imaging techniques. In Bogumi GP, Fleeger EJ, editors: *Tumors of the hand and upper limb,* London, 1993, Churchill Livingstone.

50. Leung PC: Tumours of the hand, *Hand* 13:169, 1981.

51. Litt JL: Don't excise-exorcise treatment for subungual and periungual warts, *Cutis* 22:673, 1978.

52. Louis DS: Peripheral nerve tumors in the upper extremity, *Hand Clin* 3:311, 1987.

53. Mankin HJ: Principles of diagnosis and management of tumors of the hand, *Hand Clin* 3:185, 1987.

54. Maurer A, et al: Three phase radionuclide scintigraphy of the hand, *Radiology* 146:761, 1983.

55. McPhee M, et al: Soft tissue sarcoma of the hand, *J Hand Surg* 24A:1001, 1999.

56. Milon SJ, Garbes AD, Bush DC: Fibroma of tendon sheath in the hand, *J Hand Surg* 19A:788, 1994.

57. Mohs FE: Origin and progress of Mohs micrographic surgery. In Mikhail GR, editor: *Mohs micrographic surgery,* Philadelphia, 1991, WB Saunders.

58. Moore JR, Weiland AJ, Curtis RM: Localized nodular tenosynovitis: experience with 115 cases, *J Hand Surg* 9:412, 1984.

59. Moyer RA, Bush DC, Harrington TM: Acute calcific tendonitis of the hand and wrist: a report of 12 cases and a review of the literature, *J Rheum* 16:198, 1989.

60. Nagington J, Rook A, Highet AS: Virus and related infections. In Rook A, et al, editors: *Textbook of dermatology,* London, 1986, Blackwell.

61. Oster LH, Blair WF, Steyers CM: Large lipomas of the deep palmar space, *J Hand Surg* 14:700, 1989.

62. Osterman AL, Raphale J: Arthroscopic resection of dorsal ganglion of the wrist, *Hand Clin* 11:7, 1995.

63. Owens JC, et al: Soft tissue sarcomas of the hand and foot, *Cancer* 55:2010, 1985.

64. Owens N, Stephenson KL: Hemangioma: an evaluation of treatment by injection and surgery, *Plast Reconstr Surg* 3:109, 1948.

65. Palmeri TJ: Subcutaneous hemangiomas of the hand, *J Hand Surg* 8:201, 1983.

66. Peimer CA, et al: Epithelioid sarcoma of the hand and wrist: patterns or extension, *J Hand Surg* 2:275, 1977.

67. Phalen GS: Neurolemomas of the forearm and hand, *Clin Orthop* 114:219, 1976.

68. Posch JL: Soft tissue tumors of the hand. In Jupiter JB, editor: *Flynn's hand surgery,* Baltimore, 1991, Williams & Wilkins.

69. Ransom JL, Pratt CB, Shanks E: Childhood rhabdomyosarcoma of the extremity: results of combined modality therapy, *Cancer* 40:2810, 1977.

70. Rosenburg AF, Schiller AL: Soft tissue sarcomas of the hand, *Hand Clin* 3:247, 1987.

71. Rosson JW: The natural history of ganglia in children, *J Bone Joint Surg* 71B:707, 1989.

72. Santa-Cruz DJ, Uitto J: Basal cell carcinoma of the palm, *Cutis* 22:223, 1978.

73. Schiavon M, et al: Squamous cell carcinoma of the hand: fifty-five case reports, *J Hand Surg* 13:401, 1988.

74. Smith RJ: Tumors of the hand. Who is best qualified to treat tumors of the hand, *J Hand Surg* 2:251, 1977.

75. Stout AP, Lattes R: Tumors of the soft tissues. In *Armed Forces Institute of Pathology atlas of tumor pathology,* Washington, DC, 1967.

76. Strickland JW, Steichen JB: Nerve tumors of the hand and forearm, *J Hand Surg* 2:285, 1977.

77. Strong ML: Bowen's disease in multiple nail beds: case report, *J Hand Surg* 8:329, 1983.

78. Uribu IJF, Levey VD: Intraosseous ganglia of the scaphoid and lunate bones: report of 15 cases in 13 patients, *J Hand Surg* 24A:508, 1999.

79. Uriburu IJ, Levy VD: Intraosseous growth of giant cell tumors of tendon sheath of the digits, *J Hand Surg* 23:732, 1998.

80. Vasconez L, Morris WJ, Owsley JQ Jr: Skin tumors. In Dunphy JE, Way LW, editors: *Current surgical diagnosis,* Los Altos, 1979, Lange Medical.

81. Ward WA, Labosky DA: Ruptured epidermal inclusion cyst of the palm presenting as a collar-button abscess, *J Hand Surg* 10:899, 1985.

82. Watson HK, Rogers WD, Ashmead D IV: Reevaluation of the cause of the wrist ganglion, *J Hand Surg* 14:812, 1989.

83. Weiner M, et al: Adjuvant chemotherapy of malignant fibrous histiocytoma of bone, *Cancer* 51:25, 1981.

84. Whitworth PW, et al: Extremity epithelioid sarcoma: amputation vs local resection, *Arch Surg* 126:1485, 1991.

85. Wolfe SW, et al: Computed tomographic evaluation of fatty neoplasms of the extremities, *Orthopedics* 12:1351, 1989.

86. Wright PH, et al: Synovial sarcoma, *J Bone Joint Surg* 64A:112, 1982.

87. Wu KK, Guise ER: Metastatic tumors of the hand: a report of six cases, *J Hand Surg* 3:271, 1978.

88. Yaremchuk MJ, et al: Sweat gland carcinoma of the hand: two cases of malignant eccrine spiradenoma, *J Hand Surg* 9:910, 1984.

89. Zubowicz VN, Ishii CH: Management of ganglion cysts by simple aspiration, *J Hand Surg* 12:618, 1987.

Chapter 57

DUPUYTREN'S DISEASE

Robert M. McFarlane
Joy C. MacDermid

Dupuytren's disease (DD) is thought to be a genetic disease because it is most common among people of northern European descent and often runs in families.[24] However, it is not uncommon in Orientals[9] and has been reported in Africans[29] and East Indians.[41] Either there is a mixture of the races or other factors are causative. The clues to the cause of DD rests with the cells involved and the collagen produced by those cells. Fortunately, this disease has attracted the attention of many investigators, and it is likely that the cellular mechanism that produces this disease will be better understood in the near future.

Despite our lack of fundamental knowledge, our treatment of DD continues to produce better results. This improvement is attributable to an appreciation of the natural course of the disease, a more realistic expectation of treatment, improved training of surgeons and therapists, and refinement of instruments and technique.

TYPES OF DISEASE PRESENTATION

The typical patient is a male of northern European descent and about 50 years of age. He first noticed thickening in one or other palm about 5 years earlier and presents now with disease in both hands, but more severe in one. The metacarpophalangeal (MP) joint of the ring or small finger is flexed, and the proximal interphalangeal (PIP) joint may also be flexed. This patient will be otherwise healthy and not likely to recall any relatives with DD.

The female patient often has less severe disease. It appears later (about age 60) and progresses more slowly; therefore many women with DD are not seen by a surgeon. However, when contracture occurs, the problems are similar and both sexes should be treated similarly. It has been suggested that the results of treatment in women are less satisfactory, but this is not true. Women have a higher

prevalence of reflex sympathetic dystrophy (RSD), but otherwise they do as well as men.

Patients with severe disease should be informed that their disease will be difficult if not impossible to control. These patients usually have a family history of one or more close relatives affected. Their disease begins in the third or fourth decade, and they have ectopic deposits in knuckle pads, plantar fibromatosis, and occasionally penile fibromatosis. The disease is usually bilateral and affects more than two rays of the hand, and these patients are likely to have disease on the radial side of the hand, affecting the thumb, thumb web, and index finger. Hueston[18] was the first to identify these patients with an increased diathesis to the disease.

Many diseases have been associated with DD in the past, such as gout, pulmonary tuberculosis, and cardiovascular disease, but there is no statistical evidence to support such an association. However, epilepsy, alcoholism, and diabetes mellitus seem to have more than a coincidental relationship with DD. Patients with both idiopathic and acquired epilepsy have a higher incidence of DD, suggesting that barbiturate medication is the causal factor.[2,7] Similarly, recent studies suggest that the association with alcoholism is related to the volume of alcohol ingested rather than liver disease.[3] Thus the DD in these patients is at least partly drug induced. On the other hand, the relationship with diabetes does not appear to be related to medication or the type or severity of diabetes, but rather to the duration of the disease, not unlike other complications of diabetes.[33] DD is extremely common in diabetic persons but usually does not progress to joint contracture and thus is not often seen by a surgeon.

Both manual work and a single injury to the hand have been implicated causally with DD. Epidemiologic studies have failed to establish a significant relationship with manual work, although attempts have been made to associate DD with the use of vibrating tools and heavy manual work. Occasionally, an individual will develop DD at the site of an injury shortly after that injury (within 1 or 2 years). A sufficient number of such cases have been reported, so a causal relationship seems likely when the injury and the onset of the disease are closely related anatomically and in time.[23]

The nature of DD in Orientals, East Indians, black Africans, and North American Indians is similar to that of whites in its clinical course, appearance, and histologic features. However, the disease is less aggressive, similar to that seen in women and diabetic persons. Further research should determine whether there are cytologic features that differentiate the various types of DD.

PATHOLOGY

The pathognomonic clinical feature of DD is a firm nodule just deep to the skin of the palm on either side of the distal palmar crease. Nodules also occur elsewhere, such as the base of the thumb, in the thumb web, in the proximal segment of the finger, or on the ulnar side of the palm near the base of the small finger (Fig. 57-1).

Histologically, the pathognomonic nodule is a nonencapsulated but well-demarcated area about the size of a low-power microscopic field (Fig. 57-2). The nodule consists of active fibroblasts demonstrating occasional mitosis and producing abundant collagen. In the later and more quiescent stage of the disease, the cellularity is decreased and the tissue appears more tendonlike, with abundant collagen and a few flattened fibrocytes.

INDICATIONS FOR TREATMENT

Because DD is a benign process, the indications for treatment are relative. A patient should never be persuaded that treatment is mandatory.

The painful nodule

It is common for a person to complain of pain in a nodule that has been noticed recently. However, most patients accommodate to the nodule and do not need more than reassurance about its nature. Occasionally, a nodule is unusually painful. In this case, patients are sometimes helped by an injection of steroid into the area (Ketchum LD: *Personal communication,* McFarlane RM 1994). An injection is preferable to excising the nodule because more Dupuytren's tissue is likely to form around the area of excision.

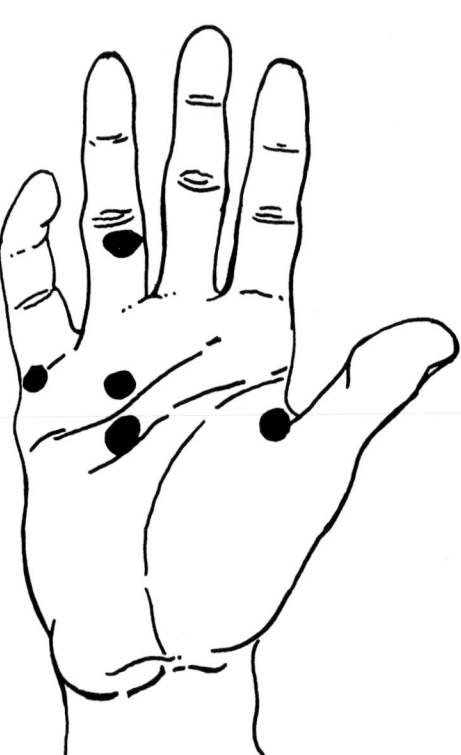

Fig. 57-1. The common location of nodules.

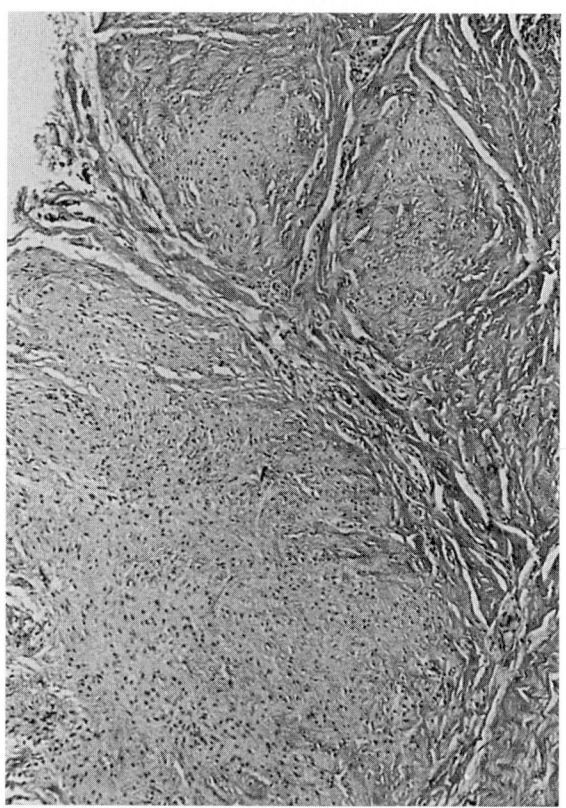

Fig. 57-2. Lower-power microscopic view of fibromatosis of Dupuytren's disease. Note the nodular configuration of the proliferating fibroblasts. There is also abundant new collagen, and special stains reveal many new capillaries (hematoxylin and eosin, 10×).

Skin involvement

The pretendinous bands of the palmar aponeurosis normally insert into the skin just distal to the distal crease of the palm, and vertical fibers of fascia attach to the skin throughout the palm. In some patients, these fibers are diffusely involved and distort the skin of the distal palm into folds and pits without joint contracture. This induration can be uncomfortable and occasionally is an indication for excision of the diseased fascia in the absence of joint contracture.

Joint flexion contracture

Joint contracture is the most common reason for surgery. The MP joint is most commonly contracted and most readily corrected because the only fascial structure that causes MP joint contracture is the pretendinous band of the palmar aponeurosis. About 30 degrees of contracture becomes a nuisance to the patient. It is embarrassing to shake hands and difficult to put one's hand into a pocket or a purse. There is no urgency for operation because MP joint contracture can be corrected regardless of the duration of contracture.

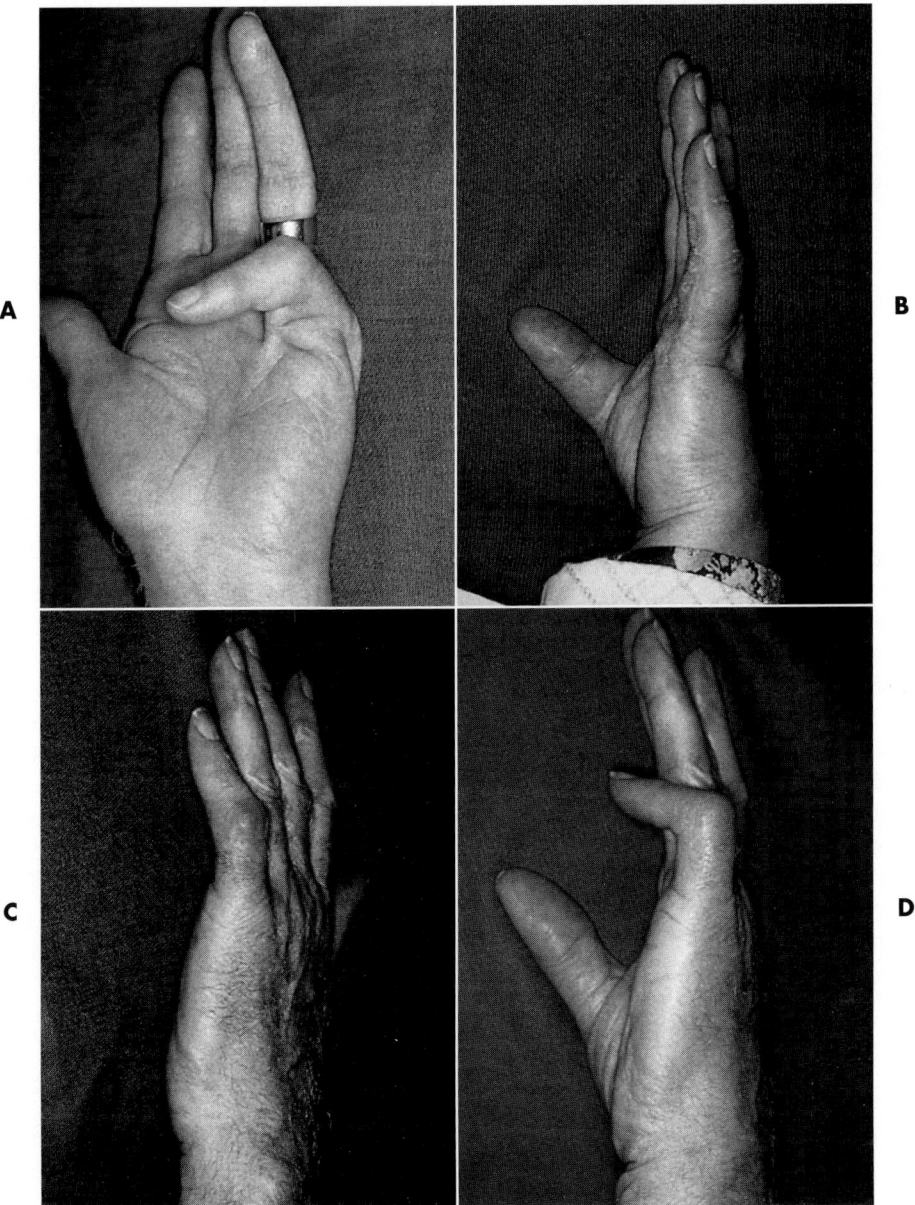

Fig. 57-3. An example of postoperative scar contracture affecting the proximal interphalangeal (PIP) joint but not the metacarpophalangeal (MP) joint. **A,** Severe, preoperative contracture at both joints. **B, C,** and **D,** The gradual increase of the PIP joint contractures from 6 weeks to 3 months and 2 years in spite of prolonged splinting. There is no sign of recurrent Dupuytren's disease.

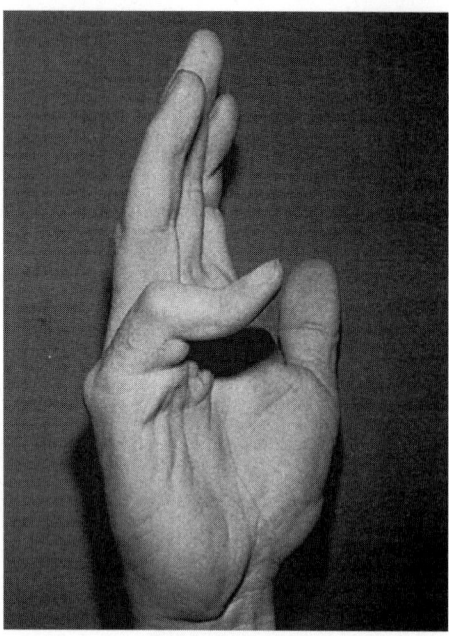

Fig. 57-4. Distal joint hyperextension occurs only with severe proximal interphalangeal joint flexion. Occasionally, it is overcome by correcting the proximal joint contracture.

Proximal interphalangeal joint flexion contracture

A PIP joint flexion contracture is more difficult to correct because more than one fascial band causes this contracture. It can be contracted alone or in combination by the central spiral, lateral, and retrovascular cords. The longer the joint is contracted, the more difficult it is to fully correct; nevertheless, one is advised to wait until the patient has about 30 degrees of flexion contracture present before advising operation. Lesser degrees of contracture are unlikely to be corrected simply because the operation itself produces sufficient scar tissue to cause some postoperative contracture. A patient should be warned that a PIP joint contracture can be improved but probably not completely corrected (Fig. 57-3).

Distal interphalangeal (DIP) joint flexion contracture is not common but is difficult to correct because the strands of fascia contracting the joint pass between the terminal branches of the vessels and nerves. Distal joint hyperextension is also difficult to correct. It is not caused by fascial contracture but rather is postural, similar to other boutonnière deformities (Fig. 57-4).

Web space contracture is common and troublesome because it prevents separation of the fingers and encourages the development of an intertrigo infection. It is caused by disease in the natatory ligament. Thumb web contracture is common and occasionally so severe that the thumb can neither abduct nor extend. This contracture is caused by a combination of cords from the pretendinous band to the thumb, the termination of the transverse fibers of the palmar aponeurosis, and the termination of the natatory ligament (Fig. 57-5).

VARIATIONS IN SURGICAL TREATMENT

The treatment of DD is empirical because the cause is unknown. As a result, many methods of treatment are advocated, depending on the surgeon's concept of the disease.[31] Is it a reaction to biomechanical stresses? If so, the appropriate treatment is to alter those stresses by incising or partially removing the contracting tissue. Is it like a neoplasm, as the term *fibromatosis* suggests? If so, the lesion should be excised to prevent recurrence and extension of the disease. There are no definite answers to these questions, so there is no one way to treat DD.

The surgeon is advised to have several treatment options in mind. If the type of incision, how the fascia is managed, and how the wound is closed are considered individually, the surgeon has great latitude in designing an operation for a given patient.

The incision can be longitudinal or transverse in the palm or in the digit. Most incisions are longitudinal, and a zigzag incision is most popular. If the disease is extensive in the palm, a single transverse incision in or near the distal crease provides exposure to remove much of the palmar aponeurosis. The diseased fascia can be incised or excised, and the surrounding, apparently normal, fascia can be left or removed. The wound can be sutured, left open to close by second intention, or skin grafted.

TYPES OF OPERATION

There are four basic types of operation, to which many variations have been added.

Fasciotomy

Fasciotomy is an appealing procedure because it is a minor operation performed under local anesthesia with an immediate result.[6] The patient not only regains extension but also does not lose flexion, even temporarily, as happens with more extensive procedures. Classically, a fasciotomy is done subcutaneously by inserting a small blade through a stab wound and cutting the contracted fascia blindly. This procedure was designed in an era when sepsis was a major problem. That is not so today. A fasciotomy can be performed more thoroughly by making an incision over the diseased cord and dividing every strand of diseased fascia under direct vision. Fasciotomy is effective in correcting MP joint contracture, but it is less satisfactory in correcting PIP joint contracture. It is a good procedure in older patients in whom the disease is quiescent and recurrence is unlikely.

Regional fasciectomy

Regional fasciectomy is an operation in which only the diseased fascia is removed, on the assumption that the fascia that is left undisturbed will not become diseased. This is the operation commonly performed in the palm, where the

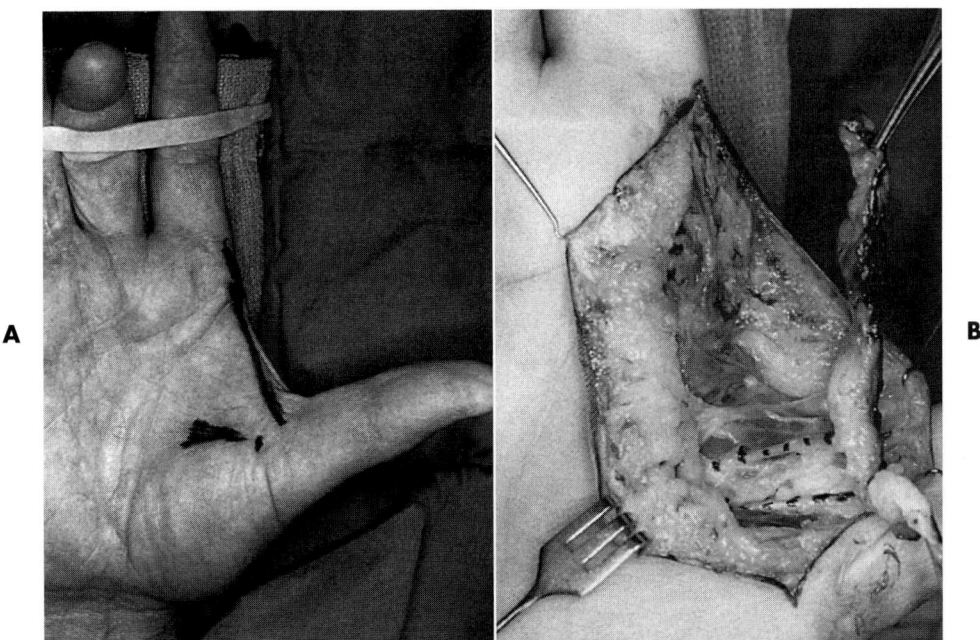

Fig. 57-5. A, Disease in the thumb web arising from the termination of the transverse fibers of the palmar aponeurosis and the natatory ligament. **B,** The digital nerves are not displaced by the displaced cords but lie immediately deep to them. The *dotted lines* indicate the course of the two digital nerves to the thumb and the radial digital nerve to the index finger.

disease is usually confined to the ring and small finger rays. These are excised, but the pretendinous bands to the uninvolved thumb, index, and long fingers are not. Regional fasciectomy is less satisfactory in the finger than in the palm because recurrent contracture is more likely if certain fascial structures remain.

Extensive fasciectomy

Extensive fasciectomy implies a more radical operation in which the potentially diseased as well as the obviously diseased fasciae are removed. This concept applies particularly to the finger, where several fascial structures can cause PIP joint contracture, and if all of them are not removed, recurrent contracture is more likely. Because of the surgical insult to the hand and the inevitable scarring that results from an extensive dissection, the morbidity is prolonged and the chance of complications is greater.

Dermofasciectomy

Dermofasciectomy is a procedure that was introduced by Hueston[17] to reduce recurrent contracture, in which not only the offending fascia is excised but also the overlying skin. The skin defect is covered by a full-thickness skin graft. Hueston noted that the disease does not recur beneath a skin graft and considered this an empirical observation. We believe there is an anatomic reason for this. In certain locations in the hand, the fascia is intimately attached to the dermis. This is especially so over the proximal phalanx of the finger, that is, between the distal crease of the palm and

middle crease of the finger, as illustrated in Fig. 57-6, *B*. The fascia in this location cannot be removed completely from the skin, even by sharp dissection under magnification. This residual fascia is the origin of recurrence and can be removed only by excising the skin.

MY PREFERRED METHODS OF TREATMENT[27]
Fasciotomy

Under local anesthesia, a longitudinal incision about 2 cm in length is made over the prominent cord and converted into a Z-plasty. Reflecting the triangular flaps of the Z-plasty provides good exposure of the cord. This is especially important when attempting to correct a PIP joint contracture because the Z-plasty allows both neurovascular bundles to be exposed before the fascia is incised. The patient is asked to straighten the finger. At the MP joint, full extension should be possible, but at the PIP joint, improvement and incomplete correction of the flexion contracture is the usual outcome. Transposition of the Z-flaps overcomes some longitudinal skin tension.

Contracture of a single ray

The most common operation performed for DD is that for contracture of a single ray. A longitudinal incision is made over the prominent cord from the proximal palm, along the midline of the finger to the distal crease (Fig. 57-6, *A*). With the aid of loupe magnification, the incision is deepened to the level of the fascia, and then the skin is undermined laterally by scalpel dissection. In the proximal palm, the separation of

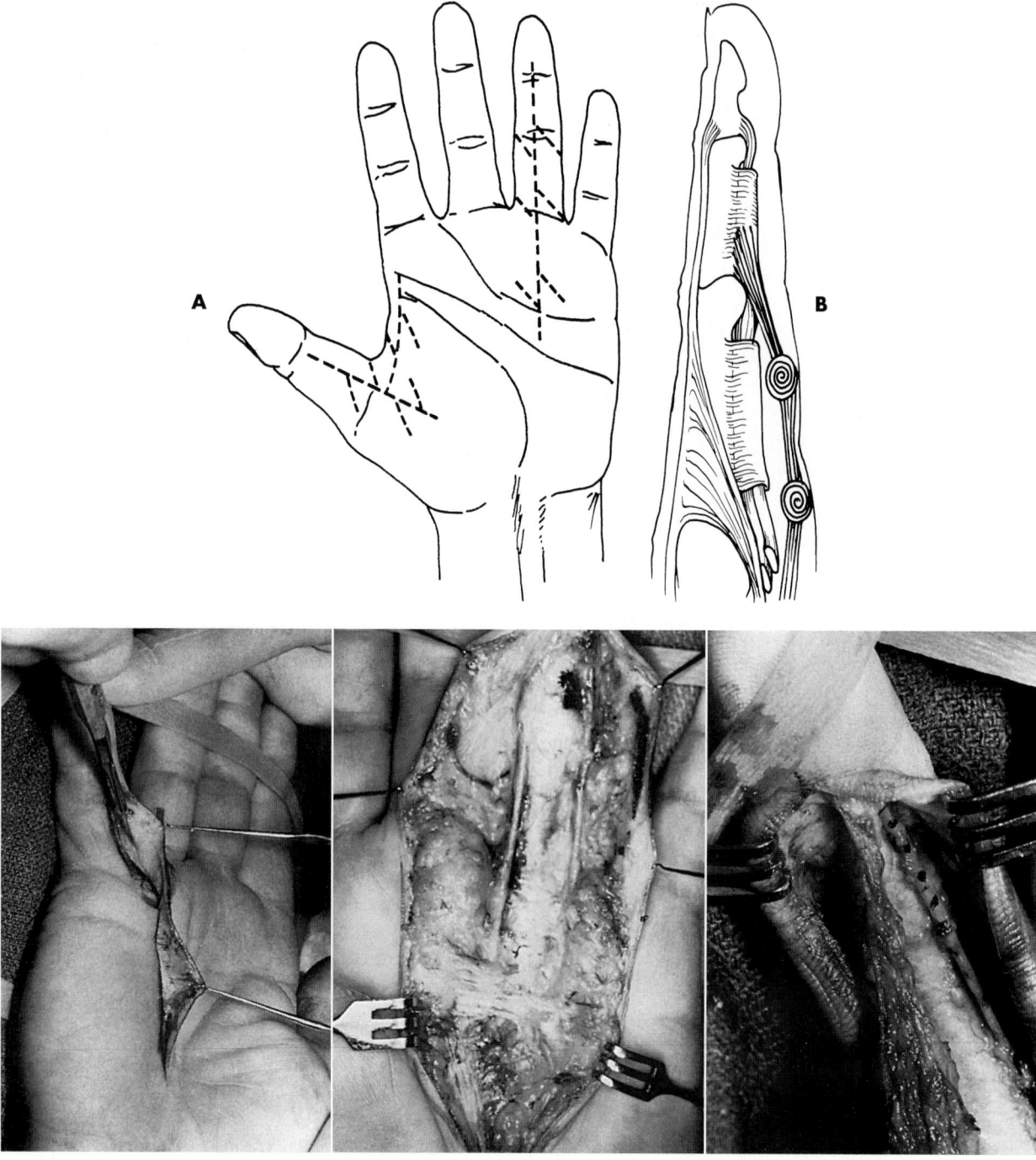

Fig. 57-6. Operation on a single ray. **A,** A longitudinal midline incision extends from the proximal palm to the distal crease of the finger. **B** and **C,** The varying relation of the dermis to the fascia. In the proximal palm and over the middle segment of the finger, this layer does not exist. **D,** The generous exposure provided by a midline incision. The disease fascia has been removed and both neurovascular bundles exposed. **E,** The need for exposure to the distal crease of the finger. The digital nerve is marked by the dots, and the diseased fascia is seen extending beyond the distal crease.

Continued

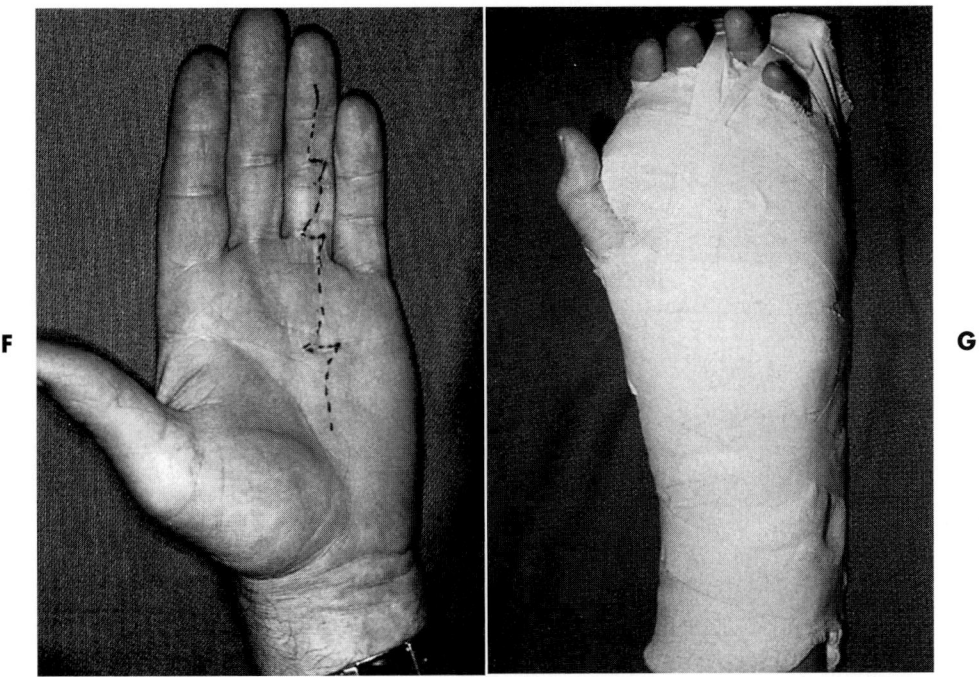

Fig. 57-6, cont'd. F, The appearance of the hand 1 year after operation showing the size and location of the Z-plasties. **G,** The postoperative dressing holds the fingers in a comfortable position of extension. A few degrees of wrist flexion permit more finger extension.

diseased fascia from overlying tissue is easy and leaves a thick, vascular layer of subcutaneous tissue on the skin. As one approaches the distal palm, the subcutaneous layer disappears and the diseased tissue must be separated from the dermis (Fig. 57-6, *B* and *C*). This plane can be found only by sharp dissection aided by magnification. At the web space, the fingers should be abducted to place the natatory ligament on tension so that this tissue can be identified for later removal. Stretching of the fingers also places the neurovascular bundles on tension in the web space, making them less likely to be damaged during dissection in this area. Over the proximal segment of the finger, the skin and fascia are intimately adherent and difficult to dissect. However, over the middle segment of the finger, the fascia is more related to the flexor tendon sheath and, as in the proximal palm, the skin can be reflected with a layer of vascular subcutaneous tissue. The dissection extends to the distal crease of the finger, or even beyond, to create a good exposure of the fascia that attaches to the flexor tendon sheath beyond the PIP joint. In the finger, the skin flaps are reflected to about the midlateral line. At this point, both neurovascular bundles are exposed. It is easiest to find the bundle at the distal crease of the finger and follow it proximally. One should try to keep the digital nerve and artery together. Volar branches of both nerve and artery must be cut to free the neurovascular bundle from the diseased fascia.

The small vessels are best coagulated during the dissection using a bipolar coagulator about 2 mm away from the main vessel. With both neurovascular bundles in view, the surgeon can remove the fascia between and on each side of the bundles without fear of damaging either the vessel or nerve (Fig. 57-6, *D*). In the palm, a regional fasciectomy is performed, although this exposure permits one to remove the pretendinous band on either side of the diseased cord as well. In the finger, not only is the diseased fascia removed, but also the potentially diseased fascia is removed; therefore this part of the operation is an extensive fasciectomy (Fig. 57-6, *E*).

Within the finger, the neurovascular bundle is often displaced toward the midline of the finger. The mechanisms of displacement are shown in Fig. 57-7. If one understands how these displacements occur, inadvertent division of vessel or nerve is less likely. In addition, it is reassuring to know that there is always a plane of dissection between the diseased fascia and the neurovascular bundle, although often this plane is difficult to develop.

The tourniquet is released and bleeding is controlled with bipolar cautery. The bleeding will be minimal if the many small vessels were coagulated during the dissection. The longitudinal wound must be broken by Z-plasties to avoid postoperative scar contracture. They are placed at the middle and proximal creases of the finger and the distal crease of the palm (Fig. 57-6, *F*). They are not planned until the tourniquet has been released so that they can be moved a bit proximally or distally to take advantage of well-vascularized skin. The Z-flaps need not be more than 1 cm in length, and thus even thin flaps will survive. They are only long enough to break up longitudinal tension in the scar and do not overcome skin

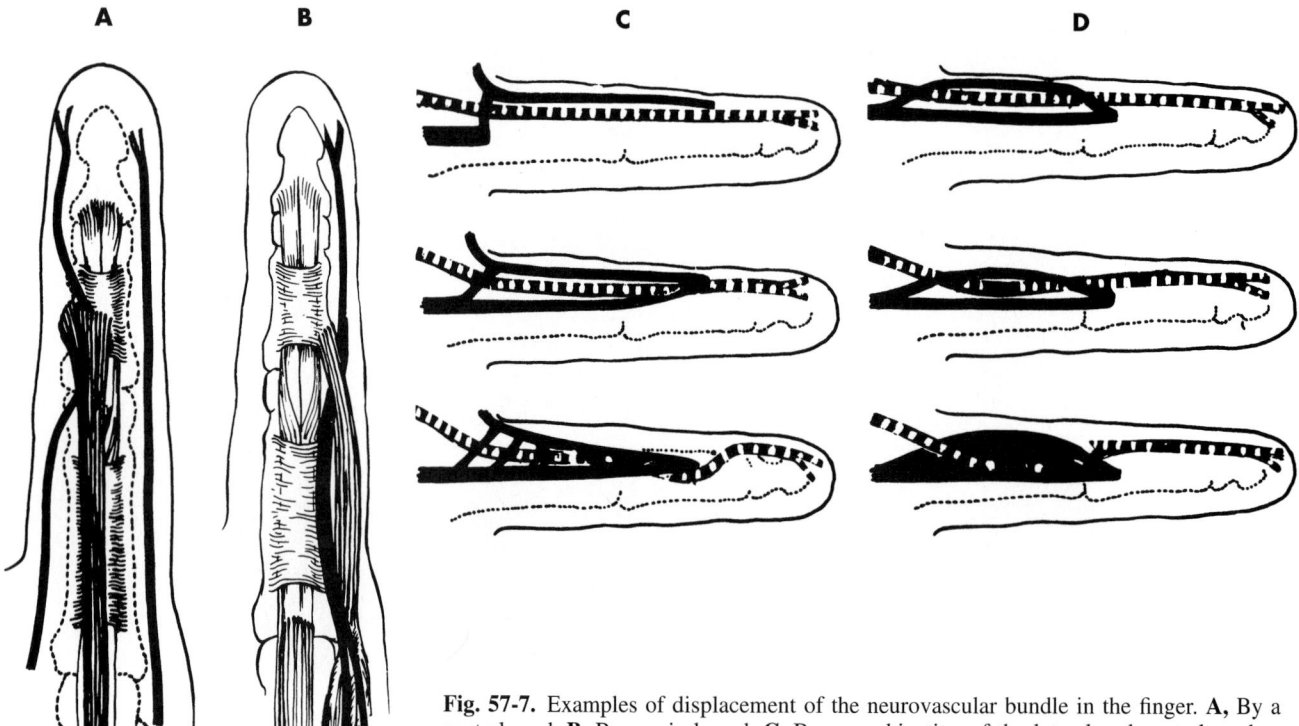

Fig. 57-7. Examples of displacement of the neurovascular bundle in the finger. **A,** By a central cord. **B,** By a spiral cord. **C,** By a combination of the lateral and central cord. **D,** By a combination of a central and spiral cord.

deficiency in the longitudinal axis of the digit to any extent. Full-thickness skin grafts are preferable to closing the wounds under tension.

At the completion of the operation, the MP joint should be straight and the PIP joint contracture improved, if not completely corrected. A dressing and splint are applied with the finger extended but not forced into extension (Fig. 57-6, *G*).

Contracture of two or more rays

If two or more rays are involved, a transverse incision is made in the palm, through which a regional fasciectomy is performed, although an extensive fasciectomy can be done through this one incision in the occasional patient who has widespread disease. The disease in the fingers is exposed through longitudinal incisions and removed as described earlier (Fig. 57-8, *A* and *B*). It is often difficult to remove the diseased fascia in the distal palm through an intact skin bridge. Adequate exposure is possible if the longitudinal incision is extended proximally to join the transverse incision in the palm.

The finger wounds are closed with appropriate Z-plasties, but the palmar wound is left open as described by McCash[26] (Fig. 57-8, *C* and *D*). The open palm method has great value in preventing a hematoma and thus avoiding swelling of the hand with residual stiffness of the fingers. However, our recent studies have revealed that the correction of PIP joint contracture is less satisfactory with the open-palm method

unless skin grafts are used in the fingers (Fig. 57-8, *E*). Therefore, if the open-palm method is to be used when severe PIP joint contracture has been corrected, it is best to apply skin grafts to the digits rather than close the wounds by suture (Fig. 57-9).

Dermofasciectomy

The indications for dermofasciectomy have increased since Hueston's original description. It remains the appropriate operation for recurrent contracture, but it is also advocated for primary contracture in patients who have an increased diathesis (Fig. 57-10) and in some patients when the palm is left open as described previously (see Fig. 57-9). A relative indication for dermofasciectomy is severe PIP joint contracture, especially at the small finger (Fig. 57-11). Recurrent and persistent contracture at this joint is consistently worse than in other digits.

Some technical points unique to dermofasciectomy deserve emphasis: (1) An extensive fasciectomy is performed in the usual way; (2) a triangular or rectangular skin defect is created, depending on the location of the defect and severity of contracture; (3) both neurovascular bundles should be in view while excising the skin; (4) a full-thickness graft, cut to pattern, is advised to lessen postoperative scar contracture; and (5) therapy can proceed in the usual way because the graft will be firmly attached within 10 days (Fig. 57-11, *C*).

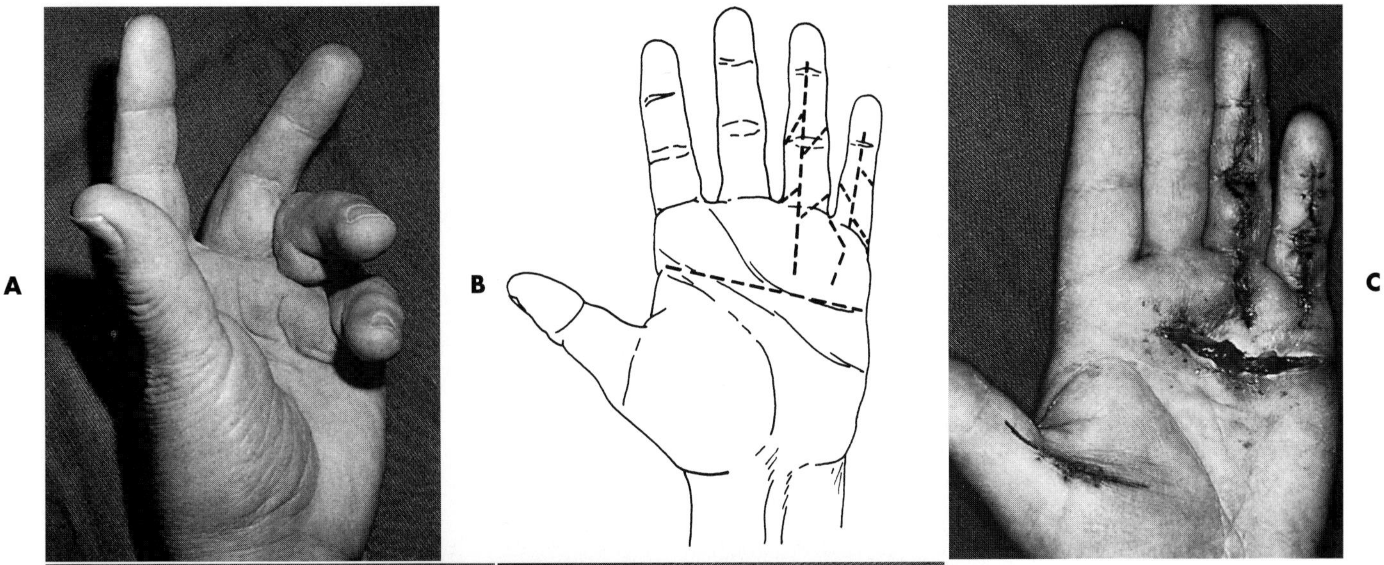

A

B

C

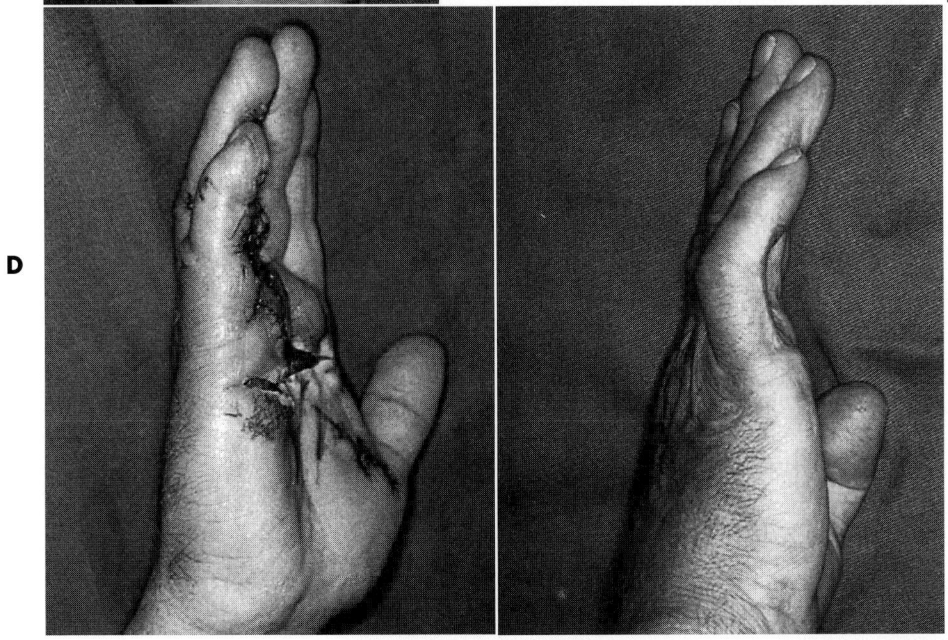

D

E

Fig. 57-8. **A** and **B,** Contracture of two rays exposed by a transverse incision in the palm and longitudinal incisions in the fingers. **C** and **D,** The early postoperative appearance of the hand showing the palmar wound left open. **E,** Two years later, there is recurrent proximal interphalangeal joint contracture caused by scar contracture. This patient should have had skin grafts applied to ring and small fingers. (From Green DP, editor: *Operative hand surgery,* ed 3, New York, 1993, Churchill Livingstone.)

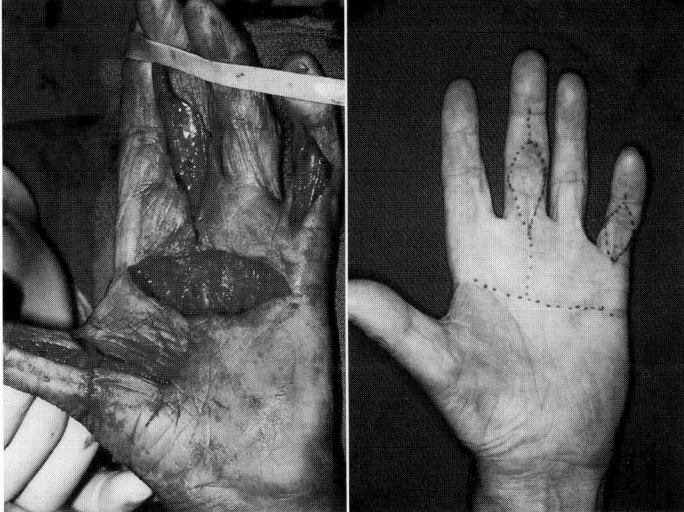

Fig. 57-9. With correction of severe proximal interphalangeal contracture using an open-palm technique, skin grafts are applied to the digits.

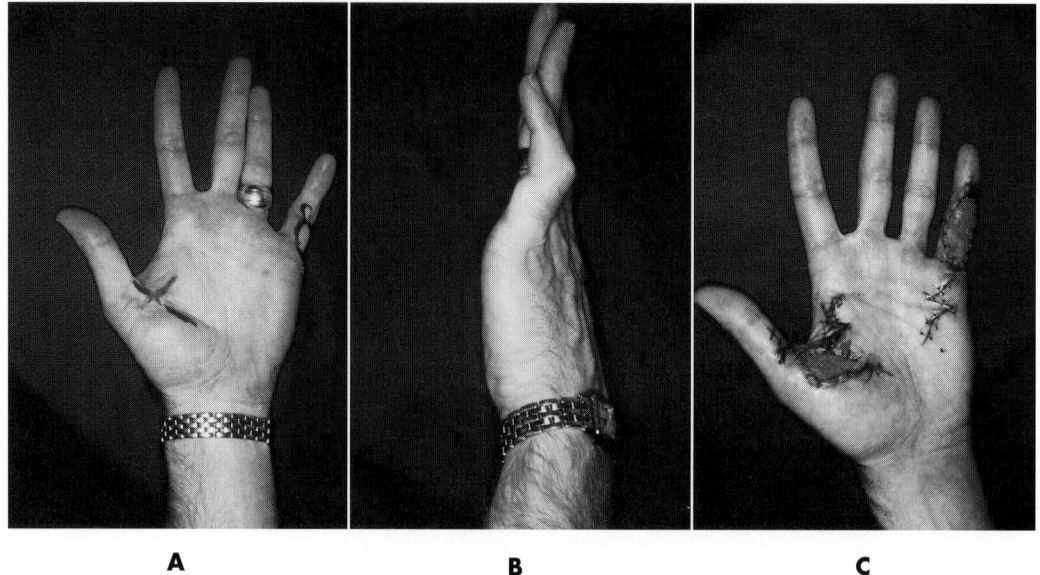

Fig. 57-10. A patient with increased diathesis evidenced by radial disease (**A**) and marked proximal interphalangeal flexion contracture of the small finger (**B**) is a candidate for dermofasciectomy (**C**).

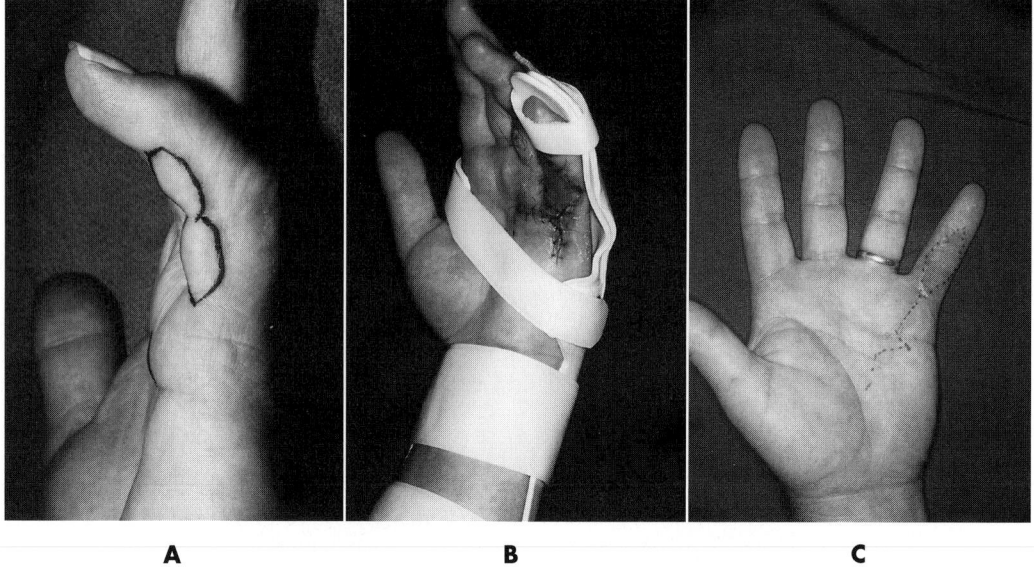

Fig. 57-11. Severe preoperative flexion contracture (**A**) treated with dermofasciectomy (**B**) with a good result (**C**).

COMPLICATIONS

Complications are most likely to occur with severe disease and an extensive operation. Thus there is a tendency to perform less extensive operations. However, operations of less magnitude are more likely to permit recurrence and extension of disease. Thus the surgeon faces the dilemma of doing too little or too much. Complications will occur in some 20% of operations, but most are minor and simply prolong the period of morbidity for 2 or 3 weeks.[28] The most

severe complications are gangrene of a digit and RSD, which cause permanent disability.

Infection, hematoma, and skin loss are a triad and usually appear together. Infection per se is not common but often follows skin loss or hematoma. Skin loss of triangular flaps or Z-plasties can usually be avoided by careful planning. If the loss is large, the wound should be debrided and the skin grafted. Small areas of loss of the tips of triangular flaps usually heal with no contracture. Hematoma is a feature of the closure of transverse incisions over the concavity of the palm. They are difficult to avoid, even with careful hemostasis. A palmar hematoma is best prevented by either leaving the wound open or applying a full-thickness skin graft.

Digital nerve and artery injury are not only annoying to the patient but likely contribute to postoperative joint stiffness and cold intolerance. The common sites of injury are in the web space and at the PIP joint, where the dissection is most difficult. Both structures should be repaired if divided, although arterial repair may be difficult when a severely contracted digit is straightened. Damage to both arteries may result in gangrene of the finger, so one or both vessels should be repaired. When treating recurrent disease, it is difficult to dissect the neurovascular bundles from the combination of scar and Dupuytren's tissue. It is prudent to leave a cuff of scar tissue around the neurovascular bundle. If a patient with recurrent disease has anesthesia on either side of the fingertip, the surgeon must assume that the digital artery, as well as the nerve, has been divided and take great care to protect the other vessel.

RSD is a serious complication of operations for DD because the patient is likely to be left with permanent limitation of movement of the digits. This complication occurs after about 5% of operations and is twice as common in women than in men.[28] It is more likely to occur after an extensive operation, so preventive measures are advised under these circumstances. Operation under regional block anesthesia using a long-acting anesthetic agent will provide a sympathetic effect for about 24 hours postoperatively, and close supervision is helpful to ensure that the hand is elevated and the patient receives adequate sedation.

HAND THERAPY MANAGEMENT

Preoperative hand therapy management of Dupuytren's contracture, such as application of ultrasound,[42] other modalities, or splinting of the diseased tissue, is not supported by scientific evidence or expert opinion.[1] Only rarely will a surgeon and therapist be presented with a patient with contracted fingers related to inadequate prior surgery or therapy. For this select group of patients, therapy may be beneficial to maximize range of motion (ROM) before any further surgery. Therefore the role of hand therapy in management of Dupuytren's contracture is largely in postoperative management.

Postoperative management of the patient with DD is designed to maintain the gains in extension obtained by the surgical procedure, minimize the effects of postoperative edema and scarring, and restore preoperative flexion and strength to the hand. The therapist's intervention with the patient includes splinting, ROM exercises and passive mobilizations, scar and edema management, wound care, education, and strengthening.

Although data from case series support the role of hand therapy in achieving optimal results after surgery, there is little evidence to differentiate which specific hand therapy techniques are most effective. For example, static volar, ulnar gutter,[38] and dorsal splints[32,34] and continuous passive motion[36] have been reported as methods of management. Both hand-based[32,34] and forearm-based[27,38] splints have been recommended. A randomized trial is the only means to prove which method, if any, is superior. Because this level of evidence does not exist with respect to hand therapy management of patients after surgery for DD, therapy programs are based on physiotherapeutic principles and positive results in case series.

Assessment

Patients with Dupuytren's release require a customized hand therapy program based on an assessment of their physical status and knowledge of the surgical procedure performed, as well as patients' diathesis, particular medical history, capability, and compliance.

Documentation of the patient's baseline physical status should include measurement of ROM, pain, and edema; vascular status; sensory thresholds; and properties of wounds and grafts. ROM of the digits and wrist are best performed by a dorsal/volar method unless swelling or bolus dressing limit the ability to do so. In such cases, a lateral placement can be used. Consistency of goniometer placement and tester on subsequent evaluations should be ensured to minimize measurement error. Pain can easily be documented on a numeric rating scale of 0 to 10. Edema can be measured using circumferential measures (at the levels of the joint creases or the distal palmar crease) or by volumetric measures. Volumetric measures are preferable but may need to be postponed until grafts are settled. Vascular status of the digits at rest and with extension positioning should be noted. The integrity of the vascular supply to the digits can be determined by performing a digital Allen's test.[43] Further information on the integrity of the neurovascular bundles can be provided by documenting sensation. Sensory thresholds measured using either Semmes-Weinstein monofilaments or the NK PSSD or two-point discrimination can be used. The color and appearance of wounds and grafts should be documented. Grip and pinch strength can be recorded when the patient is capable of doing so. A questionnaire such as the Disabilities of the Arm, Shoulder and Hand (DASH)[45] or the Michigan Hand Outcomes Questionnaire[5] can be used to measure disability.

Woodruff and Waldren[51] described a clinical grading system for DD of the hand. The grades were as follows: (1) finger contracture only, hyperextends at MP joint, hand lies flat on the table; (2) single finger pretendinous cord, MP contracture only; (3) single finger pretendinous band, MP and PIP joint contracture; (4) same as 3 but two-finger contracture; and (5) finger stuck in palm, suitable only for amputation. They further added a number of "prefixes" to document additional prognostic factors (*A*, alcohol abuse; *D*, diabetic; *Y*, young with strong diathesis; *S*, sweaty palm; *R*, recurrent disease; and *N*, normal). Documentation of these levels of clinical severity should be incorporated into treatment planning. For example, patients with more active disease (and likely more extensive surgery) with a sweaty hand are at higher risk for RSD than other patients.

Treatment

Splinting. Postoperative splinting is a major component of the hand therapy program for most patients with DD. The splint maintains the gains in extension achieved during surgery against the opposing force of wound contracture during the healing process. The wearing schedule and length of time the splint is required are dictated by the extent of the surgical procedure and the propensity of the patient to lose range of movement.

Various approaches have been described for postoperative extension splinting.* Volar splints are advocated by some to aid with scar management by placing pressure on the wound, whereas others advocate a dorsal splint to minimize tension on the healing wound.[32] Some regimens describe mild flexion of the MPP joints[10,32] to decrease tension on the neurovascular bundles and healing wound. Our approach is to apply the "maximum safe" extension, that is, the maximum extension of the digit that can be applied without compromising neurovascular bundles or inciting excessive inflammatory response. Regardless of the approach taken, therapists must remember that these patients tend to be elderly and may have shortened neurovascular bundles. Therefore observance to signs of adverse pressure on delicate tissue and excess tension on the neurovascular structures in the hand is indicated. Most of our patients are fitted with a dorsal forearm-based static extension splint on the second or third postoperative day (Figs. 57-12 and 57-13). The hand is positioned in the splint with the wrist slightly flexed. This minimizes tension on the flexor tendons and palmar skin, which have not been extended to full length because of the joint contracture. The affected fingers, and thumb if necessary, are splinted in maximum safe extension. The splint is often fabricated to accommodate full extension even if full PIP extension has not been obtained. This allows patients to progress their positioning between therapy visits.

The therapist must ensure that the splint has a proper fit and the strength required to fulfill its purpose. The splint should be two thirds the length of the forearm to provide stability for the finger extension component of the splint. Regular splint rechecks are required to ensure that the splint continues to provide the proper positioning as the patient progresses. For example, changes in swelling or the gradual

*References 20, 27, 32, 34, 36, 38.

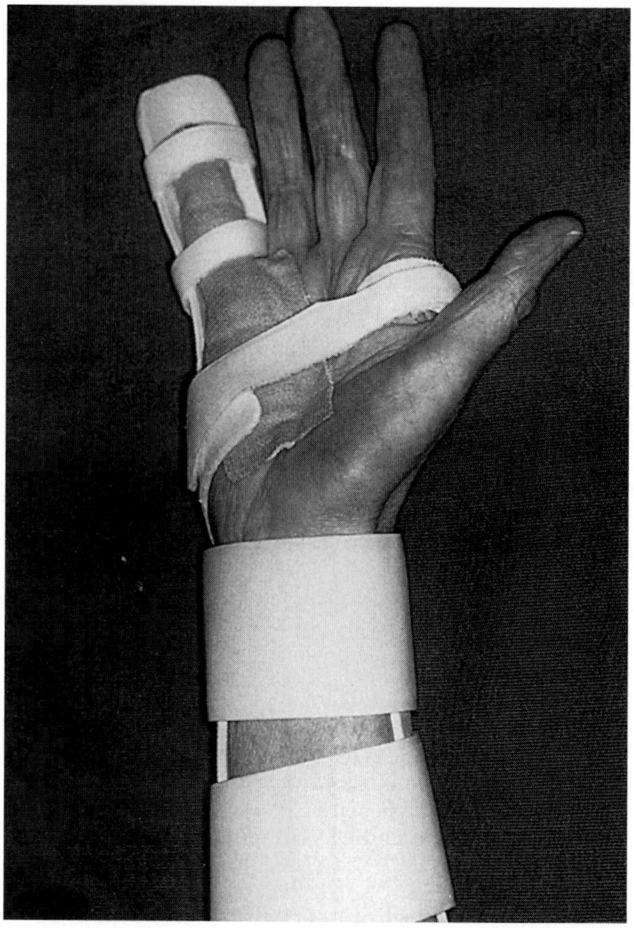

Fig. 57-12. This type of thermoplastic splint is applied within a week of surgery. A few degrees of wrist flexion relax the palmar skin and help finger extension. It is worn most of the time for 3 weeks and then removed for increasing periods to allow flexion exercises. Ideally, the patient should wear this splint every night for 3 months and for occasional periods during the day if the fingers tend to flex.

deformation of an insufficiently rigid splint may result in a loss of proper positioning.

In patients with large hands or for those who have a tendency to continually pull into a flexed position, additional reinforcement may be required to ensure that full MP and PIP extension is maintained throughout the required life of the splint. Splint reinforcement is most effective when the reinforcing component has a raised column (i.e., the reinforcing strip is arched). When a column of splinting material is created in the center of a reinforcement, the strength of this component will be proportional to the height of the column. This allows control of the reinforcement rigidity, which is necessary to support the finger, while limiting size of the splint to allow movement of adjacent fingers (Fig. 57-14).

Occasionally, a patient who required only correction of MP joint deformity and presents to the therapist with full extension postoperatively may forgo extension splinting.

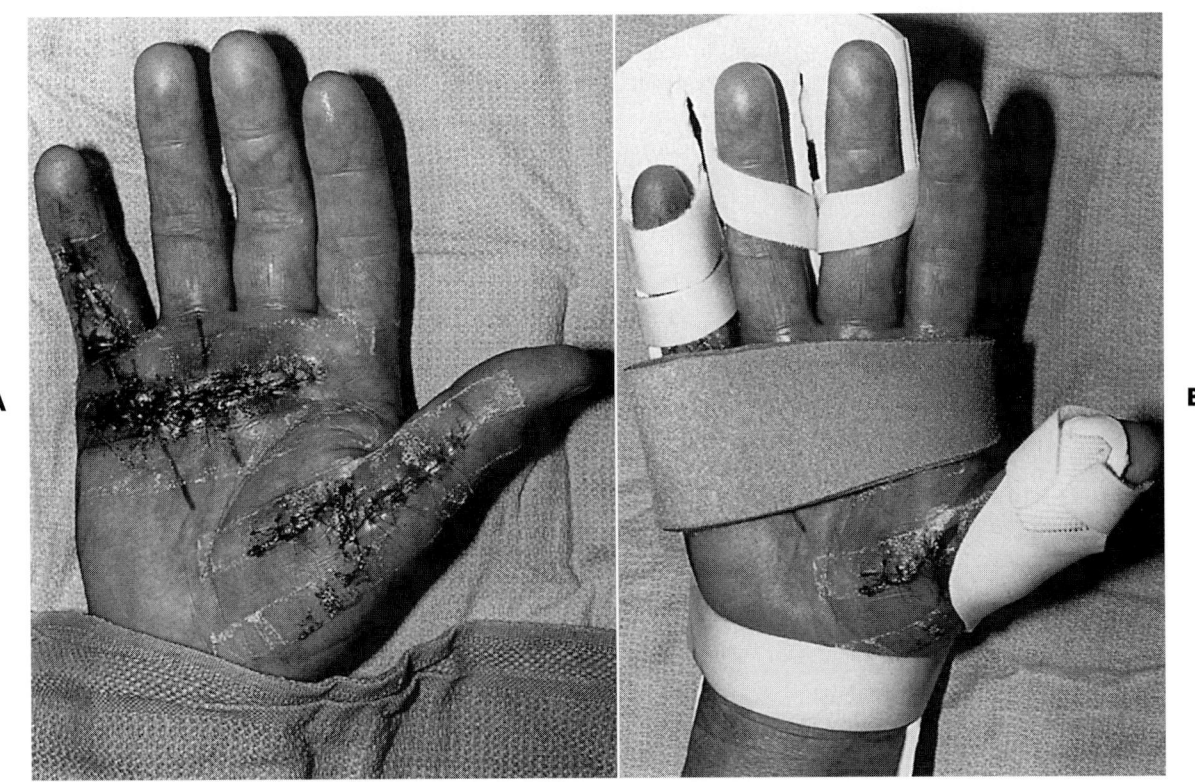

Fig. 57-13. A and **B,** This patient had extensive disease in the palm with contractures of the thumb and small fingers. The splint maintains extension of the thumb and small finger but also holds the metacarpophalangeal joints of the long and ring fingers in extension during healing of the palmar wound. Note that the proximal interphalangeal joint of the small finger is not fully extended. A smaller splint was later applied to this finger to maintain the correction obtained at operation. It was worn for varying periods up to 6 months.

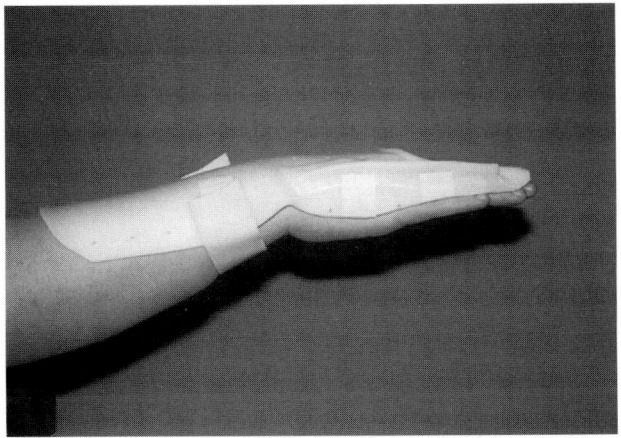

Fig. 57-14. When extra rigidity is required of the dorsal extension, a reinforcing section of splinting material can be used to augment the splint. A stronger mechanical advantage is attained by creating a column in the center of the reinforcement.

However, these patients should be followed to avoid the disappointment of a gradual loss of extension as the incisions mature. After correction of a flexion contracture at the PIP joint, loss of extension will occur unless the joint is splinted during the phase of wound contraction. These patients should be provided with a PIP joint extension splint to prevent recurrence of the contracture.

Patients with less extensive involvement of the MP or PIP joints may obtain satisfactory positioning with a hand-based extension splint to maintain the finger joints in maximum extension. We prefer a dorsal splint because it minimizes pressure on the surgical wound while maintaining extension of the digit during the early postoperative period. It also allows the patient to gradually pull the fingers back to the splint to improve extension. Others have used a palmar-based hand splint with the thought that increased pressure to the surgical site is useful as a method of scar management.[32]

The wearing schedule varies and requires the regular attention of the therapist to ensure that it is altered to suit the changing status of the patient. Removing the splint too soon or without gradual weaning may result in loss of extension, whereas excessive splinting will inevitably result in loss of flexion. Loss of flexion after surgery for DD has been reported to occur in as many as 40% of patients.[37] During the first 3 weeks, the splint is worn continuously, except for exercise and hygiene. Thereafter the patient is instructed to remove the splint for gradually increased intervals. Patients are instructed to monitor their own fingers for loss of ability to fully extend and to reapply the splint if this should occur. The time interval out of the splint is increased until the patient is able to maintain full extension throughout the day. Splinting at night is continued for at least 3 months to facilitate extension throughout the period of scar maturation. Patients with more risk factors often require more extensive surgery and are advised that commitment to a splinting program for 6 months may be required to achieve optimal results. Some patients are willing to forgo the last few degrees of extension in order to discard their splint earlier than recommended by their surgeon or therapist.

After 3 weeks, when the patient is in the remodeling phase, the therapist will need to modify the splinting regimen to accommodate the tendency of the patient to lose flexion with immobilization and the need to regain extension, particularly at the stiff PIP joint. Frequent, but brief exercise throughout the day during the first 3 weeks can go a long way in preventing problems with loss of flexion. Thus, in our experience, dynamic flexion splinting is usually required only for the RSD patient. However, stiffness of the PIP joint is a common problem because it is preexistent in many cases. Series casting and static or dynamic splinting can be used to try to regain this motion.[35] Preoperative flexion deformity may give rise to central slip attenuation, which should be addressed in the postoperative splinting regimen.[40]

Exercise. Although the purpose of a splinting program is to maintain extension, the therapist must balance this influence with regular active and passive exercise to prevent loss of flexion. These patients usually have full flexion preoperatively. Thus loss of flexion may result in functional difficulties that the patient did not have preoperatively and must be avoided. Active exercises are initiated on the first or second postoperative day. A customized exercise program taking into consideration the patient's physical status, risk of complications, and ability to comply with prescribed treatments is required.

Active exercise is usually started within the first 3 postoperative days. Flexion exercises are required to prevent loss of preexistent motion, whereas extension exercises are used to retain movement potential gained by surgery. The therapist teaches the patient to perform these exercises in the therapy session and continue them at home as a home program. Some patients will remember to perform only one exercise correctly. In such a case, the therapist may focus on

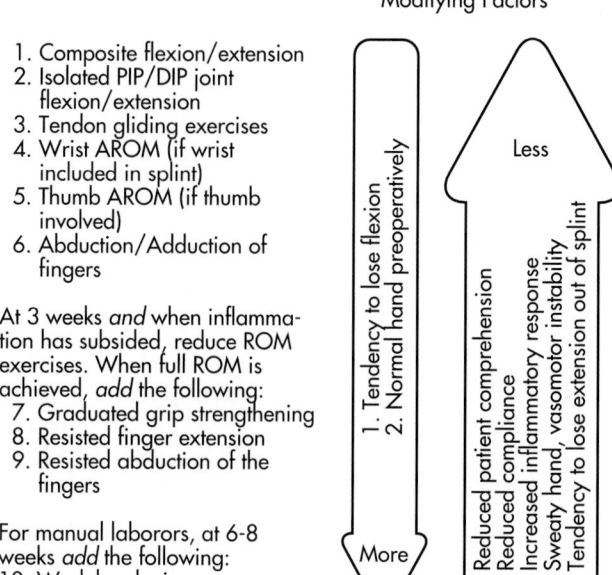

Postrelease Exercises for Patients with Dupuytren's Disease

1. Composite flexion/extension
2. Isolated PIP/DIP joint flexion/extension
3. Tendon gliding exercises
4. Wrist AROM (if wrist included in splint)
5. Thumb AROM (if thumb involved)
6. Abduction/Adduction of fingers

At 3 weeks *and* when inflammation has subsided, reduce ROM exercises. When full ROM is achieved, *add* the following:
7. Graduated grip strengthening
8. Resisted finger extension
9. Resisted abduction of the fingers

For manual laborors, at 6-8 weeks *add* the following:
10. Work hardening

Modifying Factors

More / Less arrow (left):
1. Tendency to lose flexion
2. Normal hand preoperatively

More / Less arrow (right):
1. Reduced patient comprehension
2. Reduced compliance
3. Increased inflammatory response
4. Sweaty hand, vasomotor instability
5. Tendency to lose extension out of splint

Number and intensity of exercises in the home program are modified on the basis of the factors listed in the arrows.

Fig. 57-15. A patient-specific home program is important to maximizing outcome from postoperative rehabilitation. Exercises are listed in order of their importance for inclusion in the home program. *Arrows* indicate factors that influence the intensity of the home program prescribed. Intensity is modified by altering the number of exercises selected, the number of repetitions performed in a session, the number of sessions per day, and the rate at which new exercises are introduced.

composite flexion as a home program and work on the other exercises during therapy sessions. Other patients may be given a more complete home program, including tendon gliding[48-50] exercises for the digits, wrist, and thumb ROM, as well as extension exercises.

The therapist must design the exercise program based on an assessment of the patient's impairments, physical status, physical demands, psychosocial status, and competency. The exercises selected and their frequency and intensity are modified to maximize motion and minimize the potential for complications such as excessive swelling and pain. Reduced comprehension and observations that suggest increased risk for a flare/RSD response would cause the therapist to reduce the intensity of exercise. A tendency to lose extension out of the splint may cause one to minimize the time spent out of the splint performing exercises. On the other hand, some patients start to lose flexion more easily with immobilization and thus must be taken out of the splint and exercised more frequently to avoid a loss of flexion. Patients with normal movement and function preoperatively are usually more suitable for a more progressive exercise program postoperatively (Fig. 57-15).

The therapist uses passive motion, including isolated PIP joint stretches and composite extension stretches, judiciously in the first few weeks after surgery. Carefully applied, they can assist with regaining maximal ROM, but caution must be exercised to prevent increasing the inflammatory response or compromising vascular structures through overly aggressive stretching techniques. Passive movement performed by the therapist can be initiated on the first postoperative day and progresses according to patient tolerance. Slow passive stretching techniques are most useful in restoring tissue extensibility, particularly when preceded by a preconditioning heat treatment such as whirlpool or fluidotherapy. Isolated MP and PIP joint stretches are required. Because the collateral ligaments of the MP joint are maintained to length despite flexion contracture, restoration of full movement of the MP joint is expected. However, the PIP joint collateral ligaments are held in a shortened position with flexion, and thus the PIP joint requires particular attention postoperatively to regain optimal extension. Isolated and composite stretches and joint mobilization techniques are usually required. Shortening of the extrinsic flexor muscles also should be anticipated in the DD patient; this requires stretching of the entire musculotendinous unit. The extent of "hands-on" treatment required by the DD patient depends on the severity of the disease, the type of surgery, the amount of edema, the presence of complications, and most important, the compliance of the patient with the home exercise program.

If active exercise can be performed correctly and independently by the patient, passive stretches may also be added to the home program. Passive stretches into PIP extension are used to obtain motion where it is most difficult to attain.[8]

It is important that patients demonstrate the exercises that they are performing at home upon return visits to the therapist. This will ensure that the exercises are performed correctly and that the therapist has not overloaded the patient with tasks beyond his or her capability. It will also encourage compliance by emphasizing the importance of the home program.

More strenuous use of the hand is instituted when the inflammatory response has decreased. Thus patients are encouraged to gradually resume normal use of the hand.

Scar management. Typically, the open palm heals to a linear scar across the palm and does not result in either functional or cosmetic impairment. For this reason, scar management techniques such as silicone gel and elastomer are not routinely necessary. Uneven or tight scars are more common in wounds that are skin grafted or undergo primary closure. Because patients are often concerned that these bumps indicate recurrence of DD, they should be instructed in the difference between the diseased tissue and scar tissue. Although extension splinting and scar massage are often sufficient to manage these scars, pressure therapy or silicone gel may be used as necessary. Pressure inserts made of Otoform or silicone elastomer with or without supplemental prosthetic foam can be used to modify scar appearance and texture and may be used in conjunction with splints.

Silicone or mineral oil gel sheets may be more costly than pressure inserts, but they do not require custom fitting and are easily accommodated in splints. Silicone gel sheets have been accepted by therapists for use with a variety of surgical hand scars and appear to be effective, safe,[44] and well accepted by patients. Scar management is more rigorous when surgery has involved the thumb web because these scars tend to contract to form a tight rigid band, which can be a definite functional disability.

Strengthening. Gradual progressive strengthening is added to the postoperative treatment program after wounds are healed, typically 3 to 4 weeks postoperatively for the primary closure, 6 weeks for the open palm, and 4 weeks with Coban protecting the graft for the patient with a skin graft. Return of functional grip strength is not a problem for most DD patients and can often be accomplished through a gradual increase in activity at home. Occasionally, patients who are returning to heavy manual work will require more extensive strengthening and work reconditioning. Throughout the strengthening program, the patient should perform activities that put pressure on scars or grafts (i.e., distributing pressure throughout the entire contact surface) so that a perception of weakness is not generated by failure to use the hand normally. A strengthening program that emphasizes performing functional activities and that uses a work simulator to simulate specific tasks requiring pressure through the surgical site will allow simultaneous strengthening and desensitization and thus maximize functional strength and endurance. Where the extension apparatus has been stretched from prolonged flexion deformity, patients may have limited extensor power in their digits. Digital strengthening of the long extensor, interossei, and lumbricals should be performed to restore a more normal balance to the hand.

Procedures performed for severe contracture. Occasionally a longstanding, severe joint contracture cannot be corrected surgically. Surgical solutions for these results of severe disease include fusion of the PIP joint, joint replacement, or amputation.[21,47] This problem invariably occurs at the PIP joint of the small finger.

Amputations for DD are usually at the level of the proximal phalanx. This allows the patient some ulnar grip strength to assist with cylindrical grasp. The therapist will have to ensure maximum flexion extension at the MP joint. The shortened proximal phalanx tends to contract into a flexed position, which will interfere with functional activities. Because of the short lever arm of the amputated digit, a palmar-based splint may be more effective in positioning the digit in extension. A night splint may be needed for 6 months to prevent MP joint flexion contracture. Because the disease has already diminished the cosmetic appearance and function of the digit, the patient with an amputation secondary to Dupuytren's contracture usually has a less severe psychosocial component to rehabilitation than does a patient with a traumatic injury. Patients are typically willing and able to resume functional activity soon after surgery.

Postoperative rehabilitation after joint fusion or replacement is similar regardless of whether the surgery was performed as a result of DD or for other indications. The aim is to regain full flexion and extension of the DIP joint and maximal stability and function at the PIP joint.

Factors affecting progress in postoperative rehabilitation. Close communication and cooperation among the therapist, surgeon, and patient are required to design and achieve realistic treatment goals for the DD patient. The rehabilitation program must be designed to meet these goals by including a therapy program that addresses the unique postoperative experience of each patient. In addition to the severity of the disease and associated risk factors,[51] patient characteristics and surgical management will affect rehabilitation options and expectations.

Patient progress varies with tolerance to the postoperative therapy. However, slower progress in regaining mobility should be anticipated in patients who experience either a "flare reaction" or RSD. RSD[39] and flare responses[52] are reported to occur more often in women (24.5% of women and 12.5% of men). The onset of RSD is insidious and may not be obvious until several weeks postoperatively. Early signs of RSD may be difficult to distinguish from normal postoperative pain, swelling, and stiffness. The therapist, by monitoring patient progress and response to therapy, may be the first to observe the signs of RSD. For this reason, it is important to be alert, with each patient, to the symptoms of RSD, as described in Chapters 104 and 105. Patients with RSD require more intensive hand therapy management with careful attention to prevent pain and swelling while increasing movement.

More common than RSD, the so-called flare reaction occurs in patients exemplified by a greater-than-expected inflammatory response with redness and some swelling. Pain is less intense and movement less restricted than in RSD. Differentiation of postoperative symptoms between those indicative of a flare response and those characteristic of RSD requires repeated observation; differentiation is essential to ensure that patients who require more intensive intervention are identified at the earliest stage, when treatment can be most effective in interrupting the cycle of pain, stiffness, swelling, and loss of motion.

Edema has a detrimental effect on movement postoperatively and, if not resolved promptly, leads to periarticular fibrosis and permanent contracture. Active exercise in elevation, string wrapping, Coban, and retrograde massage are often used to control edema. Pressure gloves may be used for persistent edema problems. Persistent edema is most problematic in the RSD patient, and for these patients, traditional methods of managing edema must be combined, with caution that the hand therapy program is not overly intense and contributing to edema.

Types of wound closure. Perhaps more influential on the course of hand therapy is the choice of wound closure. Primary closure, open-palm technique, and skin grafting each have a role in the surgical management of the DD patient, and each presents its own unique challenges and opportunities to the hand therapist.

Primary closure tends to be selected for less radical procedures and for patients with less severe disease. Small, dry dressings are usually sufficient and do not interfere with movement. The dressing should be removed at each therapy session to detect wound infection or hematoma. Wound infection is unusual in the DD patient. When it does occur, it is most often related to skin loss or hematoma. Proper wound care will allow the attention of the therapist to be more appropriately focused on early movement in the patient with primary closure.

If the palm or digit received a skin graft, a bolus dressing will cover the graft site.[4,14-16,22] It is usually removed within a week. If the graft has taken, it is covered by a thin protective dressing that allows some joint movement. A dorsal extension splint is applied, and therapy is continued as described for the primarily closed wound. A wound closed by skin grafting will heal in the same time as a wound closed by sutures. After the graft is secure, heat may be used to improve tissue extensibility before exercising and massaging the graft. Fluidotherapy appears to be particularly useful for patients with grafts because heat can facilitate movement and a dependent position can be avoided. Resisted activities such as kneading light putty can be started 1 month after surgery. A few patients will continue to protect the graft site beyond the mature stage and may need desensitization treatment to encourage normal use of the digit.

The open-palm technique has several advantages that facilitate early mobilization. The open wound minimizes the risk of hematoma, reduces edema, and minimizes postoperative pain.[12,13,19,25] Because these factors are significant contributors to hand stiffness, the open palm allows easier movement in the early postoperative period. Motion can be initiated on the first postoperative day. If the full benefit of the open palm is to be realized, the patient should be warned about the appearance of the palm. The patient is bound to be apprehensive about the appearance of the gaping open wound and may be afraid to move the hand. The therapist must reassure the patient about the healing process and the importance of maintaining movement throughout the process. The use of the whirlpool has been described by Fietti and Mackin[11] as a useful adjunct to hand therapy after the open-palm technique. The whirlpool provides heat to improve tissue elasticity before exercise and gentle debridement of exudate, which maintains a clean wound and has a desensitizing effect on patients who are reluctant to move their fingers. Additional debridement, by the therapist, is best performed immediately after whirlpool treatment. The whirlpool is kept at a temperature of 98° to 100° F so as *not* to provoke edema.[46] Povidone-iodine (Betadine) has been commonly used as an antiseptic in whirlpool treatment, although we have discontinued its use because of preliminary evidence that it reduces epithelialization.[30] A clear rinse and exercises in elevation are recommended after whirlpool treatment to minimize wound contamination and edema. The whirlpool is cleaned with disinfectant (i.e., Savlon) before and immediately after use by any patient with an open wound to prevent any cross-contamination between patients. This procedure obviates the need for disinfectant in the whirlpool during treatment, although a mild chlorine solution is acceptable. Patients should be informed of these sterilization procedures to prevent anxiety about their risk of infection.

Most of our patients are seen in the therapy department two to three times per week during the first few weeks, so limited home wound care is not required. Patients who cannot be seen regularly in the first few weeks can be taught to do saline soaks at home and change their own dressings. Saline soaks, using a teaspoon of salt in a quart of lukewarm water, can be performed daily and should be combined with active ROM exercises. Elderly patients may also be eligible for home care services to assist with dressing changes. A dressing impregnated with an antibiotic cream is useful to prevent infection and ease dressing changes.

RESULTS OF TREATMENT

The overall result of an operation for DD should consider the early result, within 1 year of operation, and the late result over a period of several years.

The early result pertains to the degrees of correction of joint contracture and the ability of the patient to regain full flexion. The hand therapist contributes to the success of the early result. It is well known that any type of operation is likely to result in complete correction of MP joint contracture. However, contractures at the PIP joint do not fair as well, and certain mitigating factors have been identified. The worst results occur at the PIP joint of the small finger. Less than 25% of PIP joint contractures are completely corrected, regardless of the severity of the contracture or the method of treatment. When the palm is left open, the correction to the PIP joint contracture is not as complete as when the palm is skin grafted or sutured. In the finger, a better correction is obtained at the PIP joint if the wound is closed by a full-thickness skin graft rather than by suture.

Loss of finger flexion is seen with all types of operations but is more likely to be permanent after extensive fasciectomy both in the palm and in the digit.

Long-term results are expressed by the severity of extension and recurrence of disease. Because DD is a progressive disease, some loss of extension is inevitable and extension or recurrence of the disease is likely. However, it

is uncommon for either extension or recurrence to cause sufficient joint contracture to warrant a further operation (less than 10% of patients). The factors associated with recurrence and extension are not those associated with a good or a bad early result. Rather, they are the uncontrollable features of early age of onset of disease, a strong family history, knuckle pads, plantar fibromatosis, and disease involving the radial side of the hand. Conversely, Evans[10] challenged therapists to consider whether overly aggressive hand therapy management could contribute not only to poorer immediate results but also to extension of the disease. Regardless, even the late results at the MP joint are good, and any problem contracture is likely to appear at the PIP joint. The late results are worst in the small finger.

CONCLUSION

The cause and the course of DD remain incompletely understood, but the results of treatment continue to improve because of careful selection of treatment for the given patient and improved technical aids. Consistent correction of PIP joint contracture remains the greatest challenge.

REFERENCES

1. Abbott K, et al: A review of attitudes to splintage in Dupuytren's contracture, *J Hand Surg* 12B:326, 1987.
2. Arafa M, et al: Dupuytren's and epilepsy revisited, *J Hand Surg* 17B:221, 1992.
3. Bradlow A, Mowat AG: Dupuytren's contracture and alcohol, *Ann Rheum Dis* 45:304, 1986.
4. Brotherston TM, et al: Long term follow-up of dermofasciectomy for Dupuytren's contracture, *Br J Plast Surg* 47:440, 1994.
5. Chung KC, et al: Reliability and validity testing of the Michigan Hand Outcomes Questionnaire, *J Hand Surg* 23A:575, 1998.
6. Colville J: Dupuytren's contracture: the role of fasciotomy, *Hand* 15:162, 1983.
7. Critchley EM, et al: Dupuytren's disease in epilepsy: result of prolonged administration of anticonvulsants, *J Neurol Neurosurg Psychiatry* 39:498, 1976.
8. Crowley B, Tonkin MA: The proximal interphalangeal joint in Dupuytren's disease, *Hand Clin* 15:137, 1999.
9. Egawa T, et al: Epidemiology of the oriental patient. In McFarlane RM, McGrouther DA, Flint MH, editors: *Dupuytren's*, Edinburgh, 1990, Churchill Livingstone.
10. Evans RB: Eleventh Nathalie Barr Lecture: the source of our strength, *J Hand Ther* 10:14, 1997.
11. Fietti VG, Mackin EJ: Open-palm technique in Dupuytren's disease. In Hunter JM, et al, editors: *Rehabilitation of the hand: surgery and therapy*, ed 3, St Louis, 1990, Mosby.
12. Foucher G, et al: A modified open palm technique for Dupuytren's disease: short and long term results in 54 patients, *Int Orthop* 19:285, 1995.
13. Gelberman RH, et al: Wound complications in the surgical management of Dupuytren's contracture: a comparison of operative incisions, *Hand* 14:248, 1982.
14. Gonzalez RI: The use of skin grafts in the treatment of Dupuytren's contracture, *Hand Clin* 1:641, 1985.
15. Hall PN, et al: Skin replacement in Dupuytren's disease, *J Hand Surg* 22B:193, 1997.
16. Hueston JT: The control of recurrent Dupuytren's contracture by skin replacement, *Br J Plast Surg* 22:152, 1969.

17. Hueston JT: Dermofasciectomy for Dupuytren's disease, *Bull Hosp Jt Dis* 44:224, 1984.

18. Hueston JT: Diathesis as a guide to the timing and extent of surgery in Dupuytren's disease. In Hueston JT, Tubiana R, editors: *Dupuytren's disease: GEM monograph,* ed 2, Edinburgh, 2000, Churchill Livingstone.

19. Jacobsen K, Holst-Nielsen F: A modified McCash operation for Dupuytren's contracture, *Scand J Plast Reconstr Surg Hand Surg* 11(suppl):231, 1977.

20. Jain AS, Mitchell C, Carus DA: A simple inexpensive post-operative management regime following surgery for Dupuytren's contracture, *J Hand Surg* 13B:259, 1988.

21. Jensen CM, Haugegaard M, Rasmussen SW: Amputations in the treatment of Dupuytren's disease, *J Hand Surg* 18B:781, 1993.

22. Ketchum LD, Hixson FP: Dermofasciectomy and full-thickness grafts in the treatment of Dupuytren's contracture, *J Hand Surg* 12A:659, 1987.

23. Ledingham WM, et al: On immediate functional bracing of Colles' fracture, *Injury* 22:197, 1991.

24. Ling RSM: The genetic factors in Dupuytren's disease, *J Bone Joint Surg* 45B:709, 1963.

25. Macnicol MF: The open palm technique for Dupuytren's contracture, *Int Orthop* 8:55, 1984.

26. McCash CR: The open palm technique in Dupuytren's contracture, *Br J Plast Surg* 17:271, 1964.

27. McFarlane RM: Dupuytren's disease. In Green DP, editor: *Operative hand surgery,* New York, 1993, Churchill Livingstone.

28. McFarlane RM, McGrouther DA, Flint MH, editors: *Dupuytren's disease,* Edinburgh, 2000, Churchill Livingstone.

29. Mennen U: Dupuytren's contracture in the negro, *J Hand Surg* 11B:61, 1986.

30. Menton DN, Brown MB: The effects of commercial wound cleansers on cutaneous wound healing in guinea pigs, *Phys Ther* 72:S38, 2000.

31. Messina A: La T.E.C. (Tecnica di Estensione Continua) nel Morbo di Dupuytren Grave, *Riv di Chirugie della Mano* 26:253, 1989.

32. Mullins PA: Postsurgical rehabilitation of Dupuytren's disease, *Hand Clin* 15:167, 1999.

33. Noble LS, Heathcote JG, Cohen H: Diabetes mellitus in the in patients from the Indian subcontinent, *J Bone Joint Surg* 66B:322, 1984.

34. Peterson-Bethea D: A static progressive splint for Dupuytren's release, *J Hand Ther* 10:312, 1997.

35. Rives K, et al: Severe contractures of the proximal interphalangeal joint in Dupuytren's disease: results of a prospective trial of operative correction and dynamic extension splinting, *J Hand Surg* 17A:1153, 1992.

36. Sampson SP, et al: The use of a passive motion machine in the postoperative rehabilitation of Dupuytren's disease, *J Hand Surg* 17A:333, 1992.

37. Schneider LH: The open palm technique, *Hand Clin* 7:723, 1991.

38. Schunk C, Reed K: Wrist/hand. In Schunk C, Reed K, editors: *Clinical practice guidelines: examination and intervention for rehabilitation,* Gaithersburg, Md, 2000, Aspen.

39. Sennwald GR: Fasciectomy for treatment of Dupuytren's disease and early complications, *J Hand Surg* 15A:755, 1990.

40. Smith P, Breed C: Central slip attenuation in Dupuytren's contracture: a cause of persistent flexion of the proximal interphalangeal joint, *J Hand Surg* 19A:840, 1994.

41. Srivastava S, Nancarrow JD, Cort DF: Dupuytren's disease in patients from the Indian subcontinent, *J Hand Surg* 14B:32, 1989.

42. Stiles P: Ultrasonic therapy in Dupuytren's contracture, *J Bone Joint Surg* 48B:452, 1966.

43. Taras JS, Lemel MS, Nathan R: Vascular disorders of the upper extremity. In Hunter JM, Mackin EJ, Callahan AD, editors: *Rehabilitation of the hand: surgery and therapy,* St Louis, 1999, Mosby.

44. Thurston AJ: Safety of silicone liquid in the postoperative management of Dupuytren's contracture, *Aust NZ J Surg* 67:347, 1997.

45. Upper Extremity Collaborative Group: *The DASH outcome measure: user's manual,* Toronto, 1999, Institute for Work and Health.

46. Walsh M: Relationship of hand edema to upper extremity position and water temperature during whirlpool, *J Hand Surg* 9A:609, 1984.

47. Watson HK Lovallo JL: Salvage of severe recurrent Dupuytren's contracture of the ring and small fingers, *J Hand Surg* 12A:287, 1987.

48. Wehbe MA: Tendon gliding exercises, *Am J Occup Ther* 41:164, 1987.

49. Wehbe MA, Hunter JM: Flexor tendon gliding in the hand. Part I. In vivo excursions. *J Hand Surg* 10A:570, 1985.

50. Wehbe MA, Hunter JM: Flexor tendon gliding in the hand. Part II. Differential gliding, *J Hand Surg* 10A:575, 1985.

51. Woodruff MJ, Waldram MA: A clinical grading system for Dupuytren's contracture, *J Hand Surg* 23B:303, 1998.

52. Zemel NP: Dupuytren's contracture in women, *Hand Clin* 7:707, 1991.

Part XIII

CUMULATIVE TRAUMA DISORDERS

Chapter 58

CUMULATIVE TRAUMA DISORDERS: FACT OR FICTION?

Peter A. Nathan
Kenneth D. Meadows

And science, we should insist, better than any other discipline,
can hold up to its students and followers
an ideal of patient devotion to the search for objective truth,
with vision unclouded by personal or political motive.

SIR HENRY HALLETT DALE

From the inception of modern medical practice, physicians have endeavored to adhere to the principles of the scientific method, which are based on the interplay of objective evidence and hypothesis. Application of the scientific method to the practice of medicine requires objective evidence of injury or disease for development of legitimate and specific diagnoses. In this process, there must be strong clinical correlations between specific sets of symptoms and objective evidence of an organic pathologic condition.

In recent years, some clinicians have moved away from requiring objective evidence of an organic pathologic condition and toward defining subjective soft tissue discomfort as a diagnosable condition. This has led to progressive acceptance of a symptom-based concept of disease and injury. Barsky and Borus[3,4] have studied this trend and state that in the last several decades our society has reclassified a growing array of uncomfortable and undesirable aspects of life, including musculoskeletal conditions, as diseases for which we increasingly seek medical consultation.

The movement toward redefining injury and disease has escalated through subtle adaptations of language, substituting descriptive labels for diagnostic terms. This process typically involves insertion of hypothetical etiology within terminology used to describe broad categories of discomfort, which may or may not be associated with objective evidence of disease. The descriptive label *cumulative trauma disorder* (CTD) appeared in the medical literature as early as 1966.[41] A sibling label, *repetition strain injury* (RSI), was used widely in Australia in the 1970s and 1980s to describe an outbreak of upper extremity complaints in telephonists and related occupations.[16,17]

The ambiguity of the term *CTD*, coupled with the lack of scientific evidence to support a cumulative trauma hypothesis, has caused some proponents of a symptom-based model to substitute the term *work-related musculoskeletal disorders* (WRMSD) or *musculoskeletal disorders* (MSD), as described by Hales and Bernard.[15]

Medical professionals agree that some diagnosable neuromusculoskeletal conditions can be linked to identifiable work and avocational physical stressors. De Quervain's syndrome and rotator cuff tear/tendinitis of the shoulder are examples. Most often, however, conditions classified within the CTD family involve clusters of nonspecific symptoms with little or no objective evidence of organic pathologic conditions. There is no historical, clinical, or scientific precedent for giving diagnostic status to the majority of conditions considered CTDs. The designation CTD may appeal to specific constituencies, but the scientific foundations of the medical tradition are undermined by application of descriptive labels that erroneously imply the presence of organic disease.

HISTORICAL PERSPECTIVE

An illustrative historical example is provided by an epidemic of RSI in Australia in the 1980s.[17] The epidemic manifested itself in a rapid, dramatic outbreak of arm symptoms associated with keyboard use. These symptoms resulted in time loss from work and spawned adversarial relationships between workers and employers. The epidemic appeared to have been accentuated by worker anxiety resulting from widespread media coverage. Nonspecific symptoms and epidemiologic inconsistencies frustrated efforts to address the problem diagnostically. This disease outbreak might be viewed as a phenomenon in which the means of disease transmission is psychosocial and informational in nature, rather than physiologic. By 1987, the epidemic largely subsided, as suddenly as it had begun, in the absence of objective diagnoses and proven medical cures. The literature confirms that psychosocial phenomena involved in the Australian epidemic far outweighed physiologic manifestations.[17] There have since been reported outbreaks of similar conditions (labeled CTDs) in scattered U.S. workplaces.

A CLINICAL PERSPECTIVE OF CTDs

Traditional studies of anatomy and physiology provide a basis for understanding human physical tolerance, injury, and disease. Physicians, by virtue of their training and experience, can assess the nature and magnitude of physical stresses anticipated to result in pathologic changes in human neuromusculoskeletal structures. The basic human tolerance to withstand resistive and repetitive activities has not changed over the years, even though the language and philosophic parameters describing physiologic responses to activity have evolved significantly. The mandate of the Occupational Safety and Health Administration (OSHA) has changed from that of regulating jobs that cause injury or illness to a program of workplace intervention designed to alleviate even benign, nondebilitating forms of soft tissue discomfort. This mandate has changed in the absence of objective evidence linking most forms of soft tissue discomfort with organic pathology. OSHA's altered direction does not acknowledge that soft tissue symptoms are common in nonwork settings and often resolve spontaneously, without formal medical intervention.[43] One study, for instance, showed that during a 6-week period, 50% of all people surveyed had a musculoskeletal problem and each person had an average of 4 days of musculoskeletal symptoms.[43]

The pervasiveness and the nonobjective nature of the symptom-based concept of disease and injury is underscored by OSHA's stated position that "for MSD's, on the other hand, micro-anatomic injury and repair is often sub-clinical and generally invisible to clinical testing or surveillance

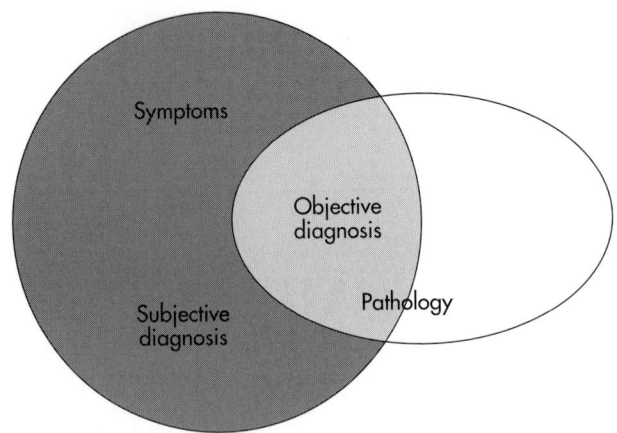

Fig. 58-1. The Venn diagram illustrates the traditional medical model of injury and disease. The union *(light gray)* of symptoms *(circle)* and disease *(ellipse)* sets the boundaries for objective diagnosis, the focus of a traditional scientific medical model. The entire circle represents cumulative trauma disorders, which predominately rely on subjective diagnosis and only a portion of which relies on objective diagnosis.

measures."[31] Although seemingly plausible, statements such as this coincide with the current trend for the progressive medicalization of physical distress wherein bodily discomfort and isolated symptoms are reclassified as diseases for which medical treatment is sought.[3] From this perspective, even the most generic forms of benign exertional myalgia can be elevated to a level of injury.

The Venn diagram in Fig. 58-1 illustrates a paradigm of the traditional medical model of injury and disease. It is based on a union of symptoms and objective findings, represented by the intersection *(light gray)* of the circle and the ellipse. This overlap of symptoms and disease sets the boundaries for clinical disease, the focus of a traditional scientific medical model. The entire circle represents CTDs, only a portion of which is represented by clinical disease. The predominating area represents nonspecific symptoms without associated disease. This is the clinical presentation most often considered to represent CTDs.

The CTD or symptom-based model not only assigns diagnostic significance to symptoms but also permits clinicians to ascribe etiologic considerations to complaints unsupported by pathologic alteration to muscle, tendon, nerve, or bone. The arbitrary clustering of symptoms under a classification system limited to descriptive terminology serves to systematize and validate as pathology many of the transient aches and pains that are a normal physiologic response to vocational and avocational activity.

CTD CONCEPT LACKS SCIENTIFIC VALIDATION

The symptom-based model ascribes causation based on temporal associations between symptoms and occupational exposure. In contrast, the traditional medical model of disease and injury ascribes an activity-related causation for soft tissue conditions only when objective evidence of disease corresponds directly to the physical forces generated by a specific set of activities.

The term *CTD* implies that upper extremity neuromusculoskeletal complaints in the workplace are caused by microtrauma inflicted over time. Two recent studies investigating peripheral nerve disease report dose-response relationships between industrial exposure and symptoms, but neither identifies a statistically significant link between exposure and objectively confirmed nerve disease.[1,19] Without an objectively determined dose-response relationship between activity and disease, assigning causation to physical activity is based on assumptions and may be fraught with error. Physicians determining etiology lack objective information to determine whether repetitive hand use constitutes an injury hazard.[12,13]

Peer-reviewed literature on the subject remains divided, despite growing acceptance for the symptom-based model and the idea that these complaints are generally work related. The literature contains case reports and cross-sectional studies that link symptoms to self-reported ergonomic hazard exposure.[5,15,20,30] Some studies link objectively confirmed medical diagnoses to self-reported ergonomic hazard exposure or self-reported symptoms to objectively measured ergonomic hazard exposure.[9,34] Arguments based on biologic plausibility abound and inconsistencies are explained as examples of selection bias or survivor bias.[5,14,15,20,30,35]

Reviews of the literature concerning relationships between repetitive work exposure and CTDs of the upper extremities reveal that most studies interpreted to show a significant, positive relationship lack specific criteria for validity.[5,21,39,42] Gerr, Letz, and Landrigan,[11] for instance, found few such studies that used rigorous assessments of exposure or well-defined objective measures of outcomes. It also has been pointed out that the literature lacks prospective, longitudinal studies that can demonstrate a consistent, positive relationship between objective measures of repetitive work exposure and objectively confirmed diagnoses.[12,21] In general, cross-sectional studies cannot demonstrate causation; they can only generate hypotheses to be tested.[13,21] Longitudinal studies give the critical dimension of time and allow demonstration that cause preceded effect and that there is a consistent, time-dependent dose effect.

We are aware of no peer-reviewed longitudinal studies that confirm statistically significant, independent, positive relationships between work and the development of most conditions considered to represent CTDs. A recent longitudinal study of risk factors for neck and upper limb disorders from Sweden failed to isolate specific work factors as a primary cause for hand and wrist conditions.[10] The authors state their findings may point to psychosocial factors ("total overload" and "dissatisfaction with life as a whole") as critical to development of upper extremity disorders.

THE IMPORTANCE OF PERSONAL AND LIFESTYLE FACTORS

In addition to excluding consideration of psychosocial factors, much of the literature has failed to consider personal and lifestyle factors such as heredity, age, gender, race, height, weight, body mass index, avocational activities, medical history, use of legal drugs, general health, and mental health, which, along with other factors, have been shown to be significant risk factors for the conditions under discussion.* In the search for etiologic relationships, those that adhere to the CTD classification almost always consider the physical aspects of work but do not consider deleterious personal and lifestyle factors.

Carpal tunnel syndrome (CTS) is the most commonly cited example of CTDs involving the upper extremity. CTS is diagnosed in the presence of an objectively defined pathologic condition (median neuropathy) and a specific, reproducible set of symptoms. There is an established, growing body of literature that demonstrates that personal, lifestyle, and genetic factors are major components in the development of CTS. This literature is based on peer-reviewed investigations that confirm that obesity, inactivity, smoking, family history, and wrist dimensions are important risk factors for the development of CTS.† Longitudinal studies that support the idea that work activity is a major cause for the underlying condition (median neuropathy) responsible for CTS are absent from the literature. Nevertheless, there remains a powerful bias toward considering CTS and a broad group of other musculoskeletal conditions to be work related.

A complete consideration of the historical and societal forces that have converged to both develop and support a symptom-based model of CTD is beyond the scope of this chapter. However, in general, there appears to be a misapplied effort to protect workers by impugning work for the development of CTDs, a practice that ultimately may be counterproductive to the general working population. Strategies that prejudicially exclude or minimize personal and lifestyle factors from etiologic discussion can have the effect of withholding or delaying development of effective preventative interventions. This practice is particularly unfortunate because a substantial majority of the overall disease burden in the United States and other developed countries is a consequence of modifiable risk factors. Obesity, for instance, now affects almost one fourth of all U.S. adults, and our population also has become more sedentary.[22] Cigarette smoking and abuse of alcohol remain prominent in the United States. Obesity, inactivity, and use/abuse of legal drugs have all been shown to increase the risk for CTS and perhaps other neuromusculoskeletal conditions.[23,25,27]

These personal and lifestyle factors can be influenced positively by wellness and health education programs.

---

*References 2, 6-8, 23-29, 32, 33, 36-38, 40, 44.
†References 18, 23, 25, 27, 33, 36.

Interventions of this nature also can affect a wide range of medical conditions outside the scope of soft tissue and musculoskeletal problems. The focus on work-related activity, common in governmental programs assessing causation, comes at the expense of programs with greater applicability and the potential for a broader impact on workplace health.

CONCLUSION

In the realm of objective scientific medicine, most CTDs do not meet the criteria for the diagnosis of injury or disease. The term *functional somatic syndrome* refers to a growing number of "related syndromes that are characterized more by symptoms, suffering, and disability than by disease-specific, demonstrable abnormalities of structure or function."[4] Most of these syndromes, including RSI and CTD, must be considered "fiction" within the black-and-white choices made available by the diagnostic constraints of objective medical science.

Although it may be scientifically accurate to say there is no pathologic basis for musculotendinous discomfort resulting from physical exertion, this knowledge does little to palliate symptoms caused by physical exertion. In this circumstance, a rigorous clinical approach can result in frustration, hostility, and wasted time and resources in an attempt to validate the complaints. Similarly, the clinical approach of those who believe that subjective symptoms alone represent a pathologic condition can be counterproductive. This approach can provoke anxiety and inhibit willingness for the affected worker to put forth physical effort in the workplace. Those labeled with "work-related cumulative trauma" may enter into a medical-legal tug-of-war with negative outcome for both employee and employer.

It may be more equitable to seek answers to issues regarding etiology within the more conciliatory shades of gray, rather then from the adversarial postures of "fact or fiction." Prompt recognition and treatment of conditions in which there is clear evidence of injury and disease are essential. Careful explanation of the nature of benign musculotendinous discomfort is also essential. Assuring patients that symptoms do not necessarily represent injury or disease can do much to alleviate anxiety.

Resolution of controversies relating to the validity of CTDs is approachable through a process of education, understanding, and discussion. Continued debate as to the measure of "fact or fiction" in the diagnostic process will do little to treat the worker, which is the unchanging mandate of those involved in occupational medicine.

REFERENCES

1. Armstrong TJ, et al: A conceptual model for work-related neck and upper-limb musculoskeletal disorders, *Scand J Work Environ Health* 19:73, 1993.
2. Atcheson SG, Ward JR, Lowe W: Concurrent medical disease in work-related carpal tunnel syndrome, *Arch Intern Med* 158:1506, 1998.
3. Barsky AJ, Borus JF: Somatization and medicalization in the era of managed care, *JAMA* 274:1931, 1995.
4. Barsky AJ, Borus JF: Functional somatic syndromes, *Ann Intern Med* 130:910, 1999.
5. Bernard B, et al: Musculoskeletal disorders and workplace factors: a critical review of epidemiologic evidence for work-related musculoskeletal disorders of the neck, upper extremity, and back, 2nd printing. USDHHS, PHS. July 1997, DHHS (NIOSH) Publication No. 97-141.
6. DeKrom MCTFM, et al: Risk factors for carpal tunnel syndrome, *Am J Epidemiol* 132:102, 1990.
7. Dereberry VJ: Etiologies and prevalence of occupational upper extremity injuries. In Kasdan ML, editor: *Occupational hand and upper extremity injuries & diseases,* ed 2, Philadelphia, 1997, Hanley & Belfus.
8. Dzwierzynski WW, et al: Psychometric assessment of patients with chronic upper extremity pain attributed to workplace exposure, *J Hand Surg* 24A:46, 1999.
9. English CJ, et al: Relations between upper limb soft tissue disorders and repetitive movements at work, *Am J Indust Med* 27:75, 1995.
10. Fredriksson K, et al: Risk factors for neck and upper limb disorders: results from 24 years of follow up, *Occup Environ Med* 56:59, 1999.
11. Gerr F, Letz R, Landrigan PJ: Upper-extremity musculoskeletal disorders of occupational origin, *Ann Rev Publ Health* 12:543, 1991.
12. Gerr F, Marcus M, Ortiz DJ: Methodological limitations in the study of video display terminal use and upper extremity musculoskeletal disorders, *Am J Indust Med* 29:649, 1996.
13. Hadler NM: Repetitive upper-extremity motions in the workplace are not hazardous, *J Hand Surg* 22A:19, 1997.
14. Hagberg M, Morgenstern H, Kelsh M: Impact of occupations and job tasks on the prevalence of carpal tunnel syndrome, *Scand J Work Environ Health* 18:337, 1992.
15. Hales TR, Bernard BP: Epidemiology of work-related musculoskeletal disorders, *Orthop Clin North Am* 27:679, 1996.
16. Hocking B: Epidemiological aspects of "repetition strain injury" in Telecom Australia, *Med J Aust* 147:218, 1987.
17. Ireland DCR: Repetition strain injury: the Australian experience—1992 update, *J Hand Surg* 20A:S53, 1995.
18. Johnson EW, et al: Wrist dimensions: correlations with median sensory latencies, *Arch Phys Med Rehabil* 64:556, 1983.
19. Latko WA, et al: Cross-sectional study of the relationship between repetitive work and the prevalence of upper limb musculoskeletal disorders, *Am J Indust Med* 36:248, 1999.
20. Mackinnon SE, Novak CB: Clinical perspective: repetitive strain in the workplace, *J Hand Surg* 22A:2, 1997.
21. Moore JS, Prezzia C: Considerations in determining the work-relatedness of carpal tunnel syndrome. In Erdil M, Dickerson OB, editors: *Cumulative trauma disorders, prevention, evaluation, and treatment,* New York, 1997, Van Nostrand Reinhold.
22. Must A, et al: The disease burden associated with overweight and obesity, *JAMA* 282:1523, 1999.
23. Nathan PA, Keniston RC: Carpal tunnel syndrome and its relation to general physical condition, *Hand Clin* 9:253, 1993.
24. Nathan PA, Keniston RC: Carpal tunnel syndrome: personal risk profile and role of intrinsic and behavioral factors. In Kasdan ML, editor: *Occupational hand and upper extremity injuries and diseases,* ed 2, Philadelphia, 1997, Hanley & Belfus.
25. Nathan PA, Keniston RC, Meadows KD: Carpal tunnel syndrome in the workplace, *Hippocrates' Lantern* 2:1, 1993.
26. Nathan PA, et al: Longitudinal study of median nerve sensory conduction in industry: relationship to age, gender, hand dominance, occupational hand use, and clinical diagnosis, *J Hand Surg* 17A:850, 1992.
27. Nathan PA, et al: Obesity as a risk factor for slowing of sensory conduction of the median nerve in industry. A cross-sectional and longitudinal study involving 429 workers, *J Occup Med* 34:379, 1992.

28. Nathan PA, et al: Tobacco, caffeine, alcohol, and carpal tunnel syndrome in American industry, *J Occup Environ Med* 38:290, 1996.

29. Nathan PA, et al: Natural history of median nerve sensory conduction in industry: Relationship to symptoms and carpal tunnel syndrome in 558 hands over 11 years, *Muscle Nerve* 21:711, 1998.

30. National Research Council: *Work-related musculoskeletal disorders. Report, workshop summary, and workshop reports,* Washington, DC, 1999, National Academy Press.

31. Occupational Safety and Health Administration. Ergonomics program: proposed rule. Federal Register, Proposed Rules, 29 CFR Part 1910, Volume 64 (225), November 23, 1999, p. 65868.

32. Phalen GS: The carpal tunnel syndrome: seventeen years' experience in diagnosis and treatment of six hundred fifty-four hands, *J Bone Joint Surg* 48A:211, 1966.

33. Radecki P: The familial occurrence of carpal tunnel syndrome, *Muscle Nerve* 17:325, 1994.

34. Silverstein BA, Fine LJ, Armstrong TJ: Occupational factors and carpal tunnel syndrome, *Am J Indust Med* 11:343, 1987.

35. Silverstein B, Fine L, Stetson D: Hand-wrist disorders among investment casting plant workers, *J Hand Surg* 12A:838, 1987.

36. Stallings SP, et al: A case control study of obesity as a risk factor for carpal tunnel syndrome in a population of 600 patients presenting for independent medical exam, *J Hand Surg* 22A:211, 1997.

37. Stevens JC, et al: Carpal tunnel syndrome in Rochester, Minnesota, 1961 to 1980, *Neurology* 38:134, 1988.

38. Stevens JC, et al: Conditions associated with carpal tunnel syndrome, *Mayo Clin Proc* 67:541, 1992.

39. Stock SR: Workplace ergonomic factors and the development of musculoskeletal disorders of the neck and upper extremity: a meta-analysis, *Am J Indust Med* 19:87, 1991.

40. Tanaka S, et al: Prevalence and work-relatedness of self-reported carpal tunnel syndrome among U.S. workers: analysis of the occupational health supplement data of 1988 National Health Interview Survey, *Am J Indust Med* 27:451, 1995.

41. Tischuer ER: Some aspects of stress on forearm and hand in industry, *J Occup Med* 8:63, 1966.

42. Vender MI, Kasdan ML, Truppa KL: Upper extremity disorders: a literature review to determine work-relatedness, *J Hand Surg* 20A:534, 1995.

43. Verbrugge LM, Ascione FJ: Exploring the iceberg: common symptoms and how people care for them, *Med Care* 25:539, 1987.

44. Vessey MP, Villard-MacIntosh L, Yeates D: Epidemiology of carpal tunnel syndrome in women of childbearing age: findings in a large cohort study, *Int J Epidemiol* 19:655, 1990.

Chapter 59

APPROACH TO MANAGEMENT OF WORK-RELATED MUSCULOSKELETAL DISORDERS

Ann E. Barr

The number of cases of work-related musculoskeletal disorders (WMSDs) in the United States has been gradually declining since its peak of 332,100 in 1994 (Fig. 59-1). However, according to the U.S. Bureau of Labor Statistics database, illnesses in the workplace resulting from repeated trauma have continued to account for approximately 4% to 4.5% of all reported injuries and illnesses in U.S. private industry since 1992 (Fig. 59-2). Recent studies of a subset of worker's compensation insurance claims to Liberty Mutual Insurance Company of upper extremity WMSD (UE WMSD) show the same trends as all illnesses resulting from repeated trauma (see Fig. 59-2).[4,12] A further subset of the Liberty Mutual database also showed a similar trend in the number of computer-related UE WMSD (see Fig. 59-2). These trends were explained by improved reporting and classification procedures, increased awareness of UE WMSD by public and medical practitioners, the expansion of worker's compensation laws to include UE WMSD, increasing productivity demands, a shift to service-industry jobs, a growing proportion of women in the work force, and an increased use of computer workstations in U.S. workplaces.

According to a recent study of approximately 186,000 federal workers during the period from 1993 to 1994, mononeuritis (93% carpal tunnel syndrome [CTS]) and enthesopathy (48% lateral epicondylitis) were the most common UE WMSD diagnoses, accounting for 43% and 31% of such claims, respectively.[11] Disorders related to tendon, synovium, and bursa (73% tenosynovitis of the hand) accounted for 24% of claims. The remaining 2% were categorized as "other" or miscellaneous, and included diagnoses such as osteoarthritis and myalgia. The age of most claimants ranged from 31 to 50 years, and they were predominantly female. CTS and enthesopathy of the elbow were the most costly claims. CTS accounted for 67% of all direct medical costs and averaged $2948 per case. Of the CTS costs, 43% were for surgical services, 16% were for nonsurgical therapies (including 12% for physical therapy), and the remainder were for diagnostic, evaluation, and management services. Enthesopathy of the elbow accounted for 16% of all direct medical costs and averaged $1771 per case. Physical therapy services accounted for 25% of elbow enthesopathy costs, evaluation and management for 20%, and surgical and diagnostic services for the remainder. The mean number of lost workdays for CTS cases was 84, and for enthesopathy cases it was 79. The average indemnity costs for CTS were $4941, and $4477 for enthesopathy. Most of the costs for CTS were incurred by a relatively small proportion of the total cases, which explains the comparable average per case costs for these two diagnoses.

Although the decline in absolute numbers of reported cases of WMSD since 1994 is encouraging, WMSDs continue to represent a small but significant proportion of worker's compensation claims. These work-related injuries may incur high direct medical costs as well as lost workdays, lost worker productivity, and diminished quality of

Cases of WMSD due to Repeated Trauma

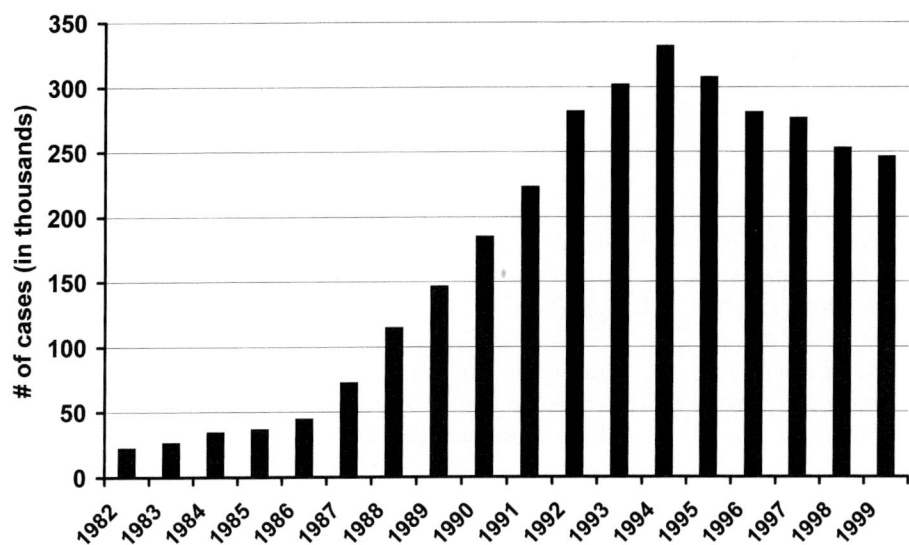

Fig. 59-1. Histogram showing the number of cases of work-related musculoskeletal disorders (WMSDs) resulting from repeated trauma reported by U.S. private industry from 1982 to 1999. Cases peaked at 332,000 in 1994 and declined slightly to 249,000 in 1999. (Data provided by the U.S. Bureau of Labor Statistics, www.stats.bls.gov/.)

Percent of WMSD due to Repeated Trauma

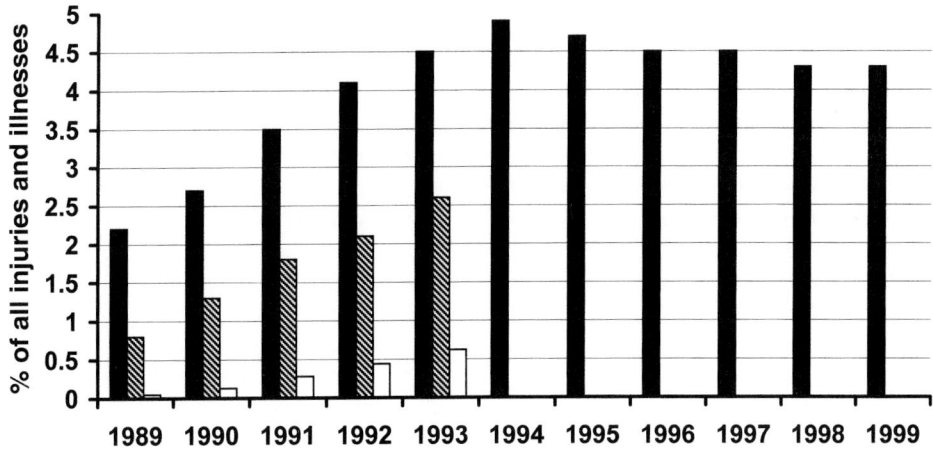

Fig. 59-2. Histogram showing proportion of work-related musculoskeletal disorders (WMSDs) resulting from repeated trauma for all body regions, the upper extremity only, and for computer-related upper extremity disorders expressed as a percentage of all workplace injuries and illnesses. Data for all body regions are shown in *black* from 1989 through 1999 and were provided by the U.S. Bureau of Labor Statistics (www.stats.bls.gov/). Data for the upper extremity only *(diagonal stripes)* and for computer-related upper extremity disorders *(white)* are shown from 1989 to 1993 and were provided by Liberty Mutual Insurance Company.[4,12] It is not known whether upper extremity WMSD trends have continued to mirror those of all body regions through the latter half of the 1990s. Despite the gradual decline in total numbers of repeated-trauma WMSD cases from 1994 through 1999, the proportion of these injuries has remained between 4% and 4.5% of all workplace injuries and illnesses.

life.[15,21,24] These injuries have the potential to develop into chronic health problems if they are not detected and managed early.[21] Unfortunately, the criteria by which individual patients enter the U.S. worker's compensation health care system favor a clear diagnosis suggestive of a definitive plan of care. In the case of work-related health problems, health care delivery within the worker's compen-

sation system is further complicated by the need to assign injury causation to the workplace and to quantify employee disability to determine reimbursement for care and lost wages. WMSDs may be of insidious onset with vague early symptoms, are of multifactorial etiology, and frequently are exacerbated by nonworkplace factors. As a result, clinicians frequently do not intervene until the advanced stages of the development of these disorders, which diminishes treatment prognosis and contributes to long-term disability.

The Occupational Safety and Health Administration (OSHA) devised its Ergonomics Program Rule for U.S. manufacturing industries and other affected U.S. workers to mandate reduction of the effects of workplace risk factors associated with WMSD.[35] Despite its emphasis on primary prevention, the OSHA Ergonomics Program Rule was repealed before it went into effect by the U.S. Congress in March of 2001 under the Congressional Review Act of 1996. However, it is likely that OSHA will reintroduce such workplace regulation in the future. In this chapter, recent clinical research data concerning the effectiveness of such ergonomic programs are presented, the various components of effective workplace ergonomics programs are summarized, and the role of health care providers in the clinical management of these disorders is emphasized.

CLINICAL RESEARCH EVIDENCE FOR EFFECTIVE WORKPLACE MANAGEMENT OF UE WMSD

Two major contemporary reviews of the scientific literature concerning WMSDs help define a framework for the workplace management of these disorders. The first was conducted under the auspices of the National Institute of Occupational Safety and Health (NIOSH) and was concerned with epidemiologic investigations of workplace risk factors that contribute to the development of WMSD.[3] Six hundred epidemiologic studies were reviewed, and evidence for relationships between specific workplace risk factors and WMSDs were stratified. Strong evidence for work-relatedness was found for neck and neck and shoulder WMSD resulting from posture; for hand-arm vibration syndrome as a result of vibration; for elbow WMSD, for CTS, and for hand and wrist tendinitis resulting from risk factor combinations. Evidence for work-relatedness was found for neck and neck and shoulder WMSD caused by force or repetition; for shoulder WMSD resulting from posture or repetition; for elbow WMSD caused by force; for CTS resulting from force, repetition, or vibration; and for hand and wrist tendinitis caused by force, repetition, or posture. Insufficient evidence for work-relatedness was found for neck and neck and shoulder WMSD resulting from vibration; for shoulder WMSD resulting from force; for elbow WMSD caused by repetition or posture; for CTS caused by posture; and for hand and wrist tendinitis resulting from force, repetition, and posture. None of the 600 studies reviewed provided evidence of no effect of work factors. In the executive summary of this review, the editor[3] noted that the amount of detailed and quantitative information concerning the relationship between risk factor exposure and WMSD was limited and depended on a variety of factors, both physical and nonphysical, and both work-related and non–work-related. This review assisted NIOSH in setting the WMSD portion of the National Occupational Research Agenda, in which federal funding priorities were determined for research concerning the physical and psychosocial risk factors contributing to the development of WMSD.[32]

Following the NIOSH review, the National Institutes of Health asked the National Research Council (NRC) to assemble a steering committee of experts to conduct an independent review of the literature relevant to WMSD of the lower back, neck, and upper extremities.[33] The conclusions of this review were similar to the NIOSH review in terms of the causal relationship between physical risk factors and WMSD. The NRC review further examined the literature concerning clinical interventions. Many studies did demonstrate that various types of interventions, including exercise, employee education, and engineering controls, do help prevent the development of WMSD.[37] The NRC steering committee also pointed out that many studies demonstrated effectiveness of multicomponent interventions in the prevention and management of WMSD. Like the NIOSH review, the NRC review indicated the need for additional research into the mechanisms of disorder development; the exposure-response relationships between workplace risk factors and WMSD; and development of targeted interventions for workplace prevention, detection, and management of these potentially disabling conditions.

Epidemiologic studies continue to find positive relationships between work-place risk factors and the development and severity of UE WMSD. These risk factors include, for example, awkward postures, task repetition, task force, duration of exposure, job stress/dissatisfaction and other psychosocial factors, and risk factor combinations.* Clinical research studies are beginning to report more long-term treatment effects regarding the various components of intervention programs.

Feuerstein et al.[9] conducted a prospective, controlled clinical trial of the effects of a multidisciplinary rehabilitation program in 34 patients suffering from UE WMSD. Nineteen patients underwent the multidisciplinary treatment and 15 received usual care. The two groups were matched for duration of work disability, severity of pain, fear of reinjury, psychologic distress, perceived work environment, age, and educational level. The diagnoses represented in this study included CTS and enthesopathy of the elbow, and lateral and medial epicondylitis; however, a total of 16 diagnoses were represented. Some cases carried more than one diagnosis, which is common in UE WMSD cases. The multidisciplinary rehabilitation program consisted of five components: (1) warm-up period (30 minutes), (2) physical conditioning (55 minutes), (3) work conditioning (55 minutes), (4) stress management (45 minutes), and (5) ergonomic consultation. Components 1 through 4 were conducted daily for 4 to 6 weeks. The usual care group was managed by a primary

*References 5, 8, 11, 13, 14, 16, 18, 23, 26, 36, 38, 39.

care physician and possibly a rehabilitation nurse. The study outcomes measured were return to work at 3 to 18 months and return to full- or part-time work. Seventy-four percent of the multidisciplinary treatment group returned to work or enrolled in state-supported vocational training as compared with only 40% of the usual treatment group. Of those who returned to work, 91% of the multidisciplinary group returned to full-time employment as compared with only 50% in the usual treatment group. The authors[9] of the study concluded that multidisciplinary treatment programs with medical management as well as ergonomic and psychosocial components improved treatment success. However, they cautioned that longer-term studies are needed to assess the occurrence of reinjury and prolonged disability.

In another study investigating a multidisciplinary approach to WMSD management, Barthel et al.[2] retrospectively reviewed 24 cases of patients with UE WMSD. The investigators categorized these patients' symptoms into 4 groups: (1) diffuse tenderness of the proximal finger flexor tendons, the lateral and medial epicondylar regions, the proximal extensor muscle mass, and the supinator trigger point; (2) focal dystonia; (3) radial tunnel syndrome; and (4) myofascial pain. Interestingly, all of the patients had symptoms falling into category 1 (tenderness of the wrist extensors and wrist and finger flexors), but many had additional symptoms from one or more of the other categories. Of the 24 patients, 20 reported that their symptoms resulted from computer-related work. Of these cases, 90% presented with bilateral involvement. A three-point outcome rating scale was used to determine treatment outcome. Of the 24 cases, 6 received the highest rating of III, indicating substantial improvement in symptoms and return to work. Thirteen patients received a rating of II, indicating a modest or partial improvement in symptoms and return to regular or modified work. Five patients received a rating of I, indicating only mild improvement in symptoms with no change in work status after treatment. The overall result was that 79% of these cases were able to continue work with total or partial resolution of symptoms and, in many cases, modified work tasks. These findings illustrate the importance of considering workplace ergonomic factors in the management of UE WMSD.

Chan et al.[6] conducted a clinical trial of a standardized 6-week intervention for work-related lateral epicondylitis. This program consisted of three components: (1) educational sessions, (2) a home exercise program, and (3) progressive work-hardening training. Fifteen female patients were enrolled in this study. Pretreatment and posttreatment measurements of pain intensity, isometric strength and endurance, self-perceived performance competence, and satisfaction with performance showed significant improvement over the 6-week treatment period. This study showed that a multifaceted rehabilitation program could improve

both the physical capacity and psychologic well-being of patients with this common UE WMSD diagnosis. The investigators suggest that controlled clinical trials with long-term outcomes need to be conducted.[6]

These three studies illustrate some important issues in the current state of clinical research in the area of UE WMSD. First, many patients suffering from UE WMSD present with multiple diagnoses or symptoms involving multiple regions of the upper limb and cervical spine. Therefore it is difficult and unrealistic to select distinct diagnostic groups to study (see reference 7 for a discussion of diagnostic criteria for UE WMSD). Management programs that address workplace risk factors, both physical and psychosocial, show better treatment outcomes than those that are restricted to usual clinical practices. Finally, patients may not experience complete resolution of symptoms, rather they often will need to participate in the long-term management of their disorder. This requires effective communication and collaboration between affected employees, their employers, and their health care providers. One of the shortcomings of the three programs described is that they were conducted in a clinical setting. It would be advantageous for workplaces to establish WMSD management programs on site. Fortunately, recent literature suggests possible structures for such programs and research to support their effectiveness.

Feuerstein et al.[10] investigated the effects of a multicomponent intervention program on UE WMSD in sign language interpreters. They conducted a prospective, uncontrolled group outcome study in which subjects were followed for 3 years after the intervention. Fifty-three subjects, 35 symptomatic and 18 asymptomatic, participated in this workplace intervention program. The program had 5 components: (1) reduce physical work load and improve flexibility and endurance through exercise, (2) train employees in job stress management, (3) change work organization and work style to reduce biomechanical risk exposure, (4) improve managerial skill in addressing UE WMSD and increase supervisor support through training, and (5) educate workers and supervisors regarding optimal health care utilization. The intervention was delivered in eleven 1.5-hour sessions over a period of 10 weeks and was conducted by various team members consisting of a clinical psychologist, a physical therapist, an exercise physiologist, and a physician with board certification in occupational medicine and rehabilitation medicine. In the 3 years following the intervention, there was a 69% reduction in the number of UE WMSD cases reported as compared with the 3 years before the intervention (24 and 78 cases, respectively). Workers' compensation health care costs were reduced 30% in the 2 years following the intervention as compared with the 2 years before the intervention ($68,000 and $97,000, respectively). Workers' compensation indemnity costs declined 64% in the 3 years following the intervention. Finally, the number of work hours logged

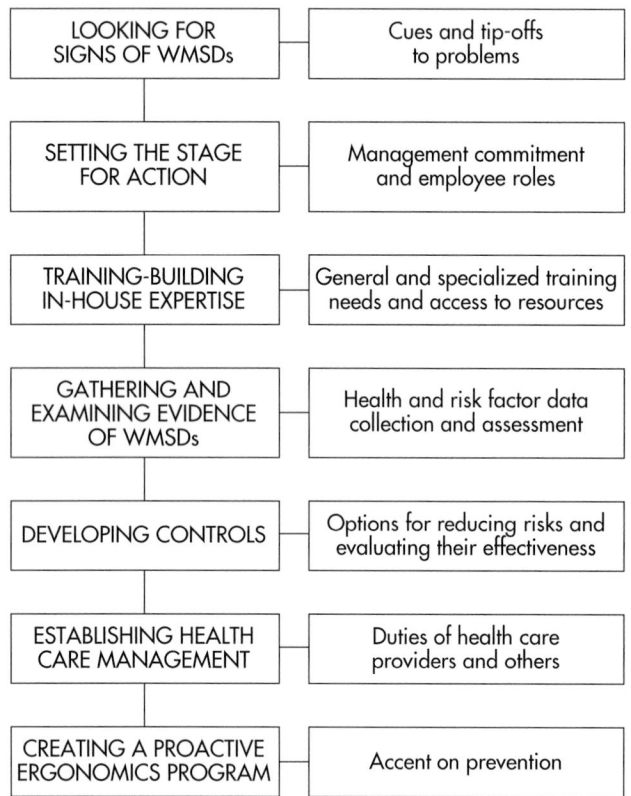

A Pathway to Controlling Work-Related Musculoskeletal Disorders (WMSDs)

Fig. 59-3. National Institute of Occupational Safety and Health (NIOSH) pathway through the seven elements of an effective workplace ergonomics program.[30] Step 1 entails looking for signs of potential musculoskeletal problems in the workplace, such as a high frequency of injury reports or the identification of jobs that expose workers to one or more known risk factors. In step 2, the employer must show management commitment in addressing possible work-related musculoskeletal disorders (WMSDs) and encourage worker involvement in problem-solving activities. Step 3 involves offering training to expand management and worker ability to evaluate potential WMSDs. In step 4, the gathering of data to identify jobs or work conditions that are most problematic is conducted. Sources of data might include injury and illness logs (i.e., OSHA 200 logs), occupational health records, symptom surveys, and job analyses. Step 5 requires identification of effective controls for high-risk tasks and then evaluation of their effectiveness once they have been implemented. In step 6, a health care management scheme should be instituted that emphasizes early detection and treatment of WMSD to prevent impairment and long-term disability. Step 7 focuses on minimizing risk factors for WMSD during the planning of new work processes and operations. Not only does such planning prevent the occurrence of WMSDs, but it also avoids costly work redesign in response to control of future WMSD incidents. (From National Institute of Occupational Safety and Health: Elements of ergonomics programs: a primer based on workplace evaluations of musculoskeletal disorders, DHHS [NIOSH] Publication No. 97-117, 1997.)

increased after the intervention, which coincides with the decreased number of reported cases of UE WMSD. This study not only demonstrated the effectiveness of a multidisciplinary approach to WMSD management but also illustrated the feasibility of a workplace management program tailored to the needs of the specific employer and employees, and is one of the few studies to analyze health care cost and indemnity outcomes. The latter findings illustrate clearly the cost benefits of workplace ergonomics management in terms of both cost savings and increased worker productivity.[10]

GUIDELINES FOR WORKPLACE MANAGEMENT OF UE WMSD

NIOSH published a compendium of presentations from industry representatives who have established successful workplace ergonomics programs.[31] Additional examples of such programs have been described in the literature.[17,19,22,25,27-29] Based on the epidemiologic and clinical research, OSHA, NIOSH, and the National Safety Council individually have developed guidelines for workplace ergonomics programs.[30,34,35] Although the regulation of UE WMSD through an OSHA work rule is presently uncertain, each of the ergonomics program guidelines from these governmental and quasi-governmental agencies embrace the same basic program components, which were delineated in the OSHA ergonomics program guidelines as follows: (1) management leadership, which consists of an effective reporting system; prompt responses to reported cases of WMSD; clear program responsibilities for participants; and regular communication between program participants; (2) employee participation, which requires employee cooperation in the early reporting of WMSD and active involvement in the development and implementation of the program; (3) job hazard analysis and control, which requires the means to identify hazards or risk factors, analyze their impact, modify jobs or equipment to reduce risk and evaluate the effectiveness of hazard control measures; (4) training of managers, supervisors, and employees in the risks and detection of WMSD and the procedures required to respond to an WMSD incident; and (5) regular program evaluation in which quantifiable measures, such as number and severity of WMSD, are determined.[35]

NIOSH schematized these major program components in its Primer on the Elements of Ergonomics Programs (Fig. 59-3).[30] This schematic emphasizes not only the importance of an effective response to cases of WMSD, but also that of prevention of these disorders in presently unaffected employees. It also emphasizes the need for the program to become an integral part of the workplace culture to be successful. It has been my experience that the commitment shown by employers who spearhead the development of a workplace ergonomics program has a positive effect on employee morale and therefore on job satisfaction. In other words, the mere presence of a company-based ergonomics program may, in and of itself, reduce one of the risk factors for WMSD.

ROLE OF HEALTH CARE PROVIDERS IN WORKPLACE MANAGEMENT OF WMSD

Health care providers who participate in workplace ergonomics programs must interact with other program team members to ensure the optimum therapeutic management of affected employees. This participation goes well beyond isolated diagnosis and treatment in the clinic. The health care provider must also understand the risk factors to which an affected employee is exposed in his or her job. This may require that the health care provider interview both the employee and the supervisor, or even perform a job or workstation analysis. When hazard controls are needed, the health care provider may be required to recommend the nature and extent of those controls. This requires an understanding of the engineering options available and effective communication with those members of the team who will order and install any necessary equipment. The health care provider must follow up with employees to ascertain the effectiveness of treatment and workplace controls. This latter point was illustrated recently in a study that showed that only 52% of 537 worker's compensation claimants in the state of Maryland reported employer actions to investigate or reduce risk factors for UE WMSD as recommended by their health care providers.[20] With proper follow-up by health care providers, such poor compliance situations may be avoided.

An algorithm describing one approach to medical management in a company-based ergonomics program is depicted in Fig. 59-4. This algorithm is based on the development of a workplace ergonomics program at a music and entertainment company with approximately 1500 employees where computer work was highly prevalent.[1] The health and safety department, which staffed three full-time nurses, a case manager, a part-time ergonomics consultant, and a part-time physician, was the central department for the ergonomics program. Aside from the clinical facilities of the health and safety department, there was also an on-site fitness facility with staff that participated in the medical management of WMSD. As part of this program, a clinical algorithm was established in which an employee-initiated report of WMSD was handled in a triage procedure. Full-time nursing staff performed an initial screening examination that helped determine the appropriate level of care. Three levels of care were available: level I (or conservative nursing management), level II (on-site physician diagnosis and management), and level III (specialist diagnosis and management). For all levels of care, exercise programs could be overseen by the

fitness facility staff, which also received training in the detection, risk reduction, and medical management of WMSD. This program used the existing health and safety department personnel of the company and empowered them to intervene in the case of affected employees. This was accomplished, first and foremost, through employer commitment to establishing a proactive program to reduce employee risk and morbidity. Consultation with clinical and ergonomics experts enabled this employer commitment to be realized in the form of a streamlined and effective workplace ergonomics program.

Other models for such programs exist and are successful. Each workplace has its own unique qualities and needs. Therefore it is necessary that any outside consultants asked to assist in the development of workplace medical management programs familiarize themselves with the company's idiosyncrasies. In addition, health care providers who are asked to provide clinical services to employees should make an effort to become an integral member of the workplace ergonomics program team even if they are not employees of that company. Finally, health care providers involved in the management of WMSD should approach these patients holistically as warranted by the multifactorial etiology of these disorders.

SUMMARY AND CONCLUSIONS

Epidemiologic studies continue to find positive relationships between physical and nonphysical, and workplace and nonworkplace, risk factors and the development and severity of musculoskeletal disorders. These disorders account for approximately 4% to 4.5% of all injuries and illness in U.S. private industry annually and result in lost work days, lost worker productivity, high medical care costs, and a negative effect on worker quality of life. Clinical intervention studies have demonstrated that risk reduction through multifactorial ergonomics programs can reduce the impact of these disorders on both the worker and the workplace. Such programs most often target physical risk control, but those that also include stress management have better outcomes than those that do not. The key components to a comprehensive workplace ergonomics program include management commitment and leadership, employee participation, hazard analysis and control, training, and program evaluation. Medical management can be provided through external health care providers or by existing workplace employee health services. Regardless of the WMSD medical management model used by a company, participating health care providers must communicate with other ergonomics program team members as well as with the affected worker to ensure that recommendations for risk reduction are properly implemented and effective. Finally, employers should recognize that effective management of WMSD contributes to a healthier and more productive work force while at

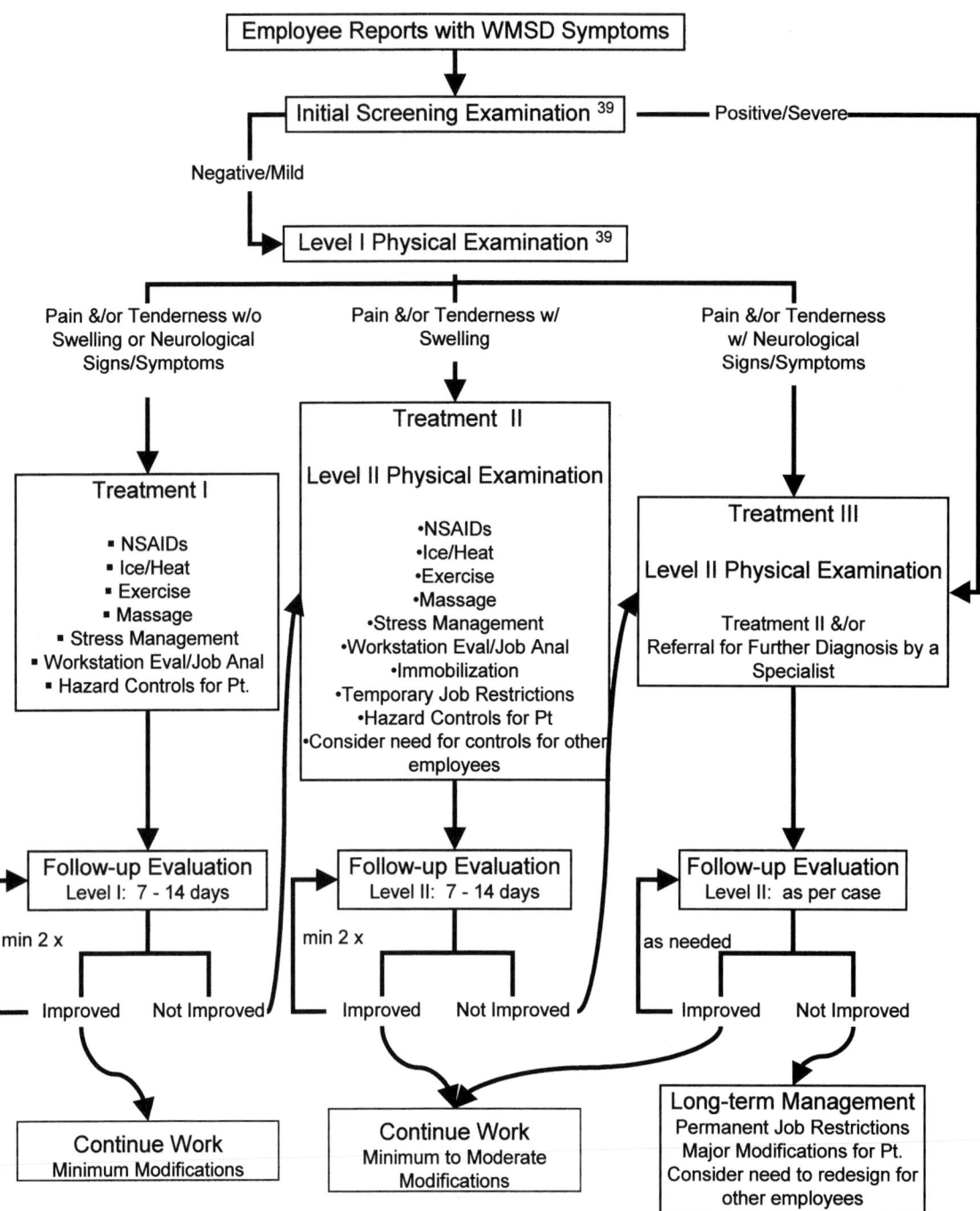

Fig. 59-4. Algorithm for a company-based upper extremity work-related musculoskeletal disorder (UE WMSD) medical management program.[1] The algorithm is triggered by an employee report of UE WMSD symptoms. An on-site occupational health nurse conducts an initial screening examination, which takes approximately 10 to 15 minutes. Based on the result of the screening, the employee proceeds to either level I physical examination, which is a more thorough nursing examination, or to level II physical examination, which is conducted by an occupational health physician. In the case of level I physical examination, employees with mild signs and symptoms may be treated conservatively by nursing and fitness center staff (treatment I). For moderate to severe signs and symptoms, employees will go on for level II physical examination. Based on the level II examination results, employees will be recommended for either treatment II, in which temporary job restrictions may be imposed, or treatment III, which may require specialist care for further diagnosis and treatment outside the company health and safety department and/or permanent job restrictions or redesign. In all three treatment options, the algorithm includes at least two time points for follow-up over the first 1 to 2 months of care. In cases in which the employee's condition either does not improve or worsens, the employee can be referred for the next highest level of care in the algorithm. The use of such an algorithm empowers health care providers within the company to clearly identify and track progress of affected employees and provides guidelines for clinical decision making. *NSAIDs,* Nonsteroidal antiinflammatory drugs.

the same time reducing the medical care and indemnity costs associated with these disorders. In this light, their specific cause, or percentage thereof, relative to particular work tasks may not be as important as the benefits of preventing and managing WMSD.

WEBSITES

Bureau of Labor Statistics: www.stats.bls.gov/
National Institute of Occupational Safety and Health: www.cdc.gov/niosh
Occupational Safety and Health Administration: www.osha.gov/

REFERENCES

1. Barr AE, et al: Development of a physical examination for a company-based management program for work-related upper extremity cumulative trauma disorders, *J Occup Rehabil* 9:63, 1999.
2. Barthel HR, et al: Presentation and response of patients with upper extremity repetitive use syndrome to a multidisciplinary rehabilitation program: a retrospective review of 24 cases, *J Hand Ther* 11:191, 1998.
3. Bernard BP: Musculoskeletal disorders (MSDs) and workplace factors: a critical review of epidemiologic evidence for work-related musculoskeletal disorders of the neck, upper extremity, and low back. Department of Health and Human Services (DHHS) (National Institute of Occupational Safety and Health [NIOSH]) Publication No. 97-141, 1997.
4. Brogmus GE, Webster B, Sorock G: Recent trends in cumulative trauma disorders of the upper extremities in the United States, *J Occup Env Med* 38:401, 1996.
5. Burdorf A, Riel M, Brand T: Physical load as a risk factor for musculoskeletal complaints among tank terminal workers, *Am Ind Hygiene Assoc J* 58:489, 1997.
6. Chan CCH, et al: A standardized clinical series for work-related lateral epicondylitis, *J Occup Rehabil* 10:143, 2000.
7. Davis TRC: Diagnostic criteria for upper limb disorders in epidemiological studies, *J Hand Surg* 23B:567, 1998.
8. Dzwierzynski WW, et al: Psychometric assessment of patients with chronic upper extremity pain attributed to workplace exposure, *J Hand Surg* 24A:46, 1999.
9. Feuerstein M, et al: Multidisciplinary rehabilitation of chronic work-related upper extremity disorders: long term effects, *J Occup Med* 35:396, 1993.
10. Feuerstein M, et al: Multicomponent intervention for work-related upper extremity disorders, *J Occup Rehabil* 10:71, 2000.
11. Feuerstein M, et al: Occupational upper extremity disorders in the federal workforce, *J Occup Env Med* 40:546, 1998.
12. Fogleman M, Brogmus G: Computer mouse use and cumulative trauma disorders of the upper extremities, *Ergonom* 38:2465, 1995.
13. Fredriksson K, et al: Risk factors for neck and shoulder disorders: a nested case-control study covering a 24 year period, *Am J Ind Med* 38:516, 2000.
14. Haufler AJ, Feuerstein M, Huang GD: Job stress, upper extremity pain and functional limitations in symptomatic computer users, *Am J Ind Med* 38:507, 2000.
15. Herbert R, Janeway K, Schechter C: Carpal tunnel syndrome and workers' compensation among an occupational clinic population in New York state, *Am J Ind Med* 35:335, 1999.
16. Hess D: Employee perceived stress: relationship to the development of repetitive strain injury symptoms, *AAOHN J* 45:115, 1997.
17. Hochanadel CD, Conrad DE: Evolution of an on-site industrial physical therapy program, *J Occup Med* 35:1011, 1993.
18. Holness DL, Beaton D, House RA: Prevalence of upper extremity symptoms and possible risk factors in workers handling paper currency, *J Occup Med* 48:231, 1998.
19. Kemmlert K: Economic impact of ergonomic intervention: four case studies, *J Occup Rehabil* 6:17, 1996.
20. Keogh JP, et al: Patterns and predictors of employer risk-reduction activities (ERRAs) in response to a work-related upper extremity cumulative trauma disorder (UECTD): reports from workers' compensation claimants, *Am J Ind Med* 38:489, 2000.
21. Keogh JP, et al: The impact of occupational injury on injured worker and family: outcomes of upper extremity cumulative trauma disorders in Maryland workers, *Am J Ind Med* 38:498, 2000.
22. Keyserling WM, Brouwer M, Silverstein BA: The effectiveness of a joint labor-management program in controlling awkward postures of the trunk, neck, and shoulders: results of a field study, *Int J Ind Ergonom* 11:51, 1993.
23. Latko WA, et al: Cross-sectional study of the relationship between repetitive work and the prevalence of upper limb musculoskeletal disorders, *Am J Ind Med* 36:248, 1999.
24. Levenstein C: Economic losses from repetitive strain injuries, *Occup Med* 14:149, 1999.
25. Lutz G, Hansford T: Cumulative trauma disorder controls: the ergonomics program at Ethicon, Inc, *J Hand Surg* 12A:863, 1997.
26. Macfarlane GJ, Hunt IM, Silman AJ: Role of mechanical and psychosocial factors in the onset of forearm pain: prospective population based study. *Br Med J* 321:1, 2000.
27. Mattila M: Improvement in the occupational health program in a Finnish construction company by means of a systematic workplace investigation of job load and hazard analysis, *Am J Ind Med* 15:61, 1989.
28. McKenzie F, et al: A program for control of repetitive trauma disorders associated with hand tool operations in a telecommunications manufacturing facility, *Am Ind Hyg Assoc J* 46:674, 1985.
29. Moore JS, Garg A: Participatory ergonomics in a red meat packing plant part II: case studies, *Am Ind Hyg Assoc J* 58:498, 1997.
30. National Institute of Occupational Safety and Health (NIOSH): Elements of ergonomics programs: a primer based on workplace evaluations of musculoskeletal disorders, Department of Health and Human Services (DHHS) (NIOSH) Publication No. 97-117, 1997.
31. National Institute of Occupational Safety and Health (NIOSH): Ergonomics: effective workplace practices and programs. Transcripts of Presentations for Conference Sponsored by NIOSH and OSHA, Chicago, Illinois, 1997. (www.cdc.gov/niosh/homepage.html)
32. National Institute of Occupational Safety and Health (NIOSH): National occupational research agenda for musculoskeletal disorders: research topics for the next decade, Department of Health and Human Services (DHHS) (NIOSH) Publication No. 2001-117, 2001.
33. National Research Council: *Work-related musculoskeletal disorders: report, workshop summary, and workshop papers,* Washington, DC, 1999, National Academy Press.
34. National Safety Council: Management of work-related musculoskeletal disorders. Accredited Standards Committee Z365, Working Draft, 2000.
35. Occupational Safety and Health Administration (OSHA): Ergonomics Program: Final Rule: 29 CFR Part 1910, Department of Labor, Occupational Safety and Health Administration, *Federal Register* 64:68262, 2000.
36. Silverstein B, et al: Claims incidence of work-related disorders of the upper extremity: Washington state, 1987 through 1995, *Am J Public Health* 88:1827, 1998.

37. Smith MJ, Karsh BT, Moro FBP: A review of research on interventions to control musculoskeletal disorders. In National Research Council: *Work-related musculoskeletal disorders: report, workshop summary, and workshop papers,* Washington, DC, 1999, National Academy Press.

38. Stoy DW, Aspen J: Force and repetition measurement of ham boning: relationship to musculoskeletal symptoms, *AAOHN J* 47:254, 1999.

39. Weigert BJ, et al: Neuromuscular and psychological characteristics in subjects with work-related forearm pain, *Am J Phys Med Rehabil* 78:545, 1999.

Chapter 60

THERAPIST'S EVALUATION AND TREATMENT OF UPPER EXTREMITY CUMULATIVE TRAUMA DISORDERS

Mary C. Kasch

OVERVIEW

A number of terms are used throughout the world to describe chronic musculoskeletal injuries, including *overuse syndromes, repetitive strain injuries, cervicobrachial disorders, repetitive motion injuries,* and in the United States, *cumulative trauma disorders* (CTDs). CTDs of the upper extremity, such as tendinitis, nerve entrapment syndromes, and myofascial pain, are common ailments in many occupations.[2]

The incidence of CTDs in the United States has increased tremendously from 50,000 cases in 1985 to 281,800 cases in 1992. Between 1981 and 1992, CTDs increased from 18% to 62% of all worker's compensation claims filed.[6,19] The cost of CTDs is alarming. The National Council on Compensation Insurance estimates that average costs for medical care and lost wages are $29,000 per claim, about 50% more than any other work-related illness or injury.[13] Liberty Mutual found that in 1989, the mean cost per case of upper extremity disorders was $8070; the total compensable cost for upper extremity CTDs was estimated to be $563 million.[37] Trends in the workplace (e.g., advances in technology, postural loads, longer work hours, increased production demands),[33] in the nature of the work performed (e.g., repetitive, static, and highly detailed work),[33] in the workforce (e.g., age and gender of workers), and in society (e.g., changes in the medicolegal environment in worker's compensation)[27] all have contributed to the rise in CTDs. Other significant factors are improved accuracy of reporting,

greater awareness of the problem by employees and employers, and advances in diagnosis.[31]

The term *CTD* should be viewed as a description of the mechanism of injury, not as a diagnosis. Even when the presenting symptoms are confusing, attempts to define a specific diagnosis are necessary because "each disorder has a different cause, treatment, and prognosis."[31] Box 60-1 lists many of the common diagnoses that are seen as CTDs.

RISK FACTORS

Work-related risk factors for CTDs include the following[2]:

- Repetition
- High force
- Awkward postures
- Direct pressure
- Vibration
- Prolonged static positioning

Exposure to risk factors may result in an adaptation (e.g., strengthening from the training effect) or an injury, which is usually manifested first as fatigue and pain. Intervention before the development of a chronic condition may be possible if the factors that contribute to the problem are understood.

A number of theories have been proposed to explain the development of pain and dysfunction associated with repetitive movement. Perhaps the most widely accepted

---

Box 60-1 Types of cumulative trauma disorders

Nerve compression syndromes

Cervical radiculopathy
Thoracic outlet syndrome
Cubital tunnel syndrome
Anterior interosseous syndrome
Posterior interosseous syndrome
Pronator teres syndrome
Carpal tunnel syndrome
Guyon's canal syndrome

Tendinitis/tenosynovitis

Extensors
de Quervain's
    Intersection syndrome
    Extensor indicis proprius
    Extensor carpi ulnaris
Flexors
    Flexor carpi radialis
    Flexor carpi ulnaris
    Trigger digits

Pain syndromes

Reflex sympathetic dystrophy
Myofascial pain syndrome
Fibrositis
Fibromyalgia

Other

Vibration white finger
Arthritis

---

hypothesis is that high levels of repetition lead to tissue microtrauma and muscle fatigue, as proposed by a variety of authors.[2,27,29,30,33]

Muscle fatigue develops when work is performed over a prolonged period. Muscle fatigue is "the point at which a specific job or work can no longer be performed with the same intensity."[30] Chronic muscle fatigue that develops in response to work tasks is not relieved by rest. The amount of fatigue is proportional to the amount of force and the duration of force application. Fatigue occurs more quickly with high force. If force is maintained, repetitions must be reduced to allow recovery. Therefore, if the force is decreased while repetitions are maintained and recovery time is adequate, harm is less likely to occur. The combination of repetitions without adequate recovery time and high force establishes an environment that is likely to lead to injury.[27] It has been found that jobs requiring the highest repetition with the least rest per cycle had the highest impairment ratings in workers who were evaluated on the basis of both subjective symptoms and objective measures.[15]

Mechanical and chemical factors may contribute to work-related pain.[30] The mechanical forces that occur in the muscles depend on muscle fiber recruitment and the type of contraction used (static versus dynamic or concentric versus eccentric).[30] If the force development is high (but not high enough to cause tissue failure), microtrauma can occur, especially during eccentric contraction. Repeated microtrauma can result in degeneration and inflammatory processes in the tendons or paratenon, muscles, and joints. Even low contraction levels can diminish muscle function and result in increased adverse reactions such as intramuscular resting pressure, muscle edema, and muscle enzymes in the blood. Diminished muscle function is experienced as muscle soreness and stiffness.

Increased intramuscular pressure leads to decreased blood flow, especially during static contractions. Insufficient blood flow can lead to a muscle energy crisis and pain.[30] In addition, there is a close relationship between fatigue and depletion of glycogen in individual muscle fibers, which may be a risk factor in the development of muscle pain.[30] Accumulation of lactic acid, accompanied by a fall in pH, may also play a role in fatigue and pain. If sufficient recovery is permitted after microtrauma, the result may be stronger tissue (the training effect). If recovery is insufficient, muscle injury may occur.[30] Recommended treatment includes rest, splinting, and antiinflammatory medications.

Higgs and Mackinnon[14] have hypothesized that maintenance of abnormal or prolonged posture, positions, or movement results in muscle imbalance (overuse/underuse and muscle shortening/lengthening) that leads to weakness and pain. These positions may also cause pressure around or stretch on a nerve, leading to nerve compression.[14] Recommended treatment includes ergonomic modifications, breaks, alternate sleeping postures, and improved fitness.

Psychologic factors may also play a role in the development of cumulative trauma. Millender[22] and Millender and Conlon[23] suggested that a comprehensive approach to treatment is ideal because of the "myriad of physical, psychological and social problems that affect patients and impede their ability to manage a work-related disorder." It has been found that perceived stress may be associated with repetition, job dissatisfaction, anxiety, depression, and pain complaints, but the relationship is difficult to quantify because of the complexity of measuring psychosocial phenomena.[35] Psychologic problems are difficult to treat within the context of a work-related injury and are often not addressed. However, it has been my clinical experience that providing treatment that is goal directed and strongly educational will often provide the patient with a sense of control and relief about his or her symptoms, which often facilitates increased cooperation with the treatment program.

Patients often report an almost immediate return of symptoms when they return to work or to the task associated with the injury, which makes CTDs especially difficult to treat. Byl et al.[10] have proposed a hypothesis that symptoms return because of a memory associated with a specific task. She and a group of research collaborators at the University of California, San Francisco, have found that repetitive hand

Health History

General information

Name _____ Birthdate _____ Today's date_____
Occupation_____ Employer _____
Highest level of education _____ High school _____ College _____ Postgraduate

Detailed personal medical history

Have you ever had: | *Circle yes or no* | *Please describe*

Allergies . . . . yes no _____
Cancer . . . . yes no _____
Chest discomfort with exertion . . . . yes no _____
Diabetes . . . . yes no _____
Epilepsy. . . . . yes no _____
Heart disease. . . . . yes no _____
High blood pressure . . . . yes no _____
Light-headedness or fainting. . . . . yes no _____
Migraine . . . . yes no _____
Orthopedic problems, arthritis . . . . yes no _____
Peripheral vascular disease . . . . yes no _____
Phlebitis, emboli . . . . yes no _____
Pulmonary disease . . . . yes no _____
Recent illness, hospitalization, or surgery . . yes no _____
Stroke. . . . . yes no _____
Tuberculosis . . . . yes no _____
Unusual shortness of breath . . . . yes no _____
Present illnesses: _____
Past and present injuries: _____
Restrictions/limitations: _____
Medications: _____

Family history

Has a blood relative ever had: | *Circle yes or no* | *Who?*

Cancer . . . . yes no _____
Coronary or heart disease . . . . yes no _____
Sudden death. yes no (at what age) _____

Personal habits

Do you exercise? _____ How often? _____
What type of exercise do you do? _____
Do you smoke? _____ How much? _____
Average hours of sleep each night? _____ Sleep problems? _____
Alcoholic beverages (circle one):   never   rarely   moderate   daily
Beverages with caffeine (including cola)   never   rarely   moderate   daily # _____
Work (job): _____ Hours per day _____ Circle one: indoors outdoors
Do you like your job?   yes   no   Comment: _____
Please list your recreational activities and hobbies: _____
_____

Fig. 60-1. Health history form.

opening and closing may lead to motor control problems and the development of focal hand dystonias through a degradation of cortical representation.[10] The learning hypothesis is that "highly attended, goal directed, rapid, repetitive, flexion and extension movements of the digits lead to simultaneous sensory stimulation of adjacent digits."[8] This may disrupt the sensory motor feedback loop and lead to awkward movements when performing a specific task. In contrast, nonsimultaneous and slow repetitive movements do not appear to cause movement dysfunction or sensory degradation.[8] Cumulative trauma, whatever the causative factors, affects a worker's functional capacity and quality of life. Keogh et al.[20] reported that 53% of respondents reported symptoms that were severe enough to interfere with work as well as difficulty in performing even simple activities of daily living 1 to 4 years after injury. Many authors have reported improved long-term results with early intervention from physicians and therapists.

HAND THERAPY EVALUATION

As the incidence of CTDs has increased, many hand therapy clinics have experienced a corresponding rise in referrals of patients with CTDs. In a practice analysis survey of Certified Hand Therapists performed by the Hand Therapy Certification Commission in 1994, CTDs represented 26% of the diagnoses treated.[32] Managing these conditions can be deceptive in that early on they may appear simple, but as chronicity develops, they are more complex to evaluate and treat. The effect of a combination of factors, including accurate diagnosis and medical management, job satisfaction, pain, and the degree of support or nonsupport at work and at home,[17] may result in feelings of helplessness or anger on the part of the patient, with subsequent development of a quagmire of signs and symptoms that appear contradictory and unexplainable.

CTDs require a systems approach in the clinic and in the workplace. A series of steps should be followed when the patient with cumulative trauma is referred to therapy. First, a health history form (Fig. 60-1) should be completed and reviewed by the therapist with the patient. A review of the progression of the injury with attention given to the nature, location, and duration of the symptoms experienced is important to identify. What is the relationship between activity and pain, tingling, or numbness? What relieves the pain? What exacerbates it? How quickly does the pain return when activity is resumed? A body pain chart and visual analog scale (Figs. 60-2 and 60-3) will assist the therapist in objectively charting the information given by the patient.

Standard measurements of range of motion (ROM), grip and pinch strength, and hand/arm volume should be recorded, although limitations in standard measurements do not always correlate well with functional limitations. Palpation of the tendons and muscles for swelling, trigger points, and passive limitations should be performed. Body posture should be analyzed. Screening examination of the cervical neck and shoulder regions should be included in evaluation of hand conditions to determine whether these areas are contributing to the patient's symptoms or limitations in function. Active movements of the neck should be conducted, with attention paid to complaints of upper extremity symptoms during cervical extension or lateral flexion to the same side. Complaints during these movements may be suggestive of nerve root irritation. Hand symptoms with opposite side bending may be a sign of adverse neural tension. Table 60-1 summarizes the components of the evaluation process.

TREATMENT OVERVIEW

Various treatment programs have been recommended for CTDs. No one approach appears to work for all patients because of the complexity of causative factors and patient response. An algorithm for evaluation and treatment of upper extremity CTDs (Fig. 60-4) may assist the therapist in evaluating symptoms and developing an appropriate treatment plan. The evaluation results will lead to a treatment program designed to reduce the symptoms.

In a new approach to treatment, Byl and Melnick[9] have demonstrated that appropriate sensory input is necessary to translate neural information into coordinated, voluntary movement. The somatic sensory cortex is mapped by body part as well as function. For example, writing activates the same area of the brain whether it is performed with the hand or the foot.[9] Byl and Melnick[8,9] hypothesize that if the brain cortex is highly plastic and highly attended repetitive behaviors lead to degradation of the representation of the hand, then specific, attended sensory retraining should be able to restore sensory representation and therefore improve motor control. Byl et al.[10] propose a clinical treatment program of specific sensory and motor retraining, including comprehensive stress reduction, mental imaging, mirror practice, and biofeedback to restore normal sensory motor processing.

In observing patients with CTDs, it is often noted that they breathe shallowly, using the upper chest, and take quick, shallow breaths rather than deep, diaphragmatic breaths. This can be documented by observing/palpating the scalene muscles while the patient inhales and exhales; during diaphragmatic breathing, the scalene muscles and upper chest should exhibit minimal movement. An important component of treatment for these patients is to instruct in proper deep-breathing techniques to increase oxygenation to the body. Deep breathing is also an effective stress reduction technique that is easily taught and can be performed at any time during the workday.

In my experience, the diagnoses associated with cumulative trauma usually fall into one of three categories: (1) tendon disorders (e.g., tendinitis, tenosynovitis, tendinosis), (2) nerve compression syndromes (e.g., carpal tunnel syndrome [CTS], cubital tunnel syndrome), or (3) myofascial pain. Each type of disorder has its own hallmarks that

Body Pain Chart

Name

Date

Time

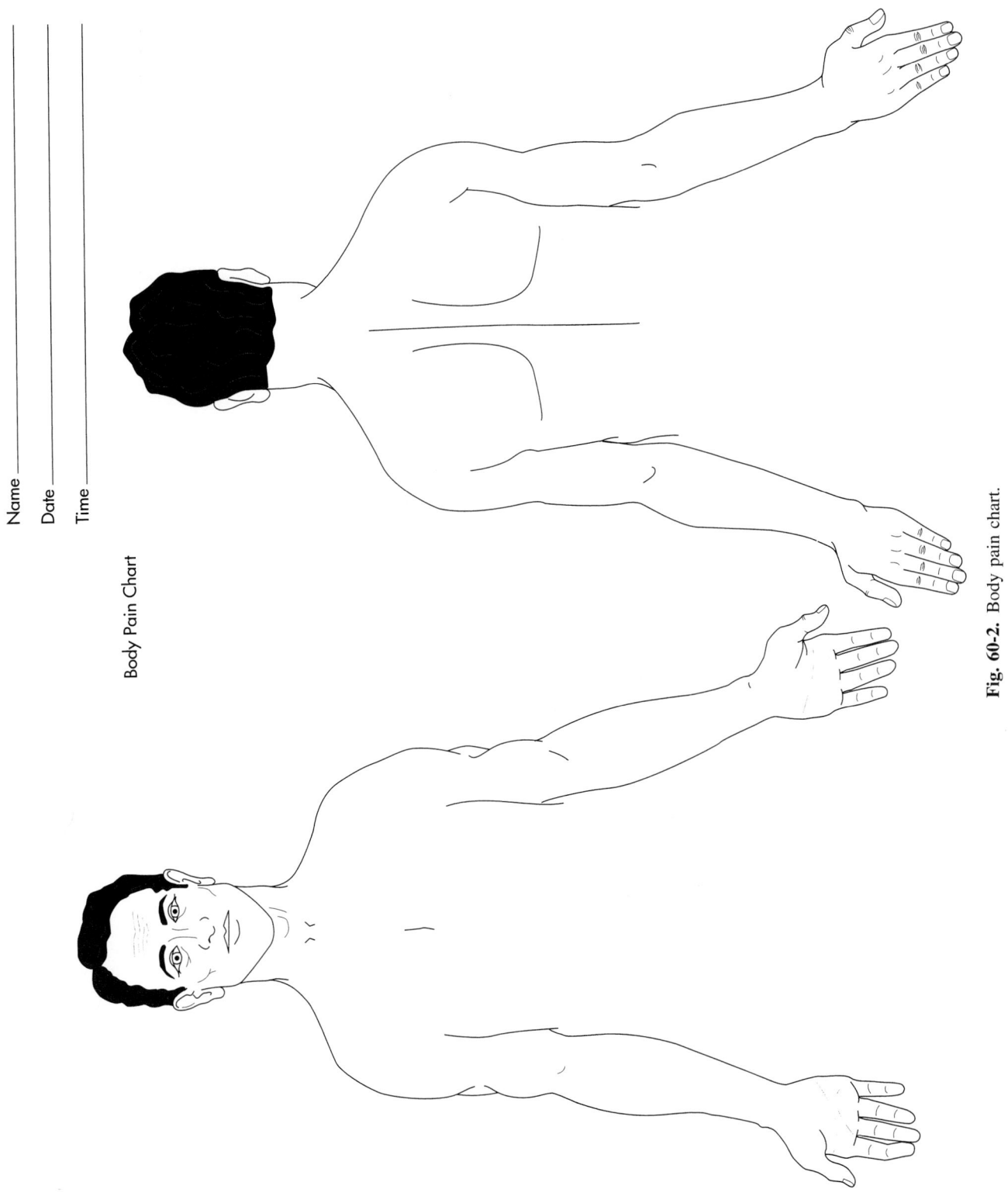

Fig. 60-2. Body pain chart.

Name _____

Date _____

Time _____

Visual Analogue Scale (VAS)

No pain

Most intense

Fig. 60-3. Visual analog scale (VAS).

Table 60-1. Components of the evaluation process

History	Subjective	Objective	Sensory
Health history form	Current symptoms	Cervical screening	Provocative tests
History of employment injury	Pain status	Postural analysis	Semmes-Weinstein test
Avocation/leisure activities	Activity of daily living status	Range of motion	Vibrometry
		Strength	Stress tests
		Palpation for trigger points, nodules, swelling	
		Work simulation	

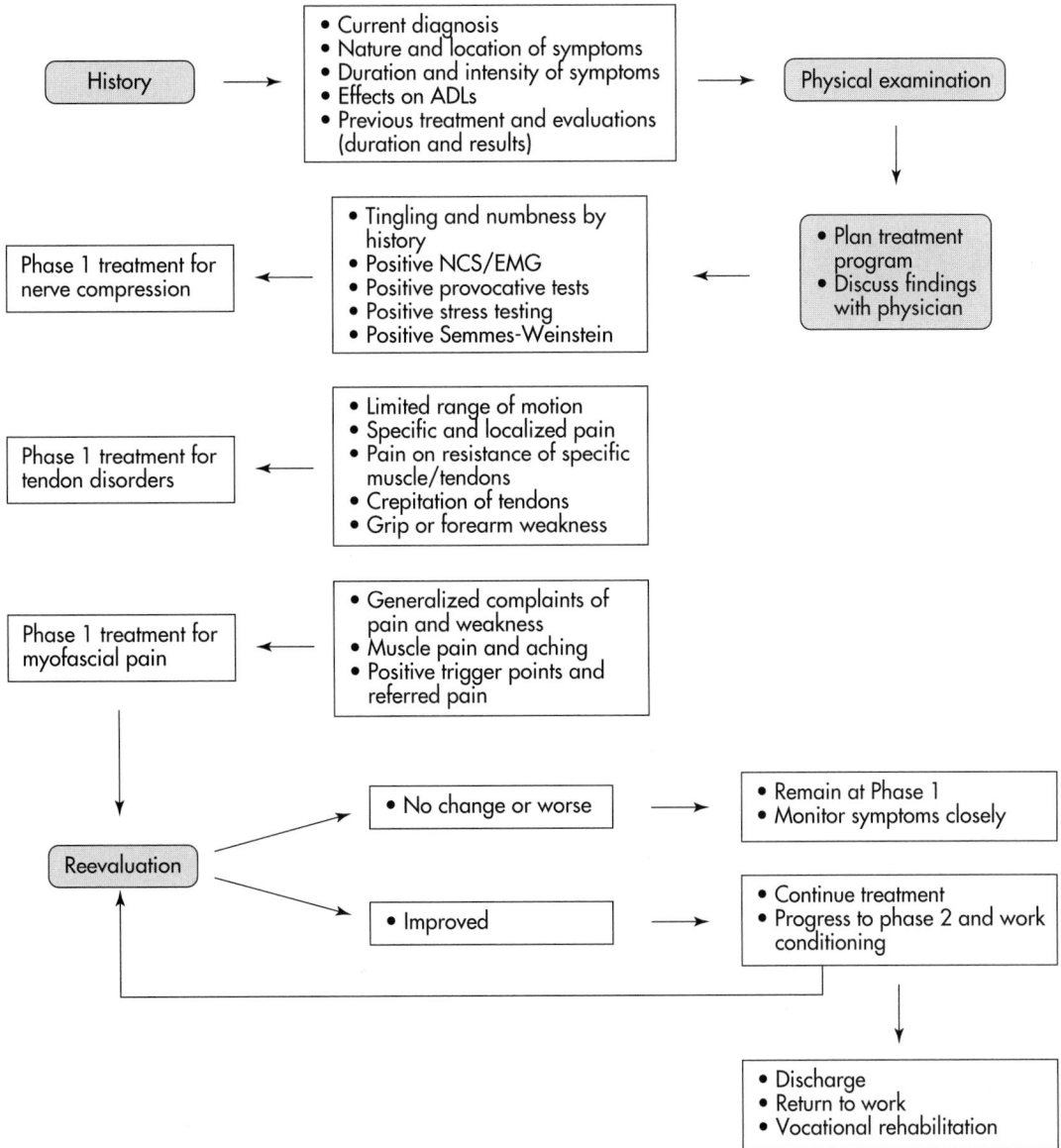

Fig. 60-4. Algorithm for evaluation and treatment of upper extremity cumulative trauma disorders. *ADLs,* Activities of daily living; *EMG,* electromyogram; *NCS,* nerve conduction study.

set it apart from other types. For example, if the patient has thoracic outlet syndrome, treatment will be geared toward correcting posture, reducing overhead reaching, altering biomechanics at work, and stretching tight structures in the upper quarter and chest. Treatment for forearm tendinitis might include splinting, stretching, icing, and rest. The specific findings should be used to guide treatment.

Further complicating the situation, therapists often discover new findings, such as trigger points in the trapezius muscles or tendinitis in the long head of the biceps. Many patients with myofascial pain have symptoms that are referred distally from a more proximal location. Patients with a diagnosis of one type of CTD may have other concurrent CTDs that will influence their care. Often, these

conditions are proximal. One should not assume that a diagnosis of a distal problem, such as CTS, excludes an additional diagnosis that is often in the cervicobrachial area.

Therapists are in a unique position to acquire and share information about CTDs. They take an active role in investigating the relationship between the injury and activity by replicating the symptoms experienced at work through work simulation, activity, and exercise. At the same time, they assess consistency of effort, document objective data and observations, and communicate findings to the treating physician. Although the therapist does not make a diagnosis, the information gleaned during evaluation will be of great value to the physician, and the diagnosis may change based on the results of therapy evaluation.

Table 60-2. Functional grading of cumulative trauma disorders

Grade	Characteristics
Grade I	Pain after activity; resolves quickly with rest. No decrease in amount or speed of work. Objective findings usually absent.
Grade II	Pain in one site while working. Pain is consistent while working but resolves when activity stops. Productivity may be mildly affected. May have objective findings.
Grade III	Pain in one or more sites while working. Pain persists after activity is stopped. Productivity affected, and multiple breaks may be necessary to continue working. May affect other activities away from work. May have weakness, loss of control and dexterity, tingling, numbness, and/or other objective findings. May have latent or active trigger points.
Grade IV	All common uses of hand/upper extremity cause pain, which is present 50%-75% of the time. May be unable to work or works in limited capacity. May have weakness, loss of control and dexterity, tingling, numbness, trigger points, and/or other objective findings.
Grade V	Loss of capacity to use hand because of chronic, unrelenting pain. Usually unable to work. Symptoms may persist indefinitely.

Adapted from Lowe C: *J Hand Ther* 5:84, 1992; modified from Fry HJH: *Med Probl Perform Art* 1:51, 1986.

Table 60-2 presents a grading system that describes the functional severity of the impairments that have resulted from the injury. Combining the objective findings with the grade of functional severity should result in a clear overall picture of the patient's degree of current impairment. The information is used to develop a treatment program that is appropriate for the condition. Emphasis should be placed on teaching coping skills and self-management techniques (e.g., training in stretching, minibreaks, icing, deep breathing, relaxation) to avoid prolonged therapeutic intervention. Treatment is not a cure in the sense of eliminating the condition, but rather it is a change in lifestyle that allows the patient to control the symptoms. Frequent reevaluation will determine whether symptoms are subsiding, which will guide the therapist in making changes and progressing the patient's therapy. If there is no improvement or if symptoms have plateaued, consideration should be given to ergonomic modifications, return to modified work on a permanent basis, or vocational rehabilitation.

CHARACTERISTICS OF THREE TYPES OF DISORDERS
Tendon disorders

Tendinitis and tenosynovitis are commonly seen in cumulative trauma. The cycle of overuse, leading to microtrauma, swelling, pain, and limitations in movement, is followed by rest, disuse, and weakness. Cortical sensory degradation may also play a role in recurrent pain associated with the resumption of a specific activity.[10]

Patients with tendon disorders usually present with some combination of localized pain, swelling, pain with resisted motion of the affected musculotendinous unit, limitations in motion, weakness, and crepitation of the tendons. Symptoms are reproduced with activity or work simulation. Isometric grip strength may be normal, but wrist and forearm strength is often decreased and out of balance. Dynamic grip strength

may be more limited because tendon gliding is more likely to increase inflammation and pain. For example, if there is tendinitis of the extensor carpi ulnaris, wrist extension strength will be out of balance with wrist flexion and will be less than the uninvolved wrist extensor strength. This muscle imbalance leads to positioning and substitution patterns that may lead to worsening or spreading of symptoms.

Nerve compression syndromes

Entrapment or compression occurs in specific anatomic areas where nerves pass under a restrictive pulley or retinacular restraint that produces compression.[11] Inflammatory changes resulting in thickening of the tendon or nerve sheaths can compress a nerve or its vascular supply.[28] Sensory fibers are particularly sensitive to ischemia, but persistent compression also will affect motor fibers. Compression can be secondary to hormonal changes associated with pregnancy, birth control pill use, menopause, diabetes, and hypothyroidism. Dynamic changes may occur in the tunnel during daily activity. These changes may cause traction or compression of a nerve, which can restrict the mobility of the nerve within the tunnel.[28] Butler[7] has described a system for testing the tension of the nerves followed by mobilization procedures, which he has found effective in reversing adverse neural tension disorders.

Symptoms of nerve compression syndromes may be vague but usually include some combination of pain, tingling, numbness, and weakness. Pain may be sharp and burning with accompanying paresthesias over a dermatome or sensory distribution area. Hyperesthesia or hypesthesia may occur. Symptoms may be seen both proximal and distal to the compression.

Stress testing, as described by Braun et al.,[4] is an effective way to reproduce the symptoms. Threshold sensibility testing should be performed before and after stress testing (see Chapter 13).

Myofascial pain

Myofascial pain syndrome may occur more often than it is recognized. One survey found that 73% of the patients referred with musculoskeletal problems displayed myofascial symptoms.[21] Overuse of a muscle causes hyperirritability, the focal point of which is the trigger point. "Trigger points display reproducible pain patterns that are usually at a site distal to or away from the locus of stimulation/pain. Trigger points have been explained as local inflammatory response, muscular hardness, local ischemia, and connective tissue irritation."[24] Conventional evaluation for musculoskeletal injuries often does not include assessment of the myofascial system for the presence of trigger points. In addition to trigger points, the muscles in myofascial pain syndrome often have a "ropey" feeling when palpated.[25]

Myofascial pain should be considered when there is generalized, diffuse pain and weakness or when traditional treatment for tendinitis has failed. The therapist can quickly check for the presence of trigger points that are known to refer pain to predictable locations throughout the body.[34] Treatment of myofascial pain is well documented. Examples of specific connective tissue treatment techniques are as follows: ischemic pressure to the trigger points, friction massage, knuckling, skin rolling, use of a vapor coolant spray or light rubbing with ice popsicles combined with stretch, transcutaneous electrical nerve stimulation (TENS), and interferential electrical stimulation around the trigger point.[24,25,34] Stretching of the muscle-tendon unit also is performed. Trigger points must be deactivated before beginning a strengthening program to prevent flare-ups resulting from exercise.

PHASE 1 TREATMENT—SYMPTOM CONTROL

Rehabilitation of individuals with CTDs requires a progressive program that is individualized according to the patient's tolerance for activity and his or her level of symptoms. The first goal in treatment is to reduce the symptoms while teaching the patient self-management techniques for long-term control. This serves to "interrupt the positive feedback loop of the pain-spasm-pain cycle."[21] The first phase of treatment is similar to that for tendon disorders, nerve compressions, and myofascial pain. The patient will be able to tolerate strengthening and conditioning only when the symptoms are under control. Moving too fast can exacerbate symptoms, which will ultimately prolong the rehabilitation process.

During the symptom-control phase of treatment, it is important to evaluate the appropriateness of rest and time off work. For the most part, if the symptoms can be controlled through splints, a modified work schedule, ergonomic aids, or modified tasks, it is better to continue work. Occasionally, a short period of complete rest is necessary, but it should not be prolonged. Splinting to provide rest to the injured structures usually begins with rigid supports and progresses

to soft supports made of neoprene or other flexible materials as symptoms begin to resolve. Ice is used several times a day, in the form of ice packs, water/alcohol slushes, ice massage, or cold wraps. The Cryostim Ice Probe (Pelton Shepherd Industries, 2721 Transworld Drive, P.O. Box 30218, Stockton, California 95213), used with transmission gel to avoid overcooling, also is effective for treating trigger points or painful tendons. Other modalities commonly used in the acute phase are iontophoresis (for inflammation), TENS, and interferential electrical stimulation. Gentle ROM and stretching of the muscles may be started within a patient's pain tolerance.

"Oxygen (through good circulation) is the key to repetitive, prolonged use of muscles."[27] Poor circulation appears to be a factor in the development of cumulative trauma, and restoration of good circulation appears to be crucial to its resolution. Therefore factors that increase circulation are encouraged, and those that decrease circulation are discouraged. At this phase, it is important to begin counseling the patient about lifestyle behaviors that may adversely affect or even contribute to the injury. Patients are asked to decrease the consumption of caffeine, nicotine (which both act as vasoconstrictors), and alcohol while beginning or increasing light aerobic exercise.

Relaxation techniques to increase blood flow and deep breathing to increase oxygen exchange begin at this point. Surface electromyographic biofeedback can be used effectively for relaxation training and self-monitoring. Relaxation tapes also can be used. Therapeutic massage may be effective, especially if proximal structures, such as the shoulder and neck muscles, are involved. Manual edema mobilization[3] may also be effective in increasing lymphatic flow and reducing edema. The therapist also must know how much and what type of medication is being used to avoid overmedication and masking of symptoms.

If a somatosensory approach is used, it can be started during the early phase of treatment.

PHASE 1 TREATMENT—STRENGTHENING

A progressive strengthening program can be started in phase 1 treatment as soon as the symptoms begin to subside. At first, three to five repetitions of static exercise at low resistance should be performed. Increases should be made only if the symptoms do not increase or if they resolve quickly when exercise is stopped. People with CTDs typically experience no symptoms immediately after activity but experience an increase in symptoms 12 to 24 hours later. Therefore symptom response to activity must be monitored carefully to avoid overexertion.

The patient is moved to phase 2 treatment (conditioning) when acceptable strength has been restored but greater endurance is required. Patients should not progress to conditioning until their symptoms have completely subsided.

Exercise principles and definitions

Muscles require five conditions to provide maximal movement, strength, and positioning[27]:

- Good circulation to provide a constant source of oxygen while eliminating waste products (which result in soreness and reduced capacity)
- Regular movement
- Leverage and efficient force exertion (good biomechanics)
- Use of the right muscle for the task
- Adequate recovery time, especially for both forceful and prolonged static exertions, which require more circulation

When these conditions are present, the muscle will work efficiently, with greater strength and endurance, reducing the risk of injury or reinjury.

Exercise terms[1,5,12]

Isometric (static). *Isometric* means the application of force without movement:

- Isometric exercise does not increase strength throughout the ROM of a joint but rather is specific to the joint angle at which the training is being effected.
- Isometric training does not improve (and may hamper) the ability to exert force rapidly. Isometrics can help overcome "sticking points" in the ROM of a joint.
- Most of the benefits of isometrics seem to occur during the early stages of training. Maximal contraction is essential for the optimal effect, and the duration of the contraction should be long enough to recruit as many fibers in a muscle group as possible. Greatest gains in strength occur when isometrics are practiced several times a day, but care must be taken not to overtrain.

Isotonic (dynamic). *Isotonic* means force with movement:

- *Concentric contraction:* Contraction of muscle results in shortening (e.g., of the biceps when the elbow is flexed).
- *Eccentric contraction:* The muscle contracts while in a lengthened state (e.g., the triceps when manually closing a garage door from overhead).
- *Constant loading:* The load remains constant, but the difficulty in overcoming the resistance varies with the angle of the joint (e.g., barbells, dumbbells).
- *Variable loading:* Specially designed machines impose an increasing load throughout the ROM so that a more constant stress is placed on the muscles (e.g., Nautilus machine).
- *Plyometric loading:* Muscles are loaded suddenly and forced to stretch before they can contract and elicit movement (e.g., catching, then throwing a ball). The involved muscles are often used to absorb shock. This

is an effective training method when used in rehabilitation, but the patient must be symptom free.

Isokinetic. *Isokinetic* is the same as isotonic variable resistance except the rate of muscle shortening is controlled (e.g., Cybex machine).

- Also called *accommodating resistance* because the exerted force is resisted by an equal force from the isokinetic dynamometer
- Allows the training of injured joints with a lower risk of injury and provides a speed-specific indication of the absolute strength of a muscle group

Strengthening. *Strengthening* involves gradually increasing resistance but not duration (direct relationship to muscles only). Muscles are strengthened by increasing their size and by enhancing the recruitment and firing rates of their motor units. Muscle strength is acquired either by dynamic high-tension, low-repetition exercises or through isometric contractions.

Conditioning. *Conditioning* involves gradually increasing both intensity and duration.

- *Muscular conditioning:* increase resistance and duration
- *Cardiorespiratory conditioning:* increase duration at an intensity that raises heart rate to 60% to 90% of maximal rate
- *General conditioning:* increase resistance, speed, and duration

In strengthening and conditioning, *intensity* usually refers to a combination of resistance and speed.

Progression. *Progression* can be performed by increasing duration, intensity, frequency, or any combination.

Stretching. *Stretching* increases the flexibility of a muscle by gently elongating it passively. It is important to stretch before exercise because the greater the initial length of a muscle, the greater the tension capability of that muscle. Benefits are as follows:

- The efficiency of the muscle in doing work is increased, and the chance of injury is decreased.
- Stretched muscles can exert greater tension and sustain heavier loads.
- Stretching can improve and maintain ROM.
- Moderate static stretching may be useful in relieving neuromuscular tension.

Warm-up and cool-down. Warm-ups and cool-downs should be performed before and after any exercise program. They consist of the following:

- Stretching and flexibility exercises
- Light resistive continuous exercises such as cycling, jogging, or working on the upper extremity ergometer until the muscles feel "loose and warm," but not to the point of exertion

Closed-chain kinematics. *Closed-chain kinematics* refers to load-bearing exercises performed for stability. These exercises transfer forces across more than one joint (e.g., upper extremity involvement in pushing a cart or doing a push-up). These exercises work on the timing of muscle recruitment.

Open-chain kinematics. *Open-chain kinematics* are exercises performed for mobility in which one joint or muscle group is isolated (e.g., isolated wrist flexion and extension).

Strengthening guidelines by diagnosis

Tendinitis. A diagnosis of tendinitis is usually considered acute if the following are present:

- Recent injury or onset
- Significant swelling
- Significant and specific pain
- Limitations in ROM

Stages sometimes are difficult to differentiate. From the perspective of exercise, *subacute* means either (1) the stage directly after a course of splinting and rest or (2) increased symptoms of pain and swelling within a chronic condition. If the condition is subacute, isometric strengthening usually is begun first. If an isotonic strengthening program is started and pain increases, the program should be modified.

Strengthening begins in the subacute phase and consists of the following:

- Warm-up on an upper body ergometer
- ROM and/or dexterity exercises
- Stretching program* of both upper extremities from the shoulder to the hand
    1. Although tendinitis may be in a specific area, a more holistic approach may prevent the formation of additional problems that sometimes develop when the patient is using compensatory positional and/or substitution patterns.
- Static strengthening program that may include grip, pinch, wrist flexion/extension/deviation, forearm rotation, elbow flexion/extension, and shoulder flexion/extension/abduction/adduction/rotation
    1. Contractions should be submaximal only because maximal effort may cause more microtrauma to the musculotendinous unit.
    2. Strengthening should be started with one set of 10 repetitions, and effort should be applied for no longer than 2 seconds per repetition, working up to 5 seconds.
- Ice, ultrasound, and/or electrical stimulation (may be used after exercise)

When progress has plateaued and symptoms are not increasing with exercise, the patient is in the chronic phase. A patient may be symptom free in the chronic phase, or

*Stretching instructions available from Stretching, Inc., P.O. Box 767, Palmer Lake, Colorado 80133.

symptoms may persist. If symptoms persist, they are stable and do not change significantly in response to activity. Conditioning can be started in the chronic phase. The conditioning program is discussed later in this chapter.

Tenosynovitis. The exercise protocol for tenosynovitis is the same as for tendinitis, except that dynamic exercises in which there is repetitive resisted tendon excursion through the affected sheath is contraindicated because this may increase irritation. Therefore only isometric grip exercises are performed. Dynamic resistance may be added during conditioning if it does not increase the symptoms.

Nerve compression syndromes. "Nerves, with their high metabolic rate, are particularly sensitive to anoxia."[6] Therefore it is especially important to maintain circulation during exercise in the presence of a nerve injury. Adequate recovery time and deep breathing should be stressed during exercise.

Nerve impingement can result from traction of the nerve, pressure over a bony structure, or hypertrophied muscle. After the source of compression is diagnosed, designing an exercise program for these patients is relatively uncomplicated. The general guidelines are as follows:

- Avoid stretching a nerve during exercise, especially if stretching is the causative factor. For example, a patient with cubital tunnel syndrome should avoid full elbow flexion while exercising the arm. Nerve gliding exercises and mobilization should be performed, with care taken not to exacerbate the symptoms.
- Bony structures should be padded for exercise or activity, and weight should not be placed on that area for stabilization. Watch body positioning and posture. Padding can be provided by wearing elbow pads or placing padding on a surface. Elbow pads that can be placed on a table or edge are available (Rolyan Elbow Pads, Smith & Nephew, Inc., One Quality Drive, P.O. Box 578, Germantown, Wisconsin 53022).
- If compression is the result of a hypertrophied muscle, do not increase the hypertrophy through exercise. For example, if the supinator is compressing the radial nerve, work on stretching the supinator and strengthening the pronator to achieve muscle balance.

Myofascial pain. The same general guidelines described for tendinitis apply to exercise for myofascial pain, except that trigger points must be neutralized before the patient will tolerate exercise. An aggressive trigger point treatment program[24,34] must be performed before the muscles can be strengthened. If that has been completed, the exercise program can progress, but careful attention must be given to increases in symptoms. Points to be considered with myofascial pain include the following:

- Isometric exercises do not seem to be as effective as a combination of stretching and dynamic exercise.
- Closed-chain exercises work well for these patients.

PHASE 2 TREATMENT—CONDITIONING

Strength, muscle balance, and general fitness are not enough to protect against cumulative trauma. When strength is acceptable, an endurance or conditioning program should be started. What sets conditioning in CTDs apart from conditioning in acute injuries is that flare-ups can occur at any time in CTDs. In the chronic stages, muscles may have lost flexibility and are not only weak but atrophied. Conditioning must progress slowly, and flare-ups must be controlled.

A daily warm-up on the upper extremity ergometer at 20 Watts and 30 to 60 rpm for 1 minute should start the program. The patient should gradually work up to a 10-minute session.

The weight well, Thera-Band, or similar devices are used to maintain flexibility by working against the involved muscles (e.g., working into flexion for the extensors) at low resistance for one set (about 50 turns of the handle on the weight well). The patient should progress to working concentrically with the involved muscle.

A variety of activities and work simulations should be used during the conditioning phase. Examples are dexterity activities, keyboarding, writing, lifting, carrying, and using tools. Whatever works to cause improvement is usually fairly comfortable to the patient. Dynamic stabilization, using a large therapy ball, is particularly effective for scapula protraction/retraction and anterior shoulder and chest tightness, which is common in office workers. The ball gives a stretch that is gravity assisted.

Surface electromyographic biofeedback is an effective modality for many situations. It can be used to train muscle efficiency with myofascial pain. For example, with a computer operator, the electrodes are placed on the trapezius muscles to monitor tension. The sensitivity level is set one level up from the baseline for relaxation. Different positions and ergonomic devices are used to find those that work best and where relaxation can be maintained. Keyboard combinations that produce "beeps" help the operator learn which combinations are easy and can be performed quickly and which produce tension and should be performed slowly. Biofeedback also can be used to detect trigger points. In my experience, muscle fibers around the trigger points produce spike waves, rather than the sustained high contractions that are seen in tendinitis.

Ergonomic assessment and recommendations

Despite the federal government's recent action to rescind the Occupational Safety and Health Administration's (OSHA) ergonomics standard, many therapists provide ergonomic assessment services to industry with excellent results. This type of intervention is especially effective when an injury is in the acute stage. Alterations in height of work surfaces, padding of sharp edges, and the addition of adjustable keyboard trays can be made very cost-effectively.

Inexpensive ergonomic keyboards are now available and easily obtained; guidelines are available for their selection.[26] There is evidence that some keyboard users experience a reduction in hand pain after several months of use of an alternative keyboard.[36] Increased comfort while working facilitates good posture, reduces muscle tension, and tends to increase a worker's satisfaction with the employer. Ergonomic modifications may permit an employee to continue working rather than taking time off for recovery.

Return to work

Return-to-work issues in cumulative trauma are somewhat different from those faced after recovery from acute trauma, such as tendon lacerations and amputations. The most striking difference is that the patient's physical status may change from day to day, with less pain and greater tolerances on some days and poor tolerances on others. Ideally, a job will allow tasks and methods, at least those under the control of the worker, to be modified. The patient often must negotiate certain restrictions with the employer. A flexible attitude on the part of the supervisor is essential because of the chronic nature of many of these conditions. However, many of the patients have a long, successful work history, and their knowledge of the job will make them appealing for rehire. Often, it is the employees with the greatest productivity levels, not the poorest, who develop CTDs, and they are valuable workers.

The first step in return to work is to obtain a detailed job analysis of the proposed job.[18] This may be performed by a therapist or other vocational specialist. The therapist should review the job analysis, with special attention to the tasks required of the upper extremity (e.g., handling, fingering, grasping, lifting).

A physical capacity evaluation (PCE) or functional capacity evaluation performed when strengthening or conditioning has reached maximal levels, and based on the requirements outlined in the job analysis, will assist in delineating potential problem areas. Ideally, the evaluation is performed over several days while the symptoms are monitored.

Team problem solving with the injured worker, physician, vocational rehabilitation professionals, employer, labor union representative, and therapist may result in employment options that are acceptable to all parties. Assisting the worker to take responsibility for control of symptoms with creativity and flexibility is the key to successful reemployment.

INTERVENTION MODELS
Vocational model

In the medical model, the injured worker is referred to as a *patient*, but in the vocational model an injured worker is a *client*. This distinction is important when communicating with rehabilitation counselors and industry. In the vocational model, the therapist will be working with a variety of rehabilitation professionals, such as vocational rehabilitation counselors, vocational evaluators, work-adjustment specialists, job developers, ergonomists, and others whose job is to find appropriate employment for a specific injured worker. The therapist may be the person who keeps the physician updated on progress in identifying employment. It is often the therapist who acts as the bridge between the medical community and the work community. To facilitate this communication, the therapist should be familiar with terms used in industry and minimize the use of medical terminology. To a therapist, the presence of de Quervain's tendinitis implies a range of symptoms and treatments. However, to a line supervisor, "painful thumb" may be more relevant and understandable. Change in productivity, job rotation, and other factors may be part of the ergonomic solution. The therapist must communicate in understandable terms if the intervention is to have the desired effect.

As the rehabilitation professionals develop job options, the therapist may review them for their physical appropriateness while suggesting supports and adjustments to fit the job to the worker. A therapist's understanding of the functional implications of injury is critical to this process.

Case management

Some therapists have developed expertise as case managers. In this role, they work as consultants for the insurance company, following the injured worker through the medical and rehabilitation phases. They coordinate services between medical professionals, making appropriate referrals and recommendations. They stay in close communication with the patient, overseeing the timely provision of financial and social benefits to the injured worker. They facilitate the progression of the patient through the worker's compensation system so that time is not wasted and the worker returns to gainful employment as soon as possible. The therapist recommends services such as work hardening, on-site evaluation, and PCE. The therapist also works with the rehabilitation professionals.

Industrial model

Intervention in industry begins with the injured worker or the at-risk worker. The intervention team may include the occupational health or rehabilitation nurse, risk manager, company or community physician, supervisor, ergonomist, industrial hygienist, and various company managers whose input or approval is needed. Programs may include ergonomic training of employees and supervisors and on-site evaluation of, or consultation on, prevention of injury. Other, more extensive, on-site services such as screening of new employees, compliance with the Americans with Disabilities Act, design and implementation of a prevention program, and operation of a first-aid center or on-site therapy clinic may be requested.[16]

The therapist will submit a proposal for such services. Ideally, the company will provide the space, equipment, and support staff for these services. The therapist or therapy clinic will provide the professional staff. The contract must be written carefully so that services can be provided in a cost-effective manner with both sides benefiting from the intervention.

In summary, hand therapists play a crucial role in the management of upper extremity cumulative trauma. Intervention may occur at any point in the process, including prevention programs, acute treatment, conditioning, and reemployment. Therapists' training in anatomy, physiology, biomechanics, evaluation and treatment techniques, psychosocial issues, activity analysis, fabrication and use of splints and ergonomic equipment, and communication skills provides the fundamental theory and knowledge needed to address these challenging problems.

ACKNOWLEDGMENT

Special thanks to Andrea Hankins, Certified Exercise Specialist, for her assistance in writing the sections on strengthening and conditioning in both the fourth and fifth editions of this book.

REFERENCES

1. American College of Sports Medicine: *Guidelines for exercise testing and prescription,* ed 3, Philadelphia, 1986, Lea & Febiger.
2. Armstrong TJ: Cumulative trauma disorders of the upper limb and identification of work-related factors. In Millender LH, Louis DS, Simmons BP, editors: *Occupational disorders of the upper extremity,* New York, 1992, Churchill Livingstone.
3. Atrzberger S: *Manual edema mobilization,* Presented at the annual meeting of the American Society of Hand Therapists, Orlando, September 1999.
4. Braun RM, Davidson K, Doehr S: Provocative testing in the diagnosis of dynamic carpal tunnel syndrome, *J Hand Surg* 14A:195, 1989.
5. Brooks GA, editor: *Exercise physiology: human bioenergetics and its applications,* ed 3, Mountain View, Calif, 2000, Mayfield Publishing.
6. Bureau of Labor Statistics: *Survey of occupational injuries and illness,* Washington, DC, 1992, US Department of Labor.
7. Butler DS: *Mobilisation of the nervous system,* New York, 1991, Churchill Livingstone.
8. Byl NN, Melnick M: The neural consequences of repetition: clinical implications of a learning hypothesis, *J Hand Ther* 10:160, 1997.
9. Byl NN, Melnick M: *The neural consequences of repetition: implications for focal hand dystonia and chronic pain,* Presented to the Northern California Hand Therapy Study Group, San Francisco, November 15, 2000.
10. Byl N, et al: Sensory dysfunction associated with repetitive strain injuries of tendinitis and focal hand dystonia: a comparative study, *J Orthop Sports Phys Ther* 23:234, 1996.
11. Eaton RG: Entrapment syndromes in musicians, *J Hand Ther* 5:91, 1992.
12. Gowitzke BA, Milner M: *Understanding the scientific basis of human movement,* ed 2, Baltimore, 1984, Williams & Wilkins.
13. Heilbroner D: The handling of an epidemic, *Working Woman* February, 1993.
14. Higgs PE, Mackinnon SE: Repetitive motion injuries, *Annu Rev Med* 46:1, 1995.
15. Higgs PE, et al: Upper extremity impairment in workers performing repetitive tasks, *Plast Reconstr Surg* 90:614, 1992.

16. Isernhagen SJ, editor: *The comprehensive guide to work injury management,* Rockville, Md, 1995, Aspen Publications.

17. Johnson RK: Psychologic assessment of patients with industrial hand injuries, *Hand Clin* 9:221, 1993.

18. Kasdan AS, McElwain NP: Return-to-work programs following occupational hand injuries. In Kasdan ML, editor: *Occupational hand injuries: occupational medicine—state of the art reviews,* Philadelphia, 1989, Hanley & Belfus.

19. Kelsey J, et al: *Upper extremity disorders, frequency, impact and cost,* New York, 1997, Churchill Livingstone.

20. Keogh JP, et al: The impact of occupational injury on injured worker and family: outcomes of upper extremity cumulative trauma disorders in Maryland workers, *Am J Ind Med* 38:498, 2000.

21. Lowe C: Treatment of tendinitis, tenosynovitis, and other cumulative trauma disorders of musicians' forearms, wrists, and hands: restoring function with hand therapy, *J Hand Ther* 5:84, 1992.

22. Millender LH: Occupational disorders of the upper extremity: orthopaedic, psychosocial, and legal implications. In Millender LH, Louis DS, Simmons BP, editors: *Occupational disorders of the upper extremity,* New York, 1992, Churchill Livingstone.

23. Millender LH, Conlon M: An approach to work-related disorders of the upper extremity, *J Am Acad Orthop Surg* 4:134, 1996.

24. Moran CA: Myofascial pain in the upper extremity. In Hunter JM, et al, editors: *Rehabilitation of the hand,* ed 3, St Louis, 1990, Mosby.

25. Moran CA: Using myofascial techniques to treat musicians, *J Hand Ther* 5:97, 1992.

26. NIOSH, Alternative Keyboards, Publication 97-148, available by calling 800-35-NIOSH or on the Internet at www.cdc.gov/niosh.

27. Parker KG, Imbus HR: *Cumulative trauma disorders current issues and ergonomic solutions: a systems approach,* Boca Raton, Fla, 1992, Lewis Publishers.

28. Pecina MM, Krmpotaic-Nemanic J, Markiewitz AD: *Tunnel syndromes,* Boca Raton, Fla, 1991, CRC Press.

29. Putz-Anderson V: *Cumulative trauma disorders a manual for musculoskeletal diseases of the upper limbs,* New York, 1988, Taylor & Francis.

30. Ranney D: *Chronic musculoskeletal injuries in the workplace,* Philadelphia, 1997, WB Saunders.

31. Rempel DM: Work-related cumulative trauma disorders of the upper extremity, *JAMA* 267:838, 1992.

32. Roth LP, et al: Practice analysis of hand therapy, *J Hand Ther* 9:203, 1996.

33. Sanders M: *Management of cumulative trauma disorders,* Boston, 1997, Butterworth-Heinemann.

34. Simons DG, Travell JG, Simons LS: *Travell & Simons' myofascial pain and dysfunction: the trigger point manual,* ed 2, Philadelphia, 1998, Lippincott Williams & Wilkins

35. Strasser PB, et al: Perceived psychological stress and upper extremity cumulative trauma disorders, *AAOHN J* 47:22, 1999.

36. Tittiranonda P, et al: Effect of four computer keyboards in computer users with upper extremity musculoskeletal disorders, *Am J Ind Med* 35:647, 1999.

37. Webster BS, Snook SH: The cost of compensable upper extremity cumulative trauma disorders, *J Occup Med* 36:713, 1994.

BIBLIOGRAPHY

Bing R, Danches MW, Jacobs K: *Work in progress: occupational therapy in work programs,* Rockville, Md, 1989, American Occupational Therapy Association.

Blair SJ, editor: Special supplement on cumulative trauma disorders, *J Hand Surg* 12A:821, 1987.

Chaffin DB, Andersson G: *Occupational biomechanics,* ed 3, New York, 1999, John Wiley & Sons.

Eastman Kodak Company: *Ergonomic design for people at work,* vol 1, New York, 1989, John Wiley & Sons.

Eastman Kodak Company: *Ergonomic design for people at work,* vol 2, New York, 1989, John Wiley & Sons.

Isernhagen SJ, editor: *Work injury management and prevention,* Rockville, Md, 1988, Aspen Publishers.

Jacobs K, editor: Industrial rehabilitation, *Work* 1:5, 1990.

Jacobs K, editor: Cumulative trauma disorders, *Work* 2:1, 1992.

Kasdan ML, editor: Occupational diseases, *Hand Clin* 9:195, 1993.

King JW, editor: Management of upper extremity problems in the workplace, *J Hand Ther* (special issue) 3:45, 1990.

Linden P: *Compute in comfort,* Upper Saddle River, NJ, 1995, Prentice Hall.

Nordin M, Andersson G, Pope MH: Musculoskeletal disorders in the workplace: principles and practice, St Louis, 1997, Mosby.

Pasacarelli E, Quilter D: *Repetitive strain injury: a computer user's guide,* New York, 1994, John Wiley & Sons.

Quilter D: *The repetitive strain injury recovery book,* New York, 1998, Walker and Company.

Part XIV

STIFFNESS OF THE HAND

Chapter 61

THERAPIST'S MANAGEMENT OF THE STIFF HAND

Judy C. Colditz

THE CHALLENGE OF THE STIFF HAND

Clinical experience confirms certain risk factors for stiffness in the hand. The more tissue traumatized, the greater the likelihood of stiffness.[48] Multiple tissue trauma often requires longer periods of immobilization to regain skeletal stability. The decrease in tissue elasticity that accompanies increasing age creates less tolerance to the insult of trauma.[130] Infection that extends the wound beyond its mechanically created boundary creates adherence between multiple remote tissue planes. However, many questions about stiffness in the hand remain unanswered: Why do some patients have great difficulty regaining motion long after others with the same diagnosis have returned to normal function? How can we identify what amount of motion, at what frequency, with what duration will maximize individual patient results? One thing we do know, as did Sir Charles Bell in 1883, "The mechanical properties of the living frame, like the endowments of the mind, must not lie idle, or they will suffer deterioration."[16]

DEFINITION OF STIFFNESS

The term *stiff* is used commonly when describing the hand lacking full mobility. Although it is usually a term reserved to describe the physical property of matter whose close molecular structure makes it rigid, resisting deformation when an external force is applied, stiffness of the hand is not an increased rigidity of the tissues themselves.[126] Rather, stiffness is the constraint created by cross-linking the previously elastic configuration of the collagen fibers.[53]

Collagen provides most of the tensional strength of tissue in the hand. Collagen fibers themselves are inelastic and have a tensile strength greater than steel, but movement between the collagen fibers imparts elasticity to the tissue.

Normal hand motion occurs when these strong, dense connective tissue structures glide relative to one another.[87] Stiffness is caused by the fixation of the tissue layers so that the usual elastic relational motion is restricted by cross-links binding the collagen fibers together.[6,20,53,61,90,105]

Peacock and Cohen[105,106] provide an excellent analogy of the strength and elasticity of normal collagen. They compare it with the strength of the relatively inelastic nylon thread used to make stockings, with the significant elasticity of the stocking fabric itself created by the weave of the nylon threads. Collagen cross-linking does not change the collagen (the nylon thread), but it does restrict the movement of one thread in relation to another (Fig. 61-1).

STIFFNESS AND THE STAGES OF WOUND HEALING

Tissue injury creates a relatively extended period of heightened collagen synthesis, degradation, and deposition within a wound as compared with normal tissue.[106] Healing tissue progresses through three stages: inflammatory, fibroplastic, and remodeling (or maturation). During the inflammatory stage, the wound prepares to heal, the tissue structure is rebuilt during the fibroplastic stage, and the final tissue configuration develops during the remodeling stage.[66] In the ideal circumstance, a healing wound progresses through these stages in an orderly and timely manner. Wounds resulting in massive tissue injury, infection, delayed healing, repeated surgery, or poor wound toileting extend these stages of healing far beyond the ideal time frame. Therapists treating complex injuries cannot follow the chronology of a wound and assume a certain stage, but rather must be able to evaluate the characteristics of the wound or healing scar and determine its stage to devise appropriate therapy.

INTRAMOLECULAR CROSS-LINKS

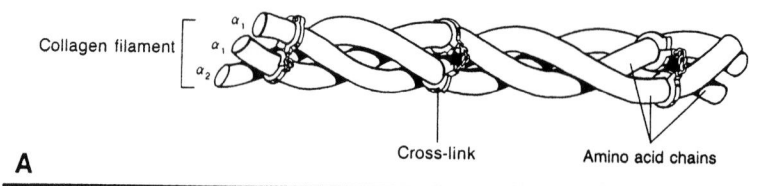

A

INTERMOLECULAR CROSS-LINKS

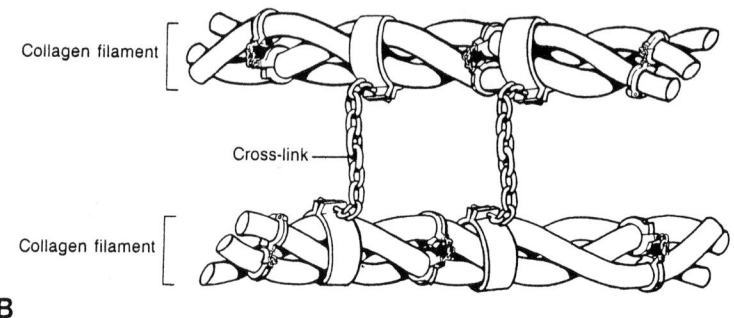

B

Fig. 61-1. Collagen cross-linking occurs between amino acid chains within one collagen filament (weak cross-links) **(A)** and between collagen filaments, locking them to one another (strong cross-links) **(B)**. (From Hardy MA: *Phys Ther* 69:1014, 1989.)

In the uncomplicated wound, the initial inflammatory phase of wound healing is completed within a few days. Because the intercellular forces are weak, wounds may be disrupted with ease during this stage,[87] and most surgical wounds are rested via immobilization until the wound healing has begun. Randomly oriented, matted collagen fibrils unite the injured structures during the early phase of healing, although fibers cannot be visualized through the light microscope until the fourth or fifth day after injury.[87]

In the uncomplicated wound, the fibroplastic stage begins at the end of the first week of healing, when the fibroblast begins replacing the macrophage as the most common cell type. About 2 days later, fibroblasts begin the process of collagen synthesis and outnumber the granulocytes and macrophages in the wound. The fibroblasts evolve into myofibroblasts and are responsible for fiber synthesis and concurrent contraction of the wound edges. Capillaries reestablish within the wound, forming a dense network. Collagen fibers are laid down between the capillaries, forming the scar needed to keep the wound closed. By the end of the second week, the wound is filled with newly synthesized but disorganized collagen fibers invading all areas of the wound.[4,5,87] Although the strength of the wound remains diminished (at 3 weeks an incised and sutured wound has less than 15% of its ultimate tensile strength[87]), the random orientation of the collagen fibers limits the ease of motion. At this stage, the scar is not strong and cannot tolerate excessive stress. If wound circumstances are ideal,

the proliferative stage occurs within the first week after the wound is created. However, in complex wounds, this period is much longer.

Joint stiffness and tissue adherence palpated during this stage can be described by a soft end-feel at the limitation of motion. This tissue responsiveness occurs because the cross-linking of the collagen fibers is weak and stress causes the collagen fibers to align themselves with the direction of stress. Because of the diminished strength of the healing tissue, excessive force can tear the fibrils, causing more injury and reviving the inflammatory process. Any force applied must be slow, gentle, and sustained. In the fibroplastic stage, intermittent active motion is the ideal means of applying stress to the disorganized collagen to encourage it to realign. More resistive motions can be coaxed by the application of a gentle sustained force applied via mobilization splinting. Young scars can be altered morphologically by conditions of stress that are ineffective in older scars.[12]

In the uncomplicated wound, the maturation stage begins between 3 and 6 weeks. In the hand with delayed healing, infection, multiple tissue trauma, or multiple surgery, the maturation phase may be delayed many weeks or months. As the cell population decreases, scar collagen fibers increase.[87] The total collagen accumulation then stabilizes and remains constant. At this stage, collagen deposition is accompanied by collagen degradation, creating equilibrium. Alternations in the architecture of scar collagen fibers occur as the scar matures. These physical changes are caused by changes in

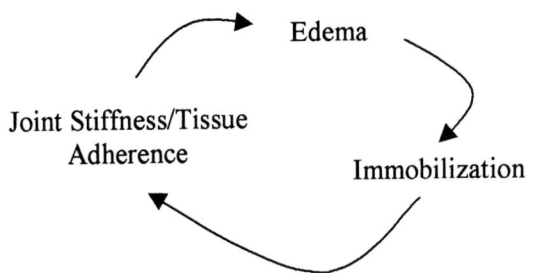

Fig. 61-2. In the early stiff hand, three factors interplay to create stiffness. Changing any one factor alters the cycle of stiffness.

the number of covalent bonds between collagen molecules. Scars remain metabolically active for years, slowly changing in size, shape, color, texture, and strength.[87]

Wounds that are well into the maturation stage exhibit a hard end-feel to passive joint motion. The joint feels as if it will not yield to force, but stops abruptly. This type of response to palpation requires more consistent application of force. In the early part of the maturation stage, intermittent serial static or static progressive splinting can be effective. More complex and resistive stiff hands require a different approach (discussed subsequently in the chronically stiff hand section).

EVALUATION AND TREATMENT OF EARLY STIFFNESS

The line that demarcates the early stiff hand from the chronically stiff hand is difficult to pinpoint. However, in the following sections, the early stiff hand is discussed separately from the chronically stiff hand because the treatment approaches I suggest differ greatly. Regardless of the type of stiffness, manual examination is required to determine which structures are limiting motion. The early stiff hand that is past the acute stage of healing but continues with edema, joint stiffness, and/or tissue adherence remains relatively immobile. The immobility may result from lack of functional use, pain, fear, or continued immobilization of healing tissue. A cycle is established in which inactivity leads to stiffness and adherence, which leads to edema, which leads to continued inactivity (Fig. 61-2). In most postsurgical hand patients, changing one of the three factors readily breaks this cycle. For example, reducing edema allows greater potential for movement, which decreases inactivity, and in turn decreases stiffness and tissue adherence. As the therapist and patient work together on each of the three factors, the other factors are directly influenced and the mobility of the hand returns.

Edema

Treatment of the injured hand cannot begin without a thorough understanding of the causes of edema and the factors that influence it. Because its presence is a primary cause for immobility of the injured hand, edema reduction to

create potential for motion is always a primary component of treating the stiff hand.

Although the reader will find other chapters about edema and the lymphatic system (see Chapters 12, 53, and 54), key points are briefly reviewed here to reinforce recommendations made later in this chapter for edema reduction techniques, which may differ from some long-held treatment beliefs.

Edema is excess fluid in the interstitium (the spaces between cells).[31,55,62,94] Because one sixth of the body consists of spaces between cells,[63,64] the interstitium provides a great deal of room for expansion when filled with edema. The injured hand develops edema as a result of increased capillary permeability, which allows leakage of fluid and protein into the tissue spaces.[62] The presence of mild postoperative edema actually facilitates wound healing by causing a moderate increase in the strength of the healing wound and an increase in macrophages and fibroblasts.[13,31] Greater amounts of edema destroy the continuity of the wound, breaking the fibrin seal and the integrity of the sutures.[31]

The lymphatic system is an intricate network of lymphatic channels that drains excess fluid and other substances, including cells, proteins, lipids, microorganisms, and debris, from the tissues to maintain homeostasis.[62,63,94]

When the lymphatic system is overwhelmed by the rate of capillary filtration and cannot carry the volume of fluid as fast as it is produced, edema develops. This edema is to be clearly differentiated from lymphedema, caused by lymphatic obstruction, which causes protein to accumulate in the tissue spaces and therefore causes osmosis of fluid out of the capillaries.

The movement of lymph fluid through the system is aided greatly by external forces: adjacent muscle contraction, tissue compression (e.g., massage, bandaging), and general stimulation (e.g., arterial pulsations, body movement). If wound healing progresses without complication, edema begins to subside and motion is regained. However, injured hands that develop significant stiffness do not follow this path, and prolonged inflammation and edema persist.

Pitting versus nonpitting edema. Before the development of visible pitting edema, the interstitial spaces must first become filled with fluid. This filling of the interstitium with fluid eliminates ease of movement. Interstitial edema is not appreciated or measured as easily as pitting edema, but it plays a large role in preventing full motion.

Most of the interstitial fluid is trapped within the interstitial tissue gel. When edema exists in pockets of free fluid outside the interstitial spaces, it "pits" with pressure. These pockets of free fluid can hold more than half of the volume of the interstitial fluid.[65] One example is the loose dorsal skin pocket of the hand. When one places pressure on the pocket, the fluid moves, leaving an indention (or pit) (Fig. 61-3).

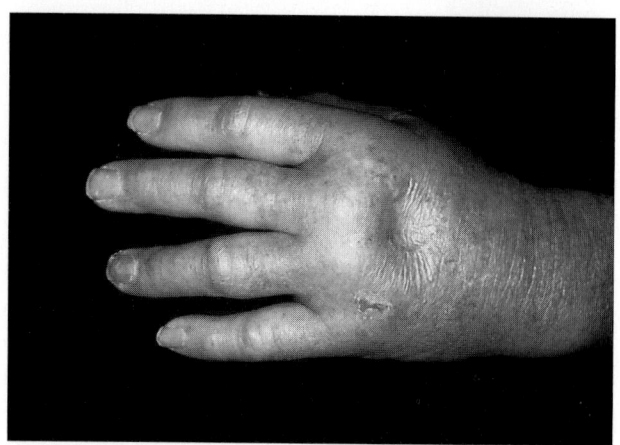

Fig. 61-3. Pitting edema is best observed on the dorsum of the hand after sustained pressure with the thumb.

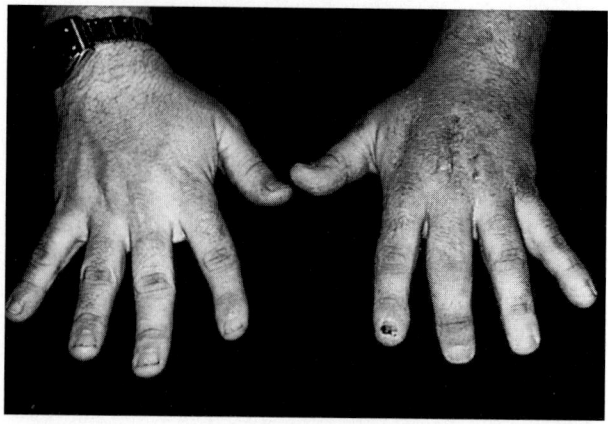

Fig. 61-4. Visual comparison of the injured and uninjured hands shows differences in skin wrinkles and creases, metacarpal head definition, and prominence of dorsal extensor tendons.

Evaluation of edema. Pitting edema can be measured accurately via water displacement.[21,127] Measurement of pressure created by interstitial edema is impossible to accurately measure externally. A precise observational evaluation is far more useful in appreciating the level of interstitial edema.

Careful inspection of both hands (Fig. 61-4), comparing their general appearance, gives a more insightful view of the presence of interstitial edema. Loss or diminution of normal small skin wrinkles, tautness or obliteration of the dorsal finger joint creases, obscurity of metacarpal head definition, and oblivion of the dorsal finger extensor tendons are recordable observations of the presence of interstitial edema.

The presence of interstitial edema can be felt if the examiner palpates both hands simultaneously with eyes closed. A fullness in the tissues is present, which creates diminished tissue mobility, especially when contrasted with the uninjured hand. (In contrast, pitting edema is felt as fluctuant.) Active and passive joint motion is limited by a palpable fullness of the space, creating a soft feel to the end-range. An experienced clinician can learn by palpation whether edema is the primary cause for limited passive joint motion.

Unfortunately, such palpation is difficult to quantify in order to allow accurate comparison in subsequent examinations to document progress. Some therapists use circumferential measurements of a digit, palm, or wrist, but the lack of reliability makes such measurements useful only as an approximate indicator of progress. If such measurements are used, the anatomic location of the measuring tape must be recorded and a repeatable amount of force must be used.

Edema control techniques. Minimizing the negative effects of immobilization caused by edema is the single most useful treatment that can be offered for the injured hand. Elevation, active muscle contraction, external pressure from various sources, and gentle stimulation via massage can influence the accumulation of edema. Understanding which edema reduction technique to use when and the optimal type of force or pressure to use throughout the stages of healing is the key to successful prevention of the stiff hand.

Elevation. Immediately following injury and surgical repair, immobilization of the tissues is necessary to allow the inflammatory phase of healing to be complete without disrupting the healing wound.

Interstitial fluids tend to accumulate in dependent parts because the increased intravascular pressure increases capillary filtration.[55,124] Even a normal hand can develop edema if it is immobile and dependent.[116] Thus elevation of the hand minimizes edema. In addition, the postcapillary blood pressure that facilitates venous return is less than 15 mm Hg of hydrostatic pressure. If the hand is in a dependent position, the pressure opposing the venous return is approximately 35 mm Hg of hydrostatic pressure.[65]

Elevation of the extremity—hand above the elbow, elbow above the heart—is the single most useful postoperative instruction to decrease the hydrostatic pressure in the vessels.[124] Patients must be instructed carefully on the precise definition of elevation. The concept of a drop of water being able to run downhill to the heart without ever encountering an uphill run helps patients visualize adequate elevation.

Maintaining the arm in a sling is not adequate elevation and encourages the extremity to become quiescent. It is far more productive to instruct the patient to maintain elevation during the day by using pillows or books and reserve the use of a sling for brief periods of ambulation. During this time, intermittent active motion of the proximal joints should be encouraged to ensure that joint motion is maintained and large muscle groups are recruited to assist return venous and lymphatic flow.

When the surgical dressing is removed and intermittent active motion of the injured part is begun, intermittent elevation is still necessary until the edema begins to subside. There is often a practical quandary. The hand is swollen and active motion is encouraged, but the patient is also instructed to elevate the hand, which is in an inactive position for the extremity. A balance can be achieved by instructing the patient to do active pumping exercises intermittently with the hand and arm elevated and to elevate the hand when not using it actively. Prolonged periods of using the hand in a dependent position with minimal active motion are to be avoided at this stage because the pumping balance is difficult to maintain.

Active motion: pumping versus gliding motion. Active muscle pumping is the single most important stimulus for increasing lymphatic flow.* However, active motion across the site of injury during the initial acute period immediately after surgery disrupts healing. In a randomized study of patients who started range of motion (ROM) immediately versus 7 days after axillary dissection for cancer, those waiting 7 days had less wound drainage, fewer days of drainage, and earlier postoperative discharge than patients who started early after surgery, although there was no difference in the outcome of ROM.[86]

Digital edema provides an unusual quandary. Because there are no muscles within the digits, skin movement and tissue compression from active movement is the stimulus required for increased lymphatic flow. When digital motion must be limited to protect healing structures, gentle pressure to the digit, elevation, and active muscle contraction in adjacent uninjured areas must substitute for active motion of the digit itself. With many digital injuries, the metacarpophalangeal (MP) joint may safely be allowed full motion. This permits the patient to perform pumping exercises of digital adduction and abduction, and MP joint flexion and extension, which contract the adjacent intrinsic muscles.

Proximal to the wrist, the muscles are larger and thus more effective stimulators of the lymphatic system. As long as the vascular status of the hand is stable, intermittent active motion of proximal muscles is begun as early as possible following surgery. Waste products that are evacuated from the injured hand are more effectively moved through the lymphatic system with this intermittent active motion. Passive range of motion (PROM) does not stimulate muscle contraction and, for that reason, cannot be substituted for active motion to reduce edema.[96]

When active motion of the injured part is allowed, elevation and proximal pumping must be continued until enough motion is present at the injury site to allow local pumping that is sufficient for adequate lymphatic flow. Patients who exercise the injured part of the hand in an elevated position see a dramatic edema reduction as they gain motion at the site of injury.

Compression. In addition to active muscle contraction that provides internal compression to the lymphatic conduits,

*References 31, 55, 62, 63, 71, 94, 110.

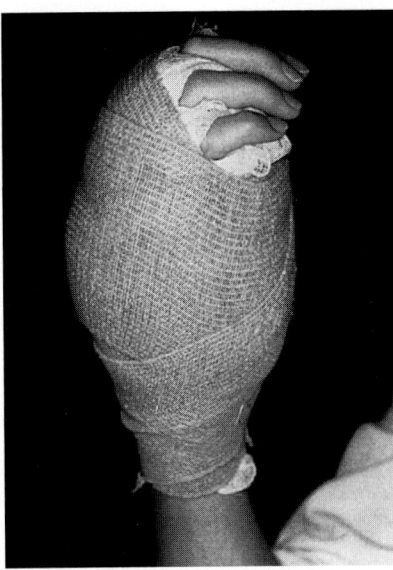

Fig. 61-5. A bulky dressing may be used overnight or a few days to provide prolonged compression for effective edema reduction.

external pressure also aids in lymphatic flow. For this reason, large compressive bandages are applied postoperatively to maintain gentle pressure to the hand. As one would expect, the use of external pressure alone, in the absence of active pumping, provides little long-term change. However, the use of external pressure as an adjunct to active motion often can break the edema cycle, allowing potential for full active motion.

External wraps or elastic garments, external splints or bandages, or gentle external massage provide external pressure treatment. In the past, recommendations have been made for firm retrograde pressure to "push" the edema out of the hand. This concept should be abandoned and a concept of gentle external pressure should be adopted to facilitate lymphatic flow.

Compressive bandage. Surgical dressings and other forms of immobilization are used early after trauma to provide necessary rest so the newly injured tissues can rest from external forces and begin the healing process. When a wound has delayed healing, some form of bandaging that continues to supply gentle compression is advisable.

When a patient presents with significant pitting edema, regardless of the stage of healing, the quantity of edema present in the tissues is so great that mobilization of the joints is futile until the edema is reduced. Although the foremost goal is mobilization of the hand, a brief period of immobilization in a bulky compressive dressing that distributes pressure to all tissues is a wise initial treatment (Fig. 61-5). The bandage is composed of multiple layers of fluffed gauze squares placed between the digits and applied dorsally and palmarly. The gauze is compressed with wraps of cast padding and gauze wraps. Elastic bandages and/or plaster of Paris slabs may be added to the exterior of the bandage for more specific support and compression. In significant pitting edema, the consistency of pressure provided by a nonremovable dressing can assist in dramatic reduction in edema overnight. If the edema is a result of excessive manipulation of the hand causing a prolonged inflammatory response, a short period of rest and immobilization in a compressive bandage reduces both edema and inflammation. This approach allows a better starting point for upgrading motion and the use of other edema reduction techniques. It may seem contradictory to immobilize a stiff swollen hand. The immobilization is necessary because it is the most effective way to provide conformed pressure that will reduce the edema to a level at which productive active motion is possible.

Splints. Immobilization decreases initial edema, reduces pain, and permits tissue repair without the stress of external forces. The use of immobilization splints during the acute stages of wound healing can provide effective rest and compression in addition to accurate positioning to protect healing structures or to maintain a balanced position. If straps are applied too snugly either dorsally or volarly, the complex of lymphatic vessels can be occluded by the pressure of the strap.[117] Pitting edema distal or proximal to a strap is a sign that the pressure of the strap is impeding lymphatic flow. A safer alternative is the use of a wide elastic wrap over the entire surface to distribute pressure rather than localize it as the strap does.

A removable immobilization splint made from dorsal and volar plaster of Paris slabs provides the most precise positioning, intimate fit, and even distribution of pressure possible[118] (Fig. 61-6). As edema subsides, if the position of the hand needs changing, a new splint is applied. Either type of immobilization splint can assist in optimal positioning and provide gentle distributed pressure while still protecting healing tissues from stress.

External wraps. Compressive wraps must be constant when applied following the acute stage, but must not restrict motion. Coban and other self-adherent elastic wraps are commonly used to control edema in the hand, especially in the digits. Use of any self-adherent elastic wrap must be done with particular caution for light application. It is the consistency of pressure, not the intensity of pressure, that is important. It is particularly important to explain this concept to patients and have them demonstrate independent application of the self-adherent elastic wrap before leaving the clinic.

A single layer of the self-adherent elastic wrap can be applied by wrapping either a 3- or 4-inch width around the digit and gently pinching it together on the dorsum of the finger and then trimming a narrow seam (Fig. 61-7). This application also allows easier adjustment of the tension with the one hand the patient has available than does the wrapping of multiple overlapping layers. One or two layers of tubular stockinette sized to fit the finger and applied underneath the

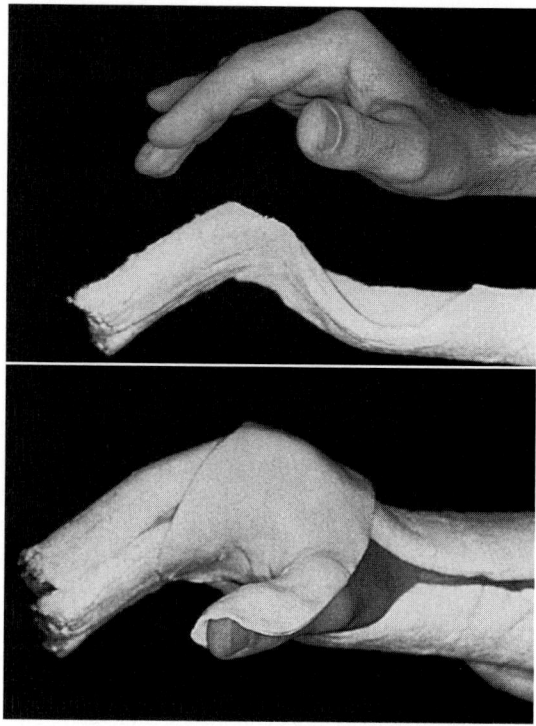

Fig. 61-6. Dorsal and volar plaster slabs provide well-distributed pressure and precise positioning of the hand joints.

self-adherent elastic wrap will offer a more gentle contact with the skin during movement of the digit.

Gloves. Elastic gloves are a convenient and inexpensive means of providing external pressure. The glove should fit like a loose second skin, providing a very gentle traction to the skin when the hand is moved within it. U.S. suppliers now market various brands of inexpensive edema gloves that are appropriate for use with the edematous hand.

Gentle external massage. All hand therapists should become thoroughly familiar with the gentle massage approach of manual lymphatic therapy techniques (see Chapter 53). Originally developed as a means of facilitating lymphatic flow in patients with chronic lymphedema, this gentle facilitatory massage can be helpful with many hand trauma patients.

After the acute phase has subsided, patients with isolated injuries may require only a short period of gentle massage. Patients with extensive crush injuries or large wound areas where the anatomy of lymphatic drainage has been altered are ideal candidates for longer-term manual edema mobilization techniques (see Chapter 53) to facilitate lymphatic flow around these injury areas until lymphatic flow has been reestablished. Above all else, vigorous, forceful massage recommended by many in the past should be abandoned. Superficial lymphatic vessels are thin, fragile structures that may be further destroyed by such vigorous therapy.[110]

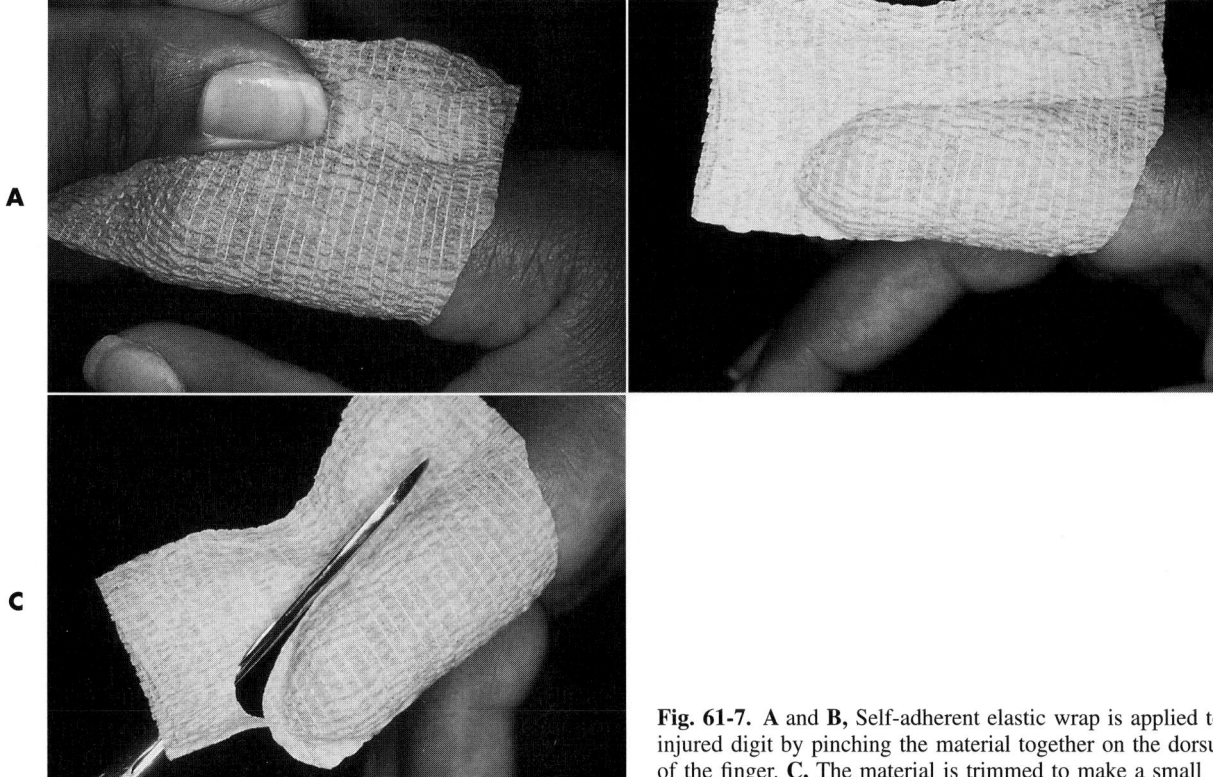

Fig. 61-7. A and **B,** Self-adherent elastic wrap is applied to the injured digit by pinching the material together on the dorsum of the finger. **C,** The material is trimmed to make a small unobtrusive seam.

Mobilizing the early stiff hand

Although many treatment techniques have been developed to mobilize the stiff hand, no basic research supports any particular exercise treatment regimen to regain mobility.[61,90] Two basic principles for postoperative rehabilitation are imperative: The effects of immobilization must be minimized and healing tissue must not be overloaded.[74]

Benefits of early motion. After injury, early movement reestablishes tissue homeostasis, increases venous and lymphatic flow, increases tensile strength of the wound, and directs the alignment and orientation of collagen fibers.[5,6,40,57,62,63,98]

In the early postoperative period, the beneficial effects of motion can be provided either by active or continuous passive motion (CPM), but active motion must quickly assume the dominant role if the patient is to resume functional use. The challenge is to allow enough motion to nullify the negative effects of immobilization but not too much motion to prevent normal healing.

Beginning with Arem and Madden,[12] many studies have validated the concept of controlled stress to promote favorable collagen orientation and to increase tensile strength of the healing tissue.* Unknown, however, is how much, how many repetitions, how often, how long, and to

*References 5, 9, 58, 87, 98, 120, 134.

what extent motion needs to be carried out for optional stress application to influence the tissue. If we knew how to precisely apply stress, postoperative therapy would be more efficient and productive.[87] At this time, the guideline for the parameters of stress application must be the observation of a positive influence on the tissue and the absence of a renewed inflammatory response.

Early active motion should be precise. Substitution motions using the uninjured joints should be avoided. Active motion needs to be to maximum range and repeated intermittently throughout the day, but frequent repetitions are not indicated. A general guideline is the more acute the injury and the more inflamed the tissues, the more intermittent the motion. As edema subsides and active motion is tolerated without an increasing inflammatory response, more frequent motion is indicated. The schedule for the balance between rest and motion depends on the tolerance of the tissue for increased frequency of motion, which can be determined only by a gentle trial-and-error method.

Balance of exercise and rest. The primary guideline for progression of exercises should be the status of the hand after exercise. If the edema, pain, and stiffness increase after exercise (or any treatment), the hand is not yet ready for that level of stress. Conversely, if the patient experiences sustained increased comfort and mobility, the amount of exercise is appropriate for the stage of recovery and may be slowly upgraded. Most patients can sense a positive tissue response versus a negative one and modify their exercise regimen to maintain the positive response.

Benefits of CPM. Because joint motion is needed to preserve joint lubrication,[6,134] the use of CPM often is used postoperatively for joint pathology. Neither laboratory nor clinical studies have shown that CPM is useful for treating joint stiffness once it has occurred.[90,111] Therefore CPM is appropriately reserved for the immediate postoperative period to prevent complications rather than to resolve stiffness. Treatment parameters for CPM are described in Chapter 108.

Blocking motions. Unlike most of the large joints in the body, the small joints of the hand are moved by muscles crossing multiple proximal joints. Because muscle pull results in the movement of the joints with the least resistance, muscle excursion will affect proximal mobile joints before affecting stiffer distal joints. Manual blocking transfers the muscle force to the targeted stiff joint, enabling the patient to experience glide at the site of restriction. For example, when the MP joint is blocked during finger flexion, extrinsic flexor glide is directed across the interphalangeal (IP) joints rather than allowing MP flexion by the intrinsic muscles (Fig. 61-8). If blocking is an early part of treatment, many patients require only manual blocking exercise to regain rebalanced motion. If joint stiffness and/or tissue adherence is persistent, a blocking-exercise splint offers a longer period of opportunity to regain balanced motion (see Fig. 61-8).

Proprioceptive feedback. When working to regain finger flexion, proprioceptive feedback is essential. Although muscle isolation must precede muscle strengthening, providing enough resistance to finger flexion to increase the patient's proprioceptive sense of digital motion is beneficial. This is particularly critical in the presence of diminished sensibility. This type of feedback can be accomplished by the patient holding an object slightly smaller than the available range of finger flexion. Use of a padded handle that demands some effort to be held firmly will allow use of the hand for eating and self-care activities while demanding slightly more finger flexion than is readily available. The size of the handle is decreased as the patient gains flexion range.

Low-load prolonged stress. It often is stated that therapy should apply a low-load, prolonged stress to accomplish plastic deformation of the tissues.[17,52,85] Early in the fibroplastic stage of healing before collagen cross-linking is well established, intermittent active motion is usually enough stress to favorably alter the cross-linking. Later in healing, when excess collagen cross-linking limits motion, low-load, prolonged stress favorably modifies the cross-links and the collagen microfils slip over each other.[128,134] This slippage is accomplished by exercises that hold the maximum range of joint motion and soft tissue glide to allow slippage of the cross-links to occur. If the tissues do not mobilize in response to this type of active exercise,

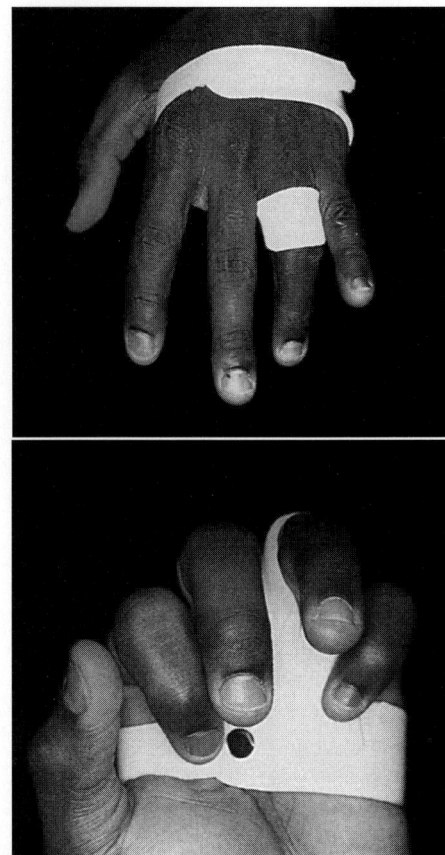

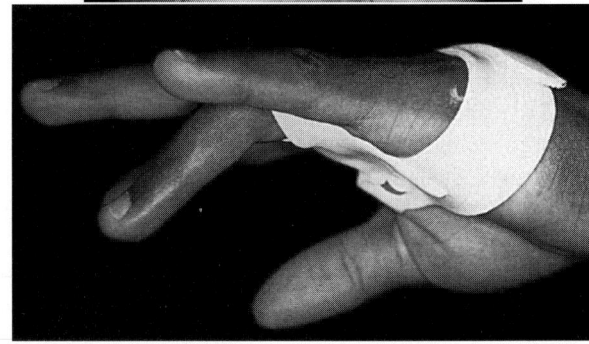

Fig. 61-8. After a proximal phalangeal fracture, a small splint to block the metacarpophalangeal joint transmits glide of the flexor and extensor tendons across the stiff proximal interphalangeal joint.

mobilization splinting that provides a gentle force for a longer period increases the passive potential to allow greater active motion.

Passive range of motion. Although joint motion can be maintained by either active or passive motion,[53] passive motion does not glide the tissue planes other than the periarticular structures. Therefore increasing passive motion does not necessarily increase active motion.

As with other therapeutic techniques, there is no empiric information to dictate the ideal beneficial force, speed, and duration of passive motion.[53] Although passive joint motion often is prescribed to overcome posttraumatic joint stiffness, no research supports the efficacy of either intermittent passive motion or CPM.[61] We do know that aggressive passive motion of the hand is detrimental and should be avoided.[20,96]

The only appropriate application of PROM to the small joints of the hand is early in the postoperative stage when the joint is gently positioned slightly beyond the available joint range to assist the patient in isolating the correct muscle. Correct passive motion technique in the injured hand should be defined as the gentle encouragement of tissues to reach a maximum available length. The amount of force should respect the resistance of the tissues, and the position should be increased only when the tissues relax and decreased resistance can be felt. Until there is control of postoperative edema, no joint should be passively flexed. When edema is diminished, any gentle passive joint motion should be done with accompanying traction to the joint to allow room for one joint surface to glide over the other without compression. One gentle, prolonged hold will allow the motion to be repeated actively more effectively than many repeated quick sudden stretches. Quick, forceful stretches result in tissue damage and should be avoided at all times.

In the hand with more mature stiffness caused by increased collagen cross-linking, the brief intermittent nature of passive motion is ineffective. Mobilization splinting that provides a more prolonged gentle force should be applied.

Joint mobilization. Although manual joint mobilization is advocated by many for the treatment of stiff joints, manual mobilization of the hand joints is best reserved for specific capsular tightness with no accompanying inflammation, rather than being used early when room for motion is limited as a result of edema. Joint mobilization without accompanying edema reduction does not increase the available room for movement.

Muscle isolation/pattern of motion. Patients who experience stiffness of the hand following injury invariably feel that a strong muscle pull is required to overcome the stiffness. Unfortunately, this excessive effort recruits the strongest muscles, overpowering the weaker, in which glide is limited (Fig. 61-9). Co-contraction of muscles is a common result of excessive effort. The patient must be taught a gentle pull that isolates the desired muscle, understanding that exercise for strengthening will come later in therapy. The patient learns a clear difference between a strong global pull that is ineffectual and a gentle but sustained precise pull that helps reestablish muscle balance. Understanding this difference ensures that the patient repeats the exercise correctly at home. It may be helpful to have the patient pull intensely and let the stronger muscles overpower to appreciate the contrast with the gentle isolation exercises.

Patients whose limbs have been immobilized in a cast following a distal radius fracture provide a useful example. The weakened wrist extensors cannot stabilize the wrist sufficiently, so the finger flexor muscles can effectively flex

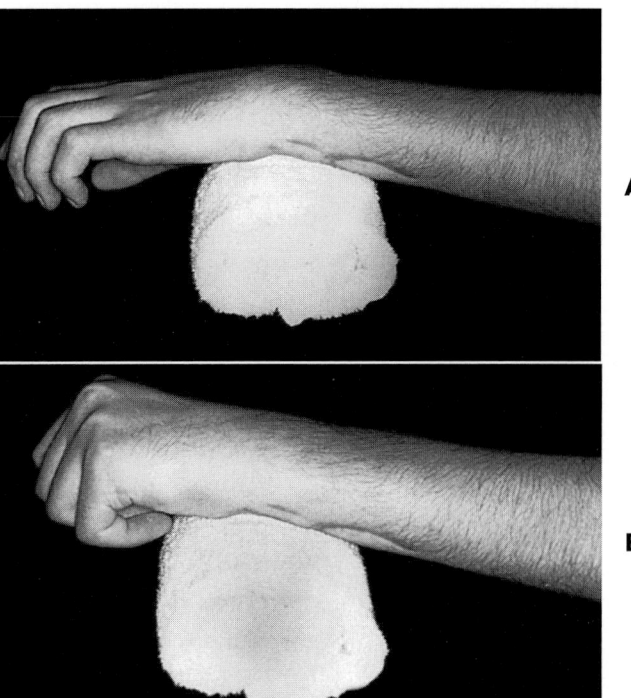

Fig. 61-9. A, After Colles' fracture, patient attempts wrist extension but uses extrinsic finger extensors. **B,** Patient maintains full finger flexion that assists in isolation of wrist extensor muscles.

the digits. When the patient is asked to extend the wrist, he or she substitutes with the finger extensor muscles because they have been unrestrained in the cast and are stronger than the wrist extensor muscles (see Fig. 61-9). If edema and finger stiffness are accompanying complications, little progress can be made with finger motion until the patient can stabilize the wrist with the wrist extensor muscles.

Pathologic patterns of motion in the early stiff hand

Loss of wrist tenodesis pattern. The exquisite balance of muscle forces crossing the wrist and fingers creates a reciprocal motion called *tenodesis*. Finger extension occurs with wrist flexion as a result of the increased tension on the extrinsic extensor muscles. Conversely, when the wrist extends, tension is increased in the extrinsic flexor muscles that cause the fingers to flex. This reciprocal action establishes the normal grasp and release pattern of the hand.

When any joint motion is restricted, the tenodesis balance is altered. In a minor injury, tenodesis is regained as motion at the injury site improves. In more severe injuries requiring long periods of immobilization, many joints may be stiff and the muscles crossing them weak, totally eradicating the reciprocal balanced motion.

The wrist is the key joint to reestablishing the tenodesis balance in the hand, because without the ability to stabilize the wrist in extension, the finger flexor muscles cannot transfer enough power to gain finger flexion. Usually, the primary goal is to regain digital flexion for grasp and

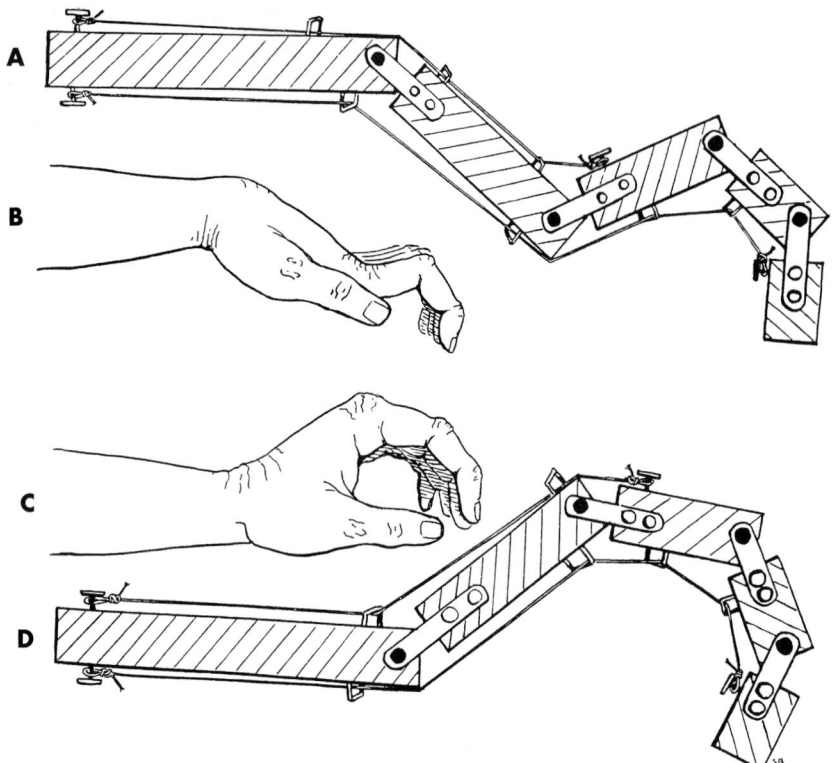

Fig. 61-10. A and **B,** Loss of wrist extension creates tension on the extrinsic extensor muscles and finger flexion is lost. **C** and **D,** With the wrist in extension, the tension on the finger flexors facilitates digital flexion. (From Bunnell S: *Surgery of the hand,* ed 2, Philadelphia, 1948, JB Lippincott.)

manipulation of objects. However, when the fingers and the wrist all have limited motion, active finger flexion is not possible without some wrist extension (Fig. 61-10).

Intrinsic-plus pattern. In normal finger flexion, IP flexion dominates before significant MP flexion begins.[11] If the hand is edematous and extrinsic flexor glide is limited (e.g., immobilization of wrist fractures or flexor tendon repair), the patient will initiate finger flexion with MP joint flexion and little IP joint flexion occurs. In this pattern of motion, the intrinsic muscles are never elongated to their maximum length and they adaptively shorten, making the mobilization of the IP joints even more difficult.

Early treatment consisting of activities, exercises, and/or splints that block MP joint flexion and require IP joint flexion (unless contraindicated by the surgical procedure) can convert global finger flexion into specific glide across the IP joints (see Fig. 61-8). In the chronic stiff hand, longer periods of intervention may be necessary to change the pattern of motion (see the section on the chronically stiff hand).

Intrinsic-minus pattern. When the intrinsic muscles are not actively participating in digital flexion, MP joint flexion is absent and all flexion occurs at the IP joints from the pull of the extrinsic flexor muscles. This may result from denervation of the intrinsic muscles, but in the stiff hand, it is more commonly a result of isolated capsular tightness of the MP joints or the restraint created by adherence of the

extensor tendons on the dorsum of the hand. Some type of MP joint flexion mobilization force is required to allow the intrinsic muscles to participate in the digital flexion.

Evaluation and treatment of joint stiffness and decreased tissue glide

Joint tightness
Evaluation. Joint tightness is discerned by manually examining the joint PROM to determine whether the range changes as proximal and distal joint positions are altered. If the joint ROM does not change, isolated joint tightness is present (Fig. 61-11).

Clinical reality usually provides a combination of joint tightness and other external constraints, such as muscle-tendon unit tightness or tendon adherence. An experienced therapist can determine the balance and mix of the many tissues that are limiting motion. Accurate appraisal of the potential may be limited until certain joint motions have been regained. For example, proximal interphalangeal (PIP) joint flexion must be gained before the true extent of intrinsic muscle tightness can be determined.

Accurate, repeated ROM measurements must be the means of monitoring improvement.[7] If there is a large discrepancy between the active range of motion (AROM) and PROM, the emphasis should lie on active pull-through. If the AROM and PROM are equal, concentration on gaining

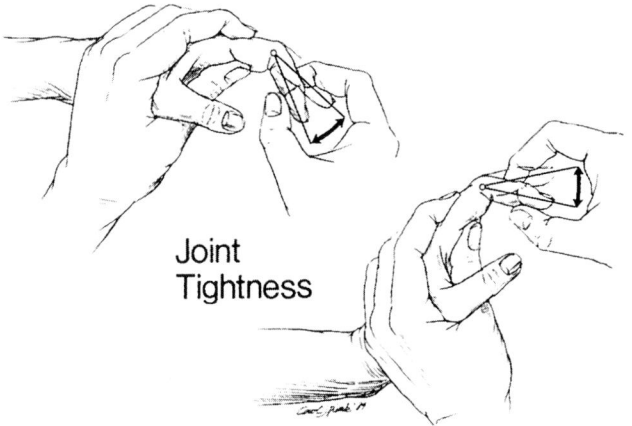

Fig. 61-11. Joint capsular tightness is defined when the range of passive joint motion is the same regardless of the position of proximal and distal joints.

passive motion via mobilization splinting will create the potential for greater active motion.

Manual treatment. The degree of trauma to the joint capsule and the stage of healing determine whether the observed resistance of the joint is the expected amount of joint stiffness. When joint tightness is being evaluated, a distinction should be made between a joint with a soft end-feel and a hard end-feel. The *soft* end-feel refers to a joint whose stiffness is characterized by a soft and springy end to the joint motion. This soft end-feel describes joint tightness resulting from edema and early stages of collagen cross-linking. With active motion and prolonged low-load stress, the capsular structures of the joint can regain independent glide. A *hard* end-feel joint is one with little edema present and more mature cross-linking. When moved to its maximum ROM, there is an abrupt well-defined endpoint to the passive test. The resistance is such that the examiner feels as if the endpoint of motion has been reached. This type of end-feel to a joint requires more prolonged periods of mobilization splinting to gain motion (see the following section on treatment of the chronically stiff hand).

Joints with a soft end-feel are the only joints appropriate for application of manual PROM. If the joint edema is minimal, gentle prolonged passive stretching to joints with a soft end-feel may enable more active motion to be transmitted across the stiff joint. In many cases, this is enough to resolve the joint stiffness. In the joint with minor trauma, early splinting with intermittent gentle passive motion may produce full active motion without further intervention.

Joint mobilization via splinting. If active and passive joint mobilization techniques are not successful or if the joint resistance is significant on the initial evaluation, mobilization splinting to regain capsular length in one direction may be essential to regaining motion. It is reasonable to splint to gain the motion that has the most resistance to passive stretch. This is the least likely to be gained with only active

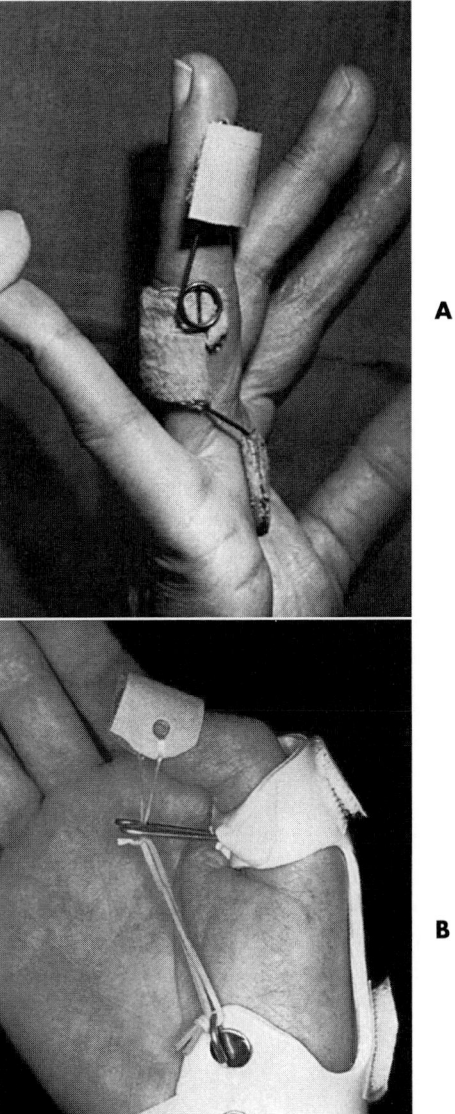

Fig. 61-12. A, A dynamic proximal interphalangeal (PIP) extension mobilization splint effectively gains PIP joint extension without including other joints. **B,** A splint stabilizes the metacarpophalangeal joint of the thumb while dynamically mobilizing the interphalangeal joint into flexion.

and intermittent passive stretching. Wrist extension, MP joint flexion, and IP joint extension are most often the stiffest joint motions and must be given splinting priority to balance the strength of the opposing muscles.

Mobilization splinting for isolated joint tightness requires that only the involved joint is included in the splint because proximal joint motion and muscle pull is not relevant to the problem (Fig. 61-12, *A*). Splints may be applied that provide a dynamic, serial static, or static progressive force. Dynamic

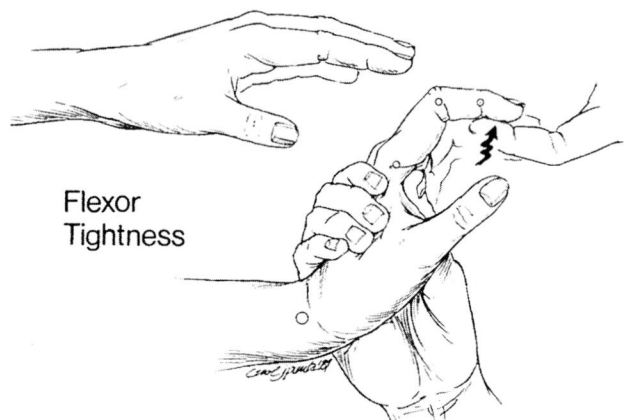

Fig. 61-13. Tightness of the extrinsic flexor muscles is seen when finger extension is limited when the wrist is extended but unimpeded when the wrist is neutral or flexed.

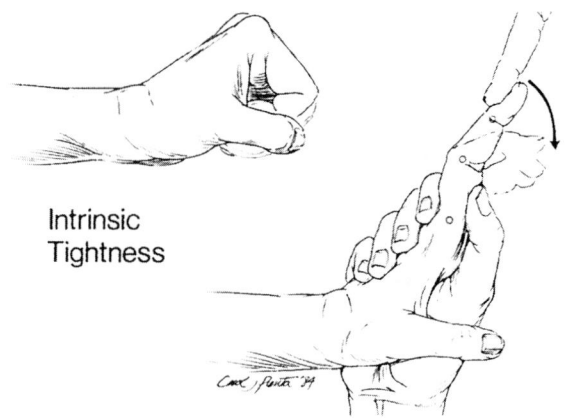

Fig. 61-14. Interosseous muscle tightness is noted when interphalangeal joint flexion range is less and resistance is greater when the metacarpophalangeal joint is extended or hyperextended than when it is flexed.

forces applied by rubber band or spring traction is a soft application of force appropriate for joints with a soft end-feel. If joint edema is present, joint motion can be gained concurrent to gentle joint compression with the application of serial static splinting. Joints that demonstrate greater resistance respond to the prolonged application of serial static splinting, or may respond to static progressive splinting. A dynamic force seems more comfortable in the end-range of joint flexion than does the unyielding force of static progressive splints because flexion dramatically increases intraarticular pressure[102] (Fig. 61-12, *B*).

Muscle-tendon unit tightness. Muscle-tendon unit tightness is shortening of the muscle-tendon unit from origin to insertion that commonly occurs secondary to immobilization in the presence of edema. In contrast, specific tendon adherence limiting glide usually is associated with direct trauma to the tendon or the tendon bed/sheath. Such an injury may allow the point of adherence to be isolated, whereas the muscle-tendon unit tightness limits the full length.

Evaluation. Tendon adherence and/or muscle-tendon unit tightness both are demonstrated by a distinct difference between the ease of passive distal joint motion when the proximal joints are positioned in flexion versus extension (Fig. 61-13).

The most proximal joint crossed by the muscle-tendon unit is the key to appraising tightness. For example, with tightness of the extrinsic extensor muscles, the fingers will be unable to flex as far when the wrist is in flexion as when the wrist is in extension. The opposite is true for extrinsic flexor muscle tightness. With wrist extension, finger extension is limited by the shortness of the flexor muscle-tendon unit. When the wrist is dropped, the fingers can extend. To achieve an effective stretch of the extrinsic flexor muscles, the wrist must be held in extension while the fingers are being extended.

The same principle holds for the interosseous muscles in the hand, with the MP joint being key to evaluating tightness. Because the interosseous tendons run palmar to the axis of the MP joint and dorsal to the axis of the PIP joints, the maximum stretch of this muscle-tendon unit occurs when the MP joints are held in maximum extension (e.g., hyperextension) and the PIP joints are passively flexed. If the range of PIP joint flexion is less and demonstrably tighter when the MP joint is held in full extension, the interosseous muscles are tight (Fig. 61-14). Examining the patient's uninjured hand for interosseous tightness gives the examiner a clear feel for the normal tightness of the individual's muscle-tendon units. This can vary considerably among individuals.

Treatment: tightness. Because muscle-tendon unit tightness most often results from immobility of the hand, active motion with intermittent prolonged passive stretching often alleviates mild muscle unit tightness. This stretch must be prolonged[78] and followed by active use of the muscle through the stretched range. If a muscle-tendon unit is left in a short position in the presence of tissue inflammation, the tendon will become adherent along its entire path. There need not be trauma directly to the tendon or the tissue bed for this adherence to occur. If seen in its early stage, this adherence usually can be eliminated by a prolonged stretch of the tendon through its maximum range. If, when stretching tightness, the therapist feels a palpable release of the adherence, the stretched position should be held in increments until this response is no longer appreciated. This sudden slipping of the tissue layers (slipping of the cross-links) can be felt as the gentle force is sustained. It should be strongly emphasized that this prolonged manual stretching uses sustained force, but it is a slowly applied force and is continued based only on a positive tissue response. The therapist can feel the resistance in the tissues

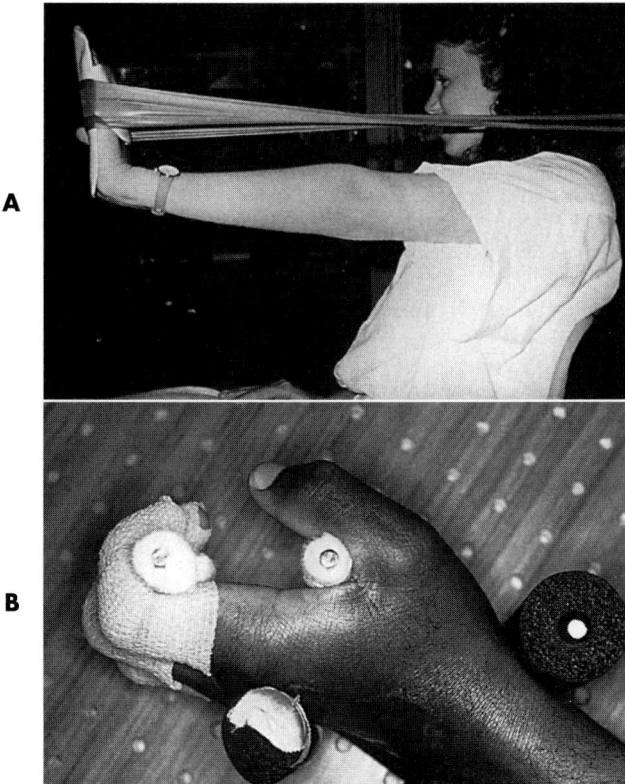

Fig. 61-15. **A,** Stretching of long flexor tightness may combine a splint to hold the fingers in extension while elastic stretches the wrist into extension. **B,** A pegboard stabilizes various joints to allow the patient to apply prolonged active stretch for interphalangeal joint tightness and intrinsic muscle tightness.

diminish. The patient should be comfortable throughout this procedure, feeling pulling and perhaps slight discomfort, but never pain. Patients with early tendon adherence may experience a dramatic improvement in motion after such a prolonged stretch. More commonly, one does not see this sudden dramatic response but sees improvement over a longer period with repeated stretching instead.

Both exercise and mobilization splints can help with elongation of muscle-tendon tightness (Figs. 61-12 and 61-15). Splints to diminish muscle-tendon unit tightness require that all joints crossed by the tightness be included in the splint and held at maximum length concurrently. Splints for muscle-tendon unit tightness should be easily adjustable or replaceable as gains are made. Splinting is discussed more fully later in this chapter.

Treatment: adherence. A tendon may be adherent anywhere along its path. Motion to decrease the adherence is accomplished only by joint motion distal to the adherence. This insight both allows correct positioning for exercise and determines the joints to be included in any splint. Mobilization splinting to decrease tendon adherence is effective only in regaining distal glide of the adherence of either a

flexor or extensor tendon. To gain proximal glide, the patient must learn to isolate and strengthen the correct muscle to regain full excursion of the adhered or tight unit.

Adherence after flexor tendon repair provides a good example of the type of active motion necessary to gain proximal glide of an adherent tendon. Commonly, after flexor tendon repair the patient flexes strongly with the unimpeded intrinsic muscles, preventing glide of the long tendons. When tendon healing permits, blocking the MP joint in extension to demand flexor tendon excursion more distally is mandatory (see Fig. 61-8, *B*). Tendon gliding exercises[129] that require independent gliding of the profundus and superficialis tendons relative to one another and the profundus relative to bone must be included. Early resistance provides helpful feedback to ensure correct motion and begins to strengthen the muscle unit that is the weakest. Neuromuscular electrical stimulation may be added both to boost the feedback effect and to recruit maximum firing of muscle fibers.

Mobilization splinting. Splinting to decrease adherence need include only the joints distal to the site of adherence. An example would be dorsal adherence of an extensor tendon on the hand secondary to a metacarpal fracture. Splinting of the finger joints in flexion to glide the tendon distally would not require inclusion of the wrist because the adherence is distal to the wrist. In contrast, if the problem is tightness of the extrinsic extensor muscles, the wrist would need to be positioned in some flexion within the splint to effectively stretch the unit.

Skin and scar tightness and adherence. All wounds heal with internal and external scar. Depending on the size, location, and direction, external scarring (especially linear scars) may limit joint motion. Even if the scar is not adherent to the underlying joints, the length of the scar may not be enough to allow multiple joints to move in the same direction at the same time. For example, a split-thickness skin graft on the dorsum of the hand can tether the skin so that either IP joint flexion or MP joint flexion is possible, but concurrent MP and IP joint flexion may not be possible.

Evaluation. Skin tightness is assessed by positioning joints so that the involved scar must transverse the maximum distance. Blanching, palpable tightness, or immobility of the scar or skin displays the extent of tightness (Fig. 61-16). If the skin tightness is limiting joint motion, placing the skin in its shortest position allows increased joint motion proximally or distally. This motion is diminished as the proximal joint is positioned to elongate the involved skin. This limitation may be difficult to determine in a severe injury causing both skin tightness and joint tightness.

Manual treatment. Scars are visually evident but must be palpated to determine their mobility and character. All new external scars will be adherent to the underlying bed and will have decreased oil and sweat present. In large scars, the lack of lubrication and adherence causes the scar to be dry

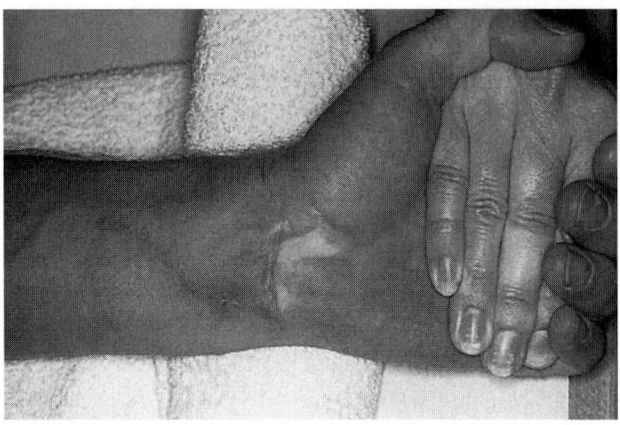

Fig. 61-16. Blanching of the skin at the wrist shows scar adherence and tightness.

and intolerant to frictional forces. As the scar reaches the stage of maturity to tolerate friction, gentle direct massage while using a lubricant is the treatment of choice.

Mobilization splinting for skin tightness. Unlike other tightness often alleviated by intermittent stretch, skin tightness requires prolonged periods of holding the skin at its maximum length. Splinting is usually mandatory to accomplish this. Prolonged serial static splinting with a positive-pressure interface mold provides the best force for realigning the collagen fibers. Any splint to elongate skin and scar tightness must position the joints at the proximal and distal ends of the tightness to allow elongation of the tissue.

Such prolonged positioning with the skin in the longest position is difficult to achieve in the hand. The need for increased mobility and strengthening must be balanced with the need for prolonged scar elongation. As a minimum, such mobilization splinting should be worn during sleep. In the initial stages of contraction, the splint may be required 23 of 24 hours if the graft or scar covers a large area. As tissue matures, the amount of splint wear may be slowly decreased to nighttime only. The rigid effect of a splint counteracts myofibroblast pull[109] and decreases scar proliferation and contraction.[128]

General principles of mobilization splinting of the early stiff hand

Therapists must have a wide spectrum of treatment skills to mobilize stiffness in the hand. If the patient is seen early after a simple injury, often no mobilization splinting is required. However, patients with greater tissue damage commonly require mobilization splinting to optimize functional motion. It must be emphasized that splinting alone is not adequate treatment but must always be in conjunction with a precise exercise program.[128] Because scar can be modified by stress application,[12] mobilization splinting may be an important part of regaining mobility of the severely injured hand. Unfortunately, all splints, even mobilization splints, impose immobilization and constriction, and the

good of the splint must far outweigh the negative effects of restriction and immobilization.[20] Early mobilization splinting that repositions joints with serial application is the safest early means of mobilizing healing tissue.

Each splint applied to the injured hand must be designed based on the purpose needed for the limitations in that hand.[14,128] Therapists must possess analytical skills, manual construction skills, and biomechanical knowledge to apply well-fitting and well-designed splints. Adequate discussion of splinting far exceeds the scope of this chapter, but important points are discussed in the following sections.

Tissue response to mobilization splinting. Human tissue responds to the application of mechanical force. Because collagen tissue is elastic by virtue of the weave configuration of the larger subunits,[105] short-duration force applied to collagen fibers elongates the tissue but provides no alteration of the collagen fiber construct. This is the elastic response.[17,24] If the force is applied over a prolonged period via a mobilization splint, the plastic response occurs. The tissue retains all or part of the elongated position.* The amount of temporary versus long-term change of tissues depends on the intensity and duration of the applied load.[40,52]

Optimal deformation is with the application of a low-load, prolonged stress.[17,40,78,88] One can understand this principle by thinking about how a rubber band, when quickly stretched, returns to its original length; however, a rubber band held stretched for a long period does not return to its original length as quickly or as completely.

The dilemma is that prolonged positioning imposes immobilization. The challenge is to balance periods of mobilization splinting with periods of active movement to ensure that passive gains can be maintained. Mobilization splinting must apply a low magnitude of force to avoid stimulation of the inflammatory response that increases edema and fibrosis.

Force application in mobilization splinting. Although it is possible to measure the amount of force being applied with a splint, there is currently no way of measuring either the optimal amount of stress needed or the optimal application time of the stress to bring about the most rapid agreeable modification of scar tissue.[128] The critical question is not about the amount of force we are applying but about the pressure exerted on the skin where the force is applied.[20] This point of force application becomes the limiting factor. Although one can measure how much pressure can be tolerated before skin necrosis occurs, this is of indirect value only because mobilization splints are applied intermittently. Pressure becomes relatively unimportant in the presence of intermittent application.[19,20,128] Fess[50] has demonstrated that experienced therapists consistently choose greater amounts of force for application to more mature scar. Flowers and LaStayo[52] have introduced the idea of total

*References 17, 20, 24, 78, 135, 136.

end-range time (the amount of time a restricted joint is held at maximum length), suggesting that, in the future, splint prescriptions will specify both the amount and duration of force application. Until we have a means of measuring the amount of resistance in the tissues and developing a rationale for the maximum desirable force, the patient's tissue response to the force application remains the primary guideline to force application.

The patient must understand that the goal is not to tolerate increasing amounts of tension but rather to tolerate low tension for longer periods. After an initial adjustment period, a patient's tissues should comfortably increase tolerance to the prolonged mobilization force. The patient should be aware of the sensation of stretching while in the splint, but pain should not be experienced. A motivated patient will eagerly wear an effective, well-fitting splint.

Types of mobilization splints. A therapist may choose from three types of mobilization splints: serial static, dynamic, and static progressive. Understanding the different mechanical effect of each type of splint allows the therapist to choose the most effective means of regaining motion while facilitating healing.

Serial static mobilization splints. A serial static splint immobilizes joints in a stationary position. The splint is applied with the tissue at its maximum length and is worn for long periods of time to allow the tissue to adapt[20,60] (Fig. 61-17). After a period of tissue accommodation, either a new splint is applied or the old splint is remolded to hold the tissue at a new maximum length. Although the splint is stationary, the repeated repositioning of the tissues mobilizes the tissues.

Dynamic mobilization splints. A dynamic splint applies force to a specific joint or joints. A stretched rubber band, spring, or wire coil generates the continuous force (see Fig. 61-12). As joint motion changes, the force of the splint continues. Although the force is constantly pulling while the splint is applied, the application of force is intermittent because the splint is removed periodically.[34] In the early stiff hand where collagen cross-linking is not mature, intermittent dynamic splinting effectively regains tissue mobility. In the hand with more mature stiffness, the intermittent nature of the force application may be inadequate to cause change.

For dynamic splints to be applied to mobilize the tightest structures, the hand must at times be positioned awkwardly in the splint. The intermittent nature of dynamic splinting allows such awkward positions to be tolerated because active therapy combines with the splinting program to regain the balance of motion. Dynamic splinting is the technique of choice when passive motion of the joints is responsive to manual stretch and inflammation has subsided.[7,23,24,121]

A period of therapy to gain active pull-through and edema reduction while increasing the tolerance to the tissue stress readies the hand for dynamic mobilization splinting. If the splint is applied too early, it can escalate the inflammatory response.

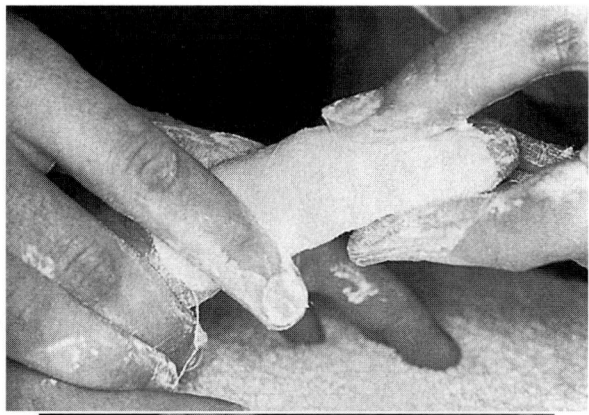

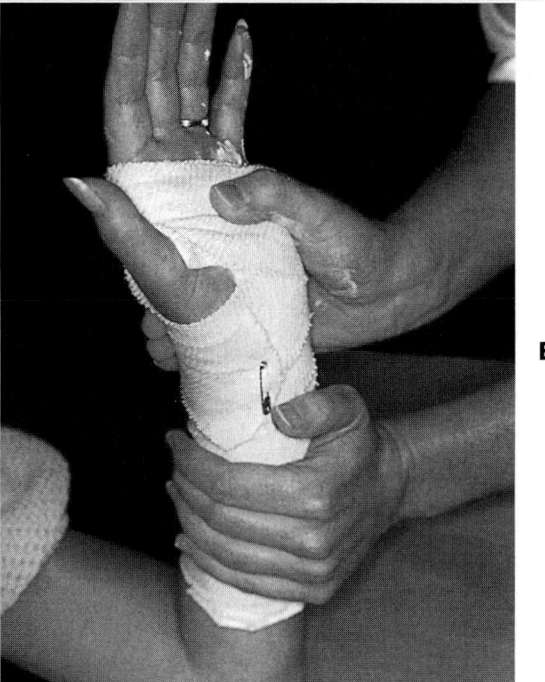

Fig. 61-17. A, A stiff proximal interphalangeal joint can be resolved effectively by a series of serial extension mobilization casts to the finger. **B,** Wrist extension is regained by serial application of dorsal and volar plaster slabs.

Static progressive mobilization splints. Static progressive mobilization splints may appear identical to dynamic mobilization splints, but the applied force is not dynamic (Fig. 61-18). Instead of the constant pull of a rubber band or spring, the tension on the joint is an adjustable static force. The force may be applied via hook and loop fastener or with commercially available components that adjust in small increments. When tension is applied, the joint is positioned at its maximum range. The force is adjusted when the tissue response allows repositioning to a new length.

Static progressive splinting is effective for joints with limited motion when there is significant resistance at the end of the passive stretch, especially when the range to be gained is at the end of the normal maximum (see Fig. 61-18). As

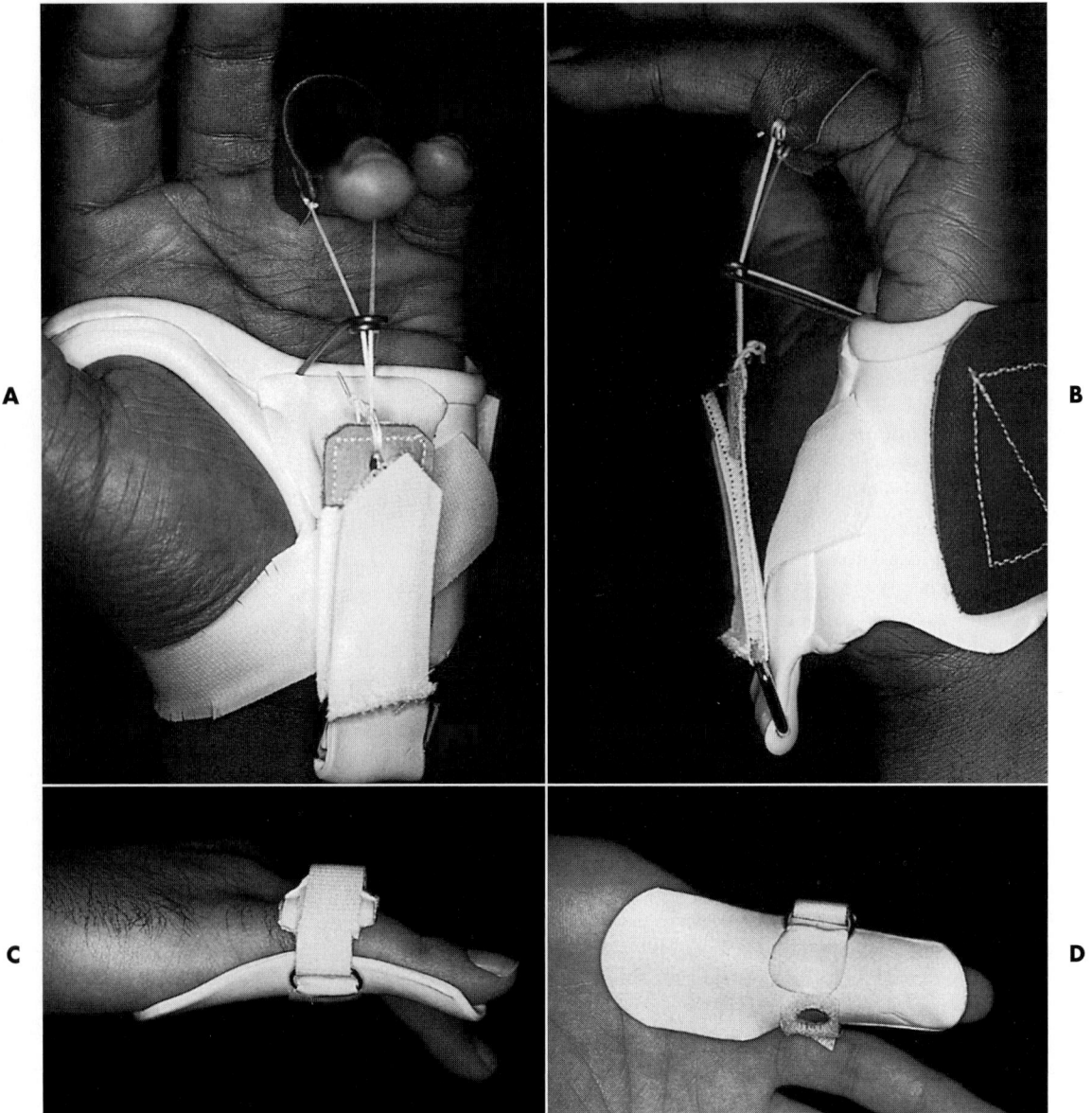

Fig. 61-18. A and **B,** Static progressive splint gains flexion of the metacarpophalangeal joint. **C** and **D,** Serial static splint for proximal interphalangeal extension mobilization where the volar piece is molded in greater extension than is available to the joint. (From Colditz JC: *Br J Hand Ther* 5:65, 2000. Copyright 2000.)

with other mobilization splints, the patient removes the splint and works on active glide and exercises or may use another splint to gain another direction of motion. Prolonged stretch at the end of the range is what gives the joint its full easy motion in both directions. The earlier the hand is ready for static progressive splinting, the shorter the time required to gain motion. The longer the time since injury, the longer the need for splinting to regain motion.

Choosing mobilization splints based on the stage of healing. The stress appropriate to mobilize tissues differs in each clinical stage of healing. Static immobilization splints rest inflamed tissues during initial healing to provide

protection and to allow inflammation to subside. If the desired position of immobilization cannot be obtained initially, serial static mobilization splints can safely reposition joints of the hand without providing undue stress to healing tissues. When injury is extensive and inflammation is prolonged, the rest provided by the splint is of continuing value. The process of tissue healing and maturation proceeds at variable rates in individuals, and many patients may have a prolonged inflammatory response.[23]

After the initial inflammation subsides, the injured tissues begin the proliferative stage of healing. Cells are multiplying at a rate greater than normal. During this stage, correctly

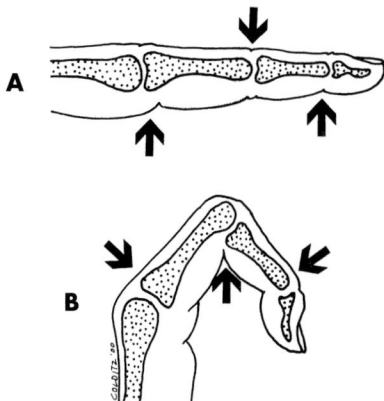

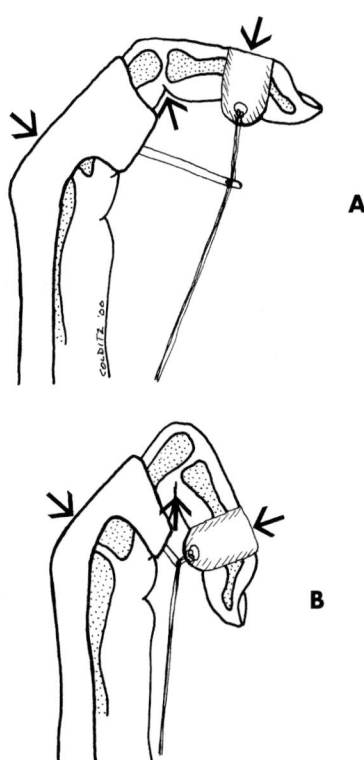

Fig. 61-19. A, The three points of force for proximal interphalangeal (PIP) extension splinting places the middle point of force directly on the extensor surface of the joint and the two opposite forces palmarly as far from the joint as possible. **B,** The three points of force for PIP flexion splinting are in the same location, but on opposite surfaces as those for extension. (From Colditz JC: *Br J Hand Ther* 5:65, 2000. Copyright 2000.)

Fig. 61-20. A and **B,** The line of force in proximal interphalangeal joint flexion mobilization changes based on the angle of maximum flexion of the join. (From Colditz JC: *Br J Hand Ther* 5:65, 2000. Copyright 2000.)

applied stress has its optimal benefit in determining the length, orientation, and relationship of the collagen fibers. If patients do not respond sufficiently to gentle manual stretching and active exercise, the gentle force of dynamic splinting is usually all that is required. If there is any indication of a continuing inflammatory response (e.g., fluctuant edema, reddened joints, pain with joint motion), serial static splinting should be chosen to provide a balance of rest while also repositioning joints.

As the tissue matures and joint motion has a hard end-feel with significant resistance, the prolonged force of serial static splinting or static progressive splinting is necessary. A truly resistive joint is best treated with a serial static splint that is not removed by the patient. Although the static progressive splint also provides prolonged positioning at the maximum passive length, its periodic removal allows the tissue to resume the original resting length. A new technique that I developed, casting motion to mobilize stiffness (CMMS), is appropriate for the chronically stiff hand that is unresponsive to traditional therapy techniques. This is discussed in a subsequent section.

Basic principles of mobilization splinting. Because mobilization splinting is an integral part of the effective therapy for the stiff hand, the basic principles of mobilization splinting are discussed in this section. The reader is directed to the in-depth information on this topic available from numerous sources.[26,27,33-35,39,47,51,75,89,119,122,132]

The effectiveness of any mobilization splint is limited by the accuracy of the design, fit, and force application. Every splint that immobilizes or mobilizes a joint must use three points of pressure.[35] The middle force is applied directly at the axis of the joint. Without crossing another joint, the two opposite forces are placed as far away from the middle force as possible for maximum efficiency (Fig. 61-19).

Extension mobilization or immobilization splinting places the middle force over the dorsum of the joint axis and the opposing forces are placed on the palmar or volar surface (see Fig. 61-19, *A*). Because there is little natural padding on the dorsal aspect of the hand, the pressure over the joint must be carefully placed and well molded to be comfortable.

The three points of pressure for flexion mobilization splinting are the reverse of extension splinting: palmarly over the axis of the joint with the two opposing forces applying pressure dorsally as far away from the joint as is practical (see Fig. 61-19, *B*). The difficulty in flexion mobilization splinting is the impossibility of applying force directly over the palmar aspect of a joint while also allowing room for the joint to fully flex.

Unlike extension mobilization splinting where the forces are almost in direct opposition, the splinting forces may be almost at right angles in flexion mobilization splinting, especially of the digits (Fig. 61-20). If the forces are at a right angle, the splint base shifts distally before the joint moves unless the splint base is adequately secured.

Distributing pressure evenly. The palmar surface of the hand, with its thicker and more adherent skin and the presence of the thenar and hypothenar muscles, can tolerate pressure more easily than can the dorsum of the hand. The skin on the dorsum of the hand is thin and highly mobile. The dorsum of the hand also has multiple bony prominences that tolerate pressure poorly. For example, in low-profile dynamic or static progressive PIP joint extension mobilization designs, the splint is molded contiguously over the MP joints to distribute pressure over as much surface area as possible. The leading edge of the block ends exactly at the joint axis so that all the force is specifically directed to the precise anatomic location.[35] Pressure on the neurovascular bundles of fingers can be minimized by constructing finger loops of a firm material and attaching string to both sides.[33]

Another example of pressure distribution is the use of dorsal and volar plaster slabs for serial repositioning of the wrist. The volar and dorsal pieces distribute pressure over both surfaces, and the three points of pressure (two volarly and one dorsally over the wrist) are distributed widely (see Fig. 61-17). This is in contrast to the use of a volar slab with only one strap concentrating the force over the dorsal wrist area.

Providing constant prolonged tension. Even distribution of pressure is the primary factor to ensure comfort with prolonged force application. Avoiding sharp edges or ill-fitting molded shapes will enhance comfortable prolonged wear. Attention to construction detail coupled with listening to the patient and modifying the splint readily in response to the patient's comments will ensure maximum wear and comfort.

The tolerance to the force of dynamic or static progressive mobilization splints usually relates to the amount of force application. Using the minimum force the patient can tolerate for increasing amounts of time is preferable to using increasing amounts of force. The patient's goal should be increased wearing time before force is increased. Conversely, if the patient cannot comfortably wear the splint beyond a few minutes and the splint fits well, the force should be decreased.

Ease of adjustment. Any mobilization splint must be easy to remold, inexpensive to replace, and quick to adjust. Because the goal is increased motion, the splint must be adaptable to the anticipated change. Low-temperature thermoplastic materials allow quick remolding and adjustments to adapt to new positions, decreased edema, or relief of unwanted pressure. The use of plaster of Paris for specific clinical applications allows quick construction of a new splint with minimal materials cost.

Brass rods used as outriggers for dynamic or static progressive mobilization splints allow adjustments to be made by bending the wire (Fig. 61-21). For example, as finger joint flexion increases, the line of pull of the finger loop needs to be directed closer toward the palm. Alternatively, as finger extension improves, the dorsal outrigger needs to be shortened and placed more proximally.

Providing a force perpendicular to the long bone axis. The construction of a dynamic or static progressive mobilization splint requires attention to a few additional mechanical principles. To mobilize a joint, one must provide a pull at a 90-degree angle to the axis of the long bone that is the distal articulation of the joint in question[33] (Fig. 61-22). The outrigger is located as close to the force application as

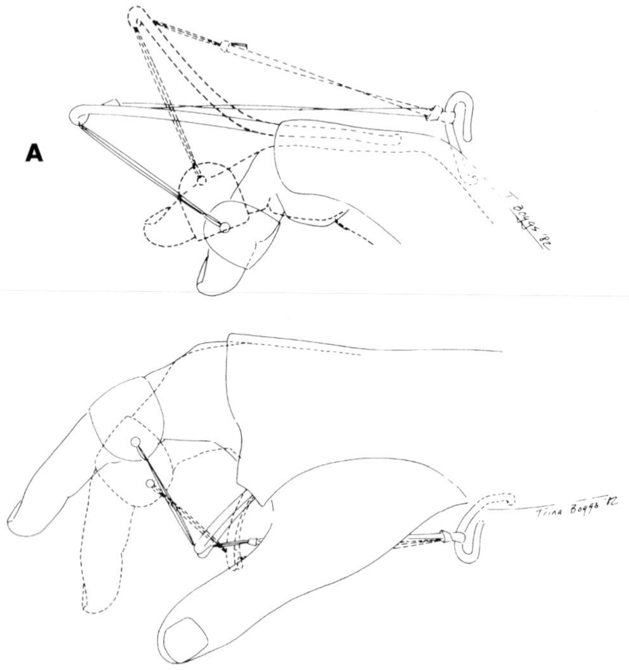

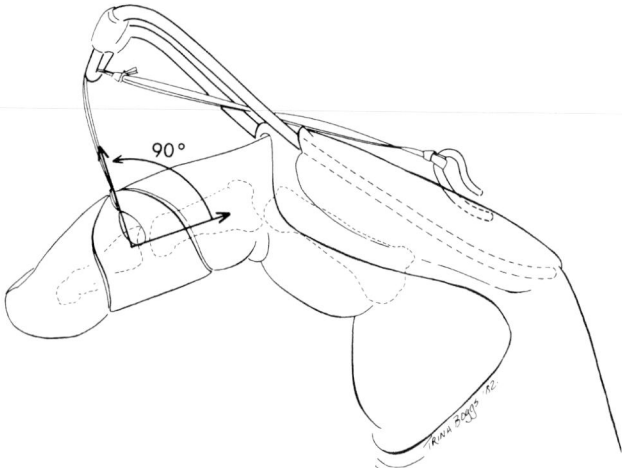

Fig. 61-21. Ease of adjustment of low-profile wire outrigger system is accomplished by bending of the wire outrigger. This allows maintenance of a 90-degree line of pull when either extension (**A**) or flexion (**B**) is accomplished. (From Colditz JC: *Am J Occup Ther* 37:182, 1983. Reprinted with the permission of the American Occupational Therapy Association, Inc. Copyright 1983.)

Fig. 61-22. Low-profile dynamic (or static progressive) splint provides a 90-degree line of pull to the distal end of the middle phalanx to extend the proximal interphalangeal joint. (From Colditz JC *Am J Occup Ther* 37:182, 1983. Reprinted with the permission of the American Occupational Therapy Association, Inc. Copyright 1983.)

possible. The outrigger redirects the line of pull and keeps the line close to, and parallel with, the splint base. This system is of value only if a secure splint base has been applied that is intimately conformed, has well-distributed pressure areas, and accurately stabilizes the proximal joints.

The outrigger will deform before the tissue elongates if either the outrigger or its attachment to the splint base is unstable. Outrigger stability is directly correlated to length of the outrigger and the manner of attachment to the base. Attaching the outrigger over a large area of the splint base to the distal edge of the splint contributes to maximum outrigger attachment stability.

Wearing tolerance. When applying a mobilization splint, one must observe two areas of progress. First, the patient must be able to tolerate the splint comfortably for increasing periods. If this does not occur, the splint either needs adjustment or is the wrong type. Intolerance also may suggest that the splint has been applied at the wrong time in the healing process. Second, precise goniometric measurements must be taken before application of the splint. If there are no measurable gains for a few weeks after splint application, the splint is not effective. Reevaluation of the type of splint, the fit, and the patient's tolerance is merited.

Many patients are encouraged by the rapid gains of motion in response to splint application. They become discouraged when they remove the force of the splint and the deformity recurs. Patients need to be instructed that maintenance of gains of motion will require prolonged use of the splint and exercises to be able to maintain the gains made in the splint.

EVALUATING AND TREATING THE CHRONICALLY STIFF HAND

Based on clinical experience and literature review, I believe that three factors interplay to perpetuate stiffness in the chronically stiff hand. (Fig. 61-23). First, there is stiffness in multiple joints, including uninjured joints. Tissue adherence is palpable and resistance to passive joint motion

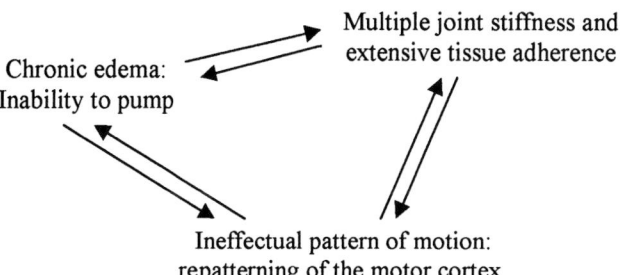

Fig. 61-23. In the chronically stiff hand, three factors are interdependent on one another and effective mobilization requires that all factors are addressed simultaneously.

is significant. Intermittent manual mobilization or mobilization splinting provides only temporary reduction of the stiffness. Second, the lack of active motion has diminished the lymphatic pumping ability and chronic edema permeates all tissue planes, even in sites remote from original injury. Results from edema reduction are temporary because the stiffness limits active motion and the lymphatic pumping cannot be maintained. Third, because an awkward and ineffectual pattern of movement has been repeated continually for a long time, it has become a dominant motion in the motor cortex. Even if the patient wants to move in a balanced normal pattern, the resistance in the tissues from tissue adherence and the chronic edema make it mechanically impossible to do so. The patient continually repeats the ineffectual pattern of movement; therefore it remains dominant.

In the chronically stiff hand, these three factors of tissue adherence and stiffness, chronic edema, and motor cortex patterning are interdependent. Changing one factor alone will not change the other factors. If mobility of the stiff hand is to be regained, all of the factors must be altered simultaneously (see Fig. 61-23). Such chronic stiffness can be reduced dramatically by using a technique that I developed, called *CMMS*.

Casting motion to mobilize stiffness

CMMS is the use of plaster of Paris casting to selectively immobilize proximal joints in an ideal position while constraining distal joints so that they move within a desired direction and range.[36] Unlike more traditional treatment methods, the CMMS technique simultaneously mobilizes stiff joints, reduces edema, and directs a new pattern of motion to revive the cortical representation of productive motion. Traditional manual mobilization techniques and mobilization splinting are less effective in the chronically stiff hand than in the newly stiff hand because these techniques are intermittent and address only one problem at a time.

The CMMS technique contradicts traditional treatment theory in a number of ways. First and most dramatically, active motion regains both active and passive joint motion. No PROM, modality, or manual treatment is applied. Because the cast immobilizes proximal joints and allows only the stiff joints to move in the range and direction needed, motion is isolated and part of the hand is immobilized. Typically, therapists believe that immobilization of any joint is to be avoided and motion in all directions should be gained concurrently. CMMS focuses on gaining the motion that is needed most, which may temporarily cause of loss of motion in the immobilized joints. This approach also contradicts the common assumption that one should never allow gains in one direction of motion at the expense of the other directions. In the chronically stiff hand, the balance of motion is overwhelmingly in favor of the stiff pattern. If the opposite pattern of motion is allowed to be the

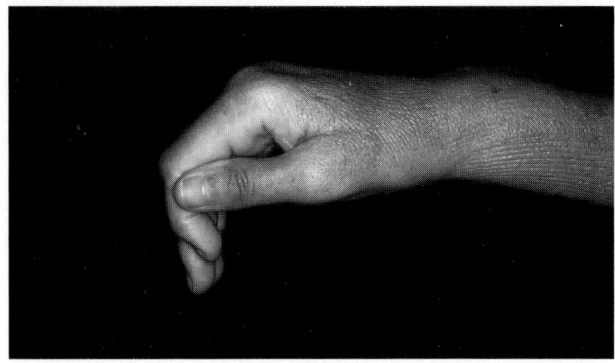

Fig. 61-24. A chronically stiff hand shows an absence of a normal tenodesis pattern and the resulting ineffectual pattern of motion.

dominant motion until tissues are mobilized, edema is evacuated, and motor relearning occurs, the opposite motion will return with time. In cases of altered anatomy following injury, one must be assured that the reconstructed anatomy has the potential to return to the balanced motion before applying the CMMS technique. The same concern is not applicable to the stiffness in uninjured joints resulting from immobilization.

CMMS can be successful with severe stiffness that is unresponsive to traditional treatment. Because the patient is mobilizing only with active motion, treatment is not painful. Therapy sessions consist of reevaluation, cast changes, and home instructions, creating a cost-effective approach. As functional motion is gained, a slow weaning process is begun and the functional use of the hand continues the progression of mobilization.

To accurately convey the appropriate application of the CMMS technique, the rationale of the technique is discussed, followed by discussion of the clinical application of the technique.

Joint stiffness and tissue adherence

Unlike other therapy approaches for stiff joints in the hand, CMMS uses only active motion to mobilize stiff joints. One does not expect active motion alone to have the ability to mobilize a stiff joint that has an abrupt hard end to passive motion. Perhaps this disbelief arises from the assumption that, if active motion could resolve joint tightness and tissue adherence, it would have been done already. However, without the constraint of the cast directing movement to the stiffest joints only, the patient will unavoidably move the more mobile joints first, leaving the stiff joint with the least power and excursion during active motion. The fact that active movement mobilizes significant joint stiffness is the most persuasive aspect of the CMMS technique.

The relative immobility of the chronically stiff hand allows the well-known negative effects of immobilization to develop (Fig. 61-24). In particular, the lack of stress to the tissues allows excess cross-link formation within the colla-

gen matrix, creating mechanical resistance to motion.* When the hand is positioned within the cast, cyclical motion across the stiff joints applies positive stress to the tissues, altering the cross-linking, and tissue resistance diminishes.[4,44,98] Because the only motion that occurs at the joint is the motion needed within the range needed, all active movement reinforces gains in ROM. In the acutely injured hand, intermittent blocking exercises are enough to accomplish this, but in the chronically stiff hand, the nonremovable cast provides the constancy needed for active motion to successfully mobilize stiff joints.

Mobilization splinting of the chronically stiff hand applies a prolonged but intermittent force at the end of the joint ROM. Unfortunately, the mobilization splint also imposes immobilization because there is no aspect of active tissue gliding when the splint is applied. When the splint is removed, the patient reverts to the ineffectual pattern of motion, thereby nullifying the gains of passive motion made while in the splint. The negative aspects of mobilization splinting in the chronically stiff hand are compared with the positive aspects of the CMMS technique in Table 61-1.

As discussed previously in this chapter, CPM has proven the effectiveness of long-term cyclical loading applied acutely after injury[102,111,123]; however, its usefulness for reducing stiffness has not been proven.[90,111] Undoubtedly, this is because the patient with a stiff hand reverts to the nonfunctional pattern of movement upon removal of the CPM, providing no reinforcement to improved joint mobility. The CMMS technique combines stiffness reduction with repatterning of the active motion simultaneously (see the following discussion).

Because of its intermittent nature, manual PROM is ineffective in changing joint stiffness in the chronically stiff hand. Although the effects of stress deprivation on the connective tissues can be prevented by both passive and active joint motion,[53] there is no proven correlation of the application of passive motion to increased active motion in the chronically stiff hand. Applied repeatedly and forcefully, PROM prolongs the inflammatory response.

To make gains in passive motion, it has been assumed that joints must be held at length by applying a low-load, prolonged stress with a mobilization splint.[20] The positive relationship between the total time that a joint is held at end-range and the decreased tissue resistance has been demonstrated.[52] However, a positive relationship between active motion and increased total end-range time has not been proven. End-range active cyclical loading[131] across stiff joints offered by the CMMS technique provides an effective low-load prolonged force, although cyclical in nature. Not only does motion occur in the range needed, but the constraint of the cast restricts the joints from returning to the position of adaptive shortening.

---

*References 2, 5, 6, 53, 61, 90, 96, 108, 134.

Table 61-1. A comparison of the disadvantages of mobilization splinting with the advantages of the CMMS technique in the chronically stiff hand

Disadvantages of mobilization splinting in treating chronic stiffness	Advantages of CMMS in treating chronic stiffness
Mobilization of stiff joints	
1. Immobilizes stiff joint(s) at end-range	1. Active motion mobilizes joint at end of range
2. Applies force in one direction only	2. Active motion allowed in two directions
3. Prevents excursion of the soft tissues and tendon(s) across the joint	3. Active motion allows repeated excursion
Reduction of chronic edema	
1. Applies constrictive force	1. Applies sustained pressure and provides pseudo-massage
2. Can apply excessive force	2. Active motion never applies excessive force
3. Lack of active lymphatic pumping	3. Active motion maintains lymphatic pumping
4. Possible prolongation of the inflammatory response	4. Directs active motion within cast; diminished observable joint inflammation
Repatterning of motor cortex	
1. Allows no active motion	1. Places hand in position so that desired motion occurs
2. Intermittent use of mobilization splints allows pattern of motion to revert each time the splint is removed	2. Nonremovable cast allows cortical repatterning
3. No effort is directed toward regaining normal tenodesis motion	3. Weaning proceeds only as patient can maintain tenodesis motion

CMMS, Casting motion to mobilize stiffness.

The principle of using a cast to limit motion in one direction to increase active motion in the other direction has been used only in the larger joints of patients with spastic muscles. King[76] reports the use of a drop-out elbow cast for spastic elbow contracture of −90 degrees. In 12 days, the contracture was reduced to −12 degrees. Others report similar improvement in motion and also report a calming effect on the spasticity as a result of cast application.[79]

Edema

The chronically stiff hand is characterized by atrophic, shiny skin with diminished or absent joint creases, mild pitting (or nonpitting) edema, and firmness to palpation of the tissues throughout the hand as compared with the contralateral uninjured side (see Fig. 61-24). Edema in the joints limits joint motion. Pain with motion dictates that it is desirable to hold the joints immobile in the most comfortable position.[31,41,66,138]

The prolonged presence of edema continues because limited active motion restricts the pumping ability of the lymphatic system. Excess fibrosis from the prolonged presence of high-protein edema further impedes the flow of fluid and proteins through the tissue channels to the initial lymphatics,[31,32,94] resulting in a low-grade chronic inflammation.[65] Although patients with trauma may have injury to the local lymphatic system, the proximal lymphatic system is normal. Lack of motion in the hand reduces the distal pumping that moves the lymphatic fluid to the more proximal lymphatic vessels. I believe that the CMMS technique resembles the effects of bandaging and gentle superficial massage used in manual lymphatic therapy techniques[38] to move lymphatic fluid.

Active motion is the single most effective stimulator of the lymphatic system.* The CMMS technique reduces edema by redirecting active motion to the stiffest area. The absence of muscles in the digits requires that skin motion and tissue compression created by digital flexion provide physical stimulation of the superficial lymphatics. The concurrent contraction of the intrinsic muscles then helps move the lymphatic fluid proximally. Active movement of unconstrained proximal joints continues the distal to proximal pumping.

In addition to active motion, light compression of the tissues and movement of the skin stimulates lymphatic flow.[81,110] The intimately molded contour of the cast provides consistent gentle pressure. The cast provides constant but minimal tissue pressure to facilitate lymphatic fluid movement in the delicate initial lymphatics of the skin.

Movement of the hand within the cast provides a pseudomassage of the skin as the hand moves against the padded but unyielding contour of the cast. Because the initial lymphatics are thin, fragile structures, they are collapsed easily by vigorous massage,[31,110] and such gentle but frequent facilitatory movement provides the appropriate amount of force and movement while eliminating the possibility of overly vigorous and destructive edema reduction techniques. The fact that the cast is nonremovable provides constant stimulation during frequent active motion. Gilbert[59] describes the lymphatic network of the palm and fingers as much more abundant than its dorsal counterpart. The firmness of the plaster of Paris in the palm during active finger flexion may provide a more effective means of lymphatic stimulation than other approaches.

The insulating quality of the cast provides neutral warmth, retaining body heat.[76,79] Because a direct relationship exists between ambient temperature and the permeabil-

*References 31, 71, 81, 94, 96, 110.

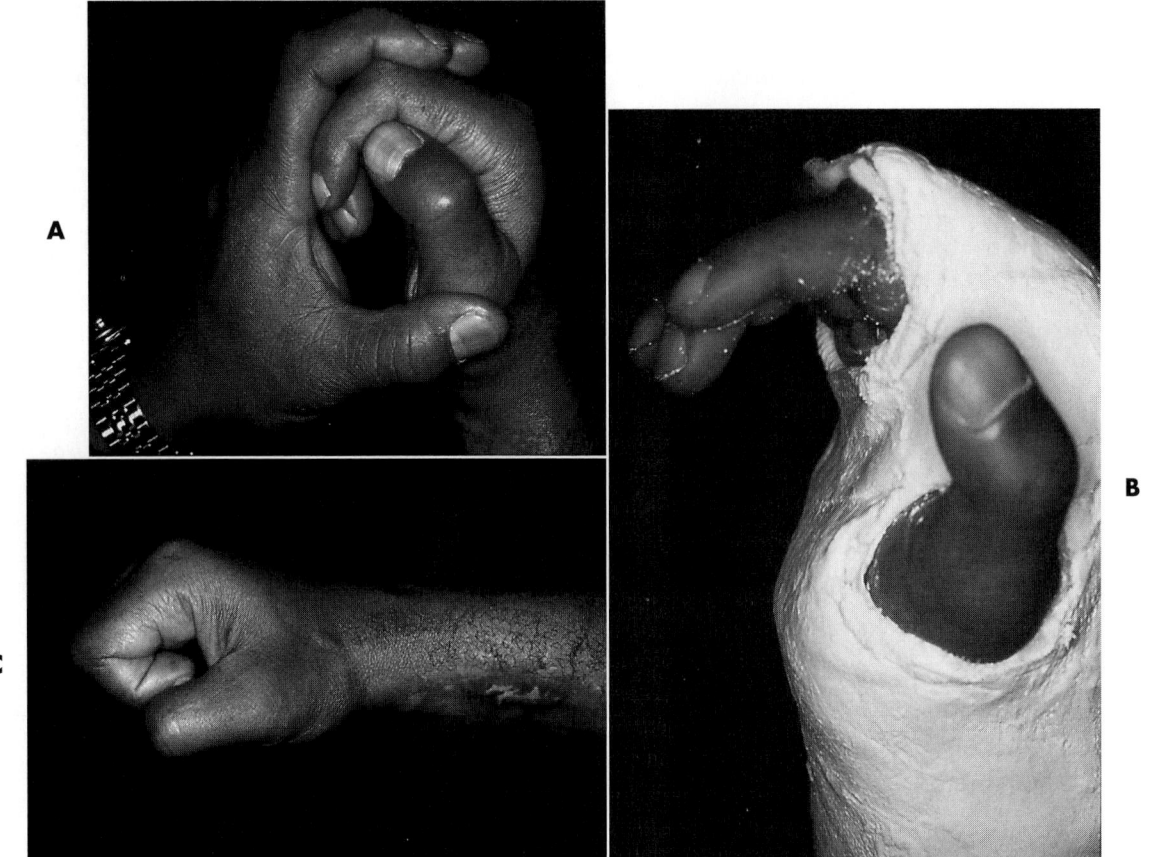

Fig. 61-25. **A,** Chronically stiff hand 7 months after injury shows limited passive motion. **B,** Cast provides optimal position for mobilization into flexion. **C,** Resulting range and pattern of flexion (note tenodesis is present) after a few weeks of cast wear.

ity of the initial lymphatics,[103,137] this factor may also assist in increasing lymphatic flow. In addition, neutral warmth may assist in general tissue relaxation and/or facilitate tissue elongation.[76,79,97] During the weaning phase, patients have elected to wear the bivalved cast, stating that the warmth, comfort, and ability to move correctly within the cast helps them feel that their hand is moving normally.

Because the accumulation of plasma proteins is a cause of chronic inflammation,[31] stimulation of the lymphatic system by the movement within the cast reduces the observable redness and pain with motion of the joints. Pain is reduced and active joint motion becomes both easy and comfortable.

Change in the pattern of motion

Perhaps the most significant but least appreciated difference between the recently injured hand and the chronically stiff hand is the change in the pattern of active motion of the hand (Fig. 61-25). Local tissue adherence and/or joint tightness prevents normal synergistic motion. This altered pattern has been present long enough that the definition of movement in the cerebral motor cortex has been altered. This altered pattern of motion restricts both the motor and sensory

feedback input and this restriction creates feedback deprivation similar to rigid immobilization.[42,83]

Neuroscience literature has proven that animals and humans trained in movement combinations magnify the cortical representations of the motor areas predominantly used, and that lack of use decreases the cortical area.* For example, squirrel monkeys given a repetitive fine motor task increased cortical representation of the small muscles of the hand with a concurrent decreased representation of the larger proximal muscles.[100] The first dorsal interosseous in the reading hand of braille readers has a larger cortical representation than in the nondominant hand of the same person or in the hands of control subjects.[104]

Therefore it is logical that the change of motion created by tissue adherence in the chronically stiff hand provides the opportunity for diminished cortical representation of the previous normal pattern of motion. At the same time, the cortical area controlling the newly dominant muscles enlarges. The constrained motion within the CMMS cast demands repetition of correct muscle movement, providing prolonged active movement necessary to repattern the

*References 25, 45, 73, 77, 83, 99, 100, 104.

somatosensory cortex. Although cortical representation changes rapidly based on use, for repatterning to become an ingrained automatic dominant motion, the motion must be repeated for long periods during the day and over many days or weeks.[72,84,92] Repatterning is enhanced by conscious, close attention to the desired motion. Unattended repetitive motion and passive motion drive weak or no significant plasticity changes in the cortex.[25,91] In the absence of permanent peripheral injury (i.e., amputation or denervation), the altered pattern can be quickly retrained to the original "normal" because the original cortical connection patterns persist and can easily be reactivated.[72]

Because of the longstanding feedback deprivation that has caused abnormal movement pattern changes in the somatosensory cortex, regaining motion is both a complex mechanical and a cerebral issue. All too often, hand therapists assume the problem is only mechanical and are frustrated when traditional mobilization techniques are not successful.

The same dysfunctional patterns of motion are seen in the chronically stiff hand as in the newly injured hand. Wrist tenodesis pattern usually is absent or altered. Wrist flexion is commonly observed when finger flexion is attempted. The key to directing normal digital movement with the CMMS cast is stabilization of the wrist in slight (20 to 30 degrees) extension. Even when the stiffness is localized to a single PIP joint, the wrist must be included in the cast to direct the force and excursion to the stiff joint. Because the wrist is the largest joint crossed by the extrinsic muscles, its position has more to do with directing excursion than do the smaller joints. Positioning the wrist in slight extension takes stretch off the weakened wrist extensors[60] and positions them so that they can fire synergistically with the finger flexors. If passive wrist extension is limited, a period of serial casting to bring the wrist into slight extension is required before application of the CMMS cast.

The mechanical problems of joint stiffness and tissue adherence are well described in the previous section on evaluation and treatment of early stiffness and are described here only in relation to the desired design of the CMMS cast.

Dominant intrinsic flexion pattern. One of the most common altered patterns in the stiff hand is digital flexion dominated by the intrinsics muscles. Flexion is initiated primarily at the MP joints before IP joint motion occurs. The patient may have difficulty initiating motion with the flexor digitorum profundus (FDP) muscles, which reinforces the intrinsic muscle dominance. Because the normal arc of digital flexion shows relatively more IP joint flexion before MP joint flexion,[11] the patient's MP joints are often immobilized in the cast to recreate the correct initial phase of digital flexion (Fig. 61-26). This facilitates profundus glide and prevents the dominant intrinsic flexion pattern. A slightly flexed position of the MP joint is desired because full extension would demand concurrent stretching of the intrinsic muscles, possibly creating too much resistance

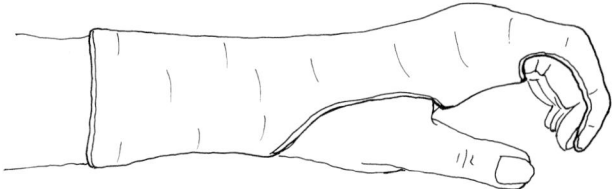

Fig. 61-26. Initial cast to facilitate long flexor glide to mobilize interphalangeal joints often includes the metacarpophalangeal joints.

initially. Full MP joint flexion makes the initiation with the extrinsic flexors more difficult and should be avoided. A position of MP joint extension also reinforces extrinsic flexor tendon glide, whereas a position of full MP joint flexion (with wrist extension) provides minimal active tension on the flexor tendons.[115] When the profundus glide and IP joint motion have improved, the MP joint immobilization may be discontinued and full composite finger flexion allowed (Fig. 61-27). This should be considered only when the patient is able to spontaneously initiate flexion with the FDP muscles.

Almost all surgical and therapy texts stress the importance of positioning the MP joints in flexion to maintain the maximum length of the collateral ligaments. Inclusion of the extended MP joints in the cast is contradictory to this traditional teaching. It is the increased IP active motion resulting from this position that reduces edema and demands glide of the intrinsic tendons across the MP joint, two factors that appear to outweigh the temporary immobilization of these joints. It is my opinion that much of the cause of limited MP joint flexion is edema within the joint capsule that is loose in extension but compressed in flexion. Because the edema within the joint is reduced and the muscle power is restored across the joint, MP joint flexion can often be regained without further specific intervention toward mobilizing the MP joints into flexion.

If the patient cannot initiate IP flexion with the profundus muscles even when the MP joints are stabilized, a dorsal hood of plaster of Paris is placed over the IP joints (Fig. 61-28). This hood simply positions the distal interphalangeal (DIP) joints in relatively greater flexion than the PIP joints, so when the patient pulls away from the dorsal hood, the motion is initiated with the FDP. It must be stressed that the purpose of the dorsal hood is not to serially push the joints into more flexion. Rather it is simply to position the joints in the ideal relationship to one another to facilitate initiation of motion with the FDP muscles.

The inability to initiate finger flexion with the profundus muscles is commonly seen in the stiff hand following immobilization for a distal radius fracture. In the initial CMMS cast, the desired relational position of DIP and PIP joint flexion may not be attainable because of joint stiffness. After a few days in the cast, the patient will gain digital flexion, but it is usually with the flexor digitorum superficialis muscles

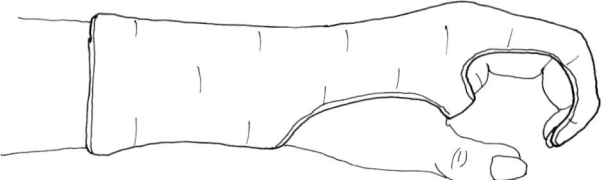

Fig. 61-27. After profundus glide is regained and interphalangeal (IP) joints are mobilized into flexion, the position of the hood can be changed and the metacarpophalangeal joints may be left free to move in concert with the IP joints.

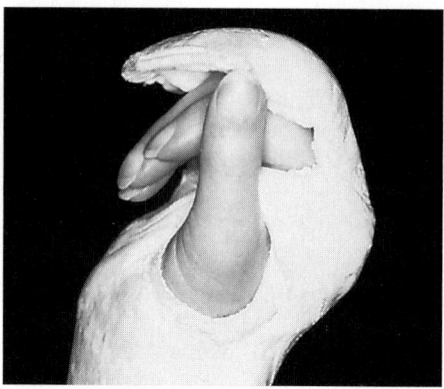

Fig. 61-28. Dorsal plaster of Paris hood is placed over the fingers to facilitate flexion at the interphalangeal joints.

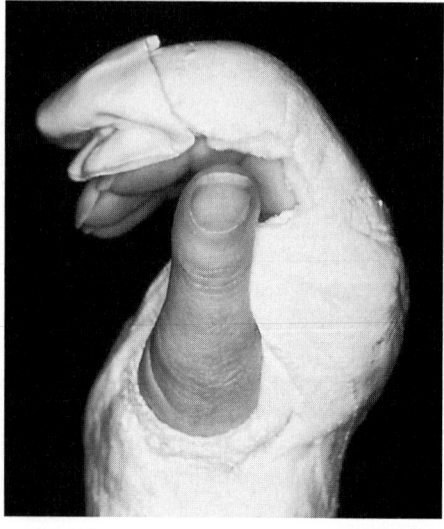

Fig. 61-29. After glide of the flexor digitorum superficialis is regained, plaster of Paris or thermoplastic is added over the distal phalanges to position the distal interphalangeal joints in greater flexion to aid in the pull-through of the flexor digitorum profundus.

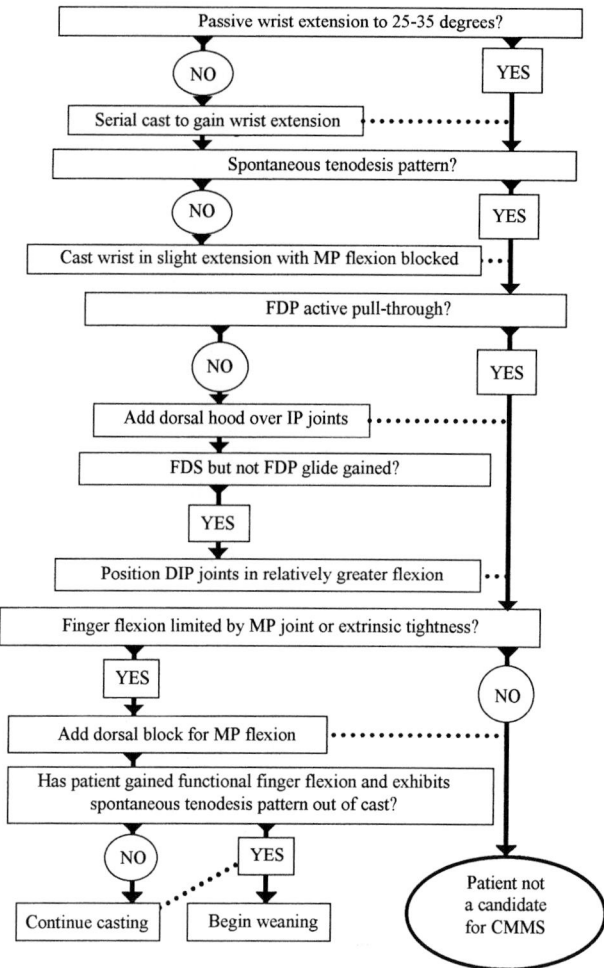

Fig. 61-30. Algorithm outlines the decision-making process for the application of the casting motion to mobilize stiffness *(CMMS)* technique to the chronically stiff hand. *DIP,* Distal interphalangeal; *FDP,* flexor digitorum profundus; *FDS,* flexor digitorum superficialis; *IP,* interphalangeal; *MP,* metacarpophalangeal.

rather than with the FDP (see Fig. 61-28). If this occurs, the addition of a small piece of plaster of Paris or thermoplastic distally on the dorsal hood just over the distal phalanx will aid in greater DIP joint flexion (Fig. 61-29). The patient is instructed to concentrate on first seeing the fingernails move

away from the dorsal hood before moving the PIP joint. The complex decision-making process of applying the CMMS technique for regaining digital flexion in the chronically stiff hand is illustrated in Fig. 61-30.

Dominant intrinsic tightness. The limited digital motion present in all chronically stiff hands will cause the intrinsic muscles to become tight. After the patient has gained digital flexion using the profundus muscle, or if finger flexion is present but not full, a cast to position the MP joints in maximum extension (or hyperextension) but to allow full IP joint flexion is applied so that cyclical active digital flexion elongates the intrinsic muscles. Active elongation of the intrinsic muscles is preferable to passive stretching. The lumbrical muscle is in its longest position when the profundus muscle is actively contracting (as a result of the moving origin of the lumbrical on the profundus tendon) while the MP joints are in extension and the IP joints are flexed.

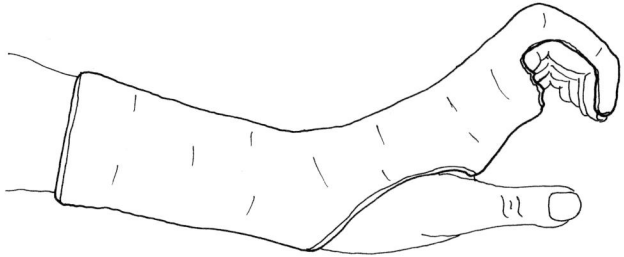

Fig. 61-31. After flexor digitorum profundus glide is regained, the hand is positioned in the cast with the metacarpophalangeal joints in full extension to allow cyclical active motion to reduce tightness of the intrinsic muscles of the fingers.

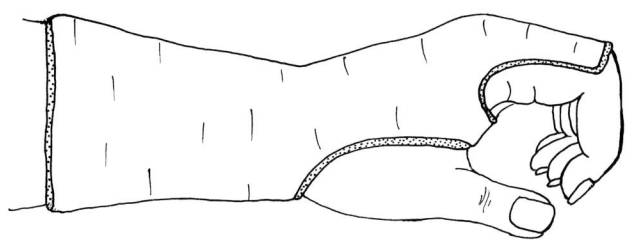

Fig. 61-32. Metacarpophalangeal (MP) flexion is regained by positioning the MP joints so that they can be exercised in the available end-range of flexion.

If the muscles are extremely tight or the patient had great difficulty in regaining profundus glide, a dorsal hood may also be attached to this cast (Fig. 61-31).

Dominant extrinsic flexion pattern. When MP joint flexion is limited either by capsular tightness or by adherence of the extrinsic extensor system, extrinsic muscles rather than intrinsic muscles control IP joint movement (also called *intrinsic-minus pattern*). The intrinsic muscles cannot get into position to provide the dominant force for digital control.

To regain MP joint flexion, the wrist is casted in slight extension and a dorsal hood is placed over the proximal phalanges, positioning them at their easy maximum flexion range (Fig. 61-32). The patient works to actively pull the proximal phalanx away from the dorsal hood without simultaneous IP joint flexion. This exercise isolates the intrinsic muscles and the cyclical motion increases the range of MP joint flexion. As flexion increases, the cast may be changed or a small pad inserted to position the MP joints in greater flexion. The purpose is not to serially position the MP joints in maximum flexion and hold them there, but rather to position the MP joints in slightly greater flexion so that the range in which the MP joints are moving is in greater flexion. The cast never holds the MP joint immobile because there is always room for the movement into end-range.

Dominance of isolated joint tightness. When injury is at or near a joint, the capsular tightness that develops prevents the stiff joint from receiving excursion force. The

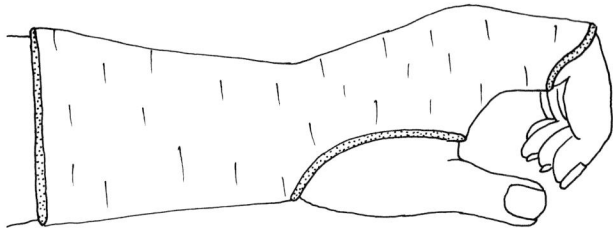

Fig. 61-33. Stiff interphalangeal joints are mobilized by immobilizing the proximal joints in the CMMS cast.

CMMS cast is applied to block all proximal joint movement (Fig. 61-33). The wrist and all digits are included so that the overflow from the adjacent digital movement will assist in helping the patient isolate the joint motion needed. In extreme cases (seen primarily in children), the distal joints may also need to be constrained. If the patient has difficulty initiating active motion because of the severity of the joint stiffness, a dorsal block may be needed to direct the desired range and direction of motion.

Clinical application of CMMS

General principles. The wrist must always be included in the cast, positioned in slight extension. It is this position that facilitates the most effective transmission of force to the joints of the hand to mobilize them into flexion. Even if the stiffness is limited to only one digit, the other digits should be included in the cast to allow the cortex representation of the uninjured digits to assist with accurate motion.[72] The only exception to this may be to allow slightly greater freedom of motion in the index finger if the stiffness is isolated in the ulnar digits.

In my opinion, it is important to use plaster of Paris for the CMMS technique because of its inherent molding ability.[37] Other synthetic casting materials are more rigid and have sharp edges. Thermoplastic splinting materials should not be substituted for the plaster of Paris because they are readily removed and provide poor skin tolerance to prolonged wear. Only in cases in which the stiffness is not yet chronic and shorter periods of exercise may be effective can the principles of the CMMS technique be applied with thermoplastic materials.

To regain joint mobility, significant time is required. In Noyes' study[98] of immobilization of the knees in monkeys, it took 1 year to fully resolve flexion contracture. This is perhaps the most difficult principle for hand therapists. When more acute injuries are being treated, tissue responds rapidly to intervention. In the chronically stiff hand, change takes much longer. Patients with chronic stiffness may wear the cast for many weeks with few or no cast changes.

Treatment protocols. It is difficult to communicate treatment protocols for the CMMS technique because each sequence is based on the patient's individual diagnosis, response to the CMMS, and pattern of motion observed at the time of reevaluation. General guidelines are given in the following sections, but the therapist must be able to intuitively decide what pattern is dominant and what position will create the most useful pattern and range of active motion within the cast.

Cast design. The design of the CMMS cast is determined by the pattern of motion (see Figs. 61-26, 61-27, 61-31, 61-32, and 61-33). The position for immobilizing proximal joints is not arbitrary. For example, if the PIP joint of the little finger is primarily lacking extension, one might choose to immobilize the MP joint in flexion to facilitate intrinsic muscle excursion across the joint. Conversely, if both flexion and extension are limited in the little finger PIP joint, a midposition between flexion and extension of the MP joint would give the best mechanical advantage for mobility of the PIP joint in both directions.

An arbitrary time period for cast wear is chosen. The cast is removed and the active pattern of motion is observed. It is the observation of this pattern that determines the exact position of the proximal joints and the position of any dorsal blocks. Only the position of the MP and IP joints is changed, the wrist is recast in the same slightly extended position.

Time in the cast. The most difficult aspect of the CMMS concept is the amount of time needed in the cast. Initial gains will be rapid and the therapist will be tempted to begin the weaning process. My experience has proven that this approach is fruitless because the patient immediately reverts to the old imbalanced pattern of motion and the stiffness returns. One should be aware of the time the hand has moved in the stiff pattern. The longer the stiffness has been present, the longer the time required in the cast for the change to be enduring. Most patients require a minimum of 2 to 4 weeks of full-time casting, although the design of the cast may be changed during this time. Patients with extreme chronic stiffness may require 6, 8, or more weeks of full-time casting. Although this seems like a protracted period for the treating therapist, one must keep in mind that it is really a short period relative to the time the stiffness has been present.

Weaning process. After a prolonged period of full-time cast wear, a slow period of weaning must occur to ensure that the patient can retain the motion gained. Because of weakness from the chronic stiffness and from partial immobilization in the cast, the patient will quickly fatigue and revert to the previous nonproductive pattern of movement.

When the patient can display the desired ROM out of the cast while demonstrating a spontaneous tenodesis pattern, weaning can begin. The cast is sawed on the radial and ulnar aspects, but the padding and stockinette underneath are cut only on the radial side. The edges of the sawn cast are covered with adhesive tape to secure the padding and stockinette and to cover the raw edges of the plaster of Paris. Circumferential hook and loop straps are then applied. The cast can then be removed and reapplied (Fig. 61-34).

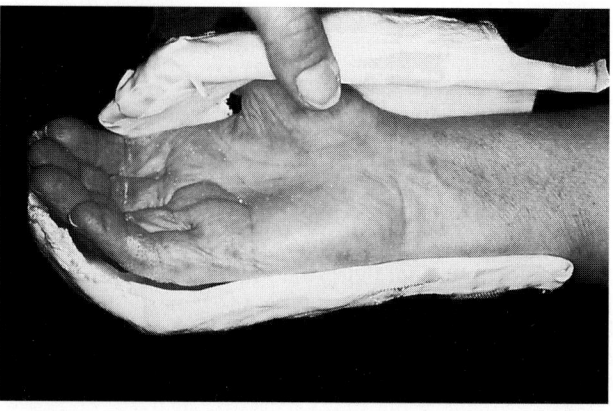

Fig. 61-34. When the patient is ready to begin weaning from the CMMS cast, it can be made removable by bivalving it and applying hook and loop straps.

The weaning process starts with brief (about 15-minute) periods out of the cast a few times a day. The patient works actively on nonresistive tasks that use the tenodesis pattern and he or she concentrates on moving in the correct active pattern. After 1 or 2 weeks of slightly increasing the time out of the cast, functional activities are added that productively use the desired motion but do not provide excessive resistance. The patient learns to identify when the pattern of motion is disintegrating, and returns to the cast. Awareness of how the hand is used ensures that all motions out of the cast are reinforcing the gains made while in the cast.

Therapists are cautioned at this time to avoid focusing on regaining motion in the opposite direction. Flexion contractures will be present. If efforts are directed toward eliminating the flexion contractures as the weaning begins, that effort will cancel the effectiveness of the time in the cast. Only when the desired motion has been regained and the patient can maintain the motion out of the cast should any effort be directed toward regaining motion in the opposite direction. Therapists also should be cautioned that, during the weaning period, it is futile to revert to the temporary intervention of manual treatment techniques. The focus should remain on functional active motion.

Invariably, patients who are weaned too quickly will require a period of repeat casting. The treatment principles of the CMMS technique are so contradictory to traditional teaching that it will require a dramatic change in thinking to become comfortable with this treatment technique.

Contraindications. The CMMS technique should not be used unless the therapist has skill in the application and removal of plaster of Paris casts. The cast must be applied perfectly, with well-distributed pressure that affords comfort. Precision is required to adequately block the small joints of the hand while allowing full motion of the adjacent joints. Excessive exothermic reaction of the hardening plaster of Paris must be avoided.[15,54,67,133] Claustrophobic patients may not be able to tolerate the confines of the cast and the technique should be applied judiciously to this population. The circumferential cast should never be applied to acute injuries, especially if vascular instability is present. It may be used in select postsurgical cases such as flexor tenolysis to facilitate correct tendon glide, but only after a few days in the compressive surgical dressing.

This technique should not be indiscriminately applied to all cases of chronic stiffness. In the cases of severe trauma, the anatomic changes caused by the injury may eliminate the potential for regaining balanced motion, and the loss of motion created by the CMMS casting may not be regained. Elderly patients with significant osteoarthritis may have some residual extension loss of the IP joints, and they should be treated with more caution.

Historically, a great deal of time, effort, and pain endurance is required to restore motion to the chronically stiff hand.[20] In the era of increasing cost-benefit analysis, the amount of motion regained relative to the time and energy expended on treatment must be an efficient return. The CMMS treatment method simplifies the treatment approach and even a severely stiff hand can be mobilized with only a few therapy visits and cast changes.

SUMMARY

Understanding the causes of stiffness in the hand and choosing the type and timing of intervention is fundamental to successful mobilization of the stiff hand. A gentle approach to the tissues of the hand aimed at reducing edema and not stimulating the continuation of inflammation is required. The ability to influence and improve motion of the hand is the result of appropriate responses to the processes occurring in the hand. Manual stretching, active motion, and use of the hand in conjunction with timely mobilization splinting can effectively transform the newly stiff hand into a mobile one. When the stiffness is prolonged and chronic joint tightness and tissue adherence limit motion, when chronic edema prolongs the inflammatory effect, and when the stiffness allows only a nonfunctional pattern of motion, these complex interrelated problems can be addressed with a new approach of CMMS.

The delicate balance between tissue glide and freedom of motion can be restored, even after severe hand injuries, if the therapist provides a program of treatment based on a sound understanding of, and respect for, tissue response and the healing continuum.

REFERENCES

1. Reference deleted in proofs.
2. Akeson WH: An experimental study of joint stiffness, *J Bone Joint Surg* 43A:1022, 1961.
3. Reference deleted in proofs.
4. Akeson WH, Amiel D, Woo SLY: Immobility effects on synovial joints: the pathomechanics of joint contracture, *Biorheology* 17:95, 1980.
5. Akeson WH, et al: Collagen cross-linking alterations in joint contractures: changes in the reducible cross-links in periarticular connective tissue collagen after nine weeks of immobilization, *Connect Tissue Res* 5:15, 1977.
6. Akeson WH, et al: Effects of immobilization on joints, *Clin Orthop* 219:28, 1987.
7. American Academy of Orthopaedic Surgeons: *Joint motion, method of measuring and recording*, Edinburgh, 1965, Churchill Livingstone.
8. Reference deleted in proofs.
9. Amiel D, et al: The effect of immobilization on collagen turnover in connective tissue: a biochemical-biomechanical correlation, *Acta Orthop Scand* 53:325, 1982.
10. Reference deleted in proofs.
11. Arbuckle JD, McGrouther DA: Measurement of the arc of digital flexion and joint movement ranges, *J Hand Surg* 20B:836, 1995.
12. Arem AJ, Madden JW: Effects of stress on healing wounds: I. Intermittent noncyclical tension, *J Surg Res* 20:93, 1976.
13. Asboe-Hansen G, Dyrbye M, Moltke E: Tissue edema: a stimulus of connective tissue regeneration, *J Invest Dermatol* 32:505, 1959.
14. Barr N: *The hand: principles and techniques of simple splintmaking in rehabilitation*, Boston, 1975, Butterworth.
15. Becker DJ: Danger of burns from fresh plaster splints surrounded by too much cotton, *Plast Reconstr Surg* 62:436, 1978.
16. Bell C: The hand: its mechanisms and vital endowments as evincing design. In *The Bridgewater Treatise*, London, 1833, Wm Pickering.
17. Bonutti PM, et al: Static progressive stretch to reestablish elbow range of motion, *Clin Orthop* 303:128, 1994.
18. Reference deleted in proofs.
19. Brand PW: The forces of dynamic splinting: ten questions before applying a dynamic splint to the hand. In Hunter JM, et al, editors: *Rehabilitation of the hand*, ed 3, St Louis, 1990, Mosby.
20. Brand PW, Hollister AM: *Clinical mechanics of the hand*, ed 3, St Louis, 1999, Mosby.
21. Brand PW, Wood H: *Hand volumeter instruction sheet*, Carville, La, United States Public Health Service.
22. Reference deleted in proofs.
23. Bryant W: Wound healing, *Clin Symp* 29:9,1977.
24. Bunch WH, Keagy RD: *Principles of orthotic treatment*, St Louis, 1976, Mosby.
25. Byl NN, Merzenich M, Jenkins WM: A primate genesis model of focal dystonia and repetitive strain injury: I. Learning-induced dedifferentiation of the representation of the hand in the primary somatosensory cortex in adult monkeys, *Neurology* 47:508, 1996.
26. Callahan AD, McEntee P: Splinting proximal interphalangeal joint contractures: a new design, *Am J Occup Ther* 40:408, 1986.
27. Cannon NM, et al: *Manual of hand splinting*, New York, 1985, Churchill Livingstone.
28. Reference deleted in proofs.
29. Reference deleted in proofs.
30. Reference deleted in proofs.
31. Casley-Smith JR, Casley-Smith JR: *High-protein oedemas and the benzo-pyrones*, Philadelphia, 1986, JB Lippincott.
32. Casley-Smith JR, Gaffney RM: Excess plasma proteins as a course of chronic inflammation and lymphoedema: quantitative electron microscopy, *J Pathol* 133:243, 1981.
33. Colditz JC: Low profile dynamic splinting, *Am J Occup Ther* 37:182, 1983.
34. Colditz JC: Principles of splints and splint prescription. In Peimer CA, editor: *Surgery of the hand*, New York, 1996, McGraw-Hill.
35. Colditz JC: Efficient mechanics of PIP mobilisation splinting, *Br J Hand Ther* 5:65, 2000.
36. Colditz JC: Preliminary report of a new technique for casting motion to mobilize stiffness, *J Hand Ther* 13:72, 2000 (abstract).

37. Colditz JC: Plaster of Paris: the forgotten splinting material, *J Hand Ther* (in press).

38. Consensus Document of the International Society of Lymphology Executive Committee: The diagnosis and treatment of peripheral lymphedema, *Lymphology* 28:113, 1995.

39. Coppard BM, Lohman H: *Introduction to splinting,* St Louis, 1996, Mosby.

40. Cyr L, Ross R: How controlled stress affects healing tissue, *J Hand Ther* 11:125, 1998.

41. deAndrade J, Grant C, Dixon A: Joint distension and reflex muscle inhibition in the knee, *J Bone Joint Surg* 47A:313, 1965.

42. Dehne E, Torp RP: Treatment of joint injuries by immediate mobilization, *Clin Orthop* 77:218, 1971.

43. Reference deleted in proofs.

44. Donatelli R, Owens-Burkhart H: Effects of immobilization on the extensibility of periarticular connective tissue, *J Orthop Sports Phys Ther* 3:67, 1981.

45. Donoghue JP, Sanes JN: Peripheral nerve injury in developing rats reorganizes representation pattern in the motor cortex, *Proc Natl Acad Sci USA* 84:1123, 1987.

46. Reference deleted in proofs.

47. Duncan RM: Basic principles of splinting the hand, *Phys Ther* 69:1104, 1989.

48. Duncan RW, et al: Open hand fractures: an analysis of the recovery of active motion and of complications, *J Hand Surg* 18A:387, 1993.

49. Reference deleted in proofs.

50. Fess EE: Rubber band traction: physical properties, splint design and identification of force magnitude, *J Hand Surg* 9A:610, 1984.

51. Fess EE, Philips CA: *Hand splinting: principles and methods,* ed 2, St Louis, 1987, Mosby.

52. Flowers KR, LaStayo P: Effect of total end range time on improving passive range of motion, *J Hand Ther* 7:150, 1994.

53. Frank C, et al: Physiology and therapeutic value of passive joint motion, *Clin Orthop* 185:113, 1984.

54. Gannaway JK, Hunter JR: Thermal effects of casting materials, *Clin Orthop* Dec:191, 1983.

55. Ganong WH: *Review of medical physiology,* ed 18, Stamford, Conn, 1997, Appleton & Lange.

56. Reference deleted in proofs.

57. Gelberman RH, et al: The influence of protected passive mobilization on the healing of flexor tendons, *J Hand Surg* 7A:170, 1982.

58. Gelberman RH, et al: Tendon. In Woo SL-Y, Buckwalter JA, editors: *Injury and repair of the musculoskeletal soft tissue,* Park Ridge, Ill, 1988, American Academy of Orthopaedic Surgeons.

59. Gilbert A: Anatomy of the lymphatics of the upper limb. In Tubiana R, editor: *The hand,* vol 1, Philadelphia, 1981, WB Saunders.

60. Gossman M, Sahrmann S: Review of the length-associated changes in muscles: experimental evidence and clinical implications, *Phys Ther* 62:1799, 1982.

61. Grauer D, et al: The effects of intermittent passive exercise on joint stiffness following periarticular fracture in rabbits, *Clin Orthop* 220:259, 1987.

62. Guyton AC: *Human physiology and mechanisms of disease,* ed 4, Philadelphia, 1987, WB Saunders.

63. Guyton AC: *Human physiology and mechanisms of disease,* ed 5, Philadelphia, 1992, WB Saunders.

64. Guyton AC, Hall JE: *Textbook of medical physiology,* ed 9, Philadelphia, 1996, WB Saunders.

65. Guyton AC, Hall JE: *Human physiology and mechanisms of disease,* ed 6, Philadelphia, 1997, WB Saunders.

66. Hardy MA: The biology of scar formation, *Phys Ther* 69:1014, 1989.

67. Hedeboe J, et al: Heat generation in plaster-of-Paris and resulting hand burns, *Burns* 9:46, 1982.

68. Reference deleted in proofs.

69. Reference deleted in proofs.

70. Reference deleted in proofs.

71. Junquerira LC, Carneiro J, Kelley RO: *Basic histology,* ed 8, Norwalk, Conn, 1995, Appleton & Lange.

72. Kaas JH: Plasticity of sensory and motor maps in adult mammals, *Annu Rev Neurosci* 14:137, 1991.

73. Kaas JH: How cortex reorganizes, *Nature* 375:735, 1995.

74. Kasperczyk WJ, et al: Influence of immobilization on autograft healing in the knee joint, *Arch Orthop Trauma Surg* 110:158, 1991.

75. Kiel JH: *Basic hand splinting,* Boston, 1983, Little, Brown.

76. King TI: Plaster splinting as a means of reducing elbow flexor spasticity: a case study, *Am J Occup Ther* 36:671, 1982.

77. Kleim JA, Barbay S, Nudo RJ: Functional reorganization of the rat motor cortex following motor skill learning, *J Neurophysiol* 80:3321, 1998.

78. Kottke FJ, Pauley DL, Ptak RA: The rationale for prolonged stretching for correction of shortening of connective tissue, *Arch Phys Med Rehabil* 47:345, 1966.

79. Law M, et al: Neurodevelopmental therapy and upper-extremity inhibitive casting for children with cerebral palsy, *Dev Med Child Neurol* 33:379, 1991.

80. Reference deleted in proofs.

81. Leduc O, Peeters A, Bourgeious P: Bandages: scintigraphic demonstration of its efficacy on colloidal protein reabsorption during muscle activity, *Prog Lymphol* XII:421, 1990.

82. Reference deleted in proofs.

83. Liepert J, Tegenthoff M, Malin J-P: Changes of cortical motor area size during immobilization, *Electroencephalogr Clin Neurophysiol* 97:382, 1995.

84. Liepert J, et al: Treatment-induced cortical reorganization after stroke in humans, *Stroke* 31:1210, 2000.

85. Light KE, et al: Low-load prolonged stretch vs. high-load brief stretch in treating knee contractures, *Phys Ther* 64:330, 1984.

86. Lotz M, Duncan M, Gerber L: Early versus delayed shoulder motion following axillary dissection, *Ann Surg* 193:288, 1981.

87. Madden JW: Wound healing: the biological basis of hand surgery, *Clin Plast Surg* 3:3, 1976.

88. McClure PW, Blackburn LG, Dusold C: The use of splints in the treatment of joint stiffness: biologic rationale and an algorithm for making clinical decisions, *Phys Ther* 74:1101, 1994.

89. McKee P, Morgan L: *Orthotics in rehabilitation,* Philadelphia, 1998, FA Davis.

90. Meals RA: Posttraumatic limb swelling and joint stiffness are not causally related experimental observations in rabbits, *Clin Orthop* 287:292, 1993.

91. Merzenich M, Jenkins WM: Reorganization of cortical representation of the hand following alterations of skin inputs induced by nerve injury, skin island transfer and experience, *J Hand Ther* 6:89, 1993.

92. Merzenich M, et al: Progression of change following median nerve section in the cortical representation of the hand in areas 3b and 1 in adult owl and squirrel monkeys, *Neuroscience* 10:639, 1983.

93. Reference deleted in proofs.

94. Mortimer PS: Therapy approaches for lymphedema, *Angiology* 48:87, 1997.

95. Reference deleted in proofs.

96. Namba RS, et al: Continuous passive motion versus immobilization, *Clin Orthop* 67:218, 1991.

97. Newton MJ, Lehmkuhl D: Muscle spindle response to body heating and localized muscle cooling: implications for relief of spasticity, *Phys Ther* 52:725, 1972.

98. Noyes FR: Functional properties of knee ligaments and alterations induced by immobilization, *Clin Orthop* 123:210, 1977.

99. Nudo RJ, Jenkins WM, Merzenich MM: Repetitive microstimulation alters the cortical representation of movements in adult rats, *Somatosens Mot Res* 7:463, 1990.

100. Nudo RJ, et al: Use-dependent alterations of movement representations in primary motor cortex of adult squirrel monkeys, *J Neurosci* 16:785, 1996.

101. Reference deleted in proofs.
102. O'Driscoll SW, Kumar A, Salter RB: The effect of the volume of effusion, joint position and continuous passive motion on intraarticular pressure in the rabbit knee, *J Rheumatol* 10:360, 1983.
103. Ohkuma M: Skin and lymphatic system, *Prog Lymphol* X-II:45, 1990.
104. Pascual-Leone A, et al: Modulation of motor cortical outputs to the reading hand of Braille readers, *Ann Neurol* 34:33, 2000.
105. Peacock EEJ: Some biochemical and biophysical aspects of joint stiffness: role of collagen synthesis as opposed to altered molecular bonding, *Ann Surg* 164:1, 1966.
106. Peacock EEJ, Cohen IK: Wound healing. In McCarthy JG, editor: *Plastic surgery,* Philadelphia, 1990, WB Saunders.
107. Reference deleted in proofs.
108. Putnam MD: Posttraumatic stiffness in the hand, *Clin Orthop* 327:182, 1996.
109. Rudolph R: Contraction and the control of contraction, *World J Surg* 4:279, 1980.
110. Ryan TJ, Mortimer PS, Jones RL: Lymphatics of the skin, *Int J Dermatol* 25:411, 1986.
111. Salter RB: The biologic concept of continuous passive motion of synovial joints: the first 18 years of basic research and its clinical application, *Clin Orthop* 242:12, 1989.
112. Reference deleted in proofs.
113. Reference deleted in proofs.
114. Reference deleted in proofs.
115. Savage R: The influence of wrist position on the minimum force required for active movement of the interphalangeal joints, *J Hand Surg* 13B:262, 1988.
116. Simons P, et al: Venous pumps of the hand, *J Hand Surg* 21B:595, 1996.
117. Sorenson MK: The edematous hand, *Phys Ther* 69:67, 1989.
118. Taams KO, Ash GJ, Johannes S: Maintaining the safe position in a palmar splint: the "double-T" plaster splint, *J Hand Surg* 21B:396, 1996.
119. Tenney CG, Lisak JM: *Atlas of hand splinting,* Boston, 1986, Little, Brown & Co.
120. Tipton CM, et al: The influence of physical activity on ligaments and tendons, *Med Sci Sports Exerc* 7:175,1975.
121. US Surgeon General's Office: *Hand surgery in World War II,* Washington, DC, 1955, US Surgeon General's Office.
122. Van Lede P, Van Veldhoven G: Therapeutic hand splints: a rational approach, Antwerp, Belgium, 1998, Provan.
123. Van Royen BJ, et al: A comparison of the effects of immobilization and continuous passive motion on surgical wound healing in mature rabbits, *Plast Reconstr Surg* 78:360, 1986.
124. Vasudevan SV, Melvin JL: Upper extremity edema control: rationale of the techniques, *Am J Occup Ther* 33:520, 1979.
125. Reference deleted in proofs.
126. Watson N: What is stiffness? *J Hand Ther* 7:147, 1994.
127. Waylett-Rendall J, Seibly D: A study of the accuracy of a commercially available volumeter, *J Hand Ther* 4:10, 1991.
128. Weeks PM, Wray RC: *Management of acute hand injuries,* ed 2, St Louis, 1978, Mosby.
129. Wehbe MA: Tendon gliding exercises, *Am J Occup Ther* 41:164,1987.
130. Weinzweig N, Weinzweig J: Basic principles and techniques in plastic surgery. In Cohen M, Goldwyn RM, editors: *Mastery of plastic and reconstructive surgery,* vol 1, Boston, 1994, Little, Brown.
131. Weisman G, Pope MH, John RJ: Cyclic loading in knee ligaments, *Am J Sports Med* 8:24, 1980.
132. Wilton J: *Hand splinting,* London, 1997, WB Saunders.
133. Woo K: Techniques in surgical casting and splinting, Philadelphia, 1987, Lea & Febiger.
134. Woo SL-Y, et al: Connective tissue response to immobility: correlative study of biomechanical measurements of normal and immobilized rabbit knees, *Arthritis Rheum* 18:257, 1975.
135. Wynn Parry CB: *Rehabilitation of the hand,* ed 3, London; Boston, 1978, Butterworth.
136. Wynn Parry CB: Stretching. In Rogoff JB, editor: *Manipulation, traction and massage,* Baltimore, 1980, Williams & Wilkins.
137. Xujian S: Effect of massage and temperature on the permeability of initial lymphatics, *Lymphology* 23:48, 1990.
138. Young A, Stokes M, Iles JF: Effects of joint pathology on muscle, *Clin Orthop* 219:21, 1987.

Chapter 62

SURGICAL MANAGEMENT OF THE STIFF HAND

Peter C. Innis

Any discussion of the surgical management of the stiff hand must begin with its prevention. The following principles should be followed: (1) elevation of the injured extremity, (2) mild compression dressing, (3) elimination of pain, (4) prevention of hematomas, (5) prevention of infection, and (6) understanding of the underlying emotional factors that occur with hand injuries. Bunnell[8] has stated that all uninjured parts should be kept unrestrained and free to move. Contraction of the muscles pumps the tissue fluids through the limb, preventing edema and stasis and keeping the tissues nourished. The importance of a high index of suspicion for reflex sympathetic dystrophy (RSD) was well stated by Bunnell[8]: "One should be alert to recognize early those cases that will go on to the edematous, immobile osteoporotic hand, by recognizing the signs of trophic disturbance and the disposition on the part of the patient to hold his hand completely immobile." A pressure point produced by the dressing or cast will lead to edema and swelling of the injured or postoperative hand. For this reason, a properly fitted dressing of cotton or gauze is preferred. One should avoid constrictive wraps, elastic bandages, or tight circumferential plaster or fiberglass casts after surgery or injury.

Any point where the patient complains abnormally about pressure and pain should be checked. Pain out of proportion to the surgery or injury may be a sign of excessive pressure or neurovascular compromise and should be evaluated immediately.

Peacock[32] has stated, on the basis of his clinical and experimental studies, that the stiffness that follows simple immobilization is attributable to fixation of the joint ligaments to bone in areas normally meant to be free from such fixation and shortening of the ligaments by new collagen synthesis. The main advantage of rigid internal fixation is that it immobilizes only the essential area while allowing early motion to minimize stiffness of adjacent joints and musculotendinous units.

CONSERVATIVE METHODS OF TREATING STIFFENED JOINTS

There are several general principles and practices in the preoperative and postoperative treatment of stiff joints.

Elevation

Elevation of the injured part to at least the level of the heart is important in that it minimizes the degree of swelling. This should be used immediately after all surgery on the hand, and one should be sure that the patient, when ambulatory, keeps the hand elevated as well.

Dynamic splints and dynamic traction

Dynamic splints and traction should be used early and continuously; the amount of tension used should not produce swelling or excessive discomfort and may operate by springs or rubber bands.[33]

Molded serial plaster splints or casts

Molded serial plaster splints or casts can be applied and changed at regular intervals (daily if possible) to gradually stretch the finger joints or wrist joint into flexion or extension. These are especially helpful with proximal interphalangeal (PIP) joint flexion contractures and boutonnière deformities.

Intermittent compression unit

Intermittent compression therapy (with the Jobst Intermittent Compression Unit) has been very helpful in reducing swelling in the posttraumatic and postoperative hand and in mobilizing the stiff interphalangeal (IP) joints. The hand is placed in the sleeve with the fingers in extension for 10 minutes, under pressure, and then in flexion for 10 minutes. The amount of pressure that can be easily tolerated by the patient is used, with the time in the pneumatic sleeve being gradually increased from 30 minutes to 1 hour, one or more times a day, and with the pressure (in mm Hg) in the sleeve also being gradually increased.

The fact that the extracellular fluid is pressed out of the hand by the intermittent pressure and that the tight capsular ligaments are stretched first into extension and then into flexion makes it possible to mobilize some joints where splinting and other methods of treatment have failed.

Constant compression

Constant or static compression can be maintained by several methods, including nonconstrictive Coban or Ace wraps, compressive garments such as Jobst or Isotoner gloves, or static air splints. These methods are integral to edema management, and the patient can be taught to use these at home.

Local heat therapy

Warm water soaks or whirlpool baths are helpful, as is hot wax therapy.

Microdyne

Microdyne or high-voltage pulsed galvanic stimulation can aid in edema, pain control, and wound healing. The electrical stimulus parameter—polarity—can be used to retard or repel fluid from the area. The basis for this is that all blood cells and plasma proteins are negatively charged at normal blood pH of 7.4.[35]

Iontophoresis, phonophoresis

Iontophoresis and phonophoresis can help with pain, stiffness, swelling, and scarring. They involve transdermal drug delivery facilitated by galvanic current *(ionto)* or by ultrasound *(phono)*. Anesthetics such as lidocaine and analgesics such as hydrocortisone and dexamethasone disodium phosphonate are the most widely used.

Stellate ganglion blocks and local nerve blocks

Blocks with local anesthesia of the painful trigger areas may be helpful. When indicated in sympathetic-mediated pain, the stellate ganglion block, intravenous (IV) Bier block, or sympathectomy can be an aid in relieving pain and decreasing edema. In general, we favor stellate blocks initially and switch to IV Bier blocks with steroid or guanethidine for residual hand stiffness with RSD. Indwelling axillary or peripheral catheters for postoperative local blocks can be helpful.

TENS

TENS, or transcutaneous electrical nerve stimulation, can aid in overcoming pain to allow better compliance and mobilization with physical therapy, to decrease narcotic dependency, and to treat chronic pain.

Active exercise

The need for active use of the hand in mobilizing stiff joints cannot be overemphasized. Functional use of the hand for light activities of daily living should be encouraged.

Passive exercise

Passive exercises can be used to improve the range of motion (ROM) in the stiff joints of the hand. The force applied must not increase the swelling or pain in the joints that are stiff.

Continuous passive motion

Continuous passive motion (CPM) machines have been developed for the hand and wrist.[3] They are more effective for wrist and metacarpophalangeal (MP) joint motion than for IP joint motion.[34] Like TENS, they can be evaluated in therapy and a home unit rented or purchased after the patient is instructed in its use.

Medical treatment

Various drugs are available for systemic use that may be helpful. Two of the most effective are the nonsteroidal antiinflammatory drugs (NSAIDs) and prednisone. The NSAIDs, rather than narcotics, should be used for pain control when possible. Their antiinflammatory properties also should be helpful. A brief 7- to 10-day course of oral prednisone is often helpful with severe stiffness or refractory RSD. Triamcinolone also may be used in an amount of 2 mg injected intraarticularly into the small finger joints. Antidepressants such as amitriptyline (Elavil), as well as α-blockers such as nifedipine, also can aid in the management of RSD.

Factitious disorders

Factitious edema[38] (Secrétan's disorder) and stiffness such as the "clenched fist syndrome" can be difficult to diagnose and treat and are absolute contraindications to surgery.[37,39] These problems are often complex, and affected patients benefit from a multidisciplinary approach involving psychiatry and social work support. These problems require understanding and patience, and direct confrontation is often counterproductive.

METACARPOPHALANGEAL JOINTS
Anatomy

The MP joints of the four fingers can be flexed and extended. When the hand is open in extension, the fingers also can be abducted and adducted; thus they perform the four movements that make up circumduction and are called *condyloid joints.* When the joints are completely flexed, neither abduction nor adduction is possible because the heads of the metacarpals, although rounded at their ends, are flattened in the front. Another reason is that the collateral ligaments, although slack on extension, are taut on flexion because of their eccentric attachments to the sides of the heads of the metacarpals and because the metacarpal head is broader volarly. The collateral ligament is attached to a pit in front of the eccentrically placed tubercle on the head of the metacarpal; it consists of two parts: (1) a dorsally placed portion or "cord" ligament and (2) a fan-shaped volar portion—the accessory collateral ligament, which extends from the metacarpal to the sides of the palmar or volar plate.

For allowance of flexion and extension, the anterior and posterior parts of the capsule must be lax. Dorsally, there is an elastic capsule over which the extensor or dorsal expansion of the extensor tendons glides. The synovium of the joint closes the joint dorsally. Anteriorly, the capsule is replaced by the fibrocartilaginous plate, the palmar ligament, or "volar accessory ligament." This plate is firmly united to the front edge of the phalanx and loosely attached to the metacarpal by areolar tissue.

Consequently, with a dorsal MP joint dislocation, the platelike palmar ligament will part from the metacarpal and remain attached to the phalanx. Fibers of the collateral ligaments radiate to the sides of this plate and keep it firmly applied to the front of the head of its metacarpal, in a visor fashion.

The palmar or volar ligaments of the fingers are united to each other by ligamentous bands, the deep transverse metacarpal ligaments of the palm, which help prevent the metacarpals from spreading.

Ankylosis

Anatomic structures that limit MP joint flexion are (1) insufficient skin coverage or scar of the skin over the dorsum of the hand, as in a burn; (2) adhesions of the extensor tendons over the dorsum of the hand or adhesions of the extensor hood mechanism over the MP joints; (3) thickening of the dorsal capsule of the MP joints; (4) contracture of the collateral ligament (cordlike portion); and (5) bony block within the joint.

Immobility of the MP joints for any reason, particularly if there is swelling with the deposition of edema fluid in the ligamentous tissue, leads to adhesions of the extensor mechanism, contracture and adhesions of the collateral ligaments, thickening of the entire capsular ligamentous structure, and the ankylosis so commonly seen in the MP joints. This immobility may have many causes. It can be seen with infection, especially those secondary to human bites and abscesses caused by intravenous drug abuse. It occurs after trauma of all types but most commonly follows metacarpal fractures splinted in inadequate flexion. Colles' fractures are a common cause. Poor cast technique with volar extension past the distal palmar crease will block full MP joint flexion. Excessive wrist flexion or excessive distraction

in a fixator will cause an MP joint extension contracture. Inadequate rehabilitation after a Colles' fracture often leads to this deformity. Burns of the hand with burn-scar contracture over the dorsum of the hand and digits are best managed by immediate excision and skin grafting with supervised mobilization by 72 hours if possible. Systemic diseases such as rheumatoid arthritis, systemic lupus erythematosus, scleroderma, and dermatomyositis; central nervous system disorders resulting in spasticity or paralysis such as cerebral palsy or stroke; and various congenital conditions such as congenital aplasia of the MP joint all can cause this immobility and stiffness.

The prevention of this very disabling MP joint stiffness is of primary importance. It can best be prevented by (1) elimination of plaster casts or splints, which immobilize the MP joint; (2) when splinting at the MP joint is required, MP joint splinting in 70 degrees of flexion to place the dorsal capsule and collateral ligament under tension; (3) early motion of the MP joint; (4) elevation of the injured extremity with prevention of edema; or (5) early dynamic traction in patients who are developing this clinical entity. In patients seen early after injury, attempts should be made to carry out dynamic flexion splinting or serial progressive static splinting, worn 12 to 24 hours a day, to determine what can be achieved with such conservative treatment.

The flexion glove tensioned by elastic bands or adjustable Velcro, or composite flexion splinting with the use of monofilament line and Merit components also works well. Static progressive splinting is especially helpful for more chronic MP joint extension contractures. The concept of applying low-load, prolonged stress to soft tissue through consecutive advancing adjustments is not new.[16,26,30] Brand[7] notes that slow, prolonged tension will alter cell proliferation and positively influence tissue growth. This tension needs to be delivered with the joint held at the end of available passive range with controlled stress for long periods.[7] The therapist or patient can adjust the amount of tension for day and night use by turning the thumb screw or guitar key (Fig. 62-1). This type of therapy can be coupled with various forms of hand therapy. Alternating positive pressure with a compression unit can be of great help in reducing edema of the hand and mobilizing the joints. In addition, active exercise should be carried out, and functional use of the hand in light and moderate activities should be encouraged.

If one is making progress with this form of treatment, the operative release should be delayed. Weeks et al.[45] found that 87% of MP joint/PIP joint contractures presenting to a hand rehabilitation center were successfully treated nonoperatively. If after several months of this type of conservative treatment there is no progress in the range of active or passive motion in the MP joints, then there is an indication for surgical release. It is important to point out that in most normal hands, the MP joints passively flex 90 degrees. However, when one flexes the fingers for grasp, as in a closed fist, the index finger actively flexes 75 degrees, the middle

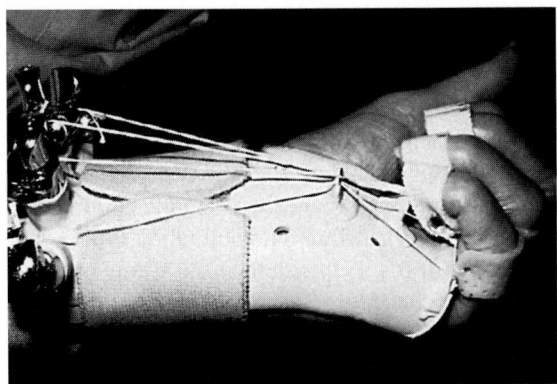

Fig. 62-1. Static progressive flexion splint for metacarpopha-langeal joint extension contractures using the MERIT components (Upper Extremity Technology, Glenwood Springs, Colo.).

finger flexes 75 degrees, the ring finger flexes 80 degrees, and the little finger flexes 80 to 85 degrees. It is not necessary to achieve 90 degrees of active flexion in the MP joints to have a useful hand, and we do not perform capsulectomies on the MP joints if the patient flexes as much as 65 degrees. With less than 65 degrees of flexion, sufficient improvement in ROM can be expected to warrant operative intervention. Bunnell[8] has stated that the essentials for success of capsulectomy are the presence of good surrounding tissue, good nerve supply and nutrition, redundant dorsal skin, good working muscles about the joints, and free extensor and intrinsic muscles or some correction for them to furnish strong flexion. An unstable dorsal burn scar or skin graft first should be replaced with satisfactory tissue such as a pedicle groin flap or free tissue transfer before capsulectomy.

The choice of arthroplasty or capsulectomy when there is an ankylosis in the MP joint will in part depend on the appearance of the metacarpal head and the base of the phalanx on the roentgenogram. Often, it is possible to salvage good ROM in the MP joint even in instances in which the roentgenogram demonstrated considerable joint destruction. One should remember that the average MP joint flexion after arthroplasty is only 50 degrees.[4,5]

Capsulectomy

Operative technique. (Fig. 62-2) A longitudinal skin incision centered over the MP joint exposes the extensor mechanism. Alternatively, a transverse incision can be used for multiple MP joints. The extensor tendon is then splint longitudinally for approximately 2.5 cm on either side of the MP joint. The extensor hood is then retracted to either side, and the attachments of the extensor tendon to the base of the proximal phalanx are severed when they are present. The dorsal capsule of the joint between the base of the phalanx and the head of the metacarpal is excised from one collateral ligament across to the opposite collateral ligament because this may be greatly thickened in severe cases.

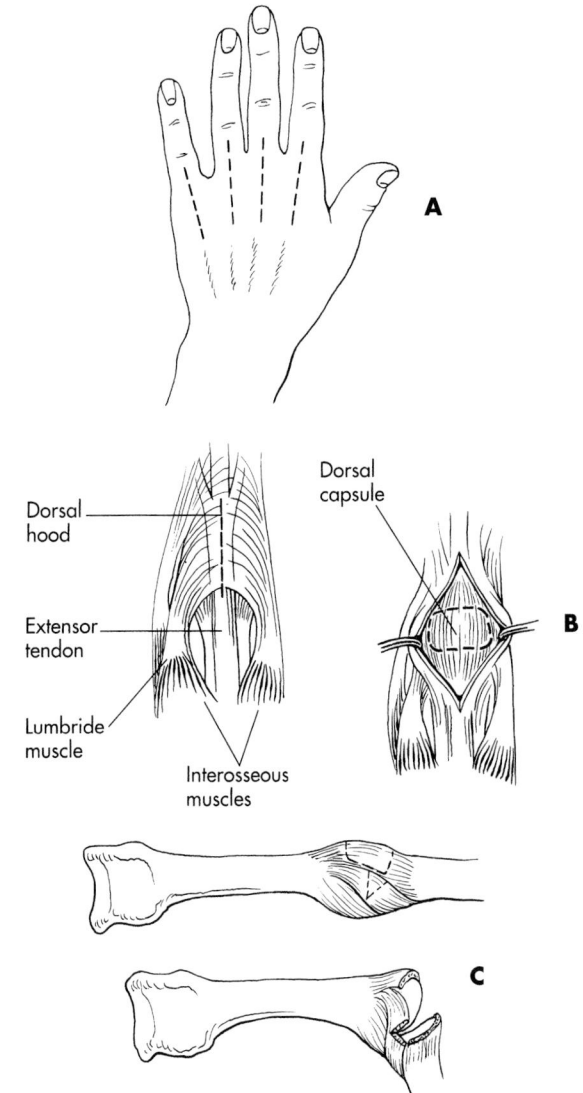

Fig. 62-2. Technique for metacarpophalangeal joint capsulectomy. **A,** Longitudinal skin incision. **B,** Splitting of the extensor tendon and retraction to expose dorsal capsule. **C,** Excision of dorsal capsule and cord portion of collateral ligament. An elevator can release adherent volar capsule and re-create the normal pouch beneath the metacarpal head.

Because the cordlike portion of the collateral ligament limits flexion, this can be released from its attachment just beneath the tubercle on either side of the head of the metacarpal, leaving it attached to the accessory collateral ligament but freeing any adhesions that may have formed between the cord portion of the collateral ligament and the head of the metacarpal.[9] Pressure against the base of the proximal phalanx will then carry the proximal phalanx into flexion beneath the head of the metacarpal.

In patients with much thickening in the collateral ligament, a section of the cordlike portion of the ligament should be removed near the tubercle on either side of the head of the metacarpal. The remainder of the cordlike portion of the collateral ligament should be left attached to the accessory collateral ligament. This will prevent ulnar deviation of the finger, which is seen when too much of the cord portion of the collateral ligament and its accessory ligament are removed. This deviation is likely to occur in the patient with ulnar-nerve palsy. One also must take care not to sever the attachment of the interosseous tendon into the base of the phalanx just distal to the attachment of the collateral ligament to the phalanx because this also may lead to ulnar deviation of the fingers. If the phalanx does not drop into flexion beneath the head of the metacarpal, a curved periosteal elevator should be inserted around the head of the metacarpal to re-create the volar pouch beneath it. In longstanding cases, this pouch becomes obliterated when the volar plate becomes adherent to the metacarpal head.

The excursion of the extensor tendons over the dorsum of the hand should be checked. If these are not gliding freely, they should be tenolysed over the dorsum of the hand and, if necessary, over the dorsum of the wrist and into the forearm. In addition, it may be necessary to free the extensor hood well onto either side of the MP joint. One may place 2 mg of triamcinolone acetonide (Kenalog) into each joint before closing the extensor tendon and distribute another 10 mg beneath the extensor tendons on the dorsum of the hand if they have been tenolysed. Some surgeons avoid this, citing concerns with wound healing and the potential for infection.

The extensor tendon is closed with a running 4-0 non-absorbable suture. The hand is dressed in a bulky dressing with the MP joints in moderate flexion, but not in such severe a degree of flexion as to cause the extensor tendons to open over the MP joint. We generally do not pin these joints, although this is favored by some authors.[18,48] This pressure dressing is left in place for 72 hours, at which time it is removed and a volar Orthoplast splint applied so that one may begin a dynamic traction by leather loops about the proximal phalanges for flexion. The initial therapy appointment should be made when the surgery is scheduled. The passive range of motion (PROM) obtained at the time of surgery is approximately the active range of motion (AROM) that can be expected with postoperative wound healing.[17] Dynamic splints are used during the day as an adjunct to the patient's active exercise program and to protect weakened structures. Static progressive splints with the MP joints placed near the limit of obtainable flexion with the wrist in extension are used at night to maintain gains in ROM and provide a prolonged gentle stretch to the soft tissues.

All splints are monitored and adjusted frequently. If an extension lag is present, dynamic flexion splinting should be alternated with dynamic extension splinting. This is continued until the patient is able to maintain the ROM present postoperatively with AROM and PROM (generally 3 to 5 months). When passive motion exceeds active motion, the

emphasis on active exercise should be increased to overcome tendon weakness or adherence.[17]

Complications

Certain complications may occur after the operative procedure of capsulectomy and may be attributable to surgical technique, postoperative therapy, patient selection and compliance, or surgical timing with inadequate tissue equilibrium. Even under ideal circumstances, the procedure may be complicated by infection, hematoma, or RSD. Problems must be treated early if a satisfactory result is to be achieved. Several problems relating to surgical technique warrant discussion.

1. Ulnar deviation of the fingers as a result of a too-radical resection of the collateral ligament on the radial side, particularly in the presence of ulnar nerve palsy, may occur. In addition, if one inadequately releases the collateral ligament on the ulnar side of the joint, ulnar deviation may result.
2. Disruption of the extensor tendons over the MP joint may occur in patients in whom one has not adequately tenolysed the extensor tendons. It may also occur in patients in whom there has been considerable shortening of the extensor muscles themselves. This latter complication usually can be prevented if the MP joints are not forced into full flexion immediately postoperatively and instead flexing with rubber band traction as the tight extensor tendons gradually loosen.
3. The ankylosis may recur where the abnormality was inadequately corrected at surgery or where adequate dynamic traction was not maintained after surgery. If a good result is not obtained, the procedure can be repeated after 4 to 6 months.

Arthroplasty

Arthroplasty with the use of a joint prosthesis may be the procedure of choice for patients who have such severe destruction of the metacarpal head or the base of the proximal phalanx that release of the capsular ligament may not provide satisfactory ROM. It is indicated in the rheumatoid arthritic patient in whom there has been severe destruction of the metacarpal head. In addition, it is used in osteoarthritic patients, in whom there is pronounced deformity in this joint, and in destruction of the joint after trauma.

With the success of silicone arthroplasty, there are limited indications for the soft tissue arthroplasty such as described by Vainio and Pulkki.[43] These may include patients with previous infection or silicone allergy and some traumatic injuries with bone loss. Joint allografts and autografts still must be considered experimental.[10] Cemented metal or ceramic hinged prostheses have not yet gained acceptance because of problems with loosening and breakage.[15] Arthrodesis of the MP joint is a significant disability but may be required in some circumstances, such as in young laborers. There are significant forces acting on this joint, and solid internal fixation such as a plate or tension-band construct should be used.

PROXIMAL INTERPHALANGEAL JOINTS

When the surgeon treats a crippled hand, he or she is often confronted with a hand that fails to function properly because of limitation of flexion or extension in the IP joints. Bunnell[8] noted that it is the narrow joint space present in the IP joints that produces limitation of motion when there is even the slightest shortening of the capsular ligaments, as might be produced by nonuse or edema of the ligaments and subsequent fibrosis. This limitation in motion may occur despite the most rigid attention to proper splinting and physical and occupational therapy and with proper reduction of fractures or dislocations.

Anatomy

The PIP joint is constructed on essentially the same plan as the MP joint. It possesses collateral ligaments, a palmar fibrocartilage, and a loose dorsal capsule or synovial tissue guarded by an extensor expansion.[6] This is considered a hinge joint because movements are restricted to flexion and extension by the anteroposterior flattening of the ends of the bones.

An important fascial structure covers the collateral ligaments on either inside of the joint. Landsmeer[28] has described this in detail as being composed of a transverse portion extending from the extensor tendon dorsally to the lateral border of the volar plate. The oblique portion of the ligament passes from the proximal phalanx and A_2 pulley to the extensor tendon over the middle phalanx.

SPRAINS

Sprains may occur with varying amounts of injury to the capsular ligaments about the joint, from minute tears of the ligament to more extensive damage. The usual history is that of a patient having twisted or jammed the finger. There may be a hemarthrosis associated with the ligament injury. After the injury, there may be months of painful swelling of the joint, with stiffness on both flexion and extension.

These injuries should receive careful attention in the acute stage: They should be splinted in slight flexion for 1.5 to 3 weeks and treated with modalities to prevent swelling. If possible, the splint should be removed periodically with careful flexion and extension, guarding against forced flexion and extension. If ligamentous laxity is present, Velcro buddy taping should be maintained during activity for an additional 3 to 4 weeks. This is especially important in the border digits, which are more prone to reinjury. Local injection of the joint with triamcinolone acetonide may help relieve pain in chronic cases and aid in mobilizing the joint.

In those cases seen late, with thickened capsular ligaments and stiffness on flexion and extension, the most careful splinting will be required to stretch the joint into full

flexion and extension. For a severely ankylosed joint in extension or flexion, a capsulectomy may be needed to restore function. Many of the same conditions that cause MP joint stiffness also affect the PIP joint. Some of the most common causes are fractures and their sequelae, RSD, and Dupuytren's contracture. The stiffness resulting from fracture can be minimized by appropriate control of pain and swelling and anatomic reductions with appropriate internal fixation and early motion when possible. Care must be taken to avoid impairment of joint motion and tendon gliding with the fixation devices.

Ankylosis in extension

The surgeon about to correct a limitation of flexion of the PIP joint must have in mind the various anatomic structures in the finger that may limit this motion. These structures are (1) scar contracture of the skin over the dorsum of the finger; (2) contracted long extensor muscle or adherent extensor tendon; (3) contracted interosseous muscle or adherent interosseous tendon; (4) contracted capsular ligament, particularly the collateral ligament; (5) retinacular ligament adherent to capsular ligament; (6) bone block or exostosis; and (7) adherence of the flexor tendons within the finger.

Before surgically correcting the lack of flexion of the IP joint, one must first determine by clinical examination and roentgenogram which anatomic structures are limiting flexion and be certain that a true ankylosis or bony fusion is not present. Bunnell, Doherty, and Curtis[9] have described various test positions of the hand and fingers to determine which structures are to blame. When the PIP joint may be actively flexed to 75 degrees or more, it is better judgment to rely on conservative measures such as hand therapy and special splinting to achieve further flexion. In patients who have a lessor degree of flexion, even in those whose fingers that are held in rigid extension but without bony ankylosis, one can expect to improve flexion by this operative procedure.

Operative technique (Fig. 62-3). The PIP joint is approached by a dorsal curvilinear incision as described by Curtis,[11,12] although bilateral midaxial incisions can also be used. The incision is deepened throughout the skin and subcutaneous tissue to expose the transverse retinacular ligament. The retinacular ligament is retracted proximally and distally to expose the collateral ligament, which is totally excised. A Beaver blade can be placed into the joint just volar to the extensor tendon to incise the dorsal capsule if necessary.

In some longstanding cases, the volar synovial pouch will have become obliterated and must be reformed with a small curved elevator or by forcing of the base of the middle phalanx into flexion. When there is an associated contracture of the interosseous muscle and a positive "intrinsic tightness test," the interosseous tendon is lengthened by tenotomy at the point where the longitudinal fibers join the middle slip of

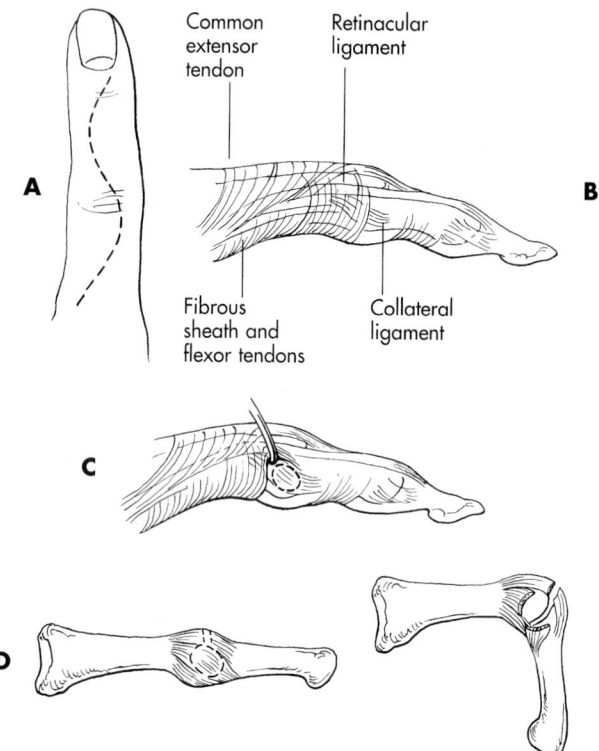

Fig. 62-3. Capsulectomy of the proximal interphalangeal joint. **A,** Dorsal incision. **B,** Skin retracted to expose lateral retinacular ligament. **C,** Elevation and retraction of retinacular ligament exposes collateral ligament. **D,** Excision of collateral ligament and incision of dorsal capsule. Preserved lateral retinacular ligament (not shown) maintains joint stability.

the extensor tendon, allowed to slide proximally, and then resutured to the extensor aponeurosis. One also can overcome this interosseous contracture by excision of a triangle, including the longitudinal fibers from the interosseous and lumbrical muscles, as recommended by Littler in the Littler release procedure.[19]

If there is severe contracture of the interosseous muscle with flexion deformity at the MP joint, it may be necessary to tenotomize this tendon proximal to the MP joint and divide the volar capsular ligament of the MP joint. If necessary, the extensor tendon mechanism should be freed over the dorsum of the finger.[36] The dissection and the freeing of all contracted tissues must continue until there is a free ROM of the middle phalanx about the distal end of the proximal phalanx. This may necessitate freeing the extensor tendon from the phalanx, opening the dorsal synovium of the joint, resecting the collateral ligaments, and releasing the contracted interosseous tendon mechanism. One may elect to place cortisone into the IP joint after this procedure.

The hand is placed in a dorsal plaster splint, using bulky cotton or gauze and mild compression, with the fingers in moderate flexion at the PIP joints. We disagree with those who routinely pin these joints for 2 weeks.[18,48] Within 48 to 72 hours, dynamic traction can begin either by leather loops

over the fingertips or by traction through the fingernail, pulling the fingers gradually into the flexed position. It may be necessary to alternate between dynamic traction for flexion at the IP joints and dynamic traction for extension of the fingers together with active exercise.

The ratio of dynamic flexion and extension splinting will be determined by the available ROM. Dynamic splinting is continued until the patient is able to maintain by active and passive exercise the ROM obtained at surgery. In some cases, therapy and part-time splinting are necessary for 3 or 4 months. The static night splint position is determined by the available range and the anatomic structures involved.[17]

When the PIP joint may be actively flexed to 75 degrees or more, it is better judgment to rely on conservative measures such as hand therapy and special splinting to achieve further flexion. In patients who have a lesser degree of flexion, even in those whose fingers are held in rigid extension but without bony ankylosis, one can expect to improve flexion by this operative procedure. This was true in a series of patients even though capsulectomy had to be combined with other operative procedures when other anatomic structures were limiting flexion.

The results of PIP capsulectomy seem to indicate that the more anatomic structures involved in the limitation of motion, the poorer the result.[11] Although not specifically studied, age appears to exert a negative influence on capsulectomy results.

If the only limiting factor for flexion in the IP joint was a capsular ligament, capsulectomy of the collateral ligaments would produce a good result for both flexion and extension. However, if it was necessary to free the extensor tendon over the proximal phalanx to perform a tenotomy of the interosseous tendons and a capsulectomy of the collateral ligaments to obtain flexion of the PIP joint, the result achieved by surgery was not as successful. This was particularly true of the finger bound by cicatrix, as in a crush injury, especially with fracture or with circumferential burn. In some of these patients, the increase in motion was only 20 to 30 degrees, but in others, the increase in motion was as much as 80 degrees beyond what existed before the operation. In many of these patients, this increase meant the difference between a hand that could be used for work and one that could not. One cannot expect that function will be restored completely by this procedure, but one can expect function to improve.

This approach is applicable to a joint stiff in extension, whether secondary to trauma, rheumatoid arthritis, or any other cause, if the joint surfaces are not too badly destroyed. When there is extensive joint-surface damage, an arthroplasty with a joint prosthesis is the procedure of choice in most situations, although arthrodesis is occasionally required.

Sprague[40] and Harrison[20] reported their results of the surgical treatment of the stiff PIP joint. Harrison[20] recommends division only of the main collateral ligament and the dorsal capsule for the joint stiff in extension utilizing Kaplan's[23] lateral approach. Others favor the dorsal approach outlined here.[14,18,48] Sprague[40] noted that as much as 50% of the initial surgical improvement was often lost by 6 months after surgery. Wisnicki et al.[46] have used a percutaneous sectioning of the collateral ligaments followed by joint manipulation for MP and PIP joints stiff in extension, with results comparable to those achieved with open capsulectomies. The authors believe that the minimization of surgical trauma permits a more aggressive mobilization but point out that this technique is not applicable to stiffness caused by problems other than fixed edema.

Ankylosis in flexion

The anatomic structure that limits extension of a finger at the PIP joint may be caused by the following structures: (1) scar of the skin over the volar surface of the finger; (2) contraction of the superficial fascia in the finger, as in Dupuytren's contracture; (3) contracture of the flexor tendon sheath within the finger; (4) contracted flexor muscle or adherent flexor tendon; (5) contraction of the volar plate of the capsular ligament; (6) adherence of the retinacular ligaments of Landsmeer to the collateral ligaments; (7) adherence of the collateral ligaments with the finger in the flexed position; and (8) bony block or exostosis. Often, more than one structure is involved in this flexion contracture.

In congenital flexion contracture of the finger, such as camptodactyly, all tissues from the skin to the joint capsule, and even the joint itself, may be involved. Interosseous function may be absent. Abnormal insertions of the lumbrical muscles have been reported.[31] The role of surgery and the specific procedure indicated will vary with the cause of the deformity. In the patient with Dupuytren's contracture that has existed for a long time and in whom there is pronounced flexion contracture of the PIP joints, the skin is contracted, there is a thick strand of contracted superficial fascia, the flexor superficialis tendon may be contracted, and the volar capsule and accessory collateral ligaments shorten in such a way as to prevent extension. The value of capsulectomy in longstanding PIP joint Dupuytren's contractures is still debated. The correction in the small finger varies from 50% to 100%.[29,42,44] With more severe contractures, secondary damage in the extensor mechanism probably accounts for the poor results in this joint.[1]

Serial casting and static splinting, as well as dynamic extension splinting, are the mainstay of conservative therapy. There are many splint designs for this problem, including the dynamic PIP extension splint, the reverse knuckle bender splint, the Capener splint, the spring wire splint, the LMB wire-foam splint, the safety-pin splint, the joint jack splint, and the belly gutter splint.[47] Therapy should be continued until a clear plateau has been reached. In general, patients with a PIP joint contracture of more than 40 degrees will benefit from surgical release. Age again appears to negatively influence results.

Operative technique. Operative release of the finger in an acutely flexed position is usually through a midlateral incision although a volar Bruner incision is preferred by some. Our initial approach is to excise a portion of the flexor tendon sheath distal to the A$_2$ pulley and see whether this simple excision will allow any extension. Next, the flexor tendons are checked for adhesions or contractures. If they are severely contracted, it may be necessary to tenotomize and lengthen the flexor tendons in the forearm. The retinacular ligament is freed from the lateral capsular ligament, and the volar plate is incised from the proximal phalanx. When necessary, the accessory collateral ligament is incised on either side of the PIP joint. Subluxation of the middle phalanx may occur if the cord portion of the ligament is completely severed. The surgical release of the contracted structures will then allow extension of the PIP joint. We avoid K-wire fixation across the PIP joint when possible and splint the hand in the intrinsic-plus position until hand therapy begins in 3 to 5 days. Active motion for flexion and extension is begun with dynamic traction and static splinting to improve the degree of extension and maintain the gain that was achieved operatively.

If a Dupuytren's contracture is present, a partial volar capsulectomy may be performed with excision of the accessory collateral ligaments when excision of the thickened fascial band does not achieve complete extension of the joint. Watson et al.[44] have reported complete intraoperative correction in 110 of 115 joints without either collateral ligament release or capsuloplasty but by volar checkrein resection. The checkreins run from thick broad attachments along the proximal edge of the volar plate, diverge, and insert separately along the volar lateral periosteum of the proximal phalanx (Fig. 62-4). The paired arterial branches running between the proximal phalanx and the checkreins supply the vinculae to the flexor tendons and should be preserved.

Compass PIP Hinge

The Compass PIP Hinge (Smith & Nephew, Inc., Memphis, Tennessee) was developed by Hotchkiss and is modeled after his Compass Elbow dynamic fixator (Fig. 62-5). It is a radiolucent unilateral hinged fixator that maintains joint stability and has a worm gear to provide controlled passive movement. Distraction can be applied across the joint if necessary, and the gear can be disengaged to allow active motion. The Compass PIP Hinge can be helpful in acute and chronic complex PIP fracture-dislocations. It is relatively low profile, easy to apply, and well tolerated by patients.[13,27] The compass elbow fixator has been a useful adjunct to elbow capsulectomy with patient-controlled passive movement and mechanical advantages similar to those of a turnbuckle splint.[22,25] The same advantages exist with the Compass PIP Hinge, and Hotchkiss and others have used this to correct joint contracture and to complement capsulectomy.[21,24] The results are preliminary, and complications such as pin-tract infections are not uncommon. The true role

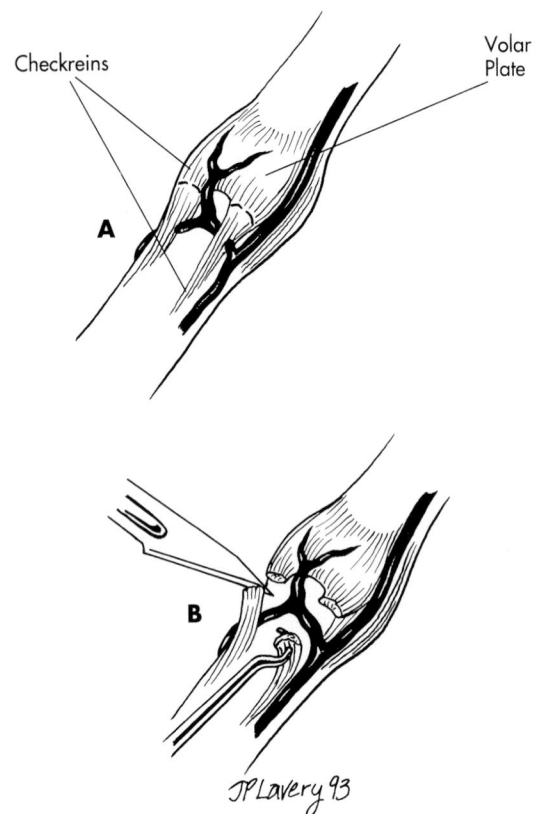

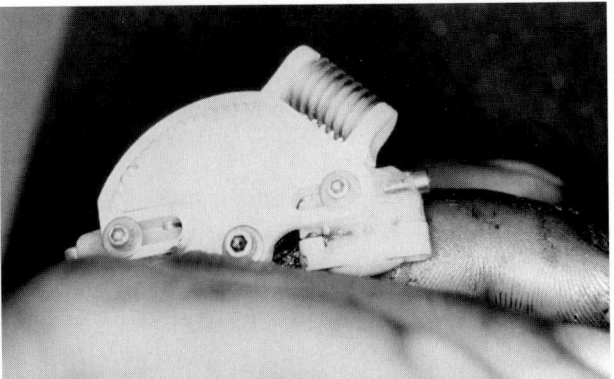

Fig. 62-5. The Compass PIP Hinge. The worm gear in the upper right corner is turned to allow passive motion and can be disengaged to allow active motion.

Fig. 62-4. Capsulectomy for proximal interphalangeal flexion contracture with checkrein release. **A,** Insertion of checkreins at neck of proximal phalanx. **B,** Excision of checkreins while preserving "ladder" vessels from digital artery. (Adapted from Watson HK: Stiff joints. In Green DP, editor: *Operative hand surgery,* New York, 1982, Churchill Livingstone.)

of the Compass PIP Hinge in the postoperative management of PIP joint capsulectomy has not yet been defined.

Complications

The complications seen after PIP joint capsulectomy are similar to those seen at the MP joint. These include overcorrection and instability, inadequate correction and recurrence of the contracture, and damage or disruption to the extensor or flexor system. Damage to the neurovascular bundle may occur with flexion contracture release. Ischemia may result if a longstanding PIP flexion contracture is splinted or pinned in full extension immediately after surgery.

Salvage

With severe contracture and extensive joint damage, salvage procedures such as arthroplasty or arthrodesis will be required. Arthroplasty of the PIP joint can be performed via the dorsal, volar, or lateral approach, with an average ROM of 40 degrees.[41] We prefer the lateral approach with release and reattachment of the radial collateral ligament. Arthrod-

esis is often preferred for young laborers, for joints after infection, and for patients with progressive diseases such as scleroderma. The position of fusion varies from 30 degrees in the index finger to 50 degrees in the small finger. Fixation may be with K-wires, tension banding, 90-90 wiring, screws, or plates. Arthrodesis of the PIP joint in the ulnar digits is a greater disability than on the radial side of the hand.

SUMMARY

This chapter represents a broad overview of the surgical management of the stiff hand. Raymond M. Curtis wrote this chapter for the first edition. One of his great interests was the stiff hand. His surgical techniques and posttreatment therapy regimens remain valid today. Variations and combinations of treatment modalities and surgical techniques will often lead to success in the restoration of joint motion and hand function. This requires the individual motivation of the patient and the combined skills of the therapist and surgeon.

REFERENCES

1. Andrew JG: Contracture of the proximal interphalangeal joint in Dupuytren's disease, *J Hand Surg* 16B:446, 1991.
2. Bain GI, et al: Dynamic external fixation for injuries of the proximal interphalangeal joint, *J Bone Joint Surg* 8B:1014, 1998.
3. Bentham J, et al: Continuous passive motion device for hand rehabilitation, *Arch Phys Med Rehabil* 68:248, 1987.
4. Bieber EJ, Weiland AJ, Volenec-Dowling S: Silicone-rubber implant arthroplasty of the metacarpophalangeal joints for rheumatoid arthritis, *J Bone Joint Surg* 68A:206, 1986.
5. Blair WF, Shurr DG, Buckwalter JA: Metacarpophalangeal joint implant arthroplasty with Silastic spacer, *J Bone Joint Surg* 66A:365, 1984.
6. Bowers WH, Wolf J, Bittinger S: The proximal interphalangeal joint volar plate. I: anatomic and biomechanical study, *J Hand Surg* 5:79, 1980.
7. Brand PW: *Clinical biomechanics of the hand,* St Louis, 1985, Mosby.
8. Bunnell S: *Surgery of the hand,* ed 3, Philadelphia, 1948, JB Lippincott.
9. Bunnell S, Doherty EW, Curtis RM: Ischemic contracture, local, in the hand, *Plast Reconstr Surg* 3:424, 1948.

10. Bury T: Repair of the proximal interphalangeal joint with a homograft, *J Hand Surg* 14A:657, 1989.
11. Curtis RM: Capsulectomy of the interphalangeal joints of the fingers, *J Bone Surg* 36A:1219, 1954.
12. Curtis RM: Management of the stiff proximal interphalangeal joint, *Hand* 1:32, 1969.
13. Dennys LJ, Hurst LN, Cox J: Management of PIP joint fractures using a new dynamic traction splint and early active movement, *J Hand Ther* 5:16, 1995.
14. Diao E, Eaton RG: Total collateral ligament excision for contracture of the proximal interphalangeal joint, *J Hand Surg* 18A:395, 1993.
15. Doi K: Alumina ceramic finger implants: a preliminary biomaterial and clinical evaluation, *J Hand Surg* 9A:740, 1984.
16. Flowers KR, Michlovitz SL: Assessment and management of loss motion in orthopaedic dysfunction, *Postgrad Adv Phys Ther* APTA, 1988:1.
17. Gorman RJ: Metacarpal and proximal interphalangeal joint capsulectomy. In Clark G, et al, editors: *Hand rehabilitation: a practical guide*, New York, 1993, Churchill Livingstone.
18. Gould JS, Nicholson BG: Capsulectomy of the metacarpophalangeal and proximal interphalangeal joints, *J Hand Surg* 4A:482, 1979.
19. Harris C Jr, Riordan DC: Intrinsic contracture in the hand and its surgical treatment, *J Bone Joint Surg* 36A:10, 1954.
20. Harrison DH: The stiff interphalangeal joint, *Hand* 9:102, 1977.
21. Hotchkiss R: Treatment of complex fracture dislocation of the PIP joint with dynamic hinged external fixation, Proceedings of the ASSH 50th Annual Meeting, San Francisco, 1995.
22. Hotchkiss R: *Compass universal hinge, surgical technique*, Memphis, 1998, Smith + Nephew.
23. Kaplan EB: *Functional and surgical anatomy of the hand*, Philadelphia, 1953, JB Lippincott.
24. Kasabian A, McCarthy J, Karp N: Use of a multiplanar distractor for the correction of a proximal interphalangeal joint contracture, *Ann Plast Surg* 40:378, 1998.
25. Kasparyan NG, Hotchkiss RN: Dynamic skeletal fixation in the upper extremity, *Hand Clin* 13:643, 1997.
26. Kottke FJ, Pauley DL, Ptak RA: The rationale for prolonged stretching for correction of shortening of connective tissue, *Arch Phys Med Rehabil* 10:345, 1966.
27. Krakauer JD, Stern JD, Stern PJ: Hinged device for fractures involving the proximal interphalangeal joint, *Clin Orthop* 327:29, 1996.
28. Landsmeer JMF: The proximal interphalangeal joint, *J Hand Surg* 7B:30, 1975.
29. Leege L, McFarlane R: Prediction of results of treatment of Dupuytren's disease, *J Hand Surg* 5:608, 1980.
30. Light KE, et al: Low-load prolonged versus high-load brief stretch in treating knee contractures, *J Am Phys Ther* 20:93, 1976.
31. McFarlane RM, et al: The anatomy and treatment of camptodactyly of the small finger, *J Hand Surg* 17A:35, 1992.
32. Peacock EE Jr: Some biochemical and biophysical aspects of joint stiffness: role of collagen synthesis as opposed to altered molecular, their treatment, *Trauma* 16:259, 1976.
33. Pratt DR: Joints of the hand and fingers: their stiffness, splinting and surgery, *Calif Med* 66:22, 1947.
34. Sampson SP, et al: The use of a passive motion machine in the postoperative rehabilitation of Dupuytren's disease, *J Hand Surg* 17A:333, 1992.
35. Sawyer P: *Biophysical mechanisms in vascularhomeostasis and intravascular thrombosis*, New York, 1965, Appleton-Century Crofts.
36. Schneider LH: Tenolysis and capsulectomy after hand fractures, *Clin Orthop* 327:72, 1996.
37. Simmons BP, Vasile RG: The clenched fist syndrome, *J Hand Surg* 5A:420, 1980.
38. Smith RJ: Factitious lymphedema of the hand, *J Bone Joint Surg* 57A:89, 1975.
39. Spiegel D, Chase R: The treatment of contractures of the hand using self-hypnosis, *J Hand Surg* 5A:428, 1980.
40. Sprague BL: The proximal interphalangeal joint contractures and their treatment, *Trauma* 16:259, 1976.
41. Swanson A: Flexible implant arthroplasty in the proximal interphalangeal joint of the hand, *J Hand Surg* 10A:796, 1985.
42. Tonkin MA, Burke FD, Varian JPW: The proximal interphalangeal joint in Dupuytren's disease, *J Hand Surg* 10B:358, 1985.
43. Vainio K, Pulkki T: Surgical treatment of arthritis mutilans, *Ann Chir Gynaecol Fenniae* 48:361, 1959.
44. Watson HK, Light TR, Johnson TR: Checkrein resection for flexion contracture of the middle joint, *J Hand Surg* 4A:67, 1979.
45. Weeks PM, Wray RC Jr, Kuxhaus M: The results of non-operative management of stiff joints in the hand, *Plast Reconstr Surg* 61:58, 1978.
46. Wisnicki JL, et al: Percutaneous desmotomy of digits for stiffness from fixed edema, *Plast Reconstr Surg* 80:88, 1987.
47. Wu SH: A belly gutter splint for proximal interphalangeal joint flexion contracture, *Am J Occup Ther* 45:839, 1991.
48. Young VL, Wray RC Jr, Weeks PM: The surgical management of stiff joints in the hand, *Plast Reconstr Surg* 62:835, 1978.

Chapter 63

POSTOPERATIVE MANAGEMENT OF METACARPOPHALANGEAL JOINT CAPSULECTOMIES

Nancy M. Cannon

HISTORIC OVERVIEW

A review of the literature shows that some of the earliest reports of metacarpophalangeal (MP) joint capsulectomy were performed by Shaw[30] in 1920 and Fowler[11] and Pratt[27] in the 1940s. This reconstructive procedure was often performed secondary to severe hand trauma from war injuries. Since then, other authors have written on the subject.[24-26,28] Most of the articles have a limited review of the surgical procedure, and only a few, at best, address the course of postoperative rehabilitation.

This chapter focuses primarily on the rehabilitation associated with dorsal MP joint capsulectomies. As an introduction, the definition of capsulectomy is reviewed. This is followed by the indications for the procedure, the anatomy surrounding the MP joint, and an overview of the surgical procedure. Volar MP joint capsulectomies are performed less frequently and are discussed at the close of this chapter.

CAPSULECTOMY

A *capsulectomy* is excision of a capsule and, in this case, a joint capsule.[9] The Latin derivation is *capsul,* meaning "the joint capsule," and *ectomy,* meaning "cutting, excision." Thus, with a capsulectomy, there is surgical excision of a portion of the joint capsule along with the soft tissue structures intricately associated with the joint. *Capsulotomy,* on the other hand, is an incision, but not excision or removal, of soft tissue structures. It is not uncommon, however, for these terms to be used interchangeably.

INDICATIONS

This procedure is recommended primarily for stiff joints in which the surfaces of the head of the metacarpal and base of the proximal phalanx of the MP joint are relatively normal and the anatomic relationship of the bones has been preserved.[11,23,27,29,32] However, other authors[5-8] believe that the procedure can be performed even when radiographs reflect considerable joint damage.

The procedure is thought to be of considerable value in a limited number of cases of joint stiffness, particularly at the MP joint level.[29] If 60 to 75 degrees of active and/or passive range of motion (ROM) already has been achieved before capsulectomy, a number of authors believe it is unlikely that the procedure will add valuable function to the hand.[6-8,23,32] Through the years, I have observed a large number of patients with approximately 60 degrees of passive MP flexion before surgery who ultimately obtained significant improvement in functional use of the hand after the procedure.

Dorsal MP capsulectomies are indicated when the MP joint has an extension contracture with significant functional limitation in MP flexion secondary to thickening and contracture of the dorsal capsule, adhesions of the extensor tendons over the dorsum of the hand or the MP joint, contracture of the collateral ligaments (primarily the cord portion), skin contracture or scarring over the dorsum of the hand as seen with burns, and conditions in which there is adherence of the volar plate to the metacarpal head.[6-8,12]

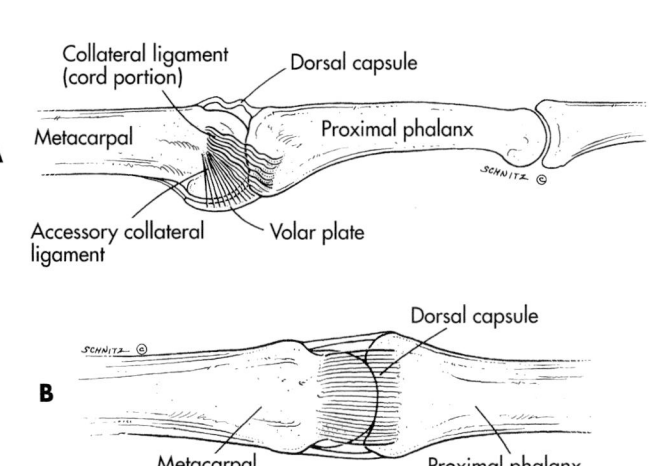

Fig. 63-1. **A,** Lateral view illustrates the relationship of the collateral ligaments, dorsal capsule, and volar plate at the metacarpophalangeal (MP) joint with the MP joint in a neutral position of 0 degrees of extension. **B,** Dorsal view illustrates the bony configuration and relationship of the metacarpal and proximal phalanx. The bony relationship between the metacarpal head and the base of the proximal phalanx differs slightly at each digit.

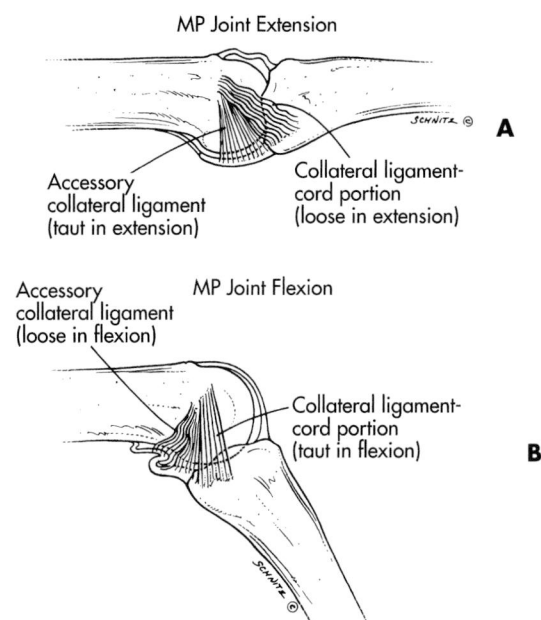

Fig. 63-2. **A** and **B,** The laxity and redundancy of the collateral ligaments in metacarpophalangeal joint extension and tautness in full flexion. The cord portion of the collateral ligament is loose in extension and becomes increasingly taut as 45 degrees of flexion is achieved. The accessory collateral ligament actually has its greatest tension through the initial 45 degrees of flexion and thereafter has slightly less tension.

Some of the more common diagnoses requiring dorsal capsulectomy are metacarpal fractures, proximal phalanx fractures (primarily at the base), crush injuries, nerve palsies, Volkmann's contracture, burns, and distal radius fractures with secondary pain and stiffness of the hand and wrist.

ANATOMY

A thorough understanding of the bony and soft tissue anatomy at the MP joint level is essential for appreciating the surgical procedure and establishing an effective postoperative treatment regimen (Fig. 63-1).

The MP joint is a diarthrodial joint with two freedoms of motion in flexion and extension and abduction and adduction.[19] Unlike the proximal interphalangeal (PIP) and distal interphalangeal (DIP) joints, which have a consistent degree of stability throughout the arc of motion, the MP joint has a relatively significant amount of lateral and rotational mobility, which is at its greatest in extension and is relatively eliminated in full flexion. This is because of its bony anatomy and surrounding soft tissue structures.[4]

Bony

The bony anatomy of the metacarpal head is configured slightly differently between each of the metacarpals.[15] The metacarpal heads have a smooth and asymmetric shape. In the index finger, the metacarpal joint surface rotates in a slightly ulnar direction, whereas the ring and small finger

metacarpal heads are rotated slightly radially, which allows the fingers to converge toward the middle finger with a common resting point for grasping. This is an important anatomic relationship to be honored with dynamic splinting in flexion. Within the joint itself, the spherical convex contour of the metacarpal head articulates with the concave articular surface of the proximal phalanx. As flexion occurs at the MP joint, the potential for direct contact between the two bones increases. In part, this is because the surface of the metacarpal head is twice as wide on the volar surface as compared with the dorsal portion.

Soft tissue

Ligaments. The ligamentous support of the MP joint is comprised of a main collateral ligament and an accessory collateral ligament arising eccentrically off the metacarpal head on the radial and ulnar sides of the joint. The main collateral ligament (cord portion) originates on the metacarpal head and inserts on the volar and lateral base of the proximal phalanx.[4] The accessory collateral ligament originates on the metacarpal head and inserts primarily into the volar (palmar) plate. The main collateral ligaments are redundant in MP extension and taut in MP flexion. As the MP joint flexes, these ligaments must stretch over the wide tubercles and volar base of the metacarpal head. The main collateral ligament in particular becomes increasingly taut as the MP joint reaches 45 degrees of flexion (Fig. 63-2).

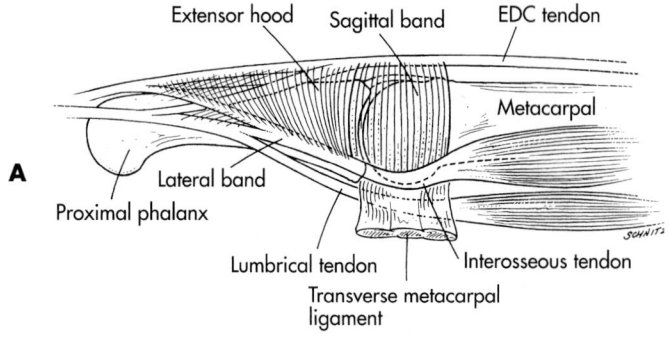

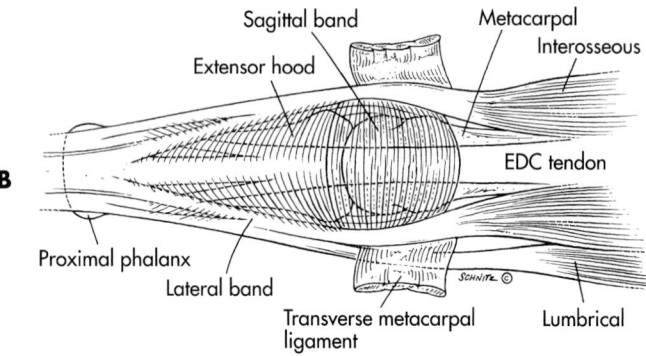

Fig. 63-3. A, The lateral view reflects the soft tissue structures that surround and support the metacarpophalangeal (MP) joint dorsally, volarly, and laterally. **B,** The dorsal view shows the intricate relationship of the extensor mechanism to the dorsal capsule and MP joint. *EDC,* Extensor digitorum communis.

Volar plate. The volar plate, or palmar plate, is a fibrocartilaginous structure on the volar surface of the MP joint. Distally, the structure is firmly secured to the proximal phalanx and is reinforced by fibers from the accessory collateral ligaments. Proximally, its attachment with the metacarpal head is loosely secured. This permits the laxity necessary for MP joint hyperextension. The deep transverse metacarpal ligament acts as an added soft tissue support structure for the volar plate and MP joint.[4]

Dorsal capsule. The dorsal capsule consists of dense connective tissue. The structure is relatively redundant in extension and becomes taut in flexion. The capsule serves as a support structure for the MP joint.

Muscles/tendons. In extension, the MP joint inherently maintains stability through the intrinsic muscles. To a lesser degree, added stability is provided through the extrinsic flexors and extensors crossing the MP joint. Both the extrinsic and intrinsic muscles assist with active flexion and extension at the MP level (Fig. 63-3).

Tendon excursion of the extensor digitorum communis (EDC) is important to keep in mind, particularly when an extensor tenolysis accompanies the MP capsulectomy[10] (Table 63-1). With the proper exercises, maximum excursion of the EDC can be obtained, thereby preventing adherence of the EDC to adjacent soft tissue and/or bony structures.

Table 63-1. Extensor digitorum communis tendon excursion—metacarpophalangeal joint

	Index	Long	Ring	Small
Bunnell, 1948[10]	15 mm	16 mm	11 mm	12 mm

Beyond the EDC, it is valuable to recognize the added contribution of the extensor indicis proprius (EIP) and extensor digiti quinti (EDQ). Both of these muscles are innervated by the radial nerve.

SURGERY

A thorough understanding of the operative procedure is essential to effectively manage the postoperative therapy. The following is an overview of one surgical approach for dorsal MP capsulectomies.[7,18,29]

- A longitudinal incision is made along the dorsal aspect of the affected joint or joints (Fig. 63-4, *A*).
- The extensor hood is incised, and the extensor tendon is either retracted laterally to the joint or split longitudinally to gain visual exposure of the joint (Fig. 63-4, *B*).
- The synovium and the dorsal capsule are exposed and excised (Fig. 63-4, *C*).
- The collateral ligaments are excised in a balanced fashion along the cord portion just beneath and on both sides of the tubercle of the metacarpal head. The distal portion of the cord is left attached to the accessory portion of the collateral ligament (Fig. 63-4, *D*).
- As passive flexion is attempted, if the MP joint opens like a book instead of the proximal phalanx gliding along the head of the metacarpal (as seen with normal joint biomechanics), then a periosteal elevator or curved dissector is passed around the volar aspect of the metacarpal head to free the adhesions between the metacarpal head and the volar plate (Fig. 63-4, *E*). This will correct the problem.
- The wound is closed. If the extensor tendon has been split longitudinally, it is reapproximated and sutured before skin closure.
- In cases of extensive dissection, consideration may be given to placing drains along the surgical area to enhance drainage and secondarily reduce postoperative edema, risk of hematoma, and ultimate scar tissue formation.
- In severe cases, where a certain degree of rebound or tendency to resist passive flexion occurs, consideration may be given to percutaneous pinning of the joint in flexion for a limited time before initiating therapy.[13,33]
- A bulky compressive dressing is evenly applied, positioning the MP joints in 45 to 75 degrees of flexion.
- If postoperative pain is a concern (based primarily on preoperative pain level after the initial injury or

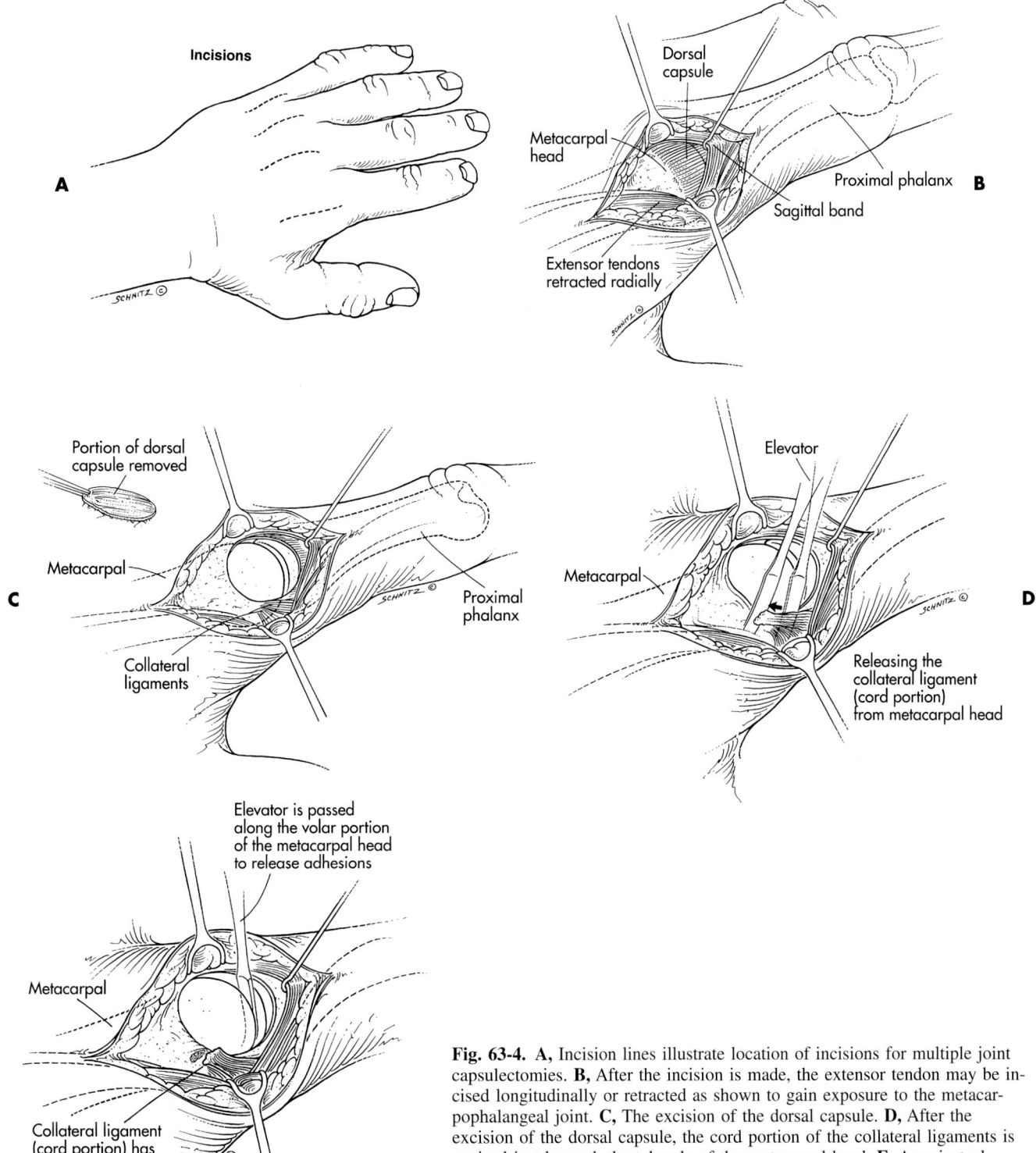

Incisions

A

Dorsal capsule

Metacarpal head

Proximal phalanx   **B**

Sagittal band

Extensor tendons retracted radially

Portion of dorsal capsule removed

Metacarpal

C

Proximal phalanx

Collateral ligaments

Elevator

Metacarpal

D

Releasing the collateral ligament (cord portion) from metacarpal head

Elevator is passed along the volar portion of the metacarpal head to release adhesions

Metacarpal

E

Collateral ligament (cord portion) has been released

Fig. 63-4. **A,** Incision lines illustrate location of incisions for multiple joint capsulectomies. **B,** After the incision is made, the extensor tendon may be incised longitudinally or retracted as shown to gain exposure to the metacarpophalangeal joint. **C,** The excision of the dorsal capsule. **D,** After the excision of the dorsal capsule, the cord portion of the collateral ligaments is excised just beneath the tubercle of the metacarpal head. **E,** A periosteal elevator or curved dissector may be passed around the volar aspect of the metacarpal head to free remaining adhesions to permit normal joint motion.

surgery) consideration may be given to postoperative transcutaneous electrical nerve stimulation (TENS) along the appropriate peripheral nerve distribution.

If an extensor tenolysis is needed, it would be the initial surgical procedure, followed by the capsulectomy. In certain cases, extensor tendon adhesions may be the primary restriction to passive flexion, and extensor tenolysis alone may prevent the need for capsulectomy.

HAND THERAPY

A limited number of articles have been contributed to the literature related to rehabilitation for MP capsulectomies. The strongest contributions have come from Laseter,[20,21] Gould et al.,[13] and Gorman.[12] Few other authors have addressed the therapy, and what mention is made is relatively brief.[6,29,31-33]

Preoperative assessment

Hand surgeons should consider including an assessment by the hand therapist as part of their initial evaluation process for patients referred with stiff hands. The hand therapist can evaluate the patient's past therapy regimen and determine whether additional therapy can positively influence the stiff MP joints and preclude the need for surgery. Conversely, the therapist can reinforce the need for the elective procedure through the objective evaluation and assessment of the patient's therapy program.

The preoperative assessment should include (1) active and passive ROM of all digits and the wrist; (2) functional performance level of the hand in activities of daily living (ADLs) and vocational and avocational activities; (3) patient's current pain level and history of pain; (4) integrity of the skin; (5) notation of any previous infection; (6) a manual muscle test of the extrinsic flexors, extensors, and intrinsic muscles; and (7) evaluation for possible intrinsic tightness and extrinsic extensor tightness.

Postoperative therapy

To establish an effective postoperative course of rehabilitation, the therapist and surgeon should thoroughly discuss the patient's surgery. The therapist must have a complete understanding of the extent of surgery performed, any residual limitations to full passive flexion, potential concerns related to joint stability, and any additional surgical procedures (e.g., tenolysis, intrinsic releases). Based on this information, the initial postoperative therapy program can be established.

Evaluation

In complement to the preoperative assessment, an objective evaluation should be performed during each treatment session after surgery. It is critical to monitor active and passive ROM, edema with circumferential measurements along the distal palmar flexion crease (DPFC), pain

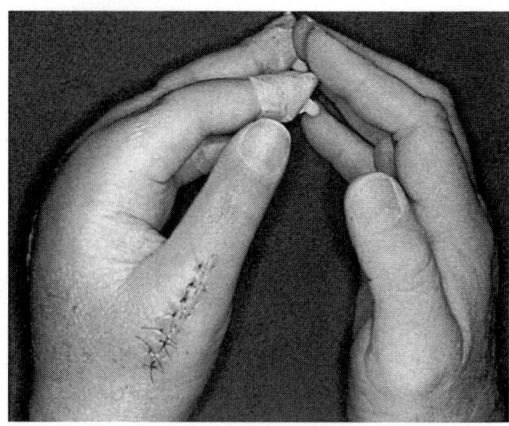

Fig. 63-5. Moderate edema is noted in the left hand, which underwent dorsal capsulectomies to the index through small finger metacarpophalangeal (MP) joints along with the thumb MP joint, compared with the right hand. Dorsal edema is common after MP capsulectomies for the initial 10 to 14 days after surgery.

with a visual analog scale or by rating the pain on a scale of 0 to 10, and the wound (size and appearance). The objective evaluation is essential to monitor the patient's progress and the effectiveness of each treatment method.

EDEMA MANAGEMENT

Control of postoperative edema during the initial 10 to 14 days after surgery is of great importance (Fig. 63-5). Effective edema management is key to a successful outcome. During the initial inflammatory phase and, more important, during the fibroplasia phase of wound healing, the fibroblasts and fibrin effectively lay down collagen, affecting the suppleness of the soft tissue structures and forming restrictive adhesions. Effective edema management minimizes the formation of adhesions, decreases the pressure and resistance to passive joint motion, and favorably influences the orientation of collagen fibers as active and passive ROM exercises are incorporated in the therapy program.

When excessive edema is present, there is heightened pain and increased risk of wound separation and subsequent infection. It is critical to effectively limit and manage the edema so that it will not interfere with the course of rehabilitation.

I believe that the most effective method for controlling postoperative edema in the hand and forearm is a carefully and evenly applied light compressive dressing (Fig. 63-6). The dressing is changed at each therapy visit and is worn for the initial 10 to 14 days after surgery. After the light compressive dressing is discontinued, elastic stockinettes may be worn on the hand and forearm along with an Isotoner glove to assist with managing any persistent edema.

In addition to the light compressive dressings and elastic stockinettes, elevation and interdigital massage (between the metacarpals and along the length of the volar and dorsal

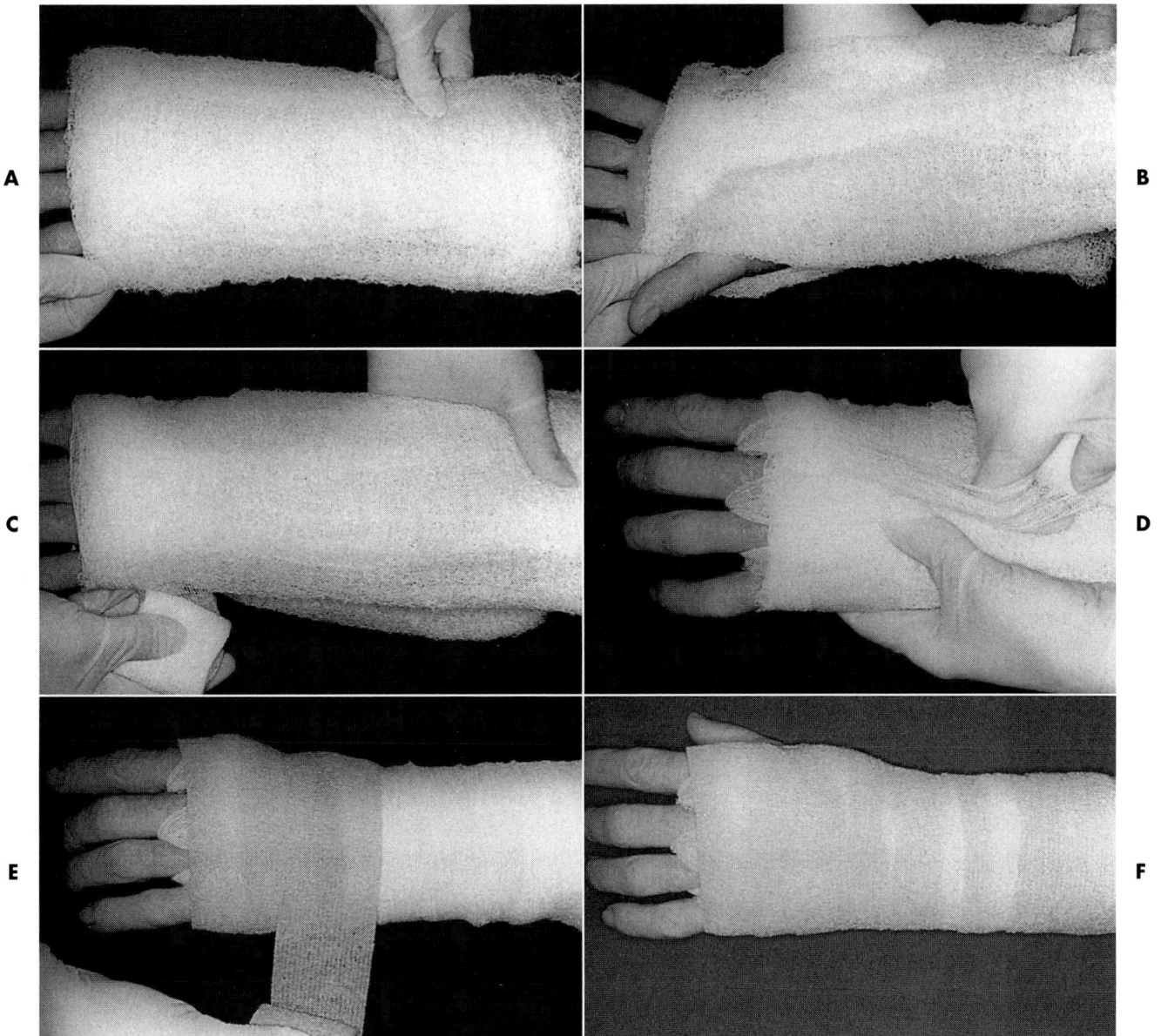

Fig. 63-6. Steps for applying a light compressive dressing. **A** and **B,** The initial step consists of "Kerlix fluffs" (a term I use) applied both dorsally and volarly. Kerlix fluffs consist of 4-inch Kerlix unfolded into approximately a 32-inch length and then carefully refolded into a rectangular segment 12 inches long by 4 inches wide. Care is taken to be sure the dorsal and volar segments overlap evenly on the medial and lateral borders of the hand and forearm. **C,** Two-inch gauze is applied distally to proximally. **D,** The 2-inch gauze is applied between the digits to secure the dressing and control interdigital edema. **E** and **F,** Two-inch Coban is evenly applied distally to proximally in single layers. Coban is preferred because it secures the dressing in place and will not lose its shape.

aspect of the hand) are effective for managing the boggy edema often noted after surgery. With the massage, it is important to avoid direct contact with the sutures and to avoid skin separation along the suture line.

To manage digital edema, finger socks or Coban are applied and worn between exercise sessions (Fig. 63-7). The edema at this level will generally subside within 2 to 3 weeks.

PAIN MANAGEMENT

Effective edema management is one means for controlling the postoperative pain associated with MP capsulectomies. In addition, TENS has proven to be beneficial in reducing the postoperative pain (Fig. 63-8). High-rate, conventional TENS, with electrode placement along the peripheral nerve distribution of the surgical area, has repeatedly proven effective for me and my colleagues.[3]

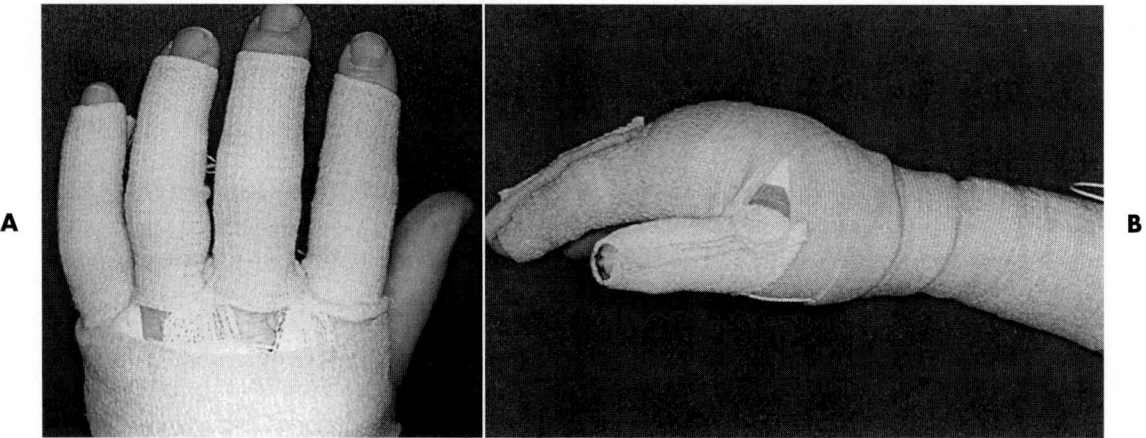

Fig. 63-7. A, "Finger socks" consist of 3-inch elastic bandages cut in 2½-by-3-inch segments sewn together in a tapered fashion to accommodate the diameter of the edematous digit. These finger sleeves also are commercially available. **B,** Coban is shown being used on the index finger with finger socks on the remaining digits and thumb.

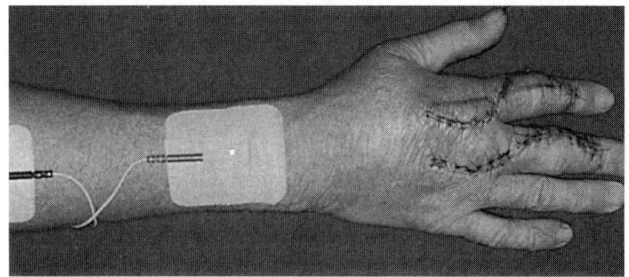

Fig. 63-8. Transcutaneous electrical nerve stimulation (TENS) is shown along the radial nerve distribution of a patient who underwent dorsal metacarpophalangeal and proximal interphalangeal capsulectomies of the index and middle fingers. Using the MEDA brand of TENS unit, I have found the following parameter settings to be effective: pulse width, 150 to 175 ms; pulse rate, 80 to 100 pps; and intensity, within the patient's comfort level. The unit is worn continually and generally is discontinued within 2 to 4 weeks.

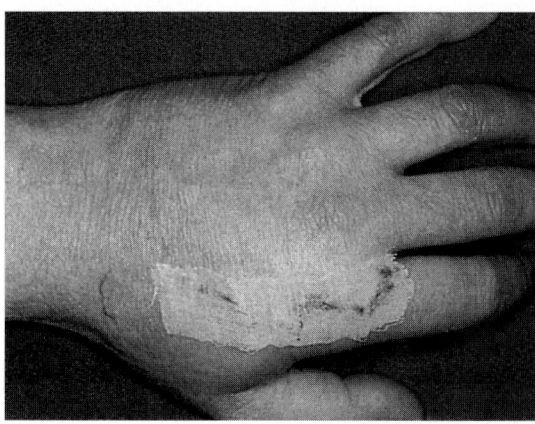

Fig. 63-9. Xeroform serves as an effective barrier to reduce the likelihood of an infection. It is left in place as the bulky dressing is removed and the new dressing is applied.

WOUND CARE

In most instances, wound care can be accomplished through the use of postoperative light compressive dressings. The dressings serve as the sterile barrier between the wound and contaminants in the environment. When possible, the Xeroform, which is often placed over the sutures before the bulky dressing is applied, is left in place to provide added wound protection (Fig. 63-9).

Occasionally, when extensive surgery is required, significant dorsal edema may create a limited degree of wound separation. These wounds generally have an uneventful course and heal readily by secondary intention.

On occasion, a hematoma will occur. In these instances, it is important to express the hematoma to prevent an environment for infection. With the use of sterile technique, hematomas may be manually expressed by slightly separating the sutured skin edges and applying pressure or by the physician aspirating the hematoma with a needle and syringe. After expression of the hematoma, the wound must be monitored carefully for signs of infection. A course of prophylactic antibiotics is not uncommon.

EXERCISES

The bulky compressive dressing should be removed within the initial 24 to 36 hours after surgery to initiate ROM exercises. It is important to begin the exercises before the close of the inflammatory phase of wound healing and before active participation of the fibroblasts in laying the framework for the formation of new collagen. Initiating early controlled motion will aid in the alignment and orientation of the newly forming collagen and will ultimately affect the final arc of motion.

Important to include in the postoperative exercise regimen are the following active, active-assisted, and passive ROM exercises (Fig. 63-10):

- Composite flexion and extension of the digits
- MP joint flexion/extension with the interphalangeal (IP) joints extended
- MP joint flexion/extension with the IP joints flexed
- Abduction/adduction of the digits

When capsulectomies have been performed to the index and small fingers, it is important to isolate the EIP and EDQ through independent extension of the index and small fingers. In addition, ROM exercises for the wrist should be performed. Wrist exercises should include isolated active and passive ROM along with simultaneous wrist and finger flexion, followed by wrist and finger extension. These exercises will provide for independent and maximum excursion of the extrinsic extensors and are especially necessary to include when extensor tenolysis accompanies the capsulectomy.

Exercising for 10 to 15 minutes each hour or two has proven effective on a clinical basis. The rest period between exercise sessions allows the wound to "quiet down" and the inflammation to somewhat subside before the initiation of the next exercise session. In addition, the muscles have more than an adequate recovery period before the next exercise session.

Patients need to understand that the ROM achieved in the first 10 to 14 days after surgery is easier to maintain than at 3 to 4 weeks. This is related to the wound healing process and proliferative nature of the new collagen following the initial 2 weeks after surgery. Patients will be more understanding and less likely to be discouraged if this has been explained in advance.

Occasionally, patients will have a sluggish start with the postoperative therapy program. Factors such as nausea secondary to anesthesia or the pain medications, postoperative pain, and edema may play a part in the slow start. In these cases, the initial therapy program may need to include an exercise session at some point during the night, in complement to the daily exercise schedule. This may be necessary to ensure that the patient continues to makes gains in motion each day.

Functional activities should be stressed along with the ROM exercises early in the postoperative therapy program. Unlike many other surgical procedures in which protection of anatomic structures is essential, this procedure can permit relatively normal use of the hand without risk of damage to soft tissue or bony structures. Therefore the earlier the hand begins performing functional activities, the sooner the hand will have restored functional use in normal daily activities. In the clinic, functional exercises that emphasize MP joint flexion with IP joint extension should be encouraged.

Strengthening exercises for the long flexors, extensors, and intrinsics may be initiated after the edema and pain have subsided. This is generally 3 to 4 weeks after surgery. Putty, hand exercisers, and hand weights are effective for enhancing the overall strength of the hand and forearm. As for initiating a work-conditioning program, it tends to be more effective when initiated approximately 6 weeks after surgery. The delay allows residual inflammation and edema to resolve before commencing repetitive lifting and heavy use of the hand.

SPLINTING

With dorsal MP capsulectomies, splinting serves three basic and important purposes: (1) immobilization to reduce inflammation and thus decrease pain and edema, (2) immobilization of the surgical area in a position that maximizes the passive flexion achieved in surgery and maintains lengthening of the soft tissue structures, and (3) dynamic mobilization to passively enhance ROM.

Clinically, I have found it effective to position the hand in a safe-position splint between exercise sessions and at night during the initial 3 to 4 weeks after surgery (Fig. 63-11). This places the MP joint collateral ligaments on optimal stretch. Occasionally, the MP joints can be positioned in as much as 90 degrees of flexion, but more commonly, the hand is positioned in approximately 75 degrees at the MP level.

Immediately after surgery, the MP joints may not achieve the desired level of flexion because of the postoperative dressing, edema, and/or discomfort. It is important to serially adjust the splint in increased flexion at each treatment session until maximum flexion is achieved.

When it is difficult to achieve full flexion of the MP joints, a dynamic flexion splint may be added to the therapy program (Fig. 63-12). The splint may be added as early as the first postoperative day if necessary. The degree of limitation in passive flexion determines the daily time requirements for wearing the splint. In severe cases in which the hand is resistant to full passive flexion, the dynamic splint may be worn between exercise sessions during the day. Rarely is it worn at night because of potential discomfort, bulkiness of the splint, and risk of heightened edema or circulatory problems.

Because immobilization can quickly lead to heightened joint stiffness, splinting should be gradually eliminated at the earliest reasonable time. This should be done as each splint has fulfilled its intended purpose. The time frame will vary, but usually within the initial 3 weeks, the splint-wearing time may be decreased each day until the splint is no longer needed. The safe-position splint is usually continued at night for 8 to 10 weeks.

Another form of passive stretching that has proven effective and that may negate the need for dynamic splinting is a simple procedure referred to as *taping* (Fig. 63-13). Either dorsal taping or composite taping may be performed. Both are effective for limbering up the hand before an exercise session.

SCAR MANAGEMENT

A valuable method of scar management after MP capsulectomies is scar massage and scar retraction with

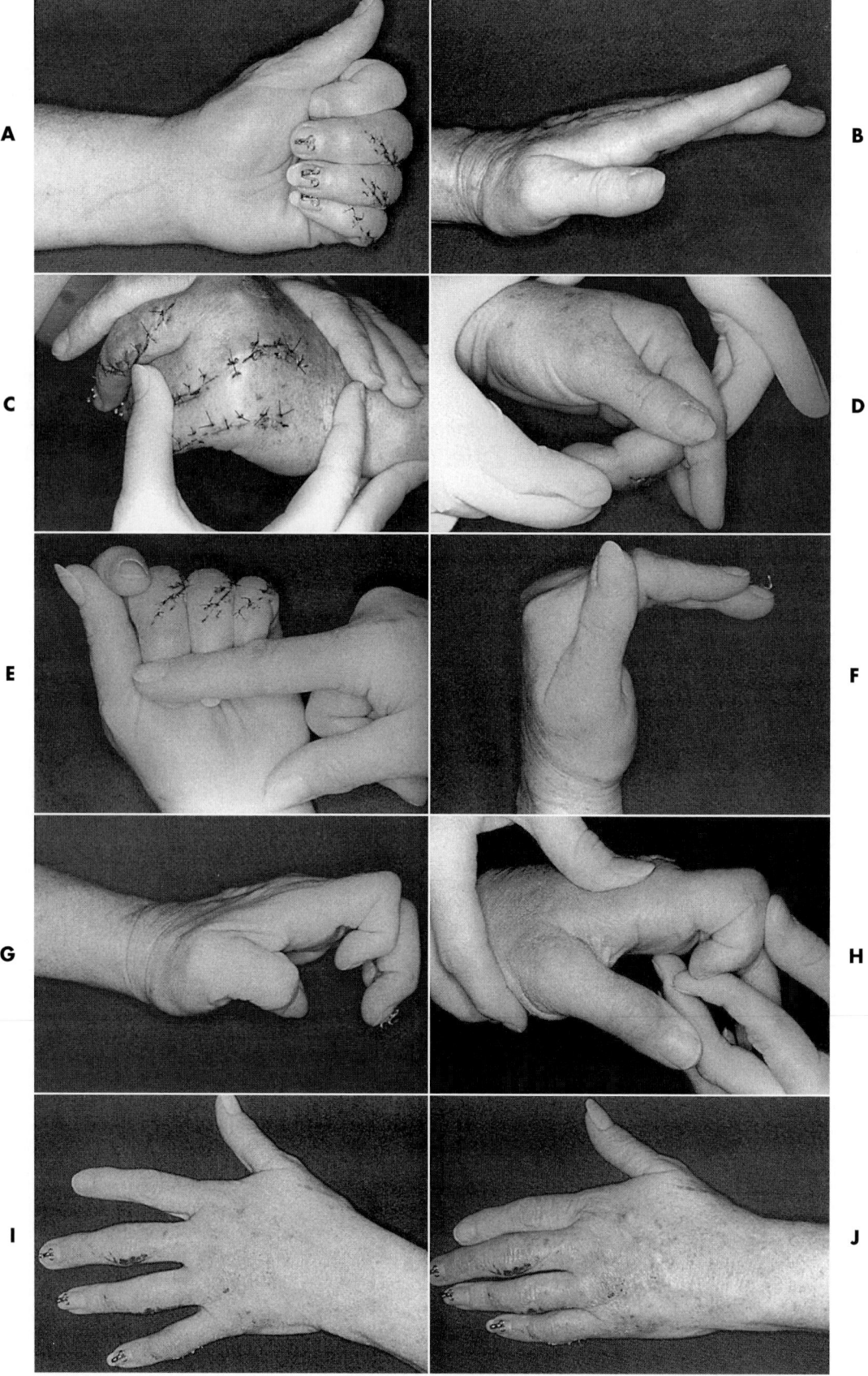

Fig. 63-10. Active and passive range-of-motion exercises are initiated within the inflammatory phase of wound healing with occasional exception. Exercises valuable to include in therapy are demonstrated. **A,** Active flexion. **B,** Active extension. **C,** Passive metacarpophalangeal (MP) flexion. **D,** Composite passive flexion. **E,** Composite passive flexion. **F,** MP flexion with the interphalangeal (IP) joints extended. **G** and **H,** MP extension with IP flexion (active/passive). **I,** Abduction of the digits. **J,** Adduction of the digits.

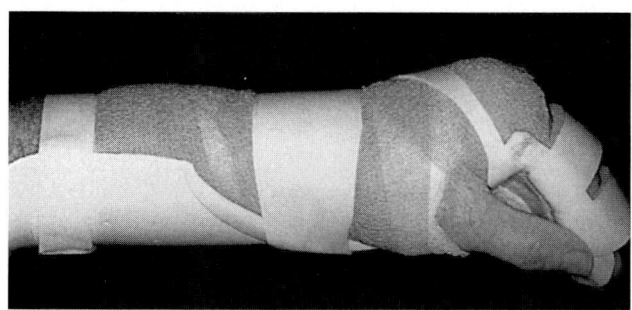

Fig. 63-11. A safe-position splint secures the metacarpophalangeal (MP) joints in maximum flexion with the interphalangeal (IP) joints in neutral. The collateral ligaments are on optimal stretch in this position. Using the American Society of Hand Therapists splinting nomenclature system, this splint is classified in the following manner: wrist extension, index-small MP flexion, IP extension, immobilization.

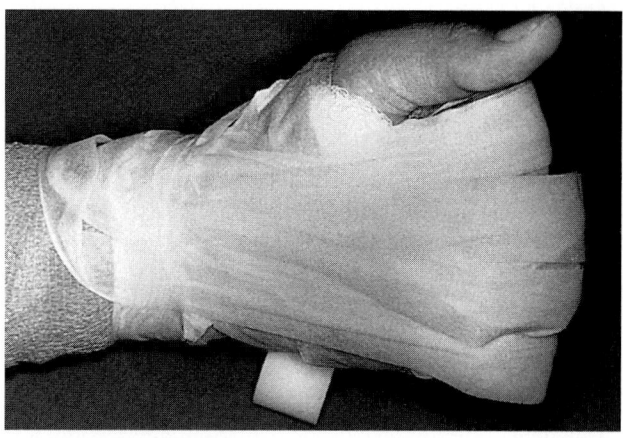

Fig. 63-13. *Taping* is a term I use to describe a method to increase passive flexion of the digits. To perform dorsal taping, a thin cotton glove is applied to the hand and ½-inch paper tape or ¾-inch masking tape is applied dorsally along the metacarpals and digits and then secured to the volar side of the wrist. Additional layers of tape are periodically added for 20 to 30 minutes to gradually gain more flexion.

A

B

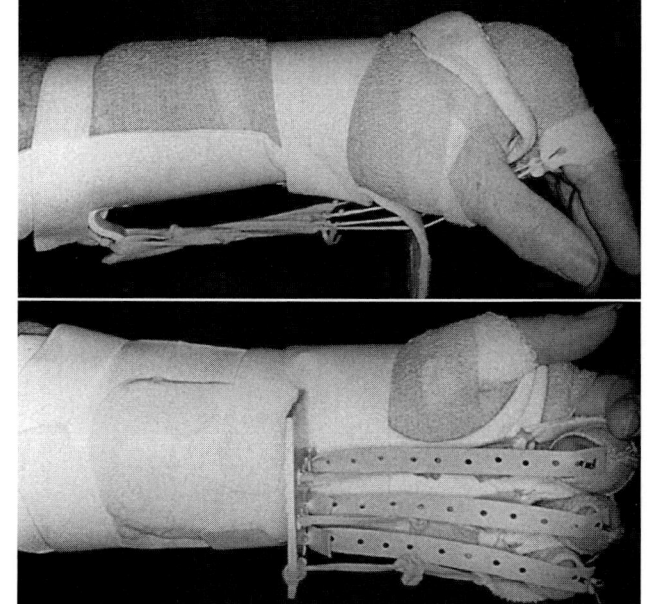

Fig. 63-12. Dynamic flexion splinting may focus on the metacarpophalangeal (MP) joints alone **(A)** or may be applied in a composite fashion when extrinsic extensor tightness is present or when dorsal capsule tightness is present at both the MP and proximal interphalangeal joint levels **(B)**. Dynamic traction in this composite flexion splint is applied by using No. 83 rubber bands attached to fingernail hooks.

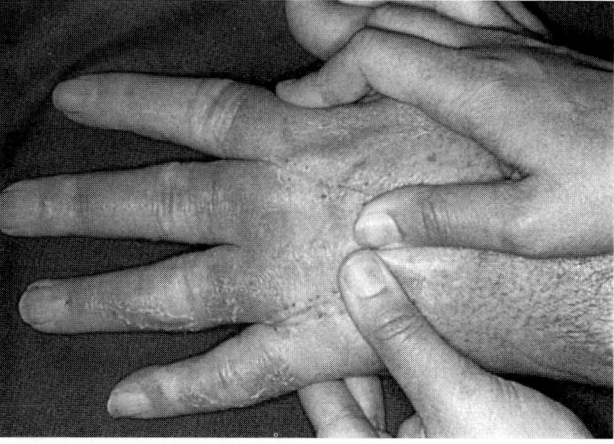

Fig. 63-14. Scar retraction may be valuable in mobilizing the skin from the underlying subcutaneous soft tissue structures.

lotion. Scar massage includes deep massage along the length of the scar, horizontally across the scar, and in circular clockwise and counterclockwise motion. Scar retraction also may be performed to mobilize the soft tissues (Fig. 63-14). With scar retraction, the patient performs active ROM while

the therapist (or the patient after being taught) mobilizes the skin in the direction opposite the active motion. The goal is to mobilize the skin and free subcutaneous adhesions. In addition, Dycem may be used with scar retraction to better stabilize the skin.

Silicone products such as Elastomer, Otoform, and 50/50 may be applied under splints or dressings to remodel the dorsal scar and aid in remodeling the orientation of the collagen fibers.

MODALITIES
Neuromuscular electrical stimulation

Neuromuscular electrical stimulation (NMES) may be used to assist with active ROM at the MP level in both flexion and extension (Fig. 63-15). With MP joint capsulectomies, it is more frequently used to maximize the proximal excursion of the EDC and the long flexors with the goal of maximizing MP joint ROM. Muscle stimulation also may be used for the intrinsics to facilitate isolated MP joint flexion.

Effective treatment parameters that I have used include the following: pulse rate, 30 to 40 pps; rise time, 2 seconds; on time, 10 seconds; off time, 20 seconds; intensity, set at a level that creates a strong motor response yet is well within the patient's comfort level; and time, 15-minute session. It is common for the NMES to be used three to four times a day as a part of the home exercise program.

Ultrasound

Occasionally, when patients heal quickly and form dense scar after surgery, it becomes difficult to maintain supple joints and tendon gliding. In these instances, ultrasound has been especially beneficial.

The ultrasound serves as a deep heating agent, elevating the temperature of the soft tissue structures.[22] The deep heat allows for greater passive suppleness and elasticity of the soft tissues. Clinically, the following parameters for using the ultrasound have met with positive success: frequency, 3.0 MHz; intensity, 0.7 to 1.2 W/cm^2, continuous mode; and treatment time, 5 to 8 minutes. Typically, the ultrasound will be continued for six to eight treatment sessions.

Continuous passive motion

Continuous passive motion (CPM) units have proven to be clinically effective in reducing postoperative pain and

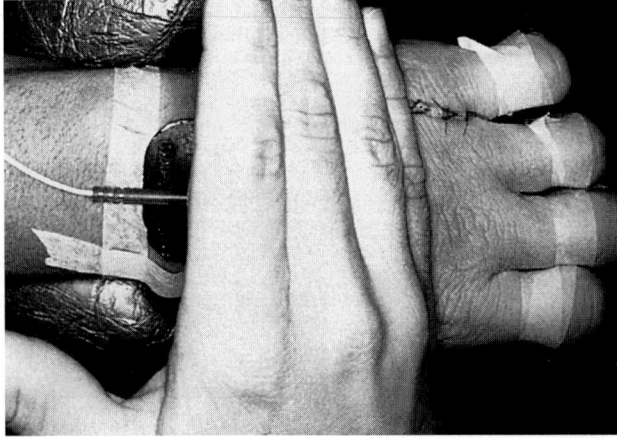

Fig. 63-15. Neuromuscular electrical stimulation is being shown to stimulate the extensor digitorum communis. The interphalangeal joints are taped in flexion to isolate extension to the metacarpophalangeal joints.

edema and ultimately may increase joint ROM. Recognizing that there are a variety of hand CPM units on the market, it is important to determine which unit will effectively produce the desired result. In the case of MP capsulectomies, the goal is to decrease pain and edema and maximize ROM at the MP joint level.

It is important to realize few CPM units, if any, create a full arc of motion with composite flexion to the DPFC and full extension. This is because of the anatomic length differences between the digits. That the CPM unit may not achieve a complete arc of motion need not preclude its use. CPM units have repeatedly proven effective in reducing pain and edema. Therefore it should be considered for the initial week to 10 days following surgery. After this time, the therapy program should be reevaluated. The CPM unit may have accomplished its intended purpose. This allows the therapy program to place greater emphasis on ROM exercises, splinting, and alternative edema management and pain management methods.

MOTIVATION

To maximize the success of the procedure, the patient must be self-motivated and have specific goals in mind for the procedure (i.e., improvement in performing specific functional tasks). These goals should be charted and the patient advised as to whether the goals are realistic and achievable.

In addition to the patient's self-motivation, the therapist must play an active role in motivating the patient to achieve the desired goals. The patient's overall success may depend on the therapist's ability to keep him or her actively involved in the early postoperative therapy regimen and to maintain that active participation 6 to 8 weeks later.

RESULTS

A limited number of articles can be found in the literature relating to the results after MP capsulectomy. Gould et al.[13] reported a series of 100 patients with dorsal MP capsulectomies in 1979. In their series, the MP joints were pinned in flexion for 10 to 14 days. With all diagnostic categories, the authors achieved a mean gain of 21 degrees of active and 29 degrees of passive MP joint motion secondary to the procedure. The greatest gains were seen in those 11 to 20 years of age. From a diagnostic perspective, greater gains were seen with the one stroke patient in their series (51.5 degrees passively) and with the five burn patients (36 degrees and 42 degrees passively). The least gains were seen with reflex sympathetic dystrophy (3 degrees actively and 28 degrees passively) and with fractures and crush injuries (18 degrees actively and 20 degrees passively). The authors stated that most patients could be flexed to 90 degrees intraoperatively, but this was rarely maintained postoperatively.

Young et al.[33] reported on 10 patients with 24 dorsal MP capsulectomies in 1978. After the procedure, the MP joints were placed in flexion and pinned for 14 days before ROM was begun at this level. The overall increase in passive ROM at the MP level was 48 degrees. The greatest gain was seen in the lacerations and other category (71 degrees in each category and closed fractures 60 degrees passively). The least gain was seen in the open fracture category (a gain of 37 degrees passively).

Buch,[1] in his series, reported a minimum average increase of 30 degrees passively in MP joint ROM. Results were significantly less notable when skin grafting was performed in association with the capsulectomy.

In 1947, Fowler[11] described his results as "excellent with 80% to 90% of motion confidently expected if local tissues are good and the mechanics of the hand satisfactory." Fowler did not include compiled clinical results with the article. Postoperative management consisted of rigid splinting or traction with the MP joints in flexion for 3 weeks before ROM was begun at the MP level.

I have found dorsal MP joint capsulectomies to be a reliable and effective procedure for enhancing overall functional performance of the hand in the majority of cases. The superior results are seen in young patients (up to 25 years old), in patients requiring exclusively capsulectomy in a single or multiple digits, and where the articular surfaces of the MP joint are relatively normal. Maintaining the results achieved in surgery is certainly a challenge, however, and becomes increasingly difficult with crush injuries to the dorsum of the hand that require extensive extensor tenolyses along with the MP capsulectomies. PIP joint capsulectomies may even be necessary concurrently with the MP joint capsulectomies. In such cases, the ring and small fingers tend to be the greater challenge in maintaining the MP flexion, and yet functionally they are the most critical.

The goal need not be to achieve a complete arc of motion from 0 to 90 degrees. The goal may be to simply make the arc of motion more functional for the patient. Crush injuries are a good example of this point. In these cases, there may be a certain degree of destruction to the articular surface of the MP joint, and it may be unrealistic to anticipate restoring full motion. What can be accomplished, however, is for the arc of motion to be altered in increased flexion and thus be of greater functional value to the patient.

FUNCTIONAL RANGE OF MOTION

It is helpful to remember what is considered functional ROM for the joints of the hand. Functional flexion averages 61 degrees at the MP joint level, 60 degrees at the PIP joint level, and 39 degrees at the DIP joint level.[17] In the thumb, functional flexion is 21 degrees at the MP joint level and 18 degrees at the IP joint level. These arcs of motion are based on common ADLs. Although they do not specifically address individual vocational and avocational pursuits, they do provide a basic guideline for functional performance measures of the hand. One should assess the individual and special needs of each patient in considering the surgery, and

in cases in which the surgery is performed, the goal must be to strive for the highest functional performance levels.

Case report

A 72-year-old man presented to the office 3 months after his initial surgery and rehabilitation for a crush injury, which included a fourth metacarpal fracture. There were significant limitations in ROM restricting the patient in daily activities and avocational interests. In particular, he had the most difficulty carrying objects in his hand and was unable to play golf because he could not grip the club. Preoperative active and (passive) ROM revealed the following:

	Index	Long	Ring	Small
MP joint	0/45	15/50	20/35	10/30
	(0)/(55)	(0)/(60)	(0)/(45)	(0)/(40)

Surgery consisted of dorsal MP capsulectomies of the index through small fingers, along with extensor tenolyses. The patient was placed in a bulky compressive dressing postoperatively and was referred to therapy the following day.

Once the bulky dressing was removed, an initial evaluation was performed, consisting of ROM measurements, wound and pain assessment, edema measurements, and the obtaining of information on his previous medical history. Based on the physician's orders, surgery performed, and initial evaluation, the following treatment program was established:

- Edema control for the forearm and hand with a light compressive dressing and digital level edema control with finger socks
- Active and passive ROM exercises, emphasizing isolated MP joint motion; composite passive flexion and extension; isolated tendon excursion of the EDC, EIP and EDQ; and intrinsic stretches
- Dynamic flexion splint for the MP joints, to be worn four times a day for 45 minutes (Fig. 63-16, *D*)
- Safe-position forearm-based splint positioning the MP joints in maximum flexion, to be worn between exercise sessions and dynamic splinting

On the third postoperative day, the patient presented with significant edema, notably on the dorsum of the hand (Fig. 63-16, *A*). A hematoma was present and manually expressed with sterile technique (Fig. 63-16, *B* and *C*). Draining of hematomas is critical to minimizing the risk of infection and excessive scar formation.

By the third postoperative week, the patient's wound had healed uneventfully. There were dense adhesions along the dorsum of the hand. Scar mobilization techniques, including scar massage with lotion, scar retraction using Dycem to mobilize the skin opposite the direction of the tendon gliding (Fig. 63-16, *E*), and ultrasound for deep heat to enhance the elasticity of the underlying soft tissue structures (Fig. 63-16, *F*), were added to the therapy program.

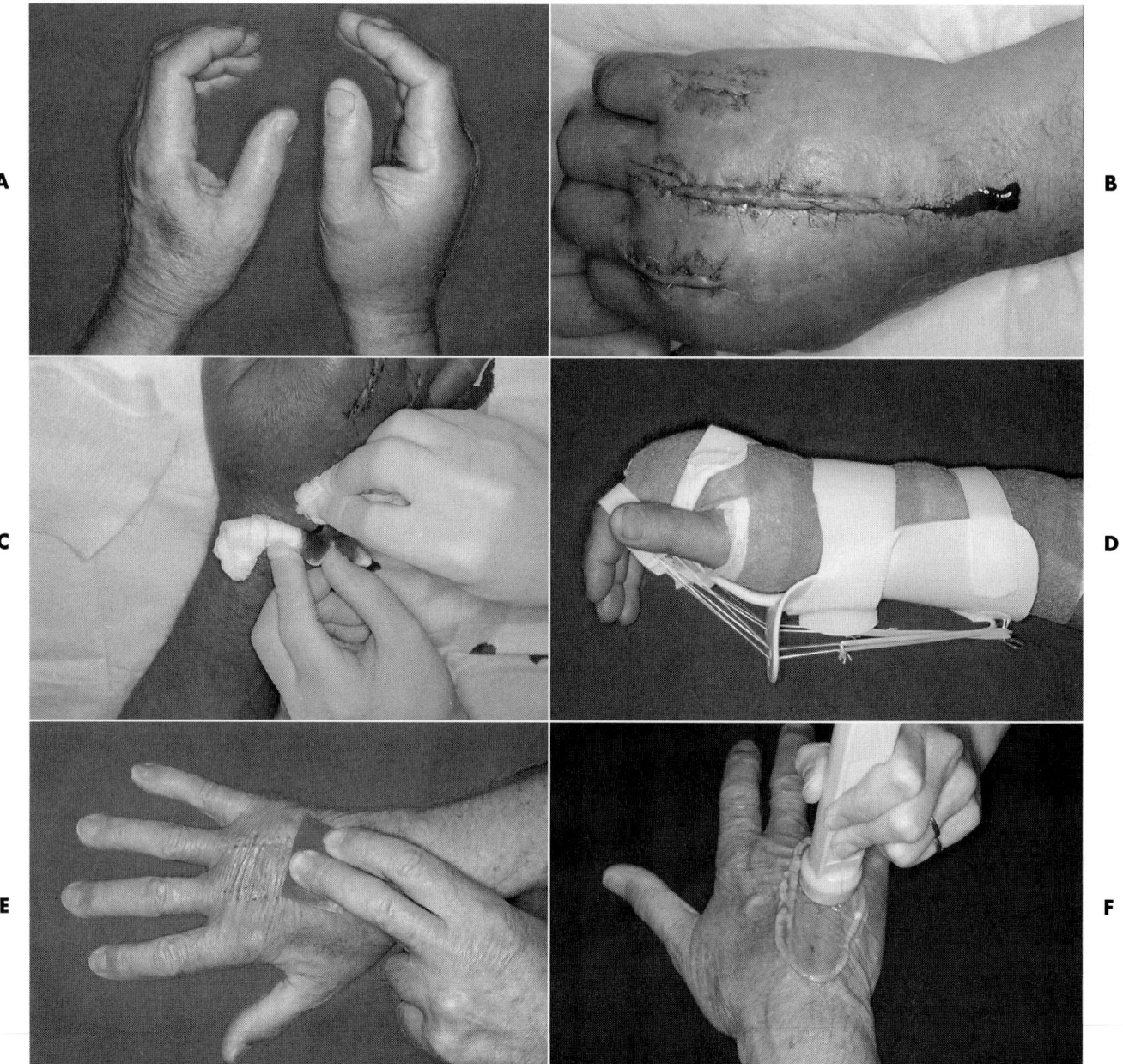

Fig. 63-16. Case example. A 63-year-old man underwent dorsal metacarpophalangeal (MP) capsulectomies and extensor tenolyses of the index through small fingers. **A,** On the first postoperative day, moderate edema was noted and typical for the extent of surgery. **B,** A hematoma present on the dorsum of the hand the third postoperative day. **C,** The hematoma was manually expressed using a sterile technique. **D,** A wrist immobilization splint with dynamic MP flexion was added to the therapy program within the first week to enhance passive flexion of the MP joints. **E,** Dycem was used to assist with scar mobilization in the area where the skin was densely adherent to the underlying scar tissue. **F,** Ultrasound was used as a deep heat to enhance the elasticity of the adhesions and secondarily increase motion with the hand in extension, as well as in flexion.

Continued

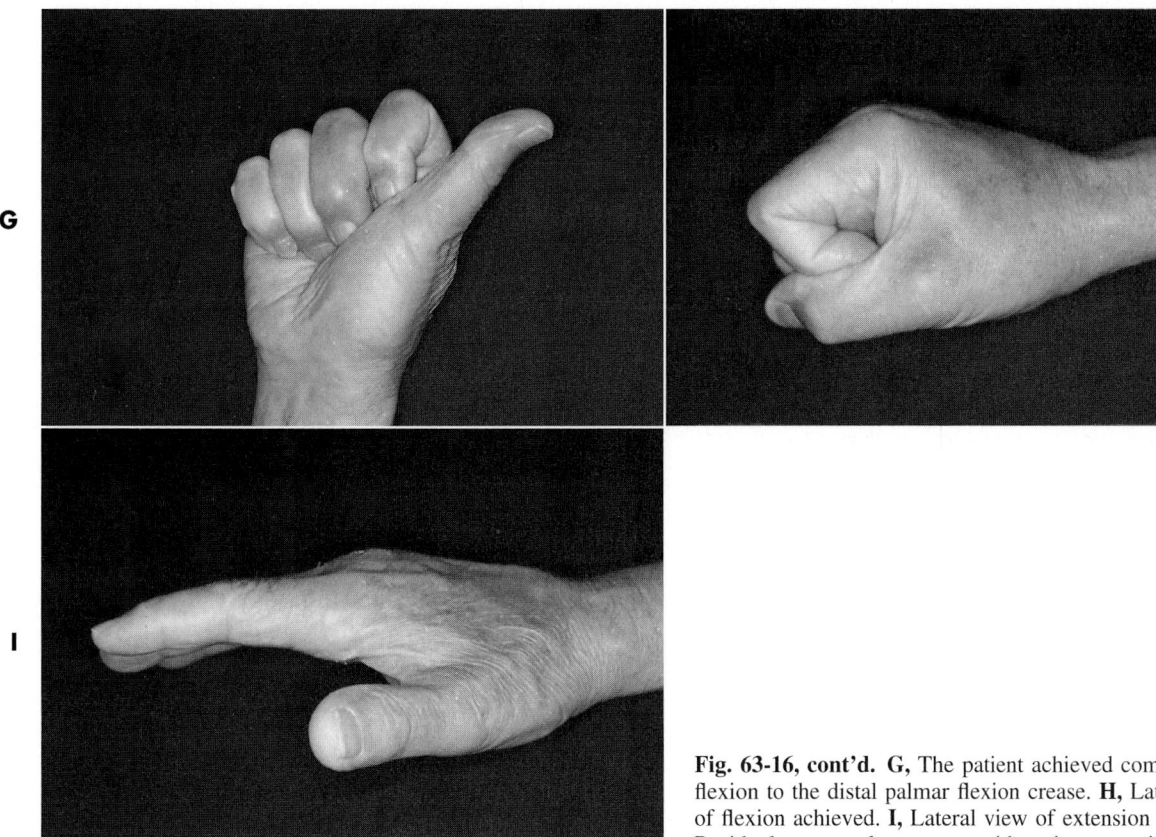

Fig. 63-16, cont'd. G, The patient achieved composite flexion to the distal palmar flexion crease. **H,** Lateral view of flexion achieved. **I,** Lateral view of extension achieved. Residual extensor lag present with active extension.

Interval therapy visits continued for 10 weeks. The patient presented with a successful final outcome (Fig. 63-16, *G* to *I*). He was able to use his hand successfully in functional activities, including golf. A reassessment at 5 months revealed the following active and (passive) ROM:

	Index	Long	Ring	Small
MP joints	0/75	30/80	20/80	15/80
	(0)/(75)	(0)/(85)	(0)/(85)	(0)/(80)

With elective surgeries such as this, it is important to keep in mind the functional goals the patient desires from surgery. Therapy should focus on continually upgrading and modifying the treatment program to meet these objectives.

Equally important, the splinting used during the course of therapy to maximize and maintain MP joint flexion must be *gradually* eliminated, or the patient may lose key motion achieved in therapy.

VOLAR METACARPOPHALANGEAL CAPSULECTOMIES

Volar MP joint capsulectomies are performed less frequently. Some of the more common diagnoses or conditions requiring volar capsulectomy are longstanding intrinsic contractures with secondary contracture of the volar plate,

burns, Volkmann's contracture, Dupuytren's contracture, crush injuries, spasticity, prolonged immobilization, soft tissue contractures along the volar surface of the MP joints, and burst injuries to the palm.[2,14,16]

In most cases, postoperative therapy may be initiated within 24 hours after surgery. Edema and pain control measures, as previously described, may be used throughout the course of therapy. Splinting of choice will be in extension. For night wear, a splint positioning the MP and IP joints in full extension is recommended. During the day, between exercise sessions, a dynamic extension splint positioning the MP joints in extension should prove effective. Exercises may consist of unrestricted active and passive ROM, including emphasis on intrinsic stretches both actively and passively. The intrinsic stretches are important because intrinsic releases are generally needed along with the volar capsule release. Within 4 to 6 weeks, the extension splinting may gradually be eliminated, with the goal of completely discontinuing the splints between weeks 8 and 10.

The overall prognosis is good for restoring MP joint extension without risking loss of MP joint flexion. The greatest difficulty is in patients with longstanding, chronic intrinsic contracture and poor soft tissue on the volar surface that may require grafting and delayed therapy intervention.

SUMMARY

Excellent ROM at the MP joint level affords patients enhanced functional use of the hand. By carefully assessing the patient's preoperative status, one can determine the added functional value surgery offers the patient. After a decision is made to perform the procedure, the motivated patient most likely will have an outcome that meets the his or her functional needs. This assumes the postoperative treatment plan is carefully orchestrated and monitored by the physician and therapist in conjunction with the patient.

REFERENCES

1. Buch VI: Clinical and functional assessment of the hand after metacarpophalangeal capsulotomy, *Plast Reconstr Surg* 53:452, 1974.
2. Bunnell S, et al: Ischemic contracture, local, in the hand, *Plast Reconstr Surg* 3:424, 1948.
3. Cannon N, et al: Control of immediate postoperative pain following tenolysis and capsulectomies of the hand with TENS, *J Hand Surg* 8:626, 1983.
4. Craig SM: Anatomy of the joints of the fingers, *Hand Clin* 8:693, 1992.
5. Curtis RM: Joints of the hand. In Flynn JE, editor: *Hand surgery,* Baltimore, 1966, Williams & Wilkins.
6. Curtis RM: Management of the stiff hand. In Lamb DW, et al, editors: *The practice of hand surgery,* Oxford, 1981, Blackwell Scientific.
7. Curtis RM: Management of the stiff hand. In Lamb DW, et al, editors: *The practice of hand surgery,* ed 2, Oxford, 1989, Blackwell Scientific.
8. Curtis RM, et al: Joints of the hand. In Jupiter JB, editor: *Flynn's hand surgery,* ed 4, Baltimore, 1991, Williams & Wilkins.
9. *Dorland's illustrated medical dictionary,* ed 29, Philadelphia, 2000, Saunders.
10. Evans RB, et al: A study of the dynamic anatomy of extensor tendons and implications for treatment, *J Hand Surg* 11A:774, 1986.
11. Fowler SB: Mobilization of metacarpophalangeal joints: arthroplasty and capsulotomy, *J Bone Joint Surg* 29:193, 1947.
12. Gorman RJ: Metacarpal and proximal interphalangeal joint capsulectomy. In Clark GL, et al, editors: *Hand rehabilitation: a practical guide,* New York, 1993, Churchill Livingstone.
13. Gould JS, et al: Capsulectomy of the metacarpophalangeal and proximal interphalangeal joints, *J Hand Surg* 4:482, 1979.
14. Green DP, et al: A transpositional skin flap for release of volar contractures of the finger at the MP joint, *Plast Reconstr Surg* 64:516, 1979.
15. Hakstian RW, et al: Ulnar deviation of the fingers: the role of joint structure and function, *J Bone Joint Surg* 49A:299, 1967.
16. Harris C, et al: Intrinsic contracture in the hand and its surgical treatment, *J Bone Joint Surg* 36A:10, 1954.
17. Hume MC, et al: Functional range of motion of the joints of the hand, *J Hand Surg* 15A:240, 1990.
18. Idler RS: Capsulectomies of the metacarpophalangeal and proximal interphalangeal joints. In Strickland JW, editor: *The hand,* Philadelphia, 1998, Lippincott-Raven.
19. Kapandji IA: The metacarpo-phalangeal joints. In *The physiology of the joints,* ed 5, New York, 1982, Churchill Livingstone.
20. Laseter GF: Postoperative management of capsulectomies. In Hunter JM, et al, editors: *Rehabilitation of the hand,* ed 2, St Louis, 1984, Mosby.
21. Laseter GF: Postoperative management of capsulectomies. In Hunter JM, et al, editors: *Rehabilitation of the hand,* ed 3, St Louis, 1990, Mosby.
22. Michlovitz SL: *Thermal agents in rehabilitation,* ed 2, Philadelphia, 1990, FA Davis.
23. Milford L: Reconstruction after injury. In Milford L, editor: *The hand,* ed 3, St Louis, 1988, Mosby.
24. Peacock EE: Some biochemical and biophysical aspects of joint stiffness: role of collagen synthesis as opposed to altered molecular bonding, *Ann Surg* 164:1, 1966.
25. Peacock EE, et al: Reconstructive surgery of hands with injured central metacarpophalangeal joints, *J Bone Joint Surg* 38A:291, 1956.
26. Phipps AR, et al: A possible new operative method for the treatment of metacarpophalangeal joint stiffness, *J Hand Surg* 11B:237, 1986.
27. Pratt DR: Joints of the hand and fingers: their stiffness, splinting and surgery, *CA Med* 66:22, 1947.
28. Rank BK, et al: Re-establishment of joint mobility. In *Surgery of repair as applied to hand injuries,* ed 4, Edinburgh, 1973, Churchill Livingstone.
29. Reid DAC: Capsulectomy of the metacarpophalangeal and proximal interphalangeal joints. In Rob & Smith's operative surgery: the hand, ed 4, St Louis, 1983, Mosby.
30. Shaw CG: Ankylosis of the metacarpo-phalangeal joints, *Med J Aust* 2:549, 1920.
31. Watson HK, et al: Stiff joints. In Green DP, editor: *Operative hand surgery,* ed 3, New York, 1993, Churchill Livingstone.
32. Wright PE: Special hand disorders. In Crenshaw AH, editor: *Campbell's operative orthopaedics,* ed 8, vol 5, St Louis, 1992, Mosby.
33. Young VL, et al: The surgical management of stiff joints in the hand, *Plast Reconstr Surg* 62:835, 1978.

Part XV

THE MIND-HAND CONNECTION: PSYCHOLOGIC ASPECTS OF HAND INJURIES

Chapter 64

PSYCHOLOGICALLY BASED HAND DISORDERS

Paul W. Brown

The late Guy Pulvertaft wrote on *Psychological Aspects of Hand Injuries* for the first three editions of this text. It was my humble privilege to follow him with a modified version of the same topic in the fourth, and now in the fifth, edition. In his writing, as in his practice, my friend and mentor, Pulvertaft, stressed the importance of communication between the physician and his or her patient, or as he put it, "the art of rapport." He was a master surgical technician who spoke eloquently on nontechnical matters and practiced what he preached. He recognized that the surgeon must deal as effectively with the psychologic effect of injury and disease on the patient as he or she does with the mechanical, anatomic, and functional aspects of the ailment. His writings on this are laced with advice that, although known to all effective healers, bears repeating:

"There are ways in which we can combine sympathy with truth."

"It is our duty to see that the infirm are supported spiritually as well as physically."

"The spirit in man can rise above the evils that can harm the body."

"Beware of false pride!" Guy Pulvertaft warned us. He argued that a surgeon must be self-confident and yet maintain a balance between surgical enthusiasm and common sense, saying that the desire to operate must not override other considerations such as the psychologic aspect of the patient's injury, the patient's emotional state, or the patient's desires.

As Pulvertaft would be quick to say, these ideas were not original. Most are at least Hippocratic in origin and have been the basis for sound medical practice for as long as history records. Nevertheless, Pulvertaft had the gift, the talent, and the sensitivity to impart this ethic in an effective and lasting manner to his many students and admirers.

MIND-BRAIN-HAND COMMUNICATION

What does mind-brain-hand communication have to do with the topic of this chapter? Plenty. The Greeks were among the first to tell us that no distinct demarcation exists between the body and the mind, that the psyche and the soma are inseparably entwined, and that each has its effect on the other. So, too, must the surgeon's psyche interact with the patient's soma, just as the patient's somatic and psychologic problems affect the emotions of the physician. If the patient's physical and psychologic problems overstress the physician's gastric mucosa, there may indeed be meaningful intercourse between the psyche and soma of both parties.

The hand's prominence in the brain is made obvious by the concept of the homunculus that is superimposed on the somatosensory portion of the brain. The brain sends messages to the hand, and generally, these messages are perceived clearly by the hand. At the same time, the hand sends messages to the brain, and generally, the brain receives and interprets the messages properly. Thus outgoing and incoming messages are pulsing back and forth between hand and brain. In the normal state, this is a smoothly orchestrated and coordinated balance of the afferent and efferent impulses; an unimpaired brain coupled with an intact hand served by a normal complement of peripheral nerves results in a *closed-loop communications system.* The net result is that the message received is the message that was sent (Fig. 64-1).

The message becomes distorted or is not received at all if something is wrong with either the transmitter or the

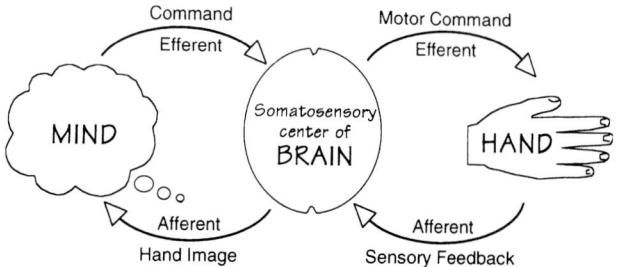

2 CLOSED LOOPS
Each of the three elements is both a
transmitter and a receiver

Fig. 64-1. The mind-brain-hand relationship.

receiver; thus the communication loop is broken, diseased, or warped. The severed sensory nerve will break the afferent loop. The nonconducting motor nerve will result in a severed efferent loop. Similarly, transmission or reception problems may occur within the somatosensory area of the brain because of any number of pathologic intracranial processes such as tumor, infection, or degeneration.

Superimposed on this basic closed communication loop between brain and hand is another closed loop, between the psyche and the somatosensory portion of the brain. No one is certain where the psyche dwells, whether it is in the prefrontal areas or diffusely throughout the cranial contents is not known, but for the purposes of this chapter it is not important to know. However, this portion of the persona constitutes the personality and emotion center, and its interplay with the loop between hand and brain will influence how the hand reacts and how the brain perceives that reaction.

Many other communication loops may influence the psyche and thereby the hand. These are *extracorporeal loops,* those communications that exist between the owner of the hand and his or her spouse or employer or others in his or her social environment. The communication loop between the patient and the physician is, or should be, a special loop, in that it should be a closed loop with both parties clearly understanding the other's transmitted messages. Sadly, all too often it is an open loop in which messages are not received or their reception is distorted.

All parts of the body are affected by these communication loops, but the hand is particularly so: Many authors, artists, and poets have seen the hand as a very special part of the body and have portrayed it as an extension of the brain—physiologically, psychologically, and esthetically.

The hand is influenced by many psychic stimuli from the mind. If these stimuli—these transmissions—deviate from the norm, as in psychosis or neurosis, the hand may reflect those abnormalities. Conversely, this communicative loop may be affected by the hand itself so that the anatomic or physiologic abnormalities of the hand may significantly

affect the owner's psyche or even the extracorporeal loops. The net result of all of these afferent and efferent messages and their reception may be a healthy hand and a sane mind, an abnormal mind and a normal hand, an abnormal mind and an abnormal hand, or an imperfect hand and a normal mind, or many nuances and combinations of any of these.

CLASSIFICATION OF PSYCHOLOGIC DISORDERS

Following is a hand surgeon's conception of the psyche and the hand. I make no pretense at understanding the mind from the psychiatrist's point of view. My credentials as a psychologist are strictly pragmatic and definitely nonacademic: They are based on interest, experience, observation, and past mistakes.

The traditional classification of psychic aberrations is complex, arbitrary, and nonscientific. The classification given in the fourth edition of the *Diagnostic and Statistical Manual of Mental Disorders* (DSM-IV) is designed primarily for psychiatrists and psychologists. The system presented here is much simpler, but it also is arbitrary and nonscientific. It is also useful. Although mental health professionals may cavil and quibble with this system, it will serve hand surgeons and hand therapists as a tool they may apply in their practice and in communication with other physicians, including psychiatrists and clinical psychologists.

Psychologically based hand disorders fall into three categories: the *psychoses,* the *neuroses,* and the *psychosocial problems.*

The boundaries of each are indistinct, and many combinations of the attributes of each are possible. There is much semantic confusion in our discussion of these disorders, and the basis for this confusion lies with the inability to define what is "normal" with any degree of agreement. We do fairly well in recognizing normalcy in the hand but do poorly in defining the normal psyche. There is little argument with classifying the severe catatonic patient as psychotic; however, the definitions for normal become increasingly blurred as we attempt to define what is neurotic, and our definition of a normal psychosocial state is impossibly indistinct. What is seen as neurotic in one person may appear to be a personality aberration in another. A psychosocial problem such as depression may wreak havoc with normal hand function in one patient, whereas the same degree of depression in another may represent an appropriate response to emotional trauma and not have somatic manifestations. The definition of *normal* is subjective.

Rather than trying to pigeonhole each of the mental disorders to make them conform to a specific classification, it is more useful to picture them as a spectrum, extending from the obvious and severe psychoses, shading with decreasing order of severity through the neuroses to the psychosocial disorders and common personality quirks and maladjustments, recognizing that the patient may combine aspects of several types.

The psychoses

Psychosis is a mental disorder in which the patient departs from what most of us define as reality. Psychosis is manifested by a serious disorganization of the personality and is sometimes accompanied by bizarre, dysfunctional problems with the hand. There are three subgroups of psychoses: organic, functional, and dementia.

Organic psychosis. When the psychosis is caused by a pathologic process such as infection, tumor, toxin, or trauma, the condition is labeled an *organic* psychosis. Hand problems with these conditions are tremor, incoordination, weakness, and palsy. Little can be done to improve the hand unless the central lesion is reversible.

Functional psychosis. Characterized by a lack of apparent organic cause, functional psychosis is separated into two basic types: schizophrenia and manic-depression.

Schizophrenia is a psychosis manifested by withdrawal, indifference, hallucinations, paranoia, and sometimes, multiple personalities. Hand symptoms may or may not be present. When present, they are often bizarre and manifested by meaningless motions or positions.

With *manic-depressive psychosis,* the patient experiences either mania, a wild state manifested by exaggerated ideas of well-being and excessive activity, or the opposite, a state of depression and melancholia. The patient may exist in only one of these states, *unipolar,* or may fluctuate between the two contrasting conditions, a *bipolar psychosis.* Hand problems are not particularly common in either, although either may present hands that are dysfunctional or symptomatic.

Dementias. Somewhere between the organic and the functional psychoses are the states of involutional mental deterioration, sometimes called the *dementias:* These are Alzheimer's disease and senile dementia. The demarcation between the two is indistinct, and either may demonstrate the same type of symptoms seen with the organic psychoses. The hands of patients with Alzheimer's do not show any obvious physical abnormalities but are often badly affected by loss of meaningful function.

The neuroses

The neuroses are mental disorders that are less serious than the psychoses. They are a psychologic reaction to stress, either real or perceived, and they are expressed in emotional behavior that is inappropriate for the stressful situation. Manifestations may be both psychic and somatic. In extreme forms, the neuroses tend toward the psychotic, whereas the less severe types are more like the psychosocial disorders. Although neuroses are given specific names, the neurotic patient often presents with a combination of several types of neuroses.

The psychiatric texts present many different classifications of the neuroses. I have borrowed from several of them, and tempering them with my own clinical experience, I have divided them into the following types, remembering that any of them may contain elements of the others and that some may be rather mild reactions to psychosocial stress and others may deviate more from reality (i.e., toward psychosis). The psychiatric diagnosis is seldom clear-cut.

Personality disorders

The personality disorders is a good class with which to start examining the neuroses because it well illustrates how the normal mind may subtly move to the abnormal. Each of us has certain personality traits that we consider normal but, if carried to extremes, are capable of disorganizing our lives; if the disorganization is significant enough, those traits may be classified as neurosis. None of us is free of some personality quirk, which if exaggerated enough, might be considered a disorder.

Narcissism, the love of one's self, is a common trait and does not become a neurosis until it is carried to extremes. The patient who is unduly concerned with the appearance of his or her hands is an example. The wearing of unusual types or numbers of hand jewelry, rings, or bracelets, particularly in inappropriate places, is typical of the narcissist. Abnormally long fingernails, real or artificial, is another narcissistic stigma, as is abnormal concern about cosmesis of the hands in general. Refusal to elect well-indicated surgery because of the dread of a surgical scar or electing to suffer discomfort or loss of function in lieu of a scar that most would consider inconsequential is a manifestation of narcissism (Fig. 64-2).

The *obsessive-compulsive personality* is somewhat similar to the narcissistic type in that the person is often unduly concerned with cosmesis and is often dissatisfied with the treatment result, no matter how good others may see it. This personality type demands perfection and accepts compromise only grudgingly.

Paranoia in its severe form is often a trait of the schizophrenic. The patient with the neurotic form may seem unduly suspicious of the motives of the surgeon, his or her employer, or a third-party payer. The neurotic paranoid patient often will accuse his or her company of not caring about him or her and will often blame the employer for the accident that crippled the hand. Paranoid personalities make rehabilitation of the injured hand difficult because rapport between patient and physician is often impossible to establish.

The *antisocial personality* is similar to the paranoid personality. He or she is suspicious of others' motives and shows it. Rapport is difficult to achieve because the patient often seems to actively court dislike. This type of patient sorely tries physicians and therapists; it is difficult to develop empathy for the patient who conveys dislike for those trying to provide help. These patients often have tattoos on the hands or fingers. A common attitude of people with antisocial personalities is that a *perfect* result is to be expected from any therapy, and if one is not attained, the obvious reason is that they have been maltreated (Fig. 64-3).

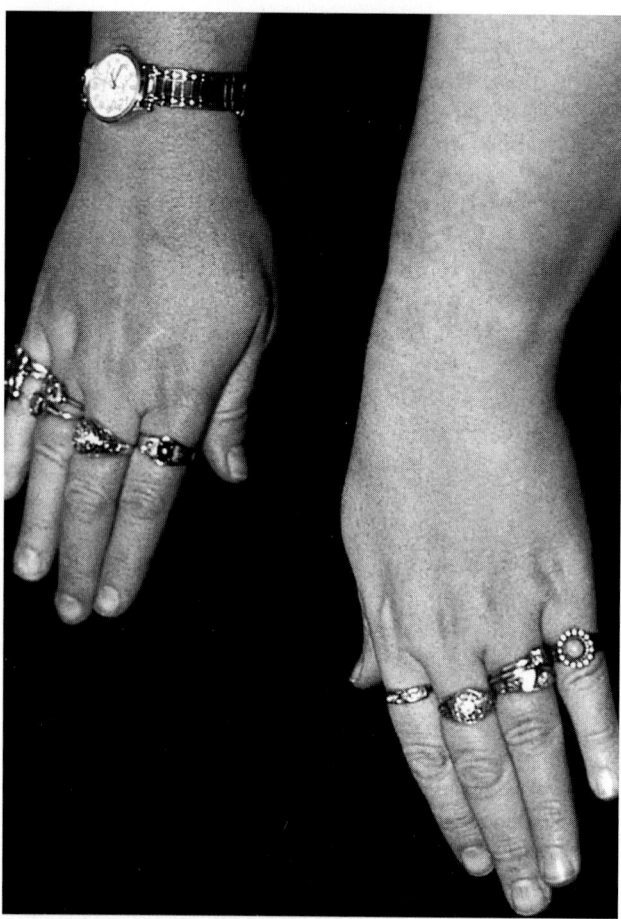

Fig. 64-2. Overdecoration of the hands often reflects a personality disorder such as narcissism, dependency, the histrionic personality, or combinations of these. (Courtesy M.L. Kasdan, MD.)

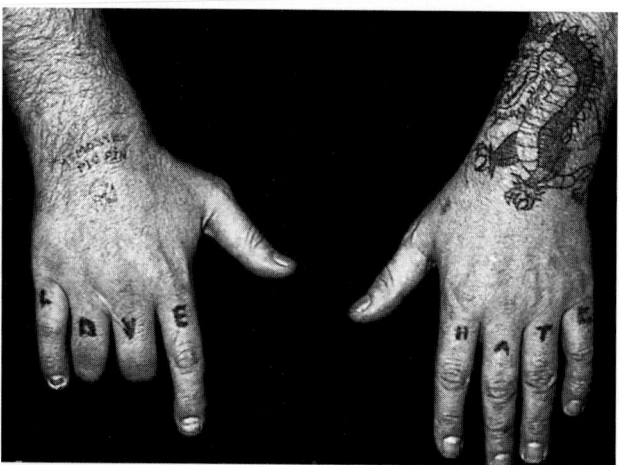

Fig. 64-3. Tattoos on fingers and hands often reflect paranoia and a sociopathic personality. (Courtesy M.L. Kasdan, MD.)

The *dependent personality* generally will be extremely passive and will not contribute actively to his or her own rehabilitation. He or she likes attention and will often exaggerate or even invent symptoms to garner it. The patient with a dependent personality is loath to admit to cure because the prospect of discontinuing treatment and taking responsibility for his or her own hand is unpleasant and even frightening. The young male dependent personality is often a gang member and may exhibit the same type of tattoos on the hands that the antisocial types do.

The *histrionic personality* overreports and overreacts, often in a dramatic manner. Minor hand problems are related as serious. The patient describes symptoms in great detail. Mild discomfort is reported to be agonizing. A small cyst is described as "huge." An accurate history is difficult to obtain, both before and after treatment. The bright side to these patients is that after treatment, they often report how truly wonderful the result is and how great their physicians and therapists are.

Anxiety neuroses

Anxiety is a common, and usually normal, reaction in the patient with a hand that is painful, diseased, or traumatized. However, anxiety can be carried to neurotic extremes, and when it is, the patient requires constant explanation and reassurance.

Panic attacks. Panic attacks are abrupt spells of fear and extreme anxiety. These patients may present many types of hand complaints, such as weakness, tremor, and profuse sweating, and may even tend toward conversion-like symptoms, such as stocking anesthesia.

Posttraumatic stress syndrome. One type of anxiety neurosis that is fairly common when the hand has been subjected to severe trauma by a weapon or a machine is posttraumatic stress syndrome. The patient often relives the traumatic event and is loath to return to the scene of the injury or to again use the machine that was responsible. Such an anxiety poses special problems in return-to-work rehabilitation.

Adjustment disorders

Psychosocial stress. Often the cause of maladjustment, problems with psychosocial stress at home or in the workplace may contribute to the development of real or imaginary upper extremity complaints or may aggravate existing somatic conditions. These disorders often have a psychosomatic element. The therapy team sometimes can manage these complaints effectively by working with the patient's employer to improve the workplace atmosphere. However, hand problems caused by domestic adjustment problems seldom can be handled effectively by the hand surgeon or hand therapist. These problems fall within the purview of the marriage counselor.

Symptom magnification syndrome. Symptom magnification syndrome is manifested by a magnification of complaints of pain or dysfunction disproportionate to the objective physical findings. The syndrome may be deliberate, bordering on malingering; partially deliberate; or subliminal. It almost always is accompanied by some prospect of secondary gain, such as a compensation reward, an escape from an unpleasant or dangerous job, or manipulation to deal with a marital maladjustment. Where there is symptom magnification, there is often an element of paranoia, with the patient blaming his or her employer or "the other driver" for all of his or her woes. People who have incurred the same or worse injuries in athletics seldom have the same complaints, and they recover much more quickly than those injured under circumstances in which litigation is likely.

An experienced clinical eye is needed to detect symptom magnification. When suspected, it is both difficult and unpleasant to deal with because the patient may have convinced himself or herself that the symptoms are real. If the physician is convinced that the patient is magnifying the symptoms beyond reason, the physician may be wading into a medical-legal swamp. If the physician commits his or her diagnosis to the record, the patient will be incensed; the patient-physician relationship may deteriorate; and if the patient has paranoid tendencies, the situation may be potentially dangerous for the physician. In addition, the attorney for the patient—and symptom magnification syndrome patients almost always have one—is sure to cry foul or even slander, and may even provoke further litigation, this time directed at the physician. Nevertheless, in view of our society's tremendous expenditure for compensation and liability claims, physicians must strive dispassionately for accuracy of diagnosis and straightforward reporting, even if it puts them in the uncomfortable position of reporting unfavorably on their patients.

In patients in whom the upper extremity is the target of symptom magnification, the lateral humeral epicondyle and the first dorsal extensor compartment are most commonly involved. Most tennis elbow and de Quervain's stenosing tenosynovitis patients respond favorably to conservative and/or surgical treatment; for those who do not and who have the prospect of receiving a reward, symptom magnification syndrome should be suspected.

Patients who exaggerate their complaints often are overtreated by hand therapists. This usually is not the fault of the therapist, but rather of the prescribing physician, who, failing to achieve a symptomatic cure within a reasonable time, insists that the therapist persist with his or her efforts. In such cases, it is often the therapist who makes the tentative diagnosis of symptom magnification, in which case clear communication between therapist and physician are essential.

Malingering. There is a wide spectrum of falsification of symptoms ranging from rationalization and wishful thinking to outright faking. Some forms of malingering probably fall within the category of adjustment disorders. In its most blatant form, malingering is fraud, but this is difficult to

prove without the aid of a private investigator. More commonly, the problem may start as fraud, or perhaps only exaggeration, but as time passes the patient succeeds in convincing himself or herself that the symptoms are real, and then of course, it is no longer fraud. The more the patient has had to describe the symptoms, the more convinced he or she becomes that they exist, and if there is a possibility of monetary gain or relief from an unpleasant situation, then the patient's conscience is gradually stifled and the symptoms convert from feigned to real. The finger that "won't bend," the hand that has lost its strength, and the tendonitis that remains painful after physical signs have subsided are examples. Because it is unpleasant and potentially dangerous to label a patient a "faker," the term *symptom magnification* is a useful euphemism.

Alexithymia

The term *alexithymia* means "no words for mood." This condition is not named in the current DSM-IV, but it is a useful designation for the surgeon. People with this neurosis lack an ability to verbalize their feelings, but instead describe multiple physical symptoms for which there seems to be no reasonable explanation. In a sense, they express their mood by a recitation of somatic problems. The hand is a common source of complaint, although any portion of the anatomy may be involved. The points of reference within the hand are vague and generally fit neither a recognized clinical nor anatomic pattern. The patient may state, "I have this aching pain throughout my hand. I can't really describe it, but it hurts." The description is invariably vague, and the harder the examiner tries to establish a pattern or a specific localization, the more elusive the patient's description becomes.

Patients with other types of neuroses may have multiple unexplained physical complaints but present themselves differently. The histrionic personality describes his or her symptoms in great detail, as does the hypochondriac neurotic, whereas the alexithymic patient is usually quiet, passive, and nonabrasive. The patient follows all therapeutic directions, but nothing ever seems to work despite the patient's diligent conformance to advice.

Factitious disorders

Factitious disorders are neuroses considered by some to be conversion disorders and by others to be psychoses. They are dramatic when they are finally recognized, but the diagnosis is often hard to establish. Hand surgeons and hand therapists are generally pragmatists used to dealing with observed details and striving for a specific diagnosis that leads to straightforward treatment with fairly predictable results. It is difficult for us to believe that anyone would deliberately inflict damage to one's own hand, and thus the patient who does so is capable of misleading and confusing us for a long time. We are not trained in the art of psychiatric diagnostic personality analysis and therefore are unsuspecting and gullible when the self-mutilator presents with a

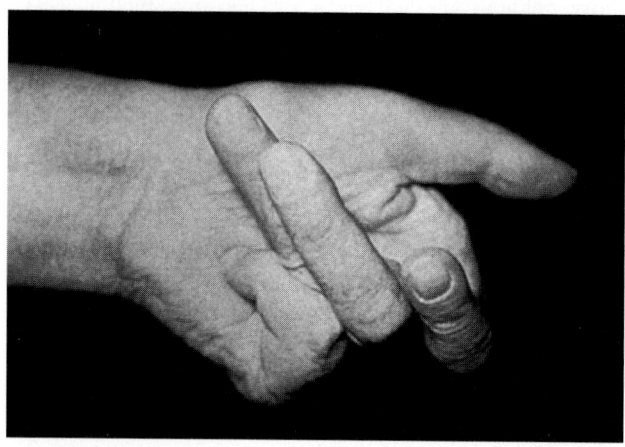

Fig. 64-4. Clenched fist syndrome. A variant in that the thumb and index finger remain conveniently functional. (Courtesy D.S. Louis, MD.)

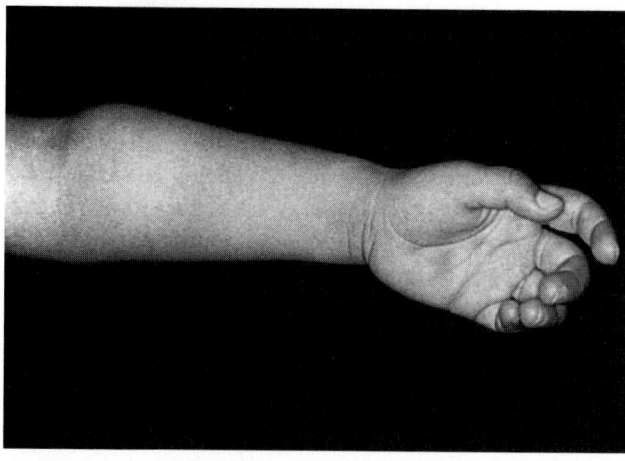

Fig. 64-5. Factitious edema of the forearm resulting from self-application of a tourniquet at the elbow. (Courtesy D.S. Louis, MD.)

damaged hand. The injury these neurotics, sometimes psychotics, do themselves is undoubtedly deliberate, but that does not necessarily mean that it is consciously deliberate; there is often a fine line between conscious and subconscious actions.

Clenched fists, unexplained swelling, sores that will not heal despite our best efforts, and bizarre posturing are among the more dramatic signs in this type of neurosis. Particularly frustrating is the uncomplicated operation that mysteriously goes awry, including unexplained wound dehiscence, infections that seem to have no reasonable explanation, or sutures that disappear without cause. It is infuriating to discover that the patient that one has been laboring to help is intent on destroying the results. Obviously, the physician cannot allow himself or herself the luxury of the anger of frustration, but self-restraint in such cases does not come easily.

The *clenched fist* is one of the more common of the factitious disorders. Sometimes it is truly a clenched fist, with all five digits involved, but more commonly it is only one, two, or three fingers that are tightly flexed. Often, the index finger and thumb are not involved, thereby neatly allowing the patient to retain fairly useful hand function. When suspected, the diagnosis is easily confirmed by anesthetizing the extremity or the patient and demonstrating that there is no fixed contracture, that the fingers are quite supple under anesthesia. The same may be demonstrated by hypnosis, although this is not usually a therapeutic tool for the hand therapist or hand surgeon. Establishing the diagnosis solves the problem for the surgeon, but not for the patient. If the patient is confronted with the diagnosis, he or she will either deny it or manifest his or her neurosis in some other form. Treatment for the clenched fist and most other neuroses should be reserved for the psychiatrist. A variation on this theme is the stiff index finger that "won't bend" except under anesthesia (Fig. 64-4).

Unexplained swelling of the hand or arm may be a result of the patient's surreptitious application of a tourniquet to the extremity. The tight band may be an Ace bandage, a sphygmomanometer cuff, a rubber band, or a piece of string. Placing the extremity in a plaster cast allows the swelling to subside and prevents further application of the constricting band, but again, confrontation will not be therapeutic; that should be left to the psychiatrist (Fig. 64-5).

Voluntary self-inflicted wounds often have an obvious origin. Cigarette burns, stab wounds, subcutaneous injection of feces and other noxious substances, and even bite wounds are seen in these neurotic patients. Deliberate amputation of a finger or two is not unknown, although this is sometimes more a ritualistic gesture of mourning (as with some aboriginal tribes) or a symbol of fealty (as with some members of the Japanese underworld). The clinician must discriminate between the *deliberate* self-inflicted wound of the neurotic and the *accidental* self-inflicted wound in patients with other types of mental problems such as the hand that is damaged by accidental intraarterial injection by a drug addict (Figs. 64-6 and 64-7).

Sometimes deliberate self-infliction of a wound does not represent neurosis. For the soldier, for whom life-threatening combat becomes unbearable, the self-inflicted gunshot wound or the deliberate shooting off of a finger seems a perfectly logical way of avoiding a greater evil.

Delicate self-cutting is rare but can be quite spectacular, with dozens, sometimes hundreds, of lacerations or scars on the forearms and hands. The lacerations usually involve only the epidermis but occasionally are deeper. The wounds are usually longitudinal or oblique and are most common on the dorsum of the hand and forearm. Shallow transverse wounds on the volar aspect of the wrist are more typical of the depressed pseudosuicide patient, and this too should be considered a psychologically based hand disorder.

Secretan's syndrome is probably a self-inflicted condition caused by the patient repeatedly striking the dorsum of the

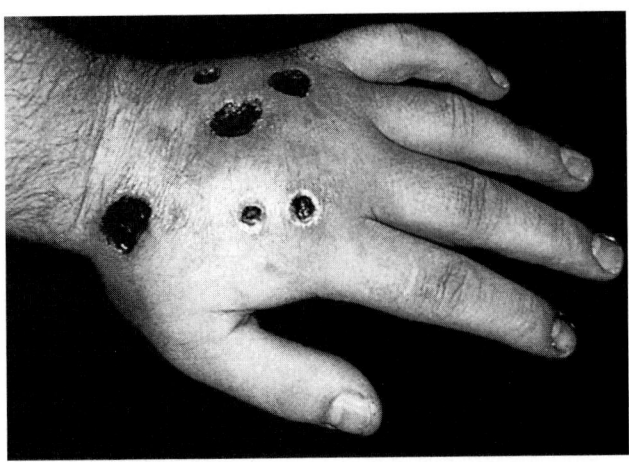

Fig. 64-6. Self-inflicted cigarette burns. The patient denied any knowledge of their cause. (Courtesy D.S. Louis, MD.)

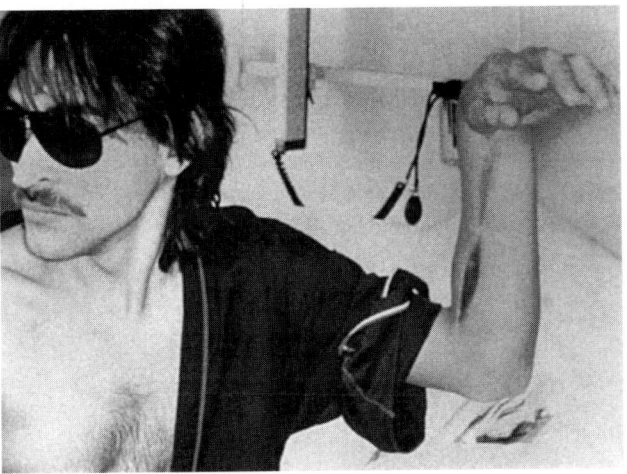

Fig. 64-7. This man had at least 16 operations on his forearm to drain abscesses that were the result of self-inflicted injections of fecal material. Note the dark glasses: When worn inappropriately, they are often a stigma of neurosis. (Courtesy D.S. Louis, MD.)

hand with a blunt object or against a blunt object, causing diffuse swelling as a result of a peritendonous fibrosis of the extensor tendons. Secretan, who first described the condition, observed that he had never seen a patient with this condition who did not have a possible claim for occupational injury.

Munchausen syndrome is appropriately named for a famous fabricator of outrageous lies. Patients with this neurosis present themselves as sufferers of all sorts of symptoms and ailments involving any and all parts of the body, including the hand. They often have a long history of many illnesses and treatments, including multiple operations. They are often migratory, going from one medical facility after another, giving detailed histories of specific ailments and begging for yet another operation. These people are generally well read in the medical literature and often know more about the ailment they are projecting than does

the physician they are consulting. When found out, they simply transfer their medical attentions to another part of the country. The patient who has had multiple carpal tunnel operations may well be a variant of this condition.

The patient with *SHAFT syndrome* may have a multitude of hand problems, real and unreal. These people are *s*ad, *h*ostile, *a*nxious, *f*rustrating, and *t*enacious. They are difficult to treat, and it is difficult to be nice to them because them seem to deliberately court anger. They are impossible to satisfy, and it is difficult to get rid of them. Suggesting to them that their personality and psyche may have something to do with their problem only accentuates their unpleasant characteristics.

Occupational cramp, although not deliberately imposed by the patient, is a problem included under the factitious disorders because it is caused by the patient. Although not necessarily neurotic in origin, there may be neurotic overtones in that these patients are usually inflexible, compulsive, and aggressive in their personalities. Musicians who develop cramping pain in their upper extremities that interferes with their artistic performance are the most difficult patients in this category. Their symptoms and findings are usually typical of commonplace disorders such as tendonitis, epicondylitis, and the like, but their response to usually effective treatments is often unrewarding; symptoms persist and interfere with their performance, and pressure is applied to the physician or therapist to "do something." Something *is* usually done, such as surgery or some other drastic treatment, and the problem often persists or worsens.

The same type of problems may involve the professional writer, either handwriter or keyboard writer, wherein the hand cramps or becomes painful, weak, or unresponsive. For these patients, just as with musicians, a frank and open discussion of the tensions and occupational pressures that are contributing to the problem is warranted. Prescribing frequent breaks in the manual activity that is symptomatic is helpful, as are relaxation techniques.

Somatization neuroses

Somatization disorders are the most common of the psychologically based hand disorders, and they are just as difficult to treat as any of the aforementioned disorders. Their nomenclature is confusing because their categorization is indistinct, with much overlapping of their boundaries. Many combinations of the various types are possible. It is useful, although perhaps arbitrary and simplistic, to consider them in four different classifications.

Briquet's syndrome. Also called the *somatization syndrome,* and perhaps more appropriately so, Briquet's syndrome is closely allied to alexithymia and to personality and adjustment disorders. It is more common in women, is usually chronic, and is characterized by multiple somatic complaints not caused by physical illness. The complaints are vague, lacking in specific detail, but are presented in a dramatic and exaggerated manner. These patients generally have seen many physicians, and they tend to be exhibitionistic, manipulative, and seductive. They often manifest anxiety and depression, which they tend to mask with antisocial behavior. Marital problems are common in their background. In its milder forms, Briquet's syndrome is not even considered to be a neurosis, but merely a personality disorder.

Conversion neurosis. The term *conversion neurosis* has been around for a long time, periodically falling into disrepute and then again being resurrected. It was often called *hysteria*. Conversion neurosis is the most useful term for the greatest number of psychologically based hand disorders a hand surgeon or hand therapist is likely to encounter. Patients in this category complain of symptoms that suggest physical disease but are without a somatic cause; the symptoms have only, or mainly, a psychologic basis. Sometimes the symptoms may have begun with a bona fide physical condition but have remained long after the physical cause has subsided. The patient has found that retention of the complaints has served a useful function, perhaps to avoid returning to an unpleasant job or home situation. Conversion neurosis is most common with the patient with chronic low back pain, but it is also present in patients with upper extremity complaints, as with the slightly damaged hand that simply "will not get well."

Another example of conversion neurosis is the patient who is convinced that he or she has painful and stiff finger joints despite the absence of physical findings. Such a patient often has a close relative with rheumatoid arthritis affecting the hands and is convinced that he or she, too, is fated to develop the same type of deformities as the relative. In the consultation, and on repeated visits, the patient will stretch out normal-appearing hands to the physician, saying, "Look how swollen they are, doctor." This poses a problem for the physician. The physician is at first inclined to wonder if he or she is missing something. If convinced that his or her observations are accurate, particularly after repeated visits, the physician may be tempted to disagree with the patient. When this happens, the patient with a conversion neurosis will ignore the physician's opinion and reasoning and will insist that the swelling and stiffness are real. When that impasse is reached, the hand surgeon should suggest psychiatric counseling. Unfortunately, this is not the usual course; more commonly, the patient is passed to another hand surgeon or is subjected to ever-more-complicated tests and screenings. All of this becomes expensive and serves to convince the patient that something truly is physically wrong with his or her hands.

The conversion neurotic also may have other neuroses and character disorders. This patient may have schizophrenic traits and may be depressed. Despite the classification presented herein, there is so much overlapping of these various psychologic problems that, for most of us in the field of hand surgery, it would be simpler and probably just as useful to lump all patients with somatic complaints without

physical findings into this category of conversion reaction. If the therapist is fortunate enough to have a working relationship with a psychiatrist or clinical psychologist who has an interest in these problems, much can be done to help these patients.

Psychogenic pain disorders. Psychogenic pain disorders are usually conversion neuroses and are the physician's despair and the quack's delight. Persistent pain without objective evidence of disease is a dilemma for physicians, therapists, and third parties such as insurance carriers and governmental compensation commissions, although with this type of neurosis, the prospect for monetary gain is often absent.

Attempting to discriminate between psychogenic pain and "real" pain is pointless. Pain is subjective and thus can be measured only by the person complaining of it. It is useless to tell the complainant that it is "all in your head." The patient's response is likely to be, "I feel it in my hand and my brain tells me that's where it is." The patient in this instance is correct; the pain centers are indeed in the brain, and for him or her, the pain is real.

The pain of these patients is often a response to environmental stress, and as with conversion reactions, the complaint may be useful to the patient in handling that stress. Sometimes there is a lesion or some other somatic basis for the pain, but the patient's response to the stimulus is disproportionate to what ordinarily would be expected from that particular lesion.

Patients with psychogenic unremitting or crippling pain are often unresponsive or antagonistic to psychiatric treatment. When the degree of pain is severe enough to interfere with a normal, productive way of life, it must be considered a true neurosis, not to be confused with adjustment disorders or malingering, wherein the pain can be eased by compensation or disability awards.

Hypochondriasis. In its various guises, hypochondriasis is common. It may be either a personality disorder or a neurosis, depending on how disruptive it is to a normal life style. It obviously overlaps the other neuroses with elements of psychogenic pain disorders and the conversion reactions. It is not difficult to diagnose after the physician is familiar with the patient, but it is extremely difficult to cure. Complaining of pain with little or no somatic basis is almost a way of life for these patients. They use their complaints to garner sympathy and attention and to manipulate family and friends to their own ends.

HAND PROBLEMS INCIDENTAL TO PSYCHOLOGIC PROBLEMS

As stated in the beginning of this chapter, there is a close relationship between hand and psyche in every patient, not just in those in whom the hand problems are *primarily* psychologic. There are those patients whose hand problems are secondary to an already existing psychologic disorder. The psychologic problems of the patient may cause behavior that causes unintended damage to the hand. Examples of this are the slashed wrist of a bungled suicide attempt, the chronic alcoholic who has mangled his or her hand in a drunken driving accident, or as already mentioned, accidental intraarterial injection of a controlled substance by a drug addict. The hands of patients in this category generally are far easier to treat than those whose hand problems are based on maladjusted psyches. The dividing line between the two categories is often indistinct.

HAND-BASED PSYCHOLOGIC PROBLEMS

Hand-based psychologic problems are hand problems that, in themselves, cause psychologic problems and thus are the opposite of all the aforementioned, in which the psychologic problem is primary. Most common of all is profound depression resulting from an incurable, chronically painful, crippling, or grotesque hand condition that threatens the patient's livelihood or seriously disrupts his or her adjustment to life. A normal psyche may be perverted or damaged by an acquired somatic hand condition, or latent psychologic problems may be brought to light by the newly developed hand disorder.

Chronic pain problems. When pain is severe enough to interfere with happiness and a satisfactory life style, chronic pain problems arise. They are among the most difficult disorders that physicians or therapists encounter.

Reflex sympathetic dystrophy. The most severe of the chronic pain problems, reflex sympathetic dystrophy (RSD), starts with a somatic insult such as a nerve injury or fracture; pain from the injury escalates, often to agonizing levels; as it progresses, sympathetic changes develop, and ultimately, there is psychologic involvement. The pain is described as a frightful burning sensation that is aggravated by any extraneous touch, even a breeze, and is severe enough to prevent the hand from being used for any function. The patient often retreats into a depressed, reclusive, "don't touch me" state. First and best described by Weir Mitchell in the nineteenth century, RSD usually develops gradually and may be aborted early if its probability is recognized. Correction of the offending sensory lesion (e.g., neuroma resection), if possible, is the first step. Sympathetic blocks followed by sympathectomy are effective if performed early in the development of the condition. Patients with RSD need a good deal of emotional support; both surgeon and therapist must supply this through empathy and rapport with the patient. The patient must be encouraged to retain some useful function of the hand if at all possible.

Neuromas. Neuromas can be another cause of chronic pain. If severe enough, neuroma pain may severely curtail any useful function of the hand. The pain, if severe, is called *causalgia* and is similar to the type of pain experienced with RSD. Surgical management of painful neuromas generally is effective. The operations range from simple excision, to capping the nerve end, to burying the nerve end in bone or muscle. As with RSD, rehabilitation

of the hand must start early. The patient who is deprived of hand function by neuroma pain is prone to develop psychologic problems such as social withdrawal, personality changes, and dependency.

Phantom limb pain. The pain that is felt in a lost limb, or *phantom limb pain,* can destroy the use of the extremity if it is not treated promptly, or better yet, aborted. Phantom limb pain is a pathologic condition; phantom limb *sensation* is a normal phenomenon experienced by all amputees, regardless of the site of amputation. If the physician explains to the amputee as soon as possible after his or her loss that the sensation in the part will remain for an indefinite time, he or she will be influenced to accept the sensation as normal. This prophylactic educational technique was aggressively applied by those of us who treated many hundreds of combat amputees during the Vietnam War. In contrast to previous wartime amputee experiences, problems with phantom limb pain were seldom. Education, patient communication, and early rehabilitation prevented the problem.

Occupational chronic hand pain. Resulting from an on-the-job injury, *occupational chronic hand pain* may cause severe psychologic problems if the injured employee tends to blame the employer or workplace for the injury. Brooding about his or her pain and loss of function, particularly if aggravated by feelings of abandonment, may nurture latent paranoid tendencies. A desire for compensation and revenge then leads to litigation and an escalation of emotions. Research has established that the longer the patient is out of work, the less is the chance that he or she will return to work. A *chronic pain cycle* may be established by unnecessarily prolonged treatment and by protracted or frivolous litigation. Although the hand injury may have been primary, it is the secondary psychologic problems that make the problem serious for the patient and expensive for society. Sunderland warns us that personality changes may be the result and not the cause of chronic pain and that physicians must be careful not to ascribe the patient's behavior to primary psychologic problems.

Congenital deformities. Congenital deformities of the hand and upper extremity may have a profound psychologic effect on the patient if they are particularly grotesque or dysfunctional. If parents are counseled early that their attitude will affect favorably or adversely how their child will accept his or her anatomic aberration, the child will accept it in the same manner as the parents. Hand surgeons and hand therapists have a great opportunity to influence the child, parents, and siblings to accept the problem for what it is and to engender a philosophical and functional approach to it.

Psychologic sequelae to severe hand injury have been discussed under anxiety neurosis and posttraumatic stress syndrome. They may be manifested by denial, nightmares, problems with concentration, and flashbacks. For most, time is the great healer, but all patients with this type of problem warrant understanding, empathy, and communication.

The *rheumatoid personality* is an exception to all of the aforementioned personalities. Rheumatoid arthritis is a disease whose cause is not understood; whose treatment is inexact and often ineffective; whose course is usually progressive; and that is characterized by pain, deformity, and loss of function. One would think that people who develop such a malady would be morose, pessimistic, depressed, and withdrawn, but such is usually not the case. More often, rheumatoid patients develop personality traits, an inner strength, that enables them to deal with their problems in a positive manner. These patients are realists; they are aware that their disease will probably progress and that there is no cure, but nevertheless they are determined to adapt to their misfortune without letting it figuratively cripple them. They tend to emphasize the positive and find many ingenious means of dealing with their decreasing hand function. Whatever psychic damage may be caused by their somatic problems is rarely displayed. Their motivation to continue to function with a minimum of complaint makes working with these remarkable people a privilege. They should be an inspiration to all the malcontents, shirkers, and neurotics who are "disabled" by far lesser ailments, but sadly, the unmotivated are seldom inspired by the highly motivated.

MANAGEMENT OF PSYCHOLOGICALLY BASED HAND DISORDERS

Hand surgeons and hand therapists cannot substitute for the psychiatrist or clinical psychologist in treating the more severe psychologic hand problems, but they can definitely play a supportive therapeutic role by supplementing their technical abilities with empathy and the practical psychology that any good physician or therapist should be able to apply. We have a chance to improve, if not cure, the less involved cases if we resolve the hand problem and render educational and emotional support as well. Our patience will be sorely tried, and we will probably be unsuccessful with many of the types of problems discussed in this chapter, but if we do not try, we are just technicians.

The following is an outline of a basic approach to the recognition and treatment of these challenging problems. As an example, consider the approach one might take with a patient with a conversion neurosis prompted by extreme anxiety (e.g., an intelligent 26-year-old female secretary with a strong family history of crippling rheumatoid arthritis). She is convinced that her dominant hand has developed joint pain, swelling, and stiffness and that she is fated to lose complete use of her hand, "just as my mother did."

First, one conducts as thorough an assessment of the patient's complaints as possible. One then takes a careful history, repeated if necessary, followed by a thorough physical examination of the upper extremities. If no objective findings correlate with the patient's complaints, one begins to suspect a psychologic problem. The suspicion should increase if the patient insists that the hand is swollen, even

though there is no overt evidence. The conscientious physician then begins to worry whether he or she is missing something. The examination should be repeated several times and, if possible, when the patient feels that her problem is at its worst.

Lacking any corroborative physical findings and unable to make a specific diagnosis, one then turns to the laboratory findings, including at least, blood chemistries and x-ray films of the hand. When the results are found to be negative and the patient insists that the physician is missing something, one is tempted to become more technical and to order bone scans, computed tomographic scans, magnetic resonance imaging scans, and more sophisticated blood studies, as well as consulting with rheumatologists and neurologists. Expenses and frustrations mount, and often the patient will turn to alternative methods of medical practice such as acupuncture, chiropractic, holistic medicine, vitamin faddists, faith healers, and the like; it is possible that any of these will obtain results as good as or better than more orthodox methods.

As one's suspicion mounts that the patient's problem may be primarily psychologic, it is time to suggest psychiatric consultation and psychometric testing with the Minnesota Multiphasic Personality Inventory (MMPI). If the patient rejects this, as most will, one then faces difficult choices. One can treat with medications, physical medicine modalities, splints, and the like, but if one is convinced now that the problem is mainly psychologic, the longer the physical treatment persists, the more the physician's integrity is tested. Although nontherapeutic medications and treatments may have a placebo effect, the longer the underlying problem is evaded, the less chance that it will be resolved.

Suggestive techniques, behavioral management, biofeedback, hypnosis, autohypnosis, and interviews with the patient using amobarbital (Amytal) are some of the techniques used by psychiatrists. Mood-modifying drugs, antidepressants, and the like are potentially dangerous, and their prescription should be left to the experts. It is often difficult to locate and establish a liaison with a psychiatrist or psychologist who is skilled and interested in psychologic problems with somatic ramifications. Once established, such a relationship with this colleague is to be cherished and nurtured.

Medications, surgery, and occupational and physical therapy may have a place if the patient has an identifiable physical lesion, but caution is important. It is a sad mistake to embark on a surgical expedition in search of an unknown. When in doubt, the physician should not operate. Similarly, protracted courses of nonsurgical therapy without objective evidence of their validity may serve only to convince the patient that his or her somatic complaint is the main problem.

The patient's somatic complaints may be protecting him or her from something worse. If our "cure" of the hand problem deprives the patient of this protection, the resulting psychic deluge may provoke a much more serious situation, both emotionally and physically. The cure may deprive the patient of something important to his or her psyche, and the physician may then be expected to compensate the patient with something of equal value, such as continued and unending support for yet another set of psychologically based symptoms.

Finally, no matter how wonderful we find the hand in its fabulous function and beauty, it behooves us to never forget that it is but an extension of the person and of the person's mind. If we become so entranced with technical details, important though those minutiae may be, that we lose our communicative and empathetic skills, we deservedly will be classed as mechanics and not healers.

BIBLIOGRAPHY

Amadio PC: Pain dysfunction syndromes, *J Bone Joint Surg* 70A:944, 1988.

American Psychiatric Association: *Diagnostic and statistical manual of mental disorders,* ed 4, Washington, DC, 1998, American Psychiatric Association.

Berne E: Games people play: the psychology of human relationships, New York, 1964, Grove Press.

Black RG: The chronic pain syndrome, *Surg Clin North Am* 55:999, 1975.

Brown PW: The role of motivation in the recovery of the hand. In Kasdan ML, editor: *Occupational hand & upper extremity injuries and diseases,* Philadelphia, 1991, Hanley & Belfus.

Cone CP, Hueston JT: Psychological aspects of hand injury. In Tubiana R, editor: *The hand,* vol 1, Philadelphia, 1981, WB Saunders.

Cooper MA, Davies DM: Charcot's oedeme bleu des hysteriques, *J Hand Surg* 10B:399, 1985.

Cullen CH: Causalgia: diagnosis and treatment, *J Bone Joint Surg* 30B:467, 1948.

Grant GH: The hand and the psyche, *J Hand Surg* 5:417, 1980.

Grunert BK, et al: Early psychological aspects of severe hand injury, *J Hand Surg* 13:177, 1988.

Grunert BK, et al: Treatment of posttraumatic stress disorder after work-related hand trauma, *J Hand Surg* 15A:511, 1990.

Grunert BK, et al: Classification system for factitious syndromes in the hand with implications for treatment, *J Hand Surg* 16A:1027, 1991.

Grunert BK, et al: Effects of litigation on maintenance of psychological symptoms after severe hand injury, *J Hand Surg* 16A:1031, 1991.

Grunert BK, et al: Predictive value of psychological screening in acute hand injuries, *J Hand Surg* 17A:196, 1992.

Haese JB: Psychological aspects of hand injuries, their treatment and rehabilitation, *J Hand Surg* 10B:283, 1985.

Ireland DCR: Psychological and physical aspects of occupational arm pain, *J Hand Surg* 13B:5, 1988.

Ireland P, et al: Munchausen syndrome, *Am J Med* 43:579, 1967.

Kaplan HI: Treatment of psychosomatic disorders. In Kaplan HI, Sadock BJ, editors: *Comprehensive textbook of psychiatry/IV,* vol 2, ed 4, Baltimore, 1985, Williams & Wilkins.

Kilgore CS, Graham WP: *The hand: surgical and non-surgical management,* Philadelphia, 1977, Lea & Febiger.

Lazare A: Current concepts in psychiatry conversion symptoms, *N Engl J Med* 305:745, 1981.

Lesser IM: Current concepts in psychiatry: alexithymia. *N Engl J Med* 312:690, 1985.

Louis DS, Lamp MK, Greene TL: The upper extremity and psychiatric illness, *J Hand Surg* 10A:687, 1985.

Matheson LN: *Symptom magnification syndrome,* vol 2, no 3, Huntington Beach, Calif, 1984, Westwork West.

Millender LH: Occupational disorders—the disease of the 1990s: a challenge or a bane for hand surgeons, *J Hand Surg* 17A:193, 1992.

Mitchell SW: *Injuries of nerves and their consequences,* Philadelphia, 1872, Lippincott.

Moldofsky H: Occupational cramp, *J Psychosom Res* 5:439, 1971.

Pao P-N: The syndrome of delicate self-cutting, *Br J Med Psychol* 42:195, 1969.

Pulvertaft RG: Psychological aspects of hand injury. In Hunter JM, et al, editors: *Rehabilitation of the hand: surgery and therapy,* ed 3, St Louis, 1990, Mosby.

Reading G: Secretan's syndrome: hard edema of the dorsum of the hand, *Plast Reconstr Surg* 65:182, 1980.

Rosenthal RJ, et al: Wrist-cutting syndrome: the meaning of a gesture, *Am J Psychiatry* 128:1363, 1972.

Secretan H: Oedeme dur et hypoplasie traumatique du metacarpe dorsal, *Rev Med Suisse Romande* 21:408, 1901.

Simmons BP, Vasile RG: The clenched fist syndrome, *J Hand Surg* 5:420, 1980.

Sims ACP: Psychogenic causes of physical symptoms, accidents and death, *J Hand Surg* 10B:281, 1985.

Smith RJ: Factitious lymphedema of the hand, *J Bone Joint Surg* 57A:89, 1975.

Spengler DM: Games patients play: recognition and management, *Contemp Orthopaedics* 7:29, 1983.

Spiegel D, Chase RA: The treatment of contractures of the hand using self-hypnosis, *J Hand Surg* 5:428, 1980.

Thompson TL II: Chronic pain. In Kaplan HI, Sadock BJ, editors: *Comprehensive textbook of psychiatry/IV,* vol 2, ed 4, Baltimore, 1985, Williams & Wilkins.

Wallace PF, Fitzmorris CS Jr: The S-H-A-F-T syndrome in the upper extremity, *J Hand Surg* 5A:492, 1978.

Wynn Parry CB: *Rehabilitation of the hand,* ed 3, London, 1973, Butterworths.

Chapter 65

PSYCHOLOGIC EFFECTS OF UPPER EXTREMITY DISORDERS

Brad K. Grunert
Cecilia A. Devine

Hand and upper extremity injuries are often accompanied by a variety of perceived psychologic reactions related to the function of the extremity and to the social acceptance of the individual, particularly if the patient has sustained a mutilating type of injury. The hands and the face are the most socially visible portions of any person's body. Because the hand is often used as a medium of nonverbal communication, disfigurement to the hand often results in loss of positive self-image and perceptions of impaired social competence. The patient's frequent concerns of cosmesis are often related to whether the injury is abnormal enough in appearance to be conspicuous and disturbing to others. In addition, the patient's perception of disfigurement is often more important than the actual degree of disfigurement present. Barely perceptible injuries often result in profound changes in self-image. Even for patients who have no mutilating injury to the upper extremity, psychologic factors can still exert a profound influence over the course of recovery when chronic pain and/or chronically debilitating conditions such as cumulative trauma disorders (CTDs) are present. However, upper extremity disorders can also be caused by psychologic factors, as evidenced by patients with conversion and factitious disorders. This chapter examines the psychologic effects accompanying acute traumatic injury to the hand, psychologic changes resulting from chronic upper extremity pain and dysfunction, and psychologic factors precipitating psychogenic hand conditions.

ACUTE TRAUMATIC INJURIES

According to statistics compiled by the U.S. Department of Health and Human Services,[23] the hand is one of the most commonly injured parts of the body. Hand injuries accounted for nearly 22% of all industrial injuries during 1990. Despite the high incidence of such injuries, little had been published at that time on the psychologic status of individuals sustaining hand injuries. Since then, a number of articles have been published dealing with psychologic adjustment to traumatic hand injury.[1,5-7,11,14] These studies document that injuries often result in a wide range of psychologic changes.

Addressing the psychologic aspects of upper extremity injuries often involves more than allowing the patient to adjust at his or her own pace. The patient needs to know that there are concerned, qualified health care professionals present to assist with this process. The appropriate health care providers include a hand surgeon, counselor, and hand therapist. To address all of the psychologic aspects, it may be necessary to recruit additional members to the rehabilitation team, including a representative of the patient's employer and a rehabilitation specialist from the workers' compensation company if the injury occurred in the work setting. By addressing all components of effective rehabilitation in a multidisciplinary manner, the patient is able to recover in an efficacious and timely manner.

Acute stress disorder

One of the earliest psychologic manifestations accompanying a traumatic hand injury is acute stress disorder.

Patients sustaining acute stress disorders often experience a variety of psychologic symptoms. The most prevalent and frightening are episodes of intrusive thoughts, including flashbacks and nightmares. Other reactive psychologic symptoms include affective lability, which is evidenced by arousal whenever the accident or injury is discussed. A grief or generalized depressive reaction is often present in conjunction with this.

For patients sustaining amputation, preoccupation with phantom limb pain can trigger frustration and irritation. At first, the role of phantom limb pain may be to help the patient deny the extent of the injury. However, it later hinders the development of a new body image that incorporates the amputation by presenting incongruent tactile and visual sensations to the patient. Concentration and attention problems are often present and result in difficulty concentrating on such common activities as watching television or reading a newspaper for even a few brief minutes. The patient is often easily distracted and has poor short-term recall. Cosmetic concerns are characterized by pronounced aversion of gaze to the point where the patient will not look at the injured extremity. They are also manifested by the constant covering of the injured part in public and by reluctance to have medical staff view the injured extremity. Many patients experience an initial fear of death, and a few have more persistent fears of dying that extend beyond the stabilization of their condition. In a study of a series of patients with traumatic hand injuries, we observed that ongoing fear of death was noted only with patients sustaining amputations proximal to the wrist. Most of these patients believed that they would bleed to death, and this belief often triggered their acute stress disorder. Gaze aversion, although common during the initial dressing changes, was considered significant only when coupled with denial of the injury. Such denial of the injury is best described by statements from patients that the upper extremity has not sustained an amputation when in fact it has. Preoccupation with cosmesis and phantom limb pain tended to increase from the time of the initial injury for the first 2 months and then decrease, whereas concentration problems, fear of death, and denial of amputation were generally eliminated by the 2-month follow-up.[14]

With intervention within the first 3 to 5 days following injury, many acute stress disorders can be addressed through a combination of imaginal exposure techniques[21] accompanied by education regarding the nature of such symptomatology. With imaginal exposure, patients go through the entire trauma using recollected images and memories that allow them to emotionally process the accident. This normalization of symptoms and structured reexposure to thoughts and memories of the trauma sustained will often desensitize patients and lead to complete recovery within a very short time after injury. The benefits of early intervention have been well demonstrated by Weis[25] in her doctoral dissertation comparing early versus delayed treatment

groups following hand trauma. When early intervention is not provided for acute stress disorders, posttraumatic stress disorder (PTSD) often results.

As stated earlier, the most prevalent and frightening psychologic symptom of acute stress disorder is the occurrence of intrusive imagery in the form of flashbacks or nightmares. Flashbacks are the recollection of the trauma resulting in a variety of emotional states against which the patient must present a psychic defense. They are often described as a combination of visual, tactile, and auditory recollections of the trauma that the person experienced. They occur when the patient is awake and are always accompanied by a fear response. Various classifications of flashbacks have been delineated.[5] The first of these categories is a *replay flashback*, which involves a replaying of the events immediately preceding the accident and continuing through the time of injury. An *appraisal flashback* consists of an image, often described by patients as being photographic in nature, of the hand immediately after the trauma. For patients experiencing a *projected flashback*, the injury images they see are actually worse than the injury they sustained. Each of these components can be combined with other components to result in more complex types of flashback experiences. One of the commonly occurring combinations is the *appraisal/projected* flashback in which the patient reexperiences the injury in a photographic manner but also sees the injury as being much more severe than it actually was. In *replay/projected* flashbacks, the patient experiences events leading up to the injury and then sees an injury that was much more severe than that which actually occurred. Although a number of patients will experience a reduction in frequency and severity of flashbacks over time, others will experience a significant number of flashbacks for months and even years following the injury.[7] Over time, flashbacks usually become more stimuli specific; that is, thoughts about the incident or exposure to various aspects accompanying the incident will trigger them. This specificity accounts for much of the avoidance that patients have for returning to situations, such as work, that are similar to that in which the injury originally occurred.

The second form of intrusive thought for most patients is the nightmare. Nightmares occur when the patient is asleep and reflect a preoccupation with further injury or anticipated incapacity resulting from the injury. They are typically most prevalent during the first or second month after injury and tend to subside significantly following that period.

POSTTRAUMATIC STRESS DISORDER

PTSD is a combination of symptoms occurring after a specific traumatic event. For a diagnosis of PTSD to be made, a variety of criteria must be present, including (1) intrusive thoughts, (2) avoidance of stimuli associated with the injury, (3) physiologic arousal, and (4) symptoms must persist for at least 30 days after the injury. The hallmark of PTSD is the persistent reexperiencing of the traumatic

---

Box 65-1   Issues to address with the patient (screening tool)

Injury

How did the injury happen?

What is the patient's job?

How long has the patient worked at place where he or she was injured?

Where does the patient place blame for his or her injury (remember this may change from right after injury to months later)?

Intrusive thoughts

Does the patient have flashbacks or nightmares?

Have the patient describe the flashbacks—their content and occurrence.

Does the patient have difficulty sleeping?

Support system

Does the patient live alone or with family or friends?

How is the patient's family handling the injury?

Is the patient able to talk to family and friends about the injury/feelings?

Have relationships between patient and family and friends changed since the injury?

Pain

Does the patient have significant pain (more than expected)?

Has the pain been decreasing or increasing?

How does the patient handle pain (what does he or she do to decrease it)?

Concentration/memory problems

Does the patient remember directions?

Assess short-term memory: For example, Can the patient read newspaper article or watch a show and remember the content? Does the patient forget appointments? Does the patient go into a room and forget his purpose for being there?

Avoidance

Is the patient engaging in preinjury activities?

Has the patient been back to work to visit?

Has the patient been to the work site where the injury occurred?

Is the patient seeing friends?

Is the patient staying home more?

Is the patient drinking or using drugs?

Cosmetic

Does the patient avoid looking at the hand?

Does the patient keep the hand hidden when entering or leaving the clinic?

Does the patient keep the hand hidden in public?

Does the patient use the injured hand?

Does the patient report that people stare at the injured hand?

Has the patient gained excessive weight?

Can the patient comfortably touch the injured hand? Are family members and friends allowed to touch the hand?

---

event. This often results in patients avoiding stimuli associated with the trauma and a generalized numbing of responsiveness in the environment. Persistent symptoms of increased arousal are also present and maintain the concentration and short-term memory deficits previously described for acute stress disorder. People with PTSD generally have flashbacks or nightmares, exaggerated startle responses to any reminders of the original traumatic event, significant disturbance of sleep, avoidance of close interpersonal relationships, high levels of anxiety and depression, and hypervigilance for any events in which they may sustain an injury in the future. Additional symptoms accompanying PTSD include depression, anxiety, fear of death, impulsive behavior, substance abuse, body preoccupation, cosmetic concerns, and reduced self-esteem.

Virtually all of the effective treatment modalities for PTSD rely on some component of exposure. Whether this is done imaginally or through direct environmental exposure does not matter as much as the success of the progressive desensitization the patient goes through. A variety of strategies for environmental exposure have been researched,[8,9,12] including returning patients to their work site shortly after their injury, on a graded basis, or accompanied by their counselor. Each technique proved helpful in

assisting various patient population groups to effectively return to work. Imaginal exposure techniques have also been successfully used with this patient population, as documented by Weis,[25] in which patients were asked to go back and imagine the entire accident again as a means of emotionally reintegrating their experience. Additional strategies for imaginal exposure include imagery rescripting,[15] which has proven quite effective in those injuries in which another person actually triggered the events resulting in the injury to the patient. Imagery rescripting uses imaginal exposure to relive the accident but also has the patients imagine themselves walking into the event as they are today to confront the person responsible for causing their injuries. This technique facilitates the patient's transition from "victim" to "survivor" of the accident. The hallmark of successful exposure techniques is the emotional reintegration that occurs as the patient desensitizes to exposure to previously feared reminders of the trauma.

THERAPIST INVOLVEMENT

The hand therapist is often the only person who sees the patient on a frequent, one-on-one basis, and therefore plays an important role in helping the patient return to preinjury physical and emotional functioning. The accompanying screening tool in Box 65-1 should be used as a guide throughout the therapy process.

During the first few sessions, the therapist should elicit pertinent information from the patient regarding the injury and the patient's support system. This information should include how the injury occurred, how long the patient has worked at his or her current place of employment, the presence of flashbacks or nightmares, any tendency to avoid discussing the injury or viewing the wounds, and the availability of a family member or friend for support. The therapist can help the patient adjust to the injury in a variety of manners. To do so, the therapist must be honest and supportive regarding the hand's appearance and the future prognosis for restoring function. Even the most "simple" injuries cannot be minimized. It is easy to become desensitized if the therapist sees a wide spectrum of injury severity. The therapist must concentrate on the entire upper extremity and not just the wound if the patient is going to incorporate the injured part of the body back into his or her total body image. The patient must be assured that initial responses such as denial, flashbacks, nightmares, and physical reactions are normal. Family members should be included in treatment sessions as appropriate. Family members can often offer invaluable support and may be called upon to assist with dressing changes or an exercise program. Some may have even had the same reactive symptoms as the patient and may require assistance in processing them during this difficult time. The therapist can teach the patient various means of pain control, including deep breathing, relaxation techniques, distraction, and pacing. It is important for the therapist to demonstrate caring, but objectivity must be maintained to help the patient progress through the physical and emotional healing process. A referral to a mental health professional should be made whenever the therapist notes problems that seem to be more severe than expected.

Early in treatment, more information should be obtained from the patient. It is important to ask the patient if any contact has been initiated with the employer or fellow employees. Conversation should be initiated regarding return to work, changes in attribution of blame for the cause of the accident, or significant avoidance. Discussion of activities of daily living (ADLs) and avocational activities to determine the patient's current level of function is also pertinent at this time. In addition, questions regarding sleep problems, memory or concentration problems, and the status of personal relationships should be initiated. It is important to be aware of continued high levels of pain and multiple requests for pain medication because these are often a means of masking emotional distress and eliciting supportive behaviors. During this early phase of treatment, the therapist must encourage the patient to have contact with the work setting and fellow employees. Care should be taken by the therapist not to become the middle person in these contacts. It is important

to help the patient resume independent ADLs and to return to previous avocational activities as much as possible. It is also important to evaluate and facilitate the appropriate use of adaptive equipment to return the patient to functioning as normally as possible. The continued assessment of pain medications, in conjunction with the patient's hand surgeon, is also important.

As the wound heals, the patient should begin to initiate normal activities. It is important to continue to assess avoidance behaviors in the areas of avocational activities, personal relationships, and return to work. The therapist needs to be proactive in this phase of physical and emotional healing. It is important to continue to increase the patient's involvement in independent avocational activities and ADLs. As healing progresses, early work conditioning should be considered. This can be initiated in conjunction with continued acute care treatment. Early return to one-handed duty or light duty can be considered before any final surgeries. An on-site job evaluation can be conducted if there are any concerns regarding the patient's ability to return to work. If the patient is included in the visit, this may actually help overcome initial fears of returning to the site of injury. Rehabilitation specialists hired by the insurance company should be used to help mediate between the medical and employment arenas. The therapist should continue to monitor the patient's level of pain and effective use of pain-control techniques and refer the patient for psychologic intervention as appropriate.

CUMULATIVE TRAUMA DISORDERS

Marked contention exists concerning the etiology of CTDs. Although the underlying cause of these injuries are not addressed here, the psychologic manifestations accompanying such injuries are apparent.[10] The key to evaluating a patient with chronic CTD is a careful psychologic assessment.[3,4] People with these types of disorders often experience widespread lifestyle changes and significant emotional consequences from their ongoing disability. Of concern is whether such patients have a primarily psychologic or primarily physical basis for their disorder. A psychologic assessment consisting of three basic processes is necessary to differentiate between physical and psychologic bases for these disorders. These three components are (1) a clinical interview, (2) a psychometric assessment, and (3) a final diagnostic statement.

The clinical interview

The clinical interview should evaluate the patient's history of the onset of symptoms. Particular factors to be addressed here include the patient's assessment of personal responsibility versus employer's responsibility for the onset of symptoms. In addition, an assessment should be made as to whether the patient is aware of personal health factors versus occupational risk factors that may have contributed to the development of symptoms.

It is important during the interview to assess the impact of the problem on the patient's personal life and recreational activities in addition to job performance. Peer appraisal of the patient's condition is often significant in terms of social adjustment within the workplace. The patient's perceptions regarding future health and employability need to be assessed carefully.

Disfiguring injuries often have a significant effect on family relationships, so these need to be evaluated as well. Affectively, an assessment of the patient's mood is also highly pertinent. The next major area of concern in the clinical interview is the patient's coping abilities. It is important to assess whether the person tends to be stoic or somatizing in the strategies selected for coping with the disorder. Physiologic factors affecting psychologic adjustment include the amount of sleep disruption present and symptoms such as numbness, tingling, weakness, and fatigue. The careful interviewer will garner much information regarding the patient's perception of problems and his or her underlying ability to cope with the disorder. By integrating this information with the physical findings of the hand surgeon and the hand therapist, a multidisciplinary treatment program can be formulated.

Psychometric assessment

Psychometric assessment is also a critical component of the psychologic assessment of a patient with CTD. The Minnesota Multiphasic Personality Inventory-II[16] is a test that is very sensitive to patients displaying somatization to an excessive degree. It is also useful in the detection of depression, anxiety, and a variety of other psychologic symptoms. Of particular concern is the patient who presents with the classic "conversion V," which identifies people who tend to sublimate psychologic difficulties by presenting physical symptoms. The conversion V is a V-shaped profile on scales 1, 2, and 3. The elevations are on the conversion and hypochondriasis scales, with the low-point occurring on the depression scale. Patients presenting with conversion V find it easier to address underlying psychic conflicts through exaggeration of physical complaints than to address them in a more direct manner. However, some evidence indicates that people sustaining physical injury do in fact have some elevation on these scales, so caution needs to be used when interpreting a conversion V.

The Pain Anxiety Symptoms Scale[18] can also be helpful in assessing patients with CTD. This scale has four subscales revealing how a person reacts to pain. Individuals are asked to rate statements regarding pain and the nature of any anxiety they experience relative to pain. Subscale 1 assesses the amount of *fear* the person has relating to the experience of dread of pain. People with high levels of fear often feel immobilized by pain and have significant difficulties implementing pain coping strategies that may be of benefit to them. *Cognitive anxiety,* the second subscale, assesses reaction to pain. People with high scores often become so preoccupied with pain that they spend a great deal of time thinking about it, which only exacerbates their pain experience. The third subscale is the *escape/avoidance* subscale. People scoring high on this scale typically try to escape or avoid situations in which their pain occurs; they do not actively attempt to cope with the pain, but rather try to remove themselves from the stimuli that produce pain. The final scale is the *physiologic anxiety* scale, which assesses a variety of physiologic conditions that may accompany the experience of pain, including rapid heart rate or excessive sweatiness.

For patients who sustain an occupational injury, the Occupational Stress Inventory—Revised[19] is used. This instrument allows assessment in three domains: occupational roles, personal strain, and personal resources. The occupational roles domain focuses on factors of role overload, insufficiency, ambiguity, boundaries, and responsibility, as well as on the amount of physical strain present in the environment. The personal strain domain evaluates vocational, psychologic, interpersonal, and physical strain as perceived by the respondent. The personal resources domain focuses on skills and resources available to the patient to help with adjustment, including recreational outlets, self-care skills, social support resources, and rational/cognitive coping skills. When combined with the previous instruments, this questionnaire gives specific information related to the work setting and how workers view themselves within it.

Final diagnostic statement

Following the clinical interview and the psychometric assessment, the clinician must synthesize all of these results to provide a final diagnostic statement. This statement should certainly influence the patient's course of treatment and may delineate the need to provide specific training in areas such as coping resources, strategies for dealing with interpersonal conflicts within the work setting, or specific strategies to decrease physiologic arousal in the face of discomfort. By synthesizing all of these factors, a comprehensive multidisciplinary rehabilitation program can be developed for each patient.

PSYCHOGENIC HAND DISORDERS

Psychogenic hand conditions present in three major varieties: *malingering, factitious disorders,* and *conversion disorders.* From a psychologic standpoint, the differentiating factors among these three diagnoses is whether symptom production is a conscious act and whether the motivation for producing symptoms is conscious to the patient. In the case of malingering, symptom production is a conscious act and the motivation is conscious to the person producing the symptoms. Quite simply, people who malinger know what they are doing and why they are doing it. Patients with factitious disorders, however, are aware that they are consciously producing the symptoms but are unaware of their motivation for doing so. The third case, the conversion disorder, occurs in patients who are neither conscious of producing the symptoms nor conscious of their motivation for doing so.

Malingering

People who malinger produce their symptoms intentionally. There is virtually always a readily recognizable goal for their symptom production. In fact, there are certain circumstances in which their behavior may actually be protective in that it keeps them from being reexposed to the cause of their original injury (e.g., machinery). Contrary to the belief that people with psychogenic hand conditions should not be confronted, confrontation is actually a very effective means of addressing the malingerer. If the therapist suspects a patient of malingering, extra care should be taken in appropriate documentation. This should include the patient's ongoing status, verbal comments, follow-through in home exercise program, and appointments missed. The therapist should document all instructions given to the patient and keep a copy of all written instructions. All conversations with workers' compensation insurance representatives, the employer, the rehabilitation specialist, and family members should be documented. The goal is to identify discrepancies or inconsistencies. Suspicions should be discussed with the physician. All discussions with the patient should be coordinated to ensure clarity and consistency. A written contract may be necessary listing specific goals and tasks, including a timeline that the patient needs to complete. Services of a psychologist should be enlisted. As soon as documentation is in place and the pattern of malingering is verified, the patient should be confronted. This is best done jointly with the doctor, therapist, and psychologist. By pointing out the inconsistencies in the patient's behavior, the hand surgeon and therapist can facilitate a return to normal daily activities and an elimination of symptoms.

Factitious disorders

Factitious disorders are generally found in people who feel a need to assume the sick role. They typically fabricate a variety of subjective complaints. It is important to note that all of these conditions are self-inflicted and that the patients rarely have external incentives for the maintenance of these behaviors. Patients with factitious disorders often present with dramatic symptoms and tend to be somewhat disruptive in their behavior within the clinic setting. They generally have extensive knowledge of medical terms and often have had multiple treatment interventions with a very fluctuating clinical course and rapid onset of complications. Of concern is the fact that many of these patients have a coexisting substance abuse problem. Patients with factitious disorders generally show improvement during the initial phases of treatment, but improvement is reliably followed by significant relapses as treatment progresses. Their symptoms often exceed the objective pathology that can be documented and they appear able to predict exacerbations in their condition.

In addition, many of them are unlucky or accident prone over their life history and may have previous suspicious physical injuries. Strikingly, many of these patients have worked in the health care system. Some of the typical presentations of chronic factitious disorder are lymphedema, nonhealing wounds, self-inflicted wounds, and chronic injection injuries.

Factitious disorders can be more difficult for the therapist to deal with than malingering. Whereas early confrontation is important with the malingerer, confrontation to a patient with a factitious disorder will result in profound depression and may cause the patient to leave treatment. The therapist should exercise the same attention to detail that was described with the malingerer. This includes thorough documentation, consistency in approach among all medical staff working with the patient, and the formulation of a time-limited and goal-oriented contract. Casting may be necessary to protect the area of suspected self-injury; casting prevents access to the area by the patient. If the wound heals while being protected and opens when again unprotected or if while the wound is protected by a cast a new wound appears in another area, this should heighten the therapist's suspicions.

Conversion disorders

The third major variant of psychogenic disorders is conversion disorders. Conversion disorders generally affect voluntary motor or sensory function. There are always psychologic factors associated with this condition, although they may not be readily apparent. The patient does not intentionally produce the symptoms, and the symptoms often cannot be fully explained by a medical condition. In extreme cases, these disorders can cause significant disability and even lifetime impairment. Common presentations of conversion disorders include such things as glove anesthesia, postural deformities, clenched fist deformities, hyperextension deformities, and movement deformities such as "ratchet hand."

The same techniques of thorough documentation, consistency of approach, and use of a contract should be used when dealing with conversion disorders. These patients are often not aware of their posturing. If confronted, they are confused because of this unawareness. Psychologic intervention is necessary.

Physical presentation of psychogenic hand disorders

The physical presentation of psychogenic hand disorders can cross all three of the psychologic diagnoses described earlier and includes postural hand deformities, movement disorders, edematous conditions, nonhealing self-inflicted wounds, and sensory conditions.[13]

Postural hand deformities. The most widely documented postural deformities are those caused by contractions. Simons and Vasile[22] first described the clenched fist syndrome. The psycho-flexed hand described by Frykman et al.[2] is a similar type of condition. Both conditions are characterized by individuals who have at least the ulnar three digits in their hand contracted into the palm. Some patients have the use of their thumb and index finger, allowing them to maintain a fair amount of functionality. Others, however, have contracted the index finger into the palm of the hand, too. As the course of these disorders becomes protracted, the fingers actually are clenched into the fist and maceration of the skin in the palm is often seen. Range of motion (ROM) is markedly restricted, and the patient often cannot volitionally extend the fingers in the later stages.

A second type of postural deformity is the extension deformity, in which the patient often has hyperextension of the joints of the hand. We have seen this condition only rarely. However, it is similar in terms of treatment to that of contraction deformities.

The third type of postural deformity is a cocontraction deformity. With the cocontraction deformity, the digits are fixed in rigid positions that, anatomically, often fail to make sense. The assessment of a patient with cocontraction deformity is fairly straightforward. When the patient is asked to move either into extension or flexion, a marked cocontraction of both the flexors and extensors is noted. There also is some contraction within the small musculature of the hand, which maintains the type of deformity seen. It is often helpful in the early stages to administer general anesthesia to these patients, which often allows the fingers to spontaneously extend so that the hand can be examined more completely. Patients with conversion disorders in conjunction with contraction deformities have benefited from behavioral shaping and hypnosis. They also benefit from long-term psychotherapy to address the underlying factors leading to the maintenance and production of these symptoms. All of these postural deformities require ongoing psychotherapy if they are conversion disorders.

Movement disorders. Movement disorders are the second major classification for the presentation of psychogenic hand disorders. The first of these consist of dystonic movement such as writer's cramp and the various dystonias that afflict performing musicians. Although probably not psychogenic in origin, psychologic factors often exacerbate dystonias. In most cases, the type of movement disorder is related to a particular task. A variety of treatments have been used with these disorders, including Botox injections and varieties of splinting (see also Chapter 126). What is often the most helpful method is to work with the patient to actually change the way he or she proceeds with a particular task. Biofeedback can be a useful adjunct treatment modality for this approach.

The second type of movement disorder is the ratchet hand. In this disorder, the patient moves in a very robotic fashion, almost as if clicking through various ratchet type movements in order to move the digits. The movement is quite jerky rather than smooth and flowing. Although we

have seen this clinically, there is no real literature on this type of disorder at present.

Edematous conditions. Psychogenic hand disorders also present in the form of edematous conditions. One subtype is Secrétan's syndrome, which is really an impact type of edema[20] first described in the early 1900s. Patient's with Secrétan's disease develop a hard edema over the dorsum of the hand. However, we have also seen edema over the dorsum of the wrist and on the radial and ulnar aspects of the wrist. This type of edema is caused by repeated impact with a variety of surfaces. Typically, when radiographs are reviewed, there is significant swelling; however, there is no actual cyst or other physical pathologic condition. People with Secrétan's syndrome tend to be characterized by the SHAFT syndrome, in which they are *s*ad, *h*ostile, *a*ngry, *f*rustrating, and *t*enacious.[24] They are difficult to deal with and often very recalcitrant in response to any intervention.

A second type of edematous condition is factitious lymphedema. This has been extensively discussed by Louis et al.[17] and by Grunert et al.[13] Patients with tourniquet edema often display massive swelling of the extremity. There is generally a point at which the swelling stops, which is the point where the tourniquet has been applied. However, patients do move tourniquets to different levels of their upper extremity, which can produce a somewhat more confusing presentation. Factitious lymphedema is best diagnosed and treated initially with casting to prevent the placement of tourniquets. Hospitalization with observation can also be beneficial in obtaining a diagnosis. In addition, we have used sodium Amytal interviews for diagnostic purposes as well as treatment interventions. Hypnosis and behavioral shaping can sometimes be of assistance. Most of these patients require prolonged psychotherapy to address some of the underlying issues that have given rise to their condition.

Nonhealing self-inflicted wounds. Psychogenic hand disorders can also present as nonhealing wounds. Factitious nonhealing wounds are easily diagnosed because they require recurrent injury to be maintained. As a result, when the patient presents, the wounds are often in various stages of healing. These patients tend to display a significant amount of depressive symptoms and generalized disruption in their lives. A common coexistent psychologic diagnosis for patients who self-inflict wounds is *borderline personality disorder*. These patients tend to be very untrusting and have great difficulty establishing ongoing relationships. Diagnosis of recurrent self-infliction often requires use of an occlusive dressing, such as a cast, to limit access to the wound. With such a dressing in place, the wound typically heals fairly rapidly. Observation while hospitalized is also of benefit in many cases. In addition, use of tetracycline to determine whether someone reaches under an occlusive dressing in an attempt to manipulate and maintain the wound can be helpful. The tetracycline will build up under the nails and can be seen under ultraviolet light, thus confirming the diagnosis.

In addition to patients with nonhealing wounds, there are others who recurrently self-wound. These patients are often in severe emotional distress and will use wounding as a way of distracting themselves from their underlying emotional upset. They typically require lengthy psychotherapy to help them learn how to manage these symptoms.

Sensory conditions. A final presentation of psychogenic hand disorders is that of sensory conditions. Sensory conditions present in one of two extremes. The first of these is the hypersensitive hand. These patients react dramatically to any minute stimulus applied to the hand. The most common presentation is pain, and from a psychologic standpoint, psychogenic pain disorder is a common diagnosis accompanying this type of presentation. Patients with hypersensitive hands tend to keep them in a rather guarded position. However, when distracted, they will occasionally do things with their hands that would not be expected based on their presentation. As such, they lack the consistency of the presentation observed in patients with true reflex sympathetic dystrophy. They also fail to have the accompanying dystrophic features present.

The other type of sensory condition we have seen is the nonsensate hand, which has been described in the literature as *glove anesthesia*. With these patients, there is no response to any stimulation to the hand. They seem to be impervious to pain, heat, and cold. Nonsensate hands tend to occur primarily as conversion disorders. People will unconsciously avoid painful stimuli if they are able to; however, these patients often present with burns and varying types of injuries that accompany their disorder. Treatment again tends to be quite protracted and consists of long-term psychotherapy augmented with hypnosis and, at times, sodium Amytal interviews.

All psychogenic hand conditions tend to be difficult to treat and are stressful for the entire rehabilitation team. It is often difficult to believe that people would willfully harm themselves or create conditions that would produce disability. Intervention itself is often very time-consuming and frustrating for the professionals involved because patients often progress only to regress in their symptoms. Nevertheless, the most effective way of managing these conditions is through a multidisciplinary team approach.

Case study—factitious disorder

L.W. was injured in January 1992. She worked for 5 years in a window factory and crushed her right hand while pushing a cart up a small incline. No surgical repairs were necessary. Patient had complaints of severe pain that continued to worsen. She was diagnosed with reflex sympathetic dystrophy and received three stellate ganglion blocks in 1992 and eight in 1993. No improvement in her condition prompted a referral to Froedtert Hand Center Multidisciplinary Team.

The patient met with the hand surgeon and psychologist on April 19, 1993. She reported that her hand was usually swollen and that the dorsum of her hand would turn black while the digits turned purple, blue, or white. At times she had "electric-type" pain extending from her hand into her arm, but she reported that her hand was usually numb. On visual examination, the patient's hand color was comparable to her contralateral hand but was cool to touch, had bracelet edema, and had limited ring finger extension and no index or middle finger extension. The patient was informed that treatment would include thermal feedback and relaxation training and that her condition should improve within 2 months. Diagnosis—psychologic factors affecting physical condition.

The patient was seen by the psychologist for 3 weeks with inconsistent results. On May 27, she presented with her hand wrapped in a tight Ace wrap, which she was instructed to remove and not reapply. A referral was made to the hand therapist. Volumetric measurements were taken: right, 550 ml; left, 440 ml. Her right arm was placed in a cast positioning the elbow in position of comfort, wrist in minimal extension, metacarpophalangeal (MP) joint flexed, interphalangeal (IP) joint in extension, and thumb in palmar abduction.

The patient did not show up for her next appointment but was next seen on June 10. Volumetric measurements showed decreased edema: right, 460 ml; left, 435 ml. Hand temperature had increased. ROM exercises were completed, and the patient was sent to see the psychologist. The patient left office to go to the restroom and returned a few minutes later with noted increased edema and a red ring around her upper arm. After the appointment with the psychologist, the arm was recast.

On June 18, the cast was removed with noted good temperature and color and decreased edema. ROM was completed, and the patient again excused herself to go to the restroom before her appointment with the psychologist. Her surface digit temperature varied by only $^3/_{10}$ of a degree, which is unusual. The hand surgeon was called to examine the patient, but she suddenly reported being sick and needed to vomit. When she returned, she was asked to don a gown for a full examination. Two distinct red circumferential lines were noted just distal to her shoulder. Her hand temperature had risen, and her skin had a blush reaction throughout the entire upper extremity. A complete home exercise program, including active range of motion (AROM) and light use, was issued. The patient was cautioned against use of compression garments.

Sodium pentothal was administered on July 13. The patient was able to freely move the digits and wrist through full AROM. No stiffness was noted in any joints of her entire upper extremity. Distinct signs of banding were noted just distal to the elbow. Normal temperature was noted. The patient was told during induction that she had full ROM. As she was coming out of the block, she questioned whether she would need further blocks and was reassured that she would not. A home exercise program was reinforced, and therapy was arranged closer to the patient's home.

The patient was evaluated on August 12 and was noted to have improved ROM and grip strength. A functional capacity evaluation was completed and a return-to-work form with restrictions was written. This was the first time patient had returned to work since her injury. Follow-up appointments on January 24, 1994, and March 31, 1994, showed continued improvements. The patient was seen for the last time on July 5 with good ROM and strength. She was to return to the clinic on an as-needed basis.

SUMMARY

In summary, there are a variety of psychologic reactions that occur in conjunction with acute traumatic injuries, cumulative trauma injuries, chronically painful conditions of the upper extremity, and psychogenic hand conditions. We have provided an overview of diagnosis and treatment strategies for these conditions. Because the hand therapist is often the primary contact for patients with upper extremity disorders, recognition and referral of appropriate patients is an important part of the therapist's role. Through the relationship engendered during therapy, the suggestions of the therapist often carry a significant impact with the patient and allow an easier transition to appropriate mental health professionals when this is required.

REFERENCES

1. Dzwierzynski WW, et al: Psychometric assessment of patients with chronic upper extremity pain attributed to workplace exposure, *J Hand Surg* 24A:46, 1999.
2. Frykman GK, Wood VE, Miller EB: The psycho-flexed hand, *Clin Orthop* 174:153, 1983.
3. Grunert BK: Psychological assessment of chronic upper extremity disorders. In Ranney D, Ranney A, editors: *Chronic musculoskeletal injuries in the workplace,* Philadelphia, 1997, WB Saunders.
4. Grunert BK: When chronic pain is the problem: chronic musculoskeletal injuries in the workplace. In Ranney D, Ranney A, editors: *Chronic musculoskeletal injuries in the workplace,* Philadelphia, 1997, WB. Saunders.
5. Grunert BK, Dzwierzynski WW: Prognostic factors for return to work following musculoskeletal symptoms of unknown etiology, *Techniques Hand Upper Extremity Surg* 1:245, 1997.
6. Grunert BK, Weis J, Rusch MD: Imagery rescripting for PTSD following failed imaginal exposure after industrial injury (in press).
7. Grunert BK, et al: Early psychological aspects of traumatic hand injury, *J Hand Surg* 13B:177, 1988.
8. Grunert BK, et al: Flashbacks following traumatic hand injury: prognostic indicators, *J Hand Surg* 13A:125, 1988.
9. Grunert BK, et al: Sexual dysfunction following traumatic hand injury, *Ann Plast Surg* 21:46, 1988.
10. Grunert BK, et al: On-site work evaluations: desensitization for avoidance reactions following hand trauma, *J Hand Surg* 14B:239, 1989.
11. Grunert BK, et al: Treatment of posttraumatic stress disorder after work related hand trauma, *J Hand Surg* 15A:511, 1990.
12. Grunert BK, et al: A classification system for factitious hand syndromes with implications for treatment, *J Hand Surg* 16A:1027, 1991.
13. Grunert BK, et al: Graded work exposure to promote work return after severe hand trauma: a replicated study, *Ann Plast Surg* 29:532, 1992.
14. Grunert BK, et al: Predictive value of psychologic screening in acute hand injuries, *J Hand Surg* 17A:196, 1992.
15. Grunert BK, et al: Psychological adjustment following work-related hand injury: 18-month follow-up, *Ann Plast Surg* 29:537, 1992.
16. Hathaway SR, McKinley JC: *Minnesota Multiphasic Personality Inventory-2,* Minneapolis, 1989, National Computer Systems.
17. Louis DS, Lamp MK, Greene TL: The upper extremity and psychiatric illness, *J Hand Surg* 10A:687, 1985.
18. McCracken LM, Zayfert C, Gross RT: The pain anxiety symptoms scale (PASS): a multimodal measure of pain specific anxiety reactions, *Behav Ther* 16:183, 1995.
19. Osipow SH, Spokane AR: *Occupational stress inventory,* Odessa, Fla, 1987, Psychological Assessment Resources.
20. Reading G: Secrétan's syndrome: hard edema of the dorsum of the hand, *Plast Reconstr Surg* 65:182, 1980.
21. Rusch MD, et al: Imagery rescripting for recurrent distressing images, *Cognitive Beh Pract* 7:173, 2000.
22. Simmons BP, Vasile RG: The clenched fist syndrome, *J Hand Surg* 5:420, 1980.
23. US Department of Health and Human Services: *Injury control: setting the national agenda for injury control in the 1990s,* Washington, DC, 1991, DHHS.
24. Wallace PF, Fitzmorris CS: The S-H-A-F-T syndrome in the upper extremity, *J Hand Surg* 3:492, 1978.
25. Weis J: *Early versus delayed imaginal exposure for the treatment of posttraumatic stress disorder following accidental injury,* doctoral dissertation, Marquette University.

INDEX

Page numbers followed by f indicate figures; t, tables; b, boxes.

I-1